I0867132

Clinical Medicine of the Dog and Cat

Third Edition

Clinical Medicine of the Dog and Cat

Third Edition

Michael Schaer DVM, DipACVIM (SAIM); DipACVECC
Emeritus Professor of Small Animal Medicine;
Adjunct Professor in Small Animal Emergency and Critical Care
College of Veterinary Medicine
University of Florida
Gainesville, Florida, USA

Frédéric Gaschen Dr.med.vet., Dr.habil., DipACVIM (SAIM), DipECVIM-CA (IM)
Professor of Companion Animal Medicine
School of Veterinary Medicine
Louisiana State University
Baton Rouge, Louisiana, USA

CRC Press
Taylor & Francis Group
Boca Raton London New York

CRC Press is an imprint of the
Taylor & Francis Group, an **informa** business

CRC Press
Taylor & Francis Group
6000 Broken Sound Parkway NW, Suite 300
Boca Raton, FL 33487-2742

© 2016 by Taylor & Francis Group, LLC
CRC Press is an imprint of Taylor & Francis Group, an Informa business

No claim to original U.S. Government works

Printed and bound in India by Replika Press Pvt. Ltd.

Printed on acid-free paper
Version Date: 20160401

International Standard Book Number-13: 978-1-4822-2605-8 (Pack - Book and Ebook)

This book contains information obtained from authentic and highly regarded sources. While all reasonable efforts have been made to publish reliable data and information, neither the author[s] nor the publisher can accept any legal responsibility or liability for any errors or omissions that may be made. The publishers wish to make clear that any views or opinions expressed in this book by individual editors, authors or contributors are personal to them and do not necessarily reflect the views/opinions of the publishers. The information or guidance contained in this book is intended for use by medical, scientific or health-care professionals and is provided strictly as a supplement to the medical or other professional's own judgement, their knowledge of the patient's medical history, relevant manufacturer's instructions and the appropriate best practice guidelines. Because of the rapid advances in medical science, any information or advice on dosages, procedures or diagnoses should be independently verified. The reader is strongly urged to consult the relevant national drug formulary and the drug companies' and device or material manufacturers' printed instructions, and their websites, before administering or utilizing any of the drugs, devices or materials mentioned in this book. This book does not indicate whether a particular treatment is appropriate or suitable for a particular individual. Ultimately it is the sole responsibility of the medical professional to make his or her own professional judgements, so as to advise and treat patients appropriately. The authors and publishers have also attempted to trace the copyright holders of all material reproduced in this publication and apologize to copyright holders if permission to publish in this form has not been obtained. If any copyright material has not been acknowledged please write and let us know so we may rectify in any future reprint.

Except as permitted under U.S. Copyright Law, no part of this book may be reprinted, reproduced, transmitted, or utilized in any form by any electronic, mechanical, or other means, now known or hereafter invented, including photocopying, microfilming, and recording, or in any information storage or retrieval system, without written permission from the publishers.

For permission to photocopy or use material electronically from this work, please access www.copyright.com (http://www.copyright.com/) or contact the Copyright Clearance Center, Inc. (CCC), 222 Rosewood Drive, Danvers, MA 01923, 978-750-8400. CCC is a not-for-profit organization that provides licenses and registration for a variety of users. For organizations that have been granted a photocopy license by the CCC, a separate system of payment has been arranged.

Trademark Notice: Product or corporate names may be trademarks or registered trademarks, and are used only for identification and explanation without intent to infringe.

Visit the Taylor & Francis Web site at
http://www.taylorandfrancis.com

and the CRC Press Web site at
http://www.crcpress.com

Dedications

To MJ, my wife, who has supported me through thick and thin throughout my entire career; to my colleagues and contributing authors who have provided me encouragement and who have instilled their wisdom throughout this textbook; and to my house officers and students who have provided me with endless inspiration - I thank you all for allowing me to make my career my everyday passion. Lastly but certainly not least, I offer my special thanks to Drs. Bill Kay, Glen Hoffsis, Jim Lloyd, Tom Vickroy, Boyd Jones, and Rowan Milner, who provided me with the opportunity and encouragement to propel myself forward toward a continuing productive life during the golden years of my career.

Michael Schaer

"If you decide to become a veterinary surgeon you will never grow rich, but you will have a life of endless interest and variety" (James Herriot)

To Lorrie, Alec, Betty, Gaston, and Louis with my love and gratitude for their support and encouragements at different times of my life - I know I owe them everything.

To those who have taken the time and energy to mentor me at different times of my career - with my never ending appreciation for your selfless investment

To the residents, interns, and students I had or currently have the privilege to work with for being a constant source of motivation and energy

To James Herriot for first opening my eyes on this great profession of ours.

And finally to Mike Schaer, for inviting me to share the helm for the 3rd edition of his book, and to all the authors who worked hard to make its content so relevant to our readers.

Frédéric Gaschen

Contents

Preface		ix
Contributors		xi
Abbreviations		xv
Part 1	**General approach**	**1**
Chapter 1	Medical history and client communication *Stephanie W. Johnson*	3
Chapter 2	Common clinical problems	11
2.1	Dyspnea (*Elizabeth Rozanski*)	11
2.2	Syncope, episodic weakness, and collapse (*Boyd R. Jones*)	17
2.3	Pigmenturia (*Michael Schaer*)	23
2.4	Vomiting (*Frédéric Gaschen*)	27
2.5	Polydipsia and polyuria (*Michael Schaer*)	33
2.6	Diarrhea (*Frédéric Gaschen*)	39
2.7	Icterus (*Julien Dandrieux*)	47
2.8	Cough (*Elizabeth Rozanski*)	53
2.9	Epistaxis (*Christine Iacovetta*)	57
2.10	Fever of unknown origin (*Robert Armentano*)	61
2.11	Dysuria (*Isabelle Cattin*)	69
2.12	Pallor (*Elisa M. Mazzaferro*)	77
Part 2	**Diseases of specific organ systems**	**81**
Chapter 3	Diseases of the oral cavity and teeth *Erin P. Ribka & Brook A. Niemiec*	83
Chapter 4	Respiratory disorders *Cécile Clercx*	105
Chapter 5	Diseases of the pleural space *J. Brad Case*	139
Chapter 6	Approach to thoracic radiographs *L. Abbigail Granger*	157
Chapter 7	Cardiovascular disorders *Romain Pariaut & Carley Saelinger*	195
Chapter 8	Digestive diseases (pharynx to anorectum) *Frédéric Gaschen*	253
Chapter 9	Liver disorders *Joseph Taboada*	333

Chapter 10	Pancreatic disorders *Michael Schaer*	361
Chapter 11	Endocrine disorders *Michael E. Herrtage*	387
Chapter 12	Nephrology/urology *Mark J. Acierno*	449
Chapter 13	Approach to abdominal radiographs *L. Abbigail Granger*	511
Chapter 14	Disorders of the nervous system and muscle *Simon R. Platt*	545
Chapter 15	Bone and joint disorders *Steven M. Fox*	637
Chapter 16	Hematologic disorders *Katie M. Boes & Rose E. Raskin*	681
Chapter 17	Disorders of hemostasis *Bobbi Conner*	745
Chapter 18	Dermatologic disorders *Diane T. Lewis*	769
Chapter 19	Ocular manifestations of systemic diseases *Dennis E. Brooks & Megan L. Sullivan*	821
Part 3	**Multisystemic disorders**	**877**
Chapter 20	Clinical toxicology *Lisa A. Murphy & Kenneth J. Drobatz*	879
Chapter 21	Infectious diseases *Richard B. Ford & Annette Litster*	909
Chapter 22	Immunologic disorders *Michael J. Day*	985
Part 4	**Elements of therapy**	**1009**
Chapter 23	Fluid therapy *Gareth Buckley & Travis Lanaux*	1011
Chapter 24	Pain management *Steven M. Fox*	1025
Chapter 25	Nutrition of the critically-ill dog and cat *Justin Shmalberg*	1059
Chapter 26	Management of the obese dog or cat *Alexander J. German*	1079
Appendix	**Clinical cases**	**1095**
Index		1129

Preface

Before the first edition of *Clinical Medicine of the Dog and Cat* was published, no other comprehensive small animal veterinary medicine textbook was available with a comparable amount and quality of relevant illustrated materials. The information in the 1st and 2nd editions was carefully selected so that it would be a great resource offering clinically applicable information for the veterinary student, the small animal intern, and the general practitioner. It complemented our belief that clinical observation and the cognitive sense of the clinician are essential professional qualities that contribute to our clinical acumen.

In the 1st and 2nd editions, the editor (MS) carefully selected experienced specialists from North America, Europe, and Australasia with the distinctive objective of providing the book with quality material that would have a truly international appeal. Soon after the publication of the 1st edition there were requests for additional topics, and the 2nd edition was expanded to include sections covering pain management, clinical nutrition, clinical toxicology, fluid therapy, and clinical immunology, and authored by recognized experts in their field.

Because of the overall success of the first two editions, it was decided to publish a 3rd edition. This time, however, it was deemed essential to appoint a co-editor (FG) who would be a resource for new ideas regarding the contents. The new team of editors has brought forth fresh ideas, which include new chapter topics and several new outstanding authors.

This new 3rd edition is composed of two main sections. The first elaborates on the medical approach to solving common medical problems. These additional short topics, written by experts, include medical history taking, polydipsia and polyuria, pigmenturia, vomiting, diarrhea, weakness, dyspnea, cough, fever of unknown origin, epistaxis, and pallor. The practical application of the information in these sections is presented with text, tables, and algorithms. The objective of this clinical problems section is merely to emphasize the logical clinical approach to the selected clinical signs.

The second section contains detailed medical information covering most organ systems. The Appendix contains selected clinical case material that applies some of the principles of medicine discussed in this textbook. The new chapters are authored by experienced specialists, and cover new topics or provide a completely rewritten approach to chapters included in previous editions of the book. They include diseases of the oral cavity and teeth, respiratory diseases, approach to thoracic radiographs, approach to abdominal radiographs, neuromuscular disorders, cardiovascular disorders, digestive diseases, uro-nephrology, and disorders of hemostasis. Other chapters from the 2nd edition have been revised by their authors with the inclusion of additional text and images.

The editors adhered to the original organizational plan of *Clinical Medicine of the Dog and Cat*, which was to cover disorders of all organ systems as well as the associated subspecialties of veterinary internal medicine. However, in order to make this a practical text for our projected audience, we omitted certain valuable topics such as genetics, preventive medicine, and coverage of the reproductive system. These areas are instead included as a part of the organ systems chapters where indicated. Ophthalmology and dermatology certainly have enough information to fill books in their own right. Therefore, the editors requested that the information provided be restricted to what would most likely impact on internal medicine.

The updated chapter covering pain management was deemed essential because it is now a major component of patient management. This is especially true for cats and dogs with neurologic and orthopedic diseases associated with acute or chronic pain. However, pain management is also of central importance in the treatment of acute pancreatitis and many other conditions that can cause visceral pain.

As in the first two editions, each chapter of this text is arranged to provide the definition of each disorder, its clinical features, the differential diagnoses, the diagnostic methodology, and the treatment and prognosis. The aim remains to achieve brevity and clarity in order to provide the practicing veterinarian with a readily available resource of important clinical information. The numerous illustrations fulfill the main philosophy of this textbook, namely that 'a picture is worth a thousand words', which is especially useful in the practice of veterinary medicine. Each author was requested to restrict his or her content to the more commonly seen clinical disorders, but was allowed to exercise as much freedom of choice as possible. A limited list of recommended references is offered in this latest edition. With today's readily available access to literature search engines, we feel that the reader can easily find unlimited information for further detailed reading.

We would like to express our sincere appreciation to the several talented people who helped organize this text. First, Ms. Jill Northcott, our publisher's coordinator, whose guidance enabled the various contributors to work harmoniously together in order to design the content of a book that would provide the broadest possible coverage of small animal internal medicine. We would also like to thank the production staff at CRC Press, led by the project manager, Ms. Kate Nardoni, who worked behind the scenes to provide the reader with the best possible page layout and the easiest possible access to the important information contained therein. We express our very special thanks to Mr. Peter Beynon and Mr. Paul Bennett, whose medical literary expertise provide the fine tuning necessary for making the book's content clearly understandable and balanced. Finally, we express our sincere gratitude to our wonderful and gifted authors for taking valuable time out of their very busy days to share their expertise with the readers of this 3rd edition.

The authors and editors acknowledge and appreciate the patience and understanding of their families and other important people in their lives. We thank them for providing the moral support and accepting the sacrifices that were necessary for successful completion of this new edition. We are also indebted to all of the helpful individuals who provided time and assistance with each author's respective assignments.

We hope that you, the readers, will truly enjoy using this textbook, and that the information provided will be of assistance in your day-to-day practice of veterinary medicine.

Michael Schaer and Frédéric Gaschen

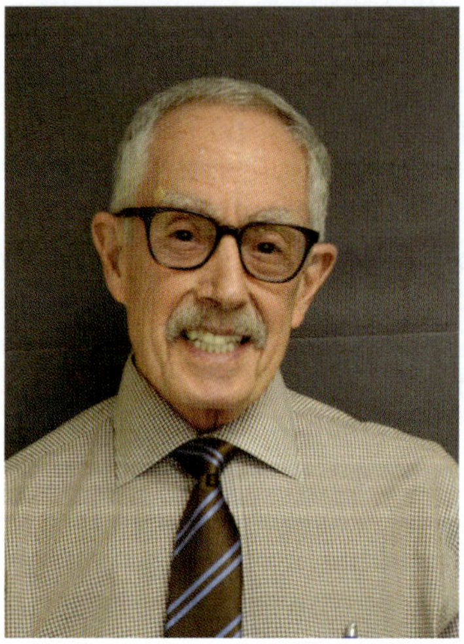

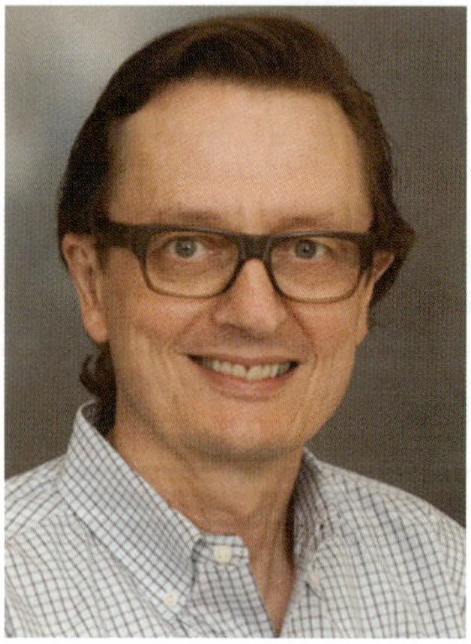

Contributors

Mark J. Acierno MBA, DVM, DipACVIM(SAIM)
School of Veterinary Medicine
Louisiana State University
Baton Rouge, Lousiana, USA

Robert Armentano DVM, DipACVIM(SAIM)
Veterinary Specialty Center
Small Animal Internal Medicine
Chicago, Illinois, USA

Katie M. Boes DVM, MS, DipACVP
Department of Biomedical Sciences and Pathobiology
Virginia Polytechnic Institute and State University
Blacksburg, Virginia, USA

Dennis E. Brooks DVM, PhD, DipACVO
University of Florida
College of Veterinary Medicine
Gainesville, Florida, USA

Gareth Buckley MA, VetMB, DipACVECC, DipECVECC
University of Florida
College of Veterinary Medicine
Gainesville, Florida, USA

Jessica Bullock DVM
University of Florida
College of Veterinary Medicine
Gainesville, Florida, USA

Sheila Justiz-Carrera DVM, DipACVIM(Neurology)
University of Florida
College of Veterinary Medicine
Gainesville, Florida, USA

J. Brad Case DVM, MS, DipACVS-SA
University of Florida
College of Veterinary Medicine
Gainesville, Florida, USA

Isabelle Cattin Dr.med.vet., DipACVIM(SAIM)
VET'Interne
Epalinges, Switzerland

Cécile Clercx DVM, PhD, DipECVIM-CA
Faculté de Médecine Vétérinaire
Université de Liège
Liège, Belgium

Bobbi Conner DVM, DipACVECC
University of Florida
College of Veterinary Medicine
Gainesville, Florida, USA

Julien Dandrieux Dr.med.vet., BSc, DipACVIM(SAIM)
Faculty of Veterinary Science
Small Animal Hospital
University of Melbourne
Werribee, Victoria, Australia

Rachel B. Davy DVM
University of Florida
College of Veterinary Medicine
Gainesville, Florida, USA

Michael J. Day BSc, BVMS(Hons), PhD, DSc, DipECVP, FASM, FRCPath, FRCVS
School of Veterinary Sciences
University of Bristol
Langford, Bristol, UK

Kenneth J. Drobatz DVM, MSCE, DipACVIM, DipACVECC
School of Veterinary Medicine
Department of Clinical Studies
University of Pennsylvania
Philadelphia, Pennsylvania, USA

Richard B. Ford DVM, DipACVIM, DipACVPM
Emerywood Drive
Raleigh, North Carolina, USA

Steven M. Fox MS, DVM, MBA, PhD
Fox Third Bearing Inc.
Forest Ave
Clive, Iowa, USA

Frédéric Gaschen Dr.med.vet., Dr.habil., DipACVIM(SAIM), DipECVIM-CA (IM)
School of Veterinary Medicine
Louisiana State University
Baton Rouge, Louisiana, USA

Alexander J. German BVSc, PhD, CertSAM, DipECVIM-CA, MRCVS
School of Veterinary Science
University of Liverpool
Neston, Cheshire, UK

L. Abbigail Granger DVM, DipACVR
School of Veterinary Medicine
Louisiana State University
Baton Rouge, Louisiana, USA

Michael E. Herrtage MA, BVSc, DVSc, DVR, DVD, DSAM, MRCVS, DipECVIM, DipECVDI
Department of Veterinary Medicine
University of Cambridge
Cambridge, UK

Christine Iacovetta BVetMed, DipACVECC
BluePearl Veterinary Partners
Forest Hills
New York, USA

Stephanie W. Johnson LCSW
School of Veterinary Medicine
Louisiana State University
Baton Rouge, Louisiana, USA

Boyd R. Jones BVSc, FACVS, DECVIM, MRCVS
Kauri Point
Katikati, New Zealand

Travis Lanaux DVM, DipACVECC
University of Florida
College of Veterinary Medicine
Gainesville, Florida, USA

Amandine LeJeune DVM
University of Florida
College of Veterinary Medicine
Gainesville, Florida, USA

Diane T. Lewis DVM, DipACVD
University of Florida
College of Veterinary Medicine
Gainesville, Florida, USA

Annette Litster BVSc, PhD, FANZCVSc, MMedSci
Emerywood Drive
Raleigh, North Carolina, USA

Leo Londoño DVM
University of Florida
College of Veterinary Medicine
Gainesville, Florida, USA

Elisa M. Mazzaferro MS, DVM, PhD, DipACVECC
Cornell University Veterinary Specialists
Stamford, Connecticut, USA

Lisa A. Murphy BS, VMD, DABT
School of Veterinary Medicine
Department of Clinical Studies
University of Pennsylvania
Philadelphia, Pennsylvania, USA

Brook A. Niemiec DVM, DipAVDC, DipEVDC, FAVD
Veterinary Dental Specialties & Oral Surgery
San Diego, California, USA

Romain Pariaut DVM, DipACVIM(CA), DipECVIM-CA
College of Veterinary Medicine
Cornell University
Ithaca, New York, USA

Simon R. Platt BVM&S, DipACVIM(Neurology), DipECVN
College of Veterinary Medicine
University of Georgia
Athens, Georgia, USA

Rose E. Raskin DVM, PhD, DipACVP
College of Veterinary Medicine
Purdue University
West Lafayette, Indiana, USA

Erin P. Ribka DVM
Gulf South Veterinary Dentistry & Oral Surgery
New Orleans, Louisiana, USA

Elodie Roels DVM
Faculté de Médecine Vétérinaire
Université de Liège
Liège, Belgium

Elizabeth Rozanski DVM, DipACVIM(SAIM), DipACVECC
Tufts University
North Grafton, Massachusetts, USA

Carley Saelinger VMD, DipACVIM(CA)
Animal Specialty and Emergency Center
Los Angeles, California, USA

Michael Schaer DVM, DipACVIM(SAIM), DipACVECC
University of Florida
College of Veterinary Medicine
Gainesville, Florida, USA

Justin Shmalberg DVM, DipACVN, DAVSMR, CVA, CVCH, CVFT
University of Florida
College of Veterinary Medicine
Gainesville, Florida, USA

Joseph Taboada DVM, DipACVIM(SAIM)
School of Veterinary Medicine
Louisiana State University
Baton Rouge, Louisiana, USA

Abbreviations

AA	arachidonic acid
α_2AP	alpha$_2$-antiplasmin
ACE	angiotensin-converting enzyme
ACEI	angiotensin-converting enzyme inhibitor
ACM	arrhythmogenic cardiomyopathy
AChR	acetylcholine receptor
ACP	acepromazine maleate
ACTH	adrenocorticotrophic hormone
AD	atopic dermatitis
ADE	adverse drug event
ADH	antidiuretic hormone
ADP	adenosine diphosphate
AF	atrial fibrillation
AGDD	agar gel double diffusion
AHDS	acute hemorrhagic diarrhea syndrome
AKI	acute kidney injury
albB	bilirubin covalently bound to albumin
ALD	acral lick dermatitis
ALP	alkaline phosphatase
ALT	alanine transaminase
AML	acute myeloid leukemia
AMPA	alpha-amino-3-hydroxy-5-methyl-isoxazole-4-proprionic acid
ANA	antinuclear antibody
APC	antigen-presenting cell
AR	aldose reductase
ARD	antibiotic-responsive diarrhea
ARVC	arrhythmogenic right ventricular cardiomyopathy
ASD	atrial septal defect
ASIC	acid-sensing ion channel
ASIT	allergen-specific immunotherapy
AST	aspartate transaminase
AT	antithrombin
ATP	adenosine triphosphate
AV	atrioventricular
AZT	azidothymidine
BAL	bronchoalveolar lavage
BAOS	brachycephalic airway obstructive syndrome
BCR	B-cell receptor
BCS	body condition score
BEF	bronchoesophageal fistula
BMI	body mass index
bpm	beats per minute/breaths per minute
BUN	blood urea nitrogen
CAPC	Companion Animal Parasite Council
CAV	canine adenovirus
cB	conjugated bilirubin
CBC	complete blood count
CCV	canine coronavirus
CD	cluster of differentiation
CDI	central diabetes insipidus
CDV	canine distemper virus
CE	chronic enteropathy
CGRP	calcitonin gene-related peptide
CH	chronic hepatitis
CHD	congenital heart disease
Che	cholinesterase
CHF	congestive heart failure
CHOP	cyclophosphamide, hydroxydaunorubicin [doxorubicin], Oncovin [vincristine], and prednisone
CIDP	chronic inflammatory demyelinating polyneuropathy
CILBD	chronic idiopathic large bowel diarrhea
CIRD	canine infectious respiratory disease
CIV	canine influenza virus
CK	creatine kinase
CKCS	Cavalier King Charles Spaniel
CKD	chronic kidney disease
CLAD	canine leukocyte adhesion deficiency
CLE	cutaneous (discoid) lupus erythematosus
CLL	chronic lymphocytic leukemia
CLMS	Chiari-like malformation syndrome
CMI	cell-mediated immunity
CNS	central nervous system
COPV	canine oral papillomavirus
CoT	coagulopathy of trauma
COX	cyclo-oxygenase
CPiV	canine parainfluenza virus
CPnV	canine pneumovirus
CPV	canine parvovirus
CRCoV	canine respiratory coronavirus
CRH	corticotropin-releasing hormone
CRI	constant rate infusion
CRP	corrected reticulocyte percentage

CRT	capillary refill time
CRTZ	chemoreceptor trigger zone
CSD	cat scratch disease
CSF	cerebrospinal fluid
CT	computed tomography
cTnI	cardiac troponin I
c-TSH	canine thyroid-stimulating hormone
CVP	central venous pressure
DAWS	disk-associated wobbler syndrome
DCM	dilated cardiomyopathy
DEA	dog erythrocyte antigen
DEXA	dual-energy X-ray absorptiometry
DIIHA	drug-induced immune hemolytic anemia
DJD	degenerative joint disease
DM	degenerative myelopathy
DMSO	dimethyl sulfoxide
DOC	disorder of cornification
DOI	duration of immunity
2,3-DPG	2,3-diphosphoglycerate
DRD	diet-responsive diarrhea
DRG	dorsal root ganglion
DTM	dermatophyte test medium
EACA	epsilon aminocaproic acid
EBDO	extrahapatic bile duct obstruction
EBP	eosinophilic bronchopneumopathy
ECG	electrocardiogram/electrocardiography
EE	energy expenditure
EEG	electroencephalogram
EGC	eosinophilic granuloma complex
EIC	exercise-induced collapse
ELISA	enzyme-linked immunosorbent assay
EM	erythema multiforme
EMG	electromyogram/electromyography
EPI	exocrine pancreatic insufficiency
EPO	erythropoietin
ER	exertional rhabdomyolysis
EU	ectopic ureter
FB	foreign body
FCEM	fibrocartilaginous embolic myelopathy
FCP	fragmented coronoid process
FCV	feline calicivirus
FDA	(US) Food and Drug Administration
FDP	fibrin degradation product
FECV	feline enteric coronavirus
FeLV	feline leukemia virus
FHV	feline herpesvirus
FIC	feline idiopathic cystitis
FIP	feline infectious peritonitis
FIV	feline immunodeficiency virus
FLAIR	fluid-attenuated inversion recovery
FLUTD	feline lower urinary tract disease
FPL	feline panleukopenia
fPLI	feline pancreatic lipase (test)
FPV	feline panleukopenia virus
FS	shortening fraction
FUO	fever of undetermined origin
GABA	gamma-aminobutyric acid
GAG	glycosaminoglycan
GC	granulomatous colitis
GCS	Glasgow Coma Scale
G-CSF	granulocyte colony-stimulating factor
GDV	gastric dilatation volvulus
GFR	glomerular filtration rate
GGT	gamma-glutamyltransferase
GH	growth hormone
GI	gastrointestinal
GM-CSF	granulocyte/macrophage colony-stimulating factor
GME	granulomatous meningoencephalomyelitis
GN	glomerulonephritis
GP	glycoprotein
GS	glucagonoma syndrome
HARD	heartworm associated respiratory disease
HCM	hypertrophic cardiomyopathy
HCS	hepatocutaneous syndrome
Hct	hematocrit
HGAL	high-grade alimentary lymphoma
Hgb	hemoglobin
HGE	hemorrhagic gastroenteritis
HH	hiatal hernia
HIV	human immunodeficiency virus
HOD	hypertrophic osteodystrophy
HP	pulmonary hypertension
HUC	histiocytic ulcerative colitis
IAC	intracranial arachnoid cyst
IBD	inflammatory bowel disease
ICH	infectious canine hepatitis
ICP	intracranial pressure
IDAT	intradermal allergy testing/test
IDST	intradermal skin test
IFA	immunofluorescent antibody (test)
IFN	interferon
IGF-1	insulin-like growth factor-1
IL	interleukin
IM	intramuscular/intramuscularly
IMHA	immune-mediated hemolytic anemia
IMNP	immune-mediated neutropenia
IMTP	immune-mediated thrombocytopenia
IPF	idiopathic pulmonary fibrosis
IPPV	intermittent positive pressure ventilation
IV	intravenous/intravenously
IVDD	intervertebral disk disease

KCS keratoconjunctivitis sicca
LA/Ao left atrium to aortic ratio
LCAT latex cryptococcal antigen agglutination test
LDDST low-dose dexamethasone suppression test
LDH lactate dehydrogenase
LES lower esophageal sphincter
LGAL low-grade alimentary lymphoma
LH luteinizing hormone
LMN lower motor neuron
LMWH low molecular weight heparin
LRT lower respiratory tract
LVIDd left ventricular diameter in end-diastole
LVIDs left ventricular diameter in end-systole
LVOTO left ventricular outflow tract obstruction
MABP mean arterial blood pressure
MAP mean arterial pressure
MAT microscopic agglutination test
MBW metabolic body weight
MCH mean cell hemoglobin
MCHC mean cell hemoglobin concentration
MCP mucocutaneous pyoderma
MCS muscle condition score
MCT mast cell tumor
MCV mean cell volume
MDS myelodysplastic syndrome
ME megaesophagus
MER maintenance energy requirement
ME-RSAT 2–mercaptoethanol rapid slide agglutination test
MG myasthenia gravis
MH malignant hyperthermia
MHC major histocompatibility complex
MIC minimum inhibitory concentration
MLV modified live virus (vaccine)
MM multiple myeloma
MMA methylmalonic acid
MMM masticatory muscle myositis
MN membranous nephropathy
MPGN membranoproliferative glomerulonephritis
MPN myeloproliferative neoplasia
MPS mucopolysaccharidosis
MRI magnetic resonance imaging
MSM methyl-sulfonyl-methane
MST median survival time
MTP membrane transfer protein
MVD mitral valve dysplasia
NAPQI N-acetyl p-benzoquinoneimine
NDI nephrogenic diabetes insipidus
NGF nerve growth factor
NI neonatal isoerythrolysis
NK natural killer (cell)
NMDA N-methyl-D-aspartate
NME necrolytic migratory erythema
NNT number needed to treat
NO nitric oxide
nRBC nucleated red blood cell
NSAID nonsteroidal anti-inflammatory drug
NT-proBNP nonbiologically active fragment of the B-type natriuretic peptide
OA osteoarthritis
OCD osteochondritis dissecans
OE otitis externa
OMI otitis media/interna
OP organophosphate
PAI-1 plasminogen activator inhibitor 1
2-PAM protopam chloride or pralidoxime chloride
PAMP pathogen-associated molecular pattern
PAS periodic acid–Schiff
PCD primary ciliary dyskinesia
PCR polymerase chain reaction
PCT proximal convoluted tubule
PCV packed cell volume
PDA patent ductus arteriosus
PDH pituitary-dependent hyperadrenocorticism
PFK phosphofructokinase
PGE_2 prostaglandin E_2
PH pulmonary hypertension
PIVKA proteins induced by vitamin K antagonism or absence
PK pyruvate kinase
PKD polycystic kidney disease
PLE protein-losing enteropathy
PLI pancreatic lipase immunoreactivity (test)
PLN protein-losing nephropathy
PMEA phosphonylmethoxy-ethyladenine
PMI point of maximal intensity
PO per os/orally
POI postoperative ileus
PNS peripheral nervous system
PNST peripheral nerve sheath tumor
PP psychogenic polydipsia
PPDH peritoneopericardial diaphragmatic hernia
PPI proton pump inhibitor
PPR pattern recognition receptor
PRAA persistent right aortic arch
PRCA pure red cell aplasia
PS pulmonic stenosis
PSS portosystemic shunt
PT prothrombin time
PTE pulmonary thromboembolism
PTH parathyroid hormone
PTHrP parathyroid hormone-related peptide

PTT partial thromboplastin time
PV polycythemia vera
qPCR quantitative PCR
RAAS renin–angiotensin–aldosterone system
RBC red blood cell
RCM restrictive cardiomyopathy
RD retinal detachment
REE resting energy expenditure
RER resting energy requirement
RF rheumatoid factor
rHuEPO recombinant human erythropoietin
RMSF Rocky Mountain spotted fever
RPE retinal pigment epithelium
rT3 reverse triiodothyronine (T3)
RT-PCR reverse transcriptase PCR
RVESP right ventricular end-systolic pressure
SAA serum amyloid A
SAMe S-adenosylmethionine
SAS subaortic stenosis
SC subcutaneous/subcutaneously
SCC squamous cell carcinoma
SCID severe combined immunodeficiency
SD sorbitol dehydrogenase
SFG spotted fever group
SG specific gravity
SIRS systemic inflammatory response syndrome
SJS Stevens–Johnson syndrome
SLE systemic lupus erythematosus
SM syringomyelia
SNA sinonasal aspergillosis
SOA sino-orbital aspergillosis
SRI serotonin reuptake inhibitor
SRID single radial immunodiffusion
SRMA steroid-responsive meningitis–arteritis
T3 triiodothyronine
T4 thyroxine
TAFI thrombin activatable fibrinolysis inhibitor
TAT tube agglutination test
Tc T cytotoxic (cell)
TCA tricyclic antidepressant
TCR T-cell receptor
TEN toxic epidermal necrolysis
TENS transcutaneous electrical nerve stimulation
TF tissue factor
TgAA thyroglobulin autoantibodies
Th T helper (cell)
THO thrombopoietin
TLI trypsin-like immunoreactivity (test)
TLR Toll-like receptor
TMJ temporomandibular joint
TNCC total nucleated cell count
TNF tumor necrosis factor
TOF tetralogy of Fallot
tPA tissue-type plasminogen activator
Treg T regulatory cell
TRs tooth resorptions
TRH thyrotropin releasing hormone
TRPV1 transient receptor potential vanilloid-1
TS total solids
TSH thyroid-stimulating hormone
TVD tricuspid valve dysplasia
TW tracheal wash
TXA tranexamic acid
UAP ununited anconeal process
uB unconjugated bilirubin
UES upper esophageal sphincter
UH unfractionated heparin
UMN upper motor neuron
uPA urokinase/urine-type plasminogen activator
UPC urine protein:creatinine (ratio)
URT upper respiratory tract
USG urine specific gravity
UTI urinary tract infection
UV ultraviolet
VAS vaccine-associated sarcoma
VHCT veterinary health care team
VHS vertebral heart scale
VSD ventricular septal defect
VS-FCV virulent systemic feline calicivirus
vWD von Willebrand disease
vWF von Willebrand factor
VKH Vogt–Koyanagi–Harada
WBC white blood cell
WHO World Health Organization
X-SCID X-linked severe combined immunodeficiency

Part 1

General approach

Chapter 1 **Medical history and client communication**
Stephanie W. Johnson

Chapter 2 **Common clinical problems**
2.1 Dyspnea (*Elizabeth Rozanski*)
2.2 Syncope, episodic weakness, and collapse (*Boyd R. Jones*)
2.3 Pigmenturia (*Michael Schaer*)
2.4 Vomiting (*Frédéric Gaschen*)
2.5 Polydipsia and polyuria (*Michael Schaer*)
2.6 Diarrhea (*Frédéric Gaschen*)
2.7 Icterus (*Julien Dandrieux*)
2.8 Cough (*Elizabeth Rozanski*)
2.9 Epistaxis (*Christine Iacovetta*)
2.10 Fever of unknown origin (*Robert Armentano*)
2.11 Dysuria (*Isabelle Cattin*)
2.12 Pallor (*Elisa M. Mazzaferro*)

Chapter 1

Medical history and client communication

Stephanie W. Johnson

INTRODUCTION

A good history contributes 60–80% of the data needed to make an accurate diagnosis. Information obtained from conversations/history taking between the veterinarian and the client is the basis for a clinical diagnosis. The history contains the biomedical information and background information about the pet. It is also vital to understand the 'story' or the client's perspective. Many times the story the client shares about their pet is just as important as the biomedical history. It gives the veterinarian a basis for what to ask next and a chance to understand/appreciate where clients are coming from and what concerns them most. In order to get an effective history, the veterinarian needs to be able to elicit the story from the client, therefore he/she needs to be a good communicator. Practicing good communication is essential to practicing good medicine.

Communication is the act or process of using words, sounds, signs, or behaviors to express or exchange information or to effectively express your ideas, thoughts, feelings, etc. to someone else. Communication skills are critical to eliciting information and understanding each other. In human medicine, effective doctor–patient communication has been shown to improve diagnostic accuracy, health status, patient compliance, and patient satisfaction. It also decreases malpractice risk; 'breakdown of communication' is the main reason for veterinary malpractice claims. Good communication also enhances supportiveness, relationships, and coordination of care. It makes it possible to enlist the client as a member of the veterinary health care team (VHCT). The more the clients feel a member of the team, the more motivated and invested they will be in participating in their pet's care. The better the communication, the more satisfied the veterinarian. Research has shown that veterinarian satisfaction is achieved through relationship building with clients.

The most important role of the VHCT is to elicit and understand the client's story. Without this understanding, the veterinarian cannot do what needs to be done for the pet or the client. The most basic form of communication is nonverbal. Sometimes it is not just what you say but how you say it. Any problems the client might be having relative to the VHCT will be exhibited through nonverbal cues regardless of whether he/she agrees verbally with the treatment/discussion. Correct interpretation of nonverbal communication will add depth to the veterinarian's ability to communicate. This stresses the importance of the team member looking at the pet owner instead of a computer screen so that body language is used to assist with interpreting the verbal message.

In order to obtain the story, members of the VHCT must be able to engage and empathize with the client. Learning to use open-ended questions and reflective listening skills is important to client engagement. Acknowledgment of what is seen, removal of barriers, imagining the experience through the eyes of the client, and use of nonjudgmental/normalizing language are the skills needed to convey empathy to clients. It is revealing that client satisfaction is more highly correlated with how the owner is treated as opposed to how the animal is treated. The desire of the owner to be treated and respected as an individual and the veterinarian's need for information suggest that clients should also be thought of as patients.

THE HISTORY

When taking a history, the objective is to obtain a chronological narrative from the client including all the actions, events, and behaviors of the pet leading up to the current presenting problem. A good history includes biomedical data, the client's perspective, and background information relative to the pet and the client. Biomedical data includes the presenting complaint, timing of events, defining of clinical signs, and a review of body systems. The client's perspective includes concerns, which may not be the same as the veterinarian's; ideas and beliefs; expectations, which again may not be the same as the veterinarian's; repercussions on daily and future living; and feelings about it all. The background history includes all previous medical

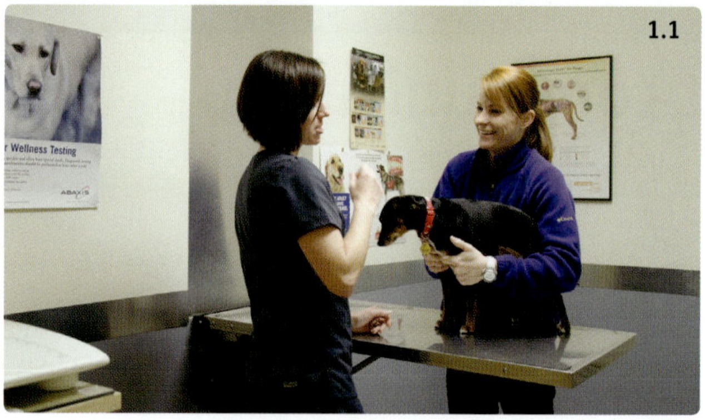

Figure 1.1 The consultation. (Courtesy White Oak Veterinary Hospital)

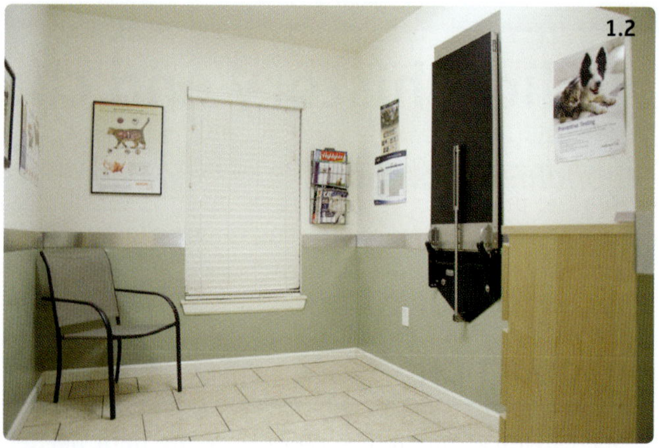

Figure 1.2 The examination room. (Courtesy White Oak Veterinary Hospital)

history including surgeries, medications, preventive medicine, and lifestyle/husbandry information. In order to gather all this information, the veterinarian must employ a thoughtful communication approach. The veterinarian needs to pay attention to his/her surroundings and set the stage. He/she also needs to pay attention to nonverbal behavior (his/her own and the client's), utilize engagement and enlistment skills, and provide a structure and organization to the meeting that will aid in the closing and negotiation relative to contracting the next steps in the treatment plan (**Figure 1.1**).

Basic communication skills

Setting the stage

Before the client enters the examination room, the veterinarian should take stock of himself/herself and the surroundings. Pet owners can learn much about you based on the physical space that surrounds you. A clinic can claim to be 'bond-centered', but if the VHCT neglects to convey the importance of the human–animal bond through the appearance of the clinic, the communication will be much less believable. Setting the stage starts with the outside of the clinic, which should present as clean and professional. Inside, the waiting area should be clean, comfortable, and well lit. Soothing colors should adorn the walls. A display of staff along with their roles is helpful to clients; it makes it easy to place a face with a name and creates an additional welcome. Information pamphlets should be made available along with perhaps a computer with access to websites recommended for educational information.

The examination room should be kept simple yet comfortable (**Figure 1.2**). Too much clutter is distracting and appears disorganized. Tables, equipment, computers, and other technology sometimes create a distance that may be desirable to the VHCT member because it provides a sense of safety through a physical barrier. Unfortunately, too much distance makes it difficult to connect with the client. If the veterinarian wants to engage with the client, the barriers need to be eliminated or, at the very least, one must learn to work around them. Standing on the same side of the table as the client, sitting on the floor with the client and his/her animal, and even using a tablet instead of a stationary computer are good examples of minimizing physical barriers. Whenever possible, the VHCT member should be at the same or below the client's height (**Figure 1.3**).

Veterinarians also need to consider their physical appearance when setting the stage. A coat and tie are not indispensable, but the veterinarian should be dressed neatly, with crisp clothes free of stains. A white coat is practical because if it becomes soiled during an encounter with an animal, the coat can be changed instead of changing clothes. The coat also sets a person as the veterinarian. Many veterinarians wear variations of 'white coats' such as a fleece pullover or polo shirt with their name and the clinic's name embroidered on

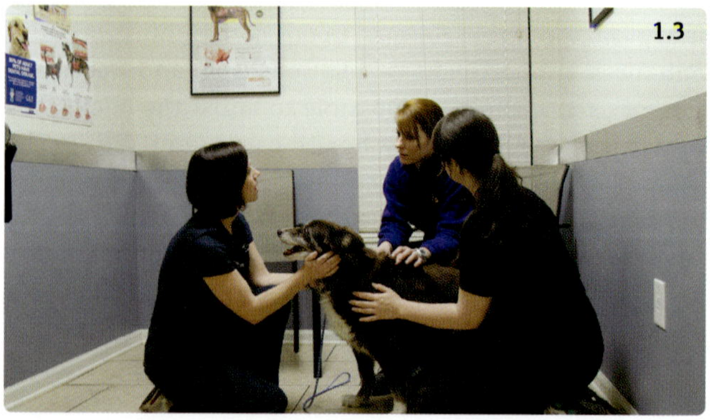

Figure 1.3 Vertical height example. (Courtesy White Oak Veterinary Hospital)

the front. Coats stained with blood, urine, feces, and any other body fluids should be changed before entering a room with a client, as this often reflects negatively in the client's mind. Veterinarians should also minimize personal distractions when they are spending time with a client. Cell phones or digital pagers must be turned off, and staff should be instructed only to interrupt if necessary. If an interruption is anticipated, whether business or personal, the client should be alerted to this possibility up front. Enough time should be allotted for the consultation so that the veterinarian can focus on the client's story rather than what they need to do, could be doing, or their next appointment or surgery.

Nonverbal behavior

Nonverbal communication is the process of communicating through sending and receiving wordless messages. Important information is exchanged at all times, much of it involuntarily. Since approximately 80% of communication is nonverbal, it is imperative that VHCT members pay attention to their client's nonverbal cues as well as their own. Nonverbal communication is conveyed through gesture and touch, by body language or posture, and by facial expression and eye contact. Cues also include voice quality, emotion and speaking style, as well as features such as rhythm, intonation, and stress. Nonverbal behavior reflects a person's feelings more accurately and adds meaning to what is being said. Nonverbal communication can:

- Repeat the message the person is making verbally.
- Contradict a message the individual is trying to convey.
- Substitute for a verbal message.
- Add to or complement a verbal message.
- Accent or underline a verbal message.

It is important to be able to identify/read nonverbal behavior in order to recognize when communication is effective or when the veterinarian is missing something. There are four categories of nonverbal communication: kinesics, proxemics, paralanguage, and autonomic change:

- Kinesics includes facial expressions, body tension, gestures, and body positioning and body movement. These are behaviors over which each person has some control.
- Proxemics includes how space is shaped between interacting individuals. This 'space shaping' looks at spatial relationships such as height differences, interpersonal distance, and angles of facing. Barriers are also included in the proxemics category, covering issues such as charts, examination tables, and perhaps the animal itself. Space shaping was discussed earlier (Setting the stage).
- Paralanguage involves all the elements of voice. These elements include voice tone, rate, rhythm, volume, and emphasis. All of these elements can be used to deliver very different messages with the same words. People 'read' each other's voices as they listen to their words. For example, a tone of voice can imply sarcasm, anger, affection, or confidence.
- Autonomic changes include those behaviors driven by the autonomic nervous system, over which a person has little or no control: flushing, blanching, tearing, sweating, changes in breathing, changes in pupil size, or involuntary swallowing. These changes often indicate that the person being observed is experiencing strong feelings relative to the present conversation. When a client displays these signs, it might be best to stop and ask how they are doing.

When considering nonverbal behavior, four basic premises are important:

- All behavior of a person is communication.
- Involuntary nonverbal communication more accurately reflects a person's feelings.
- The meaning of a communication is the response a message evokes, rather than what was intended to be communicated.
- All behavior is adaptive.

Safety is a basic human need. Clients need to feel safe with the VHCT, so they can share their real concerns and fears, and safe enough to be vulnerable. Much of what veterinarians ask clients to do involves changing something, to seemingly take a risk. Clients need to feel safe in order to make these changes and take these risks for their animal companions. Otherwise, they will respond with fight or flight behaviors. Both fight and flight have distinct nonverbal elements of kinesics, proxemics, paralanguage, and autonomic changes (**Table 1.1**).

It is important to look at the overall pattern of nonverbal behaviors and not just any one sign. Some body postures can have more than one meaning. For instance, folded arms could simply mean that the client is chilly. The rest of the cues should also be assessed to find the meaning of the behavior. If the arms are crossed, but everything else fits into the 'safe' category, the chances are that this is a reaction to the cold temperature in the

Table 1.1 Fight or flight nonverbal behaviors.

Safety	Fight	Flight
Body engaged, leaning forward	Body engaged at a distance	Body disengaged/ pushing back
Arms and legs uncrossed	Fist/jaw clenched	Arms and legs crossed
Decreased body tension	Increased body tension	Head turned away, eyes widened
Variety to gestures and voice	Voice volume increased, staccato	Voice strained, hesitant, volume low
Normal skin color and even breathing	Face flushed, breathing deeper	Skin blanched, breath shallow or held

examination room. Additionally, fight and flight are often seen together; the client may be upset with the VHCT but afraid to compromise the relationship and so prefers to stay silent.

Nonverbal behaviors do not all have the same meaning in various cultures. The main intercultural differences often revolve around eye gaze, interpersonal distance, and touch. However, issues of safety are cross-cultural as expressed through body tension, autonomic responses, and the universal facial expressions of fear, anger, grief, surprise, disgust, and joy. While Eckman found facial expressions to be the same throughout diverse cultures, Darwin also found them to be similar between species.

It is important for the VHCT to recognize expressions of confusion and helplessness, although they are not defined as universal. Confusion is depicted in rising of the eyebrows, furrowing of the brows, and sometimes a cocking of the head to one side or opening of the mouth. It is best to stop and provide clarification and answer questions when clients display this behavior. Helplessness includes a gesture of turning the hands into a palm-up position. When this gesture is observed, clients likely feel at a loss regarding the current discussion. It is important to acknowledge this feeling and provide an opportunity for the client to express this verbally.

Helping clients move from a 'not-safe' to a 'safe' place creates a helping relationship. In doing so, quality information can be gathered relative to their current situation, including the animal, assessing their readiness to accept recommendations, and gaining their collaboration in treatment. To move the client to a 'safe' place it is necessary to identify and address mixed messages.

Mixed messages can be defined as a situation in which a person is receiving verbal or nonverbal cues that seem to contradict each other, when verbal content and nonverbal behaviors do not match up. This could result from an intent to deceive, but more often mixed messages occur when a client is not feeling safe enough to tell the VHCT what is truly going on. Perhaps the client disagrees or is uneasy with what the team is recommending. In order to address these mixed messages the incongruence needs to be noticed and the disparity acknowledged through direct reflection or through the use of the third person. For instance, direct reflection would sound like, "Ms. Smith, I hear you say you agree with my recommendation to begin this medication to treat the diagnosed Cushing's, but I sense some hesitation". Using third person language would sound like, "I had someone in my office earlier with a similar situation who was concerned about this medication". Use of the third person might help create even more safety by saving face. Both methods are effective; however, direct acknowledgment is best if the situation allows.

Verbal communication

Communication skills are critical to eliciting information and understanding each other. Owners need to tell their 'story' so that the veterinarian can understand the current situation and what they need. The veterinarian needs to obtain the client's story in order to gather the required information to decide what needs to be done for the pet. In order to obtain that story it is necessary to engage the client and empathically respond to their needs. John C. Maxwell said, "People don't care how much you know, until they know how much you care". Clients assume their veterinarian cares for their animal almost as much as they do; otherwise, he/she would not have received his/her degree. How clients feel as they leave the clinic is based on how the VHCT responded to their needs as well as their pet's needs.

People working in medicine, human or animal, are comfortable with biomedical skills and good at asking the right questions in order to 'find it' and 'fix it'. Clients expect more than this from their veterinarian; they want the problem to be understood from their perspective. In order to be able to do this, the VHCT must learn how to obtain the required information. The client is going to have an emotional reaction to each situation, and the VHCT needs to respond to these emotions. In short, both biomedical and the client–animal connection information are needed to provide good care to the animal. Many times the information gleaned from the client's 'story' is just as helpful to you as the specific clinical signs when generating a list of differentials. There are specific skills that can be utilized in order to engage and empathize with a client in an effort to elicit the information the veterinarian needs.

Engagement skills

To engage is defined as: 'to occupy the attention or efforts of; to attract or please'. Engaging with a client requires establishing or re-establishing a connection with them as a partner in the care of their animal at the beginning of and throughout a visit. Engagement works at a person to person level and at a professional level. This allows the person to be seen as a person and not just an owner, while maintaining the professional partnership necessary for the well-being of the animal.

The VHCT is the voice of expertise and experience in veterinary medicine. The client is the voice of expertise and experience with their animal. Both voices need to be heard and considered for engagement to be successful. Clients want to tell a story. They are concerned with the meaning of their animal's illness. They want to explain and speak in terms of the human–animal bond with their pet. The VHCT wants to obtain the story as quickly as possible. The team is concerned with the facts and often think in terms of differential diagnoses. These different goals may be challenging. If the VHCT focuses only on the biomedical, the story can become an inquiry and feel to the client like continuous interruptions. If the veterinary care provider moves too quickly, important information may be missed. The interests of the client and the veterinarian are both equally important when gathering the necessary information to do what is best for the animal involved.

Engaging with a client necessitates an invitation requesting that the client tell their story. One of the easiest ways to do this is through the use of open-ended questions. It is easy, but it is not something most veterinarians are used to. Instead of asking closed-ended questions to direct the fact-finding mission, open-ended questions will garner much more information. Examples of open-ended questions are:

- "Tell me about..."
- "What happened next..."
- "What thoughts or feelings did you have when..."
- "Tell me more about..."
- "What was that like for you..."

When only closed-ended questions are asked, the veterinarian only gets answers to the questions he/she has asked. The client will answer what was asked and possibly not elaborate further. It is quite possible that the veterinarian did not ask the correct question in order to get the best answers. Clients will often remark, "He/she didn't ask that". Once an open-ended question is asked, it is important to sit back and listen. Allow the client to complete a thought without being interrupted. A recent study published in the *Journal of the American Veterinary Medical Association* found that veterinarians interrupt clients within 15.3 seconds into their response to questions. Listening without interruption and with thoughtful intention demonstrates interest and gives time to think and process the next question or steps. To listen with thoughtful intention, it is important to pay attention and focus on the conversation at hand. As the client responds to the open-ended questions, it may still be necessary to ask closed-ended questions to ensure that the required information is communicated. These closed-ended questions are helpful to clarify the details of the investigation:

- "Is he eating?"
- "Is the vomiting right after he eats?"
- "Any diarrhea?"

Another engagement skill is that of reflective listening, also known as parallel talk, parroting, or paraphrasing. Reflective listening presents a two-way mirror to the client; they hear what they are saying, but also hear it after it was processed by the veterinary care provider. The technique can be used to check for understanding, create empathy, and build a positive rapport. The veterinarian's reflection comes from listening, observing, and interpreting verbal and nonverbal cues as he/she tries to appreciate the client's perspective. Someone who listens reflectively expresses their desire to understand how the other person is thinking and feeling, and their willingness to help and not to judge the other person.

There are three kinds of reflective listening: a simple repeat of the client's words, a summary and interpretation, and a hypothesis test. Some examples of reflective listening are listed below:

- "I wonder if ..."
- "In your experience ..."
- "Let me see if I understand. You ..."
- "It sounds like ..."

Note the use of 'I' and 'you'. It is important to ensure that these two words are utilized to probe for understanding and to avoid them coming across as intimating blame.

Empathy skills

It is clear that an understanding of the situation the client is experiencing/has experienced is necessary. It is also important to appreciate what the experience was/ is like for the client. This can be done through empathic responses. Empathy is defined as: 'identification with and understanding of another's situation, feelings, and motives'. This understanding creates a safe environment for the client where they feel seen, heard, and accepted. Empathic responses require empathic nonverbal responses as well. These include facial expressions, awareness of physical space, using appropriate touch, matching the tone of one's voice with that of the conversation, and being comfortable with silence if that is what the moment calls for.

In order for the client to 'feel seen' it is necessary to share one's observations. This can be done by simply acknowledging the facial and body expressions of the client. Two examples of acknowledgement are: "You look very worried"; "When I said that your face changed". It is important to remove as many physical barriers as possible when using empathy. With barriers, the ability to read body language is diminished, as is the connectivity with the client. The veterinarian needs to share his/her appreciation of the situation with the client. Two examples of empathic appreciation are: "This little guy really scared you and your mom"; "It sounds like you were really worried that Fluffy wouldn't make it through the night".'

Finally, the client needs is to feel accepted by the VHCT. Avoiding being judgmental can be difficult depending on the circumstances. Empathic responses that help clients feel accepted by the VHCT include: "You were caught between a rock and a hard place"; "I think anyone who loves their animal the way you do would have reacted that way"; "It's never easy, even when we know it's right". Some self-disclosure from the veterinarian might be appropriate when trying to help a client feel accepted.

Structure and organization

It is helpful to the veterinarian and client to provide some structure when getting a history. The client has come to the clinic with a concern, the presenting problem for the pet. The opportunity for rapport building begins the moment the client walks into the clinic with their pet. Introductions, to the pet and the owner, and small talk are a good way to begin. After getting the client's answer to "what brings you in today?", the VHCT member can either continue exploring the presenting complaint or tell the client that they will first gather some general history information. Depending on the client, it may be easiest to allow him/her to direct the conversation and redirect when necessary. It may also be upsetting to a client to begin with generalities about their pet when they are very concerned about the present issue.

The transition from one line of inquiry to the next is best achieved by summarizing at the end of each line of inquiry. This allows the client to correct and/or clarify any information and it allows the veterinarian to organize his/her thoughts. The structure of the discussion should be logical, and it is important to keep the interview on track.

Once the necessary information has been gathered, and a thorough physical examination has been performed, the next steps need to be approached. The rationale of the diagnostic and treatment plans should be explained to the client before obtaining their permission to proceed both verbally and in writing, including an estimate of the projected costs. It is important to make sure that the client is involved in the planning of the next steps. It is also strongly recommended to check the client's feelings by asking what they are thinking. This allows the veterinarian to incorporate the client's perspective and to find out what type of client education should be offered. Client education is very important and alleviates fear of the unknown.

As the consultation comes to an end, the veterinarian must make sure there is nothing else the client has concerns about. Questions such as: "Have I missed anything?", "Do you have any other questions for me?", "Do you have any other concerns?" can be very helpful to the client's feelings of contentment with the consultation (**Figure 1.4**).

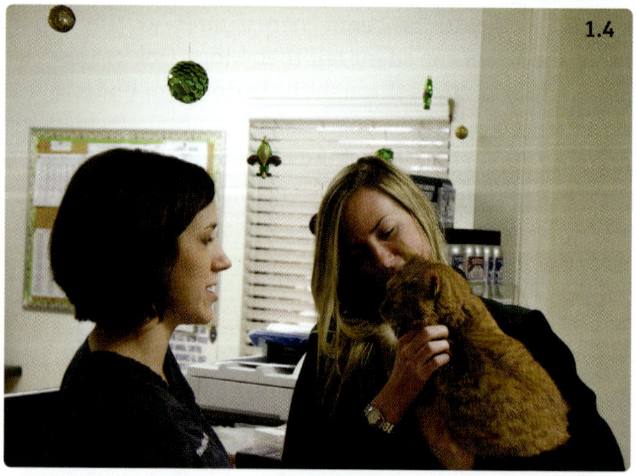

Figure 1.4 The closing. (Courtesy White Oak Veterinary Hospital)

SUMMARY

The typical veterinarian will have approximately 200,000 client consultations over a 40-year career. These consultations can be a source of both fulfillment and stress. The measures of success self-reported by veterinarians include working with animals and restoring health, and working with clients and building relationships. Good communication skills are necessary to build these strong veterinarian–client relationships. These skills are indispensable to effective consultations and include ensuring increased accuracy, efficiency, and supportiveness, enhancing client and clinician satisfaction, improving outcomes of care, and promoting collaboration and partnership. Many in veterinary medicine fear that 'good communication' takes longer; paying attention to everything mentioned above increases the consultation time. Research in the human medical field has shown that it does not take any more time to utilize these skills and that good communication increases efficiency. Mastering the art and science of communication will allow the veterinarian to provide the best possible care to animals and their owners.

RECOMMENDED FURTHER READING

Dalgleish T, Powers M (1999) (eds.) *Handbook of Cognition and Emotion*. Wiley & Sons, Chichester, pp. 21–45.

Dysart L, Coe J, Adams C (2011) Analysis of solicitation of client concern in companion animal practice. *J Am Vet Med Assoc* **238:**1609–1615.

Hampton JR, Harrison MJG, Mitchell JR *et al.* (1975) Relative contributions of history taking, physical examination and laboratory investigation to diagnosis and management of medical outpatients. *Br Med J* **2:**486–489.

Keller VF, Carroll JG (1994) A new model for physician–patient communication. *Patient Educ Couns* **23:**131–140.

Kurtz S (2006) Teaching and learning communication in veterinary medicine. *J Vet Med Educ* **33:**11–19.

Kurtz SM, Silverman J, Draper J (2005) *Teaching and Learning Communications Skills in Medicine*, 2nd edn. Radcliffe Medical Press, Abingdon.

Lagoni L, Butler C, Hetts S (1994) *The Human–Animal Bond and Grief*. WB Saunders, Philadelphia, pp. 124–131.

Marvel MK, Doherty WJ, Weiner E (1998) Medical interviewing by exemplary family physicians. *J Fam Pract* **47:**343–348.

Maxwell JC (2004) *Winning with People: Discover the People Principles that Work for You Every Time*. Thomas Nelson, Inc., Nashville, p. 91.

Osborne CA (2001) What are veterinarians worth? *J Am Vet Med Assoc* **219:**302–303.

Shaw J (2006) Four core communication skills of highly effective practitioners. *Vet Clin North Am Small Anim Pract* **36:**385–396.

Shaw J, Adams C, Bonnett BN *et al.* (2012) Veterinarian satisfaction with companion animal visits. *J Am Vet Med Assoc* **240:**832–841.

Chapter 2 Common clinical problems

2.1 Dyspnea

Elizabeth Rozanski

INTRODUCTION

Difficulty breathing, or 'dyspnea', requires prompt attention in dogs and cats. Some authors prefer to avoid the term dyspnea, as it defines a sensation of breathlessness in people, which dogs and cats are unable to describe, and substitute respiratory distress or shortness of breath. No matter the name, respiratory distress of any origin represents a true emergency, and rapid attention is warranted to identify the underlying cause, to limit the sensation of difficulty breathing, and to provide diagnostic and therapeutic information for clients of affected animals.

Localization of the source of the distress will provide useful clues as to the cause of the distress and may help direct therapeutic options. Respiratory distress may be localized to the upper airways, lung parenchyma, or pleural space. Occasionally, pain or severe acidosis may result in tachypnea, which may look similar to respiratory distress. It is particularly important to recognize upper airway obstruction or partial obstruction and pleural space disease (pneumothorax or pleural effusion), as these are particularly amenable to urgent interventions, such as intubation or thoracentesis. Success in patient management revolves around developing a solid knowledge base of potential causes of respiratory distress and 'pattern recognition' of common emergent or urgent problems affecting dogs and cats. The goals of this chapter are to provide guidelines for emergent management and to highlight common emergent conditions resulting in respiratory distress.

Any client calling to report respiratory distress or possible respiratory distress should be advised to bring the patient into the hospital immediately for evaluation. While an understanding of all potential causes of respiratory distress is helpful, the first steps in the clinical evaluation of a patient presenting with respiratory distress are to provide a supplemental source of oxygen and to obtain a brief history from the client. Respiratory distress is often acute, although some chronic medical conditions may present with new-onset respiratory distress. Common causes of new respiratory distress in patients with chronic diseases include: cardiogenic pulmonary edema associated with chronic valvular disease; pulmonary thromboembolism from a variety of causes including glomerulonephritis or hemolytic anemia; pulmonary metastatic disease, most commonly from hemangiosarcoma or carcinoma; and aspiration pneumonia associated with megaesophagus, laryngeal paralysis or other pharyngeal dysfunction.

All hospitals should have a form of supplemental oxygen available. Supplemental oxygen may be provided via a variety of options, including flow-by, face mask, nasal oxygen, e-collar and cellophane wrap ('oxygen hood'), oxygen cage, and intubation with intermittent positive pressure ventilation (IPPV). Flow-by oxygen is provided by holding an oxygen source near the mouth and nostrils of the affected patient. Flow-by oxygen is an easy and rapid solution; however, the actual increase over room air's oxygen content may be minimal, particularly with an anxious or uncooperative pet. Oxygen may also be provided with a face mask, with the oxygen tubing attached to a cone that is placed over the nose and mouth of the patient. The oxygen concentration achieved with a face mask is also variable, although with very weak animals a high percentage (>80%) may be reached. Both flow-by and face mask oxygen may require veterinary personnel to hold both the pet and the oxygen supply. Nasal oxygen involves placement of a flexible catheter into the nasal passages and insufflation of humidified oxygen, typically at 50–100 ml/kg/min. Nasal oxygen is particularly useful in pets that are neither panting nor open-mouth breathing, as high inspiratory flow rates associated with panting will result in relative decreases in the percentage inspired oxygen. Nasal oxygen is commonly placed after patient stabilization, rather than urgently in the emergency setting. Nasal catheters may also be advanced into the trachea, by-passing the upper airways. A home-made oxygen hood may be created with an Elizabethan collar and cellophane wrap, or may be commercially purchased. An oxygen cage is also frequently used to provide supplemental oxygen. Oxygen cages are commonly well-tolerated by both cats and dogs, and are also capable of reaching a high concentration of oxygen; however, if the cage door is open for patient manipulation, the oxygen concentration will rapidly equilibrate with the room air. Finally, heavy sedation and intubation plus IPPV are the best options for providing high levels of supplemental oxygen, removing respiratory fatigue, and eliminating patient fear and anxiety.

During the initial stabilization of the pet, a history should be obtained from the owner. In some cases, the precipitating cause of the respiratory distress is straightforward, such as with traumatic injuries, while in other cases the onset may be subtle. Owners should be questioned as to past medical conditions, history of routine veterinary care, including heartworm prophylaxis, and finally, the progression of the signs of respiratory distress should be described. Peracute signs are frequently associated with trauma, aspiration pneumonitis, major vascular abnormalities such as emboli or thrombosis, neurogenic pulmonary edema, and cardiogenic pulmonary edema when associated with a major cordae tendineae rupture. In less acute disease, and especially in cats, the development of respiratory distress may be preceded by anorexia, lethargy, or abnormal behavior (such as hiding and refusing to jump on furniture).

Ideally, following history and physical examination (PE), the source of the respiratory distress may be localized and further diagnostics and therapeutics pursued as indicated. Owners should be advised that the prognosis is dependent on the underlying disease, and that it is difficult to predict the outcome in any individual patient. Many animals with moderate to severe respiratory distress recover with supportive and specific care. It is easy to stereotype certain breeds of dyspneic animals to particular disorders, but it is important to avoid tunnel vision and to consider all the possibilities. However, clinical guidelines may be useful to the clinician for common causes of respiratory distress (**Table 2.1.1**) and examples are discussed in the sections below. (See also **Figure 2.1.1**.)

Table 2.1.1 Main causes of acute respiratory distress in the dog and cat.

Dog	Cat
Brachycephalic syndrome and all causes of upper airway occlusion	Pneumonia, allergic bronchitis
Laryngeal paralysis	Neurogenic pulmonary edema
Collapsed trachea and main stem bronchi	Congestive heart failure
Pneumonia	Upper airway obstruction: tumors, foreign bodies
Acute respiratory distress syndrome/acute lung injury	Acute respiratory distress syndrome/acute lung injury
Congestive heart failure	Pyo-, hemo-, chylothorax; other effusions
Neurogenic pulmonary edema	Chest trauma
Chest trauma	Pulmonary fibrosis
Spontaneous pneumothorax	
Pulmonary thromboembolism/ thrombosis	
Pulmonary metastatic disease	
Pulmonary fibrosis	
Pleural effusion (pyo-, hemo-, chylothorax)/ pleural space disease	

EXAMPLES OF TYPICAL CAUSES OF DYSPNEA IN CATS

Feline allergic bronchitis

Signalment: Young adult to middle aged cats.
PE findings: Cough/wheeze; normal rectal temperature.
Thoracic radiographs: Bronchial pattern on radiographic evaluation; hyperinflation/air trapping, collapse of a lung lobe (classically the right middle lung lobe).
Other testing: Exclude heartworm and lungworm infection; possible transtracheal aspirate for cytologic evaluation and aerobic culture; consider evaluation for *Mycoplasma* spp.
Emergent therapy: Oxygen, systemic glucocorticoids, bronchodilators (albuterol by inhalation or terbutaline [0.01 mg/kg SC or 0.1–0.2 mg/kg PO q12h (in practice ¼ of a 2.5 mg tablet)]).
Clinical course: Expect significant improvement within 12 hours of steroids and bronchodilators; rapid discharge.

Congestive heart failure

Signalment: Any age cat; hypertrophic cardiomyopathy is more common in larger cats.

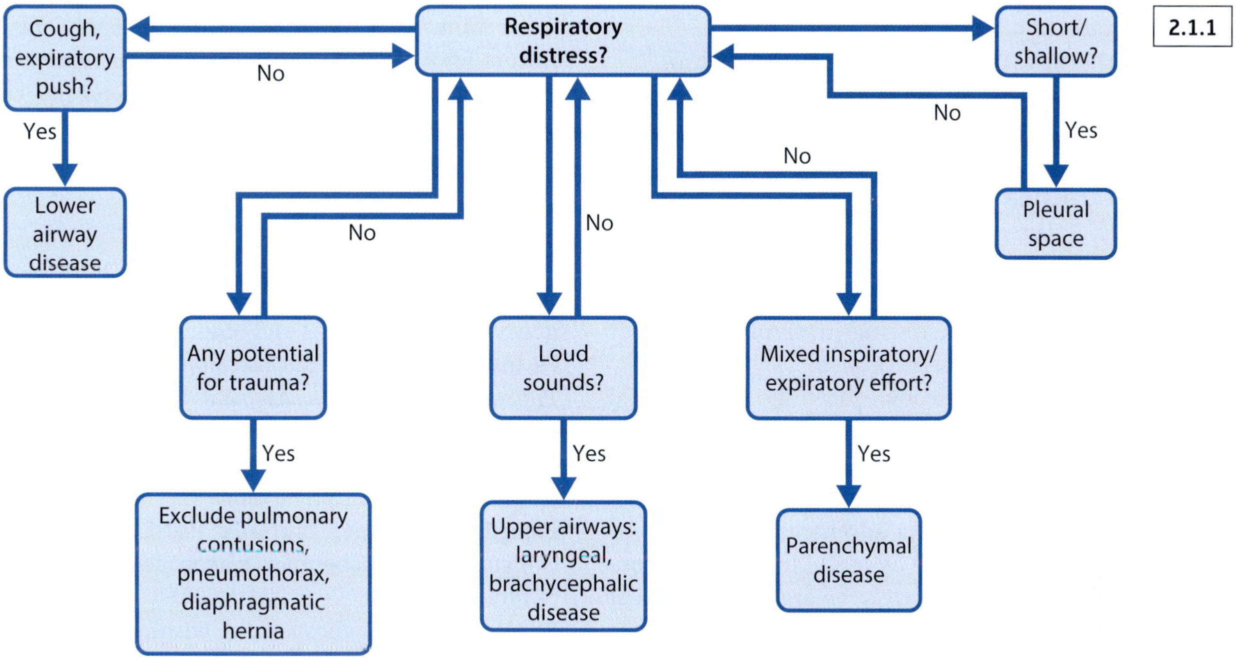

Figure 2.1.1 Diagnostic algorithm for dyspnea.

PE findings: Murmur/gallop in many but not all; jugular venous distension, hypothermia.
Thoracic radiographs: Cardiomegaly; patchy interstitial to alveolar infiltrates.
Other testing: Echocardiography; NT pro-BNP snap test may be useful.
Emergent therapy: Oxygen, furosemide (1–4 mg/kg IV or IM q2–8h).
Clinical course: Expect improvement within 12 hours; hospitalization course may extend for 2–4 days and excessive diuresis may result in dehydration and anorexia.

Upper airway obstruction

Signalment: Any age cat; younger cats are more commonly affected with polyps, foreign bodies, or infection; older cats more commonly affected with laryngeal neoplasia.
PE findings: Loud respiration, prolonged inspiratory time, anxiety, sometimes cervical extension.
Thoracic radiographs: Generally unremarkable.
Other testing: Oral examination under sedation; be prepared for a difficult intubation.
Emergent therapy: Tracheostomy.
Clinical course: Variable, depends on the cause.

Pleural space disease

Signalment: More common in older cats; younger cats may have pyothorax or mediastinal lymphoma.
PE findings: Short, shallow respiration, muffled lung sounds, increased abdominal effort.
Thoracic radiographs: Pleural space disease (fluid, air, or mass lesions) is readily apparent.
Other testing: Screening (T-FAST) ultrasound, echocardiography, thoracentesis with cytology and bacterial culture; infections may be anaerobic.
Emergent therapy: Thoracentesis; thoracostomy tube placement.
Clinical course: Variable, depends on the cause. Prognosis tends to be guarded.

EXAMPLES OF TYPICAL CAUSES OF DYSPNEA IN DOGS

Upper airway obstruction

Signalment: Brachycephalic or older large breed dogs are most commonly affected. Any dog can be affected with a foreign object (ball/rawhide).
PE findings: Loud respiration, prolonged inspiratory time; hyperthermia.
Thoracic radiographs: Generally unremarkable; may show concurrent disease such as megaesophagus, hiatal hernia, or noncardiogenic pulmonary edema.
Other testing: Oral examination under sedation. Be prepared for a difficult intubation and also be prepared to complete any surgical procedure that is warranted,

such as arytenoid lateralization (laryngeal paralysis) or soft palate resection.

Emergent therapy: Tracheostomy, sedation, cooling.

Clinical course: Variable, depends on the cause and if concurrent pneumonia or noncardiogenic edema.

Collapsed trachea

Signalment: Toy breeds.

PE findings: Typical 'honking'-type cough, but can present as dyspneic without cough.

Thoracic radiographs: Narrowing involving cervical or thoracic trachea, or main stem bronchi.

Other testing: Bronchoscopy showing intraluminal tracheal narrowing.

Emergent therapy: Oxygen, mild sedation with acepromazine, and cough suppressants. Bronchodilator (aminophylline, theophylline, or beta adrenergic drugs such as albuterol or terbutaline) may be useful in dogs with concurrent chronic bronchitis. Rarely, emergent insertion of a tracheal stent.

Clinical course: Always guarded for the first 24 hours; recurrences common.

Pneumonia

Signalment: Young puppies with or without respiratory disease, dogs with pharyngeal/esophageal disease, any condition associated with altered consciousness or that can lead to aspiration of gastric contents into the airway; hunting breeds in areas with endemic fungal disease.

PE findings: Tachypnea, fever, cough.

Thoracic radiographs: Alveolar infiltrates, particularly cranial ventral lung lobes. Fungal pneumonias may appear nodular or military.

Other testing: CBC for signs of systemic inflammation, tracheal wash for culture and cytology evaluation (while noting the associated risks with this procedure).

Emergent therapy: Prompt institution of broad-spectrum antibiotics, supplemental oxygen. Antifungal therapy.

Clinical course: Improvement within 2–3 days in most cases; respiratory failure/death are possible. Hospitalization for 3–5 days. Fungal pneumonias have more protracted course with more guarded prognosis.

Acute lung injury/acute respiratory distress syndrome

Signalment: Any age; always associated with another primary insult (pulmonary or extrapulmonary).

PE findings: Tachypnea with severe distress.

Thoracic radiographs: Alveolar infiltrates; all lung lobes affected.

Other testing: Echocardiography to exclude congestive heart failure and pulmonary thromboembolism; airway culture for pneumonia (may occur concurrently).

Emergent therapy: Supplemental oxygen; consider positive pressure ventilation.

Clinical course: Guarded prognosis; lengthy course for resolution.

Congestive heart failure

Signalment: Older small breed dogs with long-standing murmurs; Dobermanns and other large breed dogs.

PE findings: Tachycardia, tachypnea, murmur, gallop.

Thoracic radiographs: Alveolar infiltrates, particularly in the perihilar region; cardiomegaly.

Other testing: Echocardiography; NT pro-BNP if echocardiography not promptly available.

Emergent therapy: Diuretics (furosemide 2–4 mg/kg IV); consider pimobendan, nitroprusside; supplemental oxygen.

Clinical course: Improvement within 1–2 days in most cases; hospitalization for 2–4 days.

Thoracic trauma

Signalment: Any age; young dogs more commonly affected.

PE findings: Tachypnea, distress, other signs of trauma.

Thoracic radiographs: Patchy interstitial to alveolar infiltrates (contusion), pneumothorax, rib fractures, and diaphragmatic hernia are all possible. Anticoagulant rodenticide intoxication can cause alveolar infiltrates and pleural effusion without evidence of trauma.

Other testing: As clinically indicated.

Emergent therapy: Thoracentesis, correction of hernia, pain relief; avoid large volume fluid boluses; supplemental oxygen.

Clinical course: Improvement within 2–3 days in most cases; mortality usually due to associated injuries.

Spontaneous pneumothorax

Signalment: Large breed dogs, northern breeds (Akita, Alaskan Malamute, American Eskimo, and others) and Golden Retrievers appear overrepresented.

PE findings: Tachypnea, muffled lung sounds.

Thoracic radiographs: Large volume pneumothorax.

Other testing: As clinically needed; clinicians debate if CT scanning provides useful information.

Emergent therapy: Thoracentesis.

Clinical course: Recommend prompt surgical therapy for resection of bullae via a median sternotomy. Exclude (rare) neoplasia or infectious cause.

Pulmonary thromboembolism

Signalment: Any age; older dogs more likely affected with co-morbidities that are associated with pulmonary thromboembolism, such as Cushing's syndrome, protein-losing nephropathy, immune-mediated hemolytic anemia.

PE findings: Tachypnea, loud S2.

Thoracic radiographs: Oligemia, patchy infiltrates, pleural effusion may or may not be present.

Other testing: Echocardiography, CT angiogram. Laboratory testing for hypercoagulability, urine protein: creatinine ratio.

Emergent therapy: Anticoagulation with heparin or low-molecular-weight heparin, supplemental oxygen.

Clinical course: Improvement within 2–3 days in most cases; sudden death is possible.

Pulmonary fibrosis

Signalment: Older dogs; terriers (especially West Highland White) and Chihuahuas appear overrepresented.

PE findings: Tachypnea, exercise intolerance.

Thoracic radiographs: Diffuse interstitial infiltrates, possible right-sided cardiac enlargement.

Other testing: Echocardiography, CT, bronchoalveolar lavage.

Emergent therapy: Supplemental oxygen. No specific therapy known to be helpful.

Clinical course: Gradual progression over weeks to months.

Pulmonary metastatic disease

Signalment: Older dogs more commonly affected; may or may not have a known history of neoplasia.

PE findings: Tachypnea (common when bronchi are compromised), cough occasionally with hemoptysis.

Thoracic radiographs: Nodular, may have a miliary component; spontaneous pneumothorax may occur.

Other testing: Search for the primary may be undertaken, but may also be appropriate to focus on palliative care.

Emergent therapy: Supplemental oxygen.

Clinical course: Progressive disease.

RECOMMENDED FURTHER READING

Campbell VL (2011) Respiratory complications in critical illness of small animals. *Vet Clin North Am Small Anim Pract* **41(4)**:709–716,

Corcoran BM, Cobb M, Martin MW *et al.* (1999) Chronic pulmonary disease in West Highland white terriers. *Vet Rec* **144(22)**:611–616.

Epstein SE, Hopper K, Mellema MS *et al.* (2013) Diagnostic utility of D-dimer concentrations in dogs with pulmonary embolism. *J Vet Intern Med* **27(6)**:1646–1649.

Fine DM, DeClue AE, Reinero CR (2008) Evaluation of circulating amino terminal-pro-B-type natriuretic peptide concentration in dogs with respiratory distress attributable to congestive heart failure or primary pulmonary disease. *J Am Vet Med Assoc* **232(11)**:1674–1679.

Goggs R, Benigni L, Fuentes VL *et al.* (2009) Pulmonary thromboembolism. *J Vet Emerg Crit Care* **19(1)**:30–52.

Goggs R, Chan DL, Benigni L *et al.* (2014) Comparison of computed tomography pulmonary angiography and point-of-care tests for pulmonary thromboembolism diagnosis in dogs. *J Small Anim Pract* **5(4)**:190–197.

Powell L, Rozanski EA, Tidwell A *et al.* (1999) A retrospective analysis of pulmonary contusion secondary to motor vehicle accidents in 143 dogs: 1994–1997. *J Vet Emerg Crit Care* **9**:127–136.

Rozanski E, Chan DL (2005) Approach to the patient with respiratory distress. *Vet Clin North Am Small Anim Pract* **35(2)**:307–317.

Sigrist NE, Adamik KN, Doherr MG *et al.* (2011) Evaluation of respiratory parameters at presentation as clinical indicators of the respiratory localization in dogs and cats with respiratory distress. *J Vet Emerg Crit Care* **21(1)**:13–23.

Sumner C, Rozanski E (2013) Management of respiratory emergencies in small animals. *Vet Clin North Am Small Anim Pract* **43(4)**:799–815.

Chapter 2 Common clinical problems

2.2 Syncope, episodic weakness, and collapse

Boyd R. Jones

INTRODUCTION

Syncope, episodic weakness, and collapse are clinical signs that are often easily recognized, but sometimes confirmation of their cause may be difficult. Owner descriptions of what they see may be confusing or what they have seen may be misinterpreted. Syncope, weakness, or collapse may occur at rest but occur more frequently with exercise and activity.

Syncope ('fainting') refers to the sudden loss of consciousness resulting from paroxysmal episodes of impaired cerebral blood flow, which deprives the brain of energy substrates, oxygen, and glucose. True syncope is most often related to cardiac disease but can be associated with coughing ('cough syncope'), hypoglycemia, severe anemia, polcythemia, acid–base imbalance, and other causes.

Episodic weakness or exercise intolerance is weakness that occurs with activity and exercise and improves after rest. There is weakness and fatigue after mild exercise but occasionally more prolonged exercise is needed to cause clinical signs. The degree of weakness may vary from mild hindlimb ataxia to complete collapse. Most animals are normal in between episodes. Collapse may be acute with seizures, narcolepsy/catalepsy, or syncope, but also as a component of more chronic and progressive metabolic or neurologic disorders.

CLINICAL SIGNS

Syncope is characterized by a short period of flaccid collapse and loss of consciousness. Most dogs are motionless with relaxed skeletal muscles. Sometimes there is involuntary urination and vocalization. Recovery is rapid but there may be confusion for a short time afterwards.

Signs of episodic weakness are often intermittent and include a degree of weakness, stiff stilted walk, ventroflexion of the neck and head, and reluctance to continue walking or exercising. Animals may lie down and refuse to move or collapse when they attempt to get up and walk. They may be alert or obtunded and sometimes pant as they appear to be, and are, apprehensive. Muscle strength improves after rest, and between episodes the animal may appear normal. There may be key events that precipitate the clinical signs, such as exercise, feeding, or excitement; these 'triggers' must be identified by careful and complete questioning of the owner.

Relying on the owner's description of clinical signs can be misleading. Their description of what they see may not give a true indication of the clinical signs. Most digital cameras and smart phones have movie capacity so that owners can be asked to record the event to confirm what they see. The clinician can then view the event to determine its true nature and have an accurate record of the clinical signs, which is essential to aid differential diagnosis and direct the next investigations. Furthermore, the video can be sent to a specialist clinician for interpretation and specialist advice if that is required.

A complete history and clinical examination are also essential to help localize the cause to a body system and, in the case of a neurologic disease, to localize the lesion(s). Some of the important questions to ask the owner of an animal with syncope, collapse, or weakness are included in **Table 2.2.1**, along with the object of the questioning. Clinical experience, the history, and findings from a physical examination may enable the clinician to characterize the condition so that the diagnosis only needs to be confirmed. However, especially with episodic weakness, the animal may be examined when it is, or appears to be, normal, making further investigation essential. A plethora of diagnostic tests and procedures may be considered, therefore it is best to delay full investigation until an episode is viewed. For additional investigation there needs to be a high index of suspicion as to whether the condition is neuromuscular, metabolic, or cardiovascular in origin. The investigation required for each is different. An approach to working up a case with syncope or episodic weakness is shown in **Figures 2.2.1, 2.2.2** and in **Table 2.2.2**. More information about each condition can be sought from other chapters in this book.

Table 2.2.1 Questions for clients and their object, with specific outcomes related to syncope, episodic weakness, and collapse.

History	Object and outcome
What did you see?	Try to determine from the description of the clinical signs if they are cardiac or neurologic in origin.
How often have the signs occurred?	Increased frequency may suggest a progressive disease.
Are the clinical signs always the same?	Episodic conditions usually show repeatable clinical signs.
Is the animal normal immediately after an episode?	With syncopal causes and neuromuscular diseases there are often no significant signs, in contrast to seizures.
Is the animal normal in between episodes?	There may be no signs, but with some neuromuscular diseases clinical signs can be detected.
Is there anything that initiates an episode?	Exercise/coughing may induce syncope. Feeding may induce narcolepsy; exercise is a trigger for weakness and collapse with neuromuscular diseases (e.g. myasthenia gravis).
Is there vomiting/regurgitation?	Regurgitation frequently occurs with metabolic and neuromuscular disease (e.g. myasthenia gravis, Addison's disease).
Have you seen the dog vomit or regurgitate?	Try to establish if esophageal signs are present suggesting muscle disease.
Are litter mates affected?	Breed related conditions that result in weakness and syncope are well known.
Is the animal stiff or floppy during an episode	Stiffness may be present with seizures or some myopathies but often not with cardiac and metabolic causes.
What color are the tongue/gums?	Pale or cyanotic mucous membranes may indicate cardiovascular disease.
What are the heart/pulse rates?	Detection of arrhythmias indicates cardiac disease.

DIAGNOSTIC INVESTIGATION

Minimum database

Hematology, biochemistry including values for all electrolytes (sodium, potassium, calcium, phosphate, creatine kinase), and urinalysis are the minimum required for most cases and the results may provide a diagnosis or give an indication for further diagnostic tests (e.g. adrenocortical function, thyroid function, fasting blood glucose/insulin).

An electrocardiogram (ECG) should be performed if cardiac disease (especially an arrhythmia) is suspected. Owners can be taught how to check and determine the heart rate and rhythm during an attack if the animal is normal at the time of examination. An ECG is often normal and therefore ambulatory ECG (Holter) monitoring may be required. Blood pressure should be determined if cardiac disease and/or hypertension is suspected.

Lactate and pyruvate analysis can assist with some rare metabolic muscle diseases that are classified as mitochondrial myopathies. These disorders are genetic in nature and are characterized by accumulation of vacuoles of lipid, glycogen, and other metabolites within certain muscle fibers, abnormal urine organic acid and blood amino acid profiles, lactate and pyruvate elevations, and abnormal lactate and pyruvate ratios.

Endocrine

Adrenal and thyroid function tests may be indicated in some cases; measurement of insulin (with glucose) after fasting or at the time of an event is required if insulinoma or another hypoglycemia causing tumor (e.g. gastric leiomyoma) is suspected.

Serology

Measurement of acetylcholine receptor antibodies is essential in dogs with suspected myasthenia gravis (MG) or in those with acquired megaesophagus. Serology may also be of value if specific infectious diseases are suspected.

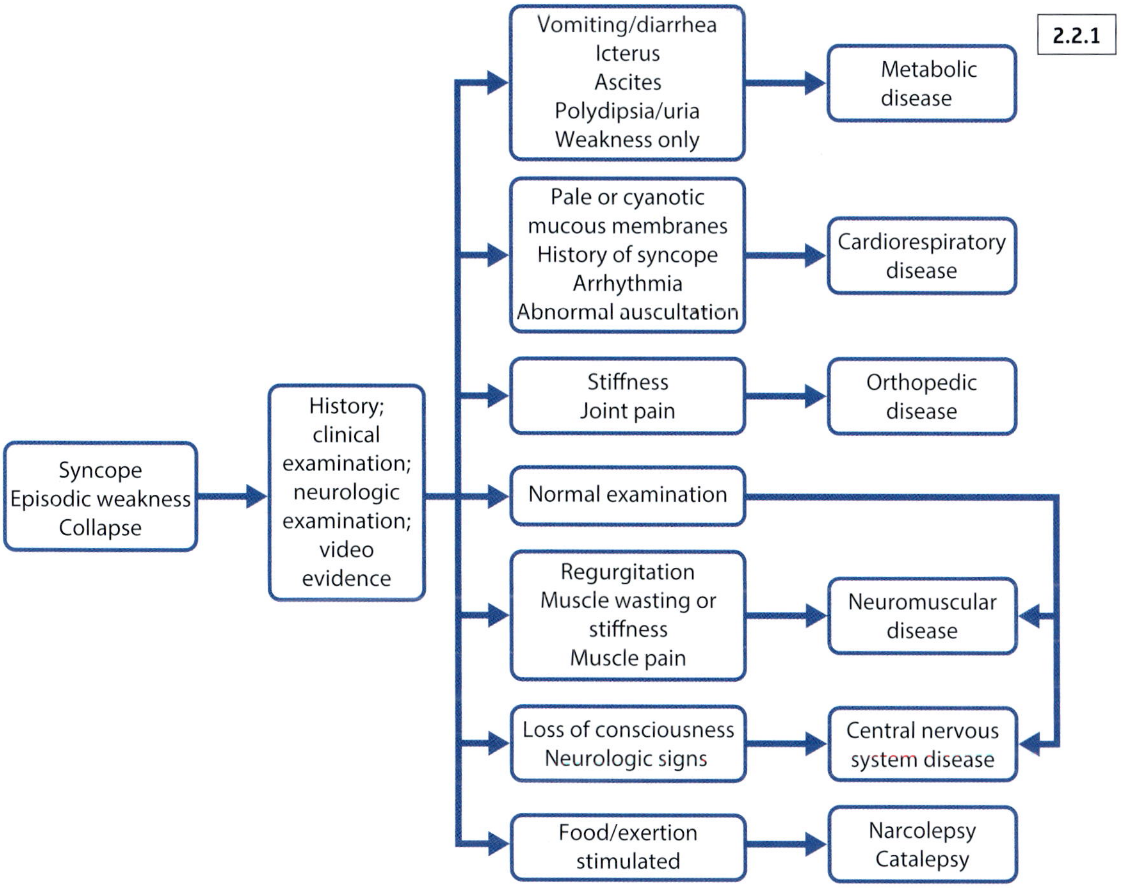

Figure 2.2.1 Algorithm for the general approach to the differential diagnosis of syncope, episodic weakness, and collapse.

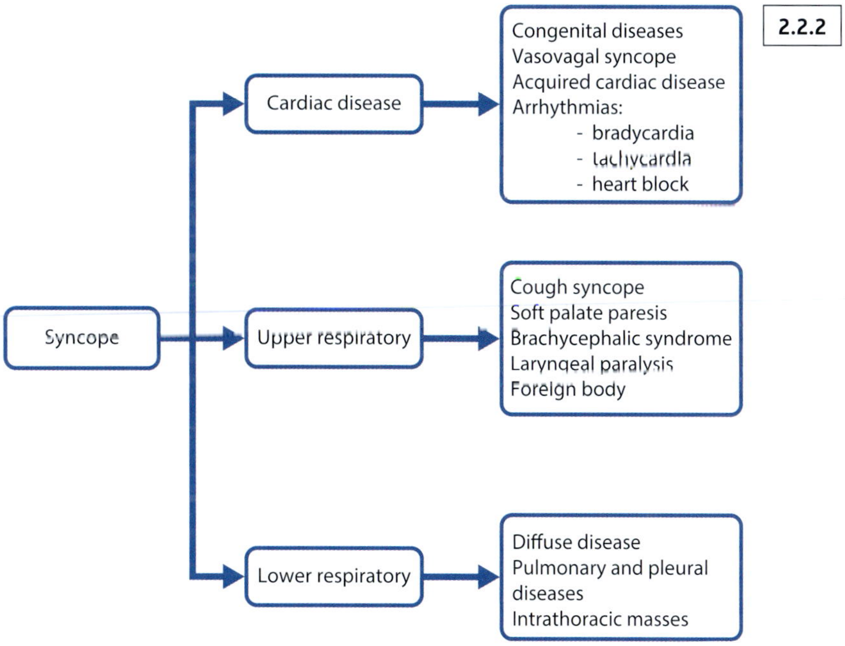

Figure 2.2.2 Algorithm for syncope.

Table 2.2.2 Differential diagnosis of weakness.

Endocrine diseases	Insulinoma Hypoadrenocorticism Hyperadrenoocorticism (Cushing's myopathy) Hypothyroidism (myopathy) Hypoparathyroidism Pheochromocytoma Diabetes mellitus/ketoacidosis
Orthopedic diseases	Degenerative joint disease (hips, stifles, spondylosis) Polyarthritis – various types
Hematologic diseases	Anemia – all causes Myeloproliferative disease Polycythemia Hemoglobinopathies
Metabolic diseases	Uremia (encephalopathy and hypokalemia) Hyperglycemia/hypoglycemia Hypernatremia/hyponatremia Hypokalemia/hyperkalemia Hypercalcemia/hypocalcemia Acidosis Hyperthermia Hypoxia
Myopathies	Inherited: • Labrador Retriever mypopathy • Sex-linked muscular dystrophies (dystrophin defects): Golden Retriever, Japanese Spitz • Devon Rex cat myopathy • Burmese cat hypokalemic myopathy • Metabolic myopathies (e.g. pyruvate dehydrogenase deficiency) • Myotonia • Muscular dystrophies Polymyositis: • Infection: protozoal, viral, etc. • Immune-mediated Exertional myopathy Malignant hyperthermia Paraneoplastic (Lambert–Eaton syndrome associated with myasthenia gravis) Nutritional Endocrine: steroid, hypothyroid, hyperthyroid (cats) Lipid storage myopathy Miscellaneous: • Exercise-induced collapse (Labrador Retrievers) • Ischemic myopathy (cat thromboembolism)
Neuromuscular junction	Myasthenia gravis: acquired, congenital Organophosphate toxicity Tick paralysis Snake bite (Elapidae and pit viper) Botulism

Neurologic	Episodic falling (Cavalier King Charles Spaniel) Scottie cramp (also other breeds: Jack Russell, Norwich Terrier) Narcolepsy/catalepsy (breed association) Polyradicular neuritis (Coonhound paralysis) Inherited breed specific neuropathies Motor neuron diseases Endocrine (hypothyroid, insulinoma/hypoglycemia, hyperlipidemia) Neoplastic/paraneoplastic diseases Distal denervating diseases Lysosomal storage diseases Axonopathies (e.g. Boxer)

Cerebrospinal fluid analysis

Cerebrospinal fluid (CSF) analysis is of limited value unless there is a high index of suspicion of a neurologic disease. CSF analysis rarely contributes unless there is a diffuse infectious or inflammatory disease of the central nervous system.

Electrophysiology

If neuromuscular disease is suspected, electrophysiologic investigation may help confirm the suspicion. Electromyogram (EMG) insertion activity can help confirm muscle or nerve disease and help differentiate muscular from axonal disease. Nerve conduction velocity might provide more definitive information with neuropathies.

Imaging

Dogs with suspected cardiac disease require echocardiography; plain radiographs of the thorax can help if cardiorespiratory disease or megaesophagus is suspected. Contrast radiography or fluoroscopy can determine esophageal dilatation/function. Individual cases may have indication for CT/MRI investigation.

Muscle/nerve biopsy

Muscle biopsy is of particular value for the diagnosis of the inherited myopathies. Nerve biopsy can confirm axonal degeneration/regeneration, demyelination, and fibrosis, findings that have diagnostic and/or prognostic significance.

Edrophonium response

Slow intravenous administration of an ultrashort-acting anticholinesterase (0.1–1.0 mg edrophonium hydrochloride [Tensilon®]) is used for the diagnosis of MG. In dogs and cats with MG there is a rapid improvement in the ability to exercise for several minutes.

Blood gas analysis

Blood gas analysis can assist with some cardiorespiratory diseases (hypoxemia) and some metabolic myopathies (metabolic acidosis with exercise).

Genetic tests

Molecular (DNA) diagnostic testing is available for some inherited diseases (e.g. Burmese cat hypokalemic polymyopathy, Labrador Retriever myopathy, Japanese Spitz myopathy, narcolepsy). Your diagnostic laboratory should be consulted or an internet search made for information on what diagnostic tests are available for that breed if you suspect a familial link.

RECOMMENDED FURTHER READING

Platt SR, Olby N (2011) (eds.) *BSAVA Manual of Canine and Feline Neurology*, 3rd edn. British Small Animal Veterinary Association, Gloucester.

Vite CH, Braund KG (2003) (eds.) *Braund's Clinical Neurology in Small Animals: Localization, Diagnosis and Treatment*. Ithaca, New York. www.ivis.org/advances/vite/toc.asp

Chapter 2 Common clinical problems

2.3 Pigmenturia

Michael Schaer

INTRODUCTION

Under normal circumstances, the color of urine ranges from clear pale yellow to dark yellow or amber depending on the concentration of the urochrome (a product of bilirubin metabolism). Dilute urine is clear and light yellow while concentrated urine is dark yellow. Pigmenturia relates to urine that is discolored because of a pathologic process or as a result of some ingested chemical found in food or drugs. Certain foods are known to cause discolored urine and these include beetroot (red), senna and rhubarb (yellow to brown or red), and carotene (brown). Various drugs that can cause pigmenturia in humans are listed in **Table 2.3.1**. An example of drug-associated pigmenturia is shown in **Figures 2.3.1a, b**, which depicts methylene blue-induced blue pigment change involving oral mucosa and blue–green pigmenturia in a cat.

The main endogenous causes of pigmenturia include red blood cells (**Figure 2.3.2**), hemoglobin (**Figure 2.3.3**), bilirubin (**Figure 2.3.4**), myoglobin (**Figure 2.3.5**), and chyle. Sometimes, crystalluria can cause a color change that is dependent on the specific type of crystal, which can be formed from errors in metabolism (alkaptonuria in humans) or from the ingestion of certain drugs (e.g. sulfa drugs and others). The main pathologic concerns in dogs and cats involve hemoglobin and myoglobin because they can cause acute kidney injury (AKI). Crystalluria derived from the metabolism of certain drugs can also cause injury to renal tubules. Although bilirubinuria and chyluria represent potentially serious underlying disorders in the body, most clinicians focus their main concerns toward the tubulotoxicity associated with hemoglobinuria and myoglobinuria. The algorithm (**Figure 2.3.6**) shows the differential features of pigmenturia.

Table 2.3.1 Some drugs that can cause pigmenturia in humans, dogs, and cats.

Drug	Urine color
Deferoxamine	Red
Rifampin	Red
Hydroxycobalamine	Red
Methylene blue	Blue, green

Adapted from: Aycock RD, Kass DA (2012) Abnormal urine color. *South Med J* **105(1)**:43–47 and Plum DC (2011) *Plumb's Veterinary Drug Handbook*, 7th edn. PharmaVet Inc, Wisconsin.

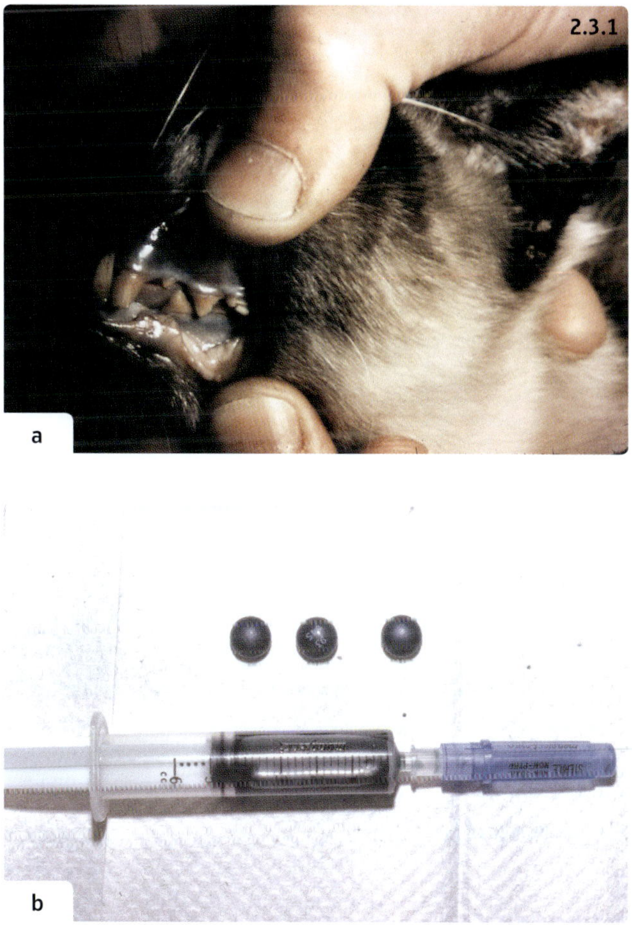

Figures 2.3.1a, b This cat's oral mucous membranes were discolored from the methylene blue contained in its medication for urinary tract disease (a). The cat's urine sample was a blue–green color (b). This product is no longer used in cats because of the associated Heinz body hemolytic anemia that it can cause.

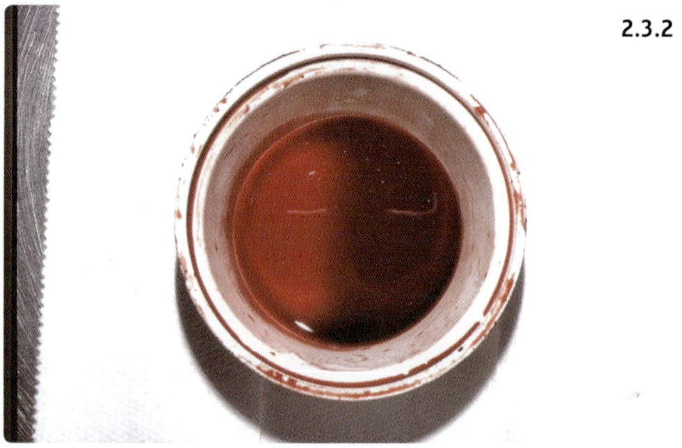

Figure 2.3.2 This urine sample shows hematuria. The bright red color is characteristic. Centrifugation of this sample would yield a clear amber supernate and a red button on the bottom of the tube representing the spun red blood cells.

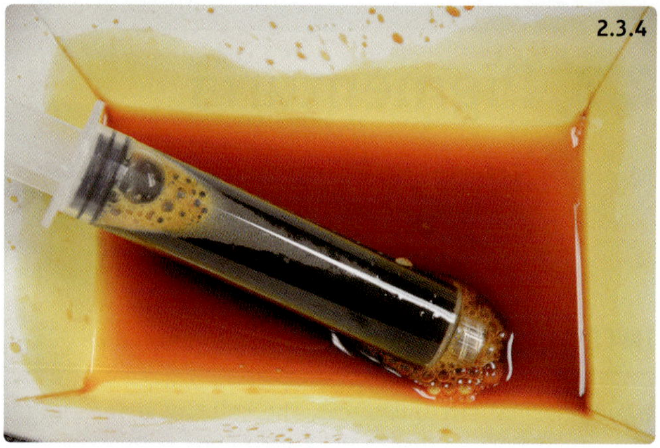

Figure 2.3.4 This sample depicts bilirubinuria from an icteric dog with severe cholangiostatic liver disease.

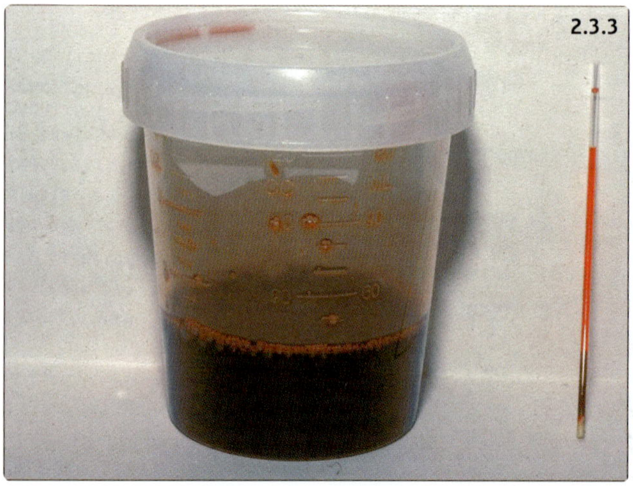

Figure 2.3.3 This sample shows hemoglobinuria and its characteristic dark red color. Centrifugation will not produce a red button representing precipitated red blood cells. The color of the supernate will remain the same dark red.

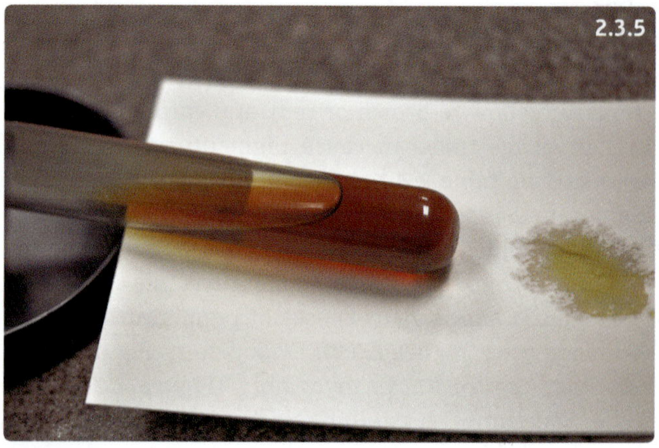

Figure 2.3.5 Myoglobinuria represents rhabdomyolysis. It is typically acellular and tea colored.

HEMOGLOBINURIA AND MYOGLOBINURIA

PATHOPHYSIOLOGY

Hemoglobin

Heme protein can cause oxidative stress, leading to systemic toxicity. The red blood cell membrane acts as a protective barrier against the proinflammatory effects of heme protein. The body offsets the toxic effects of any heme that is normally released into the circulation through mechanisms involving haptoglobin, the oxidation of ferrous heme to ferric heme, and the ability of nitrous oxide to oxidize hemoglobin to more soluble methemoglobin. These protective mechanisms are overwhelmed with massive hemolysis and the subsequent increase of hemoglobinuria.

The exact mechanism for the tubulotoxicity caused by hemoglobin is unclear. The heme proteins are thought to precipitate cast formation and cause obstruction of the kidney tubule, resulting in acute tubular necrosis of the proximal renal epithelial cells. Hemoglobinuria imparts a dark red color to the urine, which is not due to red blood cells, as confirmed after urine centrifugation.

2.3.6

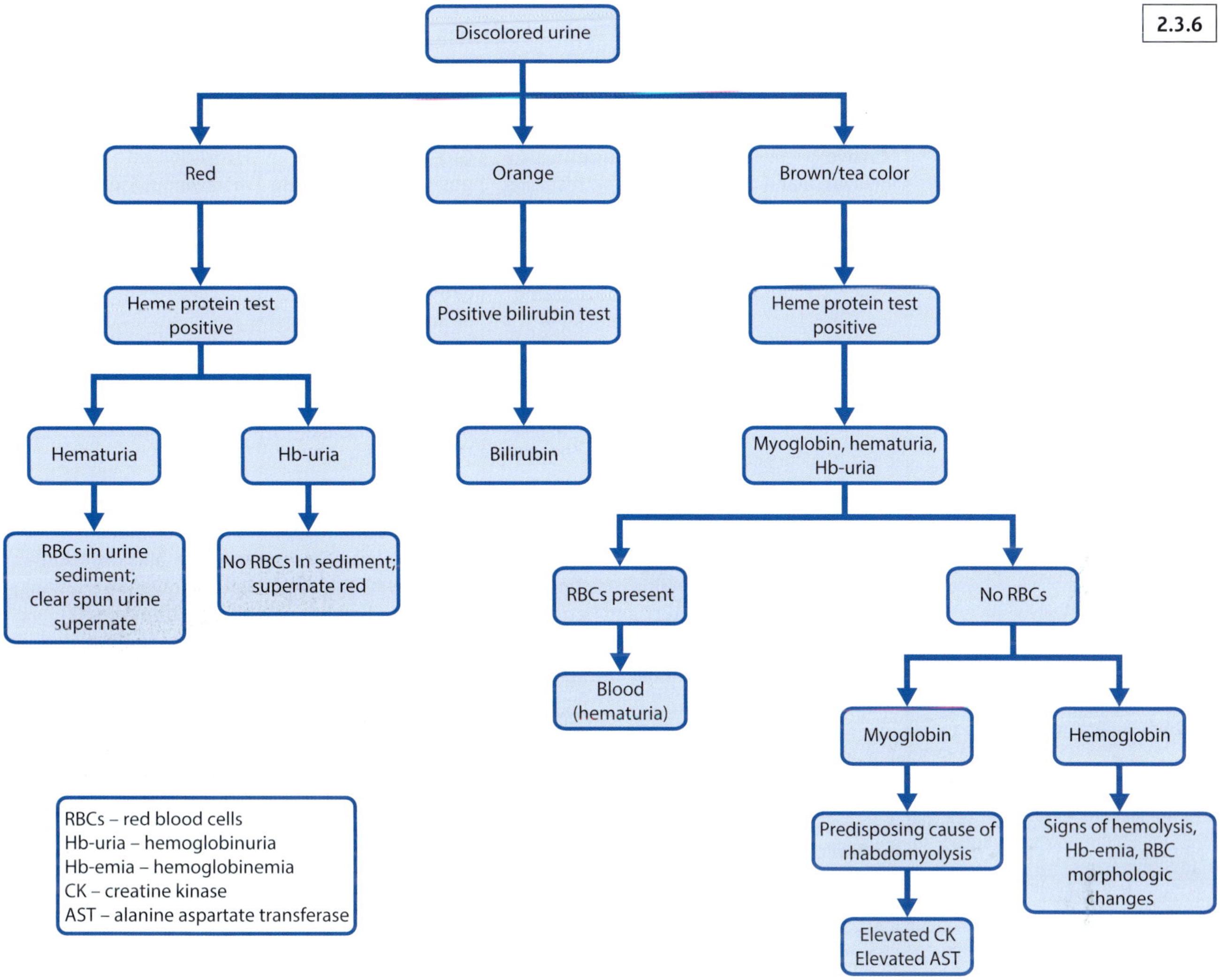

Figure 2.3.6 Algorithm showing the differential features of endogenous pigmenturia.

Myoglobin

This muscle protein accumulates in the circulation as a result of rhabdomyolysis. It appears in the urine as reddish-brown ('tea-colored') urine. Kidney injury is thought to result from intrarenal vasoconstriction, direct and ischemic tubule injury, and tubular obstruction. Myoglobin becomes concentrated along the renal tubules and precipitates when it interacts with Tam–Horsfall protein, a process that is favored by acidic urine. Distal renal tubular obstruction and proximal tubule toxicity are the main consequences. Myoglobin tubular toxicity does not occur unless the urine is acidic, and this requirement has therapeutic implications.

CLINICAL FEATURES AND MANAGEMENT

The main clinical features and general treatment recommendations are outlined in **Table 2.3.2**. Although AKI in the dog and cat is a rare complication associated with hemolysis and rhabdomyolysis, the clinician should be diligent in assessing their patients with these disorders for early signs of AKI. Damage will be indicated with elevations in blood urea nitrogen (BUN) and serum creatinine and the presence of tubular casts in the urine sediment. The damage is maximized by co-existing metabolic acidosis, dehydration, and other causes of decreased renal perfusion. The most important

Table 2.3.2 Endogenous pathologic causes of pigmenturia.

Pigment name	Physical features	Associated disorder	Pathophysiology	Diagnostic features	Treatment
Hemoglobinuria	Dark red	Massive intravascular hemolysis; acute blood transfusion reaction	Red blood cell destruction resulting from immune, chemical or drug damage to the RBC membrane allowing for the release of heme protein into the circulation and its eventual accumulation in the renal tubule	Grossly red color; positive heme protein test with urine dipstick; no RBCs in the urine sediment. Gross evidence of hemolysis. Macroagglutination of RBCs if associated with immune hemolytic disease	Hydration with intravenous isotonic crystalloid solution; intravenous sodium bicarbonate; hemodialysis
Myoglobin	Reddish-brown; tea colored	Rhabdomyolysis	Kidney injury is thought to result from intrarenal vasoconstriction, direct and ischemic tubule injury, and tubular obstruction	Markedly elevated serum enzyme tests (CK, AST). Urine dark brown with no RBCs in sediment. Clinical signs of disease causing the rhabdomyolysis	Hydrate with intravenous isotonic crystalloid solution; alkalinization with intravenous sodium bicarbonate, sometimes with added mannitol. Hemodialysis has been shown to help. Antioxidants such as vitamins E and C and pentoxiphylline might help
Hematuria	Red	Systemic bleeding disorder from drugs or disease; urinary calculi; renal and urinary bladder neoplasia; urinary tract trauma/infection	Specific to the particular cause	History and physical examination; coagulogram; diagnostic imaging when indicated; urine culture	Depending on cause: • Stop all drugs that promote bleeding. • Antidotes when indicated; • Surgery where indicated. Not renal tubulotoxic
Bilirubinuria	Orange	Hemolysis and liver disease	Prehepatic, hepatic, and posthepatic disorders	Elevated liver enzyme tests; diagnostic imaging abnormalities; hemolysis and associated features	Treat primary disorder. Not renal tubulotoxic.

therapeutic objectives entail replacing dehydration deficits and providing for increased maintenance doses of isotonic intravenous fluids. Once rehydration and improved urine output are established, diuresis can be provided.

Although parenteral fluid administration will not prevent AKI, it decreases its severity. Patients who do not respond to treatment and those who become oliguric will often require hemodialysis while still facing a very guarded prognosis until the patient shows a decrease in the serum BUN and creatinine that can be sustained without dialysis.

RECOMMENDED FURTHER READING

Bosch X, Poch E, Grau JM (2009) Rhabdomyolysis and acute kidney injury. *N Engl J Med* **361:**62–72.

Wolfson AB (2010) Renal failure. In: *Rosen's Emergency Medicine*, 7th edn. (eds. JA Marx, RS Hockberger, RM Walls *et al.*) Mosby Elsevier, Philadelphia, pp. 1257–1281.

Chapter 2 Common clinical problems

2.4 Vomiting

Frédéric Gaschen

INTRODUCTION

Vomiting is characterized by the forceful oral ejection of gastric content with or without addition of small intestinal content.

The vomiting response can be divided into three sequential phases. The *prodromal phase* is characterized by nausea with licking of the lips, yawning, hiding, and depression, and occurs with hypersalivation and excessive swallowing. This is associated with relaxation of the lower esophageal sphincter and proximal part of the stomach. The second phase is *retching*, with retrograde giant small intestinal contractions that bring jejunal and duodenal chyme (and bile) back into the gastric lumen if the pylorus is patent, followed by rhythmic retching, inhibition of salivation, activation of the intercostal muscles, protection of the airways by laryngeal elevation, and increased upper esophageal sphincter tone. Finally, during the final *expulsion phase*, the cervical esophageal and pharyngeal tones decrease, the lower esophageal sphincter relaxes, the rectus abdominis muscle contracts, and the diaphragm squeezes the stomach. Breathing is momentarily inhibited and the glottis closed while the gastric content is propelled into the esophagus and ultimately out of the mouth.

Regurgitation, dysphagia (associated with oral and pharyngeal diseases), and coughing/gagging may be misinterpreted as vomiting by pet owners. Regurgitation is the passive oral evacuation of esophageal content associated with esophageal dysmotility, obstruction, and/or dilation. Typically, retching does not occur with regurgitation. Moreover, esophageal diseases are less prevalent than disorders causing vomiting. Regurgitation is therefore less commonly observed overall than vomiting.

PATHOPHYSIOLOGY

The vomiting or emetic center is a conglomerate of nuclei located in the medulla oblongata. Vomiting can be elicited by activation of neural or humoral pathways. The emetic center is closely associated with the chemoreceptor trigger zone (CRTZ), an area lacking a blood–brain barrier where receptors are in direct contact with circulating blood. Stimulation of the CRTZ by blood-borne emetogenic substances (e.g. uremic toxins, endotoxins, drugs) is the basis of the humoral pathway of emesis. The emetic center may also be stimulated by the vestibulocochlear nucleus (e.g. motion sickness) and cortical centers. Additionally, it receives direct input from the peritoneum and abdominal organs via nerve fibers traveling with the vagus nerve, the neural pathway of vomiting (**Figure 2.4.1**). The emetic center is responsible for the coordination of the vomiting effort through efferent pathways. Numerous receptors are involved in the stimulation of vomiting and are the targets of antiemetic drugs (**Table 2.4.1**).

DIFFERENTIAL DIAGNOSES

A wide range of diseases may cause vomiting in dogs and cats through direct stimulation of the emetic center via afferent vagal branches or indirectly via stimulation of the CRTZ (**Table 2.4.2**). Diseases of the gastrointestinal (GI) tract generally act directly on the vomiting center through the neural pathway, while systemic disorders such as kidney diseases often stimulate the CRTZ via the humoral pathway.

2.4.1

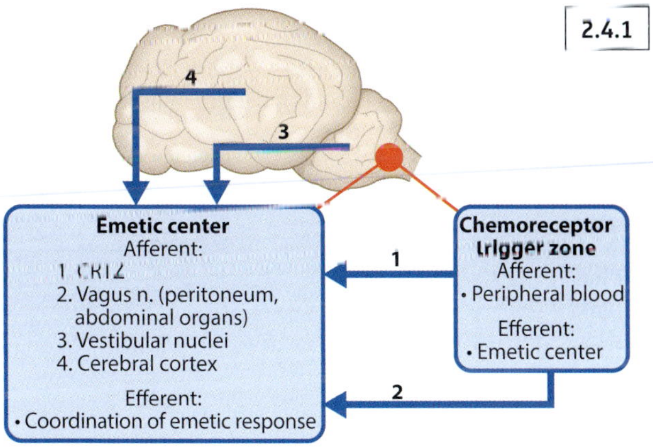

Figure 2.4.1 Afferent and efferent pathways to and from the emetic center and chemoreceptor trigger zone.

Table 2.4.1 Antiemetic drugs used in dogs and cats and their target receptors.

Antiemetic drug	Target/antagonism	Dose and route	Other effects
Maropitant	NK1-receptors: substance P antagonist	1 mg/kg/day SC or IV in dogs and cats. IV use is off-label: dilute the drug 1:5 with saline and administer slowly	
Metoclopramide	Dopamine-2 receptor (D)	0.3–0.5 mg/kg SC q8h or 1–2 mg/kg CRI q24h	Prokinetic effects on gastric antrum
Odansetron	5-HT_3 receptors in the CRTZ (D, C) and afferent nerves (D)	0.5–1 mg/kg IV, PO q12h	
Dolasetron		0.6–1 mg/kg IV, PO q12h	
Chlorpromazine	α_2 receptors, dopamine-2 receptors, histamine-1 receptors, muscarinic-1 receptors	0.2–0.4 mg/kg SC, IV q8h	Hypotensive, sedative
Prochlorperazine		0.1–0.5 mg/kg SC, IM q6–8h	Hypotensive, sedative
Yohimbine	α_2 receptors		Hypotensive, sedative

D, dog; C, cat. If not specified, applies to both dogs and cats.

Table 2.4.2 Common causes of vomiting in dogs and cats.

Gastrointestinal	Outside gastrointestinal tract
Stomach Obstructive: gastric foreign body, space-occupying lesion in pylorus Adverse reaction to food including dietary indiscretion Infectious: viral, bacterial, parasitic Toxic: drugs, plants, chemicals Chronic gastritis Gastric neoplasia Gastric ulcer Gastric motility disorder	**Abdominal** Acute and chronic recurring pancreatitis Diseases of liver and biliary tree Peritonitis Diaphragmatic hernia Neoplasia Pyometra
Small bowel Infectious: viral, bacterial, parasitic Obstructive: foreign body, intussusception, space-occupying lesion Adverse reaction to food including dietary indiscretion Toxic: drugs, plants, chemicals Inflammatory disease Intestinal neoplasia Paralytic ileus	**Metabolic** Uremic syndrome Electrolyte disorders Acid–base disorders Endocrine diseases: hyperthyroidism, diabetic ketoacidosis, hypoadrenocorticism Toxins: drugs, plants, chemicals Sepsis, endotoxemia
Colon Colitis Severe constipation	**Neurologic** Motion sickness Vestibular disorders Encephalitis/meningitis Increased intracranial pressure Psychogenic (excitation, fear, pain) Dysautonomia

D, dog; C, cat. If not specified, applies to both dogs and cats.

CLINICAL APPROACH

It is likely that many dogs and cats that experience a few episodes of acute vomiting are not presented for veterinary examination because the problem is self-limiting. If presented to a veterinarian, acutely vomiting animals should be assessed for the severity of disease. A few episodes of vomiting in the absence of complications such as dehydration in an otherwise healthy animal may not require any further investigations or treatment, even though a bland diet and possible empirical prescription of antiemetics may be of benefit. However, dogs and cats that are ill need to undergo more detailed examination and investigations

The most relevant differential diagnoses may differ on the basis of the animal's signalment. Younger animals are more prone to infectious diseases, such as parvovirus infection in dogs, and to ingestion of foreign objects (**Figures 2.4.2, 2.4.3**).

A detailed history should be obtained. Important questions include: diet, environment, duration and frequency of vomiting, relationship to eating, description of the vomiting process, appearance of the vomitus (e.g. presence of bile [**Figure 2.4.4**], hairballs [**Figure 2.4.5**], hematemesis [see Chapter 8, Digestive diseases, **Figure 8.33**], frank blood [**Figure 2.4.6**]), behavioral changes, and co-existing clinical signs, as well as previous illnesses, deworming history, and current medications. This information helps confirm the existence of vomiting, assess the disease severity, and may yield valuable data about any underlying disease(s).

A thorough physical examination should be performed. In cats particularly, it is important to visualize the lingual frenulum by applying gentle pressure in the intermandibular space with the thumb, searching for a piece of string looping around the base of the tongue at the

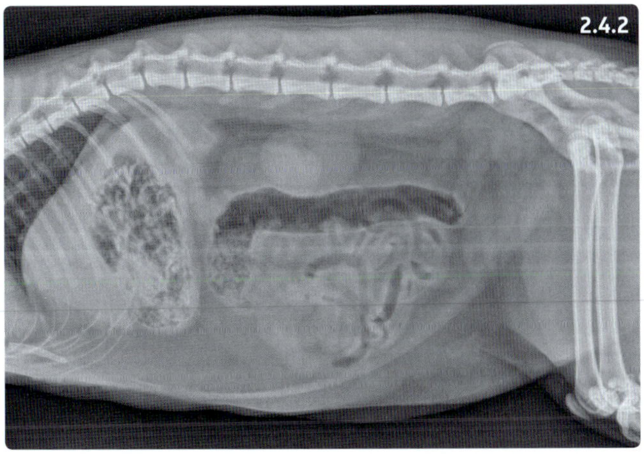

Figure 2.4.2 Right lateral abdominal radiograph from a 4-year-old male neutered cat with vomiting of 1-week duration. The stomach is moderately distended with mixed gas and soft tissue opacities that are clumped together and linear in shape. The pyloric antrum contains gas and the duodenum and remainder of the small intestine are fluid/gas filled.

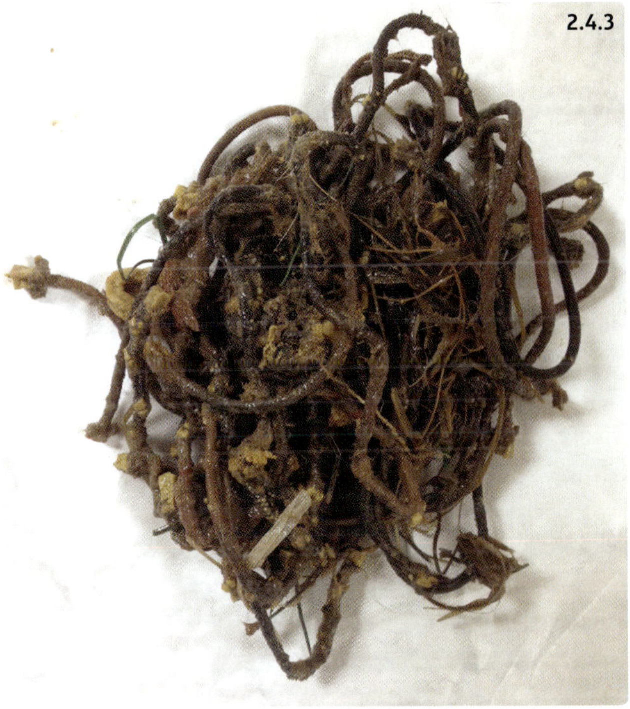

Figure 2.4.3 Same cat as in Figure 2.4.2. Hair bands extracted endoscopically from the stomach. It is likely that they were ingested over a prolonged period of time, even though the history indicated a recent problem.

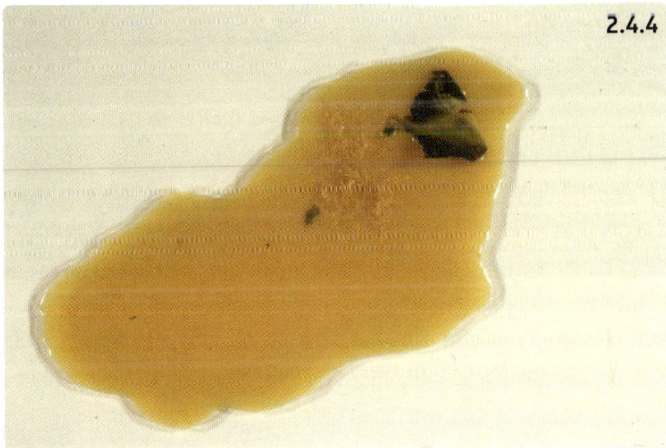

Figure 2.4.4 Canine vomit admixed with bile. (Courtesy M. Schaer)

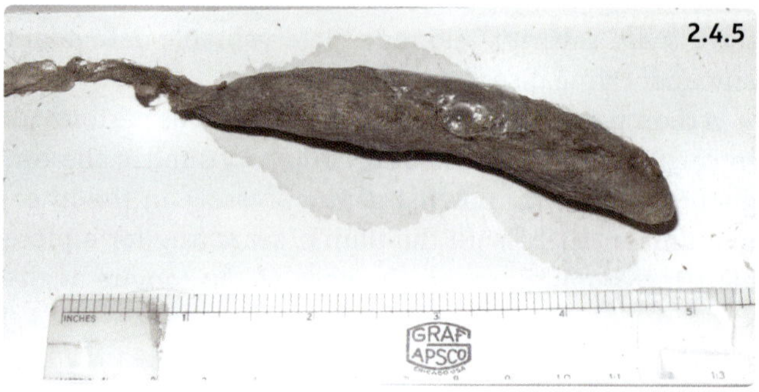

Figure 2.4.5 Hairball vomited by a cat. (Courtesy M. Schaer)

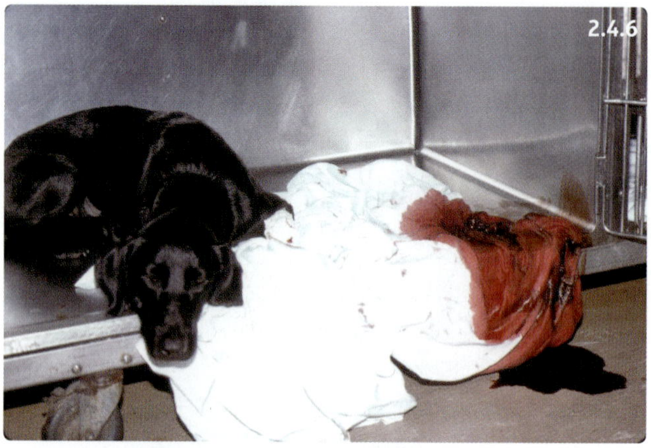

Figure 2.4.6 Hematemesis with frank blood in a young Labrador Retriever. (Courtesy M. Schaer)

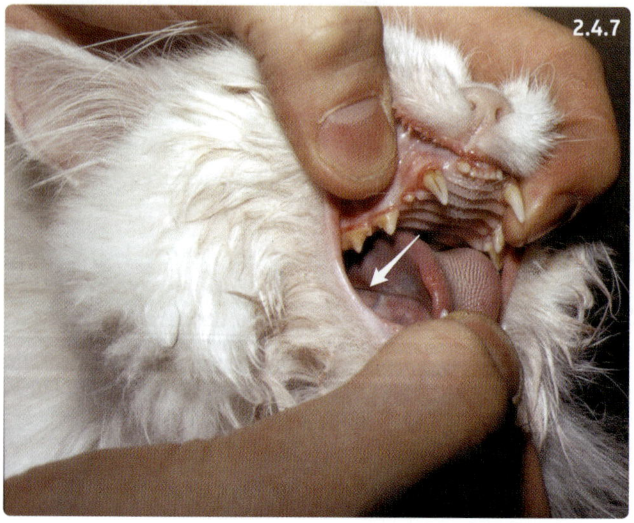

Figure 2.4.7 A piece of thread (arrow) looped around the base of the tongue in a vomiting cat with a radiographic diagnosis of a linear foreign body. (Courtesy M. Schaer)

origin of a linear foreign body (**Figure 2.4.7**). Abdominal palpation may reveal discomfort or pain (gastroenteritis, pancreatitis), or abdominal masses (foreign body, intussusception, granuloma, neoplasia). Hydration and cardiovascular status are important to guide the planning of fluid therapy.

In dogs presented with acute vomiting, dietary indiscretion, GI foreign body, ingestion of toxic substances, and acute pancreatitis are the top four differential diagnoses and should be the focus of the initial diagnostic investigations (**Figure 2.4.8**). Gastric dilatation volvulus (GDV) may be associated with vomiting, although the efforts are often unproductive. Moreover, abdominal distension with gastric tympany is often present and easily noticed. Abdominal radiographs are useful to evaluate gastric position and confirm the diagnosis of GDV. They are also necessary to rule out GI obstruction (one or two lateral views and a ventrodorsal view). Cats may ingest foreign bodies or chew on toxic plants; however, dietary indiscretion is less prevalent in this species, and pancreatitis is less commonly associated with significant vomiting.

Animals with chronic or chronic intermittent vomiting commonly have diseases affecting the digestive tract (including stomach and intestine, liver, and pancreas) or other organ systems such as the kidneys or the endocrine system. Therefore, the search for an underlying cause is best started with a minimal database consisting of bloodwork (CBC, chemistry panel) and urinalysis to assess the function of various organ systems. Abdominal imaging (radiographs, ultrasound) can be carried out to assess the appearance of abdominal organs. Then, based on the information obtained from the initial database, additional more specific tests can be performed in order to identify the primary problem. Cats may vomit chronically in the absence of any other problems ('healthy' chronic vomiters); this is sometimes associated with hairballs (**Figure 2.4.5**), but the cause often remains unknown. In these cats, increases in the vomiting frequency and onset of additional clinical signs such as hyporexia justify further investigations.

Treatment of vomiting dogs and cats needs to focus on three points: (1) stopping the vomiting process with judicious use of antiemetics (**Table 2.4.1**), (2) correcting the fluid and electrolyte deficits resulting from vomiting, and (3) addressing the underlying disease at the origin of vomiting.

2.4.8

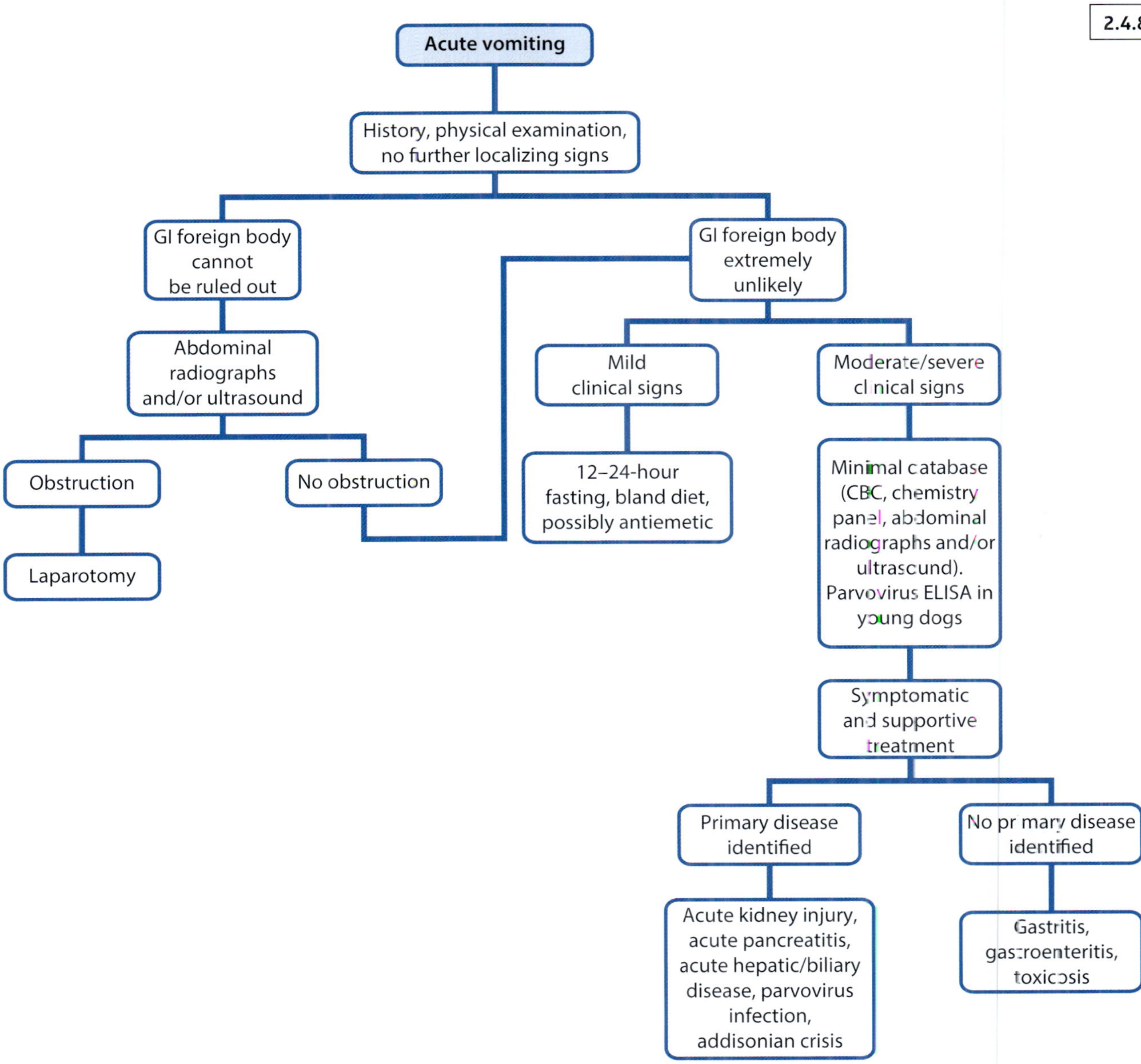

Figure 2.4.8 Algorithm for the clinical approach to acute vomiting in a dog after gastric dilatation volvulus has been initially ruled out.

RECOMMENDED FURTHER READING

Baral RM (2012) Approach to the vomiting cat. In: *The Cat: Clinical Medicine and Management*. (ed. SE Little) Elsevier Saunders, St. Louis, pp. 426–431.

Elwood C, Devauchelle P, Elliott J *et al.* (2010) Emesis in dogs: a review. *J Small Anim Pract* **51(1)**:4–22.

Twedt DC (2010) Vomiting. In: *Textbook of Veterinary Internal Medicine*, 7th edn. (eds. SJ Ettinger, EC Feldman) Saunders Elsevier, St. Louis, pp. 195–200.

2.5 Polydipsia and polyuria

Michael Schaer

INTRODUCTION

Polydipsia is defined as increased thirst. Normal water consumption in dogs should not exceed 90 ml/kg per day (**Figure 2.5.1**) while normal water intake in a cat should not exceed 45 ml/kg per day (**Figure 2.5.2**). Any water intake that exceeds these amounts is described as polydipsia. Normal urine production in the dog and cat ranges from 20 to 45 ml/kg per day, and an amount that exceeds this range is described as polyuria.

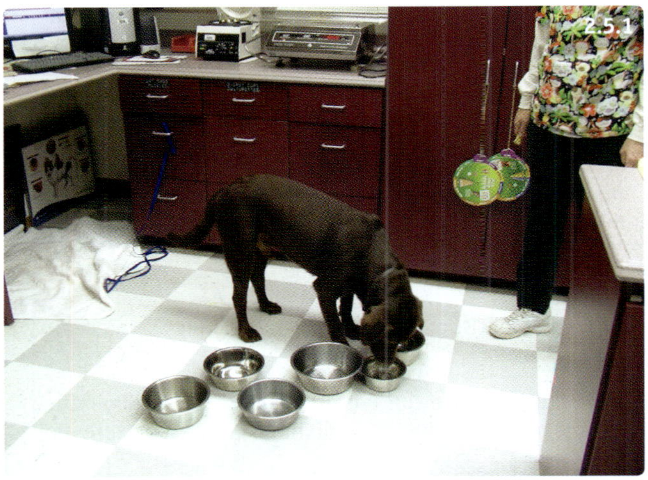

Figure 2.5.1 This polydipsic dog was diagnosed with psychogenic polydipsia. He was able to concentrate his urine to 1.025 with the water deprivation test.

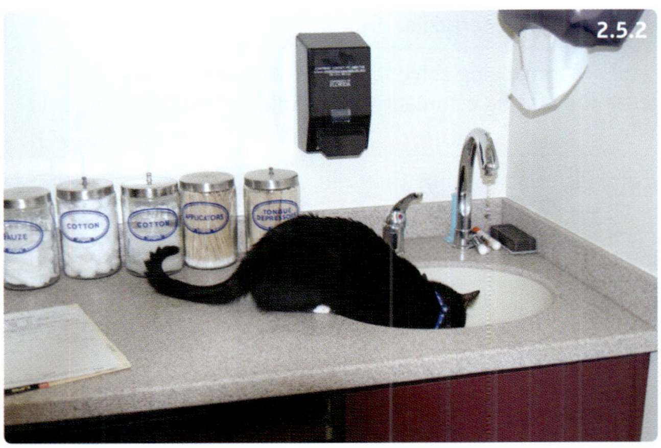

Figure 2.5.2 This cat was obviously polydipsic during its physical examination.

ETIOLOGY

The two main causes of polydipsia and polyuria (PD/PU) syndromes include primary disorders of excessive water intake and those that involve excessive urine production. There are approximately 14 endogenous causes of PD/PU and three exogenous causes. These and their main mechanisms are shown in **Table 2.5.1**. Many of the endogenous causes of PD/PU are accompanied by several other clinical features that characterize the specific disorder (**Table 2.5.2**). Also, there are certain conditions that can characteristically progress to eventually make the patient overtly ill when dehydration and any associated toxin accumulation occurs (**Table 2.5.3**).

PATHOPHYSIOLOGY

The pathophysiology underlying each PD/PU disorder varies and depends on the particular syndrome at hand (see **Table 2.5.1**). Any animal that is able to concentrate its urine to >1.025 will usually not qualify as having a PD/PU syndrome unless the increased thirst and urination are periodic, which might characterize psychogenic polydipsia (**Figure 2.5.3**). A patient that shows no evidence of any major underlying disease and no response to the water deprivation test might be suspect for having diabetes insipidus (**Figure 2.5.4**).

CLINICAL SIGNS

Several disorders, such the syndromes of psychogenic polydipsia, diabetes insipidus, and hyperadrenocorticism, will not characteristically result in a clinically ill patient so long as water is available and the animal can successfully imbibe and retain the water. Other conditions that will eventually worsen to cause a clinically ill patient

Table 2.5.1 The causes and mechanisms of polydipsia and polyuria.

Disease	Mechanism of polydipsia/polyuria
Endogenous causes	
Diabetes mellitus	Osmotic diuresis; hyperosmotic stimulation of the hypothalamic thirst center
Chronic kidney disease	Decreased nephron mass; dysfunctional renal medullary countercurrent multiplier
Hypoadrenocorticism	Renal sodium loss and impaired renal countercurrent multiplier
Hyperthyroidism	Hyperdynamic renal blood flow causing increased renal water filtration and impaired medullary concentrating ability. Other factors: aquaporin downregulation and decreased renal filtration fraction
Hyperadrenocorticism	Increase renal plasma blood flow; central thirst stimulation, distal renal tubular resistance to ADH
Hypercalcemia	Nephrocalcinosis; renal distal tubular resistance to ADH
Pyometra	Uterine *E. coli* bacterial endotoxins impairing distal renal tubular response to ADH. In some cases, antigen–antibody deposits along with impaired renal perfusion causing acute kidney injury
Diabetes insipidus	Decreased ADH release from posterior pituitary or absent distal renal tubular and collecting duct response to ADH
Chronic liver disease	Decreased urea synthesis impairing function of renal medullary countercurrent multiplier; central thirst stimulation
Postobstructive (and postoliguric kidney injury) diuresis	Solvent drag associated with the accumulated osmoles in the blood subsequently being able to filter through the kidney. Polydipsia due to the excessive water loss stimulating the hypothalamic osmoreceptors and the thirst mechanism
Hypokalemia	Primary stimulation of thirst; diminished urine concentrating ability due to diminished renal tubule response to ADH. The reason for the latter might be decreased expression of aquaporin 2
Psychogenic polydipsia	Psychologically induced disturbance involving the hypothalamic thirst center
Exogenous causes	
Diuretics	Various mechanisms affecting the absorption of electrolytes and water at specific points along the nephron, depending on particular drug
Hyperosmotic solution infusions	Increased renal perfusion and accompanying solvent drag as seen with mannitol. Hypertonic saline can increase the plasma osmolality and stimulate the thirst center in the hypothalamus
Excessive parenteral fluid administration	Increased renal blood flow and filtration causing water diuresis
Glucocorticoid drugs	Increased renal plasma flow causing increased glomerular filtration rate
Increased sodium chloride ingestion	Increased plasma space tonicity, increased thirst, and increased urination

ADH, antidiuretic hormone.

Table 2.5.2 Typical clinical features of the polydipsia/polyuria syndromes. (See specific chapters for details. Note that exact clinical signs are subject to individual patient variation.)

Disease	Classic clinical features (not all signs necessarily present depending on stage of disease)
Diabetes mellitus	PD/PU, eventually dehydration, weight loss, and vomiting, varying urine SG; hyperglycemia, glycosuria, +/- hyperketonemia/hyperketonuria; other serum chemistry abnormalities (hypokalemia, hyponatremia, hypophosphatemia); metabolic acidosis; azotemia
Chronic renal disease	PD/PU with isosthenuria, weight loss, and dehydration at moderate and late stages, vomiting, urine SG isosthenuric (1.008–1.012); azotemia; hyperphosphatemia, other electrolyte abnormalities (hyper-, eu-, or hypokalemia, hyper- or hypocalcemia); nonresponsive anemia
Hypoadrenocorticism	Progressive weakness and poor appetite, vomiting, diarrhea, weight loss and dehydration, decreased vitality, hypovolemic shock in late stages, varying urine SG, hyperkalemia, hyponatremia, hypochloremia, mild anemia, hypoproteinemia and hypocholesterolemia, hypocortisolemia, ACTH stimulation test cortisol <1.0 μg/dl, ECG abnormalities
Hyperthyroidism	Progressive weight loss despite increased appetite, heart rate normal or increased; increased serum thyroxin; sometimes mild increased liver enzymes; sometimes mild anemia
Hyperadrenocorticism	PD/PU, panting, dermatologic changes, abdominal distension, elevated liver enzymes (especially serum alkaline phosphatase in dogs), lipid abnormalities, increased serum cortisol to creatinine ratio, increased response to ACTH stimulation, impaired response to dexamethasone suppression; increased plasma ACTH levels with pituitary origin and low ACTH concentration with functional adrenal tumor origin
Hypercalcemia	PD/PU, lethargy, weakness, dehydration, vomiting, vague abdominal discomfort, urinary calculi, hypercalcemia, hyper- or hypophosphatemia, increased or normal serum PTH with primary hyperparathyroidism, low serum PTH with hypercalcemia of malignancy, eventually azotemia and hyposthenuria or isosthenuria
Pyometra	PD/PU, dehydration, decreased appetite, purulent vaginal discharge with open pyometra, uterine enlargement , leukocytosis, sometimes renal dysfunction, sometimes overt sepsis and septic shock
Diabetes insipidus (DI)	Marked PD/PU, hyposthenuria (urine SG <1.008); no response to water deprivation. Central DI will respond to ADH (**Figure 2.5.4**); nephrogenic form has no response to ADH
Chronic liver disease	Decreased appetite and weight loss. Increases in serum liver enzyme tests, hyperammonemia, decreased liver size, sometimes coagulopathy and anemia, sometimes icterus
Hypokalemia	Low serum potassium (<3.5 mEq/l), skeletal and smooth muscle weakness, ECG changes, features of underlying disease (diabetes mellitus, hyperaldosteronism, metabolic alkalosis and its cause [gastric outflow obstruction], chronic kidney disease)
Postobstructive and postoliguric kidney injury	Features of the underlying urinary tract disease, marked PD/PU
Psychogenic polydipsia	PD/PU; no other signs of organic disease; able to concentrate urine with water deprivation test

ACTH, adrenocorticotropic hormone; PTH, parathyroid hormone.

Table 2.5.3 PD/PU disorders that can rapidly progress to cause severe clinical illness*.

Chronic renal disease
Diabetes mellitus
Hypoadrenocorticism
Pyometra
Hypercalcemia
Chronic liver disease
Extreme hypokalemia (serum K^+ <2.5 mEq/l)

* These disorders can progress to cause sick, dehydrated, anorectic animals unlike other PD/PU disorders such as diabetes insipidus, psychogenic polydipsia, and hyperadrenocorticism.

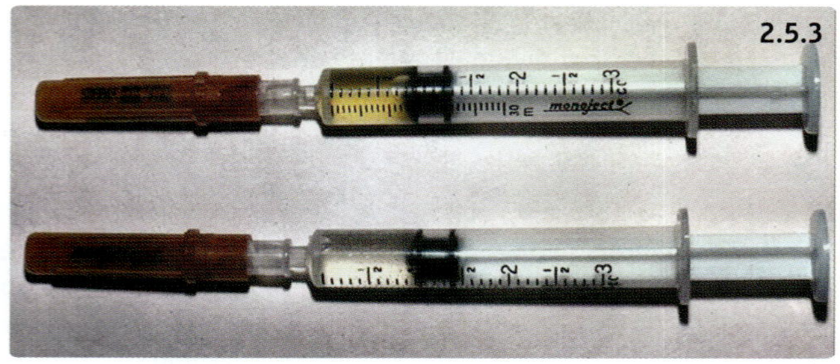

Figure 2.5.3 These two urine samples show urine concentration ability after an 8-hour water deprivation test. The diagnosis was psychogenic polydipsia. It is important to realize that actual measurement of the urine SG is the only way to lend credence to this empirical visual impression.

include renal failure, diabetic ketoacidosis, pyometra, hypercalcemia, hypoadrenocorticism, and chronic liver disease. Some conditions can worsen to involve multiple organ systems, which can cause the patient's demise. One of these is illustrated with diabetic ketoacidosis being accompanied by AKI and sepsis.

Primary polydipsia occurs because of a defect involving the thirst center in the hypothalamus. In humans, there can be underlying diseases such as mental disorders or diseases such as sarcoidosis that can impair hypothalamic function and disrupt the thirst center. Most of these patients, including dogs, are able to maintain normal serum sodium concentrations because they are able to excrete the extra water that they have imbibed. In rare situations in humans, the polydipsia can overwhelm the kidney's ability to excrete the excess water, and this can result in water retention and hyponatremia.

The characteristic features of each disorder are provided in **Table 2.5.2.** Urine SG determination is useful to help identify the cause of PD/PU (**Figure 2.5.5**), although its accurate application must always be used in light of the accompanying clinical findings.

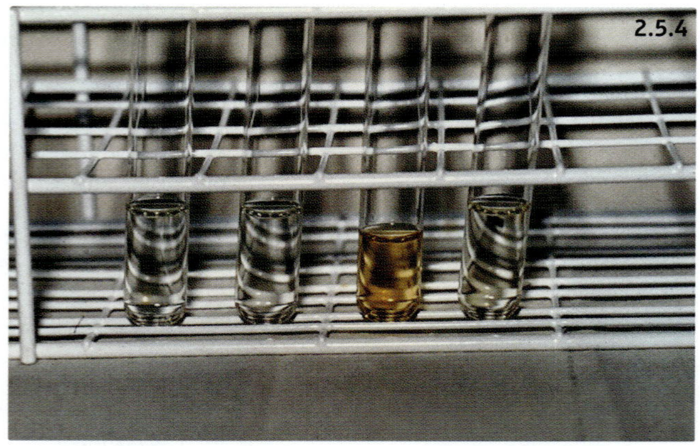

Figure 2.5.4 This series of urine-filled tubes show the results of a positive ADH response test in a dog with central diabetes insipidus. The most pale colored urine sample was the most dilute while the progressively darker colored urine was more concentrated when measured with a refractometer.

MANAGEMENT AND PROGNOSIS

A disorder such as psychogenic polydipsia has a very good prognosis because it lacks any life-threatening pathophysiology as compared with other causes of PD/PU, such as renal failure and diabetic ketoacidosis, which can progress to a clinically decompensated stage and lead to the ultimate demise of the patient. A water deprivation test should not be done until the patient is first evaluated for other disorders causing PD/PU because it can cause a negative water balance that can have adverse effects on blood pressure and tissue perfusion.

RECOMMENDED FURTHER READING

Dibartola SP (2012) *Fluid, Electrolyte, and Acid–base Disorders in Small Animal Practice*, 4th edn. Elsevier Saunders, St. Louis.

Rose DR, Post TW (2001) *Clinical Physiology of Acid-base Disorders*, 5th edn. McGraw-Hill, New York.

Wang W, Li C, Summer SN *et al.* (2007) Polyuria of thyrotoxicosis: downregulation of aquaporin water channels and increased solute excretion. *Kidney Int* **72(9):**1088–1094.

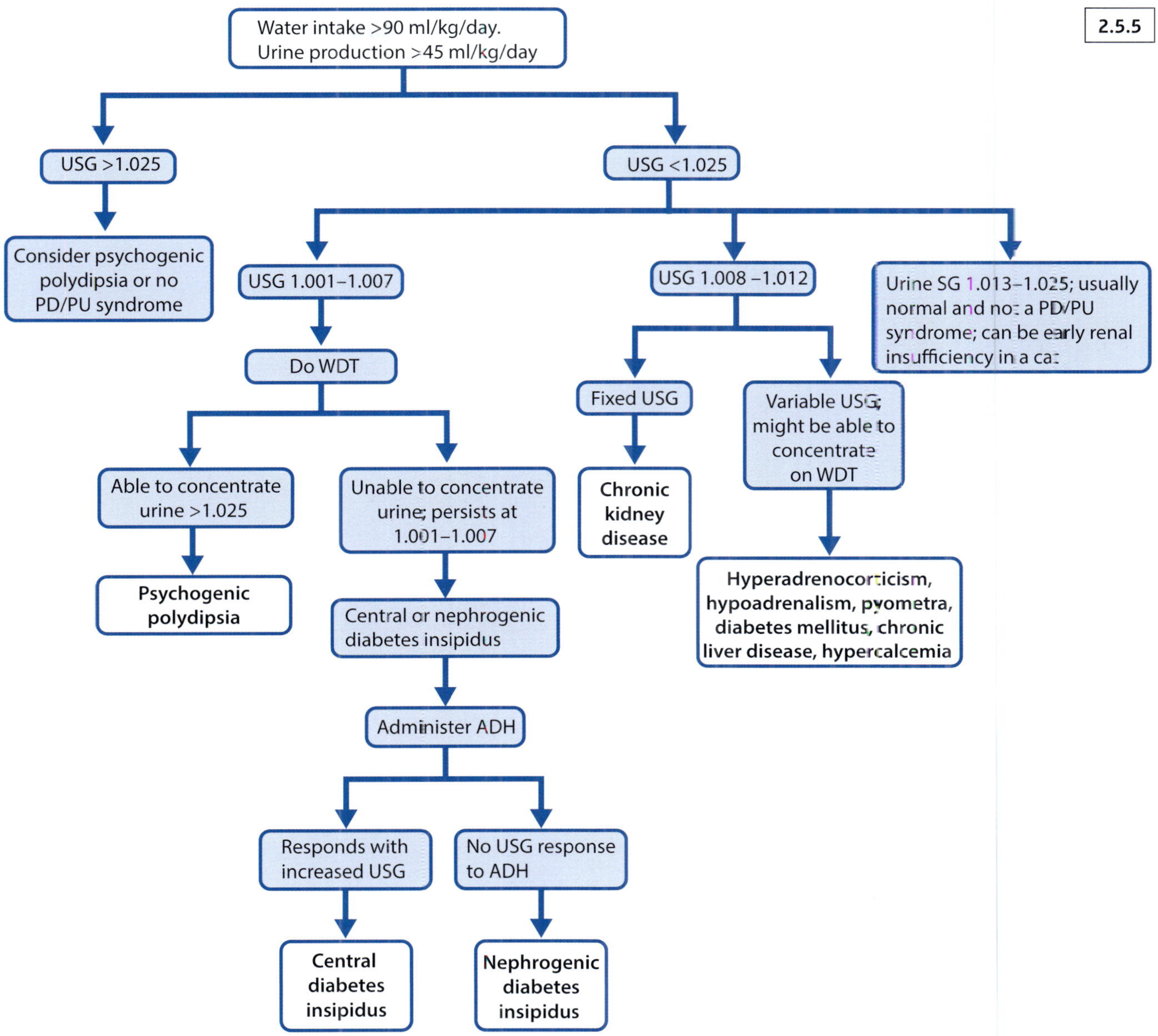

Figure 2.5.5 This algorithm demonstrates how to identify the polydipsia/polyuria syndromes using urine SG determination. WDT, water deprivation test; USG, urine specific gravity; ADH, antidiuretic hormone.

Chapter 2 Common clinical problems

2.6 Diarrhea

Frédéric Gaschen

INTRODUCTION

Diarrhea is characterized by decreased fecal consistency, increased fecal volume, and/or increased defecation frequency.

Animals with diarrhea all have intestinal dysfunction due to primary intestinal disease or secondary intestinal involvement associated with disorders originating outside the intestine. The clinical signs vary depending on whether the disease primarily originates in the small intestine or in the colon (**Table 2.6.1**, **Figures 2.6.1–2.6.6**). However, in some instances, diarrhea may not be observed even if the animal suffers from intestinal disease. This occurs frequently in cats with inflammatory bowel disease (IBD) or alimentary lymphoma affecting the small intestine. They may present with weight loss, dysorexia, lethargy, and/or vomiting without diarrhea in spite of significant involvement of their intestinal mucosa.

Secondary signs that may occur in diarrheic animals include dehydration, lethargy, dysorexia, abdominal pain, borborygmi, flatulence, hematochezia, melena, and anal/perianal irritation. Animals with chronic small intestinal diarrhea may present with weight loss (including loss of muscle mass) and possibly ascites in case of significant intestinal protein loss.

Table 2.6.1 Clinical signs associated with small and large bowel diarrhea.

Clinical sign	Small intestinal disease	Large intestinal disease
Frequency of defecation	Normal or only slightly increased	Moderately to severely increased
Fecal volume per defecation	Normal to large	Small
Presence of mucus	No	Common
Presence of blood	Melena (digested blood); possibly hematemesis	Hematochezia (fresh blood)
Steatorrhea	Possible	No
Tenesmus	No	Common
Urgency	No	Common
Dyschezia	No	Common
Flatulence, borborygmi	Possible	Uncommon
General condition	May be decreased (lethargy)	Usually unchanged
Appetite	Dysorexia common	Usually unchanged
Abdominal discomfort	Possible	Possible
Vomiting	Relatively common	Possible but occasional
Weight loss	Common (if chronic)	Uncommon

Note: Commonly, the disease process may involve both the small and large intestine and affected animals present with a mixture of clinical signs indicating small and large bowel diarrhea.

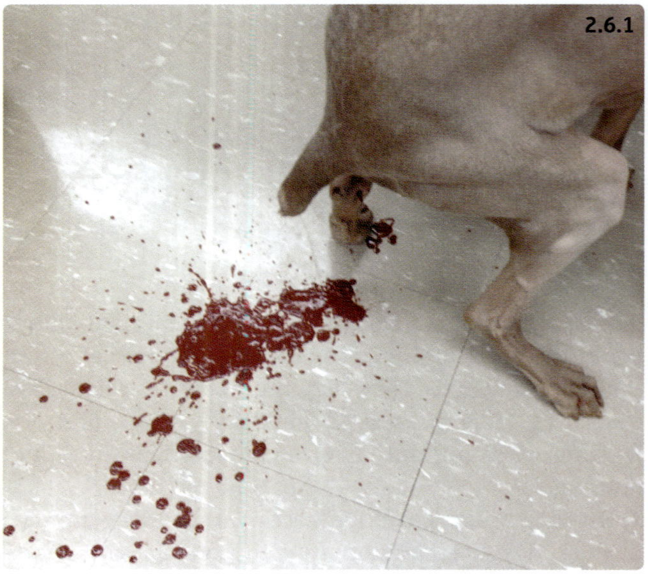

Figure 2.6.1 A 4-year-old male neutered Weimaraner with dietary indiscretion and bloody diarrhea.

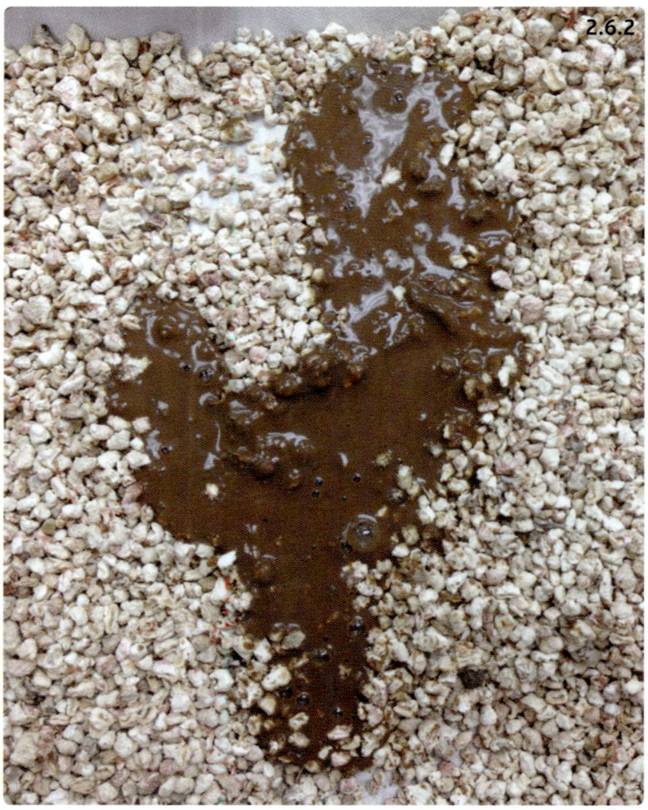

Figure 2.6.2 Liquid diarrhea of small bowel origin in a cat with inflammatory bowel disease.

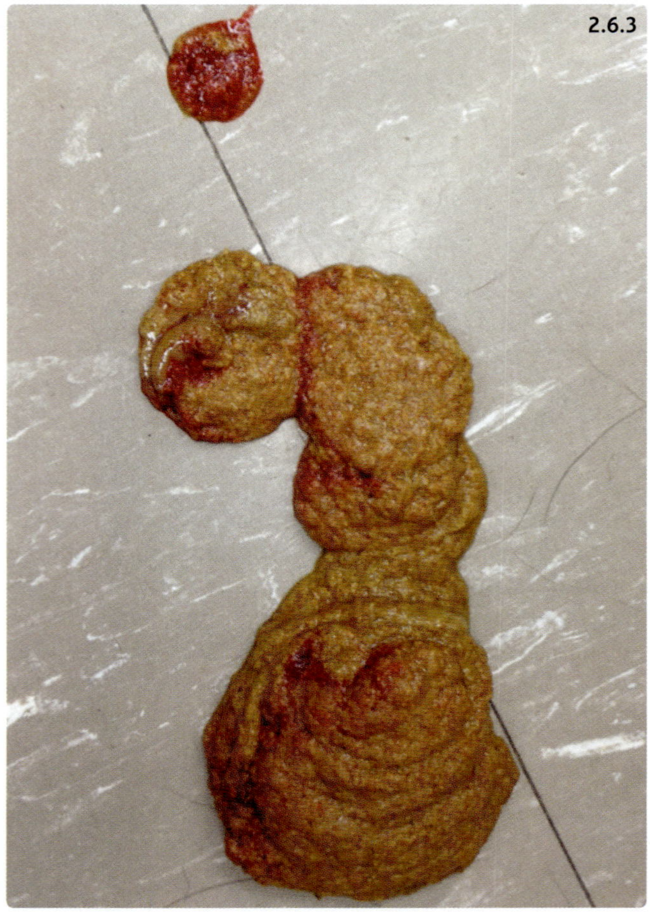

Figure 2.6.3 Hematochezia with soft stool in a dog with diet-responsive chronic enteropathy.

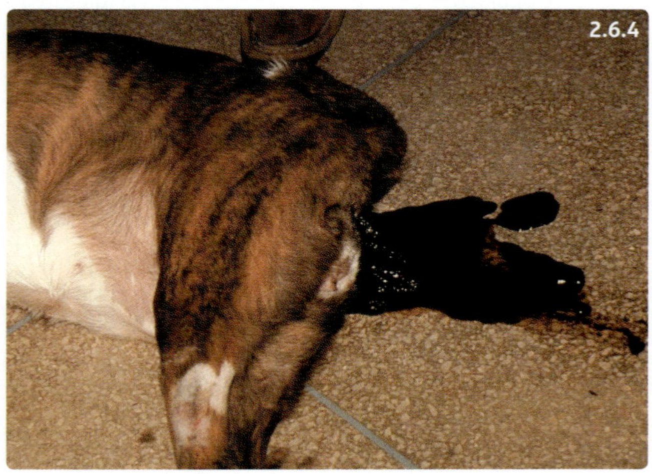

Figure 2.6.4 Melena and diarrhea in a Boxer with GI bleeding secondary to duodenal adenocarcinoma. (Courtesy M. Schaer)

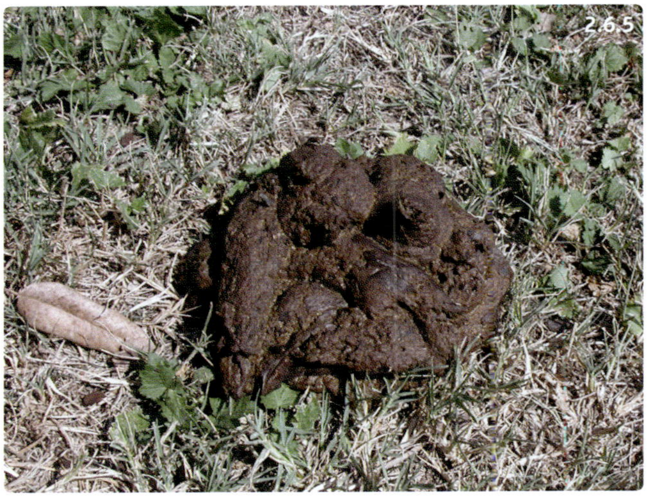

Figure 2.6.5 Cow-pat-like feces from a 9-month-old Mastiff with exocrine pancreatic insufficiency.

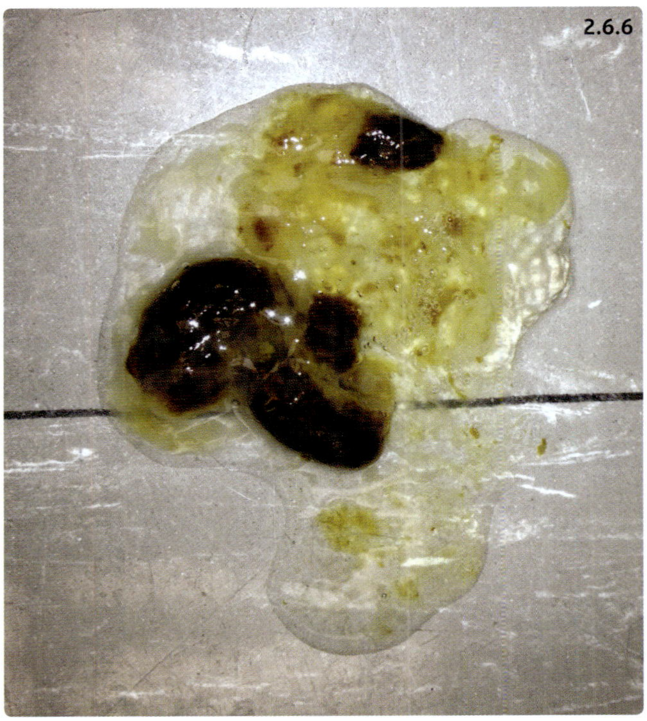

Figure 2.6.6 Mucoid feces from a dog with chronic idiopathic colitis.

PATHOPHYSIOLOGY

The following mechanisms are commonly involved in the pathogenesis of diarrhea. In many instances, several mechanisms contribute concurrently to the onset of diarrhea in intestinal diseases.

Osmotic diarrhea

Osmotic diarrhea occurs in the presence of large, poorly absorbable osmotically active molecules such as undigested carbohydrates, solutes that may additionally undergo fermentation by intestinal microbiota. These molecules ultimately result in a lack of water absorption and loss of water and nutrients in the feces. Osmotic diarrhea may occur following dietary indiscretion and with maldigestion secondary to exocrine pancreatic insufficiency or severe intestinal mucosal inflammation. Unlike most other forms of diarrhea, it typically resolves after the affected animal is fasted.

Secretory diarrhea

Secretory diarrhea is the result of activation of cellular pathways leading to the secretion of electrolytes and water by the enterocytes. Inflammatory cytokines, fatty acids, bile acids, and bacterial endotoxins may trigger this pathway. IBD and enteropathogenic *E. coli* may elicit diarrhea through this pathway.

Increased mucosal permeability

This results from a loss of integrity of the intestinal mucosal barrier, which may occur through loss of enterocytes (erosive or ulcerative intestinal disease) or compromise of paracellular structures such as the tight junctions connecting the enterocytes. Examples of diseases include parvovirus infection, IBD, alimentary lymphoma, and protein-losing enteropathy (PLE).

Abnormal intestinal motility

This develops in the presence of mucosal inflammation. Giant aboral contractions (small intestine) and giant migrating contractions (colon) are common and may severely shorten intestinal transit times.

DIFFERENTIAL DIAGNOSES

There are a myriad of possible causes for diarrhea in dogs and cats. Therefore, it is meaningful to differentiate acute from chronic diarrhea and young from adult animals when preparing a list of differential diagnoses. In addition, the environment plays an important role: dogs and cats in group housing are more susceptible to developing infectious diseases (animal shelters, boarding facilities, breeding facilities). Common differential diagnoses for dogs and cats with acute and chronic diarrhea are summarized in **Tables 2.6.2** and **2.6.3**.

Table 2.6.2 Common causes of acute diarrhea in dogs and cats.

	Dog	Cat
Infectious		
Viral	Parvovirus*, coronavirus*	Parvovirus*, FeLV, FIV
Bacterial	*Campylobacter* spp., *Clostridium perfringens*, *Clostridium difficile*, *E. coli*, *Salmonella* spp., *Neorickettsia heminthoeca*[@]	*Campylobacter* spp., *E. coli*, *Salmonella* spp., *Clostridium perfringens*, *Clostridium difficile*
Parasitic	Nematodes (roundworms, hookworms, and whipworms)	Nematodes (roundworms and hookworms)
	Protozoa: coccidia (*Isospora* spp.*, *Cryptosporidium* spp.), *Giardia* spp.	Protozoa: coccidia, (*Isospora* spp.*, *Cryptosporidium* spp.), *Giardia* spp., *Tritrichomonas fetus*[#]
Diet	Dietary indiscretion, abrupt diet change	Abrupt diet change, dietary indiscretion
Toxins, drugs	Numerous plants, drugs (especially antimicrobials), chemicals	Numerous plants, drugs, chemicals
Idiopathic	Hemorrhagic gastroenteritis, also known as acute hemorrhagic diarrhea syndrome	
Diseases originating outside the intestine	Pancreatitis, liver disease, kidney disease, toxemia, sepsis	Pancreatitis, liver disease, kidney disease, toxemia, sepsis

*, puppies and kittens;
[@], in endemic areas;
[#], young cats, multi-cat housing.

Table 2.6.3 Common causes of chronic diarrhea in dogs and cats.

	Dog	Cat
Bacterial	*Campylobacter* spp., *Clostridium perfringens*, *Clostridium difficile*, *E. coli*, *Salmonella* spp., *Neorickettsia helmintheca*[@]	*Campylobacter* spp., *E. coli*, *Salmonella* spp., *Clostridium perfringens*, *Clostridium difficile*
Fungal, algal	*Histoplasma capsulatum*[@], *Prototheca* spp.[@]	
Parasitic	Nematodes (round, hook and whipworms), *Heterobilharzia americana*[@]	Nematodes (round and hookworms)
	Protozoa: coccidia (*Isospora* spp.*, *Cryptosporidium* spp.), *Giardia* spp.	Protozoa: coccidia, (*Isospora* spp.*, *Cryptosporidium* spp.), *Giardia* spp., *Tritrichomonas fetus*[#]
Diet	Diet-responsive diarrhea	Diet-responsive diarrhea
Dysbiosis	Antibiotic-responsive diarrhea	

	Dog	Cat
Chronic inflammation	Inflammatory bowel disease, granulomatous colitis°	Inflammatory bowel disease
Neoplasia		Low-grade alimentary lymphoma
Idiopathic diseases	Idiopathic intestinal lymphangiectasia, lymphoma	
Diseases originating outside the intestine	Atypical hypoadrenocorticism, exocrine pancreatic insufficiency, chronic pancreatitis, liver disease, kidney disease	Exocrine pancreatic insufficiency, chronic pancreatitis, liver disease, kidney disease

*, puppies and kittens;
#, young cats, multi-cat housing;
@, in endemic areas;
°, Boxers and Bulldogs.

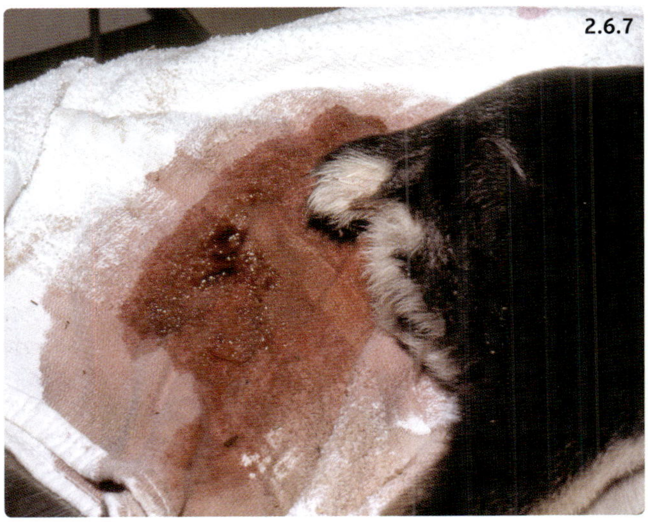

Figure 2.6.7 Liquid bloody diarrhea from a puppy with parvovirus infection. (Courtesy M. Schaer)

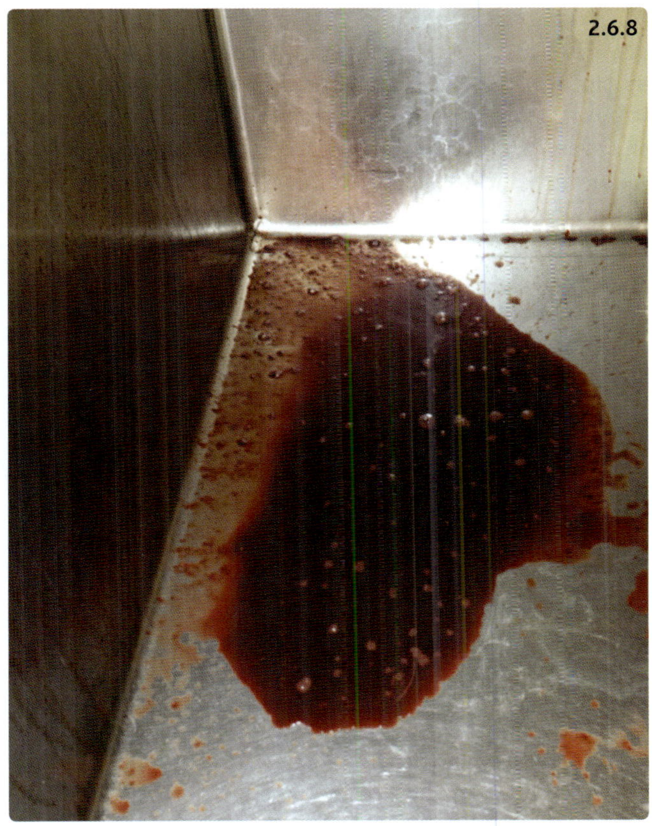

Figure 2.6.8 Liquid bloody diarrhea from a mixed-breed dog with hemorrhagic gastroenteritis/acute hemorrhagic diarrhea syndrome.

Acute diarrhea

In young dogs and cats, acute diarrhea is often caused by enteric infections, and parvovirus infection is an obligate initial rule out in puppies/kittens presenting with acute-onset vomiting and bloody diarrhea (**Figure 2.6.7**). Additionally, parasitic infestations with nematodes (e.g. roundworms, hookworms, whipworms) or protozoa (e.g. various coccidia, *Giardia*) are very frequent causes of acute diarrhea. Alternatively, diarrhea may also be dietary in origin (dietary overload, dietary indiscretion, abrupt change in diet).

In adult dogs and cats, parasitic and dietary causes of diarrhea are also very common and need to be ruled out early in the diagnostic process. Acute flare-ups of chronic recurring diarrhea should be differentiated from truly acute disease. Hemorrhagic gastroenteritis (HGE), also called acute hemorrhagic diarrhea syndrome (AHDS), is a disease of unknown etiology that typically affects middle aged dogs of small and toy breeds (**Figure 2.6.8**), but large-breed dogs can be affected as well. Severe cases may have a fatal outcome without aggressive treatment.

The role of bacterial enteropathogens is difficult to establish definitely since these bacteria and their toxins have been detected in similar amounts in the feces of young and adult healthy and diarrheic animals. However, bacterial infections should be considered in animals held in groups (kennels, cattery, breeder) and in cases that are refractory to usual treatment.

Chronic diarrhea

As is the case with acute diarrhea, parasites (nematodes and protozoa) are also very frequently involved, and the precise role of bacterial enteropathogens remains unclear (see above).

Chronic enteropathies (CEs) are associated with intestinal mucosal inflammation. A complex relationship exists between the intestinal microbiota and the host immune system in the gut. This equilibrium is disrupted in chronic intestinal diseases, and additional factors such as dietary antigens may also contribute to the resulting inflammation. Considerable and long-lasting changes in the composition of the microbiota have been documented in dogs and cats with CE. The differential diagnoses of canine CE include diet-responsive diarrhea, antibiotic-responsive diarrhea (most common in young large breed dogs such as German Shepherd Dogs), and IBD. Diet-responsive disease and IBD are also very common causes of feline CE, and must be differentiated from low-grade alimentary lymphoma, which may present with similar clinical signs.

CLINICAL APPROACH

A thorough history should be obtained that includes a description of the onset and duration of diarrhea, appearance of the feces, description of defecation, including frequency, and clinical course of the disease. Acute and new problems should be differentiated from recurrent or chronic issues. Additionally, the presence of factors that may trigger the development of diarrhea, such as dietary changes or administration of drugs such as antibiotics or non-steroidal anti-inflammatory drugs (NSAIDs), should be discussed. Anthelmintic treatment and vaccination history should be obtained. The owner should also be asked if other animals in the household have the same signs and if the diarrheic dog/cat also shows additional signs such as hyporexia, vomiting, weight loss, polydipsia, and polyuria.

Acute diarrhea

At the time of initial presentation, puppies and kittens that could have highly contagious parvovirus infection should be identified on the basis of clinical signs and absent/incomplete vaccination status. They should be immediately triaged and screened for the presence of viral antigen in the feces. Cage-side fecal tests have excellent specificity, and positive animals should be isolated from the rest of the hospital population while they receive treatment. However, fecal antigen test sensitivity is good but not perfect, and a negative result does not rule out the presence of virus. Consequently, in unvaccinated or incompletely vaccinated animals, suggestive clinical signs are sufficient to justify isolation.

In adult animals, acute diarrhea is often self-limiting, particularly if the underlying problem (parasites, diet) can be eliminated. Feces should be collected for parasitological testing (e.g. direct smear, zinc sulfate flotation, *Giardia* ELISA). Alternatively, a broad-spectrum anthelmintic drug such as fenbendazole can be administered empirically (50 mg/kg PO q24h for 3 days). Further diagnostic tests such as screening for additional infectious diseases may be indicated in kennel, cattery, or shelter situations.

Treatment is supportive and focused on fluid therapy to address dehydration, the most common complication of acute diarrhea. Dogs and cats with limited systemic repercussions of diarrhea and mild dehydration may benefit from oral and SC fluids; however, lethargic, anorexic, and moderately to severely dehydrated animals require IV fluid therapy designed to rapidly and efficiently correct existing fluid and electrolyte deficits. In severe cases, significant protein loss into the intestinal lumen may occur because of the severely compromised intestinal barrier and may justify the use of IV colloids.

All animals with acute diarrhea generally benefit from a 12-hour fasting period followed by frequent small meals consisting of easily digestible food (commercial 'intestinal' diet or home prepared boiled chicken breast and rice) for 3–5 days before being progressively reintroduced to their regular diet. Importantly, young puppies and kittens should not be systematically fasted as they may become hypoglycemic if not fed regularly. Antidiarrheal drugs are rarely necessary in small animals with acute diarrhea. Loperamide, an opiate agonist that does not cross the blood–brain barrier, may be considered (0.1–0.2 mg/kg PO q8h as needed) in animals with particularly severe disease and significant abdominal pain. Antimicrobials are generally not recommended in the treatment of acute diarrhea, except in the presence of severely compromised mucosal barrier and evidence of severe systemic repercussions such as severe depression, marked leukocytosis, or leukopenia, or in shelter animals. In a few clinical studies, probiotics have been documented to shorten the time to passage of normal feces and the time to discharge. A 2–4-week week treatment extending well beyond expected clinical recovery is generally recommended.

Chronic diarrhea

Dogs and cats with small or large bowel diarrhea and absent or minimal systemic repercussions (e.g. lethargy, dysorexia, weight loss) benefit from a sequential approach using various empirical treatment trials (**Box 2.6.1**). First and foremost, intestinal parasites must be eliminated using a broad-spectrum anthelmintic drug such as fenbendazole (50 mg/kg PO q24h for 3 days). Then a dietary trial using either a novel protein or a hydrolyzed peptide commercial diet should be implemented. Clinical studies have shown that 50–65% of dogs and cats with chronic diarrhea respond to such a dietary trial within 1–2 weeks. The proportion of responders is even higher among young large breed dogs with mostly large bowel diarrhea. Animals that do not respond to the dietary trial should receive antimicrobials in an attempt to correct chronic idiopathic dysbiosis, which represented approximately 10–15% of all dogs with chronic CE in one clinical study. Tylosin (10–20 mg/kg PO q12h) or metronidazole (10–15 mg/kg PO q12h) is often used for the treatment of antibiotic-responsive diarrhea (ARD). Recently, concerns have been raised regarding the rising resistance of fecal bacteria to metronidazole, and the author currently recommends tylosin as the best first-line option for ARD. Additionally, while there are still only a few clinical studies documenting the benefits of probiotics in the treatment of canine CE, the results are promising, and probiotics should be considered in the treatment of clinical cases. Prolonged administration is generally recommended (4–8 weeks). Finally, if empirical treatment is not successful, a full work up is indicated (see below).

In sick dogs and cats with chronic diarrhea and dysorexia, lethargy, weight loss, or ascites, a more aggressive approach is recommended. This includes a minimal database with CBC, biochemical profile, and urinalysis, as well as abdominal ultrasound if available. Depending on the severity of disease, these tests may reveal an inflammatory leukogram, panhypoproteinemia (hypoalbuminemia and hypoglobulinemia), and increased liver enzymes. Abdominal ultrasound may document intestinal wall lesions in all or select segments of the intestine. In parallel to the diagnostic plan, correction of fluid and electrolyte deficits may be required. Ultimately, intestinal mucosal biopsies may need to be collected endoscopically or surgically and evaluated histologically. In severely debilitated patients that are poor anesthetic risks or in cases with financial limitations, a carefully designed treatment trial for the most likely cause of the chronic diarrhea can be initiated if indicated (for further details see Chapter 8, Digestive diseases [pharynx to rectum]).

The recommended approach to chronic large bowel diarrhea is illustrated in the algorithm (**Figure 2.6.9**).

Box 2.6.1 Approach to chronic diarrhea in dogs with minimal or absent systemic signs. While a sequential application of the following steps is theoretically preferable, they can also be combined (e.g. parasiticide and diet initiated at the same time).

1. **Rule out intestinal parasites**
   Repeated parasite screenings and/or treatment with broad-spectrum anthelmintic drug (e.g. fenbendazole 50 mg/kg q24h for 3 days).
2. **Rule out diet-responsive enteropathy**
   Elimination trial with 'hypoallergenic' diet; a response should be seen within 2 weeks. In case of failure, some cases may benefit from a second trial with a different diet:
   - Novel protein diet (based on patient's dietary history) or
   - Hydrolyzed peptide diet.
3. **Rule out antibiotic-responsive enteropathy**
   Administer tylosin (10–20 mg/kg PO q12h), or metronidazole (10–15 mg/kg PO q12h), or other antibiotic of choice; a response should be seen within 2 weeks. If successful, treatment should be pursued for 4–8 weeks.
4. If none of the above approaches works, **obtain a minimal database** with CBC, biochemistry panel, urinalysis, and abdominal ultrasound. Finally, endoscopy and intestinal biopsy or full-thickness surgically obtained intestinal biopsies might be required for a histopathologic diagnosis.

RECOMMENDED FURTHER READING

Baral RM (2012) Approach to the cat with diarrhea. In: *The Cat: Clinical Medicine and Management*. (ed. SE Little) Elsevier Saunders, St. Louis, pp. 459–465.

Marks SL (2013) Diarrhea. In: *Canine and Feline Gastroenterology*. (eds. RJ Washabau, MJ Day) Elsevier Saunders, St. Louis, pp. 99–108.

Willard MD (2010) Diarrhea. In: *Textbook of Veterinary Internal Medicine*, 7th edn. (eds. SJ Ettinger, EC Feldman) Saunders Elsevier, St. Louis, pp. 200–202.

2.6.9

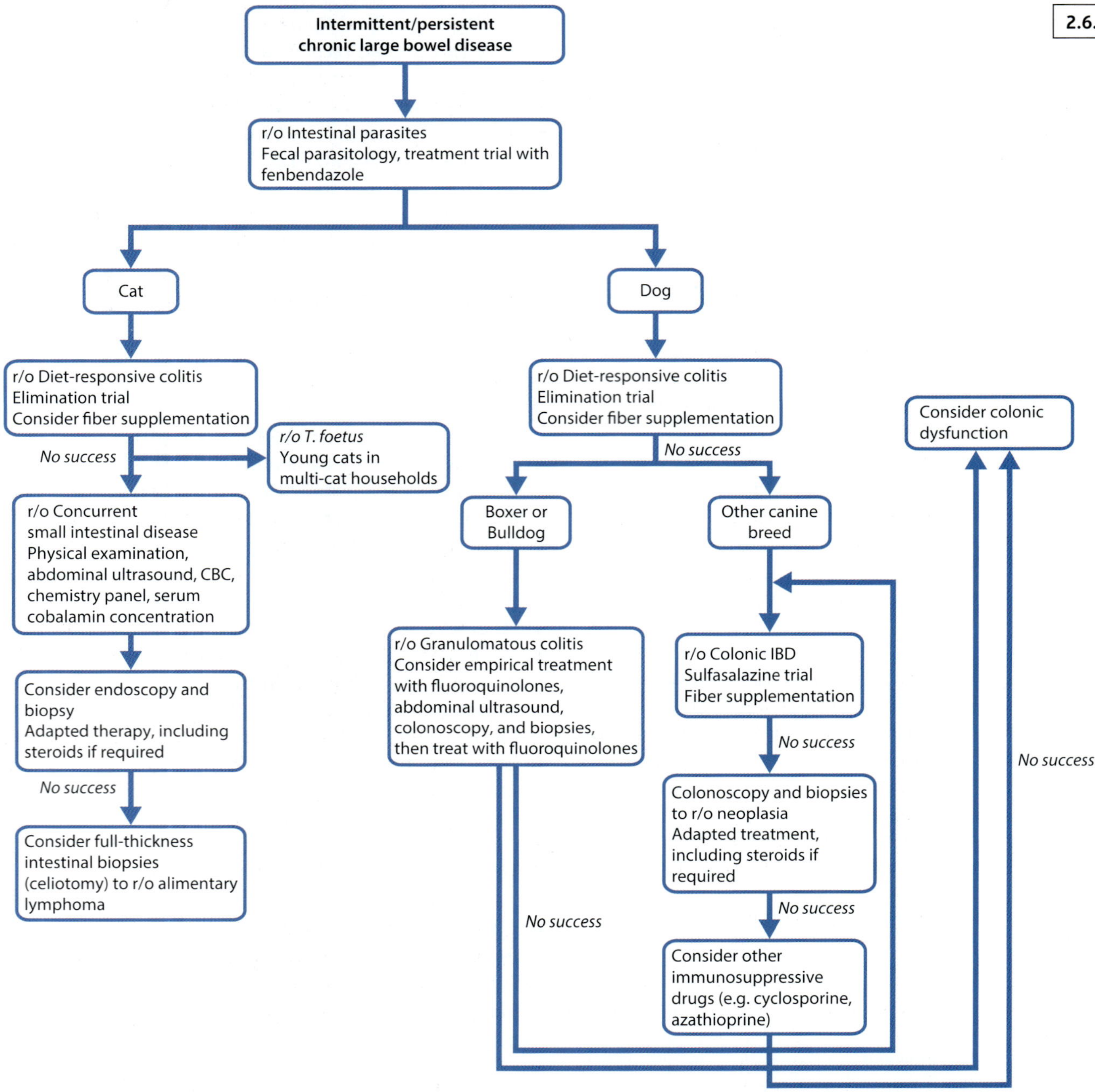

Figure 2.6.9 Clinical approach in cats and dogs with intermittent or persistent chronic large bowel diarrhea. r/o, rule out.

2.7 Icterus

Julien Dandrieux

INTRODUCTION

Icterus (or jaundice) is a clinical finding that is characterized by the yellow discoloration of tissues (including sclerae, mucous membranes, and skin) and body fluids (such as plasma and urine) secondary to hyperbilirubinemia and bile pigment deposition. The following text will outline the diagnostic approach to the icteric patient; the reader is referred to the chapters discussing anemia and liver and biliary disease for an in-depth discussion of the different diseases or their treatment.

In the normal physiologic state, bilirubin is constantly produced from the degradation of heme (contained principally in hemoglobin, but also in other hemoproteins) by phagocytes in the liver, spleen, and bone marrow. Hydrophobic unconjugated bilirubin (uB) is produced and transported in the plasma noncovalently bound to albumin. Bilirubin is taken up by the hepatocytes and conjugated to a hydrophilic form (cB), which can then be excreted through the biliary system into the intestinal lumen. The excretion of cB is the rate-limiting step. cB is further metabolized by intestinal bacteria and is the origin of the normal color of feces (stercobilin). Acholic feces (pale to white in color) can sometimes be seen in animals with lack of cB secretion in the intestine due to complete extrahepatic bile duct obstruction (EBDO).

If cB cannot be excreted into the biliary system, it will backflow in the blood and be excreted in the urine. Renal tubular resorption of bilirubin in dogs is very limited, which explains why bilirubinuria can precede hyperbilirubinemia. Furthermore, dogs (male more than female) have the capacity to process heme in the renal tubules to uB, and then cB. For this reason, mild bilirubinuria is often detected in healthy dogs with a urine SG of 1.025–1.040 (1+) or moderate levels with a SG higher than 1.040 (up to 2+). Cats have a higher capacity for tubular resorption and are not able to process bilirubin in their kidneys; for these reasons bilirubinuria is always considered pathologic in this species.

Bilirubin can be found in a third form: covalently bound to albumin (albB, also called delta-bilirubin or biliprotein). This form occurs spontaneously in disease, but is not present in healthy animals. The half-life of albB is the same as albumin (about 8 days in dogs) and can be the reason why jaundice may persist in some animals after resolution of the cause. It needs to be considered in a patient that is clinically improving despite persistent icterus.

Urobilinogen is a colorless compound formed from the degradation of bilirubin in the intestine and passively absorbed by the small bowel mucosa. The fraction that is not removed from the portal blood by hepatocytes enters the blood and is excreted in the urine. Urobilinogen is detected in the urine with a dipstick reagent. Increased levels can accompany hemolytic and hepatobiliary diseases, but the test is not commonly used because of its nonspecific interpretation.

In summary, bilirubin in a healthy animal predominantly consists of uB with negligible concentrations of cB and albB.

ETIOLOGY

Hyperbilirubinemia can occur either when the rate of uB production exceeds the rate of uB uptake in the hepatocytes (hemolysis), when uB is not converted to cB or transported into the biliary tract (hepatic insufficiency), or when the rate of cB formation exceeds the rate of cB excretion in the bile (biliary tract disease). The main causes for icterus can be summarized as follows:

- Prehepatic icterus: increase in red blood cell destruction.
- Hepatic icterus: liver insufficiency.
- Posthepatic icterus: obstruction at the level of the biliary system (intra- or extrahepatic) or rupture of the biliary tree.
- Other causes: sepsis (cholestasis induced by tumor necrosis factor alpha and endotoxin), resorption of large hematomas (rare).

CLINICAL APPROACH TO THE ICTERIC PATIENT

The icteric patient can be identified on physical examination or by the color of its plasma or serum (**Figures 2.7.1, 2.7.2**). Concentrations at which jaundice become visible in different locations are summarized in **Table 2.7.1**.

The first step after detection of icterus on physical examination is to inquire about possible toxic or infectious causes with a thorough history including vaccination status and travel history (common causes are listed in **Table 2.7.2**).

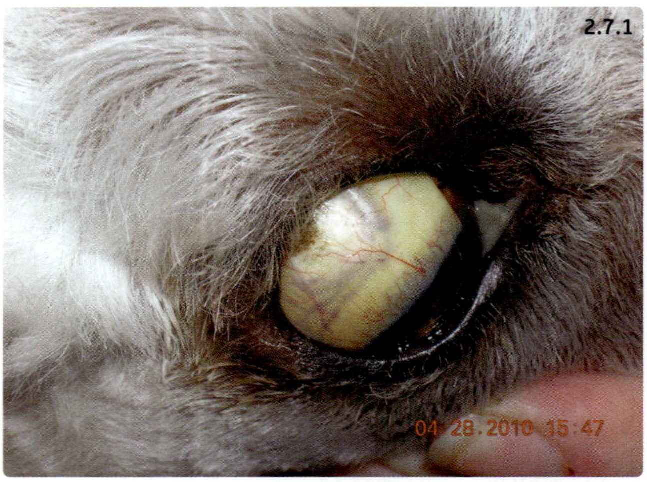

Figure 2.7.1 Icteric sclera in a dog with immune-mediated hemolytic anemia secondary to lymphoma. Note the bright yellow color of the sclera.

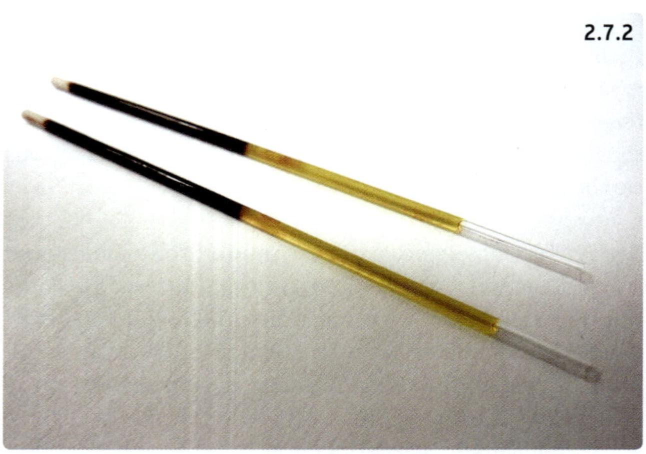

Figure 2.7.2 Icteric plasma. Picture of microhematocrit tubes from the same dog as in Figure 2.7.1 after centrifugation. The yellow discoloration of the serum is evident and is detectable at lower bilirubin concentrations than are necessary to detect icteric sclera.

The second step is to determine whether other abnormalities are present on physical examination. A good body condition score is suggestive of an acute disease (e.g. acute cholangiohepatitis, hemolytic anemia, hepatic toxic insult) whereas a poor body condition score suggests chronic disease (e.g. chronic cholangiohepatitis, neoplastic process, end-stage liver disease). Generalized peripheral lymphadenomegaly is suggestive of infectious disease or lymphoma and fine-needle aspiration and cytologic evaluation can help in reaching a diagnosis. If ascites is present, fluid sampling for analysis should be done. Findings such as septic peritonitis or bile peritonitis secondary to biliary tree rupture are strong indications for exploratory laparotomy. Splenomegaly and hepatomegaly are common findings with prehepatic icterus secondary to extramedullary hematopoiesis, which can accompany immune-mediated diseases, but it can also be seen with neoplastic or infectious diseases.

Laboratory testing, including hematology, biochemistry, and urinalysis, is the next step to determine the cause of the icterus and typical findings are outlined in **Figure 2.7.3**. If liver disease or complete EBDO is suspected, a coagulation profile including fibrinogen concentration is recommended prior to taking biopsies, as coagulopathies may develop secondary to these conditions. Moderate to marked anemia is expected with prehepatic icterus, and should become regenerative within 3–5 days, whereas anemia is usually only mild and nonregenerative with primary hepatic or posthepatic causes. In an animal with icterus of hepatic origin, hepatocellular enzymes (ALT and AST) are expected to be increased to a higher magnitude than biliary epithelium enzymes (ALP

Table 2.7.1 Interpretation of bilirubinuria and plasma thresholds for detection of icterus.

Where	Concentration/degree of bilirubinuria or bilirubinemia*
Urine	Cat: any degree is abnormal. Dog: up to 2+ bilirubin with SG >1.040 can be normal. Bilirubinuria can precede hyperbilirubinemia
Serum or plasma	>0.9 mg/dl (15 μmol/l)
Sclera	>1.5 mg/dl (25 μmol/l)
Mucous membrane (nonpigmented)	>2.6 mg/dl (45 μmol/l)

* These are not absolute values and the threshold for visual detection of icterus varies between individuals.

Table 2.7.2 Common causes of icterus in dogs (D) and cats (C).

Type	Toxin	Infection	Others
Prehepatic → hemolysis	Copper; drugs (acetaminophen/paracetamol [C, HB]; fenbendazole); onions (HB); zinc (HB)	*Dirofilaria* (caval syndrome [D]); *Cytauxzoon felis* (C)	DIC; erythrocyte congenital defect (e.g. PFK); hypophosphatemia (C>D); neoplasia (e.g. hemangiosarcoma)
Prehepatic → immune-mediated hemolysis	Drugs (cephalosporin, penicillin, potentiated sulfonamides)	*Babesia* (D); *Ehrlichia* (D); FeLV (C); hemotropic *Mycoplasma* spp. (C)	Blood transfusion; idiopathic IMHA (D>C); neoplasia (e.g. lymphoma); inflammation (e.g. pancreatitis, prostatitis)
Hepatic	Aflatoxins; mushrooms (*Amanita* spp.); blue–green algae; copper accumulation; drugs (acetaminophen/paracetamol [C>D], diazepam [C], ketoconazole, itraconazole, lomustine, methimazole [C], NSAIDs [D], phenobarbital, trimethoprim–sulfonamide); sago palm; xylitol (D)	Virulent calicivirus (C); coronavirus (C); canine adenovirus (D); *Histoplasma capsulatum; Leishmania* (D); *Leptospira* (D); *Toxoplasma* (C>D)	End-stage chronic liver disease; heat stroke; hepatic lipidosis (C); hepatitis/cholangiohepatitis; neoplasia (carcinoma, lymphoma)
Posthepatic		Liver flukes (C)	Cholecystitis; cholelithiasis; gallbladder rupture; gallbladder mucocoele (D); neoplasia (biliary adenocarcinoma); pancreatitis

DIC, disseminated intravascular coagulation; FeLV, feline leukemia virus; HB, formation of Heinz bodies; IMHA, immune-mediated hemolytic anemia; PFK, phosphofructokinase deficiency.

and GGT), whereas the opposite is expected with a posthepatic icterus. Liver functional parameters (albumin, urea, cholesterol, and glucose) might also be decreased with significant loss of liver function. These parameters are expected to be normal with posthepatic obstruction, with the exception of cholesterol, which will be increased (cholestatic disease). Although these changes can help determine the origin of the icterus they have many limitations. For example, prehepatic icterus often causes hepatic hypoxia with increases in ALT and AST. The serum activity of these two enzymes might normalize in end-stage liver disease because of the decrease in functional tissue. Additionally, hepatocytes will often be affected by processes causing posthepatic icterus over time, resulting in increases in ALT and AST. Therefore, all abnormal test results must be interpreted within the context of the patient and its stage of disease.

Prehepatic icterus should be suspected in the presence of moderate to severe anemia, which is usually regenerative within 3–5 days of onset. The next diagnostic step is to determine its origin. Immune-mediated hemolytic anemia (IMHA) is a common cause of hemolysis. Dogs are more prone to primary (idiopathic) IMHA and cats to secondary IMHA from a variety of primary diseases. Imaging and testing for different infectious diseases, depending on the travel history and geographic location of the animal, is indicated.

Imaging modalities, particularly abdominal ultrasound, are very useful for differentiating hepatic from posthepatic icterus (**Figure 2.7.4**). Abdominal ultrasound can help confirm the location of the problem and suggest possible causes such as microhepatica in end-stage liver disease, changes in liver echogenicity or outline with infiltrative disease (**Figure 2.7.5**), or dilation of the common bile duct with long-standing posthepatic obstruction (**Figures 2.7.6, 2.7.7**). Abdominal ultrasound is also useful for collecting samples for cytology, histology, and culture, as indicated, to obtain a final diagnosis (**Figure 2.7.8**),

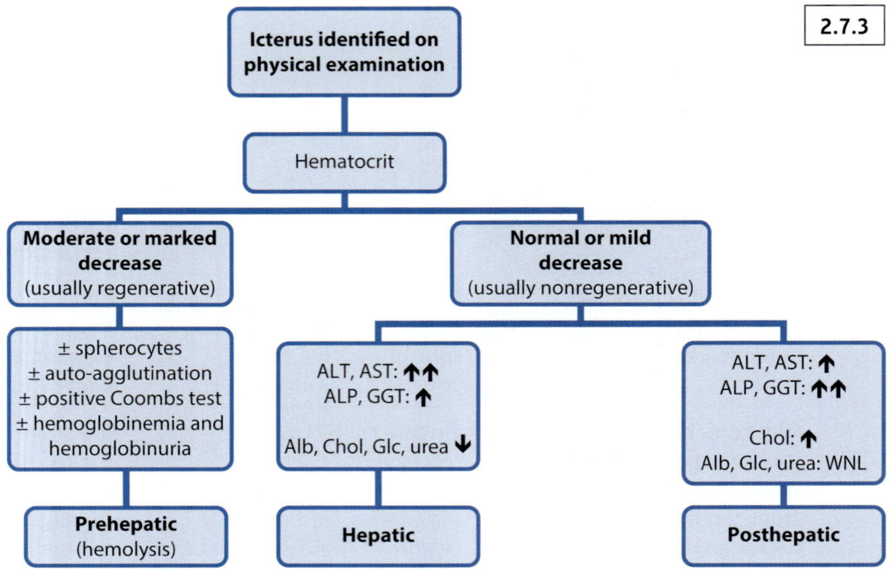

Figure 2.7.3 Flow chart showing the findings on laboratory blood work that can help determine the origin of icterus. Alb, albumin; ALP, alkaline phosphatase; ALT, alanine transaminase; AST, aspartate transaminase; Chol, cholesterol; GGT, gamma-glutamyltransferase; Glc, glucose; WNL, within normal limits; ↑, relative increase; ↓, relative decrease. See text for limitations in the interpretation. Further work up is then needed to determine the disease process.

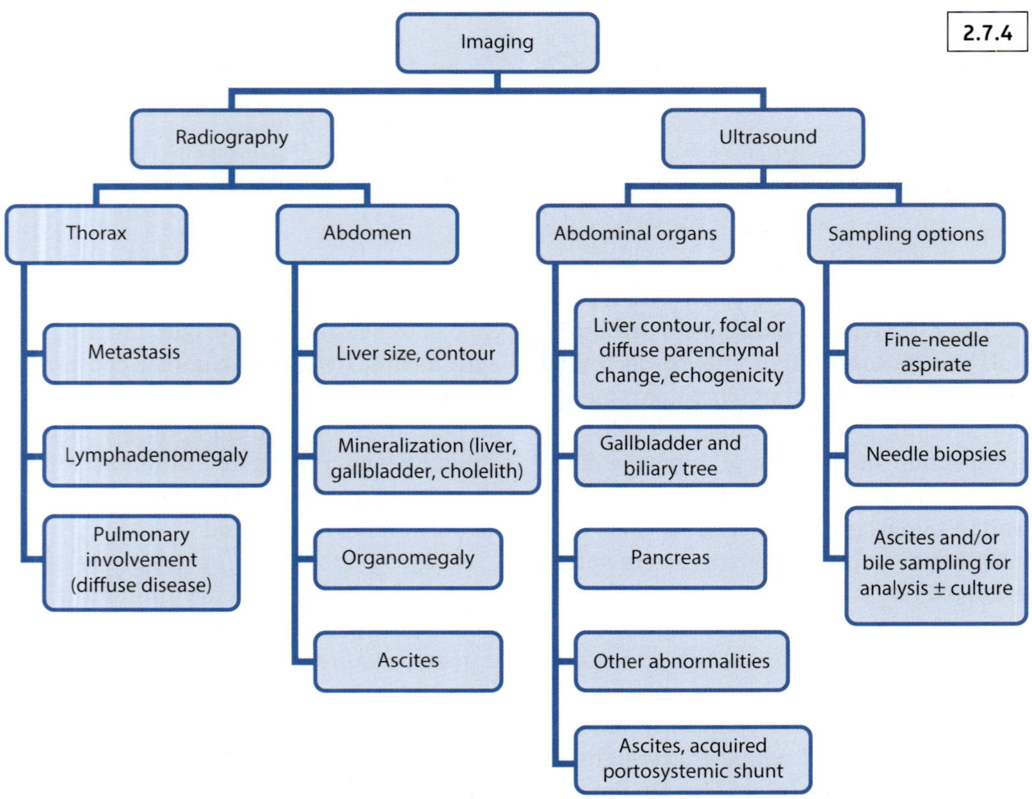

Figure 2.7.4 Flow chart showing the imaging modalities for the work up of the icteric patient. Radiographs are an adequate first step to get an overview of the abdominal organs and the chest, if a systemic disease is suspected. Ultrasound can be very helpful, but yields are dependent on machine quality and operator. It allows targeted sampling.

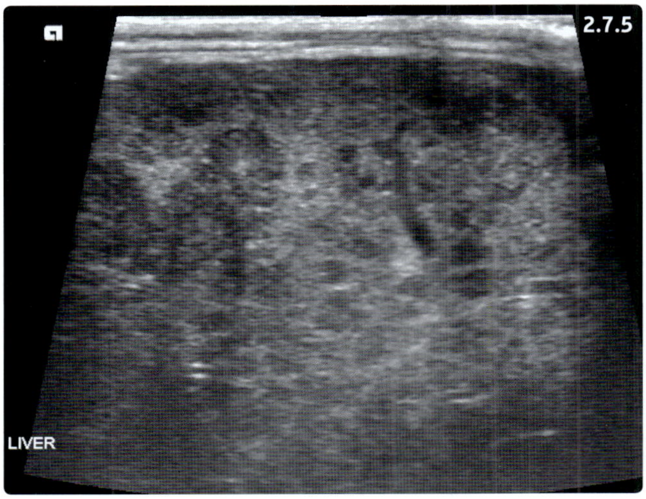

Figure 2.7.5 Ultrasonographic appearance of the liver in a dog presented with icterus. The parenchyma is heterogeneous with hyper- and hypoechoic nodules. (Courtesy D. Tyrell) Fine-needle aspirates were taken and the cytology is depicted in Figure 2.7.8.

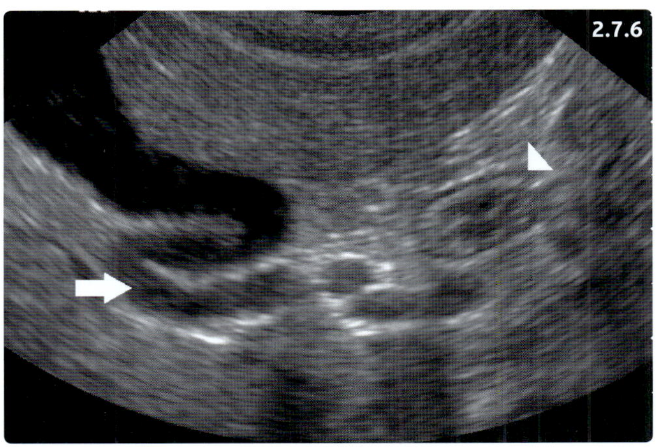

Figure 2.7.6 Ultrasound image of the liver in an icteric cat. The neck of the gallbladder is on the left hand side of the picture with the common bile duct (CBD) extending towards the right (arrow). The duodenum can also be seen on the right (arrow head). The dilation of the CBD is consistent with a posthepatic obstruction. (Courtesy D. Tyrell)

although in some cases surgical biopsies are preferred. Other modalities such as CT, nuclear imaging, and MRI may be helpful in complex cases if these options are available.

If neoplasia is high on the list of differentials, chest radiographs or CT should be considered to screen for metastasis.

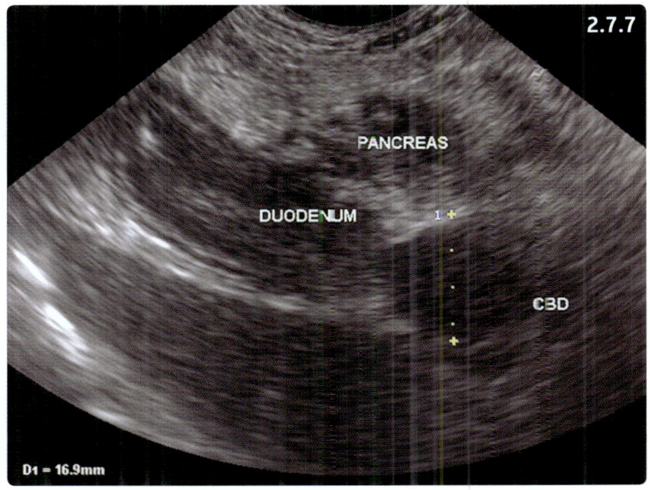

Figure 2.7.7 Ultrasound image of the common bile duct in an icteric cat. Anatomically, the duodenum, pancreas, and common bile duct (CBD) are in close contact with each other, as can be appreciated on this ultrasound picture. This explains how a severe pancreatitis can lead to development of icterus. Note in this patient that the CBD is markedly enlarged (16.9 mm, normal is less than 3 mm). (Courtesy C. Beck)

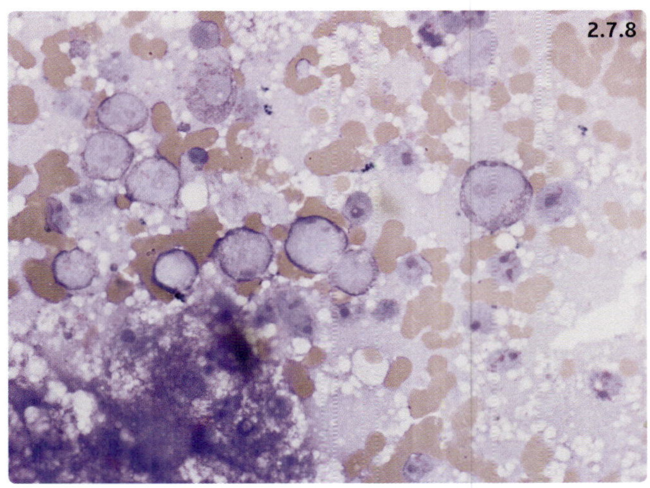

Figure 2.7.8 Cytologic slide from a fine-needle liver aspirate in an icteric dog (from the dog in Figure 2.7.5). Hepatocytes can be seen in the bottom left corner displaying marked vacuolation. A population of large atypical round cells with round nuclei containing fine chromatin and a thin rim of cytoplasm is also present. These cells are consistent with lymphoma. (Courtesy C. Connolly)

RECOMMENDED FURTHER READING

Stockham SL, Scott MA (2008) Erythrocytes. In: *Fundamentals of Veterinary Clinical Pathology*, 2nd edn. (eds. SL Stockham, MA Scott) Blackwell Publishing, Ames, p. 114.

Stockham SL, Scott MA (2008) Urinary system. In: *Fundamentals of Veterinary Clinical Pathology*, 2nd edn. (eds. SL Stockham, MA Scott) Blackwell Publishing, Ames, pp. 466–467.

Stockham SL, Scott MA (2008) Liver function. In: *Fundamentals of Veterinary Clinical Pathology*, 2nd edn. (eds. SL Stockham, MA Scott) Blackwell Publishing, Ames, pp. 681–690.

Watson PJ (2014) Diagnostics tests for the hepatobiliary system. In: *Small Animal Internal Medicine*, 5th edn. (eds. RW Nelson, CG Couto) Elsevier Mosby, St. Louis, pp. 512–535.

Webster CRL (2010) History, clinical signs, and physical findings in hepatobiliary disease. In: *Textbook of Veterinary Internal Medicine*, 7th edn. (eds. ST Ettinger, EC Feldman) Elsevier Saunders, St. Louis, pp. 1612–1625.

Chapter 2 Common clinical problems

2.8 Cough

Elizabeth Rozanski

INTRODUCTION

Cough is a common presenting complaint for dogs and, to a lesser extent, cats. Cough is a sign of an underlying disorder, not a primary disease. Therefore, the cause of the cough should be identified and the underlying disease, not just the cough, should be treated if possible. In some cases the cause of cough may be simple to identify and easy to correct, such as kennel cough. In other cases, the cough may be multi-factorial or relatively resistant to therapy.

Cough is defined as a sudden expiratory effort producing a noisy expulsion of air from the lungs. A cough usually signals an effort to clear the lungs of real or imagined foreign material. Cough can be productive or dry, although it may be at times hard for owners to determine if the cough is productive, as animals rarely expectorate and tend to swallow any mucus that is produced. A cough can be classified as acute or chronic. A cough is considered chronic if it lasts for 2 months or longer.

Most coughing in animals is presumed to be an involuntary response. Stimuli to cough include pressure on the outside of the airway, presence of foreign material or perception of foreign matter, excessive secretions, or recurrent aspiration. Coughing can become apparently habitual in some dogs. Interestingly, and in contrast to people, cough is hard to induce in healthy dogs. Cough serves as an important function both by aiding in the clearance of foreign debris and by enhancing the actions of the mucociliary elevator. The cough reflex is the primary defense mechanism to prevent aspiration of large particles or debris.

ETIOLOGY/PATHOPHYSIOLOGY

Historical information and a description of the cough may help to pinpoint the etiology. The patient's geographic history is important when considering certain of the systemic mycoses (e.g. coccidioidomycosis [western arid United States]; blastomycosis and histoplasmosis [midwestern and southeastern United States]). The status of heartworm prevention is extremely important to know in heartworm endemic regions. Cough may also be classified as to a specific time of day (e.g. night, morning) or coupled with an event such as drinking, eating, running, or pulling on a leash. Coughing at night time may result in more complaints due to inference with the owner's own sleep, especially for owners that are away during the daytime. Postnasal drip can be a cause of coughing at night or when the animal is recumbent. In cats, cough may be confused with retching or attempts to vomit hairballs. Many small-breed dogs cough frequently and owners may not interpret that as abnormal unless questioned. In this population of dogs, earlier management of cough is more likely to be successful than after years of unrelenting cough.

Kennel cough (or canine infectious respiratory disease complex [CIRD]) is common in dogs, and even brief exposure to other apparently healthy dogs can result in infection. As always, questions about prior therapy and any apparent benefit may help improve the diagnostic and therapeutic options.

PHYSICAL EXAMINATION

Pets that are presented for evaluation of cough should be immediately assessed as 'stable' or 'not stable'. Congestive heart failure most commonly presents as tachypnea and/or respiratory distress, but occasionally signs are misinterpreted to be only cough, particularly when large volumes of pulmonary edema are present. Tracheal collapse may result in severe respiratory distress due to airflow obstruction, although the initial signs may be cough. Other 'not stable' causes of cough include pneumonias and pleural space disease, such as spontaneous pneumothorax or chronic pleural effusion. Unstable pets should be rapidly administered supplemental oxygen and diagnostic testing should be pursued at an efficient, yet unstressful, pace.

In stable patients, a complete physical examination of the cardiopulmonary system is warranted, including examination of the oral cavity, palpation of the neck for masses or lymphadenopathy, auscultation of the upper and lower airways and heart, and abdominal palpation. Dogs with a visible expiratory 'push' commonly have obstructive lower airway disease. Chronic bronchitis with obstructive lower airways and asthma associated with hypersensitivity lung disease are common examples of this disorder. Pets should be evaluated for weight loss or loss of muscle mass, which may accompany primary or metastatic neoplasia, heart disease, or severe obstructive pulmonary disease. Esophageal (megaesophagus) and laryngeal dysfunction may lead to recurrent pneumonias due to aspiration.

(See algorithm [**Figure 2.8.1**].)

DIAGNOSTIC IMAGING

Thoracic imaging is recommended for evaluation of the patient with cough. Chest radiographs are useful for evaluation of lung parenchyma and airways, as well the cardiac size and pleural space. CT may be used as well for pulmonary diagnostics, and may provide additional information about the airway and lung parenchyma.

At a minimum, dogs and cats with cough should have chest radiographs performed for evaluation as to the possible cause, and to direct appropriate therapeutics.

SAMPLING

Airway sampling for collection of samples for cytology, aerobic culture and sensitivity testing, and/or PCR testing should be considered in dogs and cats without a clear diagnosis from the history, physical examination, and radiographs. Airway cytology can be obtained with bronchoscopy, transtracheal wash, or endotracheal tube passage and wash procedures. It is useful to document infection, inflammation, or eosinophilic infiltrates. It is important to recall that the normal upper airway structures are not sterile, and aerobic culture results should always be interpreted in light of the cytological findings.

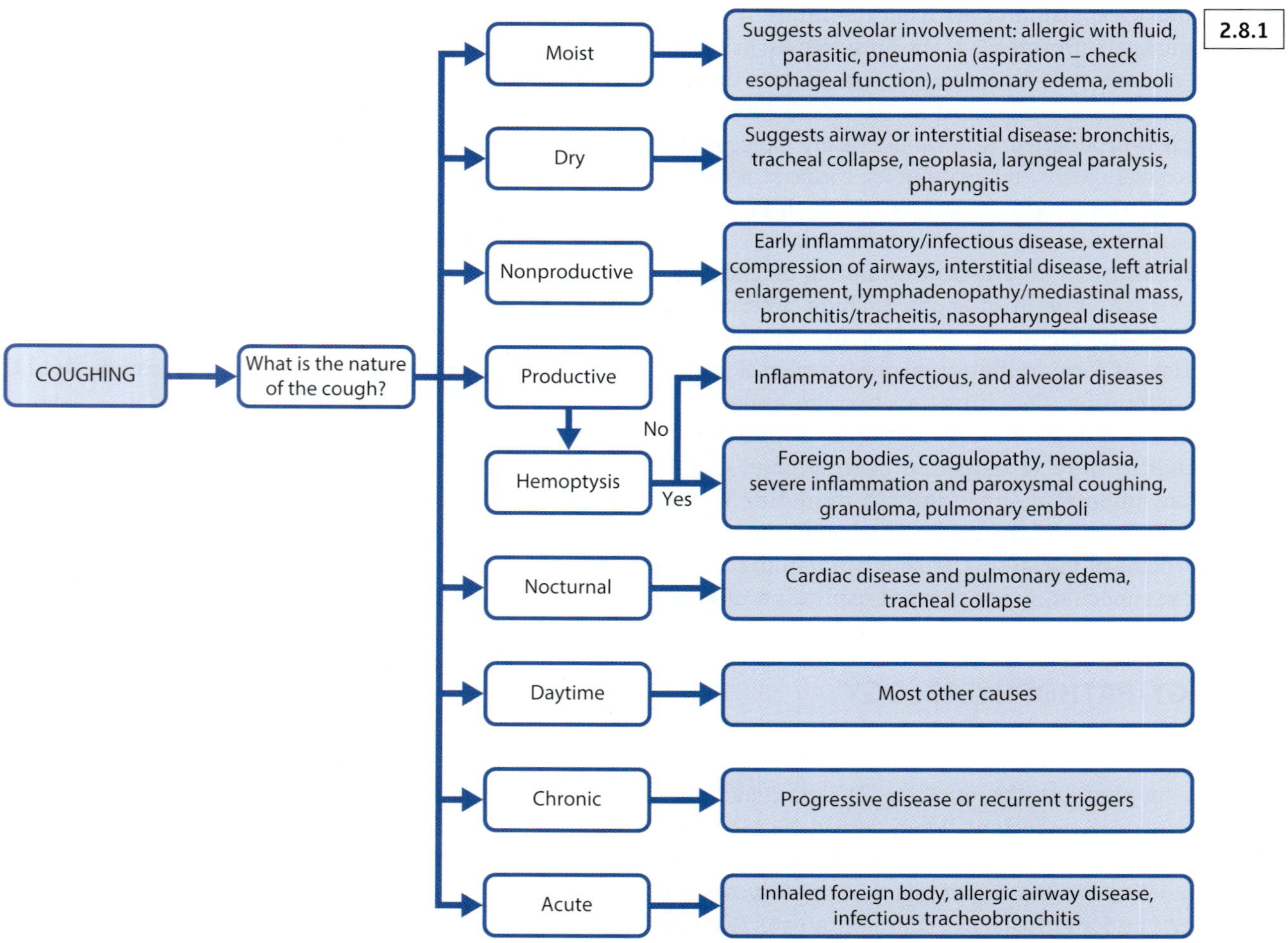

Figure 2.8.1 Diagnostic algorithm for cough.

MANAGEMENT

Treatment of cough is varied depending on the identified underlying cause. The most common cause of chronic cough in dogs is chronic bronchitis, and in cats it is feline lower airway disease/asthma. If possible, specific therapy is more likely to be useful than simple supportive care. If no specifically treatable cause is found, supportive care should be used. Lifestyle changes may help significantly with cough; these include switching to a harness from a collar, avoiding excessive excitement (and accompanying barking), and avoiding indoor air pollutants such as cigarette smoke and perfumes. Additionally, contact with dogs that may have infectious respiratory disease such as kennel cough complex should be avoided.

Many dogs that cough are overweight or obese, and as cough or exercise intolerance may limit activity, further weight gain may occur. Meaningful improvements in cough may occur with weight loss, and a weight loss plan should be prescribed and carefully followed in affected dogs.

Controlling inflammation is helpful in dogs with chronic bronchitis, and is most often achieved through oral or aerosolized glucocorticoids. Glucocorticoids decrease airway inflammation, which subsequently decreases cough. They are usually extremely effective against cough, but may have side-effects such as weight gain, panting, polyphagia, and polydipsia and polyuria, which preclude long-term high dose use. Oral glucocorticoids may be tapered to the lowest dose that controls signs. Inhaled glucocorticoids (e.g. fluticasone) are gaining in popularity for treatment of airway disease, and may be very useful for long-term control.

While chronic bronchitis is not primarily an infectious disease, treatment with antibiotics may be warranted during exacerbations. In people with chronic obstructive pulmonary disease, treatment with macrolides (e.g. azithromycin) reduces hospitalizations. The fluoroquinolones and doxycycline are also useful. In most cases, duration of treatment will range from 1 to 2 weeks, but frequent recurring disease might require repeated antimicrobial treatment.

Cough suppressants are also used for treatment of chronic bronchitis. In general, the cough reflex is essential to help clear secretions or trapped foreign particles. Chronic cough may be very tiring for both the dog and the family. Antitussives may be divided into centrally acting and locally acting substances. Centrally acting drugs act at the cough center in the brain by depressing the sensitivity of the cough centers to the various stimuli. Opioids are effective centrally acting antitussives. They may have additional properties such as sedation or constipation. In some animals, one opioid may be clearly more effective than another. Thus, if significant coughing is still occurring, it may be useful to try another medication or to increase the dose, as tolerance may develop after prolonged usage. It is particularly helpful to give the cough suppressant to the dog before bedtime, to help both the pet owner and the pet sleep through the night.

Centrally acting cough suppressants used in veterinary medicine include codeine, butorphanol, and hydrocodone. Tramadol may be helpful in some dogs, and has the added benefit of being less expensive. Dextromethorphan is available over the counter in many human cough medications, and is occasionally effective in dogs.

Recently, maropitant and gabapentin have been proposed for cough, although clinical trials have not been performed. In people, gabapentin has been effective in chronic cough.

RECOMMENDED FURTHER READING

Bexfield NH, Foale RD, Davison LJ *et al.* (2006) Management of 13 cases of canine respiratory disease using inhaled corticosteroids. *J Small Anim Pract* **47**:377–382.

Boyle TE, Hawkins EC, Davis JL *et al.* (2011) Failure of nebulized irritant, acidic, or hypotonic solutions or external mechanical stimulation of the trachea to consistently induce coughing in healthy, awake dogs. *Can J Vet Res* **75(3)**:228–232.

Ferasin L, Crews L, Biller DS *et al.* (2013) Risk factors for coughing in dogs with naturally acquired myxomatous mitral valve disease. *J Vet Intern Med* **27(2)**:286–292.

Hawkins EC, Clay LD, Bradley JM (2010) Demographic and historical findings, including exposure to environmental tobacco smoke, in dogs with chronic cough. *J Vet Intern Med* **24(4)**:825–831.

Maggiore AD (2014) Tracheal and airway collapse in dogs. *Vet Clin North Am Small Anim Pract* **44(1)**:117–127.

McKiernan BC (2000) Diagnosis and treatment of canine chronic bronchitis. Twenty years of experience. *Vet Clin North Am Small Anim Pract* **30(6)**:1267–1278.

Padrid P (2000) Feline asthma. Diagnosis and treatment. *Vet Clin North Am Small Anim Pract* **30(6)**:1279–1293.

Peeters DE, McKiernan BC, Weisiger RM *et al.* (2000) Quantitative bacterial cultures and cytological examination of bronchoalveolar lavage specimens in dogs. *J Vet Intern Med* **14(5)**:534–541.

Ryan NA, Birring SS, Gibson PG (2012) Gabapentin for refractory chronic cough: a randomized, double-blind, placebo-controlled trial. *Lancet* **380**:1583–1599.

Yamaya Y, Sugiya H, Watari T (2014) Tobacco exposure increased airway limitation in dogs with chronic cough. *Vet Rec* **174(1)**:18.

2.9 Epistaxis

Christine Iacovetta

PATHOPHYSIOLOGY

Epistaxis refers to hemorrhage originating from the nose. The nose itself encompasses the external nasal planum, the paired nasal cavities, and the paranasal sinuses. Turbinate bones covered by mucosa fill a large portion of the nasal cavities, whose main blood supply originates from the maxillary branch of the external carotid artery. The presence of vascular plexuses throughout the mucosa provides a large blood supply that, when damaged, can lead to significant bleeding. Venous blood exits the nose via the dorsal nasal and sphenopalatine veins, eventually emptying into the external jugular vein. Hemorrhage from the nose often occurs due to local destruction by neoplastic, infectious, or inflammatory processes. In some cases, traumatic events or inhalation of foreign material may be the primary cause. Systemic infections or defects in hemostasis are other potential causes of epistaxis. Less commonly, hypertension or hyperviscosity syndromes secondary to polycythemia, hyperlipidemia, hyperglobulinemia, or neoplasia occur (**Tables 2.9.1, 2.9.2**).

CLINICAL PRESENTATION

Epistaxis is readily visible (**Figure 2.9.1**) and often disturbing to owners; therefore, pets usually present with nasal bleeding as a primary complaint. Occasionally, epistaxis can be covert if blood only flows into the nasopharynx and is subsequently swallowed or inhaled. A detailed history is important in determining the possible underlying cause of the epistaxis and in some cases the breed of the patient may also be helpful (e.g. Dobermanns and von Willebrand deficiency) (**Table 2.9.3**). The owner should be questioned as to the presence of any other type of discharge (e.g. purulent), if there is sneezing, hemoptysis, hematemesis, hematuria, or hematochezia present, and if the bleeding is acute or chronic. Sometimes, knowing if the epistaxis is unilateral or bilateral is helpful in distinguishing intranasal versus systemic causes; however,

Table 2.9.1 Causes of epistaxis in the dog and cat.

Intranasal	Extranasal
Mycotic infection Trauma Foreign body Oronasal fistula Nasopharyngeal polyp Dental abscess Lymphoplasmacytic rhinitis Eosinophilic rhinitis Parasites: *Pneumonyssoides caninum* Viral: parainfluenza, adenovirus, distemper	Thrombocytopenia Thrombocytopathia Coagulation factor deficiency Hypertension Hyperviscosity Systemic infection

Table 2.9.2 Systemic infections leading to epistaxis in the dog and cat.

Ehrlichia and *Anaplasma* spp.
Hepatozoonosis
Rocky Mountain spotted fever
Feline leukemia virus
Feline immunodeficiency virus
Leishmaniasis
Leptospirosis
Septicemia
Heartworm disease

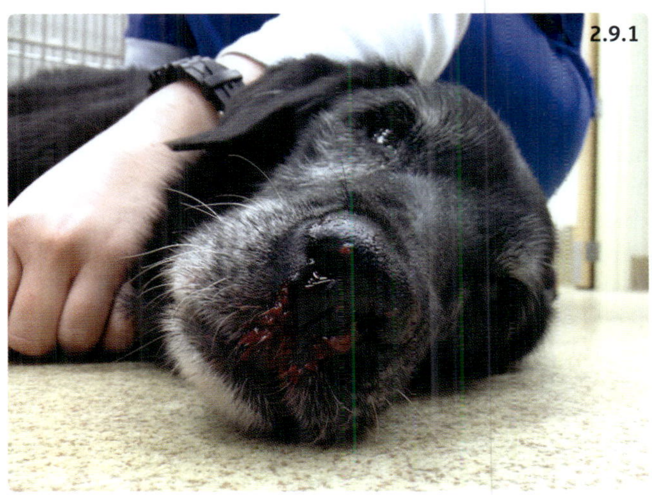

Figure 2.9.1 The bilateral epistaxis in this dog was due to a systemic coagulopathy.

Table 2.9.3 Clinical signs typically associated with intranasal versus extranasal causes of epistaxis in the dog and cat.

Signs associated with intranasal disease	Signs associated with extranasal disease
Unilateral discharge Ocular discharge Decreased ocular retropulsion Rubbing or pawing at face Other types of nasal discharge Violent sneezing Pain Depigmentation of the nose Deformity of the palate	Bilateral discharge Ecchymosis Petechiation Hematuria Hematochezia Systemic signs (e.g. anorexia, vomiting)

this is not always accurate. Obtaining a travel history will help determine exposure to certain infectious diseases. A history of running in tall grass or rooting in the ground with or without pawing at the face may increase suspicion for a foreign body. It is helpful to know if the owner has noticed any changes in cognition or behavior at home. Lastly, the general health of the pet should be considered (e.g. appetite, vomiting) as well as any medications they receive (e.g. tick preventives used, NSAIDs).

DIAGNOSIS

Epistaxis is a clinical sign and not a diagnosis; determination of the underlying etiology requires diagnostic tests. The first step in any diagnostic plan should always be a thorough physical examination. This should begin with visually assessing facial symmetry, palpation of the muzzle, and assessing for ocular retropulsion when evaluating a patient for nasal disease. These steps will help determine if there is pain, deformities of bony structures, and exophthalmos, all of which are suggestive of a highly destructive process. Placing a small piece of cotton in front of each nostril can help determine airflow and the extent of obstruction, as can looking to see if the animal has open-mouth breathing. The oral cavity should be examined, in particular the dental arcade, for any discharge or evidence of periodontal disease, and both the hard and soft palate should be assessed for any structural changes. Neurologic function should be tested as changes can alert the clinician to possible intracranial extension of nasal disease. The patient should also be closely examined for any evidence of bleeding elsewhere, specifically the epidermis, oral mucosa, pinnae, joints, retina, and anterior chamber of the eye. A rectal examination for the assessment of melena is recommended. Completion of a good history and physical examination may or may not give the clinician a suspicion of the underlying cause. In cases of epistaxis, it is usually best to start with a coagulation assessment before doing further diagnostic tests (**Figure 2.9.2**).

MANAGEMENT

As with any patient, the first step in treatment is stabilization. A patient with significant epistaxis may require blood products to replace lost red cells as well as provide clotting factors. Ideally, blood for coagulation testing should be obtained prior to transfusion if time allows. Occasionally, uncontrolled nasal hemorrhage may occur that cannot be managed with transfusions alone. Initially, intranasal applications of vasoconstrictor drugs such as epinephrine or phenylephrine might temporarily decrease the bleeding. If this is unsuccessful, the patient should be anesthetized, endotracheally intubated, and the nasal cavity packed with absorbent material to provide direct pressure (umbilical tape works well for this purpose). Having suction equipment available to visualize the oropharynx for intubation is advised. Nasal packing material is left in place for 30 minutes prior to slowly attempting unpacking. If there is no recurrence of bleeding, anesthesia can be stopped and the patient allowed to wake up in a calm controlled manner.

Treatment of epistaxis is dependent on the underlying cause and in a stable patient begins with discontinuation of any possible contributing medications (e.g. aspirin). Foreign bodies can often be removed nasally at the time of discovery, nasal neoplasia may require surgery and/or radiation, mycotic infections are ideally treated with intranasal antifungal infusions, polyps may be removed with traction, and rhinitis is treated medically to reduce the inflammatory response. Most trauma cases can just be monitored and treated supportively. Systemic infections should be treated accordingly, hypertension managed, and any coagulation disorders addressed. Uncontrolled recurrent nasal bleeding can be managed by carotid artery ligation or, in some cases, local vascular embolization as salvage procedures. More specific therapies can be found in the relevant chapter in this book (Chapter 4, Respiratory disorders).

RECOMMENDED FURTHER READING

Bissett SA, Drobatz KJ, McKnight A *et al.* (2007) Prevalence, clinical features, and causes of epistaxis in dogs: 176 cases. *J Am Vet Med Assoc* **231(12)**:1843–1850.

Weisse C, Nicholson ME, Rollings C *et.al.* (2004) Use of percutaneous arterial embolization for the treatment of intractable epistaxis in three dogs. *J Am Vet Med Assoc* **224(8)**:1307–1311.

2.9.2

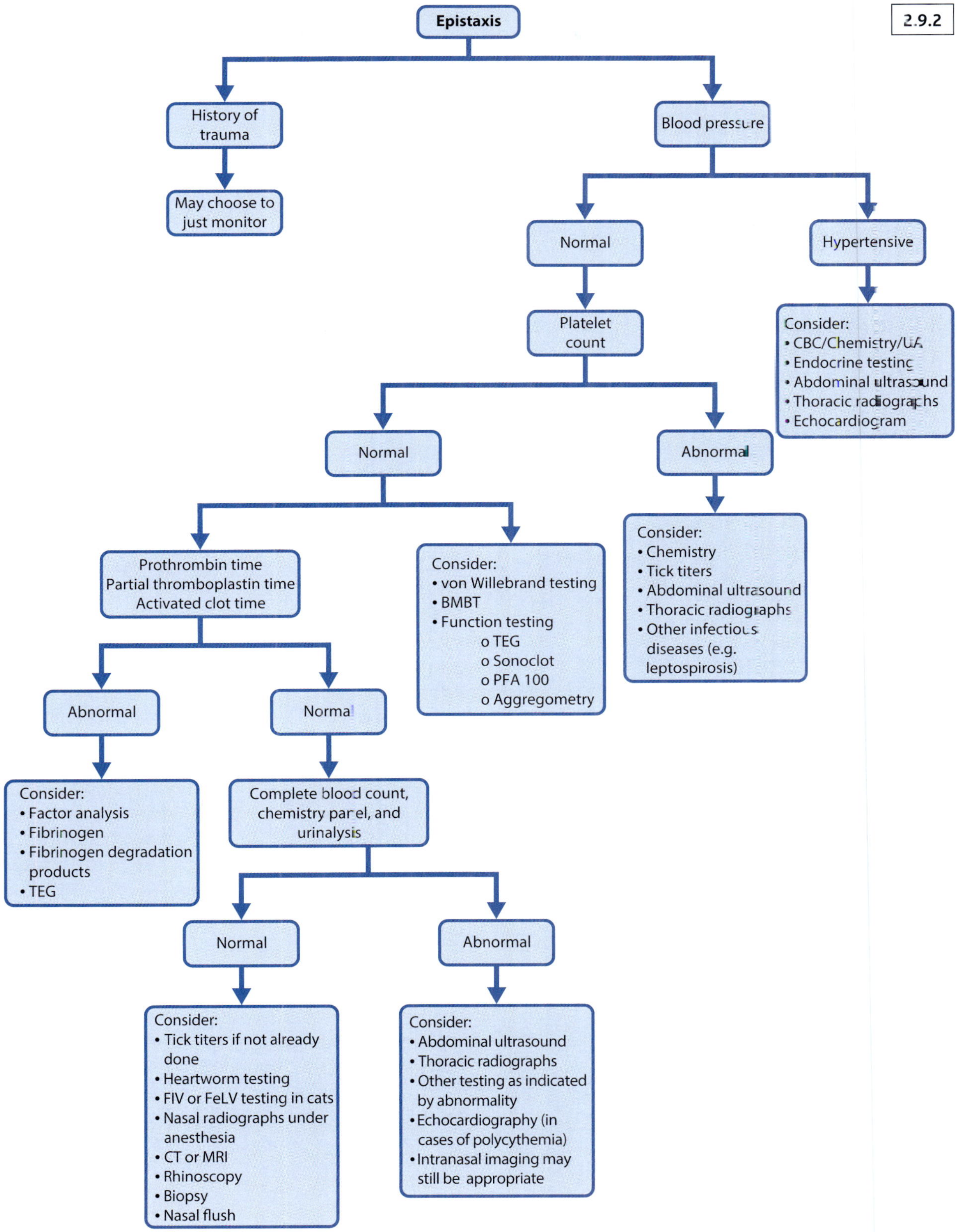

Figure 2.9.2 Diagnostic algorithm for epistaxis. BMBT, buccal mucosal bleed time; UA, urinalysis; CBC, complete blood count; TEG, thromboelastography; PFA 100, platelet function analyzer 100.

Chapter 2 Common clinical problems

2.10 Fever of unknown origin

Robert Armentano

INTRODUCTION

The classic definition of 'fever of unknown origin' (FUO) provided for humans by Beeson and Petersdorf involves an illness of at least 3 weeks' duration, fever (continuous or fluctuating temperature of >104°F [40°C]), and no established diagnosis after at least 1 week of hospital investigation. There is no accepted definition of this term in veterinary medicine, except that the term FUO is used to define any febrile animal patient for which there is no obvious cause after 'routine' diagnostic tests have been done. What constitutes 'routine' will vary amongst different authors. The main diagnostic categories for FUO include infections (local, systemic), neoplasms, and immune-mediated diseases. Other less common causes include: granulomatous diseases; noninfectious, inflammatory diseases such as pancreatitis, steatitis, and tissue necrosis (ischemic insults); and drugs. It is only after a search for the above causes that the clinician is left with the diagnosis of FUO. Generally, the etiology of FUO is not a rare disease but is rather a common disease presenting in an atypical fashion.

PATHOPHYSIOLOGY

Normal body temperature is regulated within a fairly narrow range and is a balance between heat producing and heat dissipating mechanisms of the body. Fever is an increase of body temperature above the circadian variation as the result of a change in the thermoregulatory center located in the hypothalamus. Substances that cause fever are called pyrogens and may be either exogenous or endogenous. The majority of exogenous pyrogens are microorganisms, their products, or toxins. Endotoxin (lipopolysaccharide) is the best characterized exogenous pyrogen, derived from the cell wall of gram-negative and gram-positive bacteria. Exogenous pyrogens can act directly on the brain to cause fever, but they act primarily by inducing the formation of endogenous products. These endogenous pyrogen-producing substances include antigen–antibody complexes with complement, complement cleavage products, steroid hormone metabolites, bile acids, and some cytokines.

The term 'cytokine' is used to describe the endogenous pyrogens that consist of several interleukins (IL), cell-derived inflammatory polypeptides, and growth promoting peptides. The major pyrogenic cytokines include IL-1β, IL-1α, tumor necrosis factor (TNF)-α, TNF-β, interferon α and IL-6. These cytokines circulate to the anterior hypothalamus where prostaglandin E2 and other arachidonic acid metabolites are produced. These in turn induce the formation of secondary messengers such as cyclic adenosine monophosphate, which cause the rise in the thermoregulating set point leading to increased heat conservation, heat production, and fever.

ETIOLOGY

The true incidence of FUO is unknown. A study by Feldman noted the cause of FUO in dogs to be 40% infectious, 20% neoplastic, 20% immune-mediated disease, 10% miscellaneous disease, and 10% true FUO. A true FUO is diagnosed as a fever in which the underlying etiology is never determined and that either spontaneously resolves or responds to a combination of antibiotics and/or steroids.

There are few retrospective papers documenting FUO in dogs (**Table 2.10.1**). There are no large published studies in cats but, anecdotally, infectious etiologies are much more common than neoplastic and immune-mediated diseases. The conclusions from three recent retrospective reviews in dogs were that immune-mediated was the most commonly diagnosed category of disease, with immune-mediated polyarthritis as well as steroid-responsive meningitis–arteritis being the most common diagnoses (**Tables 2.10.1, 2.10.2**). These studies also concluded that imaging (radiographs and ultrasound) and cytology had the highest diagnostic yield.

In a recent paper describing the causes of FUO in humans, the distribution of the causes was infectious 16%, neoplasia 7%, noninfectious inflammatory disease 22%, miscellaneous 4%, and no diagnosis 51%.

Table 2.10.1 Review of diagnoses in dogs with fever of unknown origin (FUO) (prevalence).

Retrospective study			
Disease category	Dunn and Dunn (1998)	Battersby *et al.* (2006)	Chervier *et al.* (2012)
Immune mediated	22%	34.8%	48%
Bone marrow	22%	NA	NA
Infectious	16%	5.8%	18%
Neoplasia	9.5%	7.6%	6%
Miscellaneous	11.5%	9.1%	0%
True FUO	19%	22.7%	28%

Dunn KJ, Dunn JK (1998) Diagnostic investigation in 101 dogs with pyrexia of unknown origin. *J Small Anim Pract* **39(1)**:574–580.
Battersby IA, Murphy KF, Tasker S *et al.* (2006) Retrospective study of fever in dogs: laboratory testing, diagnoses and influence of prior treatment. *J Small Anim Pract* **47(7)**:370–376.
Chervier C, Chabanne L, Godde M *et al.* (2012) Causes, diagnostic signs, and the utility of investigations of fever in dogs: 50 cases. *Can Vet J* **53(5)**:525–530.

Table 2.10.2 Common differential diagnoses (not all inclusive) and common tests available.

Category	Disease	Dog	Cat	Tests available
Infectious disease				
Bacterial				
Systemic	Infectious endocarditis	X		Echocardiogram, blood cultures
	Meningitis	X	X	Cerebrospinal fluid tap for cytology, cultures
	Bacteremia	X	X	CBC, blood culture
Localized	Pyelonephritis	X	X	Urine culture, AUS, pyelocentesis
	Cholangitis/ cholecystitis	X	X	Serum liver enzymes, ultrasound, cholecystocentesis, liver biopsy
	Pyothorax	X	X	TXR, thoracentesis, culture
	Peritonitis	X	X	AUS, abdominocentesis, culture, glucose/lactate blood:fluid comparison
	Discospondylitis	X	X	Radiographs, CT/MRI, FNA
	Infectious arthritis	X	X	Joint tap for cytology and culture
Specific	Leptospirosis	X		MAT serology, urine PCR
	Borreliosis	X		4DX, C6 antibody
	Brucellosis	X		Serology
	Mycobacteriosis	X	X	Culture, PCR
	Bartonellosis	X	X	Serology, PCR, BAPGM culture/PCR

(*Continued*)

Category	Disease	Dog	Cat	Tests available
	Plague		X	Serology, cytology, IFA
	Mycoplasmosis	X	X	Culture, PCR
Viral	Feline leukemia		X	Serology(antigen), IFA
	Feline infectious peritonitis		X	Histopathology, IFA of macrophages, cytology, Rivalta test
	Feline immunodeficiency virus		X	Serology (antibody)
	Calicivirus		X	PCR
	Distemper	X		IFA, serology
Vector-borne	Ehrlichiosis	X	X	Serology, PCR, blood smear
	Anaplasmosis	X		Serology, PCR
	Rocky Mountain spotted fever	X		Serology, PCR
	Hemotropic mycoplasmosis	X	X	PCR, blood smear
Fungal	Blastomycosis	X	X	Urine antigen, cytology/histopathology
	Cryptococcosis	X	X	Serology (latex agglutination)
	Coccidioidomycosis	X	X	Serology
	Histoplasmosis	X	X	Urine antigen, cytology/histopathology
	Aspergillosis (other)	X		Cytology/histopathology, fungal culture, PCR, galactomannan serology
Protozoal	Toxoplasmosis	X	X	Serology (IgG/IgM), histopathology
	Neosporosis	X		Serology, histopathology, PCR
	Hepatozoonosis	X	X	PCR, histopathology
	Babesiosis	X	X	PCR
	Leishmaniasis	X	X	Serology, cytology, PCR
Immune/ inflammatory				
Immune mediated	Systemic lupus erythematosus	X		Cytology/histopathology, ANA
	Immune-mediated polyarthritis	X	X	Cytology, rheumatoid factor
	Steroid-responsive meningitis	X		CSF cytology
	Vasculitis	X	X	Histopathology
	Immune-mediated neutropenia	X		CBC, bone marrow cytology/histopathology

(Continued)

Table 2.10.2 Common differential diagnoses (not all inclusive) and common tests available. (*Continued*)

Category	Disease	Dog	Cat	Tests available
Inflammatory	Nodular panniculitis	X	X	Histopathology
	Lymphadenitis	X	X	Histopathology
	Steatitis	X		Histopathology
	Pancreatitis	X	X	AUS, PLI, histopathology
	Granulomatous	X	X	Cytology, histopathology
	Hypereosinophilic	X	X	Histopathology, CBC
Neoplasia				
Solid tumors	Any, hepatic, GI, pulmonary	X	X	TXR, AXR, AUS, cytology, histopathology
Hematopoietic	Lymphoma	X	X	TXR, AXR, AUS, cytology, histopathology, PARR, flow cytometry
	Leukemia	X	X	CBC, bone marrow cytology, flow cytometry
	Myeloma	X	X	Globulin, radiographs, Bence-Jones proteinuria, bone marrow cytology
	Malignant histiocytosis	X	X	Histopathology
Miscellaneous	Portosystemic shunt	X	X	Chemistry, bile acids, AUS, abdominal CT, nuclear scintigraphy
	Drug reaction	X	X	Eliminate medications
	Amyloidosis	X	X	Histopathology

TXR, thoracic radiography; AXR, abdominal radiography; AUS, abdominal ultrasound; MAT, microscopic agglutination test; FNA, fine-needle aspiration; BAPGM, Bartonella alpha Proteobacteria Gowth Medium; IFA, immunofluorescent antibody; PARR; PCR for antigenic rearrangement; ANA, antinuclear antibody; PLI, pancreatic lipase immunoreactivity.

The paper compared the causes in 2013 with those listed in 1961, which was infectious 36%, neoplastic 19%, noninfectious inflammatory 17%, miscellaneous 19%, no diagnosis 9%.

Infections should always be considered first in the search for the etiology of FUO because of their frequency and potential response to treatment. It is helpful to categorize infections as either localized or systemic in order to allow for an eventual well-focused approach to the patient's problem. In the cat, viral agents such as parvovirus, herpesvirus, or calicivirus usually cause fairly classical clinical signs and rarely persist long enough to fit the definition of true FUO. Feline infectious peritonitis coronavirus infection is a common cause of FUO because it produces insidious, chronic illness and frequently defies easy diagnosis. Fever is often associated with retroviral infections (FeLV, FIV) as a direct result of the virus infection, but more often due to an opportunistic infection occurring secondary to the immunosuppressive effects of the viral disease.

For bacterial and fungal infections in the dog and cat that are easy to recognize, treatment success will vary according to a whole host of factors such as age, underlying organ dysfunction, immune status, and type of organism. Localized bacterial infections in an occult location (e.g. metritis, low-grade pleuritis, osteomyelitis, tooth root abscess) or those caused by fastidious organisms that are not sensitive to treatment with commonly prescribed antimicrobial agents (e.g. *Mycobacterium*, *Nocardia*, *Mycoplasma*, L-form bacteria) are the most likely to cause persistent fever in the infectious category. Systemic mycotic diseases (e.g. histoplasmosis, blastomycosis, coccidioidomycosis) cause fever unresponsive to antibiotics and should be included in the differential list for patients residing in or having traveled through regions endemic for these agents. *Cryptococcus neoformans* rarely produces a febrile response unless infection is generalized or involves the CNS. Infections with *Mycoplasma haemofelis* (*Haemobartonella felis*), *Toxoplasma gondii*, aberrant helminth migration, and pulmonary embolization by *Dirofilaria immitis* may also cause fever.

The urinary and pulmonary systems must be thoroughly assessed in any patient with a fever that cannot be localized on physical examination, and this especially applies to acquired infections in patients that are hospitalized for more than 7 days. All too often, these are the sites of origin for disseminated infection. Other disorders, such as infective endocarditis and localized abdominal abscesses, might be difficult to diagnose without the aid provided by imaging techniques such as ultrasound, CT, and MRI. Only after the site of the infection is localized can a definitive therapeutic plan be devised.

Neoplasia is a fairly common cause of fever. FeLV-related cancers (e.g. lymphoma, myeloproliferative disease) in cats are the most common cause of fever in this particular disease class. The fever can be a paraneoplastic syndrome associated with the tumor itself, or it can be due to secondary complications from the cancer such as infections occurring as a result of myelophthisic disease. Solid tumors such as pulmonary adenocarcinoma can also cause fever as the result of the host's immune response to the tumor, damage to adjacent tissue from the expanding tumor mass, or because of avascular tumor necrosis.

As mentioned earlier, noninfectious inflammatory diseases, including immune-mediated diseases, are not so rare. Some immunologic diseases, such as IMHA, the pemphigus family of dermatoses, and systemic lupus erythematosus, can be readily identified. Others such as the polyarthropathies, sterile meningitis, and polymyositis are other examples of immune-mediated inflammatory disease.

There are many other causes of noninfectious inflammatory fevers. In the dog and cat these include noninfectious inflammatory diseases such as cholangiohepatitis, inflammatory bowel disease, pancreatitis, and pansteatitis. Drug-associated fever is most common with tetracycline but has also been reported with sulfonamides, penicillins, quinidine, novobiocin, nitrofurantoin, amphotericin B, barbiturates, iodine, propylthiouracil, atropine, cimetidine, salicylates, prednisone, antihistamines, and procainamide. Metabolic and endocrine diseases, including hyperthyroidism, pheochromocytoma, hyperlipemia, and hypernatremia, and primary neurologic diseases causing CNS inflammation or impinging on the hypothalamic thermoregulatory center may occasionally cause fever. This information is summarized in **Table 2.10.2**.

DIAGNOSIS

The key to obtaining a diagnosis includes a systematic approach for the work up of FUO in both dogs and cats. The most important steps prior to implementing a diagnostic plan include a thorough history and physical examination. The physical examination should include orthopedic, neurologic, funduscopic (**Figure 2.10.1**), and rectal examinations. A staged diagnostic approach should be implemented in patients with vague clinical signs and no definitive lesion identified (**Table 2.10.3**).

Stage one testing includes the history and physical examination as well as screening laboratory testing. Routine tests should include a serum chemistry panel, CBC with pathologist review, and a complete urinalysis. Screening infectious disease testing such as a 4DX in dogs (heartworm, Lyme, *Anaplasma*, and *Erhlichia* ELISA Snap test) and FeLV/FIV testing in cats should also be done. Evaluation of blood cells microscopically may assist in the diagnosis of hemoparasites, as well as a review of white cells for cytotoxicity. If the physical examination findings indicate a body cavity lesion, such as lung crackles, or long bone pain, radiographs should be included in stage one testing. Occasionally, there is enough diagnostic

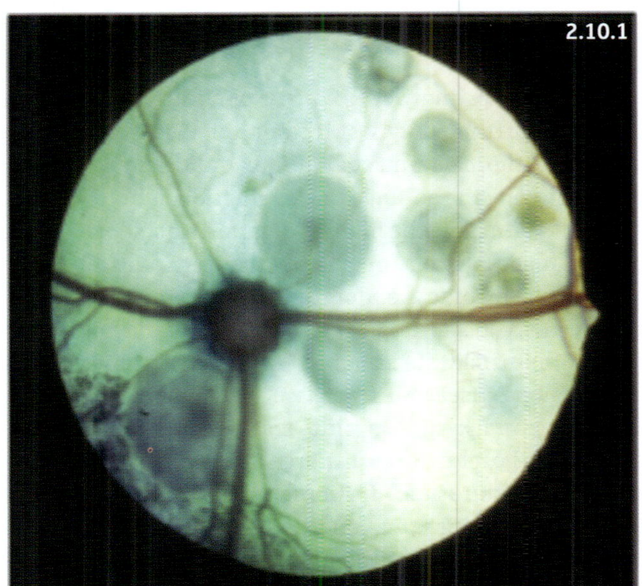

Figure 2.10.1 Fundic examination lesion in a cat with *Cryptococcus* spp. infection. (Courtesy M. Schaer)

Table 2.10.3 Systematic diagnostic approach for fever of unknown origin.

Stage	Recommended testing
1	History, physical examination Screening blood testing CBC, chemistry, urinalysis Infectious disease screening: • '4DX' (heartworm, Lyme, *Anaplasma*, *Ehrlichia*) • FeLV/FIV +/- Thoracic radiographs +/- Abdominal ultrasound
2	Chest, abdominal, skeletal radiographs Tissue/fluid cultures (urine, blood) Urine, blood Urine protein:creatinine Serum bile acids Infectious disease testing Vector-borne disease serology/PCR +/- Immune testing (ANA, RF) Abdominal ultrasound +/- Echocardiography
3	Arthrocentesis Bone marrow cytology/biopsy Advanced imaging (e.g. CT, MRI) Cerebrospinal fluid analysis Bronchoscopy Laparoscopy Thoracoscopy Exploratory laparotomy

information from stage one to start treatment as indicated below.

Stage two testing would consist of additional imaging tests and further diagnostic sampling. Imaging should consist of thoracic and abdominal radiography if they were not done in the stage one evaluation. Cytology samples will often have the highest diagnostic yield if a lesion is identified. Further diagnostic imaging is also helpful and often includes abdominal ultrasonography and, potentially, echocardiography, particularly if a new heart murmur is auscultated.

Infectious disease testing is a key component to the diagnostic work up. Specific tests should be selected based on the clinician's differential diagnoses, patient signalment, duration of clinical signs, and geographic locale. Bacterial culture and sensitivity testing should be done on urine, specific abnormal tissues, and blood if sepsis is suspected. Blood cultures, if indicated, should be performed early in the diagnostic phase since it often takes days for results to become available (**Figure 2.10.2**).

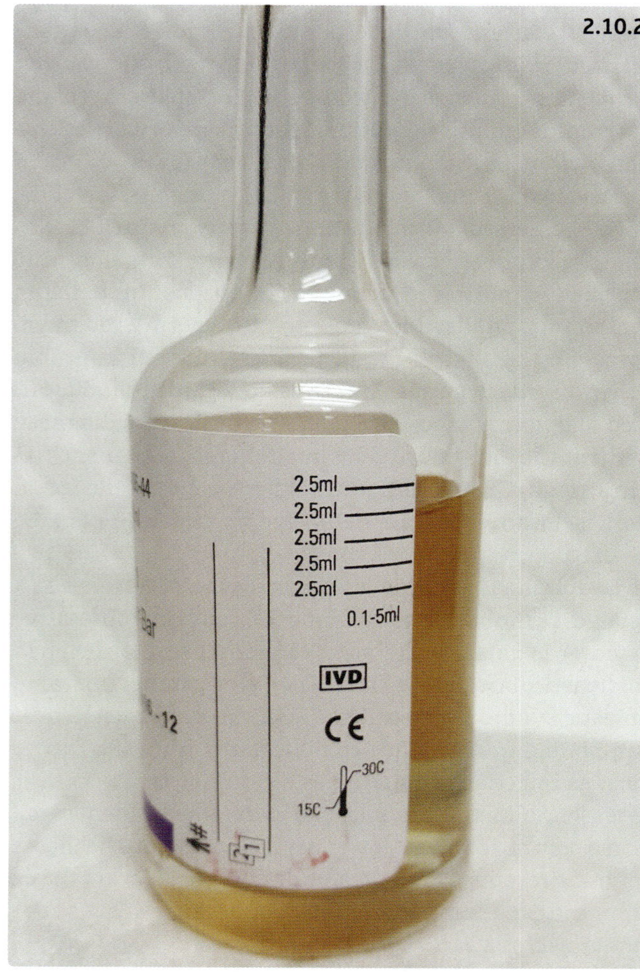

Figure 2.10.2 Blood culture vials. To maximize culture utility, a large sample volume is recommended (16–20 ml in large dogs, 5 ml in small dogs and cats), as well as using vials with antibiotic binding beads and aerobic and anaerobic culture media. Sterile collection is required, ideally at 2–3 venous (+/- one arterial) sites.

Stage three diagnostic testing includes advanced imaging or more invasive tissue sampling techniques. Testing is chosen based on prior test results and physical examination findings or to begin searching for more unusual causes of FUO. These tests include arthrocentesis, echocardiography, and bone marrow analysis even if a lesion is not identified (no apparent murmur, normal CBC, no joint effusion), as diseases in these locations can remain sequestered and asymptomatic early in the disease process.

MANAGEMENT

Medications used for empiric treatment of the febrile patient often include antibiotics and/or antipyretics. Broad-spectrum antimicrobials are targeted against a multitude of different bacterial agents or, more specifically, toward vector-borne disease. Doxycycline or azithromycin are often used in cases of the latter etiology. Antipyretics should not be used in the acute phase of disease unless temperatures exceed 106°F (41.1°C). Anti-inflammatory medications will often mask the underlying disease and can compromise the patient. NSAID side-effects such as GI ulceration, as well as hepatic and renal damage, must be considered when prescribing these medications in debilitated and dehydrated patients. If the patient's body temperature exceeds 106°F (41.1°C), IV fluid therapy should be administered. NSAID therapy may be considered if the risks of adverse reactions are minimal. External cooling, such as fans, is not recommended, as this will only combat the thermoregulatory mechanisms, causing compensatory shivering to maintain the hypothalamic set point. Depending on the status of the patient, it is often appropriate to forgo an empiric medication trial and pursue staged diagnostic testing as noted in order to identify the underlying etiology. Steroids, and other immunosuppressive medications, are frequently used but only if an autoimmune disease is diagnosed and/or infectious disease has been deemed highly unlikely. The prognosis for FUO is dependent on the underlying etiology and the ability to implement an early and appropriate treatment plan.

RECOMMENDED FURTHER READING

Flood J (2009) The diagnostic approach to fever of unknown origin in dogs. *Compend Contin Educ Vet* **31(1)**:14–20.

Horowitz HW (2013) Fever of unknown origin or fever of too many origins. *N Eng J Med* **368**:197–199.

Lunn KF (2012) Fever. In: *Infectious Diseases of the Dog and Cat*, 4th edn. (ed. CE Green) Elsevier, St. Louis, pp. 1115–1123.

Miller JB (2010) Hyperthermia and fever of unknown origin. In: *Textbook of Veterinary Internal Medicine*, 7th edn. (eds. SJ Ettinger, EC Feldman) Elsevier, St. Louis, pp. 41–45.

Chapter 2 Common clinical problems

2.11 Dysuria

Isabelle Cattin

INTRODUCTION

Dysuria is defined as difficulty urinating. It is often combined with pain during urination, although this is not always the case. Other urination abnormalities can be seen with dysuria, such as pollakiuria (frequent urination), stranguria (extreme difficulty in passing urine [**Figure 2.11.1**]), and the presence of hematuria (blood in the urine [**Figure 2.11.2**]). Dogs and cats with dysuria are at risk for developing potentially life-threatening complications associated with urinary obstruction and inability to urinate. Therefore, a thorough and timely evaluation of the patient is essential.

EVALUATION OF THE PATIENT WITH DYSURIA

The initial evaluation of a dog or cat presented with dysuria should include signalment, a thorough history, and a physical examination (**Figure 2.11.3**). A detailed signalment can be helpful as some conditions associated with dysuria might be seen more readily at a certain age or in specific breeds. For example, cystitis occurs commonly in both adult and young animals, whereas a neoplastic process will be higher on the list of differential diagnoses in a geriatric patient. A complete history should be taken, including duration of clinical signs and general health of the patient, and description of the urination pattern including appearance of the urine. Pigmenturia such as bilirubinuria or hemoglobinuria will signal other disorders elsewhere in the body and the pattern of urination can help localize a urinary tract disorder, where stranguria reflects pathology involving the lower urinary tract. Drugs and concurrent diseases that could potentially make the animal more susceptible to urinary disorders should be ruled out. The evaluation of the urination pattern includes voiding frequency and urine volume, ability to pass urine (normal stream versus dripping), pain, urination in inappropriate places, as

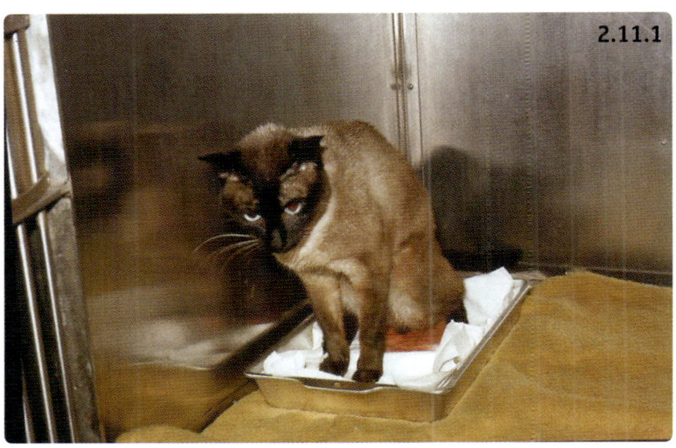

Figures 2.11.1 Cat with stranguria and hematuria associated with urethral obstruction and cystitis. (Courtesy M. Schaer).

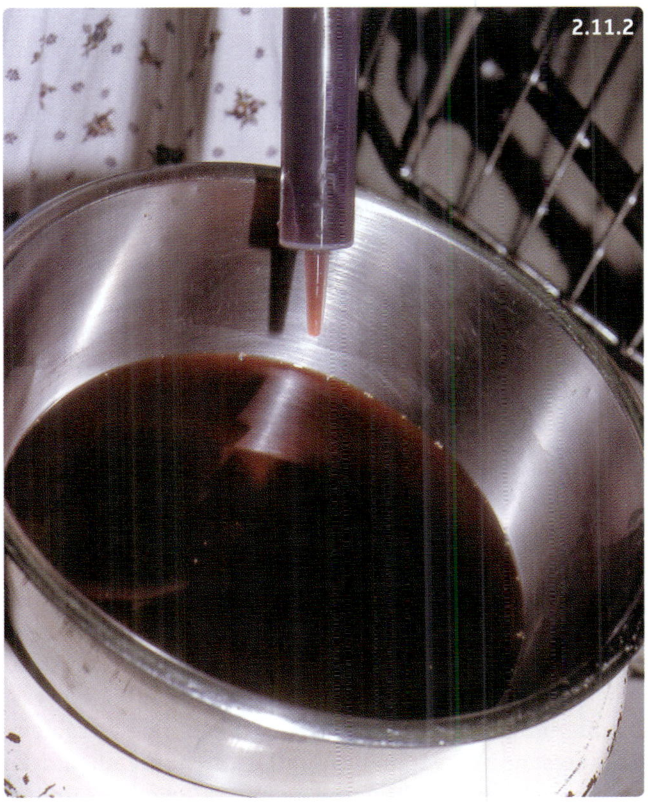

Figure 2.11.2 Hematuria in a sample taken from a dog with an atonic bladder and secondary *E. coli* cystitis. (Courtesy M. Schaer)

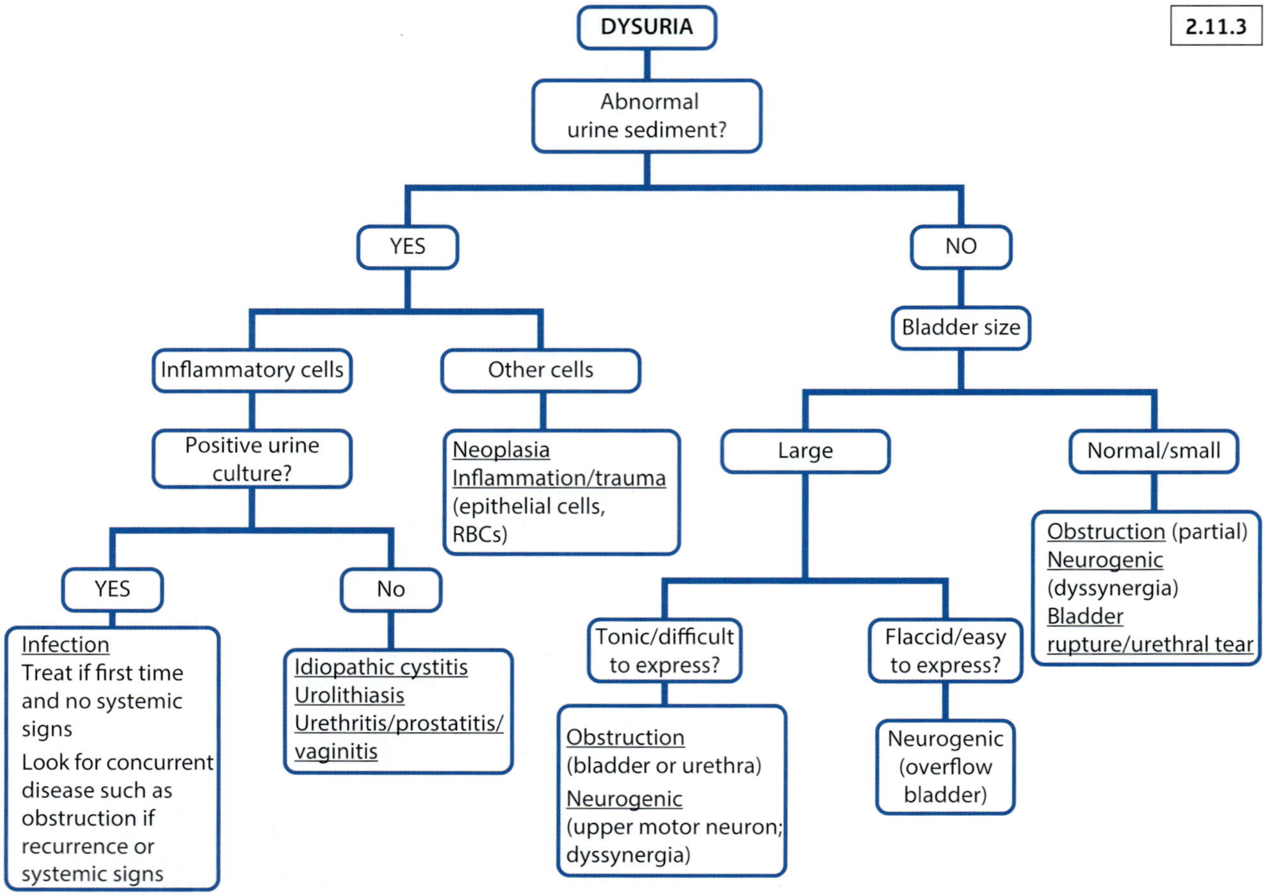

Figure 2.11.3 Algorithm for the clinical approach to dysuric dogs and cats.

well as passing discolored/bloody urine. The presence of systemic signs should also be assessed, as they may reveal the existence of an underlying disease that needs to be addressed and the need for urgent care. While discussing clinical signs, care should be taken to differentiate dyschezia and tenesmus from straining to urinate, especially with feline patients, in order to avoid misdiagnosing a urinary obstruction. Physical examination should encompass a routine examination and temperature taking. The clinician should then especially focus on palpation of the urinary bladder to assess the following aspects: size, shape, and tonicity of the bladder wall. These simple elements will be very helpful in the initial assessment of the ongoing process. For example, a large, tonic, painful bladder in a cat suggests acute urethral blockage, whereas a large, flaccid (and easy to express) bladder might rather point toward a neurologic problem. The presence of vaginal/preputial discharge should be assessed as well. An attempt to pass a urinary catheter with caution in male dogs can help confirm the presence and severity of a urethral obstruction.

ETIOLOGY

Causes of dysuria can be divided into several categories: inflammatory/infectious, obstructive, neurogenic, and traumatic. The first two are the most prevalent in dogs and cats. These categories can be further separated into various conditions, which are discussed below.

Inflammatory/infectious causes

Bacterial or, less commonly, fungal urinary tract infections can be seen in both cats and dogs and will commonly result in dysuria and pollakiuria. Urinalysis and a urine culture are necessary to confirm the presence of infection and select an appropriate treatment. In intact male dogs, prostatic infections (prostatitis, prostatic abscess) should be ruled out. In less common instances, congenital malformations (e.g. remnant urachus) can be the cause for recurrent/persistent urinary infections. While inflammation is frequently found in correlation with an ongoing infectious process, noninfectious, inflammatory conditions can occur in various locations of the urinary or genital tract, and result in dysuria. Cystitis, urethritis, and vaginitis can occur without a concurrent infectious cause. 'Idiopathic' (or interstitial) cystitis is a very common disease in cats, and has a multi-factorial origin. Behavioral issues play an important role in the etiology of feline idiopathic cystitis, and a thorough history should be collected from all cases with suggestive clinical signs. Inflammatory (granulomatous) urethritis is a proliferative disease seen mostly in female dogs.

Obstructive causes

Obstructive processes in any area of the lower urinary tract can result in dysuria, stranguria, or even inability to pass any urine. Intraluminal obstructions can be caused by urolithiasis, urethral blood/mucus plugs, urethral strictures, or neoplastic processes. While dysuria can result from discomfort associated with bladder wall inflammation secondary to urinary bladder stones, urethral obstruction should always be ruled out because it requires immediate care. In cats, blood clots or mucus plugs are a frequent cause of urethral obstruction (**Figure 2.11.4**). Urethral strictures can occur with severe urethritis or secondary to local trauma such as occurs with urethral stones, traumatic catheterization, or urethral surgery. Neoplastic processes in the urinary bladder or the urethra can cause dysuria secondary to inflammation or be due to partial or complete obstruction. This should be considered especially in older animals, but can occur at any age. Extraluminal obstructions of the urethra can commonly be seen with prostatomegaly in conditions such as prostatitis, prostatic abscess (**Figures 2.11.5a, b**), prostatic cyst, or prostatic neoplasia. Benign prostatic hyperplasia rarely causes urinary outflow obstruction in dogs and cats because of anatomic differences and the failure of hyperplastic tissue to invade the urethra. Extraurinary masses impinging on the urinary tract are less common causes of extraluminal obstruction.

Neurogenic causes

Upper or lower motor neuron diseases can cause either a loss of ability to contract the bladder or an increased spasticity of the external urethral sphincter, both resulting in difficulty urinating. A full neurologic examination and palpation of the urinary bladder are important steps in evaluating neurologic causes of dysuria. Increased urethral sphincter tone can cause a dynamic obstruction with inability to pass urine, while a decreased bladder tone can result in pollakiuria or even incontinence ('overflow bladder'). In animals experiencing prolonged difficulty in emptying the bladder secondary to urethral obstruction, neurogenic dysuria can occur as a result of

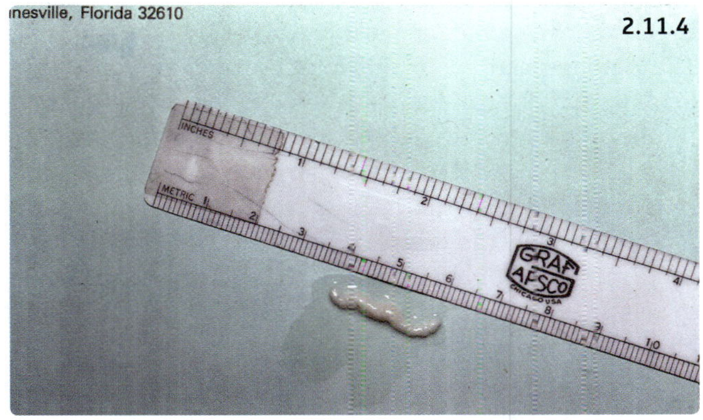

Figure 2.11.4 A large mucocrystalline plug digitally removed from a male cat with urethral obstruction. (Courtesy M. Schaer)

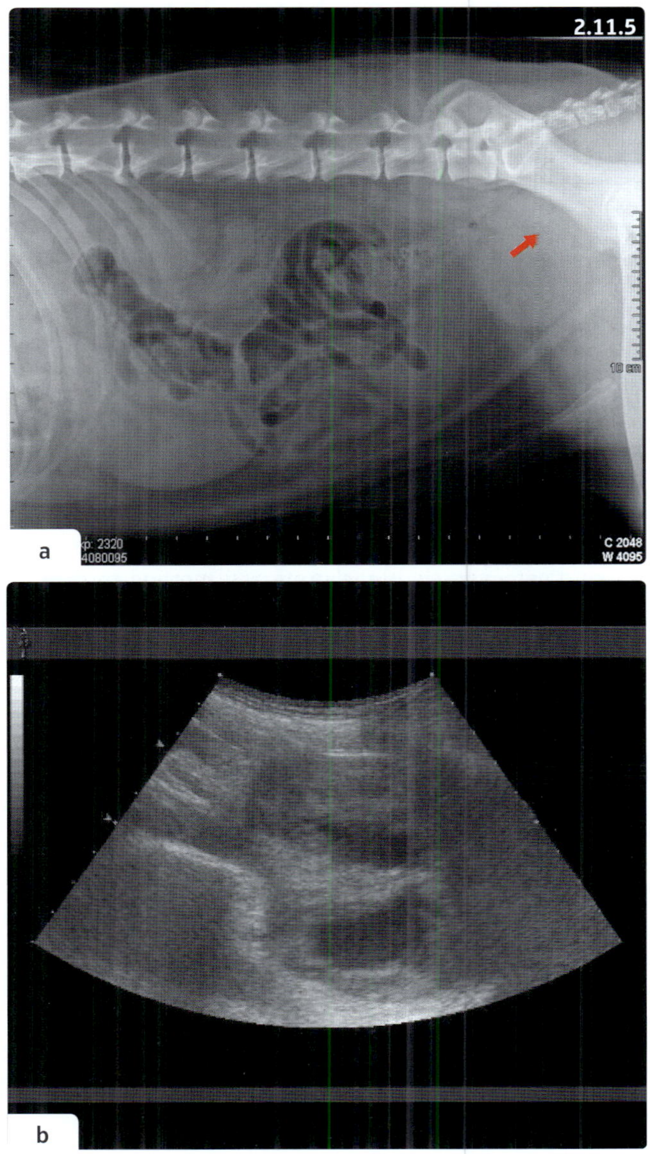

Figures 2.11.5a, b A lateral radiograph (a) and an ultrasound image (b) of a dog with a prostatic abscess. (Courtesy M. Schaer)

the chronically distended urinary bladder (**Figure 2.11.6**). The damage caused to the muscles and nerves of the urinary bladder can be irreversible if the problem is not promptly recognized and the obstruction not relieved in a timely manner. Reflex dyssynergia is a condition seen in large breed dogs that results from inadequate coordination between the detrusor muscle in the bladder and urethral sphincter musculature. The urethral muscle fails to relax when the bladder contracts, thus impairing the ability to urinate.

Traumatic causes

Tears or rupture of the urinary bladder or urethra may occur following trauma and lead to dysuria. Causes include road traffic accidents, gunshots, blunt abdominal trauma, iatrogenic rupture by palpation or instrumentation (**Figure 2.11.7**), or urinary calculi (**Figure 2.11.8**).

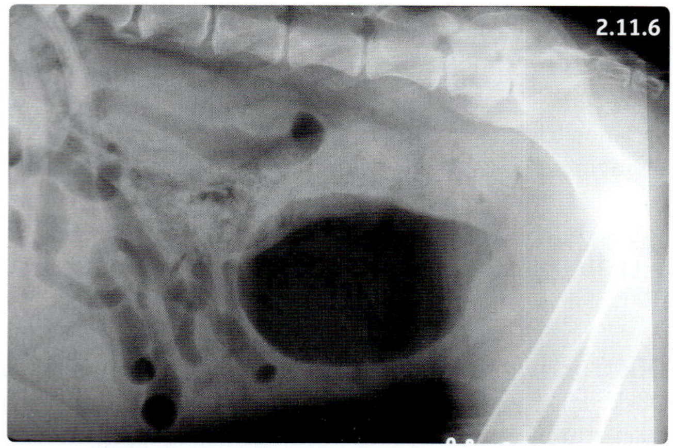

Figure 2.11.6 This plain radiograph shows emphysematous cystitis in a dog with an atonic urinary bladder from a lumbosacral intervertebral stenosis. Note the similarity to a pneumocystogram, but no such procedure was done in this patient. (Courtesy M. Schaer)

FURTHER INVESTIGATIONS

Diagnostic tests are generally necessary to make a precise diagnosis. Laboratory tests and diagnostic imaging can be very helpful in patients with dysuria. However, some more specialized methods, such as endoscopy or cystometry/urethral pressure profile, might be of benefit in specific cases, thus requiring referral to a specialist.

Laboratory testing

Urinalysis and urine culture are helpful to rule out urinary tract infections or inflammation. Urinalysis should include urine SG and cytologic analysis of the urine sediment. Cystocentesis is the preferred method to sample urine for culture and sensitivity. Catheter samples are adequate as well. Voided samples may be contaminated by cells and bacteria from the lower genital tract (vagina, prepuce). Sediment analysis may reveal the presence of red and/or white blood cells, crystals, infectious organisms, parasite ova (*Capillaria* [*Pearsonema*] spp., *Schistosoma* spp.), and neoplastic cells (**Figure 2.11.9**). It is helpful to remember that the absence of crystals does not rule out the presence of uroliths and that the presence of crystals does not imply the presence of calculi. Additionally, different types of uroliths and urinary crystals can be present together in the urinary tract.

A urine culture should be performed to document an infection and assist in the choice of appropriate antibiotic treatment. The urine sediment of immunosuppressed animals may not show any signs of inflammation,

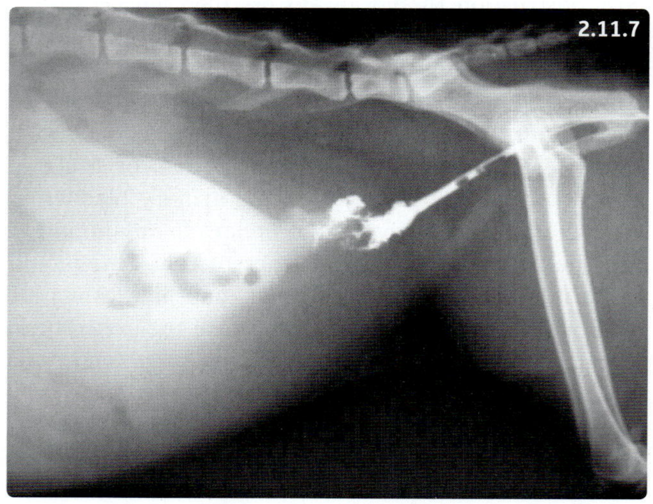

Figure 2.11.7 Cystogram showing a ruptured urinary bladder caused by excessive palpation. (Courtesy M. Schaer)

therefore a urine culture should always be performed in immunosuppressed patients. Blood chemistry analysis can help detect kidney disease or life-threatening electrolyte imbalances, for example in the case of complete urethral obstruction. A CBC can be helpful in documenting a systemic inflammatory response (e.g. pyelonephritis) or anemia in patients with chronic or significant hematuria. In male dogs with an abnormal prostate, cytologic analysis of an ultrasound-guided fine-needle aspiration biopsy of the prostate can help document the nature of prostatic changes.

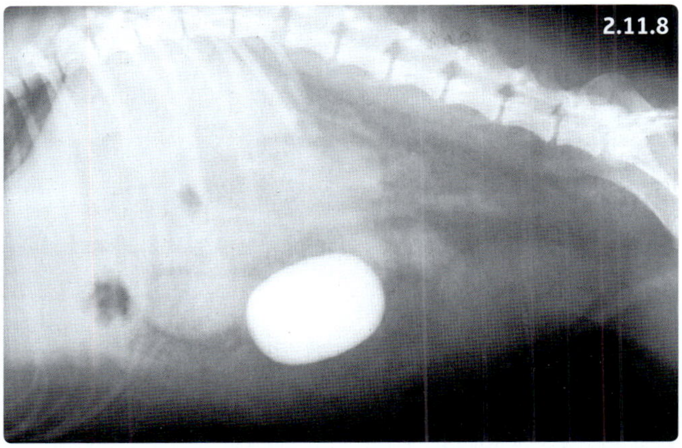

Figure 2.11.8 Lateral radiograph showing a large bladder calculus in the peritoneal space resulting from a spontaneous rupture of the bladder. This dog was systemically sick as a result of the uroperitoneum. She recovered well with surgery. (Courtesy M. Schaer)

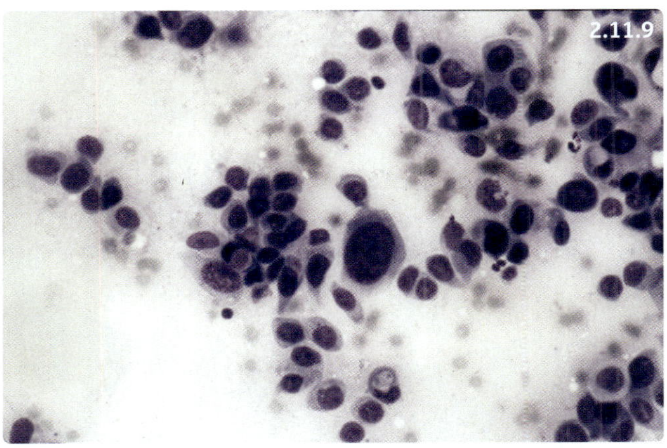

Figure 2.11.9 Cytology sample (obtained by 'urethral massage') from a dog with transitional cell carcinoma, showing many typical neoplastic round cells.

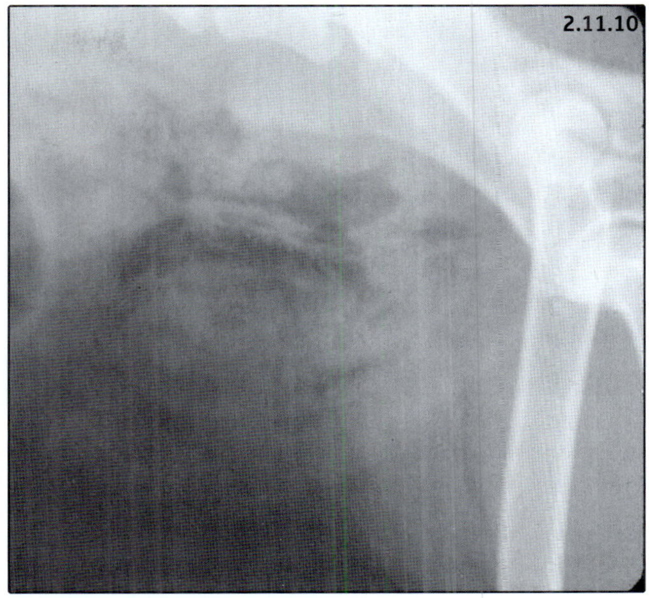

Figure 2.11.10 A plain lateral abdominal radiograph showing emphysematous cystitis in a dog with diabetes mellitus and glycosuria. The air in the bladder mucosa is caused by bacterial fermentation of the glucose. (Courtesy M. Schaer)

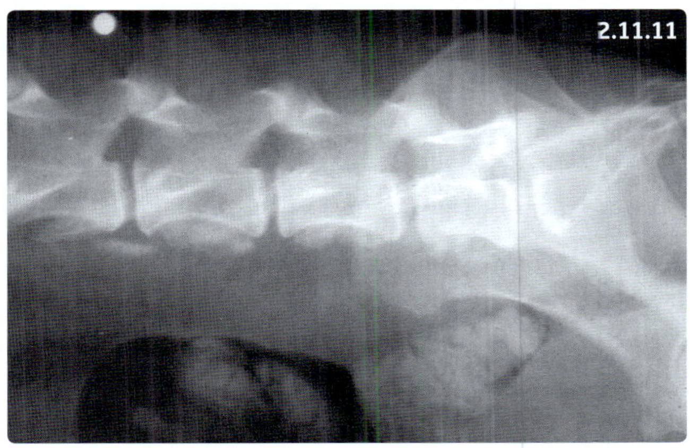

Figure 2.11.11 A lateral dorsal caudal abdominal radiograph of a dog with prostatic carcinoma and lumbar metastases as evidenced by the proliferation of bone on the ventral vertebral bodies of L4 to L7. (Courtesy M. Schaer)

Imaging

Radiography (survey films, studies with contrast agents) and ultrasonography are very useful assets to diagnose causes of dysuria (**Figure 2.11.10**).

Radiography is helpful to evaluate the size and position of the urinary bladder and can document the presence of uroliths, although not all types of uroliths are radiopaque. Extraurinary structures can be assessed, such as the prostate, sublumbar lymph nodes, and bony structures (pelvis, spine). Radiography can also provide evidence of any vertebral abnormality that might represent a neurologic cause of the urinary problem (diskospondylitis, lumbosacral stenosis (**Figure 2.11.6**), intervertebral disks, and other forms of pathology such as spinal neoplasia [**Figure 2.11.11**]). Radiographic contrast studies (double contrast cystogram, retrograde urethrogram) can provide further help in identifying causes of urinary obstruction that cannot readily be seen on survey films, such as radiolucent stones, narrowing of the urethral lumen (as in urethral strictures or spasms), or mucosal abnormalities (inflammation) in the urinary bladder or urethra (**Figures 2.11.12, 2.11.13**). The appropriate use of contrast agents can also help document abnormalities of the bladder mucosa (inflammation, masses) or the presence of urinary leakage.

Ultrasonography is mostly helpful to evaluate the urinary bladder (mucosa, presence of stones, or masses

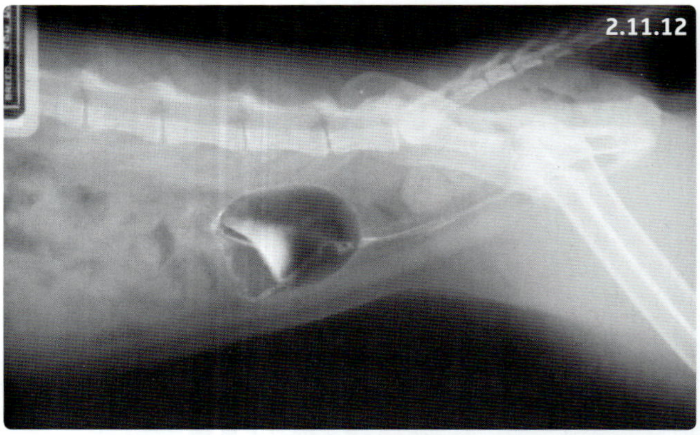

Figure 2.11.12 A double contrast cystogram in a cat with a transitional cell carcinoma in the urinary bladder that caused a radiographic filling defect. (Courtesy M. Schaer)

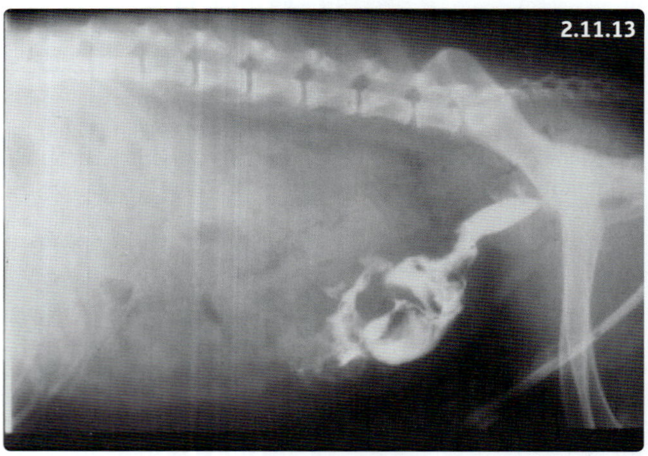

Figure 2.11.13 Cystogram of a dog with transitional cell carcinoma of the urinary bladder showing mucosal filling defects caused by the tumor and a uroperitoneum caused by spontaneous rupture of the weakened wall of the urinary bladder. (Courtesy M. Schaer)

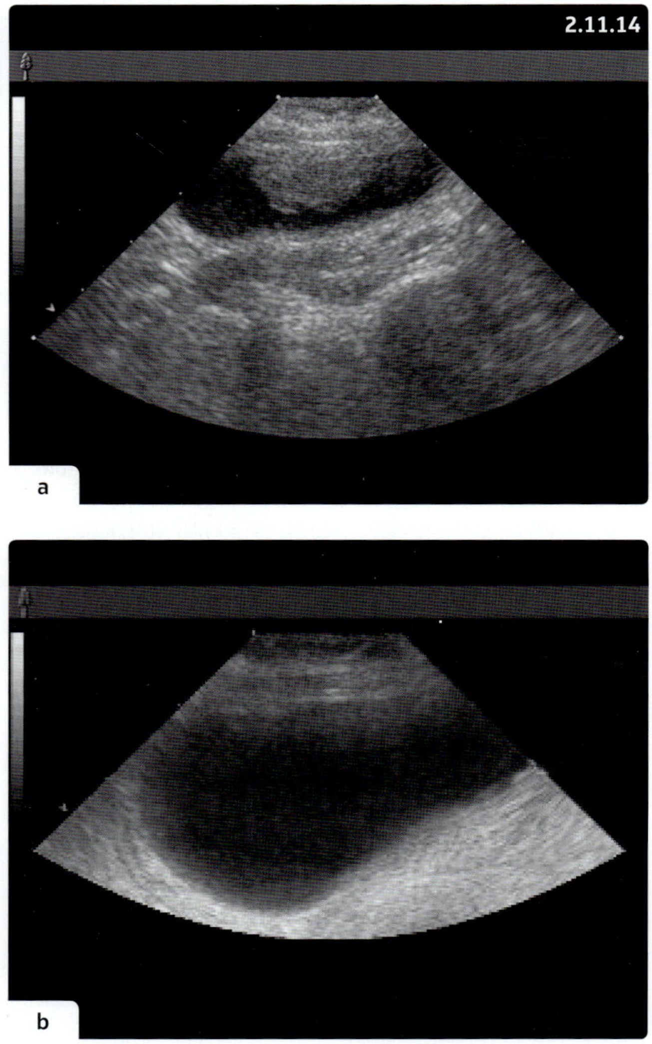

Figures 2.11.14a, b (a) Ultrasound image of a cat with *E. coli* cystitis that caused urinary bladder mucosal thickening that resembled that caused by bladder neoplasia. The fine-needle aspirate cytology showed only neutrophils and bacteria. (b) The same cat 2 weeks later after antibiotic treatment showing regression of the thickened bladder mucosa. (Courtesy M. Schaer)

[**Figures 2.11.14a, b**]), the prostate, and the surrounding organs (kidneys, lymph nodes). Evaluation of the urethra is more difficult due to the intrapelvic location and limited visibility, although an experienced ultrasonographer can easily identify many forms of urethral pathology (**Figure 2.11.15**).

Other diagnostic methods

Urethroscopy and cystoscopy allow direct visualization of the urinary tract mucosa. Endoscopy can be a very useful diagnostic tool for confirming urethral strictures and mucosal abnormalities (**Figure 2.11.16**). Additionally, it allows the operator to collect mucosal biopsies in order to differentiate inflammatory from neoplastic processes. Furthermore, successful endoscopic removal of bladder stones using lithotripsy has been reported.

Cystometry and urethral pressure profilometry are specialized techniques used to assess the function of the urinary bladder and urethral muscles in cases of suspected neurogenic dysuria (for example reflex dyssynergia); these are best done by individuals well trained with the appropriate instrumentation required. A review of the indications for the different diagnostic tests used in dysuria is shown in **Table 2.11.1**.

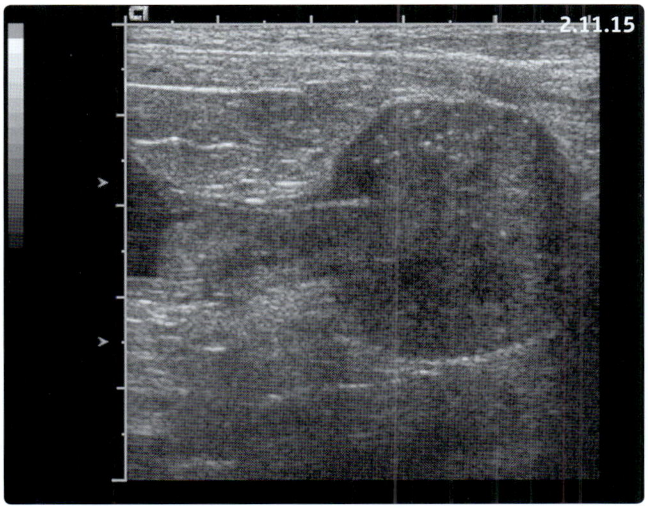

Figure 2.11.15 Ultrasound image of a dog with prostatic carcinoma showing urethral pathology caused by tumor invasion. (Courtesy M. Schaer)

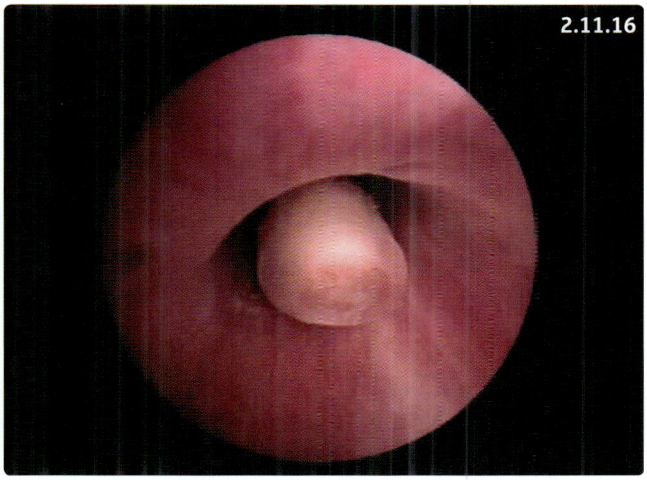

Figure 2.11.16 Cystoscopic view of a urethral foreign body. (Courtesy University of Florida Small Animal Internal Medicine Service)

Table 2.11.1 Clinical usefulness of various tests in dysuric cats and dogs.

Test	Indication/suspected process	Advantages	Disadvantages
Urinalysis	Any case of dysuria	Fast and cheap Can be helpful to document infection, crystalluria, possibly neoplasia	Non-specific Some causes can be missed (neoplasia, urolithiasis)
Urine culture (usually aerobic)	Abnormal urinalysis Recurrent signs Underlying disease with risk of 'silent' infection Evaluation of treatment success	Readily available Reasonable cost Allows targeted treatment	Delayed results (48–72 hours) Does not always preclude further testing (an infection can be secondary to other causes)
Radiography (plain)	Urolithiasis Extraurinary diseases Posterior abdominal extraluminal masses	Readily available Easily performed Evaluation of extraurinary/bony structures	Radiolucent uroliths not seen Mucosal abnormalities rarely visible
Radiography (with contrast)	Mucosal abnormalities Urolithiasis Urethral disease	Minimally invasive Allows evaluation of urethral content/mucosa	Requires technical skills Sedation or anesthesia usually necessary
Ultrasound	Urolithiasis Bladder wall abnormalities Extraurinary diseases Diseases of the proximal urethra	Frequently available Excellent image of bladder mucosa Allows sampling Can show all types of uroliths	Requires technical skills Urethra cannot be fully viewed
Endoscopy	Urethral disease Urolithiasis Bladder wall abnormalities	Allows direct visualization of mucosa Allows sampling Therapeutic in some cases (urolithiasis, polyps)	Only available in limited facilities Needs experienced operator Anesthesia necessary Increased cost

SUMMARY

A systematic stepwise approach to dysuria cases is necessary to localize the problem, as well as to assess the urgency of the care needed. Dysuria may lead to potentially serious complications and dysuric dogs and cats should always be evaluated without delay. History taking and a complete physical examination are essential to localize the origin of the problem. Knowledge of the different diseases and their clinical expression helps in choosing further diagnostic steps and identifying underlying diseases. Treatment recommendations for the different conditions mentioned in this chapter are discussed in Chapter 12 (Nephrology/urology).

RECOMMENDED FURTHER READING

Adams LG, Syme HM (2010) Canine ureteral and lower urinary tract diseases. In: *Textbook of Veterinary Internal Medicine*, 7th edn. (eds. SJ Ettinger, EC Feldman) Saunders Elsevier, St. Louis, pp. 2086–2115.

Labato MA, Acierno MJ (2010) Micturition disorders and urinary incontinence. In: *Textbook of Veterinary Internal Medicine*, 7th edn. (eds. SJ Ettinger, EC Feldman) Saunders Elsevier, St. Louis, pp. 160–164.

Lane IF (2009) Urinary diseases. In: *Kirk's Current Veterinary Therapy XIV*. (eds. JD Bonagura, DC Twedt) Saunders Elsevier, St. Louis, pp. 844–971.

Westropp JL, Buffington CAT (2010) Lower urinary tract disorders in cats. In: *Textbook of Veterinary Internal Medicine*, 7th edn. (eds. SJ Ettinger, EC Feldman) Saunders Elsevier, St. Louis, pp. 2069–2086.

2.12 Pallor

Elisa M. Mazzaferro

INTRODUCTION

Pallor is defined as an extreme or unnatural paleness of the skin. Pallor can be caused by anemia, peripheral vasoconstriction, hemorrhage, stress, or death. In humans, pallor is most readily observed in the skin and mucous membranes. In animals with fur and pigmented mucous membranes, pallor may be less easily identified. In general, pallor is a subjective visual index of tissue perfusion and oxygen delivery to the skin and mucous membranes, including the conjunctiva.

ETIOLOGY/PATHOPHYSIOLOGY

A clinician's index of suspicion as to the cause of a clinical problem, including pallor, starts with a thorough patient signalment and history. Could an animal have ingested any toxins, including a vitamin K antagonist rodenticide, or zinc-containing objects including USA pennies minted after 1982? Is there a potential history of trauma? Is there a travel history outside of the patient's normal location? Have there been recent vaccinations or medications including over-the-counter or homeopathic remedies? Has there been a change in appetite, vomiting, diarrhea, weight loss, or apparent weight gain? Has there been a change in the color of the feces or the urine? Has there been any coughing, hemoptysis, or gingival or other bleeding? Do the clients use flea and tick preventatives?

Oxygen delivery is a function of cardiac output, peripheral vascular resistance, and arterial oxygen content (**Figure 2.12.1**). Cardiac output is a function of the heart rate and the stroke volume. The latter involves the cardiac preload (the amount of blood that is delivered

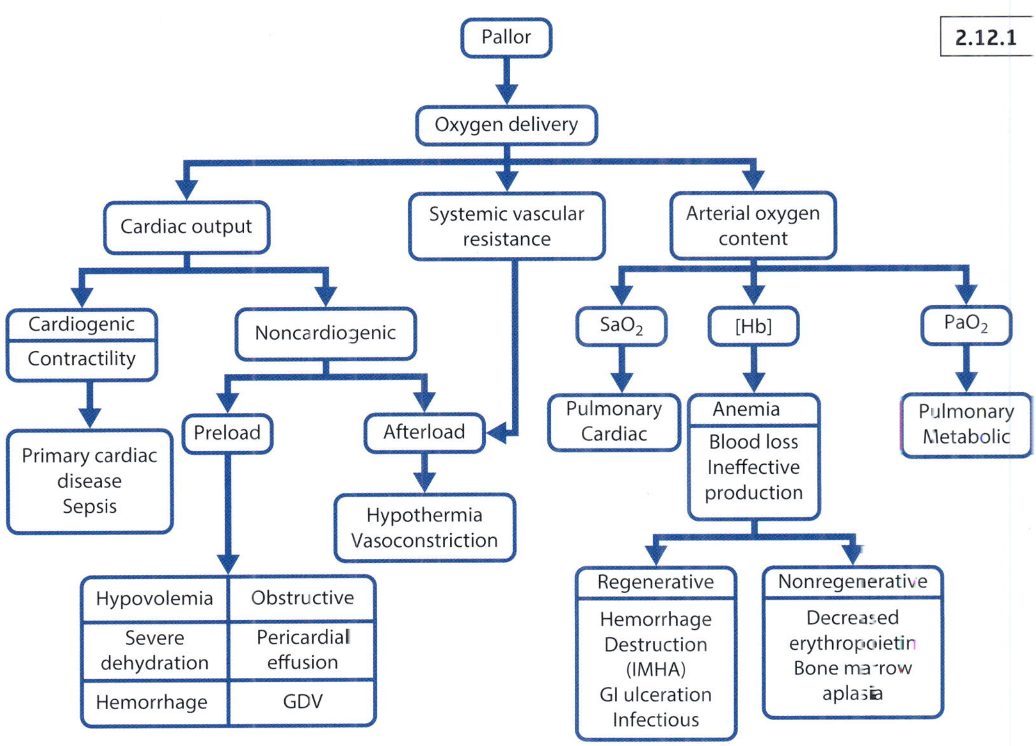

Figure 2.12.1 Algorithm for the pathophysiology of pallor.

to the heart), cardiac afterload (the force against which the heart must contract), and myocardial contractility. Hemorrhage and hypovolemia, including that caused by severe dehydration, in addition to obstructive causes such as pericardial effusion/tamponade and/or GDV or large masses within the abdominal cavity, can result in impaired cardiac preload. Hypothermia, as well as the release of catecholamines to promote vasoconstriction as an adaptive mechanism to maintain perfusion during states of hypovolemia, can increase cardiac afterload. Finally, primary cardiac disease such as dilated cardiomyopathy, end-stage mitral insufficiency, as well as impaired contractility due to circulating inflammatory cytokines with sepsis, can all result in impaired myocardial function and decreased cardiac output.

The second important contributor to pallor or lack thereof is red blood cell mass and saturation of hemoglobin. Conditions associated with blood loss, such as hemorrhage, body cavity effusions/bleeding, GI ulceration, and immune-mediated destruction of red blood cells, can result in regenerative anemia. Inadequate erythropoiesis, as observed with end-stage renal disease, or inadequate production at the level of the bone marrow, as observed with myelophthisis or bone marrow aplasia, can also result in inadequate production of red blood cells. Iron deficiency can result in inadequate production of hemoglobin and a microcytic, hypochromic anemia. Finally, lack of adequate saturation of hemoglobin with oxygen, due to primary or secondary pulmonary disease, can also result in clinical signs of pallor.

CLINICAL APPEARANCE

Once a thorough history is obtained, the physical examination should be performed, with careful attention paid to perfusion parameters: heart rate, capillary refill time (CRT), pulse rate, synchrony and quality, body temperature, and peripheral extremity warmth. The CRT normally should be 1–1.5 seconds in a small animal patient. A brisk CRT (<1 second) may be observed with compensatory shock or sepsis, whereas a prolonged CRT (>2 seconds) is observed in decompensatory shock or hypothermia. Extreme tachycardia (>160 bpm in dogs, >220 bpm in cats) or cardiac dysrhythmias may be observed with compensatory hypovolemic shock, anemia, or due to primary cardiac disease or other conditions such as GDV. In addition, extremely low bradyarrhythmias, such as that observed with sick sinus syndrome, 3rd degree AV block, or end-stage decompensatory shock, can also result in the clinical signs of pallor. Although perfusion parameters are very different to hydration parameters, marked eye retraction within the globe, dry mucous membranes, and extreme skin turgor are also physical examination signs of severe dehydration, which can result in hypovolemia. Careful attention should be paid to auscultation of the heart and the lungs. Muffled heart sounds may be present with pericardial tamponade, severe hypovolemia, or pleural effusion. The presence of both muffled heart and muffled lung sounds should lead the clinician to consider pleural space disease such as pleural effusion or pneumothorax. Harsh lung sounds may be present with pulmonary contusions, pneumonia, or hemorrhage, for example.

DIAGNOSIS

At the time a physical examination is being performed, the patient's blood pressure should be measured and ECG performed to rule out systemic hypo- or hypertension and cardiac dysrhythmias (**Table 2.12.1**). Pulse oximetry should be considered to determine whether the patient is hypoxemic. Initial diagnostic blood work should include a packed cell volume (PCV) and total solids (TS), as well as a CBC. If a patient is anemic (low PCV) with a concomitant low TS, a source of whole blood loss should be considered. If, however, the PCV is low with a normal TS, destruction of red blood cells or lack of production should be considered. That is where the CBC, with a reticulocyte count, is important, to determine if the anemia is regenerative or nonregenerative. If an automated CBC is not possible, performing a saline agglutination test and peripheral blood smear to evaluate for the presence of spherocytes, red blood cell parasites, anisocytosis, red blood cell pallor, and thrombocytopenia can be useful in an emergency situation. Tests of coagulation, particularly the prothrombin time, can be useful as a screening test for vitamin K antagonist rodenticide intoxication. Thoracic and abdominal radiographs may be useful to investigate for dilated cardiomyopathy, pericardial effusion, pulmonary parenchymal disease, pneumothorax, pleural effusion, abdominal effusion and masses, metallic foreign material, GDV, or peritoneal effusion. Finally, a focused assessment using sonography of the abdomen and thorax may prove to be useful in scanning for pericardial or peritoneal effusion or pneumothorax.

RECOMMENDED FURTHER READING

Ortega-Simpson T (2010) Pallor. In: *Textbook of Veterinary Internal Medicine*, 7th edn. (eds. SJ Ettinger, EC Feldman) Saunders Elsevier, St. Louis, pp. 278–283.

Table 2.12.1 Differential diagnosis for pallor.

Anemia

- Regenerative:
  - Blood loss:
    - Hemorrhage:
      - Trauma
      - Neoplasia
      - Toxin (vitamin K antagonist rodenticide)
    - GI ulceration
    - Body cavity effusion
    - Destruction:
      - Immune mediated
      - Infectious
      - Toxin (zinc, *Allium* spp.)
- Nonregenerative:
  - Decreased erythropoietin – renal disease
  - Bone marrow aplasia
  - Anemia of chronic disease

Decreased oxygen delivery

- Decreased cardiac output:
  - Decreased preload:
    - Hemorrhage/hypovolemia
    - Abdominal mass/effusion/GDV
    - Pericardial mass or effusion/tamponade
    - Pleural effusion
    - Pneumothorax/tension pneumothorax
  - Increased afterload:
    - Peripheral vasoconstriction:
      - Compensatory from cardiogenic or hypovolemic shock
      - Increased catecholamines (pheochromocytoma)
      - Hypothermia
- Depressed myocardial contractility:
  - Primary cardiac disease:
    - Dilated cardiomyopathy
    - End-stage mitral insufficiency
    - HCM/HCOM/RCM/unclassified
  - Secondary to circulating myocardial depressant cytokines:
    - Sepsis
    - Systemic inflammatory response

Decreased saturated hemoglobin

- Pulmonary disease:
  - Pulmonary hemorrhage
  - Pulmonary contusions/trauma
  - Pulmonary edema
  - Pneumonia
  - Neoplasia
  - Pulmonary hypertension
- Pleural space disease:
  - Pleural effusion
  - Pneumothorax
- Metabolic/toxic:
  - Methemoglobinemia

GDV, gastric dilatation volvulus; HCM, hypertrophic cardiomyopathy; HOCM, hypertrophic obstructive cardiomyopathy; RCM, restrictive cardiomyopathy.

Part 2

Diseases of specific organ systems

Chapter 3 **Diseases of the oral cavity and teeth**
Erin P. Ribka & Brook A. Niemiec

Chapter 4 **Respiratory disorders**
Cécile Clercx

Chapter 5 **Diseases of the pleural space**
J. Brad Case

Chapter 6 **Approach to thoracic radiographs**
L. Abbigail Granger

Chapter 7 **Cardiovascular disorders**
Romain Pariaut & Carley Saelinger

Chapter 8 **Digestive diseases (pharynx to anorectum)**
Frédéric Gaschen

Chapter 9 **Liver disorders**
Joseph Taboada

Chapter 10 **Pancreatic disorders**
Michael Schaer

Chapter 11 **Endocrine disorders**
Michael E. Herrtage

Chapter 12 **Nephrology/urology**
Mark Acierno

Chapter 13 **Approach to abdominal radiographs**
L. Abbigail Granger

Chapter 14 **Disorders of the nervous system and muscle**
Simon R. Platt

Chapter 15 **Bone and joint disorders**
Steven M. Fox

Chapter 16 **Hematologic disorders**
Katie M. Boes & Rose E. Raskin

Chapter 17 **Disorders of hemostasis**
Bobbi Conner

Chapter 18 **Dermatologic disorders**
Diane T. Lewis

Chapter 19 **Ocular manifestations of systemic diseases**
Dennis E. Brooks & Megan L. Sullivan

Chapter 3

Diseases of the oral cavity and teeth

Erin P. Ribka & Brook A. Niemiec

INTRODUCTION

Veterinary dentistry and oral surgery is a growing field. Over the past decade, veterinarians and pet owners alike are learning the importance of good oral health for companion animals. Thanks to this and other medical and nutritional improvements, pets are living longer, healthier lives. Dental disease is more common in our aging pet populations and, without proper care throughout their lives, extensive treatment is increasingly necessary. Recent research supports the connection between oral and systemic health, including diabetes, cardiac, hepatic, renal, and pulmonary diseases, and an increased incidence of certain neoplasias (particularly oral). In this chapter, we aim to provide a basic overview of normal oral anatomy and physiology as well as some of the most common issues encountered in small animal clinical practice. The entire breadth of oral diseases cannot be covered completely in a single chapter, therefore resources for more detailed information are provided at the end of this chapter.

ANATOMY

A basic understanding of the oral anatomy and terminology is essential. The accepted dental formulas for the dog and cat are as follows:

- Canine deciduous (total = 28):
  - Maxilla (2×) - 3 incisors, 1 canine, 3 premolars
  - Mandible (2×) - 3 incisors, 1 canine, 3 premolars
- Canine permanent (total = 42):
  - Maxilla (2×) - 3 incisors, 1 canine, 4 premolars, 2 molars
  - Mandible (2×) - 3 incisors, 1 canine, 4 premolars, 3 molars
- Feline deciduous (total = 26):
  - Maxilla (2×) - 3 incisors, 1 canine, 3 premolars
  - Mandible (2×) - 3 incisors, 1 canine, 2 premolars
- Feline permanent (total = 30):
  - Maxilla (2×) - 3 incisors, 1 canine, 3 premolars, 1 molar
  - Mandible (2×) - 3 incisors, 1 canine, 2 premolars, 1 molar

Several tooth numbering systems exist for efficient written or verbal communication regarding the oral cavity. The most commonly used system is the modified Triadan system. Each quadrant of the mouth is given a number, as is each tooth. The right maxillary quadrant is the 100 arch (500 for deciduous teeth), left maxillary is 200 (600), left mandibular 300 (700), and right mandibular is 400 (800). Teeth are numbered beginning with the first incisor and moving distally (or caudally) as 01–10 in the canine maxilla and 01–11 in the canine mandible. Therefore, the permanent right maxillary canine tooth would be termed 104. The maxillary fourth premolars are 108 (right) and 208 (left), and the mandibular first molars are 309 (left) and 409 (right). These teeth are typically referred to as the carnassial teeth (**Figures 3.1a, b**).

Cats do not have a full complement of premolars and molars and so are 'missing' several teeth (**Figures 3.2a, b**).

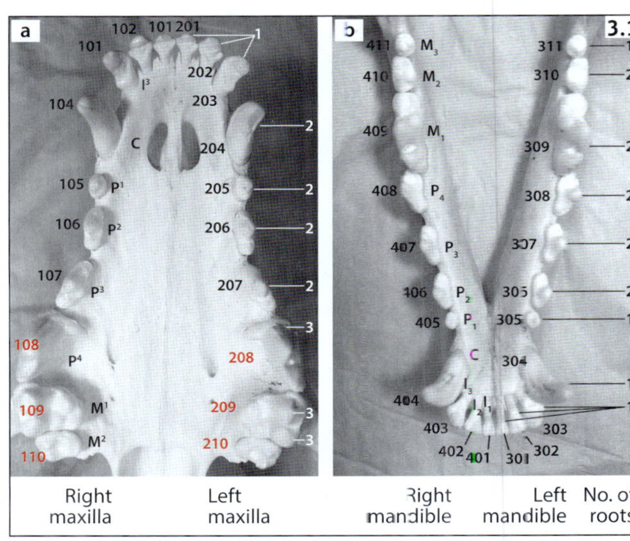

Figures 3.1a, b Modified Triadan numbering system in the dog. (a) Maxilla (3-rooted teeth numbered in red); (b) mandible. (From Niemiec BA (2011) *Small Animal Dental, Oral & Maxillofacial Disease: A Color Handbook*. CRC Press, London, with permission)

	Dogs				Cats			
	Incisors	Canines	Premolars	Molars	Incisors	Canines	Premolars	Molars
Deciduous (weeks)	3–4	3	4–12	-	2–3	3–4	3–4	-
Permanent (months)	3–5	4–6	4–6	5–7	3–4	4–5	4–6	4–5

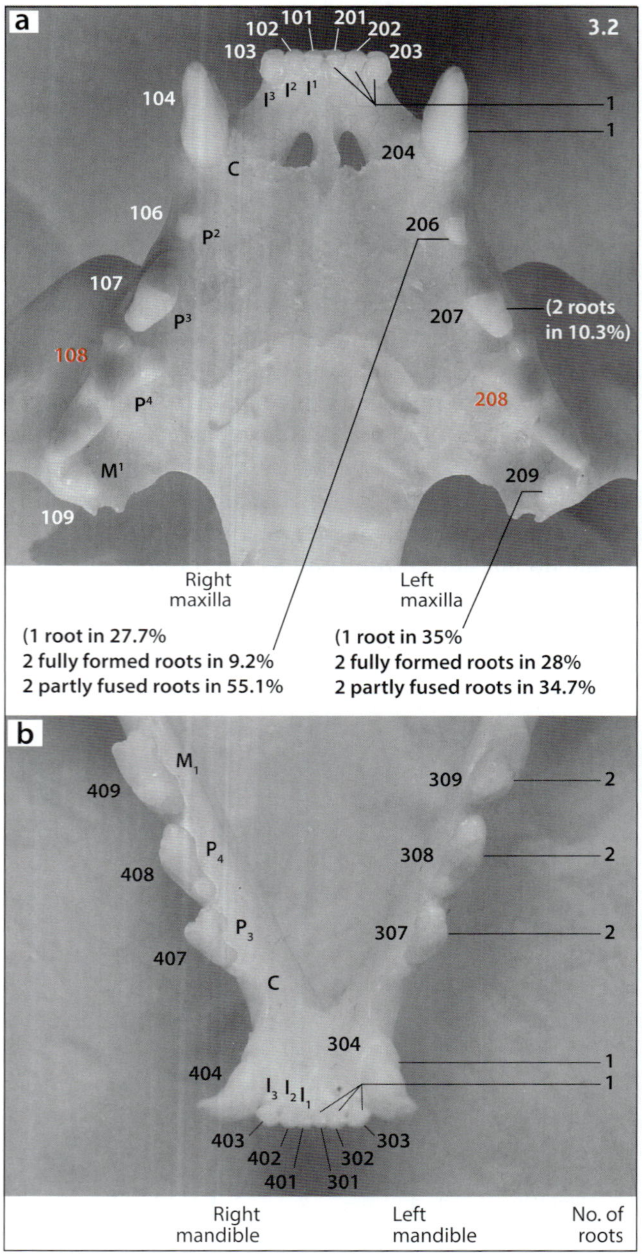

Figures 3.2a, b Modified Triadan numbering system in the cat. (a) Maxilla (3-rooted teeth numbered in red); (b) mandible. (From Niemiec BA (2011) *Small Animal Dental, Oral & Maxillofacial Disease: A Color Handbook*. CRC Press, London, with permission)

The eruption times of deciduous and permanent teeth in the dog and cat are shown above:

Directionally, surfaces of teeth are referred to as (**Figures 3.3a, b**):

- Mesial: nearer the rostral midline.
- Distal: away from the rostral midline.
- Buccal surfaces face the inside of the cheeks.
- Labial surfaces face the lips.
- Lingual surfaces are next to the tongue.
- Palatal surfaces face the palate.

It is also important to understand tooth structure and development. The crowns of teeth are covered in enamel, which is the hardest substance in the body. Enamel cannot be regrown once it is lost and is much thinner in dogs and cats (<1 mm) than in humans. Beneath the enamel is dentin, which has a mineral content similar to bone. It is comprised of numerous microscopic dentinal tubules (**Figure 3.4**). Each dentinal tubule contains an odontoblastic process, which is essentially an extension of the root canal system. Dentin is produced throughout life and this accounts for the decreasing width of the pulp canal evident on dental radiographs as patients age. Dentin is porous and irritation or injury may incite its component cells to protect the tooth by forming reparative or tertiary dentin. Vessels and nerves enter and exit the teeth through the tip of the root or the apex. The entire root structure (in normal teeth) is surrounded and supported by the periodontal ligament, which holds teeth in place in the surrounding alveolar bone. The periodontium consists of the gingiva, periodontal ligament, cementum, and alveolar bone. The gingiva is part of the specialized mucosa that protects the tooth and supporting structures from infection and detachment. Cementum covers the root much as enamel covers the crown of the tooth, increasing with age.

ORAL EXAMINATION

Conscious visual examination may be limited or fairly detailed, depending on the patient's temperament and the skill of the examiner. It may be possible to diagnose persistent deciduous teeth, fractured teeth, caries, tooth resorptions, masses, and malocclusions/orthodontic

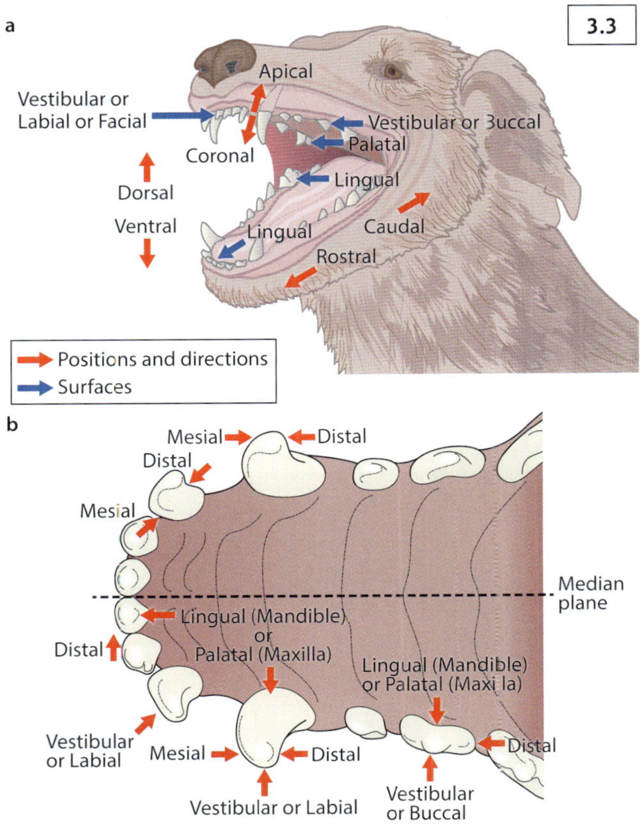

Figures 3.3a, b Dental anatomic terminology. (a) Extraoral view; (b) intraoral view. (From Niemiec BA (2011) *Small Animal Dental, Oral & Maxillofacial Disease: A Color Handbook*. CRC Press, London, with permission)

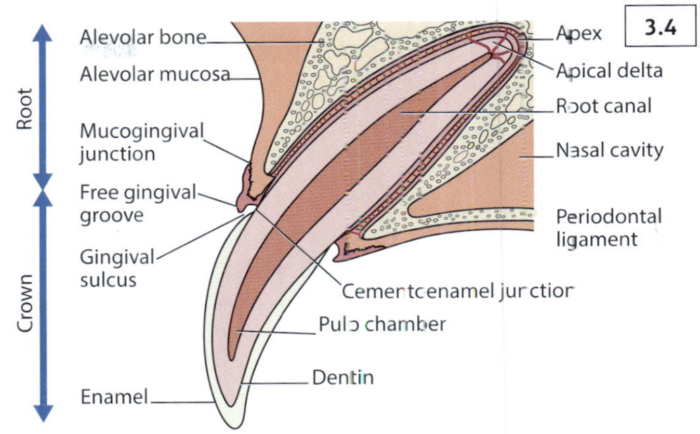

Figure 3.4 An adult maxillary tooth and its peridontium. (From Niemiec BA (2011) *Small Animal Dental, Oral & Maxillofacial Disease: A Color Handbook*. CRC Press, London, with permission)

problems and to develop a preliminary sense of the level of periodontal disease. (**Note:** The conscious evaluation is not a replacement for an anesthetized examination.) There are many factors that make a complete examination impossible in an awake animal, not least of which are pain and aggression. An anesthetized examination should include a complete visual assessment of the entire oral cavity, including all soft and hard tissues, periodontal probing and exploring of all aspects of individual teeth and gingival sulci, and intraoral radiography of any abnormalities. Further, many veterinary dentists recommend full mouth radiographs be obtained for all dental patients. Therefore, all anesthetized patients should receive an oral examination (**Figures 3.5–3.8**).

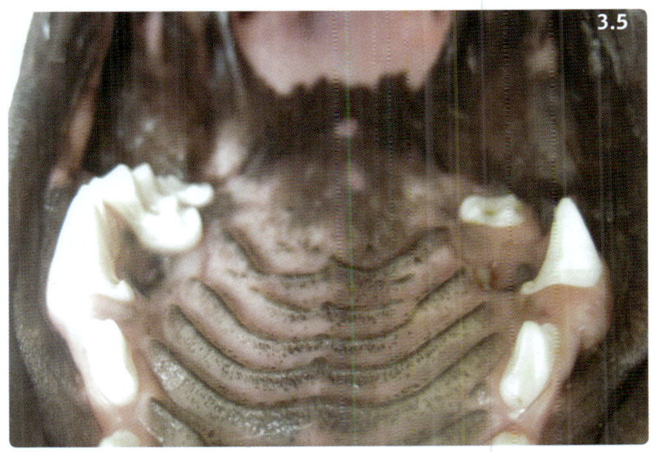

Figure 3.5 Impacted right maxillary first molar (109) in a 7-month-old Golden Retriever presented for routine orchiectomy.

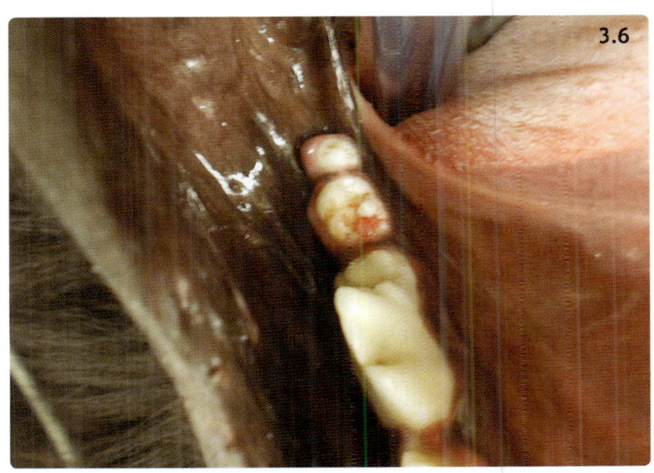

Figure 3.6 Complicated crown fracture with exposed pulp of the left mandibular second molar (310). This injury was noted by the technician monitoring anesthesia during a routine, elective ovariectomy in a 7-month-old mixed breed dog.

PERIODONTAL DISEASE

Definition/overview

Periodontal disease is the most common disease affecting small animal patients. It has long been established that 70% of cats and 80% of dogs exhibit some level of periodontal disease by 3 years of age. However, current

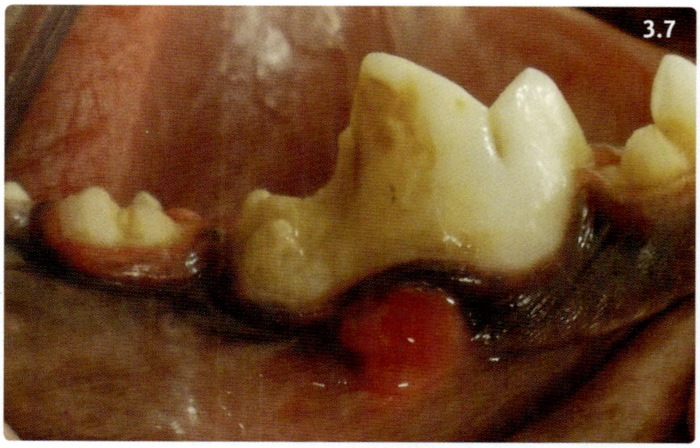

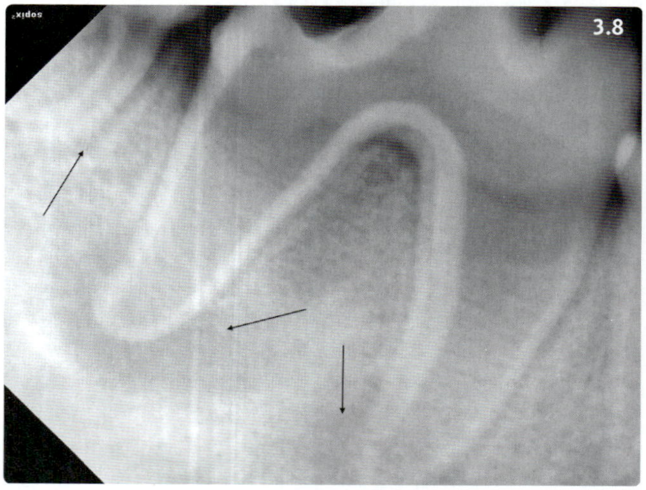

Figures 3.7, 3.8 (3.7) Evidence of developmental enamel abnormality and tooth root abscess was noted in the area of the tooth adjacent to the fractured molar. (3.8) Dental radiographs were exposed and the first molar was found to be non-vital. The teeth were deemed unsalvageable and surgically extracted during the same anesthetic episode. Note the periodontal lucency around tooth roots in the radiograph (black arrows). This is the same dog as in Figure 3.6.

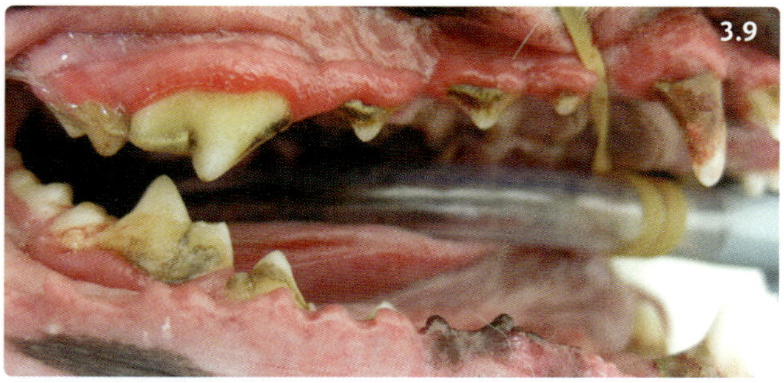

Figure 3.9 Canine periodontal disease. Note the red, swollen gingiva. The significant calculus buildup does not equate to severity of periodontal disease.

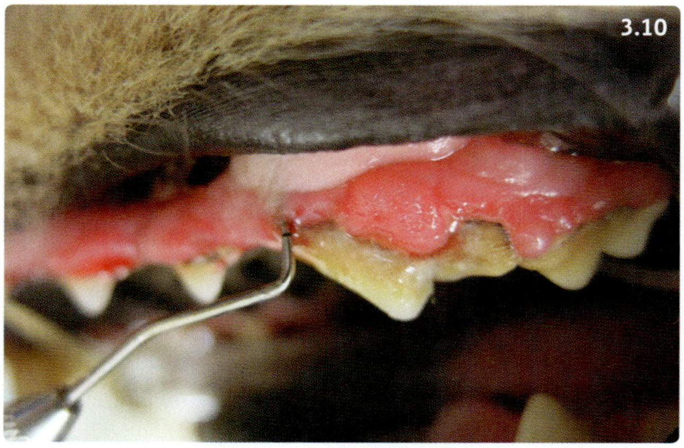

Figure 3.10 Canine periodontitis. The probe is inserted to a depth of 11 mm. This is a deep periodontal pocket, requiring radiographs to rule out periodontal–endodontic disease and open curettage or extraction.

research suggests that 90% or more of dogs have some degree of periodontal disease by just 1 year of age (**Figure 3.9**).

Periodontal disease encompasses gingivitis and periodontitis, which each represent a stage in the progression of the disease complex. Gingivitis is the earlier, reversible stage of inflammation confined to the gingival tissues. Once the inflammation reaches the deeper tissues of the periodontium (periodontal ligament and alveolar bone), it becomes periodontitis. Periodontal inflammation may result in osteoclastic resorption of the alveolar bone (**Figures 3.10, 3.11**). This bone loss is considered irreversible without advanced periodontal surgeries and guided tissue regeneration. Therefore, prevention is critical. There are numerous significant local/regional consequences of advanced periodontal disease, including: ocular disease or damage; pathologic mandibular fractures; osteomyelitis; oral cancers; and periodontal–endodontic infections/abscesses.

In addition, recent research has linked periodontal disease to many deleterious systemic effects such as: hepatic inflammation and disease; glomerulonephritis and renal insufficiency; valvular endocarditis and heart disease; cerebral infarction (strokes); diabetes mellitus; and early mortality.

Etiology

Plaque is the cause of periodontal disease. Plaque is a biofilm of oral bacteria. A biofilm is a unique compilation of organisms (bacteria), minerals, and proteins that develops into a complex structure, significantly more resistant to antibiotics and antiseptics than any of the individual bacteria themselves.

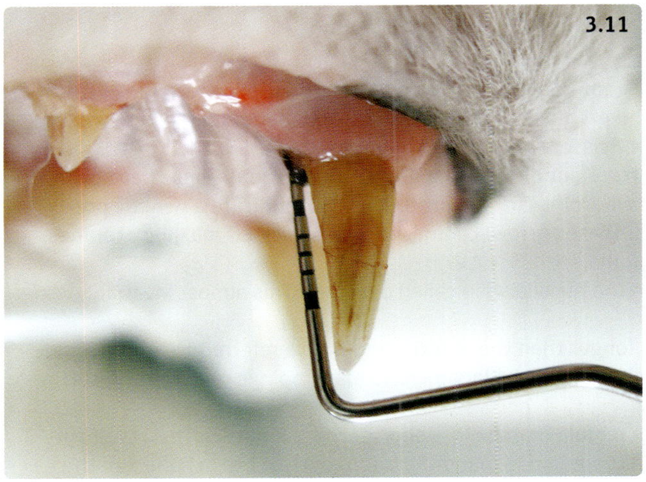

Figure 3.11 Feline periodontal disease. The probe reaches to a depth of 4–5 mm, necessitating radiographs, closed root planing, and perioceutic administration at a minimum.

Pathophysiology

The development of periodontal disease begins with the adherence of plaque to oral structures, particularly teeth. The first step in the adherence of plaque to teeth is pellicle formation, followed by an initial adhesion and attachment and, finally, colonization and plaque maturation. There are a variety of conditions that result in roughened tooth surfaces and may increase plaque retention, including enamel hypoplasia, enamel defects, crown fractures, crowding, tooth resorptions, and malocclusions.

The rate and degree of progression of periodontal disease are determined by a combination of bacterial infection and host (patient) response. Systemic diseases (such as diabetes mellitus, endogenous or exogenous hypercortisolemia) that increase host susceptibility to infection and/or decrease wound healing also contribute to periodontal disease. It is more common in small and toy breed dogs, probably because of tooth crowding, extended life spans, and other genetic factors.

Clinical presentation

The vast majority of patients with periodontal disease show no outward signs of disease. Patients with advanced disease may present with halitosis, ptyalism, pain, pawing at the mouth, tooth exfoliation, or even pathologic jaw fractures. Periodontal disease may be noted on routine conscious oral examination, but is best diagnosed during anesthetized oral examination with probing and intraoral dental radiographs.

Differential diagnosis

Neoplasia, immune-mediated disease, resorptive lesions, foreign bodies, candidiasis (thrush).

Diagnosis

Gingival inflammation (redness and swelling) is the first outward sign of periodontal disease. However, bleeding on probing or brushing is actually the first sign of periodontal disease, therefore diagnosis is often delayed. These signs – redness, swelling, and bleeding – are enough to warrant a diagnosis of gingivitis. It is critical to note that while dental calculus (tartar) is typically associated with periodontal disease, it is not the source of the disease. Therefore it should not be relied on to determine a need for professional therapy. Orastrip® (PDx Biotech), a relatively new product, can be used quickly and easily in the awake patient to test for the presence of thiol compounds, metabolic products of the subgingival biofilm that are the cause of periodontal disease. This will provide a diagnosis earlier in the disease process as well as an objective measure as to the level of periodontal disease. This knowledge may improve client compliance and allow earlier intervention.

Gingivitis may be diagnosed in the conscious patient by the gross appearance of red or swollen gums or in the owner's reporting of bleeding on brushing. Periodontitis generally requires anesthetized examination with probing and dental radiographs for diagnosis, unless there is marked gingival recession.

Periodontal probing of the circumference of each tooth during the anesthetized examination may reveal pocket depths greater than the normal gingival sulcular depth (generally 0–3 mm in dogs, 0–0.5 mm in cats). A normal probing depth does not necessarily indicate a disease-free state, as teeth affected by gingivitis can have normal sulcular depth or gingival recession. A simple color coded probe (Niemiec periodontal probe, Dentalaire Products) has been developed to allow easy diagnosis of pathologic periodontal pockets. Periodontal disease may also be identified on dental radiography.

Management

Thorough anesthetized professional periodontal therapy and consistent home care are vital to the management of periodontal disease. Gingivitis can be reversed with such treatment. Pathologic pockets less than 6 mm are best treated with closed root planing and perioceutic treatment (Doxirobe, Zoetis; Clindoral, Trilogic Pharma). Deeper pockets, or teeth with class II or III furcation, must be treated with periodontal flap surgery and open curettage (+/- guided tissue regeneration), or extracted. Following these additional therapies, regular professional periodontal therapy and diligent home care are required. Teeth often become unsalvageable and require extraction. Examples include significantly mobile teeth

Table 3.1 Malocclusion classifications.

• **Class 0.** Normal (orthoclusion). The mandibular canines are equidistant between the maxillary third incisor and canine, the mandibular incisors sit just caudal to the maxillary incisors, and the premolars of the maxillary and mandibular arches interdigitate in a manner reminiscent of pinking shears, hence the term scissors bite.
• **Class I.** Normal jaw lengths (scissors bite) where one or more teeth are out of proper alignment (occlusion). These have been considered nonhereditary. However, the high incidence of certain syndromes in specific breeds does indicate a genetic predisposition. Class I malocclusions include linguoversed mandibular (base narrow) canines and mesioversed maxillary canines (lance effect). The former typically results in significant palatal trauma.
• **Class II.** Mandibular brachygnathism; the mandible is shorter than the maxilla. Also called overshot. This almost invariably causes significant palatal or tooth trauma.
• **Class III.** This is a jaw length discrepancy in which the mandible is longer than the maxilla, and is also referred to as undershot. This class of malocclusion does not typically create significant trauma, but maxillary incisors may impinge on opposing soft and hard tissues and should be carefully examined.
• **Class IV.** 'Wry bite'. This is a jaw length discrepancy in which one mandible or maxilla is shorter than the other. This results in a shift of the mandibular midline. A true class IV malocclusion occurs when one mandible is longer than the maxilla and the other mandible is shorter than the maxilla.

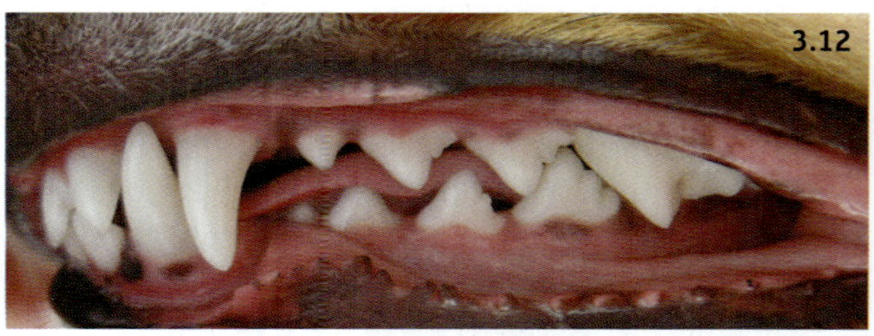

Figure 3.12 Normocclusion. Scissors bite.

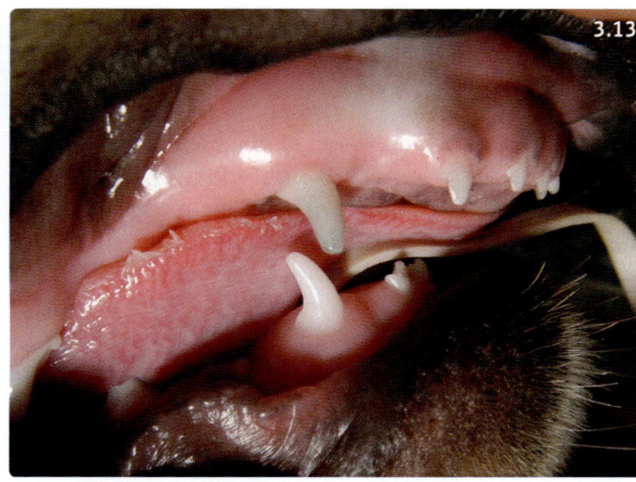

Figure 3.13 Class II malocclusion. Also termed overbite or overshot, the mandible is shorter than the maxilla. This malocclusion often requires interceptive orthodontia to relieve trauma and allow the mandible to develop to its full potential.

or periodontal–endodontic lesions. Small teeth may also be sacrificially extracted to better access and treat more strategic teeth.

Prognosis

Outcomes depend much on severity of disease, quality of treatment and client commitment. Prognosis therefore ranges from good to guarded to poor.

MALOCCLUSION

Definition/overview

A malocclusion is a deviation of one or more teeth and/or jaws from normal alignment. Malocclusions may be cosmetic only, or result in slight to significant oral trauma. Malocclusions are categorized by class (**Table 3.1; Figures 3.12–3.14**).

Etiology

Most malocclusions are considered hereditary in nature, in particular the jaw length malocclusions (class II, III, IV). They may result from inbreeding to produce desirable head size or shape, or from matings of parents with dissimilar jaw lengths. Mesiocclúded or 'lance' canines are also considered genetic (seen commonly in Shetland Sheepdogs and Persian cats). Nongenetic causes of malocclusions include trauma or systemic influences such as severe illnesses, nutritional disturbances, or endocrine diseases. In general, these nongenetic causes have historical or other clinical support.

Clinical presentation

Patients often show no overt clinical signs, but may present for oral pain, bleeding, ptyalism, aggression, 'mouth shyness', halitosis, periodontal disease, or even an oronasal fistula.

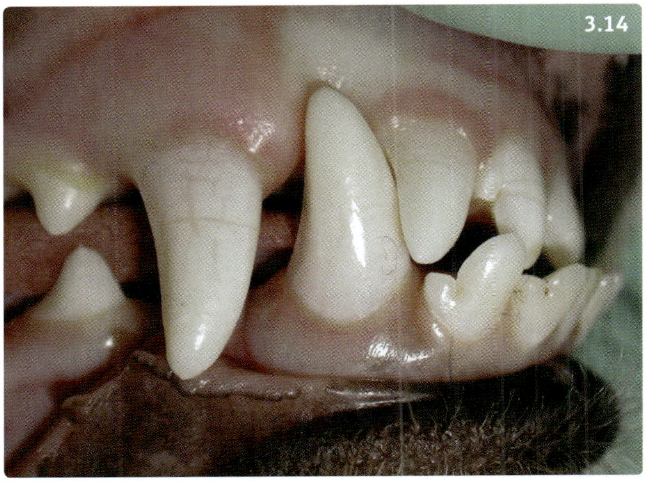

Figure 3.14 Class III malocclusion in an adult dog. Also termed underbite or undershot, the mandible is longer than the maxilla and the mandibular incisors are rostral to the maxillary incisors.

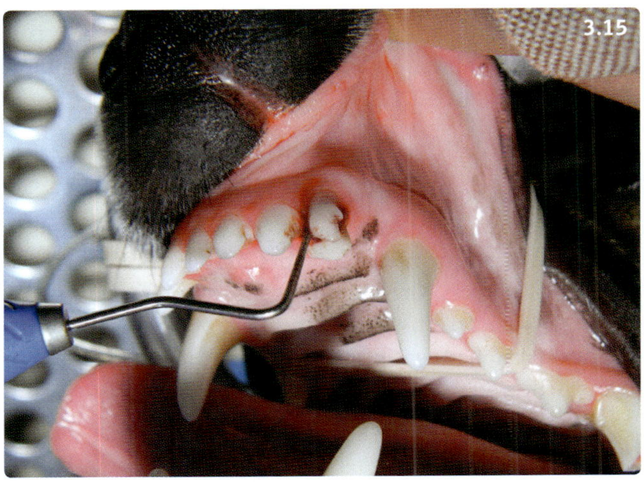

Figure 3.15 A persistent deciduous maxillary incisor tooth (603) in an adult dog. Note the associated periodontal disease demonstrated by the placement of the probe.

Differential diagnosis

Trauma, temporomandibular joint dislocation, mandibular fracture, normal bite for the breed.

Diagnosis

Diagnosis can usually be made with visual examination. Some malocclusions may require sedation for accurate and complete evaluation and diagnosis. Dental radiographs should be made to evaluate the involved teeth for periodontal or endodontic disease.

Management

Treatment depends on type and severity. If the malocclusion is purely cosmetic, intervention is neither warranted nor recommended, as orthodontic correction can be a long and uncomfortable process. If a malocclusion is diagnosed in the deciduous dentition, interceptive orthodontics can be attempted. This involves extraction of the deciduous dentition that is causing the trauma and/or resulting in an adverse dental interlock (not allowing the jaws to grow to their full genetic potential).

Orthodontic treatment should never be performed in patients destined for breeding or showing. Malocclusions resulting in oral trauma or prevention of normal mandibular growth should be treated early and aggressively. This may be achieved by extraction of the offending tooth or teeth, coronal reduction and vital pulp therapy, or orthodontic appliances. All clients should receive genetic counseling.

Prognosis

Successful treatment is dependent on early diagnosis and appropriate intervention. Clients should receive counseling on the genetic basis of most malocclusions. Neutering is generally recommended.

PERSISTENT DECIDUOUS TEETH

Definition/overview

A deciduous tooth is considered persistent if it remains present in the oral cavity after the corresponding permanent tooth has erupted to any degree.

Etiology

The most common cause of this condition is an aberrant eruption path of the permanent tooth. Lack of a permanent tooth as well as nutritional or hormonal imbalances may also result in persistent deciduous teeth

Pathophysiology

As the permanent tooth erupts along its natural path, the pressure it places on the apex of the root of the deciduous tooth results in resorption of the deciduous tooth root. As the permanent tooth continues its coronal advancement, the root continues to resorb and eventually exfoliates and the permanent tooth assumes its place. When the permanent tooth fails to follow its natural path, the deciduous tooth root does not receive the proper pressure to result in adequate resorption for exfoliation.

Clinical presentation

While they typically occur in toy and small breed dogs, persistent deciduous teeth may occur in any breed as well as in cats. The condition is often bilateral and most commonly affects the canine teeth, followed by the incisors and premolars (**Figure 3.15**).

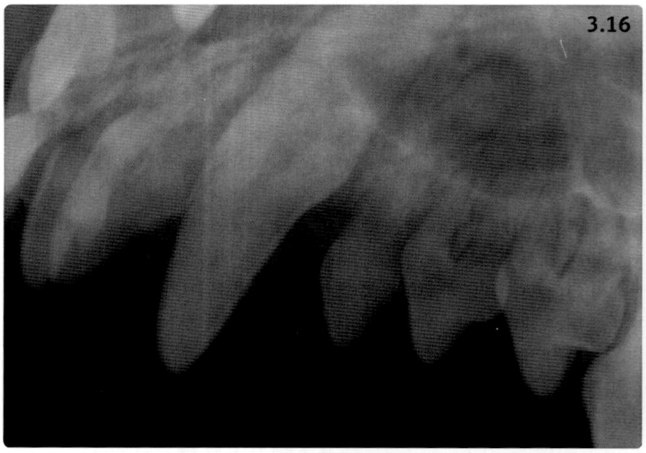

Figure 3.16 Dental radiograph of a persistent deciduous tooth with periapical lucency in an 8-year-old dog.

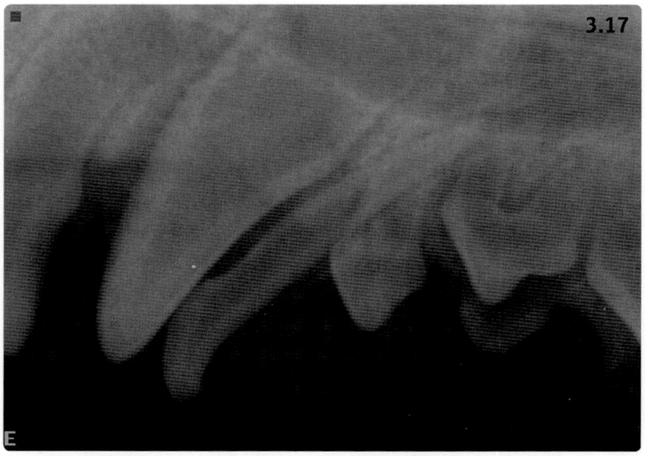

Figure 3.17 Persistent deciduous maxillary canine tooth (604). Note the thin, fragile walls.

Differential diagnosis

Supernumerary teeth, lack of associated permanent tooth, crown malformation.

Diagnosis

Conscious oral examination is usually sufficient for diagnosis of persistent canines; however, since the deciduous maxillary fourth premolars are palatal to the permanent ones, anesthesia may be required. Sedated or anesthetized examination and intraoral radiographs may be necessary to accurately distinguish between supernumerary teeth, crown malformation, and lack of permanent dentition.

Management

Early detection and extraction of offending teeth is critical. Two teeth of the same type should never occupy the same place at the same time, as periodontal and orthodontic damage can occur very quickly. The authors recommend enlisting clients in monitoring for the appearance of this condition, instructing them in home care from the time of the first puppy (or kitten) visit and evaluating the oral cavity thoroughly at each vaccine booster appointment. The deciduous tooth should be extracted as soon as the permanent begins to erupt, unless the deciduous tooth is significantly mobile. Intraoral radiographs should be exposed prior to and following extraction, as these teeth can be quite difficult to remove because of their long roots and thin, fragile walls. In addition, partial and complete root resorption may further complicate extraction (**Figure 3.16**). Patience and great care must be taken to avoid damaging the unerupted permanent tooth. Root remnants should not be left behind if at all possible, as they may become infected and/or act as a foreign body and result in significant inflammation and discomfort (**Figure 3.17**).

Prognosis

Prognosis is good if detected and treated very early and carefully. Permanent teeth damaged during extraction of deciduous teeth or retained roots may exhibit evidence of enamel defects. Orthodontic consequences may occur within 2 weeks of the first sign of eruption of secondary dentition and irreversible periodontal disease may begin even earlier.

MISSING TEETH

Definition/overview

Hypodontia is the congenital absence of one to five permanent teeth. Oligodontia is the congenital absence of six or more permanent teeth. Anodontia is the congenital lack of all permanent teeth.

Etiology

May be congenital or developmental.

Pathophysiology

Permanent teeth are formed from buds of the deciduous teeth with the exception of the molars and first premolars, which have no corresponding deciduous. A truly missing deciduous tooth will result in lack of a permanent tooth. Hypodontia of deciduous dentition is extremely rare; more often, a deciduous tooth is prematurely lost to trauma.

Genetic conditions resulting in defects of tooth development are the most common cause of missing teeth. Developmental disturbances can also have a profound effect on tooth development. In addition, trauma, medications, and gestational problems can also result in significant tooth anomalies and defects.

Clinical presentation

Most often an incidental finding, most patients are not clinically presented solely for missing teeth. However, they show signs of pain or discomfort, swelling, or mandibular fracture.

Differential diagnosis

Previous extraction, avulsion, or fracture; retained tooth root, impaction/embedded/unerupted tooth.

Diagnosis

Unless the practitioner has previous information from prior examination or surgery (including postoperative radiographs) that the tooth was extracted or otherwise not present, diagnosis must be confirmed with intraoral radiography. Missing teeth are generally diagnosed on awake examination. However, sedation or anesthesia is often required to diagnose missing molars (**Figures 3.18, 3.19**).

Management

All 'missing' teeth should be radiographed to rule out impacted teeth or retained roots. These should be extracted once diagnosed unless the patient is geriatric, the tooth has undergone significant replacement resorption, and/or the extraction would be challenging, in which case referral to a veterinary dentist is recommended. A 'wait and see' approach in a young patient is generally considered inappropriate. Congenitally missing teeth do not require intervention beyond intraoral radiography for diagnosis. Genetic counseling may be warranted.

Prognosis

Prognosis is good if appropriate surgical intervention is taken when necessary. Impacted teeth that are not removed may develop dentigerous cysts, which can have significant consequences, such as tooth displacement, which may lead to malocclusion, tooth and/or bone resorption, or a pathologic fracture (see Appendix: Clinical case 1.) Rarely, dentigerous cyst lining has been reported to undergo malignant transformation. Retained tooth roots can become infected and cause significant pain as well as local and systemic infection.

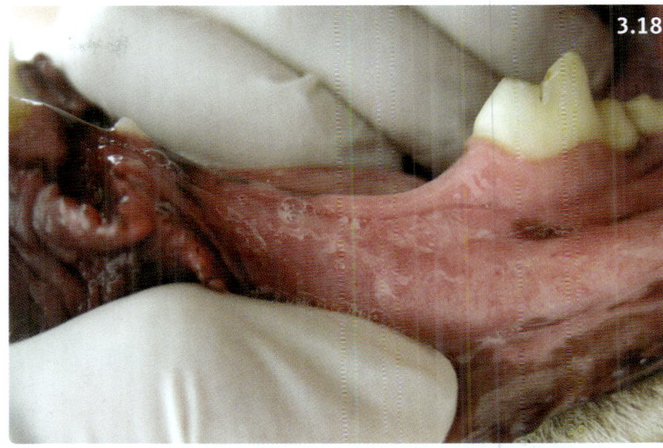

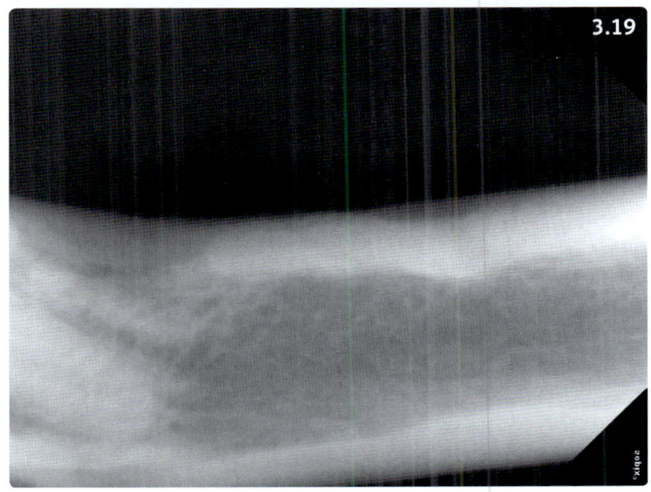

Figures 3.18, 3.19 Missing mandibular premolars in a 6-year-old male neutered Catahoula Leopard Dog. Congenital oligodontia was confirmed with intraoral radiography.

FRACTURED TEETH

Definition/overview

Fractured teeth are classified by location of the fracture (crown, root, or both) and whether or not the pulp is exposed. Tooth fractures that result in pulp exposure are referred to as complicated; those that do not result in pulp exposure are termed uncomplicated.

Etiology

Tooth fractures occur as a result of excessive force applied to a tooth or stresses that act on a tooth in a nonphysiological direction. They commonly occur secondarily to biting or chewing on rocks, bones, hard chew toys, and even hard rawhides. They may also be the result of impact trauma (e.g. automobile accidents, running into walls, horse kicks, falls) (**Figures 3.20, 3.21**).

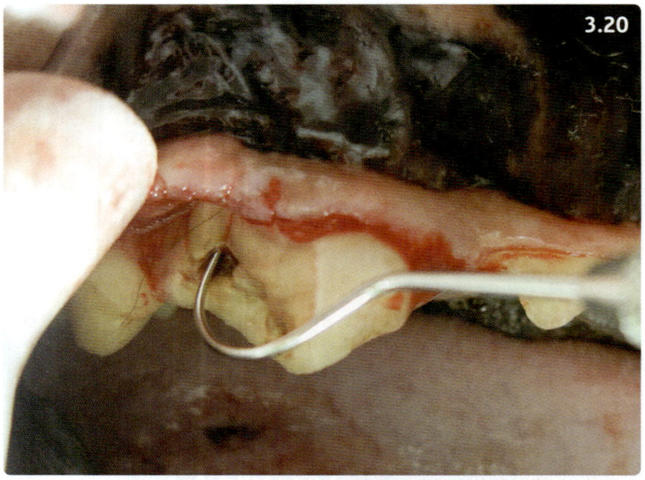

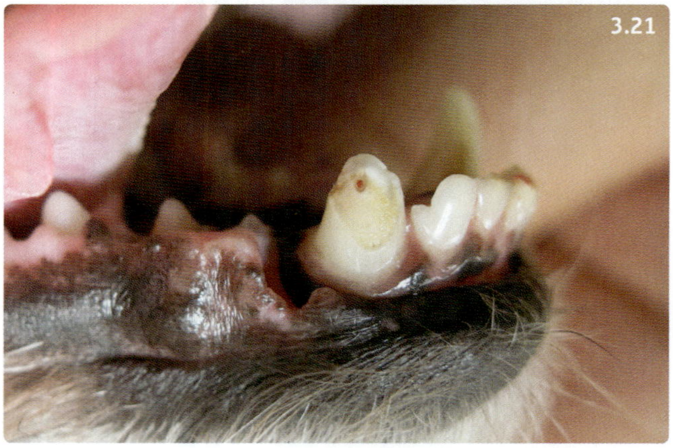

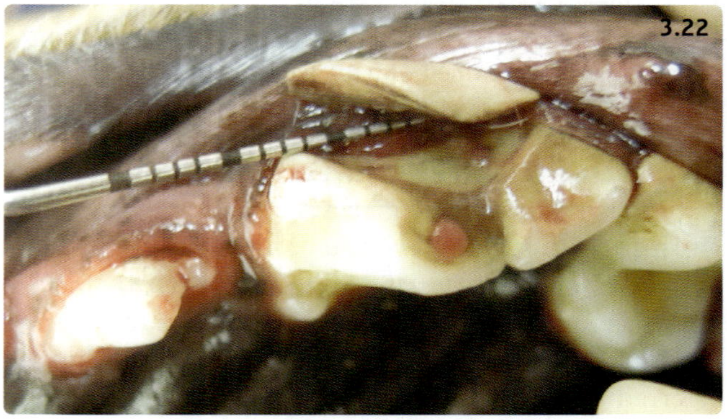

Figures 3.20–3.22 (3.20, 3.21) Complicated crown fractures of the right maxillary 4th premolar (108) and mandibular canine (404). Note the darkened, necrotic pulp and the explorer within the pulp cavity of 108 (3.20) and the fresh, hemorrhagic pulp of 104 (3.21). (3.22) This is a slab-type fracture of the left maxillary 4th premolar (208). This particular tooth has a complicated crown-root fracture, but slab fractures are very common in dogs and may be complicated or uncomplicated.

Pathophysiology

Enamel is the extremely hard, smooth, impervious substance covering the crowns of normal teeth. Underlying the enamel is dentin, a softer, rougher substance made up of dentinal tubules that lead directly to the dental pulp.

When a crown fractures and the pulp is exposed, it is initially exceedingly painful. In addition, an open path to the blood vessels and nerves of the tooth is created, leading quickly to pulpitis, infection, and pulp necrosis. Following pulp necrosis, bacterial invasion of the periapical area occurs, which may create systemic spread of the infection.

Uncomplicated crown fractures result in direct dentinal exposure, which is considered indirect pulp exposure, as the dentinal tubules contain extensions of the root canal system called odontoblasts. These fractures may also result in significant pain for the patient. Furthermore, there is an opportunity for eventual infection of the pulp through the dentinal tubules. How long that process takes is unknown and is likely affected by the amount of damage inflicted on the pulp and other tissues during the initial insult. Typically, the tooth will eventually respond to this exposure and seal off the tubules via tertiary dentin, but this process takes months and may not be effective. Finally, all fractures result in a roughened tooth surface increasing plaque adhesion and hastening the onset of periodontal disease.

Clinical presentation

If the inciting cause is significant traumatic impact (i.e. hit by car/fall), patients may be presented with other injuries (e.g. facial or jaw fractures, head trauma, pulmonary contusions, abdominal bleeding). These patients must be stabilized and treated appropriately prior to complete oral examination, assessment, and treatment. Owners may notice swelling or drainage in the area of the affected tooth, most commonly in the maxilla just ventral to the eye, but it may also occur in the ventral mandible.

The majority of the time tooth fractures are incidental findings, as pets very rarely show signs of oral pain. However, it is known that these conditions are very painful. Animals may present with some degree of pain, halitosis, reluctance to chew, or changes in eating behaviors (bear in mind that cats and dogs generally do not stop eating because of dental disease, except in very limited cases such as caudal stomatitis).

Differential diagnosis

Abrasive wear, attrition (tooth on tooth wear), developmental malformation, oral tumor.

Diagnosis

Fractured teeth are generally simple to diagnose on awake examination or incidentally during professional periodontal therapy. Freshly fractured teeth are identified by an abnormally shaped area of the tooth and a roughened surface (dentin) compared with the surrounding tooth (enamel) if uncomplicated, and by a central area of pink or red (pulp) if complicated (**Figure 3.21**).

Older fractures may be more difficult to identify if they have been covered in plaque and calculus. Pulp necrosis may be evident as a dark brown, gray, or black central area of the tooth in an older, complicated, crown fracture. Root fractures may not be apparent until sedated examination and radiographs are possible.

Management

All fractured teeth should be radiographed to evaluate for evidence of endodontic disease. Fractured deciduous teeth should be extracted urgently to prevent damage to the underlying permanent tooth bud. Uncomplicated crown fractures should be managed with bonded sealants if there is no radiographic evidence of endodontic disease and the pulp chamber cannot be accessed with a fine dental explorer. This will relieve the pain, block off the pathway of infection, and smooth the tooth. Crown/root fractures that are uncomplicated may be treated with bonded sealant if the gingiva is first repositioned apically so that the sealant does not extend below the gingival margin (**Figure 3.22**). Some root fractures may be managed with benign neglect if no portion of the fracture extends into the oral cavity, the tooth is stable, and there is no evidence of endodontic disease. Complicated crown fractures and uncomplicated crown fractures with evidence of endodontic disease on intraoral radiographs must be treated either with root canal therapy or by complete extraction. Root fractures and teeth treated with bonded sealants or root canal therapy must be rechecked radiographically at 9–12 months and annually thereafter. Toys and chews should be checked for hardness, in order to avoid risk of tooth fracture. Proper items should be easily indented with a fingernail. Owners must be warned about the causes of tooth fractures and changes implemented at home if fractures are secondary to chew toys, treats, or housing. The inciting cause should be removed and replaced with softer, less dangerous options if at all possible. Owners should also be counseled that bonded sealants are only effective for as long as they remain on the tooth; in other words, until the tooth breaks again. Referral to a veterinary dentist for crown placement should be considered, especially for working dogs and those extreme chewers that are at high risk for recurrent tooth fractures.

Prognosis

Early, appropriate treatment after complete examination, probing, and intraoral radiography provides the best outcome. Referral to a veterinary dental specialist for endodontic treatment, crown therapy or to manage complicated or multiple tooth fractures when necessary is recommended. Fractured teeth are painful to the patient, although they will not complain. Recovery from surgical extraction is approximately 2 weeks; recovery from endodontic treatment is nearly immediate (1–2 days). In either case, prognosis is very good if the pet receives timely, appropriate treatment.

TEMPOROMANDIBULAR JOINT LUXATION

Definition/overview

Temporomandibular joint (TMJ) luxation is usually a rostrodorsal displacement of the condylar process of the mandible from the articular surface of the mandibular fossa of the temporal bone. The TMJ may sometimes separate caudally, and this displacement is usually accompanied by a fracture of the retroarticular process.

Etiology/pathophysiology

TMJ luxation is uncommon in cats and rare in dogs. It is usually traumatic in nature. It is therefore also often accompanied by other oromaxillofacial injuries. It may also be a result of TMJ dysplasia or disease.

Clinical presentation

Patients often present with an open or dropped jaw appearance, an inability to close (or sometimes to open) the mouth, and lateral deviation of the lower jaw towards the side opposite the luxation. Joint pain, dysphagia, or ankylosis may accompany chronic TMJ luxations, as well as TMJ fractures or ramus fractures.

Differential diagnosis

Mandibular fracture, maxillary fracture, TMJ dysplasia/fracture, periodontal disease, foreign body, idiopathic trigeminal neuritis, craniomandibular osteopathy.

Diagnosis

The classical dropped jaw appearance and inability to close the mouth is suggestive, although this may also be seen with idiopathic trigeminal neuritis or bilateral caudal mandibular fracture. Properly positioned dorsoventral radiographs may show an increased TMJ space. CT is also useful to confirm the diagnosis. Radiographs should be exposed to evaluate for concurrent maxillary or mandibular fractures.

Management
Under general anesthesia, a fulcrum of an appropriate size for the patient (e.g. pencil, dowel, toothbrush, syringe) is placed between the maxillary fourth premolar and mandibular first molar teeth on the affected side and the mouth is gently forced closed to lever the condylar process back into the mandibular fossa. A return to normal dental occlusion is indicative of successful reduction. The joint should then be stabilized with a loose fitting nylon or tape muzzle, or with interarcade wiring for 1–2 weeks, especially if it easily reluxates. Unstable, refractory, or chronic luxations can be treated with open reduction and suture imbrication of the joint or, more commonly, with a condylectomy procedure.

Prognosis
Acute, uncomplicated luxations that are properly reduced and managed have a good prognosis. Those associated with chronicity, recurrence, underlying disease, dysplasia, or ramus fractures carry a less favorable prognosis and frequently result in condylectomy.

MAXILLOFACIAL/JAW FRACTURES

Definition/overview
Oromaxillofacial fractures are usually the result of traumatic injury but may also occur secondary to a pathologic process. In the case of trauma, patients may have significant injury to other body systems or other serious complications and should be stabilized prior to treatment for oromaxillofacial injury. Pathologic fractures can be difficult to treat because of issues related to delayed healing or underlying neoplastic or infectious conditions.

Etiology/pathophysiology
There is a wide variety of types and causes of maxillofacial and mandibular fractures. In the cat, symphyseal separation is the most common oral 'fracture' and mandibular ramus fractures are more common than those of the mandibular body. Fractures to the body of the mandible are most commonly seen in dogs and may be termed stable (**Figure 3.23a**) or unstable (**Figure 3.23b**) depending on the angle of the fracture line, with stable fractures running in a caudodorsal direction. The large muscles of the jaw insert at the caudal aspect of the mandible and compress the fragments of favorable fractures.

In the dog, mandibular ramus fractures are less common than either symphyseal separation or mandibular body fractures, and repair can be very difficult because of the large amount of overlying musculature. TMJ fractures are uncommon. Maxillary fractures are often minimally displaced because of the inherent stability of the maxilla. Midline palatal features are commonly a result of high-rise syndrome in cats. Like mandibular symphyseal separation, these are not true fractures, but a separation of the interincisive suture or the median palatine sutures. Pathologic fractures are not uncommonly seen and are usually the result of chronic, severe, untreated periodontal disease or, rarely, a neoplastic process.

Clinical presentation
Patients may present with an obvious malocclusion or fracture, particularly of the mandible, or with symphyseal separation. Swelling, pain, soft tissue trauma, and ptyalism are common. Inability to open or close the mouth may be noted. Maxillary fractures in particular may present more subtly, with minimal displacement.

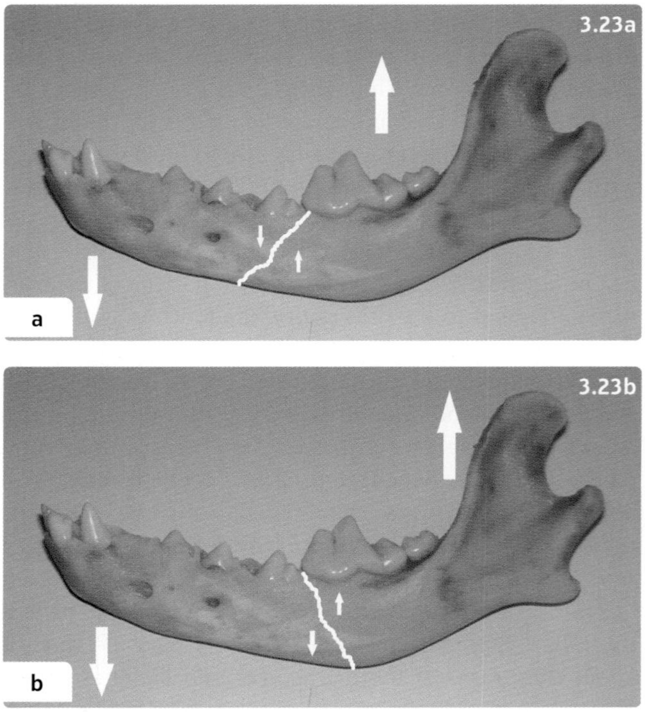

Figures 3.23a, b A left mandible demonstrating a stable (a) and an unstable (b) fracture line. The large white arrows indicate the directional pull of the masticatory muscles. Small white arrows illustrate the subsequent forces placed on the fracture line. In 3.23a, the muscular forces keep the fracture in place; in 3.23b, the unstable direction of the fracture leads to distraction of the fracture line.

In some patients, the maxillofacial or mandibular fracture is not noticed for a day or several days after the initial traumatic incident, when the owner notes that the animal is reluctant or unable to eat, drops food from the mouth, or is malodorous. Patients with pathologic jaw fractures tend to be nonpainful and often lack an obvious history of trauma. This is because the weakened bone took minimal force to fracture. Further, these fractures are typically seen in the areas of the mandibular first molars or canines of small and toy breed dogs. This is because their teeth are proportionally larger than those of large breed dogs and comprise a significant amount of the mandible.

Differential diagnosis

Trauma, severe periodontal disease, neoplasia, TMJ luxation, osteomyelitis, hypoparathyroidism (rare).

Diagnosis

Careful examination under sedation or general anesthesia (if the patient is stable) and intraoral and skull radiography may all be utilized to determine the exact nature and extent of the injury. Depending on presentation, thoracic and abdominal radiographs, abdominal ultrasound, or CT may be indicated as well as CBC/chemistry panel/urinalysis, T4, and parathyroid hormone level. Histopathology and bacterial culture and sensitivity may also be warranted in unusual cases.

Pathologic jaw fractures require intraoral dental radiographs to properly diagnose and treat. The subtle loss of bone is often not seen on skull radiographs. The classic appearance of a pathologic fracture is one located at the mandibular first molar or canine in a small breed dog with associated periodontal disease.

Management

Symphyseal separation can generally be treated with simple circumferential wire stabilization. Generally, mandibular body fractures are best repaired with intraoral splinting and either interdental or interosseous wiring techniques to recreate proper occlusion of the teeth. However, unstable or comminuted fractures often require greater fixation. Plates and external fixation techniques are occasionally indicated, but great care must be taken to avoid damaging tooth roots and neurovascular structures. Fractures of the mandibular ramus, condylar, coronoid, and angular processes are usually managed conservatively due to the great difficulty in performing internal repair. Many of these fractures are managed by interarch bonding or with loose nylon muzzles for 2–3 weeks (if a unilateral fracture dorsal to the condylar process) or 4–5 weeks (if below the condylar process). Maxillary fractures are often minimally displaced and more stable than mandibular fractures, and so require no more than digital reduction and soft tissue repair. However, more significant fractures require reduction and stabilization (typically an acrylic splint).

Pathologic jaw fractures carry a guarded prognosis for healing due to the lack of remaining bone, the low oxygen tension in the area, and the difficulty in rigidly fixating the caudal mandible. It is important to realize that a pathologic fracture will not heal (no matter how good the fixation is) if the diseased tooth root is not removed from the area of the fracture line. This is because a diseased root acts as a nidus of infection, which prevents healing. Extraction of the diseased root associated with the area of fracture is necessary, but unfortunately creates a large defect in the bone, which makes alignment more challenging and increases healing time.

Prognosis

Oromaxillofacial fractures often occur concurrently with other serious injuries and patients must be well stabilized prior to treatment of maxillary or mandibular fractures. Malocclusion is a serious potential complication of oromaxillofacial fracture and repair Invasive fixation methods are only rarely necessary and often result in further damage to surrounding oral structures such as teeth and neurovascular tissues. There is a concern with mandibular ramus fractures for callus formation, which results in restriction of normal jaw movement. In addition, there is often damage to teeth during the initial insult that may not be immediately apparent. Recheck examination and radiographs are always indicated for jaw fractures.

Pathologic fractures caused by severe periodontal disease or neoplastic processes carry a guarded prognosis. These can be extremely difficult if not impossible to repair and, especially in the case of neoplasia, often result in mandibulectomy or maxillectomy. The underlying cause of any pathologic fracture must be investigated and addressed prior to attempting fixation. Stabilization or fixation of fractures caused by neoplastic processes should not be attempted; mandibulectomy, maxillectomy, radiation, and/or chemotherapy may be appropriate in such situations. Consultation with a veterinary dentist, surgeon, and/or oncologist is recommended.

ORAL MASSES AND NEOPLASIA

Definition/overview

Oral masses are quite common in dogs and cats. In fact, the oral cavity is the fourth most common location for a tumor/neoplasm in the body in both canine and feline patients. Oral masses may be either benign or malignant. Like masses elsewhere, gross examination is generally insufficient for accurate diagnosis. All oral masses, no matter how small, should be biopsied and evaluated histopathologically. While most oral masses are benign, aggressive neoplasms are fairly common in the oral cavity.

Etiology

Oral tumors may be odontogenic or nonodontogenic, but a true etiology is unknown in most cases. An exception is canine squamous cell carcinoma (SCC), which is frequently associated with papillomavirus.

Clinical presentation

Presentation is variable depending on the type of tumor. Many masses are found incidentally during routine oral examination. Others may be erosive or ulcerated and secondarily infected or inflamed, causing discomfort, dysphagia, halitosis, or ptyalism.

Differential diagnosis

Gingival hyperplasia (enlargement), granuloma, dentigerous cyst, abscess, eosinophilic granuloma.

Diagnosis

Intraoral dental radiographs and histopathology are required for accurate diagnosis of any oral mass. Palpable lymph nodes should be aspirated or excised in cases of malignant neoplasia. If cytopathology or histopathology is consistent with malignancy, standard clinical staging should be performed, including 3-view thoracic radiography, CBC, chemistry panel, urinalysis, +/- abdominal ultrasound.

Management

In general, surgical excision is the treatment of choice, with required margins (see below) and follow-up chemotherapy or radiation treatment dependent on histopathologic diagnosis.

Prognosis

Prognosis for benign tumors is excellent with adequate surgical resection. Malignant oral tumors may have a good prognosis if diagnosed and definitively treated very early. Advanced malignancies carry a poor to grave prognosis even with radical surgical excision and chemo or radiation therapy. (**Note:** Individual tumor types are discussed below.)

PERIPHERAL ODONTOGENIC FIBROMA/FOCAL FIBROUS HYPERPLASIA (PREVIOUSLY TERMED EPULIS)

Epulis is not a diagnosis, but a clinical description that includes neoplasia, fibromas, and odontogenic tumors. It refers to any swelling of the gingiva. Peripheral odontogenic fibroma is a benign neoplasm, previously classified as fibromatous or ossifying epulis. These are slow growing and usually found around maxillary premolars. They exhibit no evidence of bony involvement on radiographs but may show mineralized areas. The majority of gingival growths are histopathologically focal fibrous hyperplasia, frequently seen in Boxers. Marginal surgical excision of the tumor is generally curative.

ACANTHOMATOUS AMELOBLASTOMA

Previously known as acanthomatous epulis, these masses are now termed canine or peripheral acanthomatous ameloblastoma (**Figure 3.24**). They most often occur around the incisors in large breed dogs and are fleshy and proliferative masses. These tumors are locally aggressive but do not metastasize. Radiographs typically reveal local bone infiltration and tooth displacement. Since local recurrence with marginal excision is common, wide (0.5–1 cm of normal tissue) surgical excision is recommended. Another treatment option is radiation therapy, which has a 90% control rate.

PAPILLOMATOSIS

These are generally pedunculated or cauliflower-like in appearance and white, gray, or flesh colored. Further, their appearance is benign mucosal thickening with finger-like projections. They may be solitary or multiple. They are of viral origin (papillomavirus), with a 2–6-month incubation, and are spread usually through direct, but sometimes indirect, contact. Generally self-limiting, they resolve in weeks to months and the patient is generally immune in the future. They are only cause for concern if they are large enough to interfere with mastication, are infected, or inflamed. They can mimic more aggressive tumors and there are reports of transformation to SCC. No treatment is usually recommended; however, atypical appearance, failure to regress in the expected time period, and infection all are indications for excisional biopsy and

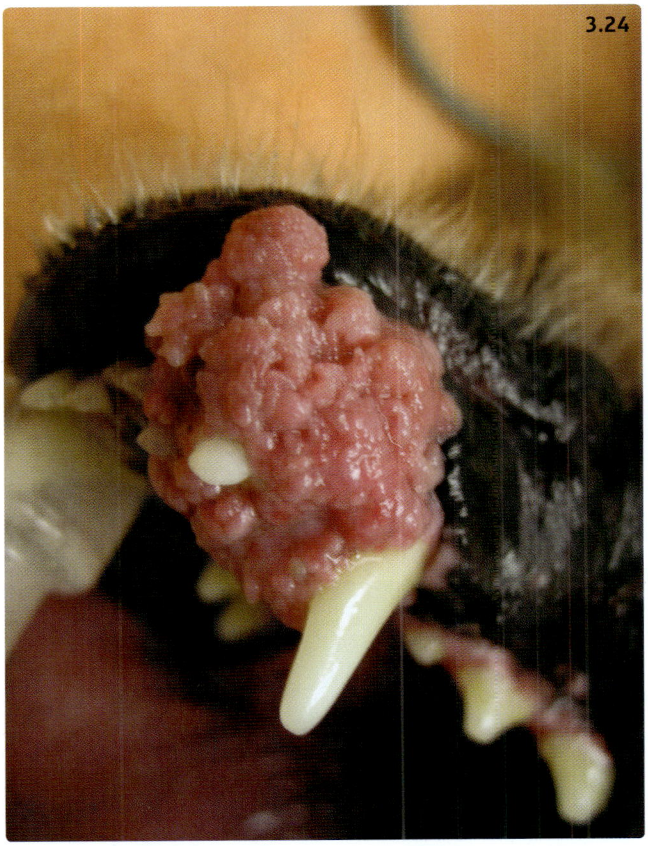

Figure 3.24 Acanthomatous ameloblastoma associated with the maxillary left 3rd incisor (203) and affecting the second incisor (202) and canine tooth (204).

histopathology. Removal may also be indicated if they are large enough to interfere with mastication. Excision may be accomplished with standard sharp excision, cryosurgery, electrocautery, or laser surgery. Vaccination, traumatic crushing, and chemotherapy have also been utilized, but are generally no longer recommended.

ORAL MALIGNANT MELANOMA

Oral malignant melanoma (OMM) **(Figure 3.25)** is the most common malignant oral cavity tumor in dogs. They may be pigmented or amelanotic and are highly aggressive, with early metastasis to lymph nodes (less frequently to lungs and other organs). Palpable lymph nodes should be aspirated or excised at the time of diagnosis. Standard clinical staging after confirmatory cytopathologic or histopathologic diagnosis (3-view thoracic radiographs, CBC, chemistry panel, urinalysis, +/- abdominal ultrasound) should be performed prior to wide surgical excision (2–3 cm normal tissue). Follow-up chemotherapy, immunotherapy, or radiation therapy may also be

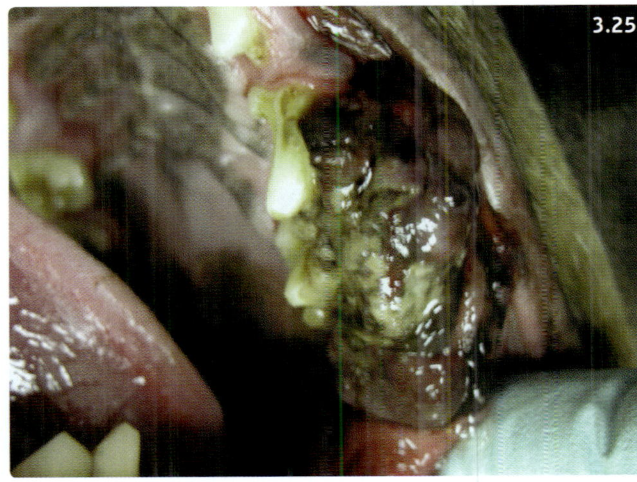

Figure 3.25 Malignant melanoma affecting the left maxillary 4th premolar and molar teeth of a dog. Note the irregular, pigmented appearance. These are highly aggressive tumors that may or may not be pigmented.

indicated, as distant dissemination of disease is common, as is local recurrence. If complete resection is not possible, radiation therapy should be considered as a primary treatment. Prognosis is generally poor, but a fair to good response may be achieved with early diagnosis and aggressive treatment and follow up.

FIBROSARCOMA

This is a malignant mesenchymal tumor, most often seen in young (4–5-year-old) large breed dogs and older (~8-year-old) small breed dogs. Fibrosarcomas are locally invasive with a high postsurgical recurrence rate. Prognosis is variable, depending on location, size, grade, and stage at time of diagnosis. The maxilla is the most common site. This tumor can present as an innocuous, lobulated, sessile mass or, alternatively, as a rapidly growing, hemorrhagic, ulcerated lesion. They are often noted at dental margins and the palate, but may also originate from nasal cartilages and the lateral surface of the maxilla or palate. Well-differentiated masses are best treated with wide surgical excision (2 cm margin). Poorly differentiated tumors require radical excision and postoperative radiation treatment.

A subcategory of fibrosarcoma, termed histologically low-grade, biologically high-grade, is most common in large breed dogs, particularly Golden Retrievers. These tumors are characterized by rapid growth, bony invasion, and high metastatic potential. Treatment for these tumors has not yet been optimized and local recurrence is very common.

SQUAMOUS CELL CARCINOMA

SCC (**Figure 3.26**) is the most common oral neoplasm in cats and the second most common in dogs. These are large, locally aggressive tumors that exhibit lymph node and lung metastasis late in the course of disease. Feline maxillary and lingual SCC carries a poor prognosis, mandibular tumors a somewhat better prognosis, and rostral mandibular locations a fair prognosis. Cure is possible with very early lesions and wide surgical excisions. Papillomavirus DNA has been frequently associated with canine oral SCC. These are erosive, fleshy lesions and with local bony invasion dental displacement may occur. There may be chronic, nonhealing ulcers of the associated skin. Wide surgical excision (2 cm) is recommended, including glossectomy for dogs with lingual tumors. Radiation treatment may be considered for local control or palliation, but is fairly ineffective in cats. Chemotherapy is also an option for microscopic disease.

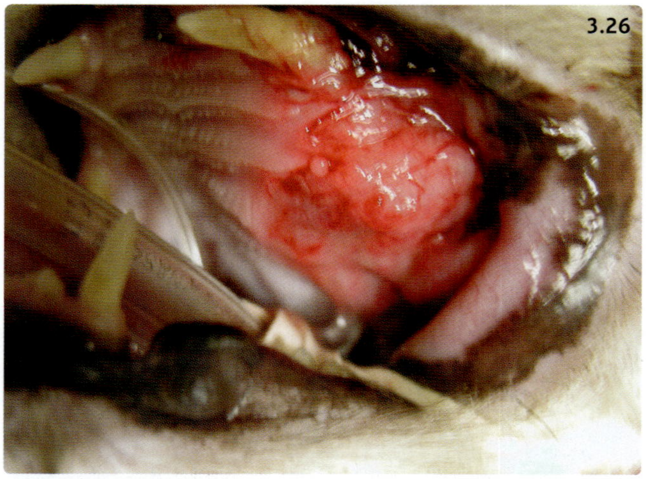

Figure 3.26 Squamous cell sarcoma in the left maxilla of a cat.

OSTEOSARCOMA

Osteosarcoma (OSA) may occur in either the mandible or maxilla. It is much less common in cats than in dogs. These tumors are locally aggressive, but have less metastatic potential than appendicular OSA. Mandibular OSA carries a more favorable prognosis than maxillary, with a reported median survival time of 7 months, whereas the median survival of maxillary OSA is 5 months. It may be identified as a fleshy expansile mass that may or may not be ulcerative in the early stages. The significant tissue destruction and locally aggressive bony swelling frequently lead to subsequent facial swelling and may be associated with pain and discomfort on opening or closing the mouth. Wide or radical surgical excision is recommended depending on stage, and radiation treatment should be considered for microscopic disease.

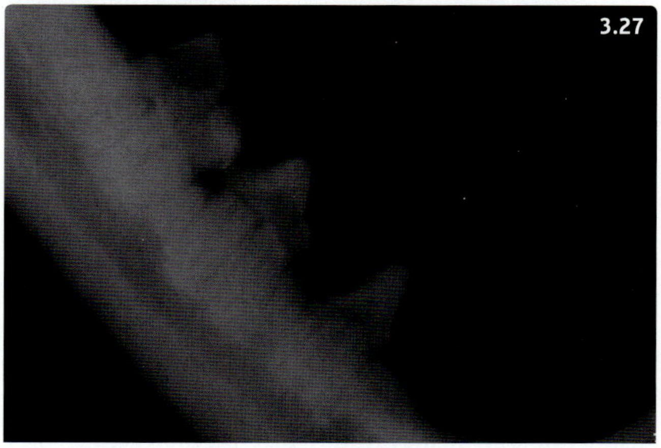

Figure 3.27 Radiograph of the right mandible of a cat, demonstrating type 1 tooth resorption in all three teeth. Note the varying degrees of lucency, most obvious in the molar tooth (409). Complete extraction of crowns and all roots is the recommended treatment.

TOOTH RESORPTION

Definition/overview

Previously called neck lesions, cervical line lesions, feline odontoclastic resorptive lesions, and several other names, these lesions are currently referred to as tooth resorptions (TRs). They represent noncarious odontoclastic destruction of teeth. There are two types of feline TR: type 1 and type 2. Type 1 resorptions do not result in the replacement of roots by bone (**Figure 3.27**) while in type 2 resorptions, the lost root structure is replaced by bone (**Figure 3.28**). An individual tooth may exhibit both type 1 and type 2 resorption, and is then classified as type 3.

TR typically begins externally, and may occur in the crowns, roots, or both (see **Table 3.2** for AVDC classification). TR occurs in dogs and humans, but is most commonly seen in cats and may represent different disease processes or etiologies in the different species. (**Note:** Internal resorption can also occur, but is rare and more common in dogs than cats.)

Etiology

Although there are several theories, the cause of tooth resorption remains unknown. Different theories have suggested either excess levels of dietary vitamin D or that feline teeth were not developed to masticate hard, dry kibble diets, leading to abfraction injuries (see below). Type 1 TRs in cats are more commonly associated with oral

3.28

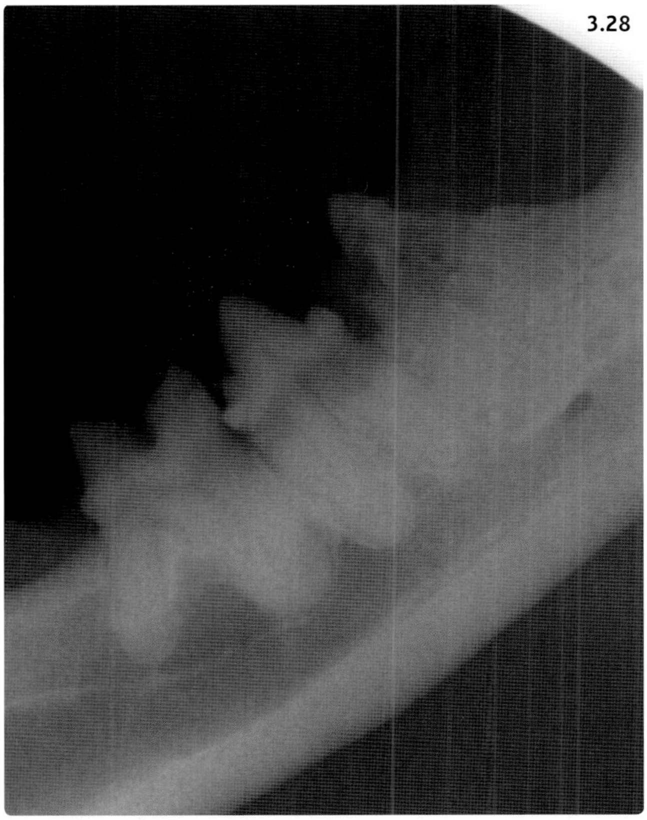

Figure 3.28 Type 2 tooth resorption in the right mandibular 3rd premolar of a cat. Note the lack of a visible periodontal ligament and how the roots have an appearance similar to that of the surrounding bone.

inflammation (gingivitis, periodontitis, or stomatitis) than are type 2, but no clear cause and effect has been shown. Type 2 TRs are not as commonly associated with significant oral inflammation, but the lesion itself may create mild gingivitis. Neither form of TR has been shown to be related to the retroviral status of cats. In humans, abfraction (lateral forces that result in microflexure of the crown of the tooth) is a proposed cause of TR and although not proven, this could also be a cause of TR in cats and other species.

Pathophysiology

As stated above, type 1 TRs are typically associated with oral inflammation, especially in younger cats. There is an increasing likelihood for developing TRs (especially type 2) with age. Odontoclastic destruction of cementum usually begins in the apical third of the root and generally extends into dentin. The dentinal destruction may eventually extend under the enamel and undermine it, at which point the enamel flakes off exposing the underlying dentin. This creates a significantly painful area of exposed tooth structure. Clinically, they are generally first noticed in the area of the cementoenamel junction. The tooth structure is damaged and eventually weakened to a point at which the crown of the tooth fractures, leaving roots behind. In type 1 lesions these roots have intact endodontic systems and can create pain and/or infection, whereas in type 2 lesions the roots have partially or completely been replaced by bone. In cases of complete replacement by bone, they are known as 'ghost roots'.

Table 3.2 American Veterinary Dental College Tooth Resorption Classification.

Tooth resorptions are classified by radiographic type as well as stage of resorption:

- **Type 1.** Focal or multifocal radiolucency is present in the tooth with otherwise normal radiopacity and normal periodontal ligament space.
- **Type 2.** Radiographic narrowing or disappearance of the periodontal ligament space in at least some areas and decreased radiopacity of part of the tooth.
- **Type 3.** Radiographic features of both type 1 and type 2 are present in the same tooth. A tooth with this appearance has areas of normal and narrow or lost periodontal ligament space, and there is focal or multifocal radiolucency in the tooth and decreased radiopacity in other areas of the tooth.

- **Stage 1.** Mild dental hard tissue loss (cementum or cementum and enamel).
- **Stage 2.** Moderate dental hard tissue loss (cementum or cementum and enamel with loss of dentin that does not extend to the pulp cavity).
- **Stage 3.** Deep dental hard tissue loss (cementum or cementum and enamel with loss of dentin that extends to the pulp cavity); most of the tooth retains its integrity.
- **Stage 4.** Extensive dental hard tissue loss (cementum or cementum and enamel with loss of dentin that extends to the pulp cavity); most of the tooth has lost its integrity:
  - **Stage 4a.** Crown and root are equally affected.
  - **Stage 4b.** Crown is more severely affected than the root.
  - **Stage 4c.** Root is more severely affected than the crown.
- **Stage 5.** Remnants of dental hard tissue are visible only as irregular radiopacities and gingival covering is complete.

It is possible that type 1 TRs are an early form of type 2 and that some type 1 lesions may progress to type 2 resorptions. However, the exact cause of TR is unknown at this time. In cats, it has also been proposed that type 2 lesions commonly seen in their canine teeth may not be related to inflammation, but rather to ankylosis and age-related bone replacement.

Clinical presentation

Type 1 lesions are often, but not always, accompanied by oral inflammation (gingivitis, stomatitis, and/or periodontal disease). In both type 1 and type 2 resorptions there is often an associated area of gingival enlargement, which may or may not be inflamed, that covers or fills the lacuna that results from the resorption (**Figures 3.29, 3.30**). Cats typically show no clinical signs even with advanced lesions, but they rarely may exhibit pain, dysphagia, decreased appetite, halitosis, depression, or other signs. (**Note:** One author [ER] has treated a cat whose only clinical sign was inappropriate urination that resolved with definitive treatment of the TR.) The mandibular 3rd premolars are often the first teeth affected, but TRs can occur in any tooth. Cats with one/any TR are at increased risk for developing future lesions. Dogs may present for pain or suspected tooth fracture or resorptions, but typically TRs are incidental findings during routine dental prophylaxis or intraoral radiographs.

Differential diagnosis

Gingivitis or periodontitis (without resorption), bone loss/furcation exposure in multirooted teeth, gingival hyperplasia or mass, fractured tooth, caries.

Diagnosis

Visual examination and subgingival exploration are often sufficient for identifying a clinical TR. However, intraoral radiography is essential for proper classification of the type and stage of the lesion and appropriate therapy planning, as well as finding incipient subgingival lesions.

Management

Extraction is the treatment of choice for TR. Crown amputation is only appropriate for type 2 lesions under the following conditions:

- No evidence of caudal stomatitis.
- No clinical or radiographic evidence of periodontal disease in the area of the root to be left.

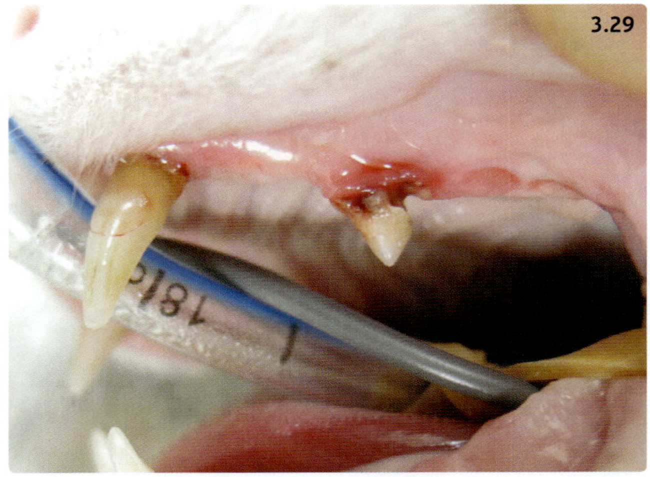

Figure 3.29 Tooth resorption of the left maxillary 3rd premolar (207) in a cat. Although the mandibular 3rd premolar is the most common location for tooth resorptions, they may occur in any tooth.

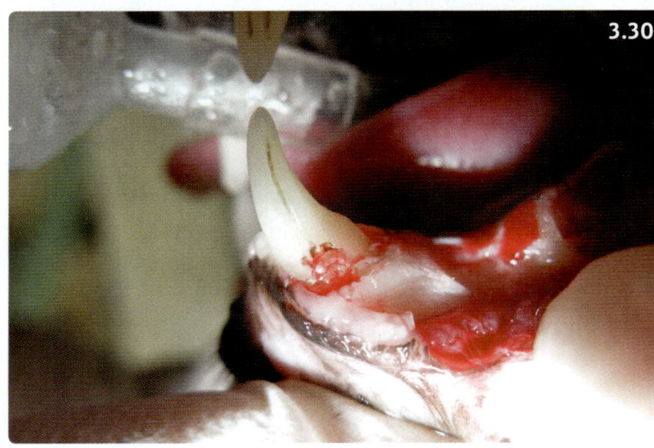

Figure 3.30 Tooth resorption in the left mandibular canine tooth (304) of a cat.

- No identifiable tooth root structure, periodontal ligament, or root canal.
- There must be no evidence of endodontic disease.

If any of these criteria are not met, complete extraction is required. This may be very difficult due to root ankylosis. Radiographs must be obtained prior to and following extraction or crown amputation. Resorption that is completely subgingival and does not extend into the oral cavity may be monitored if there is no evidence of periodontal or endodontic disease, no stomatitis, and the patient is not showing clinical signs of pain, dysphagia, or inappetence. While there are no studies to this effect, crown amputation may be recommended for extremely advanced cases of TR in dogs. However, if at all possible, teeth and roots should be removed completely and complete extraction verified radiographically.

Prognosis

With appropriate diagnosis and treatment prognosis is good. However, animals with a single TR lesion are at greater risk of developing lesions in other teeth. Some cats require full or near full mouth extractions to alleviate their discomfort.

FELINE CAUDAL STOMATITIS

Definition/overview

Stomatitis refers to inflammation and proliferation of the oral mucosa, while gingivitis more specifically refers to inflammation and proliferation of the gingival tissues. Gingivostomatitis is a clinical descriptive term, while lymphoplasmacytic stomatitis is the histopathologic diagnosis most commonly associated with this condition. It may range from mild to severe and generally increases with chronicity. The current terminology for this condition is caudal stomatitis, which is when the inflammation extends to the caudal oral tissues (caudal mucositis).

Etiology

The cause of caudal stomatitis is unknown, and is possibly multifactorial. Suggested inciting causes or cofactors include an exaggerated inflammatory response to plaque, viral infection (particularly calicivirus), *Bartonella henselae* infection, and altered immune status.

Pathophysiology

Feline calicivirus (FCV) has been isolated from cats with caudal stomatitis and cats exhibiting signs of the disease are more likely to be shedding FCV and feline herpesvirus-1 (FHV-1) from the oral mucosa. However, there is no evidence that FCV causes caudal stomatitis. Additional research is being done to more fully understand the role of FCV in chronic caudal stomatitis. Neither are FIV and FeLV implicated directly in cases of caudal stomatitis, but infection with either virus may contribute to its development in individual cats. While cats that are positive for FIV and *B. henselae* exhibit increased levels of mandibular lymphadenopathy and gingivitis compared with noninfected cats, *B. henselae* is not currently believed to be a significant contributing factor in caudal stomatitis. An exaggerated response to bacterial plaque has been speculated to play a role in this disease, as cats with chronic caudal stomatitis exhibit significantly lower salivary IgA and higher serum IgA, IgG, and IgM levels than healthy cats. It has been proposed that the decreased salivary IgA in affected cats may have a contributing role in the development of chronic caudal stomatitis.

Clinical presentation

It is not uncommon for affected cats to present for anorexia (complete or partial), dysphagia, pain, and ptyalism. They may also exhibit halitosis, pawing at the mouth, weight loss, vocalization, and an unkempt appearance due to lack of grooming (**Figure 3.31**). Paws and perioral areas may be stained with saliva, blood, and/or purulent material. Affected cats may have undergone behavior changes, becoming either more aggressive or more withdrawn than usual. Chronic caudal stomatitis is the oral disease most likely to result in anorexia. These patients are often extremely painful and oral examination may prove very difficult, as opening the mouth can cause great discomfort. If oral examination is possible, the practitioner may note varying amounts of tissue inflammation, ulceration, and proliferation. The key clinical sign that differentiates this condition from periodontal disease is the caudal location of the stomatitis (**Figure 3.32**).

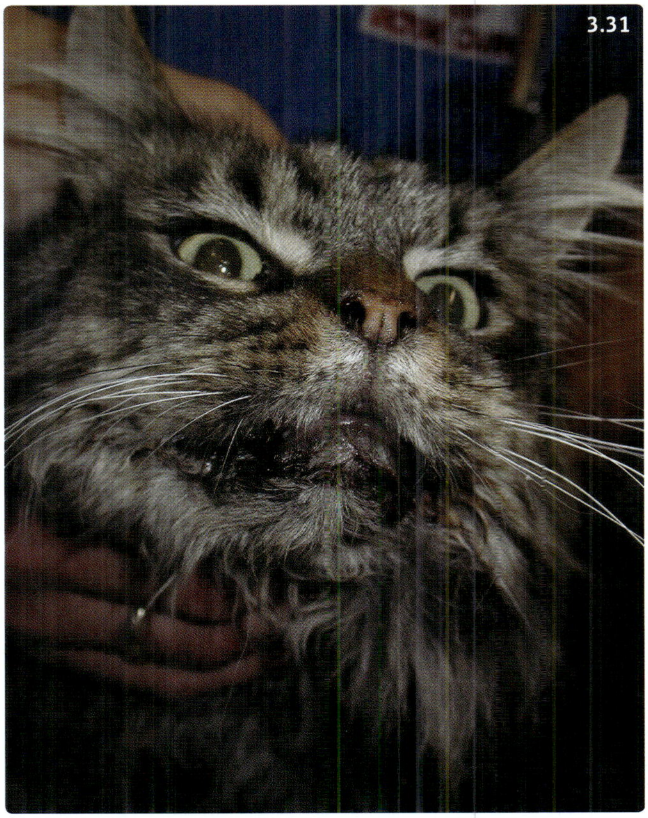
3.31

Figure 3.31 A cat with caudal stomatitis. Note the excessive ptyalism and unkempt coat.

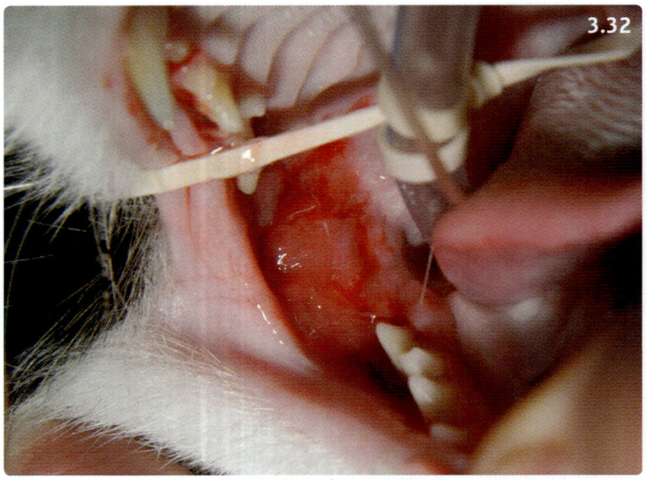

Figure 3.32 Caudal stomatitis in a cat. The severe erythema and inflammation in this area is pathognomic for this condition.

Differential diagnosis

Neoplasia (especially SCC), periodontal disease, eosinophilic granuloma complex (EGC), autoimmune disease, foreign body mucosal entrapment.

Diagnosis

As described above, caudal stomatitis represents a clinical syndrome rather than a specific etiology or diagnosis. Therefore, diagnosis of caudal stomatitis is primarily a clinical one, based on visual identification and testing for underlying contributing factors. A thorough visual examination under anesthesia, as well as dental radiographs to identify any retained root tips, periodontal disease, or any bony changes consistent with neoplasia, is crucial. In addition, CBC and blood chemistry screening, including retroviral testing for FeLV and FIV status, are all indicated. Hyperglobulinemia may be present as a result of chronic antigenic stimulation. Testing for FCV and *B. henselae* may also be considered, but is not generally recommended. In addition, biopsies for histopathology should be collected if there is asymmetry in inflammation or ulceration, a nonclassical appearance to the inflammation, or if radiographs are suspicious for neoplasia.

Management

The goal of treatment is complete resolution of the oral inflammation. It has now been fairly well established that prolonged medical treatment with extensive or chronic use of steroids or NSAIDs results in poorer long-term responses than when early, aggressive surgical treatment is performed. Many if not most cats will respond best if all teeth and tooth remnants caudal to the canines are removed early in the course of the disease. Extraction of the canine and incisor teeth should also be considered, especially if the inflammation extends to the gingiva covering them. Aggressive management of periodontal disease is vital to treatment success. Some veterinary dentists are advocating CO_2 laser ablation of proliferative tissues following caudal mouth extractions; however, there is minimal research to support this procedure at this time. Patients may require some medical therapy with steroids or NSAIDs during the course of treatment, but these drugs are not a replacement for aggressive tooth extractions. Esterified fatty acid complex supplements have also shown some promise.

Prognosis

Extraction of all teeth and tooth remnants caudal to the canines (or full mouth extractions if canine and incisor teeth are clinically abnormal) results in improvement in approximately 80% of affected cats. Of these, about 20% still show some signs of inflammation, but do not appear to be in pain. The remaining 20% require additional care, which may include laser or surgical ablation, interferon therapy (used often in Europe, but not widely available in the USA), or medical therapy (typically cyclosporine, but also possibly steroids, NSAIDs, or fatty acid supplementation [1-TDC]). (**Key point:** Early tooth extractions are indicated. Prolonged, repeated use of steroids not only has many undesirable side-effects, it also decreases the likelihood of resolution and worsens outcomes.)

EOSINOPHILIC GRANULOMA COMPLEX

Definition/overview

EGC is, as the name suggests, a group of conditions that share a common etiology and some histopathological features. Seen most frequently in cats, EGC can also occur in dogs (Cavalier King Charles Spaniels, Siberian Huskies, and Malamutes in particular).

Etiology

The true etiology remains unknown, but it is suspected to be a hypersensitivity or immune-mediated reaction. Most likely EGC occurs in response to flea and/or food allergy or atopy. However, it should be noted that lesions have also been found in cases where infectious and allergic diseases have been essentially ruled out. Finally, there may be a genetic predisposition to EGC.

Pathophysiology

Inflammation and necrosis are seen and thought to be the result of the inflammatory agents released by accumulations of eosinophils in the lesions.

Clinical presentation

The most common presentation is an indolent or rodent ulcer seen as a reddish brown lesion at the philtrum or around the maxillary canine teeth (**Figure 3.33**). Indolent ulcers may be uni- or bilateral, and females appear to be overrepresented. Linear granulomas (**Figure 3.34**) are the second most common presentation and may be single or multiple. They are typically found on the lips, tongue, gingiva, and palate, but can occur in any location in the mouth. These granulomas are yellow–pink, lobulated, raised masses and are generally nonpainful, although they may become secondarily infected and/or ulcerated. Occasionally, they can severely damage oral mucosa and even bone. There are reported cases of severe periodontal disease, oronasal fistulas, and even pathologic fractures as a result of eosinophilic granulomas. These lesions should not be taken lightly and should be on the differential list for any aggressive appearing oral lesion. Another manifestation of EGC is the collagenolytic granuloma, a firmly swollen rostral mandibular lip lesion most commonly seen in young female cats. Eosinophilic plaques may also be found (rarely) in the oral cavity, where they appear much like a linear granuloma. These are more commonly seen as a dermatologic lesion. In fact, oral EGC very often occurs concurrently with dermatologic manifestations of the syndrome.

Differential diagnosis

Neoplasia; gingival hyperplasia; uremic stomatitis; immune-mediated disease; trauma; periodontal disease; thermal, electric and chemical burns; foreign body mucosal entrapment.

Diagnosis

A minimum data base (CBC, biochemical profile, urinalysis) should be obtained to rule out underlying disease. Histopathology should be performed to confirm the diagnosis. A thorough allergy evaluation (diet trial, serum, or intradermal testing) should be performed on histologic confirmation.

Management

Treatment is directed at the underlying cause of the disease, generally by controlling allergies. This may include strict flea control, hypoallergenic diets, and short-term (for acute control) steroids, but most often long-term medical management is with cyclosporine or corticosteroids. Cyclosporine has proven effective for therapy of oral eosinophilic diseases and a veterinary product is approved for use in dogs and cats for allergic disease. Weaning to the lowest effective dose at the longest interval that provides patient relief and disease control is recommended. Surgical removal has been occasionally successful, including cryosurgery and laser surgery. Finally, radiation therapy has been used in some cases.

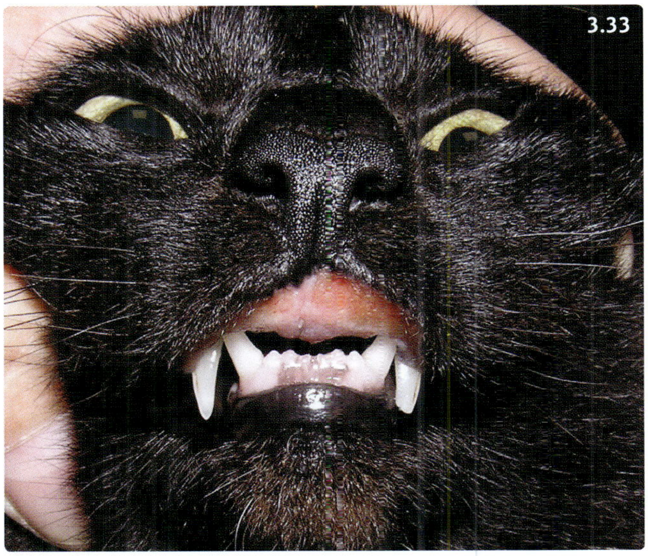

Figure 3.33 Typical 'rodent ulcer.' This lesion is pathognomonic for eosinophilic granuloma complex in a cat.

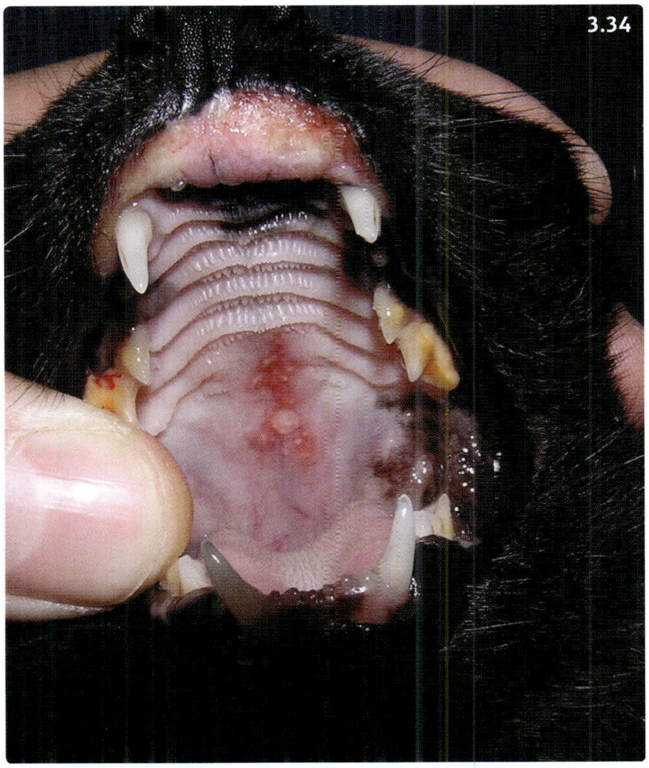

Figure 3.34 Palatal linear granuloma associated with eosinophilic granuloma complex. A rodent ulcer is also visible at the rostral maxillary lip. This is the same cat as in Figure 3.33.

RECOMMENDED FURTHER READING

Bellows J (2010) *Feline Dentistry: Oral Assessment, Treatment, and Preventative Care*. Wiley-Blackwell, Ames.

Niemiec BA (2010) *Small Animal Dental, Oral and Maxillofacial Disease: A Colour Handbook*. Manson Publishing, London.

Niemiec BA (2010) *Veterinary Endodontics*. Practical Veterinary Publishing, Tustin.

Niemiec BA (2012) *Veterinary Orthodontics*. Practical Veterinary Publishing, Tustin.

Niemiec BA (2013) *Veterinary Periodontology*. Wiley-Blackwell, Ames.

Niemiec BA (2014) *Veterinary Restorative Dentistry for the General Practitioner*. Practical Veterinary Publishing, Tustin.

Verstraete FJ (2012) *Oral and Maxillofacial Surgery in Dogs and Cats*. Saunders Elsevier, St. Louis.

Chapter 4

Respiratory disorders

Cécile Clercx

INTRODUCTION

Respiratory diseases are common clinical problems in small animal practice. Some are readily diagnosed on the basis of history and clinical signs while others can prove difficult to diagnose. Upper airways generally refer to the nasal cavities and frontal sinuses, naso- and laryngopharynx, larynx, and extrathoracic trachea, while lower airways include organs inside the thoracic cage, including (1) the intrathoracic part of the trachea, the airways or 'conducting pipes' (i.e. the bronchi and bronchioli) and (2) the lung parenchyma, composed of functional units (i.e. the alveoli, surrounded by capillaries, where gas exchange takes place, and interstitial tissue). Pleural disorders, and diseases involving other intrathoracic organs, such as the heart and vessels, and mediastinal organs will cause clinical signs similar to those encountered in parenchymal diseases.

Clinical history is of great importance since a good description of the complaints can help determine the segment of the respiratory tree involved. A physical examination is essential and will often be very helpful in the diagnosis of upper airway diseases, while in respiratory diseases of intrathoracic origin, diagnosis is much more challenging and several ancillary diagnostic tests, mainly imaging, will always be needed.

The clinical signs encountered in disorders of the different affected areas are summarized in **Table 4.1**.

UPPER AIRWAY DISORDERS

NASAL, SINUS, AND/OR NASOPHARYNGEAL DISORDERS

Nasal, sinus, and/or nasopharyngeal diseases will be presented together since differentiation, based on clinical signs alone, is challenging and because in most diseases all three regions can be involved. Although the clinical signs (e.g. sneezing, discharge, reverse sneezing, stertor) localize the disease to this area, confirmation of the etiology depends on additional diagnostic tests, primarily imaging (mainly CT) and rhinoscopy (direct and retrograde). Direct rhinoscopy can be performed using a rigid scope (**Figures 4.1a. b**), but investigation of the frontal sinus and nasopharynx usually requires a flexible endoscope (**Figures 4.2a, b**). These procedures require general anesthesia. When CT is indicated, it should precede rhinoscopy, if performed during the same anesthetic procedure. During rhinoscopy, other procedures, such as brushing, biopsies, nasal lavage, and sampling for microbiologic examination, can be performed.

Disorders of the nasal cavities must be differentiated from nasal planum (planum nasale) disorders. Indeed, some disorders of the nasal cavities induce changes on the nasal planum (e.g. hyperkeratosis, erosions, and ulcerations, together with local oozing or bleeding) that can be confused with nasal discharge. However, diseases of the nasal cavities are often accompanied by sneezing and discharge coming from inside the nasal cavity. These include skin or mucocutaneous junction disorders (e.g. tumors, immune-mediated diseases, or leishmaniasis), which can be associated with coagulopathy in addition to being associated with epistaxis unrelated to coagulopathy. In these cases, a full clinical examination must be performed before considering other diagnostic procedures such as rhinoscopy, nasal/ sinus radiographs, or CT under anesthesia.

Stenosis of the nares (**Figure 4.3**) causes a decrease in the intranasal opening, resulting in a stertorous breathing during normal attempts to breathe. This pathology is encountered mainly in brachycephalic breeds of dogs and is often associated with the clinical signs reported in dogs with brachycephalic airway obstructive syndrome (BAOS) (see below). If stenosis of the nares is encountered alone, which is uncommon, the noisy respiration can be associated with some degree of serous nasal discharge.

MYCOTIC RHINOSINUSITIS (DOGS)

Definition/overview

Sinonasal aspergillosis (SNA) is a common disease and affects between 12% and 34% of dogs evaluated for chronic sinonasal disease. The term 'nasal aspergillosis', which was used in the past to describe this condition, is better replaced

Table 4.1 Clinical signs in respiratory tract diseases.

	Major signs	Less common signs
Upper airway disorders		
Nasal cavities, sinuses, nasopharynx	Sneezing Nasal discharge Reverse sneezing Alterations of the nasal plane Change in nostril patency Stertor	Facial deformity (tumor) Systemic signs of illness (aspergillosis) (e.g. lethargy, inappetence, weight loss) Seizures
Pharynx	Stertor Open-mouth breathing Sneezing, nasal discharge Cough	Upper digestive symptoms Gagging, retching Dysphagia Ptyalism
Larynx	Exercise intolerance Stridor Difficult breathing/respiratory distress Cough Hypoxemia/cyanosis	Modified barking sounds Gagging or coughing with eating
Extrathoracic trachea	Cough (mainly in dogs, not in cats) Stridor (mainly in cats) Retching, gagging	Exercise intolerance Dyspnea (when severe obstruction)
Lower airway disorders		
Intrathoracic trachea	Cough (mainly in dogs, not in cats) Stridor Gagging	Exercise intolerance Difficult breathing (when severe obstruction)
Bronchi	Cough Dyspnea	Exercise intolerance Systemic signs of illness
Pulmonary parenchyma	Exercise intolerance Tachypnea Dyspnea (obstructive or restrictive)	Systemic signs of illness (depending on the cause) Hypoxemia
Pleural space	Exercise intolerance Orthopnea Dyspnea	Varies with cause
Mediastinal	Exercise intolerance Orthopnea Dyspnea	Cough Digestive signs

by the term 'sinonasal' aspergillosis, since the infection involves the nasal cavity and frontal sinus in most cases. Aspergillosis in dogs typically causes destructive rhinitis and sinusitis. Most affected dogs are young to middle aged and of mesencephalic and dolichocephalic breeds.

Etiology

In most instances, *Aspergillus fumigatus* is the etiologic agent but *A. niger*, *A. nidulans*, *A. flavus*, as well as *Penicillium* spp. may also be involved. *A. fumigatus* is a filamentous saprophyte and ubiquitous fungus.

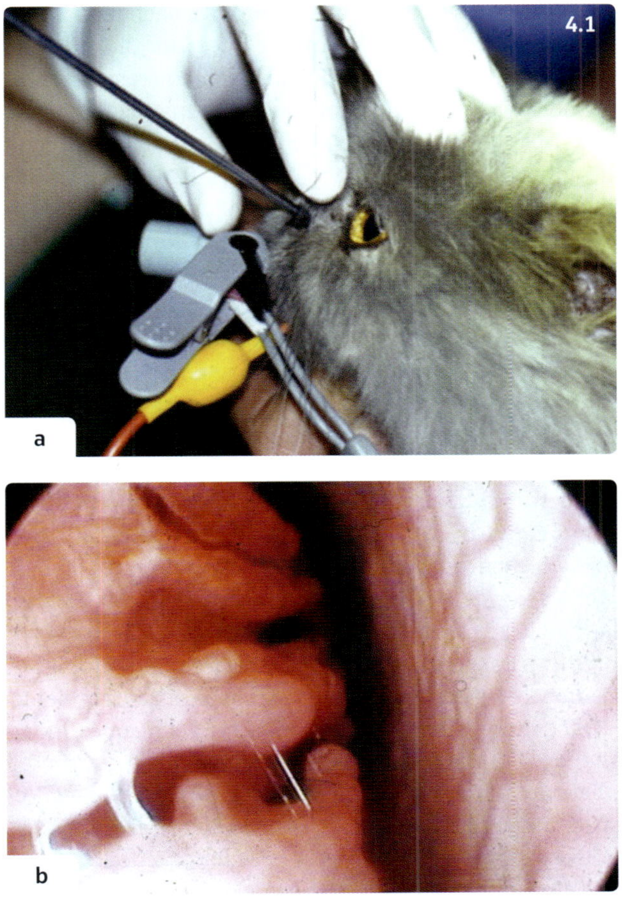

Figures 4.1a, b Direct rhinoscopy. (a) Use of a rigic scope in a Persian cat. (b) Rhinoscopic view of the turbinates in a dog.

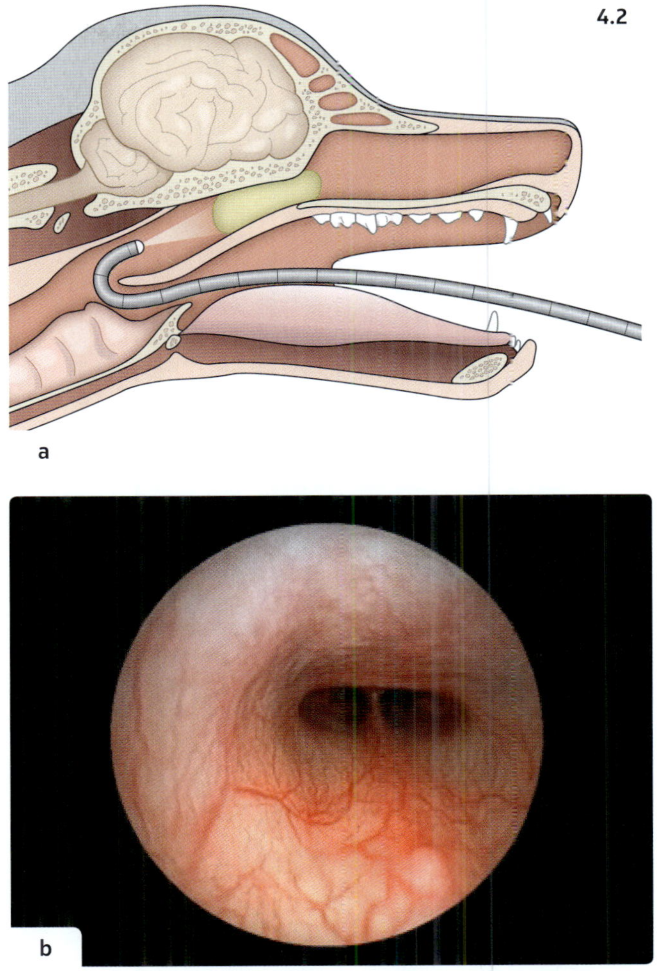

Figures 4.2a, b Retrograde rhinoscopy. (a) Diagram showing the use of a flexible endoscope. (b) Normal aspect of the choanae in a dog.

Pathophysiology

Despite numerous investigations, the pathogenesis is, to date, poorly understood. As the disease usually affects systemically healthy dogs, and as *A. fumigatus* is a ubiquitous fungus, a local immune deficiency in affected dogs has been suggested. The fungus invades the nasal cavity and sinus and causes necrosis of the turbinates, which is painful. The fungus can also induce lysis of the medial septum and invade the contralateral nasal cavity/sinus, or cause lysis of the cribriform plate.

Clinical presentation

Clinical signs associated with the disease include, in decreasing frequency:

- Profuse nasal discharge, unilateral when the disease begins, then possibly bilateral when the disease progresses, due to septal erosion. The discharge can be mucopurulent, although more often it is sanguinopurulent or bloody.
- Sneezing and reverse sneezing.
- Signs of nasal and frontal sinus pain, as evidenced by restriction of head movements, lethargy, and decreased appetite.
- Hyperkeratosis of the planum nasale and ulceration of external nares (**Figure 4.4**).
- Increased nasal airflow, as shown by placing a thin piece of cotton wool in front of each nostril alternately, related to the destruction of the turbinates (this abnormality is easily demonstrated from early in the course of the disease).
- Enlarged mandibulary lymph node(s), probably related to secondary bacterial infection of the nasal cavities and/or frontal sinus.

In advanced cases, other clinical abnormalities that can occur include facial deformity due to frontal bone hyperostosis, epiphora secondary to extension of the pathologic process into the orbit, or signs of forebrain

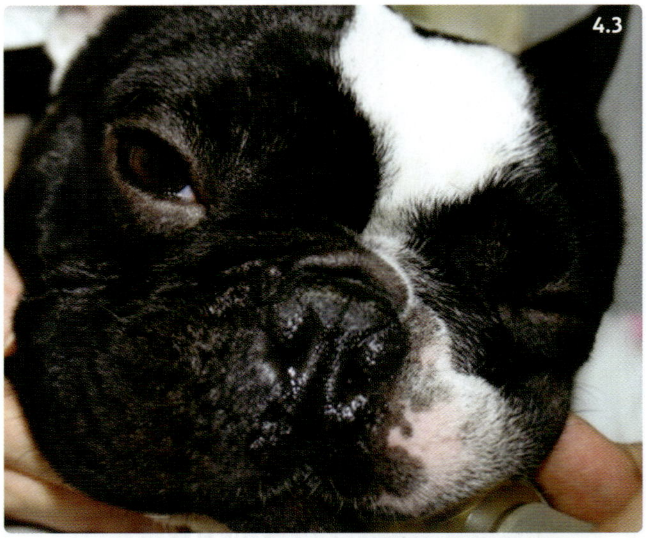

Figure 4.3 Stenotic nares in a French Bulldog.

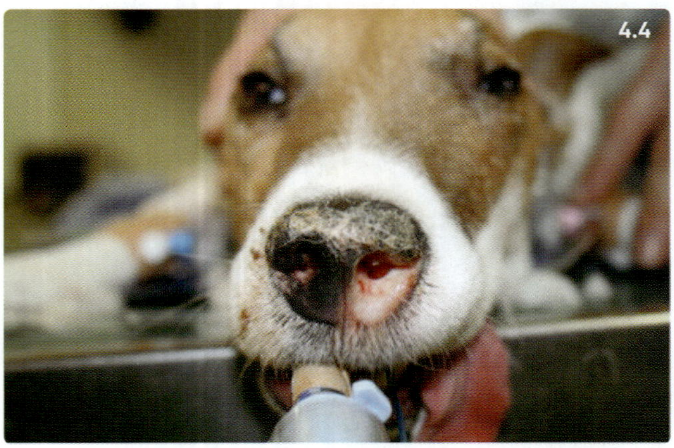

Figure 4.4 Ulceration of the external nares, hyperkeratosis and discharge in a dog with sinonasal aspergillosis.

dysfunction (e.g. seizures, dullness) if there is cribriform plate destruction.

Differential diagnosis

Includes lymphoplasmacytic rhinitis, early nasal tumor, chronic nasal foreign body, bacterial rhinitis due to dental disease, and fungal rhinitis.

Diagnosis

SNA may be suspected based on signalment, history, and clinical signs but reaching a definitive diagnosis remains a clinical challenge. Medical imaging (CT or MRI), endoscopy, cytology/histology, fungal culture, serology, and fungal DNA quantification have been reported to help in the diagnosis of canine SNA. However, there is no single consistently reliable diagnostic method as false-positive and false-negative results can occur with each test. Direct rhinoscopy may detect turbinate lysis in the affected cavity(ies) in addition to any fungal plaques with their associated accumulation of necrotic material in the affected cavity (**Figure 4.5**). In early cases, rhinoscopy may not detect the presence of typical fungal colonies because the plaques might not yet be formed.

Radiographic signs of fungal rhinitis consist of a loss of the normal intranasal trabecular pattern together with an increased lucency of the affected nasal cavity(ies). High-resolution CT is much more useful. Typical features of nasal aspergillosis include cavitary destruction of the turbinates with abnormal soft tissue within the nasal cavity, a rim of soft tissue along the frontal and sinus bones, and thick reactive bone (**Figure 4.6**). The value of MRI for the diagnosis of aspergillosis is very similar to that provided by CT because of the greater detail they provide compared with radiography.

Rhinoscopy is required for a definitive diagnosis because it is the only technique that is able to show the presence (active overt aspergillosis) or absence of fungal colonies. It also allows access to the plaques for surgical debridement.

Direct endoscopic visualization of fungal plaques, along with biopsy of the pathologic tissue, have become accepted as the gold standard for the diagnosis of SNA. Referral of suspect patients to veterinary centers that have the diagnostic expertise can be a great service for practices that are not equipped for such diagnostic testing.

Agar gel double immunodiffusion (AGDD) is the most commonly used serologic test for diagnosing SNA. This method is cheap, simple, and easy to perform. Although fungal culture of nasal specimens is highly specific for the diagnosis of SNA, nasal secretions sampled blindly with swabs are an unreliable source for fungal culture in contrast to fungal plaque and mucosal biopsy samples. Incubating samples for fungal culture at 98.6°F (37°C) improves the chance of fungal isolation in the laboratory.

Rarely, hyphae or conidia can be seen on cytologic or histopathologic preparations.

Management

Effective treatment of SNA in dogs is very challenging. Treatment options include systemic oral therapy, topical antimycotic therapy, and more invasive surgical procedures. The reported success rates and short-term and long-term outcome are variable.

Systemic oral treatments (ketoconazole, 5 mg/kg q12h or itraconazole 5 mg/kg q12h) are noninvasive but require prolonged administration (more than 4 weeks in all cases) because of poor efficacy and may have significant side-effects, especially on liver function.

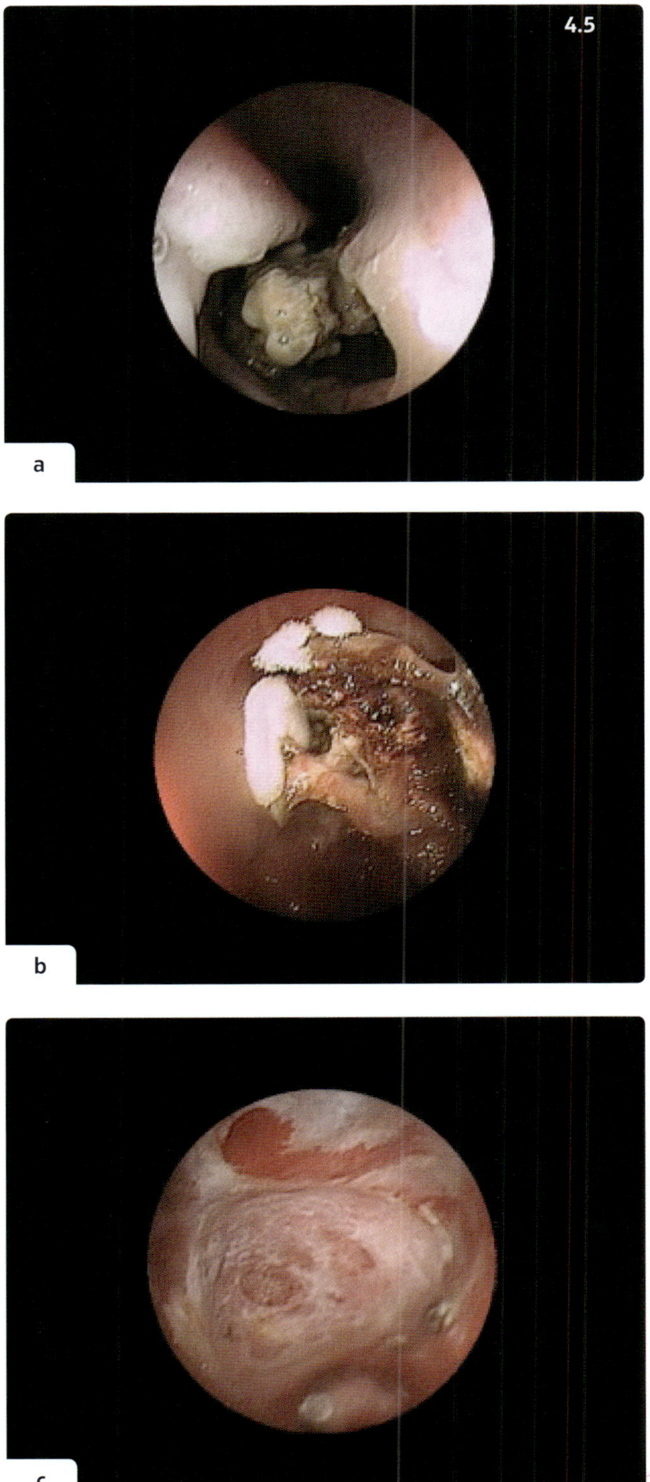

Figures 4.5a–c Rhinoscopy in a dog with SNA showing (a) important turbinate lysis and presence of necrotic material in the nasal cavity; (b) presence of typical fungal plaques and collection of necrotic material in the nasal cavity, and (c) a cleaned frontal sinus after debridement.

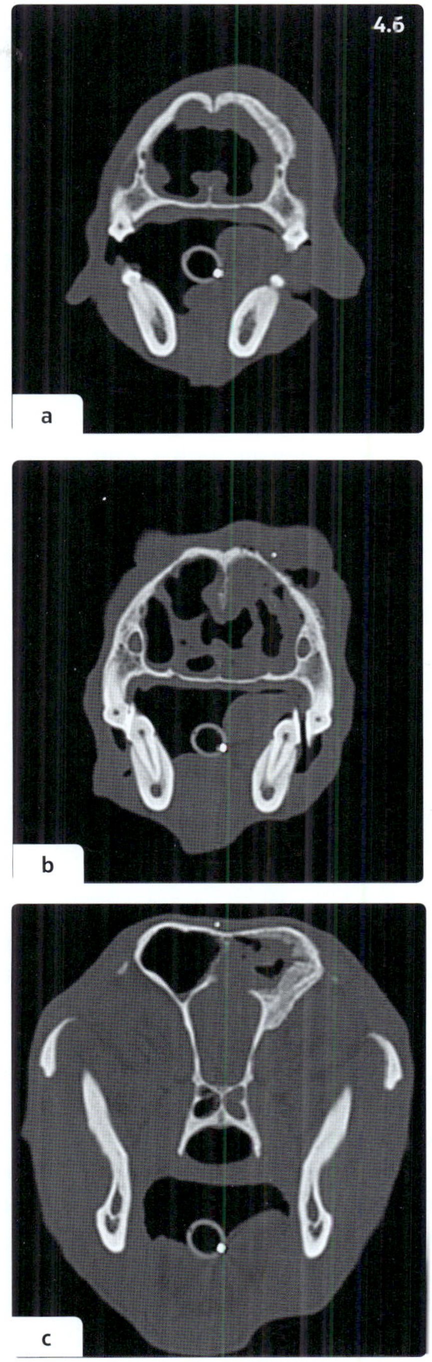

Figures 4.6a–c Transverse high-resolution CT images of a dog with severe nasal aspergillosis, showing (a) bilateral cavitary destruction of the turbinates with abnormal fluid/soft tissue within the nasal cavities and L>R frontal sinuses; (b) thickening of the mucosa along the inner surface of the bones of the left frontal sinus and nasal cavities; and (c) thick reactive maxillary, incisive, nasal, and frontal bones (hyperstosis) as well as lysis of the maxillary, nasal, and incisive bones, nasal septum, frontal crest, and cribriform plate. Note the swelling of the dorsal subcutaneous tissue on the left side. (Courtesy G. Bolen)

Currently, the most rewarding therapies include topical treatments. They have been associated with greater success and have improved the management of SNA. Various procedures have been developed to administer medication topically, and these procedures vary in invasiveness and ease of performance. Extensive débridement prior to infusion is a critical and essential step. Topical therapy includes mainly the use of enilconazole and clotrimazole, at a concentration of 1–2%. These methods have shown good efficacy and reach success rates of up to 80–90%. Although the use of topical agents via noninvasive methods is well tolerated and shows a high success rate, these procedures are time-consuming and require general anesthesia. Infusion of 1% clotrimazole cream through bore holes into the frontal sinus, which acts as a depot agent to minimize anesthesia time while providing an extended period of drug contact, has been described.

Prognosis

Despite all these treatment procedures, some dogs remain refractory to any treatment and the prognosis is then very poor. The inability to predict first-treatment success rate is frustrating. Severity of disease, experience of the treating clinician, and the ability and extent to which débridement is performed are contributing factors to treatment response. Recurrence after apparent remission is not uncommon and has been demonstrated to occur several years after an initial successfully treated episode of SNA.

Mycotic rhinosinusitis (cats)

Definition/overview

In contrast to canine SNA, aspergillosis in cats is rare, but is considered an emerging condition. In cats, upper respiratory tract (URT) aspergillosis can be divided into SNA and sino-orbital aspergillosis (SOA), with SOA being the most common and invasive form. In contrast to canine SNA, purebred brachycephalic cats, predominantly of Persian or Himalayan breeds, account for most cases. The disease affects young to middle aged cats, with evidence of immunocompromise in some cases, but not in most. Previous viral URT infection or recurrent antimicrobial therapy might be additional risk factors.

Etiology

A diverse range of *Aspergillus* species has been identified in cats with URT aspergillosis.

Clinical presentation

Feline SNA is characterized by more local signs of chronic nasal infection (e.g. sneezing, uni- or bilateral serous to mucopurulent nasal discharge) and, sometimes, epistaxis. Soft tissue masses protruding from the nares and bone lysis are less frequent abnormalities. SOA probably represents an extension of SNA to orbital and subcutaneous tissues, caused by more invasive *Aspergillus* species. It is characterized by signs of orbital and surrounding tissue invasion, including unilateral exophthalmos, third eyelid prolapse, conjunctival hyperemia, and keratitis. In some cases, a mass in the pterygopalatine fossa or an ulceration of the hard palate can be seen. The CNS can also be involved, leading to neurologic signs.

Differential diagnosis

Includes mainly viral upper URT infections, neoplasia (lymphoma, carcinoma), and severe chronic rhinosinusitis (idiopathic or secondary to polyp, nasopharyngeal stenosis or atresia, or palatal defect), cryptococcosis, foreign body.

Diagnosis

Confirmation of the diagnosis relies on advanced imaging (CT or MRI) and rhinoscopy. Biopsy or a nasal lavage specimen can be used for histology, cytology, culture, and even molecular identification when a negative fungal culture is suspected. In SOA, CT-guided biopsy of orbital or other paranasal mass lesions can be performed.

Management

Evidence-based treatment protocols are not available. Only small numbers of reported treated cases exist and very little follow-up information is available. Successful treatment regimens have been described using systemic antifungal therapy alone or with topical intranasal antifungal infusion. As with canine SNA, débridement of fungal lesions appears to be a very important step in any treatment protocol. To date, optimal treatment regimens have not been investigated, confirmed, or identified.

Prognosis

SNA carries a favorable prognosis with treatment, whereas the prognosis for SOA is poor.

Cryptococcosis

Definition/overview

Cryptococcus is a dimorphic fungus that exists in the yeast form in the animal. In nature it is found in bird guano. Various species exist (*Cryptococcus neoformans* var *grubii* or var *neoformans*, *Cryptococcus gattii*) with various geographic distributions. Cryptococcal infection is reported much more commonly in cats than in dogs, and the disease is much less frequent than aspergillosis.

Clinical presentation

Clinical signs include facial distortion, sneezing, and chronic mucopurulent nasal discharge, and can be accompanied by skin lesions, chorioretinitis, or CNS signs such as seizures.

Diagnosis

Diagnosis involves cytologic identification of the organism in nasal smears, exudates, aspirates, or impression smears. The organism is characteristic (3–8 microns round, surrounded by a clear capsule ranging in size from 10 to 30 microns). There is also a serum latex agglutination test that has shown reliable accuracy in detecting the cryptococcal antigen.

Management/prognosis

Itraconazole (50–100 mg/cat/day) is reportedly efficacious in most cases

Tumors (dogs)

Definition/overview

Nasal and paranasal tumors account for 1–2% of canine neoplasms. Dolichocephalic breeds and medium to large breeds of dogs are more often affected. Older dogs are predominantly affected. The tumors are mostly malignant and include mainly carcinomas, but sarcomas also occur. Nasal lymphomas are infrequent in dogs, but are not rare in cats. Benign tumors are very rare. Nasal tumors are locally invasive; systemic metastasis is infrequent, while local lymph node involvement can be seen.

Clinical presentation

Dogs exhibit chronic nasal discharge, which is at first unilateral and can then become bilateral. The discharge is serous to mucopurulent and/or hemorrhagic. Epistaxis is common. Other clinical features include stertor, sneezing, and reverse sneezing. Ocular discharge, facial deformity, alteration of the nasal plane, weight loss, and CNS signs are less frequently encountered.

Diagnosis

History and clinical signs lead to a presumptive diagnosis in most cases. A very easy and interesting test is the airflow passage test, which is measured by placing a thin piece of cotton wool in front of each nostril alternately. Airflow passage is always decreased or absent when associated with nasal cavity tumors. Diagnostic imaging is useful to define the extent of the disease and provide a presumptive diagnosis. CT is the imaging modality of choice for diagnosing nasal neoplasia, although radiographs are often adequate. CT is superior for staging and is required before any surgical and/or radiotherapeutic treatment is started. MRI is more sensitive for identifying intracranial involvement.

Rhinoscopy is an important diagnostic procedure because it allows not only visualization of the mass, but also the opportunity to take selective biopsies in order to confirm the diagnosis and determine the histopathologic type of the tumor.

A number of different techniques have been described for obtaining cytology or biopsy tissue samples from the nasal cavity. These include nasal flush, traumatic core biopsy, and rhinoscopy-assisted biopsy. Retrograde rhinoscopy allows for visualization of the posterior nasal cavity (**Figure 4.7a**). Imprint and/or brush cytology can be diagnostic for nasal tumors, but deep biopsy and histopathology are recommended since biopsies that are too superficial may fail to confirm the neoplastic nature of the mass. Fine-needle aspiration of the submandibular lymph node is a simple, inexpensive, minimally invasive technique that can help detect metastasis.

Differential diagnosis

Includes inflammatory rhinitis, aspergillosis, and intranasal foreign bodies.

Diagnosis

The diagnosis of intranasal neoplasia is complicated by the difficulty in obtaining a representative biopsy and many neoplasms are initially diagnosed as inflammatory disease.

Management/prognosis

In dogs, regardless of the chosen therapeutic procedure, prognosis is poor. Chemotherapy will provide varying results with nasal lymphoma in dogs and cats, but is not otherwise recommended with other tumor types.

Surgery alone is ineffective since local recurrence is a consistent outcome, resulting in survival times comparable to those observed in untreated dogs. However, surgery may be used to achieve cytoreduction, but it must be associated with other treatment modalities. Radiation alone or after cytoreductive therapy has been the standard of care for treating nasal tumors. The most common therapy currently used in veterinary medicine is high-voltage radiotherapy using megavoltage x-ray or cobalt-60, because this method has reportedly improved outcomes compared with other treatments.

Various treatments have been used in dogs for nasal tumors, including cryosurgery, iridium-192 brachytherapy, cisplatin chemotherapy, cyclo-oxygenase inhibitors (piroxicam), tyrosine kinase inhibitors, and some others, all without noteworthy improvement.

Tumors (cats)

Overview

Lymphoma in cats normally carries a guarded prognosis; however, nasal lymphoma is prognostically the best variant, with a good chance of long-term remission and even a possibility of cure. Response rates to treatment (chemotherapy and/or radiation therapy) average 66–75%, with reported median survival times of 12–30 months, even when chemotherapy is delivered intraperitoneally. The disease is often localized and the cats are often still eating well and are usually FeLV negative. Negative prognostic factors for nasal lymphoma (**Figure 4.7b**) include anorexia, anemia, and involvement of the cribriform plate as seen with CT.

Foreign body

Etiology

Most intranasal foreign bodies are of vegetable origin. Foreign material can be aspirated into the nasal cavity. It can also be stopped at the entrance of the larynx or regurgitated from the esophagus and misdirected toward the nasopharyngeal area where it lodges in the nasopharynx, above the soft palate, behind the choanae. Dogs are more commonly affected than cats, and young animals are more frequently affected than older dogs, but the disease can be found in any breed and at any age (**Figure 4.8**).

Clinical presentation

Clinical signs are quite suggestive and include sudden onset of sneezing bouts, nasal pruritus (the animal rubs his nose against the ground or with his paw), and a serous nasal discharge, which can become mucopurulent or even bloody with time. When the foreign body is blocked in the nasopharyngeal area, clinical signs will occur suddenly, and consist of reverse sneezing, stertor if the choanal opening is reduced, ptyalism, and gagging. Later, nasal discharge, sneezing, anorexia, and halitosis can occur.

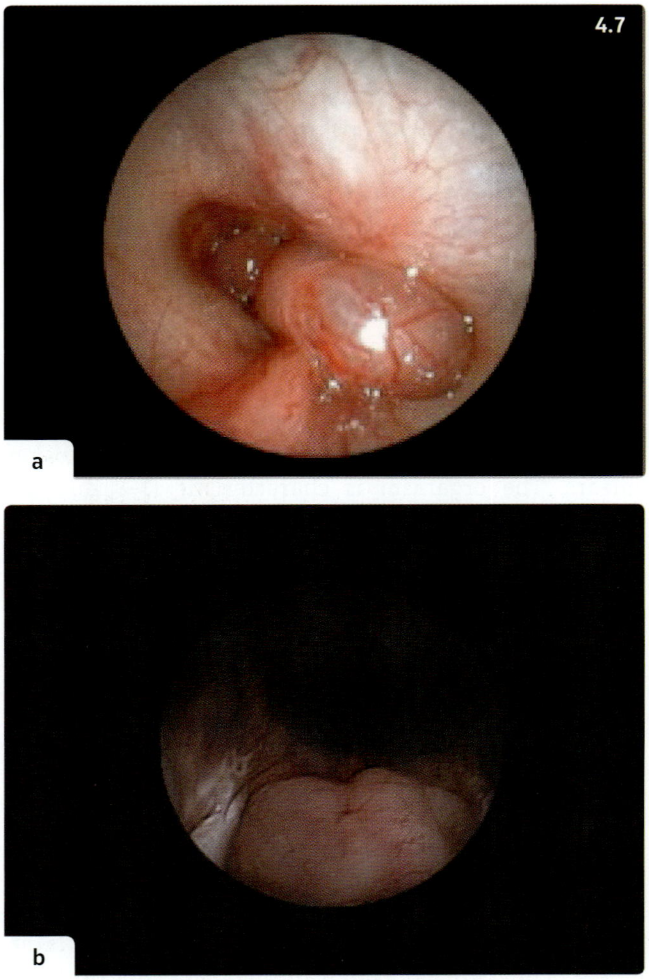

Figures 4.7a, b (a) Retrograde rhinoscopy in a dog, showing a nasal tumor invading and obstructing both choanae. (b) Retrograde rhinoscopy in a cat, showing an enlarged nasopharyngeal tonsil, infiltrated with a lymphoma.

Diagnosis

Diagnosis is confirmed by direct or retrograde rhinoscopy. If performed very early, the nasal foreign body can sometimes be visualized in the anterior nasal cavity and retrieved with the help of an otoscope. This approach will not be feasible if the foreign body has migrated to the caudal nasal cavity. In this case, a rhinoscope is needed. For detection and retrieval of nasopharyngeal foreign bodies, retrograde rhinsocopy is essential.

Management/prognosis

Early removal is advised. No other treatment is warranted, unless severe inflammation and/or turbinate lysis have occurred. In this case, nasal drops containing antibiotics can be prescribed and given intranasally 3–4 times a day for 1 week. The antibiotics can be given orally as well.

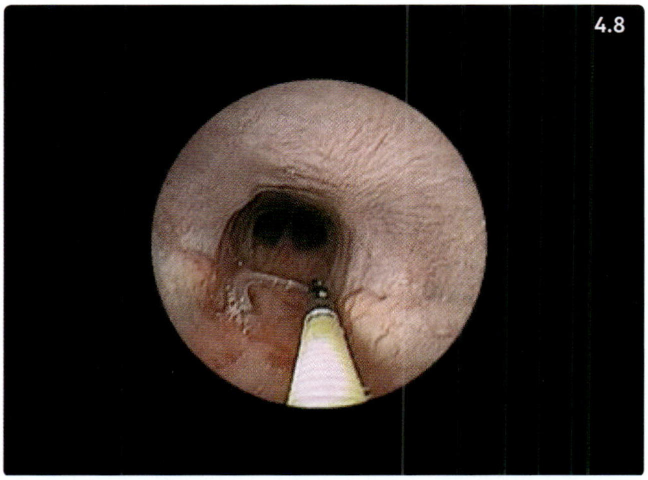

Figure 4.8 Retrograde rhinoscopy showing a foreign body in the nasopharynx.

Unless the foreign body has caused chronic mucosal inflammatory changes, the prognosis is excellent. However, nasopharyngeal ulceration can potentially lead to secondary nasopharyngeal stenosis (see below).

Parasitic rhinitis ('Nasal mite')

Etiology
This is a rare disease, associated with the presence of the nasal mite *Pneumonyssoides caninum*. This nasal cavity parasite of dogs has been reported worldwide; however, details of the parasite's life cycle remain to be elucidated.

Clinical presentation
Clinical signs include daily repeated episodes of reverse sneezing, sneezing, and mild nasal discharge.

Diagnosis
Diagnosis is based mainly on clinical signs and rarely on visualization of the mites during retrograde or direct rhinoscopy. There is no valid serologic test to confirm the diagnosis.

Management
Treatment is with milbemycin oxime (0.5–1.0 mg/kg PO once a week for 3 consecutive weeks). Selamectin (6 mg/kg SC) or ivermectin (0.2 mg/kg SC or PO, given twice during 3 weeks) is generally successful as well.

Nasopharyngeal stenosis and choanal atresia

Definition/overview
Nasopharyngeal stenosis is acquired and results from excessive formation of scar tissue in the nasopharynx secondary to a local inflammatory process of infectious, caustic (e.g. passage of acid gastric fluids during regurgitation and vomiting), or traumatic (e.g. foreign body, surgery) origin.

Choanal atresia is a congenital anomaly that results from failure in the development of the communication between the posterior nasal cavities and the nasopharynx (i.e. the formation of the choanae). Atresia can be unilateral or bilateral, partial or total, and bony or membranous.

Clinical presentation
Both nasopharyngeal stenosis and choanal atresia lead to decreased nasal patency (obstruction of airflow through the nose). Progressive stertor and possibly secondary nasal discharge are present; sometimes, open-mouth breathing is observed, with subsequent respiratory discomfort and inappetence.

Diagnosis/management/prognosis
Retrograde rhinoscopy is required for both diagnosis and treatment.

The best therapeutic approach is balloon dilation of the stenosis. This gives favorable results for nasopharyngeal stenosis (**Figures 4.9a–d**), but a less favorable prognosis for choanal atresia.

Nasopharyngeal polyp

Etiology/pathophysiology
Nasopharyngeal polyps usually affect young cats. Their etiology is unknown. They are made of pedunculated fibrous inflammatory tissue that originates in the eustachian tube and invades the nasopharyngeal area. The polyp may also grow into the middle ear and invade the external auditory tube.

Clinical presentation
Because they can lead to unilateral or bilateral nasal obstruction, polyps in the nasopharynx cause stertorous breathing and inspiratory dyspnea. A chronic serous or mucopurulent nasal discharge may be present. Polyps in the middle ear may cause vestibular signs and Horner's syndrome. In advanced cases, permanent open-mouth breathing progressively leads to inappetence and poor general condition.

Diagnosis, management, and prognosis
The rostral part of the soft palate may be depressed by the polyp, which can be visualized, under anesthesia, after rostral retraction of the soft palate. Retrograde rhinoscopy can facilitate polyp visualization in the posterior nasal cavity. Ear canal examination will identify any polyp in

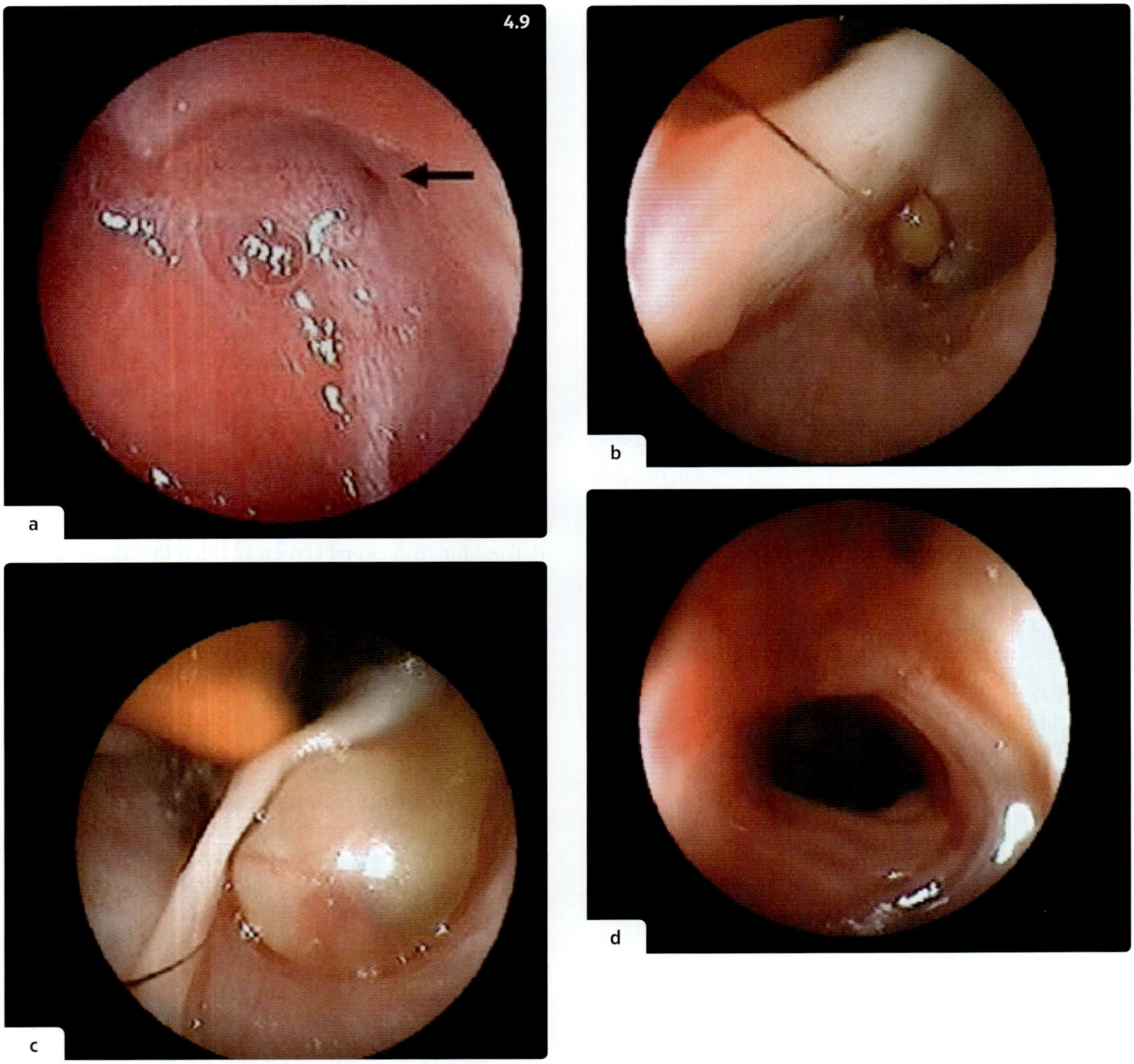

Figures 4.9a–d Retrograde rhinoscopy in a cat with left nasopharyngeal stenosis before (a), during (b, c), and after ballooning (d).

this particular location. This is important since surgery, along with tympanic bulla curettage, is the preferred treatment option, leading to cure without recurrence. Radiographic examination of the bullae or high-resolution CT of the skull should be performed if the polyp cannot be visualized on direct examination prior to planning surgery (**Figure 4.10**).

Recurrent infectious rhinitis in dogs

Definition/overview

Primary acute rhinitis is rare in dogs. Canine distemper virus is the only virus able to induce rhinitis in dogs and is always accompanied by other, more severe, clinical signs.

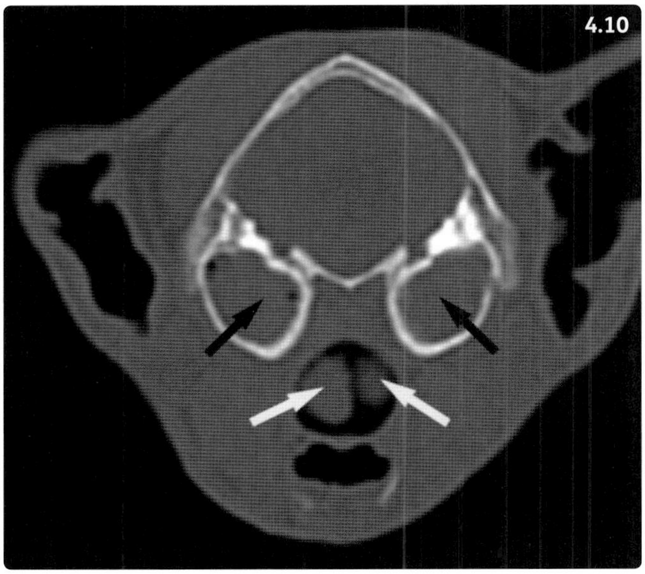

Figure 4.10 Transverse CT image of the skull of a cat with bilateral nasopharyngeal polyps showing both tympanic bullae totally filled with soft tissue attenuating masses (black arrows) and the presence of two soft tissue images in the nasopharyngeal lumen (white arrows). (Courtesy G. Bolen)

Etiology, clinical presentation, and differential diagnosis

A primary etiology should be looked for when clinical signs of mucupurulent rhinitis improve with antibiotic therapy but recur after discontinuation of therapy. Tooth root infection as well as silent bacterial pneumonia must be ruled out as possible causes. Tooth root infection leading to chronic or recurrent mucopurulent rhinitis is most commonly encountered in middle aged to old small breed dogs (e.g. Poodles, Yorkshire Terriers) with stomatitis associated with dental tartar. An oronasal fistula can be found in some cases and the discharge can be malodorous and have a whitish granular appearance. If clinical signs appear at a very young age, a severe metabolic problem such as immune deficiency (e.g. rhinitis/bronchopneumonia syndrome in Irish Wolfhounds) or a primary ciliary defect should be suspected. In such cases, the nasal discharge is mostly associated with other clinical signs, mainly related to lower airway recurrent infection (see below).

Acute feline upper respiratory tract disease

Definition/overview

Acute feline URT disease is very common in cats. Young kittens are most commonly affected, but older cats can become infected when exposed to high concentrations of pathogens (e.g. in a shelter environment).

Etiology/pathophysiology

The most commonly implicated organisms include FHV-1, FCV, *Chlamydophila felis*, and *Bordetella* spp. Viral infection predisposes to bacterial infection, which can also act as a primary pathogen. Viral infection usually resolves within 10 days, but it is highly contagious since viral shedding can persist for up to 3 weeks. Moreover, affected cats can become carriers and viral shedding may be reactivated during periods of stress. Virulent strains of FCV have been described, leading to pneumonia with a high mortality rate.

Clinical presentation

Clinical signs are dominated by sneezing and a serous to mucopurulent oculonasal discharge, while fever and systemic illness (lethargy, anorexia, dehydration) are common. *C. felis* is often associated with uni- or bilateral conjunctivitis and chemosis, and FCV causes lingual ulcers and, sometimes, pneumonia.

Diagnosis

Viral and bacterial confirmation using isolation or PCR, or bacterial cultures are rarely necessary in acute cases in practice unless the disease is associated with high morbidity and mortality in a community of cats (shelters, cattery or multi-house environments).

Management and prognosis

Supportive care and systemic antibiotic therapy against secondary bacterial infection are indicated. Many antibiotics can be used. *Chlamydophila* is best treated with doxycycline (10 mg/kg/day for 6 weeks). The efficacy of novel treatments such as lysine and antiviral therapy have not yet been proven in large clinical settings.

Most kittens survive but mortality is still quite high. Vaccination against viruses may reduce the clinical signs and limit the spread of the disease.

Chronic nonspecific lymphoplasmacytic rhinitis in dogs

Definition/overview

Idiopathic lymphoplasmacytic rhinitis is a common, chronic, and gradually progressive inflammatory nasal disease of unknown etiology associated with varying severity of clinical signs. It is characterized by lymphoplasmacytic to mixed inflammation of the nasal mucosa.

Etiology

The pathogenesis of this disease remains unknown. An aberrant immune response to inhaled organisms or allergens, but not to fungi, is suspected.

Pathophysiology

In chronic conditions, persistent inflammation of the mucosa leads to loss of epithelium and squamous metaplasia, which reduces the population of ciliated cells present in the distal third of each nasal cavity. Furthermore, hyperplastic subepithelial glands secrete increasingly viscid mucus, which also impedes normal ciliary clearance. As a consequence, mucus plugs accumulate and entrap inhaled bacteria and irritating particles within the nasal cavities, thus perpetuating the inflammation. When this material accumulates in the distal part of the nasal cavities, it obstructs the choanae and tends to induce reverse sneezing as well as heavy efforts to clear the throat and nose.

Clinical presentation

Clinical signs include sneezing, reverse sneezing, and chronic uni- or bilateral serous or mucopurulent nasal discharge that is characterized as tenacious and sometimes hemorrhagic in nature. The patient's general condition is usually unaffected.

Differential diagnosis

Before a diagnosis of chronic nonspecific lymphoplasmacytic rhinitis can be made, other underlying causes such as a nasal or nasopharyngeal foreign body, soft palate defects (where an increased opening between the oro- and the nasopharynx leads to misdirection of food/saliva), nasopharyngeal atresia or stenosis, or nasopharyngeal cysts or polyp must be excluded. Any chronic inflammatory disease of the nasal cavities caused by bacteria or fungi can give rise to progressive chronic lymphoplasmacytic rhinitis. Xeromycteria (dry nose) can also cause mild signs of chronic rhinitis.

Diagnosis

Diagnosis cannot rely on clinical signs. Diagnostic imaging and gross rhinoscopic findings are variable and nonspecific. A nasal mucosal biopsy taken during rhinoscopy shows epithelial and glandular hyperplasia, lymphoplasmacytic infiltration, and sometimes fibrosis. It is important to perform these examinations in order to eliminate other potential causes, such as aspergillosis, tumors, chronic foreign body, tooth root infection, or anatomic abnormalities, which could be treated specifically.

Management

In all chronic nasal diseases with epithelial hyperplasia and glandular hyperplasia, treatment should include local therapy with saline and mucolytics, since the physiological mucociliary clearance protective mechanism is impaired. This can be administered intranasally or by aerosol therapy. Nebulization devices used in human medicine can be used. Treatment entails the intranasal instillation of saline or mucolytic drops 2–4 times daily. Sometimes, the addition of nasal antibiotics becomes necessary in case of secondary bacterial infection. Improvement should occur after 1–3 weeks in most cases; other cases can remain refractory. Some authors advise treatment with prednisone (1 mg/kg q12h for 1–2 weeks, followed by a gradual taper) in refractory cases, although this recommendation will vary amongst different authors.

Prognosis

Although the condition is benign, treatment is unrewarding in some dogs, where clinical signs will fluctuate and require prolonged treatment.

Feline idiopathic chronic rhinosinusitis

Definition/overview

Chronic rhinitis or rhinosinusitis is one of the most common chronic disorders in cats and is characterized by chronic and/or recurrent nasal discharge and sneezing.

Etiology

Although the underlying pathogenesis is unclear, the disease is likely multifactorial. Some chronic forms are presumed to be caused by FHV-1, FCV, *Chlamydophila felis*, or a combination of these agents. FHV-1 is most commonly implicated in the chronic form of disease since more than half of the cats exposed to the virus remain latent carriers. Secondary bacterial infections and poorly regulated or improper immune responses also play a role in the pathogenesis. There is some evidence that *Bordetella bronchiseptica* is also a cause of chronic respiratory disease in cats. The low prevalence of FeLV and FIV infection in affected cats suggests that these viruses are not responsible for the disease.

Clinical presentation

Clinical signs include sneezing and chronic uni- or bilateral nasal discharge of a serous to mucopurulent nature, stertor, and intermittent open-mouth breathing. The cat's general condition can be affected.

Diagnosis

Rarely, a primary defect can be identified (nasopharyngeal foreign body, soft palate defects, nasopharyngeal stenosis, or nasopharyngeal cysts or polyps). Imaging and/or rhinoscopy can reveal mild to severe turbinate remodeling. Microbiologic identification of microorganisms does not usually help manage the disease since they are usually secondary infections. The signs are mostly related to irreversible remodeling of intranasal lesions rather than to bacterial infections.

Management

Currently, treatment is supportive and aims at the consequences of nasal and sinus dysfunction, decreasing inflammation, and eliminating secondary bacterial infections. Cats with chronic rhinosinusitis often have a transient response to antimicrobial treatment. Many antibiotics can be used orally for prolonged periods (from 3 up to 8 weeks or more). When *Chlamydophila* is suspected, doxycycline (10 mg/kg/day for 6 weeks) can be used. The use of azithromycin (10–15 mg/kg q24h followed by 5 mg/kg q48h or even q72h) is helpful for treating cats that are difficult to pill and need prolonged treatment.

Intranasal administration of drugs is difficult in most cases because cats are usually intolerant of this treatment method.

Prognosis

Chronic rhinosinusitis is frustrating to manage. Owners must be informed that cure is unlikely and that clinical signs will probably not resolve. Treatment aims at reducing the frequency and severity of clinical signs.

BRACHYCEPHALIC AIRWAY OBSTRUCTIVE SYNDROME

Definition/overview

The term BAOS refers to a disorder resulting from multiple anatomic abnormalities commonly found in brachycephalic canine breeds, mainly the English and French Bulldog and the Pug. It is also recognized in Persian cats.

Etiology

Conformational anomalies in brachycephalic dogs are related to breeding selection of 'hypertypes', which leads to progressive shortening of the face and nose, with subsequent shortening of the bony structures of the skull without concurrent reduction in surrounding soft tissues.

Pathophysiology

Primary inherited abnormalities include stenotic nares, elongated soft palate, hypoplastic trachea, and, sometimes, protrusion of the nasal turbinates into the nasopharynx. In some dogs the soft palate can be too long in addition to being exceptionally thick; macroglossia can also occur. Secondary lesions develop as a consequence of increased pressures on the pharyngeal, laryngeal, and intrathoracic structures during breathing. These lesions include everted laryngeal saccules, progressive laryngeal collapse, and probably bronchial collapse (mainly collapse of the left main bronchus). In addition, subepiglottic cysts, severe edema of the dorsal aspect of the laryngopharynx, and laryngeal granulomas ('kissing lesions') all further narrow the air passage at the laryngeal inlet. The severity and the combination of these abnormalities will vary. To complicate matters even further, these same dogs can have various accompanying gastrointestinal abnormalities involving the distal esophagus, stomach, and duodenum including inflammatory disease with co-existing functional or anatomic anomalies (cardial atony, gastroesophageal reflux, gastric retention, pyloric mucosal hyperplasia, and pyloric stenosis).

Clinical presentation

The abnormalities associated with the BAOS impair air flow through the upper airways and cause clinical signs of upper airway obstruction including noisy respiration, stridor, stertor, exercise and heat intolerance, respiratory distress, cyanosis, syncope, gagging and retching, and sometimes sleep apnea. The clinical signs are exacerbated by exercise, excitement, and high environmental temperatures. As a result, some dogs can be presented with life-threatening clinical signs of airway obstruction. Digestive signs such as regurgitation and vomiting are common. Secondary aspiration pneumonia is also a common associated finding and must be addressed.

Diagnosis

A tentative diagnosis can be based on the breed and clinical signs. Laryngoscopy (**Figures 4.11a–e**) and radiography (**Figure 4.12**) are essential diagnostics. Other procedures such as bronchoscopy and gastroscopy might be necessary in order to assess the full scope of the existing abnormalities and will be helpful in providing an accurate prognosis and the best treatment recommendation.

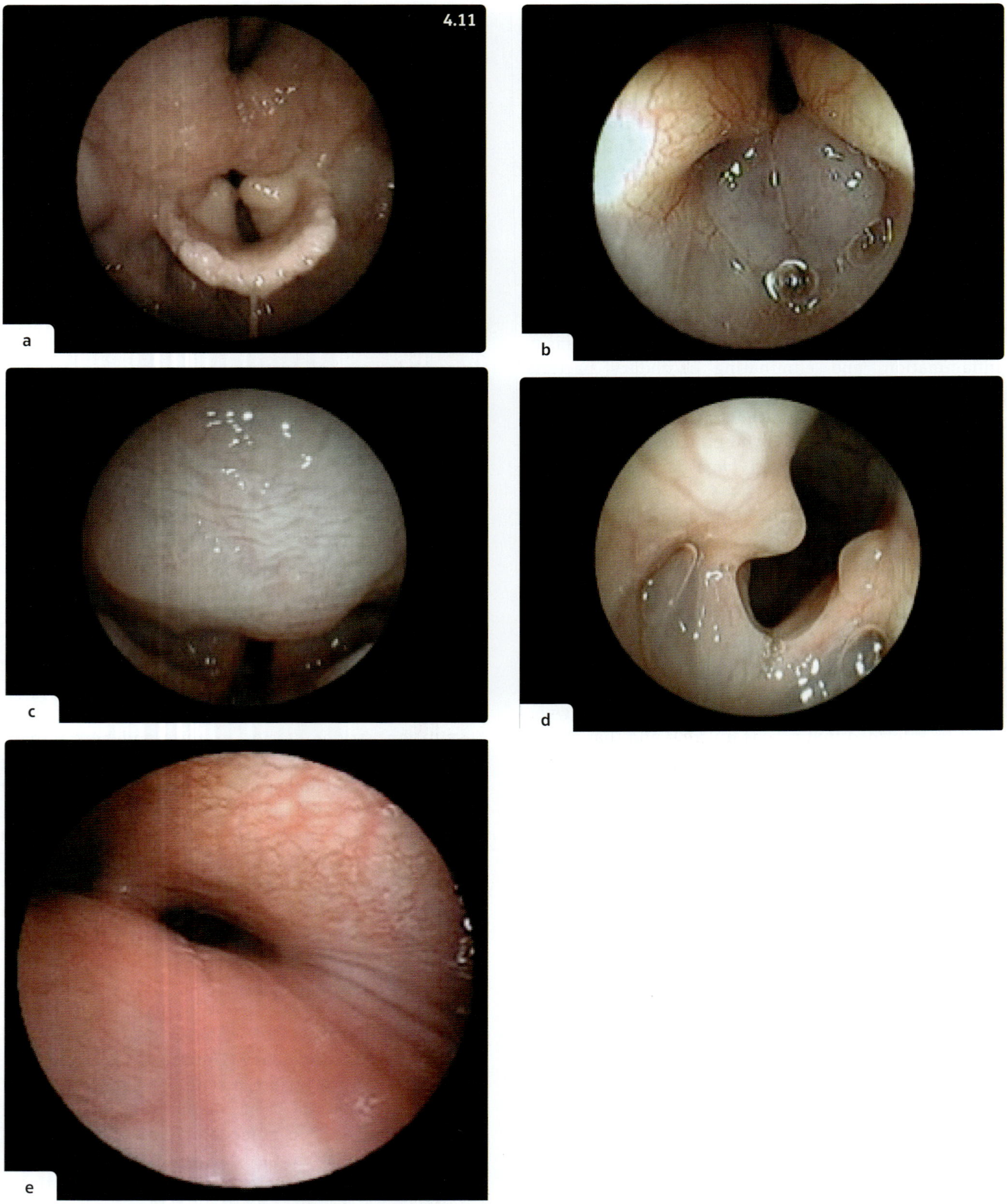

Figures 4.11a–e Laryngoscopic features of BAOS. (a) Elongated soft palate; (b) everted laryngeal saccules; (c) severe edema of the dorsal part of the laryngopharynx; (d) intralaryngeal granuloma ('kissing lesion'); (e) localized bronchomalacia at the level of the left mainstem bronchus.

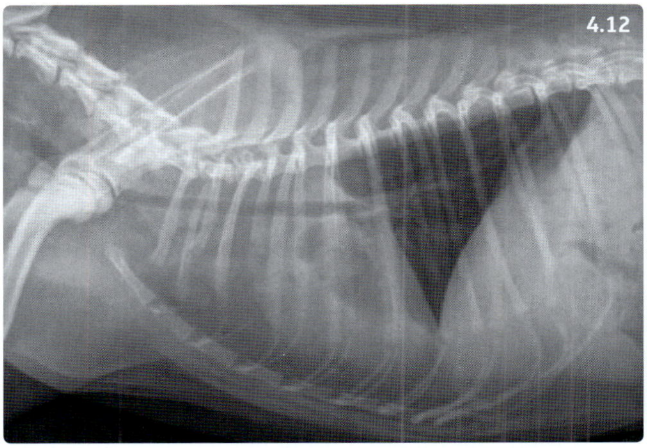

Figure 4.12 Thoracic radiograph (lateral projection) of a non-Bulldog brachycephalic dog showing tracheal hypoplasia with a ratio of 0.14 (tracheal diameter/thoracic inlet diameter ≥0.16 for Pugs) and ventral distribution of an alveolar pattern consistent with an aspiration pneumonia. (Courtesy G. Bolen)

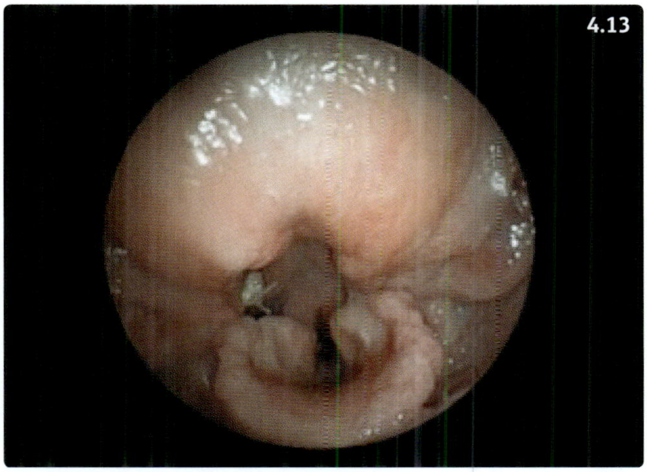

Figure 4.13 Laryngoscopic view of a BAOS dog after surgery (soft palate and ventriculectomy), showing persistance of laryngeal collapse.

Management

Animals presented with life-threatening upper airway obstruction should be cooled, oxygenated, sedated, and if necessary anesthetized and intubated. A tracheotomy might be indicated in cases of severe upper airway occlusion. In other cases medical therapy consisting of anti-inflammatory doses of short-acting glucocorticoids (prednisone, 0.5 mg/kg q12h) will suffice. Surgical widening of stenotic nares and surgical removal of excessive soft palate (**Figure 4.13**) and everted laryngeal saccules should be performed if there are no complicating abnormalities, such as laryngeal or tracheal hypoplasia, which would render treatment impossible. Corrective surgical procedures should be done as early in life as possible in order to decrease the consequences of long-term negative pressure on the airway structures (laryngeal cartilage collapse). Once severe laryngeal dysfunction occurs, successful management is much more difficult. Cricoarytenoid lateralization combined with thyroarytenoid caudolateralization, arytenoid laryngoplasty, or permanent tracheoscopy might be necessary in the setting of severe laryngeal pathology. If tracheal hypoplasia, with its associated ventilation impairment, is still severe after reaching adult size (at 1 year of age), there is nothing else that can be done to remedy the situation. Stress, excitement, and weight gain must be avoided in these animals.

Digestive tract medical treatment combined with upper respiratory surgery appears to decrease the complication rate and improve the prognosis of dogs presented for upper respiratory syndrome.

Prognosis

Prognosis depends on the severity of the abnormalities and the ability to surgically correct them. Laryngeal collapse and tracheal hypoplasia are poor prognostic indicators.

A combination of primary and secondary changes can progress to life-threatening laryngeal collapse in many brachycephalic dogs. Early recognition of the primary anatomic abnormalities is essential since it allows the clinician to make early recommendations for medical and surgical management, which can improve the quality of life in affected animals. Factors that may increase the risk and further complicate the condition include obesity, overexcitement, and exercise.

LARYNGEAL DISEASES

LARYNGEAL PARALYSIS (DOGS)

Definition/overview

Laryngeal paralysis (**Figure 4.14**) refers to lack of abduction of the arytenoid cartilages during inspiration due to loss of innervation of the intrinsic musculature of the larynx through the recurrent laryngeal nerves and resulting in inspiratory dyspnea.

Etiology

Laryngeal paralysis is most often of unknown cause (idiopathic laryngeal paralysis). This is most commonly observed in middle aged to old large breed animals (Labradors Retrievers seem to be predisposed).

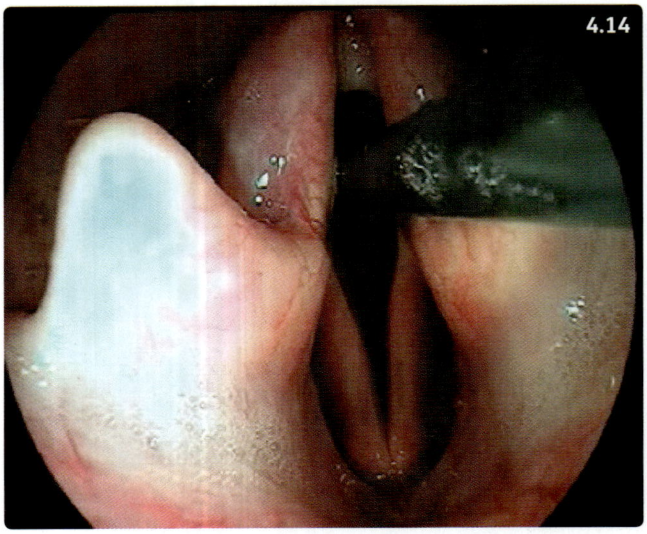

Figure 4.14 Laryngeal paralysis. Endoscopic image of the larynx during inspiration, showing a lack of abduction.

Congenital laryngeal paralysis appears to be inherited and has been reported in breeds such as the Bouvier des Flandres and Husky. Young Dalmatians, Rottweilers, and Great Pyrenees can acquire laryngeal paralysis as part of a polyneuropathy complex. Masses or trauma involving the ventral neck region or the anterior thoracic cavity can damage the recurrent laryngeal nerves and cause uni- or bilateral paralysis or paresis. Laryngeal paralysis has also been reported in dogs as a manifestation of various peripheral neuropathies or polyneuromyopathy complex, resulting from immune-mediated diseases (such as myasthenia gravis), endocrinopathies (such as hypothyroidism), or other systemic disorders.

Clinical presentation

The clinical signs vary in severity. The characteristic signs of dyspnea and stridor result from increased airflow resistance occurring during inspiration. They are initially prominent during the inspiratory phase of respiration in association with exertion, excitement, or exposure to high environmental temperatures. As the reduction in laryngeal diameter worsens, the signs can occur during both inspiration and expiration, and even at rest. Changes in bark can also occur. Cyanosis and syncope are observed in advanced cases, when secondary edema further narrows the glottis, exacerbating the signs and creating a vicious circle. As a result, some dogs may present with life-threatening upper airway obstruction. Some dogs with laryngeal paralysis exhibit gagging or coughing while eating. Secondary aspiration pneumonia is a possible complication.

Diagnosis

The clinical features of laryngeal dysfunction are easily identified. Direct laryngoscopic examination under light anesthesia allows for visualization of this disorder and differentiation from laryngeal edema, laryngeal tumor, or collapse. Weak, fluttering movements of the arytenoid cartilages and vocal folds may be observed due to changes in airway pressure and airflow and should not be confused with normal movements. Since anesthesia impairs laryngeal motion (moderate to deep planes of anesthesia result in cessation of all laryngeal movement), administration of doxapram hydrochloride (1.1–2.2 mg/kg IV), a potent respiratory stimulant, during laryngeal examination is useful for differentiating normal dogs from dogs with laryngeal paralysis. Electromyographic studies of the intrinsic laryngeal muscles, done under general anesthesia, and ultrasonographic evaluation of the larynx have also been used to assess laryngeal function. Once a diagnosis of laryngeal paralysis is established, additional diagnostic tests should be considered to identify an underlying cause.

Management/prognosis

Animals presented with life-threatening upper airway obstruction should be cooled, oxygenated, and sedated. Some may require general anesthesia and intubation, while other extreme cases require a tracheotomy. In less severe situations, initial therapy can begin with anti-inflammatory doses of short-acting glucocorticoid drugs (prednisone, 0.5 mg/kg q12h, followed by progressive tapering). This reduces the inflammatory reaction and alleviates some of the clinical signs. Surgery is inevitable and should be done as soon as possible. The recommended procedure is unilateral arytenoid lateralization. Aspiration pneumonia is the most common postoperative complication. Suture breakdown is another postoperative complication. However, most owners are ultimately pleased with the outcome. Poor outcomes are associated with underlying diseases causing a generalized polyneuropathy.

LARYNGEAL PARALYSIS (CATS)

Laryngeal paralysis appears to be infrequent in cats. Both uni- and bilateral dysfunctions have been documented, although left-sided unilateral paralysis is predominant. This condition can result from trauma or some other destructive process of the recurrent laryngeal nerves or in cases where the cause is idiopathic. Conservative management (weight loss, minimization of excitement, and anti-inflammatory therapy) and surgical treatment are mostly successful.

Laryngeal tumors

Definition/overview

Laryngeal neoplasms are rare (**Figures 4.15a–c**). They are mainly carcinomas, which affect middle aged to older dogs. However, younger dogs, especially Labrador Retrievers, can be affected with rhabdomyoma, which is a benign tumor. Tumors of tissues surrounding the larynx, such as thyroid carcinomas and lymphomas, can also compress and invade the larynx, causing similar signs of upper airway obstruction.

Clinical presentation

The clinical features of laryngeal tumors are similar to those of other laryngeal diseases and include stridor, dyspnea, changes in bark, and cyanosis.

Differential diagnosis

Includes laryngeal paralysis, foreign body, abscess, and traumatic granuloma.

Diagnosis

Primary laryngeal tumors are best identified by laryngoscopy. It is very important to make the diagnosis on the basis of histopathologic examination of a biopsy of the mass rather than on the gross appearance alone, since some tumors are benign and some growths are actually granulomas. CT can be helpful in assessing the extent of the mass and in making a decision for surgery.

Management/prognosis

Benign tumors should be excised surgically and, in case of rhabdomyoma, the prognosis is excellent when surgical excision is complete. In cases of malignant tumors, complete surgical excision is rarely achievable, and complete laryngectomy and permanent tracheostomy are the only surgical options.

Laryngeal edema

Definition/overview/etiology

Edema or infiltration of the larynx with inflammatory cells occurs frequently. It can be secondary to paralysis, tumor, or trauma, and is seen in brachycephalic dogs with BAOS. In cats, the larynx is very sensitive and edema can develop after faulty intubation technique or following an excessive application of local anesthetic agent. In some cases, the cause is not determined.

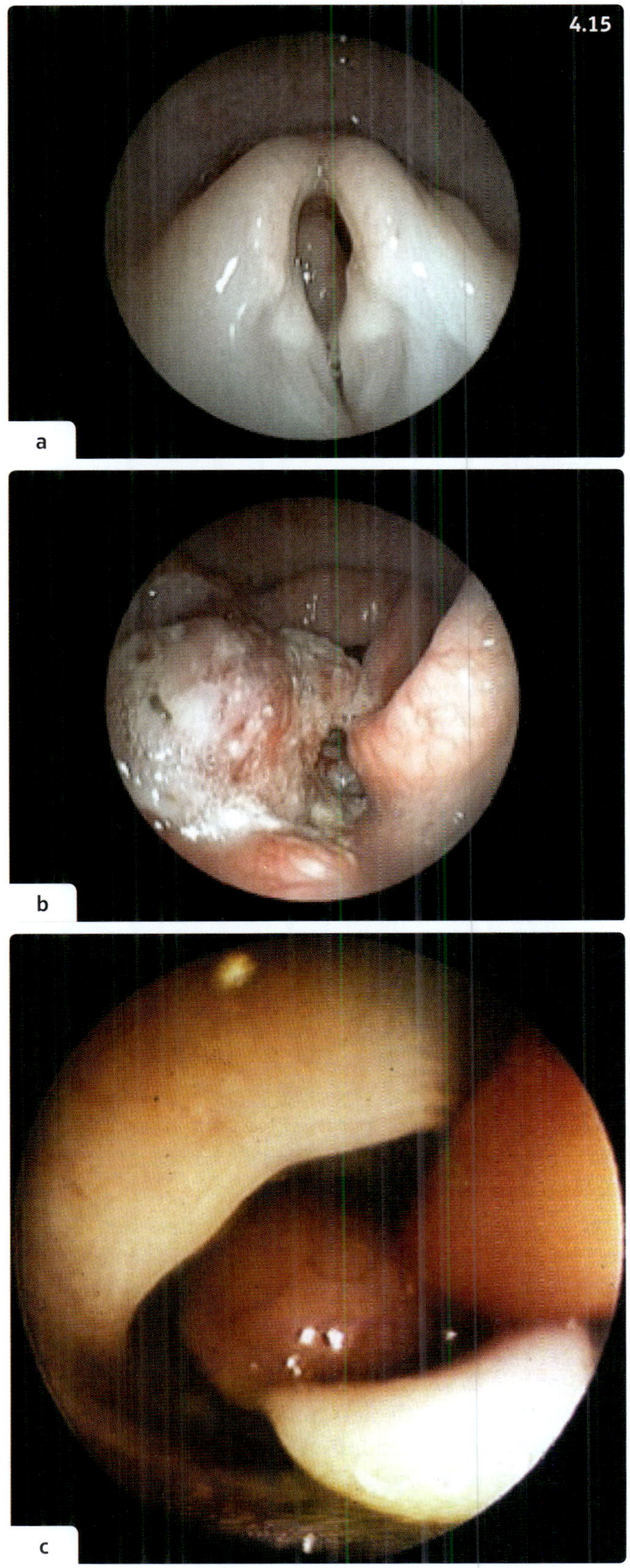

Figures 4.15a–c Laryngeal tumors in a cat (a) and two dogs (b, adenocarcinoma; c, rhabdomyoma).

Clinical presentation

Clinical signs are those typical of an upper airway obstruction, and identical to those observed in laryngeal paralysis. They range from exercise intolerance and stridor after excitement to life-threatening respiratory distress.

Differential diagnosis

Apart from the primary causes (paralysis, tumor, trauma, BAOS, intubation), chronic laryngitis, due to excessive and repeated barking, and laryngospasm ('glottis cramp') can also cause some degree of laryngeal edema. In cats, severe edema and laryngeal neoplasms can appear similar.

Diagnosis

Laryngoscopy shows irregular proliferation, hyperemia, and swelling of the larynx. Additional diagnostic procedures, such as biopsy or brush cytology or fine-needle aspiration, should not be performed when the laryngeal opening is severely reduced, unless a temporary tracheostomy is in place, especially in cats. It is prudent to first treat the patient medically before instituting any interventional procedures.

Management/prognosis

Most animals respond to glucocorticoid therapy within a couple of days. Prednisone (0.5–1.0 mg/kg q24h to q12h) is used initially. The dose can be gradually tapered over the next 3 weeks once the signs have resolved.

The prognosis is good unless the response to medical treatment is poor. In such cases, tracheostomy should be considered.

TRACHEAL DISORDERS

TRACHEAL COLLAPSE AND MALACIC AIRWAYS

Definition/overview

Tracheal collapse is a very common disorder characterized by dorsoventral flattening of the tracheal rings with laxity of the dorsal tracheal membrane. Bronchial collapse, essentially of the left cranial lobar bronchus, is often present as well. The syndrome is encountered in middle aged to older toy or miniature breeds (Yorkshire Terrier, Miniature Poodle, Chihuahua, Pomeranian, Shih Tzu, Lhasa Apso). The sound of the cough is a characteristic 'honking noise' or 'goose honk'.

Etiology/pathophysiology

The cause is complex and is best regarded as multifactorial. The development of the clinical condition requires the presence of a primary cartilage abnormality, resulting in intrinsic weakness of the tracheal rings, together with secondary factors capable of initiating progression to the symptomatic stage. These potential triggering factors include obesity, cardiomegaly, inhalation of irritants and allergens, periodontitis, respiratory infections, and recent endotracheal intubation. The dynamic changes of tracheal collapse may be confined to either the cervical or thoracic region of the trachea, or both, and are frequently more pronounced at the cervicothoracic junction. In dogs with tracheal collapse, concurrent bronchomalacia is frequently encountered and does not appear to be related to airway inflammation.

Once clinical signs occur, the syndrome is perpetuated by the cycle of chronic inflammation of the tracheal mucosa and the accompanying cough reflex.

Clinical presentation

Clinical signs include chronic cough, mild to severe panting, and varying degrees of inspiratory and expiratory dyspnea (respiratory distress). Cyanosis can occur in extreme cases. The cough is harsh, followed by a terminal retch, and is generally described as 'goose honk', which is precipitated by activity, excitement, tracheal pressure (such as caused by pulling on a leash), or drinking. This characteristic cough can be easily elicited by palpation of the trachea.

Differential diagnosis

Includes chronic mitral valvular heart disease, which can be a concurrent disease, chronic bronchitis, chronic tracheitis (both possibly secondary to tracheal collapse), and chronic pulmonary parenchymal disease such as idiopathic pulmonary fibrosis.

Diagnosis

Radiographic examination of animals with a collapsed trachea can be done with both still and motion studies. The most useful radiographic examinations include lateral projections of the thoracic inlet, a tangential (rostrocaudal) projection of the thoracic inlet, and fluoroscopic investigation to demonstrate movements of the dorsal membrane during the respiratory cycle. On lateral radiographs, a redundant dorsal tracheal membrane that invaginates into the tracheal lumen can be seen as a soft tissue opacity along the dorsal aspect of the caudal cervical tracheal lumen. During inspiration, it will cause an increased tracheal diameter. This condition can be seen in both small and large breed dogs as a consequence of coughing, and must be differentiated from a superimposed esophagus. Therefore, lateral radiographs made during both the maximal inspiratory and expiratory phases (**Figure 4.16**) of the respiratory cycle are needed

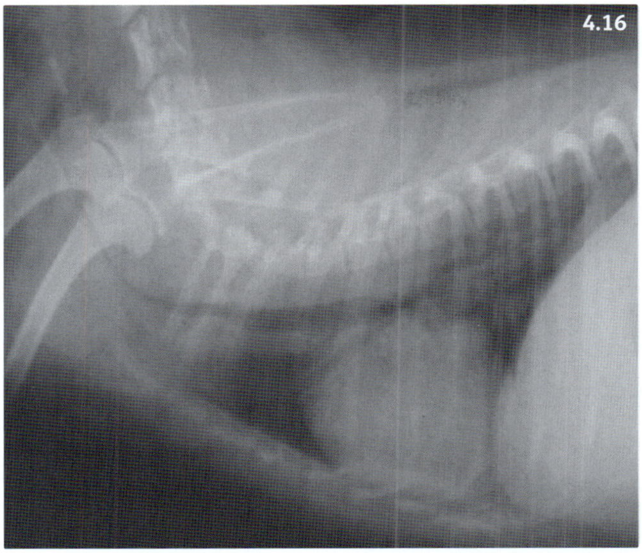

Figure 4.16 Lateral thoracic radiograph of an 8-year-old Yorkshire Terrier showing probable tracheal collapse with a decreased expiratory cervical tracheal diameter. (Courtesy G. Bolen)

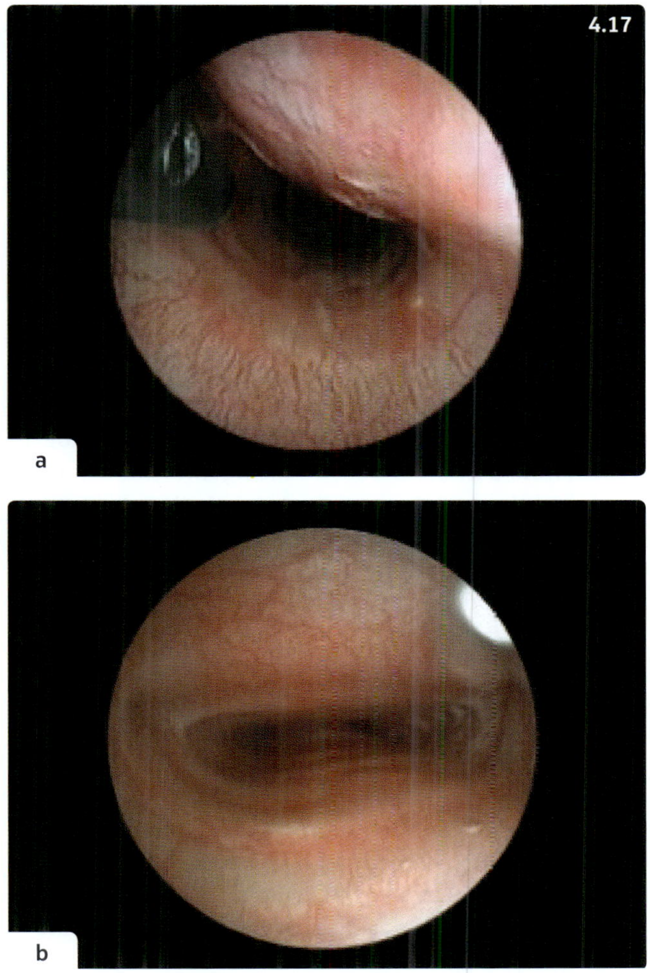

Figures 4.17a, b Endoscopic views of the trachea showing grade 2 (a) and grade 4 (b) tracheal collapse.

to demonstrate a dynamic collapse. Collapse of the cervical tracheal segment occurs in inspiration because of decreased pressure within the trachea, whereas the thoracic portion tends to collapse during the expiration phase as a consequence of increased intratracheal pressure. These dynamic changes are best viewed in real time using image-intensified fluoroscopy. In the skyline projection, the trachea is seen as an oval, 'C' or crescent shape.

Tracheoscopy, although rarely needed to confirm the diagnosis, reveals a decreased dorsoventral diameter due to flattening of the cartilagenous rings, with a pendulous dorsal membrane. A severe collapse can cause complete obstruction of the tracheal lumen (**Figures 4.17a, b**). Tracheobronchoscopy is helpful in determining the degree of severity of the tracheal and, especially, the bronchial collapse, as well as in assessing concomitant airway disease. Radiographs greatly underestimate the incidence of bronchomalacia. Therefore, bronchoscopy is recommended in all cases of suspected tracheal collapse before stent placement is considered, because the presence of severe bronchomalacia and/or lower airway disease will greatly impact on the prognosis after stent placement.

Management

In animals with marked respiratory difficulty, oxygen supplementation should be provided along with sedation and antitussive agents. Butorphanol (0.05–0.2 mg/kg q4–6h) and acepromazine (0.01–0.1 mg/kg) can be injected SC in order to allay anxiety, and prednisolone sodium succinate (15–30 mg/kg IV) can be administered to decrease acute inflammation.

Long-term treatment aims principally at decreasing potential promoting factors and the level of inflammation of the tracheal mucosa. Weight reduction in obese animals is essential. Weight loss alone can sometimes be curative in terms of dealing with the clinical signs. Likewise, removal of the neck collar and its replacement by a harness can be helpful. Removing the dog from respiratory irritants such as noxious gases, smoke, and dust is essential. It is also important to detect and treat other diseases such as chronic airway disease, cardiac disease, or Cushing's disease.

Some authors recommend short- to long-term therapy consisting of very low-dose steroids orally (prednisone, 0.2 mg/kg daily for 2 days to 2 weeks, followed by the same dose every other day, then at 3-month intervals) or by inhalation (fluticasone, 120 µg puff q12h using a face mask and spacer). Short-term administration of sedatives such as acepromazine can be useful in very excited animals to break the 'cough/excitation/cough cycle'. However, oversedation must be avoided because the animal will benefit from limited exercise as far as weight gain and airway clearance is concerned. A combination of opioid-antitussive/anticholinergic drug (diphenoxylate HCl plus atropine, 0.25 mg/kg q8–12h) is used with great success by many clinicians. Oral antitussive agents are effective in controlling symptoms (e.g. hydrocodone, 0.22 mg/kg q12h; or butorphanol, 0.55 mg/kg q12h). Bronchodilators (methylxanthines or beta agonists) can also be used, their benefits being due to a reduction in bronchoconstriction thereby reducing intrathoracic pressures and the associated collapse of the larger airways. Furthermore they improve mucociliary clearance and reduce diaphragmatic fatigue.

In dogs that do not respond to medical management, a more recent treatment involves placement of intraluminal self-expanding stenting devices. Determination of the appropriate size and type of the stent is a critical step. In some dogs, this minimally invasive technique is the only successful treatment option. Tracheal prosthetic devices are very expensive and their use is not without complications. These include stent displacement/migration, rupture, stent detachment with development of purulent pockets between the stent and the tracheal mucosa, and inflammatory granuloma (**Figure 4.18**). The inflammatory complications might respond to oral or nebulized glucocorticoid drugs. It is important to note that the tracheal stent might not benefit the dog if bronchial collapse and bronchomalacia are present together with tracheal collapse.

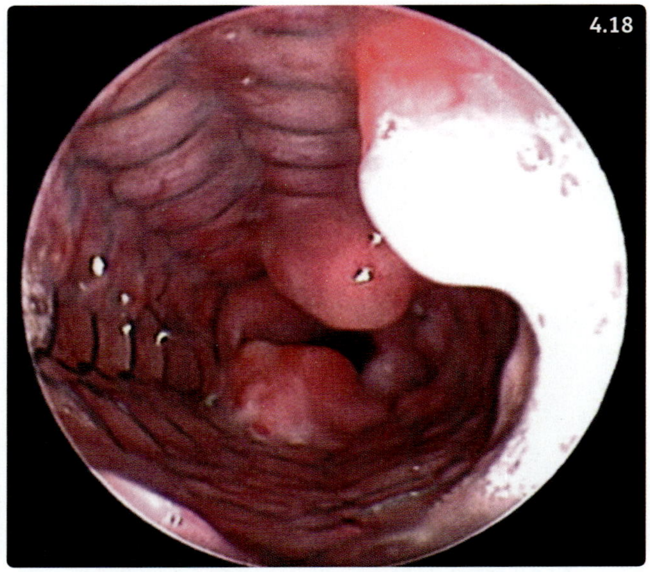

Figure 4.18 Endoscopic view of the trachea of a dog 6 months after stent placement showing exuberant granulation tissue filling most of the tracheal lumen.

Prognosis

Most animals can improve with an individualized treatment plan, but the condition is generally progressive and the long-term prognosis poor, especially when irreversible airway collapse is present.

Tracheal injuries (cats)

Definition/overview

Tracheal injuries range from small lacerations to tracheal avulsions and can be caused by intraluminal or external trauma. Intraluminal trauma is mostly associated with endotracheal intubation, while external trauma is most commonly the result of blunt trauma to the thorax. Often the diagnosis and treatment are delayed, resulting in attempted surgical repair months or even years after the injury.

Etiology

Stenosis occurs after laceration, necrosis, or rupture following endotracheal intubation associated with overinflation of the endotracheal tube cuff. A blunt traumatic incident to the neck or thorax, or both, probably includes a hyperextension injury of the head and neck. This stretches the trachea and ruptures it intrathoracically.

Pathophysiology

After the avulsion injury, the airway lumen is thought to be maintained by either intact tracheal adventitia or by thickening of mediastinal tissue, leading to the development of a pseudoairway. Rupture and avulsion of the trachea result in stenosis of the lumen at both ends of the injury.

Clinical presentation/diagnosis

Apart from some possible cough, clinical signs of inspiratory distress and tracheal stridor are delayed and are due to tracheal obstruction. In acute cases, subcutaneous emphysema can be seen over the cervical and thoracic areas due to air escaping from the trachea into the subcutaneous tissue.

Diagnosis is confirmed by thoracic radiography and tracheoscopy.

Management/prognosis

Surgical management consists of resection of the stenosed end(s) of the injured trachea and subsequent repair by anastomosis. The prognosis is good.

Tumors

Intratracheal tumors are rare. The tracheal lumen can also be reduced by an extrathoracic tumor, such as a mediastinal tumor, which will cause deviation or compression of the trachea.

LOWER AIRWAY AND LUNG DISORDERS

APPROACH TO PATIENTS WITH LOWER AIRWAY AND LUNG DISEASE

Diagnosis of lower airway disease is based on history, physical examination, blood testing, radiography, ultrasonography, CT, and on more invasive techniques (e.g. transtracheal aspiration, bronchoscopy and bronchoalveolar lavage [BAL], transthoracic fine-needle aspiration, transthoracic or open-chest lung biopsy). Pulmonary function tests are not commonly used.

Signalment, origin, present environment, vaccination, and prior medical problems must be assessed before detailing the current complaint and previous treatment. Signs typical of lower respiratory tract (LRT) disease include cough, exercise intolerance, dyspnea, hypoxemia, cyanosis, and systemic signs such as anorexia, depression, weight loss, and fever. Determination of the type of breathing pattern is provided by inspection of the thorax. Respiration should be observed for rate, depth, and regularity. Increased respiratory rate, which is sometimes the only visible sign, may be difficult to differentiate from stress-induced polypnea. Careful and symmetrical auscultation of the lung fields may indicate increased normal breath sounds, crackles, and wheezes as well as silent areas. The thorax should be percussed to assess resonance. A dull note will be obtained with significant lung consolidation and pleural effusion. Again, comparison of percussion notes obtained on the left and right sides is essential, especially in cases where there is a unilateral thoracic problem.

Noninvasive methods include radiography, ultrasonography, and CT. Radiography is still the preferred initial diagnostic test in respiratory medicine. Thoracic radiographs are absolutely essential for proper evaluation of dogs and cats with bronchopulmonary diseases. Thoracic radiographs should be obtained and interpreted before doing any other more invasive procedure. Correct radiographic technique, knowledge of thoracic anatomy, and skilled radiographic interpretation will maximize the amount of information derived from radiography.

Ultrasonography is used to evaluate pulmonary mass lesions adjacent to the body wall and consolidated lung lobes. The consistency of the lesions can often be determined (solid or fluid-filled) and vascular structures may be visible (which can help diagnose lung lobe torsion). It can also be used to guide biopsy instruments into solid masses for specimen collection.

Echocardiography helps distinguish respiratory from cardiac diseases. High-resolution CT is used for evaluation of patients with intrathoracic diseases (e.g. interstitial pulmonary diseases such as idiopathic pulmonary fibrosis or lung lobe torsion) or for determining the extent of intrathoracic mass lesions before considering surgery.

More invasive techniques for cell and tissue sampling include transtracheal wash, endotracheal tube bronchial wash, bronchoscopy with BAL, percutaneous fine-needle aspiration, and lung biopsy obtained through surgical or endoscopic thoracic exploration.

Bronchoscopy allows for examination of the tracheobronchial tree and identification and localization of structural abnormalities of the major airways. It can detect the presence of mucus, pus, or hemorrhage in the airways. It is also used to assess for intraluminal foreign bodies, granulomas, neoplasia, and parasites. It allows for the detection of abnormal mucosal surfaces (**Figure 4.19**) as well as the presence of bronchiectasis and airway patency.

Specimen collection techniques performed in conjunction with bronchoscopy include BAL and various mucosal biopy techniques. The latter include periendoscopic pinch mucosal biopsy, periendoscopic mucosal brush for cytologic smears, and transbronchial biospsy. A familiarity with the bronchoscopic anatomy of bronchopulmonary structures is helpful. An endobronchial nomenclature for a systematic evaluation of the canine and feline airway

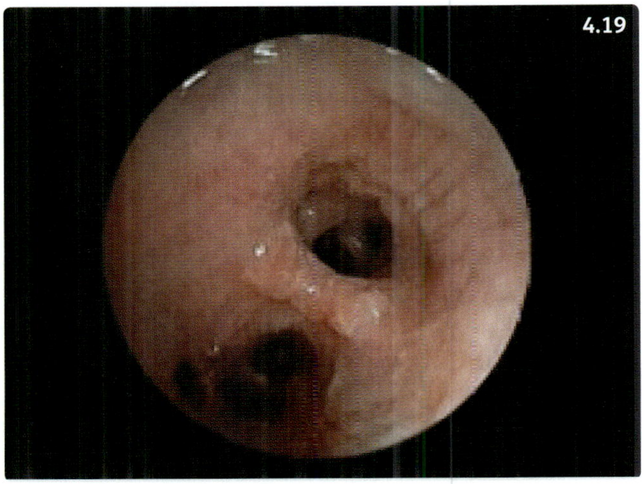

Figure 4.19 Bronchoscopic view of a dog with eosinophilic bronchopneumopathy showing the thickened and polypoid appearance of the bronchial mucosa.

systems has been proposed. The nomenclature enables the bronchoscopist to locate the lesions, to correlate bronchoscopic and diagnostic imaging findings, and to assess the lesions throughout the course of the disease. The procedure also allows for photography of the lesions. Animals undergoing bronchoscopy need general anesthesia, even though they are at increased risk of anesthetic complications. Allowing for the delivery of oxygen before, during, and after the procedure helps to avoid oxygen desaturation, but does not remove the risk of iatrogenic pulmonary decompensation. Other concerns include the expense of the equipment and the need for proper training of the bronchoscopist. A pediatric bronchoscope (diameter of about 3.6–5.0 mm) is the preferred equipment for this procedure. Bronchoscopes are expensive, delicate, and fragile, and need to be handled, used, and cleaned with the utmost care. Additional equipment for optimal sampling includes brush catheters and biopsy and retrieval forceps. If available, the endoscope should be connected to equipment with video projection capability.

In cats with chronic cough and/or dyspnea, the procedure is considered less safe than in dogs, mainly due to the small size of their airways and the greater degree of airway irritability. The procedure can be performed rapidly by a skilled, experienced endoscopist, which limits the risks to the patient.

The risk to benefit ratio should be evaluated before each endoscopy. BAL can be performed with or without an endoscope. The procedures require anesthesia, preoxygenation, and in cats premedication with a bronchodilator such as a single 100 µg puff of aerosolized albuterol, administered through an inhaler and a face mask, or terbutaline orally. Pulse oximetry should be available throughout the procedure until full recovery. When performing bronchoscopic BAL, several small aliquots of warmed sterile saline, using either weight-adjusted (2 ml/kg) or fixed-amount volumes of lavage fluid, are instilled either into the channel of the endoscope or through a sterile catheter passed into this channel. It is important that the endoscope is properly cleaned and disinfected, including the insertion and retrieval channels, prior to each procedure. Nonetheless, contamination of the endoscope by colonizing bacteria is not uncommon and this possibility should always be kept in mind while interpreting microbiological results from BAL fluid analysis.

Alternatively, endotracheal tube bronchial washing or a tracheal wash (TW) can be performed to obtain a bronchial fluid specimen. A sterile catheter is passed through the endotracheal tube or it can be inserted between two tracheal rings into the distal trachea. The recommended volume of fluid varies amongst different authors with each aliquot ranging from 5 to 15 ml. A smaller volume consisting of 0.5 ml/kg is likely to cause less bronchospasm in cats and small breeds of dogs. For medium to large sized dogs the lavage volume can range from 5 to 40 ml or approximately 2 ml/kg. The fluid is instilled through the catheter and immediately aspirated. The technique provides fluid and cells that can be used to identify diseases involving the major airways, while bypassing the normal flora and debris of the oral cavity and pharynx. The advantages of this technique compared with BAL are that the procedure is inexpensive and minimally invasive. The procedure can be performed in awake or sedated animals. Potential complications are rare and include tracheal laceration, subcutaneous emphysema, and pneumomediastinum. Disadvantages are that the lesions and site of sampling cannot be visualized and the TW fluid analysis is less likely to identify interstitial, alveolar, or focal disease processes compared with BAL fluid analysis.

Both BAL and TW fluids are evaluated cytologically and microbiologically and therefore should be collected before initiation of antibiotic treatment whenever possible. Semiquantitative bacterial culture allows for identification of organisms and antimicrobial susceptibility testing. Healthy dogs and cats have bacteria in their airways that can be cultured. Therefore, the significance of organisms must be interpreted in conjunction with the cytologic findings and other clinical data. Cells collected in BAL and TW fluids are fragile and must be quickly and meticulously processed. Nucleated cell counts and differential cell counts are performed. The cells are evaluated qualitatively for determination of the type of inflammation (neutrophilic, eosinophilic), evidence of macrophage activation, neutrophil degeneration, lymphocyte reactivity, characteristics of malignancy, and presence of infectious agents.

Transthoracic needle biopsy is very useful in identifying diffuse interstitial peripheral lesions and solitary lesions of the lung that are located adjacent to the thoracic wall. It also allows for sampling and identification of infectious agents. Samples can be collected using large-bore biopsy or fine-needle aspiration techniques. The site for sampling must be carefully selected radiographically, and the accuracy of sampling can be improved by using ultrasonographic guidance. In most cases this technique does not require general anesthesia and does not require expensive or sophisticated material. Potential complications with fine-needle aspiration, although rare, include pneumothorax, hemoptysis, and bleeding.

Open-chest biopsy is a diagnostic test of last resort because of the invasiveness, cost, degree of morbidity, and danger of mortality associated with this technique.

It is advised when exploratory thoracotomy might also be therapeutic or when it will result in confirmation of a negative prognosis (diffuse metastasis) and justification for euthanasia during surgery.

Video-assisted thoracoscopy, allowing lung biopsy as well as therapeutic procedures, is a very helpful technique since it is much less invasive than open-chest procedures, but offers the same advantages of direct visualization and sampling of the lesion. However, this technique requires special skills and expensive equipment, thus limiting its availability.

Pulmonary function tests can be useful in the diagnosis and evaluation of patients with pulmonary disease. LRT diseases can result in inadequate oxygenation due to decreased ventilation, improper matching of ventilation and perfusion within the lung (V/Q mismatching), and interference with the diffusion of gases across the alveolar membrane. Diseases in small animals can affect these two major physiological functions. Blood gas measurement and calculation of alveolar and arterial oxygen concentrations (A–a gradient) is currently available for assessment of impaired lung function with regard to gas exchange. Normal PaO_2 values range from 80 to 100 mmHg. Hemoglobin saturation with oxygen, and thus whole blood content, does not begin to decrease greatly until the PaO_2 falls below 60 mmHg. Other pulmonary function tests are difficult to apply in veterinary medicine because most of them depend on patient cooperation during the testing procedure or require expensive and sophisticated equipment. Pulmonary scintigraphy is a noninvasive technique used to assess pulmonary ventilation and perfusion, but this test is not routinely available to most veterinarians. Other noninvasive functional testing that has been developed in awake unrestrained dogs and cats includes tidal breathing flow volume loops, measurement of lung compliance, and the 6-minutes walk test.

CANINE INFECTIOUS RESPIRATORY DISEASE COMPLEX IN YOUNG DOGS ('KENNEL COUGH')

Definition/overview

Canine infectious respiratory disease (CIRD) complex is also known as 'kennel cough'. The disease is commonly seen in young dogs that have been in boarding kennels. This contagious disease is often self-limiting in dogs, but a wide range of respiratory signs can be found.

Etiology

Athough many agents have been implicated, CIRD usually results from infection by any one or more of the following pathogens: *Bordetella bronchiseptica*, canine parainfluenza virus, canine influenza virus, canine adenovirus, and canine respiratory coronavirus. *B. bronchiseptica* is a gram-negative, aerobic coccobacillus that is recognized as a primary cause of respiratory disease in dogs. It can also be a serious complicating factor in dogs simultaneously infected with a viral pathogen. *Bordetella* and canine parainfluenza virus have commonly been described as the principal pathogens recovered from dogs involved in CIRD outbreaks.

Pathophysiology

Adherence of *B. bronchiseptica* to cilia via adhesion molecules, induction of ciliostasis, and damage to ciliated epithelium have been implicated in the pathogenesis of *Bordetella* infection. Given the ability of this bacterium to regulate its virulence and the likelihood that co-infected dogs tend to experience more serious clinical disease than dogs infected with single agents, viral co-infection could influence *B. bronchiseptica* virulence and clinical manifestations of CIRD in an individual patient.

Young dogs are more susceptible, especially those housed within a high population density environment, since the viruses and *Bordetella* are highly contagious. Despite the widespread availability of *Bordetella* vaccines, the disease is still common.

Clinical presentation

CIRD is often self-limiting in dogs. In the typical infection, a mild dry cough is the only clinical symptom. However, infection with *Bordetella* can elicit a chronic cough that is more challenging to cure. Respiratory signs may range from mild illness to severe life-threatening pneumonia.

Diagnosis

Diagnosis of bordetellosis relies on positive bacterial culture or, more recently, on positive PCR from BAL fluid. Several laboratories offer PCR testing; however, studies investigating the reliability of this method are lacking. It is difficult to interpret the significance of a positive PCR test result for this disease because *B. bronchiseptica* can be commonly isolated from the URT of clinically healthy dogs, in addition to the fact that a recovered asymptomatic dog may still shed the organism for several weeks. Finding pleiomorphic cocci or coccobacilli adhering to the cilia of the epithelial cells is reported to be a characteristic cytologic feature (**Figure 4.20**).

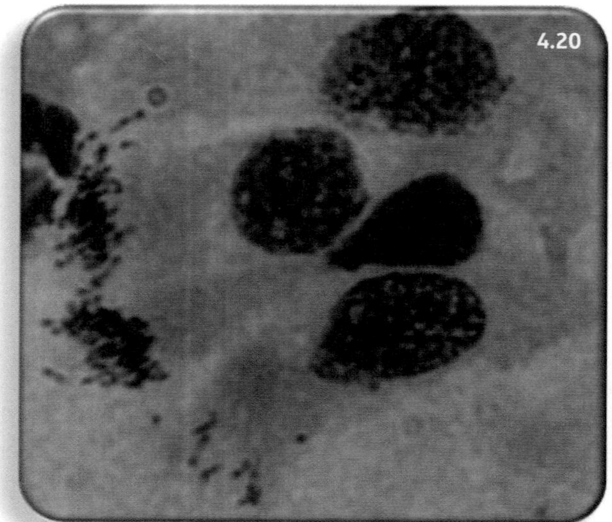

Figure 4.20 Pleiomorphic cocci or coccobacilli found adhering to the cilia of the epithelial cells in a dog with bordetellosis.

Management

Treatment generally consists of empirical antimicrobial therapy. Doxycycline is one of several drugs that can be used effectively. Dogs that are unresponsive to oral or parenteral antibiotics may respond to a nebulized form of administration. Aerosolized topically nonabsorbable antibacterials such as gentamicin have been shown to be effective in reducing the population of *B. bronchiseptica* organisms in the trachea and bronchi of infected dogs.

BACTERIAL BRONCHOPNEUMONIA

Definition/overview

Bronchopneumonia of bacterial origin is much more frequently diagnosed in dogs than in cats, although it might be underdiagnosed in cats. In dogs, many underlying problems can be associated with bacterial bronchopneumonia.

Etiology

A wide variety of bacteria can result in bronchopneumonia, mostly as opportunistic invaders. A single pathogen such as *Escherichia coli, Pasteurella multocida,* staphylococci, streptococci, or *Klebsiella pneumoniae* can be isolated in the majority of cases, but mixed infections are common. Bacteria enter the LRT primarily by inhalation or aspiration or by hematogenous routes. Whether or not a respiratory infection will develop depends on the complex interplay of many factors, such as interference with natural defense mechanisms. Multiple host defense mechanisms exist to protect the LRT from damage secondary to inhaled materials and from possible microbial invasion.These include the mechanisms of coughing and mucociliary clearance, local immunoglobulin (particularly IgA), and cellular and humoral defense mechanisms. Macrophages are responsible for phagocytosis and intracellular killing, and inhibition of macrophage function by viral infections, such as distemper, and corticosteroid use has a major role in the development of secondary bacterial infection.

Pathophysiology

The possibility of an underlying problem should not be overlooked since bacterial infection can complicate nearly any other respiratory disease. There are many clinical conditions that predispose animals to bacterial pneumonia, and these include viral, mycoplasmal, or fungal respiratory infections, metabolic disorders, immunosuppressive therapy, therapy with specific drugs (aspirin, digoxin), functional and anatomic disorders (obstruction of upper airways, tracheal hypoplasia, primary ciliary dyskinesia), immunodeficiency (phagocyte or lymphocyte dysfunction), and contaminated indwelling catheters. Diseases causing dysphagia and vomiting and reduced levels of consciousness can result in foreign material being inhaled into the lung and aspiration pneumonia.

Clinical presentation

Animals with bacterial bronchopneumonia can present with signs typical of lower respiratory disease, such as cough, exercise intolerance, dyspnea, nasal discharge, and cyanosis, in addition to systemic signs of anorexia, depression, weight loss, and fever, the degree of which will vary between patients. However, none of these signs can be used to confirm or rule out bacterial pneumonia. Animals with mild or localized disease show no obvious signs. Most dogs with bronchopneumonia will cough, but many will show only labored breathing. The severity of aspiration pneumonia will vary according to the characteristics of the inspired material and the patient's health status prior to aspiration.

Diagnosis

Diagnosis of bacterial bronchopneumonia is based on history, physical examination, blood testing, and radiographic studies. Other tests such as transtracheal aspiration, bronchoscopy and BAL, and transthoracic fine-needle aspiration are used if deemed necessary. Physical examination signs can include tachycardia and weak pulses, hyperemic oral mucous membranes, and dehydration. Determination of the type of breathing pattern is useful. An increased respiratory effort with an exaggerated abdominal component is common. Nasal flaring also occurs. Auscultation can detect absent or increased lung sounds depending on the degree of pulmonary consolidation.

Thoracic radiography is an essential component of the diagnostic evaluation. The radiographs may show only an interstitial pattern early in the disease. An alveolar pattern develops as the disease progresses. Distribution of lesions may also be helpful in identifying underlying problems. Focal lesions may be associated with foreign bodies. Involvement of the dependent lung lobes commonly occurs with pneumonia with or without aspiration (**Figure 4.21**). Hematogenous-borne infections may have a caudodorsal distribution. Diagnosis may be confirmed by microbiologic and cytologic examination of material from the tracheobronchial tree or lung through aspirates, washings, or brushing performed by transtracheal aspiration, bronchoscopy, or fine-needle lung aspiration.

A CBC may reveal a neutrophilic leukocytosis and left shift with a monocytosis. It is not uncommon to find only a stress response or even a normal leukogram.

Adequate bronchopulmonary sampling techniques for cytologic evaluation and culture of aspirates include tracheal washing, BAL, or brushing and percutaneous fine-needle aspirations. Bacterial culture is more sensitive than cytology for identifying organisms and also allows for susceptibility testing. However, bacteria can be cultured from the airways of healthy dogs. This microbacterial population has the potential to cause or complicate respiratory infections and clouds the interpretation of airway and lung cultures. Therefore, the significance of organisms must be interpreted in conjunction with the cytologic findings and other clinical data. Quantitative culture of BAL fluid is advised since the threshold to define clinically relevant bacterial growth in diagnosing LRT infection has been determined (1.7 x 10^3 colony-forming units per ml of BAL fluid).

Management

Antimicrobial therapy is essential for the treatment of lower airway bacterial infections. The most important criterion for selection of an antibiotic is identification of the bacterial organism and the results of sensitivity testing. There appears to be much variability in the *in-vitro* sensitivity of common isolates in different countries, emphasizing the importance of culture and sensitivity testing for individual patients. Broad-spectrum coverage for life-threatening infections or sepsis can be obtained using combinations of either amoxicillin–clavulanic acid and enrofloxacin or amoxicillin–clavulanic acid and an

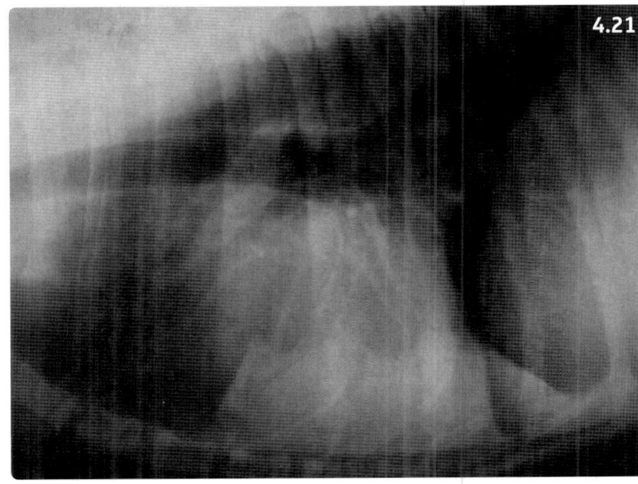

Figure 4.21 Thoracic radiograph of a dog with aspiration pneumonia showing ventral distribution of an alveolar pattern with air bronchograms and lobar signs.

aminoglycoside. Fluoroquinolones specifically achieve excellent concentrations within the lung.

Systemic oral or parenteral antibiotics should be administered in high doses for a minimum of 2 weeks and sometimes longer so that maximum concentrations are reached in lung tissue and airway secretions. Obvious clinical improvement will optimally be noted after 3–5 days of treatment. Ideally, the animal should be re-examined weekly in order to monitor the response to treatment, based on clinical and radiographic findings. Therapy may be discontinued 1 week after resolution of all clinical signs and the disappearance of the radiographic infiltrates.

Maintenance of normal systemic hydration is very important for mucociliary clearance and secretion mobilization. Airway hydration can also be achieved using saline aerosol therapy followed by physiotherapy (mild forced exercise, increasing cough frequency by chest wall coupage or tracheal manipulation, and postural drainage). The use of aerosol administration of antibacterials or other drugs should be restricted to cases of bordetellosis.

Animals with severe tachypnea, dyspnea or hypoxemia (PaO_2 <60 mmHg) require oxygen therapy. The oxygen should be humidified to prevent drying of respiratory membranes. Oxygen can be administered by oxygen cage, mechanical ventilator, intratracheal cannula, or nasal catheter. Antitussives and antihistamines that inhibit mucokinesis and exudate removal are contraindicated with bacterial pneumonia.

Although the value of expectorant therapy (saline expectorants, guaifenesin, and inhaled volatile oils that are inhaled) has not been scientifically demonstrated, their use can be beneficial.

Pulmonary lobectomy can be an alternative in the management of pneumonia in dogs, especially if a diagnosis of abscessation is suspected or if a lesion does not resolve after several months of aggressive adequate antibiotic therapy.

Prognosis

Bacterial pneumonias are generally responsive to appropriate antibiotic therapy and supportive care. The severity and chronicity of the infection, the presence of an underlying disease, and the development of complications can affect the long-term prognosis. Potential reasons for failure are many. They may be related to the organism involved (not sensitive to the antibiotic used or capable of developing resistance) or to the antibiotic itself. Failures attributable to the drug may relate to the dosage regimen, spectrum of activity, or ability to achieve effective concentration. Other causes of failure include inaccurate diagnosis or existence of an undiagnosed underlying disorder.

PRIMARY CILIARY DYSKINESIA

Definition/overview

Primary ciliary dyskinesia (PCD), previously referred to as immotile cilia syndrome, results from a heterogeneous group of inherited diseases that cause defective ciliary motility mostly associated with ultrastructural abnormalities. It is a predisposing cause of recurrent bacterial pneumonia. In dogs, as in humans, the ineffectiveness and incoordination of ciliary function result in ineffective clearance of mucus from the airways, which in turn results in chronic mucus plugging and inflammation of nasal cavities and airways. Kartagener's syndrome represents a triad of signs that includes bronchiectasis, complete transposition of viscera (situs inversus), and chronic rhinosinusitis (**Figures 4.22a, b**). This syndrome has been reported in humans and in dogs with PCD. In dogs, PCD is a rare disease that has been reported in more than 19 breeds.

Etiology

Currently, PCD-causing mutations have been identified in 20 human genes. Each causative gene can be associated with particular ultrastructural ciliary defects and these 20 genes only explain 50% of human PCD cases; more genes need to be identified. In dogs, a recent mutation in a new causative gene (*CCDC39*) has been identified in the Old English Sheepdog. This new mutation is dispersed in a significant worldwide population and is responsible for PCD in this breed. A new genetic test has been developed and is currently available for breeding purposes.

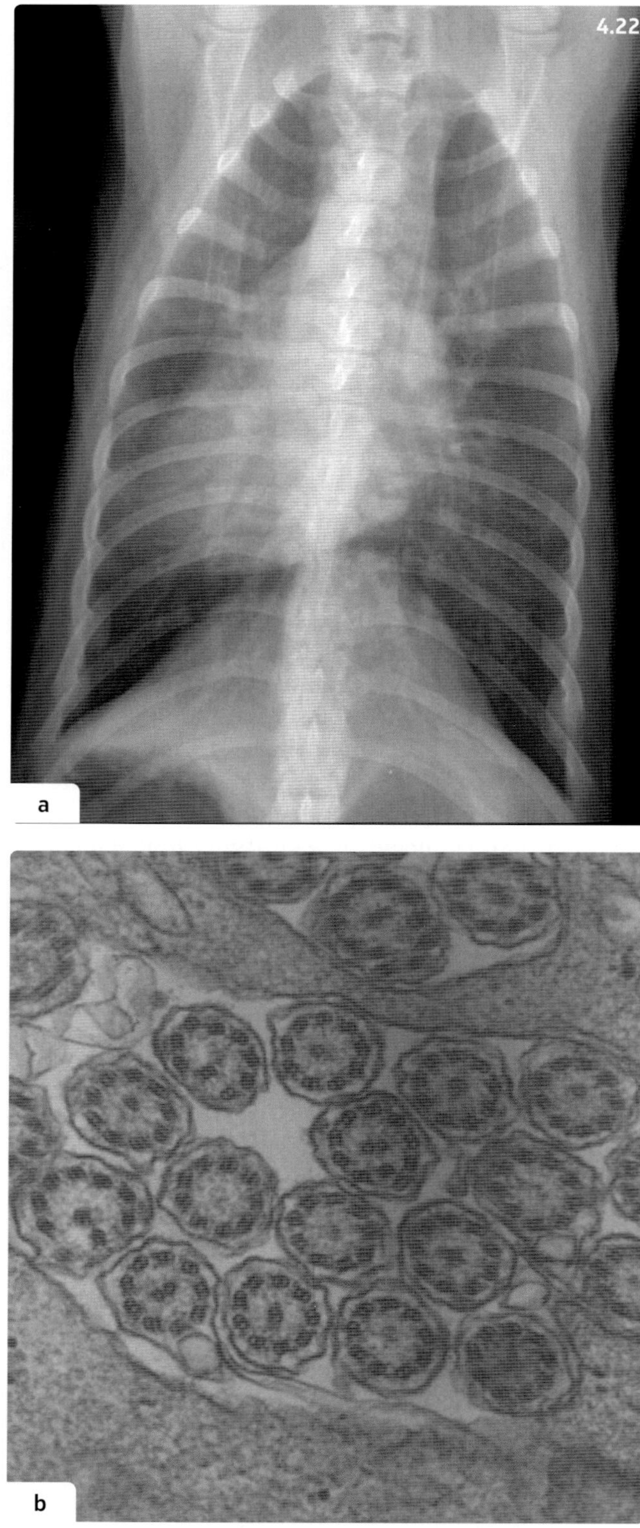

Figures 4.22a, b Old English Sheepdog with primary ciliary dyskinesia associated with situs inversus. (a) Dorsoventral thoracic radiograph. (b) Transmission electron microscope image of transverse sections of cilia showing a primary defect (absence of the central pair of doublets) and many secondary defects.

Clinical presentation

As a consequence of impaired mucociliary clearance, clinical signs include chronic respiratory abnormalities such as rhinosinusitis, bronchitis, bronchopneumonia, and bronchiectasis. Although the respiratory system signs are usually the presenting complaint, other signs related to pathology in other tissues with ciliated epithelia or microtubules can occur, such as otitis media, infertility in females, asthenoteratospermia in males, hydrocephalus, and renal fibrosis or dilation of renal tubules. The signs typically begin at an early age in a purebred vaccinated dog; however, some dogs have remained asymptomatic until several months to several years of age. Hallmark clinical features (i.e. recurrent bilateral nasal discharge and repeated episodes of bronchitis or bronchopneumonia since birth) should alert the clinician to include PCD in the differential diagnosis.

Diagnosis

Finding the hallmark clinical features in combination with situs inversus is even more suggestive. Most other potential possible causes should be excluded by a complete physical examination as well as currently available complementary tests. Confirmation of a diagnosis of PCD requires both *in-vivo* and *in-vitro* functional and ultrastructural analysis of cilia. *In-vitro* functional analysis of cilia in dogs suspected of having PCD utilizes scintigraphy as the diagnostic tool to evaluate mucociliary clearance. *In-vivo* functional analysis in PCD consistently demonstrates an uncoordinated or a dyskinetic ciliary beat. Transmission electron microscopy can reveal specific ultrastructural abnormalities, although regularly the distinction between PCD and secondary ciliary defects (caused by another primary disease) based on ultrastructural findings is difficult.

Other causes of recurrent bacterial infection of the lower airways should be investigated, such as the presence of an immune deficiency, a resistant bacterium, a bronchial foreign body, or any other predisposing cause (see above). In Irish Wolfounds, a rhinitis/bronchopneumonia syndrome characterized by transient to persistent mucoid or mucopurulent rhinorrhea, cough, and dyspnea since an early age has been described; so far PCD has not yet been formally identified as the cause of the disease in this particular breed.

Management

Even though PCD is not a curable disease, it can frequently be managed for some years. A key element in successful management is adequate monitoring of infecting microorganisms and judicious use of antibiotics over time. Moreover, a regular routine consisting of good systemic and local hydration, daily coupage, and vigorous exercise will help to clear mucus from the airways.

Prognosis

The long-term prognosis is poor, since even in cases with adequate management, the disease generally progresses over time and the response to treatment worsens. It would be very useful to have a genetic test able to identify carriers in order to prevent their use for breeding.

PARASITIC BRONCHOPNEUMOPATHY IN DOGS, ANGIOSTRONGYLOSIS (FRENCH HEARTWORM DISEASE)

Definition/overview/etiology

The nematode worm *Angiostrongylus vasorum* is an emerging disease, with reported increases in both distribution and incidence in the United Kingdom, Europe, South Africa, and Canada. The expanding geographic range might be related to the influence of the climate on parasite distribution.

The worm infects dogs and foxes and is spread through ingestion of intermediate hosts, including slugs and snails, harboring infective third-stage larvae. The adult parasites live in the pulmonary arteries and the right ventricule of the heart. The prepatent period is 40–60 days.

Respiratory disease results from the inflammatory response induced by migration of the larvae, causing granulomatous pneumonia and probably thrombotic disease.

Clinical presentation

Infection seems more common in outdoor young dogs, especially those playing with/eating slugs. Dogs are presented for a combination of signs including cough, exercise intolerance, respiratory distress, coagulopathy (hemoptysis, bleedings), lameness, neurologic signs, and syncope. However, clinical signs may be variable and range from subtle and chronic to more acute and severe.

Diagnosis

Eosinophilia, thrombocytopenia, and hyperglobulinemia are relatively common. Thoracic radiographs generally show an interstitial and/or alveolar pattern, most often present in the dorsocaudal lung fields. Definitive parasitologic diagnosis relies on observation of first-stage larvae (L1) in the respiratory tract or feces, using the Baermann test. L1 are sometimes observed on airway cytology. A major limitation of the Baermann test is that L1 excretion appears to be intermittent, and infected dogs might be negative on fecal examination. A single Baermann test is likely to detect at most 50% of infected dogs, although sensitivity can be increased by serial examination (e.g. of samples collected 3 days in succession, which is not always practical).

Improved diagnostic tests are likely to emerge. Parasite proteins or DNA can be detected in blood or BAL fluid using sandwich ELISA or PCR, respectively. Serologic ELISA tests to detect host antibodies to the parasite have also been developed.

Management

Fenbendazole (25–50 mg/kg PO q24h for 7–21 days) has been the most commonly used anthelminthic drug during the last decade. Milbemycin oxime and moxidectin (e.g. Advantage Multi®, a spot-on combination formulation of moxidectin plus imidacloprid) both prevent establishment of adult parasites when given during the prepatent period, and substantially reduce worm burdens. However, continued monitoring after treatment is advisable, with repeated treatment as necessary. Depending on the severity of clinical signs, additional therapy with corticosteroids, IV fluid support, and oxygen can be required.

Prognosis

Dogs carrying a low worm burden may remain subclinical. The prognosis is guarded in those animals with severe respiratory signs. The disease can be fatal if left untreated.

EOSINOPHILIC BRONCHOPNEUMOPATHY IN DOGS

Etiology/pathophysiology

Canine eosinophilic bronchopneumopathy (EBP) is a disease characterized by eosinophilic infiltration of lung and bronchial mucosa, considered to be manifestations of immunologic hypersensitivity. Although the etiology of EBP is still unknown, the association of eosinophilic infiltration with $CD4^+$ T cells favors a likely Th2 immune response mounted in the lower airways. Suspected and known causes of pulmonary hypersensitivities in humans and animals include fungi, molds, drugs, bacteria, and parasites. However, in many cases no underlying cause is found. The role of inhaled allergens in EBP is still unclear. EBP is mostly diagnosed in young dogs. Siberian Huskies and Malamutes are predominantly affected but many other breeds also can be affected.

Clinical presentation

Usually, the general condition of the animal is good, unless the disease is associated with concomitant bacterial bronchopneumonia. Clinical signs include mainly cough, gagging, and retching. In acute cases, gagging and retching are sometimes the main complaint, extending the differential diagnosis to dyspeptic problems. Dyspnea is a very frequent sign. Nasal discharge (about 50% of affected dogs) is less commonly encountered.

Differential diagnosis

Several parasites including *Strongyloides* spp., *Ascaris* spp., *Toxocara canis*, and *Ancylostoma* spp. can lead to eosinophilic pneumonia in humans, and probably in dogs as well; respiratory symptoms are mild and gastroenterologic signs usually predominate.

In the dog, occult heartworm disease caused by *Dirofilaria immitis* can cause eosinophilic pneumonitis. Migration of larvae of *Angiostrongylus vasorum* through pulmonary parenchyma may also result in eosinophilic pneumonia in dogs (see above). Other bronchopulmonary parasites, such as *Capillaria aerophila*, *Oslerus osleri*, *Filaroides hirthi*, *Crenosema vulpis*, or *Paragonimus kellicotti*, are also implicated in the migration of eosinophils into the airways (*O. osleri*) or lungs (other parasites) in dogs, and can mimic EBP.

Diagnosis

The diagnostic work up of dogs with pulmonary disease should include a search for parasitic disease, using BAL fluid analysis or feces examination (fecal zinc sulfate centrifugation/flotation and Baermann sedimentation procedure). However, a single negative fecal examination by either method is not conclusive. The fecal examination should therefore be repeated or, alternatively, the animal treated for potential parasites using a course of an appropriate anthelmintic (e.g. fenbendazole, thiabendazole, or levamisole). In endemic areas it is strongly advised to run a heartworm antigen test to rule out occult heartworm disease.

The diagnostic criteria for the diagnosis of EBP include anamnestic factors (breed, young age, previous response to corticosteroids), clinical signs, radiographic and bronchoscopic findings, blood eosinophilia, tissue eosinophilic infiltration as demonstrated by cytologic and histopathologic examinations, response to adequate treatment, and the exclusion of other pulmonary conditions. The most common radiographic finding is a mixed moderate to severe bronchointerstitial pattern (**Figure 4.23a**). Bronchoscopy can reveal typical macroscopic features, which include the presence of abundant yellow–green mucus or mucopurulent material, severe thickening of the mucosa with irregular or polypoid surface (see **Figure 4.19**), and in some cases partial airway closure during expiration. Peripheral blood eosinophilia is frequently found (about 60% of the cases) but not always observed. BAL fluid or brush cytology demonstrates a marked eosinophilic component

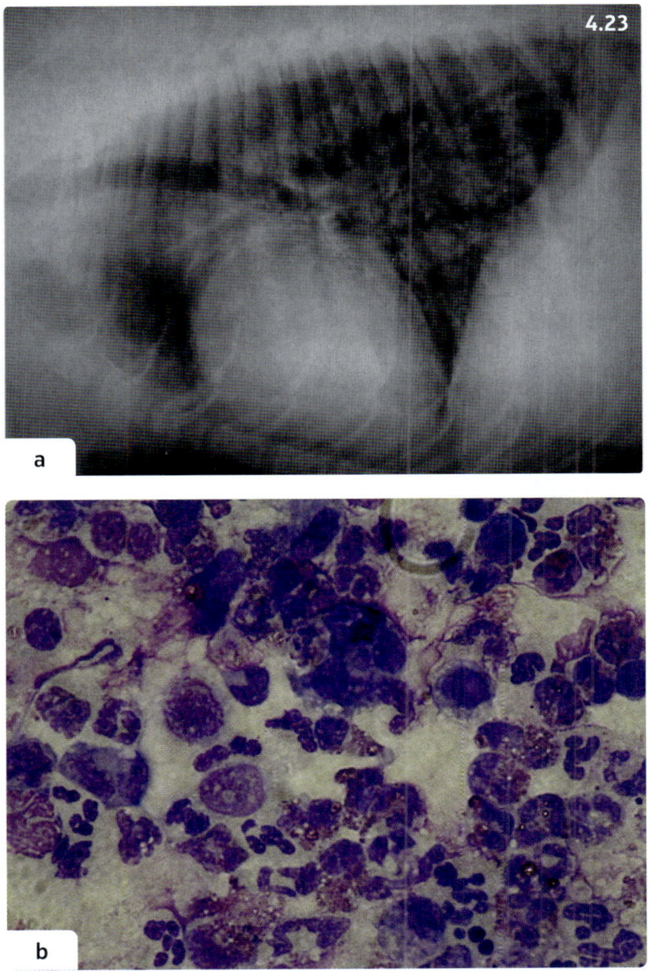

Figures 4.23a, b Four-year-old male Akita Inu with eosinophilic bronchopneumopathy. (a) Lateral thoracic radiograph showing a severe bronchointerstitial pattern with peribronchial infiltration. (b) Cytologic preparation (BAL fluid cytospin) showing 47% of eosinophils (total cell count = 7,000 cells/ml).

(**Figure 4.23b**); frequently, more than 50% of the inflammatory cells are eosinophils. In most cases eosinophilic infiltration of the bronchial mucosa can also be observed histopathologically in biopsy samples.

Management

The response to steroid therapy is generally very good (prednisone, initial dosage of 1 mg/kg q12h for the 1st week, then on alternate days during the 2nd and 3rd weeks, followed by a gradual decrease to the lowest possible maintenance dose). Inhaled glucocorticoid therapy can be considered for long-term maintenance in order to help avoid the systemic complications of chronic glucocorticoid treatment, although this might not allow for complete clinical control of the disorder. This treatment modality is well tolerated, results in improvement in clinical signs and reduction in side-effects, and allows for a reduction of oral steroid dosage in steroid-dependent animals.

Prognosis

Relapse frequently occurs within weeks to months after drug discontinuation, although some dogs may remain asymptomatic after discontinuation of glucocorticoid treatment.

CHRONIC BRONCHITIS IN DOGS

Definition/overview

Chronic bronchitis is mostly seen in middle aged to old smaller breeds of dogs, but it can occur in larger breeds. It is a chronic inflammatory airway disease that results mainly in cough.

Chronic bronchitis in dogs is defined when three diagnostic criteria can be fulfilled:

- Chronic cough.
- Evidence of excessive mucus or of mucus hypersecretion.
- Exclusion of other chronic cardiopulmonary diseases (e.g. congestive heart failure, chronic infectious bronchopneumonia, pulmonary neoplasia, eosinophilic bronchopneumopathy).

Co-existing diseases (e.g. congestive heart failure and airway collapse) may be present and complicate diagnosis and treatment. The most common sequela is chronic airway obstruction, referred to as chronic obstructive pulmonary disease, a syndrome that is well described in humans.

ETIOLOGY

Many causes of chronic bronchitis are a result of chronic airway irritation and inflammation. The condition is usually diagnosed after a protracted period (>2 months) of clinical signs that can result from exposure to passive smoking, excessive environmental perfumes, or atmospheric pollution.

Pathophysiology

Chronic bronchitis results in inflammatory changes within the bronchial mucosa, including increased mucus production. Bronchial wall thickening and progressive bronchomalacia contribute to airflow obstruction and further worsening of the inflammation and clinical signs, which consist mainly of a productive cough.

Clinical presentation

Middle aged to older smaller dog breeds are more often affected, although any dog that is exposed to chronic airway irritants or has suffered from smoke inhalation can be similarly affected. Most dogs with chronic bronchitis have a rather sonorous cough, which is followed by a retching movement.

Differential diagnosis

Chronic cough related to specific causes should be ruled out, mainly tracheal collapse, lung fibrosis, EBP, parasitic lung diseases, bronchial or lung primary or secondary tumors, mitral valve disease.

Diagnosis

Diagnostic tests are carried out to rule out other causes of chronic cough. The hemogram is usually normal and thoracic radiographs show bronchial wall thickening or generalized increased airway-oriented interstitial density, or both. BAL cytology typically has excess mucus with hyperplastic epithelial cells and increased numbers of neutrophils, goblet cells, and macrophages. Echocardiography helps to diagnose any concomitant disorders such as mitral valve disease and right heart enlargement associated with pulmonary aterial hypertension, which can occur secondary to chronic pulmonary disease.

Management

The bronchial alterations are not readily medically reversible. Therapy is based on an assessment of the nature and severity of the individual animal's problems and includes:

- Avoidance of airway irritants and neck compression.
- Control of body weight because obese dogs often show improvement associated with weight reduction.
- Relief of airway inflammation: anti-inflammatory therapy using a low dose of glucocorticosteroids, which reduces mucus hypersecretion and mucosal bronchial wall thickening. Bronchodilators (β_2 agonists, theophylline) are frequently used, although their effectiveness in the treatment of chronic bronchitis has not been widely addressed.
- Control of infection and maintaining good dental hygiene.

Prognosis

Treatment can alleviate clinical symptoms but ongoing airway disease will likely persist.

CHRONIC IDIOPATHIC PULMONARY FIBROSIS IN WEST HIGHLAND WHITE TERRIERS AND OTHER TERRIER BREEDS

Definition/overview

Chronic idiopathic pulmonary fibrosis (IPF) in West Highland White Terriers and other terrier breeds is an emerging chronic and progressive pulmonary condition. It has been described in middle aged to old West Highland White Terriers, but also in other young to middle aged terrier dogs such as the Staffordshire Bull Terrier. A similar condition exists in humans. Very little is known about IPF prevalence, pathogenesis, and prognosis in dogs.

Etiology

As in humans, the etiopathogenesis of IPF in dogs is not known. There is emerging evidence for the role of genetic factors in the development of the disease. Most cases appear to be caused by an interaction between a specific environmental exposure and a genetic predisposition. In dogs, the predisposition of related terrier breeds combined with very low incidence within non-terrier breeds also strongly suggests an underlying genetic cause.

Pathophysiology

Current prevailing hypotheses for the condition focus on dysregulated epithelial–mesenchymal interactions promoting a cycle of continued epithelial cell injury and fibroblast activation leading to fibrosis. Multiple abnormalities in a myriad of biological pathways affecting inflammation and wound repair, including matrix regulation, epithelial reconstitution, the coagulation cascade, neovascularization, and antioxidants, modulate this defective process and promote fibrogenesis.

Clinical presentation

The disease is clinically characterized by progressive dyspnea, exercise intolerance, and pronounced crackles on auscultation. General body condition is good and dogs do not lose weight. Cough is described principally in the earliest phase of the disease. The condition might also be associated with some degree of tracheal collapse that develops secondarily in some dogs.

Differential diagnosis

The disease is not easily distinguished from chronic bronchitis, which may co-exist. In IPF, cough can be attributed to tracheal collapse, which is found in a proportion of affected dogs. Crackles might suggest cardiogenic edema;

however, such a diagnosis is not compatible with other clinical findings.

Diagnosis

Radiographic, bronchoscopic, hematologic, or biochemical findings are nonspecific, but help to eliminate other possible disorders. Echocardiography may reveal signs of secondary pulmonary arterial hypertension.

Arterial blood gas analysis shows low levels of PaO_2 and a high alveolar–arterial oxygen gradient. Other noninvasive pulmonary function tests are rarely used in veterinary practice.

Lung imaging using high-resolution CT looks promising and is currently often used to evaluate IPF in humans. However, ultimate confirmation of the diagnosis requires (open-chest) lung biopsy and histopathology. Histopathologically, the predominant changes include septal and interstitial fibrosis and pneumocyte hyperplasia.

Management/prognosis

As the disease is a progressive condition, the long-term prognosis is poor. A mean survival time of about 18 months has been reported. The course of the disease is characterized by a slow progression together with episodes of worsening. Treatment of dogs with IPF is essentially symptomatic and supportive. Glucocorticoid drugs have been tried but have not proved beneficial, while subjecting the dog to potentially detrimental side-effects.

BRONCHIECTASIS

Definition/overview

Bronchiectasis is pathologically defined as an abnormal and permanent dilatation and distortion of subsegmental airways due to destruction of the elastic and muscular components of the bronchial walls. Several congenital or acquired conditions that lead to a cycle of chronic airway infection and inflammation may result in bronchiectatic changes.

Etiology/pathophysiology

Focal bronchiectasis most often results from foreign body aspiration. Diffuse bronchiectasis often occurs subsequent to aspiration or inhalation injury, primary ciliary dyskinesis, infection with *Bordetella bronchiseptica* or *Pneumocystis carinii* (in relation to immune deficiency), eosinophilic bronchopneumopathy, and chronic bronchitis. Affected airways are usually partially obstructed by purulent or viscid exudates since the dilation greatly interferes with normal airway clearance. Dysfunction of mucociliary clearance allows pooling of mucus, exudates, and microbes, which eventually leads to secondary infection and its accompanying inflammatory response, creating a vicious cycle of further damage to the airway wall and predisposition to recurrent bronchopulmonary infections.

Clinical presentation/diagnosis

There appears to be a breed predilection since bronchiectasis is more prevalent in certain breeds such as the American Cocker Spaniel, Miniature Poodle, Siberian Husky, and English Springer Spaniel. Most dogs with bronchiectasis are 7 years of age or older. The clinical signs are typical of chronic bronchial disease and include cough, gagging, tachypnea, dyspnea, and occasionally fever.

Diagnosis

Bronchiectasis can be detected by thoracic radiography, high-resolution CT, or bronchoscopy.

Management

Treatment is the same as for chronic bronchitis, but the disease is more difficult to control. The goal of therapy is to control clinical signs and eliminate any bacterial infections. Removing any likely pulmonary irritants from the dog's environment is essential to slow the progression of bronchial wall destruction. Dogs with bronchiectasis may survive for years despite substantial clinical abnormalities. Patients with focal bronchiectasis might benefit from surgical resection of the pathologic lung lobe.

PULMONARY CONTUSIONS

Etiology

Pulmonary contusion is caused by blunt trauma. It is a common finding in dogs that have received thoracic trauma and can be associated with pneumothorax, pneumomediastinum, rib fracture, and many other adverse effects of the traumatic insult. Hemorrhage into the interstitium and alveoli occurs, usually in localized lung regions.

Clinical presentation

Generally there is historical and physical evidence of trauma. Increased respiratory efforts are usually obvious, but the clinical picture will depend on the effects of other ongoing injury.

Diagnosis

Alveolar infiltrates are seen on thoracic radiographs along with other signs of thoracic injury. They include large localized areas of alveolar and interstitial opacities.

(**Editors' note:** Pulmonary hemorrhage can also occur from anticoagulant rodenticide ingestion. The history, absence of other signs of trauma, and abnormal blood clotting times will distinguish this from traumatic pulmonary contusions.)

Management

Dogs should first be treated for life-threatening trauma-related problems. Decreased physical activity and cage rest in a 40% oxygen enriched environment is advised. Oxygen can also be provided with nasal cannulation. Pulmonary contusion will begin to show radiographic resolution after 3–5 days.

Prognosis

Prognosis varies from good to guarded depending on the extent of the injuries. Progression of pulmonary injuries to acute respiratory distress syndrome is an ominous complication.

FELINE BRONCHIAL SYNDROME

Definition/overview

Cough is an infrequent clinical sign in cats. It is fairly specific for tracheobronchial disease in cats since cough of cardiac origin is rare. Feline bronchial disease (feline asthma or bronchitis) is characterized by inflammation of the lower airways without an obvious identifiable cause. Many other terms are found in the literature such as chronic bronchitis, allergic bronchitis, eosinophilic bronchitis, and bronchial asthma. It is recognized clinically with signs of cough, wheezing, exercise intolerance, and respiratory distress attributable to airway obstruction caused by bronchial inflammation.

Etiology

Feline asthma is thought to be an allergic disorder based on the associated tissue pathology and the response to glucocorticoid drugs, although it might be difficult to distinguish the condition from other types of chronic airway disease.

Pathophysiology

Clinical signs are related to reversible airway inflammation and obstruction linked to hyperreactivity and smooth muscle hypertrophy, excessive mucus production (mucous gland hypertrophy) and accumulation, and bronchial wall edema. These changes are often reversible. However, chronic inflammation can lead to severe lower airway obstruction, which causes lung hyperinflation and air trapping. Lung hyperinflation may lead to permanent pathology, evidenced by progressive airway remodeling including bronchectasis, fibrosis, or emphysema. Sometimes, reversible atelectasis can occur.

Clinical presentation

Young to middle aged cats are most commonly affected. The clinical signs are cough and increased breathing effort, which can vary in severity. The signs are often chronic or slowly progressive. Mildly affected cases may only have occasional and brief episodes of cough separated by long periods without symptoms, while in moderately or severely affected cases, cough occurs daily and cats may have a decreased quality of life with breathing discomfort. Cats with severe exacerbations (also called 'asthmatic crisis') may present acutely with open-mouth breathing, dyspnea, and cyanosis. Exacerbation may occur in association with exposure to potential allergens or irritants or after stress or exercise.

Differential diagnosis

Includes any disease that can affect the feline airway. Pulmonary parasitic diseases, including infection with *Aerulostrongylus abstrusus* and *Dirofilaria immitis* (in endemic regions), will result in similar clinical findings including eosinophilic airway inflammation.

Diagnosis

Physical examination in the asymptomatic cat can be normal at rest, but those with active disease will show a prolonged expiratory phase of breathing with auscultable wheezes or crackles. The classic radiographic pattern with established disease includes signs of bronchial wall thickening (doughnuts or railroad tracks) and air trapping (increased lucency and flattening of the diaphragm). Some cats will have a right middle or some other lung lobe atelectasis.

The hemogram can range from normal to having an eosinophilia. Other abnormalities include a stress leukogram, a secondary polycythemia, or hyperglobulinemia. Fecal examination is recommended as part of the diagnostic work up in order to exclude a parasitic origin for the eosinophilic infiltration (*Aelurostrongylus, Dirofilaria*).

Cytologic examination of airway samples, obtained by BAL or endotracheal wash, generally provides evidence of airway inflammation, with increased numbers of eosinophils and/or neutrophils. Although a preponderance of eosinophils may be found in fluids from healthy cats, the number of eosinophils and neutrophils in BAL fluid has been shown to correlate with disease severity, both in cats with spontaneous disease and in those with experimentally induced bronchial disease Feline asthmatic disease is primarily characterized by a predominance (as high as 17%) of eosinophils identified in the BAL fluid. Culture of BAL fluid and PCR for *Mycoplasma* detection can be useful, but its presence does not necessarily signify it being the cause of the airway disease. Feces examination (fecal floatation and Baermann) and heartworm antibody/antigen testing can help detect heartworm disease or *Toxocara cati* and *Aerulostrongylus abstrusus*.

Pulmonary function testing is not commonly used in the diagnostic assessment of cats with bronchial disease.

Management

Stress should be minimized and an oxygen enriched environment provided when managing any cat with acute respiratory distress. Parenteral therapy with beta-agonist bronchodilators such as terbutaline (0.01 mg/kg IV, IM, or SC) and a rapidly acting corticosteroid (e.g. dexamethasone, 0.25 mg/kg IV or IM) should be administered. Inhaled bronchodilator medication can be used as well.

Most retrospective studies involving cats with lower airway disease have documented a beneficial response to oral or parenteral glucocorticoids and/or bronchodilators. An initial dose of prednisone or prednisolone, beginning at 1–2 mg/kg q24h over a 2-week period followed by a gradual tapering dose over another 2-week period, has been shown to be a consistent, reliable, and effective treatment. Bronchodilators, such as inhaled salbutamol and albuterol, are very useful to alleviate acute clinical signs, but as they fail to control airway inflammation, they should not be used without glucocorticoid drugs.

The use of inhaled medication using a face mask and spacing chamber (**Figure 4.24**) is popular Medications given via inhalation offer the advantage of providing high drug concentrations within the the airways while attenuating systemic side-effects. Long-term treatment with inhaled corticosteroids (e.g. fluticasone propionate), and bronchodilators (e.g. albuterol) is the preferred medication.

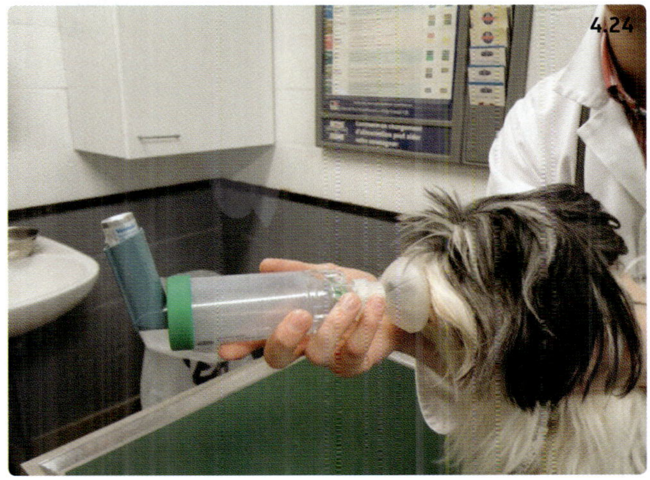

Figure 4.24 Inhaled steroid therapy for a dog with a chronic cough using a spacer and face mask (Aerokat*, Trudel. Medical International, Ontario, Canada).

RECOMMENDED FURTHER READING

Ettinger SJ, Feldman EC (2010) (eds.) *Textbook of Veterinary Internal Medicine*, 6th edn. Elsevier Saunders, St. Louis.

Johnson LR (2007) (ed.) Respiratory physiology, diagnostics and diseases. *Vet Clin North Am Small Anim Pract* **37(5)**:829–1012.

Johnson LR (2014) (ed.) Canine and feline respiratory medicine. *Vet Clin North Am Small Anim Pract* **44(1)**:1–190.

Johnson LR (2010) (ed.) *Clinical Canine and Feline Respiratory Medicine*, 1st edn. Wiley-Blackwell, Ames.

King LG (2004) (ed.) *Textbook of Respiratory Diseases in Dogs and Cats*. Elsevier Saunders, St. Louis.

Luis Fuentes V, Johnson LR, Dennis S (2010) (eds.) *BSAVA Manual of Canine and Feline Cardiorespiratory Medicine*, 2nd edn. British Small Animal Veterinary Association, Gloucester.

Chapter 5

Diseases of the pleural space

J. Brad Case

PNEUMOTHORAX

Definition/overview

Pneumothorax is a common disease among dogs and cats and is characterized by an accumulation of air in the pleural space and subsequent restriction to pulmonary inflation. The result is hypoxemia, which can be severe in many cases and eventually cause death of the animal.

Etiology

Two broad etiologic categories are recognized in dogs and cats; traumatic and spontaneous pneumothorax. Traumatic pneumothorax (closed or open chest) is seen most commonly after blunt automobile trauma but is also observed following thoracic penetrating trauma (e.g. bite, gunshot, porcupine quill wounds). In contrast, spontaneous pneumothorax is not associated with thoracic wall trauma or any observed inciting cause. Subpleural blebs (**Figure 5.1**) and pulmonary bullae are the most common causes of spontaneous pneumothorax but parasitic, infectious, and neoplastic diseases have also been documented. Disease-specific etiologies are summarized in **Table 5.1**.

5.1

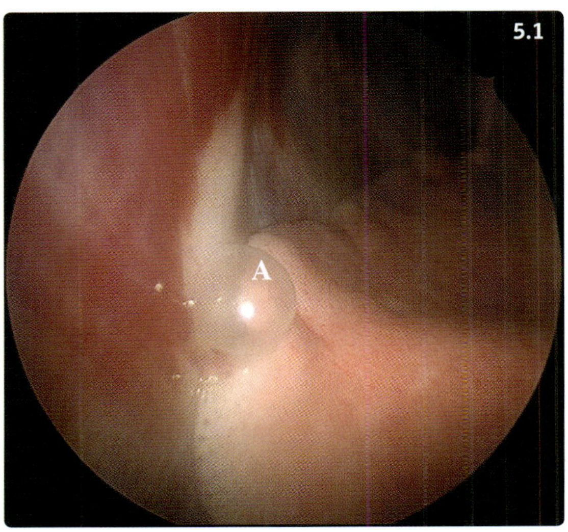

Figure 5.1 Thoracoscopic image of a subpleural bleb (A) in a dog with spontaneous pneumothorax.

Table 5.1 Causes of pleural space diseases.

Cause
Pneumothorax
Traumatic closed chest (blunt trauma)
Open chest (penetrating projectiles, bites, automobile)
Spontaneous (bullae, blebs, foreign bodies, bronchoesophageal fistula, abscess, bronchiectasis, pneumonia)
Pyothorax
Pneumonia
Bronchiectasis
Foreign body
Esophageal perforation
Trauma
Surgical
Chest drain
Feline infectious peritonitis/feline leukemia virus
Abscess (common causative agents: *Actinomyces* spp., *Nocardia* spp., *Filifactor* spp.)
Chylothorax
Idiopathic
Lung lobe torsion
Neoplasia
Traumatic
Cardiomyopathy
Pericardial disease
Heartworm disease
Lung lobe torsion
Spontaneous
Neoplasia
Pneumonia
Pleural effusion
Surgery
Diaphragmatic herniation
Traumatic
Congenital
Thoracic neoplasia
Hemangiosarcoma
Lymphosarcoma
Osteosarcoma
Chondrosarcoma
Carcinoma
Mesothelioma
Lymphoma and others

Pathophysiology

Pulmonary expansion and effective gas exchange at the blood–pulmonary interface is dependent on a negative intrapleural pressure gradient. With significant pneumothorax this pressure gradient is lost and the lungs do not expand with air. This in turn limits the transfer of oxygen and other gases to and from the systemic arterial circulation, ultimately resulting in hypoxemia.

Clinical presentation

Dogs and cats with pneumothorax typically present with varying degrees of dyspnea, tachypnea, and restlessness. Dyspnea in animals with acute trauma should raise the index of suspicion for pneumothorax and prompt support, therapy, and diagnostics should be performed. In most cases of closed traumatic pneumothorax, an obvious thoracic wound or communication with the pleural space will not be present. Furthermore, up to 50% of dogs with traumatic pneumothorax will also have significant concurrent musculoskeletal injuries. Animals with spontaneous pneumothorax often present with mild to moderate dyspnea and tachypnea with no other concurrent clinical signs.

Differential diagnosis

See **Tables 5.2** and **5.3**.

Table 5.2 Differential diagnosis of pleural versus pulmonary parenchymal and vascular diseases.

Reduction of thoracic capacity
Pleural effusions:
Hydrothorax
Hemothorax
Chylothorax
Pyothorax
Neoplastic
Inflammatory
Pneumothorax
Diaphragmatic rupture/hernia
Cardiac enlargement
Intrathoracic masses
Abdominal masses/fluid
Loss of pulmonary exchange capacity
Bronchopneumonia
Pulmonary edema
Pulmonary hemorrhage/contusion
Metastatic neoplasia
Pulmonary emphysema
Idiopathic pulmonary fibrosis
Pulmonary thromboembolism
Paraquat poisoning

Diagnosis

Diagnosis of pneumothorax is made either by visualization of a full-thickness thoracic wall lesion, thoracic radiography, or thoracocentesis. However, it important that the examining clinician prioritize stabilization of the patient prior to thoracic radiography, as sudden stress can exacerbate the condition and lead to rapid deterioration of the patient. Typical survey radiographic findings include regions of radiolucency in the pleural cavity, which abut retracted lung lobes, and dorsal elevation of the cardiac silhouette off of the sternum on the lateral projection (**Figures 5.2–5.4**). CT (**Figure 5.5**) is useful for identifying accompanying bronchiectasis, neoplasia, and, in some cases, pulmonary foreign bodies. However, in most instances of pneumothorax it is unnecessary.

Management

Initial stabilization of the patient is essential regardless of the ultimate management strategy (medical or surgical). Oxygen supplementation is administered and therapeutic thoracocentesis performed. The patient is then monitored for signs of worsening dyspnea. If dyspnea is progressive,

Table 5.3 Types and causes of pleural effusion.

Transudate
Hypoproteinemia (gut or urine loss, severe liver disease)
Modified (protein-rich) transudate
Congestive cardiac failure, particularly in cats
Neoplasia (particularly cranial mediastinum, thoracic wall)
Lung lobe torsion
Diaphragmatic rupture and incarceration of liver
Hemothorax
Trauma
Coagulopathies
Neoplasia
Anticoagulant rodenticide
Chylothorax
Trauma
Neoplasia
Congestive heart failure, especially in cats
Heartworm disease
Infections
Lung lobe torsion
Idiopathic
Pyothorax
Nocardia spp
Bacteroides spp
Tuberculosis
Actinomyces spp
Inflammatory
Feline infectious peritonitis
Acute pancreatitis
Feline pansteatitis

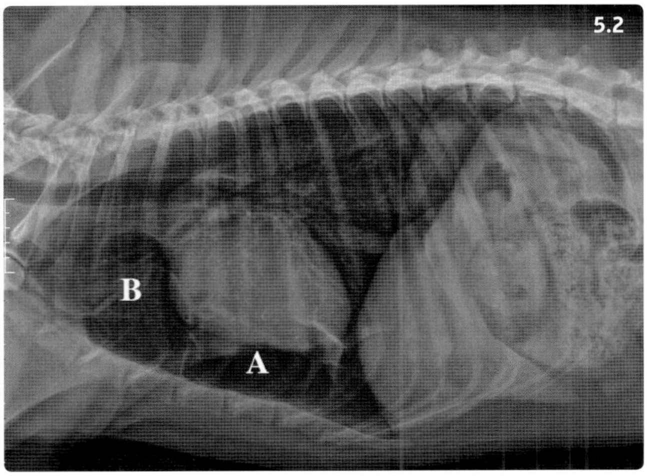

Figure 5.2 Lateral thoracic radiograph of a dog with a moderate pneumothorax showing cardiac elevation (A) and cranial lobe retraction (B).

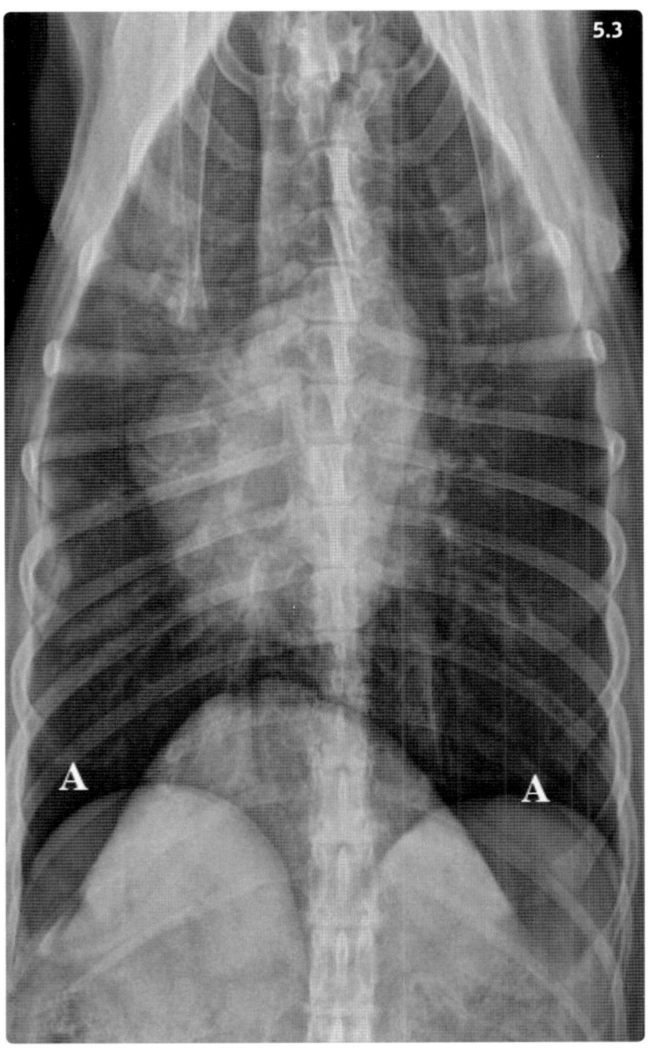

Figure 5.3 Ventrodorsal thoracic radiograph of a dog with pneumothorax demonstrating caudal lung lobe retraction (A).

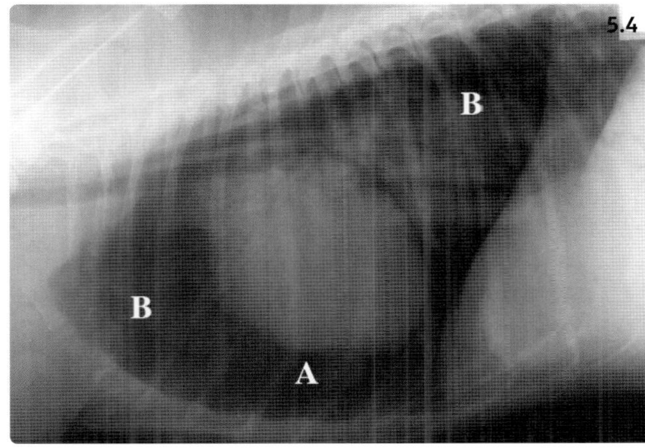

Figure 5.4 Lateral thoracic radiograph of a dog with a severe pneumothorax showing cardiac elevation (A) and minimal aeration of the pulmonary parenchyma (B).

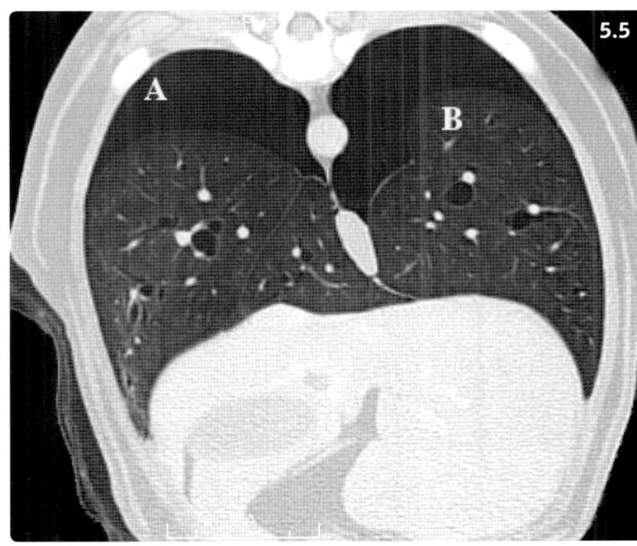

Figure 5.5 Transverse computed tomography scan of a dog with pneumothorax. Note the free gas in the pleural space (A) and retraction of the lungs (B).

a thoracostomy tube is placed. In the case of flail or open chest pneumothorax, the wound is débrided and repaired to allow stabilization of the patient. In most instances of closed traumatic pneumothorax, intermittent needle thoracocentesis is effective in resolving the pneumothorax. If frequent, repetitive aspiration of air from the pleural cavity is required, a chest tube should be placed (**Figures 5.6a, b**). Thoracostomy tubes can be aspirated intermittently or continuously depending on the production of air. The author prefers a continuous negative pressure approach if repeat aspiration is required more frequently than every 2 hours. A negative pressure

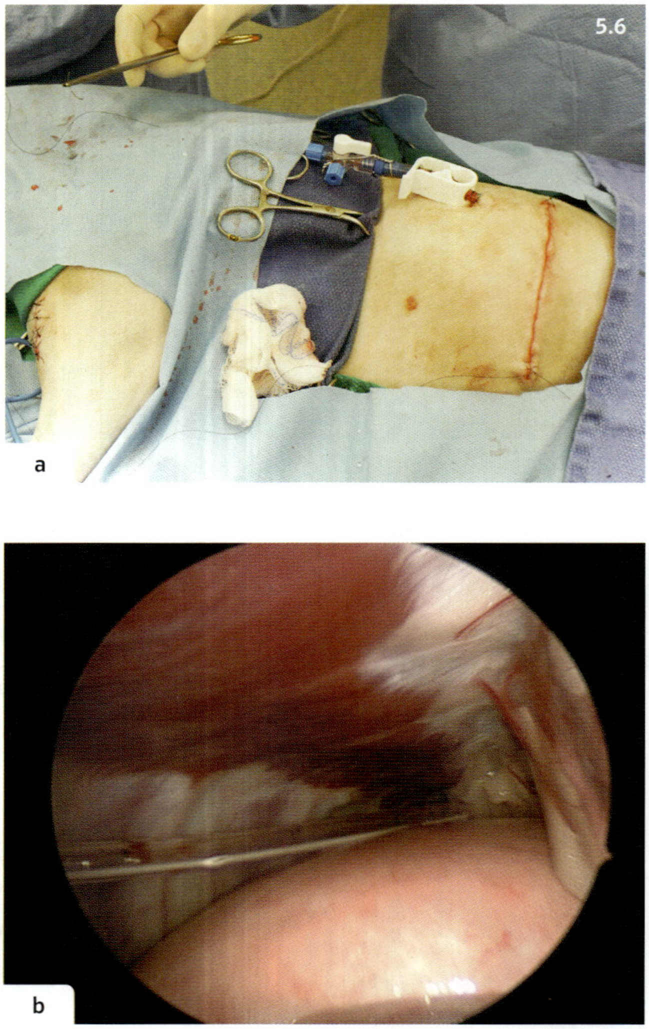

Figures 5.6a, b Extra- and intrathoracic views of appropriate chest tube placement.

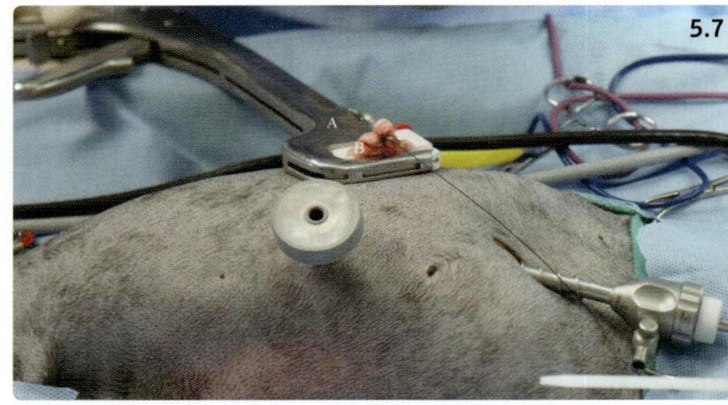

Figure 5.7 Video-assisted partial lung lobectomy from the dog in Figure 5.1.

between 2 and 4 cm H_2O is effective in most cases. If pneumothorax is continuous and persists longer than 2–3 days, surgical exploration and complete or partial lung lobectomy (**Figures 5.7–5.9**) of the pathologic lung lobe is indicated.

Dogs with spontaneous pneumothorax present a significant challenge and most often require surgical lung lobectomy for definitive resolution of the pneumothorax. Although many cases of spontaneous pneumothorax can resolve temporarily with medical treatment, recurrence is very common. Surgical exploration of the thoracic cavity is performed via a median sternotomy or exploratory thoracoscopy. Intercostal thoracotomy does not allow evaluation of both hemithoraces, which is necessary in most spontaneous pneumothorax cases.

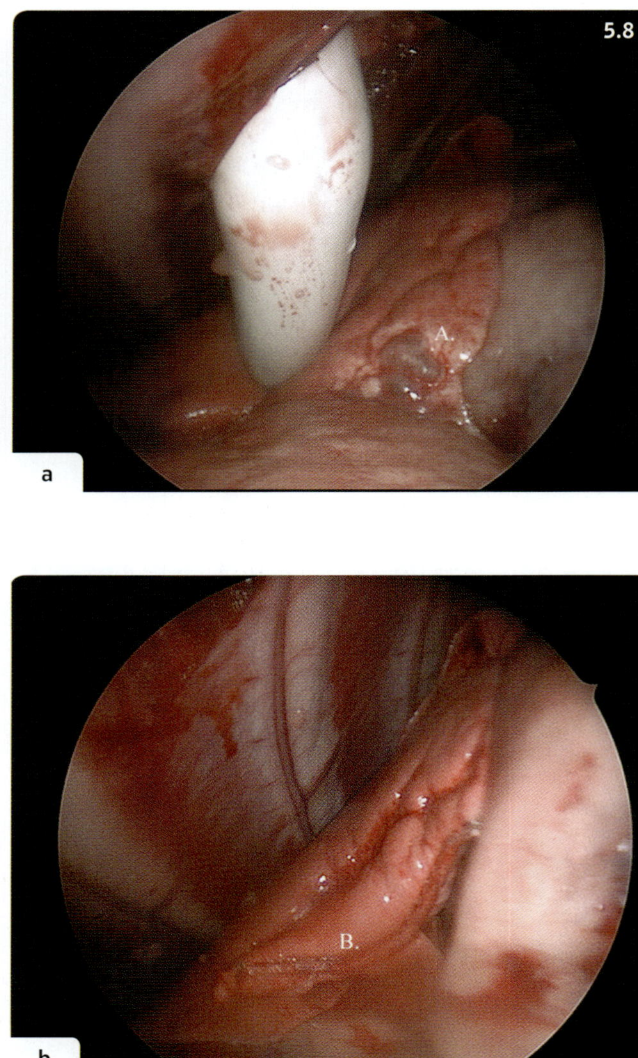

Figure 5.8 Thoracoscopic image of a pulmonary bulla before (a) and after (b) a stapled partial lung lobectomy.

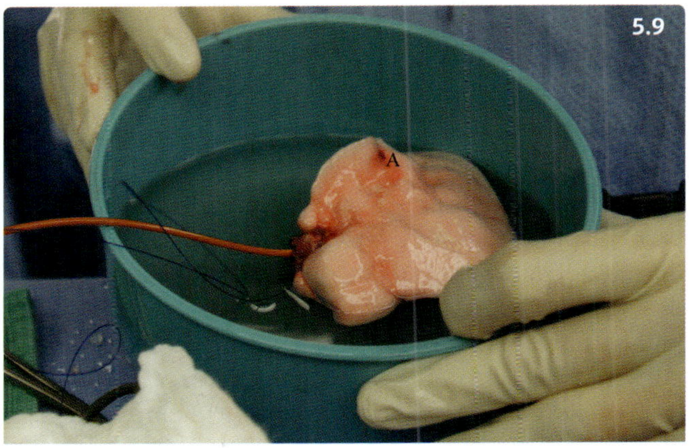

Figure 5.9 Intraoperative leak test to confirm the presence of a leaking lobe.

Prognosis

Short-term prognosis for pneumothorax in dogs and cats is generally good provided that emergent and effective treatment is instituted. Long-term prognosis is dependent on the specific pathologic condition causing the pneumothorax. Spontaneous pneumothorax treated surgically is associated with a 10% mortality and 3% recurrence rate, whereas medically treated dogs have a 50% mortality and recurrence rate.

PYOTHORAX

Definition/overview

Pyothorax, taken from the Greek word 'py', meaning pus, and 'thorac', pertaining to the chest, is a serious and life-threatening disease. The disease is characterized by accumulation of septic exudate within the thoracic cavity. Most cases of pyothorax are bacterial in origin; however, fungal pyothorax also occurs. Pyothorax is typically seen in young field dogs such as the German Shorthaired Pointer and is consistently more common in males. Pyothorax is commonly diagnosed in cats, and it can also be seen associated with a variety of diseases such as feline infectious peritonitis.

Etiology

Aerobic and anaerobic microbes are causative in most cases of pyothorax and many infections are polymicrobial. *Actinomyces* and actinomyces-like bacteria (e.g. *Nocardia* spp. and *Filifactor* spp.) are also responsible for infections and can be associated with migrating grass awns. Migrating grass foreign bodies are thought to migrate through the respiratory system after inhalation, ultimately penetrating the pulmonary parenchyma. Other mechanisms of infection include esophageal perforation, hematogenous seeding, extension from a pneumonic infection, penetrating trauma, chest tube stoma, and surgical site infections. Often, the exact mechanism of infection is not identified. Disease-specific etiologies are summarized in **Table 5.1**.

Pathophysiology

In addition to restrictive pulmonary function due to fluid build up within the pleural space, bacterial pathogens release endotoxins that act as pyrogens. This can lead to a myriad of untoward systemic sequelae including systemic inflammatory response syndrome and multiple organ dysfunction/failure. Furthermore, inoculated foreign material within the thoracic cavity presents a significant challenge for clearance of infection. Specifically, foreign bodies can wall themselves off, thus preventing penetration and clearance by the immune system. The persistence of foreign material within the chest cavity is a common cause of long-term failure and recurrence.

Clinical presentation

Most dogs and cats with pyothorax are dull, lethargic, hyporexic, often febrile, and have differing degrees of restrictive dyspnea. In severe cases, open-mouth breathing, abducted elbows, and cyanosis may be observed. Clinical examination reveals variable findings including elevated rectal temperature, diminished lung and heart sounds, and potentially penetrating thoracic wounds (e.g. dog bite).

Differential diagnosis

See **Tables 5.2** and **5.3**.

Diagnosis

The definitive diagnosis of pyothorax is made by thoracocentesis and identification of a septic suppurative exudate on cytologic examination (**Figure 5.10**). *Actinomyces* is gram positive and non-acid-fast, while *Nocardia* is gram positive and partially acid-fast. Culture and susceptibility testing are necessary for species identification and for evaluation of appropriate antimicrobial therapy. Other important clinical diagnostics include CBC, serum biochemistry, urinalysis, and 2-view thoracic radiography. Thoracic radiographs demonstrate increased radiopacity in the pleural space, with concomitant dorsal elevation and scalloping of lung lobes on the lateral view. Pleural fissure lines are easily seen and the cardiac silhouette is typically obscured (**Figures 5.11a, b**). Positive-contrast CT is also recommended when available. This is helpful in

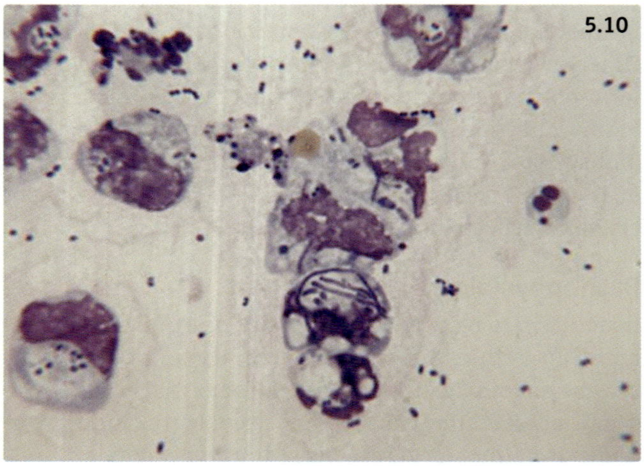

Figure 5.10 Cytologic example of a septic exudate from a dog with pyothorax. (Courtesy H. Wamsley)

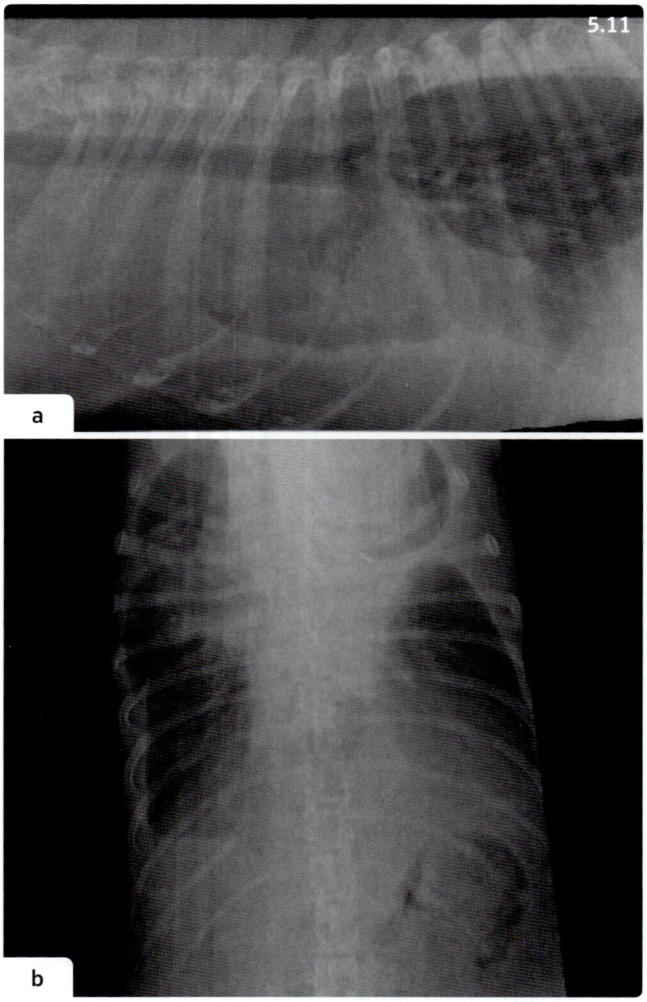

Figures 5.11a, b Lateral (a) and dorsoventral (b) thoracic radiographs of a dog with pyothorax.

cases where radiopaque foreign bodies may be present, as associated regions of tissue inflammation will typically demonstrate enhancement.

Management

Antimicrobial therapy is the cornerstone of treatment of pyothorax in dogs and cats. Broad-spectrum, empirical antibiotic therapy is indicated early and for an extended period of time (usually 6–8 weeks) in most cases. Popular and effective combinations of antibiotics include (1) a potentiated penicillin or (2) cephalosporin in conjunction with clindamycin or metronidazole. *Actinomyces* is most sensitive to penicillins while *Nocardia* is often sensitive to sulfonamides. Other antibiotics can also be used effectively, as most infections are not particularly resistant. Antibiotic susceptibility testing should be utilized to guide therapy once results are available.

In addition to antimicrobial therapy, removal of septic fluid and any foreign or necrotic material is important, as treatment failure and recurrence may result if this is not performed. Thoracostomy drain placement either unilaterally or bilaterally is necessary in the initial treatment of pyothorax. Thoracostomy drains are used to drain and lavage the pleural space, which facilitates clearance of debris and septic material. Failure to place a thoracostomy drain is associated with an unacceptable level of treatment failure. Pleural lavage is performed using sterile physiologic 0.9% saline at 10–20 ml/kg up to 4 times daily. The addition of heparin to the lavage fluid at 5–10 U/ml has been recommended and theoretically may result in diminished adhesion formation.

Surgical intervention may be important in dogs with masses or cases where a foreign body is present or highly suspected (e.g. *Actinomyces* infection). Median sternotomy is indicated for exploration of both hemithoraces in cases of bilateral pyothorax when a cause is not identified or if medical treatment failure occurs. If a mass lesion is seen or if pus is limited to a single hemithorax, an intercostal thoracotomy may be an appropriate alternative to median sternotomy. Thoracic surgery regardless of the approach is challenging and marred with potential complications and should be performed only by experienced surgeons.

The author prefers exploratory thoracoscopy (**Figures 5.12–5.14**) as a diagnostic and therapeutic procedure in most cases of pyothorax. Exploratory thoracoscopy utilizes two to three 5.5 mm portals to explore, débride, and biopsy pleural and mediastinal tissues, and is used to perform thorough lavage of both hemithoraces followed by video-assisted thoracostomy drain placement. A single thoracostomy drain is used after

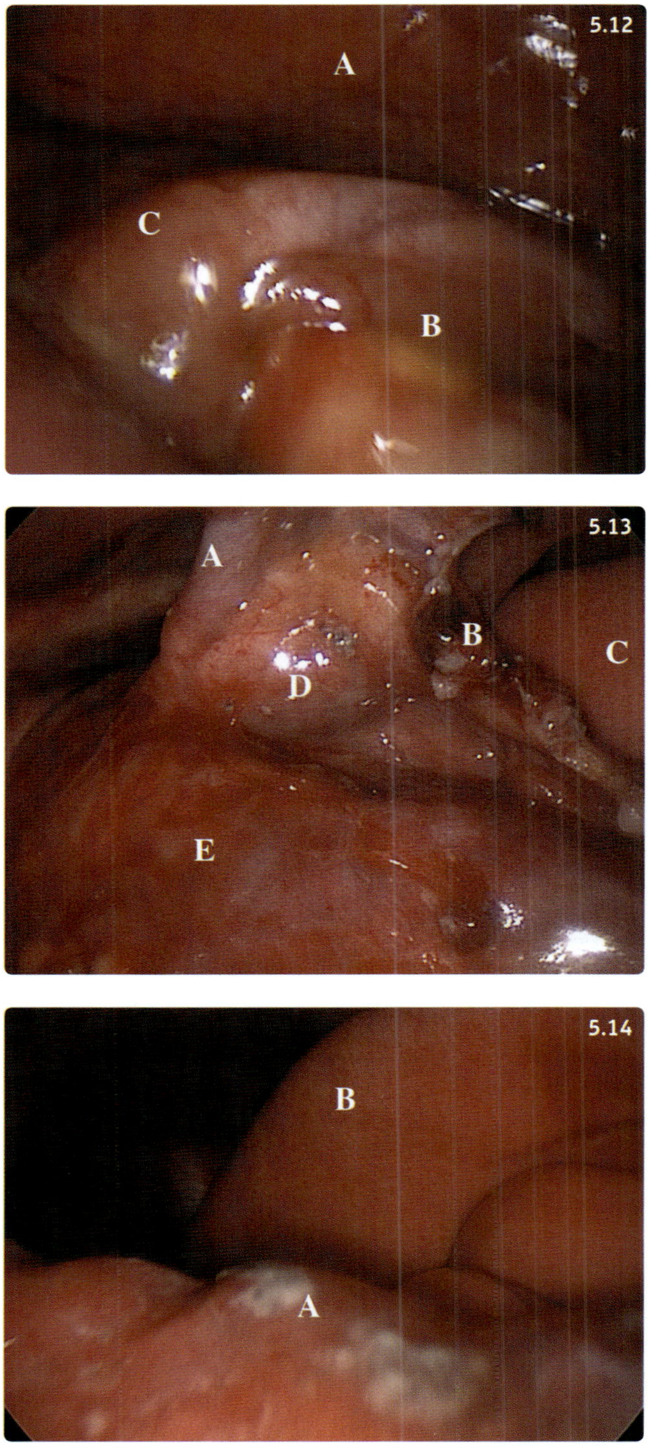

Figures 5.12–5.14 Dog undergoing thoracoscopic treatment for pyothorax. (5.12) Purulent fluid (C) and fibrin (B) in the cranial thorax. The pulmonary pleura is inflamed (A). (5.13) Thoracoscopic view of the cranial mediastinum after mediastinal débridement (B) and sternal lymph node (D) biopsy. The right internal thoracic artery (A), inflamed dorsal mediastinum (E), and left cranial lung lobe (C) are also visible. (5.14) Thoracoscopic view of the cranial mediastinum. Note the fibrinous plaques (A) and left cranial lung lobe erythema (B).

exploratory thoracoscopy as the mediastinal tissues are well débrided and therefore do not isolate one side of the thorax from the other. The efficacy of this treatment has not been reported in the veterinary literature, but experience and anecdotal reports are supportive.

Prognosis

Overall prognosis for pyothorax in dogs and cats is good as long as appropriate and prudent medical treatment is instituted. The long-term success rate for dogs managed medically ranges from 30 to 70% while dogs managed surgically experience a more consistent long-term success rate between 70 and 80%.

CHYLOTHORAX

Definition/overview

Chylothorax is defined as a pathologic accumulation of chyle within the thoracic cavity. It is a relatively rare disease in dogs and cats, but is associated with an untoward outcome in many cases, despite treatment.

Etiology

There are a number of potential causes of chylothorax including traumatic thoracic duct rupture, neoplasia, cardiomyopathy, heartworm disease, restrictive pericarditis, and lung lobe torsion. However, most cases appear to be idiopathic. Because the exact cause is often unidentified despite appropriate diagnostic testing, target-based treatment can be challenging. Disease-specific etiologies are summarized in **Table 5.1**.

Pathophysiology

Direct injury to the thoracic duct can occur secondary to trauma or neoplastic disease. Disease processes that increase right-sided cardiac pressure, such as cardiomyopathy or restrictive pericarditis, also can induce chylothorax by causing extravasation of lymph from the lymphatic system. Similarly, lymphaticovenous obstructive diseases such as mediastinal lymphoma can cause chylothorax. Chylothorax induces significant inflammation within the pleural cavity, ultimately resulting in restrictive pleural fibrosis. Consequently, early and effective treatment is indicated to minimize the risk and severity of pleural fibrosis.

Clinical presentation

Clinical signs typical of pleural effusion are seen in dogs and cats with chylothorax. Specifically, restrictive dyspnea, tachycardia, lethargy, and hyporexia are commonly reported. Reduced or absent bronchovesicular sounds on thoracic auscultation is a common finding. In chronic cases, poor body condition and cough may be observed. Among dogs, Afghan Hounds, Shetland Sheepdogs, and Shiba Inus are overrepresented.

Differential diagnosis

See **Tables 5.2** and **5.3**.

Diagnosis

Chylous fluid has a milky white-to-pink gross appearance (**Figure 5.15**) and is characterized as a modified transudate. The definitive diagnosis of chylothorax is based on pleural fluid analysis. Distinguishing between chyle and pseudochyle is typically done by measuring fluid triglyceride levels then comparing those with serum triglyceride levels. Dogs and cats with a pseudochylous effusion will have equivalent fluid and serum triglyceride values, whereas patients with true chylous effusion will have fluid triglyceride levels significantly higher than serum levels. Other bench top tests that can be performed to help differentiate a chylous effusion from a pseudochylous effusion include a positive ether clearance test and positive Sudan black uptake by chylomicrons. Cytology of pleural fluid is important to rule out other potential diseases such as neoplasia (**Figure 5.15**).

Thoracic radiographs demonstrate increased radiopacity in the pleural space, with concomitant dorsal elevation and scalloping of lung lobes on the lateral view (**Figure 5.16**). Pleural fissure lines are easily seen and the cardiac silhouette is typically obscured.

Thoracic ultrasonography (**Figure 5.17**) can also be used to diagnose the presence of free pleural fluid and may be preferred in emergent cases, as it can be performed without significant restraint in most cases. Ultrasonography also allows for diagnostic and therapeutic image-guided thoracocentesis, which can be rapidly performed in emergency situations. Pleural fluid is identified as a hypo- to anechoic signal on ultrasound. Small volumes of fluid may not be easily visible using ultrasound. Presence of a thin hyperechoic pleural fissure line immediately adjacent to the body wall with associated gas shadow is inconsistent with significant pleural effusion.

CT lymphangiography is the procedure of choice for imaging of the thoracic duct (**Figure 5.18**) and cisterna chyli (**Figure 5.19**). While it is not necessary to perform CT lymphangiography to make the diagnosis of chylothorax, it is an important diagnostic test in the presurgical evaluation of patients with chylothorax.

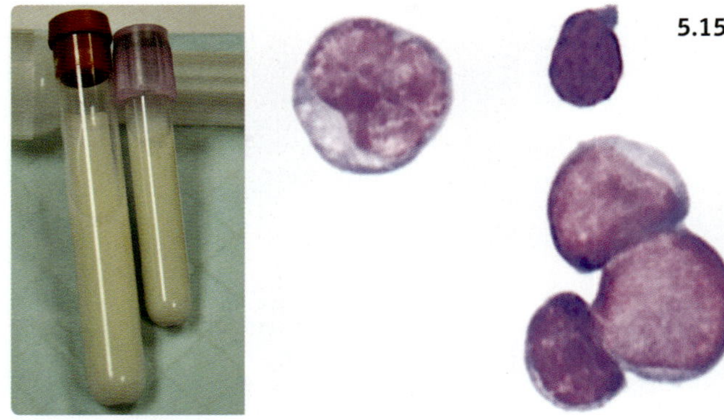

Figure 5.15 Pleural fluid. Gross appearance and cytology in a dog with chylothorax secondary to lymphangiosarcoma. Note the neoplastic characteristics of the cells: high nuclear to cytoplasmic ration, multiple nucleoli, and anisokaryosis. (Courtesy H. Wamsley)

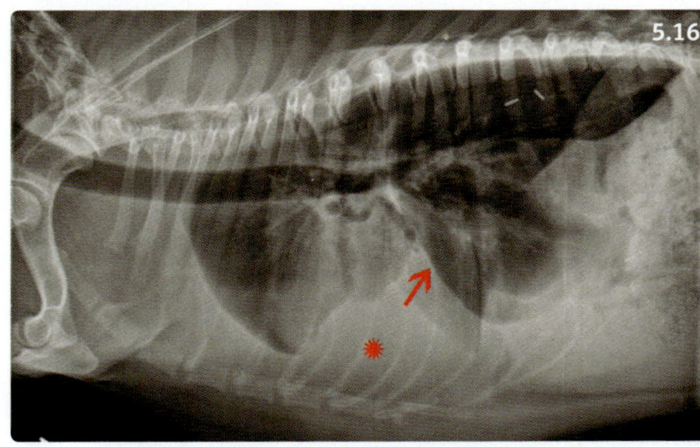

Figure 5.16 Lateral thoracic radiograph of a dog with recurrent pleural effusion 8 months after thoracic duct ligation and pericardectomy. This dog was eventually diagnosed with lymphangiosarcoma. Note the retracted lung lobes (arrow) and pleural fluid (*).

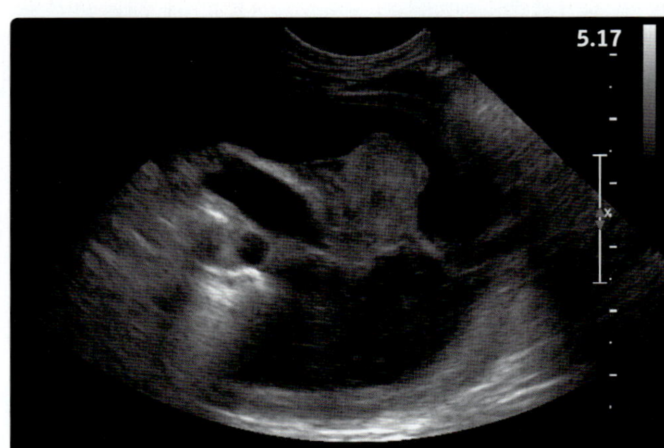

Figure 5.17 Thoracic ultrasonogram of a dog with pleural effusion. Note the hypoechoic shadow and linear hyperechoic fibrin strands indicative of pleural fluid. (Courtesy M. Winter)

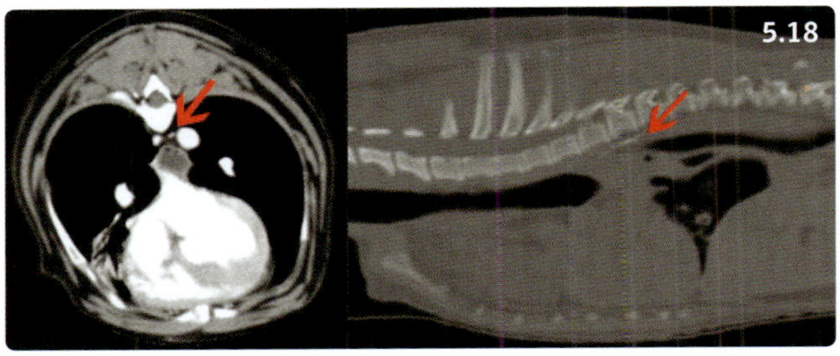

Figure 5.18 Transverse and sagittal computed tomography lymphangiography has been performed. Note the thoracic duct medial and dorsal to the descending aorta (arrows).

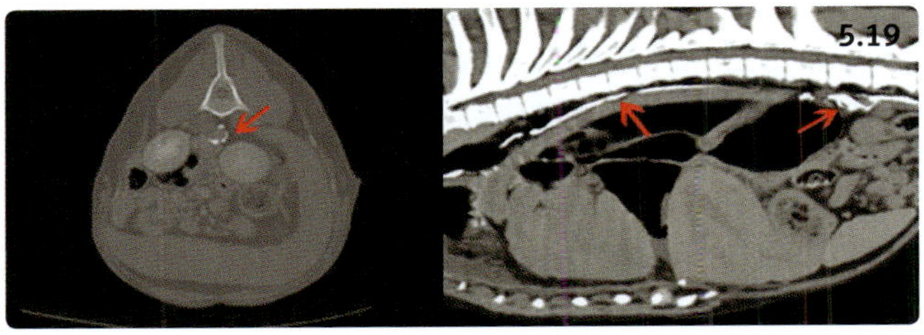

Figure 5.19 Transverse and sagittal computed tomography lymphangiography has been performed. Note the thoracic duct (sagittal view, left arrow) and cysterna chyli (both projections, right arrow on sagittal view).

Management

Conservative management of dogs and cats with chylothorax is rarely rewarding and is associated with a high degree of treatment failure. Medical options include feeding a low-fat/high-fiber diet to minimize the absorption and flow of chyle within the lymphatics. Nutraceuticals, such as bioflavonoids (e.g. Rutin, 20–50 mg/kg q8h), can also be supplemented to enhance macrophage activity. Other medications such as somatostatin and octreotide have also been used. Serial thoracocentesis is frequently required in medically managed dogs and cats with chylothorax. Because prolonged exposure of the visceral pleura to chylous fluid can result in pleural fibrosis, medical management should be attempted with caution. Owners should be counseled about the risks of pleural fibrosis at the time of diagnosis.

Surgical management is recommended in dogs and cats with idiopathic chylothorax, as it is associated with the best chance of treatment success. A number of surgical treatments have been recommended, but the most commonly performed are thoracic duct ligation (**Figure 5.20**), in combination with cysterna chyli ablation (**Figures 5.21, 5.22**) and/or pericardectomy, and thoracic cavity omentalization.

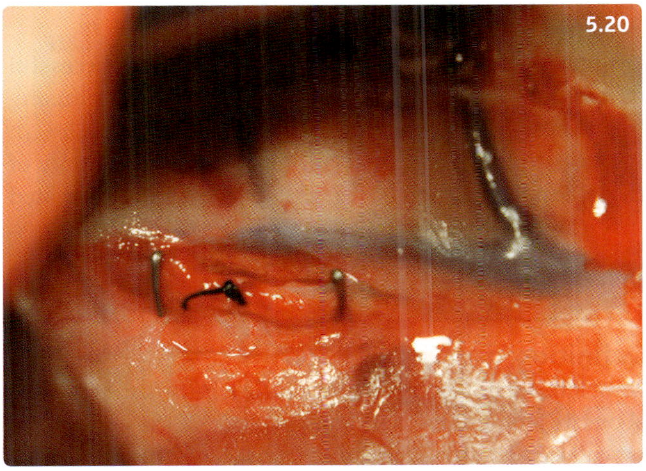

Figure 5.20 Intraoperative image of the thoracic duct subsequent to ligation. Note the azygous vein just dorsal to the ligated thoracic duct.

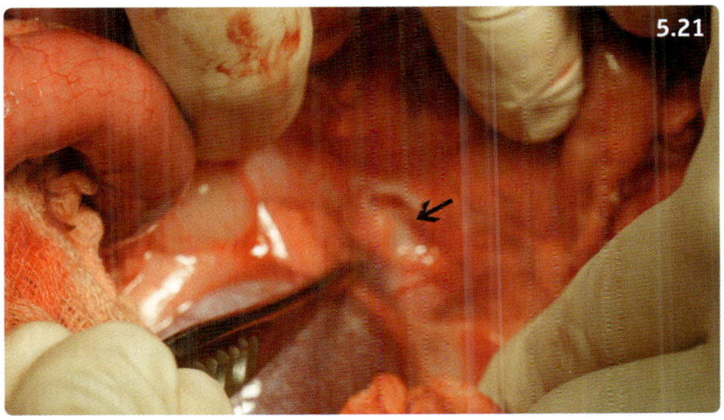

Figure 5.21 Intraoperative image of the cysterna chyli during ablation surgery. Note the dilated milky white appearance of the cysterna (arrow). This dog was fed cream prior to surgery to enhance visualization during the procedure.

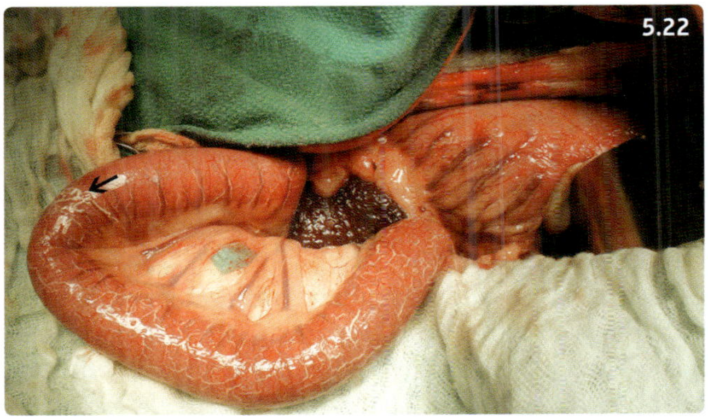

Figure 5.22 Dilated intestinal lymphatics (arrow) following oral cream administration in the dog in Figure 5.21.

Prognosis
Prognosis with medical management alone is successful in less than 25% of cases. Surgical success varies among treatments but in general ranges from 75% to 85% in the short and medium term. Long-term resolution of chylothorax is expected in about 70% of dogs treated surgically.

LUNG LOBE TORSION

Definition/overview
Lung lobe torsion occurs when a lung lobe becomes twisted about its longitudinal axis so as to obstruct the pulmonary vasculature and the bronchus. In most cases the pulmonary artery is patent. Lung lobe torsion is a relatively uncommon disease. Male dogs and those with a narrow and deep chest appear to be predisposed to lung lobe torsion. Afghan Hounds and Pug dogs appear to be overrepresented. Lung lobe torsion does occur in the cat, but it is rare.

Etiology
The precise etiology of lung lobe torsion in many cases is unknown and it is therefore referred to simply as spontaneous. In some dogs the condition may be seen in conjunction with other pathology including pulmonary neoplasia and chylothorax. Any disease process that results in collapse of the airway and which increases mobility of a particular lobe may predispose that lobe to torsion. Examples of associated diseases include bronchomalacia and bronchial collapse, pulmonary neoplasia, chylothorax, and alteration of normal anatomy due to previous thoracic surgery (e.g. lung lobectomy). Disease-specific etiologies are summarized in **Table 5.1**.

Pathophysiology
When a lung lobe undergoes torsion, the venous and lymphatic outflow becomes obstructed, resulting in fluid congestion and distension of the affected lobe. With time, the fluid accumulation becomes severe, eventually resulting in necrosis and pleural effusion formation. A low ventilation/perfusion mismatch results but may not be clinically apparent if the remaining lung lobes are healthy.

Clinical presentation
Clinical signs include coughing, respiratory difficulty, tachypnea, lethargy, and hyporexia. Respiratory signs can be severe, especially if significant pleural effusion exists. In some cases, a history of previous thoracic surgery may be known, but in many instances no significant medical history exists.

Differential diagnosis
See **Tables 5.2** and **5.3**.

Diagnosis
Diagnosis is typically made via thoracic radiography (**Figures 5.23, 5.24**) or CT (**Figures 5.25, 5.26**). Survey radiographic findings may vary depending on the presence of pleural fluid and chronicity of the disease. In early cases without significant pleural effusion, or following thoracocentesis, consolidation with or without the presence of air bronchograms may be evident. In more chronic cases, complete consolidation of the lung lobe with blunting of the pulmonary bronchus may occur. CT is useful in identifying obstructed or narrowed bronchi and is more sensitive than survey radiography for detection of lung lobe torsion.

Pleural fluid analysis typically reveals a modified transudate, which may be chylous.

Management
Surgical ligation and excision of the affected lung lobe is the recommended treatment. Dogs and cats with lung lobe torsion are stabilized prior to surgical lung lobectomy. Stabilization usually requires therapeutic thoracocentesis and IV fluid replacement. Any electrolyte or acid–base disruptions should be corrected prior to anesthesia and surgery. Dogs and cats undergoing thoracotomy should have a preoperative hematocrit of at least 30% (0.3 l/l), as hemoglobin is the most significant contributor to blood oxygen content, and hypoxemia and blood loss can be significant with thoracic surgery.

Lung lobectomy can be performed via a video-assisted thoracic approach (**Figure 5.27**), median sternotomy, or video-assisted or intercostal thoracotomy (**Figure 5.28**). Video-assisted thoracic surgery is the author's preferred approach as exploration of the pulmonary parenchyma is possible and the procedure can be performed with minimal tissue injury and postoperative pain. Regardless of the surgical approach, ligation of the vascular pedicle (without derotation of the lung lobe) using a triple-row surgical stapler or suture ligation is performed (**Figure 5.29**). Patients are monitored and supported in a critical care facility postoperatively.

Prognosis
Prognosis is dependent on the underlying disease process and the experience and ability of the anesthesia and surgery services. Mortality rates have been reported as high as 40%, but Pug dogs appear to have a much higher survival rate.

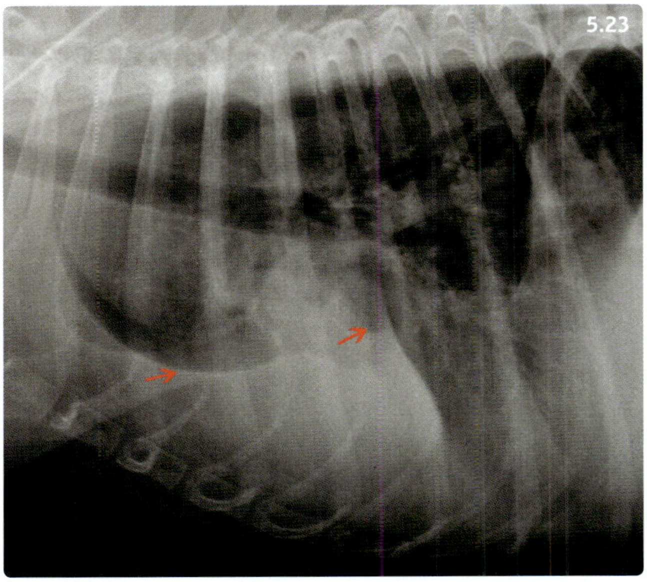

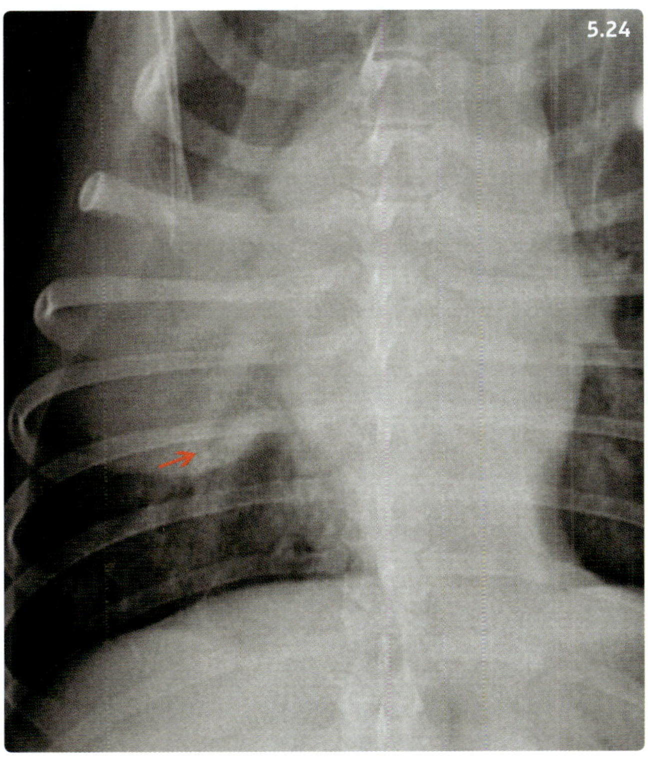

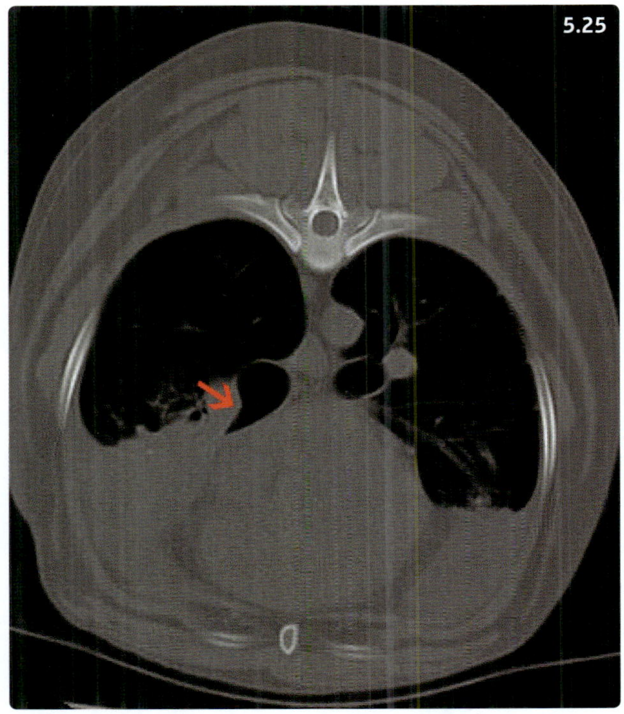

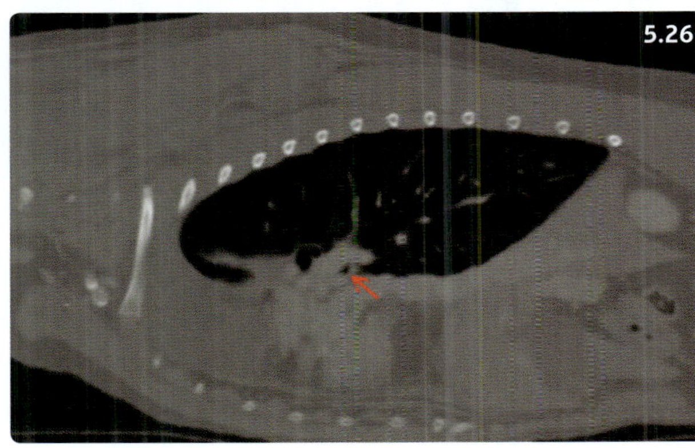

Figures 5.23–5.26 Dog with lung lobe torsion. (5.23) Lateral thoracic radiograph. Note the pleural effusion (left arrow) and blunt ended bronchus (right arrow). (5.24) Ventrodorsal thoracic radiograph. Note the consolidated right middle lung lobe with blunted bronchus (arrow). (5.25) Transverse computed tomography view. The occluded bronchus and consolidated lung lobe are easily visualized (arrow). (5.26) Sagittal computed tomography view. The occluded bronchus is demonstrated (arrow).

DIAPHRAGMATIC HERNIATION

Definition/overview

Pleural–peritoneal diaphragmatic herniation results when the diaphragm is ruptured or when an abnormal communication of the peritoneal and pleural cavities exists. The diaphragm is composed of a large central tendon, which originates from the sternal, costal, and lumbar musculature. In health, the diaphragm maintains three normal ostia: the aortic, vena cava, and esophageal hiatus. Peritoneal–pericardial diaphragmatic hernias are not true pleural–peritoneal hernias as the communication exists only between the peritoneum and pericardial spaces.

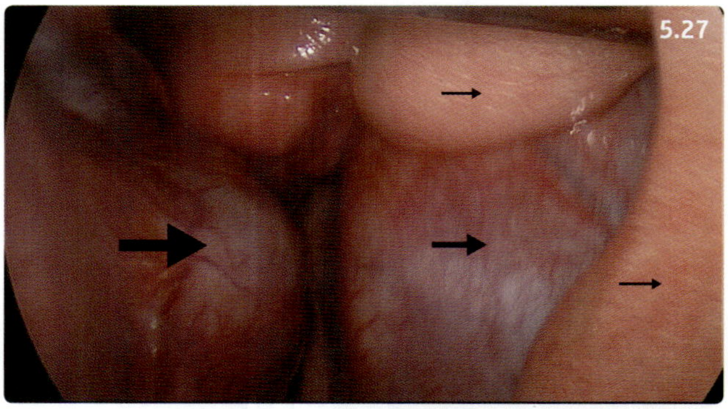

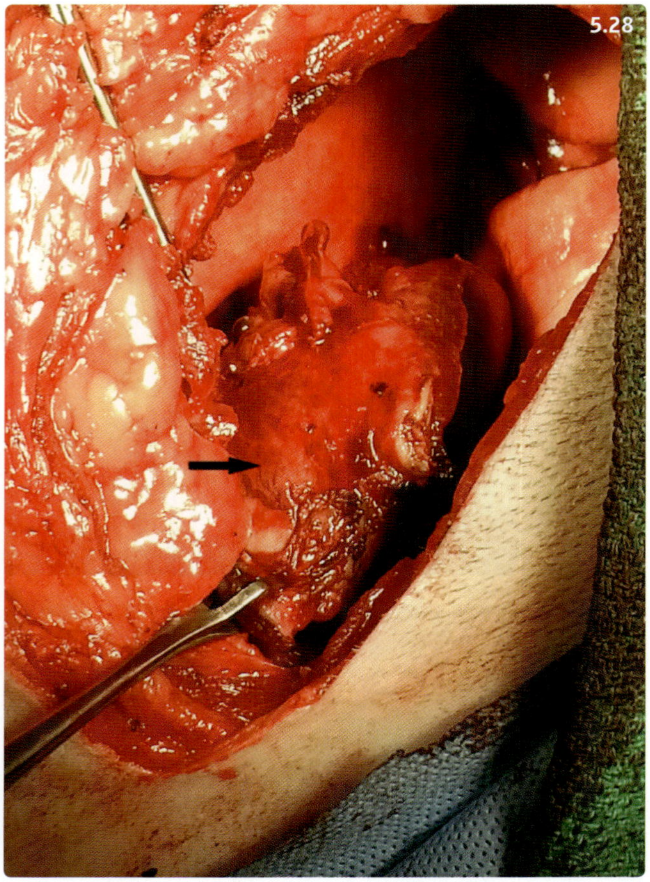

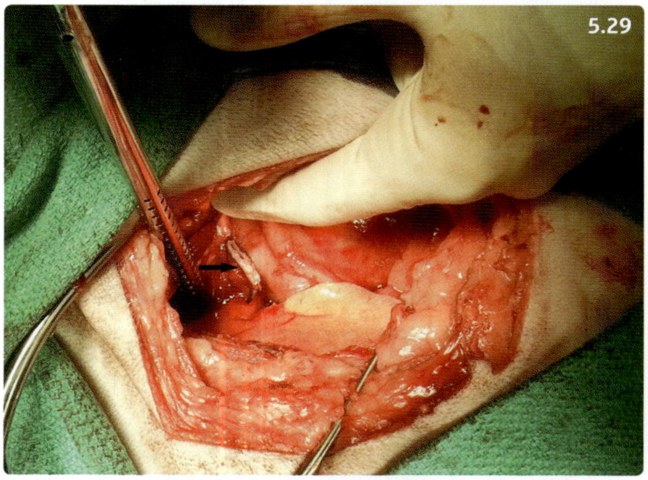

Figures 5.27–5.29 Same dog as in Figures 5.23–5.26. (5.27) Video-assisted thoracic surgical view of the consolidated right middle lung lobe (thickest arrow), which was adhered to the chest wall. The heart (middle thickness arrow) and lungs (thinnest arrows) are retracted to the right of the image. (5.28) Intraoperative view of the torsed lung lobe (arrow) during intercostal thoracotomy just prior to lung lobectomy. (5.29) Intraoperative view of the ligated bronchus (arrow) following lung lobectomy.

Etiology

Diaphragmatic hernias are broadly classified as congenital or acquired, with acquired being most common. Congenital diaphragmatic hernias are rare and typically result from failure of the lumbar musculature to fuse. These hernias are typically located in the dorsolateral region of the diaphragm. Acquired diaphragmatic hernias are seen commonly following blunt trauma such as automobile associated injury. Traumatic diaphragmatic herniation can develop in any part of the diaphragm. Tears can be multiple or single, large or small, and radial or longitudinal. Disease-specific etiologies are summarized in **Table 5.1**.

Pathophysiology

The pathophysiologic effects of diaphragmatic herniation depend on the severity of the hernia, chronicity, and presence of concurrent injuries. The diaphragm plays an integral role in ventilation and oxygenation by altering intrapleural pressure and volume during respiration. Injury to the diaphragm impairs this function. Furthermore, with herniation of viscera (liver most commonly), compression of the pulmonary pleura and pleural vasculature results in compressive atelectasia and venous impairment. The end result is hypoxemia and reduced cardiac output. Concurrent rib fractures cause pain, which further reduces ventilatory capacity and exacerbates hypoxemia. Herniation of intestine into the pleural space can result in intestinal obstruction and intestinal ischemia.

Clinical presentation

The clinical presentation for dogs and cats with diaphragmatic herniation is variable and can range from minimal or no clinical signs to severe dyspnea and hypovolemic shock. It is important to remember that small diaphragmatic tears may not elicit significant clinical signs and may go undetected until herniation of abdominal viscera occurs. This may take years in some cases. Thus, diaphragmatic injury should be considered even in dogs and cats without respiratory signs following significant thoracic trauma. Dogs with herniated gastrointestinal (GI) organs may be obstructed and will often present with vomiting and anorexia.

Physical examination may reveal concurrent soft tissue and orthopedic injuries, reduced abdominal organ content, or minimal to absent bronchovesicular and heart sounds.

Differential diagnosis

See **Tables 5.2** and **5.3**.

Diagnosis

Survey thoracic radiography is the most commonly performed diagnostic procedure and is very sensitive for diagnosing herniation of peritoneal contents into the pleural space (**Figures 5.30, 5.31**). Typical radiographic findings include retracted pulmonary parenchyma, presence of increased soft tissue opacity in the pleural cavity, loss of normal cardiac silhouette, presence of gas-filled viscera in the pleural cavity, loss of a normal hepatic shadow, and cranial gastric axis shift. Contrast abdominal radiography can be performed to help identify intestinal herniation and obstruction (**Figures 5.32, 5.33**).

CT is also useful and is more sensitive at detection of small diaphragmatic hernias with minimal or no herniation of GI viscera (**Figures 5.34, 5.35**).

Arterial blood gas analysis and calculation of the alveolar–arterial oxygen gradient is helpful in diagnosing hypoxemia.

Management

Hypoxemic and hypovolemic patients should be resuscitated and stabilized on an emergency basis. Replacement IV fluid therapy and increased inspired oxygen content can be started immediately. Most dogs and cats will respond well to fluid therapy, but response to increased inspired oxygen may be poor due to the low ventilation–perfusion mismatch that frequently exists. Reduction of herniated organs and repair of the diaphragm are required before significant improvement in oxygenation will occur.

Diaphragmatic herniorrhaphy by laparotomy (**Figures 5.36–5.38**) or laparoscopy (**Figures 5.39, 5.40**) following reduction of herniated viscera is the definitive treatment for pleural–peritoneal diaphragmatic herniation. Adjunctive surgical procedures such as resection and anastomosis of devitalized bowel or liver lobectomy for refractory hemorrhage may also be indicated.

Prognosis

Prognosis for dogs and cats with traumatic diaphragmatic herniation is good to excellent, with overall survival around 90%. Dogs and cats with traumatic diaphragmatic hernias undergoing surgery without effective resuscitation and support have a higher mortality.

THORACIC NEOPLASIA

Definition/overview

Thoracic neoplasia is common in aged dogs and cats. The result in most cases is production of malignant pleural effusion and respiratory difficulty. Space-occupying masses can also impair normal respiratory effort and function. Thoracic neoplasia is almost exclusively malignant, but effective treatment can be accomplished in many cases depending on the owner's expectations and the biology of the particular disease.

Etiology

Thoracic neoplasia is most commonly mesenchymal or epithelial and can originate from the ribs, pleura, lungs, mediastinum, thymus, lymph nodes, pericardium, heart, trachea, and esophagus. Mediastinal lymphoma and lymphangiosarcoma are also commonly diagnosed. Disease-specific etiologies are summarized in **Table 5.1**.

Pathophysiology

Thoracic neoplasia commonly results in malignant pleural effusion, while pericardial and cardiac neoplasms frequently engender pericardial effusion with or without pleural effusion. Consequently, respiratory and diastolic cardiac function are compromised in affected dogs and cats. Moderate to marked volumes of pleural space fluid cause restriction of the pulmonary parenchyma, which results in hypoxemia. Excessive pericardial effusion or mechanical compression of the right cardiac chambers by a mass results in tamponade and diastolic failure.

Clinical presentation

Dogs with thoracic neoplasms can present in significant distress depending on the location and size of the mass as well as the location and volume of malignant effusion. Common clinical signs include dyspnea, coughing, lethargy, and hyporexia. Cough is usually associated with a

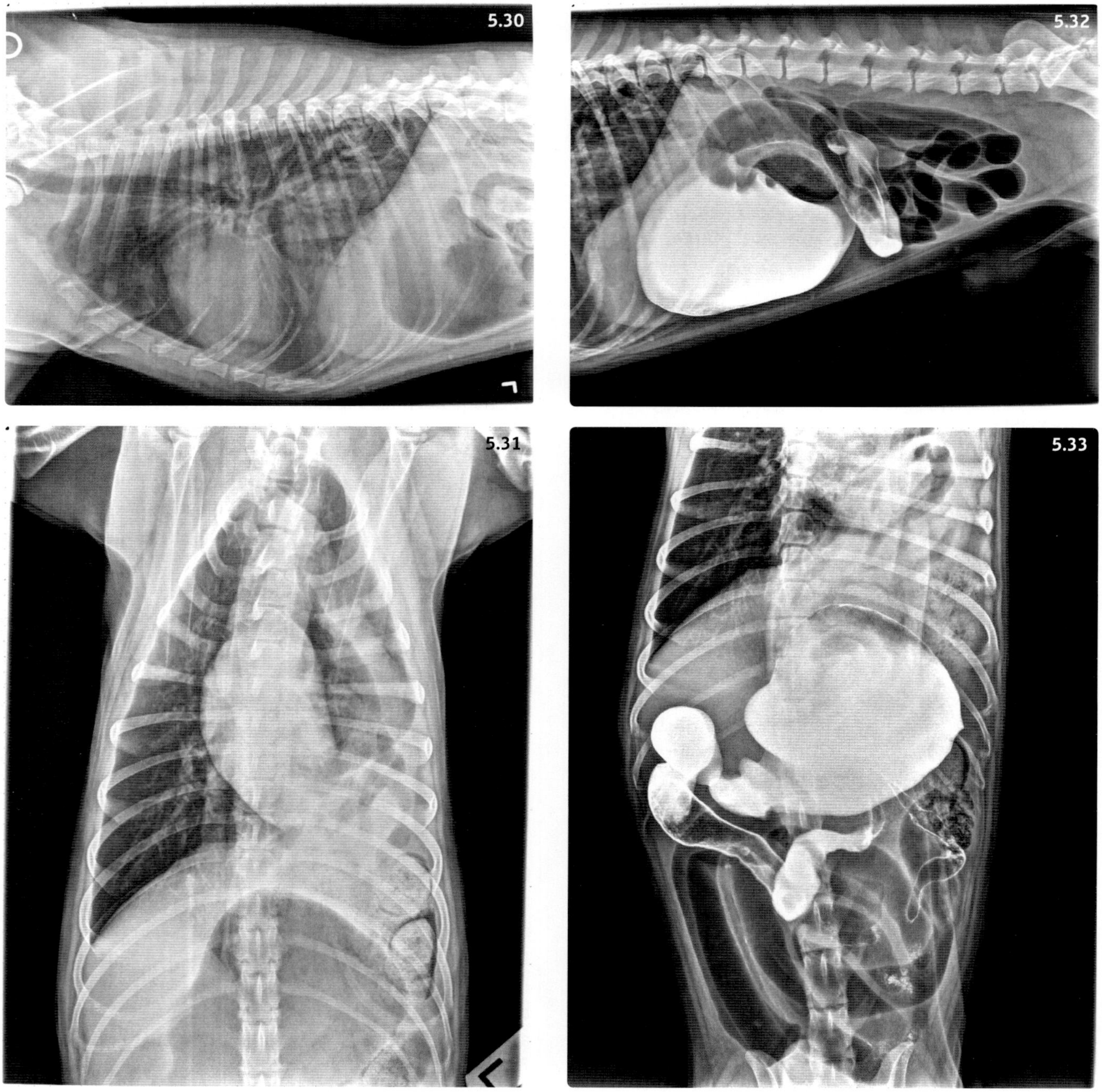

Figures 5.30–5.33 Dog with a diaphragmatic hernia. (5.30) Lateral thoracic radiograph. Note the cranial displacement of the gastric axis and gas-filled viscus in the pleural cavity. (5.31) Ventrodorsal thoracic radiograph. Note the loss of liver shadow and the gas-filled viscus in the pleural cavity. (5.32) Contrast lateral abdominal radiograph. This dog had persistent emesis, which was thought to be secondary to intestinal obstruction. Contrast was hung up in the duodenum due to herniation and occlusion of the orad jejunum. Note the absence of a splenic shadow. (5.33) Contrast ventrodorsal abdominal radiograph.

lesion that compresses a bronchus. In some cases, cyanosis and syncope may be reported. Dogs and cats with thoracic wall tumors may have a visible or palpable mass present on physical examination. Cardiothoracic auscultation may reveal diminished or absent bronchovesicular or cardiac sounds.

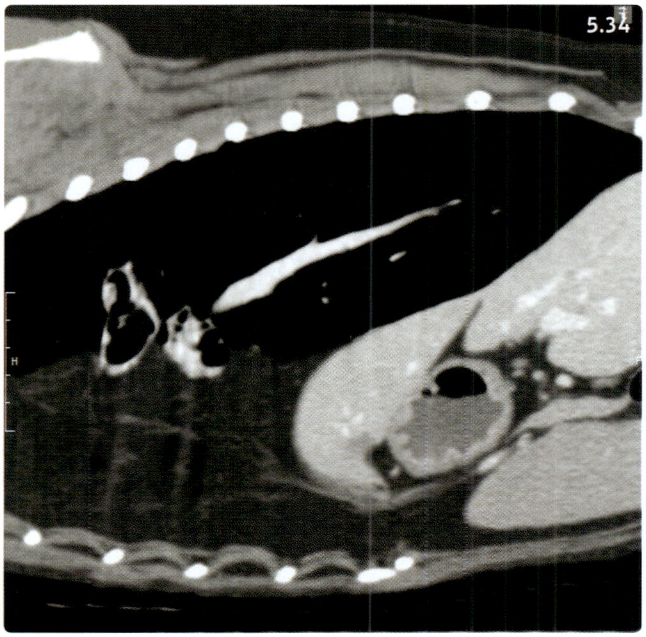

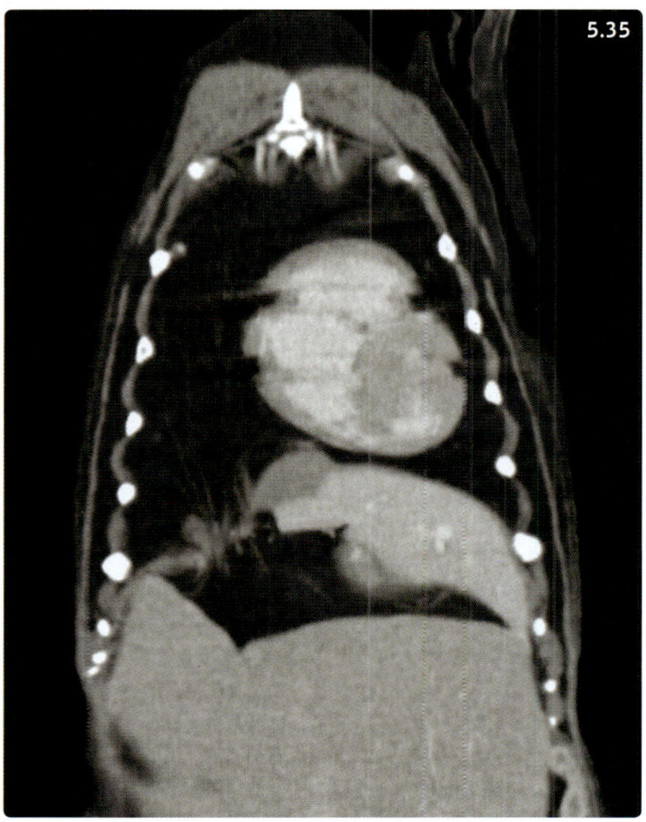

Figures 5.34, 5.35 Dog with a traumatic ventral diaphragmatic rupture. Sagittal (5.34) and coronal (5.35) computed tomography scans. Note the diaphragmatic defect and omental fat streaking into the thoracic cavity.

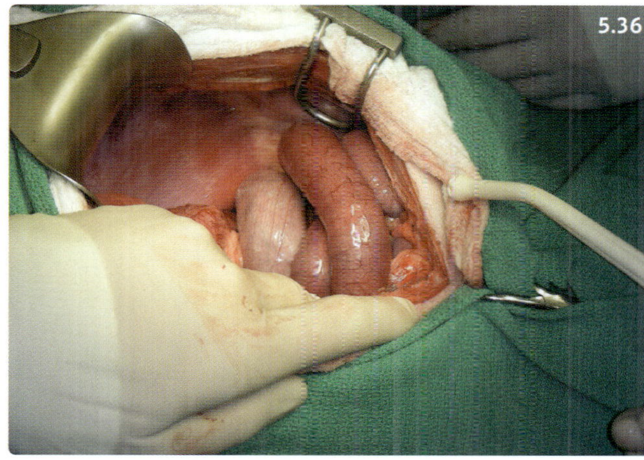

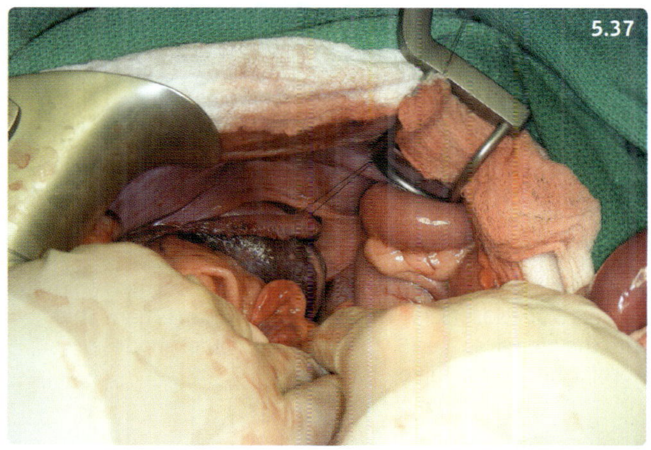

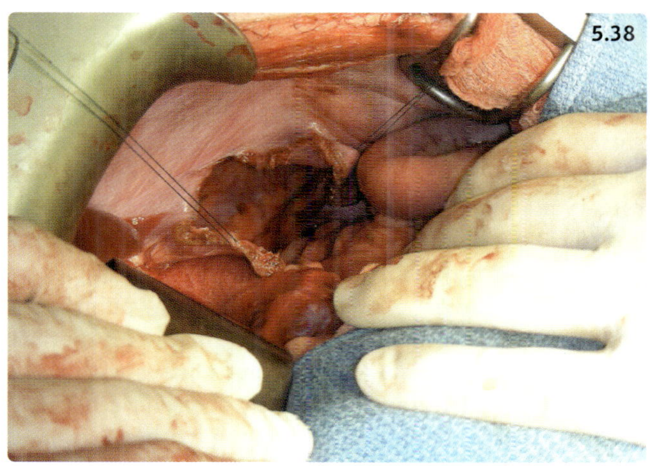

Figure 5.36–5.38 Intraoperative views of the dog in Figures 5.30–5.33. (5.36) Note the herniated colon and obstructed erythematous jejunum. (5.37) Note that the bowel has been reduced and the herniated spleen is now visible. (5.38) Note that all of the abdominal viscera has been reduced.

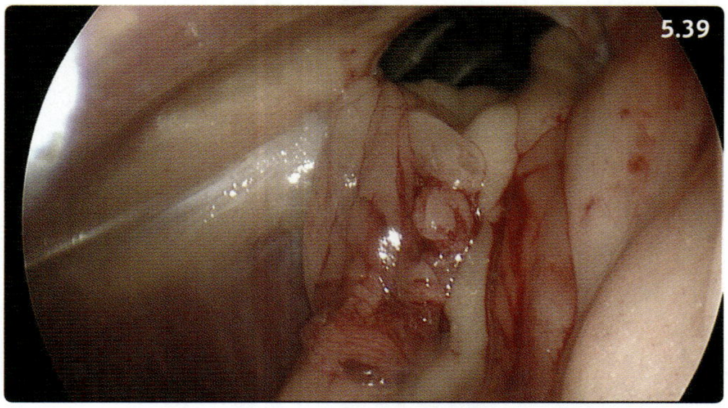

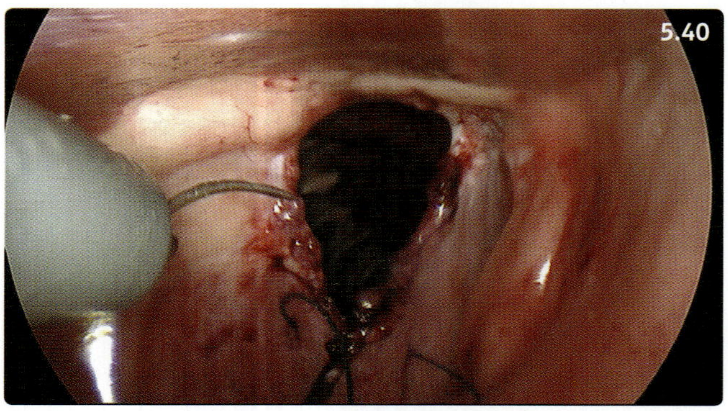

Figures 5.39, 5.40 Laparoscopic views of the dog in Figures 5.30–5.33. (5.39) The greater omentum is herniated into the pleural space. (5.40) An intracorporeal knotless herniorrhaphy is being performed.

Differential diagnosis

See **Tables 5.2** and **5.3**.

Diagnosis

Cytologic analysis of malignant effusions is often inconclusive either due to lack of representative cells in the sample or because of similarity of reactive mesothelial cells to malignant mesothelial cells. Routine blood work is typically nonspecific. Radiographic and echocardiographic imaging usually reveals the presence of pleural and/or pericardial effusion. Mediastinal, pulmonary, and thoracic wall masses can be identified with thoracic radiography (**Figures 5.41–5.44**), but masses within the pericardial space typically are only seen via echocardiography. Three-dimensional imaging with CT or MRI is ideal for imaging the thoracic cavity (**Figure 5.45**). Cytology obtained from ultrasound-guided fine-needle aspirates may be useful, but tissue biopsy and histopathology are often essential for a definitive diagnosis (**Figures 5.46–5.48**).

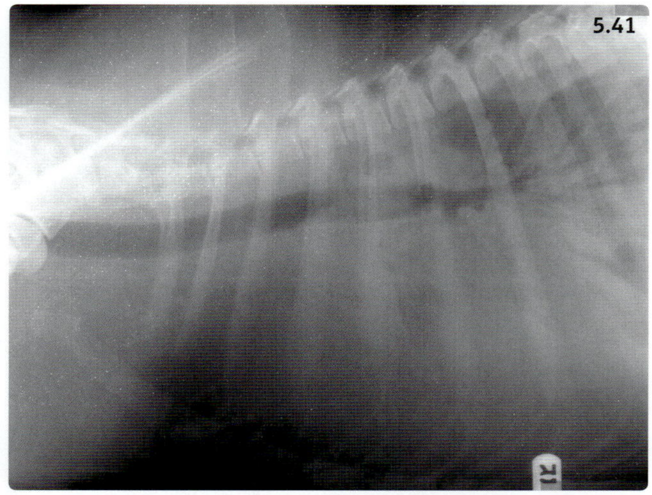

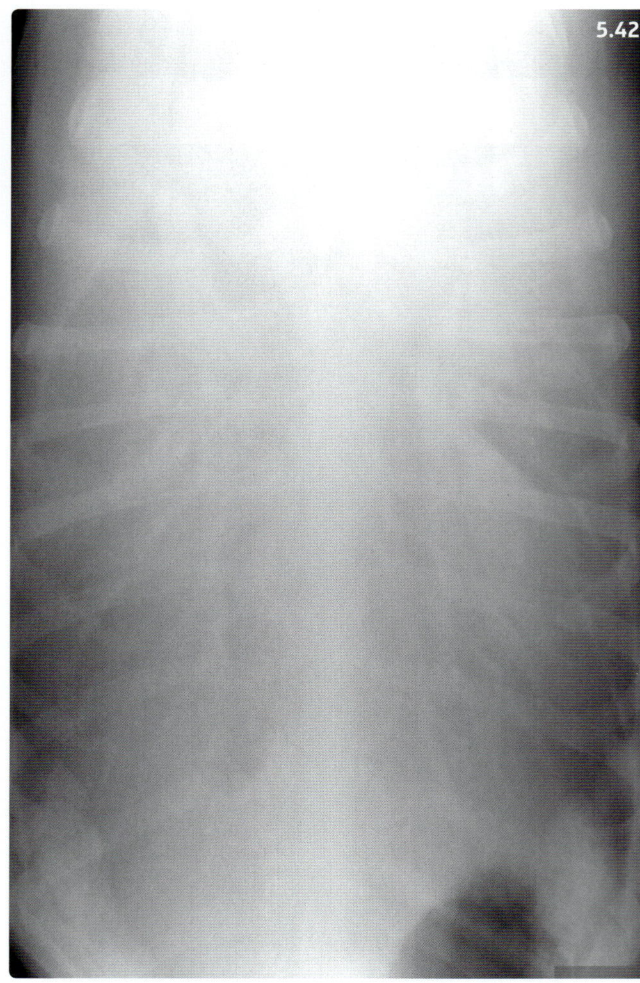

Figures 5.41, 5.42 Dog with severe malignant pleural effusion. Lateral (5.41) and ventrodorsal (5.42) thoracic radiographs. This dog was diagnosed with pleural mesothelioma.

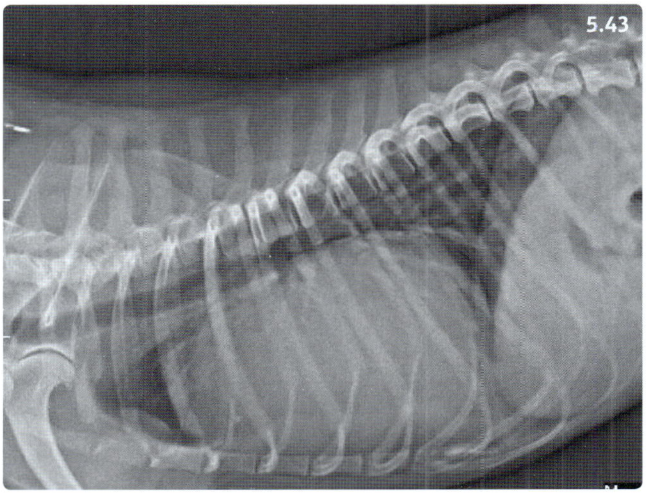

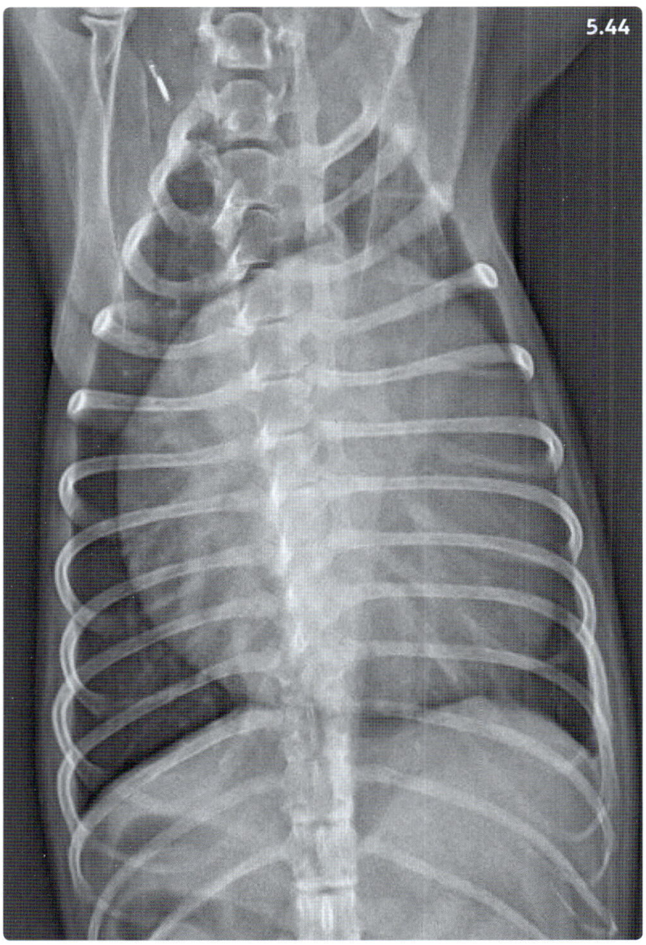

Figures 5.43, 5.44 Dog with severe malignant pericardial effusion. Lateral (5.43) and ventrodorsal (5.44) thoracic radiographs. This dog was diagnosed with a right auricular hemangiosarcoma.

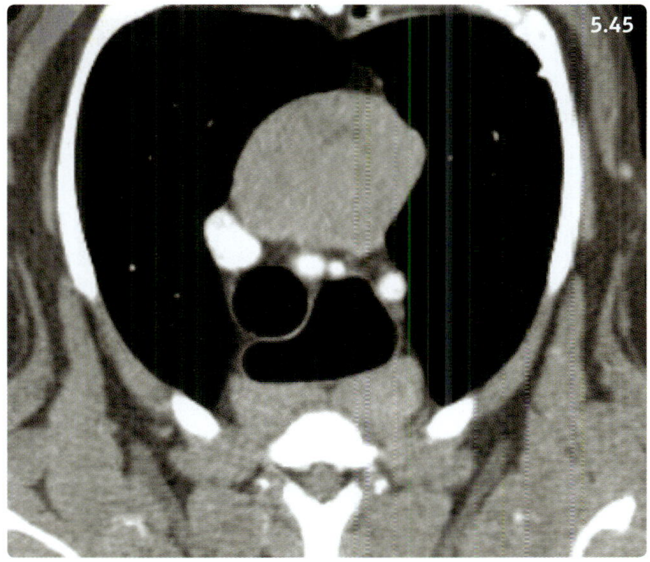

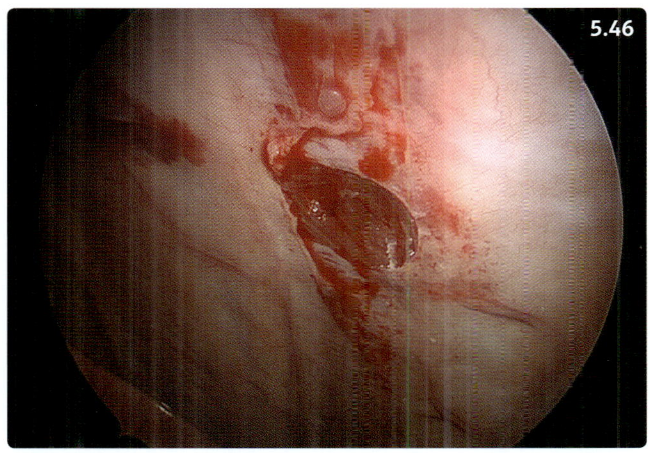

Figures 5.45, 5.46 Dog with a non invasive thymoma. (5.45) Transverse computed tomographic view. Note the thymoma (center of image), left subclavian artery, left internal thoracic artery, brachiocephalic artery, and cranial vena cava (5.46) A thoracoscopic pleural biopsy has been performed. Note the pleural nodule above the biopsy site.

Management

Initial medical treatment may include thoracocentesis, pericardiocentesis, IV fluid resuscitation, and oxygen supplementation. Tissue diagnosis and staging is recommended (although sometimes not possible) before prescribing a treatment plan. Surgery is often indicated for a variety of neoplastic processes, and chemotherapy may also be indicated depending on the biologic behavior of the cancer.

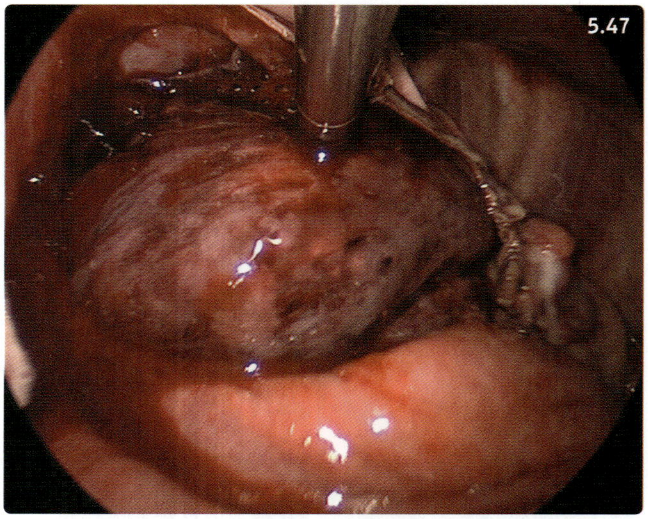

Figure 5.47 Pericardioscopic view of a massive right atrial appendage hemangiosarcoma that is compressing the right atrium.

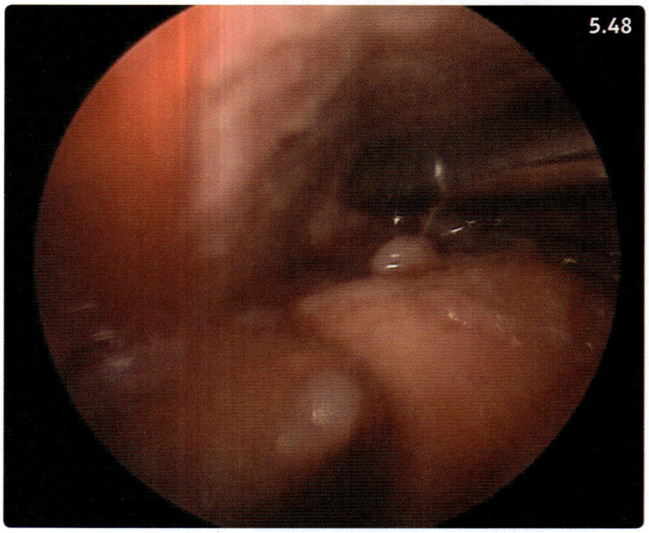

Figure 5.48 Pericardioscopic view of a dog with multiple small heart base nodules. These nodules were not seen on echocardiography or preoperative computed tomography. The diagnosis was pericardial and pleural mesothelioma.

Prognosis

Prognosis is dependent on the clinical health of the subject, the specific neoplasm, and the treatment elected. In general, thoracic neoplasms have a poor long-term prognosis, but disease-free intervals and survival times up to years can be achieved in some cases. Prognosis should be based on histopathology if possible, as some diseases (e.g. idiopathic pleural effusion) can mimic malignant thoracic neoplasms.

RECOMMENDED FURTHER READING

Monnet E (2013) *Small Animal Soft Tissue Surgery*, 1st edn. Wiley-Blackwell, Ames.

Tobias KM, Johnston SA (2012) *Veterinary Surgery: Small Animal*, 1st edn. Elsevier Saunders, St Louis.

Chapter 6

Approach to thoracic radiographs

L. Abbigail Granger

BASICS OF THORACIC RADIOGRAPHY

Technique and positioning

Choosing thoracic views

At least two orthogonal views (right or left lateral and ventrodorsal or dorsoventral views) should be obtained for each thoracic study. Evidence supports obtaining at least three views because of the effect recumbency has on lesion conspicuity. This is true especially when clinical suspicion is present for aspiration or bronchopneumonia, pulmonary bullae, any unilateral or nondiffuse pulmonary disease, or when radiographs are obtained as a screening for metastasis. As exact diagnosis is often unknown at the time of imaging due to overlapping clinical signs, many radiologists advocate three- or four-view thoracic studies as standard of care.

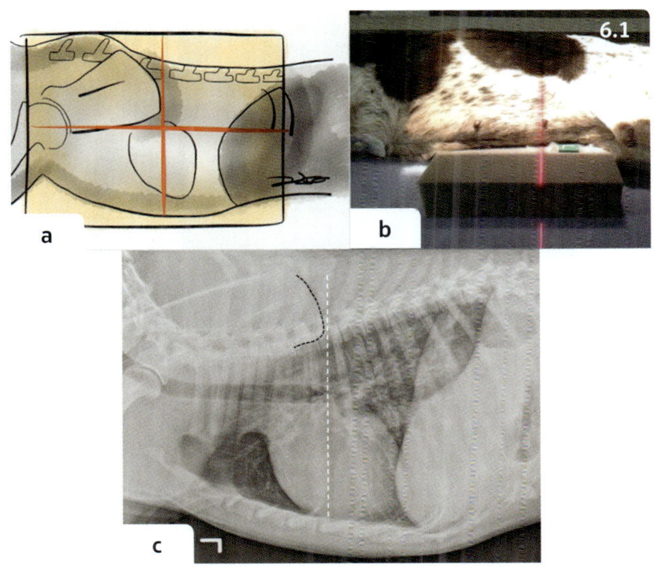

Figures 6.1a–c Palpable landmarks and positioning for a lateral thoracic view. The caudal angle of the scapula is a reliable landmark for centering the beam over the heart (a, b). To correctly use this landmark and to limit superimposition over the cranial lungs, the forelimbs must be extended (c). In most cases, a foam wedge is essential to preventing obliquity. Radiographically, the caudal angle of the scapula (dashed black line) is superimposed near the center of the heart (dashed white line).

Positioning

To obtain a lateral view, position the animal in right or left recumbency and extend the forelimbs to remove superimposition over the cranial thorax. To avoid obliquity, a radiolucent positioning device such as a foam wedge is often needed at the level of the sternum, especially in deep chested dogs. Rely on palpable landmarks to appropriately center and collimate each view. Easily palpable landmarks include the thoracic inlet and the proximal aspect of the 13th ribs, which reliably define the cranial and caudal margins of the thorax. The collimated beam should be centered at the caudal angle of the scapula, which is typically in the same plane as the central heart when the forelimbs are extended (**Figures 6.1a–c**). The ventrodorsal or dorsoventral view should also be obtained with forelimbs extended. Patients can be positioned in a radiolucent trough for a ventrodorsal view or directly on the radiology table for a dorsoventral view (**Figures 6.2a–d**). Sandbags, tape, and radiolucent wedges should be used to properly position patients and avoid personnel exposure. The entire thorax should be included in each view, including the spine and the sternum. In some cases, patients are too large to fit onto one field of view and will require a cranial and caudal view. In such cases, it is also useful to obtain a view centered at the heart, especially when cardiac disease is a concern.

Exposure and timing

Thoracic views should be exposed on peak inspiration in order to maximize inherent contrast. Because of patient respiration, there is a risk of motion unsharpness when obtaining a thoracic radiograph. Because of this, a technique using low mA or short exposure time and a high

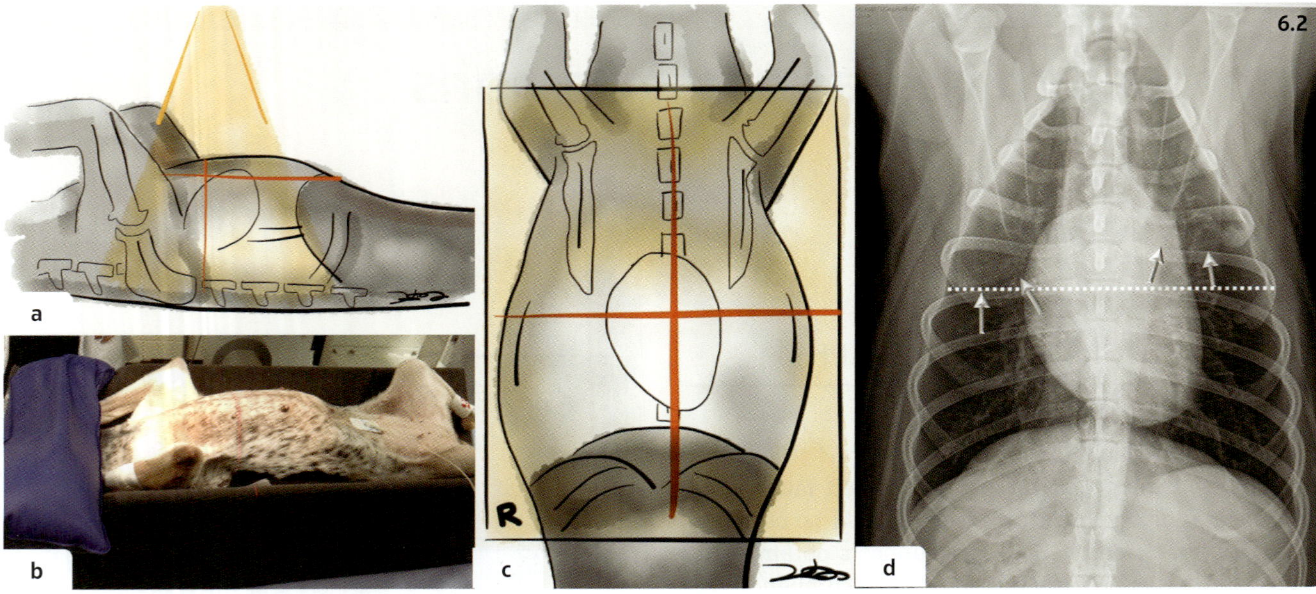

Figures 6.2a–d Positioning (a–c) to obtain a ventrodorsal view (d). The thoracic inlet and the proximal aspect of the caudal ribs should be included to ensure all lungs are in the field of view. The view should be centered at the caudal angle of the scapula, a palpable landmark for the heart when the forelimbs are extended. To avoid obliquity, a trough may be used (b). Sandbags can be used to avoid personnel exposure. On the ventrodorsal radiograph (d), the caudal margins of the scapulae (arrows) are superimposed near the plane of the center of the heart when the view is appropriately collimated and centered (dotted white line).

kV is most suitable for thoracic imaging. Motion can also be limited by use of sedation. If full anesthesia is required, the patient must be intubated and the views obtained under positive pressure in order to avoid confounding results created by atelectasis, which can occur within 5 minutes when 100% inspired oxygen is used.

READING THORACIC RADIOGRAPHS

Systematic approach

Indications for thoracic radiography are listed in **Table 6.1**. A systematic approach increases the comfort level for interpretation of radiographic studies and

Table 6.1 Indications for thoracic radiography.

Indication	Associated clinical signs or history	Some common differential diagnoses
Thoracic barrier abnormality	Palpable or visible defect; thoracic wall pain; known trauma	Rib or soft tissue thoracic wall mass: neoplasia (lipoma, sarcoma); abscess/ cellulitis (trauma, migrating foreign body) Trauma: rib fracture, hematoma Congenital malformation
Respiratory disease	Cough; dyspnea/tachypnea; cyanosis; exercise intolerance; syncope; altered respiratory sounds	Tracheobronchitis: inflammatory/allergic; infectious (viral, bacterial, parasitic) Tracheomalacia/bronchomalacia Bronchopneumonia/aspiration Bronchiectasis Tracheal hypoplasia Cardiogenic edema Noncardiogenic edema: near drowning; strangulation; electrocution; toxicity/drug reaction; neurogenic; barotrauma; acute lung injury or acute respiratory distress syndrome; re-expansion pulmonary edema; aspiration of irritant; overhydration; vasculitis; uremic pneumonitis

(*Continued*)

Indication	Associated clinical signs or history	Some common differential diagnoses
		Upper airway obstruction: tracheal/bronchial foreign body; mural abnormality; extramural compression by mass or cardiac enlargement Interstitial infiltration: pneumonitis (inflammatory/allergic, infectious); neoplasia (e.g. lymphoma) Pulmonary mass(es): neoplasia; abscess; granuloma; cyst; hematoma Pulmonary fibrosis Hemorrhage Lung lobe torsion Anomaly: Kartagener's syndrome or ciliary dyskinesia; surfactant deficiency
Cardiovascular disease	Audible murmur; dyspnea/tachypnea; exercise intolerance; syncope; cough; altered respiratory sounds; cyanosis; arrhythmia	Acquired cardiac diseases: endocardiosis; cardiomyopathy; heartworm infection Congenital cardiac diseases: intra- and extracardiac shunts (L → R or R → L); valvular malformations Pericardial disease/effusion Cor pulmonale
Pleural disease	Dyspnea/tachypnea; exercise intolerance; altered respiratory sounds (decreased); decreased audibility of heart	Pleural effusion: transudates; exudates; hemorrhage; chyle Pneumothorax Diaphragmatic rupture Pleural mass
Mediastinal disease (noncardiac)	Regurgitation/dysphagia; dyspnea/tachypnea; exercise intolerance; altered respiratory sounds	Megaesophagus (generalized): metabolic; congenital; esophagitis Focal esophageal dilation (esophageal obstruction): luminal foreign body; mural lesion; extraluminal compression; vascular ring anomaly; hiatal herniations Mediastinal mass: lymph node (lymphoma); thymus Tracheal compression/obstruction Pneumomediastinum Mediastinitis
Trauma	Dyspnea/tachypnea; altered respiratory sounds; thoracic wall pain; palpable or visible thoracic wall defect	Pulmonary contusions Rib fractures Pneumomediastinum Pneumothorax and/or pleural hemorrhage Shock Diaphragmatic rupture
Systemic disease	Fever; lethargy; weight loss; neoplasia	Numerous potential causes
Screening test	Geriatric patient; preanesthetic	Maybe none
Monitor response to treatment	Improved or worsened clinical signs	

prevents lesions being missed. To be systematic, the interpreter should have a standardized protocol of thoracic views. The influence of recumbency on the appearance of thoracic structures is detailed in **Table 6.2**. Also, each view should be oriented and reviewed the same way each time. All radiographic studies must be approached in the same way, analogous to completing a checklist of anatomic structures (**Box 6.1**).

Table 6.2 Influence of recumbency on the appearance of thoracic structures.

Lateral views	
Right	**Left**
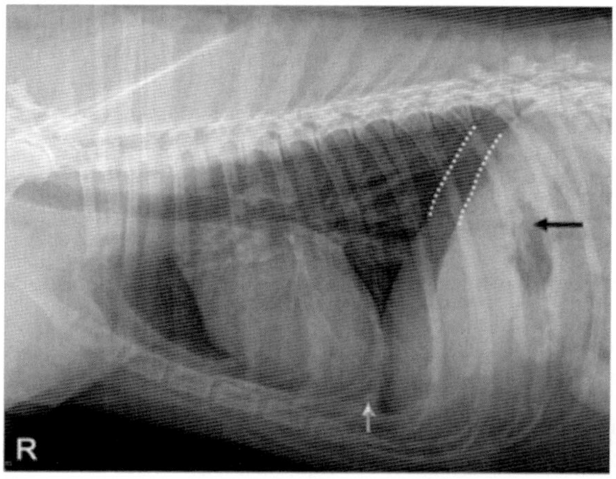	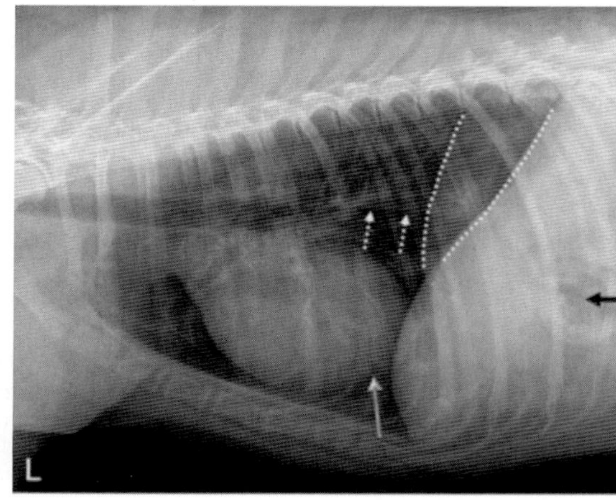
Heart more elongated (apex contacts sternum, white arrow) Diaphragmatic crura parallel (dotted line) Right crus more cranial Gas located in gastric fundus (black arrow) Esophagus often not visible Assess left-sided lungs	Heart more rounded (apex can appear elevated, white arrow) Diaphragmatic crura diverge (dotted line) Left crus more cranial Gas located in pylorus (black arrow) Esophagus more readily seen (dotted arrows) Assess right-sided lungs
Ventrodorsal/dorsoventral views	
Ventrodorsal	**Dorsoventral**
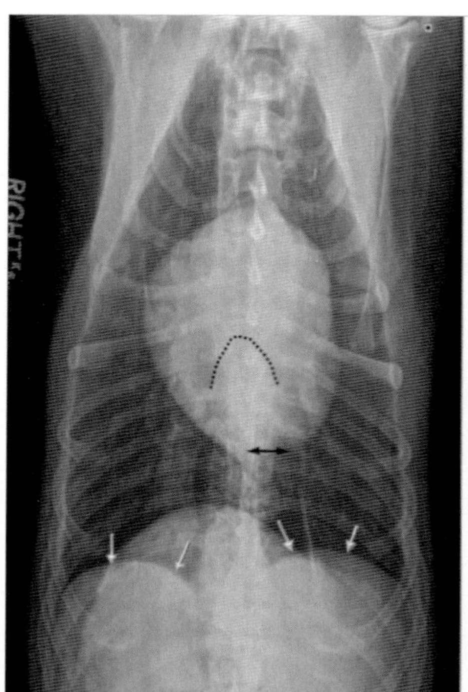	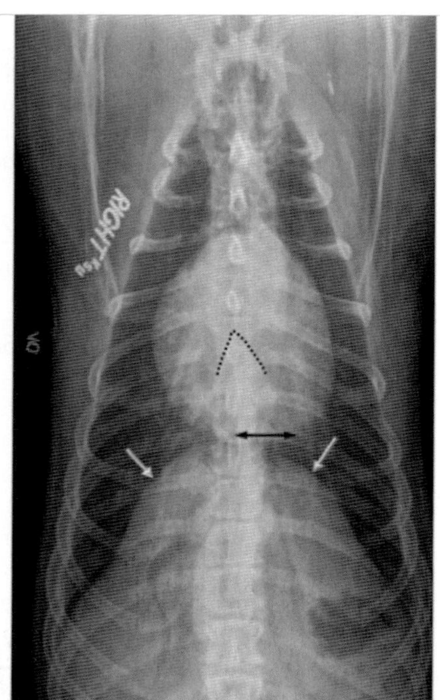

(Continued)

Diaphragmatic crura seen (white arrows) in addition to the central cupola Increased distance between cardiac apex and diaphragm Heart elongated Apex closer to midline (black double arrow) Increased apparent divergence of principle bronchi (dotted line) Accessory lung lobe better aerated and better assessed Caudal vena cava better seen	Only the cupola of the diaphragm is seen creating a dome shape (white arrows) Contact between diaphragm and cardiac apex Heart rounded Apex positioned further to left (black double arrow) Position of principle bronchi less divergent (dotted line) Caudal lung lobes better aerated and better assessed Caudal lobar vessels better seen

Box 6.1 Systematic evaluation of the thorax.

- Extrathoracic structures:
  - Superficial soft tissues (skin, fat, muscle)
  - Skeleton (spine, sternum, ribs, visible forelimbs)
  - Diaphragm
  - Visible abdomen
- Pleural space
- Noncardiac mediastinum:
  - Mediastinal reflections
  - Trachea
  - Esophagus*
  - Vascular structures (e.g. aorta, caudal vena cava, azygos*)
  - Thymus**
  - Sternal, cranial mediastinal, and tracheobronchial lymph nodes*
  - Lymphatics*
- Heart, great vessels, and pericardium
- Lungs:
  - Airway (bronchi, bronchioles*, and alveoli*)
  - Pulmonary arteries and veins
  - Interstitium (elastic fibers, collagen, fibroblasts, smooth muscle, mast cells, mononuclear cells)

*Structures not radiographically visible in a normal animal.
**Structure not normally visible in a mature animal.

Description

When an abnormality is detected during systematic evaluation, it must be described. The classic approach to radiographic description uses a list of signs: size, shape, location, number, margination, and opacity. These can be used to prompt the interpreter of characteristics to consider when describing apparent lesions. Evaluating a lesion with respect to these descriptors ensures that the interpreter processes the abnormality thoroughly and has a starting point for researching causes of any lesions. These morphologic descriptions are essential for recognizing abnormalities and differentiating their causes.

INTERPRETATION OF THORACIC ABNORMALITIES

Extrathoracic structures

Extrathoracic structures should be evaluated early during interpretation, as findings within the thorax often distract from extrathoracic lesions. The presence or lack of symmetry of the thoracic wall should be noted on the ventrodorsal/dorsoventral view. Often, enough of the abdomen is included to determine the presence of cranial organomegaly or loss of detail. Regardless of whether lesions located in extrathoracic structures are related to clinical signs, they can influence the appearance of structures within the thorax and should be noted prior to determination of intrathoracic abnormalities.

Superficial soft tissues and skeleton

Thoracic boundaries include the intercostal and paraspinal muscles, ribs, spine, diaphragm, and thoracic inlet. Opacities comprising the thoracic wall include soft tissue, fat, and mineral and the appearance can vary based on conformation and body condition score. Lesions within the thoracic wall can be categorized as congenital or acquired. Additionally, acquired abnormalities can be further categorized as traumatic or nontraumatic and as originating from the skeleton versus soft tissue.

Congenital thoracic wall abnormalities include vertebral body malformations, transitional vertebrae, and sternal anomalies such as pectus excavatum or carinatum. Most of these abnormalities do not create clinical signs requiring correction.

Differential diagnoses for thoracic wall mass are typical of a mass at any location and include neoplasia (skeletal or soft tissue), abscess/cellulitis, hematoma, granuloma, and cyst. Ranking of these differential diagnoses is based on a full description of the abnormality along with the clinical history. Neoplasia, cellulitis/abscess, and hemorrhage/hematoma formation are the three most likely causes of a thoracic wall mass.

Lipomas are the most common thoracic wall neoplasms. Most often, these are benign, slow-growing, well-demarcated nodules or masses located in the subcutaneous soft tissues and recognized by their fat opacity rather than soft tissue opacity. Nonlipomatous, focal, acquired nodules or masses associated with the thoracic wall may be soft tissue or mineral opaque. They may be broad based (sessile) or have a stalk-like attachment to the thoracic wall (pedunculated). Malignant thoracic wall lesions are most often sarcomas originating from ribs, with primary osteosarcoma and chondrosarcoma being the most common. Radiographically visible rib lysis or periosteal proliferation is seen as evidence of aggression (**Figures 6.3a–c**). Care must be taken to correctly categorize a lesion as originating within the thoracic wall rather than within lung, as differential diagnoses appropriate to the organ of origin must be assigned. Lesions extending into the thorax may be mistaken as having a pulmonary organ of origin. Lysis or periosteal proliferation of the skeleton of the thoracic wall is evidence of a thoracic wall lesion. Also, the presence of an extrapleural sign can differentiate mass lesions as being associated with thoracic wall rather than being pulmonary. An extrapleural sign occurs when the margin of a thoracic wall lesion has a broad-based contact with the wall and an obtuse angle is formed between the lesion and the normal pleural surface. This localizes a lesion to the extrapleural space, which includes any structure superficial to the parietal pleura. A lung lesion would be expected to have a more narrow point of contact, creating an acute angle between the mass and the thoracic wall. Care must be taken to view the location of the mass relative to the profile at its junction with the thoracic wall, as an extrapleural mass not located on a tangent with the wall will create an acute angle, falsely appearing pulmonary rather than extrapleural in origin (**Figure 6.3c**).

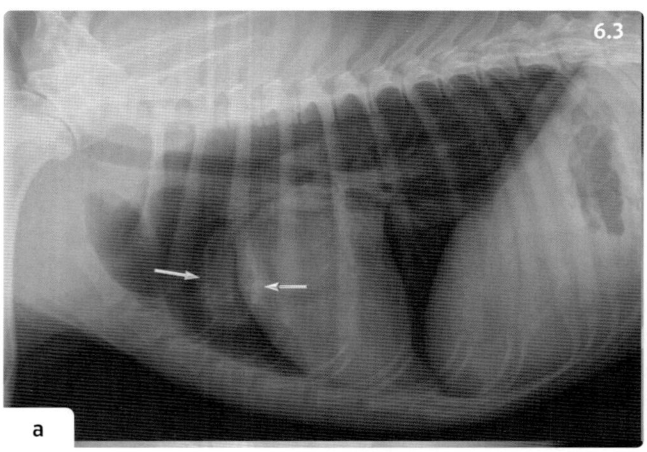

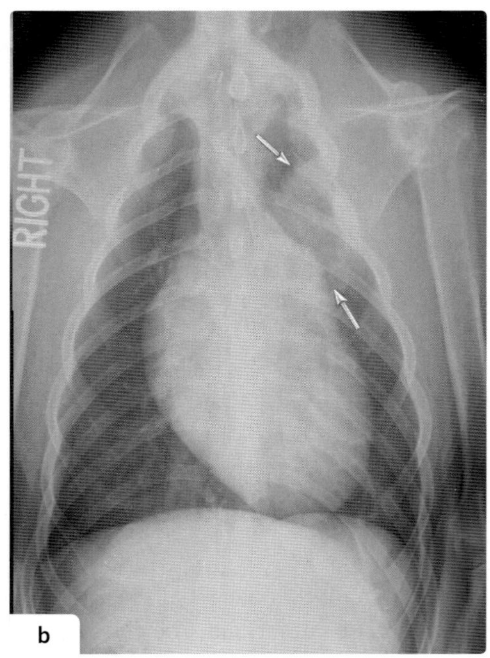

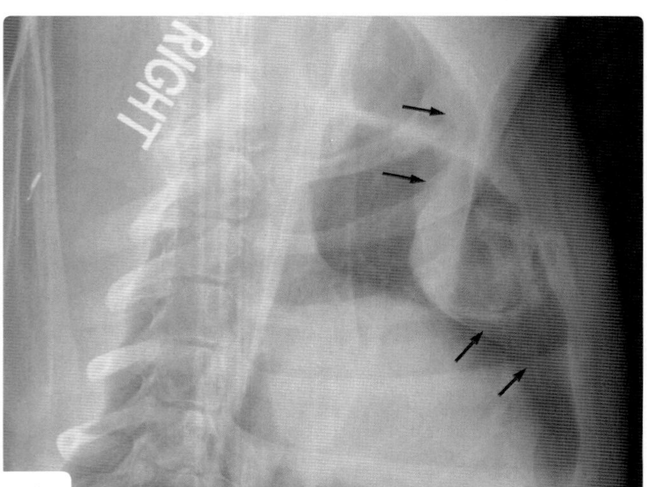

Figures 6.3a–c Extrapleural sign in a dog with chondrosarcoma of the left 3rd rib. A focal region of expansile rib lysis and surrounding mass is present within the left cranial thoracic wall (a, b, white arrows). On the lateral and humanoid ventrodorsal projections (a, b), the mass appears to have a narrow-based point of contact creating an acute angle with the thoracic wall. On an oblique image obtained to view the lesion at its junction with the thoracic wall (c), the soft tissue component of the mass is clearly broad based, creating an obtuse angle between it and the thoracic wall (black arrows). The broad-based point of contact combined with the visible rib lysis confirms an extrapleural origin for the mass.

Most thoracic wall masses associated with neoplasia or infection are palpable on physical examination. The benefit of radiographic examination is to determine opacity and, therefore, potential tissue type of the mass, involvement of bone, or presence of intrathoracic extension.

In cases of trauma, hematoma formation may result in a soft tissue mass of the thoracic wall. The presence of concurrent rib fractures overwhelms the effect of hematoma formation in deforming the thoracic wall. Serial and segmental rib fractures are most likely to create an alteration in thoracic shape on physical examination and radiographically, and may result in paradoxical chest wall movement indicative of flail chest.

Diaphragm and cranial abdomen

The diaphragm defines the caudal thoracic boundary. On a normal thoracic study, the diaphragm should be positioned near the 11th or 12th thoracic vertebra on full inspiration. A position cranial to this may indicate a technical failure to expose the view on inspiration and should be corrected. If not due to technical factors, a cranially positioned diaphragm may be categorized as a primary disturbance of the diaphragm itself or secondary to abdominal or thoracic abnormalities. Primary diaphragmatic pathology is rare and includes unilateral or bilateral paralysis and malformation of the muscle (diaphragmatic eventration). Secondary causes may be related to increased abdominal mass or abnormalities within the lungs or pleural space. A caudally positioned diaphragm is typically not associated with any technical error, although extreme inspiration can result in a diaphragm that is positioned at T13 or caudally. Additional causes of a caudally positioned diaphragm are listed in **Table 6.3**. Keep in mind that diaphragmatic malpositioning may be unilateral or bilateral.

Loss of distinction of diaphragmatic margins is most often due to border effacement associated with pleural or pulmonary disease. If the diaphragm is effaced, its integrity cannot be confirmed.

Pleural space

The thoracic boundaries (thoracic wall and diaphragm) are lined by parietal pleura. The parietal pleura reflects onto itself dorsally to surround the right and left lungs, forming a continuation called the visceral pleura that is tightly adhered to the lung surface. The two layers of pleura surrounding the right and left lungs form the pleural sacs. The pleural sacs each create boundaries of the mediastinum, which lies primarily on midline. The visceral pleura surrounds each lung lobe and extends between each lobe as the lungs exit the hilus. This creates fissures between each of the lung lobes, which can be radiographically evident in cases of pleural disease.

Soft tissue opacity in the pleural space

Pleural effusion

Pleural effusion is the accumulation of fluid within the pleural space. As the fluid volume exceeds 100 ml, it will become radiographically evident in most dogs and cats. Several radiographic signs indicate the presence of pleural effusion (**Box 6.2** and **Figures 6.4a, b)**. Often, several of these signs are present on each thoracic view, increasing the support for a diagnosis of pleural effusion. The visibility of each radiographic sign is more pronounced with increasing fluid volumes.

Box 6.2 Radiographic signs indicating pleural effusion.

- Separation of lungs from the thoracic wall by fluid opacity:
    - Secondary decreased lung volume creating interstitial or alveolar pulmonary patterns
- Presence of pleural fissure lines that widen at the periphery seen on lateral and ventrodorsal views
- Blunting of the right and left costophrenic angles seen on the ventrodorsal view
- Scalloping of ventral lung margins on the lateral view(s)
- Border effacement of the mediastinum, heart, thoracic wall, and diaphragm
- Increased thoracic diameter with severe fluid accumulations

Table 6.3 Pathologic causes of unilateral or bilateral abnormal diaphragmatic positioning.

Cranially positioned diaphragm	Caudally positioned diaphragm
Study exposed on expiration	Exaggerated inspiration
Obese patient	Air trapping (lower airway obstruction)
Abdominal mass effect	Pulmonary emphysema
Pulmonary atelectasis	Increased intrapleural/intrathoracic volume
Upper airway obstruction	Pneumothorax
Pain with inspiration	Pleural effusion
Diaphragmatic paralysis (rare)	Thoracic mass(es)
Diaphragmatic eventration (rare)	

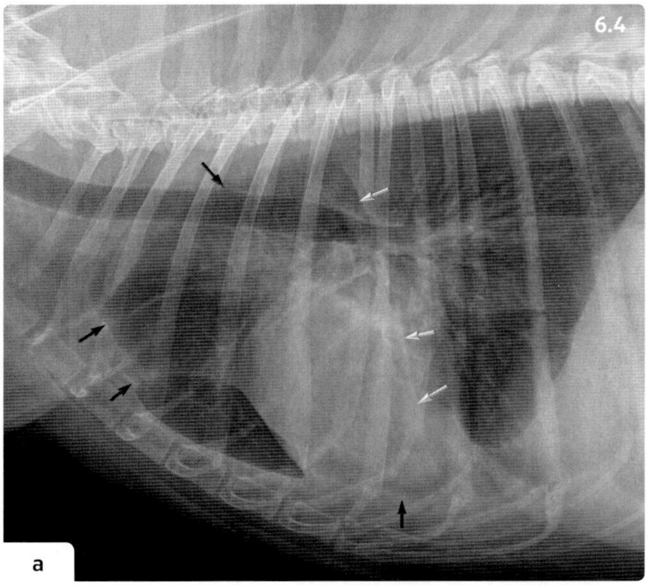

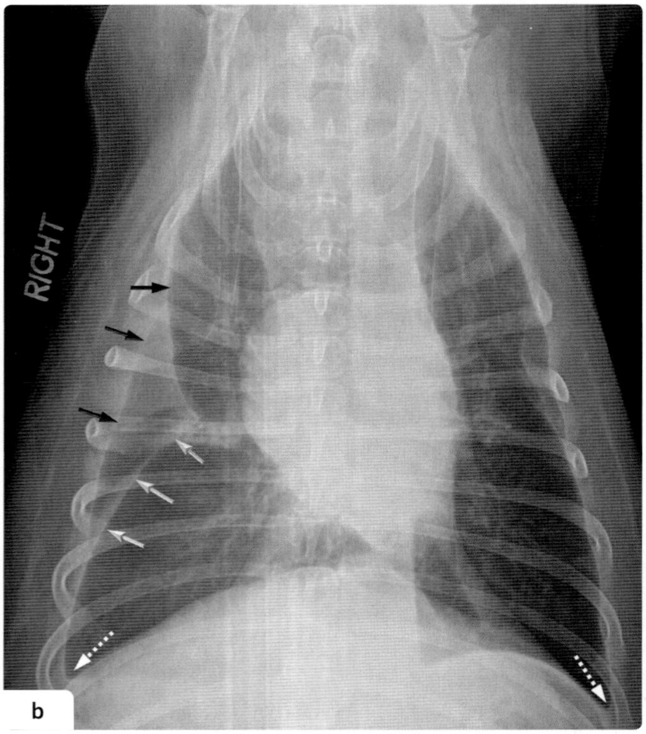

Figures 6.4a, b Right lateral (a) and ventrodorsal (b) radiographs of a dog with moderate pleural effusion. There is separation of the lungs from the thoracic wall by fluid opacity (black arrows). Pleural fissure lines are present that widen at the peripheral aspect of the thorax, further from the hilus (white arrows). The right and left costophrenic angles are blunted (dotted white arrows). Additionally, there is border effacement of the cardiac apex and ventral diaphragm on the lateral view (a). The presence of each of these findings will be more pronounced with increased fluid volumes.

The position of the animal influences the visibility of each of the radiographic signs presented in **Box 6.2**. First, pleural fissure lines are less prominently seen on the dorsoventral view than on the ventrodorsal view. Also, the visibility of the cardiac silhouette varies with sternal or dorsal recumbency (**Figures 6.5a, b**). The heart is a soft tissue opaque, ventrally located structure. When an animal is positioned in sternal recumbency, gravity-dependent fluid accumulates ventrally and surrounds the ventrally located heart. Because the heart and fluid are of identical opacity and are in direct contact with each other, margins become effaced. When an animal is positioned in dorsal recumbency, the fluid accumulates dorsally. Lungs rise to the nongravity dependent part of the thorax, which is ventral, and surround the heart, making its margins evident.

Causes of pleural effusion

Pleural effusion is most often secondary to another disease process. Pleural fluid should be considered based on the underlying cause of each of the potential fluid types: transudates including modified transudates, exudates, hemorrhage, and chyle. Causes for each of these fluid types are listed in **Table 6.4**. The most common causes of pleural effusion in both dogs and cats are pyothorax, neoplasia, and cardiac failure. In many cases, determination of the underlying cause of pleural effusion requires fluid analysis, systematic clinical work up, and advanced imaging such as thoracic ultrasound or CT.

Keys to interpreting cases with pleural effusion

Interpretation of thoracic studies showing pleural effusion can be a challenge. Especially with moderate to severe fluid volumes, the visualization of soft tissue thoracic structures such as the heart, mediastinum, and

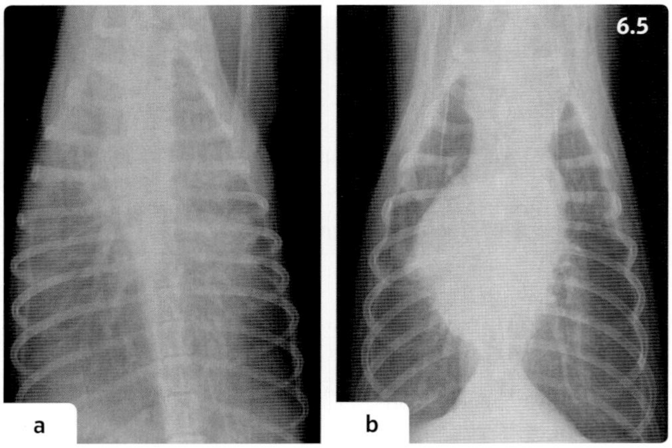

Figures 6.5a, b Mobility of fluid in the pleural space in sternal (a) and dorsal (b) recumbency.

Table 6.4 Causes of pleural effusion.

Fluid type	Underlying causes
Transudates and modified transudates	Congestive heart failure or systemic venous obstruction Hypoproteinemia Diaphragmatic translocation of peritoneal effusion Diaphragmatic rupture Neoplasia Vasculitis Lung lobe torsion Pleuritis, mediastinitis
Exudates (septic/ pyothorax or nonseptic inflammatory)	Primary lung disease (pulmonary abscess or pneumonia) Pleuritis, mediastinitis Foreign body migration (grass awn)
Hemorrhage (hemothorax)	Coagulation deficit Trauma Neoplasia
Chyle (chylothorax)	Obstruction of lymphatic return (congestive heart failure, neoplasia) Ruptured lymphatics (trauma, neoplasia)

Box 6.3 Next steps in the analysis of cases with pleural effusion.

- Obtain all four radiographic projections so that all lung fields, the mediastinum, and the cardiac silhouette can be best assessed:
  - Ensure that the entire thoracic wall, including all the ribs, is visible in the study
- When evaluating the radiographic study, pay close attention to the following:
  - Cardiac size and shape (need ventrodorsal view)
  - Tracheal positioning for evidence of a cranial mediastinal mass
  - Ribs, sternum, and spine for evidence of an extrapleural lesion
  - Lungs for evidence of masses or nodules (all four views may be needed)
  - Bronchi for alterations in position or blunting, possibly indicating lung lobe torsion
  - Presence of a mediastinal shift in the face of bilateral pleural effusion indicating a thoracic mass or diaphragmatic rupture
  - Presence of abdominal disease at the edge of the study
  - Lung margination as being sharp or rounded
- Tap the fluid and repeat radiographic views
- Perform analysis of tapped fluid
- Perform thoracic ultrasonography or CT

pleural margins can be impossible. In such cases, the interpreter should make the best of what clues are visible in order to diagnose, or at least rule out, sources of pleural effusion, keeping in mind that pleural effusion is typically a secondary process and nonpleural disease is often the cause of the pleural effusion. Some steps that can be used to investigate the causes of pleural effusion are listed in **Box 6.3**.

Mediastinal masses often result in pleural effusion and can sometimes be evident owing to an alteration in tracheal positioning, which remains air filled and readily distinct. Marked deviations or compressions of the trachea should be noted as potential signs of underlying mediastinal disease resulting in pleural effusion (**Figures 6.6a, b**). In cases of pleural effusion, the trachea will elevate to some degree, but its path should remain straight with no focal changes in direction. Also, the tracheal hilus should be located at the 5th or 6th intercostal space in a normal animal or an animal having only pleural effusion. If a mediastinal mass is large enough, caudal displacement of the hilus may result. The cranial mediastinum is best assessed on the ventrodorsal view in cases of pleural effusion, as most masses are ventrally located and are effaced by any fluid located ventrally.

Primary or metastatic neoplasms resulting in pulmonary masses or nodules can be obscured by pleural effusion. In cases of moderate to severe pleural effusion, the lung volume will be decreased. This results in a secondary atelectasis and an increase in pulmonary opacity that is typically most severe in the cranial or right middle lung lobes. When atelectasis is severe, interpretation of lungs as normal or abnormal is impossible and it can preclude visibility of masses and nodules. Additionally, border effacement of the heart, mediastinum, and thoracic wall by fluid can prevent interpretation of these structures. Removal of fluid and repeat radiographic examination can increase the visibility of mass(es) within the thorax (**Figures 6.7a, b**). As with removal of any tissue, unless a diagnosis is known, the fluid sample should be analyzed for evidence of its underlying cause.

Diaphragmatic rupture

Separation of the lungs from the thoracic wall by soft tissue opacity and border effacement of the diaphragm are most often caused by pleural fluid; however, these signs may be due to soft tissue rather than fluid. Diaphragmatic rupture must always be considered in thoracic studies where pleural soft tissue opacity is

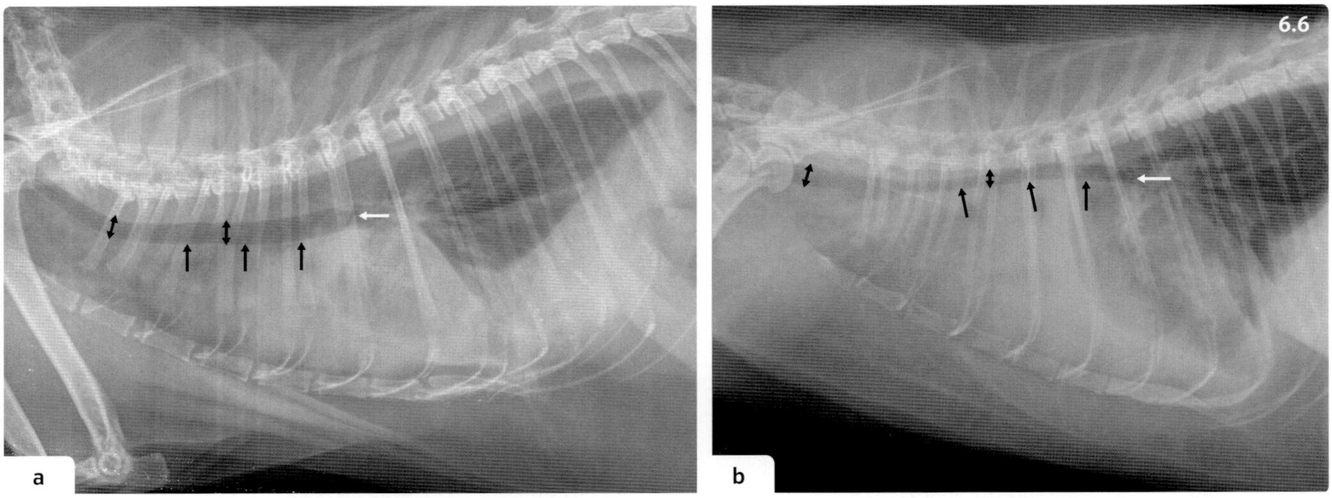

Figures 6.6a, b Lateral thoracic radiographs of a cat having only pleural effusion (a) and a cat having a mediastinal mass with concurrent pleural effusion (b). In the cat with pleural effusion, the trachea is mildly uniformly elevated (a, black arrows) due to the pleural fluid and the influence it has on lung and, subsequently, tracheal positioning. The tracheal hilus is in a normal position located at the junction between the 5th and 6th intercostal spaces (a, white arrow). Additionally, the tracheal lumen remains similar in diameter throughout its length (a, double-headed arrows). In the cat having concurrent pleural effusion and a cranial mediastinal mass, the trachea is markedly elevated and focally deviated in the region of the cranial mediastinum (b, black arrows). The trachea is compressed, as seen by a decrease in diameter at the level of the tracheal deviation (b, double-headed arrows). The tracheal hilus is also caudally displaced and is located at the center of the 7th intercostal space (b, white arrow).

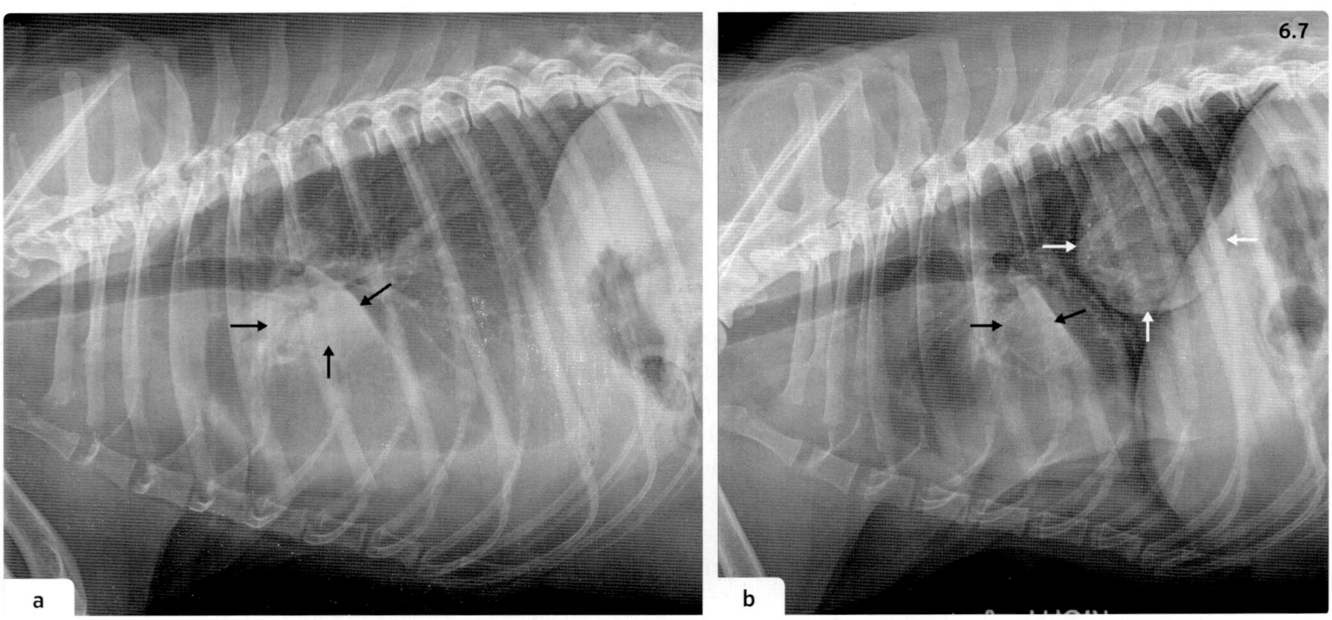

Figures 6.7a, b Right lateral radiographs of the same dog before (a) and after (b) tapping pleural effusion that was secondary to a primary pulmonary carcinoma of the right caudal lung lobe. Prior to tapping a pulmonary mass is not visible due to the presence of marked pleural effusion. A general increase in pulmonary opacity is present, which is most severe near the tracheal hilus, where an alveolar pulmonary pattern is seen (a, black arrows). This is typical of the location for atelectasis when complete lung expansion is prevented by pleural fluid. After tapping the fluid, a well-defined, round mass within the caudal lung is clearly evident (b, white arrows). Fluid analysis was consistent with carcinoma. The region of atelectasis, although not completely resolved, is diminished (b, black arrows).

present and the diaphragmatic margins are effaced such that its integrity cannot be confirmed. In many cases of diaphragmatic rupture, concurrent pleural effusion is present along with herniated abdominal organs, complicating radiographic confirmation of herniation. Several radiographic signs (**Box 6.4** and **Figures 6.8a, b**) raise suspicion of diaphragmatic rupture above that of pleural fluid occurring alone.

Pleural masses

In addition to herniated abdominal organs, neoplasia or severe pleuritis can be responsible for pleural mass lesions. Often, concurrent, mobile pleural fluid is also present in these cases, resulting in border effacement of the pleural mass and making it radiographically invisible. Similar to diaphragmatic rupture with abdominal organ herniation, pleural masses due to neoplasia or pyogranulomatous pleuritis can be large enough to create a thoracic mass effect recognized as a deviation of the heart, trachea, or lungs away from the lesion (contralateral mediastinal shift). Again, the mediastinal shift may be the only indication of a pleural mass versus mobile pleural effusion.

Box 6.4 Radiographic signs indicating diaphragmatic rupture.

- Partial border effacement of the diaphragm that is more prominent on one side versus the other
- Separation of lungs from the thoracic wall by soft tissue/fluid opacity that is more prominent in one hemithorax versus the other
- Contained tubular or round gas opacities within the thorax or crossing the diaphragm
- Decreased abdominal contents within peritoneal space:
  - Absence of visible organs
  - Wasp-waist appearance to abdominal wall
- Cranially displaced gastric axis
- Evidence of pleural mass effect:
  - Contralateral mediastinal shift with displaced heart and trachea away from the hemithorax having the most pleural opacity

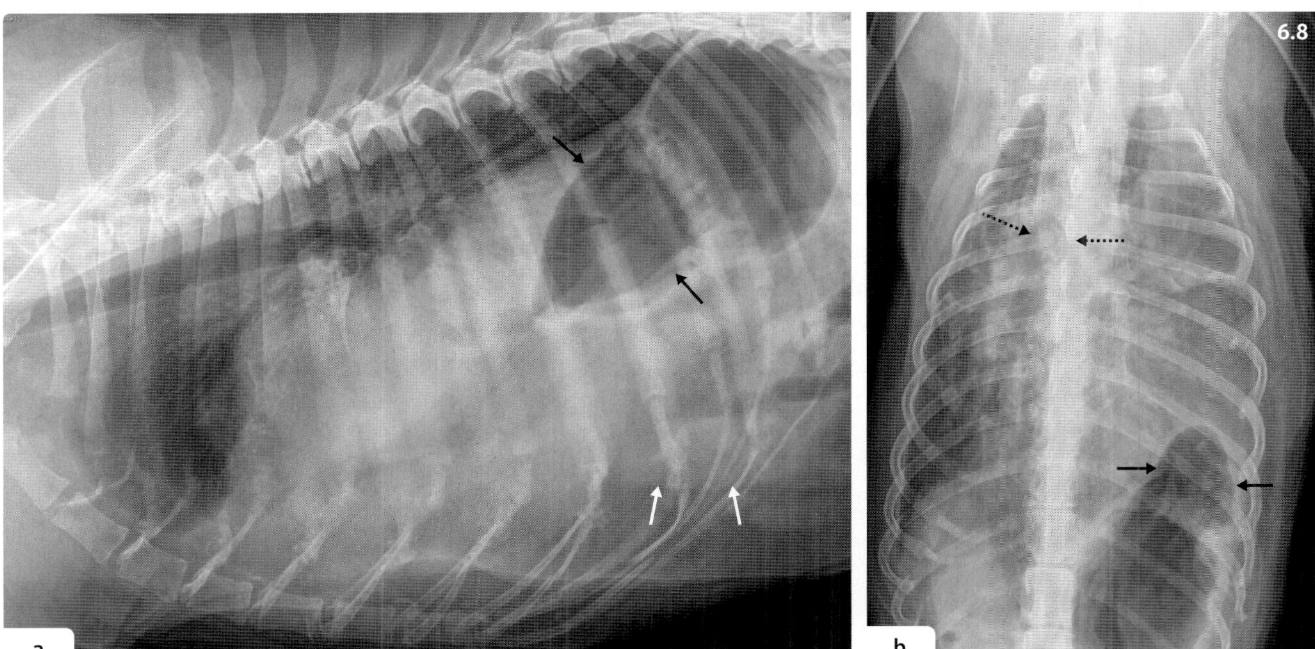

Figures 6.8a, b Lateral (a) and dorsoventral (b) radiographs of a dog presented for increased respiratory effort after vehicular trauma. A marked increase in soft tissue opacity is present within the caudal ventral thorax, which is notably located on the left side. There is border effacement of most of the cardiac silhouette and the diaphragm. The left diaphragmatic margin is effaced on the dorsoventral view. The tracheal hilus is deviated to the right hemithorax (b, dotted black arrows), consistent with a mediastinal shift away from the hemithorax containing most of the increased soft tissue opacity. The normal caudoventral liver margin is not identified and the tail of the spleen (a, white arrows) is cranially displaced. These findings support the diagnosis of diaphragmatic rupture with herniated abdominal organs. Finally, a gas-filled structure with visible rugal folds consistent with the stomach is seen crossing from the abdomen to the thorax (black arrows), confirming diagnosis of herniation.

Gas opacity in the pleural space (pneumothorax)

Pneumothorax is accumulated gas within the pleural space, between the parietal and visceral pleura. It has multiple potential causes that are categorized as traumatic, spontaneous, or iatrogenic (**Table 6.5**). Pneumothorax may also be considered open or closed. An open pneumothorax implies a penetrating or perforating trauma with extension of air from the environment into the pleural space. Closed pneumothorax occurs when the respiratory system is the source of gas within the pleural space. Trauma is the most common underlying cause of pneumothorax and is the only category that can result both closed and/or open configurations.

Spontaneous pneumothorax is always closed and results from some extension of air from the respiratory system. It can be primary or secondary. Primary spontaneous pneumothorax occurs when there is no evidence of underlying pulmonary disease. In reality, most cases are assumed to be the result of a ruptured pulmonary bulla or bleb, which, of course, implies underlying pulmonary pathology. Secondary spontaneous pneumothorax is associated with known underlying lung disease (except pulmonary bullae or blebs). Dogs most commonly have primary spontaneous pneumothorax; cats have secondary spontaneous pneumothorax.

The radiographic signs of pneumothorax are summarized in **Box 6.5**. The right lateral view is the most sensitive view for detection of pneumothorax, where separation of the heart from the sternum is often the first sign seen (**Figures 6.9a–d**). Some thin animals lack thoracic fat along the sternum thus giving a false impression of cardiac elevation. Additionally, separation of the lungs from the thoracic wall with gas opacity indicates pleural gas. The key to diagnosing pleural gas is recognizing the absence of pulmonary vascular markings in the region suspected of absent lungs. In cases of spontaneous pneumothorax, the underlying pulmonary bulla or bleb is often not evident radiographically. Compared with radiography, CT is able to detect the underlying bullae with much greater sensitivity.

Table 6.5 Categories and causes of pneumothorax.

Category	Underlying cause(s)
Traumatic	Open: penetrating or perforating wound Closed: blunt force trauma
Spontaneous	Primary: • Idiopathic • Presumed rupture of bulla or bleb Secondary: • Rupture of necrotic or cavitary lung lesions (not bullae or blebs): ◦ Pneumonia ◦ Parasitic infection ◦ Pulmonary abscess ◦ Cavitary neoplasm ◦ Congenital lobar emphysema ◦ Bronchopulmonary dysplasia ◦ Grass awn migration ◦ Interstitial pneumonitis or fibrosis ◦ Pulmonary thromboembolism
Iatrogenic	Extreme positive pressure ventilation Thoracocentesis

Box 6.5 Radiographic signs indicating pneumothorax.

- Separation of the heart from the sternum (earliest visible sign seen on lateral view):
  - Absence of pulmonary vascular markings at the region of separation
- Retraction of lungs from the thoracic wall by gas opacity:
  - Absence of pulmonary vascular markings at the region of retraction
- General increased lung opacity:
  - More evident with increasing pleural volume of gas
- Evidence of tension (only with severe gas accumulations):
  - Flattened or tented diaphragm
  - Mediastinal shift away from pleural space containing most gas
  - Barrel-shaped chest

Noncardiac mediastinum

As an entry point into the central thorax and evaluation of the mediastinum, the extrathoracic trachea should be followed, evaluating its margins until the bifurcation is reached. From this point, the mediastinum can be evaluated. Abnormalities include alterations in margination (decreased visibility due to borer effacement), position, size, or opacity of the mediastinum. The mediastinum spans from the thoracic inlet to the diaphragm and the entire dorsal to ventral dimension of the thorax. The mediastinal compartment communicates with fascial planes of the neck cranially and with the retroperitoneal space caudally (through the aortic hiatus). This communication is important when determining the underlying cause of pneumomediastinum, as discussed later. The mediastinum includes many structures that are not normally visible on thoracic radiographs due to border effacement, including sternal, cranial mediastinal, and

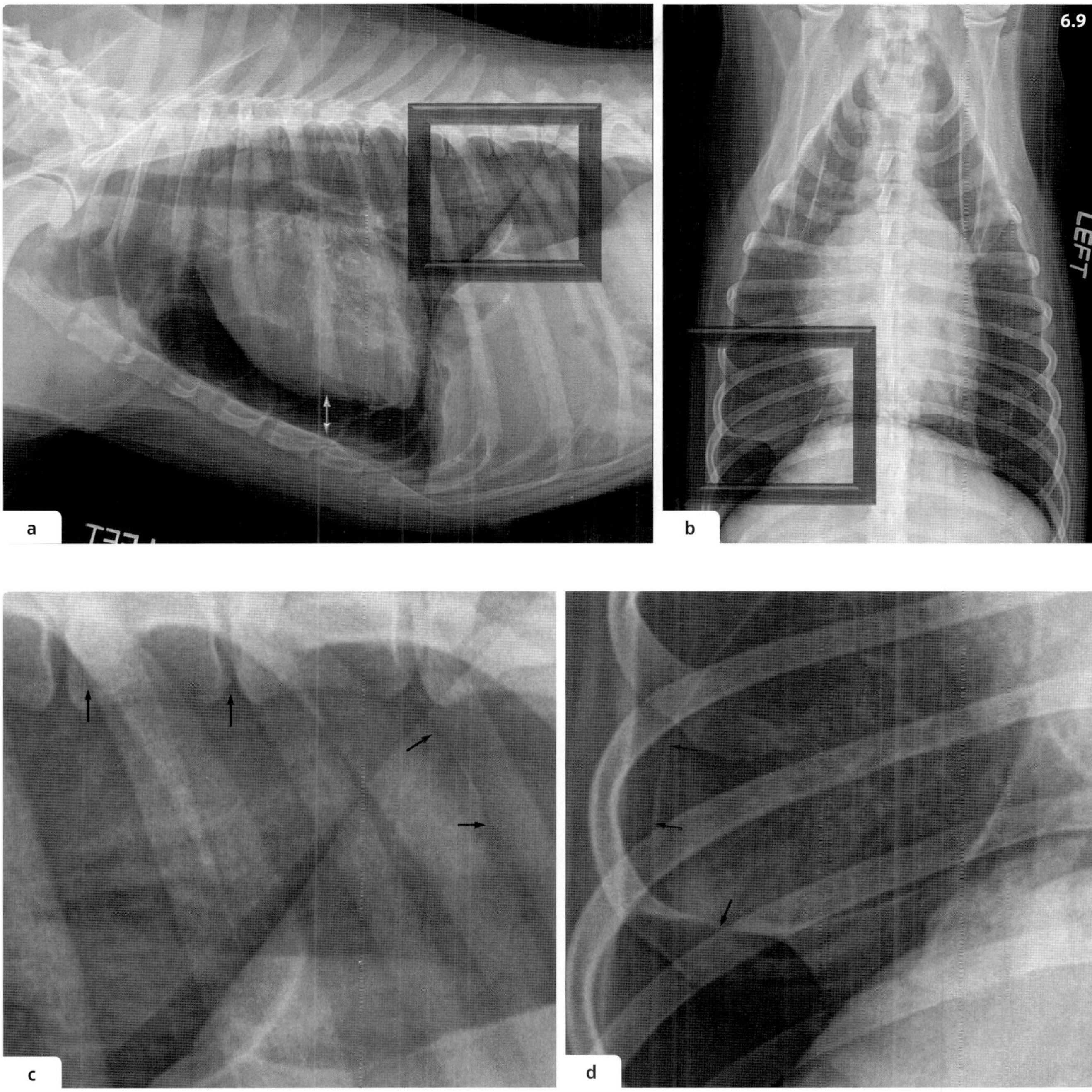

Figures 6.9a–d Lateral (a) and ventrodorsal (b) radiographs of a dog with moderate pneumothorax with accompanying magnified views of the indicated regions (c, d). Moderate separation of the heart from the sternum with interposed gas opacity is seen on the lateral view (a, white double arrow). Additionally, separation of the lungs from the thoracic wall is visible on both views (c, d, black arrows). The lungs are mildly, diffusely increased in opacity, consistent with atelectasis due to increased pleural volume.

tracheobronchial lymph nodes, thymus, esophagus, vessels (e.g. brachiocephalic trunk, left subclavian, azygos vein), nerves, and lymphatics. In the diseased state, these structures may become visible due to altered size or opacity. The main visible mediastinal structures are the trachea, heart, and great vessels. Cardiovascular mediastinal structures will be discussed in more detail in the next section. The thymus is visible only in young animals.

Mediastinal gas (pneumomediastinum)

Mediastinal gas, or pneumomediastinum, can be seen independently or concurrent with pneumothorax. Radiographically, mediastinal gas is readily distinguished from pleural gas because it acts as a contrast, increasing visibility of opaque soft tissue from margins within the cranial mediastinum that are not normally seen (**Figure 6.10**). The most commonly seen radiographic sign is increased delineation of the outer tracheal wall as it is highlighted by gas. The lateral view is typically the only view that is diagnostic for pneumomediastinum, as superimposition precludes visibility of mediastinal gas on the orthogonal view. Pneumomediastinum has several potential causes (**Box 6.6**). In many cases, the clinical history provides a clue as to the underlying cause. Trauma is the most commonly reported cause of pneumomediastinum.

Given the potential causes of pneumomediastinum, it is recommended that radiographs be obtained of the entire neck in order to assess the larynx, trachea, and other cervical structures, which may be the cause of mediastinal gas. In many cases of tracheal rupture, a lesion is not identified on radiographs and endoscopic examination may be needed to assess the integrity of the trachea and esophagus. Typically, when esophageal rupture causes pneumomediastinum, concurrent mediastinal and, therefore, pleural effusion is seen.

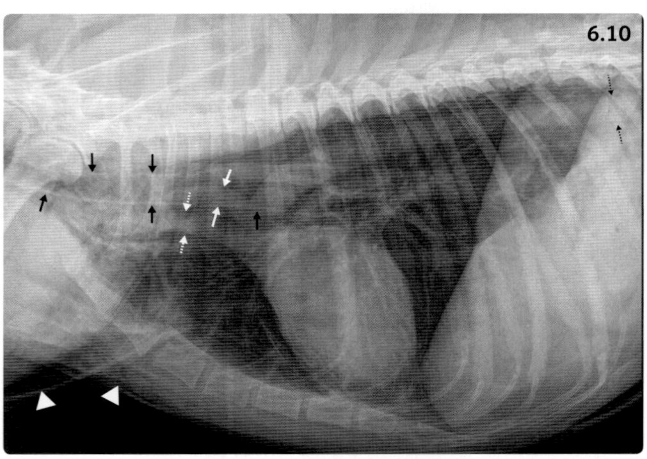

Figure 6.10 Pneumomediastinum in a dog that had received multiple bite wounds. Subcutaneous emphysema is present superimposed over the thorax and located ventrally (white arrowheads). The outer margin of the trachea is visible (black arrows) because it is surrounded by gas. The margins of the brachiocephalic trunk (dotted white arrows) and left subclavian (white arrows) are no longer effaced by surrounding soft tissue structures due to interposed gas highlighting their margins. The cranial abdominal aorta is visible (dotted black arrows) because it is surrounded by gas extending into the retroperitoneal space through the aortic hiatus.

Regardless of the cause of pneumomediastinum, gas within the mediastinal space can leak into the pleural space due to fenestrations. However, gas within the pleural space will never leak into the mediastinum, as excess pleural pressure due to the pneumothorax would be expected to collapse the mediastinum and would, in fact, be protective against gas entering the mediastinum. Also, as previously mentioned, the mediastinum communicates with the cervical fascial planes cranially and the retroperitoneal space caudally. Therefore, gas within the mediastinum can extend to these spaces and gas within these spaces can extend to the mediastinum. Pneumomediastinum that is of such severity as to cause subcutaneous emphysema after tracking through the cervical soft tissues should be assumed to occur from tracheal rupture.

Mediastinal shift

Mediastinal structures such as the trachea and heart can be displaced from their midline locations due to disease in the pleural or pulmonary space. Mediastinal shifts can be categorized as contralateral or ipsilateral. A contralateral mediastinal shift follows disease present in the right or left hemithorax that causes a push of the mediastinum away from the diseased side. An ipsilateral mediastinal shift occurs when disease within the thorax causes a pull of the mediastinum towards the diseased side, which has a decrease in volume or a physical tethering of the mediastinum towards the lesion. Some diseases that may cause a mediastinal shift have been mentioned previously in the discussion on pleural diseases. Additional causes are shown in **Table 6.6**. Recognition of a mediastinal shift can be key to differentiating the causes of pulmonary or pleural lesions seen, but it is almost never associated with mediastinal lesions alone, therefore its presence typically indicates disease outside the mediastinum.

Box 6.6 Causes of pneumomediastinum.

- Cervical trauma:
  - Penetrating wounds (e.g. bites) introducing gas into deep cervical soft tissues
- Tracheal or laryngeal rupture
- Alveolar rupture causing tracking of gas through interstitium:
  - Blunt force thoracic trauma
  - Iatrogenic pulmonary hyperinflation
- Esophageal rupture (concurrent effusion is expected)
- Extension from the retroperitoneal space (uncommon)
- Mediastinitis due to gas-producing bacteria (concurrent effusion is expected)

Mediastinal masses

Recognition of the position of the trachea is key to differentiating the most likely organ or origin for many mediastinal masses. As previously mentioned, many of the structures within the mediastinum, especially within the cranial mediastinum, are not visible in the normal animal. However, when mediastinal structures become enlarged, they create masses characteristic to their location within the mediastinum, which assists with identifying the organ of origin for the mass. The location of mediastinal masses associated with specific organs is shown in **Table 6.7**. The effect that these masses have on the trachea is also shown.

Table 6.6 Categorization and causes of a mediastinal shift.

Ipsilateral: mediastinum is pulled *towards* the abnormality	Pleural disease: • Adhesions between mediastinal and thoracic wall pleura (uncommon) • Atelectasis caused by fibrotic pleura constricting lung(s) (uncommon) Pulmonary disease: • Remaining causes of atelectasis (common): ◦ Positional/recumbency/ anesthesia associated ◦ Bronchial obstruction
Contralateral: mediastinum is pushed *away* from the abnormality	Pleural disease: • Unilateral pleural effusion or pneumothorax (common) • Pleural mass (uncommon) • Diaphragmatic rupture with herniated abdominal organs (common) Pulmonary disease: • Lung mass (common)

Mediastinal structures

Trachea

In most small animals, the normal tracheal path diverges from the thoracic spine, beginning at the thoracic inlet and extending to the tracheal bifurcation. The normal tracheal diameter should be consistent throughout and should be slightly less than the diameter of the larynx. Variations of tracheal diameter to thoracic inlet ratios according to breed are listed in **Table 6.8**.

A decrease in tracheal luminal diameter may be diffuse throughout its length or segmental/focal. Also, any tracheal narrowing can be caused by extraluminal, luminal, or mural factors (**Table 6.9**). Diffuse narrowing of the tracheal lumen is caused by mural abnormalities, specifically tracheal hypoplasia, severe tracheal collapse (**Figure 6.11**), or severe thickening of the tracheal mucosa caused by tracheitis or hemorrhage. These causes may be radiographically indistinguishable; however, tracheal

Table 6.7 Location of masses associated with mediastinal structures and their most common effect on tracheal positioning.

Organ of origin	**Mediastinal location for mass**	**Direction of tracheal deviation**
Esophagus: • Generalized enlargement • Focal enlargement	Dorsal: • Cranial, middle, and caudal mediastinum • Craniodorsal or dorsal middle, most typically	Ventral
Sternal lymph nodes	Cranioventral	Dorsal, if severe enlargement
Cranial mediastinal lymph nodes	Cranioventral	Dorsal
Thymus	Cranioventral	Dorsal +/- right
Ectopic thyroid	Cranioventral	Dorsal
Mediastinal (pharyngeal) cyst	Cranioventral	Dorsal
Heart base	Cranial or middle	Dorsal and right
Tracheobronchial lymph nodes	Middle	Ventral
Left atrium	Middle	Dorsal
Hiatal hernia	Caudodorsal	None

Table 6.8 Tracheal diameter to thoracic inlet ratios in normal dogs.

Breed type	Ratio value
Nonbrachycephalic breeds	0.20 +/- 0.03
Nonbulldog brachycephalic breeds	0.16 +/- 0.03
Bulldogs	0.13 +/- 0.04

Table 6.9 Causes of tracheal narrowing.

Length of trachea affected	Differential diagnoses
Diffuse	Mural abnormalities: • Tracheal hypoplasia • Tracheitis • Mucosal hemorrhage • Severe tracheal collapse

Focal or segmental	Mural abnormalities:
	• Tracheal collapse
	• Tracheal stricture or cicatrix
	• Neoplasia:
	  ◦ Osteochondroma, chondrosarcoma, osteosarcoma, papilloma
	• Polyp
	• Granuloma:
	  ◦ Parasitic (*Filaroides osleri*)
	  ◦ Previous tracheal irritation or trauma
	Extramural abnormalities:
	• Mediastinal mass
	• Pulmonary mass (rarely)
	Luminal abnormalities:
	• Foreign body

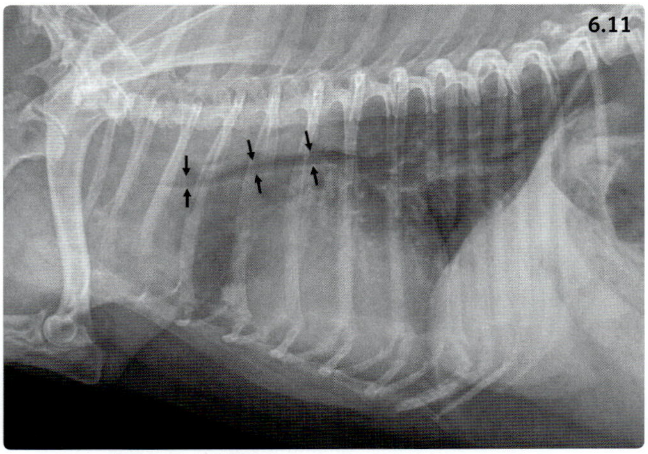

Figure 6.11 Lateral thoracic radiograph of a dog with severe tracheal collapse. The view was obtained under attempted inspiration. The trachea at the thoracic inlet is collapsed and not radiographically visible. The intrathoracic trachea is visible, but narrow. The severity of this dog's respiratory signs precluded evaluation of tracheal collapse during cough using fluoroscopy. The diaphragm is cranially positioned, overlapping with the cardiac silhouette. Also, the caudal lungs are mildly increased in opacity and reduced in size due to underaeration. These findings indicate a secondary upper airway obstruction.

Box 6.7 Radiographic signs indicating upper airway obstruction.

- Tracheal narrowing at the obstruction
- Increased tracheal diameter cranial to the obstruction
- Decreased lung volume:
  - Cranially positioned diaphragm
  - Increased opacity of caudal lungs
- Sternal elevation (most commonly seen in cats)
- Inward deviation of intercostal muscles (most commonly seen in cats)
- Hiatal herniation due to decreased intrathoracic pressure

hypoplasia is congenital and a sudden decrease in tracheal luminal diameter in an animal with a previously normal tracheal diameter would not be expected with true hypoplasia, but may occur with acquired tracheitis or hemorrhage. Tracheal hypoplasia is typically seen in Bulldogs associated with other factors comprising brachycephalic airway syndrome and is often, though not always, diagnosed in younger animals. The radiographic signs of upper airway obstruction are shown in **Box 6.7**.

Esophagus

Because of its dorsal position within the mediastinum, esophageal dilation usually causes ventral displacement of the trachea. A dilated esophagus may contain fluid, gas, or both. On occasion, mineral material can be identified. The radiographic signs and differential diagnoses for various esophageal diseases are listed in **Table 6.10**. Radiographic signs indicating esophageal dilation are listed in **Box 6.8**. Gas-filled esophageal dilation is sometimes more challenging to recognize because the gas within the esophagus creates little contrast with the lungs (**Figures 6.12a, b**). The tracheal stripe sign can be seen when the ventral esophageal wall contacts the dorsal tracheal wall and creates a thick soft tissue opaque line at the point of contact, which is surrounded by luminal tracheal and esophageal gas. Also, in a gas-dilated esophagus, soft tissue opaque lines are seen within the

Table 6.10 Radiographic descriptors and some common differential diagnoses for esophageal disease.

Radiographic descriptor	Differential diagnoses
Altered esophageal opacity	Luminal material: • Mineral, metal, or soft tissue opaque foreign body or ingesta • Megaesophagus with excess luminal gas or fluid Mural mass (concurrent with increased size): • Soft tissue mass (granuloma, abscess, or neoplasia) • Mineralized mass (e.g. malignant transformation of *Spirocerca lupi* granuloma)
Esophageal dilation	Generalized megaesophagus: • Idiopathic • Metabolic disease: ∘ Hypoadrenocorticism ∘ Hypothyroidism • Infection: ∘ Botulism ∘ Distemper • Toxicity: ∘ Lead ∘ Organophosphate • Anesthetic induced (transient) • Esophagitis • Paraneoplastic: ∘ Thymoma • Lower esophageal obstruction: ∘ Hiatal hernia ∘ Lower esophageal mass • Neuromuscular diseases: ∘ Dysautonomia ∘ Myasthenia gravis ∘ Storage diseases Focal esophageal dilation: • Obstruction (luminal, extraluminal, or mural causes): ∘ Foreign body ∘ Vascular ring anomaly ∘ Stricture ∘ Esophageal mass • Esophageal diverticulum
Pneumomediastinum (+/- pneumothrorax) and mediastinal/pleural effusion	• Esophageal perforation

Box 6.8 Radiographic signs of esophageal dilation.

- Visibility of the esophagus on plain radiographs:
  - Soft tissue opaque tube located dorsally and on midline (fluid or ingesta-filled esophagus)
  - Converging soft tissue opaque lines within the caudal mediastinum (gas-filled esophagus)
- Ventral displacement of the trachea
- Tracheal stripe sign (gas-filled esophagus)
- Secondary abnormalities:
  - Aspiration pneumonia
  - Pneumomediastinum, pleural effusion, pneumothorax, gas within cervical soft tissues (esophageal perforation)

caudal mediastinum representing the walls of the esophagus as they converge at the esophageal hiatus. These lines are visible in the expected location of the esophagus (within the caudal mediastinum, between the aorta and caudal vena cava on the lateral view and near the midline on the orthogonal view). Megaesophagus is a risk factor for aspiration pneumonia. When megaesophagus is positively identified, the lungs should be carefully evaluated.

Focal esophageal dilation may be caused by luminal, extraluminal, or mural obstructions. Luminal causes of obstruction occur with esophageal foreign bodies. Esophageal foreign bodies are most commonly confined between the heart base and diaphragm (**Figures 6.13a, b**).

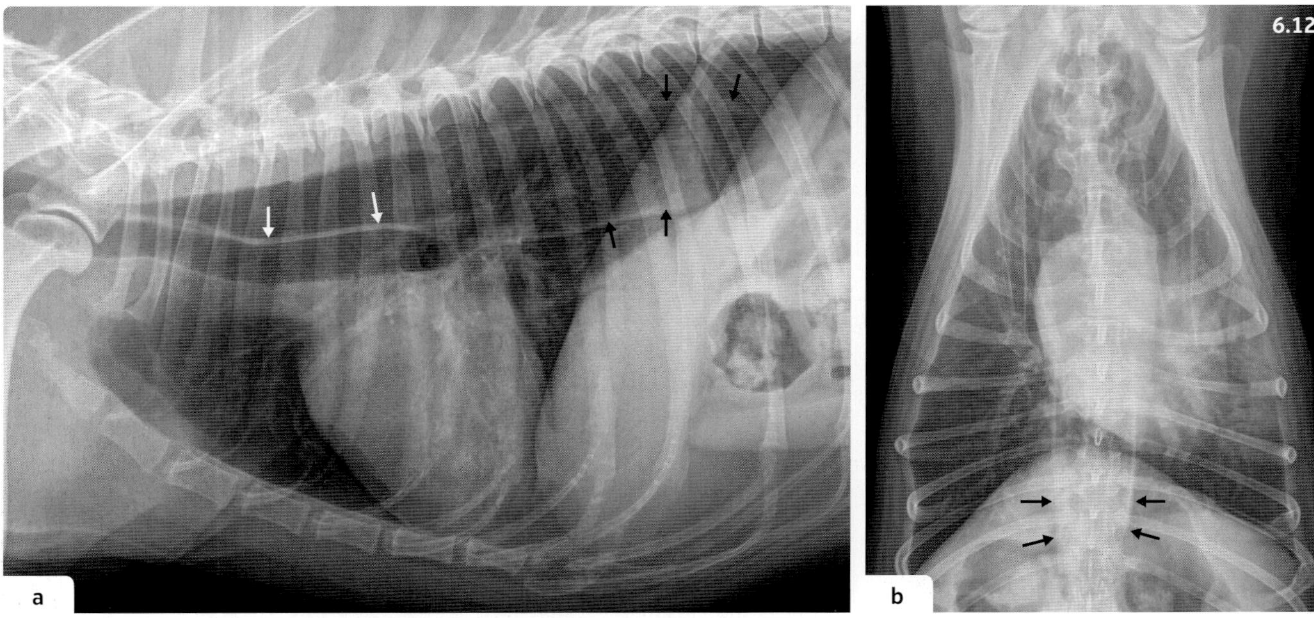

Figures 6.12a, b Lateral (a) and ventrodorsal (b) radiographs of a dog with a gas-filled megaesophagus. The thoracic trachea is ventrally displaced. A tracheal stripe sign is present (a, white arrows). Additionally, converging soft tissue opaque lines (a, b, black arrows) are visible in the caudal mediastinum between the aorta and caudal vena cava on the lateral view and on the midline on the ventrodorsal view consistent with margins of the esophageal wall, which are separated by excess luminal gas opacity. Increased left-sided pulmonary opacity consistent with alveolar disease is present due to aspiration secondary to megaesophagus.

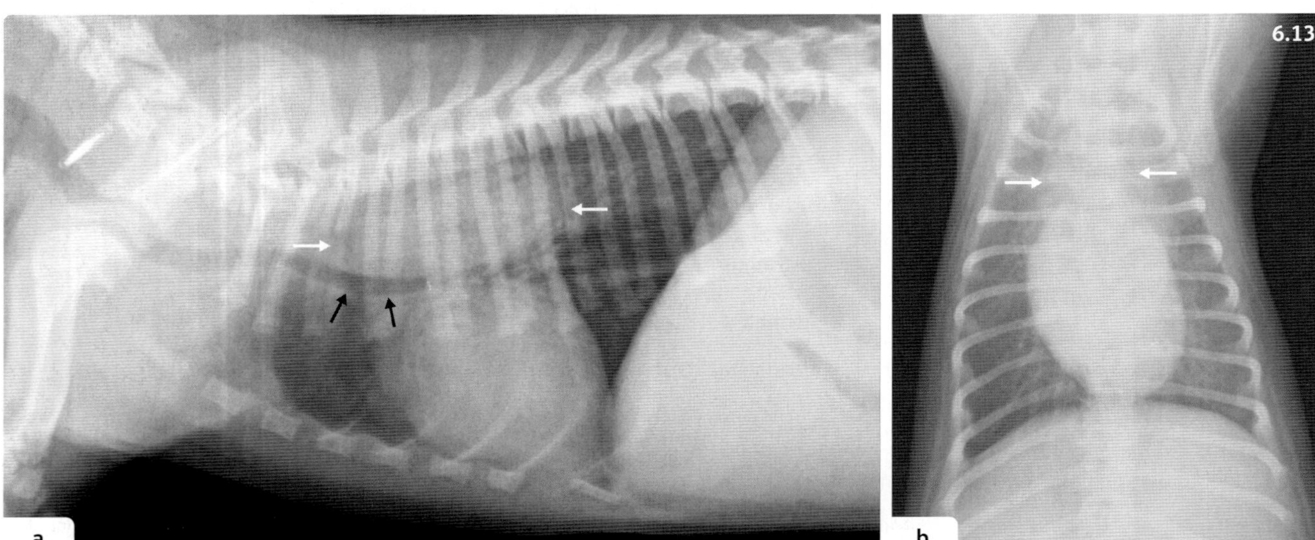

Figures 6.13a, b Lateral (a) and ventrodorsal (b) radiographs of a dog presented for retching and gagging. A poorly defined soft tissue opaque mass is present within the dorsal thorax (a, white arrows). The mass is causing focal ventral deviation of the trachea (a, black arrows) and it is located in the midline, causing widening of the mediastinum (b, white arrows). These findings confirm that the mass is mediastinal in origin, most likely originating from the esophagus. A leather belt was removed endoscopically.

Soft tissue opaque foreign bodies, such as rawhide treats, can look similar to esophageal mural masses; however, foreign bodies are more common and present more acutely than mural masses. Extraluminal causes of obstruction resulting in focal esophageal dilation are infrequent. Vascular ring anomalies are the most common cause of extraluminal obstruction. Typically, a vascular ring anomaly will cause the portion of the esophagus cranial to the cardiac base to be dilated along with focal leftward deviation of the esophagus and trachea. On some occasions, the entire esophagus may be dilated with a focal narrowing near the heart base. Mural esophageal masses caused by neoplasia, granuloma, or abscess are rare causes of esophageal obstruction that can appear similar to each other. Hiatal diseases, including sliding hiatal and paraesophageal hernias, and gastroesophageal intussusceptions also cause soft tissue opaque masses associated with the caudal mediastinum. Sliding hiatal hernias are the most common of the hiatal diseases and may be transient from one radiographic view to the other. The similarity in survey radiographic findings of the various causes of caudal esophageal masses is shown in **Figures 6.14a–c**. The similarities often necessitate use of positive contrast esophagography or endoscopy to differentiate among them.

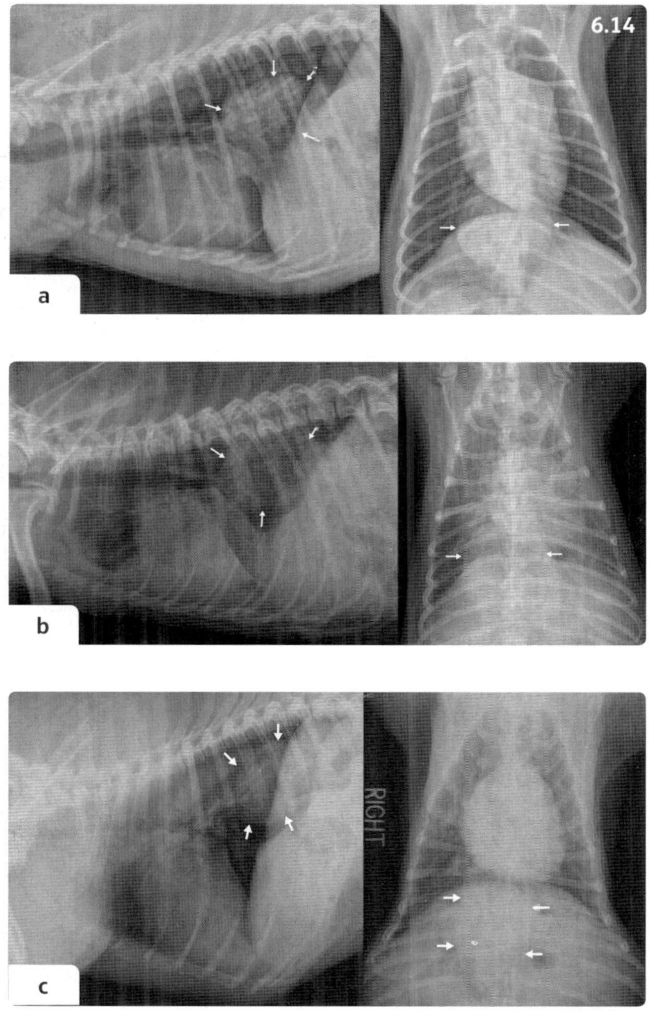

Figures 6.14a–c Lateral and ventrodorsal radiographs of caudal mediastinal masses due to esophageal diseases of different causes. In 6.14a, a mixed gas and soft tissue opaque mass is seen in the caudal mediastinum (white arrows). Endoscopy confirmed the presence of an esophageal diverticulum. In 6.14b, a soft tissue opaque mass with a central gas bubble is seen in the caudal mediastinum (white arrows). A rawhide foreign body was diagnosed endoscopically. In 6.14c, a soft tissue opacity is present in the caudal mediastinum (white arrows), which has a focal gas bubble at its caudal margin. A sliding hiatal hernia was confirmed and surgically repaired. Oral administration of contrast could be performed to further characterize the lesions; however, barium would be contraindicated in 6.14b, as concurrent pleural effusion is present, indicating potential for esophageal rupture, which was found during endoscopy.

Lymph nodes

Three main lymph node centers are present within the mediastinum that can become radiographically visible when enlarged: sternal (**Figures 6.15a, b**), cranial mediastinal (**Figures 6.16a, b**), and tracheobronchial (**Figures 6.17a, b**). Both the sternal and cranial mediastinal lymph nodes are located in the cranial mediastinum and the tracheobronchial lymph nodes are located in the middle mediastinum. In the normal animal, these lymph nodes are invisible. Most often, when lymph nodes become radiographically visible, the underlying cause is neoplastic or granulomatous disease and may be secondary to disease in locations that drain along the lymphatic system.

Thymus

The thymus is located in the caudal part of the cranioventral mediastinum, within the cranioventral mediastinal reflection. It is not radiographically visible in a normal animal more than 1 year of age, due to involution. In a young animal, the thymus may be visible, creating a soft tissue opacity within the cranioventral mediastinal reflection that is triangular in shape, appearing similar to a sail on the ventrodorsal/dorsoventral view. Thymic enlargement is more ventral in location than cranial mediastinal lymph node enlargement and is more caudal than sternal lymph node enlargement. However, when cranioventral mediastinal lesions approach massive sizes, their organ of origin is often impossible to identify with certainty. Masses associated with the thymus are typically caused by thymoma (in dogs) or thymic lymphoma (in cats). Additional potential causes of thymic enlargement include thymic cysts, hemorrhage, and amyloidosis. Thymic masses, especially those caused by thymomas, can be quite immense, causing dyspnea due to tracheal compression and decreased lung volume (**Figures 6.18a, b**).

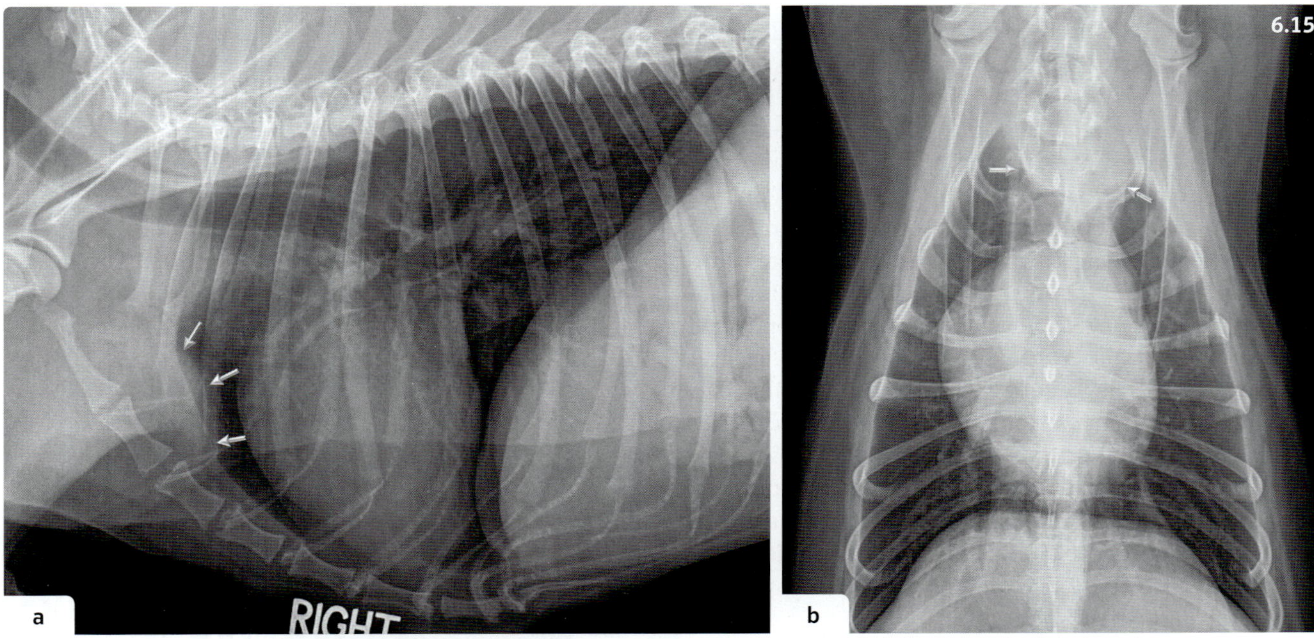

Figures 6.15a, b Lateral (a) and ventrodorsal (b) radiographs of a dog with sternal lymphadenopathy due to lymphoma. A broad-based soft tissue opacity is seen within the cranioventral thorax (a, white arrows) on the midline, creating a widened cranial mediastinum on the ventrodorsal view (b, white arrows) and confirming a mediastinal location for the lesion. The cranial mediastinum, in addition to being wide, is nonuniform in its width.

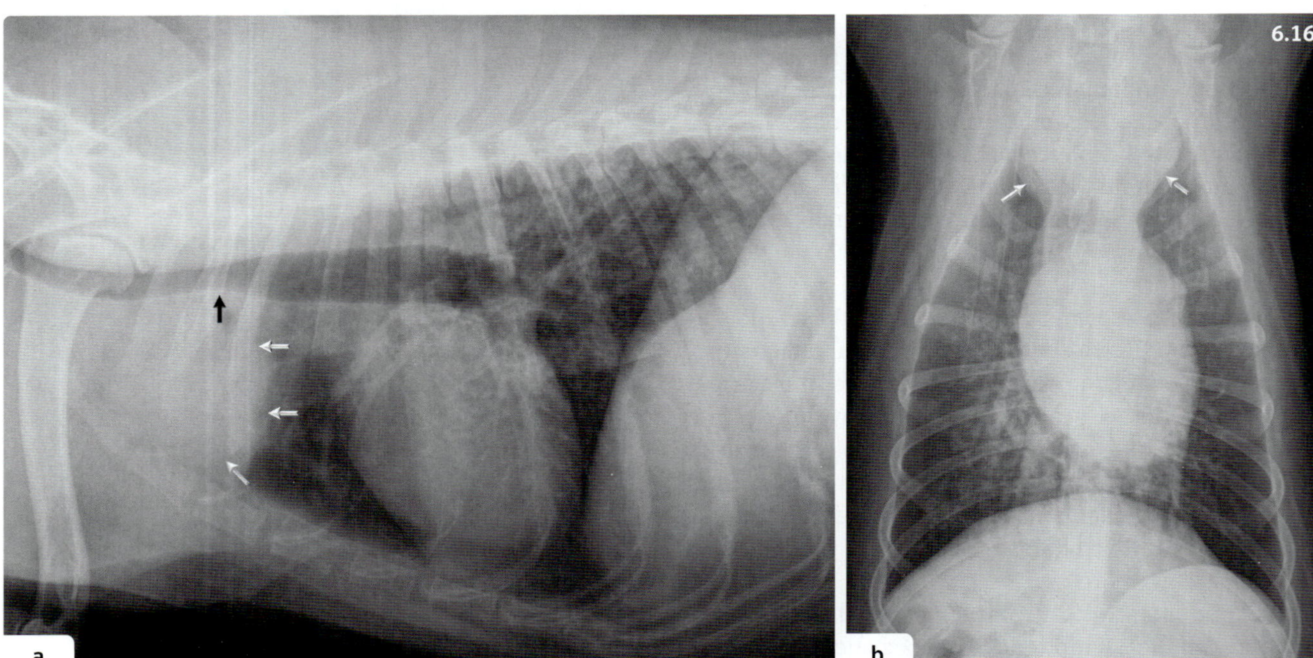

Figures 6.16a, b Lateral (a) and ventrodorsal (b) radiographs of a dog with cranial mediastinal lymphadenopathy due to lymphoma. A mass is located in the cranial and ventral aspect of the cranial mediastinum (white arrows), which is causing dorsal deviation and compression of the cranial thoracic trachea (a, black arrow) and a widened cranial mediastinum (b, white arrows). An interstitial pattern is also present, most evident in the caudal lungs, which is causing an increase in prominence of the bronchi due to pulmonary lymphoma.

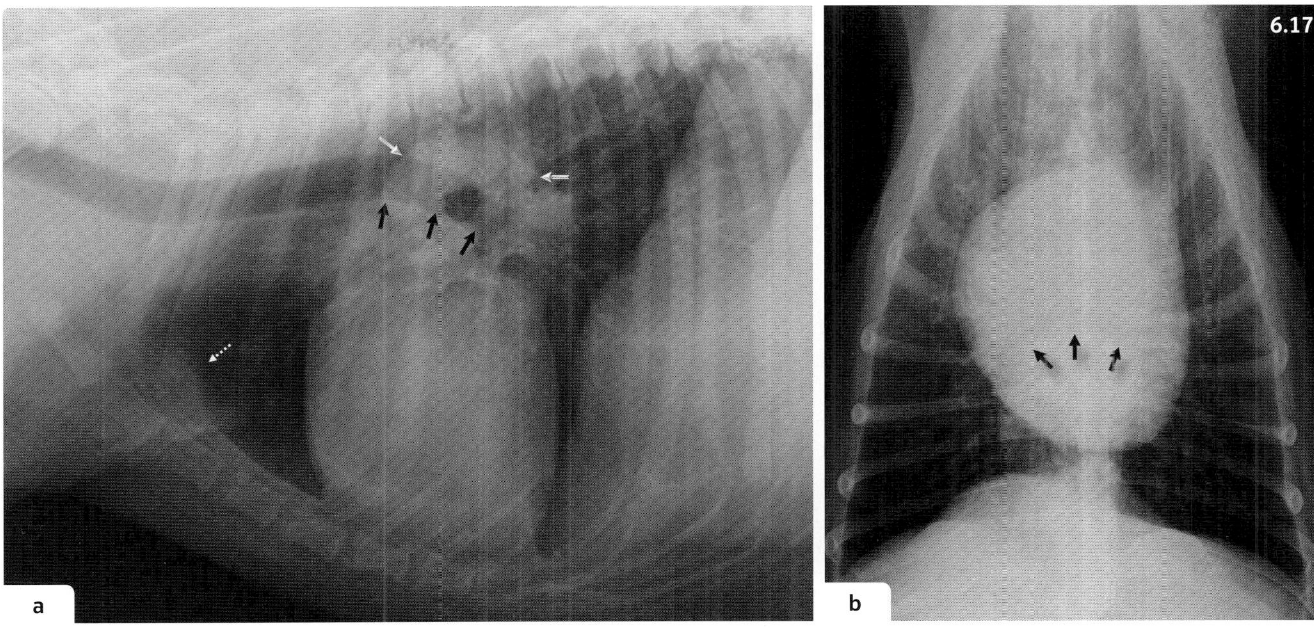

Figures 6.17a, b Lateral (a) and ventrodorsal (b) radiographs of a dog with lymphoma and tracheobronchial lymphadenopathy. The distal aspect of the trachea at the hilus and mainstem bronchi is focally ventrally deviated, giving the trachea a 'J' shape (a, black arrows). A moderately well-defined soft tissue opacity is present in the region of the hilus on the lateral view (a, white arrows). This opacity is located between the mainstem bronchi on the ventrodorsal view and is causing widening of the angle between the right and left bronchus (b, black arrows). These findings confirm a mediastinal location for a mass due to tracheobronchial lymphadenopathy. Mild concurrent sternal lymphadenopathy is present that is only visible in the lateral view (a, dotted white arrow).

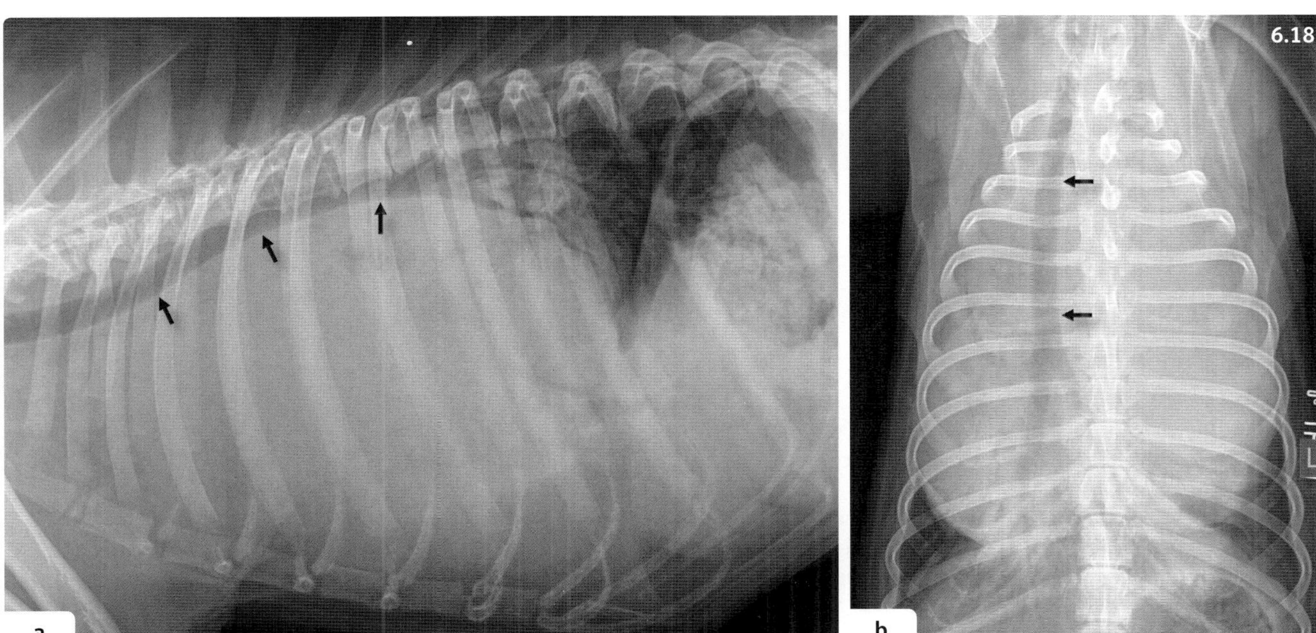

Figures 6.18a, b Lateral (a) and ventrodorsal (b) radiographs of a 2-year-old Labrador Retriever that presented for tachypnea and dyspnea. A large cranial mediastinal mass is present, which is causing marked dorsal displacement of the trachea (a, black arrows) and caudal displacement of the tracheal hilus to the level of the 7th intercostal space. A mild rightward mediastinal shift is present, as shown by the position of the trachea on the ventrodorsal view (b, black arrows). The margins of the heart are effaced and there is a marked decrease in lung volume due to the size of the mass. Thymoma was diagnosed histopathologically.

Heart, great vessels, and pericardium

Cardiac radiographic anatomy

Heart size can be subjectively determined based on the apparent size of the heart relative to the thoracic cavity and the overall shape of the heart, created by individual chambers. The indications for cardiac imaging are listed in **Box 6.9**. Keeping in mind that breed variations exist, the normal canine and feline cardiac silhouettes are described in **Box 6.10**.

Box 6.9 Indications for cardiac imaging.

- Audible murmur
- Exercise intolerance
- Coughing
- Dyspnea
- Increased lung sounds
- Cyanosis
- Syncope
- Abdominal distension/jugular pulses
- Heartworm infection
- Re-evaluation of previously diagnosed cardiac disease

Box 6.10 Cardiac size relative to thoracic cavity.

Canine	
Lateral view: • Length of the heart is less than two-thirds the dorsoventral diameter of the thorax • Width of the heart is 2.5–3.5 intercostal spaces (deep chested breeds narrower than barrel chested breeds) • Two-thirds of the width of the heart is cranial to the carina and one-third is caudal • Trachea nearly parallel to the sternum	Ventrodorsal view: • Left cardiac margin flatter than the right margin • Width of the cardiac silhouette less than two-thirds the width of the thorax • Apex positioned slightly left of midline
Feline	
Lateral view: • Length of the heart is less than two-thirds the dorsoventral diameter of the thorax • Width of the heart is 2–3 intercostal spaces • Trachea diverges from spine and is nearly parallel to the sternum • Increased tracheal divergence from spine with age	**Ventrodorsal view:** • Left cardiac margin flat • Width of the cardiac silhouette less than one-half the width of the thorax • Apex positioned moderately left of midline

A scale can also be used to measure cardiac size. On the lateral view, a line is drawn along the long axis of the heart from the level of the cardiac base (at the level of the tracheal hilus) to the cardiac apex. A second line is drawn along the short axis of the heart from the level of the ventral caudal vena cava. This line extends to the cranial cardiac margin so that the second line is orthogonal to the original line. Both of these lines are then transposed onto the thoracic spine from the level of the cranial endplate of T4 extending caudally (**Figure 6.19**). The number of vertebrae encompassed within these lines constitutes the vertebral heart scale (VHS). Most normal dogs (98%) have a VHS less than 10.6, although some normal dogs will fall above this value. To address this, breed-specific VHS values have been published for several barrel-chested small breed dogs and Greyhounds. The reported upper limit of the VHS in cats is 8.0. Regardless of the VHS obtained, the cardiac silhouette must be examined for alterations in shape and an increase in the VHS over time may indicate an abnormality, even if the measured VHS remains within normal limits.

In order to arrive at an appropriate differential list, specific chamber enlargement should be identified when cardiomegaly is identified. Bulges seen within the cardiac

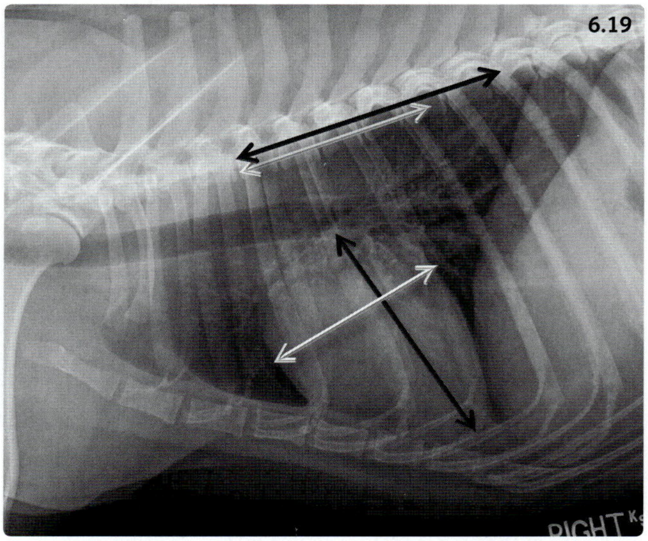

Figure 6.19 Technique for measuring the vertebral heart scale (VHS). (See text for details.)

silhouette must be anatomically differentiated within the overall shape of the heart. This can be accomplished by way of the clock-face analogy (**Table 6.11**). The chambers of the heart are located within specific 'times' along the clock. The clock-face analogy is similar in cats, except that the left atrium is located more peripherally along the left aspect of the cardiac silhouette rather than dorsally at the caudal cardiac base.

Radiographic appearance of right-sided cardiomegaly

Radiographically, right-sided cardiomegaly causes an increase in width of the cardiac silhouette on the lateral view and increased rounding of the right cardiac margin on the ventrodorsal/dorsoventral views. Bulges in the cardiac silhouette can be seen corresponding to the right atrium, right ventricle, or both, according to the clock-face analogy.

Right atrial enlargement will cause an apparent increase in soft tissue opacity between the cranial cardiac base and the cranial mediastinum on the lateral view (8:00 to 11:00 position). On the orthogonal view, a bulge at the right cranial cardiac margin in the 9:00 to 11:00 position can be seen (**Figures 6.20a, b**). Secondary to cardiac enlargement, the trachea will often be elevated, especially cranial to the hilus. On some occasions, especially with concurrent right ventricular enlargement, the cardiac apex will be displaced to the

Table 6.11 Times corresponding to specific cardiac chambers using the clock-face analogy.

Lateral view

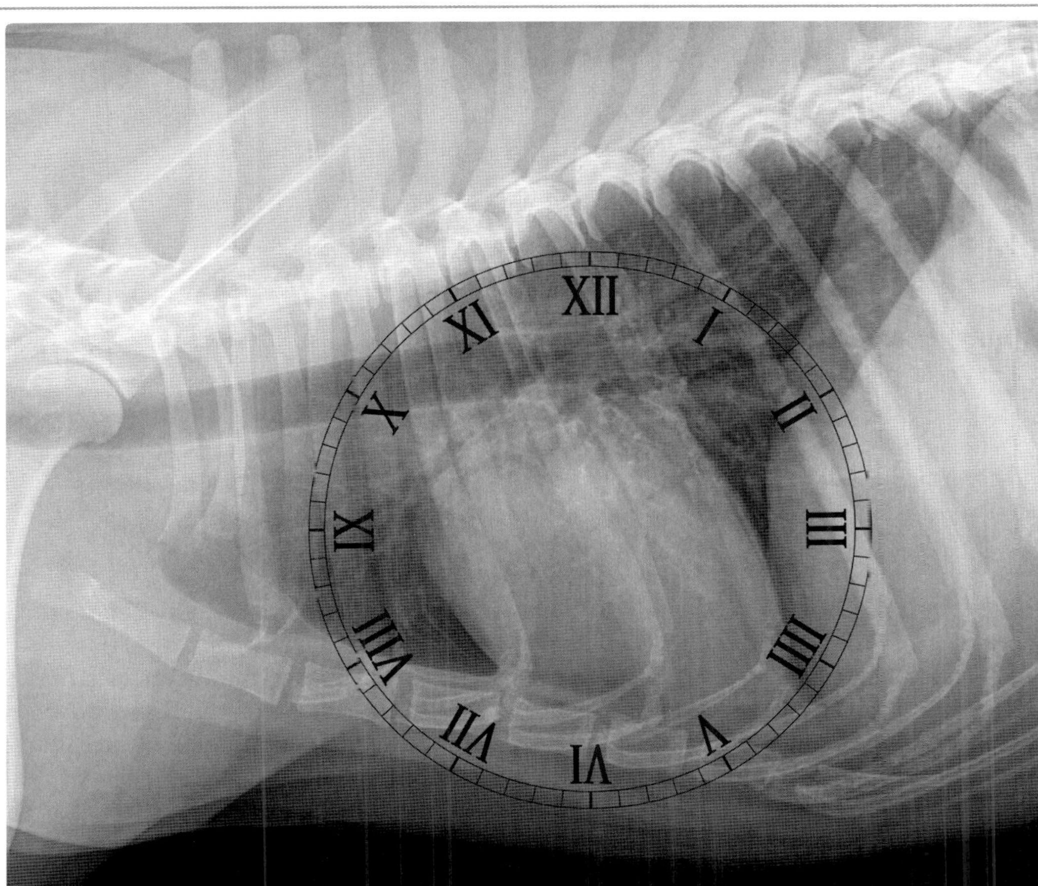

Time:	Cardiac chamber(s):
12:00 to 3:00	Left atrium
3:00 to 5:00	Left ventricle
5:00 to 8:00	Right ventricle
8:00 to 11:00	Right atrium, main pulmonary artery, ascending aorta and arch

(Continued)

Table 6.11 Times corresponding to specific cardiac chambers using the clock-face analogy. (*Continued*)

Ventrodorsal view

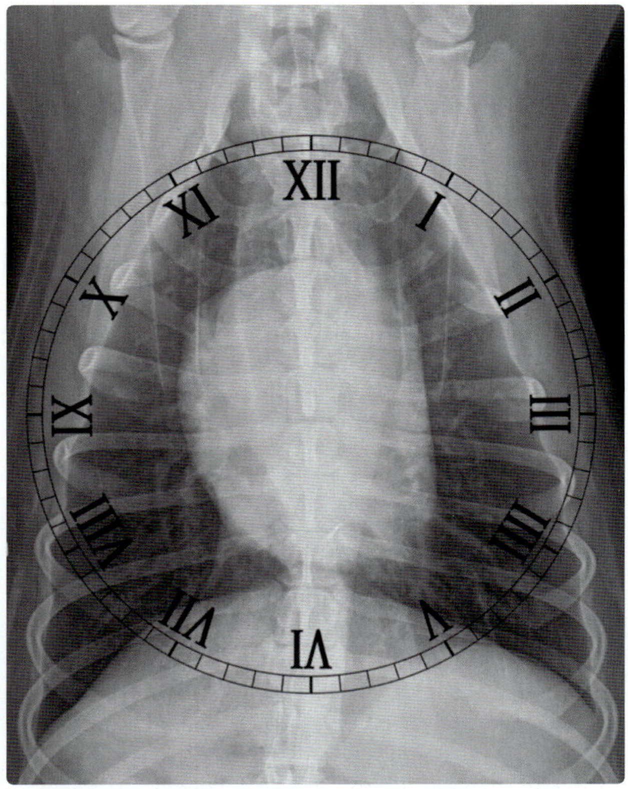

Time:	Cardiac chamber:
11:00 to 1:00	Aorta
1:00 to 2:00	Main pulmonary artery
2:00 to 3:00	Left auricle
3:00 to 5:00	Left ventricle
5:00 to 9:00	Right ventricle
9:00 to 11:00	Right atrium
Center dial (between mainstem bronchi)	Left atrium

left on the ventrodorsal/dorsoventral views. In general, right atrial enlargement is more evident on the ventrodorsal view.

Right ventricular enlargement will cause a rounded cranial margin on the lateral view that creates an increase in the apparent width of the cardiac silhouette. The heart will appear to contact an increased length of sternum, although this can be a normal finding in many breeds. A 'reverse D' shape is often described in reference to right-sided enlargement on the ventrodorsal view. This shape is more specific for right ventricular enlargement, rather than atrial enlargement. The reverse D is nonspecific for the underlying cause of right ventricular enlargement, although it is often described in cases of cardiac remodeling due to heartworm infection. When right ventricular enlargement is severe, the cardiac apex as seen on the lateral view will elevate. The enlarged cardiac silhouette will cause tracheal elevation, similar to that seen with right atrial enlargement (**Figures 6.21a, b**).

Radiographic appearance of left-sided cardiomegaly

Left-sided cardiomegaly causes increased height of the cardiac silhouette on the lateral view. Bulges in the cardiac silhouette are seen in the region of the left atrium

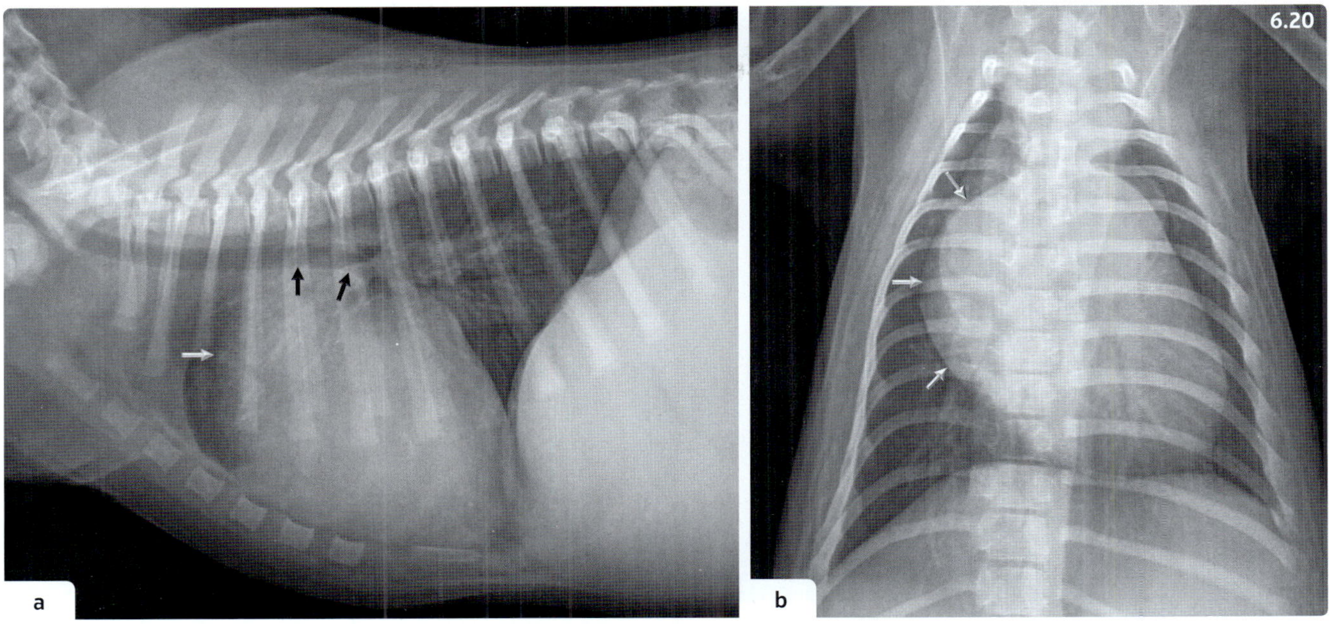

Figures 6.20a, b Lateral (a) and ventrodorsal (b) radiographs of a puppy with marked right atrial enlargement due to tricuspid insufficiency secondary to a dysplastic tricuspid valve. On the lateral view, the trachea is elevated cranial to its hilus (a, black arrows). A bulge is present at the cranial cardiac base on the lateral view (a, white arrow) in the 8:00 to 11:00 position and at the right cranial cardiac margin on the ventrodorsal view (b, white arrows) in the 9:00 to 11:00 position. Also, note the subjective decrease in size of the pulmonary arteries and veins secondary to return flow of vascular volume into the right atrium rather than forward into the main pulmonary artery and lungs.

and/or ventricle. Because of the prevalence of certain diseases in dogs and cats, left-sided cardiomegaly is more common than purely right-sided. Additionally, most cardiomyopathies, which can affect the left or right heart, tend to preferentially cause left-sided cardiomegaly.

With left atrial or left ventricular enlargement, the caudal cardiac margin is flat on the lateral view. This is often the first indication of mild enlargement. Left atrial enlargement will cause a bulge at the caudal cardiac base (12:00 to 3:00 position) on the lateral view. On the orthogonal view, the left atrium is not located at the periphery of the cardiac silhouette, but is positioned between the mainstem bronchi, being superimposed over the cardiac silhouette analogous to the center of the dial using the clock-face analogy. Left atrial enlargement will cause widening of the angle between the mainstem bronchi, creating a 'U' shape rather than the normal 'V' shape. Sometimes, the caudal margin of an enlarged left atrium will create a well-defined rounded margin parallel to the cardiac apex on the ventrodorsal view, referred to as the 'double-bubble sign'. An enlarged left auricle is peripheral in location along the cardiac silhouette on the ventrodorsal view at the 2:00 to 3:00 position. Loss of the normal flat left-sided cardiac margin will be seen due to a bulge created by left auricular enlargement. Secondary to left atrial enlargement, the trachea will be elevated, similar to that seen in right-sided cardiomegaly. However, in the case of left atrial enlargement, the caudal mainstem bronchi are additionally elevated (**Figures 6.22a, b**).

Left ventricular enlargement without concurrent left atrial enlargement is uncommon. It is less apparent radiographically than left atrial enlargement. The caudal cardiac margin will be flat, similar to left atrial enlargement; however, with severe enlargement a pronounced convexity may be seen. The heart will be tall, encompassing greater than two-thirds of the dorsoventral diameter of the thorax on the lateral view and elevating the caudal vena cava. The cardiac apex is rounded and may be displaced towards the left on the ventrodorsal view.

Generalized cardiomegaly

When the cardiac silhouette is generally enlarged (instead of predominantly right sided or left sided), pericardial disease must be considered. Most often, if the left

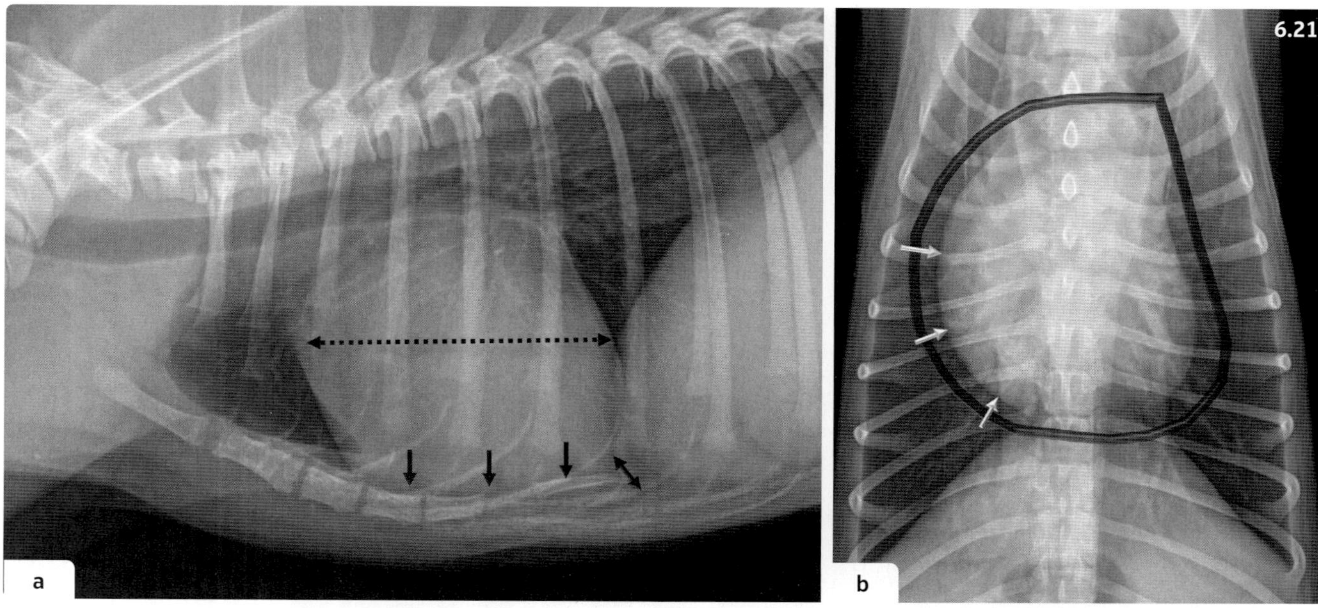

Figures 6.21a, b Lateral (a) and ventrodorsal (b) radiographs of a dog with marked right ventricular enlargement due to severe pulmonic stenosis. The trachea is elevated, being parallel to the spine. The cardiac silhouette is subjectively wide on the lateral view (a, dotted black line) encompassing over four intercostal spaces. Increased sternal contact is present (a, black arrows). The apex of the cardiac silhouette at the junction between the sternum and diaphragm is mildly elevated (a, double-headed black arrow). The contour of the left margin of the cardiac silhouette is flat. The entire right cardiac margin is rounded with the ventricle (in the 5:00 to 9:00 position) being more peripheral than the atrium (b, white arrows) and creating a silhouette whose outline is reverse 'D' in shape (b, black outline surrounding the heart).

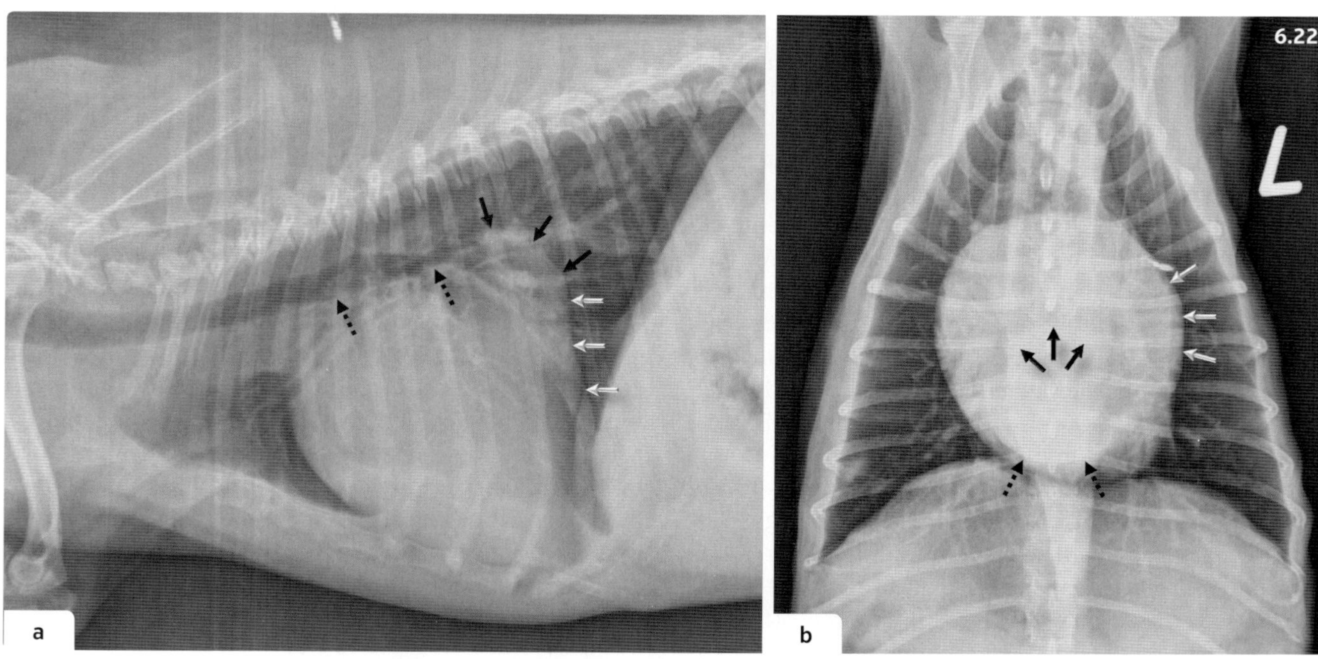

Figures 6.22a, b Lateral (a) and ventrodorsal (b) radiographs of a dog with left atrial enlargement due to mitral valvular degeneration. The heart often appears tall on the lateral view. The caudal cardiac margin is flat on the lateral view (a, white arrows). A bulge is visible in the caudal cardiac base (a, black arrows). The trachea and mainstem bronchi are elevated (a, black dotted arrows). On the ventrodorsal view, the angle between the mainstem bronchi is widened (b, black arrows). The caudal margin of the enlarged left atrium is visible parallel to the cardiac apex (b, dotted black arrows). A left auricular bulge is visible peripherally along the left cardiac margin (b, white arrows).

atrium is detected as enlarged, the cardiomegaly is due to true heart enlargement rather than pericardial disease. If the heart is markedly enlarged and globoid while a dilated left atrium is not seen, pericardial disease/effusion should be ranked first. (**Note:** Severe right-sided cardiomegaly is similar in appearance to pericardial effusion.) The various characteristics of cardiac enlargement are listed in **Tables 6.12–6.14**.

Enlarged great vessels

Enlargement of the main pulmonary artery or aortic arch can occur due to turbulent blood flow or an increase in pressure downstream in the direction of the vascular flow. Findings consistent with enlargement of great vessels should be correlated with additional abnormalities seen within the study (e.g. heart enlargement, peripheral pulmonary vascular size, signs of failure) to decide on likely differential diagnoses.

An enlarged main pulmonary artery will cause a bulge in the cranial cardiac base (8:00 to 11:00 position) on the lateral view. This is also the location of the aorta and right atrium. The ventrodorsal view must be used to distinguish these three potential causes of a cardiac bulge in this location. On the ventrodorsal view, an enlarged main pulmonary artery causes a bulge in the left cranial cardiac margin at the 1:00 to 2:00 position (**Figures 6.23a, b**). The two main causes of a dilated main pulmonary artery are turbulent flow (poststenotic dilatation secondary to pulmonic stenosis or patent ductus arteriosus [PDA]) or congestion due to pulmonary hypertension. All causes of an enlarged main pulmonary artery can result in right-sided cardiomegaly. The main distinguishing factor among the differential diagnoses is the appearance of the peripheral pulmonary vasculature (**Table 6.15**).

An enlarged aortic arch will cause a bulge in a similar location to that of right atrial and main pulmonary arterial enlargement on the lateral view at the cranial cardiac base (8:00 to 11:00 position). On the orthogonal view, enlargement of the aortic arch will appear as a bulge in the cranial cardiac margin at the 11:00 to 1:00 position. Often, aortic arch enlargement will appear as a widening of the caudal aspect of the cranial mediastinum. Enlargement of the aortic arch is most often caused by

Table 6.12 Eccentric versus concentric hypertrophy of the heart.

Eccentric hypertrophy	Concentric hypertrophy
Increased chamber volume More radiographically evident Due to: • Volume overload • Myocardial dysfunction caused by cardiomyopathy (DCM) • Coronary artery disease	Increased wall thickness/ decreased chamber volume Not seen radiographically until severe Due to: • Pressure overload • Myocardial dysfunction caused by some cardiomyopathies (e.g. HCM)

Table 6.13 Causes of right-sided cardiomegaly.

Right atrium	Right ventricle

Chamber dilation only (eccentric hypertrophy):
• Volume overload due to:
  ◦ Insufficient/dysplastic tricuspid valve
  ◦ Atrial septal defect
• Pressure overload due to stenotic tricuspid valve
Right atrial mass (e.g. hemangiosarcoma)
	Chamber dilation (eccentric hypertrophy):
	• Volume overload due to:
	  ◦ Tricuspid valvular insufficiency
	  ◦ Pulmonic valvular insufficiency
	  ◦ Atrial septal defect
	  ◦ Overhydration
	  ◦ Myocardial failure (arrhythmogenic right ventricular cardiomyopathy)
	• Chronic anemia
	• Athletic heart
	• Cardiac conduction abnormalities
	Wall thickening (concentric hypertrophy):
	• Pressure overload due to:
	  ◦ Pulmonic stenosis
	  ◦ Pulmonary hypertension (cor pulmonale)
	  ◦ Heartworm disease
	  ◦ Tetralogy of Fallot
	• Cardiomyopathy (HCM)

Table 6.14 Causes of left-sided cardiomegaly.

Left atrium	Left ventricle

Chamber dilation only (eccentric hypertrophy):
• Volume overload due to:
  ◦ Insufficient/dysplastic mitral valve
  ◦ Left-to-right shunts (PDA, VSD, ASD)
• Pressure overload (stenotic mitral valve)
	Chamber dilation (eccentric hypertrophy):
	• Volume overload due to:
	  ◦ Mitral valvular insufficiency
	  ◦ Aortic valvular insufficiency
	  ◦ Left-to-right shunts: PDA, VSD, ASD
	  ◦ Overhydration
	• Myocardial failure (cardiomyopathy [dilated])
	• Chronic anemia
	• Athletic heart
	• Cardiac conduction disturbances
	Wall thickening (concentric hypertrophy):
	• Pressure overload due to:
	  ◦ Aortic stenosis
	  ◦ Systemic hypertension
	• Cardiomyopathy (HCM)

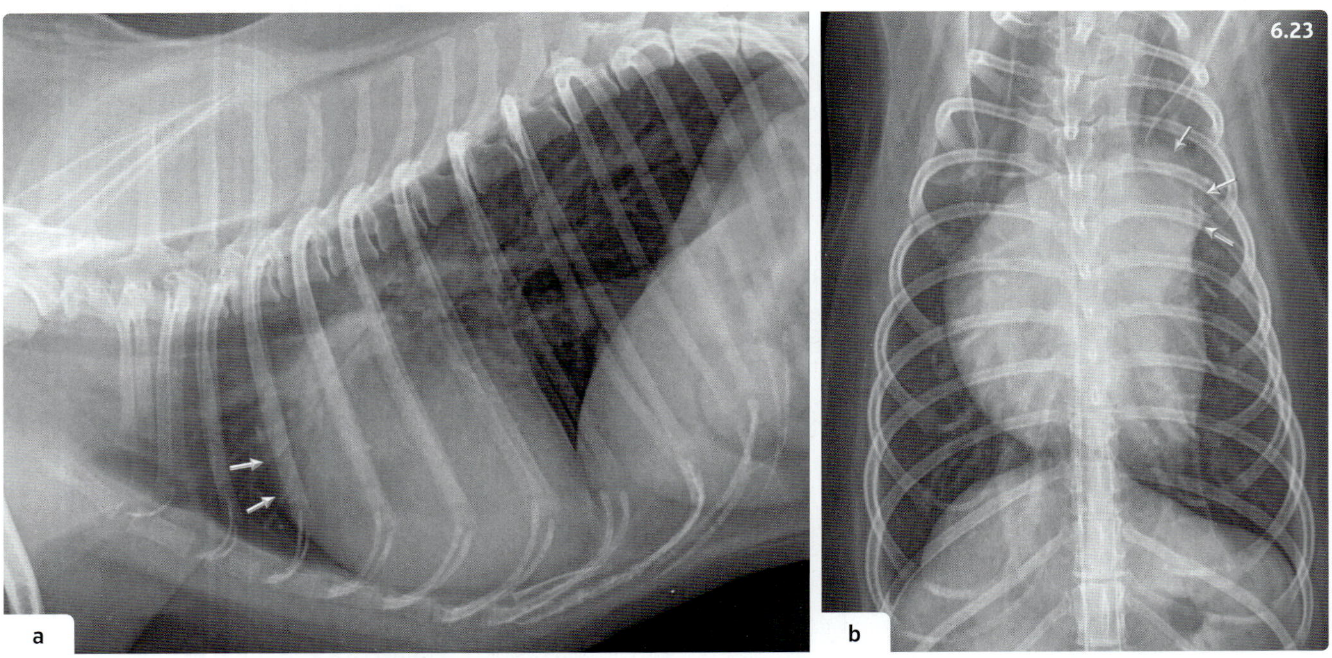

Figures 6.23a, b Lateral (a) and ventrodorsal (b) radiographs of a dog with radiographically evident main pulmonary artery enlargement. An increased convexity is present at the cranial cardiac base on the lateral view (a, white arrows). A large focal bulge is present at the left cranial cardiac margin on the ventrodorsal view in the region of the main pulmonary artery (1:00 to 2:00 position; b, white arrows).

Table 6.15 Differential diagnoses and distinguishing factors for main pulmonary artery (MPA) enlargement.

Radiographic findings	Primary differential
Dilated MPA + small peripheral pulmonary vasculature	Pulmonic stenosis
Dilated MPA + dilated peripheral pulmonary arteries	Pulmonary hypertension (primary or secondary to heartworm infection)
Dilated MPA + dilated peripheral arteries and veins	Patent ductus arteriosus

turbulent flow and poststenotic dilatation secondary to aortic stenosis (**Figures 6.24a, b**).

Aortic enlargement can also occur at the level of the proximal descending aorta. Enlargement in this location is radiographically distinct from enlargement of the aortic arch due to aortic stenosis and is almost pathognomonic for a PDA. The enlargement is due to turbulent flow caused by abnormal blood flow between the main pulmonary artery and aorta that occurs at the proximal descending aorta. This finding is most evident on the ventrodorsal view (**Figure 6.25**).

The caudal vena cava should be less than 1.5 times the width of the aorta. An enlarged caudal vena cava is most often due to congestion from right-sided heart failure. Radiographic changes consistent with right-sided cardiomegaly may be concurrently evident. The cranial vena cava is not seen as a distinct structure separate from other soft tissue opacities within the cranial mediastinum, therefore its enlargement is not radiographically visible.

Pulmonary arteries and veins

Differential diagnoses for cardiac enlargement should always be considered in combination with pulmonary vascular appearance. Pulmonary venous enlargement, pulmonary arterial enlargement, and combination pulmonary arterial and venous enlargement or hypovascularity have entirely separate differential diagnoses. The differential diagnoses for pulmonary arterial and/or venous enlargements are summarized in **Table 6.16**.

The pulmonary arteries and veins are paired and surround the lobar bronchi, creating a triad of artery, bronchus, and vein. On the lateral view, the arteries are always located dorsal to the bronchus and the veins are located ventral. The size of the cranial lobar arteries and veins is best assessed on a lateral thoracic radiograph and should be similar in diameter to each other and to the proximal aspect of the 4th rib. The caudal lobar arteries and veins are best assessed on the ventrodorsal/dorsoventral view. The caudal lobar arteries are peripherally located relative to the bronchi and veins. As such the veins are centrally located and are said to be 'central and ventral' within the triad of artery, bronchus, and vein on the radiographic views. The size of the caudal lobar pulmonary arteries and veins can be compared with the diameter of the 9th ribs as they cross on the ventrodorsal view; they should be similar in size to each other and to the 9th rib at the location of their crossing. If the pulmonary arteries and

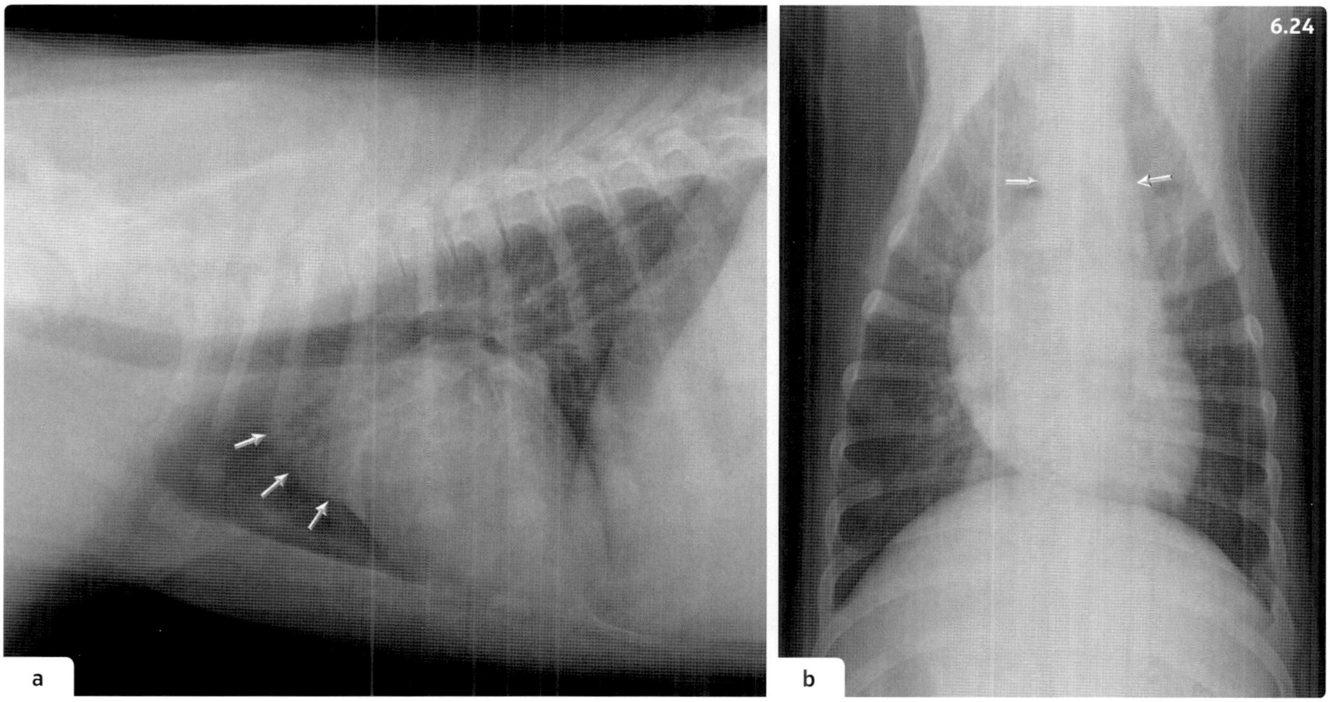

Figures 6.24a, b Lateral (a) and ventrodorsal (b) radiographs of a dog with an enlarged aortic arch due to a poststenotic dilatation from subaortic stenosis. On the lateral view, a focal bulge is seen at the cranial cardiac base in the 8:00 to 11:00 position (a, white arrows). On the ventrodorsal view, an increase in soft tissue opacity is seen at the caudal aspect of the cranial mediastinum associated with the 11:00 to 1:00 position of the cardiac silhouette (b, white arrows).

veins are normal in size, the summation of the vasculature crossing the rib will form a square.

Congestive heart failure

Right-sided congestive heart failure is the inability of the heart (specifically the right atrium) to accommodate blood volume returning from systemic circulation. Increased right atrial pressure causes those vascular structures draining into the right atrium from the systemic circulation (cranial vena cava, caudal vena cava, lymphatics) to become congested and unable to transmit blood volume forward into the heart. The compensatory mechanisms of the heart are overwhelmed and this results in congestive failure. Right-sided cardiomegaly does not automatically imply right heart failure; however, when right-sided cardiomegaly is diagnosed radiographically, the interpreter must evaluate for evidence of failure. Radiographic signs indicating right-sided heart failure are shown in **Box 6.11** and **Figure 6.26**.

Left-sided congestive heart failure is the inability of the heart (specifically the left atrium) to accommodate blood volume returning from pulmonary circulation. Increased left atrial pressure causes those vascular structures draining into the left atrium (i.e. the pulmonary

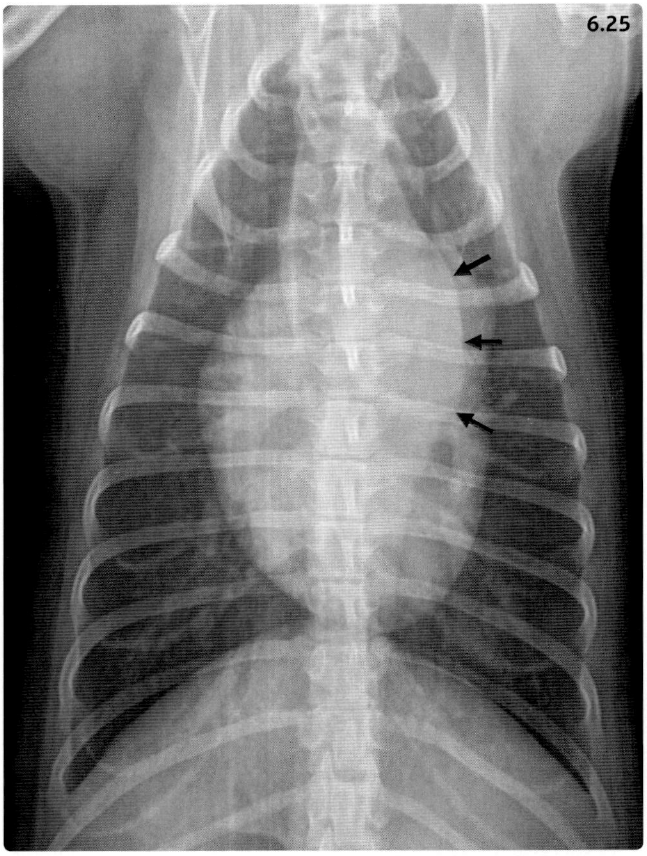

Figure 6.25 Ventrodorsal radiograph of a dog with enlargement of the proximal descending aorta secondary to a patent ductus arteriosus. The proximal aspect of the descending aorta has a focal convexity at the level of the proximal descending aorta (black arrows) that is distinct from aortic arch enlargement due to aortic stenosis. (Compare with Figure 6.24b.)

Table 6.16 Differential diagnoses for abnormal pulmonary vascular size.

Dilated pulmonary veins Elevated left atrial pressure (e.g. mitral insufficiency, cardiomyopathy)
Dilated pulmonary arteries Arteritis secondary to parasitic infection (e.g. heartworm infection) Pulmonary hypertension Pulmonary thromboembolism
Dilated pulmonary arteries and veins Left-to-right shunting of blood (PDA, VSD, ASD) Volume overload Chronic or severe mitral valvular disease (pulmonary venous dilation expected prior to arterial dilation)
Small pulmonary arteries and veins Hypovolemia Shock Severe pulmonic stenosis Tricuspid dysplasia or severe tricuspid insufficiency Right-to-left shunts: • Reverse PDA • VSD combined with pulmonic stenosis or pulmonary hypertension • Tetralogy of Fallot

Box 6.11 Radiographic findings of right heart failure include right-sided cardiomegaly or pericardial disease in combination with one or more of:

- Dilated caudal vena cava
- Generalized hepatomegaly
- Peritoneal effusion
- Pleural effusion (cats)*

* In dogs, effusion occurring in the pleural space due to right heart failure occurs only after effusion in the peritoneal space. Therefore, peritoneal effusion or bicavitary effusion has a differential diagnosis of right heart failure, but pleural effusion alone is not typically caused by right heart failure.

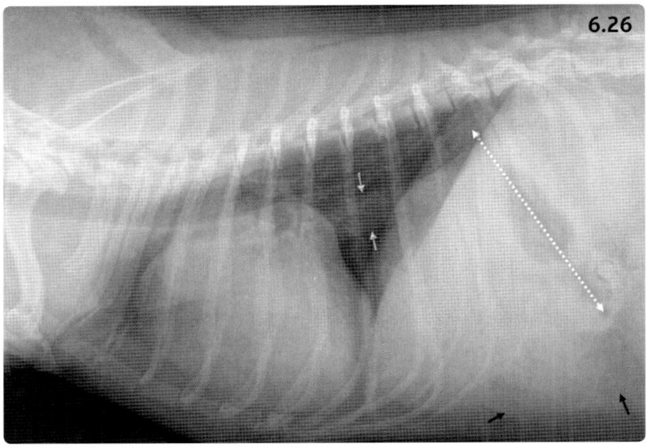

Figure 6.26 Lateral radiograph of a dog with right-sided cardiac failure due to pulmonic stenosis and tricuspid dysplasia. The caudal vena cava is dilated and fails to taper towards the diaphragm (between white arrows). The liver is enlarged, causing caudal displacement of the gastric axis (dotted white arrow). Peritoneal effusion is present, causing soft tissue opaque streaking and a decrease in detail of visible abdominal structures (black arrows). These findings combined with an enlarged, wide cardiac silhouette are indicative of right-sided heart failure.

veins) to become congested and unable to transmit blood volume forward. The compensatory mechanisms of the heart are overwhelmed and this results in congestive failure with excess blood volume in the pulmonary veins. Left-sided cardiomegaly does not imply left heart failure. The radiographic study must be specifically evaluated for indications of failure, which include dilated pulmonary veins and cardiogenic edema characterized by interstitial or alveolar pulmonary opacity typically having a perihilar/caudodorsal distribution. The edema is most often symmetrical, but can be asymmetrical as well. An asymmetrical distribution tends to occur most often secondary to mitral valvular disease. Radiographic signs indicating left-sided heart failure are listed in **Box 6.12** and **Figures 6.27a–c**. In cats, the regional distribution of cardiogenic edema is often less predictable and can be diffuse or multifocal (**Figures 6.28a, b**). Additionally, although the mechanism is unclear, pleural effusion often accompanies cardiogenic edema in cases of left-sided failure in cats. This is not a feature seen in dogs, where only right-sided heart failure causes pleural effusion.

Pericardial effusion

The most common causes of pericardial effusion are idiopathic or due to neoplasia such as right atrial hemangiosarcoma, heart base chemodectoma, or mesothelioma.

Box 6.12 Radiographic findings of left heart failure include left-sided cardiomegaly in combination with one or more of:

- Dilated pulmonary veins
- Cardiogenic pulmonary edema
  - As pulmonary venous dilation and congestion progress, the increased pressure causes edema within the pulmonary interstitium. As edema worsens, the pulmonary pattern becomes alveolar
  - Dogs: cardiogenic edema centered in perihilar/caudal lung lobe regions – symmetrical or asymmetrical
  - Cats: cardiogenic edema has multifocal distribution and can be anywhere

Pericardial fluid increases pressure within the pericardium, which can overwhelm the right atrial and ventricular pressure and result in cardiac tamponade and right-sided heart failure. The radiographic signs associated with pericardial effusion are summarized in **Box 6.13** and **Figures 6.29a, b**. Effusion within the pericardial space creates a globoid cardiac silhouette, which, when severe, precludes the visibility of normal cardiac chambers. A key feature differentiating pericardial effusion from generalized cardiomegaly is the absence of visible left atrial dilation. Severe right-sided cardiomegaly and pericardial effusion can appear radiographically similar. Smaller volumes of effusion have the potential for causing cardiac tamponade, with normal cardiac chambers still being visible radiographically, especially in acute cases. Secondary signs of right-sided heart failure are often seen at the time of diagnosis as part of the presenting complaint. Clinically significant pleural effusion that is severe enough to cause right heart failure is rare in cats. Small volumes of pericardial effusion are often seen in cats presenting with heart failure secondary to feline cardiomyopathy.

Microcardia is a small heart due to decreased systemic venous return. Causes are similar to those for small pulmonary arteries and veins and include shock, dehydration/hypovolemia, hypoadrenocorticism, overinflated lungs, pneumothorax, and obstructed venous flow. Microcardia is often accompanied by a consistently small vena cava in addition to decreased pulmonary vascular diameter.

Lungs

Alveolar pulmonary pattern

Three descriptive hallmarks are seen with alveolar disease of any cause: air bronchogram, lobar sign, and border effacement. Having any one of these three would classify the pulmonary pattern as alveolar; however, often not all

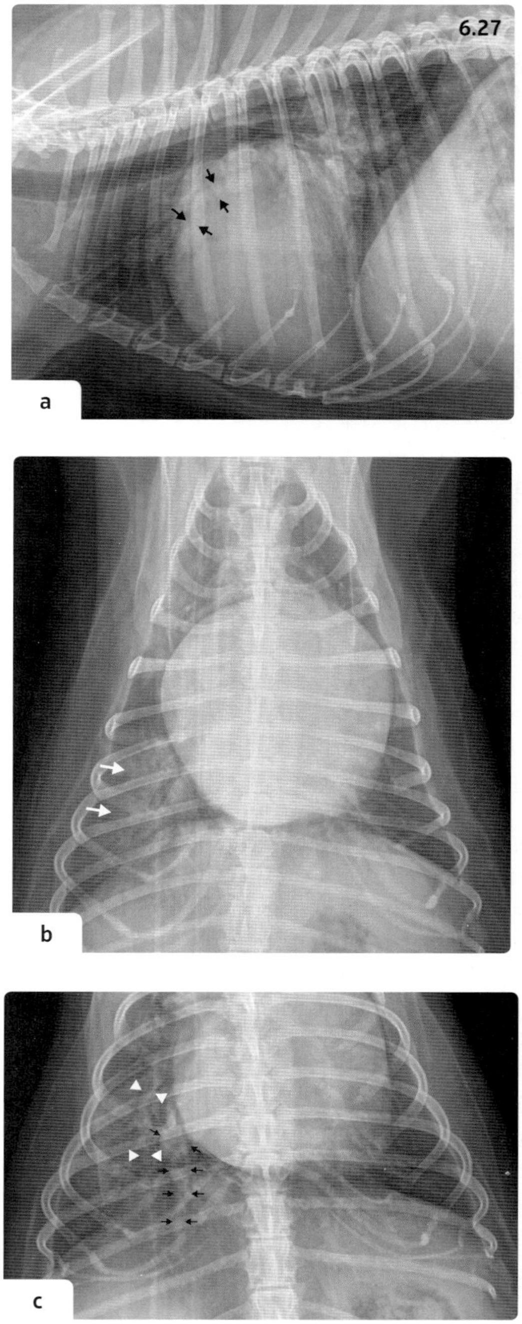

Figures 6.27a–c Lateral (a), ventrodorsal (b), and dorsoventral (c) radiographs of a dog with left-sided cardiac failure due to mitral valvular insufficiency. The cranial lobar veins are increased in size (a, between black arrows). The caudal lobar vasculature is partially obscured by an increase in pulmonary opacity located in the perihilar and caudodorsal lungs and is more severe on the right side (b, white arrows). On the dorsoventral view, the dilated caudal lobar pulmonary veins (c, black arrows) are more clearly seen relative to the normal pulmonary arteries (c, white arrowheads). These findings, combined with a tall cardiac silhouette and marked left atrial enlargement, indicate left-sided cardiac failure.

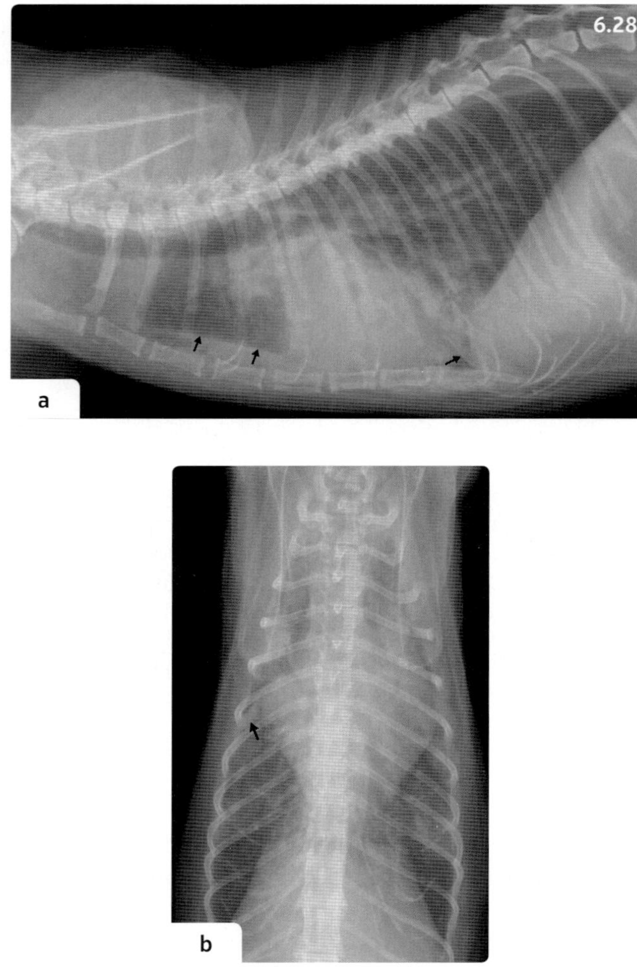

Figures 6.28a, b Lateral (a) and ventrodorsal (b) radiographs of a cat with left-sided congestive heart failure due to cardiomyopathy. The regional distribution of cardiogenic edema is multifocal and predominantly ventral, causing partial border effacement of the cardiac silhouette. Cardiac enlargement can be assumed due to dorsal elevation of the trachea and the visibility of atrial enlargement on the ventrodorsal view. Additionally, evidence of mild pleural effusion is visible where lungs are retracted from the thoracic wall and small pleural fissure lines are present (black arrows). Pleural fluid is a common finding in cats with left-sided cardiac failure.

Box 6.13 Radiographic appearance of pericardial effusion.

- Globoid cardiac silhouette.
  - Cardiomegaly without radiographic evidence of specific chamber enlargements
- Right-sided heart failure:
  - Dilated caudal vena cava
  - Generalized hepatomegaly
  - Peritoneal effusion
  - Pleural effusion

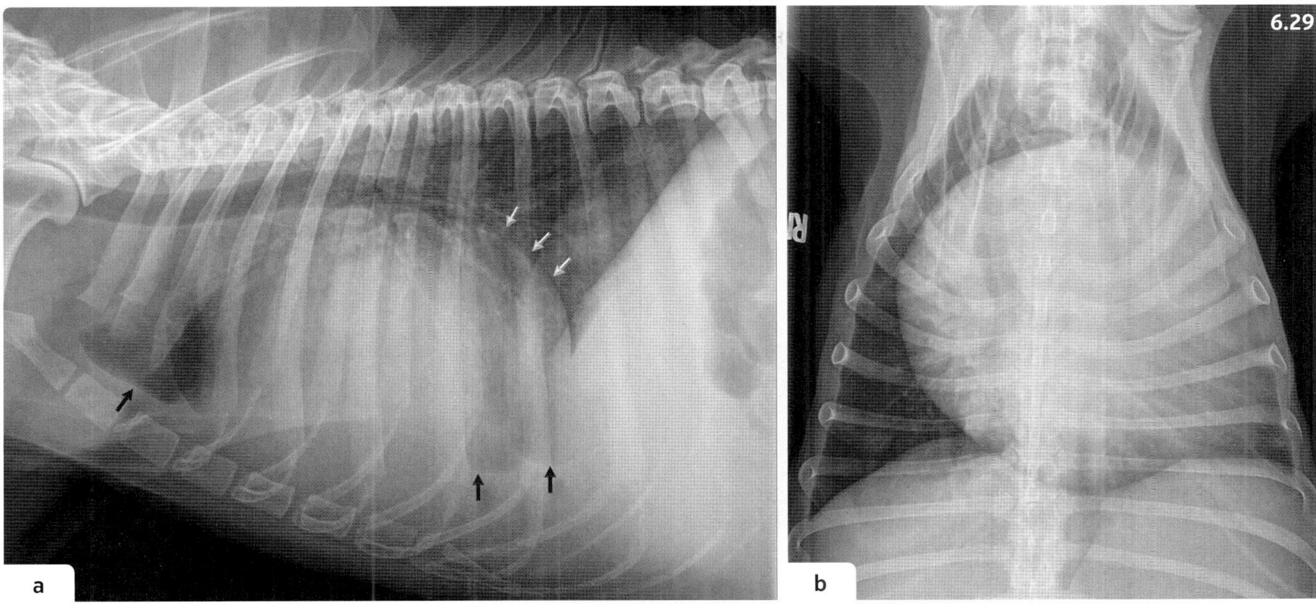

Figures 6.29a, b Lateral (a) and ventrodorsal (b) radiographs of a dog with marked pericardial effusion. The cardiac silhouette is globoid with no evidence of specific enlarged chambers. Note the absence of visible left atrial enlargement (a, white arrows). Right heart failure is also present, denoted by poor abdominal serosal detail and pleural effusion (retraction of lungs from the thoracic wall by fluid; a, black arrows).

hallmarks are present. An air bronchogram occurs when alveoli are not aerated (i.e. they contain fluid [edema, hemorrhage, pus]) or are collapsed while the bronchi remain aerated. Its appearance is likened to a 'tree in a snowstorm', where the branching lucent bronchus is evident against a white backdrop. A lobar sign occurs when alveolar disease is peripheral relative to lobar margins and inconsistent among lung lobes. This allows the margin of the lung lobe to be evident as a relatively distinct line between an affected lobe that is adjacent to a more aerated lobe. Border effacement is the most consistently present hallmark of alveolar disease. When objects are effaced, their margins can no longer be delineated. In order for this to occur, the objects have to be identical in opacity (usually both are soft tissue/fluid opaque) and they have to be in direct physical contact with each other. When alveolar disease is present, fluid within alveoli, which is identical in opacity to the heart, pulmonary vasculature, and bronchial walls, contacts any of these structures such that their margins are no longer distinguishable. The hallmarks of alveolar disease are depicted in **Figures 6.30a–d**.

The first descriptive discriminator in differentiating causes of alveolar disease is lung size. A decrease in lung size due to collapse of airways is called atelectasis. Atelectasis results in an increase in pulmonary opacity and decreased lung volume seen as a mediastinal shift towards the opaque lung (ispilateral mediastinal shift) and ipsilateral cranial positioning of the diaphragm. Atelectasis can be due to obstructive or nonobstructive causes. Obstructive (or resorption) atelectasis occurs when the diameter of the airway is reduced or blocked, most commonly from mucus plugging, bronchial wall inflammation, or a neoplastic mass. The reduction in diameter may be luminal, mural, or extramural in origin; regardless, trapped gas is resorbed and not replaced, resulting in decreased lung volume. This form of atelectasis is most commonly seen in cats with bronchial disease, resulting in mucus plugging and so-called right middle lung lobe syndrome or atelectasis of the right middle lung lobe. Nonobstructive atelectasis may be due to compression/relaxation, surfactant deficiency, or loss of pulmonary compliance due to cicatrization (e.g. fibrosis of pleura limiting lung expansion).

When not caused by atelectasis, alveolar disease is typically caused by fluid accumulation (edema, hemorrhage, or pus) or cells (granuloma or neoplasia) within alveoli. The regional distribution is the most effective means of distinguishing these, as shown in **Table 6.17**. Pulmonary edema can be caused by cardiogenic or noncardiogenic

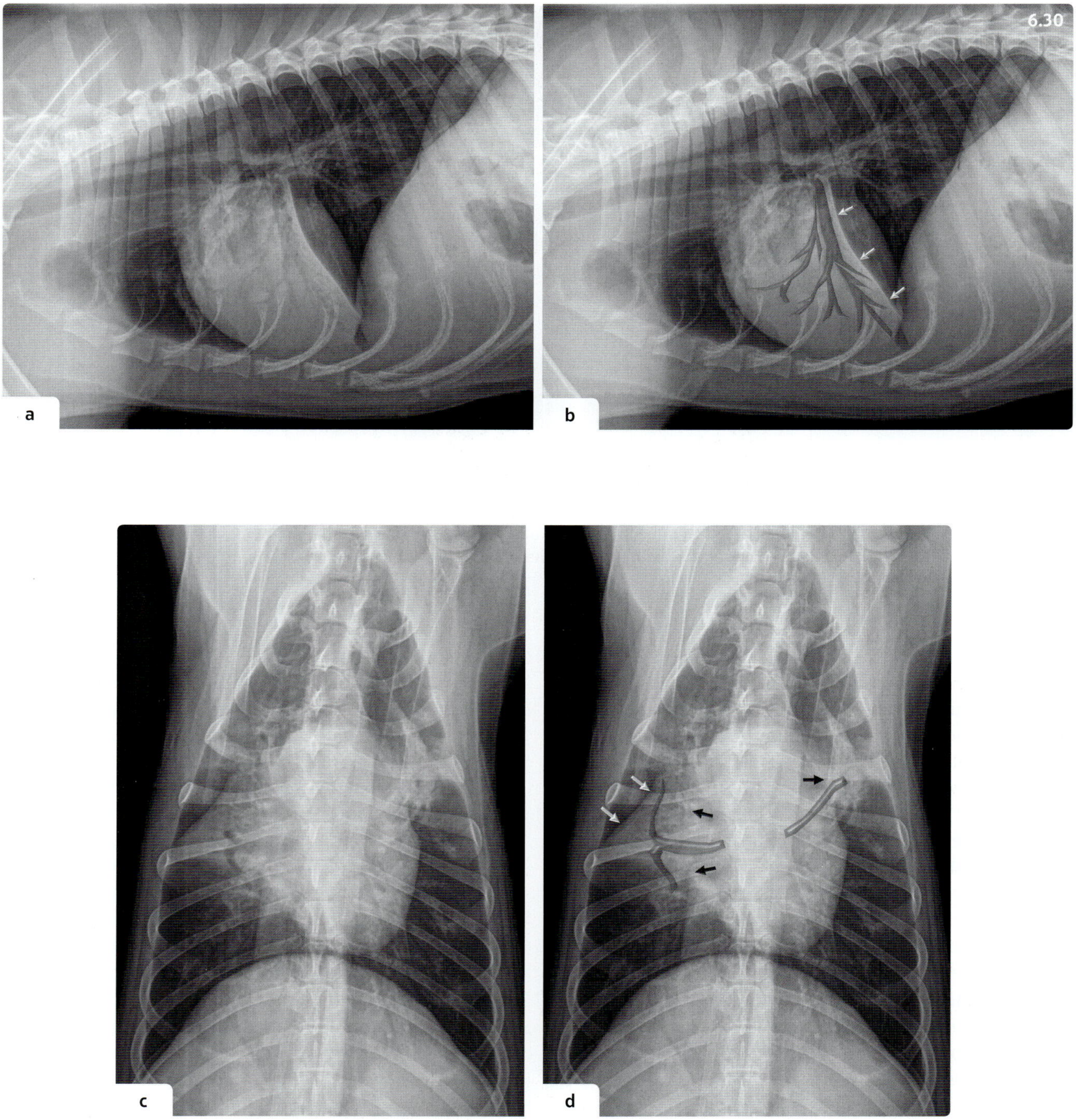

Figures 6.30a–d Lateral projection (a) with accompanying schematic (b) and ventrodorsal projection (c) with accompanying schematic (d) radiographs of a dog with alveolar pulmonary disease within the right middle and left cranial lung lobes due to aspiration pneumonia. All the hallmarks of alveolar disease are evident. Air bronchograms can be seen as gray branching structures (b, d, highlighted in gray) against a white backdrop and are visible on both projections, in this case. Lobar signs (b, d, white arrows) are visible between the right middle lung lobe and the more aerated adjacent lobes. Finally, border effacement prevents the ability to see the right and left cranial cardiac margins (b, d, black arrows) and margins of vasculature/bronchi within the affected lobes.

Table 6.17 Regional distribution of lung diseases resulting in an alveolar pulmonary pattern.

Cause of alveolar pattern	Regional distribution
Aspiration or bronchopneumonia (**Figure 6.30**)	Ventral to trachea
Cardiogenic pulmonary edema (**Figures 6.27, 6.28**)	Perihilar/caudodorsal/diffuse Multifocal in cats Peribronchial in dogs with DCM
Noncardiogenic pulmonary edema	Caudodorsal
Hemorrhage: • Trauma • Coagulopathy	 Variable Variable/caudodorsal
Interstitial pneumonia	Caudodorsal/diffuse
Pulmonary thromboembolism	Variable
Atelectasis	Often ventral to trachea/variable
Primary lung tumor	Lobar/caudal lobes/variable

mechanisms. The causes of the latter category are listed in **Box 6.14**.

Box 6.14 Causes of noncardiogenic pulmonary edema.

- Upper airway obstruction
- Head trauma
- Electrocution
- Uncontrolled seizures
- Hypoglycemia
- Thoracic trauma
- Smoke inhalation
- Near drowning
- Acute lung injury/acute respiratory distress syndrome
  - Acute interstitial pneumonia/pneumonitis
  - Systemic inflammatory response syndrome
  - Pancreatitis
  - Sepsis
  - Uremia

Interstitial pulmonary pattern

The interstitial pulmonary pattern is subcategorized into structured and unstructured. The unstructured interstitial pulmonary pattern is notoriously difficult to diagnose, as the appearance of the interstitium is greatly influenced by technical factors; additionally, it may indicate active or past disease. An unstructured interstitial pulmonary pattern is described by an increase in pulmonary opacity that is less intense per unit area when compared with alveolar disease, such that margins of vessels are less delineated but not totally effaced (**Figures 6.31a–d**). Any disease resulting in an alveolar pulmonary pattern can appear as an unstructured interstitial pulmonary pattern with a similar regional distribution. As the evolution of fluid changes from less to more severe or as resolution occurs with treatment, a shift can be seen from interstitial to alveolar and from alveolar to interstitial, respectively. Therefore, the distribution and differential diagnoses for interstitial disease can be described as given above for alveolar disease. Additionally, in cases of an unstructured pulmonary pattern that is distributed diffusely, fibrosis, neoplasia (lymphoma, hemangiosarcoma), or hematogenous pneumonitis (infectious/noninfectious inflammatory) should be considered.

The structured pulmonary pattern is reserved for any nodular or mass lesion(s) seen within the lung. This pattern can be relatively intense per unit area, depending on the size of the nodule. The difference between a nodule and a mass is strictly size – a mass is 3 cm or greater. Masses and nodules are best delineated from other lesions of high intensity per unit area (e.g. alveolar lung disease) by the rounded, sometimes well-defined margins seen with structured interstitial disease. The main differential diagnoses for this pulmonary pattern are summarized in **Table 6.18**. Granulomatous pneumonia tends to occur in younger animals and the nodules tend to be of a similar size with indistinct margins. Sometimes, nodules can appear very small, creating a miliary type of pulmonary pattern (**Figure 6.32**). Multiple nodules due to metastatic disease tend to occur in older animals. The nodules are more often variable in size with well-defined margins.

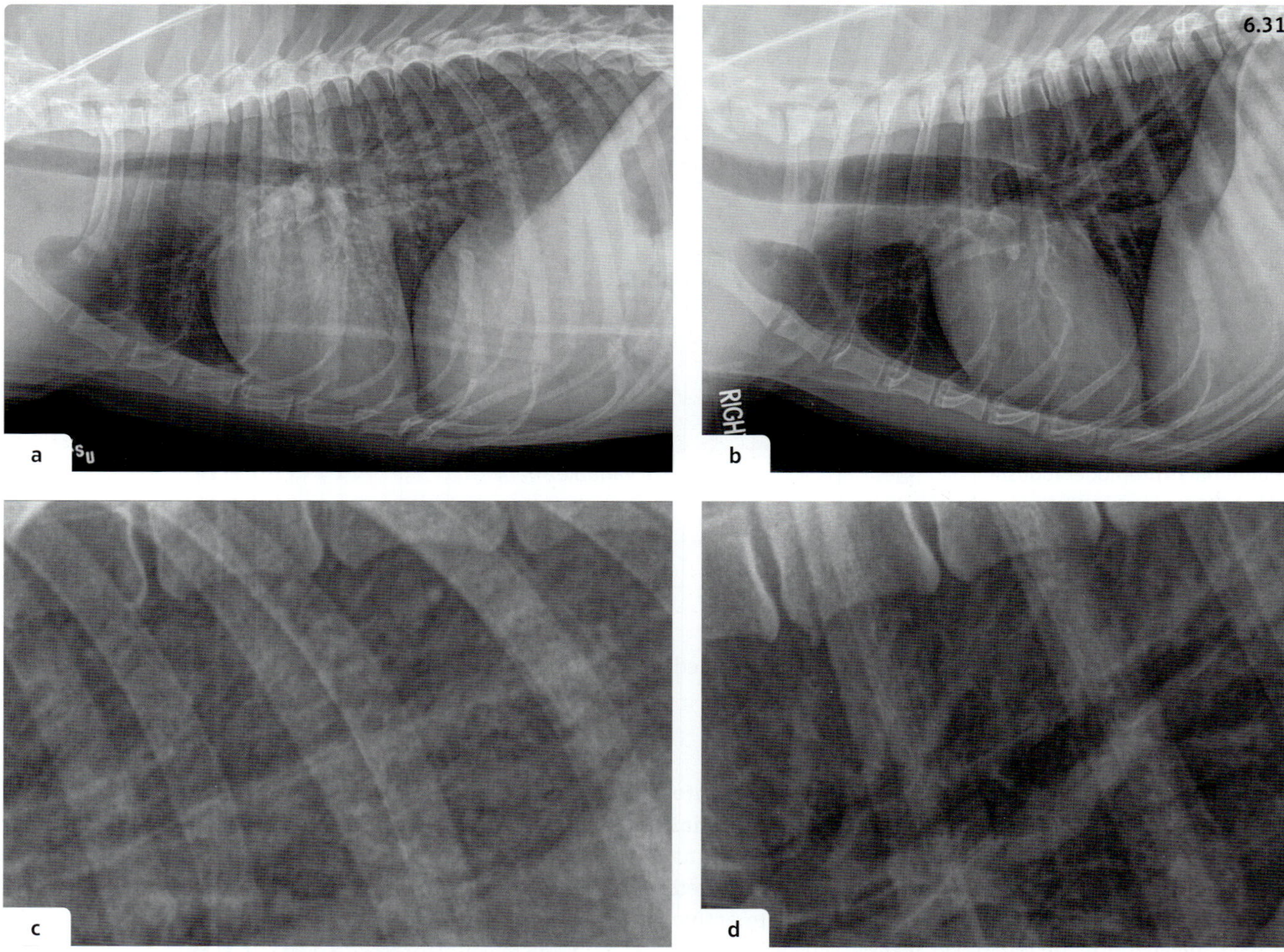

Figures 6.31a–d Unstructured interstitial pulmonary pattern. Lateral (a) and close-up (c) radiographs of a dog with confirmed uremic pneumonitis creating an interstitial pulmonary pattern. Lateral (b) and close-up (d) radiographs of a normal dog not having clinical respiratory disease are shown for comparison. The caudodorsal distribution of pulmonary opacity makes noncardiogenic pulmonary edema more likely, which is a typical appearance for acute lung injury due to uremic pneumonitis.

Table 6.18 Differential diagnoses for a structured interstitial pulmonary pattern.

Description	Differential diagnoses
Multiple soft tissue nodules	Metastasis, granulomatous pneumonia, septic emboli, parasitic (e.g. *Paragonimus kellicotti*), cysts, artifactual (end-on vasculature, superimposed superficial nipple or debris)
Solitary soft tissue nodule or mass	Primary tumor, single metastasis, granuloma (foreign body), abscess, fluid-filled cyst, artifactual (see above)
Multiple or single cavitary nodule(s)/mass(es)	Thick-walled: neoplasia (primary or metastatic), abscess, granuloma, parasitic Thin-walled: bulla, cyst, airway dilation (bronchus/bronchiectasis, alveoli/emphysema)
Single or multiple mineral nodule(s)	Pulmonary osteomas, chronic fungal granulomas, rarely parasitic nodules or neoplasia

Multiple mineralized pulmonary nodules, called pulmonary osteomas, pulmonary osteomata, or heterotopic bone, occur as a benign finding in dogs, especially Boxers and Shetland Sheepdogs. They are often in higher

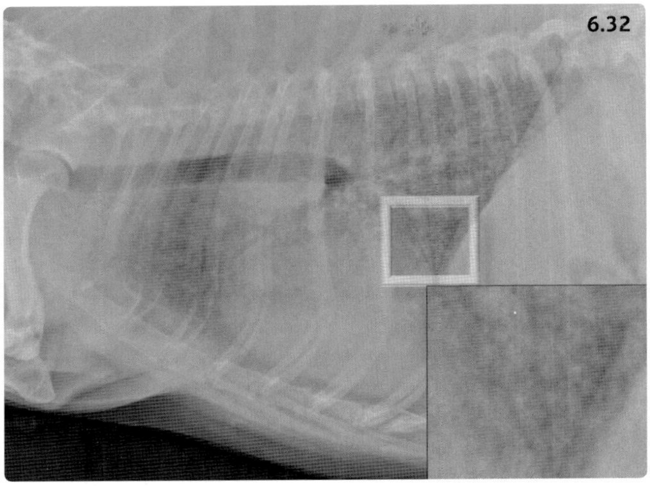

Figure 6.32 Lateral thoracic radiograph with magnified inset in a dog with a miliary structured interstitial pulmonary pattern due to blastomycosis. The nodules are very small, resembling an accumulation of millet seeds, and have very indistinct margins reflecting active inflammation. The diagnosis was achieved with lung fine-needle aspiration.

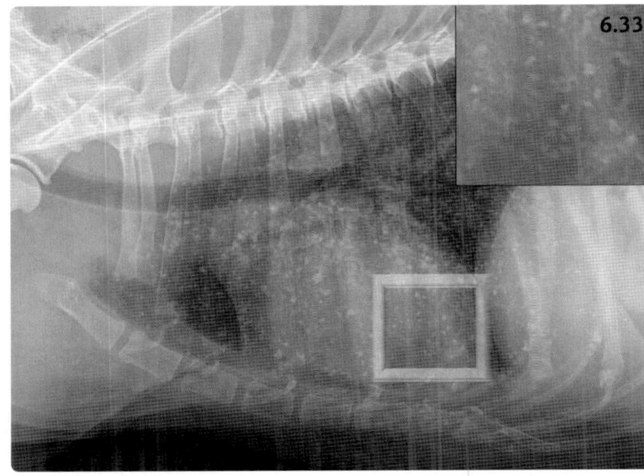

Figure 6.33 Lateral thoracic radiograph of a Shetland Sheepdog presented for a metastasis check. Numerous, well-defined mineralized nodules are present. Many of these nodules are less than 3 mm in size yet are highly visible, supporting suspicion of mineralized benign pulmonary osteomas. On close inspection of the magnified inset, the nodules are highly irregularly marginated rather than being round in shape.

numbers ventrally and only a few millimeters in size. True soft tissue opaque nodules of this size would be poorly detected on radiographs, so when a nodule that is 3 mm or less is visible on radiographs, the interpreter must consider a mineralized nodule or end-on vessel. Additionally, these mineralized pulmonary osteomas are typically irregularly marginated when inspected closely, also distinguishing them from many soft tissue opaque nodules. As mentioned, pulmonary osteomas are benign and can be quite numerous (**Figure 6.33**). Mineralized malignant nodules are extremely rare in veterinary medicine.

Regardless of whether or not the interstitial pulmonary pattern is structured or unstructured, a definitive diagnosis is most often determined via lung aspiration rather than airway sampling.

Bronchial pulmonary pattern

The bronchial pulmonary pattern implies disease that is airway related. Fluid or cells infiltrate bronchial walls and result in radiographically evident thickening. In most cases, the ailment affecting the bronchus extends into surrounding peribronchial interstitium. In some cases, the infiltration may be limited to peribronchial interstitium; however, airway-related disease remains the most common underlying cause. It is a common mistake for inexperienced interpreters to assign a bronchial pattern when normal bronchi are noticed, especially if clinical signs such as coughing are present. Seeing bronchi does not make the study abnormal. Disease can be assumed, however, when the bronchi are thickened, irregular, and/or indistinct in margination. Irregular and thickened bronchial walls create the so-called tram tracks and rings within the lungs (**Figures 6.34a, b**).

In addition to bronchial walls being thickened and irregular when radiographically visible disease is present, bronchi can fail to taper because of bronchiectasis (**Figure 6.35**). Bronchiectasis is important to recognize as an irreversible sequela of chronic airway-related disease and as a predisposing factor for future airway-related symptoms and bronchopneumonia.

Vascular pulmonary pattern

This pattern is reserved for cases where the pulmonary arteries and/or veins are too big or too small. Many do not consider this a true pulmonary pattern. If arteries and/or veins are enlarged or small, causes of cardiopulmonary vascular disease should be pursued as discussed above (Heart, great vessels, and pericardium). The most common cause of a vascular pulmonary pattern in endemic regions is heartworm infection. The characteristic radiographic changes associated with heartworm disease are described in **Box 6.15**.

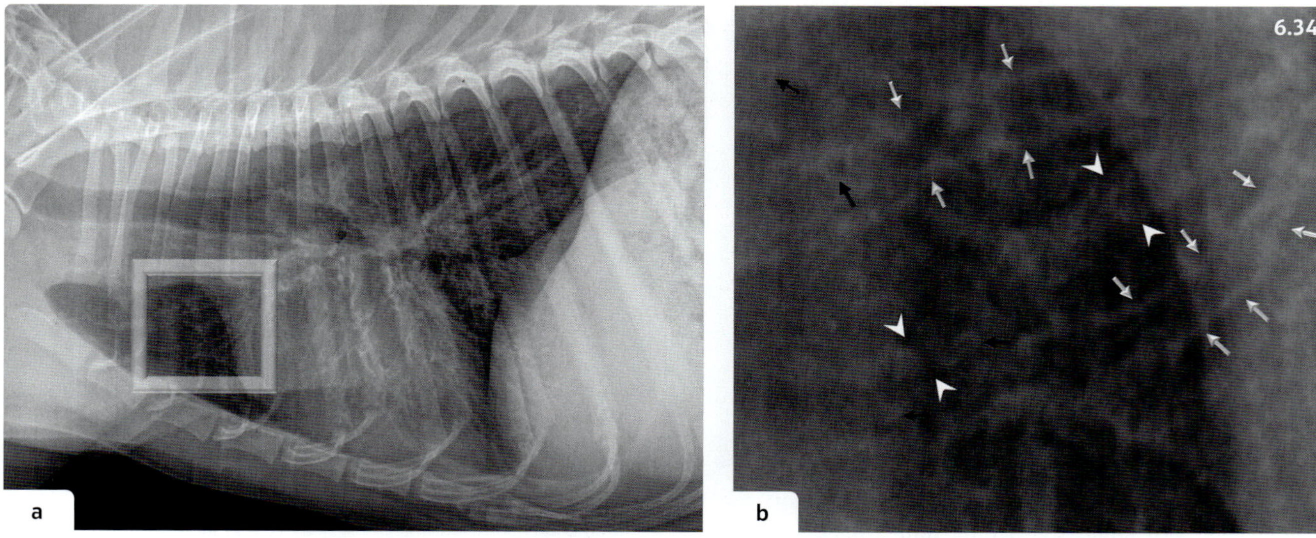

Figures 6.34a, b Lateral radiograph (a) and magnified inset (b) of a dog with chronic bronchial disease. The bronchial walls seen in the longitudinal orientation (b, white arrows) and those seen end-on (b, black arrows) are thick and irregular, creating the tram-tracks and rings expected with bronchial disease. The walls are thinner and more irregular than adjacent pulmonary vasculature (between white arrowheads). A noninfectious, inflammatory airway condition was determined based on bronchoalveolar lavage.

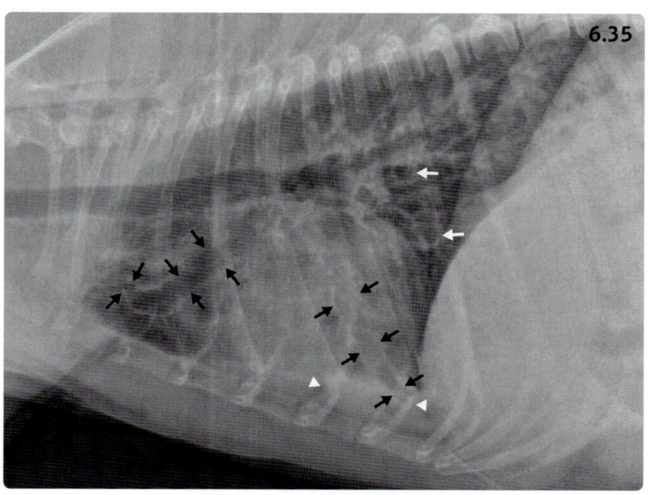

Figure 6.35 Left lateral radiograph of a dog with a chronic cough of 11 years' duration. Increased irregular, well-defined linear and ring markings are present in all lung lobes, consistent with a chronic bronchial pattern. Multiple bronchi fail to taper at the periphery of the lung (black arrows). The tubular shape of the bronchi is consistent with cylindrical bronchiectasis. Enlarged, dilated rings are also visible dorsally, consistent with bronchiectasis viewed end-on. Focal ventral alveolar disease is also present, consistent with bronchopneumonia (white arrowheads), a common predisposing factor and sequela seen in cases of bronchiectasis.

Box 6.15 Radiographic appearance of heartworm infection.

- Right ventricular enlargement:
  - Concentric nature of hypertrophy makes radiographic detection insensitive until severe
  - Lateral view: wide cardiac silhouette, increased sternal contact, elevated cardiac apex
  - Ventrodorsal view: bulge in 5:00 to 9:00 position at the right cardiac margin
- Main pulmonary arterial enlargement:
  - Lateral view: bulge in the 8:00 to 11:00 position at the cranial cardiac base
  - Ventrodorsal view: bulge in the 1:00 to 2:00 position at the left cranial cardiac margin
- Peripheral pulmonary arterial enlargement
- Pulmonary eosinophilic inflammation:
  - Peribronchial interstitial to alveolar pulmonary opacity
  - Multifocal nodular pulmonary pattern in some cases
- Right-sided heart failure:
  - Dilated caudal vena cava
  - Generalized hepatomegaly
  - Peritoneal effusion
  - Pleural effusion

RECOMMENDED FURTHER READING

Dennis R, Kirkberger RM, Wrigley RH *et al.* (2001) *Handbook of Small Animal Radiological Differential Diagnosis*. WB Saunders, London.

Kealy JK, McAllister H, Graham JP (2011) *Diagnostic Radiology and Ultrasonography of the Dog and Cat*. Saunders, St. Louis.

Suter PF (1984) *Thoracic Radiography: A Text Atlas of Thoracic Diseases of the Dog and Cat*. Wettswil, Switzerland.

Thrall DE (2013) *Textbook of Veterinary Diagnostic Radiology*. Saunders, St. Louis.

Chapter 7

Cardiovascular disorders

Romain Pariaut & Carley Saelinger

HISTORY AND PHYSICAL EXAMINATION

Introduction

Cardiovascular disease is common in dogs and cats, and a thorough history and physical examination are crucial steps in making the diagnosis of heart disease. They not only can assist in differentiating respiratory from cardiac disease, but also help determine the severity of the disease and response to therapy.

Signalment

Age, breed, and sex are useful information to establish a short list of differential diagnoses. Young animals tend to present with congenital defects, while acquired diseases should be suspected in older animals. There are known breed predispositions and males are more susceptible to certain diseases. However, there are exceptions in all of these cases and care should be taken not to exclude diseases simply from signalment. Signalment in combination with heart murmur characteristics and pulse quality are particularly useful to shorten differential lists in puppies with congenital heart disease.

History

A thorough history should include questions about onset, duration, and progression of presenting signs; current medications and the response to those medications; travel history and possible infectious disease exposure; and concurrent medical problems.

Presenting complaints

Common presenting signs of cardiac disease include tachypnea, dyspnea, cough, exercise intolerance, syncope, abdominal swelling, decreased appetite, weight loss, cyanosis, paresis/paralysis, and poor growth.

Tachypnea/dyspnea

Tachypnea is an overly rapid respiratory rate. Owners of pets with cardiac disease should be instructed to keep a resting respiratory rate log at home, and this should be reviewed as part of the history. If the resting respiratory rate is steadily increasing, or is >40 bpm, cardiogenic pulmonary edema should be suspected in animals previously diagnosed with cardiac disease. Dyspnea is labored breathing and can be caused by primary respiratory disease or decompensated cardiac disease. Caution should be taken with dyspneic animals as they may quickly become unstable if placed in a stressful environment.

Cough

Cats rarely cough with cardiac disease, although it is reported with heartworm infection. However, cough is the most common complaint in dogs with cardiac disease. It is important to differentiate cough due to cardiac disease from that due to respiratory causes. A high-pitched or honking cough is more commonly associated with tracheobronchial collapse, whereas dogs with heart disease will tend to have an intermittent, harsh, low pitched cough, which may be more prominent at night. Cough can be more specific of congestive heart failure (CHF) in large breed dogs than in small breeds.

Syncope

Syncope is a loss of consciousness associated with decreased cerebral blood flow. It is important to differentiate syncope from seizures. Syncopal episodes are generally brief and the animal is normal immediately preceding and following the episode. Syncope has a variety of causes (**Table 7.1**).

Table 7.1 Causes of syncope in dogs and cats.

Arrhythmia: • Bradyarrhythmia: high-grade second-degree atrioventricular block, third-degree atrioventricular block, sick sinus syndrome • Tachyarrhythmia: sustained supraventricular tachycardia, ventricular tachycardia
Severe pulmonary hypertension
Vasovagal syncope associated with coughing, urination, defecation
Systemic hypotension: may be induced by vasodilatory therapy
Severe decrease in cardiac output
Cardiac tamponade

Abdominal distension

Abdominal swelling is due to ascites, the cardiac causes of which include right-sided heart disease, pericardial effusion, constrictive pericardial disease, severe pulmonary hypertension (PH), and obstructions to venous return. Ascites develops secondary to congestion in the liver and spleen. It can lead to dyspnea and tachypnea because of increased pressure on the diaphragm, as well as decreased appetite due to abdominal discomfort. Increased intra-abdominal pressure impairs renal blood flow and intestinal absorption of nutrients and drugs.

Weight loss/cachexia

Cardiac cachexia is a generalized loss of muscle, bone, and adipose tissue mass secondary to CHF. It is due to a catabolic/anabolic imbalance and carries a poor prognosis. High calorie diets and more frequent feeding are often required to limit the effects of cardiac cachexia. Patients with ascites usually develop more profound and rapid cardiac cachexia.

Cyanosis

Cyanosis is associated with decreased oxygenation of blood and leads to blue-tinged mucous membranes (**Figure 7.1**). Cyanosis is most commonly seen secondary to cardiac defects leading to right-to-left blood shunting, although it can also be due to severe left heart failure or respiratory disease. There will often be a concurrent polycythemia.

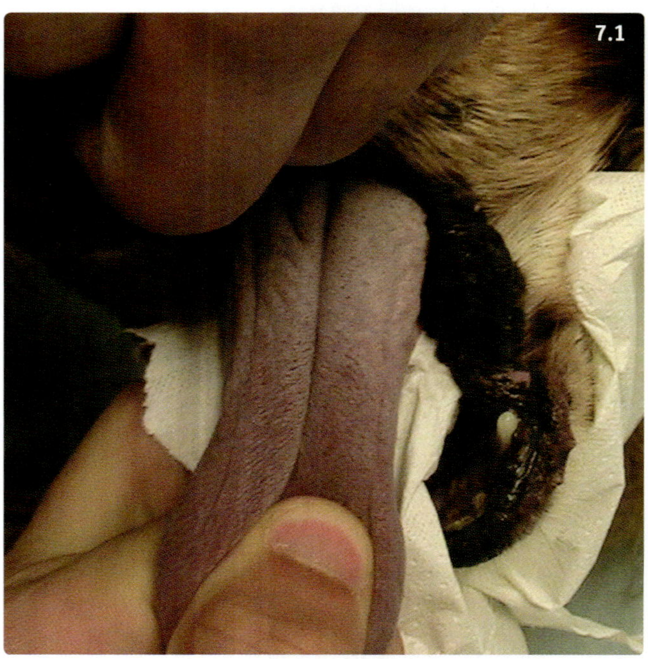

Figure 7.1 Cyanosis in a dog with a right-to-left intracardiac shunt.

Paresis

Paresis is most commonly seen in cats with arterial thromboembolic disease. The limb affected depends on the location of the thromboembolus.

Physical examination

The physical examination should begin with inspection from a distance, to collect information on respiratory status and mentation.

Examination of the mucous membranes

Mucous membrane color and perfusion should be examined. Cyanosis is due to poor ventilation or alveolar diffusion. Pallor can indicate anemia, hypoxemia, or poor perfusion, and hyperemia may indicate polycythemia or sepsis. The color of the oral mucous membranes should be compared with caudal membranes to assess for differential cyanosis, which is characteristic of a right-to-left patent ductus arteriosus (PDA). Capillary refill time (CRT) is a poor indicator of tissue perfusion. It is considered normal when it is less than 2 seconds.

Palpation of the pulses

The femoral pulse should be evaluated in every patient. The palpated pulse pressure is determined by the difference between systolic and diastolic pressures and the rate at which pressure reaches its peak systolic value. For example, a large difference between diastolic and systolic pressures, or a rapid rise of pressure, results in a 'bounding' or 'hyperdynamic' pulse. Pulse quality cannot be used to estimate actual arterial blood pressure values. Both femoral pulses should be evaluated and the pulse rate compared with the auscultated heart rate. The detection of changes in pulse quality and pattern can help establish a list of differential diagnoses (**Table 7.2**).

Examination of the jugular veins

The jugular veins should be examined while the animal is standing with its head in a neutral position. Any pulse extending above the lower third of the neck is considered abnormal and may be due to right-sided CHF, pulmonic stenosis (PS), severe PH, pericardial disease, heartworm disease, or arrhythmias. In addition to abnormal pulses, generalized jugular distension may be noted. This finding indicates increased systemic venous pressures secondary to right heart failure, pericardial disease, or cranial vena cava obstruction that can occur with mediastinal or heart base masses. The hepatojugular reflux

Table 7.2 Description of pulses and their causes.

Pulse type	Description	Cause
Bounding/hyperkinetic	'Water hammer' forceful pulse	Aortic insufficiency, PDA, thyrotoxicosis, anemia
Pulsus bisferiens (bifid)	Double pulse for each beat	HOCM, SAS, aortic insufficiency
Pulsus alternans	Alternating pulse strength with each beat	Severe myocardial disease
Pulsus paradoxus	Inspiration is associated with weakened or absent pulse	Pericardial effusion and tamponade
Pulsus parvus et tardus	Delayed onset of pulse and weak pulse	SAS
Pulsus bigeminus	Pulses come in pairs with pause between each pair and the second pulse weaker than the first	Bigeminal arrhythmias
Pulse deficits	Auscultated heart beats do not have coinciding pulse	Arrhythmias
Hypokinetic pulses	Weak and difficult to palpate	Hypotension, hypovolemia, SAS, congestive heart failure
Absent pulses	No pulse palpated	Thromboembolism

PDA, patent ductus arteriosus; HOCM, hypertrophic obstructive cardiomyopathy; SAS, subaortic stenosis.

sign, which corresponds to a distension of the jugular veins when pressure is applied to the cranial abdomen, can be seen with right-sided heart disease and occurs due to the inability of the diseased heart to compensate for the increased return of blood occurring during abdominal compression (**Figure 7.2**).

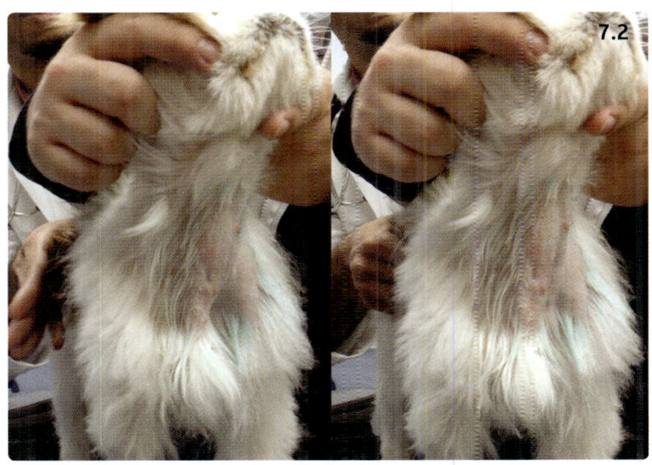

Figure 7.2 Hepatojugular reflux sign. There is marked distension of the jugular veins (right) when pressure is applied to the cranial abdomen, compared with baseline (left).

Palpation

The apex beat should be felt most strongly on the left side of the thorax between the 4th and 6th intercostal spaces. The apex beat may be shifted due to cardiac enlargement, intrathoracic masses, collapsed lung lobes, diaphragmatic hernias, or sternal abnormalities. A decreased intensity of the apex beat may be secondary to pericardial effusion, pleural effusion, pneumothorax, diaphragmatic hernia, thoracic masses, or obesity. A precordial thrill, a localized vibration of the chest caused by turbulent blood flow, can be felt when a severe murmur is present.

Auscultation

Auscultation should be performed in a quiet room with both the bell (for low-frequency sounds) and diaphragm (for high-frequency sounds) of the stethoscope. Auscultation should be performed in a systematic manner, evaluating all areas of the thorax and each valve region (**Table 7.3**). The animal should be in a standing position for auscultation. The heart and lungs should be auscultated separately to avoid confusing or overlooking abnormal sounds. Heart rate and rhythm should be noted, as well as the presence or absence of heart sounds and abnormalities. The normal heart sounds are S1, associated with closure of the atrioventricular (AV) valves, and S2, associated with closure of semilunar valves. S1 is normally longer and louder than S2. A split S1 may be auscultated and indicates asynchronous closure of the AV valves. S2 is shorter and higher pitched than S1, and is loudest over the pulmonic and aortic areas. Splitting of S2 indicates asynchronous closure of the aortic and pulmonic valves (**Table 7.4**).

Abnormal heart sounds in small animals include S3, due to rapid ventricular filling, and S4, due to atrial contraction into overly distended or noncompliant ventricle.

Table 7.3 Areas of auscultation in dogs.

Mitral area	Left hemithorax	5th intercostal space at costochondral junction
Aortic area	Left hemithorax	4th intercostal space at costochondral junction
Pulmonic area	Left hemithorax	2nd to 4th intercostal space at left sternal border
Tricuspid area	Right hemithorax	3rd to 5th intercostal space near costochondral junction

Table 7.4 Abnormal heart sounds and their causes.

Abnormal heart sound	Causes
Split S1	Normal in some large breed dogs Right bundle branch block APCs VPCs Mitral valve/tricuspid valve stenosis
Split S2	Normal during inspiration in some animals Pulmonary hypertension Right bundle branch block VPCs Pulmonic stenosis Left bundle branch block SAS Severe hypertension Aortic insufficiency
S3	DCM Decompensated AV valve disease PDA with left ventricular dilation
S4	HCM 3rd degree AV block
Mid-systolic click	Mitral valve prolapse

APC, atrial premature complex; VPC, ventricular premature complex; SAS, subaortic stenosis; DCM, dilated cardiomyopathy; AV, atrioventricular; PDA, patent ductus arteriosus; HCM, hypertrophic cardiomyopathy.

Both S3 and S4 are quiet, low pitched, and occur in diastole. An audible S3 is indicative of dilated ventricles and S4 indicates a thickened or noncompliant ventricle or atrial contraction against an already closed AV valve. When S3 or S4 is audible it is called a gallop rhythm. Systolic click is a transient sound that may mimic a gallop rhythm. It is caused by the prolapse of the AV valves, typically in the early stage of degenerative mitral valve disease in dogs. Conversely, a gallop rhythm in dogs usually results from a very enlarged left ventricle, and therefore advanced cardiac disease.

Cardiac murmurs are abnormal sounds caused by turbulent blood flow. Murmurs may be functional or pathologic. Functional murmurs are further divided into physiologic and innocent. Physiologic murmurs have a known cause unrelated to primary cardiac disease, and are associated with increased cardiac output or altered blood viscosity. Innocent murmurs occur in young animals and have no known cause or associated cardiac disease. They should be no louder than a grade 3 and should disappear by 5 months of age (**Table 7.5**). Pathologic murmurs are caused by an underlying cardiac disease (**Table 7.6**).

Murmurs should be described by their timing, duration, grade, and point of maximal intensity (PMI). Additional information includes quality and pitch of the murmur. The timing of the murmur is either systolic, diastolic, continuous, or to-and-fro. Systolic murmurs are the most

Table 7.5 Causes of functional murmurs in dogs and cats.

Physiologic:
- Anemia
- Fever
- Hypoproteinemia
- Hypertension
- Pregnancy
- Hyperthyroidism

Innocent:
- No known cause or underlying cardiac disease

Table 7.6 Causes (and location) of pathologic murmurs in dogs and cats.

Systolic murmurs:
- AV valve regurgitation (left or right apical)
- Right ventricular outflow tract obstruction; pulmonic stenosis or dynamic right ventricular outflow tract obstruction (right basilar)
- Left ventricular outflow tract obstruction; subaortic stenosis or dynamic left ventricular outflow tract obstruction (left basilar)
- Ventricular septal defect (right apical, sternal, left basilar)
- Valvular endocarditis (left apical)

Diastolic murmurs:
- Aortic insufficiency (left basilar)
- Mitral valve stenosis (left apical)
- Valvular endocarditis (left basilar)

Continuous murmurs:
- Patent ductus arteriosus

common and can be further classified into: early, mid-, or late systolic; holosystolic (murmur extends throughout systole, but heart sounds remain audible); or pansystolic (murmur extends through systole, but S2 is obscured). Diastolic murmurs are often quiet and are much less common. Continuous murmurs can be heard during all phases of the cardiac cycle. To-and-fro murmurs occur when there is a distinct systolic and diastolic murmur. Murmurs are graded on a 1 to 6 scale (**Table 7.7**). Murmur grade does not necessarily correlate with the severity of the underlying disease.

The PMI is the location where the murmur is heard loudest. If possible, it should be localized to a single valve region. However, in small dogs and cats, the distinction of apical versus basilar is acceptable. Additionally, the locations of the radiation of the murmur should be described.

ELECTROCARDIOGRAPHY AND HOLTER MONITORING

Definition

The electrocardiogram (ECG) records the electrical activity of the heart from electrodes positioned at the surface of the body. A normal ECG displays three distinct events: a P wave during atrial depolarization; followed by a ventricular complex, or QRS complex during ventricular depolarization; and finally a T wave, which corresponds to ventricular repolarization (**Figure 7.3**). The atrial repolarization is usually not detected. The duration and the amplitude of the waves can be measured from the ECG.

Table 7.7 Murmur intensity grading system.

Murmur grade	Description
1	Can only be heard after several minutes of listening in a silent room
2	Soft and only heard in a focal region of the thorax
3	Heard throughout one side of the thorax, but does not radiate to the opposite side; equal in volume to normal heart sounds
4	Heard on both sides of the thorax; no precordial thrill
5	Palpable precordial thrill; very loud murmur
6	Audible with the stethoscope slightly off the thorax

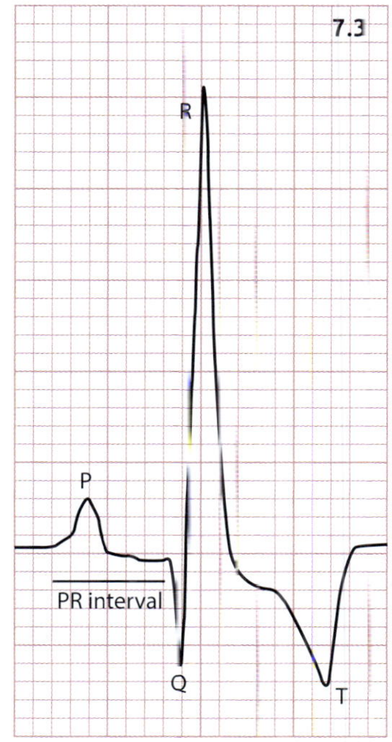

Figure 7.3 P-QRS-T illustrating the sequence of activation of the heart. Note that on this ECG there is no clearly defined S wave.

The duration (or width) of a wave depends on the time it takes for the electrical impulse to propagate within the cardiac chambers. The amplitude, or height, of a wave usually changes with the size of the cardiac chambers. All measurements should be made in lead II. The amplitude of the waves can decrease when fluid (air or liquid), fat, or a large mass interferes with the propagation of the electrical signals to the surface of the body. The P-R interval reflects the conduction time through the AV node (**Table 7.8**).

Ambulatory electrocardiography devices, known as Holter systems, allow clinicians to record a 24–72-hour ECG recording while the animal has a normal activity level in a familiar environment (**Figure 7.4**). Implantable devices are now available to collect ECG data. These devices are event recorders that can be manually triggered to save an ECG whenever clinical signs are observed by the owner of a pet. They are indicated in animals that only present with rare episodes of weakness or syncope.

Indications

The ECG is used to measure heart rate and evaluate cardiac rhythm. It is less reliable for gathering information about structural cardiac changes, such as hypertrophy. Therefore, it should be performed when an arrhythmia is detected on physical examination and when the presenting complaint may be explained by an arrhythmia.

Table 7.8 ECG features of the normal dog and cat. (Adapted from Tilley LP (1992) *Essentials of Canine and Feline Electrocardiography. Interpretation and Management*, 3rd edn. Lea & Febiger, Philadelphia.) All measurements made in lead II.

	Dog	Cat
Heart rate	70–160 bpm for adult dogs 60–140 bpm for giant breeds Up to 180 bpm for toy breeds Up to 220 bpm for puppies	Range 120–240 bpm Mean 197 bpm
Rhythm	Normal sinus rhythm Sinus arrhythmia Wandering SA pacemaker	Normal sinus rhythm
P wave	Width: maximum 0.04 sec; 0 .05 sec in giant breeds Height: maximum 0.4 mV	Width: maximum 0.04 sec Height: maximum 0.2 mV
P-R interval	Width: 0.06–0.13 sec	Width: 0.05–0.09 sec
QRS complex	Width: maximum 0.05 sec in small breeds; 0 .06 sec in large breeds Height of the R wave: maximum 2.5 mV in small breeds; 3 mV in large breeds	Width: maximum 0.04 sec Height of the R wave: maximum 0.9mV
S-T segment	No depression: not more than 0.2 mV No elevation: not more than 0.15 mV	No marked depression or elevation
T wave	Positive, negative, or biphasic Not greater than one fourth amplitude of R wave	Positive, negative, or biphasic. Most often positive Maximum amplitude 0.3 mV
Q-T interval	Width: 0.15–0.25 sec at normal HR; varies with HR	Width 0.12–0.18 sec at normal HR; varies with HR
Mean electrical axis	+40 to +100 degrees	0 to +160 degrees

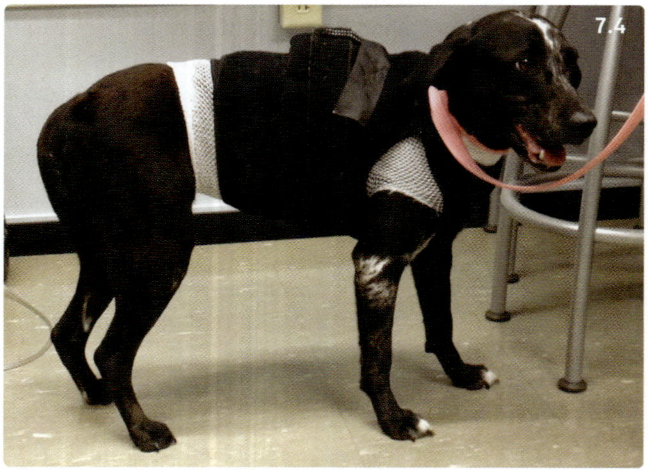

Figure 7.4 Twenty-four-hour Holter recording in a dog.

The main indications for Holter recordings are the detection of an arrhythmia as the cause for unexplained syncope, the quantification of arrhythmias, and monitoring of the response to antiarrhythmic therapies. This technique is also used to screen predisposed breeds for signs of specific cardiac diseases, in particular arrhythmogenic right ventricular cardiomyopathy (ARVC) in Boxers.

Method

Recording artifacts, caused by poor contact between the skin and the electrodes, breathing, shivering, or electrical interference, frequently interfere with the interpretation of ECG recordings. It is therefore critical to dedicate enough time and personnel to obtain a good quality ECG. First, the animal should be restrained in right lateral recumbency. Although ECGs can be recorded in a standing position or in sternal recumbency in patients in respiratory distress or that are uncooperative, it may change the appearance of the ECG tracing. The electrodes should be secured at the level of the elbows and knees, or as distal as possible on the four limbs to reduce artifacts secondary to the motion of the chest during breathing (**Figure 7.5**). Alcohol or a specifically formulated conducting gel is applied to improve contact between the skin and the electrodes. The recording sensitivity is usually selected at 10 mm/mV, but should be increased or decreased according to the amplitude of the waves on the ECG. A recording speed of 50 mm/sec is usually preferred. Some filters can be applied to the recording to reduce artifacts.

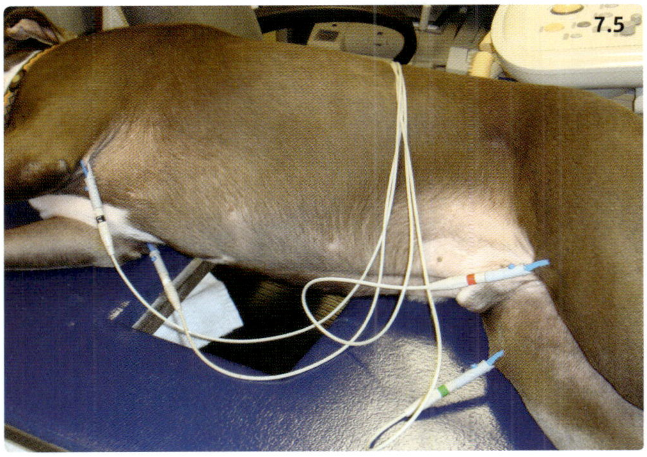

Figure 7.5 Electrode placement for good quality ECG recording.

The placement of four electrodes on the surface of the body allows recording of six leads: I, II, III, aVR, aVL, and aVF. These six leads display simultaneously the ECG from six different directions. If a wave is mostly above the baseline, it indicates that the electrical signal travels towards the recording electrode. The wave is below the baseline if the signal moves away from the recording electrode.

Tracing interpretation

First, the heart rate (in bpm) should be calculated manually, because the number displayed by some electronic ECG systems may be inaccurate. Usually, an average heart rate calculated over a few seconds is sufficient. For example, the number of QRS complexes can be calculated during 3 seconds (which corresponds to 15 cm, or the length of a regular pen, when the recording speed is set at 50 mm/s), and the number obtained is multiplied by 20 to obtain the heart rate per minute. Second, the waves should be identified on the tracing, and their duration and amplitude measured (**Table 7.8**). The P waves can be absent in some arrhythmias but the T waves are always present following QRS complexes. Next, the heart rhythm is analyzed in order to evaluate if it is regular or irregular, and if the rhythm is sinus (each P-wave related to each QRS complex with a constant P-R interval) or not. Analysis of the morphology of the QRS complexes provides information on the origin (e.g. supraventricular or ventricular) of the rhythm. QRS complexes of normal duration indicate that the electrical impulse travels through the specialized conduction system within the ventricle and, therefore, that the rhythm originated in the atrium or the AV node. Conversely, wide QRS complexes usually indicate that the electrical impulses originate within the ventricles (**Figure 7.6**). Alternatively, it may indicate a bundle branch block, which is a lesion of part of the specialized conduction system requiring the electrical depolarization to travel slowly between cardiomyocytes. Left and right ventricular hypertrophy and intraventricular conduction disturbances can change the amplitude, duration, and/or the direction of the QRS complexes during sinus rhythm. The direction of the QRS complexes is determined by calculation of the mean electrical axis. In dogs, the QRS complex in lead I should always be positive (larger amplitude R wave), indicating that the mean electrical axis of the QRS complexes is oriented towards the left. A negative QRS complex (larger amplitude S wave) in lead I indicates a right axis shift. In cats, the QRS complex in lead aVF should always be positive, indicating that the mean electrical axis is oriented caudally. When the QRS complex is negative in lead aVF and positive in lead I, it indicates a left axis shift. When it is negative in lead aVF and lead I, it indicates a right axis shift (**Figures 7.7–7.12**).

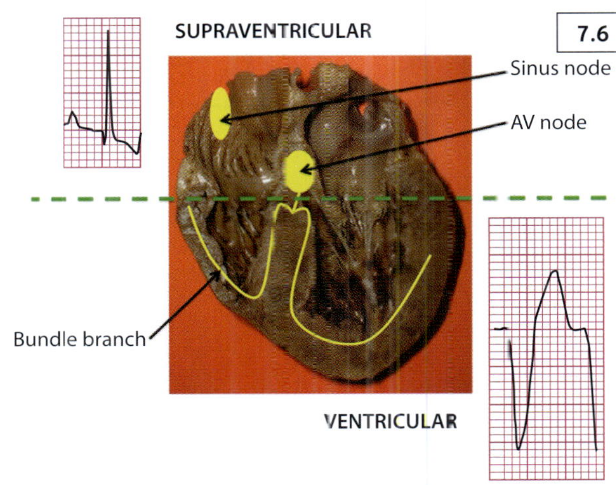

Figure 7.6 QRS complex morphology based on the origin of the electrical impulse. Electrical impulses originating at or above the atrioventricular node, that is the supraventricular area, conduct through the specialized conduction system (in yellow). Electrical impulses originating in the ventricles travel within nonspecialized tissue at a lower speed. Supraventricular QRS complexes are narrow; ventricular QRS complexes are wide.

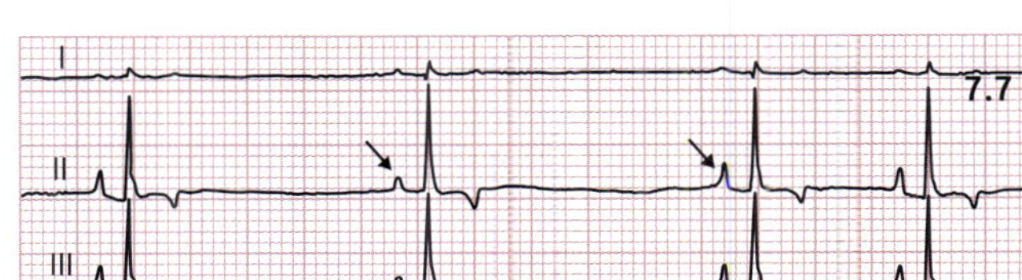

Figure 7.7 ECG showing respiratory sinus arrhythmia with wandering pacemaker (arrows) in a dog. Both result from variation of vagal tone with breathing in a healthy dog. Wandering pacemaker is a variation in the amplitude of the P waves with breathing caused by a shift of the origin of the electrical impulses within the sinus node. (Amplitude 10 mm/mV, speed 50 mm/sec)

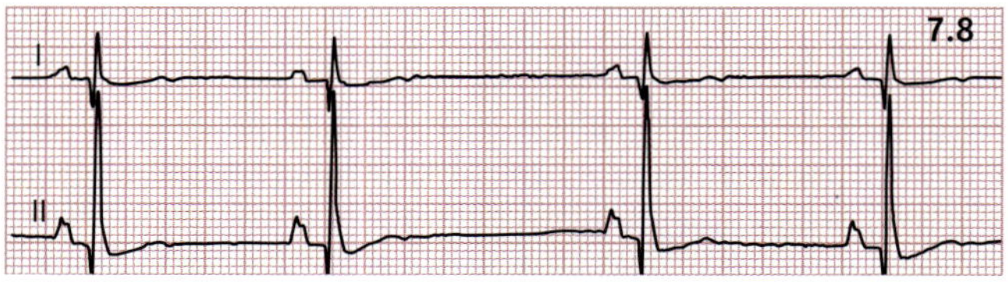

Figure 7.8 ECG showing sinus rhythm with a tall and wide P wave suggesting atrial enlargement (most likely left atrium). (Amplitude 10 mm/mV, speed 50 mm/sec)

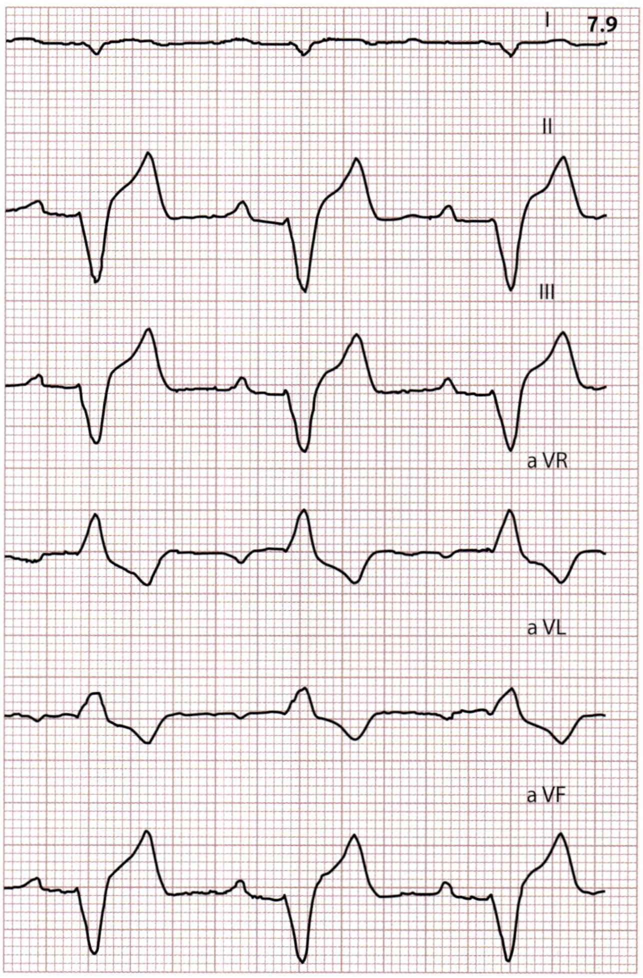

Figure 7.9 ECG showing sinus rhythm with a right-axis shift (negative QRS in lead I, II, III, and aVF) and wide QRS complexes, consistent with a right bundle branch block. (Amplitude 10 mm/mV, speed 50 mm/sec)

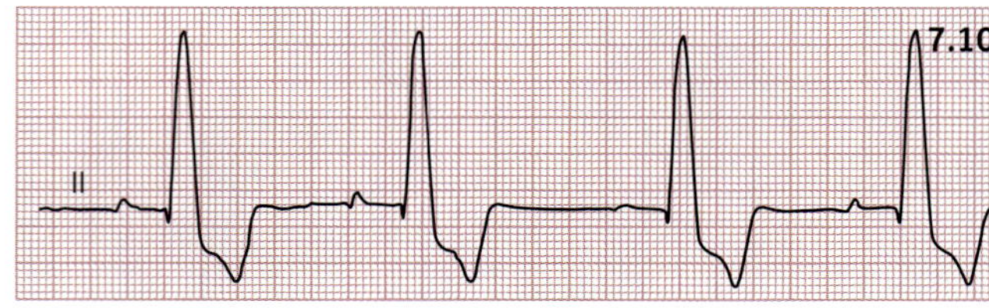

Figure 7.10 ECG showing sinus rhythm with positive and wide QRS in lead II, consistent with a left bundle branch block. (Amplitude 10 mm/mV, speed 50 mm/sec)

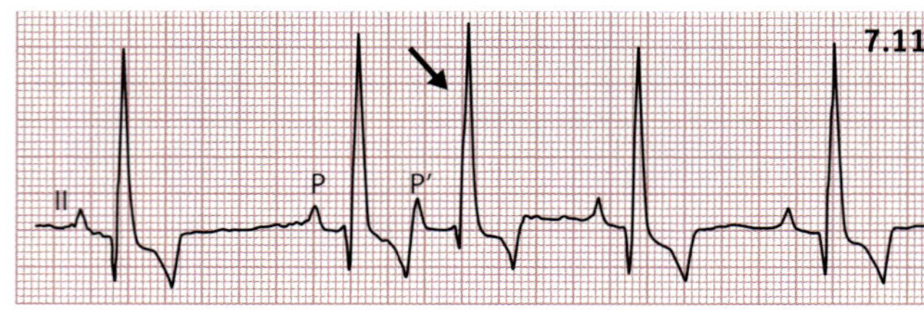

Figure 7.11 ECG showing sinus rhythm with one atrial premature contraction (APC) (arrow). The morphology of the QRS complex of APCs is similar to the QRS of sinus beats, as the electrical impulse uses the specialized conduction pathways in the ventricles. A P wave is visible just after the T wave, and its morphology slightly differs from the P wave of sinus beats. (Amplitude 10 mm/mV, speed 50 mm/sec)

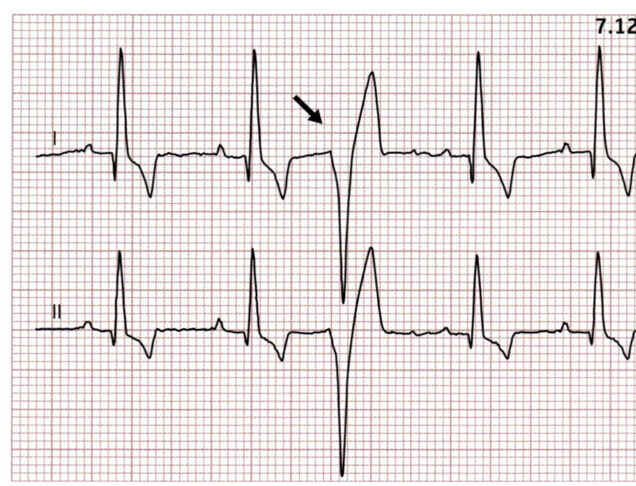

Figure 7.12 ECG showing sinus rhythm with one ventricular premature contraction (VPC) (arrow). The morphology of the QRS is 'wide and bizarre' and very different from the QRS complexes of sinus beats. It indicates the slow conduction of the electrical impulse in the ventricles.

ECHOCARDIOGRAPHY

Indications

Echocardiography is a noninvasive method of evaluating cardiac anatomy and function. Thoracic radiography and echocardiography are complementary in the evaluation of an animal with cardiac disease: presence or absence of CHF and size of the pulmonary vessels can only be evaluated from chest radiographs; information about chamber size, valve motion, and ventricular function can, however, only be obtained via echocardiography. A comprehensive echocardiographic examination requires the use of various modalities including 2-dimensional, M-mode, and Doppler echocardiography (**Figure 7.13**).

At the end of an echocardiogram, the clinician should have identified the primary lesion and its likely cause, the presence of coexisting abnormalities, the size and function of all four cardiac chambers, and the severity of the lesion (mild, moderate, severe). Finally, the initial echocardiographic examination provides baseline information for assessing the progression of the disease and monitoring the response to treatment of individual patients on follow-up examinations.

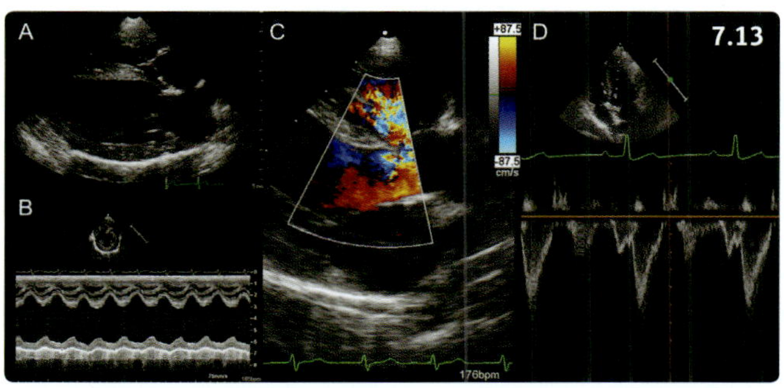

Figure 7.13 Echocardiographic modalities: two-dimensional (A), M-mode (B), color Doppler (C), spectral Doppler (D).

Imaging techniques

Echocardiographic windows

Transthoracic images of the heart can be obtained where lung tissue is not interposed between the heart and the chest wall. A parasternal window is present on the right side of the thorax between the sternal border and the costochondral junction from the 3rd to the 6th intercostal spaces. On the left side it is close to the sternal border between the 5th and 7th intercostal spaces (caudal or apical views) and between the sternum and the costochondral junction at the 3rd or 4th intercostal space (cranial views) (**Figure 7.14**).

Animal positioning

Echocardiograms are usually obtained with the patient in lateral recumbency on a 'cutout' table that allows transducer manipulation from beneath the animal. One or two assistants help restrain the patient in left and right lateral recumbency. ECG cables should be attached to the animal's limbs and an ECG tracing should be continuously displayed on the monitor. Sedation is usually not needed. Dogs and cats can also be examined in standing position.

Transducer selection

Transducers with a small contact surface are preferred. The optimal transducer frequency is therefore determined by the size of the animal: 8–10 MHz for cats and small

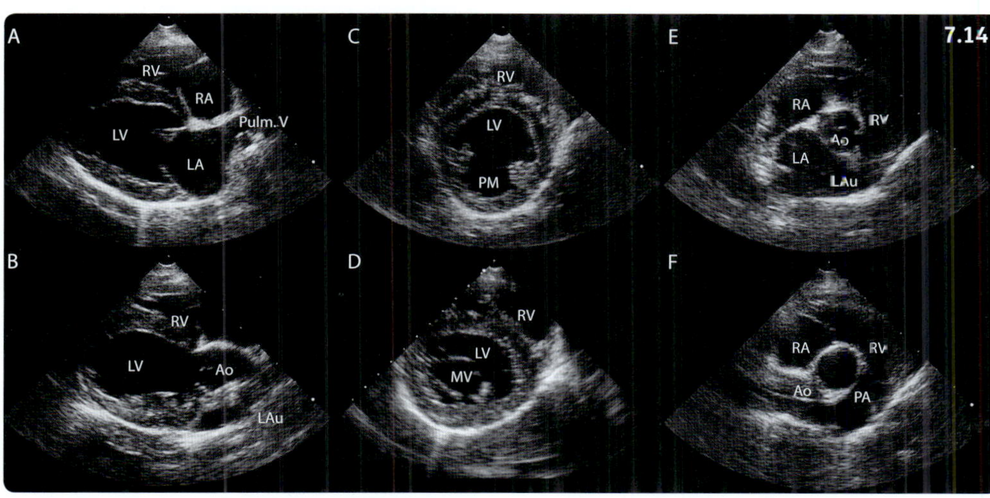

Figure 7.14 Standard two-dimensional echocardiographic views. (A) Right parasternal long-axis four-chamber view allows visualization of all four cardiac chambers. (B) Right parasternal long-axis outflow view. (C) Right parasternal short-axis view at the level of the left ventricular papillary muscles. This view is used to measure wall thicknesses and the diameter of the left ventricle in diastole and systole. (D) Right parasternal short-axis view at the level of the mitral valve; also called 'fish-mouth' view. (E) Right parasternal short-axis view at the left atrium/aorta level. This view is used to measure the diameter of the left atrium. (F) Right parasternal short axis view at the pulmonary artery level. The pulmonic valve and the diameter of the pulmonary artery and its main branches can be evaluated from this view.

breed dogs, 5–8 MHz for medium size dogs, and 2–5 MHz for large breed dogs.

Echocardiographic evaluation of cardiac chamber size and function

Every clinician should be able to evaluate left atrial size, left ventricular size and function, and the size of the right-sided cardiac chambers (**Box 7.1**).

Left ventricle

The left ventricle is the largest cardiac chamber. It is conical in shape and forms the apex of the heart. The cavity of the left ventricle is divided into an inflow and an ouflow region. The interventricular septum delimits the outflow tract medially, and the septal leaflet of the mitral valve forms an intermittent lateral boundary at the base of the heart. There is no anatomic partition of the outflow tract in the apical and mid-ventricular regions. The outflow tract is best imaged from the right parasternal long-axis outflow view and the left apical five-chamber plane. The interventricular septum separates the left ventricle from the right ventricle, and is best imaged from a right parasternal long-axis view. It is thick (thickness similar to the left ventricular free wall) and muscular for most of its length, but has a thin membranous part at the origin of the aorta.

Standard measurements include the interventricular septum thickness, the left ventricular internal diameter, and the left ventricular posterior wall thickness in end-diastole and end-systole. End-diastole is measured at the onset of the QRS complex on ECG, which also corresponds to the frame following mitral valve closure or the frame in which the left ventricular internal diameter is maximum. End-systole occurs at the end of the T wave.

Box 7.1 Qualitative echocardiographic evaluation of cardiac structure and function in the dog.

- Left and right atrium are approximately the same size
- The diameter of the left atrium is less than 1.5 times the diameter of the aortic valve annulus
- The right ventricular internal diameter is approximately one-third of the left ventricular internal diameter
- The thickness of the right ventricular wall is approximately one-third of the thickness of the left ventricular free wall
- The interventricular septum is approximately the same thickness as the left ventricular free wall
- The left ventricular internal diameter should decrease by 30–40 % in systole compared with diastole (fractional shortening = 30–40%)
- The diameter of the main pulmonary artery is the same as the aortic root diameter

In the absence of an ECG, systole coincides with the frame preceding mitral valve opening or the frame in which the left ventricular internal diameter is the smallest. Measurements are made on the right parasternal short-axis view at the chordae tendineae level, either directly with calipers on a two-dimensional still frame or on an M-mode display (**Figure 7.15**).

Qualitative assessment of left ventricular function should be complemented with quantitative measurements. In dogs and cats, left ventricular systolic function is usually determined by calculating the shortening fraction (FS) from linear measurements of the left ventricular internal diameter in end-diastole (LVIDd) and end-systole (LVIDs). FS (expressed as a percentage) is calculated from the formula:

$$FS = (LVIDd - LVIDs)/LVIDd \times 100$$

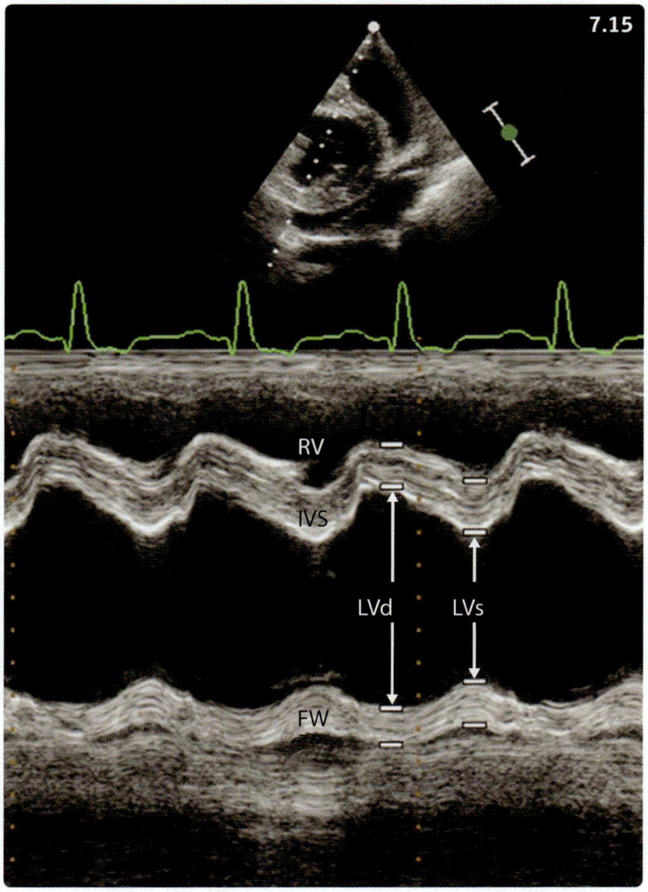

Figure 7.15 M-mode view of the left ventricle at the chordae tendineae level. The M-mode cursor is placed perpendicular to the interventricular septum and bisects the left ventricular free wall between the two papillary muscles. LVd, left ventricular internal diameter in diastole; LVs, left ventricular internal diameter in systole; RV, right ventricle; IVS, interventricular septum; FW, left ventricular free wall.

For example, a FS equal to 30% indicates that the left ventricular internal diameter is 30% smaller in systole than it is in diastole. In the authors' echocardiography laboratory, normal dogs have an FS of 30–45%. However, it seems that FS can be as low as 22–25% in normal large breed dogs. FS is around 40% in cats.

Right ventricle

The right ventricle has a complex geometry, described as crescent shaped or pyramid shaped. This, in addition to its smaller size and thinner walls, makes the echocardiographic assessment of the right ventricle difficult. Qualitatively, the right ventricular internal diameter is approximately one-third of the left ventricle, and the right ventricular free wall is equal to one-third or one-half of the thickness of the left ventricular free wall.

The right ventricle chamber is divided into an inflow and an outflow region by a ridge of muscular tissue known as crista supraventricularis. Both regions cannot be fully examined on the same echocardiographic view. The inflow region is directly beneath the tricuspid valve. It is best assessed from the right parasternal long-axis four-chamber view and the left apical four-chamber view. The outflow region extends upward and to the left. It is best imaged from the right parasternal short-axis view at the aorta level and the left cranial short-axis views. Small papillary muscles originate from the apical portion of the interventricular septum.

Left atrium

The left atrium is an oval-shaped chamber positioned caudal to the aorta and above the left ventricle. It is divided into the body of the atrium and the auricle. The auricle is heavily trabeculated. It is best imaged from a right parasternal short-axis view at the aortic valve level. Contraction of the left atrium delivers 15–30% of left ventricular filling. The left atrium receives blood from 5–8 (usually 7) pulmonary veins, which enter the craniodorsal and caudodorsal part of the chamber. They are usually not clearly visible on the echocardiogram, but pulmonary venous inflow can be identified and studied by pulsed-wave Doppler. The interatrial septum separates the left atrium and the right atrium. The flap of the foramen ovale may be seen from a right parasternal long-axis four-chamber view on the left atrial side in animals with a patent foramen ovale.

Linear measurements of the left atrium are used to calculate the left atrium to aortic ratio (LA/Ao). LA/Ao ratio is independent of body weight. In healthy dogs and cats, the LA/Ao ratio is between 1.3 and 1.5 (**Figure 7.16**). It is usually not >1.6.

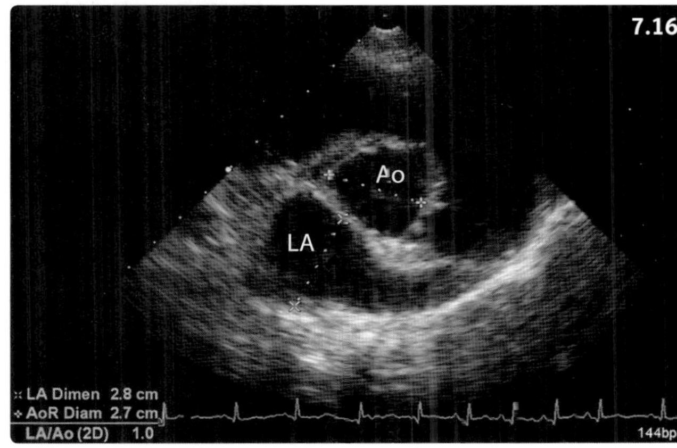

Figure 7.16 Measurement of the left atrium and aortic valve annulus from a two-dimensional right parasternal short-axis view. The LA/Ao ratio should be less than 1.5 in healthy animals. LA, left atrium; Ao: aorta.

Right atrium

The right atrium is an ovoid structure divided into a main chamber and the right auricle. The right auricle is difficult to image with transthoracic echocardiography. In clinical practice, qualitative assessment of the right atrium is made by comparing its size with the left atrium. In healthy animals, left and right atrium are of comparable size.

Doppler echocardiography

Doppler echocardiography provides information on blood flow direction and velocity. Color-flow Doppler is used to 'map' blood flow on a two-dimensional view of the heart. Blood flow velocity across valves, septal defects, and at the level of extracardiac vascular shunts is measured via pulsed-wave and continuous-wave Doppler. Pressure gradients between cardiac chambers can be calculated from blood flow velocity using the simplified Bernoulli equation (pressure gradient = 4 × peak velocity^2), which makes Doppler echocardiography a practical and noninvasive technique for estimating intracardiac chamber pressures (**Figure 7.17**).

CARDIAC BIOMARKERS

Cardiac biomarkers are biological molecules found in the blood that inform about the presence of cardiac disease.

Natriuretic peptide

Natriuretic peptides are released by the atria and ventricles in response to stretch caused by volume or pressure overload. A nonbiologically active fragment of the B-type natriuretic peptide (NT-proBNP) has been extensively studied. It has been suggested that NT-proBNP might

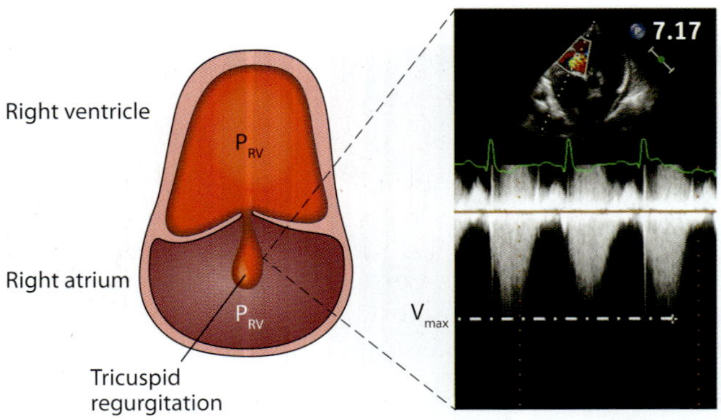

$$\Delta R = P_{RV} - P_{RA} = 4 \times V_{max}^2$$
$$P_{RV} = 4 \times V_{max}^2 + P_{RA} \text{ (mmHg)}$$

Add 5 if RA normal size
Add 10 if enlarged RA, no congestive heart failure
Add 15 if enlarged RA, no congestive heart failure

Figure 7.17 Use of Doppler echocardiography to estimate right ventricular pressure. In the presence of tricuspid regurgitation, the peak velocity of blood flow across the tricuspid valve can be obtained by spectral Doppler and depends on the pressure gradient between the right ventricle and the right atrium. The pressure in the right atrium can be approximated from its size and the presence or absence of heart failure. For example, if V = 5 m/s, $\Delta P = 4 \times 5^2 = 100$ mmHg; if the right atrium is normal size, right ventricular pressure is approximately 100 + 5 = 105 mmHg, indicating pulmonary hypertension. P_{RV}, right ventricular pressure in systole; P_{RA}, right atrial pressure; V_{max}, peak velocity.

be useful in identifying a cardiac cause for dyspnea, detecting occult cardiac disease (dilated cardiomyopathy [DCM], hypertrophic cardiomyopathy [HCM]), and predicting mortality in dogs with heart disease. However, studies have shown that NT-proBNP has limited value as a stand-alone test, but can be used to orientate a decision to pursue more advanced tests (chest radiographs, echocardiogram, Holter recording). Cut-off values vary between commercially available assays. Typically, NT-proBNP level is elevated in dogs with heart failure and increases as the heart enlarges. In cats with HCM, NT-proBNP concentration is increased. High NT-proBNP levels in a cat with pleural effusion strongly suggest a cardiac cause for the effusion. However, increased NT-proBNP concentration is also detected with hyperthyroidism, systemic hypertension and PH, and renal failure, because it is renally excreted.

Cardiac troponin I

Cardiac troponin I (cTnI) is one of the proteins involved in contraction of cardiomyocytes. Disruption of the membrane of some cardiomyocytes leads to leakage of cTnI into the circulation. Moderate to large elevations in cTnI concentration can be detected with current assays. Moderate elevations (approximately 10-fold increase compared with healthy animals) are common in the presence of CHF, third-degree AV block or subaortic stenosis (SAS). Large elevations (approximately 50–200-fold increase compared with healthy animals) are thought to indicate myocarditis if this diagnosis is supported by the history and clinical presentation. Important elevations of cTnI concentration also occur with myocardial infarction, but it is rare in dogs and cats.

HEART FAILURE

Definition/overview

Heart failure occurs when there is inadequate delivery of oxygen to the tissues of the body from impaired cardiac function and maldistribution of blood despite adequate venous return to the heart. CHF occurs with impaired cardiac function and a concurrent increase in venous and capillary pressures, which results in fluid accumulation in tissues and organs of the body.

Pathophysiology

Biomechanical, mechanical, and functional alterations occur in the failing heart. Biochemical changes are dominated by a decrease in the rate of adenosine triphosphate (ATP) hydrolysis. Cardiac contraction depends on the interaction between actin and myosin proteins, particularly the heavy meromyosin heads that repeatedly bind to actin. Decreased ATP hydrolysis leads to less interaction of heavy meromyosin heads with actin. The primary mechanical derangement in the failing heart is a reduction of the maximal velocity at which the heavy meromyosin heads can cycle, resulting in a decrease in myocardial fiber shortening. Overall, this is a decrease in contractility or pump function that is observed with heart failure. In a healthy heart, increased ventricular filling (or preload) results in a more forceful contraction. The failing heart, however, generates a lower force of contraction (systolic function) than expected despite an increased preload present prior to contraction. Hence, for any given preload, the systolic function is less than anticipated when compared with normal.

A small decrease in cardiac output is detected by high-pressure baroreceptors in the aorta and triggers an activation of the adrenergic system. Alpha and beta-adrenergic stimulation results in an increase in heart rate and cardiac contractility, as well as peripheral vasoconstriction. In addition to the stimulation of the sympathetic nervous system, renin is released from the kidneys secondary to decreased renal blood flow. Angiotensinogen is cleaved via renin to angiotensin I in the liver; angiotensin I is then cleaved by the angiotensin-converting enzyme (ACE) to angiotensin II in the vasculature. Angiotensin II activation results in: vasoconstriction; antidiuretic hormone (ADH) release from the posterior pituitary gland, which further constricts small arteries, arterioles, and veins and decreases urine production; and aldosterone release from the adrenal medulla, which results in sodium and water retention in the distal collecting duct. Moreover, over time angiotensin II stimulates myocardial hypertrophy, fibrosis, and vascular smooth muscle growth, leading to arteriolar narrowing (**Figure 7.18**).

Pulmonary edema from left-sided CHF occurs typically when left atrial pressure is above 18–22 mmHg (normally 7 mmHg) and a large volume of serum begins to weep from the pulmonary capillaries into the lung interstitium and alveolar space at a rate above the capacity of the pulmonary lymphatics to drain it in accordance with the principles of Starling's Law.

Clinical presentation

Animals with left-sided CHF (pulmonary edema) typically present with tachypnea and dyspnea depending on the chronicity and amount of edema accumulation. Thoracic auscultation most commonly reveals tachycardia; however, some cats and, rarely, dogs are bradycardic. Cardiac auscultation may also reveal the presence of heart murmurs, gallop sounds, and arrhythmias. Respiratory sounds are usually increased and crackles may or may not be present. Tachycardia with increased respiratory rate and effort in a dog is a more reliable indicator of pulmonary edema than the presence of crackles alone. Cough may be present but can commonly occur with airway disease in small breed dogs with concurrent mitral valve degeneration and tracheal collapse. Cough in a large breed dog is a more reliable indicator of pulmonary edema. Syncope may also be reported in dogs with mild pulmonary edema. More severe clinical signs include coughing up pink-tinged sputum; these animals require immediate emergency attention and exceptional measures such as intubation and mechanical ventilation (**Figure 7.19**).

Left-sided CHF in cats may differ from dogs in terms of clinical signs and fluid accumulation. Cats more frequently develop bradycardia, hypotension, and hypothermia. Additionally, left-sided CHF can also lead to pleural effusion and/or small amounts of pericardial effusion. Dual venous drainage of the pleural surfaces in cats can allow pleural effusion with left- and/or right-sided CHF. It is hypothesized that in cats with left-sided CHF, the visceral lung drainage via the pulmonary veins is impaired and pleural effusion results. Conversely,

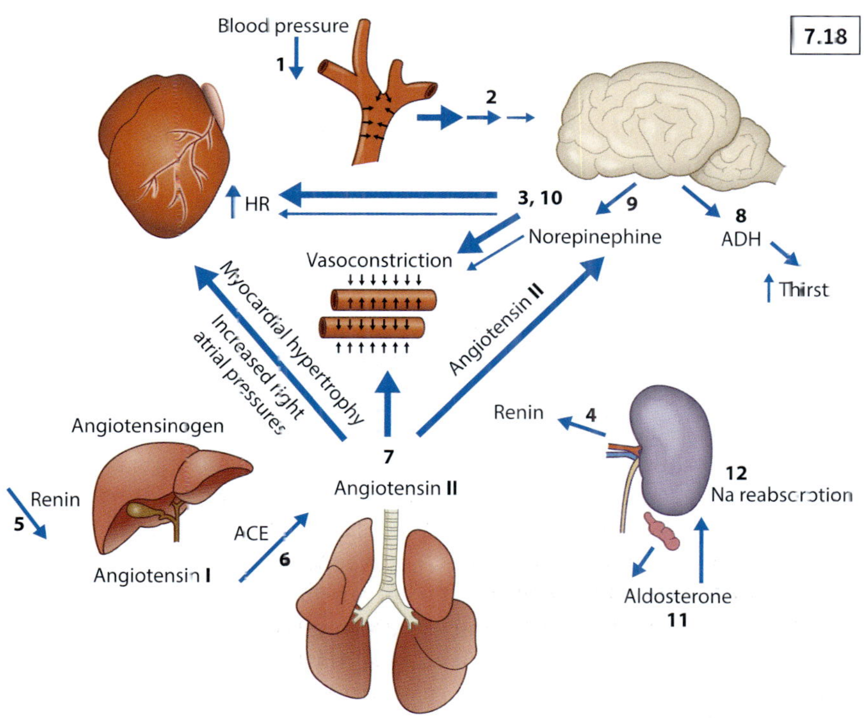

Figure 7.18 Sequence of compensatory mechanisms during heart failure. Numbers indicate the sequence of events. Vascular underfilling (1) detected by the arterial baroreceptors activates the sympathetic nervous system (2), resulting in vasoconstriction and tachycardia (3), and renin release (4). Activation of the renin angiotensin system (6) contributes to activation of the sympathetic system (9) and vasoconstriction (10). Release of ADH (8) causes thirst and aldosterone (11) is responsible for sodium and water retention (12).

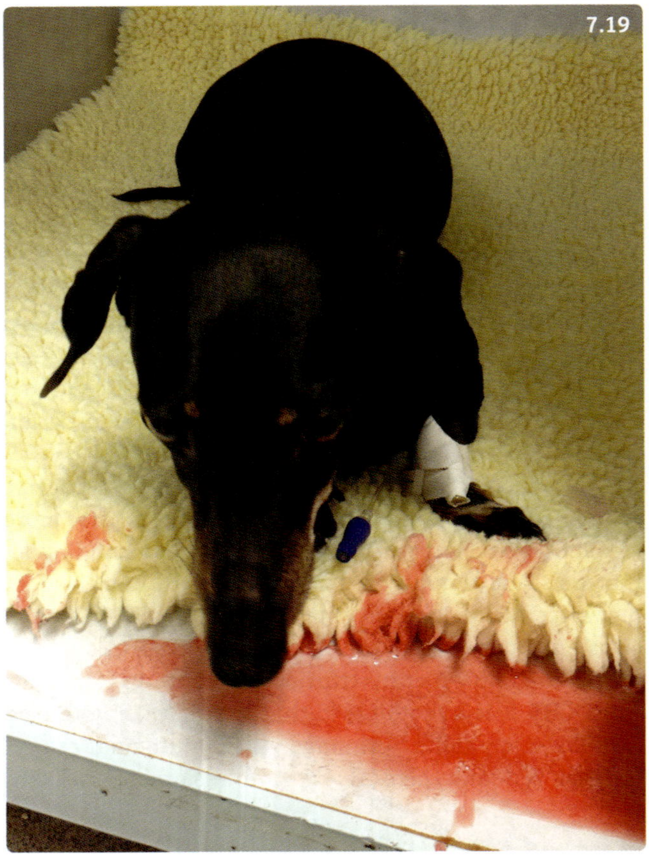

Figure 7.19 Dog with severe pulmonary edema coughing up pink, blood-tinged sputum.

pleural effusion in cats with right-sided CHF would result from impaired drainage of the parietal lung via the systemic veins.

Right-sided CHF in dogs typically causes ascites. Pleural effusion, pericardial effusion, and subcutaneous edema can also be seen, but tend to occur at a later stage of the disease than ascites. Pleural effusion alone is unusual but can be seen with tricuspid valve dysplasia (TVD)/stenosis, pericardial disease, cranial caval obstruction (functional or congenital), and supraventricular tachyarrhythmias. Signs of right-sided CHF include abdominal distension, jugular pulsation and distension, positive hepatojugular reflex, and possibly swollen subcutaneous tissue. Limb edema is most commonly seen with advanced disease and focal facial and neck swelling may suggest cranial caval obstruction or pericardial disease. Auscultation most commonly reveals tachycardia. Murmurs, gallop sounds, split S2 heart sounds, and arrhythmias may also be noted. Lung sounds and heart sounds may be decreased in the presence of a large volume of pleural effusion.

In cats, right-sided CHF is rare, and ascites alone in a cat is usually not cardiac-related. Pleural effusion is the most common presentation for right-sided CHF, albeit uncommon.

Differential diagnosis

Conditions that mimic left-sided CHF include pulmonary thromboembolism (PTE), noncardiogenic pulmonary edema (airway obstruction, strangulation, near-drowning, neurogenic), hemorrhage, neoplasia, systemic inflammatory response syndrome, and acute respiratory distress syndrome. Differential diagnoses for ascites and pleural effusion should include right-sided CHF, hypoalbuminemia, hepatic disease, vasculitis, hemorrhage, infection, and neoplasia.

Diagnosis

Diagnosis of left-sided CHF can be made readily from thoracic radiographs (see Chapter 6: Approach to thoracic radiographs). Pulmonary edema can be noted in canine patients, and pulmonary edema and/or pleural effusion may be noted in cats. In dogs, pulmonary infiltrates are most commonly seen in the caudodorsal lung lobes, and typically in the right caudal lung lobe first. Left-sided cardiomegaly will often be present, as well as pulmonary venous distension unless the patient is already being administered furosemide (**Figure 7.20**). In cats, pulmonary edema has a more diffuse distribution, and cardiomegaly may be more difficult to recognize than in dogs. Ultrasonography is a useful tool to detect pleural effusion.

Diagnosis of right-sided CHF can be made from physical examination, radiographs, and/or ultrasound. Thoracic radiographs may show pleural effusion and suggest ascites as a loss of detail in the cranial abdomen. Abdominal ultrasound shows abdominal effusion and hepatic venous congestion.

Management

Treatment recommendations are made according to a classification of the consecutive stages of heart failure (**Table 7.9**). Drugs indicated for the treatment of heart failure include diuretics, vasodilators, positive inotropes, and modulators of the autonomic tone (**Table 7.10**).

There is no consensus on the initiation of medical therapy before the onset of CHF. The initiation of ACE inhibitors in dogs with severe cardiac disease but no evidence of decompensation (late stage B2) is controversial. Dogs with stage B1 and B2 heart failure should be rechecked every 6–12 months to monitor the progression of the disease and educate the pet owner to recognize the signs of CHF. Whenever the risk of CHF is high, the pet owner should monitor the animal's resting respiratory rate on a daily basis. A resting respiratory rate above 40 bpm is a sensitive indicator of CHF and should trigger a visit to the veterinary clinic.

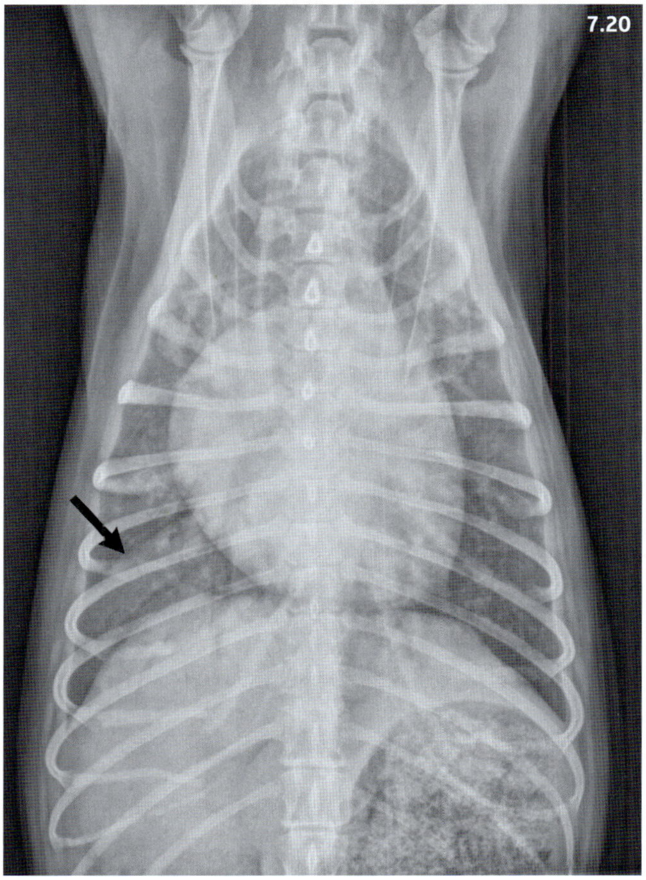

Figure 7.20 Radiograph from a dog with cardiogenic pulmonary edema. Note that the alveolar pattern is predominantly right sided (arrow).

Table 7.10 Drugs commonly used in treatment of congestive heart failure.

Diuretics	Furosemide 0.5–4 mg/kg PO, IM or IV q8–12h; usually 0.3–0.5 mg/kg/h CRI (up to 1 mg/kg/h in refractory cases) Spironolactone 0.5–2 mg/kg PO q12–24h Hydrochlorothiazide 0.5–1 mg/kg PO q12–24h Torsemide – total daily furosemide dose divided by 10 and split into PO q12h dosing
ACE inhibitors	Benazepril 0.25–0.5 mg/kg PO q24h Enalapril 0.25–0.5 mg/kg PO q12–24h
Positive inotropes	Pimobendan 0.2–0.4 mg/kg PO q12h Digoxin 0.005 mg/kg PO q12h Dobutamine 3–10 µg/kg/min IV CRI
Calcium channel blockers	Amlodipine 0.01–0.1 mg/kg PO q24h Diltiazem 0.5–2 mg/kg PO q8–12h Diltiazem extended release 2–3 mg/kg PO q12h
Beta-adrenergic receptor blockers	Atenolol 0.5–2 mg/kg PO q12–24h Propranolol (beta 1 & 2) 0.25–2 mg/kg PO q8h
Vasodilators	Nitroprusside 2–5 µg/kg/min CRI Hydralazine 0.5–3 mg/kg PO q12h
Nitrates	Nitroglycerin 0.5 inch/5 kg topically q8h Isosorbide dinitrate 0.2–2 mg/kg PO q12h
PDE-5 inhibitor	Sildenafil 1–3 mg/kg PO q8–12h

*All doses are for canines unless otherwise indicated. PDE-5, phosphodiesterase-5.

Table 7.9 Classification of heart failure stages (based on ACVIM consensus statement).

Stage of heart failure	Description
A	Animals at high risk for developing heart disease but currently have no identifiable structural disorder of the heart
B	Animals with structural heart disease (e.g. the typical murmur of mitral valve regurgitation is present), but have never developed clinical signs caused by heart failure: • **Stage B1:** Asymptomatic animals that have no radiographic or echocardiographic evidence of cardiac remodeling in response to CVHD • **Stage B2:** Asymptomatic animals that have hemodynamically significant valve regurgitation, as evidenced by radiographic or echocardiographic findings of left-sided heart enlargement
C	Animals with past or current clinical signs of heart failure associated with structural heart disease. May or may not require hospitalization and aggressive anticongestive therapy
D	Animals with end-stage disease with clinical signs of heart failure caused by CVHD that are refractory to standard therapy'. Such patients require advanced or specialized treatment strategies in order to remain clinically comfortable with their disease. As with stage C, some animals in stage D will require acute, hospital-based therapy and others can be managed as outpatients

CVHD, chronic valvular heart disease.

Treatment of left-sided CHF in dogs always involves administration of furosemide. IV, SC, or IM furosemide and oxygen therapy should be considered in patients with moderate to severe pulmonary edema and clinical signs. IV furosemide is beneficial in these patients to rapidly clear edema and cause inherent release of prostaglandins, which increase renal blood flow. Administration of furosemide as a constant rate infusion (CRI) is a good alternative to repeated boluses every few hours. However, a bolus of furosemide should always be given when the CRI is started. In hospitalized patients, IV dobutamine administration for positive inotropic support via direct beta-adrenergic stimulation can be considered, especially in patients with DCM or advanced mitral valve disease. Pimobendan is frequently administered during hospitalization as part of the management of acute heart failure. Afterload reduction with IV nitroprusside through direct vasodilatory properties can be considered, especially in cases of severe mitral valve degeneration that are refractory to standard diuretic therapy. Mild edema may be treated on an outpatient basis with possible single dose administration of furosemide (IV, SC, or IM) and continued therapy at home with oral furosemide. An ACE inhibitor should always be instituted for the long-term management of all cardiac patients with left-sided CHF as long as renal values and clinical signs related to renal disease are reasonable and the patient is eating well at home. ACE inhibitors are imperative for blunting the neurohormonal activation of the renin–angiotensin–aldosterone system (RAAS) system, which is stimulated by the continuous administration of furosemide. Administration of pimobendan has become part of the standard treatment protocol in all canine patients with left-sided CHF. Further RAAS blockade can be considered with spironolactone administration, an aldosterone blocker and weak potassium sparing diuretic. Arrhythmias that are present may also require treatment. Chronic refractory left-sided CHF can be managed by multi-nephron blockade with additional diuretics that work at different levels of the kidney (spironolactone, hydrochlorothiazide). Hydrochlorothiazide must be used very cautiously in patients with concurrent kidney disease, low sodium, and refractory CHF where ADH levels are likely high, as this diuretic will interfere with the ability of the patient to dilute urine and excrete solute free water. Torsemide, a diuretic 10 times more potent than furosemide, can be used to replace furosemide in chronic cases. Finally, sildenafil administration for treatment of severe PH can be considered, and for its possible effect of phosphodiesterase-5 inhibition in improving myocardial function in the ventricles.

Treatment of right-sided CHF in canine patients is similar to that for left-sided CHF. Typically, treatment is not as urgent, but initiation of injectable furosemide may be beneficial in cases with ascites where abdominal organs surrounded by fluid may not readily absorb oral furosemide. Body cavity fluid removal is as imperative as furosemide administration, and as much fluid as possible should be removed from the abdominal and/or pleural spaces (**Figure 7.21**). Oral administration of the medications discussed above is also recommended for right-sided CHF, with an emphasis on diagnosing and treating PH. Administering spironolactone is recommended by some, as normal aldosterone breakdown by the liver may be inhibited with a congested liver and right-sided CHF. Additionally, atrial tachyarrhythmias should also be investigated and treated, as loss of atrial contraction may worsen right-sided CHF more than left-sided CHF. Furosemide doses may also be more conservative in cases of severe PH where dramatic preload reduction may result in poor forward flow and systemic hypotension.

Treatment of cats with CHF will vary from dogs in five major ways: (1) furosemide dosage will be lower and more conservative; (2) efforts should be made to correct hypothermia and hypotension; (3) pimobendan is not indicated unless echocardiographic evidence of systolic dysfunction is noted; (4) hypokalemia is a common side-effect of furosemide therapy, therefore potassium concentration should be monitored frequently and oral supplementation initiated before signs of hypokalemia occur; (5) diuretics other than furosemide and spironolactone must be used with extreme caution.

PH, cough from bronchi compression by an enlarged heart, and syncope are also complications of heart failure that may require specific therapies (**Table 7.11**).

Prognosis

The average survival time for a patient with CHF is approximately 1–2 years with aggressive medical management. Dogs with right-heart failure and recurrent

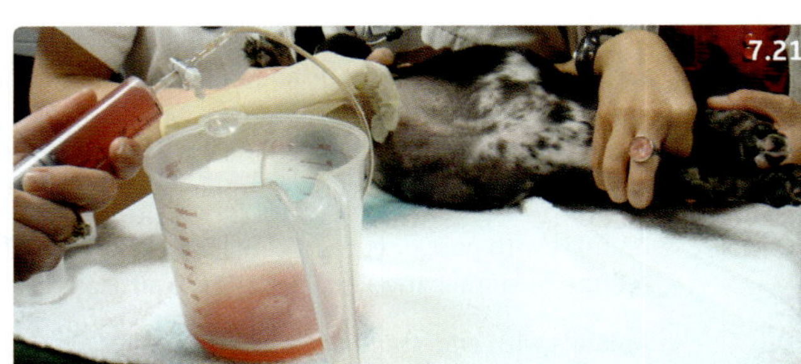

Figure 7.21 Abdominocentesis in a dog using a 16-gauge catheter. It is important to remove as much fluid as possible.

Table 7.11 Treatment of clinical signs of heart failure in the absence of congestive heart failure.

Clinical sign	Treatment
Syncope	Rule out CHF with radiographs. Start ACE inhibitor or increase current dose of furosemide or ACE inhibitor to alter loading of the heart
Pulmonary hypertension	Sildenafil 1–3 mg/kg PO q8–12h
Cough	Hydrocodone 0.25 mg/kg PO q6–12h Butorphanol 0.2–0.4 mg/kg PO q6–12h

ascites quickly develop cardiac cachexia, which significantly impairs their quality of life.

CONGENITAL HEART DISEASES

Congenital heart diseases (CHDs) are morphologic abnormalities of the heart and great vessels present at birth. CHDs are uncommon in dogs and rare in cats. The most common CHDs in the dog are SAS, PS, and PDA. The most common CHDs in the cat are atrial septal defects (ASDs) or ventricular septal defects (VSDs) and valvular dysplasias. Although many CHDs have breed predispositions and some have been shown to be heritable traits, not all CHDs are inherited (**Table 7.12**). CHDs are often diagnosed based on auscultation of a significant or unusual murmur in a young patient, leading to further cardiac work up. Swift detection may allow for treatment at an earlier stage of disease, improving patient prognosis and quality of life.

Table 7.12 Breed predisposition for congenital heart diseases.

Congenital defect	Breed predisposition	Known heritable mutation
Subaortic stenosis	Newfoundland, Rottweiler, Golden Retriever, Boxer, Great Dane, German Short-haired Pointer, German Shepherd Dog, Bouvier des Flandres, English Bulldog, Samoyed, Bull Terrier	Newfoundland
Pulmonic stenosis	English Bulldog, West Highland White Terrier, Beagle, Mastiff, Samoyed, Miniature Schnauzer, American Cocker Spaniel, Keeshond, Boxer, Chihuahua, Airedale Terrier	Beagle
Tricuspid valve dysplasia	Labrador Retriever, Golden Retriever, German Shepherd Dog	Labrador Retriever
Ventricular septal defect	Beagle, English Springer Spaniel, Keeshond, English Bulldog	Beagle, English Springer Spaniel
Atrial septal defect	Poodle, Dobermann, Boxer, Samoyed	Poodle
Mitral valve dysplasia	Bull Terrier, Rottweiler, Golden Retriever, Newfoundland, Mastiff, German Shepherd Dog	
Patent ductus arteriosus	Poodle, German Shepherd Dog, Pomeranian, Shetland Sheepdog, Collie, Maltese, Yorkshire Terrier, Chihuahua, Bichon Frise, Keeshond, American Cocker Spaniel, Rottweiler, English Springer Spaniel, Labrador Retriever, Newfoundland	Poodle
Tetralogy of Fallot	Keeshond, English Bulldog, Wire-haired Fox Terrier, Miniature Schnauzer, West Highland White Terrier	Keeshond
Persistent right aortic arch	German Shepherd Dog, Irish Setter, German Short-haired Pointer, Greyhound	German Short-haired Pointer

SUBAORTIC STENOSIS

Definition/overview

Aortic stenosis results from a narrowed left ventricular outflow tract in the region of the aortic valve, which can occur at a subvalvular, valvular, or supravalvular level. In dogs, the most common manifestation is SAS.

Etiology

A genetic mutation responsible for SAS has been identified in Newfoundlands.

Pathophysiology

Stenosis occurs from anomalous development of a fibrous band or ring of tissue at the subvalvular level, which interferes with blood flow. The induced pressure overload on the left ventricle causes left ventricular concentric hypertrophy and, sometimes, left atrial enlargement. The turbulence and increased velocity of flow through the stenotic outflow tract creates a left systolic basilar murmur. SAS predisposes to ventricular arrhythmias secondary to myocardial ischemia due to the increase in myocardial volume, diminished coronary blood flow, and subendocardial fibrosis. Less commonly, the increase in pressure in the left atrium can lead to left-sided CHF.

Clinical presentation

Animals with moderate to severe SAS often present with signs of failure to thrive, exercise intolerance, and syncope. Tachypnea or dyspnea associated with the development of CHF occurs in older dogs. Animals that develop rapid and sustained ventricular tachyarrhythmias may die suddenly. Physical examination reveals a left basilar systolic murmur whose grade correlates with the degree of SAS, weak femoral pulses when the stenosis is severe and, on occasion, arrhythmias.

Differential diagnosis

PS, VSD, physiologic murmur.

Diagnosis

Thoracic radiographs may show a poststenotic dilation of the aortic root. Definitive diagnosis is accomplished via echocardiography, which allows visualization of the location of the stenosis and the fibrous anomaly itself, as well as the severity of secondary changes, including left ventricular concentric hypertophy and atrial dilation (**Figure 7.22**). A small amount of aortic insufficiency is also habitually present. Color-flow echocardiography may show turbulent blood flow through the left ventricular outflow tract and can identify the severity of the stenosis based on the peak systolic aortic blood flow velocity. The severity of the stenosis is quantified by Doppler echocardiography (**Figure 7.23**). A pressure gradient above 80 mmHg across the stenosis is consistent with severe SAS. Boxers and Golden Retrievers, which are predisposed to SAS, can also have mild forms of the disease that result in soft murmurs that can be difficult to differentiate from physiologic murmurs. In Boxers, a narrow left ventricular outflow tract compared with similar sized dogs may explain the high prevalence of physiologic murmurs in this breed. For breeds with a high prevalence of SAS, programs that rely on auscultation and Doppler echocardiography to differentiate healthy dogs with physiologic murmurs from animals with mild SAS have usually been developed.

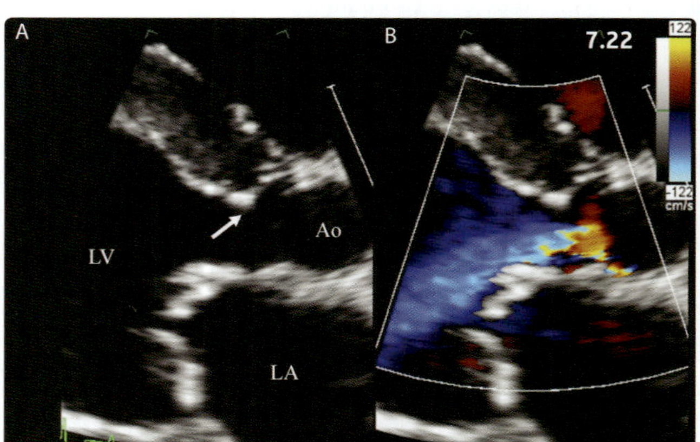

Figure 7.22 (A) Right parasternal long-axis echocardiographic view showing a subaortic ridge (arrow). (B) Color Doppler reveals turbulence in the aorta beyond the stenotic lesion.

Management

Moderate to severe SAS can be medically managed with beta-blockers (atenolol, 0.5–1 mg/kg PO q12–24h) to slow the heart rate, reduce myocardial oxygen demand, and for their antiarrhythmic properties. The goal of medical therapy is to decrease the frequency of syncopal episodes, improve exercise tolerance, and reduce the risk of sudden death. Interventional procedures to relieve the stenosis have had mixed results. Severe cases of SAS with a poor long-term prognosis may benefit from cardiac catheterization with a cutting balloon to relieve the pressure gradient across the stenosis, but this technique is as yet unproven in terms of improving quality of life and long-term outcome. The less common cases of valvular stenosis may improve with a more traditional balloon valvuloplasty technique. CHF is managed as appropriate with diuretic and ancillary medications. Antibiotics are

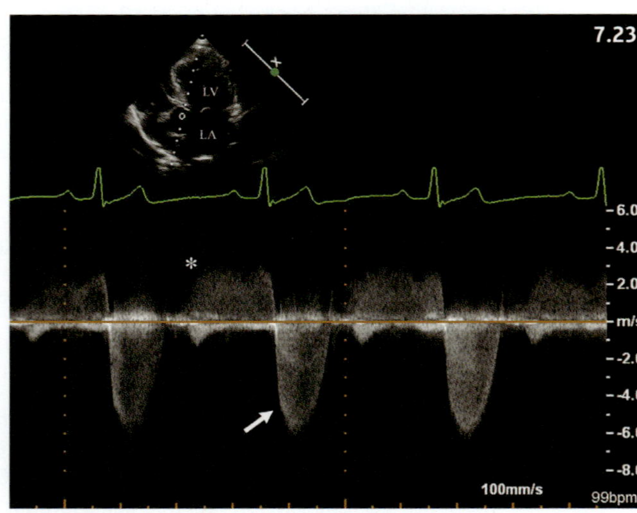

Figure 7.23 Continuous-wave Doppler recording of aortic flow in a dog with severe subaortic stenosis. The ultrasound beam has been oriented parallel to the blood flow from a left-sided apical four-chamber echocardiographic view. Peak velocity in systole is 6 m/sec (pressure gradient of 164 mmHg) and consistent with severe subaortic stenosis (arrow). There is also aortic insufficiency in diastole (*).

recommended during surgery and for dental prophylaxis procedures because of the mildly increased risk of infective endocarditis found in patients with SAS.

Prognosis
Mild SAS has a good prognosis, but cases of moderate SAS tend to develop CHF later in life. Dogs with severe SAS are at significant risk of sudden death before 3–5 years of age.

PULMONIC STENOSIS

Definition/overview
PS results from a narrowed right ventricular outflow tract in the region of the pulmonic valve, which can occur at a subvalvular, valvular, or supravalvular level. The most common manifestation in dogs is valvular. PS is less common in cats. The lesion consists of thickening or fusion of the valve leaflets, and may be accompanied by hypoplasia of the valve annulus. English Bulldogs often have an abnormal coronary vasculature, which consists of a single right coronary artery circling in front of the pulmonary artery to supply blood to the left ventricle (R2A anomaly) (**Figure 7.24**). This vessel might contribute to the stenosis, and may rupture or be occluded during balloon valvuloplasty, resulting in the dog's death. Other coronary abnormalities have been described in dogs with PS.

7.24

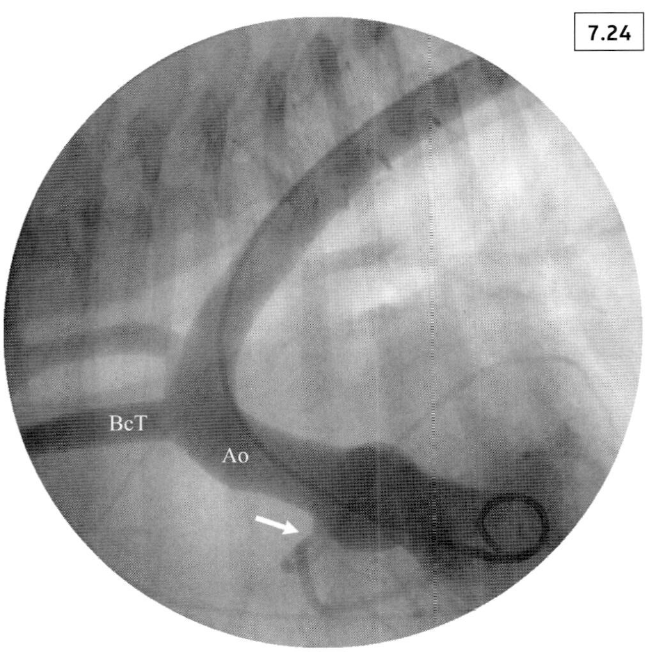

Figure 7.24 R2A anomaly in an English Bulldog. Aortogram using a pigtail catheter reveals a single coronary artery originating from the right coronary cusp (arrow). A branch crosses in front of the aorta and supplies blood to the left ventricle. Ao, aorta, BcT, brachiocephalic trunk.

Etiology
PS is heritable in Beagles.

Pathophysiology
The obstruction to flow results in an increased pressure within the right ventricle, causing concentric right ventricular hypertrophy and myocardial fibrosis with possible dilation of the right atrium. Turbulent blood flow and increased velocity through the stenotic valve result in a left basilar systolic murmur. Patients with severe PS develop right-sided diastolic dysfunction and ultimately are at risk of right-sided CHF from chronic pressure overload. Right ventricular myocardial failure may eventually result from severe PS. TVD is an occasional concurrent congenital defect and results in exacerbation of right heart dysfunction and more severe clinical signs.

Clinical presentation
Most animals with PS will have no to mild clinical signs. The approximately one-third of dogs with PS that do exhibit clinical signs often present with dyspnea, lethargy, exercise intolerance, or syncope. In later stages, signs associated with right-sided heart failure may be present. Physical examination reveals a left-sided systolic basilar murmur (with a concurrent right apical murmur if tricuspid regurgitation is present). Jugular distension is associated with an increase in right atrial pressure. If right-sided CHF is present, abdominal palpation may reveal the presence of ascites and hepatomegaly. The presence of a patent foramen ovale at the atrial level can be the site of right-to-left blood shunting, leading to cyanosis, hypoxemia, and polycythemia.

Differential diagnosis
SAS, physiologic murmur, tetralogy of Fallot (TOF), VSD.

Diagnosis
Thoracic radiographs often show the presence of poststenotic dilation of the pulmonary trunk and right-sided cardiomegaly. Echocardiography is used to determine the structure of the pulmonic valve and the severity of ventricular concentric hypertrophy and to detect the presence of tricuspid insufficiency (**Figure 7.25**). Doppler echocardiography is essential to determine the severity of the stenosis. Continuous-wave Doppler is used to determine the peak systolic pressure gradient across the stenosis. Good alignment of the Doppler beam with blood flow can usually be obtained from the right parasternal short-axis view at the level of the pulmonary artery or from a left cranial window along the sternum. The severity of the stenosis is based on peak systolic pressure gradient. It is mild when the peak gradient is between 20 and

49 mmHg (velocity of 2.25–3.5 m/sec), moderate when peak gradient is between 50 and 80 mmHg (velocity of 3.5–4.5 m/sec), and severe if the peak gradient is above 80 mmHg (velocity above 4.5 m/sec).

Management

The goal of treatment is to reduce the systolic right ventricular pressure overload. This is accomplished in cases of moderate to severe PS via surgical procedures or balloon valvuloplasty. Balloon valvuloplasty works best in cases of valvular stenosis without hypoplasia of the valve annulus (**Figure 7.26**). Generally, a reduction of 40–50% can be expected in the pressure gradient, and this reduction is maintained in the majority of cases. In cases of mild PS or those with mild clinical signs, beta-blockers can be used to reduce myocardial oxygen demand and for their antiarrhythmic properties.

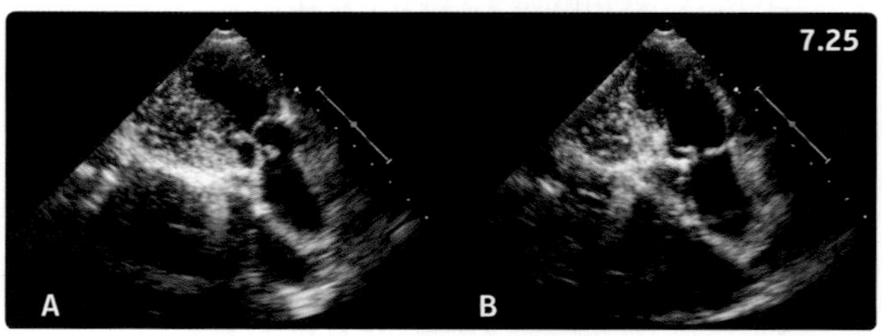

Figure 7.25 Right parasternal short-axis echocardiographic view from a dog with pulmonic valve stenosis. The valve is shown in diastole (A). In systole, the valve takes a dome-like shape (B).

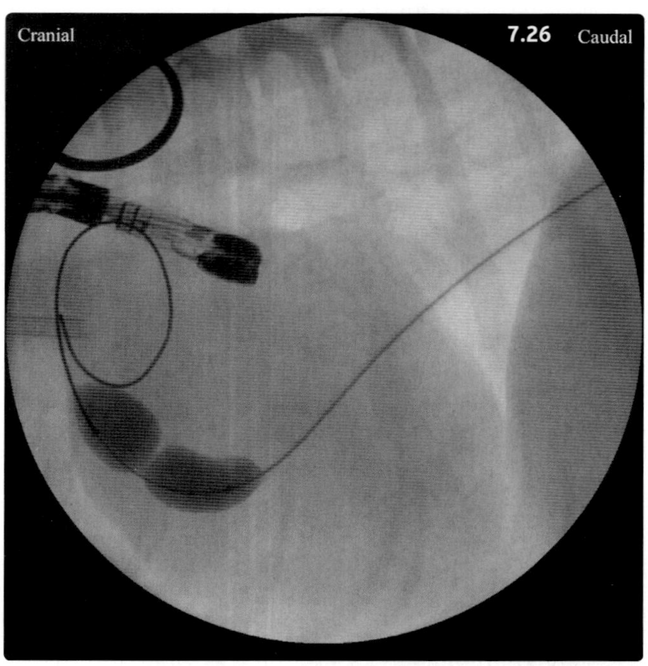

Figure 7.26 Fluroscopic view during balloon valvuloplasty. The catheter is inserted from a femoral vein and positioned at the level of the pulmonic valve. During inflation a waist is seen in the center of the balloon. Abrupt expansion of the balloon usually results in a successful procedure.

Prognosis

Prognosis varies based on the severity of the stenosis.

PATENT DUCTUS ARTERIOSUS

Definition/overview

The ductus arteriosus during fetal development serves to shunt oxygenated blood from maternal circulation away from the fetal lungs directly to the systemic circulation. When the lungs inflate at birth, reversal of the blood flow brings oxygenated blood from the aorta through the ductus and stimulates constriction of the ductus smooth muscle. Normally, the ductus closes by 7–10 days after birth. A PDA occurs when the ductus remains patent past this period, allowing blood to shunt according to the pressure gradient.

Etiology

PDA is considered heritable in Poodles.

Pathophysiology

In most cases, a PDA results in blood shunting from the aorta to the pulmonary artery (left-to-right shunt) and a left-sided volume overload. The blood shunting directly to the pulmonary circulation returns to the left side of the heart. As a result, the left ventricle and left atrium become dilated. Large shunts increase the filling pressure in the left heart and pulmonary veins, with the end result being left-sided CHF. The severity of the shunt (mostly determined by the size of the patent vessel) and the presence of other defects result in varying progression of secondary changes. In rare cases with large shunts and severe PH, shunt reversal is observed. Blood thus flows from the pulmonary artery to the aorta – a right-to-left shunt – causing a differential cyanosis, hypoxemia, and eventually polycythemia (Eisenmenger's physiology). Shunt reversal typically occurs in puppies that are a few days to a few weeks old. It is not the usual progression of a PDA in adult dogs.

Clinical presentation

Clinical signs vary based on the size of the shunt, the direction of the shunt, and the presence of CHF. Signs may include exercise intolerance, syncope, cough or dyspnea, and, in the case of a reverse shunt, hindlimb weakness or seizures. On physical examination of animals with a left-to-right PDA, a pathognomonic continuous (machinery) murmur is heard cranially in the left axillary region.

Bounding femoral pulses may be palpated due to diastolic run-off. In animals with a reverse PDA, there is no audible murmur, but careful inspection of the mucous membranes should reveal differential cyanosis, that is cyanosis limited to the caudal mucous membranes.

Differential diagnosis

Aortopulmonary window, which is a connection between the ascending aorta and the pulmonary trunk. A to-and-fro murmur from aortic stenosis and insufficiency could mimic the continuous murmur heard with a PDA.

Diagnosis

Thoracic radiographs may show left-sided cardiomegaly, pulmonary overcirculation, signs of CHF, and a ductal aneurysm of the aorta at the insertion of the ductus. Electrocardiography frequently shows a tall R wave in lead II (indicative of left ventricular enlargement). Echocardiography is necessary to confirm the presence of the shunt, evaluate the severity of left heart chamber enlargement, and identify concurrent CHDs and the presence of mild to severe PH. Measurement of the shunt is performed to determine suitable procedures for shunt closure (**Figure 7.27**).

Management

PDAs are best treated with early closure, either by surgical or cardiac catheterization procedures. Medical treatment for patients in CHF is indicated prior to closure. Small patients not amenable to catheterization are best treated surgically; surgery performed by experienced surgeons has a success rate of up to 95% (**Figure 7.28**). Other current interventional procedures used to close shunts use catheterization to place coils (coil embolization) or other devices produced specifically to interrupt blood flow across the shunt (occluder, vascular plug) (**Figure 7.29**). Residual flow after intervention, if present, may decrease over time. The risk of infection of the implants

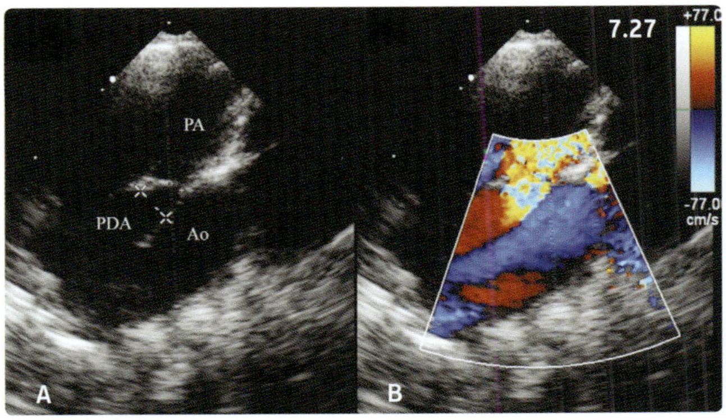

Figure 7.27 (A) Transthoracic echocardiographic view of a patent ductus arteriosus (PDA). Measurements of the PDA diameters are obtained. (B) Color Doppler reveals turbulence (mosaic of colors) in the pulmonary artery. PA, pulmonary artery; PDA, patent ductus arteriosus; Ao, aorta.

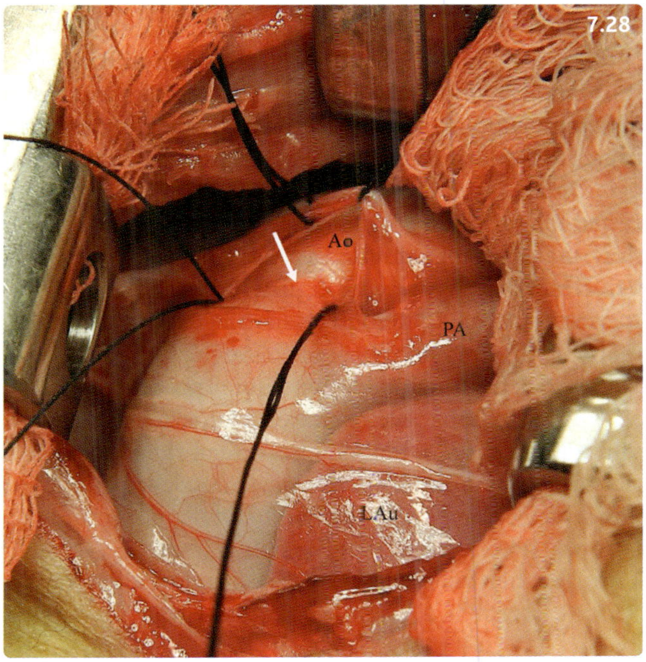

Figure 7.28 Surgical ligation for a patent ductus arteriosus (arrow) from a left thoracotomy. Ao, aorta; PA, pulmonary artery; LAu, left auricle.

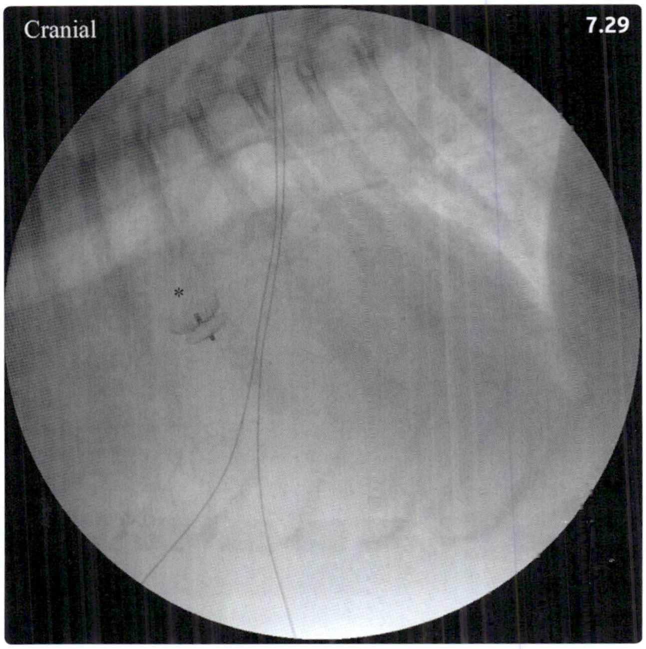

Figure 7.29 Lateral thoracic radiograph from a dog after patent ductus arteriosus occlusion with an Amplatz Canine Duct Occluder (*). (Manufacturer: Infiniti Medical, LLC)

is unknown; antibiotics are recommended during surgery and for dental prophylaxis procedures for 1 year after the implant is placed. Closure of reverse PDAs is contraindicated.

Prognosis

Secondary changes can reverse with early and successful closure of the PDA, and in these cases prognosis is excellent. Animals with a PDA that is not closed rarely live past 1 year of age, although some, albeit rare, have been known to live well into adulthood with an uncorrected PDA.

VENTRICULAR SEPTAL DEFECTS

Definition/overview

VSDs are defects that allow communication between the left and right ventricles. The most common form is a defect in the membranous, or upper, portion of the septum. It is the most common congenital cardiac defect in cats.

Etiology

VSDs are heritable defects in Keeshonds and English Springer Spaniels.

Pathophysiology

Blood shunts from left to right during systole. Because of the location of VSDs in the upper portion of the outflow tract, the increased blood flow enters almost immediately into the pulmonary artery and returns to the left heart. Therefore, VSDs in dogs and cats typically result in volume overload of the left ventricle and atrium. The outcome of a VSD depends on the size of the defect and the pressure gradient between the systemic and the pulmonary circulation. Small VSDs that restrict blood flow have minimal hemodynamic consequences. Larger VSDs can result in left-sided volume overload and, subsequently, left-sided CHF. They also have the potential to cause significant pulmonary overcirculation and lead to PH. In the presence of severe PH, right ventricular pressure may exceed left ventricular pressure during part of or the entire duration of the cardiac cycle, resulting in reversal of the shunt (right-to-left shunt) and cyanosis (Eisenmenger's physiology).

Clinical presentation

Physical examination findings associated with a VSD depend on the size of the shunt and the pressure gradient between the pulmonary and the systemic circulation. Left-to-right shunts result in a right-sided, sternal or left basilar systolic murmur depending on the location of the septal defect on the interventricular septum. Smaller VSDs often result in a greater velocity of blood flow through the shunt and may have a louder murmur, but are often associated with fewer secondary changes. Blood overflow through a VSD located in the basilar portion of the septum may damage the cusps of the aortic valve, leading to aortic insufficiency and a left basilar diastolic murmur on auscultation. A large VSD allowing pressures between the two ventricles to equalize may cause a softer murmur or no audible murmur at all. Signs associated with CHF or hypoxemia may be present.

Differential diagnosis

Mitral regurgitation, tricuspid regurgitation, SAS, PS.

Diagnosis

Diagnosis is made by visualization of the defect or the shunt with color-flow Doppler echocardiography. On echocardiography, the size of the VSD can be compared with the diameter of the aortic annulus. Small VSDs are less than 25%, moderate VSDs are between 25 and 75%, and large VSDs are more than 75% the aortic diameter. Various parameters are assessed to determine the clinical significance of VSDs. The direction and velocity of blood flow across small defects is recorded by Doppler imaging. Color Doppler technique is used to scan the surface of the interventricular septum from different views and demonstrates a left-to-right turbulent, high velocity jet during systole (**Figure 7.30**). Blood flow velocity measurements recorded by continuous-wave Doppler are used to estimate the pressure gradient across the defect using the simplified Bernoulli's equation. The normal pressure gradient between the ventricles is around 100 mmHg (which corresponds to blood flow velocity of approximately 5 m/sec). Assessment of left atrium and ventricle size and assessment of left ventricular function can be done with Doppler imaging.

The size of restrictive VSDs determines the risk of left ventricular volume overload and CHF. The clinical significance is better determined by measuring the size of the left-sided cardiac chambers. Follow-up examinations are usually necessary to determine the long-term hemodynamic consequences of a VSD.

Management

VSDs are treated based on the severity of secondary changes and clinical signs. Small VSDs may not require any intervention and have a good prognosis. Hemodynamically significant left-to-right VSDs are managed medically when signs of left-sided CHF occur. The cyanosis and polycythemia that result from right-to-left VSDs may improve with sildenafil, which targets PH.

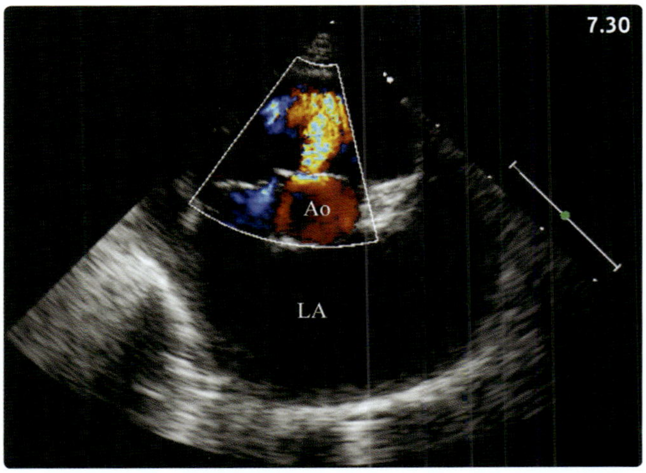

Figure 7.30 Right parasternal short-axis echocardiographic view confirming the presence of a ventricular septal defect with color-flow Doppler. Turbulent blood flow is seen entering the right ventricle from a defect located just below the aorta in the perimembranous portion of the interventricular septum. Ao, aorta; LA, left atrium.

Prognosis
Prognosis varies based on the size of the VSD.

ATRIAL SEPTAL DEFECTS

Definition/overview
ASDs are defects that occur due to malformation of the septum primum and septum secondum.

Pathophysiology
ASDs typically result in a left-to-right shunt of blood. This may cause dilation of the right heart, pulmonary overcirculation, and right heart failure. However, most shunts are small and have minimal hemodynamic consequences. When right-sided heart disease results in elevated right atrial pressures, the direction of blood flow across the ASD may change.

Clinical presentation
ASDs rarely cause a murmur because the low volume and low pressure gradient across the defect do not result in high velocity turbulent blood flow. On occasion, a soft left basilar systolic blood flow is ausculted. This is due to the increased volume of blood circulating within the right ventricular outflow tract, which becomes turbulent. Most ASDs remain asymptomatic. Large defects or those associated with another congenital defect may result in signs of right heart failure or shunt reversal with various degrees of cyanosis and hypoxemia.

Differential diagnosis
Mild SAS, mild PS, physiologic murmur.

Diagnosis
Diagnosis is made by echocardiographic visualization of the defect.

Management
Most small ASDs do not require treatment. Large defects cause right heart failure if not treated surgically, which may be difficult due to limited access and expense. Right heart failure is managed medically, if it develops.

Prognosis
Prognosis varies based on the size of the ASD. Most small ASDs have an excellent prognosis.

MITRAL VALVE DYSPLASIA

Definition/overview
Mitral valve dysplasia (MVD) occurs from malformation of the mitral valve apparatus and can include the valve leaflets, chordae tendineae, or papillary muscles. Large breed dogs are predisposed.

Pathophysiology
Severe MVD causes significant mitral regurgitation and can cause secondary changes similar to degenerative valvular disease. In dogs, valve insufficiency frequently occurs in combination with valve stenosis. Long-term complications include the development of left-sided CHF.

Clinical presentation
Physical examination findings with MVD include a left apical systolic murmur whose intensity correlates with the severity of the regurgitation. Signs associated with arrhythmias or CHF may be present.

Differential diagnosis
Mitral regurgitation from degenerative valve disease, DCM.

Diagnosis
Thoracic radiographs and echocardiography may show variable levels of left-sided heart enlargement; if CHF is present, signs of pulmonary edema in dogs or edema and/or pleural effusion in cats may be present. Echocardiography will reveal the abnormalities of the mitral valve apparatus.

Management

Medical management consists of treating heart failure and any arrhythmias.

Prognosis

Prognosis is poor due to the early onset of arrhythmias and/or CHF.

TRICUSPID VALVE DYSPLASIA

Definition/overview

TVD occurs from malformation of the tricuspid valve apparatus and can include the valve leaflets, chordae tendineae, or papillary muscles.

Etiology

TVD is the most common CHD in Labrador Retrievers and is heritable in that breed.

Pathophysiology

TVD causes significant tricuspid regurgitation and can cause elevations in right atrial pressures and development of right-sided CHF.

Clinical presentation

Physical examinations findings with TVD include a right apical systolic murmur; however, mild TVD may not result in an auscultable murmur. Signs associated with arrhythmias or CHF may be present. A common arrhythmia in dogs with TVD is atrial fibrillation (AF).

Differential diagnosis

Tricuspid regurgitation, VSD, DCM.

Diagnosis

Radiographically, dogs with TVD often have dramatic right atrial enlargement, a dilated caudal vena cava, and hepatomegaly. Cats have an enlarged right atrium and a dilated, tortuous caudal vena cava. Right heart failure in dogs may cause signs of jugular venous distension, hepatomegaly, and ascites. Electrocardiography may show supraventricular arrhythmias, and splintered QRS complexes are a common finding in dogs (**Figure 7.31**). Echocardiography reveals structural abnormalities of the tricuspid valve apparatus (**Figure 7.32**).

Management

TVD is treated medically by managing CHF and arrhythmias.

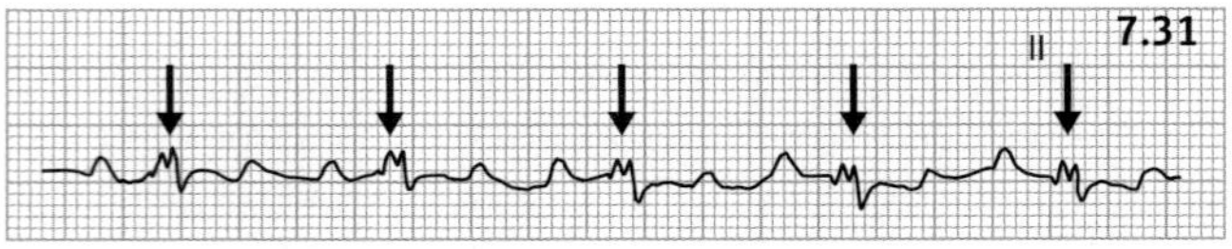

Figure 7.31 ECG from a dog with tricuspid dysplasia. There is a sinus rhythm with splintered QRS complexes (arrows). (Amplitude 10 mm/mV, speed 50 mm/sec)

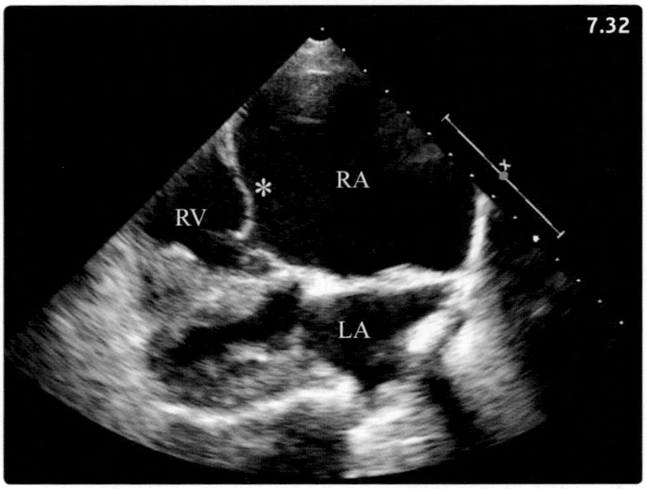

Figure 7.32 Right parasternal long-axis echocardiographic view from a dog with tricuspid dysplasia. The right atrium is markedly dilated and the parietal leaflet of the tricuspid valve is elongated (*). RA, right atrium; RV, right ventricle; LA, left atrium.

Prognosis

Prognosis is poor when tricuspid valve regurgitation is severe due to the early onset of arrhythmias and/or CHF. Dogs with mild TVD have a normal life expectancy.

TETRALOGY OF FALLOT

Definition/overview

The four defects that form the TOF consist of a VSD, dextroposition of the aorta, PS, and the resulting right ventricular concentric hypertrophy. Abnormal development of the conotruncal septum results in this combination of defects.

Etiology

TOF is heritable in Keeshonds.

Pathophysiology

PS increases the right ventricular pressures and results in various degrees of right-to-left shunting across the VSD. The consequences include cyanosis, hypoxemia, and polycythemia. Concurrent CHD may be present.

Clinical presentation

TOF is usually accompanied by a systolic murmur originating from the PS and/or the VSD. Animals with TOF may develop episodes of respiratory difficulties when the right-to-left shunting worsens, causing systemic hypoxemia.

Differential diagnosis

PS, VSD.

Diagnosis

Thoracic radiographs show right heart enlargement and pulmonary undercirculation. Echocardiography allows for visualization of the VSD, quantification of PS severity, the displacement of the aortic root towards the right side, and right ventricular hypertrophy. Color-flow Doppler is needed to visualize the shunt.

Management

Medical management is aimed at limiting right-to left shunting and hypoxemia by blunting the decrease in systemic vascular resistance in response to exercise with the administration of oral nonselective beta-blockers (propranolol). Phlebotomies are indicated when polycythemia is responsible for clinical signs (usually PCV above 70%).

Prognosis

Prognosis varies based on the severity of the shunt and right ventricular pressure overload. Most dogs with TOF reach the age of 5 years.

VASCULAR RING ANOMALIES

Definition/overview

Vascular ring anomalies occur from persistence of vessels that normally regress during development, or abnormalities in vessel formation. The most common vascular ring is a persistent right aortic arch (PRAA).

Etiology

There is evidence that PRAA is heritable in German Shorthaired Pointers and Greyhounds.

Pathophysiology

Normally, the right aortic arch develops into the brachiocephalic trunk and right subclavian artery and the left aortic arch persists as the dorsal aorta. When the right aorta persists with a left ligamentum arteriosum, a vascular ring forms around the trachea and esophagus with the heart base forming the last portion of the ring. A retroesophageal subclavian artery is the most common concurrent anomaly. PRAA alone does not result in cardiac abnormalities.

Clinical presentation

PRAA is usually suspected based on the onset of regurgitation when a puppy is introduced to solid food. This occurs due to esophageal constriction by the vascular ring. Signs of aspiration pneumonia may be present.

Differential diagnosis

Esophageal stricture, congenital megaesophagus, other gastrointestinal (GI) disorders.

Diagnosis

Diagnosis is often made based on clinical signs and thoracic radiographs. Thoracic radiographs show leftward deviation of the trachea cranial to the border of the heart in ventrodorsal views, and barium esophagrams can aid in diagnosis based on constriction of the esophagus at the heart base with cranial dilatation (see **Figures 8.15–8.17**). Definitive diagnosis may require advanced imaging or surgical exploration.

Management

Surgical ligation is the treatment of choice for PRAA and other vascular anomalies resulting in constricting vascular rings. Surgical procedures vary based on the type of vascular ring and the presence of concurrent anomalies. Early surgical treatment is recommended to prevent progressive esophageal dysfunction, although there have been reports of successful surgical treatment in adult dogs.

Prognosis

Prognosis is good with early intervention and dietary modification.

ACQUIRED VALVULAR DISEASES

DEGENERATIVE MITRAL VALVE DISEASE

Definition/overview

Degenerative mitral valve disease is the most common form of acquired cardiovascular disease in dogs, representing approximately 75% of all cardiology cases seen in practice. It particularly affects small breed, middle aged to older dogs and an earlier onset has been reported in males. There are known breed predispositions, such as the Cavalier King Charles Spaniel and Dachshund. However, large breed dogs may also develop the disease. The mitral valve is affected alone in 60% of cases, the tricuspid valve alone in 10% of cases, and both valves are affected in 30% of cases. Rarely, involvement of the aortic and pulmonic valves is seen.

Etiology

The etiology is unknown, although there is a known genetic component. It has been suggested that there are predisposing abnormalities/disruptions in the collagen and extracellular matrix components, with accumulation of proteoglycans and glycosaminoglycans in the spongiosa layer of the valve. Although the inciting factor for degenerative valve disease is not certain, high levels of circulating serotonin have been shown to cause valvular changes.

Pathophysiology

Myxomatous lesions of the valve progress over time. These abnormalities also extend to the chordae tendineae. These changes lead to thickening of the free edge of the valve leaflets and secondary fibrosis causes contracture of the valve leaflets and chordae, preventing normal coaptation. This scenario leads to various degrees of regurgitation, leading to left-sided volume overload and atrial and ventricular enlargement.

Clinical presentation

The clinical presentation varies with the severity of the disease. Very early in the disease process, the only abnormality on physical examination may be a systolic click associated with mitral valve prolapse. In most cases, the first clinical sign is a systolic murmur with a PMI in the region of the mitral valve. Worsening of the murmur intensity usually coincides with worsening disease severity. Coughing and exercise intolerance are also common presenting complaints. Often dogs will remain preclinical for long periods of time and will only show clinical signs at the onset of CHF (**Table 7.9**).

Differential diagnosis

The differential diagnoses for systolic heart murmurs are reviewed in the physical examination section of this chapter. Differential diagnoses for the respiratory signs seen include CHF, pneumonia, compression of the left mainstem bronchus by the enlarged left atrium, tracheal collapse, and primary lower airway disease such as chronic bronchitis.

Diagnosis

The diagnosis of degenerative mitral valve disease is generally easily made based on physical examination findings and patient signalment. However, it is important to confirm the diagnosis with echocardiography. Radiography should also be used to assist in assessing disease severity, presence/absence of CHF, and disease progression. Generalized cardiomegaly with left atrial and left ventricular enlargement is seen radiographically in dogs that are stage B and higher. If CHF is present, an interstitial-to-alveolar pattern is commonly seen in the perihilar and caudal lobar regions. Echocardiography will show a thickened and irregular valve (**Figure 7.33**), valvular insufficiency during systole (**Figure 7.34**), and atrial and ventricular eccentric hypertrophy dependent on the affected valve(s).

Management

Management depends on the stage of the disease present. Animals in stage A do not require therapy. There is disagreement regarding stage B dogs, as studies in humans have shown benefit of ACE inhibitor therapy, but it was unclear in veterinary clinical trials. It is possible that ACE inhibitors benefit dogs when the disease is compensated but severe left atrial enlargement is present. Stage C and D dogs should be treated with the appropriate medications to control the signs of CHF (see Congestive heart failure, Management).

Prognosis

Disease progression and prognosis are variable, with many dogs remaining asymptomatic for their entire lifetime. However, from onset of CHF, the average survival time is 12–18 months with medical management.

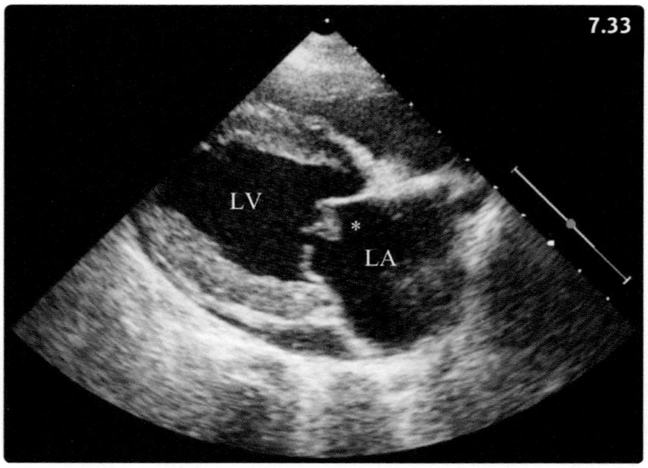

Figure 7.33 Right parasternal long-axis echocardiographic view from a dog with severe degenerative mitral valve disease. The septal leaflet of the mitral valve (*) is markedly thickened and prolapses into the left atrium. LA, left atrium; LV, left ventricle.

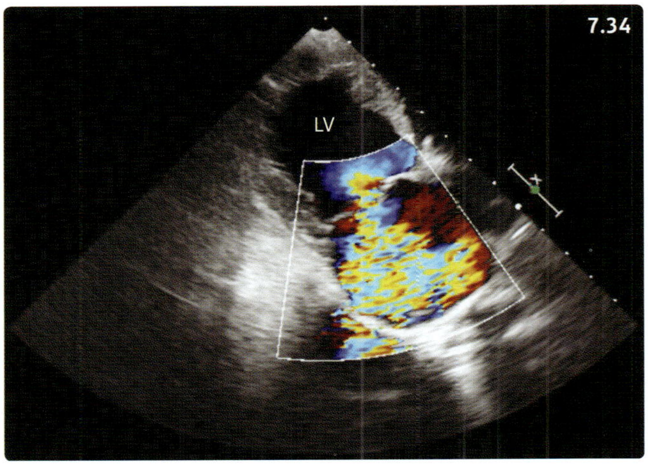

Figure 7.34 Color Doppler showing severe mitral valve regurgitation filling more than 50% of the left atrium. The mosaic of color indicates turbulent blood flow. LV, left ventricle.

BACTERIAL ENDOCARDITIS

Definition/overview

Endocarditis corresponds to an infection and secondary inflammation of the endocardial surface following a transient or persistent bacteremia. Vegetative endocarditis occurs when vegetations composed of platelets, fibrin, bacteria, and inflammatory cells are found adhered to heart valves. Clinical signs vary widely and are vague, making recognition difficult. The reported incidence of infectious endocarditis in dogs and cats is very low, with the highest incidence in male, middle aged, medium to large breed dogs, particularly German Shepherd Dogs.

Etiology

Endothelial damage in conjunction with bacteremia is required for infectious endocarditis to develop. The underlying cause of the damage to the endothelium is unproven, although patients with SAS are at increased risk. It is usually not possible to identify the origin of the bacteremia. The most common bacterial isolates are *Staphylococcus* spp. and *Escherichia coli*, with *Streptococcus* spp., *Corynebacteria* spp., and *Erysipelothrix rhusiopathiae* also reported. Recently, *Bartonella* spp. have emerged as important causative agents.

Pathophysiology

In companion animals, infectious endocarditis involves mitral and aortic valve tissue in the majority of cases. Once endothelial damage has occurred, bacteria bind and are covered by fibrin. Additional layers of bacteria and fibrin are deposited to form vegetative lesions, which lead to the destruction of normal valvular and chordal tissue, leading to valvular insufficiency and possible stenosis. Acute vegetative lesions are composed of an inner layer of platelets, fibrin, red blood cells, white blood cells, and some bacteria; a middle layer of bacteria; and an outer layer of fibrin. These vegetations are friable and commonly embolize to distant sites (**Figure 7.35**).

Clinical presentation

The clinical presentation is highly variable and nonspecific, with the most common clinical signs being waxing and waning fever, lethargy, depression, anorexia, weight loss, shifting leg lameness, dyspnea, and tachypnea. These signs can be acute or chronic and are related to the organs affected by bacteremia, septic thrombi, and secondary immune complex formation and deposition.

A new or changing murmur is considered highly suggestive for endocarditis, although lack of a murmur should not preclude the diagnosis. Both systolic (more common) and diastolic murmurs occur, along with arrhythmias. CHF, polyarthritis, and glomerulonephritis are common sequelae.

Differential diagnosis

Differential diagnoses for systolic heart murmurs are reviewed in the physical examination section of this chapter. Infectious, inflammatory, and immune-mediated causes of glomerulonephritis, polyarthritis, and fever of unknown origin should also be ruled out.

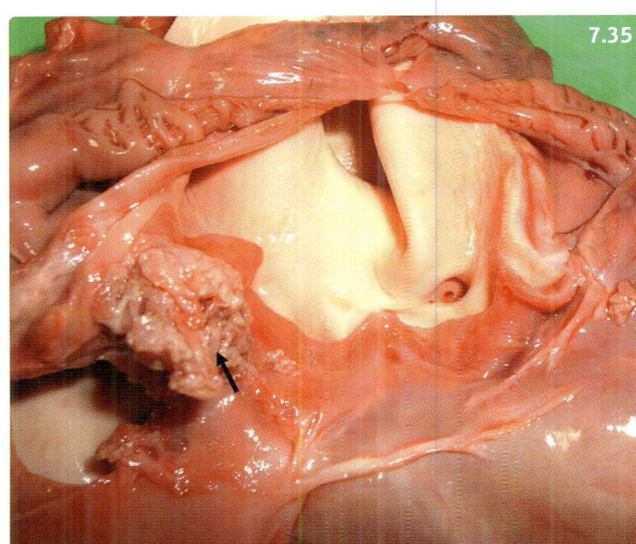

Figure 7.35 Vegetative lesion (arrow) on the aortic valve of a dog.

Diagnosis

Recognition and diagnosis of endocarditis can be very difficult, in part because of the vague clinical signs and clinicopathologic findings. Radiography may be unremarkable or may show cardiomegaly and signs of left-sided CHF. ECG will often show rhythm disturbances, with ventricular rhythms and AV block being most common. Echocardiography is the gold standard of diagnostics and will often show a hyperechoic, independently oscillating lesion on the affected valve (**Figure 7.36**). Clinicopathologic laboratory findings can help support the diagnosis, but are often nonspecific. They include leukocytosis, nonregenerative anemia, thrombocytopenia, hypoalbuminemia, an elevated alkaline phosphatase, and azotemia. Urinalysis may show changes consistent with a glomerulonephritis or bacterial infection, which may be the source of bacteremia or secondary to it. Blood cultures should be taken, although they have both a low sensitivity and low specificity. A negative culture should not be used to exclude the diagnosis of endocarditis.

Management

The goals of treatment are to sterilize the vegetative lesion and address cardiac and systemic complications. Bactericidal therapy should be instituted based on culture and sensitivity. Prior to obtaining culture results, or if culture is negative, empiric broad-spectrum coverage with penicillin, potentiated penicillin, or 1st or 2nd generation cephalosporin along with either a fluoroquinolone or an aminoglycoside should be chosen. Antibiotics at the upper end of the dosing range should be administered parenterally for 1–2 weeks followed by oral administration for 6–12 weeks. If *Bartonella* is suspected or confirmed, azithromycin (5–10 mg/kg PO q24h for 7 days, then every other day for 6–12 weeks) or doxycycline should be administered. Treatment with corticosteroids is contraindicated and confers a negative prognosis. Though anticoagulation therapy was proposed in the past, no benefit has been proven and it may increase the risk of hemorrhage. Cessation of therapy should be determined based on serial monitoring of echocardiograms, body temperature, CBC, and repeat blood and urine cultures.

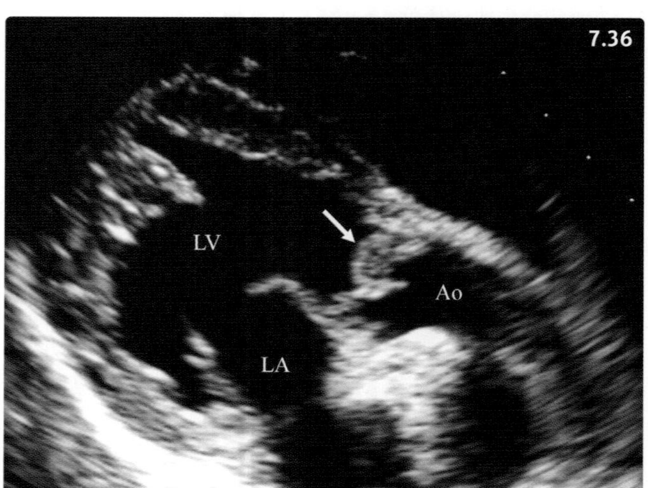

Figure 7.36 Right parasternal echocardiographic view from a dog with a vegetative lesion (arrow) on the aortic valve. LA, left atrium; LV, left ventricle; Ao, aorta.

Prognosis

Prognosis for vegetative infectious endocarditis is guarded to grave in both canine and feline patients. Aortic valve endocarditis, thrombocytopenia, and glomerulonephritis are also associated with worse prognosis.

CANINE CARDIOMYOPATHY

Cardiomyopathies are diseases that affect the heart muscle. When the cause is unknown, the term primary cardiomyopathy is used. When a cause can be identified for the heart muscle disease, the term secondary cardiomyopathy is used. The disease can then be described based on the underlying cause; for example, 'adriamycin (doxorubicin) cardiomyopathy'. Cardiomyopathy is one of the most common acquired cardiovascular diseases in dogs second only to degenerative valve disease and heartworm disease depending on the geographical location. The most common myocardial disease in dogs is DCM.

DILATED CARDIOMYOPATHY

Definition/overview

DCM is a primary myocardial disease characterized by decreased systolic function and subsequent ventricular dilation. This disease is most commonly seen in large breed dogs with Dobermanns, Great Danes, and Irish Wolfhounds being overrepresented. Some medium size breeds such as Cocker and English Spaniels may also develop the disease. Significant variation of disease presentation, progression, and prognosis can be seen depending of the breed of dog.

Etiology

The cause of DCM is not known but a genetic cause is suspected. In Dobermanns, DCM has been shown to be inherited as an autosomal dominant trait. Recently, a splice deletion in the pyruvate dehydrogenase kinase 4 gene (a gene involved in the regulation of myocardial energy utilization) has been associated with DCM in this breed.

Pathophysiology

Myocardial changes secondary to DCM lead to eccentric hypertrophy of the ventricles, which is usually more pronounced on the left side. In addition, left ventricular systolic function is markedly reduced. Over time, left ventricular enlargement leads to dilation of the mitral valve annulus and secondary mitral regurgitation. Left atrial enlargement results from volume overload, impaired ventricular filling, and secondary mitral regurgitation. Ventricular arrhythmias are caused by the disruption of the normal architecture of the ventricular myocardium, and various triggers such as increased adrenergic tone, electrolyte imbalances, and hypoxemia. AF is more likely to occur when the left atrium is markedly dilated and fibrotic.

Clinical presentation

In general, DCM has an adult onset with male dogs being affected more commonly. However, Portuguese Water Dogs often develop the disease before 12 weeks of age. Clinically, two phases of the disease can be detected: an occult or asymptomatic phase and an overt phase. In the occult phase, there are no clinical signs; however, arrhythmias or myocardial changes are present. The occult phase is variable and may last months to years. More commonly, the disease is not diagnosed until the overt stage when exercise intolerance, CHF, or syncope is noted. In some dogs, sudden death may be the first and only sign of disease. This is especially true for Dobermanns, in which sudden death can be the first sign of disease in approximately 30–50% of affected dogs.

Differential diagnosis

Other causes of left ventricular dilation in large breed dogs, including tachycardiomyopathy, cardiomyopathy secondary to taurine deficiency or doxorubicin toxicity, and myocarditis. Primary mitral valve insufficiency is associated with left ventricular systolic dysdunction, which may mimic DCM. Chronic cardiac changes of left-to-right shunt, especially PDAs in adult dogs, ressemble those of DCM.

Diagnosis

During physical examination, a grade 1 to 3/6 systolic murmur (a result of mitral insufficiency due to annular dilation) and/or an S3 gallop sound (indicating left ventricular dilation) may be noted over the left apex. A weak femoral pulse (a result of decreased stroke volume due to poor contractility) is a common finding. An irregular rhythm along with pulse deficits may be present as ventricular arrhythmias and AF are commonly seen in these dogs. Arrhythmias are often an early indication of disease and breeds predisposed should be screened with ECG and Holter monitor. Detection of ventricular premature complexes in an asymptomatic dog, particularly a Dobermann, should raise a high level of suspicion for occult cardiomyopathy. Sinus tachycardia, AF, and ventricular tachycardia are commonly seen in dogs with DCM. Giant breeds such as the Great Dane and Irish Wolfhound are more likely to develop AF, whereas Dobermanns are more likely to have ventricular arrhythmias. Arrhythmias are often noted around 2–4 years of age and can vary from single ventricular premature complexes to life-threatening ventricular tachycardia. Electrocardiographic changes suggesting left ventricular enlargement (R wave amplitude >3.0 mV) and conduction disturbances such as right or left bundle branch block may also be noted. It is important to note that a normal ECG does not rule out the presence of DCM. On radiographs, generalized cardiomegaly may be noted in dogs with DCM. However, radiographs are not sensitive to mild cardiac changes, therefore cardiomegaly is better assessed with echocardiography, particularly in the occult stage of the disease. In the overt stage, radiographs are more valuable in helping to diagnose CHF, showing pulmonary venous distension and pulmonary edema. Due to their chest conformation, the degree of cardiomegaly may be underestimated in Dobermanns. Echocardiography is essential for the evaluation of cardiac enlargement and function The classic sign of DCM on an echocardiogram is systolic dysfunction. This is seen as reduction in FS and ejection fraction (most accurately measured with the Simpson's method) along with increases in E point-to-septal separation and left ventricular end-systolic diameter. Increased left ventricular end-diastolic diameter as well as left atrial enlargement are seen as the disease progresses (**Figure 7.37**). Early in the disease, affected individuals may only have ventricular arrhythmias and normal echocardiograms. Therefore, it is important that when screening for the occult phase of the disease, both echocardiogram and Holter monitor evaluation are performed. A central jet of mitral regurgitation (secondary to annular dilation) can be found with moderate or severe left ventricular dilation. If concurrent degenerative valve disease is present, the mitral regurgitation jet will be more prominent and the degree of atrial dilation may be disproportional when compared with the degree of systolic dysfunction.

Management

In dogs with DCM and heart failure, standard CHF therapy is initiated with antiarrhythmic therapy used as needed based on the arrhythmia burden. Administration

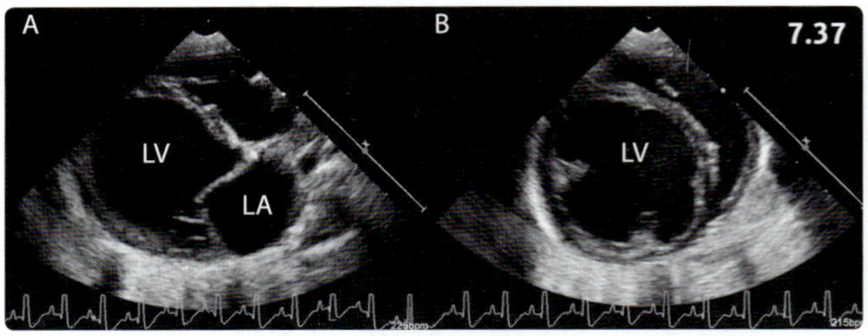

Figure 7.37 Right parasternal long-axis (A) and short-axis (B) views from a dog with dilated cardiomyopathy. The left ventricle appears markedly dilated. The ECG shows sinus tachycardia with wide QRS complexes, consistent with a left bundle branch block. LA, left atrium; LV, left ventricle.

of pimobendan delays the onset of CHF and extended survival in Dobermanns with occult DCM. Syncope is often the result of rapid ventricular tachycardia in DCM dogs. When this is seen, antiarrhythmic treatment is needed to control the syncope. Antiarrhythmic treatment does not prevent sudden death and many dogs with syncope will die suddenly, especially Dobermanns. Less likely causes of syncope in DCM include collapse due to decreased cardiac output, vasovagal syncope or, on occasion, secondary to the onset of AF. Treatment of ventricular arrhythmias includes the use of sotalol monotherapy or a combination of mexiletine and a beta-blocker.

Prognosis

Prognosis with DCM varies with breed and severity of disease but mostly is considered fair to poor, especially after the onset of CHF. The majority of dogs with DCM presenting for the development of CHF survive approximately 6–12 months. In some Cocker Spaniels, the disease may be associated with taurine deficiency and subsequent improvement may occur with supplementation. Dobermanns with DCM may carry a worse prognosis compared with other breeds. Onset of CHF at a young age and the presence of ascites and AF also carry a negative prognosis.

ARRHYTHMOGENIC RIGHT VENTRICULAR CARDIOMYOPATHY (BOXER CARDIOMYOPATHY)

Definition/overview

In dogs, ARVC is a myocardial disease dominated by ventricular arrhythmias and clinical signs of syncope. Most dogs have normal ventricular size and function at the time they develop the arrhythmia. The disease is primarily seen in Boxers but has also been documented, although less frequently, in other breeds including English Bulldogs. It is typically an adult-onset disease, but it can be diagnosed in dogs as young as 1 year of age.

Etiology

In humans, mutations in multiple genes coding for intercalated disc proteins have been associated with ARVC. In Boxers, only one genetic mutation has been associated with ARVC to date; it affects the striatin gene. Boxers positive for the striatin mutation have a higher number of VPCs on 24-hour Holter recordings.

Pathophysiology

ARVC is characterized by fatty or fibro-fatty myocardial replacement, predominantly in the right ventricle and, to a lower extent, the left ventricle and the left and right atria (**Figure 7.38**).

Clinical presentation

Clinically, the disease is characterized by ventricular tachycardia, right ventricular enlargement, syncope, and sudden death. There are three stages to the disease, which may be observed in succession as ARVC worsens: (1) initially, the patient is asymptomatic and ventricular arrhythmias are an incidental finding during physical examination for an unrelated condition; (2) the patient presents for syncope associated with the ventricular arrhythmias; and (3) the patient presents with signs of CHF secondary to systolic dysfunction and frequently a history of weakness or syncope related to the arrhythmias.

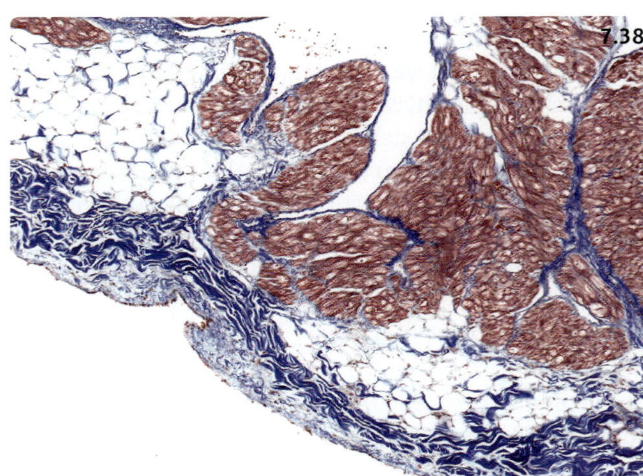

Figure 7.38 Histopathology of the myocardium of a Boxer with arrhythmogenic right ventricular cardiomyopathy revealing fatty replacement of the myocytes and interstitial fibrosis. The Masson trichrome stain shows collagen in blue. Magnification ×70.

Similar to Dobermanns with DCM, in some cases sudden death is the first and only sign of the disease.

Differential diagnosis

Myocarditis and other causes for left ventricular enlargement and arrhythmias, including tachycardiomyopathy and doxorubicin toxicitiy.

Diagnosis

The most common physical examination finding reported is the detection of an arrhythmia; this can be either single premature beats or paroxysms of tachycardia. On occasion, the arrhythmia is permanent when AF is present. Another physical examination abnormality common with ARVC is the presence of a systolic murmur on auscultation. Apical systolic murmurs result from mitral or tricuspid insufficiency caused by the annular dilation that accompanies cardiomegaly. Less frequently, a cardiac gallop is detected. Left basilar systolic murmurs may be noted in some Boxers, but these should not be linked to ARVC as they are usually physiologic or secondary to SAS. The most common electrocardiographic change noted is ventricular ectopy, in the form of ventricular premature complexes (singles, couplets, triplets, or bigeminy) or ventricular tachycardia. The ventricular ectopic beats tend to arise from the right ventricular myocardium, and are classically described as having a left bundle branch block pattern morphology with a predominantly positive deflection of the QRS complex in leads II, III, and aVF. If severe, the ventricular tachycardia can lead to syncopal episodes and potentially sudden death. The frequency of the ventricular beats can have as much as an 80% day to day variation with ARVC. To increase the possibility of identifying these arrhythmias, 24-hour Holter monitoring is recommended if there is evidence of arrhythmia on auscultation or a history of clinical signs such as syncope (**Figure 7.39**). Repeating a Holter recording or the use of an event monitor may increase the likelihood of arrhythmia detection in cases where an arrhythmia is not detected on initial evaluation. Although ARVC is a primary myocardial disease, structural changes may only be present on histopathology and not be evident on echocardiography. The expected findings on echocardiography vary depending on the stage of disease progression. The majority of asymptomatic Boxers, as well as most dogs suffering from syncopal episodes, have normal echocardiograms, but signs of depressed ventricular function and chamber dilation are reported on occasion. Atrial enlargement also develops as a result of ventricular dysfunction, and is more pronounced in dogs with CHF. Ultimately, disease progression may lead to biventricular failure, making it difficult to distinguish ARVC from idiopathic DCM.

7.39

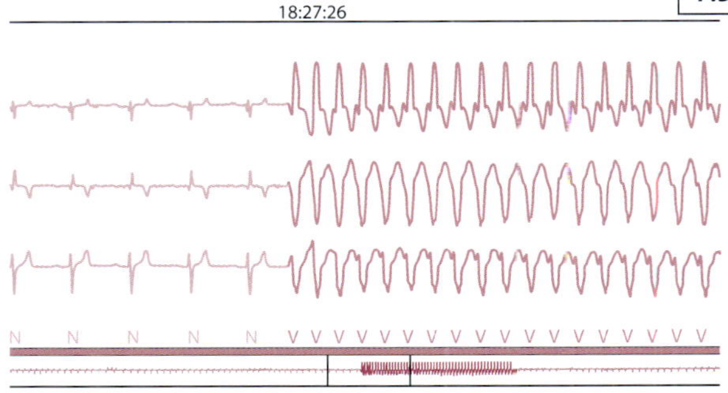

Figure 7.39 Holter recording from a Boxer with arrhythmogenic right ventricular cardiomyopathy showing a run of ventricular tachycardia.

Management

Treatment of ARVC aims at alleviating the clinical signs, as there is no specific treatment for the disease. In the absence of clinical signs and if the arrhythmia burden is mild, no treatment may be necessary. However, if the arrhythmia is of clinical concern or if there are collapsing episodes, antiarrhythmic therapy is implemented. In dogs, common protocols for the treatment of ventricular arrhythmias include the use of sotalol monotherapy or a combination of mexiletine and a beta-blocker. The response to antiarrhythmic therapy should be assessed via 24-hour Holter monitoring, since a large daily variation in the number of ventricular arrhythmias may be seen in dogs with ARVC. In cases where CHF is present, standard heart failure therapy is initiated with the need for addition of antiarrhythmic therapy determined by the patient's underlying rhythm. Administration of antiarrhythmic drugs can lead to a reduction in clinical signs and therefore improve quality of life, but the risk for sudden death from ARVC is not decreased by these medications.

Prognosis

ARVC progresses over several years and the rate of progression varies between dogs. In dogs with severe arrhythmia or syncope but normal cardiac function, a 2–3-year survival is not unusual when the clinical signs are controlled with antiarrhythmic therapy. Survival is usually less than 1 year once myocardial failure and CHF occur.

HYPERTROPHIC CARDIOMYOPATHY

Definition/overview

HCM is a rare primary myocardial disease in dogs. It is characterized by concentric hypertrophy of the left ventricle in the absence of a reason for the hypertrophy. Therefore, the diagnosis excludes valvular stenosis, hypertension, or other systemic illness that may stimulate left ventricular hypertrophy.

Clinical presentation

Most dogs with HCM are males and most are diagnosed before 3 years of age. In humans and cats with HCM, asymmetrical hypertrophy of the left ventricle is seen; however, dogs with HCM more commonly have symmetrical hypertrophy of the left ventricle. The vast majority of dogs also have systolic anterior motion of the mitral valve causing dynamic left ventricular outflow tract obstruction (LVOTO). Some dogs may have myocardial hypertrophy as a result of the LVOTO and not because of a primary myocardial disorder such as HCM. Concurrent abnormalities of the mitral valve have been described in patients with HCM and LVOTO. In addition, treatment with beta-blockers causes significant reduction of the LVOTO and may lead to improvement or resolution of the hypertrophy in some cases.

Differential diagnosis

Rule out systemic hypertension and other causes of increased afterload, such as SAS. Infiltrative myocardial disease, in particular lymphoma, may be responsible for concentric ventricular hypertrophy.

Diagnosis

Diagnosis relies on an echocardiogram to demonstrate left ventricular concentric hypertrophy in the absence of an obstruction to ejection of blood in the aorta or systemic hypertension.

Management

Treatment is primarily aimed at reducing or eliminating the LVOTO with beta-blockers (e.g. atenolol: 1 mg/kg q12–24h), which slow the heart rate and decrease contractility.

Prognosis

In most of the described cases, HCM was a fatal disease. The primary concern in these dogs is sudden death; less commonly, dogs may develop CHF secondary to diastolic dysfunction and severe left atrial enlargement.

INFILTRATIVE DISEASE

Definition/overview

Infiltrative myocardial disease is infrequent in dogs. The most commonly seen cause is a cardiac tumor. Infiltration by a tumor to the degree that it impairs myocardial diastolic or systolic function is rare.

Etiology

Lymphosarcoma is usually suspected. Lapland dogs have been reported to develop myocardial infiltration with glycogen, secondary to glycogen storage disease. These dogs had clinical signs associated with skeletal muscle disease; however, arrhythmias were also noted.

Clinical presentation

Most often dogs will present with clinical signs related to cardiac arrhythmia, pericardial effusion and, on occasion, obstruction to blood flow by the cardiac tumor.

Differential diagnosis

The degree of infiltration of the myocardium can be severe enough to resemble HCM.

Diagnosis

Diagnosis is based on a detailed echocardiographic examination. If pericardial effusion is present, a sample should be obtained via pericardiocentesis and submitted for cytologic evaluation. An abdominal ultrasound and fine-needle aspirates of enlarged organs and lymph nodes may help reach the diagnosis of lymphoma.

Management

Treatment is aimed at addressing the underlying cause for the myocardial infiltration and the use of antiarrhythmic medication determined by the underlying rhythm.

Prognosis

If cardiac lymphoma is diagnosed, survival depends on response to chemotherapy, with some dogs living more than 6 months after diagnosis.

FELINE CARDIOMYOPATHY

Definition/overview

Cardiomyopathies are diseases of the myocardium associated with cardiac dysfunction and are the most common form of cardiac disease in felines. HCM is associated with increased cardiac mass due to a hypertrophied, nondilated left ventricle in the absence of a hemodynamic load or metabolic cause. It is the most common form of cardiomyopathy in felines (60% of cases) with a higher prevalence in certain breeds (Maine Coon, Ragdoll, Norwegian Forest Cat, British Shorthair, American Shorthair, Sphynx, Siberian, and Persian), although Domestic Shorthairs are seen most commonly. Males are predisposed (65–70% of cases) possibly related to co-modifying genes or hormonal influences. Prevalence within the feline population has been reported as between 8% and 15%, although the criteria for diagnosis vary between studies and prevalence may be higher in some breeds.

Restrictive cardiomyopathy (RCM) is defined as restricted filling and reduced diastolic volume of one or both ventricles with normal or reduced systolic function and normal wall thickness. It is the second most associated with common form of cardiomyopathy (20% of cases). DCM is associated with dilation and impaired contractility of the left ventricle or both ventricles. Arrhythmogenic cardiomyopathy (ACM) is characterized by progressive fibro-fatty replacement of the myocardium that is regional or global, leading to a dilated and hypocontractile right ventricle with various arrhythmias and conduction abnormalities. It may also affect the left ventricle. Unclassified cardiomyopathy is diagnosed when there is echocardiographic myocardial disease that does not readily fit into other categories of cardiac disease.

Etiology

Familial HCM has been documented in Maine Coon cats as an autosomal dominant trait with incomplete penetrance, and a similar pattern of inheritance is suspected for other breeds. Separate mutations in different regions of the myosin binding protein C (MyBPC3) gene are considered causative of HCM in both Maine Coon and Ragdoll breeds. Importantly, these mutations have not been identified in other breeds, and it is likely that other mutations in this gene or in genes for other sarcomeric proteins exist, but have not yet been discovered. Over 1,400 mutations in 27 genes coding for sarcomeric or other structural proteins have been identified in humans with HCM. In humans, there is a correlation for some genes between the location of the mutation, severity of hypertrophy, and incidence of sudden death. Development of the HCM phenotype is not an inevitable consequence in individuals with an HCM genotype, as there is a low penetrance for the MyBPC3 mutation and it is likely age related. Additionally, co-modifier genes and environmental influences may affect phenotypic expression.

Myocardial hypertrophy can occur secondary to pressure overload (outflow obstruction, systemic hypertension), hyperthyroidism, hypersomatotropism, and infiltrative diseases of the myocardium. These causes should be excluded as soon as possible before a diagnosis of HCM is made.

The other forms of cardiomyopathy (RCM, DCM, ACM) are idiopathic and likely have a genetic basis. DCM was historically due to a taurine deficient diet and is now rare due to supplementation in commercial diets. Current cases of DCM may be found in feline patients on nontraditional diets (vegetarian diet or being fed canine food). RCM and ACM may be associated with an inflammatory process secondary to infectious, neoplastic, or immune-mediated disorders.

Pathophysiology

In HCM, it is hypothesized that the production of abnormal sarcomeric proteins creates a functional defect in the process of muscle contraction, leading to increased myocyte stress with subsequent activation of trophic factors (angiotensin II, aldosterone, insulin-like growth factor) that induce myocyte hypertrophy. Diastolic dysfunction is the primary mechanism responsible for clinical manifestations in HCM and RCM. Hypertrophy of the left ventricle wall (HCM) causes impaired or delayed relaxation and interstitial/endomyocardial fibrosis (HCM and RCM) increases myocardial stiffness and reduces distensibility. These changes impair left ventriclular filling and result in filling only at higher pressures. Elevated filling pressures inevitably lead to left atrial enlargement, pulmonary venous hypertension, and CHF. (See Congestive heart failure, Pathophysiology, for further discussion of neurohormonal activation.)

HCM generally leads to normal or increased global systolic performance of the left ventricle; however, regional systolic impairment has been documented in HCM patients using tissue Doppler imaging. Systolic dysfunction may be present in any myocardial disease due to ischemia and replacement fibrosis. Regional systolic impairment may increase regional wall stress and stimulate myocardial hypertrophy. DCM results in left ventricular or biventricular systolic dysfunction. ACM affects systolic performance primarily of the right ventricle and leads to a dilated, thin-walled, hypokinetic right ventricle and may affect the left ventricle. Tachyarrhythmias can affect diastolic performance and lead to myocardial dysfunction. Unclassified cardiomyopathy may show evidence of systolic or diastolic dysfunction.

Clinical presentation

Most cats with cardiomyopathy are diagnosed at a mean age of 5–7 years (range 3 months to 18 years), and HCM is typically diagnosed at an earlier age than other forms of cardiomyopathy. Certain breeds may present more commonly at a younger age. They may be presented in the asymptomatic phase due to the presence of auscultatory abnormalities such as a heart murmur or gallop sound. Various prevalence studies have shown that nearly 50% of apparently healthy cats with heart murmurs do not have evidence of cardiac disease; however, the presence of a heart murmur warrants further evaluation. In one study, 70% of cats with HCM did not have auscultatory abnormalities, so the absence of these findings does not exclude the presence of cardiac disease. Cats with occult cardiomyopathy (more common for RCM, DCM, ACM, unclassified cardiomyopathy) are often not identified until clinical signs are present, including dyspnea, tachypnea, lethargy, poor appetite, hindlimb paresis, collapse, or sudden death. Clinical signs are not an inevitable consequence for individuals with HCM.

Differential diagnosis

Includes cardiomyopathy secondary to systemic disease (hypertension, hyperthyroidism, hypersomatotropism), degenerative valve disease, congenital heart disease, and myocarditis. Differentials for respiratory signs include feline lower airway disease (feline asthma), pneumonia, noncardiogenic pleural effusion or pulmonary edema, hemorrhage, and PTE.

Diagnosis

Echocardiography is the gold standard for diagnosis and is an excellent noninvasive test that permits evaluation of morphologic and functional abnormalities of cardiac structures. Diagnosis of HCM is based on the identification of a diastolic wall thickness >6 mm on 2-dimensional or M-mode echo. Hypertrophy may be diffuse or segmental and may be symmetric or asymmetric (**Figure 7.40**). Other findings on echo may include papillary muscle hypertrophy, end-systolic cavity obliteration, left atrial enlargement (identified as left atrial dimension >16 mm or indexed to the aorta, LA/Ao >1.5). HCM may uncommonly affect the right ventricle. There is a subset of patients with hypertrophic obstructive cardiomyopathy due to obstruction in the left ventriclular outflow tract associated with systolic anterior motion of the mitral valve (**Figure 7.41**). It is unclear if the obstruction leads to hypertrophy of the left ventricle or if obstruction is the result of abnormalities in left ventricular geometry, the mitral valve apparatus, or loading conditions associated with hypertrophy of the left ventricle.

Thoracic radiographs may identify cardiomegaly, although it may be subtle especially if atrial enlargement is not present or the primary abnormality is concentric ventricular hypertrophy. The classic valentine shape results from severe biatrial enlargement. Pulmonary venous congestion, a patchy or diffuse interstitial to alveolar pattern, and/or pleural effusion are present in cats with CHF.

ECG may show chamber enlargement patterns, although these are not sensitive findings. Various arrhythmias and conduction abnormalities may be present. A left anterior fascicular block is the most common finding in cats with HCM (**Figure 7.42**). Supraventricular tachycardia and, rarely, AF may be present in cats secondary to severe atrial enlargement.

The sensitivity of an elevated NT-proBNP for identification of subclinical HCM may be up to 94% or higher, although its value as a screening test is still uncertain. It has been shown to discriminate between cats with respiratory signs due to CHF and cats with primary respiratory disease. An elevated NT-proBNP warrants further diagnostic evaluation. A normal value should not be used to rule out cardiac disease if other findings are supportive.

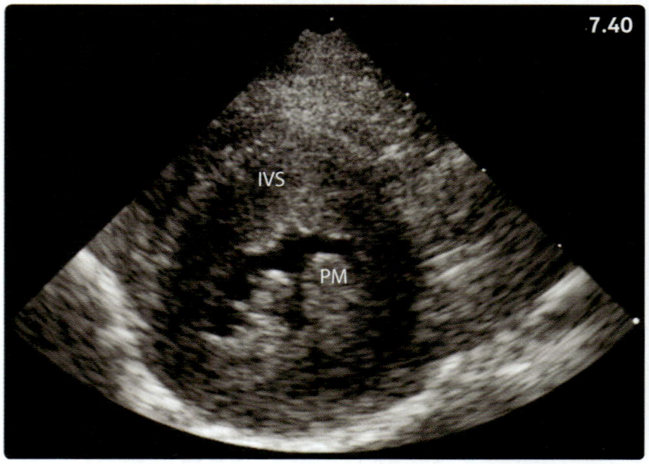

Figure 7.40 Right parasternal short-axis echocardiographic view from a cat with hypertrophic cardiomyopathy. There is concentric hypertrophy of the interventricular septum and the left ventricular free wall. The papillary muscles are prominent. IVS, interventricular septum; PM, papillary muscle.

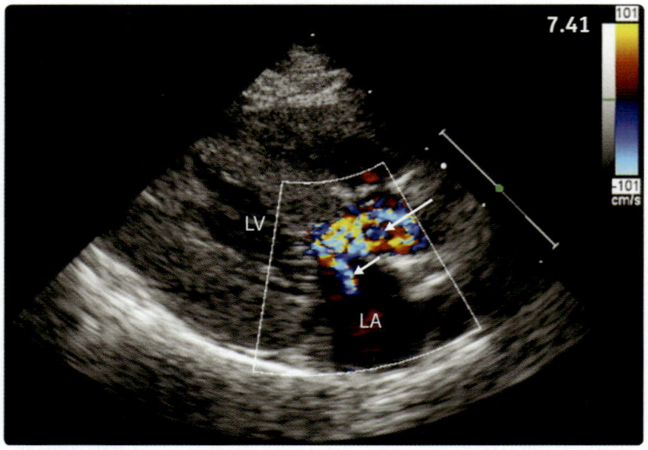

Figure 7.41 Color Doppler from a cat with hypertrophic obstructive cardiomyopathy showing two areas of turbulence: one in the left ventricular outflow tract caused by the septal leaflet of the mitral valve (long arrow); the other in the left atrium corresponds to a small amount of mitral regurgitation resulting from the incomplete closure of the mitral valve in systole (short arrow). LA, left atrium; LV, left ventricle.

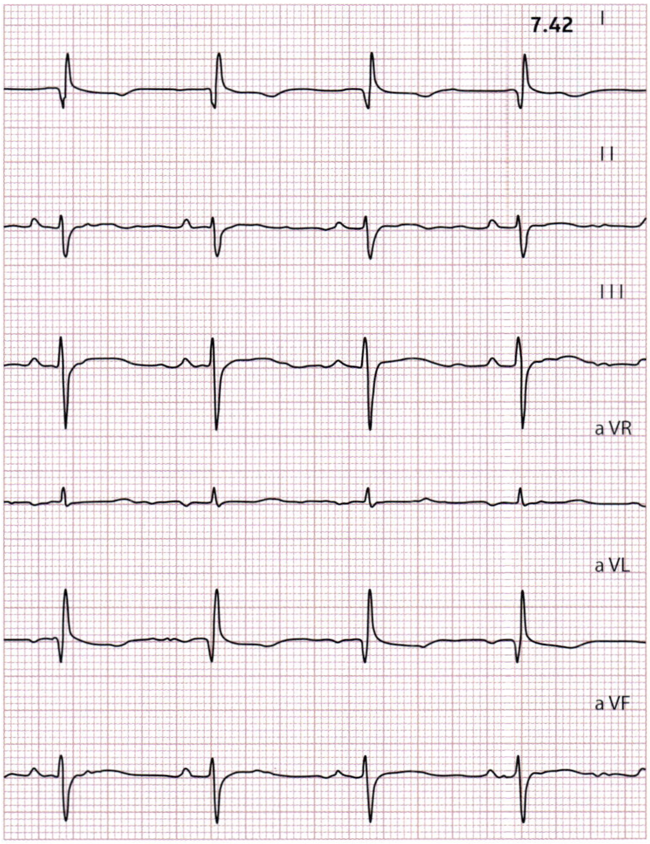

Figure 7.42 ECG from a cat with hypertrophic cardiomyopathy showing a sinus rhythm with a left axis deviation (lead I mostly positive, lead aVF mostly negative), also called left anterior fascicular block.

cTnI may also be elevated in cats with moderate to severe HCM with or without CHF.

Genetic testing for a specific genetic mutation is currently only available for Maine Coon and Ragdoll cats. These tests are most useful for identifying breeding cats that carry this mutation to assist in breeding recommendations, although cats that do not carry the mutation may still develop HCM. Due to the inability of echocardiography to determine the genotype, genetic testing should be utilized in addition to echocardiographic screening in breeding cats to avoid the production of individuals homozygous for the mutation.

Management

Standard therapy for feline patients with CHF includes administration of furosemide and an ACE inhibitor (**Table 7.13**). Patients with respiratory signs should receive supplemental oxygen, and mild sedatives may reduce stress associated with dyspnea. Pimobendan may be included if there is echocardiographic evidence of systolic dysfunction. Appropriate management of arrhythmias is important (see Arrhythmias, Management, for specific recommendations). Prevention of thromboembolic complications with antithrombotics (clopidogrel) is appropriate for cats at risk for this complication or those presenting with signs of arterial thromboembolism (**Figure 7.43**). It is important to monitor renal values and electrolyte disturbances during treatment of CHF. Hypotension, hypothermia, and bradycardia are not uncommon in patients with CHF at presentation or during treatment and cats should be monitored for their occurrence.

Currently, there is no evidence that treatment with various medications (beta-blocker, calcium channel blocker, ACE inhibitor, or spironolactone) in asymptomatic HCM patients alters the progression of the disease or delays the time to development of heart failure. Anecdotally, some cats with severe left ventricular outflow obstruction due to systolic anterior motion may clinically benefit from administration of a beta-blocker (atenolol); however, it has not been shown to significantly alter outcome or long-term prognosis.

Table 7.13 Drugs used in the management of cardiomyopathy in cats.

Drug	Dosage	Comment
Atenolol	0.5–2 mg/kg PO q12–24h	In cats with dynamic left ventricular outflow tract obstruction. Consider long-term treatment if improvement of hypertrophy. Start with low dose and increase slowly over a few weeks
Enalapril, benazepril	0.25–0.5 mg/kg PO q12–24h	Start q24h
Furosemide	1–2 mg/kg IM or IV q1–8h 1–3 mg/kg PO q8–24h	Monitor blood potassium concentration
Pimobendan	0.25 mg/kg PO q12h	Only when low-output failure confirmed by echocardiography
Clopidogrel	18.75 mg PO q24h	In cats after episode of thromboembolism, or if severe left atrial enlargement +/- visible thrombus

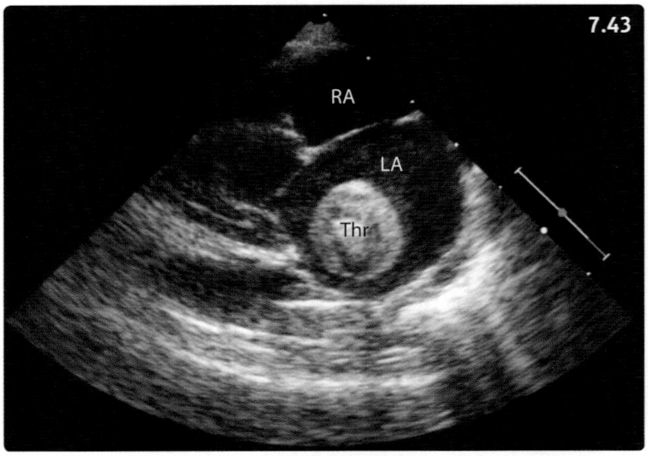

Figure 7.43 Right parasternal echocardiographic view of a cat showing a large thrombus in the left atrium. LA, left atrium; RA, right atrium; Thr, thrombus.

Prognosis

Prognosis for cats with HCM is variable. Asymptomatic patients may live several years after diagnosis and there are a modest number of felines with mild HCM that do not experience disease progression and live a normal life span. Other cats have a more aggressive form of the disease and die suddenly at a young age, develop CHF, or suffer thromboembolic complications. Extreme hypertrophy (>9 mm), decreased left ventricular systolic function (FS <30%), and decreased left atrial systolic function (↓ left atrial FS%) are associated with increasing risk of cardiac death.

In acute CHF, there is an approximate 80% survival to discharge. Patients with systolic dysfunction and CHF have historically had a poor prognosis; however, there may be improved survival with the addition of pimobendan. The prognosis from the first episode of heart failure is generally 6–12 months among the various cardiomyopathies; however, it is quite variable with some patients having shorter survival and others surviving well beyond 1 year (some up to 2–3 years). Cats with thromboembolic complications generally have a poor long-term prognosis, with an average survival of 6 months and up to 30% mortality during the immediate hospitalization period; however, some cats live for several years.

MYOCARDITIS

Definition/overview

Myocarditis is defined as an inflammation of the myocardium associated with myocyte necrosis. Although myocardial inflammation is present in all forms of cardiac disease, the term myocarditis is reserved for inflammation of the heart as the result of pathogens (viruses, bacteria, parasites), drug exposure, or immune-mediated diseases. The expression traumatic myocarditis is also used for inflammation of the myocardium after a mechanical trauma.

Etiology

Myocarditis in dogs (**Table 7.14**) and cats (**Table 7.15**) may be secondary to pathogens (viruses, bacteria, parasites), immune-mediated diseases, drug toxicity, or trauma. *Trypanosoma cruzi* (Chagas disease) is one of the pathogens most commonly recognized as a cause of myocarditis in endemic areas (particularly in the southern part of North America).

In cats, transmissible myocarditis–diaphragmitis is reported to affect adult cats in California and Florida during the summer months. Although infectious agents are thought to be involved (*Bartonella henselae*, virus), the cause of this contagious disease remains unknown. Unfortunately, identifying the cause of myocarditis remains unsuccessful most of the time.

Pathophysiology

Myocardial lesions can be a direct effect of infectious agents or drugs, but they can also be secondary to an immune response. Viruses can enter myocytes and interfere with cell metabolism, which may induce cell death,

Table 7.14 Etiology of canine myocarditis.

Infectious:
- Bacteria:
  - *Bartonella vinsonii* ssp. *berkhoffi*
  - *Bacillus piliformis*
  - *Citrobacter koseri*
  - *Borrelia burgdorferi*
- Viruses:
  - West Nile virus
  - Adenovirus type 1
  - Parvovirus
  - Canine herpesvirus
  - Canine distemper virus
- Parasites:
  - *Trypanosoma cruzi* (Chagas disease)
  - Leishmaniasis
  - *Neospora caninum*
  - *Babesia*
  - *Toxocara canis*
  - Fungal disease: blastomycosis, cryptococcosis, coccidiodomycosis, aspergillosis

Immune-mediated:
- Lymphocytic nonsuppurative myocarditis
- Myocarditis associated with polymyositis

Drug reaction:
- Anthracyclines: doxorubicin

Table 7.15 Etiology of feline myocarditis.

Infectious:
- Bacteria:
  - *Bartonella henselae*
  - Other bacteria
- Viruses:
  - Parvovirus (panleukopenia virus)
  - Other virus: herpes or calicivirus
- Parasites:
  - *Toxoplasma gondii*

Immune-mediated:
- Eosinophilic syndrome

Drug reaction:
- Anesthesia

Unknown:
- Transmissible myocarditis–diaphragmitis of cats

hypertrophy, or dysfunction. By modifying the myocyte cytoskeleton, viruses can lead to cardiac dysfunction with echocardiographic characteristics of DCM. The immune response can lead to cytokine release and enzyme activation. During the inflammatory process, activated collagenase and elastase enzymes contribute to cardiac remodeling. Activation of specific cytokines, especially transforming growth factor-beta, may predispose to pathologic fibrosis.

Chagas disease, also called American trypanosomiasis, is due to *Trypanosoma cruzi* infection. The preferential sites for reproduction in the host are the muscles, especially the myocardium (**Figure 7.44**). This tropism explains why myocarditis is the hallmark of the disease. Trypomastigotes can penetrate into the blood if the feces of the vector bug (*Triatoma* sp. – 'kissing bug') are deposited close to the bite or if the host ingests a reservoir host (armadillo, opossum, raccoon, mouse, squirrel, rat). Once in the cardiac muscle, trypomastigotes multiply and are released by cell rupture (**Figure 7.45**). This step corresponds to the acute phase of the disease (0–4 weeks after infection) and the peak of clinical signs. After the acute phase, the clinical signs decrease or disappear and the healing process mediated by the immune system induces cardiac remodeling (myocardial necrosis, fibrosis, coronary spasm). The onset of the chronic stage may appear several months to several years post inoculation. Progressive cardiac remodeling leads to systolic dysfunction, arrhythmias (most commonly second- or third-degree AV block, but ventricular tachyarrhythmias are also reported) and possibly CHF.

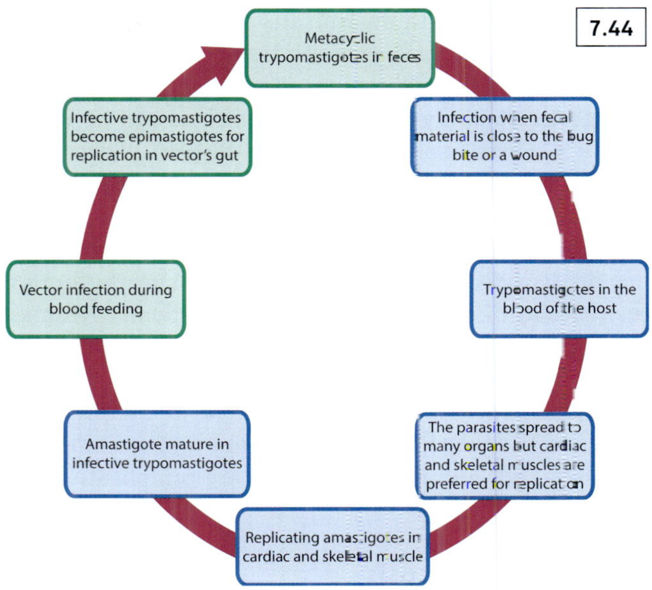

Figure 7.44 Life cycle of *Trypanosoma cruzi*. The green boxes represent the vector period; the blue boxes represent the host period.

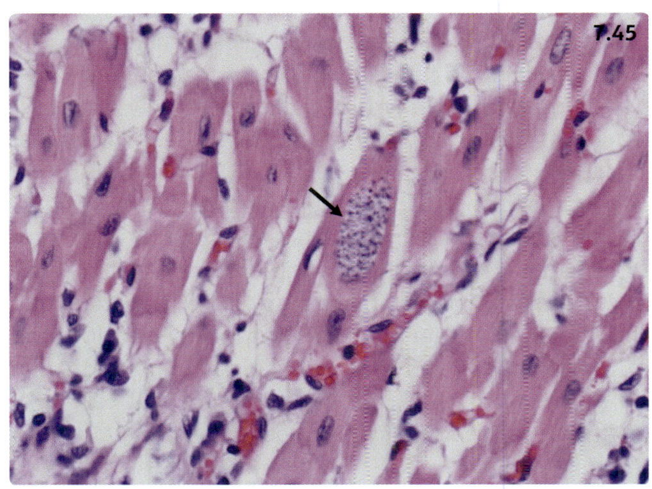

Figure 7.45 Histologic section of a canine heart. Infrequently, cardiomyocytes are expanded by protozoal pseudocysts (arrow) that contain numerous amastigotes. H&E stain. Magnification ×40.

Clinical presentation

Myocarditis can affect dogs and cats of all ages. However, several diseases are more likely in the young dog (Chagas disease, parvovirus) or in immunocompromised animals (e.g. leishmaniasis, toxoplasmosis). Obtaining a complete history is essential because living conditions or travel to endemic area may help the clinician identify an etiologic factor for a specific disease.

Dogs and cats with myocarditis are usually presented for weakness, syncope, exercise intolerance, respiratory difficulties, and/or abdominal distension. Clinical signs are most commonly acute but these signs can be insidious (e.g. chronic phase of Chagas disease). Fever and leukocytosis are unusual findings. Complex arrhythmias are frequent and should alert the clinician to the possibility of myocarditis when they occur in a breed that is not predisposed for cardiomyopathy. Tachyarrhythmias (ventricular or supraventricular) and bradyarrhythmias (most commonly second- or third-degree AV block) are reported. A low-grade left apical systolic heart murmur or a gallop rhythm can be auscultated in the presence of severe left ventricular enlargement and systolic dysfunction. Left- and right-sided CHF are complications of myocarditis.

Differential diagnosis

Myocarditis is characterized by nonspecific clinical signs, therefore differential diagnoses include other cardiac diseases and other cause of arrhythmias.

When the myocarditis is associated with both systolic dysfunction and ventricular and/or supraventricular arrhythmias, the differential diagnosis should include DCM, tachycardia-induced cardiomyopathy, and infiltrative cardiomyopathy (e.g. lymphoma). However, myocarditis is usually acute compared with other causes of systolic dysfunction.

It is suspected that in cats as in humans, myocarditis may also lead to myocardial concentric hypertrophy. Differential diagnosis for feline ventricular hypertrophy includes HCM, systemic hypertension, hyperthyroidism, acromegaly, muscular dystrophy, myocarditis, and cardiac lymphoma. Therefore, the differential diagnosis of myocarditis in cats should include all causes of ventricular hypertrophy and other cardiomyopathies (ACM, RCM, DCM).

Diagnosis

Myocarditis is usually suspected in dogs and cats (especially in young animals) with acute clinical signs consistent with arrhythmias and systolic dysfunction. A complete biochemistry profile and hemogram are necessary to assess organ dysfunction, inflammation, or the presence of blood parasites.

In all dogs and cats with suspected myocarditis, an ECG (+/- Holter recording) should be performed, especially if arrhythmias are detected during physical examination or if the reason for the consultation includes weakness, exercise intolerance, or syncope. A complete echocardiogram is essential to exclude other cardiac diseases and to evaluate systolic function. cTnI serum level increases secondary to massive myocardial cell death. A marked elevation in circulating cTNI level is common with myocarditis.

Thoracic radiography is indicated if respiratory signs are present to evaluate the possibility of pulmonary edema or pleural effusion. Any pleural or abdominal fluids removed should be submitted for bacterial culture and cytology. Any accessible lesions should be aspirated or biopsied for analysis.

Diagnosis of Chagas disease can be made by direct observation of *Trypanosoma cruzi* on a stained blood smear or buffy coat smear, on lymph node aspirates or in abdominal effusion. PCR is sensitive in the acute phase but the sensitivity decreases with chronicity. Antibody titer is usually positive by 3 weeks post infection. The most commonly used serologic tests are the indirect immunofluorescent antibody test and the ELISA test (possible cross reaction with *Leishmania*). Radioimmunoprecipitation assays, indirect hemagglutination assays, and flow cytometry are used for research purposes.

Management

Treatment should be directed at improving cardiac function, decreasing arrhythmia burden, controlling CHF, and treating the cause if possible. Inotropes are indicated to improve systolic dysfunction; pimobendan is probably the most effective oral inotrope. In combination with diuretics (especially furosemide), it helps to control CHF. Abdominocentesis and thoracocentesis should be performed in all dogs and cats with ascites or pleural effusion. High-grade second- and third-degree AV blocks do not respond to medical treatment, therefore pacemaker implantation is needed to increase the heart rate and improve cardiac output. Tachyarrhythmias are treated according to the underlying mechanism involved (see Tachyarrhythmias).

No effective treatment is currently available to treat Chagas disease in dogs. Nifurtimox and benznidazole are reserved for human use only. Albaconazole has been shown to reduce parasite proliferation but not totally eliminate the parasite. Ketoconazole, gossypol, and allopurinol have not shown sufficient efficacy. Prednisolone (0.5–1 mg/kg PO q12–24h) may increase survival. Because the immune system is involved in the mechanism of myocardial lesions even in infectious myocarditis, glucocorticoids are often recommended to reduce inflammation. Antibiotics can be effective against bacterial myocarditis and the choice should ideally be made on the basis of blood culture results.

Prognosis

Prognosis is usually guarded and unpredictable. Chagas disease is usually associated with poor outcomes because even if a dog survives the acute phase, the chronic phase may induce severe cardiac dysfunction. Young dogs have a worse prognosis (<5 months survival) than adult or old dogs (30–60 months survival), probably because of a different immune response to the disease.

Most of the time, puppies that develop myocarditis secondary to parvovirus die in a few days because of severe myocardial necrosis. However, myocarditis can also resolve in a few days or a few weeks without specific treatment. Some authors report that cats may develop myocardial hypertrophy and CHF secondary to anesthesia or surgery and occasionally recover spontaneously.

PERICARDIAL DISEASES

Definition/overview

The most common manifestation of pericardial disease is pericardial effusion. Cardiac tamponade describes pericardial effusion associated with clinical signs because a large volume of effusion is present or because fluid has accumulated very fast. Constrictive pericarditis is caused by a markedly thickened pericardial sac that prevents adequate cardiac filling.

Etiology

Pericardial effusion in dogs is frequently caused by cardiac tumors. Cardiac hemangiosarcoma is the most common tumor responsible for cardiac tamponade. Golden Retrievers and German Shepherd Dogs are overrepresented. Brachycephalic breeds are predisposed to chemodectoma. Other tumors include mesothelioma, lymphoma, and ectopic thyroid carcinoma. Idiopathic pericardial effusion is another common cause of cardiac tamponade. Unusual causes for tamponade include trauma, coagulation disorders, and an atrial tear in dogs with severe mitral valve regurgitation and a dilated left atrium. Pericardial effusion is less common in cats and is usually associated with CHF. Tamponade is rare in cats, but could result from lymphosarcoma or feline infectious peritonitis (FIP). Constrictive pericarditis can be a complication of any chronic effusion or pericarditis. It has been described as a complication of *Coccidicides immitis* infections.

Pathophysiology

Pericardial fluid has little effect on cardiac function unless the intrapericardial pressure equals or exceeds cardiac diastolic pressure. The pericardium can accommodate a moderate amount of fluid that accumulates slowly with little change in pericardial pressure. However, large amounts of fluid, or even small amounts that accumulate quickly (hemorrhage), can cause a significant increase in pericardial pressure leading to cardiac tamponade. Tamponade impedes diastolic filling As a result, cardiac output falls. When pericardial fluid accumulates over days or weeks, this decrease in cardiac output results in an activation of the adrenergic tone and neurohormonal mechanisms. This includes activation of the RAAS, leading to increased angiotensin II, aldosterone, and vasopressin. This results is an increase in heart rate and fluid retention. Renal fluid excretion is not promoted because there is no increase in secretion of atrial natriuretic peptide. Over time, right-sided CHF occur. Conversely, when hemorrhagic pericardial effusion accumulates within a few seconds, there is no time for water retention to occur and prevent a rapid drop in cardiac filling and, subsequently, an important reduction in cardiac output. Cardiogenic shock is therefore the typical consequence of acute cardiac tamponade. Reduced coronary perfusion during tamponade can also impair ventricular systolic function.

Clinical presentation

Clinical signs of cardiac tamponade are consistent with right-sided CHF and reduced cardiac output. History may include weakness, lethargy, exercise intolerance, collapse, syncope, abdominal distension, and tachypnea, as well as weight loss in chronic cases. Signs of right-sided CHF predominate. Physical examination may reveal jugular vein distension, weak femoral pulses, and muffled heart sounds (Beck's triad). Also a positive hepatojugular reflux, hepatomegaly, ascites, tachypnea, and dyspnea can be present. Pleural effusion from right-sided CHF may also muffle heart sounds and lung sounds ventrally. Sinus tachycardia, pale mucous membranes, and prolonged CRT are common due to increased sympathetic tone. A murmur may be present if there is underlying cardiac disease; however, pericardial effusion will not cause a heart murmur on its own. Pulsus paradoxus is not always present but is characteristic of pericardial effusion. It results in weaker femoral pulses during inspiration and stronger pulses during expiration.

Differential diagnosis

Congenital causes of canine pericardial disease include pericardial cysts, partial/total pericardial agenesis, and peritoneopericardial diaphragmatic hernia (PPDH). PPDH is the most common congenital pericardial disease in cats. Causes of acquired pericardial disease and pericardial effusion in dogs include: hemangiosarcoma, heart base tumor, idiopathic pericardial effusion, malignant mesothelioma, hypoalbuminemia, uremia, CHF, septic pericarditis (bacterial, fungal [coccidiomycosis], protozoal [leishmaniasis]), left atrial rupture, trauma, and hemorrhage (coagulopathy). Causes of acquired pericardial disease in cats include: CHF, FIP, hypoalbuminemia, idiopathic, and lymphosarcoma.

Diagnosis

Radiography

Radiographic findings are not always reliable for diagnosing pericardial effusion. The typical, large, globoid cardiac silhouette results when there is a moderate accumulation of chronic effusion. Acute effusions causing clinical signs of cardiac tamponade may not always be evident on a chest radiograph.

Radiographs of animals with PPDH show convergence of the cardiac silhouette and the diaphragm. GI segments may be evident as gas opacities within the pericardial space and, depending on the amount of organ displacement, the abdomen may be partially devoid of intestinal segments or other organs. Liver and omental fat are most commonly herniated through the defect. Sternal defects are often found concurrently with PPDH. Other congenital cardiovascular defects have also been reported in dogs and cats with PPDH.

Electrocardiography

Animals with cardiac tamponade are tachycardic. In addition, low amplitude QRS complexes are common in animals with a moderate amount of pericardial effusion. Electrical alternans (a beat-to-beat variation in the R wave amplitude) is less common (**Figure 7.46**).

Echocardiography

Two-dimensional echocardiography is the most sensitive, noninvasive test for confirming the presence of pericardial effusion and elucidating the cause. Pericardial effusion is seen as an anechoic space between the epicardium and pericardium (**Figure 7.47**). The amount of effusion can be roughly quantitated and signs of cardiac tamponade can be identified. The areas of the right atrium/auricle, heart base, and main pulmonary artery should be examined carefully since these are common locations for cardiac masses (**Figure 7.48**). The specific tumor type can often be predetermined based on location. Overall, echocardiography is estimated to be 90% sensitive for detecting cardiac masses. Heart base tumors are commonly found adjacent to the aorta on standard transthoracic views. Right atrial/auricular masses (commonly hemangiosarcoma) may be difficult to see, so the absence of a mass in this location does not necessarily rule it out. Transesophageal echocardiography may more easily reveal these masses, but this technique requires special equipment and general anesthesia. False-positive findings have been reported, and normal cardiac structures can be misidentifed as a mass when imaged in oblique positions, especially by inexperienced echocardiographers. In cases of cardiac tamponade, the ventricular walls may show pseudohypertrophy due to external compression and collapse of the right atrial and ventricular walls during diastole. The myocardial texture should be observed for any signs of

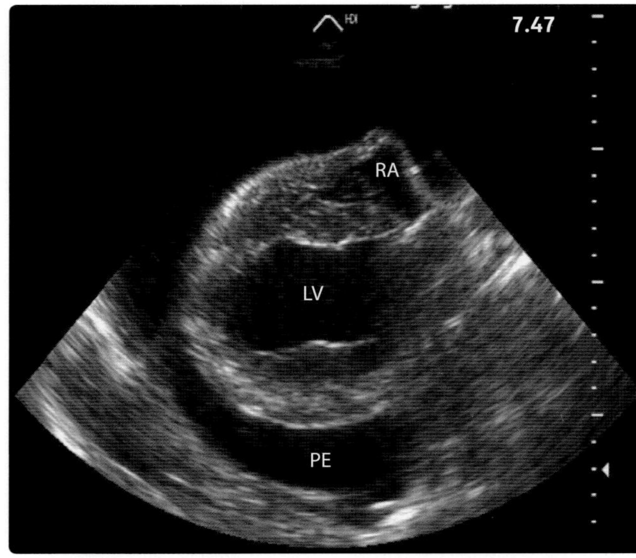

Figure 7.47 Echocardiographic view from a dog with pericardial effusion. The effusion is seen as an anechoic space around the heart. LV, left ventricle; PE, pericardial effusion; RA, right atrium.

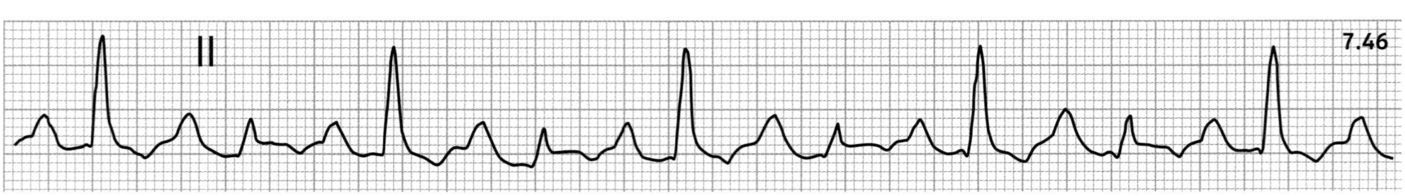

Figure 7.46 ECG (lead II) from a dog with cardiac tamponade. There is sinus tachycardia with a beat-to-beat variation in QRS complex amplitude, called electrical alternans.

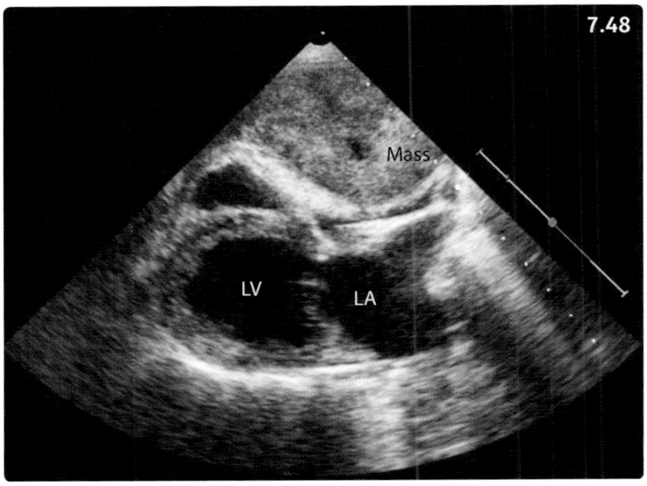

Figure 7.48 Right parasternal echocardiographic view from a dog with a large cardiac mass expanding along the right atrium and ventricle. The mass is so large that it is compressing the right atrium and ventricle. LA, left atrium; LV, left ventricle.

tumor infiltrate (primary or metastatic neoplasia such as lymphoma). In the case of a left atrial tear, a clot may be visualized in the pericardial space along with the pre-existing valvular disease.

Pericardial fluid analysis

Pericardiocentesis is frequently necessary for emergency stabilization of a patient with pericardial effusion and cardiac tamponade; however, fluid analysis is rarely diagnostic. Fluid samples are often hemorrhagic or serosanguineous sterile inflammatory exudates. Not surprisingly, hemangiosarcoma and aortic body tumors are rarely confirmed on cytologic examination of pericardial fluid. Less common causes of pericardial effusion, such as lymphosarcoma or infectious pericarditis, are more reliably diagnosed with pericardial fluid analysis.

Management/prognosis

Acute management of pericardial effusion requires pericardiocentesis in most cases. The pericardium should be approached from the right side to reduce the risk of lacerating a coronary vessel. Many animals will tolerate the procedure without sedation, but a sedative such as butorphanol can be used. The right thorax is clipped and aseptically prepared. The ideal location for entry can be determined with ultrasound. Typically, a 14- or 16-gauge over-the-needle catheter is used along with an extension set and a three-way stop-cock. The skin, intercostal muscles, and parietal pleura are infiltrated with local anesthetic. The catheter is then inserted while applying negative pressure. Once the needle enters the pericardium and fluid flows into the extension set, the catheter can be advanced. To distinguish red pericardial fluid from blood within the heart or blood vessels, a sample of fluid is collected in an activated clotting time tube. Blood should normally clot within 60–90 seconds, unlike sanguineous body cavity effusions in which clotting factors and platelets are depleted. Ventricular arrhythmias are common during this procedure, so ECG monitoring should be available. The treatment and prognosis for specific pericardial diseases are described below.

Hemangiosarcoma

Cardiac hemangiosarcoma has usually metastasized by the time of diagnosis. Commonly, palliation with pericardiocentesis alone is elected. However, the fluid and cardiac tamponade can return quickly and result in death or euthanasia. Median survival time for dogs treated with pericardiocentesis alone is approximately 2 weeks. Other aggressive therapies include tumor resection, pericardectomy, chemotherapy, and splenectomy. Some dogs live up to 3–6 months. Adjuvant chemotherapy has been shown to provide little survival advantage.

Heart base tumors

Complete surgical resection of these tumors is usually impractical because they are highly vascular and surround major blood vessels. Palliation with pericardectomy alone commonly results in prolonged survival with good quality of life, sometimes over 2 years after pericardectomy.

Mesothelioma and other cardiac tumors

There are only a few case reports of successful treatment for mesothelioma. However, complete pericardectomy followed by intracavitary cisplatin and IV doxorubicin have been reported to result in a disease-free state 2 years later. Patients may also require periodic thoracocentesis for pleural effusion. Since mesothelioma can be difficult to diagnose even with histopathology, accumulation of a large amount of pleural effusion 4–6 months after pericardectomy increases the suspicion for the disease. Cardiac lymphosarcoma, rhabdomyosarcoma, and fibrosarcoma are rare. Cardiac lymphosarcoma is treatable with chemotherapy.

Infectious pericarditis

Bacterial infections of the pericardium are thought to arise most commonly from foreign body penetration, often migrating foxtails (*Hordeum* spp.). Therefore, pericardectomy and removal of the foreign body is crucial for resolution of the disease. Therapy, including pericardectomy, removal of any foreign bodies, and long-term antibiotic therapy (up to 6 months), results in a good prognosis. Treatment for coccidioidomycosis is similar except that antifungal medications replace antibiotics. Prognosis for *Coccidioides* infection involving the pericardium is guarded as constrictive pericarditis is a common complication after the fungal infection is treated.

Idiopathic pericardial effusion and constrictive pericarditis

Idiopathic pericardial effusion is a diagnosis of exclusion and often not completely distinguishable from mesothelioma. Animals with idiopathic pericardial effusion can develop effusive–constrictive pericarditis over time with repeated thoracocentesis. For this reason, pericardectomy is recommended. Many animals go on to do well after successful surgery.

PULMONARY HYPERTENSION

Definition/overview

PH is defined as elevated blood pressure within the pulmonary vasculature with a systolic pulmonary artery pressure >30 mmHg, mean pressure >25 mmHg, or diastolic pressure >19 mmHg. Recognition of PH has increased since the widespread availability of Doppler echocardiography. It occurs most commonly in middle aged to older, small breed dogs, although it may occur in any canine patient and is less commonly identified in cats.

Etiology

Primary (idiopathic) PH is uncommon in veterinary medicine. PH occurs most commonly secondary to underlying diseases and classification may be based on location (precapillary versus postcapillary) or based on the pathophysiologic mechanism (**Table 7.16**).

Pathophysiology

The pulmonary vasculature is normally a low-pressure system with minimal resistance and high capacitance (highly distensible). Prolonged exposure of the vascular bed to significant increases in pulmonary blood flow occurs with large left-to-right shunting congenital cardiac defects. Increased flow causes vascular endothelial damage, vasoconstriction, and remodeling of small pulmonary arteries leading to the development of PH and may cause irreversible damage to the pulmonary vasculature.

Table 7.16 Etiology of pulmonary hypertension.

Pulmonary hypertension secondary to increased blood flow (congenital intra- or extracardiac systemic-to-pulmonary shunts):
- Atrial septal defect
- Ventricular septal defect
- Patent ductus arteriosus

Postcapillary (pulmonary venous hypertension):
- Mitral valve disease
- Myocardial disease
- Miscellaneous left-sided heart diseases

Precapillary:
- Pulmonary arterial hypertension with pulmonary disease or hypoxia:
  - Chronic obstructive pulmonary disease
  - Interstitial pulmonary fibrosis
  - Neoplasia
  - High-altitude disease
  - Reactive pulmonary artery vasoconstriction (e.g. hypoxia due to pulmonary edema)
- Pulmonary arterial hypertension due to vascular obstruction or destruction:
  - Thromboembolism (immune-mediated hemolytic anemia, neoplasia, cardiac disease, protein-losing disease, hyperadrenocorticism, sepsis, trauma, recent surgery)
  - Heartworm disease
  - Necrotizing vasculitis/arteritis
  - Idiopathic

Miscellaneous:
- Compressive mass lesions (neoplasia, granuloma)

Postcapillary (venous) PH occurs with left-sided cardiac diseases (e.g. mitral valve insufficiency, DCM). Increased filling pressure impedes drainage of the pulmonary capillaries and leads to a compensatory increase in pulmonary artery pressure to maintain forward blood flow. This is the most common cause of PH and tends to be mild to moderate. Hypoxic pulmonary artery vasoconstriction may worsen PH if pulmonary edema is present. Precapillary PH occurs from obstruction or destruction of the pulmonary vasculature or narrowing of the vessels without physical obstruction. Physical obstruction or destruction occurs with PTE, heartworm disease, or obliterative endarteritis. Hypoxemia and release of vasoactive substances from activated platelets causes reactive vasoconstriction, further increasing pulmonary vascular resistance. PTE is underdiagnosed in veterinary patients and is secondary to a number of disease processes. Hypoxia leads to pulmonary arteriolar constriction as an adaptive mechanism to shunt pulmonary blood flow to regions of well oxygenated lung tissue. High altitude and chronic lung diseases cause hypoxic vasoconstriction. Chronic lung diseases also distort the pulmonary vasculature such that there is narrowing of the pulmonary arterioles without causing physical destruction or obstruction of the vessels.

PH creates a pressure overload on the right ventricle leading to right heart enlargement, right ventricular dysfunction, and tricuspid valve insufficiency and may progress to right-sided CHF. PH may also limit preload (filling) to the left ventricle, decreasing cardiac output to the systemic circulation.

Clinical presentation

Clinical signs and physical examination findings are varied and are a result of the underlying primary disease process or due to PH. Presenting clinical signs may include lethargy, exercise intolerance, cough, dyspnea, tachypnea, syncope, and cyanosis. Clinical signs may only be present during exercise. Patients with mild to moderate PH are often asymptomatic. Physical examination findings may include pulmonary crackles, wheezes, a loud or split second heart sound, systolic heart murmurs (due to tricuspid or mitral valve insufficiency), diastolic heart murmur (pulmonic insufficiency if severe with PH), various arrhythmias, and a palpable right-sided apex beat. In dogs, when PH leads to right-sided CHF, ascites is present.

Differential diagnosis

Differentials for respiratory signs include PTE, pneumonia, CHF, pleural effusion, chronic bronchitis, pulmonary hemorrhage or contusions, and lung lobe torsion. Differentials for syncope or exercise intolerance include arrhythmias, cardiomyopathy, vasovagal syncope, hypotension, acute pericardial effusion, and anemia.

Diagnosis

The gold standard diagnostic test is right heart catheterization and direct measurement of pulmonary pressures; however, this technique is impractical in most clinical situations. Doppler echocardiography is an excellent, noninvasive method of estimating pulmonary pressures and is considered diagnostic in veterinary medicine. The velocity of tricuspid valve regurgitation (in the absence of PS) is used to measure right ventricular end-systolic pressure (RVESP) to estimate the systolic pulmonary artery pressures using the modified Bernoulli equation ($P = 4v^2$) where P is the pressure gradient (between right ventricle and right atrium) and v is the velocity of the regurgitant jet (**Figure 7.49**). Pulmonic valve insufficiency may be used to estimate diastolic pulmonary artery pressure (PAP). Based on systolic pressure, PH is classified as mild (RVESP 36–60 mmHg, estimated PAP 40–65 mmHg), moderate (RVESP 60–80 mmHg estimated PAP 65–90 mmHg), or severe (RVESP ≥80 mmHg, estimated PAP ≥90 mmHg). Abnormalities on 2-dimensional or M-mode echocardiography may suggest the presence of PH, including right ventricular hypertrophy (eccentric or concentric), right atrial enlargement, flattening of the interventricular septum (**Figure 7.50**), paradoxical septal motion, and dilation of the main pulmonary artery (**Figure 7.51**). These findings are not always present and PH should not be ruled out if the right heart appears structurally normal. Other findings based on pulmonary artery systolic flow profiles, right ventricular tissue Doppler imaging, and systolic time intervals may support a diagnosis of PH in the absence of direct measurement. If PH is due to left-sided heart disease, then evidence of significant structural disease should be present. If left heart disease is absent, the left ventricle may be small and underfilled.

Additional diagnostics should be performed to identify an underlying cause and should include a CBC, biochemistry, urinalysis, and thoracic radiographs. Evidence of right heart enlargement, main pulmonary artery bulge, dilation of lobar pulmonary arteries, or pulmonary disease may be identified on thoracic radiographs. Radiographic findings may be suggestive of PH, but are not diagnostic. Further diagnostic testing may be indicated based on the suspected differentials after initial evaluation and may include arterial blood gas, heartworm antigen testing, abdominal ultrasound, urine protein:creatinine ratio, fluoroscopy, bronchoscopy, bronchoalveolar lavage, CT, angiography, and a coagulation profile including D-dimers and possible thromboelastogram. An ECG may suggest right heart enlargement, although it is not a sensitive finding. Various arrhythmias may be identified.

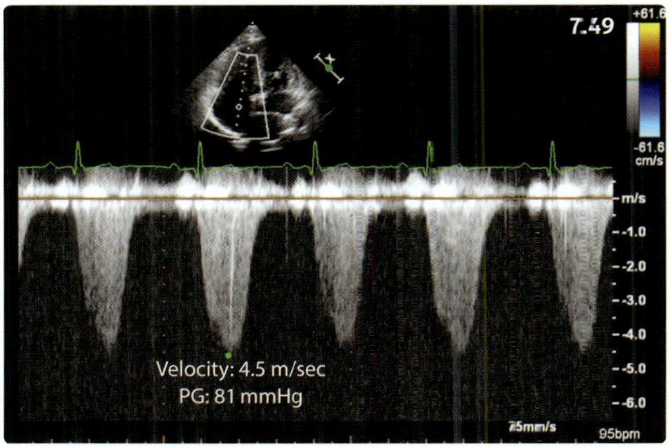

Figure 7.49 Spectral Doppler of a tricuspid valve regurgitation jet consistent with severe pulmonary hypertension.

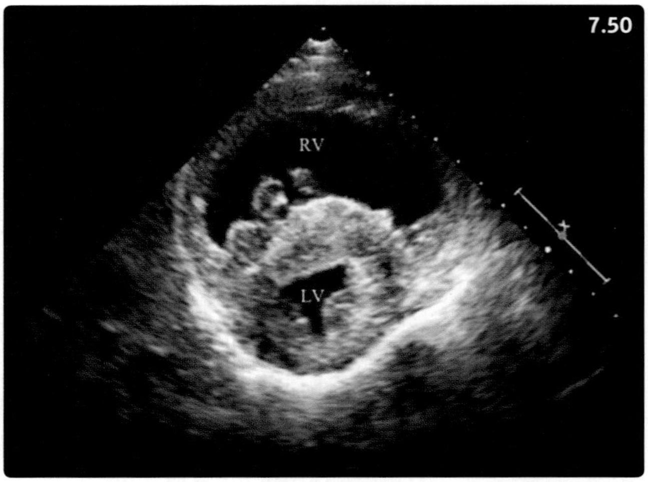

Figure 7.50 Echocardiographic short-axis view from a dog with severe pulmonary hypertension. The right ventricle is severely dilated. There is marked thickening of the interventricular septum, with prominent papillary muscles on the right side. The left ventricle is small as a result of decreased filling. LV, left ventricle; RV, right ventricle.

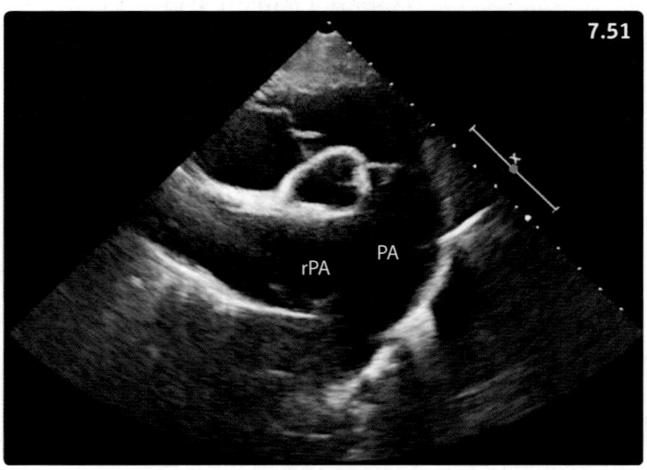

Figure 7.51 Echocardiographic view of the main pulmonary artery of a dog with pulmonary hypertension. There is severe dilation of the main and right pulmonary arteries. PA, pulmonary artery; rPA, right pulmonary artery.

Management

Treatment is directed at resolving the underlying cause if one can be identified. Supplemental oxygen and sedatives (butorphanol) should be provided if the patient is in respiratory distress. PH due to left-sided heart disease often improves with standard treatment of CHF with administration of diuretics, ACE inhibitors, and positive inotropes. Treatment directed at an underlying cause of hypercoagulability along with anticoagulant therapy (unfractionated heparin, low molecular weight heparin) for pulmonary thromboemboli is recommended. Anticoagulant therapy should be started prior to receiving coagulation test results if there is a high index of clinical suspicion or if an underlying cause cannot be easily determined, especially if the patient has known predisposing factors for hypercoagulability **(Table 7.16)**. Antithrombotics (aspirin, clopidogrel) may be used adjunctively.

Pulmonary vasodilators should be used when treatment of the primary underlying disease does not adequately control PH or in cases of idiopathic PH. Phosphodiesterase-5 inhibitors (sildenafil, tadalafil, vardenafil) cause pulmonary vasodilation associated with the nitric oxide pathway and may reduce pulmonary artery pressure, improve quality of life, reduce clinical signs, and prolong survival. Sildenafil is commonly used at a dose of 1–3 mg/kg PO q8–12h. The high end of the dosage range seems to provide the best clinical response.

Prognosis

Prognosis is related to the underlying disease process and response to treatment. PH can rarely be cured unless it is due to a left-to-right shunt that can be surgically corrected (such as PDA) before irreversible damage occurs. PH is commonly mild to moderate in patients with left-sided heart disease and infrequently causes clinical symptoms or requires specific treatment. Data regarding the effect of treatment with pulmonary vasodilators on survival for the various etiologies of PH are lacking. The prognosis for PH because of chronic lower airway disease or chronic PTE is often poor because of the chronic nature of the disease process, irreversible damage, and remodeling of the pulmonary vasculature.

SYSTEMIC HYPERTENSION

Definition/overview

Systemic hypertension is defined as a systolic blood pressure >160 mmHg or diastolic pressure >100 mmHg.

Etiology

Systemic hypertension has been documented in veterinary patients most commonly from secondary disease processes and is rarely essential/primary. Causes of secondary hypertension can be classified as volume loading hypertension or not. Diseases that result in increased circulating blood volume or peripheral vasoconstriction include hyperaldosteronism, hyperthyroidism, primary renal disease, diabetes mellitus, Cushing's disease, pheochromocytoma, hyperviscosity syndrome (polycythemia, multiple myeloma, macroglobulinemia), and acromegaly. These diseases result in either activation of the RAAS at different levels, or osmotic increases due to glucose, steroids, red blood cells, proteins, or growth hormones. Essential hypertension has been documented in a line of Siberian Husky mixed breed dogs.

Pathophysiology

Whether primary or secondary, hypertension is associated with increased systemic vascular resistance. Four organs are particularly affected by a chronic elevation in blood pressure: the heart, kidneys, eyes, and brain.

Clinical presentation

Most hypertensive dogs and cats are middle aged to older. Signs reported by the owner are usually caused by the various diseases that lead to systemic hypertension or by lesions in the organs that are most sensitive to the effects of hypertension. For example, hypertensive animals may develop acute blindness or seizures. Target organ consequences caused by uncontrolled hypertension are listed in **Table 7.17**. Physical examination may reveal epistaxis, a palpable thyroid slip, a gallop rhythm, and/or heart murmur.

Differential diagnosis

Differential diagnosis for pathologic systemic hypertension includes physiologic hypertension from stress.

Diagnosis

Diagnosis of systemic hypertension is based on invasive or noninvasive measurements of blood pressure. Invasive blood pressure measurements are made most commonly with the animal restrained in lateral recumbency and a 22–25 gauge catheter inserted into the femoral artery connected by a heparinized saline-filled tubing to a physiologic pressure transducer and hemodynamic oscilloscope recorder. Tubing should not be excessively long and should be kept at the level of the heart.

Noninvasive blood pressure measurement can be obtained by auscultation of Doppler signals with Korotkoff sounds when blood flow to a limb or the tail is obstructed with an appropriately sized and inflated cuff. The choice of cuff is based on the patient's distal limb size. Additionally, noninvasive oscillometric blood pressure measurement is a common technique that relies on detection of arterial pulsation through the use of an automatically inflating and deflating cuff that is wrapped around a distal limb or tail. The accuracy of such devices may be limited in smaller patients, where Doppler measurement is preferred.

Diagnostic tests for secondary causes of systemic hypertension are listed in **Table 7.18**.

Table 7.17 Target organ consequences of systemic hypertension.

Target organ	Consequences
Cardiovascular	Left ventricular concentric hypertrophy Aortic valve insufficiency Arteriosclerosis Atherosclerosis
Cerebrovascular	Infarcts Hemorrhage Cerebrovascular accidents (strokes) Vasospasm
Renal	Polyuria secondary to pressure diuresis Glomerulosclerosis (nephrosclerosis) Glomerular atrophy and nephron loss Tortuous intrarenal vasculature Ischemic renin release
Intraocular	Blindness Retinal detachment, hemorrhage, and/or hyphema Closed angle glaucoma Corneal ulceration

Table 7.18 Diagnostic tests for hypertensive diseases.

Disease	Test
Thyroid disease	T4, free T4, antibody panel
Hyperadrenocorticism	ACTH stimulation test, dexamethasone suppression test, urine cortisol:creatine ratio, abdominal ultrasound
Pheochromocytoma	Abdominal ultrasound, plasma/urinary catecholamine levels
Hyperaldosteronism	Serum sodium and potassium levels, aldosterone assay; abdominal ultrasound
Renal disease	CBC, chemistry, urinalysis, urine culture, urine protein:creatinine ratio, abdominal ultrasound, renal biopsy, creatinine clearance
Polycythemia	Primary versus secondary; CBC, erythropoietin assay, bone marrow biopsy, cardiopulmonary evaluation, abdominal radiographs, and ultrasound
Hyperviscosity	Chemistry, protein electrophoresis, bone marrow biopsy
Intracranial disease	MRI
Acromegaly	Growth hormone assay, clonidine stimulation test
Hyperestrogenism	Estrogen assay, abdominal ultrasound

Management

Underlying causes of secondary systemic hypertension should be treated if possible. Additionally, medical management with antihypertensive medications may be needed acutely and in the long term for treatment of hypertension. Emergency treatment for severe hypertension is described in **Table 7.19**. Drugs commonly used for treatment of hypertension are listed in **Table 7.20**.

Table 7.19 Emergency treatment of systemic hypertension.

Autonomic independent vasodilators	Nitroprusside IV CRI at 0.5–1 µg/kg/min carefully titrated to effect by increasing by 1 µg/kg/min increments every 15 minutes as long as the blood pressure decreases to desired degree (usually 2–5 µg/kg/min with upper limit of 8–10 µg/kg/min) Hydralazine 0.5–1 mg/kg PO q12h in patients administered an ACE inhibitor
Calcium channel blockers	Amlodipine 0.01–0.1 mg/kg PO q24h

Table 7.20 Treatment of systemic hypertension.

ACE inhibitors	Benazepril 0.25–0.5 mg/kg PO q24h Enalapril 0.25–0.5 mg/kg PO q12–24h
Calcium channel blockers	Amlodipine 0.01–0.1 mg/kg PO q24h Diltiazem 0.5–2.0 mg/kg PO q8–12h Diltiazem extended release 2–3 mg/kg PO q12h
Beta-adrenergic receptor blockers	Atenolol 0.5–2.0 mg/kg PO q 12–24 h Propranolol (beta1 and 2) 0.25–0.20 mg/kg PO q8h
Alpha-adrenergic receptor blockers	Prazosin 1 mg/15 kg dog PO q8–12h
Vasodilators	Hydralazine 0.5–1.0 mg/kg PO q12h in patients administered an ACE inhibitor
Diuretics	Furosemide 0.5–4.0 mg/kg PO q8–12h Spironolactone 0.5–2.0 mg/kg PO q12–24h Hydrochlorothiazide 0.5–1.0 mg/kg PO q12–24h

Prognosis

Prognosis for systemic hypertension is good if an underlying cause is identified and treated appropriately and if end-organ damage is minimal.

HEARTWORM DISEASE

Heartworm disease (or dirofilariasis) occurs worldwide. The dog is the typical host of the parasite, but cats can also develop the infection. It is critical to administer year-round chemoprophylaxis, which is highly effective at protecting dogs and cats from heartworm disease.

CANINE HEARTWORM DISEASE

Etiology

Heartworm disease is caused by *Dirofilaria immitis*, a filarial nematode that resides in its adult form in the pulmonary arteries of canids, and uses several species of mosquitoes as vector. Adequate temperature and humidity are necessary to support a viable mosquito population and allow maturation of the heartworm larvae to the infective stage.

Pathophysiology

Infected mosquitoes deposit 1-mm long stage 3 larvae on the dog's skin at the time of a blood meal. Larvae reach the dog's subcutaneous tissues and muscle from the puncture side, and then molt to stage 4 larvae by day 3. Larvae then migrate between muscle fibers where they mature to immature adult worms that enter the circulatory system, which transports them to the pulmonary artery by day 70. Worms measure 10 cm and become sexually mature by 4 months. Mature females release microfilariae, a prelarval stage, into the bloodstream where they are picked up by mosquitoes, which completes the worm's life cycle. Microfilariae first appear in the circulation 6 months post infection. Microfilariae live up to 2.5 years. Heartworms harbor an endosymbiotic bacterium, *Wolbachia* spp.. Elimination of *Wolbachia* has negative effects on *Dirofilaria immitis* fecundity and development. It is also believed that *Wolbachia* trigger an immune response in the dog, which may be responsible for some of the clinical signs associated with heartworm disease.

Live worms cause vascular inflammation with thickening of the pulmonary artery wall and pneumonitis. Additional thromboembolic lesions occur when the worms die and worm fragments obstruct branches of the pulmonary arteries. Over time, lung lesions result in the development of PH and, in severe cases, congestive right heart failure.

Clinical presentation

Most dogs with heartworm disease do not have clinical signs. When present, typical signs involve the respiratory system with cough, tachypnea, and dyspnea; exercise intolerance is also common. Rarely, syncope associated with exercise, hemoptysis, and CHF (ascites) are observed.

Caval syndrome occurs when adult worms embolize in the right ventricle and atrium, where they interfere with tricuspid valve closure (**Figure 7.52**). Caval syndrome is most likely triggered by a profound alteration in hemodynamics, such as the one that accompanies a PTE, and usually a large worm burden. Most dogs with caval syndrome usually show signs of poor perfusion (weakness, tachycardia), dyspnea and tachypnea, ascites, and hemoglobinuria.

Differential diagnosis

Other causes of PH, including PTE, and angiostrongylosis where it is prevalent (Europe, Newfoundland and Labrador provinces of Canada). *Angiostrongylus vasorum*, also referred to as the French heartworm, resides in the pulmonary arteries of dogs. Infected dogs may show respiratory signs, including chronic cough, dyspnea, and exercise intolerance. Others develop PH. Diagnosis is by detection of larvae in feces. Cross-reactions with the *Dirofilaria* antigen tests have been reported.

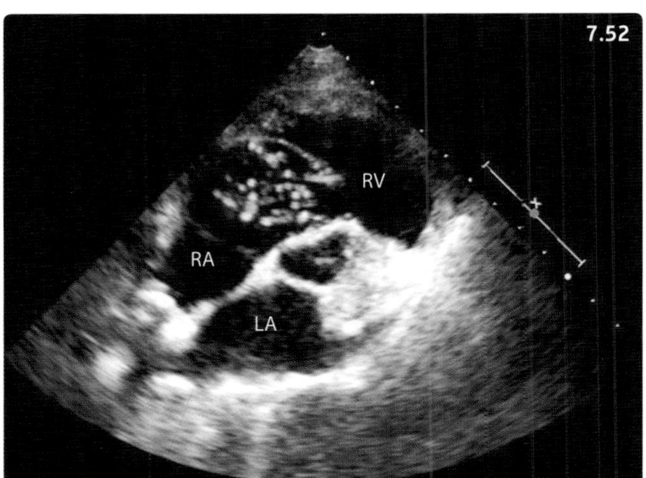

Figure 7.52 Echocardiographic view from a dog with caval syndrome. Worms are visible within the right cardiac chambers. The reflection of the ultrasound on the surface of segments of the worms give this typical image of an '= sign'. LA, left atrium; RA, right atrium; RV, right ventricle.

Diagnosis

Heartworm disease is usually detected during routine yearly screening. The heartworm antigen test, which detects circulating adult female antigens, is a very sensitive and specific test as long as it is performed at least 6 months after infection. Therefore, a test in an infected dog may be negative if it is performed too early, if only male worms are present, or if there are less than three adult worms.

Microfilariae can be detected in some dogs in the peripheral circulation on a direct blood smear or using a Knott's test. However, many dogs experience occult heartworm infections (i.e. microfilariae are not present in the circulation). This is usually the result of the regular or occasional administration of chemoprophylactic drugs that interfere with heartworm reproduction.

Thoracic radiographs, blood work, and urinalysis are usually performed in heartworm-positive dogs to determine the severity of the disease. Radiographs may reveal large and tortuous pulmonary arteries, interstitial to alveolar lung patterns, and, on occasion, right-side cardiomegaly. Eosinophilia and basophilia can be identified on CBC and proteinuria secondary to heartworm-induced glomerulonephritis may be detected on urinalysis. Echocardiography is indicated in dogs presenting with severe signs of heartworm disease. Adult worms are sometimes visible in the right and main pulmonary arteries. The presence of worms in the right cardiac chambers is diagnostic for caval syndrome. In these dogs, a loud intensity right-sided apical systolic murmur, caused by tricuspid valve regurgitation, is usually present.

Management

In infected dogs, the goal of therapy is to kill the adult worms in order to prevent additional damage to the lung vasculature. All dogs with heartworm disease should be treated, and the treatment should include adulticide therapy. The only adulticide currently available is melarsomine dihydrochloride (Immiticide®). Before treatment with melarsomine, preventive medications should be administered for 2–3 months to prevent reinfection and allow heartworm larvae to mature to a young adult stage, which is more sensitive to the effects of melarsomine. Doxycycline (10 mg/kg PO q12h) should be given for 1 month to eliminate *Wolbachia* spp.. Alternatively, minocycline can be used. Melarsomine is administered following a 3-dose protocol (1 injection followed by 2 injections 24 hours apart 1 month later) and 2 months of strict exercise restriction starting the day of the first injection in order to limit the risk of thromboembolism. Animals should be monitored for side-effects for a few hours following injection of melarsomine. Dogs should be retested with a heartworm antigen test 6–9 months later to confirm successful treatment (**Table 7.21**).

Caval syndrome is managed by surgical extraction of the heartworms. Access to the right heart chambers is obtained from a jugular vein. Wire baskets designed for endoscopy inserted in the right atrium and right ventricle under fluoroscopy guidance can be used to 'fish the worms out'. Despite surgical extraction, the mortality of dogs with caval syndrome approaches 40–50%. It is usually not necessary to extract worms that are visible in the pulmonary arteries on echocardiography. Adulticide therapy must be initiated as soon as the animal has recovered from the surgical extraction in order to eliminate the worms still present in the distal pulmonary vessels.

In all dogs that test negative for heartworm disease, macrocyclic lactones (ivermectin, selamectin, moxidectin, milbemycin) are used to prevent the development of stage 3 and stage 4 larvae after mosquito bites. Macrocyclic lactones also have adulticide properties: for example, ivermectin has been shown to kill adults in 31 months. Macrocyclic lactones may not eliminate microfilariae at preventive doses. Year-round prophylaxis is recommended and most drugs are approved for monthly administration.

Table 7.21 Adulticide treatment protocol for dogs with positive antigen test.

Timeline	Treatment
Day 0	Start monthly preventive treatment (macrocyclic lactone): pretreat with antihistamine +/- steroids if circulating microfilariae are present Start 1 month of doxycycline (10 mg/kg PO q12h); alternatively use minocycline Start short course of steroids at anti-inflammatory dose if cough or inflammatory lung lesions present on radiographs Begin exercise restriction
Day 30	Continue preventive treatment
Day 60	Administer first injection of melarsomine (2.5 mg/kg IM) Begin strict exercise restriction (crate, leash walk) Continue preventive treatment
Day 90	Administer second injection of melarsomine (2.5 mg/kg IM) Continue preventive treatment
Day 91	Administer third injection of melarsomine (2.5 mg/kg IM) Continue strict exercise restriction (crate, leash walk)
Day 120	Resume normal exercise levels Make sure year-round administration of preventive is continued
Day 271	Antigen test. If positive, repeat test 2 months later

Heartworm resistance

Most cases of drug failure to prevent heartworm infection can be traced back to poor owner compliance. However, there are convincing reports of resistance to macrocyclic lactones in some regions. One cause for resistance might be the chronic use of macrocyclic lactones in heartworm-positive dogs, which selects a resistant population of microfilariae. Results from experimental studies suggest that the resistance is heritable. It may therefore be important to not only eliminate adult worms but also eliminate microfilariae with microfilaricidal doses of macrocyclic lactones.

Prognosis

Dogs with low-burden infection and limited lung lesions may fully recover after adulticide therapy. However, dogs with severe lesions and PH may develop right-heart failure over time. Once ascites is present, survival is usually less than 1 year.

FELINE HEARTWORM DISEASE

Introduction/overview

Heartworms rarely develop to the adult stage in cats. Most commonly, the manifestations of feline heartworm disease are described as heartworm associated respiratory disease (HARD), which occurs in response to an immune response to larvae and mimics the signs of feline asthma.

Pathophysiology

In regions where canine heartworm disease is prevalent, cat exposure to heartworms is between 5% and 20%. However, in this species, development of the worms usually stops at larval stage 5 (immature worms), and the presence of adult worms is uncommon. Despite incomplete worm development and the absence of long-lasting infection, pulmonary vascular and parenchymal inflammatory lesions are responsible for clinical signs. In cats with mature infection, thromboembolism from dead worms and PH causing right-sided heart failure are major complications of the disease. Finally, aberrant larval migration is more common in cats than dogs, resulting in neurologic signs if larvae reach the central nervous system.

Clinical presentation

It is important to distinguish cats with mature heartworm infection and cats exposed to larvae that failed to develop into adult worms. HARD occurs in response to the short-lived presence of larvae in the pulmonary vasculature. Its clinical manifestations are similar to feline bronchial disease, including dyspnea and wheezes. Cough is frequent. When a small number of adult worms survive in the pulmonary circulation, cats usually develop severe respiratory signs, PH, right heart failure, syncope, and sudden death.

Differential diagnosis

It is challenging to differentiate HARD from feline bronchitis and asthma.

Diagnosis

It is difficult to establish a definitive diagnosis of heartworm disease in cats because most of the available tests lack sensitivity or specificity. Antigen tests, which only detect mature female heartworms, are rarely positive in cats, because they typically only harbor fewer than five worms and sometimes all males. Antibody tests, when positive, indicate that the cat has been exposed to heartworm disease and larvae have developed at least to stage 5 (immature worms). However, they do not indicate the presence of adult worms nor that the infection is ongoing. A negative antibody test usually rules out the presence of adult worms. It is usually recommended to start with an antibody test and perform an antigen test when the antibody test is positive. The presence of circulating microfilariae in the peripheral circulation of cats is unusual. Indirect signs of heartworm disease, such as eosinophilia and basophilia, enlarged pulmonary arteries and bronchointerstitial lung pattern on chest radiographs, and echocardiographic evidence of adult worms in the branches of the pulmonary artery, are inconsistent. Therefore, when HARD or adult worm infection is suspected, diagnosis of heartworm disease relies on suggestive clinical signs, in particular cough, and the results of laboratory tests and imaging.

Management

HARD usually responds to medications used for the treatment of feline asthma including steroids and bronchodilators. If adult worms are present, the high incidence of life-threatening complications associated with use of melarsomine limits the use of this drug in cats. Alternatively, cats can be administered monthly preventive therapy and steroids should be used to control inflammation. The authors use doxycycline for 1 month. Sildenafil can be used if severe PH is present.

Prognosis

Mortality is high in cats that harbor adult worms.

BRADYARRHYTHMIAS

Bradycardia corresponds to a heart rate less than 60 bpm in dogs and approximately 100 bpm in cats. Bradyarrhythmias can result from an increase in vagal tone, drugs, electrolyte abnormalities, inflammation or infiltration of the myocardium, and degenerative disease of the conduction system. Although the etiology frequently remains unclear, the clinician needs to determine from the ECG and the clinical signs whether extracardiac factors are the cause for the arrhythmia, if treatment is needed, and how to choose between medical and pacemaker therapy.

SICK SINUS SYNDROME (SINUS NODE DYSFUNCTION)

Definition/overview

Sick sinus syndrome is a disease of the conduction system in dogs characterized by periods of normal sinus rhythm or sinus bradycardia, interspersed with long periods of sinus arrest or block that can last up to 10–12 seconds. The pauses result from a failure of the junctional and ventricular pacemakers to initiate escape beats, indicating that this disease involves the conduction system beyond the sinus node (**Figure 7.53**). A variant of the disease, sometimes called tachy–brady syndrome,

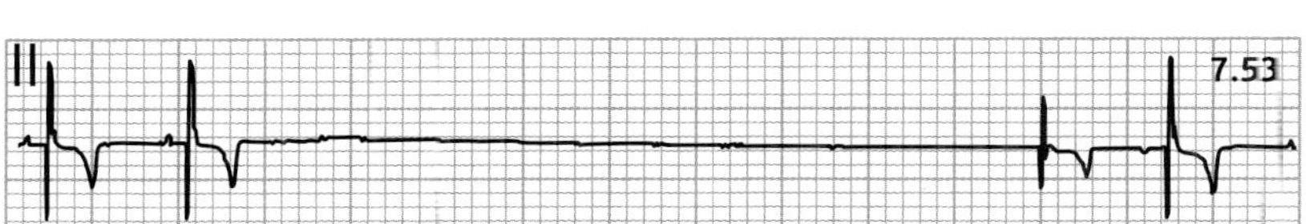

Figure 7.53 ECG (lead II) from a dog with sick sinus syndrome. The initial sinus rhythm is followed by a long period of sinus arrest that is interrupted by a junctional escape beat.

is characterized by periods of paroxysmal supraventricular tachycardia followed by a temporary failure of the sinus rhythm to resume when the tachycardia abruptly terminates.

Etiology

The cause for sick sinus syndrome is unknown. However, there is a breed predisposition, with Miniature Schnauzers and West Highland White Terriers being overrepresented, and the condition typically occurs in older dogs.

Clinical presentation

Exercise intolerance and lethargy are some of the clinical signs reported with sick sinus syndrome. Syncope occurs when periods of sinus arrest last more than 6–8 seconds. The use of opioids as sedatives frequently results in a prolongation of the periods of asystole, and it is not uncommon for dogs that were asymptomatic while awake to become hemodynamically unstable after sedation or general anesthesia.

Differential diagnosis

Other bradyarrhythmias that may cause clinical signs, in particular bradyarrhythmias resulting from high vagal tone in the presence of GI, respiratory, neurologic, and ocular diseases. Marked vagotonia may cause sinus bradycardia, pronounced respiratory sinus arrhythmia, and occasionally second-degree AV block, which may mimic a mild form of sick sinus syndrome.

Diagnosis

In older small breed dogs, the suspicion of sick sinus syndrome is usually confirmed on an ECG recording. To differentiate sick sinus syndrome from vagally-induced bradycardias, response to the administration of parasympatholytic medications can be evaluated. A rapid increase in heart rate following IV administration of atropine (0.04 mg/kg) or glycopyrrolate (0.01 mg/kg) strongly suggests the contribution of vagal tone to the bradyarrhythmia. However, an increase in heart rate may also be observed in dogs with sick sinus syndrome. It is therefore recommended to evaluate the ECG over a longer period of time using a 24-hour Holter recording.

Management

Temporary response to terbutaline (0.2 mg/kg PO q8–12h or 0.01 mg/kg IV), a selective beta2-agonist commonly used as bronchodilator, or aminophylline (10 mg/kg twice PO q12h or 10 mg/kg IV), a phosphodiesterase inhibitor and bronchodilator with mild chronotropic effect, is observed in some dogs with sick sinus syndrome. However, dogs frequently develop side-effects with chronic use of these drugs, and the clinical signs frequently reccur as the disease progresses (**Table 7.22**).

Permanent pacemaker implantation is indicated in dogs that display clinical signs. The simplest and most commonly used type of pacing in veterinary patients involves a single lead placed in the right ventricle via the jugular vein and a generator placed subcutaneously in the

Table 7.22 Drugs for the treatment of bradycardia.

Drug	Dosage	Indications
Atropine	0.02–0.04 mg/kg SC, IM, IV (D,C)	Sinus bradycardia Sick sinus syndrome First- and second-degree AV block
Glycopyrrolate	0.005–0.01 mg/kg SC, IM, IV (D,C)	Sinus bradycardia Sick sinus syndrome First- and second-degree AV block
Terbutaline	0.2 mg/kg PO q8–12h (D) 0.625 mg PO q8–12h (C) 0.01 mg/kg IV (D,C)	Sinus bradycardia Sick sinus syndrome
Isoproterenol	0.04–0.09 μg/kg/min, to effect (D,C)	Second- and third-degree AV block
Aminophylline Theophylline	10 mg/kg PO q12h (extended release) (D,C) 10 mg/kg IV (D)	Sick sinus syndrome

AV, atrioventricular; C, cat; D, dog.

cervical region. Pacemakers are able to detect spontaneous activity and stimulate cardiac contraction if the heart rate drops below a preprogramed number (usually around 80 bpm). In dogs with sick sinus syndrome the pacemaker maintains a regular rhythm and adequate cardiac output during periods of sinus arrest; because the rhythm abnormalities associated with sick sinus syndrome are intermittent, the pacemaker is usually activated less than 50% of the time in these dogs. It therefore mimics a ventricular escape rhythm, whose rate can be adjusted.

Prognosis

Clinical signs worsen as the disease progresses and without treatment some dogs experience several syncopal episodes every day. Some will eventually die suddenly, but it is common for dogs with sick sinus syndrome to experience signs for months and even years before they die. Long-term prognosis is good after pacemaker implantation if complications associated with the procedure do not occur within 1 month, and in the absence of underlying structural heart disease, such as degenerative mitral valve disease, which is also common in older small breed dogs and may lead to CHF. Major but rare pacemaker complications include lead dislodgement during the first 4 weeks following implantation, and device infection, which is more likely to occur during the first year.

ATRIOVENTRICULAR BLOCK

Definition/overview

AV block corresponds to a delay of conduction or the inability for a impulse originating from the atrium to cross the AV node. The AV node is the only pathway for electrical impulses to travel from atrium to ventricle.

Etiology

Fibrosis of the AV node is the most common cause for AV block in older dogs and cats. Inflammation and infiltration of the AV node by neoplastic cells (e.g. lymphoma) are other causes of AV block. Elevated vagal tone may delay AV node conduction. Drugs, such as beta-blockers and calcium-channel blockers, can also cause AV block.

Pathophysiology

Three forms of AV block, corresponding to different degrees of disease severity, are recognized. In the mild form of the disease, all impulses originating at the supraventricular level (usually the sinus node) cross the AV node but with some delay (first-degree AV block). As the disease progresses, some impulses are unable to reach the ventricles (second-degree AV block). In the most severe form of the disease, there is complete dissociation between impulses in the atrium and an escape rhythm originating in the ventricles that maintains a low heart rate and a decreased cardiac output (third-degree AV block). Clinical signs occur when too many supraventricular impulses are blocked in the AV node, which results in the absence of ventricular contraction for 4–8 seconds, or when the slow ventricular escape rhythm does not maintain adequate cardiac output

Clinical presentation

Animals with first-degree AV block do not display clinical signs, as all the impulses from the atrium are transmitted to the ventricles with a short delay. Clinical signs of lethargy, weakness, or syncope only occur in the severe forms of second-degree AV block and third-degree AV block. Surprisingly, some dogs with third-degree AV block and an average heart rate between 20 and 60 bpm do not show obvious clinical signs. Clinical signs are commonly absent in cats because the ventricular escape rhythm is usually around 100 bpm in this species. However, if a slow heart rate persists for several months it will progressively lead to cardiac enlargement and possibly CHF (usually right-sided).

Differential diagnosis

Other cardiac causes of syncope and lethargy

Diagnosis

Diagnosis is usually easily reached from an ECG. With first-degree AV block all the atrial impulses are conducted to the ventricles, but the PR interval is prolonged on the ECG (PR >130 ms in dogs, PR >90 ms in cats). Second-degree AV block is diagnosed when some P waves are not followed by a QRS complex on the surface ECG (**Figure 7.54**).

Two types of second-degree AV blocks are recognized. Mobitz type I second-degree AV block is characterized by a progressive increase in the PR interval duration ending with a blocked P wave, known as Wenckebach phenomenon. It usually results from a combination of AV node fibrosis and a progressive increase in vagal tone. This form of AV block is usually benign and does not require specific treatment Mobitz type II second-degree AV block is characterized by the unexpected occurrence of blocked P waves. PR intervals before and after the blocked P waves are identical. The QRS complexes of conducted beats can be wide when the area of block is below the His bundle, causing bundle branch blocks and intraventricular conduction delays. This form of block is more likely to worsen and result in clinical signs. Administration of atropine (0.04 mg/kg IV) can help the clinician differentiate between the two forms of block. Type I usually improves after atropine and type II worsens.

Third-degree, or complete, AV block is characterized by an absence of conducted P waves to the ventricles (**Figure 7.55**). The ECG displays independent atrial and ventricular activities. Cardiac output is dramatically reduced. In response, the atrial rate, which is under control of the adrenergic tone, is elevated. Electrical activation of the ventricles is dependent on an escape rhythm beyond the site of the block. The QRS complexes are generally wide and bizarre at rates of around 20–60 bpm in dogs and 60–120 bpm in cats. In addition, the ventricular rate is regular, unless ventricular premature beats originating from an ischemic myocardium are present.

A 24-hour Holter recording is sometimes necessary to identify occasional second-degree AV block as the cause for syncope. An echocardiogram is always indicated to identify a tumor as the cause for AV block and to identify concomitant structural cardiac disease. AV block is often associated with structural cardiac disease in cats. Although a mild elevation of serum cTnI concentration is common in dogs with third-degree (complete) AV block, a marked increase in concentration suggests myocarditis as the cause for the arrhythmia.

Management

Pacemaker implantation is usually the best treatment option when clinical signs are present. AV node conduction may improve in some dogs with second-degree AV block after administration of theophylline or terbutaline.

Prognosis

Good after pacemaker implantation in dogs with clinical signs. Some dogs with myocarditis spontaneously return to sinus rhythm.

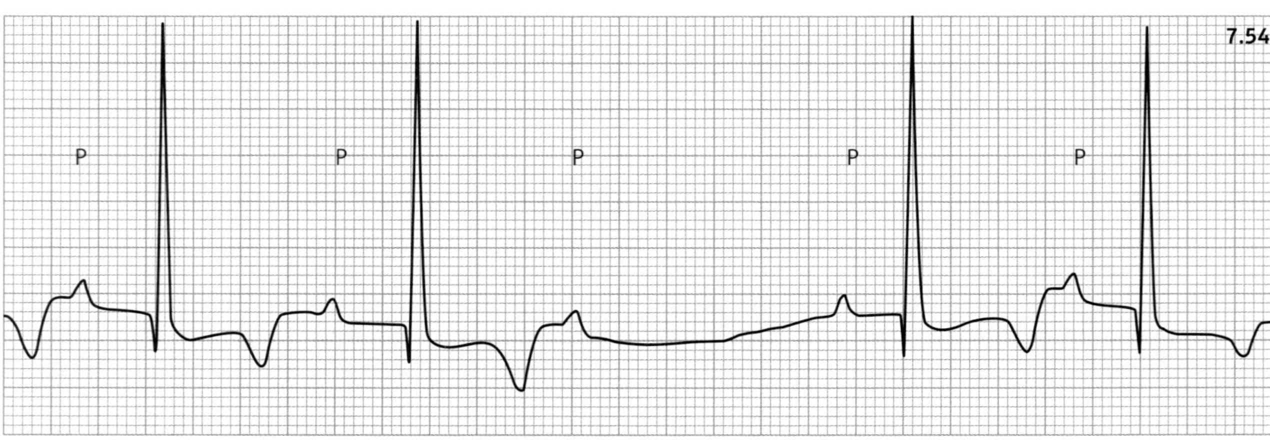

Figure 7.54 ECG (lead II) from a dog with first-degree and Mobitz type 1 second-degree atrioventricular block. The baseline PR interval is prolonged. There is one nonconducted P wave consistent with second-degree atrioventricular block. Note the variable PR interval indicating the effects of vagal tone on atrioventricular conduction.

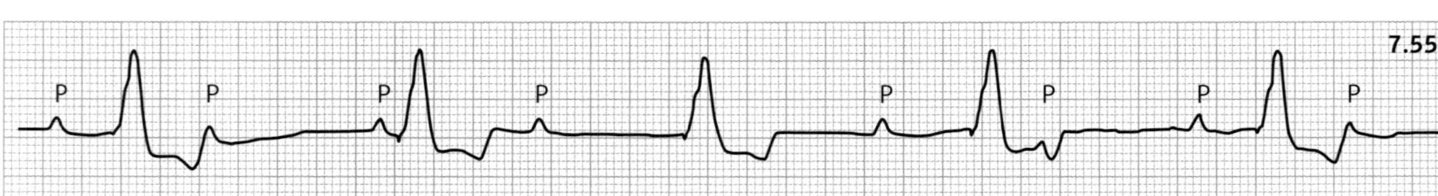

Figure 7.55 ECG (lead II) from a dog with third-degree atrioventricular block. There is complete dissociation between the P waves and QRS complexes. Some P waves overlap T waves.

ATRIAL STANDSTILL

Definition/overview

Atrial standstill corresponds to the absence of visible atrial electrical activity (and therefore contraction) on the ECG. It can be permanent or temporary. Permanent atrial standstill is rare.

Etiology

Permanent atrial standstill affects young dogs and a genetic etiology is likely. It may be more prevalent in English Springer Spaniels. Hyperkalemia is the cause for temporary atrial standstill.

Clinical presentation

Dogs with permanent atrial standstill usually present with signs associated with severe bradycardia. Animals with hyperkalemia have signs caused by the underlying disease, including Addison's disease, urinary tract obstruction or rupture, severe arterial thromboembolism in cats, and tumor lysis syndrome.

Diagnosis

Permanent atrial standstill is recognized on the ECG as a lack of P waves with a regular ventricular or AV nodal escape rhythm at rates of 20–60 bpm in dogs (**Figure 7.56**). The ECG changes of hyperkalemia include a narrowing and increased amplitude of the T wave as plasma concentration of potassium increases above 5.5 mmol/l. As potassium continues to rise, it leads to a decrease in heart rate associated with reduced P wave amplitude and a widening of the QRS complexes. P waves then become invisible, consistent with a sino-ventricular rhythm that cannot be distinguished from atrial standstill.

Management

Permanent atrial standstill requires permanent pacemaker implantation. Successful management of hyperkalemia results in return of normal cardiac rhythm and ECG trace.

Prognosis

Permanent atrial standstill carries a poor prognosis, as the disease affecting the atrium and causing a progressive replacement of the myocytes by fibrous tissue seems to progress to the rest of the myocardium.

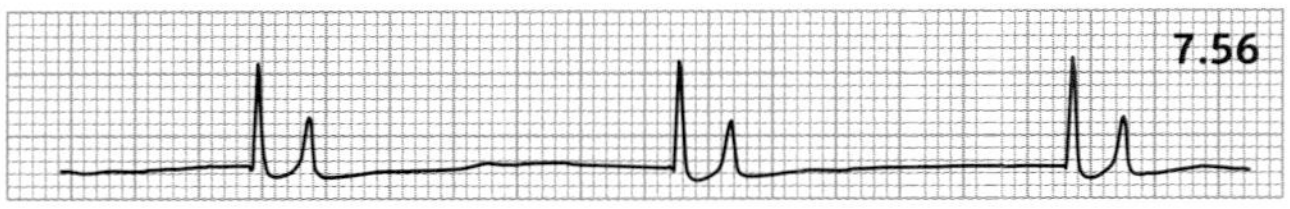

Figure 7.56 ECG (lead II) from a dog with atrial standstill. There are no visible P waves and the ventricular rhythm is regular.

TACHYARRHYTHMIAS

Tachycardia is defined by a heart rate typically >180–200 bpm in dogs and >220–240 bpm in cats. Tachyarrhythmias are divided into supraventricular tachycardia, which originates from structures above the ventricles (sinus node, atrial myocardium, AV node), and ventricular tachycardia. AF, a form of supraventricular tachycardia, and ventricular tachycardia are the most common types of tachyarrhythmias. Other types of supraventricular tachycardias are rare and can usually be managed in the same way as AF.

ATRIAL FIBRILLATION

Definition/overview

AF is characterized by uncoordinated atrial activation from multiple simultaneous electrical wavelets resulting in inadequate mechanical contraction of the atrium and an irregular ventricular response rate.

Etiology

Atrial dilation is a risk factor for developing AF. Therefore, AF commonly occurs in large breed dogs with only mild to moderate atrial dilation, but is rarely present in small breed dogs with degenerative mitral valve disease despite extreme atrial dilation. It is also rarely diagnosed in cats. Fibrosis, inflammation, and autonomic imbalances are other important contributors to the initiation of AF.

Pathophysiology

Most dogs with AF have underlying primary cardiac disease in the form of DCM or degenerative mitral valve disease. The atrial enlargement provides the substrate for maintenance of the arrhythmia. During AF, the AV node is bombarded by hundreds of impulses originating from the atria. Because the AV node has the role of a filter, only some of the impulses are able to reach the ventricles, with an irregular response to the supraventricular impulses. In the presence of heart failure, elevated adrenergic tone decreases the filtering property of the AV node resulting in tachycardia. Less commonly, 'lone' AF occurs in giant breed dogs with structurally normal hearts. In this instance, vagal tone, which is typically high in dogs in the absence of heart failure, increases the filtering effect of the AV node, resulting in a heart rate within the normal range for dogs. AF is rarely identified in cats. However, most cats with AF have underlying structural cardiac disease with atrial enlargement. Many of these cats also show signs of CHF. Once initiated, AF does not spontaneously resolve.

Clinical presentation

The vast majority of dogs with AF are giant and large breed dogs. In the giant breed group, Irish Wolfhounds, Mastiffs, Newfoundlands, Rottweilers, and Great Danes are over-represented, with a male predisposition. Cats with AF are usually older males. Most dogs with 'lone' AF are asymptomatic. Conversely, some dogs with compensated cardiac disease and AF show signs of lethargy, exercise intolerance and, rarely, anorexia, cough, or syncope. When AF occurs in the presence of CHF, generalized weakness, dyspnea, cough, and abdominal distension from ascites are usually present. Cats frequently show signs of an underlying cardiac disease, including dyspnea and arterial thromboembolism. However, AF can also be an incidental finding on auscultation in this species.

Differential diagnosis

Other permanent tachyarrhythmias. The distinctive feature of AF is that it is irregular, whereas most sustained tachyarrhythmias are regular.

Diagnosis

On physical examination, AF is identified as a sustained and 'irregularly irregular' rhythm accompanied by pulse deficits. A murmur may be ausculted, as severe underlying cardiac disease is common in dogs with AF.

On the surface ECG, AF is an irregular tachyarrhythmia, with usually narrow QRS complexes and no P waves, which can be replaced by an undulation of the baseline, or F waves (**Figure 7.57**). It is also permanent, indicating that sinus rhythm never spontaneously resumes following initiation of AF, and the average heart rate is typically >180–200 bpm. The rate is much lower with 'lone' AF, usually approaching 100–120 bpm at rest. Although AF is a supraventricular tachycardia, lesions of the ventricular conduction system (bundle branch block) may result in a widening of the QRS complexes, which may resemble those of ventricular tachycardia.

Determination of the average ventricular rate during AF provides critical information in deciding on a treatment strategy. Unfortunately, brief ECG recordings obtained in an unfamiliar environment do not adequately reflect the daily variations of heart rate. Heart rate is therefore better assessed from a 24-hour Holter recording. For reference, the average heart rate of healthy dogs varies between 85 and 100 bpm. Conversely, it is approximately 120 bpm in dogs with 'lone' AF, 155 bpm in dogs with underlying cardiac disease, and 200 bpm in dogs with CHF.

Management

A rate-control strategy is usually applied to the treatment of AF. The rate-control approach aims at slowing ventricular rate in response to the rapid supraventricular impulses. However, it does not terminate the arrhythmia. Rate control is based on using drugs to decrease the ability of the AV node to conduct impulses. Ideally, the need for pharmacologic control of the heart rate is determined from the heart rate distribution obtained from a baseline 24-hour Holter recording. The effect of rate-control drugs is then assessed on a follow-up Holter 2 weeks after treatment initiation. As for defining adequate control, an average heart rate of no more than 120–140 bpm is considered adequate to observe clinical improvement. If the average heart rate is considered too high, drug dosages are increased by small increments, with close monitoring of the animal's clinical status, as the response to antiarrhythmics varies between patients. In contrast, medical therapy is usually not needed in dogs with 'lone' AF; in these dogs, AF can be reverted to normal rhythm using DC electrical cardioversion.

Diltiazem is widely used for the management of AF. A graded dose of diltiazem results in a decrease in ventricular response rate, because of slower action potential propagation in the AV node. Oral formulations include an extended release form. A dose of 3–4 mg/kg PO q12h of the extended release formulation usually achieves satisfactory rate control. Better rate control, especially during periods associated with high adrenergic tone, can be obtained by adding digoxin to the treatment regimen. Calcium channel blockers decrease ventricular contractility and may cause hypotension when used in animals with severely depressed cardiac function.

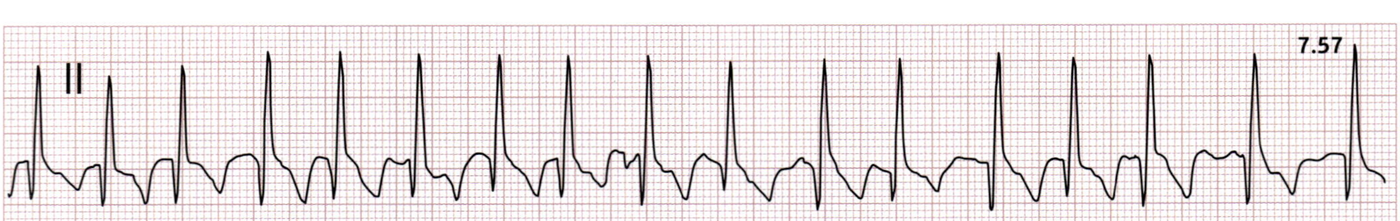

Figure 7.57 ECG (lead II) from a dog with atrial fibrillation. It is an irregular tachycardia. The QRS complexes are narrow indicating that it is supraventricular in origin. In addition, there are no visible P waves.

Table 7.23 Drugs for the treatment of supraventricular tachycardia.

Drug	Dosage	Comment
Digoxin	0.005 mg/kg PO q12h (D)	AF (rate control)
Diltiazem	0.1–0.4 mg/kg IV over 5 min (D,C) 0.05–0.15 mg/kg/h CRI (D,C) 1–2 mg/kg PO q8h (D,C) 3 mg/kg PO q12h (extended release) (D) 15–30 mg PO q12–24h (extended release) (C)	SVT (rate control or conversion) AF (rate control)
Atenolol	0.2–1 mg/kg PO q12–24h (D) 6.25–12.5 mg PO q12–24h (C)	SVT (rate control or conversion) AF (rate ontrol)
Esmolol	0.2–0.5 mg/kg IV over 1 min, repeat q5min (D,C)	SVT conversion
Procainamide	5–15 mg/kg IV over 1 min (D) 1–2 mg/kg IV (C) 20–50 μg/kg/min CRI (D)	SVT conversion
Lidocaine	2 mg/kg IV over 30 sec. Maximum 3 boluses (D) 0.25–0.5 mg/kg IV (C)	SVT conversion Vagally-mediated AF conversion
Sotalol	1–3 mg/kg PO q12h (D,C)	SVT conversion SR maintenance

C, cat; D, dog; SVT, supraventricular tachycardia; AF, atrial fibrillation; SR, sinus rhythm.

The range of indications and side-effects for beta-blockers are very similar to those of calcium channel blockers. Beta1-selective agents, such as atenolol, are preferred to nonselective agents that can cause bronchospasm (**Table 7.23**).

Prognosis

Long-term prognosis is good for dogs with 'lone' AF. However, in some breeds, in particular Irish Wolfhounds, it may be an early sign of DCM. In dogs with AF with underlying structural heart failure, median survival has been reported to be 32 months. However, it was only 5 months when CHF was present. In cats, treatment targeted at AF is rarely required as their ventricular response rate usually approaches the heart rate recorded in cats with sinus rhythm and heart failure.

VENTRICULAR TACHYCARDIA

Definition/overview

Ventricular tachycardia is a rapid rhythm originating from the ventricles. A ventricular rhythm with a rate above the typical ventricular escape rhythm seen with AV block, but slower than ventricular tachycardia, is called accelerated idioventricular rhythm.

Etiology

Ventricular tachycardia is usually diagnosed in Boxers and English Bulldogs with ARVC and in Dobermanns with DCM. It can also occur in the presence of myocarditis, infiltrative cardiac disease, electrolyte imbalances, pheochromocytoma, or hypoxemia/ischemia. Cats are rarely diagnosed with ventricular tachycardia that requires treatment. In this species, it is associated with HCM and hyperthyroidism. Accelerated idioventricular rhythm is triggered by episodes of ischemia/reperfusion involving extracardiac tissues (e.g. gastric dilatation volvulus, trauma, arterial thromboembolism, or pancreatitis).

Pathophysiology

The two factors that determine the clinical consequences of ventricular tachycardia are rate and duration. Ventricular tachycardia must be sustained (more than 30 seconds) and rapid (usually more than 220–240 bpm) to cause clinical signs. Some forms of ventricular tachycardia can degenerate into ventricular fibrillation, resulting in sudden death.

Clinical presentation

Dogs with intermittent ventricular premature contractions do not show clinical signs. It is only when the rate of the ventricular tachycardia is rapid (>250–300 bpm) that signs of poor cardiac output may be present and syncope may occur. Clinical signs will also be influenced by the degree of underlying heart disease. Thus, a patient with systolic dysfunction and ventricular arrhythmia may exhibit clinical signs at a slower rate of ventricular firing than a patient without underlying myocardial disease and ventricular tachycardia.

Diagnosis

Ventricular arrhythmias are diagnosed on ECG by the presence of wide and bizarre complexes (**Figure 7.58**). Beats originating in the ventricles are wide because the electrical impulse depolarizing the ventricles does not use the specialized cells of the conduction system. The QRS complex of ventricular beats is followed by a large T wave opposite to the direction of the QRS complex. Ventricular tachycardia is usually regular. It can last for a few seconds or be sustained for hours. A 24-hour Holter recording is indicated to evaluate the frequency of the arrhythmia and determine if its severity explains the clinical signs manifested by the animal. An echocardiogram is recommended to identify underlying structural heart disease and measure the left ventricular function. Chest radiographs and blood work are indicated to rule out any extracardiac cause for the arrhythmia, especially in the presence of an idioventricular accelerated rhythm.

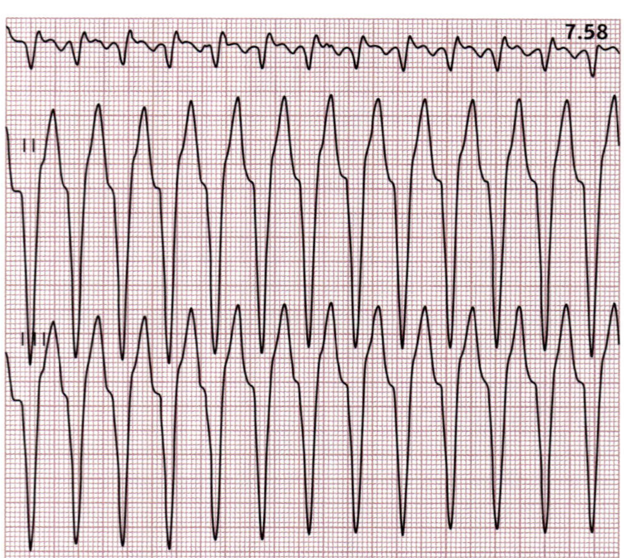

Figure 7.58 ECG from a dog with ventricular tachycardia. The QRS complexes are 'wide and bizarre' and the rhythm is regular.

Management

Treatment of ventricular tachycardia is justified when it causes hemodynamic compromise and, therefore, clinical signs. Hemodynamic compromise is typically related to the rate of the tachycardia and its duration. Sometimes treatment is initiated in apparently nonclinical animals based on the arrhythmia burden in an a Holter recording and the concern that the arrhythmia could worsen or result in sudden death. The risk of sudden death is probably higher in the presence of structural cardiac disease.

For a dog presented in an emergency with rapid sustained ventricular tachycardia, treatment is based on lidocaine boluses. It is important to measure serum potassium concentration, as lidocaine works better with normal potassium levels. Procainamide is an alternative to lidocaine when it fails to terminate the arrhythmia. Lidocaine should be used carefully in cats because they are more likely to develop neurologic side-effects.

Long-term management of ventricular tachycardia is based on oral drugs and frequent monitoring with 24-hour Holter recordings to evaluate the response to treatment. Sotalol, which shares antiarrhythmic and beta-blocking properties, is usually very effective at controlling ventricular arrhythmias in dogs. Mexiletine is another good antiarrhythmic agent, but has become increasingly difficult to obtain for veterinary patients and has several times come off the market. It is often used in combination with atenolol or sotalol for resistant arrhythmias or as an initial antiarrhythmic agent for dogs with systolic dysfunction. Amiodarone appears to be effective for arrhythmias refractory to other drugs; however, it has been reported to have significant and severe side-effects in dogs. The low end of the dosage range should be used first and titrated upwards only if necessary. Amiodarone very commonly causes adverse clinical signs with chronic use. It may cause anorexia due to elevated liver enzymes, therefore liver enzymes should be evaluated before starting and periodically while receiving amiodarone, and any time anorexia develops. It may also cause neutropenia of unknown clinical significance and neurologic signs and/or ataxia, especially at higher doses and with prolonged use. IV antiarrhythmic agents are rarely needed in the cat. Oral products, in particular atenolol and sotalol, are usually sufficient for clinical needs (**Table 7.24**).

Prognosis

Prognosis depends more on the underlying etiology than the tachycardia itself.

Table 7.24 Drugs for the treatment of ventricular tachycardia.

Drug	Dosage
Amiodarone	10–20 mg/kg PO q24h for 7–10 days then reduce to 3–15 mg/kg PO q24–48h thereafter (D)
Atenolol	0.2–1 mg/kg PO q12–24h (D) 6.25–12.5 mg PO q12–24h (C)
Esmolol	0.2–0.5 mg/kg IV over 1 min, repeat q5min (D,C)
Lidocaine	2 mg/kg IV over 30 sec. Maximum 3 boluses (D) 0.25–0.5 mg/kg IV (C) 25–80 µg/kg/min CRI (D)
Mexiletine	4–8 mg/kg PO q8h (D)
Procainamide	5–15 mg/kg IV over 1 min (D) 1–2 mg/kg IV (C) 20–50 µg/kg/min CRI (D)
Sotalol	1–3 mg/kg PO q12h (D,C)

C, cat; D, dog.

RECOMMENDED FURTHER READING

American Heartworm Society. Current guidelines for the diagnosis, prevention, and management of heartworm (*Dirofilaria immitis*) infection in dogs. http://www.heartwormsociety.org

Atkins C, Bonagura J, Ettinger S *et al.* (2009) Guidelines for the diagnosis and treatment of canine chronic valvular heart disease. *J Vet Intern Med* **23:**1142–1150.

Brown S, Atkins C, Bagley R *et al.* (2007) American College of Veterinary Internal Medicine. Guidelines for the identification, evaluation, and management of systemic hypertension in dogs and cats. *J Vet Intern Med* **21:**542–558.

Kellihan HB, Stepien RL (2012) Pulmonary hypertension in canine degenerative mitral valve disease. *J Vet Cardiol* **14:**149–164.

Oyama MA, Reynolds CA (2014) Ventricular arrhythmias in dogs. In: *Kirk's Current Veterinary Therapy XV*. (eds. JD Bonagura, DC Twedt) Elsevier Saunders, St. Louis pp. 745–748.

Pariaut R, Santilli R, Moise NS (2014) Supraventricular tachyarrhythmias in dogs. In *Kirk's Current Veterinary Therapy XV*. (eds. JD Bonagura, DC Twedt) Elsevier Saunders, St. Louis, pp. 737–745.

Chapter 8

Digestive diseases (pharynx to anorectum)

Frédéric Gaschen

Part 1: Diseases of the pharynx, masticatory muscles, and salivary glands

DYSPHAGIA

Definition/overview

The word 'dysphagia' is derived from Greek and means difficulty in eating and swallowing. A closely related term is odynophagia, which describes pain while eating/swallowing. The three phases of the normal swallowing reflex are described in **Table 8.1**.

Etiology

Three types of dysphagia are recognized.

Oral dysphagia

Oral dysphagia relates to a difficulty prehending food and forming a bolus of food. It can occur with most oral and dental diseases. Additionally, tongue atrophy or paralysis and diseases of the masticatory muscles and temporomandibular joint can also lead to oral dysphagia.

Pharyngeal dysphagia

Pharyngeal dysphagia is characterized by abnormal passage of food through the oropharynx. It may occur with pharyngeal diseases such as pharyngeal edema, trauma and foreign bodies, intraluminal masses, and extraluminal masses (e.g. grossly enlarged lymph nodes, retropharyngeal abscess, salivary gland enlargement), or result from abnormalities in the tightly regulated swallowing reflex. Affected animals may show numerous unsuccessful attempts to swallow regurgitate immediately, gag, cough, and experience nasal reflux. Aspiration pneumonia is common. Diagnosis is confirmed by fluoroscopy that shows failure of the pharynx to constrict and the upper esophageal sphincter (UES) to relax. In the absence of an obvious cause for dysphagia, rabies should be considered in unvaccinated dogs. Dogs with laryngeal paralysis or myasthenia gravis may show concurrent pharyngeal dysphagia. If no cause can be identified, the prognosis of pharyngeal dysphagia is generally poor.

Cricopharyngeal dysphagia

Cricopharyngeal dysphagia is characterized by a failure of the UES to relax (achalasia) or a lack of coordination between pharyngeal contraction and UES relaxation (dyssynchrony). This disorder is rare, and is usually observed in puppies at the time of weaning. Detailed oropharyngeal inspection yields no abnormal findings. Diagnosis is confirmed with a fluoroscopic swallowing study showing that the food remains in the pharynx in spite of normal

Table 8.1 Physiology of swallowing.

Oropharyngeal phase	Voluntary oral stage: formation of food bolus in the oropharynx, passage to the base of tongue, pharyngeal peristaltic contractions, bolus propelled to the laryngopharynx
	Pharyngeal phase: contraction of oral and tongue muscles with closure of pathway between oral cavity and pharynx, elevation of the soft palate, glottis closure, and tipping of the epiglottis after rostral displacement of the larynx
	Cricopharyngeal phase: relaxation of the UES (cricopharyngeal and thyropharyngeal muscles) to allow food bolus to be propelled into the upper esophagus
Esophageal phase	A primary peristaltic wave is generated in the pharynx and propagated through the esophagus to propel the bolus to the LES (lower esophageal sphincter). If the primary wave is not successful, a secondary wave is quickly generated by esophageal distension
Gastroesophageal phase	Relaxation of the LES and passage of the bolus into the stomach

pharyngeal motility. A congenital neurologic disorder is suspected. In the absence of complicating factors, the prognosis for dogs with confirmed cricopharyngeal achalasia is good after myotomy or myectomy of the cricopharyngeal muscle. Injection of botulinum toxin A into the muscle through an oral approach with endoscopic guidance has been anecdotally successful. However, the effect is limited to 2–4 months. The procedure may help identify patients who would most benefit from surgery.

Pathophysiology

Bouvier des Flandres dogs may be affected with a congenital pharyngeal myopathy. Golden Retrievers are overrepresented among dogs with cricopharyngeal dysphagia. Large breed dogs are also predisposed to laryngeal paralysis, a disease more commonly associated with pharyngeal and upper esophageal dysfunction

Clinical presentation

While dogs and cats with oral dysphagia are reluctant or unable to chew properly, animals with pharyngeal or oropharyngeal dysphagia are unable to swallow the food bolus in spite of repeated attempts. If the affected animal takes a quick breath of air between swallowing actions, food may enter the larynx and trachea, eliciting a cough. Dogs will try again and again, and will sometimes succeed in achieving a more adequate swallowing action. They regurgitate the food bolus, which is covered with saliva. Their ability to drink from a water bowl may be maintained or impaired as well. Animals are generally hungry and weight loss and lean body condition are common. Other signs include coughing and nasal discharge.

Diagnosis

Diagnosis relies on clinical signs (**Box 8.1**). A thorough oral and pharyngeal examination, ideally in the sedated animal, is often valuable. Radiographs of the pharynx are recommended in animals with suspect foreign body (FB) or other causes of obstruction. Fluoroscopic swallow studies can be very useful to confirm the type of dysphagia, but are only available in referral centers. If aspiration pneumonia is suspected, chest radiographs are helpful to evaluate the severity and extent of the process.

> **Box 8.1** Practical tip on the clinical approach to dysphagic dogs and cats.
>
> First, observe the animal while it is eating. Videos filmed by the owner can be helpful as well. This allows recognizing the different types of dysphagia and designing a targeted further approach

Management

Nonspecific measures include optimizing the consistency of the food (generally, moist food is best tolerated). Specific treatments correcting the primary disease are most helpful if available (see above). Additionally, in severe or untreatable cases, endoscopically or surgically placed low profile gastrostomy tubes allow bypass of the pharynx and proximal esophagus in order to provide enteral nutrition.

PHARYNGITIS AND TONSILLITIS

Definition/overview

Inflammation causes hyperemia and swelling of the pharyngeal mucosa, which may be associated with tonsillar enlargement and protrusion of the tonsils out of the palatine fossae. Tonsillitis is not uncommon in the dog, particularly in young miniature and toy breeds, but is quite rare in the cat. The inflammation is usually bilateral; however, it may be unilateral in association with FBs such as grass blades, pieces of wood, and grass seeds.

Etiology

Acute pharyngitis with or without secondary tonsillitis may occur following trauma, foreign bodies, insect stings, snake bites, allergic reactions, chemical or thermal injuries, and viral infection of the upper respiratory tract (cat). Additionally, disorders causing chronic vomiting, gagging, coughing, or regurgitation may be associated with acute tonsillitis.

Clinical presentation

Coughing, gagging, retching, or expectorating white foamy mucus (which may be confused with vomiting by the pet's owner) are commonly reported. Dysphagia, repeated swallowing attempts, odynophagia, hypersalivation, excessive licking, and pica can also be observed. Some animals can present with decreased appetite, malaise, and fever. Pharyngeal examination reveals a hyperemic (dog) or injected (cat) pharynx, possibly with enlarged tonsils protruding out of the palatine fossae. Hyperemia, mottled appearance, petechiations, and white specks are reliable signs of acute inflammation. Chronically inflamed tonsils may just be enlarged with an irregular surface.

Differential diagnosis

Tonsillitis should be differentiated from tonsillar neoplasia such as lymphoma (unilateral or bilateral enlargement [**Figure 8.1**]) or squamous cell carcinoma (SCC) (unilateral, highly malignant).

Diagnosis
Diagnosis is based on the abnormal appearance of the pharynx and tonsils in association with the existence of compatible clinical signs. Secondary tonsillitis is common, and a thorough search for a primary underlying disease should be performed. Radiographs of the pharynx and retropharyngeal area may reveal the presence of FBs or space-occupying processes (**Figures 8.2, 8.3**). Fine needle aspiration or brush cytology may help rule out neoplasia and confirm inflammation.

Management
For acute cases, treatment usually consists of a 10–14-day course of antibiotics (e.g. amoxicillin and clavulanic acid), possibly with analgesics if indicated. In chronic cases with significantly enlarged tonsils, tonsillectomy may be required if the tonsils become an obstacle preventing passage of food into the pharynx.

Prognosis
Good, although acute tonsillitis may recur. The disorder usually resolves spontaneously with time.

DISEASES OF THE SALIVARY GLANDS

The four salivary glands of dogs and cats are the submandibular (located rostrolaterally from the submandibular lymph node), sublingual, parotid (under mandibular ramus), and zygomatic (infraorbital) glands. Salivary gland diseases are uncommon in dogs and very rare in cats.

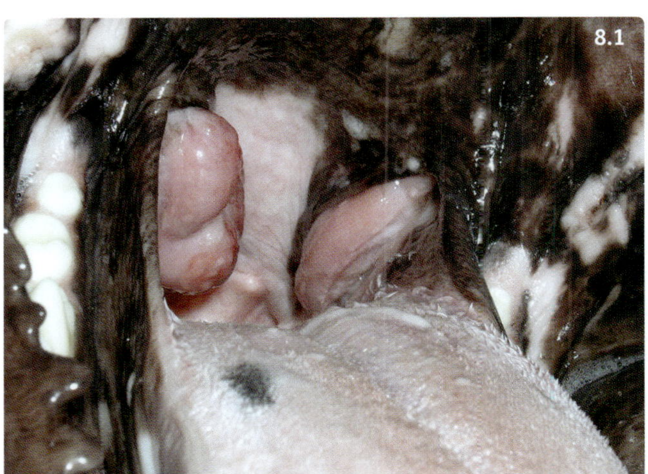

Figure 8.1 Bilaterally enlarged tonsils in a middle aged mixed-breed dog. Cytology from a fine needle aspirate revealed lymphoma. (Courtesy R. Husnik)

MUCOCELE, SIALOCELE

Definition/overview
Sialocele is the most frequently diagnosed salivary gland disorder of dogs. It consists of an accumulation of saliva in the periglandular tissues due to salivary duct obstruction and/or rupture. The wall of the mucocele is not epithelial, therefore mucoceles are not true salivary gland cysts.

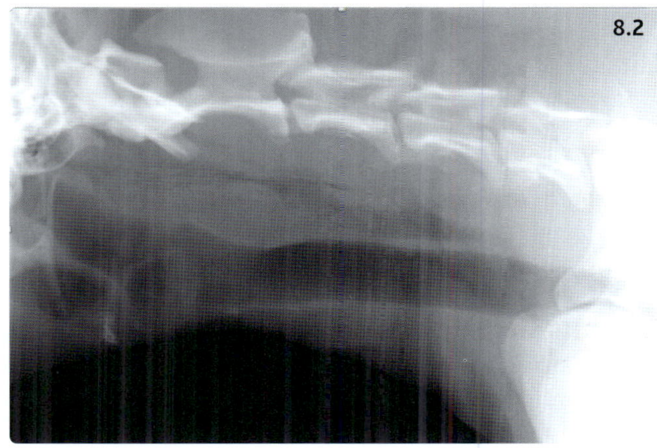

Figure 8.2 Proximal cervical radiograph from a 5-year-old Belgian Shepherd Dog taken 2 hours after the owner pulled a stick that appeared to be stuck in the dog's throat. There is retropharyngeal accumulation of air. Persistent wood fragments cannot be ruled out based on these films. Esophagoscopy was negative, and the dog recovered with antibiotic treatment.

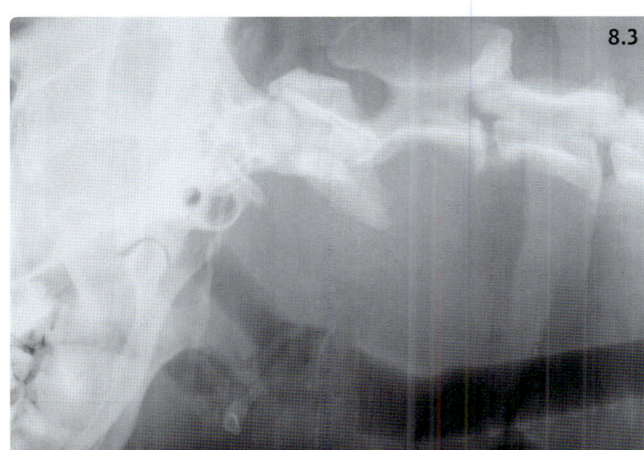

Figure 8.3 Proximal cervical radiograph of an 8-year-old Bernese Mountain Dog with dysphagia. A space-occupying lesion is pushing the pharynx, esophagus, and trachea ventrally. Fine needle aspiration revealed histiocytic sarcoma.

They can occur in the vicinity of each salivary gland; however, the sublingual and submandibular glands are the most frequently affected. German Shepherd Dogs and Poodles appear to be more susceptible to developing sialoceles.

Etiology
Trauma is thought to be the most frequent cause of sialocele (direct trauma, FB, sialadenolith), although signs of original trauma have usually resolved by the time the sialocele is diagnosed.

Clinical presentation
A large usually nonpainful mass is observed in the upper cervical region, the pharynx, or the oral cavity (**Figure 8.4**). Oral and pharyngeal sialoceles may cause dysphagia and oral bleeding following self-trauma. Pharyngeal and cervical mucoceles can occasionally cause dyspnea.

Differential diagnosis
Other causes of salivary gland enlargement such as inflammation (sialadenitis) and neoplasia.

Diagnosis
Diagnosis is based on history, physical examination, and results of fine needle aspiration of the mucocele with a large-bore needle (blood tinged, thick mucoid fluid with few neutrophils). Diagnostic imaging (ultrasound, sialography) can help confirm which gland is involved.

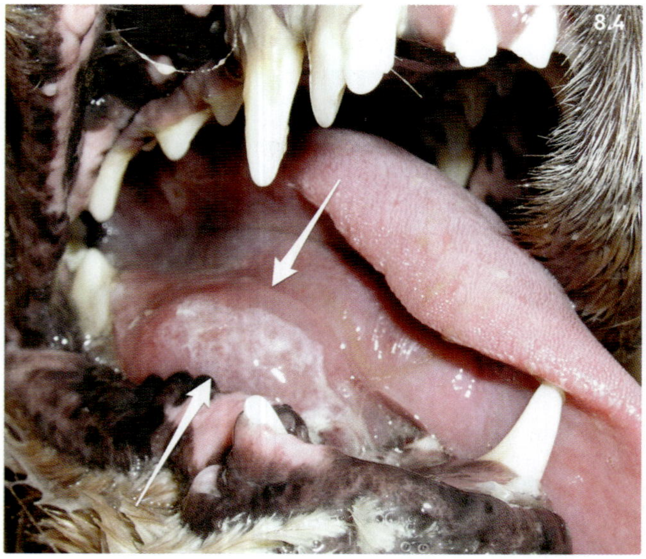

Figure 8.4 A ranula or sialocele affecting the sublingual salivary gland is visible at the base of the tongue of this dog (arrows). (Courtesy R. Husnik)

Management
Treatment consists of removal of the ipsilateral sublingual and submandibular gland as well as drainage of the fluid accumulation.

Prognosis
Prognosis is good following surgery.

SIALADENITIS

Sialadenitis describes inflammation of the salivary glands. A syndrome of inflammation and necrosis is occasionally observed in dogs. The condition leads to enlargement of one or several glands (most frequently the mandibular gland [**Figure 8.5**]). In the presence of severe inflammation, pain and dysphagia can occur. Therapy for sialadenitis is symptomatic and supportive. In severe cases, surgical removal of the gland may be indicated. A nonpainful, noninflammatory swelling has been described in association with vomiting, and seems to respond to phenobarbital therapy.

SALIVARY GLAND NEOPLASIA

Salivary gland neoplasia occurs rarely (more frequently in cats than in dogs). The submandibular gland is most commonly affected. Adenocarcinoma is the most common type.

MASTICATORY MUSCLE MYOSITIS

Definition/overview
Masticatory muscle myositis (MMM) is a common focal inflammatory myopathy of dogs. It selectively affects the muscles of mastication, including temporalis, masseter,

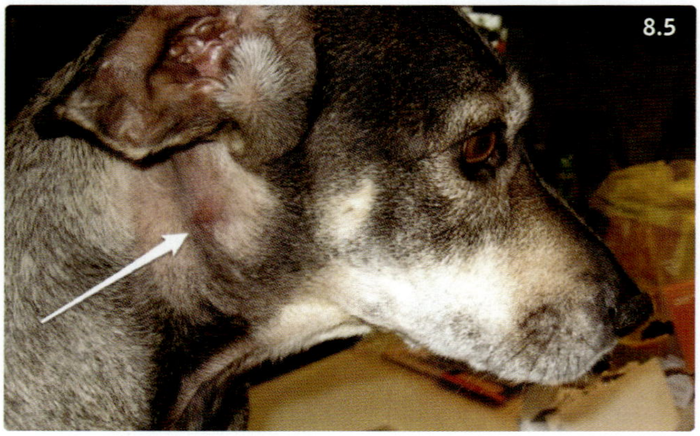

Figure 8.5 A swelling is visible in this dog with sialadenitis of the mandibular salivary gland (arrow). (Courtesy M. Schaer)

pterygoid, and rostral digastricus muscles, while sparing the spinal and limb muscles. Large breed dogs and Cavalier King Charles Spaniels are overrepresented among dogs with MMM.

Etiology/pathophysiology

MMM is caused by an autoimmune process directed against type 2M (superfast) myosin and a myofibril-associated protein, both exclusively found in masticatory muscle fibers.

Clinical presentation

In acute cases, clinical signs include acute swelling of the temporalis and masseter muscles (**Figure 8.6**), masticatory myalgia, restricted jaw movement, pain on opening of the mouth, and exophthalmos. Muscle atrophy and fibrosis with or without restricted jaw movement is present in chronically affected dogs.

Differential diagnosis

The differential diagnosis for dogs with difficulty and/or pain on opening of the mouth is listed in **Table 8.2**. Atrophy of the masticatory muscles may also occur as a result of chronic corticosteroid therapy.

Diagnosis

A serum assay with an excellent sensitivity (85–90%) and specificity (100%) allows detection of circulating autoantibodies against masticatory muscle type 2M fibers (http://vetneuromuscular.ucsd.edu). Serum creatine kinase (CK) activity may be mildly increased or normal. In acute cases, electromyography (EMG) usually reveals abnormal activity. Diagnostic confirmation is obtained with biopsy of the temporalis or masseter muscle (**Box 8.2**) with histopathology and type 2M autoantibody immunohistochemistry. The severity of inflammation and presence of fibrosis are assessed.

Management

Immunosuppressive doses of corticosteroids should be used (e.g. prednisone, 2 mg/kg/day) until the normal range of jaw motion returns and serum CK, if elevated, returns to normal. The dose should then be gradually decreased until the lowest alternate day dose is reached that will keep the dog free of clinical signs. This low dose should then be continued for at least 6 months. MMM is usually very steroid responsive; however, other immunosuppressive agents such as azathioprine may be added in dogs experiencing significant corticosteroid side-effects so that a faster weaning off of steroids is possible. Insufficient doses of corticosteroids for inadequate periods of time result in relapse of the disorder and worsening of the fibrosis.

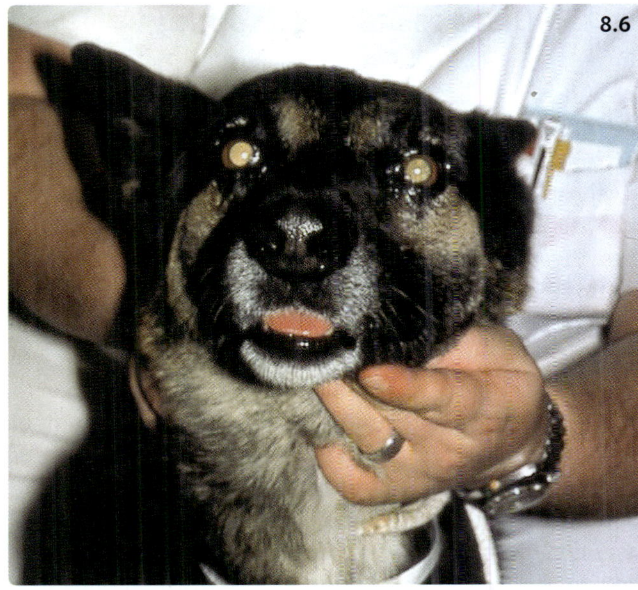

Figure 8.6 German Shepherd Dog with masticatory muscle myositis. The left masseter muscle is visibly swollen. (Courtesy M. Schaer)

Table 8.2 Diseases causing difficulty or pain on opening of the mouth in dogs.

Masticatory muscle myositis
Temporomandibular joint disorders: ankylosis, osteoarthritis
Retrobulbar masses: cellulitis, abscess, granuloma, neoplasia
Zygomatic arch, coronoid process fracture
Craniomandibular osteopathy
Tetanus

Box 8.2 Practical tip on collection of temporalis muscle biopsies.

Make sure the subcutaneous platysma muscle is incised, the thick fascia overlying the temporalis muscle is incised and retracted, and the temporalis muscle itself is exposed and biopsied. The platysma muscle does not contain type 2M fibers and is not affected by masticatory muscle myositis.

Prognosis

Prognosis is good with early diagnosis and treatment. If diagnosis and treatment are delayed until marked atrophy and fibrosis are present, prognosis is poor for return of jaw function and muscle mass. Delayed therapy and/or inadequate doses are common causes for poor clinical outcome.

Part 2: Diseases of the esophagus

Overview

The esophagus is a frequently forgotten part of the gastrointestinal (GI) tract. Esophageal diseases occur relatively commonly in dogs, but are infrequent in cats. They may have serious implications and severely debilitate affected animals. The resulting esophageal dysfunction may lead to regurgitation of undigested food with a high risk of food inhalation and aspiration pneumonia. Additionally, chronic esophageal problems may lead to undernourishment and associated complications. Foreign bodies, strictures, and neoplasia may cause intraluminal obstructions. Vascular abnormalities with compression of the esophagus may also compromise the esophageal lumen. Esophagitis is a frequent complication of esophageal diseases and of gastroesophageal reflux and vomiting. Severe cases may result in development of strictures. Congenital or acquired functional disorders cause esophageal dysmotility and may eventually result in megaesophagus (ME).

Esophageal anatomy

The UES consists of striated muscle fibers of both cricopharyngeal and esophageal origin. The two spirally arranged muscularis layers of the esophagus wind in opposite directions. In cats, they consist of striated muscle fibers in the proximal third of the esophagus (cervical segment), while they only contain smooth muscle fibers in the distal two-thirds of the esophagus (thoracic segment). In contrast, the muscularis layers of the canine esophagus are made exclusively of striated muscle fibers over the whole length of the esophagus. The lower esophageal sphincter (LES) is a thickening of the esophageal muscle located before the gastroesophageal junction.

Normal esophageal function

Esophageal motility is triggered by passage of a food bolus through the pharynx (**Table 8.1**). Afferent impulse is conducted by the glossopharyngeal and vagus nerves to the nucleus solitarius in the brainstem. The information is processed with the help of the reticular formation and the nucleus ambiguus, where the motor neurons are located. These are activated and transmit impulses to the vagus nerve.

Table 8.3 Clinical signs associated with esophageal diseases in dogs and cats.

Regurgitation
Dysphagia
Swallowing attempts 'on empty'
Halitosis
Excessive salivation
Odynophagia (esophagitis)
Anorexia/inappetence (esophagitis)
Ravenous appetite (motility disorders, megaesophagus)
Tachypnea, dyspnea, cough, exercise intolerance, fever (aspiration pneumonia)

Clinical presentation

The clinical signs consistent with esophageal disease are summarized in **Table 8.3**. Regurgitation describes passive retrograde evacuation of undigested food or liquids, and may be associated with pharyngeal or esophageal dysfunction. Differentiation of regurgitation and vomiting relies on several well-defined clinical parameters but can be challenging at times (**Table 8.4**).

Table 8.4 Parameters that help differentiate regurgitation from vomiting*.

Parameter	Regurgitation	Vomiting
Chronology	Usually occurs immediately or soon after food intake, although exceptions may occur	May occur at any time point, after ingesting a meal or in between meals
Appearance	Typically looks like undigested food covered with saliva	May have many different appearances and look more or less digested. The presence of bile or digested (dark) blood suggests gastric origin
Behavior	Usually occurs without prodromal phase	Often preceded by nausea (frequently with hypersalivation)
Abdominal contractions	Usually absent	Retching typically present
Associated clinical signs	Dysphagia, odynophagia, hypersalivation, repeated swallowing attempts, weight loss if chronic	Nausea, lethargy, anorexia, weight loss
Risk of aspiration pneumonia	High	Moderate

* **Note**: there may be considerable overlap in the signs associated with regurgitation and vomiting.

ESOPHAGEAL OBSTRUCTION

ESOPHAGEAL FOREIGN BODY

Esophageal FBs are a common problem in dogs while they are infrequently diagnosed in cats.

Etiology

In dogs, esophageal FBs are frequently observed in small breeds, but may occur in any size dog. The foreign material often consists of beef, pork, veal, or chicken bone(s) coated with various amounts of connective tissue. Dog treats swallowed with insufficient chewing have also been reported. Fishing hooks when swallowed also get stuck in the esophagus. Esophageal FBs are most often located at one of three sites: thoracic inlet, heart base, or cranial to the distal sphincter of the esophagus.

Clinical presentation

Animals are often presented with a suggestive history (e.g. ingestion of bones, toys missing). The clinical signs typically include regurgitation, dysorexia, excessive drooling, odynophagia, halitosis, and retching. Additional signs (e.g. lethargy, anorexia, dyspnea, shock associated with systemic inflammatory response syndrome [SIRS], or sepsis) may occur in association with complications such as esophageal perforation with mediastinitis or pleuritis, or aspiration pneumonia.

Differential diagnosis

Other esophageal diseases: stricture, esophagitis, ME, and esophageal tumors. Additionally, differentiation between clinical signs of esophageal FB and those of vomiting and associated diseases can be difficult at times (**Table 8.4**).

Diagnosis

The presence of an esophageal FB is best confirmed using chest radiographs that reveal a soft tissue mass in the esophagus at the level of the obstruction (**Figures 8.7, 8.8**). In most instances, the use of barium sulfate is not required, and risks associated with its use can be avoided (aspiration pneumonia, damage to endoscopic equipment if esophagoscopy is performed soon after the esophagram). It is important to evaluate radiographs for the presence of free air in the mediastinum and pleural effusion, as these may indicate esophageal perforation or rupture.

Management/prevention

Treatment consists of extracting the FB under endoscopic or fluoroscopic guidance as soon as possible (**Figure 8.9**). If extraction through the oral cavity is too difficult, the FB can be pushed into the stomach. Bone, cartilage, and fibrous tissue material can generally be digested by gastric juice and eliminated naturally. If passage through the pyloric canal seems impossible, gastrotomy and extraction of the FB is performed.

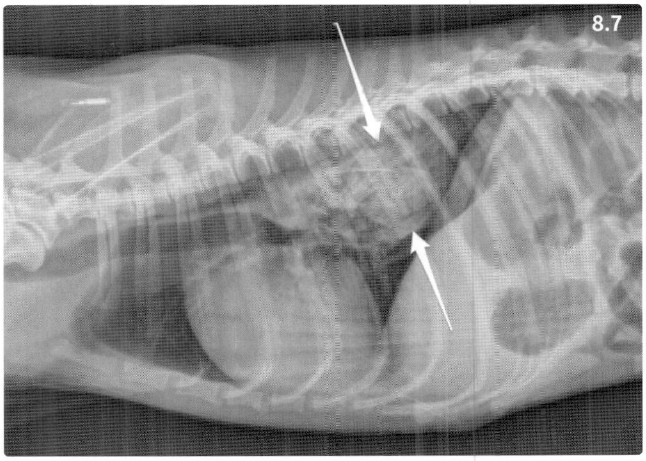

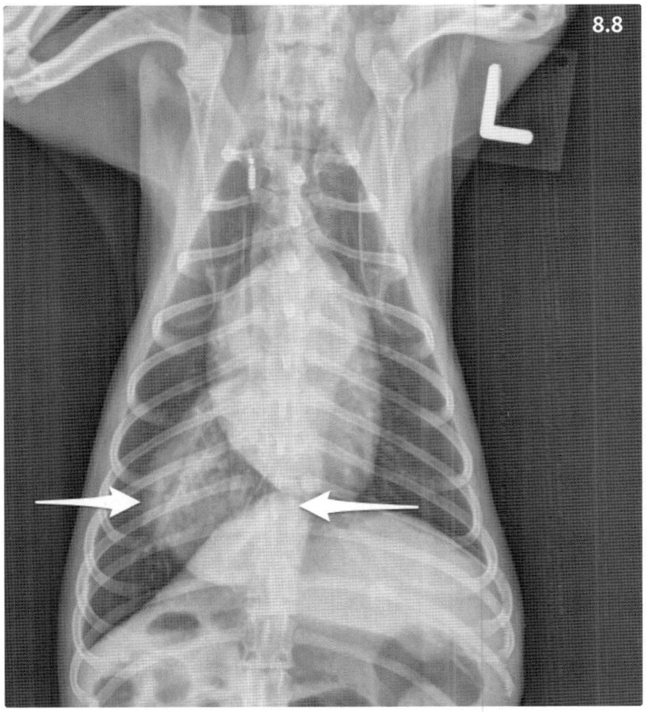

Figures 8.7, 8.8 Four-year-old male Papillon Spaniel. (8.7) Right lateral thoracic radiograph. A large soft tissue opacity is visible in the caudal half of the thoracic esophagus (dorsal and ventral limits shown by arrows). Interpretation: esophageal foreign body without indication of esophageal perforation and pleuritis. (8.8) The ventrodorsal thoracic radiograph shows the same soft tissue opacity in the esophagus caudal to the heart base (arrows).

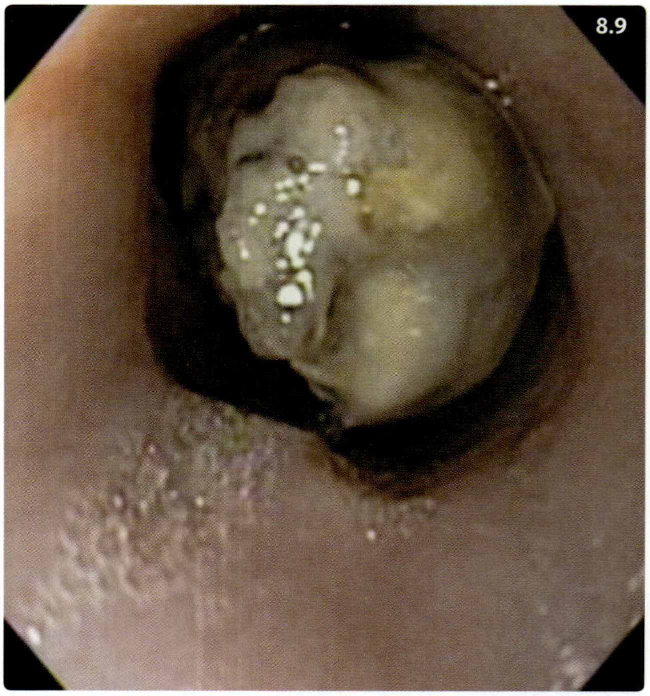

Figure 8.9 Esophagoscopy showing a bone foreign body in the caudal thoracic esophagus.

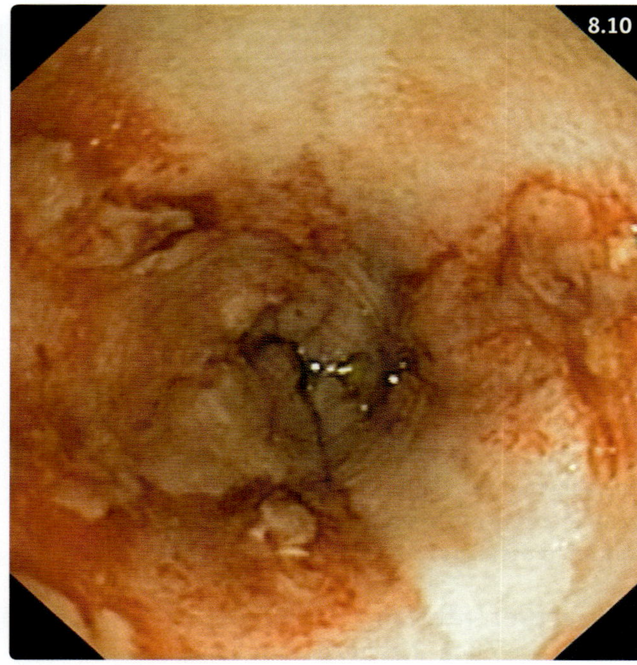

Figure 8.10 Endoscopic view of moderate esophageal mucosal lesions located cranial to the lower esophageal sphincter after removal of an esophageal foreign body in a dog. (Courtesy R. Husnik)

In case of esophageal perforation or rupture, a surgical approach is generally necessary. If severe esophageal mucosal lesions are present following extraction, a 24–48-hour fasting period is recommended. In the most severe cases, endoscopic placement of a regular or low profile gastrostomy tube is required to provide nutrition without compromising mucosal healing for the period following FB removal. Additionally, treatment of esophagitis and prevention of gastroesophageal reflux and further esophageal mucosal damage is recommended (see Esophagitis).

Access to bones or disproportionately large pieces of meat that are unlikely to reach the stomach should be limited if the dog does not chew them. Five to six ml of water should be administered with a syringe after pilling cats with any drug, but particularly doxycycline and clindamycin tablets.

Prognosis

Generally, the prognosis for esophageal FB after nonsurgical removal is good to excellent. Esophagitis is present in up to 80% of dogs after FB removal (**Figure 8.10**), but seems to resolve relatively rapidly. Esophageal strictures are a feared complication that may develop over time, particularly in dogs with severe esophageal mucosal lesions.

BENIGN ESOPHAGEAL STRICTURE

Strictures occur less commonly than FBs in dogs and in cats.

Etiology/pathophysiology

Benign strictures are a complication of severe esophagitis (FB, gastroesophageal reflux, dry swallow of pills to cats, ingestion of caustic substances). They occur with deep inflammation when lesions extend to the submucosa and muscularis layers of the esophageal wall. They are characterized by excessive scar tissue formation with narrowing of the esophageal lumen and resulting partial or total obstruction.

Clinical presentation

The history often reveals esophageal disease (for instance esophageal FB) or general anesthesia (with gastroesophageal reflux) prior to the development of signs. The animal shows frequent regurgitation, which can be associated with a particular food consistency. A dog with esophageal stricture may regurgitate dry food but not a puréed diet. Moreover, the clinical signs typical of esophagitis may also be present.

Differential diagnosis

See Esophageal foreign body.

Diagnosis

Thoracic radiographs are useful to rule out other causes of esophageal obstruction (e.g. esophageal FB, external compression). Diagnosis is confirmed either by esophagoscopy (**Figure 8.11**) or contrast esophagram. Administration of contrast agents may lead to aspiration pneumonia, and may damage endoscopic equipment if an esophagoscopy is performed soon after the contrast study. If esophageal perforation is suspected, and an esophagram is indispensable, low osmolar iodinated contrast agents are preferred over barium sulfate. It is essential to differentiate stricture of the esophageal lumen from external compression.

Management

Treatment involves dilating the stricture(s) under endoscopic or fluoroscopic control using balloons of different diameters (**Figures 8.12, 8.13**) or 'bougies' of different sizes. Multiple sessions at intervals of 1–2 weeks are often necessary. Submucosal injection of triamcinolone at the level of the stricture prior to dilation or bougienage can help reduce the number of procedures required (**Figure 8.14**). Drug therapy is similar to that for esophagitis (see below). Systemic administration of prednisone/prednisolone is ineffective. Esophageal stenting is an option to consider in cases refractory to dilation attempts.

Prognosis

Without treatment, the prognosis is poor to grave due to the risk of aspiration pneumonia and malnutrition. After stricture dilation, the prognosis is guarded to good: several dilation attempts may be required to re-establish patency of the lumen for a normal size food bolus. In some instances, patency can only be partially restored, thus requiring liquid or moist food (and not dry kibbles) to be fed. Occasional regurgitation episodes may not be avoidable.

OTHER CAUSES OF OBSTRUCTION

VASCULAR RING ANOMALIES

Vascular ring anomalies cause entrapment of the esophagus at the level of the heart base. The most common vascular ring anomaly is persistent right aortic arch (PRAA), which is characterized by the presence of a fibrous band that connects the main pulmonary artery and the anomalous aorta and causes extraluminal compression and entrapment of the esophagus. Regurgitation typically occurs when puppies or kittens are weaned to solid food, and aspiration pneumonia is a common complication. Affected puppies are generally hungry and with time become malnourished and lose weight. Diagnosis relies on the typical history and clinical signs, and is confirmed with thoracic radiographs that reveal esophageal dilation cranial to the heart base and deviation of the trachea to the left, cranial to the cardiac silhouette that is visible on ventrodorsal or dorsoventral views (**Figures 8.15–8.17**). Treatment of vascular ring anomalies consists of thoracotomy and transection of the compressive fibrous band. Prognosis of PRAA is generally good after surgery. In some cases, normal motility may not return if the cervical esophagus was very dilated or if an esophageal diverticulum was formed. While most dogs are reported to do well, some may need continuous support such as upright feeding (see Megaesophagus, Management).

ESOPHAGEAL TUMORS

Esophageal tumors occur rarely. Leiomyoma is the most common benign neoplasm in dogs, and often occurs in the caudal esophagus. Fibrosarcoma and osteosarcoma may develop in dogs infected with *Spirocerca lupi* (see below). Other tumors include leiomyosarcoma, lymphoma, and metastatic lymphoma. The most common primary esophageal neoplasia of cats is SCC. Clinical signs may be very discrete unless the tumor causes significant luminal obstruction. Diagnosis relies on radiographs, which may show esophageal dilation cranial to the mass. A contrast esophagram may be helpful. Esophagoscopy is required for final confirmation, with collection of biopsies for histopathologic analysis. Tumor excision with esophageal resection and anastomosis can be attempted, but the surgical procedure may be associated with postoperative morbidity. Esophageal stenting is a palliative option to consider.

ESOPHAGITIS

Definition/overview

Esophagitis is a disease characterized by inflammation of the esophageal mucosa. It may occur in dogs and cats, and mild cases may go unnoticed.

Etiology/pathophysiology

Noninfectious inflammation

The esophageal mucosa may easily be damaged by gastric acid and bile in gastroesophageal reflux disease, as gastric acid induces the formation of proinflammatory cytokines in the esophageal mucosa (**Figure 8.18**). Esophagitis may be a complication of LES relaxation during general anesthesia. Esophagitis may also occur in animals with frequent and severe vomiting. In addition,

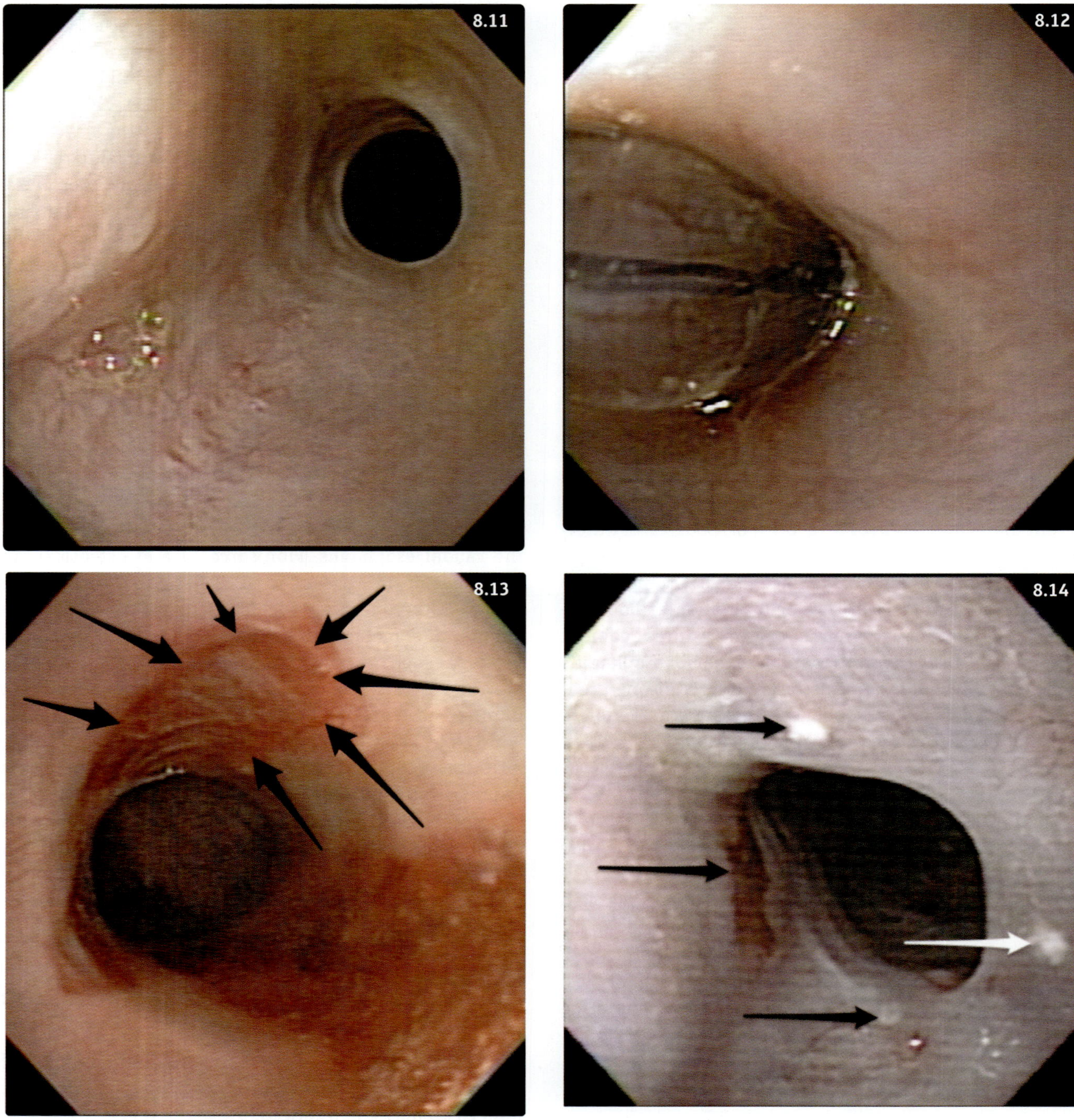

Figures 8.11–8.14 Esophageal stricture in a 3-year-old female spayed Golden Retriever with a 2-week history of regurgitation. The regurgitation was attributed to severe reflux esophagitis associated with an intestinal foreign body and concurrent pancreatitis. Note the narrowed esophageal diameter due to a fibrous ring. (8.11) A balloon catheter filled with saline is in place to dilate the stricture. (8.12) The dog after balloon dilation of the stricture. (8.13) There is a tear in the dorsal esophageal mucosa exposing the underlying structures (arrows). Esophageal tear and perforation are possible complications of stricture dilation. A conservative approach is indispensable during dilation attempts with increasing balloon sizes. (8.14) 0.5 ml triamcinolone acetate 20 mg/ml was injected submucosally in four sites at the base of the stricture (arrows).

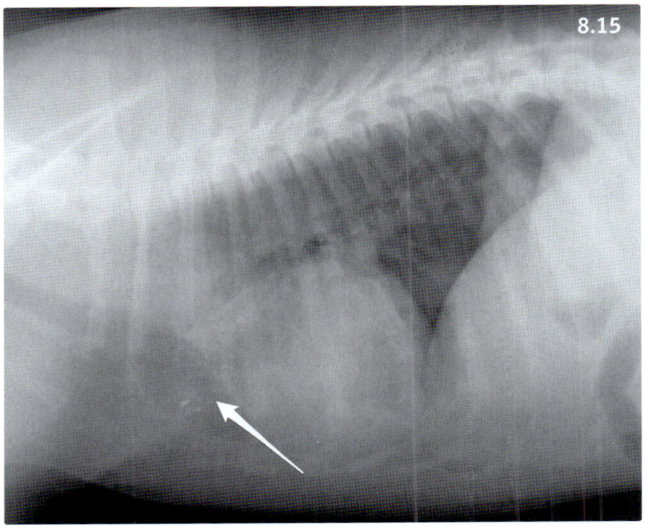

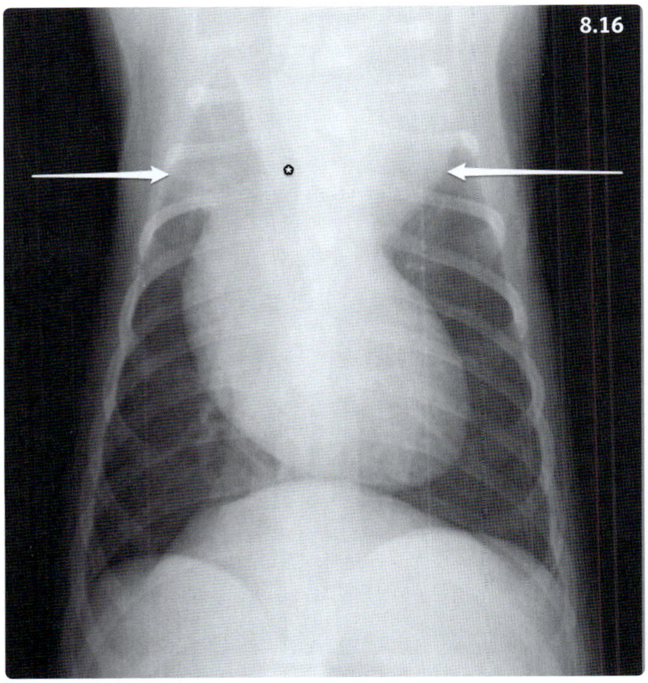

Figures 8.15, 8.16 A 3-month-old German Shepherd Dog with a persistent right aortic arch. (8.15) Lateral radiograph. The dilated esophagus is seen as a soft tissue opacity in the cranial mediastinum that displaces the trachea ventrally. Note the presence of granular material in the dilated esophagus cranial to the cardiac silhouette (arrow). (8.16) Ventrodorsal radiograph. The dilated esophagus is recognizable as a structure of soft tissue density in the cranial mediastinum (white arrows). Note the deviation of the trachea to the left cranial to the heart base (arrows).

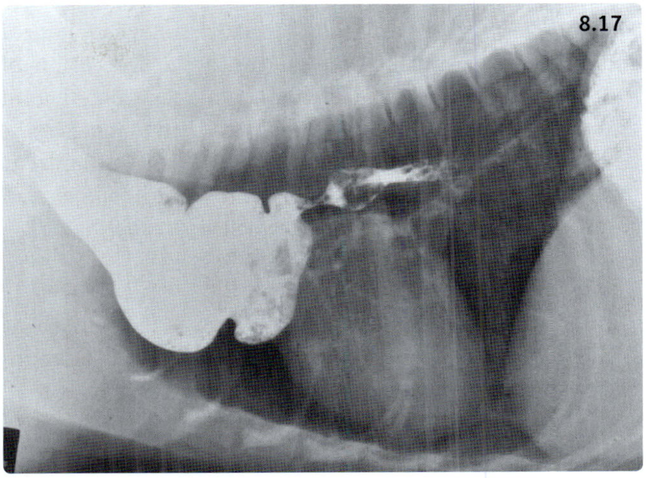

Figure 8.17 Contrast esophagram of a dog with a persistent right aortic arch. The dilated esophageal pouch located in the cranial mediastinum is clearly visible.

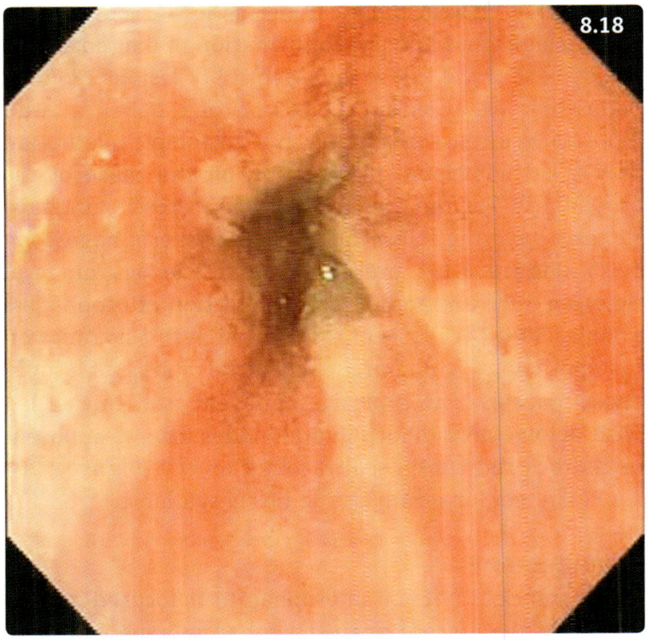

Figure 8.18 Esophagoscopy showing severely inflamed esophageal mucosa surrounding the lower esophageal sphincter due to gastroesophageal reflux. (Courtesy M. Schaer)

esophageal FBs and swallowing of caustic substances may cause esophageal mucosal inflammation. In cats, administration of doxycycline, clindamycin, and other drugs in the form of oral tablets without subsequent water flush may cause severe esophagitis and possibly esophageal stricture.

Infectious inflammation

In endemic areas (worldwide tropical and subtropical regions), *Spirocerca lupi* is a common cause of esophagitis. The ingested larvae migrate extensively and eventually mature into adults after a prepatent period of 3–9 months.

The adult worms generally inhabit the esophageal submucosa and adventitia, and cause the formation of granulomatous nodules of less than 1 cm to more than 4 cm diameter in the caudal esophageal wall. Esophageal infections with the oomycetal agent *Pythium insidiosum* occur infrequently in endemic areas (worldwide tropical and subtropical regions), and may cause severe esophagitis.

Clinical presentation

Clinical signs are characteristic of esophageal diseases (**Table 8.3**). Mild cases of esophagitis may remain subclinical or mild signs may go unnoticed by the owners.

Differential diagnosis

Includes all the other esophageal diseases described in this chapter.

Diagnosis

A tentative clinical diagnosis is made on the basis of clinical signs and history. Confirmation of diagnosis and assessment of the extent and severity of lesions requires endoscopic examination. Collection of esophageal wall biopsies is often challenging, but histologic evaluation may yield additional information on the cause of the esophagitis. For the diagnosis of spirocercosis, diagnostic tests have the following sensitivities: esophagoscopy 100% (**Figure 8.19**), presence of parasite ova on fecal flotation 80%, and radiographic detection of esophageal nodules 50%. Diagnosis of esophageal pythiosis relies on histopathology and immunochemical stains of esophageal biopsies. The typical esophageal wall thickening with involvement of local lymph nodes may be apparent on thoracic radiographs, ultrasound, and CT (**Figure 8.20**). An ELISA test for serum antibodies is available.

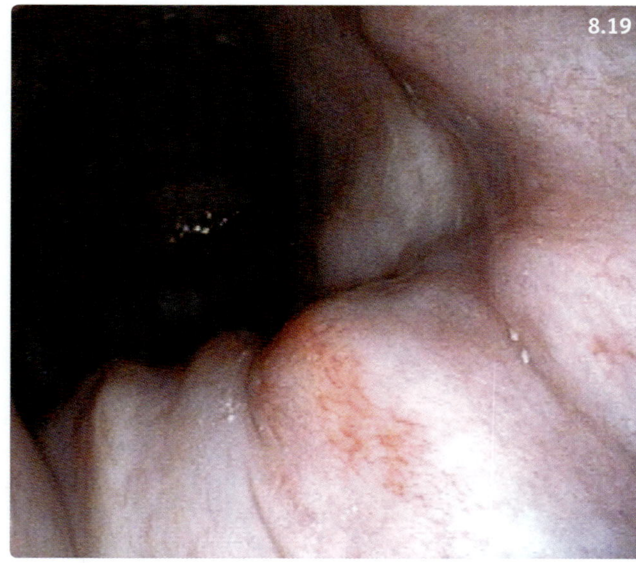

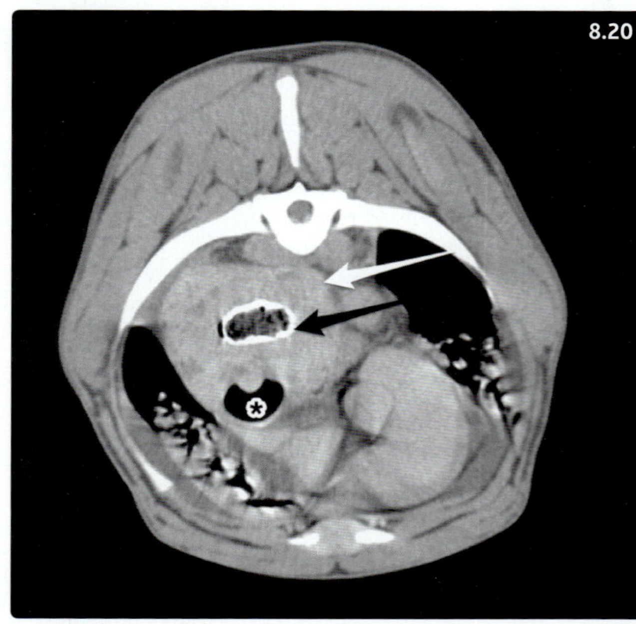

Figures 8.19, 8.20 Mixed-breed dog with dysphagia and esophageal obstruction. (8.19) Esophagoscopy shows an irregular mucosal surface. (8.20) Post-contrast CT scan of the cranial mediastinum. The esophageal wall is severely and irregularly thickened (white arrow, serosal surface; black arrow, mucosal surface covered with a fine layer of barium; asterisk, trachea). (Courtesy LSU SVM Diagnostic Imaging Service)

Management

Symptomatic treatment of esophagitis is focused on protection of the mucosa against further damage and facilitation of mucosal healing. Fasting for 24–48 hours is recommended, if feasible without compromising the dog's condition. In severe cases, placement of a gastrostomy tube via endoscopy or surgery is beneficial to provide enteral nutrition and prevent complications associated with malnutrition. A diet low in fat is recommended because high fat diets may be associated with increased episodes of gastroesophageal reflux.

Sucralfate suspension is used to promote mucosal healing (1 g q8h for large dogs, 0.5 g q8h for smaller dogs). Inhibitors of gastric acid secretion, preferably a proton pump inhibitor such as omeprazole (1mg/kg PO q12h), and a prokinetic agent that accelerates gastric emptying (metoclopramide, 0.5 mg/kg PO, SC q8h, or CRI of 1–2 mg/kg over 24h) or promotes gastric emptying and increases the distal esophageal sphincter tone (cisapride, 0.5–1 mg/kg PO q8h) should be administered, preferably 30–60 minutes before meals.

Treatment of spirocercosis consists in administration of specific parasiticides. Doramectin is an avermectin licensed for use in cattle but used off-label in dogs. Recommended protocols include 0.2–0.4 mg/kg SC every 14 days for 3–6 injections, or 0.5 mg/kg PO q24h for 6 weeks. These very high doses of avermectins must not be administered to Collies and other herding breeds that are prone to develop potentially lethal central nervous complications due to a mutation in the MDR-1 gene.

Treatment of esophageal pythiosis is challenging. Surgical excision of the lesion with safe tissue margins is the preferred treatment of GI pythiosis but is not feasible in the esophagus. Medical treatment of unresectable pythiosis is often unrewarding (itraconazole, 10 mg/kg PO q24h and terbinafine, 5–10 mg/kg PO q24h). Anti-inflammatory doses of prednisone can be used in the hope of decreasing local inflammation and to palliate clinical signs.

Prognosis

Noninfectious inflammation

Mild and moderate cases generally have a good prognosis. Severe inflammatory mucosal lesions may lead to esophageal stricture development.

Infectious inflammation

Esophageal neoplasia (osteosarcoma, fibrosarcoma) is a common complication of *S. lupi* infection and requires a surgical approach if the mass significantly obstructs the esophageal lumen. Esophageal pythiosis carries a poor to grave prognosis.

MEGAESOPHAGUS

Definition/overview

ME is characterized by generalized dilatation of the esophagus. It is the most common cause of regurgitation and a common esophageal disease in dogs, but is a rare occurrence in cats.

Etiology

Congenital ME occurs in puppies and rarely in kittens, while acquired ME is seen mostly in middle aged to older adult animals. The diseases frequently associated with ME in the dog are listed in **Table 8.5**. Among those, idiopathic ME and ME secondary to focal myasthenia gravis (MG) are most common. Acquired ME is also a feature of feline and canine dysautonomia.

Pathophysiology

With the exception of focal MG, the pathogenesis of canine and feline ME has not been fully elucidated. In dogs with MG, autoantibodies are formed against nicotinic acetylcholine receptors located at the neuromuscular junction in striated muscle. MG is discussed in further detail in Chapter 12 (Disorders of the nervous system and muscle). Congenital ME and other forms of acquired ME most likely result from malformation or changes in the complex neural network responsible for esophageal innervation.

Miniature Schnauzers, Fox Terriers, German Shepherd Dogs, Great Danes, Irish Setters, Labrador Retrievers, Shar Peis, and Newfoundlands are at increased risk for development of primary idiopathic ME.

Clinical presentation

The clinical signs are similar to those of other esophageal diseases (**Table 8.3**), and regurgitation is the most frequent complaint in dogs with ME. Secondary esophagitis is a common complication. The risk of aspiration pneumonia is high; accordingly, affected animals may present with exercise intolerance, cough, tachypnea, and dyspnea.

Differential diagnosis

Includes all the other esophageal diseases described in this chapter.

Diagnosis

The first step in the diagnostic approach is to rule out esophageal obstruction (FB, stricture) by taking a detailed history and obtaining good quality thoracic radiographs. A generalized dilatation of the esophagus is usually easily identified on the thoracic films (**Figures 8.21, 8.22**). It is important to carefully check for aspiration pneumonia in these patients. This is best done by thoroughly examining the distal parts of the lung lobes, in particular the right middle, and left and right cranial lobes for presence of interstitial or alveolar infiltrate (**Figure 8.22**).

Table 8.5 Causes of megaesophagus in the dog.

Congenital megaesophagus:
- Congenital myasthenia gravis
- Congenital neuropathy

Acquired megaesophagus:
- Idiopathic megaesophagus
- Myasthenia gravis
- Esophagitis
- Endocrine diseases (hypoadrenocorticism, possibly hypothyroidism)
- Toxicosis (e.g. lead toxicity)
- Polymyositis, polyneuropathy
- Less common causes: other neurologic diseases (botulism, tetanus, dysautonomia, rabies), systemic lupus erythematosus

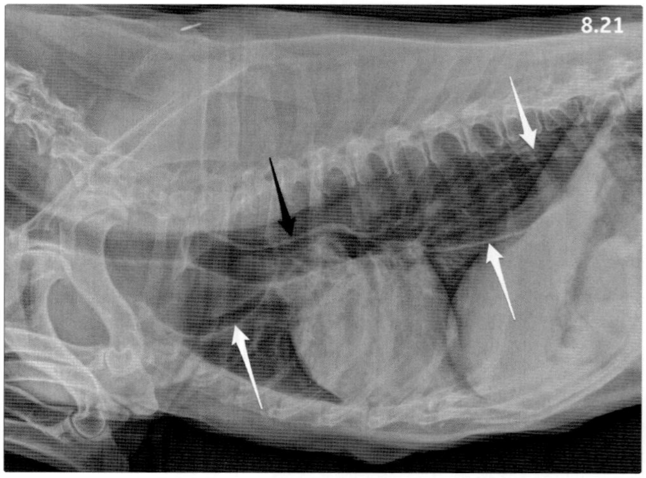

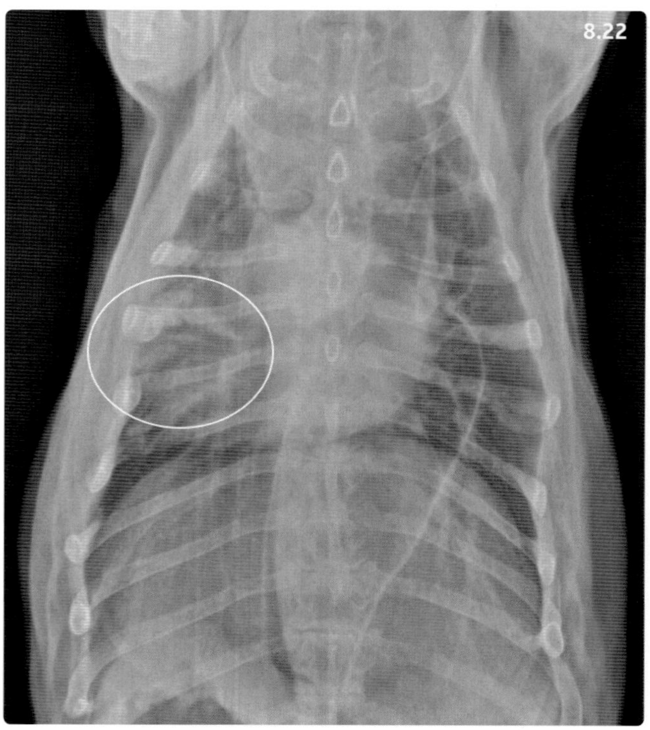

Figures 8.21, 8.22 Nine-year-old female spayed Basset Hound with megaesophagus due to focal myasthenia gravis. (8.21) Right lateral radiograph. The white arrows point to the dorsal and ventral walls of the esophagus, which are both clearly visible. The black arrow points to summation of the dorsal tracheal and ventral esophageal walls (tracheal stripe sign). (8.22) Ventrolateral radiograph. The walls of the dilated esophagus are clearly visible in the caudal mediastinum. Air bronchograms within the circle are indicative of aspiration pneumonia in the caudal subsegment of the left cranial lung lobe.

The systematic approach is continued by screening animals for primary diseases associated with secondary ME. A minimal database consisting of CBC, biochemistry panel (including serum CK), and urinalysis is recommended. Next, screening for endocrinopathies (adrenocorticotropic hormone [ACTH] stimulation test, possibly serum thyroxine and endogenous thyroid-stimulating hormone [TSH]), and a search for opacities in the cranial mediastinum (looking for possible thymoma associated with MG) are recommended. A sensitive and specific serum assay documenting the presence of autoantibodies against nicotinic acetylcholine receptors is available for the diagnosis of MG (http://vetneuromuscular.ucsd.edu). Endoscopic examination of the esophagus may be useful in unclear cases and to allow visualization of the extent and severity of the esophagitis, if present. In cases with suspected polymyositis or polyneuropathy, electrodiagnostics (EMG, nerve conduction studies) and collection of muscle and nerve biopsies for histopathologic evaluation should be considered.

Management

Dietary management is essential. It is important to try various options such as dry food kibbles, canned food formed into meat balls, and food blended with water in different consistencies (thick or thin slurry) because each animal may respond differently. Dogs and cats with ME should be fed a calorie-dense diet in a vertical position and be maintained in that position for 10–15 minutes after the meal in order to use gravity to facilitate aboral movement of the food bolus. Small dogs can be held on a person's lap for that time. Medium size and large dogs can be fed on stairs and maintained with their forelimbs higher than their hindlimbs. The Bailey chair is a useful device to keep medium size and large dogs in a vertical position during and after meals (**Figure 8.23**). This aspect of treatment can be a challenge for dogs with pre-existing orthopedic diseases such as coxofemoral arthritis.

In severe cases, placement of a gastrostomy tube may be beneficial to ensure appropriate nutrition and timely delivery of oral medications to the stomach, and to prevent aspiration pneumonia.

Identified underlying diseases need to be treated. For instance, the recommended treatment of MG includes administration of the acetylcholinesterase inhibitor pyridostigmine (1–3 mg/kg PO q12h, start with a low dose to minimize risk of cholinergic crisis) and immunosuppressive doses of prednisone or prednisolone (1–2 mg/kg PO q12h).

Cisapride and erythromycin increase LES tone in dogs; however, gastric prokinetic drugs do not significantly influence esophageal motility. Bethanechol is a cholinergic agent that has been shown to increase esophageal motility in some dogs and can be used in the management of clinical cases of idiopathic ME (5–15 mg/dog PO q8h,

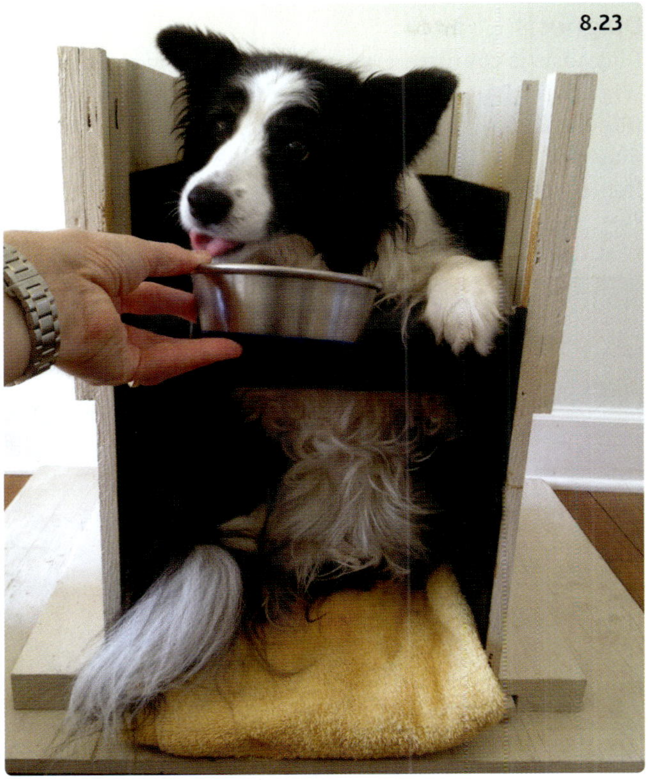

Figure 8.23 A 10-year-old female spayed Border Collie with idiopathic megaesophagus eating in a custom-made Bailey's chair. The dog is kept in an upright position in the chair for 20 minutes after each meal.

start with a low dose to minimize risk of cholinergic crisis). Because of the high prevalence of esophagitis in patients with ME, sucralfate suspension should be administered to facilitate mucosal healing (0.5–1.0 g/dog q8h, 0.25–0.5 g/cat q8–12h). Treatment of aspiration pneumonia is mostly supportive. If secondary bacterial infection is suspected, antibiotic treatment is best based on culture and sensitivity from a bronchial wash; however, empiric treatment with a broad-spectrum antibiotic may be necessary in some cases (e.g. amoxicillin and clavulanic acid, ampicillin and sulbactam).

Home management of pets with ME is complex and time-consuming. Owners may feel overwhelmed and discouraged at first. Therefore, optimal communication between the veterinary care team and the animal's owners is essential for successful management of this condition (**Box 8.3**).

Prognosis

Recent studies from Scotland and Germany reported a short median survival time of 3 months after diagnosis regardless of the etiology in dogs with ME. In the Glasgow study, only 41% of dogs survived 1 year, 31% were alive at 2 years, and 22% survived for 5 years. Identified risk factors for shorter survival were dogs older than 13 months of age at the time of diagnosis and presence of aspiration pneumonia at diagnosis. ME may be reversible when associated with endocrinopathies, but this represents only a small percentage of dogs with ME.

Box 8.3 Practical tip for support of owners of dogs with megaesophagus.

The management of dogs with megaesophagus requires considerable dedication from the pet's owners and can be overwhelming at times. Clients should be made aware of the existence of support groups on the internet (type 'megaesophagus support group' in your favorite search engine). These groups provide useful tips to optimize the quality of homecare and to make it possible for owners to include these new tasks in their busy daily routines.

LESS COMMON ESOPHAGEAL DISEASES

Esophageal diverticulum is defined as a circumscribed outpouching of the esophageal wall that may be congenital or acquired. Congenital diverticula result from abnormal embryologic development of the esophagus. Acquired diverticula are classified as either traction (resulting from periesophageal inflammation) or pulsion forms (resulting from increased esophageal luminal pressure). Esophageal diverticula generally appear in three locations: pharyngoesophageal, midthoracic, or caudal thoracic. The accumulation of ingesta within diverticula leads to esophagitis with disturbed esophageal motility and possibly obstruction. The clinical signs are typical of esophageal disease (**Table 8.3**). Plain radiographs should be evaluated for the presence of an air- or food-filled soft tissue density representing the impacted diverticulum, signs of aspiration pneumonia, and/or esophageal dilation. A positive contrast esophagram usually demonstrates a deviation or outpouching of the esophageal lumen. Small diverticula may be managed medically by feeding a soft, bland diet with the animal in an upright position to avoid food accumulation in the pouch. Large diverticula generally require excision and reconstruction of the esophageal wall. Prognosis is good if the diverticulum is uncomplicated by lung adhesions, abscesses, or bronchoesophageal fistulas.

Esophageal fistula is an abnormal communication between the esophageal lumen and surrounding structures. The most common fistula in the dog is the bronchoesophageal fistula (BEF) due to trauma caused by a retained sharp esophageal FB. Most canine BEFs due to an esophageal FB connect the esophagus with either the right caudal or the middle lung lobe bronchus. Physical examination may reveal coughing, dyspnea, respiratory crackles over affected lung regions, hemoptysis, anorexia, depression, weight loss, regurgitation, and dysphagia. Coughing associated with drinking liquids is a sign frequently associated with BEF. Survey thoracic radiographs may reveal radiopaque foreign bodies in the esophagus or bronchus, pulmonary consolidation, pleural fluid accumulation, or localized interstitial, alveolar, and/or bronchial lung patterns. Contrast esophagram or esophagoscopy is required for definitive diagnosis. Treatment consists of thoracotomy and surgical correction of the fistulous tract. Lung lobectomy may be necessary if extensive pulmonary lesions are present. Prognosis ranges from good to guarded depending on the preoperative condition of the patient, the ability to resolve pulmonary infection, and the success of surgery.

HIATAL HERNIA

Definition/overview

Hiatal hernia involves herniation of parts of the stomach through the esophageal hiatus into the mediastinum. Four types of hiatal hernias (HHs) have been described in people, and most cases documented in dogs and cats are type I or sliding HH.

Etiology/pathogenesis

Type I HHs are usually due to a congenital weakness of the esophageal hiatus. They have been reported most frequently in Shar Peis and English Bulldogs and also in cats. Acquired type I HH may occur following trauma or in combination with obstructive upper respiratory disease and abnormally high negative intrathoracic pressure during inspiration, such as may occur in dogs with brachycephalic syndrome and laryngeal paralysis.

Clinical presentation

Common clinical signs are due to the secondary reflux esophagitis and include regurgitation, hypersalivation, vomiting, dysphagia, dyspnea, anorexia, and weight loss. Puppies and kittens are presented at the time of weaning to solid food, but onset of clinical signs can also be delayed into adulthood. Aspiration pneumonia is possible and affected animals may show typical respiratory signs.

Differential diagnosis

Esophageal diseases, in particular esophageal obstruction (FB, stricture), vascular ring anomaly in puppies, and acute or chronic gastritis.

Diagnosis

Diagnosis is confirmed with survey thoracic radiographs (**Figure 8.24**) and positive contrast esophagram (**Figure 8.25**) to confirm the type of HH. Sliding hernias may not be visible at the time of the examination, and fluoroscopy may be required for confirmation. The HH

8.24

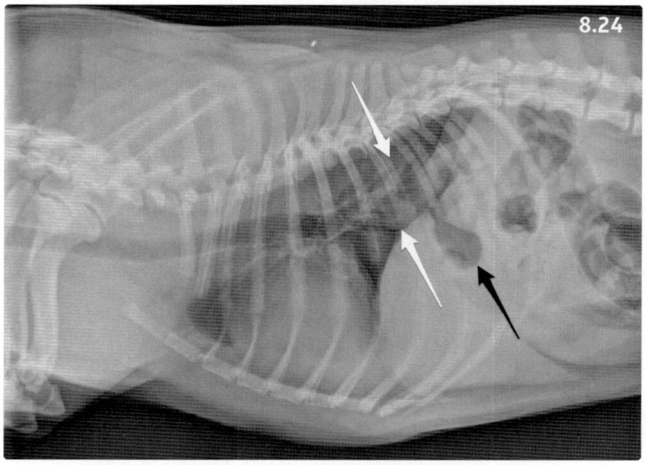

Figure 8.24 Right lateral thoracic radiograph of a 1-year-old male French Bulldog with hiatal hernia. The stomach is not in a normal anatomic position within the abdomen (black arrow) and is displaced cranially into the caudal thorax and confluent with the soft tissue opacity in the region of the esophagus (white arrows). (Courtesy LSU SVM Diagnostic Imaging Service)

8.25

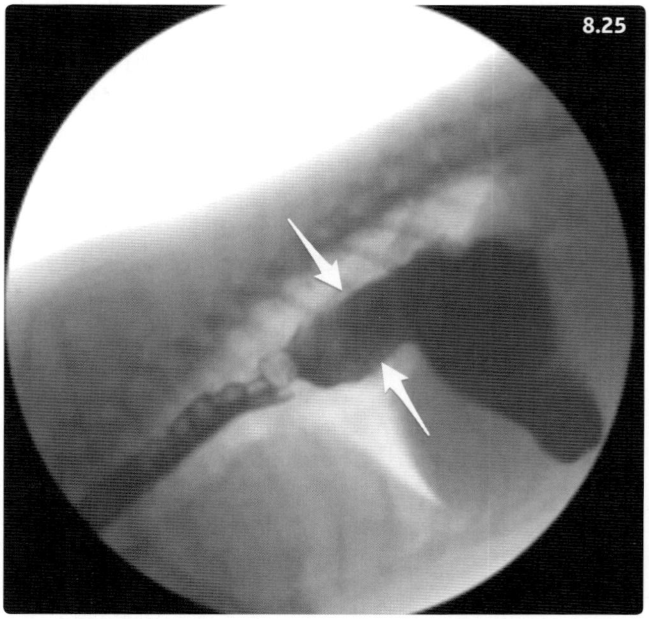

Figure 8.25 Right lateral view from a 6-year-old male neutered Welsh Corgi with dysphagia and sliding hiatal hernia. The arrows show the dorsal and ventral walls of the herniated stomach.

may also be viewed using ultrasound from an abdominal approach. Esophagoscopy allows visualization of the extent and severity of the esophagitis.

Management

Medical management is aimed at treating the secondary esophagitis and protecting esophageal mucosa from further damage (see Esophagitis, Management). A 30-day trial of medical therapy is often recommended prior to making plans for surgical correction as it may cause clinical signs to abate with restitution of adequate quality of life in a significant proportion of dogs. However, medical treatment was not successful in a series of Shar Peis presented before the age of 5 months, and surgery was recommended with no delay in such puppies. Surgical techniques include reduction of the abnormal diaphragmatic hiatus (phrenoplasty), esophagopexy, and left-sided gastropexy used alone or in combination. Clinical signs may persist after surgical reduction until resolution of secondary esophagitis.

Prognosis

Prognosis for dogs and cats with HH is generally good. Animals that respond to medical management will probably require long-term treatment (continuous or intermittent). If medical treatment fails, surgical correction has a favorable outcome in most cases.

Part 3: Diseases of the stomach

Overview

Gastric diseases are common in dogs and cats. The stomach plays a key role in the digestive process through gastric acid and pepsinogen production. It functions both as a storage organ (fundus and body) and as a grinder (antrum), reducing the size of food particles until they are small enough to pass through the pyloric sphincter, and be further processed in the small intestine.

Gastric anatomy

The stomach can be divided into five anatomic parts: cardia, fundus, body, pyloric antrum, and pylorus. The mucosa of the fundus and body folds into countless gastric glands that are lined with cells responsible for secretion of acid (parietal cells), mucus (neck cells), pepsinogen (chief cells), and GI hormones (endocrine cells) (**Figure 8.26**). The pyloric mucosa is thinner, and contains a lower density of glands. Pyloric glands mostly consist of mucous cells and endocrine cells (many of them producing gastrin).

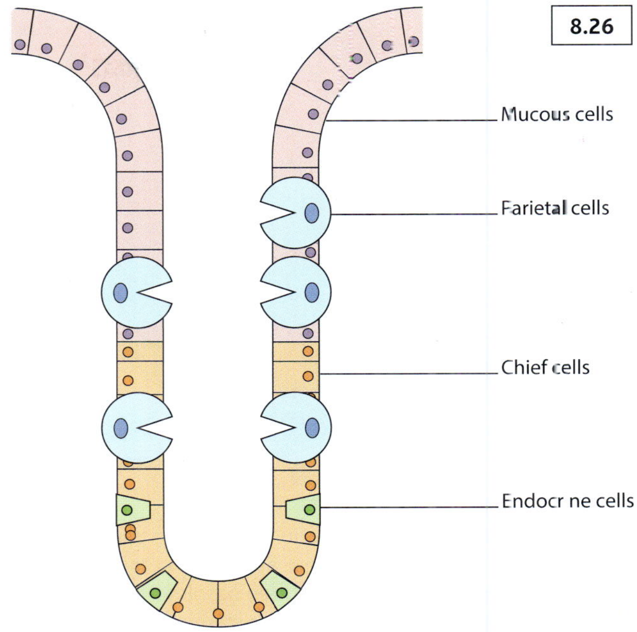

Figure 8.26 Schematic representation of the microscopic anatomy of a canine gastric gland.

Normal gastric function

Acid and enzyme production

While unstimulated gastric acid production is minimal in dogs and cats, postprandial acid production is considerable, with gastric acidity reaching a pH as low as 1 or less. Acid is produced in the parietal cells in response to three types of stimuli: activation of histamine type 2 receptors by histamine produced by neighboring enterochromaffin-like cells; muscarinic type 3 receptors activated by vagal nerve endings; or gastrin receptors (also called CCK type 2 receptors) activated by gastrin produced by antral G-cells (**Figure 8.27**). Enzyme secretion is limited to pepsinogen, released by chief cells and broken down to the proteolytic enzyme pepsin, and gastric lipase.

Gastric motility

After ingestion of solid food, the gastric antrum acts as a pump from which peristaltic waves originate while the gastric body acts as a high compliance reservoir. The mechanical action of the antral pump is divided into three phases: (1) propulsion, (2) emptying of fine particles into the duodenum and mixing, and (3) retropulsion of particles >1–2 mm for continued grinding. In dogs, complete emptying of the stomach is followed by synchronized housekeeping contractions (phase III migratory motor complexes).

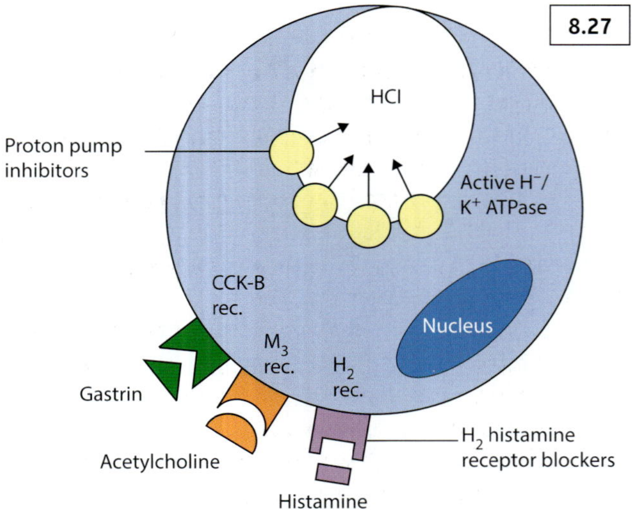

Figure 8.27 Schematic representation of a canine parietal cell. Apical proton pumps actively secrete protons into the glandular lumen under stimulation by one of three basolateral receptors: CCK-B (gastrin), M_3 (acetylcholine), and histamine type 2. The site of action of proton pump inhibitors and H_2 histamine receptor blockers is illustrated.

GASTRITIS

ACUTE GASTRITIS

Definition/overview

Acute gastritis is a clinical syndrome that occurs commonly in dogs and occasionally in cats. The diagnosis is rarely confirmed histopathologically, and affected animals are usually treated symptomatically with good success.

Etiology

The most common cause of acute gastric inflammation is dietary indiscretion or food intolerance. Other common causes include gastric FBs (including hairballs), drugs (e.g. antibiotics, nonsteroidal anti-inflammatory drugs [NSAIDs]), toxins (plant material, bleach, cleaners, heavy metals), bacteria (*Helicobacter* spp.), toxins, and viruses. Additionally, acute gastritis may also be associated with diseases primarily affecting other organs (e.g. hypoadrenocorticism, acute kidney injury, acute hepatitis, cholangitis, cholecystitis).

Clinical presentation

Sudden-onset vomiting, possibly associated with dysorexia and lethargy. Hematemesis may occur as well. The history may reveal exposure to spoiled food, drugs, or toxins. Untreated animals become dehydrated and hypovolemic. Hypokalemia may occur as well due to potassium loss associated with vomiting and metabolic alkalosis.

Differential diagnosis

Other diseases causing sudden onset vomiting such as GI FB, acute pancreatitis, endocrine diseases (e.g. hypoadrenocorticism, diabetic ketoacidosis), acute kidney injury (e.g. toxicosis with ethylene glycol or grapes/raisins, Easter lily, leptospirosis), acute hepatitis, cholangitis, or cholecystitis.

Diagnosis

History and clinical signs are usually suggestive. Abdominal radiographs should be obtained in order to rule out the presence of a GI FB. Underlying diseases should be ruled out, particularly in older animals or in atypical cases, with the help of a minimal database (CBC, serum biochemistry, urinalysis).

Management

Treatment is mostly symptomatic and consists of antiemetics, parenteral fluids to correct fluid and electrolyte deficits, and analgesia with opiates in case of abdominal pain. Animals usually benefit from a short fast (12 hours) until vomiting has subsided, followed by frequent feedings of small quantities of an easily digestible bland food (e.g. boiled chicken and rice, or commercial prescription food) for 2–3 days. Once the animal feels better, the usual diet can be reintroduced progressively over 2–3 days.

Prognosis

Most dogs and cats with acute gastritis respond very well to symptomatic treatment. In cases with severe underlying conditions, the prognosis of the primary disease is determinant.

CHRONIC GASTRITIS

Definition/overview

Chronic gastritis is a common disease in dogs with clinical signs such as chronic vomiting. Histopathologic lesions of gastric inflammation can also be present in significant numbers of asymptomatic dogs. The prevalence of chronic gastritis in cats has not been established.

Etiology

Possible causes of chronic gastritis include infectious agents or parasites, drugs (see Gastric ulcers and erosions), or chronic FBs (see Gastric outlet obstruction). In many cases, a specific cause cannot be identified and the term idiopathic gastritis is used. Food intolerance or allergy, occult parasitism, or other mechanisms are thought to play a role in the pathogenesis of idiopathic gastritis.

Ollulanus tricuspis is the small gastric worm that infests the feline stomach. It is 0.7–1 cm in length and is transmitted directly from cat to cat through ingestion of vomitus. Depending on the severity of the infestation, cats may remain subclinical or show severe signs of chronic gastritis. *Physaloptera* spp. are larger (2–6 cm long) and may be found in dogs and cats (**Figure 8.28**), although their final host appears to be the coyote. *Pythium insidiosum* is an oomycetal microorganism that may infect the canine GI tract in subtropical climates (such as the Southeast and Gulf of Mexico regions of the USA) and sporadically in other areas. Young, large breed dogs with access to the outdoors are most commonly affected and typically vomit regularly without losing their appetite. Gastric pythiosis is characterized by severe transmural antral thickening and possible gastric outflow obstruction, and may be difficult to differentiate from gastric antral neoplasia. *Helicobacter* infection is discussed in further detail below.

Clinical presentation

Chronic or chronic-intermittent vomiting of food and/or bile is the main clinical sign associated with chronic gastritis. Depending on the severity of the disease, varying combinations of hyporexia, weight loss, melena, or hematemesis may be observed.

Differential diagnosis

All diseases that may cause chronic vomiting need to be considered. These include chronic enteropathies (vomiting and hyporexia may be the only signs of inflammatory bowel disease [IBD] in cats), chronic pancreatitis, chronic diseases of the liver and biliary tree, chronic kidney disease, and endocrinopathies (dog: hypoadrenocorticism, cat: hyperthyroidism).

Diagnosis

A minimum database consisting of CBC, biochemistry panel, and urinalysis is useful to assess the presence of underlying conditions with secondary gastritis and the systemic impact of gastritis. For instance, eosinophilia may be suggestive of parasites, allergic reactions, or mast cell tumor. Hypoalbuminemia may occur with severe GI bleeding or with concurrent small intestinal involvement. Abdominal radiographs may reveal delayed gastric emptying (presence of food in the stomach after a 12-hour fast). Abdominal ultrasound is useful to assess antral wall thickness and overall gastric motility. Fecal flotation is not very helpful for diagnosis of *Ollulanus* or *Physaloptera*. In dogs with history, physical examination and abdominal imaging findings suggestive of gastric pythiosis, serum ELISA documenting the presence of specific antibodies may be helpful. In cases refractory to symptomatic treatment, gastroscopy allows visualization of the gastric lesions (**Figure 8.29**) and collection of gastric mucosal biopsies, which are evaluated histopathologically. The duodenum should also be evaluated and biopsied since gastric diseases may extend to the small intestine as well. Lymphoplasmacytic infiltrates are the most common, but infiltrates may also consist of eosinophils or other inflammatory cells. Eosinophilic gastritis may reflect the presence of parasites or allergic processes. In cats, it may be part of the feline hypereosinophilic syndrome.

Management

Symptomatic treatment is initiated with antiemetics (see Chapter 2.4: Vomiting), and protection of the gastric mucosa (**Table 8.6**). In addition, identified underlying diseases also need to be addressed. In dogs and cats with unexplained gastritis, empirical treatment with broad-spectrum anthelminthics such as fenbendazole (50 mg/kg q24h for 5 days [*Ollulanus* and *Physaloptera* spp.]) or pyrantel pamoate (5–10 mg/kg [*Physaloptera* spp.]) may be warranted.

Regardless of the cause of the chronic gastritis, a sensible dietary approach is necessary. Obtaining a good

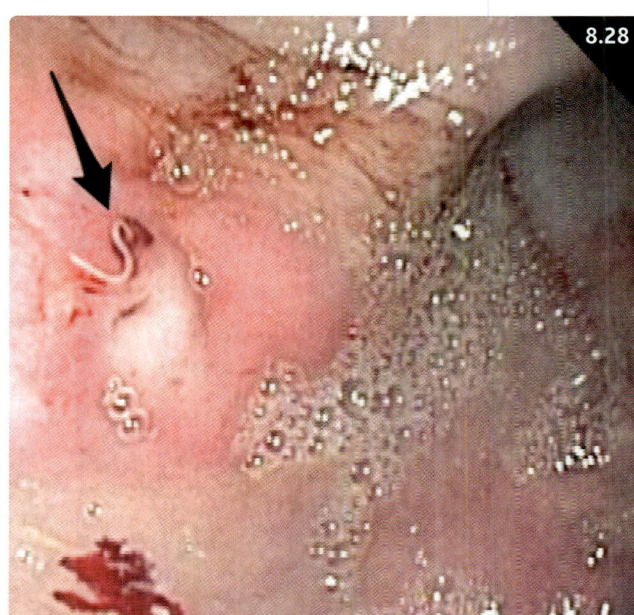

Figure 8.28 Endoscopic view of a *Physaloptera* worm (arrow) found in the gastric mucosa of a young adult male dog with chronic vomiting. (Courtesy K. Harkin)

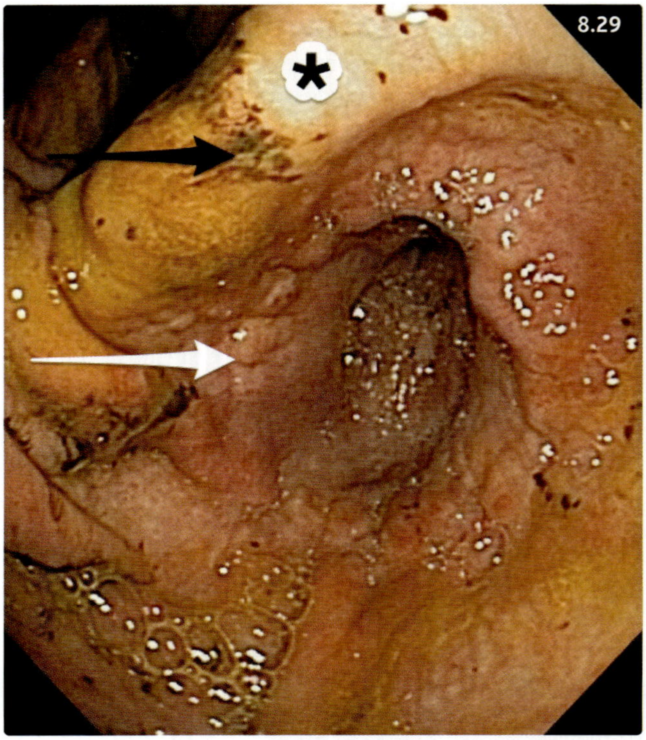

Figure 8.29 Gastroscopic view of a dog with chronic vomiting and hyporexia after endoscopic extraction of a plastic foreign body. The pyloric antrum can be seen below the incisura angularis (asterisk). The antral mucosa looks thickened (white arrow) and there are multiple mucosal erosions (black arrow). (Courtesy R. Husnik)

Table 8.6 Recommended dosages for inhibitors of gastric acid production, prostaglandin analogs, and sucralfate.

Drug	Dog	Cat
Omeprazole	0.7–1.0 mg/kg PO q12–24h	Same
Pantoprazole	0.7–1.0 mg/kg PO q12–24h	Same
Ranitidine*	1–2 mg/kg PO, SC, IV q12h; use low end of range if renal azotemia present	Same
Famotidine*	0.5 mg/kg PO, IV q12h; if renal azotemia is present q24h	Same
Misoprostol	2–5 μg/kg PO q8–12h	Unknown
Sucralfate	0.5–1 g PO q8–12h	0.25–0.5 g PO q8–12h

*H2-receptor antagonists have been shown to be inferior to proton pump inhibitors in their ability to suppress gastric acid production in dogs and cats.

dietary history is helpful. For idiopathic chronic gastritis, the recommended diets are based on novel proteins or hydrolyzed peptides. They should be easily digestible and fed in several small meals throughout the day to optimize gastric emptying. Dietary management may be sufficient in mild cases with few or no systemic signs, and improvement generally occurs within 2 weeks of receiving the new diet. If this is not the case, a different diet may be tried for another 2 weeks, or immunosuppressive therapy may be initiated. In moderate and severe cases, immunosuppressive doses of glucocorticoids are often required (e.g. prednisone, 1–2 mg/kg q24h for 2 weeks, then slowly taper in 2-week steps to every other day, or lowest effective dose over 8–12 weeks). Additional immunosuppressives may be required in refractory cases.

GI pythiosis is best managed with surgical resection of the lesion with sufficient margins. This is often difficult to achieve in the stomach. Medical treatment of unresectable pythiosis is often unrewarding (itraconazole, 10 mg/kg PO q24h; terbinafine, 5–10 mg/kg PO q24h). Anti-inflammatory doses of prednisone can be used in the hope of decreasing local inflammation and to palliate clinical signs.

Prognosis

All identifiable causes and underlying diseases should be addressed and properly managed. Idiopathic chronic gastritis generally has a fair to good prognosis.

HELICOBACTER SPP. INFECTION

Definition/overview

Helicobacter spp. are spiral-shaped gram-negative bacteria that can live in an acidic environment. While their association with peptic ulcer and gastric neoplasia in people has been clearly documented, their pathogenic potential in dogs and cats is less well defined. *H. pylori*, the most prevalent *Helicobacter* infecting people, does not represent a significant problem in small animals. *H. heilmanii* is the predominant species isolated from cats, while *H. bizzozeronii* and *H. salomonis* are the most common species in dogs. The bacteria colonize mucus in the gastric glands and cause local inflammation.

Clinical presentation

The main clinical sign is chronic-intermittent vomiting.

Diagnosis

Diagnosis is based on ruling out other causes of chronic gastritis (see above), and confirming with gastroscopy, which may show gross lesions (**Figure 8.30**). Gastric mucosal biopsies are collected and evaluated cytologically (**Figure 8.31**), histopathologically, and/or using the urease test (**Figure 8.32**).

Management

While the pathogenic potential of *Helicobacter* spp. in dogs and cats is still subject to discussion, animals presented with clinical signs of chronic gastritis, histologic evidence of gastric inflammation, and concurrent presence of spiral-shaped bacteria in the gastric mucosa and gastritis should be treated. Eradication requires treatment with different drugs usually consisting of one or more antimicrobial(s), an acid-reducing drug, and bismuth in some protocols for a duration of 14–21 days. Examples of eradication protocols are listed in **Table 8.7**.

Prognosis

Prognosis is good; however, many animals may reinfect themselves in their home environment.

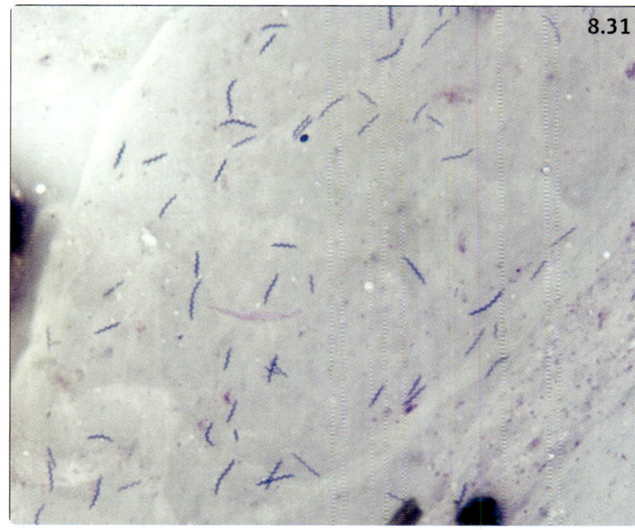

Figure 8.31 Cytology picture of a gastroscopic mucosal brushing showing multiple spiral-shaped bacteria in a dog with helicobacteriosis. (Courtesy R. Husnik)

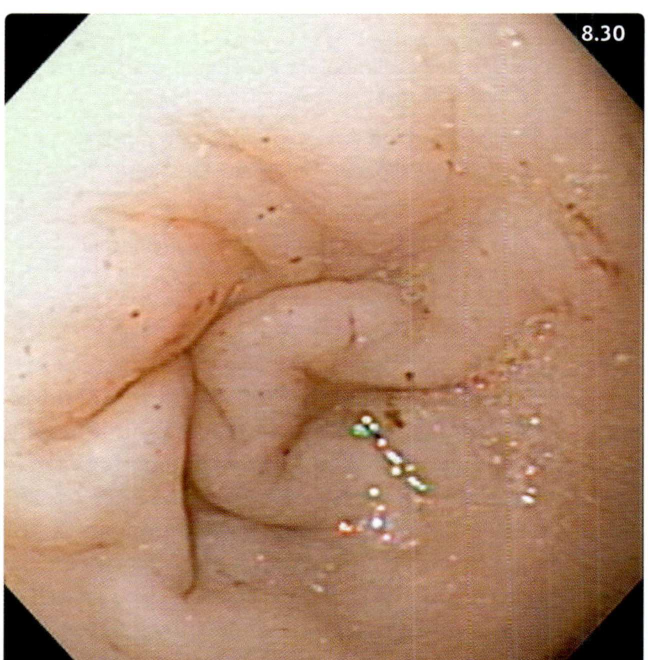

Figure 8.30 Gastroscopic view showing the pyloric antrum of a 12-year-old male neutered Domestic Shorthair cat with a 15-month history of intermittent vomiting, hyporexia, and weight loss. There are multiple erosions associated with mucosal bleeding. Histopathology revealed mild lymphoplasmacytic inflammation and numerous spiral-shaped bacteria on the mucosa. The cat responded to treatment with amoxicillin, clarithromycin, and metronidazole.

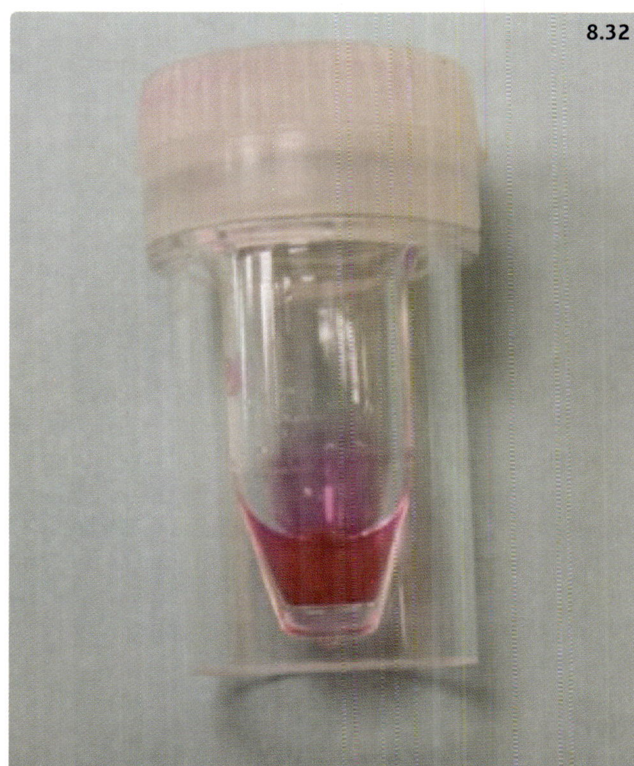

Figure 8.32 Urease test. A gastric biopsy sample was placed in this vial at the time of gastroscopy. The liquid was initially yellow and then turned red, indicating the presence of urease-producing *Helicobacter*. (Courtesy R. Husnik)

Table 8.7 Examples of oral treatment protocols for eradication of *Helicobacter* spp. in dogs and cats.

Antimicrobial	Antacid	Other	Comments
Metronidazole (10–15 mg/kg q12h) Amoxicillin (20 mg/kg q12h)	Famotidine (0.5 mg/kg q12h)		D: 2-week duration
Metronidazole (10–15 mg/kg q12h) Amoxicillin (20 mg/kg q12h)		Bismuth subsalicylate (0.22 ml/kg q6–8h)	D, C: 3-week duration
Amoxicillin (20 mg/kg q12h) Clarithromycin (7.5mg/kg q12h) Metronidazole (10 mg/kg q12h)			C: 2-week duration

D, successful use reported in dogs; C, successful use reported in cats.

Table 8.8 Causes of gastrointestinal ulceration in dogs and cats.

Dogs	Cats
Drugs NSAIDs: (1) accidental ingestion (acute toxicosis); (2) chronic administration (to treat orthopedic conditions) Steroids: (1) with intervertebral disk disease; (2) other	**Drugs**: NSAIDs; steroids
Neoplasia: gastric carcinoma, and other gastric tumors; mast cell tumor; gastrinoma	**Neoplasia**: alimentary lymphoma, and others; systemic mastocytosis; gastrinoma
Poor perfusion of gastric mucosa: hypoadrenocorticism, shock, inadequate fluid therapy during anesthesia	**Poor perfusion of gastric mucosa**: shock, inadequate perfusion during anesthesia
Other: *Helicobacter* spp. infection, inflammatory bowel disease, pancreatitis, liver disease, uremic syndrome, prolonged intensive physical activity (sled dogs), pyloric outflow obstruction, gastric dilatation–volvulus, gastric FB	**Other**: inflammatory bowel disease, hypereosinophilic syndrome, *Dieffenbachia* toxicosis, stress, gastric FB

GASTRIC ULCERATIONS AND EROSIONS

Definition/overview

Ulcers are mucosal lesions that extend to the muscularis mucosae and the deeper layers (submucosa, muscularis), and erosions are more superficial and limited to the lamina propria. While there are no reported numbers for the prevalence of GI ulcers in small animals, they appear to be uncommon in dogs and rare in cats.

Etiology

The main reported causes of gastric ulcer in dogs and cats are listed in **Table 8.8**. Long-term treatment with NSAIDs is probably the most common cause of canine GI ulcers. Administration of NSAIDs using a higher dose than that recommended by the manufacturer, or in combination with other NSAIDs or corticosteroids, significantly increases the risk of GI lesions. Dogs treated for intervertebral disk disease are also at high risk of developing ulcerative lesions in the GI mucosa. Additionally, GI ulceration may represent a complication of a variety of diseases originating in or outside the GI tract. Gastric tumors frequently ulcerate due to compromise in the blood supply required to maintain the integrity of the gastric mucosa. Finally, secretion of gastrin by gastrinomas and histamine by mast cell tumors may lead to excessive gastric acid production and disruption of the gastric mucosal barrier, with resulting erosions and ulcerations.

Pathophysiology

The gastric mucosal barrier protects the gastric mucosa from the acidic environment of the gastric lumen. The hydrophobic mucous layer produced by the mucous neck cells provides a physical barrier separating the gastric epithelium from the gastric lumen and its content. It is rich in bicarbonate, which acts as a buffer against acid.

Other factors involved in maintaining the mucosal barrier include the high mucosal blood flow providing nutrients, bicarbonate, and oxygen to the mucosa and eliminating acid residues, the local production of prostaglandin E2, and the rapid turnover of epithelial cells. Gastric ulcers and erosions occur in the presence of drugs or disease processes that weaken or disrupt the gastric mucosal barrier.

Clinical presentation

In dogs, the typical presentation revolves around vomiting with or without hematemesis (**Figure 8.33**). Cranial abdominal pain may be present. Signs resulting from fluid and possibly blood loss (dehydration, shock, anemia) may become apparent. While melena may be observed during the rectal examination (**Figure 8.34**), it is only obvious in case of significant blood loss (>2.5–3.5 ml/kg body weight). In case of perforating ulcer, septic peritonitis usually develops with systemic inflammatory response syndrome (SIRS, sepsis).

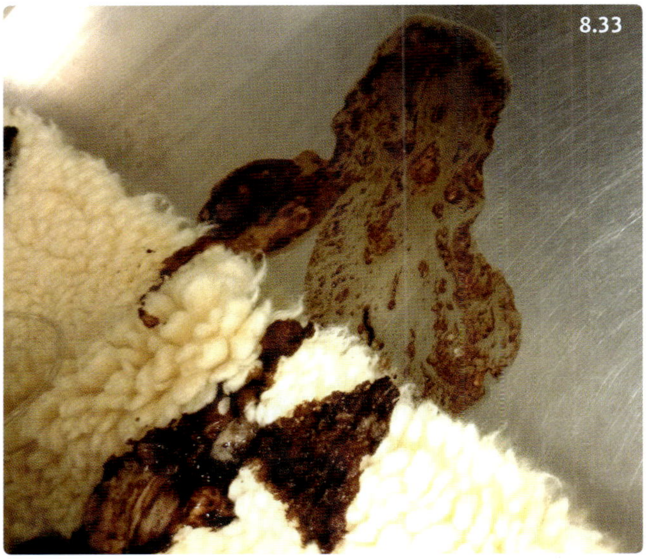

Figure 8.33 Bloody vomit with typical coffee ground appearance from a dog with a gastric ulcer due to acute NSAID toxicosis. (Courtesy R. Husnik)

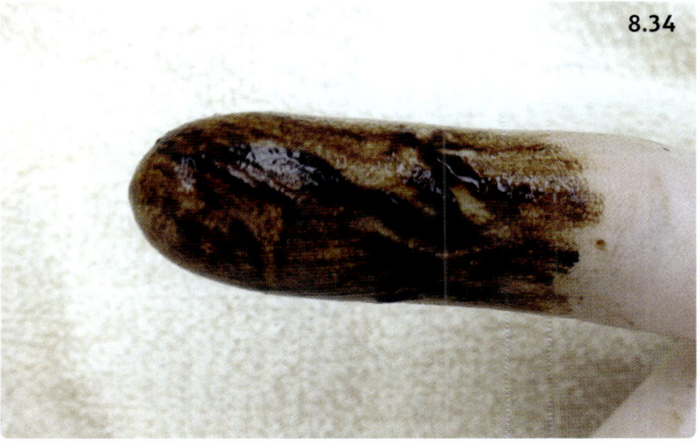

Figure 8.34 Melenic feces recovered from the rectum of a dog with gastric adenocarcinoma.

Cats with GI ulceration may also be presented with vomiting, hematemesis, abdominal pain, and melena. However, some cats may only show vomiting with nonspecific signs such as anorexia and lethargy. GI ulcers associated with neoplasia (e.g. gastric tumor, mastocytosis) tend to have a more protracted course with weight loss and other clinical signs caused by the underlying disease.

Differential diagnosis

Vomiting (see Chapter 2.4, **Table 2.4.2**). Severe gastric inflammation, duodenal ulcers, and acute pancreatitis may also cause hematemesis. Furthermore, mucosal bleeding associated with coagulopathies or platelet diseases may also lead to hematemesis and melena. Abdominal pain may be associated with acute pancreatitis, GI FBs, and gastroenteritis.

Diagnosis

In animals with suggestive evidence of GI ulceration, the diagnostic approach should focus on two objectives: (1) confirm the presence of an ulcerative GI lesion, and (2) search for an underlying disease predisposing the animal to develop GI ulcers.

A minimal database consisting of CBC, serum biochemistry, urinalysis, and abdominal imaging should be obtained. The CBC may show evidence of blood loss anemia (microcytic hypochromic anemia), which may be regenerative or nonregenerative depending on the duration of blood loss, and/or changes associated with the underlying disease. Serum biochemistry may reveal an increased BUN in an otherwise fasted patient (suggestive of GI bleeding) and/or abnormal results due to fluid and electrolyte loss or to an underlying disease. Abdominal radiographs are important to rule out a GI obstruction. Additionally, they may identify signs of perforation and peritonitis (e.g. peritoneal effusion with decreased serosal detail, pneumoperitoneum). Abdominal ultrasound allows a more detailed assessment of the gastric pylorus, antrum, and body, and is useful to confirm the presence of free fluid or gas in the peritoneum. Moreover, a full abdominal scan allows evaluation of the other abdominal organs in the search for underlying disease. Masses detected during the physical examination (e.g. skin masses [mast cell tumors]) or during the ultrasound examination should be aspirated and evaluated cytologically.

The diagnostic examination of choice to confirm GI ulceration is endoscopy. Ulcers may be disseminated throughout the gastric mucosa (long-term use of NSAIDs in dogs) or present on the lesser curvature at the entrance of the pyloric antrum (acute NSAID toxicosis, gastric tumors) (**Figures 8.35, 8.36**). Mucosal biopsies should be collected around the ulcer margins and in other areas and evaluated histologically. In cases of gastric neoplasia, an effort should be made to collect deep biopsies of the tissue surrounding the ulcer(s).

Management/prevention

Supportive treatment is essential and includes correction of fluid and electrolyte deficits and administration of antiemetics as needed. If the animal is in pain, appropriate analgesia should be provided using opioid drugs. A surgical approach is required after initial stabilization of the patient in cases of perforated ulcers and associated peritonitis.

Protection of the gastric mucosa with inhibitors of acid secretion is essential. Proton pump inhibitors (PPIs; e.g. omeprazole) are considered more effective than histamine type-2 inhibitors (H2-inhibitors; e.g. famotidine, ranitidine) for providing continuous acid suppression during their duration of action. Among H2-inhibitors, famotidine is more reliably efficacious than ranitidine and cimetidine. Inhibitors of acid secretion should be administered over a prolonged period of time to dogs and cats with GI ulcers (4–6 weeks). Additionally, sucralfate is the drug of choice to coat ulcers and promote a quicker re-epithelization and healing. It is usually administered simultaneously with an H2-receptor blocker or PPI, although there is still some debate about the value of staggering oral administration of sucralfate and these drugs. Misoprostol is an oral prostaglandin E analog that has been used with success in dogs with NSAID toxicosis (see dosage in **Table 8.6**). Additionally, treatment of identified underlying conditions should be initiated as early as possible.

Dietary support for gastric ulcers should consist of an easily digestible diet that is low in fiber and fat and promotes rapid gastric emptying. Alternatively, in some patients, the preferred diet may need to be selected on the basis of identified underlying diseases (e.g. hydrolyzed diet in IBD, 'renal diet' in chronic kidney disease).

Prevention of GI ulcers is recommended in patients at risk. First, simultaneous administration of steroid and NSAIDs or treatments involving combinations of NSAIDs should be avoided at all costs. In animals with severe joint pain that are unresponsive to single agent therapy, opioids and/or tramadol should be considered as part of the analgesic protocol. Dogs and cats with a significant burden of mast cell tumors are likely to benefit most from H2-blocker therapy. In high-risk patients such as dogs with intervertebral disk disease treated with corticosteroids or NSAIDs, PPIs or H2-blockers are often administered in the hope of limiting the extent of gastric mucosal lesions. Similarly, dogs receiving long-term NSAIDs due

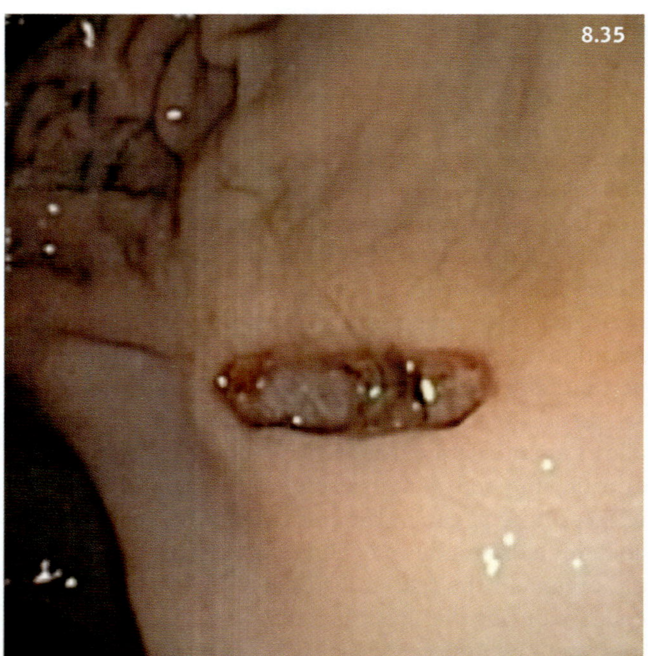

Figure 8.35 Gastroscopic view from a young Dalmatian that accidentally ingested a high dose of naproxen. A sharply delineated peptic ulcer is visible on the lesser curvature.

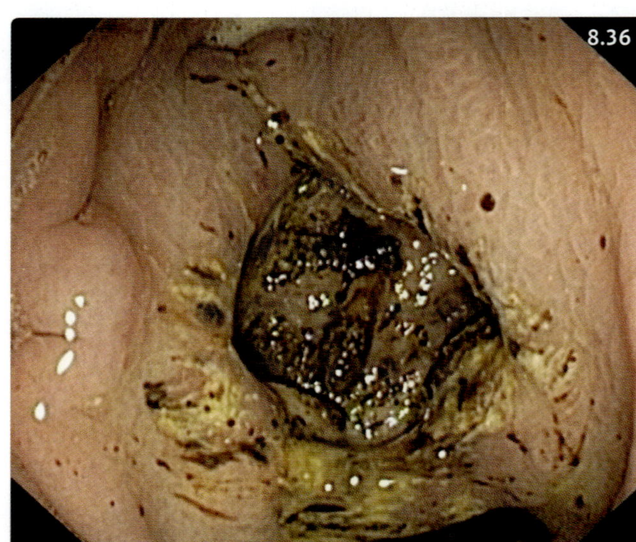

Figure 8.36 Gastroscopic view from an older mixed-breed dog showing an ulcerated gastric adenocarcinoma with a deep ulcerated center and raised edges. (Courtesy R. Husnik)

to chronic osteoarthritis or other orthopedic problems may benefit from preventive gastroprotective treatment, particularly once they have experienced signs of erosive/ulcerative gastritis. Misoprostol may be of benefit as well. Other risk situations include dogs receiving high immunosuppressive doses of corticosteroids to treat various immune-mediated diseases, although there is no documented benefit of preventive use of inhibitors of gastric acid production in these patients.

Prognosis

In the absence of perforation, canine GI ulcers are usually associated with a good outcome if their cause can be identified and eliminated (e.g. acute NSAID toxicosis). However, in many instances the underlying disease may significantly compromise the prognosis (e.g. gastric neoplasia, chronic liver failure, chronic kidney disease). Cats with GI ulcers secondary to gastric lymphoma, gastrinoma, and mastocytosis appear to have a good prognosis.

Dogs with perforated gastric or duodenal ulcers that undergo surgery usually have a reasonable survival if the underlying problem can be successfully addressed. However, only 50% of dogs with nonmalignant perforated ulcers survived in a recent study from the UK. In cats, surgically treated perforated GI ulcers appear to have a good prognosis.

GASTRIC DILATATION AND VOLVULUS

Definition/overview

Gastric dilatation–volvulus (GDV) is a syndrome that occurs in large to giant breed dogs and is characterized by rotation of the stomach on its mesenteric axis followed by gaseous gastric distension.

Etiology

The precise etiology of GDV is unknown. Identified risk factors include a narrow and deep thoracic conformation, stress, and nutritional factors that ultimately lead to rapid filling of the stomach with large quantities of food or water. For instance, once daily feeding, rapid ingestion of a meal, exercising after a meal, and eating from a raised platform all have the potential to trigger GDV.

Pathophysiology

The pylorus moves ventrally from the right to the left with a resulting rotation of 90–360 degrees, and positions itself near the gastric cardia on the left side. Gas accumulates in the stomach since neither eructation nor aboral emptying is possible. The distended stomach compresses the caudal vena cava and the portal vein, resulting in decreased venous return to the heart, decreased cardiac output, and ultimately cardiovascular collapse.

Clinical presentation

Abdominal distension with tympany, abdominal pain, retching or vomiting (often nonproductive), hypersalivation, and acute collapse are common presenting signs. Hypovolemic and/or distributive shock may be noticeable on presentation (tachycardia, weak pulses, pale mucous membranes with abnormal capillary refill time).

Differential diagnosis

Gastric dilatation secondary to overeating, mesenteric volvulus, splenic torsion, diaphragmatic tear with gastric herniation.

Diagnosis

Typical history and physical examination are suggestive; however, they do not allow differentiation between gastric dilatation and GDV. Gastric volvulus is confirmed with right lateral abdominal radiographs (**Figure 8.37**). However, aggressive shock treatment and attempts to deflate the stomach are often necessary before obtaining survey abdominal films.

Management

Aggressive treatment of cardiovascular collapse using two large bore catheters placed in each cephalic vein is life-saving and needs to be initiated immediately after

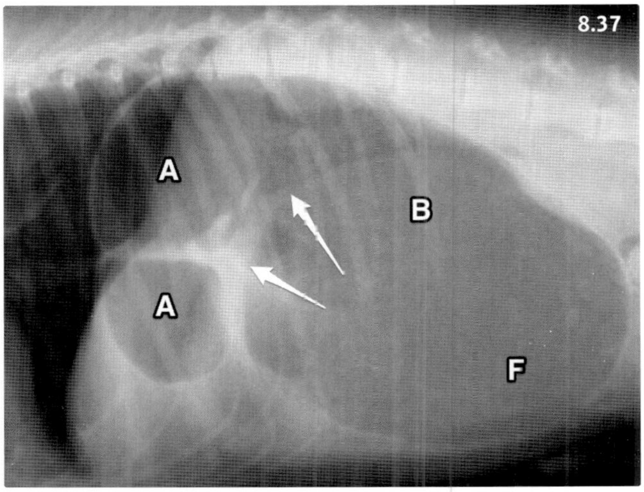

Figure 8.37 Right lateral abdominal radiograph of a dog with gastric dilatation–volvulus. The antrum (A) is visible in the dorsocranial aspect of the abdomen while the fundus (F) and body (B) are located more caudal. Compartmentalization of the stomach is visible (arrows). (Courtesy L. Gaschen)

presentation. (See Chapter 23: Fluid therapy, for proper choice of fluids and required doses.) If surgery needs to be delayed (e.g. because of fluid resuscitation), orogastric intubation is attempted in order to decompress the stomach and lavage its content (**Box 8.4**). If attempts at orogastric intubation are unsuccessful, percutaneous trocharization may be performed using a 3 inch 12–14G IV catheter that is introduced into the stomach caudally to the last rib in the left flank after the region is clipped and aseptically prepared. This usually causes some peritoneal contamination with gastric content. Ultimately, explorative celiotomy with repositioning of the stomach is followed by evaluation of gastric wall vitality (**Figure 8.38**). Partial gastrectomy may be required if segments of the stomach are devitalized; partial or total splenectomy may be necessary in the presence of splenic necrosis, infarction, or torsion. Gastropexy (pyloric antrum to right abdominal wall) is recommended to lower the likelihood of recurrence. Cardiac dysrhythmias commonly occur and need to be addressed if they significantly compromise cardiac output. Hypokalemia and hypomagnesemia need to be diagnosed and treated as they may complicate cardiac arrhythmias.

Prognosis

The overall mortality rate is currently between 10% and 27%. Negative prognostic factors include >6-hour duration of clinical signs, post-fluid therapy serum lactate concentration >6.4 mmol/l or <4 mmol/l decrease between pre- and post-fluid lactate, and devitalized gastric wall with need for gastric resection.

Box 8.4 Procedure for passage of an orogastric tube in a dog with gastric dilatation–volvulus.

1. Material. Use largest diameter smooth surfaced flexible orogastric tube possible (e.g. >9.5 mm outside diameter in large dogs). Water-soluble lubricating jelly. Canine mouth speculum (e.g. roll of 2 inch adhesive tape).
2. Sedation. With exception of recumbent or severely affected dogs, mild sedation is usually required. One option is IV administration of butorphanol (0.2–0.4 mg/kg) with diazepam (0.2–0.5 mg/kg).
3. Preparation. Mark the distance from the canine tooth to the last rib on the tube using piece of tape.
4. Introduction. Cover the end of the tube with lubricating jelly and gently introduce the tube through the speculum, pharynx, and esophagus. When the level of the tape marking is reached, the tube should be at the lower esophageal sphincter. Gently rotating the tube may be required to pass the sphincter. Passage through the lower esophageal sphincter should not require force.
5. Limit. The procedure should be aborted if the stomach cannot be intubated after a few attempts. Consider percutaneous gastric trocharization (see text).

GASTRIC OUTLET OBSTRUCTION

Causes of gastric outlet obstruction include gastric FBs, antral pyloric hypertrophy, and gastric neoplasia as well as gastric pythiosis.

GASTRIC FOREIGN BODY

Definition/overview

Young animals are more likely to play with foreign objects, but ingestion of gastric FBs may occur in animals of any age. While many dogs are indiscriminate eaters at risk for any type of GI FB, cats are more likely to ingest linear FBs.

Etiology

FBs may consist of bones, toys, socks, towels, or linear material such as string or wool. Linear FBs may lodge at the pylorus and cause intestinal perforation and peritonitis. Hair balls may be a problem, especially in long-haired cats (**Box 8.5**).

Pathophysiology

Gastric outlet obstruction may cause hypokalemic metabolic alkalosis.

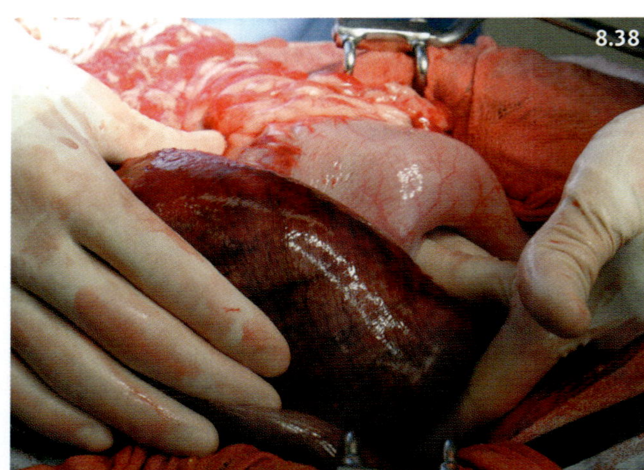

Figure 8.38 Exploratory celiotomy of a dog with gastric dilatation–volvulus after repositioning of the stomach. A devitalized portion of the stomach (antrum) is shown in the foreground and compared with the normally perfused body. (Courtesy D. Ogden)

Box 8.5 The problem of feline hairballs.

While hairballs commonly occur, particularly in longhaired cats, they do not usually cause significant health problems. Typically, affected cats vomit occasionally while remaining otherwise healthy ('healthy vomiters'). The formation of hairballs may be related to the unusual fasted digestive motility pattern displayed in cats, which may make the emptying of hair material into the duodenum more difficult. This promotes gastric retention of swallowed hair, and ultimately formation of a hairball.

In most cats, treatment involves administration of a petroleum laxative or dietary supplementation with a bulk laxative. Psyllium is sufficient to control the problem. Longhaired cats may benefit from regular clipping. In some cats, trichobezoars may form, cause chronic gastritis, and/or obstruct the gastric outlet and therefore require endoscopic or surgical extraction. Frequent vomiting of hairballs may also be an early sign of chronic enteropathies and should prompt clinicians to initiate further diagnostic tests. This is particularly true in shorthaired cats, which are usually not prone to having hairballs.

Clinical presentation

History of possible FB ingestion and acute onset vomiting in an otherwise normal animal. Anorexia and lethargy are commonly associated signs. Cranial abdominal discomfort or pain may be elicited on palpation. Dehydration and electrolyte and acid–base abnormalities are frequent complications.

Differential diagnosis

Dietary indiscretion and GI infections (e.g. parvovirus) are the most important differential diagnoses in puppies. In adult dogs, acute gastritis due to dietary indiscretion and acute pancreatitis are the top two differentials. However, any GI or systemic disease causing acute vomiting should be considered both in dogs and cats.

Diagnosis

Diagnosis is confirmed with abdominal imaging. Survey radiographs may show a dilated stomach full of food or secretions for a prolonged period after meals. In some cases, the foreign object may be visible (**Figures 8.39–8.41**). In case of doubt, contrast radiographs may help to visualize the obstruction more accurately. Alternatively, ultrasound examination of the stomach may confirm the presence of a foreign object.

Management

Gastric FBs need to be removed either endoscopically (**Figures 8.41, 8.42**) or surgically. Foreign material that has partially passed into the duodenum (e.g. socks, towels) should be removed surgically. Fluid therapy is promptly initiated to replace deficits and stabilize the patient prior to inducing anesthesia.

Prognosis

Prognosis is generally good once the foreign material has been removed. It may be guarded to poor in severely debilitated animals or in cases with gastric perforation and peritonitis. Possible surgical complications include dehiscence and peritonitis.

GASTRIC ANTRAL PYLORIC HYPERTROPHY

Definition/overview

Thickening of the antral wall may be due to hypertrophy of the mucosa, the muscularis, or both layers. Acquired pyloric antral hypertrophy is most commonly due to hyperplasia of the antral mucosa, and occurs preferentially in middle aged to older small breed dogs (e.g. Lhasa Apso, Pekingese, Maltese, and Shih Tzu). Congenital pyloric hypertrophy characterized by hyperplasia of the antral muscularis is a rare congenital disorder of brachycephalic breeds such as Boxers, Boston Terriers, and Bulldogs and has also been reported in Siamese cats.

Etiology/pathophysiology

The exact causes and pathophysiology remain unknown. Recently, an increased frequency of GI tract lesions was reported in brachycephalic dogs, and acquired pyloric antral hypertrophy was diagnosed endoscopically in >80% of examined dogs, although most of the dogs did not show any clinical signs. An association was suggested between the chronic inspiratory dyspnea seen in these breeds and chronic duodenogastric reflux, which may be the cause of the antral mucosal hypertrophy.

Clinical presentation

Chronic-intermittent vomiting that worsens progressively with severity of the mucosal hypertrophy and resulting pyloric obstruction. In puppies and kittens with the congenital form, signs start after weaning. Projectile vomiting may occur.

Differential diagnosis

Other diseases of the stomach, chronic pancreatitis, diseases originating outside the GI tract (e.g. chronic kidney disease).

Diagnosis

Survey abdominal radiographs or abdominal ultrasound may suggest delayed gastric emptying and show thickening of the antral wall. Barium contrast studies may be useful to visualize the narrowing of the pyloric passage.

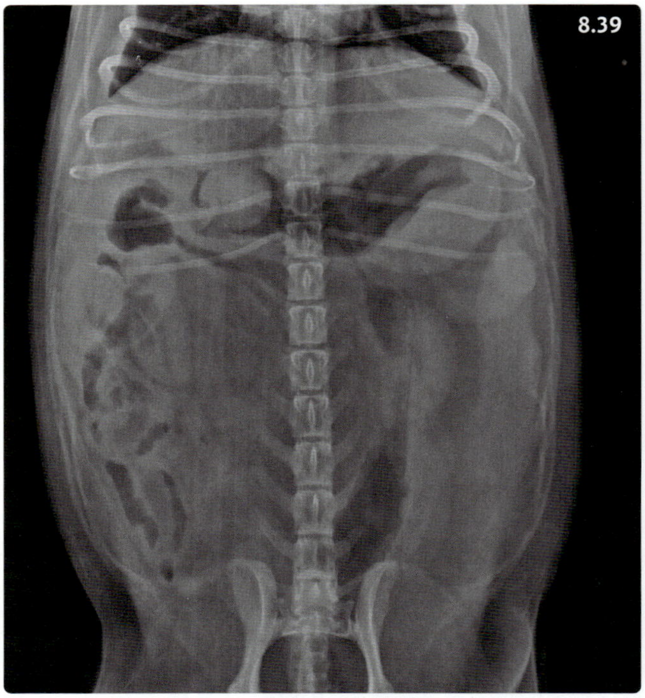

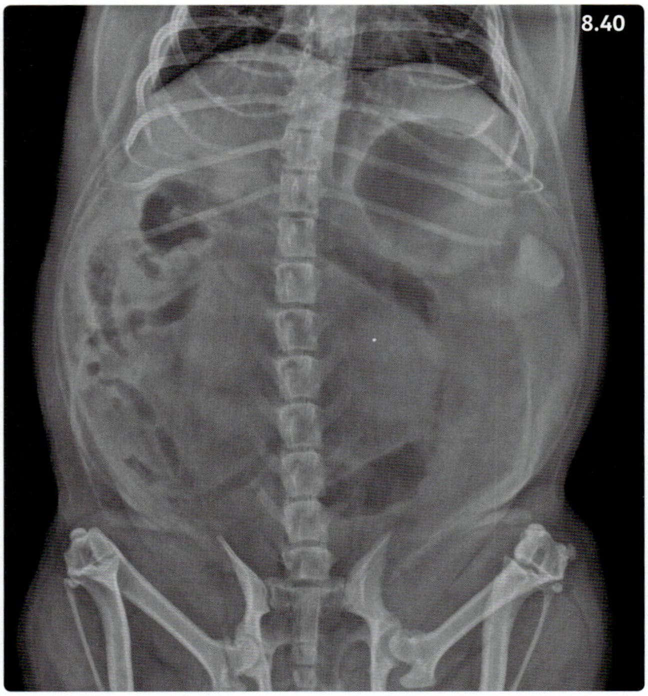

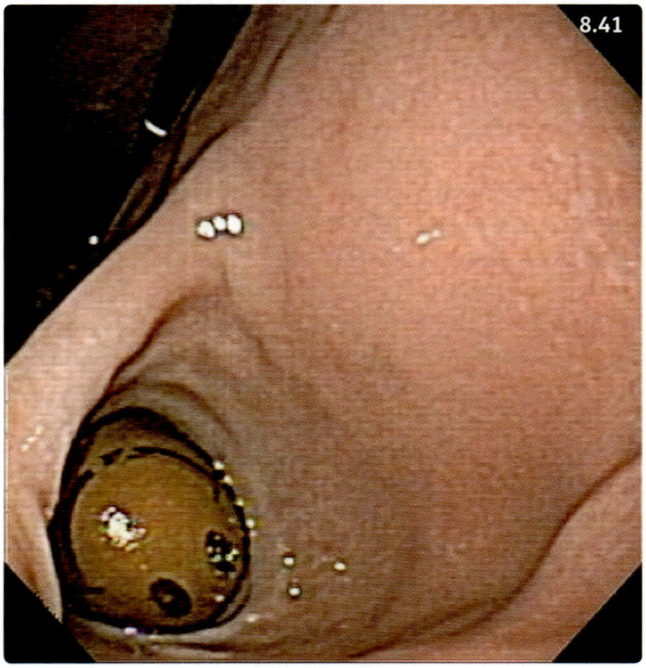

Figures 8.39–8.41 Eight-year-old male neutered Pekingese presented with a 10-day history of anorexia, vomiting, and lethargy. (8.39) Ventrodorsal abdominal radiograph. A round structure of soft tissue density is visible surrounded by gas in the pyloric antrum. (8.40) The foreign body is not visible in this dorsoventral view where gastric gas has accumulated in the fundus. This highlights the importance of obtaining both ventrodorsal and dorsoventral views for an optimal evaluation of the stomach. (Radiographs courtesy LSU SVM Diagnostic Imaging Service) (8.41) Gastroscopic view. A bouncing ball with a smiley face is visible in the pyloric antrum and could easily be extracted using an endoscopic snare.

Diagnosis is confirmed with gastroscopy or surgical exploration, and histologic evaluation of mucosal or full-thickness biopsies. Antral mucosal folds can easily be viewed on endoscopic evaluation of the stomach (**Figures 8.43, 8.44**). Histopathologic examination of mucosal biopsies confirms the mucosal hyperplasia.

Management

Treatment is surgical and consists of removing the redundant tissue and performing a Y-U pyloroplasty. Tissue specimens should be submitted for histologic confirmation. In some instances, pyloric antral resection may be required. Pyloric myotomy, while easier to perform, is usually not successful in these animals.

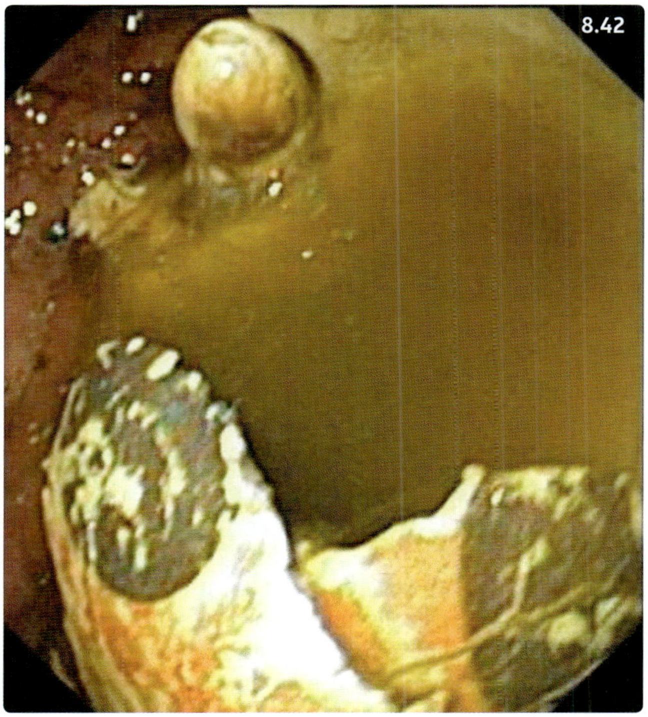

Figure 8.42 Gastroscopic view of a dog that had chewed and swallowed parts of a plastic soccer ball. Typical clinical signs had been present for 3 weeks.

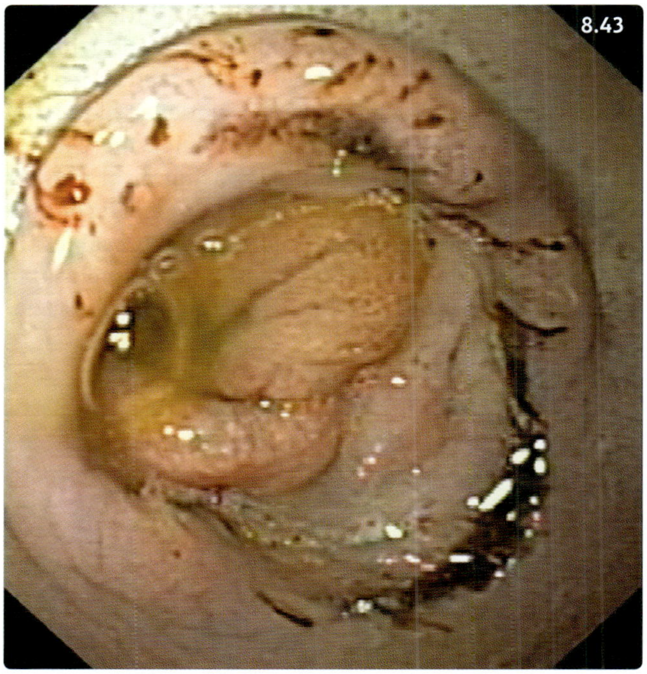

Figure 8.43 Gastroscopic view of the pylorus in a French Bulldog with gastric antral pyloric hypertrophy. Note the prominent mucosal folds surrounding the pylorus, with multiple erosions (bleeding) that may be associated with duodenogastric reflux. (Courtesy P. Lecoindre)

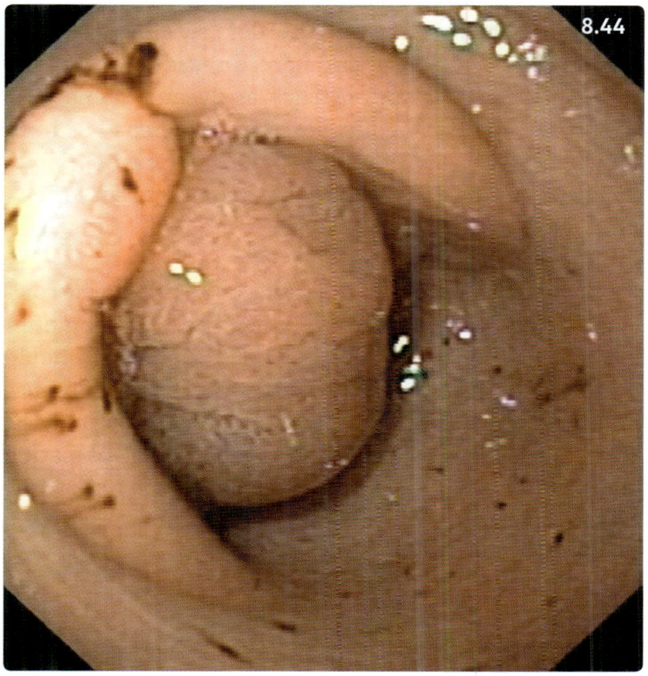

Figure 8.44 Gastroscopic view of the pylorus in a Boxer dog with gastric antral pyloric hypertrophy. Note the prominent mucosal fold obstructing the pylorus. There are multiple erosions (bleeding) surrounding the pylorus. (Courtesy P. Lecoindre)

Prognosis

Surgery is curative and the prognosis is good. Possible surgical complications include dehiscence or lack of improvement due to inappropriate surgical technique.

NONOBSTRUCTIVE GASTRIC EMPTYING DISORDERS

Definition/overview

Motility is often the 'missing link' in the complex equation of GI health in dogs and cats. The prevalence of GI motility disorders in small animals cannot be precisely documented because obtaining a definitive diagnosis is often difficult, sometimes even impossible. However, it is thought that these disorders are of significant clinical importance.

Etiology

Elucidating the origin of nonobstructive GI dysmotility is often challenging. Often, it results from diseases located outside the GI tract, including abdominal inflammation (e.g. acute pancreatitis), immune-mediated diseases, and metabolic diseases. Alternatively, motility disorders may also result from primary GI disorders such as GI inflammation or neoplasia. Furthermore, diseases affecting the autonomic nervous system, such as dysautonomia, also impact GI motility. Finally, postoperative ileus has been shown to cause a significant delay in gastric emptying of up to 48 hours in dogs undergoing abdominal surgery.

Clinical presentation

Vomiting of more or less digested food is the most common clinical sign, particularly when it occurs long after food intake (e.g. >10–12 hours), when the stomach should be empty. Projectile vomiting may occur in the absence of a prodromal phase. Additionally, the animal may be bloated and have pain on cranial abdominal palpation and/or signs of colic. Decreased appetite or anorexia, signs of nausea, increased belching, pica, and/or polydipsia may also be observed.

Differential diagnosis

Due to the relatively vague symptomatology, the list of differential diagnoses is long. It is essential to first rule out GI obstruction, which may require immediate surgical management.

Diagnosis

Since many underlying disorders may affect gastric motility, a minimal database (CBC, chemistry panel, urinalysis) plus survey abdominal radiographs are indicated to screen for underlying diseases and confirm the absence of GI obstruction (**Figure 8.45**). Accurate assessment of gastric emptying is difficult under practical conditions. Radionuclide scintigraphy is recognized as the current gold standard in dogs and cats but is only available at select referral centers. Radiographic studies are easily accessible in clinical veterinary practice. However, assessment of gastric emptying of liquid barium is an insensitive technique, with the exception of diagnosis of mechanical obstructions. Mixing barium with food may allow better evaluation of the solid phase of gastric emptying. Unfortunately, barium can easily dissociate from the test meal and cause the study to be unreliable. Barium-impregnated polyethylene spheres (BIPS™) have been used for evaluation of GI transit times in dogs and cats. However, correlation between gastric emptying of BIPS and the gold standard has been disappointing in dogs and in cats, and the use of these spheres has been limited. Abdominal ultrasound is a promising and widely available modality for the evaluation of gastric antral motility and gastric emptying.

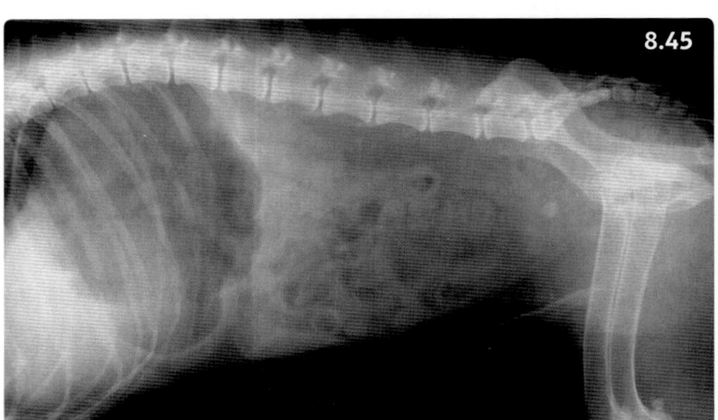

Figure 8.45 Right lateral abdominal radiograph of a 15-year-old male neutered Cocker Spaniel with recurrent episodes of bloat and colic. The stomach is dilated with gas, but there is no indication of gastric outlet obstruction. **Note:** A radiopaque cystic calculus is visible.

Management

Proper diagnosis and treatment of any underlying disease that may affect gastric motility are essential. Therapy of functional, nonobstructive disorders of gastric motility is based on dietary modification and judicious use of prokinetic drugs.

Dietary modifications designed to facilitate gastric emptying are based on knowledge of digestive physiology. First, gastric emptying of liquid food is faster than that of solid foods. Also, diets with high caloric density tend to remain longer in the stomach. In addition, gastric emptying of fat is slower than that of proteins, which is slower than that of carbohydrates. Consequently, feeding a liquid or semi-liquid diet of low caloric density low in fat and protein should maximize gastric emptying. Finally, increased meal frequency and decreasing meal size are also useful. Dietary treatment of bilious vomiting or duodenogastric reflux consists of feeding a light meal late at night. Additionally, prokinetic drugs may be beneficial in nonobstructive disorders of gastric emptying (**Table 8.9**)

Prognosis

Prognosis is good if the primary cause of delayed gastric emptying can be corrected. Idiopathic GI dysmotility can be a challenge to manage efficiently. Dysautonomia carries a poor prognosis in cats and dogs.

GASTRIC NEOPLASIA

Definition/overview

Stomach tumors are uncommon, and typically occur in older in dogs and cats. Benign canine gastric neoplasms include adenomatous polyps and leiomyomas. Adenocarcinoma and lymphoma are the most prevalent tumor types diagnosed in the dog, followed by

Table 8.9 Site of action and recommended dosage of gastrointestinal prokinetics.

Name	Site of action	Dose
Metoclopramide	Pyloric antrum, duodenum (?)	0.2–0.5 mg/kg PO, SC q8h CRI: 1–2 mg/kg/24h
Cisapride	Lower esophagus (C), lower esophageal sphincter, pyloric antrum, small intestine, colon	0.1–0.5 mg/kg PO q8–12h; dose can be progressively increased up to 1 mg/kg q8h
Mosapride	Pyloric antrum	0.25–2 mg/kg PO q12–24h (D); currently only available in Asia
Prucalopride	Pyloric antrum, small intestine (?), colon	0.01–0.6 mg/kg PO q12–24h; currently not available in the USA
Erythromycin	Lower esophageal sphincter (D), pyloric antrum, small intestine, colon	0.5–1.0 mg/kg PO or IV q8h (after dilution)
Ranitidine	Pyloric antrum (possibly small intestine, colon)	1–2 mg/kg PO q12h, or slowly IV (after dilution)
Nizatidine	Same as raniditine	2.5–5 mg/kg PO q24h

(D), dog only; (C), cat only; CRI, constant rate infusion.

leiomyosarcoma and stromal tumors. Lymphoma is the most common gastric neoplasia found in cats.

Etiology

The etiology of gastric tumors has not been elucidated. Canine breeds at risk for adenocarcinoma include the Belgian Shepherd Dog, Rough Collie, and Staffordshire Bull Terrier. A predisposition in male dogs has been reported for gastric adenocarcinoma and gastric lymphoma.

Clinical presentation

The early stages of gastric neoplasia usually remain subclinical. Hyporexia is the most common clinical sign followed by vomiting and weight loss. In advanced stages with ulceration of the gastric mucosa, hematemesis and melena may occur. Vomiting is due either to gastric outflow obstruction or to abnormal gastric motility associated with the neoplastic wall infiltration. Adenomatous polyps are usually subclinical unless they cause gastric outflow obstruction.

Differential diagnosis

Other disease processes causing gastric outflow or small intestinal obstruction (FBs, pythiosis). Other conditions associated with dysorexia and vomiting that originate from the GI tract or from other organ systems.

Diagnosis

A minimal database consisting of CBC, biochemistry panel and urinalysis is recommended to evaluate the general condition of the animal and screen for possible systemic repercussions of gastric tumors such as blood loss anemia. Diagnosis is confirmed with abdominal imaging. In some instances survey abdominal radiographs may reveal an enlarged stomach with delayed emptying (**Figure 8.46**). Filling defects or ulcerated areas may be detected on contrast studies. Abdominal ultrasound often shows thickening of the gastric wall (**Figure 8.47**). Most canine gastric adenocarcinomas are located in the antral area or on the lesser curvature, while lymphomas are often diffusely infiltrative. Enlarged lymph nodes and/or hepatic nodules suggestive of local metastases may be visible (**Figure 8.48**). Double lateral thoracic radiographs are useful to screen for pulmonary metastases. Cytologic evaluation of ultrasound-guided aspirates of the abnormal gastric wall may be helpful to diagnose lymphoma (**Figure 8.49**). Endoscopic evaluation with sampling of mucosal biopsies in and around the suspect areas (**Figures 8.36, 8.50**) and histologic evaluation are useful to confirm the tumor type. While no appearance is typical for one specific tumor type, most adenocarcinomas are ulcerated. Occasionally, tumors are located in the submucosal layers, and obtaining representative endoscopic biopsies may be challenging.

Management/prognosis

By the time animals develop clinical signs and are presented to a veterinarian, the neoplastic process is often advanced and severe. Probably due to a high prevalence of metastases at the time of diagnosis, surgical resection (antral resection and gastroduodenostomy, or Billroth type I procedure) does not significantly improve

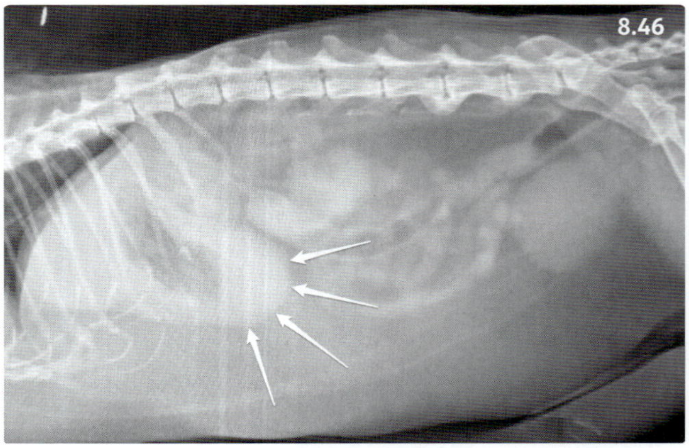

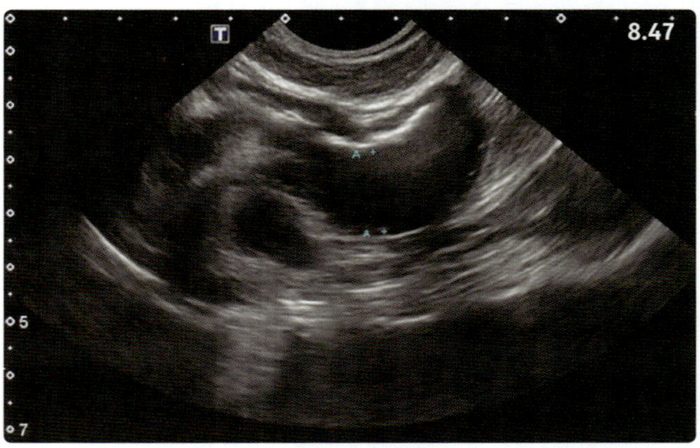

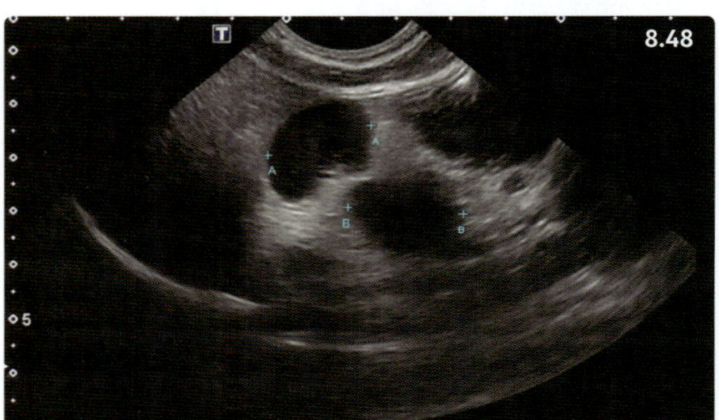

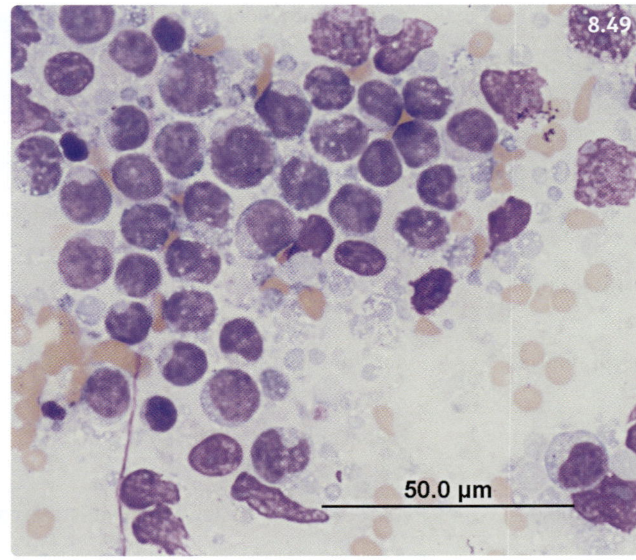

Figures 8.46–49 Twelve-year-old Domestic Shorthair cat with anorexia, weight loss, and lethargy of 4 weeks' duration. (8.46) Right lateral abdominal radiograph. The cat is severely overweight. Although the cat did not eat for 2 days, the stomach is distinctly visible and partially filled with gas (arrows). The gastric wall appears thickened at the level of the pyloric antrum (although this could also be due to summation of gastric fluid and gastric wall), and the serosal contour of the stomach is somewhat irregular. (Courtesy C. Montgomery) (8.47) Abdominal ultrasound of the same cat. The gastric wall at the level of the pyloric antrum is severely thickened (14.8 mm between the two calipers). (8.48) Abdominal ultrasound of the same cat. The gastric lymph nodes are very prominent (distance "A", 19.6 mm; distance "B", 21.2 mm). (Ultrasound images courtesy LSU SVM Diagnostic Imaging Service) (8.49) Cytologic evaluation of a fine needle aspirate from the gastric wall depicted in 8.47. A dense population of medium-sized lymphocytes and a few large lymphoblasts are visible, confirming the diagnosis of gastric lymphoma (50× objective). (Courtesy V. Le Donne)

the prognosis of dogs with gastric adenocarcinomas. However, surgery may be a successful option for canine leiomyosarcomas, with a reported median survival time of 12 months. While canine gastric lymphomas usually carry a poor prognosis, feline alimentary lymphomas may respond to specific chemotherapy protocols. Small cell feline alimentary lymphomas usually achieve prolonged remission with prednisolone (1–2 mg/kg PO daily) and chlorambucil (2 mg PO q48h) therapy. Large cell alimentary lymphomas require more aggressive chemotherapy protocols and their prognosis is less favorable.

Part 4: Diseases of the small intestine

Overview

Small intestinal diseases are common in dogs and cats. The small intestine is the intestinal segment where absorption of nutrients, electrolytes, and water takes place. Small intestinal brush border enzymes are essential for activation of pancreatic enzymes and final processing of nutrients before they can be absorbed through the mucosa using active and passive diffusion mechanisms.

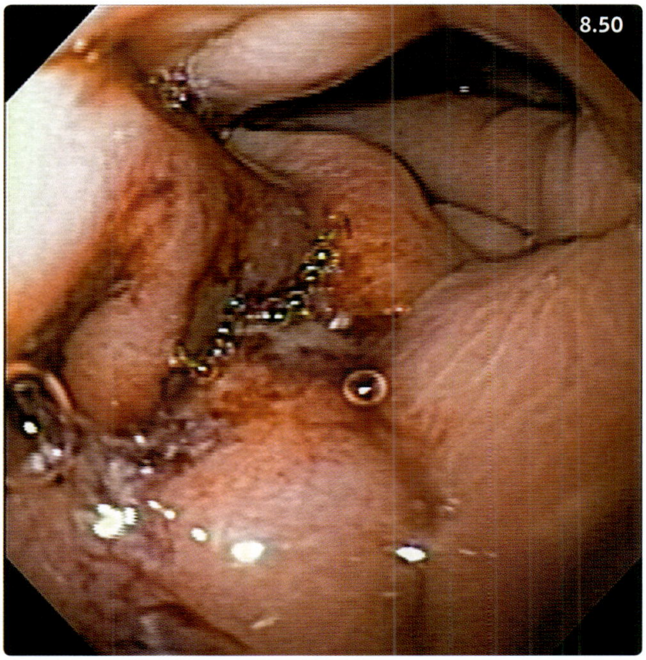

Figure 8.50 Close-up endoscopic view of a gastric adenocarcinoma in a 15-year-old female spayed Miniature Schnauzer. There are thickened mucosal folds surrounding an ulcerated area.

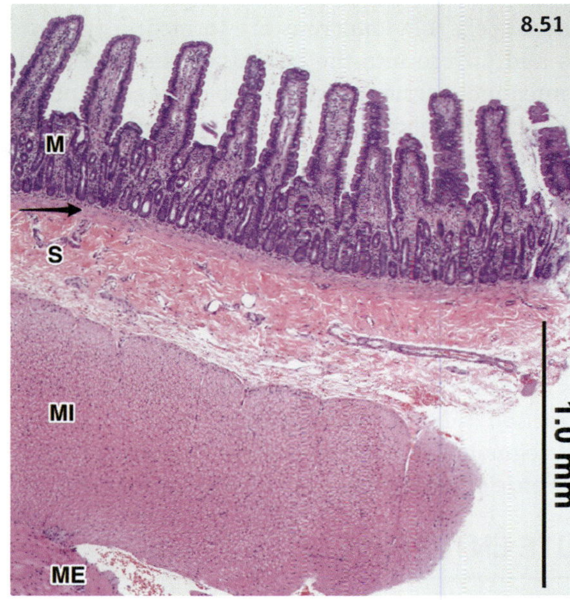

Figure 8.51 Photomicrograph of the jejunal wall in a cat at low power. M, mucosa; S, submucosa; MI, muscularis interna (circular muscle layer); ME, muscularis externa (longitudinal muscle layer); arrow (muscularis mucosae). H&E stain.

Small intestinal anatomy

The small intestine is divided into three anatomic segments: duodenum, jejunum, and ileum. The total surface of the small intestinal mucosa is multiplied by a factor of 500 through formation of mucosal villi and presence of microvilli on the luminal surface of the enterocytes. The microscopic structure consists of mucosa, submucosa, and both the internal and external muscular layers (**Figure 8.51**). The mucosa consists of villi, lamina propria, and muscularis mucosae (**Figure 8.52**). The epithelial cells multiply in the small intestinal crypts and migrate over a few days to the tips of the small intestinal villi while they are undergoing maturation.

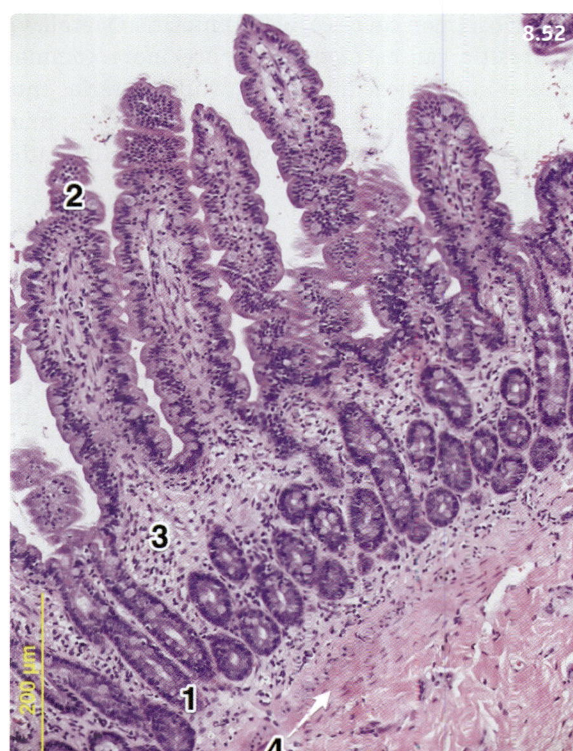

Figure 8.52 Photomicrograph of the jejunal mucosal layer in a cat. 1, jejunal crypt; 2, tip of jejunal villus; 3, lamina propria; 4, muscularis mucosae (arrow). H&E stain, 40× objective.

Normal small intestinal function

Digestion and absorption

In the small intestine, pancreatic and gastric enzymes facilitate luminal digestion, while enzymes produced by epithelial cells and located in the brush border of enterocytes are responsible for triggering the activation of pancreatic enzymes and further processing of oligo- and disaccharides, small peptides, and lipids. Carbohydrates, amino acids, and fatty acids are transported actively or passively through the epithelial barrier using transcellular and paracellular pathways. Lipids undergo complex transformations in order to be absorbed into the epithelial cells. Chylomicrons are formed in the enterocytes and diffuse into the lacteals to the thoracic duct. The intestinal barrier prevents free passage of intestinal content into the body and consists of the enterocytes with the glycocalyx that bathes their microvilli and the tight junctions that connect them on their lateral membrane.

Small intestinal motility

Three physiologic motility patterns are described in the small intestine: peristaltic waves (aboral movement of chyme over long intestinal segments), stationary contractions (leading to intestinal segmentation), and clusters of contraction (mixing and aboral movement of chyme over short segments). Diarrhea usually is associated with the occurrence of pathologic giant aboral contractions.

ACUTE ENTERITIS

Overview

Acute enteritis occurs frequently in dogs and cats and can be a sign of many diseases affecting the small intestine primarily or secondarily. The approach to diarrhea is explained in Chapter 2.6 (**Table 2.6.1** lists the characteristics of small bowel diarrhea; **Table 2.6.2** lists the various causes of acute diarrhea). This chapter provides further details on common causes of acute enteritis. Overall, viral and parasitic causes of enteritis are more commonly diagnosed in puppies and kittens, while bacterial enteritis and dietary indiscretion can occur at all ages; finally, acute hemorrhagic diarrhea syndrome (AHDS) affects middle aged to older dogs.

VIRAL ENTERITIS

CANINE PARVOVIRAL ENTERITIS

Overview

The etiology, pathogenesis, diagnosis, and prevention of canine parvovirus infection are also discussed in Chapter 21 (Infectious diseases). The virus targets rapidly dividing cells such as small intestinal crypt cells (**Figures 8.53, 8.54**). It eventually greatly diminishes the absorptive capacity of the small intestine and compromises the intestinal barrier. The risk of bacterial translocation, bacteremia, and sepsis is greatly enhanced by the concurrent neutropenia.

Clinical presentation

The following breeds are at higher risk of infection: Rottweiler, Dobermann, Labrador Retriever, American Staffordshire Terrier, German Shepherd Dog, and Alaskan Malamute. The most severe cases occur in puppies

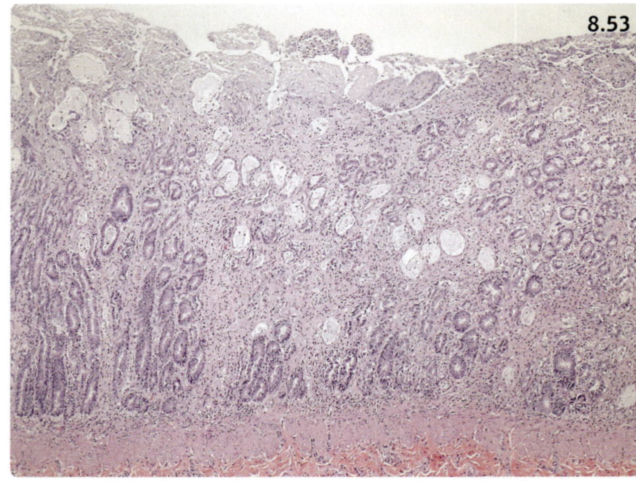

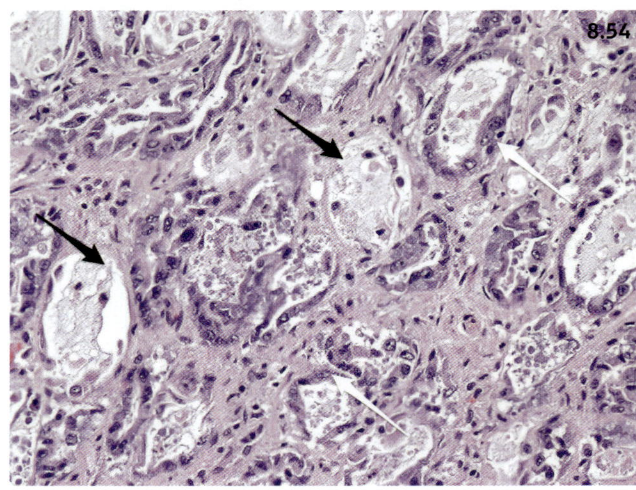

Figures 8.53, 8.54 Six-month old dog with parvovirus infection. (8.53) Photomicrograph of the jejunal mucosa. There is severe villous atrophy with necrotic crypts (see 8.54). H&E stain, 40x objective. (8.54) Photomicrograph of the jejunal crypts. Several crypts lack epithelial lining (black arrows) and are filled with necrotic material, while others show evidence of epithelial regeneration (white arrows). (Courtesy N. Wakamatsu)

between the ages of 4 and 12 weeks, at the time when maternal immunity fades away. However, parvovirus infection is prevalent in dogs until 6 months of age. Anorexia and vomiting are often the first clinical signs observed. They are followed a few hours later by foul smelling, often bloody diarrhea (see **Figure 2.6.7**). Without treatment, puppies rapidly dehydrate. Fever is generally associated with secondary bacterial infection.

Intense vomiting and diarrhea may cause metabolic acidosis that often responds well to IV fluid therapy with crystalloids and colloids, and generally does not require administration of sodium bicarbonate. Hypokalemia results from GI loss and may contribute to the occurrence of intussusception. In severe cases, severe complications, including sepsis and disseminated intravascular coagulation, may occur.

Differential diagnosis

In puppies or in young dogs presented for acute vomiting, the differential diagnosis must include GI FB and intestinal intussusception, which should be ruled out with abdominal radiographs. "Garbage can gut" and severe infestation with intestinal parasites may also cause hemorrhagic gastroenteritis.

Diagnosis

A preliminary diagnosis of parvovirus infection is made in the presence of acute hemorrhagic gastroenteritis in a young dog that is not adequately vaccinated. The probable presence of a highly contagious disease justifies drastic measures in order to prevent the spread of the infection in the veterinary hospital (isolation of the sick dog, thorough disinfection). Confirmation of diagnosis requires fecal testing for parvoviral antigen using a cageside test. The antigen test may be positive during the viral shedding period, which lasts for 10–12 days after infection. However, the result may be false negative as viral shedding may wax and wane. Also, the test can give a false-positive result in dogs that have been recently vaccinated with a modified live vaccine. In such cases, fecal PCR may be useful to differentiate vaccine and wild type virus. Neutropenia is a typical finding in dogs with parvovirus infection; however, it is not always present at the time of the initial veterinary visit. Detection of other laboratory changes may be useful to set up an adequate treatment plan. Electrolyte abnormalities, especially hypokalemia, should be corrected. Panhypoproteinemia (characterized by simultaneous presence of hypoalbuminemia and hypoglobulinemia) is due to intestinal protein loss. Depending on the severity of the problem, natural or synthetic colloids should be used to support oncotic pressure.

Management

Aggressive treatment is required and consists of rapid correction of fluid deficits and electrolyte imbalances. Crystalloids and colloids are used in adequate amounts with added electrolyte solutions as needed. However, a recent scientific abstract has suggested good success in treating dogs with parvovirus infection on an outpatient basis (**Box 8.6**).

It is essential to stop the vomiting as quickly as possible. A variety of antiemetic agents are available (see Chapter 2.4, **Table 2.4.1**). A combination of these antiemetic drugs with different modes of action is sometimes required to obtain the desired result. Recent research has shown the benefits of early feeding in very small amounts; dogs that received early nutrition after they stopped vomiting had a lower mortality and a faster weight gain during recovery.

Box 8.6 Practical tip: outpatient treatment of canine parvovirus infection.

An outpatient treatment for dogs with parvoviral enteritis was evaluated in a recent study. After initial in-hospital stabilization with IV fluids, the outpatient treatment consisted of:

- SC administration of isotonic fluids (40 ml/kg q8h after replacement of fluid deficits)
- Enteral nutrition
- Daily SC injections of maropitant (1 mg/kg)
- One SC injection of cefovecin (8 mg/kg), a proprietary long-acting 3rd generation cephalosporin.

The 80% survival rate compared favorably with the 90% recovery rate in hospitalized parvovirus patients treated with IV fluids. Also, there was no difference in time to recovery between the hospitalized and the outpatient group. The results of this study appear to document the validity of an alternative option for owners who cannot afford the costly hospitalization for puppies and young dogs infected with parvovirus.

Source: Preisner K, Sullivan L, Boscan P *et al.* (2013) Evaluation of an outpatient protocol in the treatment of canine parvoviral gastroenteritis. *J Vet Intern Med* **27(3)**:721 (Abstract)

Because of the risk of secondary bacterial infection, parenteral administration of broad-spectrum antibiotics such as amoxicillin and clavulanic acid (12.5–20 mg/kg IV q12h) is recommended. Parenteral aminoglycosides (with risk of nephrotoxicity) or fluoroquinolones (e.g. enrofloxacin, 10 mg/kg q24h, off-label in growing dogs) may be added to improve efficacy against gram-negative bacteria.

Disinfection of contaminated surfaces is essential in order to prevent spread of infection. Disinfectants with demonstrated efficacy against parvovirus include sodium hypochlorite, aldehydes, and oxidizing agents. A 1:30 dilution of commercially available bleach is efficacious after 10 contact minutes. However, bleach is a mucosal irritant and may damage metals, rubber, plastic, and cement. It is inactivated by light, thus it is preferable to prepare solutions immediately before their use. It is also inactivated in the presence of organic material such as mud or feces. Oxidizing solutions such as hydrogen peroxide (Virox®, Accel®) and potassium peroxide monosulfate (Virkon®, Trifectant®) claim extremely high efficacy within minutes with minimal corrosive effect.

Prognosis

Dogs with mild to moderate disease generally have a good prognosis if appropriate treatment is initiated early. In severe cases the prognosis is fair because complications are more common and therapy is more intensive. Overall, quick diagnosis and early and aggressive treatment optimize therapeutic success.

Other viral intestinal infections

Feline panleukopenia and canine and feline coronavirus infections are discussed in detail in Chapter 21 (Infectious diseases).

BACTERIAL ENTERITIS

Overview

The term intestinal microbiota describes all microorganisms naturally present in the intestinal lumen. The small intestinal microbiota has important functions in the preservation of anatomic structures and for the proper occurrence of physiologic processes necessary for digestion of food and absorption of nutrients. It also plays an important role in the prevention of colonization of the mucosa by pathogenic bacteria, and exerts a positive influence on the development of the enteric immune system.

Rarely, dogs and cats may develop bacterial enteritis. Responsible pathogenic agents include *Campylobacter*, *Clostridium perfringens* and *Clostridium difficile*, and *Salmonella* spp., as well as specific strains of *Escherichia coli*. However, these same bacteria can also be isolated in the feces of healthy dogs and cats. While the exact role of bacterial enteropathogens in dogs and cats with enteritis remains controversial, they may present a risk of zoonotic infection for people after contact with shedding dogs and cats. These facts have contributed to an unclear situation that renders diagnostic and therapeutic decisions difficult. If these bacteria are not the source of the animal's problems, use of antibiotics is not recommended because it may lead to development of resistant strains, which in the long term may have repercussions on public health. Additional research is necessary to more clearly define the role of enteropathogens in canine and feline intestinal diseases.

Campylobacteriosis

Etiology

Campylobacter spp. are slender, curved gram-negative bacilli with polar flagellae that generally have a spiral shape (**Figure 8.55**). According to numerous studies, *C. upsaliensis*, *C. jejuni*, *C. helveticus*, and *C. coli* may be present in the feces of healthy and diarrheic cats and dogs.

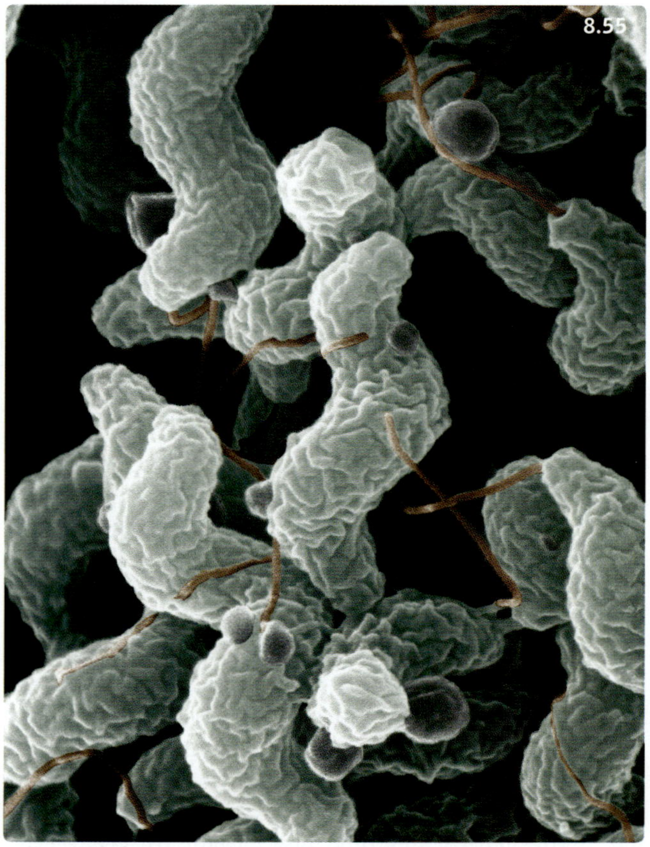

Figure 8.55 *Campylobacter jejuni*. Scanning electron microscope view. (Source: USA Department of Agriculture)

Pathophysiology

Campylobacter attach to enterocytes, invade them, and produce enterotoxin-like substances. However, the true role of *Campylobacter* as a cause of diarrhea in dogs and cats is difficult to assess, since both healthy and diarrheic animals may shed these bacteria in their feces. In people, *Campylobacter* may cause abdominal discomfort, fever, and (possibly bloody) diarrhea. The disease is often self-limiting, but may require antibiotic treatment. Risk factors for infection in people include consumption of poultry cooked at home, drinking water from a well, a lake or a river, and daily contact with a dog. Consequently, fecal excretion of *Campylobacter* in healthy pets appears to represent a possible source of infection.

Clinical presentation

Campylobacter may colonize both the small intestine (jejunum, ileum) and colon and cause enterocolitis. Therefore, clinical signs may include small and/or large intestinal diarrhea of varying severity in puppies and kittens as well as adult animals. The disease is usually self-limiting (1–2 weeks).

Differential diagnosis

Other causes of acute enteritis and/or colitis such as parvovirus infection (in puppies), parasite infestation with hookworms, whipworms, *Giardia*, *Cryptosporidium*, or *Tritrichomonas* (cats), other bacterial infections, dietary indiscretion, AHDS (see below).

Diagnosis

Clinical signs of acute enterocolitis (with possible complications such as dehydration) and positive fecal culture or PCR test are suggestive. However, *Campylobacter* may also colonize the intestine as opportunists and be retrieved in feces from healthy and sick dogs and cats. Documentation of spiral-shaped bacteria on fecal cytology is not a useful tool to confirm the diagnosis because it does not allow differentiation between *Campylobacter* and other nonpathogenic, spiral-shaped gram-negative bacteria.

Management

In animals with diarrhea, vomiting, and/or other clinical signs of enterocolitis, appropriate antibiotic treatment is often recommended even if the cause-to-effect relationship between fecal presence of *Campylobacter* and clinical disease is difficult to confirm. Antibiotics of choice for treatment of campylobacteriosis in dogs and cats include macrolides (e.g. erythromycin, 10–20 mg/kg PO q12h; azithromycin, 5–10 mg/kg q24h for 10–14 days) and fluoroquinolones (e.g. enrofloxacin, 5–10 mg/kg PO q24h for 1 week). Repeat culture or fecal PCR is recommended after completion. Use of probiotics may be beneficial (**Box 8.7**). Owners should be advised about proper hygiene.

Prognosis

Generally excellent. If an unrelated enteropathy is present, therapeutic success depends on identification and treatment of the underlying disease.

Box 8.7 Practical tip: use of probiotics in acute enteritis.

Probiotics are living microorganisms that may modulate intestinal immune function, promote epithelial cell homeostasis, exert neuromodulatory effects, block the effects of pathogenic bacteria, and have nutritional benefits.

Probiotics designed for use in dogs and cats and manufactured by reputable pharmaceutical or pet food companies are preferred, as over the counter products have been shown not to be as reliable. Some products contain one bacterial strain while others have several strains.

They have been shown to shorten the duration of acute diarrhea in shelter cats and to decrease the time to first normal feces in dogs with acute enteritis. In a recent open study of dogs with IBD, a multi-strain highly concentrated probiotic administered for 60 days appeared to be as efficient as a combination of prednisone and metronidazole.

Probiotics should be administered for 2–4 weeks to animals with acute enteritis and probably for months in dogs and cats with chronic enteritis. It may be preferable to delay the initiation of probiotic treatment in dogs with bloody diarrhea and compromised intestinal mucosal barrier until the hemorrhagic diarrhea has resolved.

Clostridial infection

Etiology

Clostridia are gram-positive anaerobic bacteria that produce endospores. *Clostridium perfringens* is broadly distributed in the environment. It has been cultivated from 70% or more feces of healthy dogs and diarrheic dogs. It produces enterotoxin, and only 5–14% of isolates from healthy dogs and 15–34% from diarrheic dogs are enterotoxigenic. Enterotoxigenic *C. perfringens* causes food-associated toxin infections in people. *Clostridium difficile* produces two toxins (toxins A and B). In various studies *C. difficile* was detected in feces from healthy puppies and their dam, from healthy adult cats and dogs, and from cats and dogs with diarrhea presented to veterinary clinics. In people, infections with toxigenic *C. difficile* are a frequent cause of nosocomial enteric infections, and are associated with antibiotic use and pseudomembranous colitis.

Pathophysiology

High concentrations of pathogenic clostridial toxins in the intestinal lumen may cause enteritis, but this hypothesis has not been confirmed.

Clinical presentation

In dogs and cats, clostridial infections have been associated with nosocomial diarrhea, hemorrhagic enterocolitis, and acute or chronic small and/or large bowel diarrhea. *C. perfringens* may also be implicated in the pathogenesis of AHDS (see below).

Differential diagnosis

See Campylobacteriosis.

Diagnosis

Confirmation of diagnosis is problematic in small animals. Fecal isolation or PCR amplification of *C. perfringens* or *C. difficile* does not confirm that clostridia are indeed responsible for the diarrhea. Similarly, a fecal endospore count performed on fecal smears is not reliable. Fecal enterotoxin and toxins A and B can be detected using immunoenzymatic methods, and the presence of toxin genes can be confirmed with PCR amplification. However, the precise value of diagnostic tests for clostridial toxins in confirming the pathogenicity of *C. perfringens* or *C. difficile* still needs to be established.

Management

Clostridial enteritis and/or colitis are generally self-limiting and respond well to supportive treatment. The necessity for antimicrobial therapy is subject to discussion. *C. perfringens* and *C. difficile* are considered to be sensitive to ampicillin, metronidazole, and tylosin. Use of probiotics may be beneficial (**Box 8.7**). In cases of hospital-associated diarrhea, the required disinfection measures must be implemented, and a good infection prevention protocol should be enforced.

Prognosis

Excellent if proper treatment can be given.

SALMONELLOSIS

Etiology

Salmonella are rod-shaped facultative anaerobic gram-negative bacteria of the Enterobacteriaceae family. The majority of *Salmonella* relevant to veterinary medicine are serovar *S. enterica* subspecies *enterica*.

Pathophysiology

Salmonella are enteroinvasive bacteria that may induce acute mucosal inflammation resulting in enterocolitis, mucosal sloughing, and secretory diarrhea. While most *Salmonella* infections remain localized to the GI tract, bacterial translocation and septicemia may occur and cause severe systemic complications. Generally, healthy adult carnivores are resistant to salmonellosis. The prevalence of healthy carriers is highest in shelters.

In people, salmonellosis is characterized by diarrhea, fever, and abdominal cramps, often mild to moderate in severity and followed by spontaneous recovery. The most common infection pathway is through ingestion of contaminated food, in particular chicken eggs and egg-based products, but also pork and chicken meat or contaminated vegetables. Even though dogs and cats are only rarely implicated in outbreaks of human salmonellosis, isolated foci have been associated with visits to a veterinary hospital. This is why excellent hygiene is recommended around dogs and cats shedding *Salmonella*, particularly if sensitive subjects such as very young children, elderly people, and immunocompromised patients may be exposed.

Clinical presentation

Fever, vomiting, small and/or large bowel diarrhea, anorexia, weight loss, and lethargy. In case of bacterial translocation, signs of sepsis and involvement of other organs.

Differential diagnosis

See Campylobacteriosis.

Diagnosis

Fecal isolation and serotyping of *Salmonella*, PCR. CBC may show changes suggestive of systemic inflammation, and biochemistry profile may indicate involvement of other organs.

Management

Treatment consists of administration of antimicrobial drugs on the basis of documented sensitivity of the isolated strain.

Prognosis

Animals recovering from clinical salmonellosis may become healthy *Salmonella* carriers for weeks after the clinical signs have subsided. This may be due to persistence of *Salmonella* in the lymph nodes. *Salmonella* may survive for long periods in the environment.

PARASITIC ENTERITIS

The Companion Animal Parasite Council (CAPC) maintains a very informative and freely accessible website on intestinal parasitoses of small animals that should be consulted for additional information (www.capcvet.org).

HOOKWORMS

Etiology

Hookworms are common in tropical and subtropical areas (*Ancylostoma caninum* – dog; *A. tubaeforme* – cat) and warm coastal regions (*A. braziliense* – dog, cat), but also in cooler climates (*Uncinaria stenocephala* – dog). Adult hookworms live in the small intestine and produce eggs that are shed with the host's feces, and develop to 3rd stage larvae (L3), which are infectious. Dogs and cats infect themselves by ingesting L3 (direct fecal–oral transmission, ingestion of infected paratenic hosts such as flies, cockroaches, and dung beetles), or through penetration of the skin by L3. In dogs, puppies can be infested by nursing an affected bitch (transmammary infection). Some larvae undergo arrested development in muscle and can be reactivated during stressful events and migrate to the intestine.

Pathophysiology

Adult hookworms ingest the host's blood and cause intestinal inflammation (**Figure 8.56**).

Clinical presentation

The clinical signs consist mainly of small bowel diarrhea. Blood loss anemia can be life threatening in puppies (**Figure 8.57**). Hyporexia, weight loss, poor hair coat, and pica may also be observed. In dogs that were infected percutaneously, pruriginous skin lesions may occur at the points of entry, particularly in the interdigital spaces.

Differential diagnosis

Other causes of acute enteritis. Acute blood loss anemia in puppies may also be caused by heavy flea infestation, which may occur concurrently to hookworm infestation in stray puppies and kittens from tropical and subtropical areas.

Diagnosis

Fecal flotation and visualization of the parasite ova (**Figure 8.58**).

Management/prevention

Treatment with pyrantel pamoate (5–10 mg/kg PO, repeat after 7–10 days) is approved for all hookworm species. Fenbendazole (50 mg/kg PO q24h for 3 consecutive days) is also efficient. The efficacy of avermectins such as moxidectin, milbemycin oxime, and ivermectin differs between species. Supportive treatment as required: for example, anemic puppies and kittens often require blood transfusion (whole blood or packed red blood cells).

Detailed preventive treatment protocols can be found on the CAPC website.

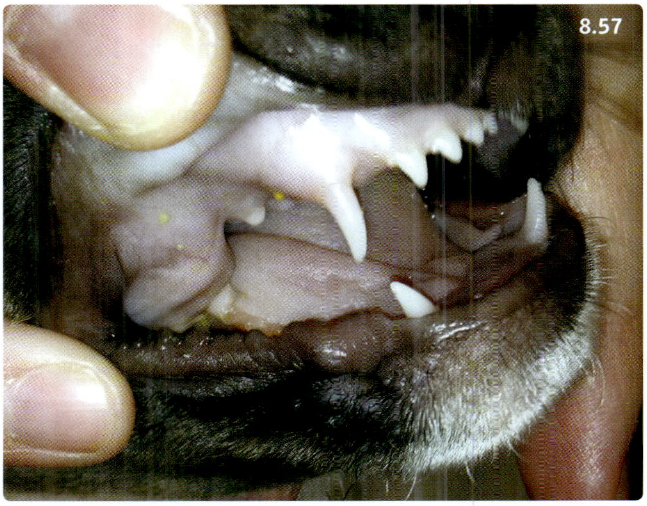

Figure 8.57 Pale oral mucous membranes in a 12-week-old mixed-breed puppy with massive hookworm infestation.

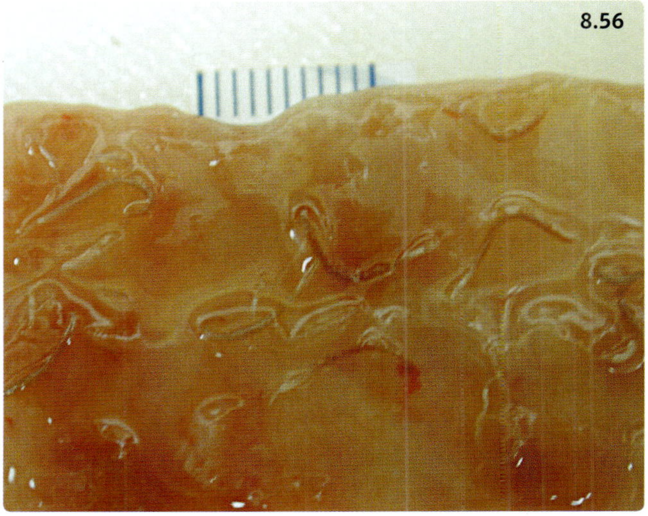

Figure 8.56 Postmortem view of hookworms causing damage to a dog's small bowel mucosa.

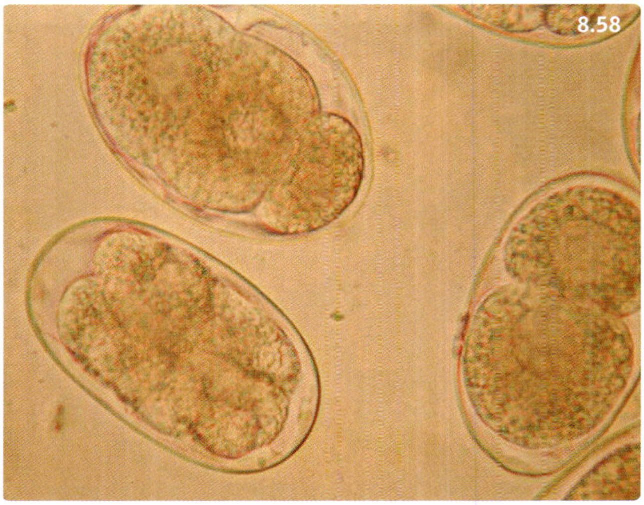

Figure 8.58 Photomicrograph of an *Ancylostoma caninum* ova. (Courtesy E. Greiner)

Public health consideration

Cutaneous larva migrans can occur when hookworm larvae penetrate human skin and result in a prurignious but self-limiting dermatitis.

Prognosis

Good to excellent.

Roundworms

Etiology

Ascarids that may infest small animals include *Toxascaris leonina* (dogs and cats), *Toxocara canis* (dog), and *Toxocara cati* (cat). Additionally, *Baylisascaris procyonis* (the raccoon roundworm) may also occasionally infest dogs in North America. Adult roundworms live in the small intestine (**Figure 8.59**) and produce eggs that are shed in the feces. Larvae are released upon ingestion of embryonated eggs and migrate to the liver and lungs. Pulmonary lesions can induce clinical signs in puppies. Larvae then undergo tracheal migration, and eventually infest the small intestine, or somatic migration, with formation of cysts in tissues with possible reactivation in stressful situations.

Pathophysiology

Adult roundworms cause enteritis, particularly in puppies and kittens.

Clinical presentation

Puppies and kittens: vomiting, small intestinal diarrhea, poor general health, and development of a potbelly are common. Heavy infestation can result in small intestinal obstruction or intussusception. It can also cause pulmonary signs such as coughing and tachypnea. Adult dogs and cats: infestation is less common, and less likely to cause clinical signs.

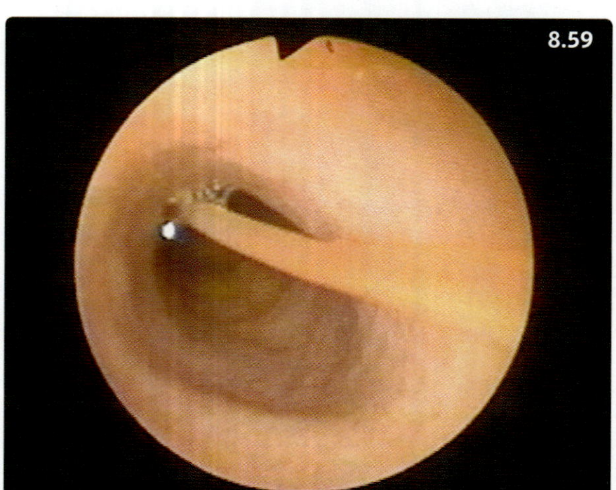

Figure 8.59 Endoscopic view of an adult roundworm in the duodenum of a cat. (Courtesy R. Husnik)

Differential diagnosis

In puppies and kittens other causes of acute enteritis; intestinal FBs if the roundworms cause bowel obstruction.

Diagnosis

Fecal flotation and visualization of the parasite ova (**Figure 8.60**).

Management/prevention

Piperazine, pyrantel pamoate, fenbendazole, and selected avermectins (e.g. milbemycin oxime, moxidectin) should be given to eliminate roundworms. Supportive treatment should be administered as required.

Detailed preventive treatment protocols can be found on the CAPC website.

Public health consideration

In people, ingestion of embryonated eggs from *Toxocara* spp. may lead to larva migrans and cause pulmonary and hepatic disease, retinitis, and neurologic disease. *Toxocara* larva migrans can have a devastating outcome in people.

Prognosis

Excellent.

Isospora spp.

Etiology

Dog – *Isospora canis, I. ohiensis, I. neorivolta, I. burrowsi*. Cat – *I. felis, I rivolta*. Sporulated oocysts are ingested

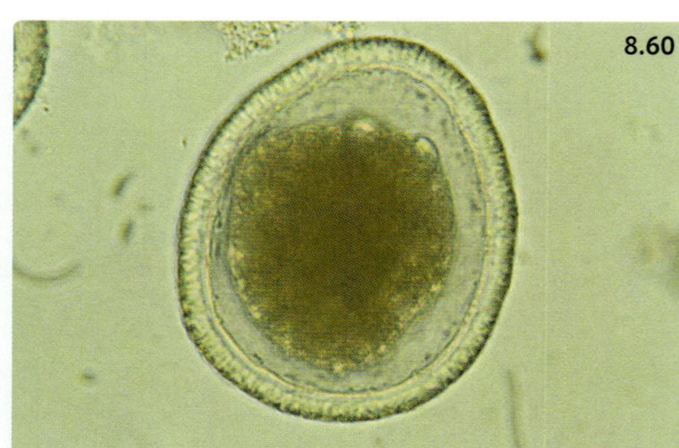

Figure 8.60 Photomicrograph of a *Toxacara canis* egg. (Courtesy E Greiner)

(directly or via paratenic hosts) and further develop in the small intestinal enterocytes (entero-epithelial cycle).

Pathophysiology

Isospora spp. replicate in the small intestine and may induce villus atrophy, lacteal dilation, and hyperplasia of the lymphatic follicles in Peyer's patches.

Clinical presentation

Clinical signs generally only occur in puppies and kittens, and may consist of vomiting, watery diarrhea, abdominal pain, and dysorexia. Dehydration and death can occur in severe cases.

Differential diagnosis

Other causes of acute enteritis in puppies and kittens.

Diagnosis

Isospora spp. oocysts are usually large and easy to detect on microscopic examination of supernatant fluid after fecal flotation.

Management

While the disease is generally self-limiting, treatment may be required in clinical situations. The poorly absorbed sulfa drug sulfadimethoxine (50–60 mg/kg PO q24h for 5–20 days) is the only approved anticoccidial drug for dogs and cats in the USA (and in the UK). Other antiprotozoal drugs, such as ponazuril (20 mg/kg PO q24h for 1–3 days), are frequently administered off-label to dogs and cats after adequate compounding. In breeding facilities and shelters, proper cleaning of the environment (prompt elimination of feces before oocysts sporulate, steam cleaning of contaminated surfaces), treatment of dams prior to parturition, and preventive anticoccidial treatment of all puppies and kittens may be required.

Prognosis

Excellent.

DIETARY INDISCRETION

Definition/overview

Dietary indiscretion is probably the most common cause of acute gastroenteritis in dogs. Overall, puppies and young dogs are more commonly affected than older dogs. Some canine breeds such as Retrievers are known to be prone to dietary indiscretion. Cats are more discriminant eaters, and dietary indiscretion is rarely diagnosed in this species.

Etiology

Ingestion of unusual food such as food prepared for human consumption, garbage that may contain food in various stages of decomposition, or any other food not usually part of the affected dog or cat's diet.

Pathophysiology

Toxins from rotting food cause small intestinal mucosal irritation and may cause osmotic and secretory diarrhea. Unusual food, such as food prepared for human consumption cannot be properly digested and absorbed and thus can cause osmotic diarrhea.

Clinical presentation

Acute diarrhea (with or without vomiting) is the most common presentation. Lethargy, hyporexia, dehydration and electrolyte imbalances, and abdominal discomfort are common accompanying signs.

Differential diagnosis

Other causes of acute gastroenteritis/enteritis such as parasite infestation and viral or bacterial enteritis. In vomiting animals, intestinal obstruction should be ruled out with appropriate abdominal imaging (**Figure 8.61**). In puppies with possible exposure and questionable immune status, parvovirus infection should be ruled out prior to hospitalization.

Diagnosis

History and presentation are often very suggestive.

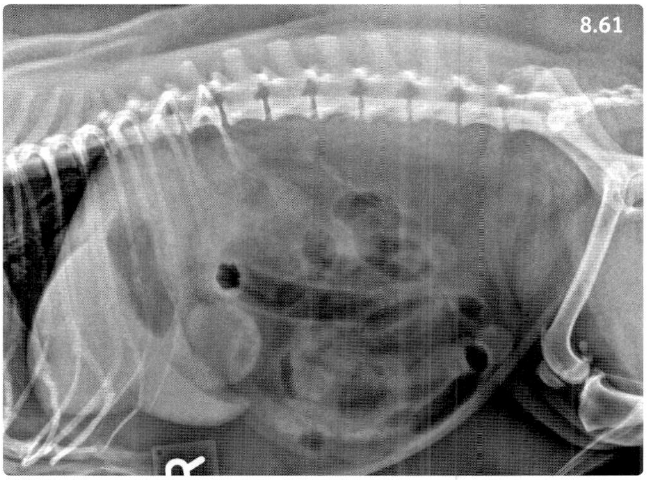

Figure 8.61 Right lateral abdominal radiograph from a adult mixed-breed dog with dietary indiscretion and functional ileus. Generalized distension of small intestinal loops is present. (Courtesy L. Gaschen)

Management

Supportive with administration of fluids (IV, SC, or PO depending on the severity of clinical signs), and antiemetics in vomiting or nauseous animals. A 12–24-hour fast is implemented (puppies will require parenteral glucose solution during fasting in order to avoid hypoglycemia), followed by offering small meals consisting of commercial or home-made, easily digestible diet for 3–5 days and progressive return to a balanced diet after that. Probiotics may be useful (**Box 8.7**). In dogs with severe diarrhea and abdominal discomfort, loperamide (0.1–0.2 mg/kg PO q8h) or diphenoxylate (0.1 mg/kg PO q8h) may be indicated for 24–72 hours, although this is only rarely necessary. Dogs that live in multi-story high-rise buildings might also be candidates for antidiarrheal drugs because of the difficult logistics for bringing them outdoors for defecation.

Prognosis

Good to excellent in most cases. Recurrences are common in dogs prone to eating offending foods.

ACUTE HEMORRHAGIC DIARRHEA SYNDROME

Definition/overview

AHDS is a new name proposed to describe the canine syndrome known for decades as hemorrhagic gastroenteritis (HGE). A recent study demonstrated that affected dogs do not have any gastric inflammation. The syndrome can affect dogs of all breeds and all ages, although middle aged dogs of small and toy breeds seem to be predisposed.

Etiology

The etiology of AHDS/HGE is not known, although abundant *Clostridium perfringens* were shown to be present in the duodenum of affected dogs. Other hypotheses include dietary or microbial toxins and severe dietary indiscretion.

Pathophysiology

It is unclear if clostridial proliferation is a cause or a consequence of the disease. Clostridial toxins do not appear to be significantly involved in the pathogenesis. In addition, acute enteritis has negative repercussions on species diversity of the intestinal microbiota, and may cause acute dysbiosis.

Clinical presentation

Acute onset bloody diarrhea (**Figure 8.62**), possibly with vomiting and anorexia. Affected dogs are usually very dehydrated and in various stages of hypovolemic shock. Lethargy and abdominal pain are also common.

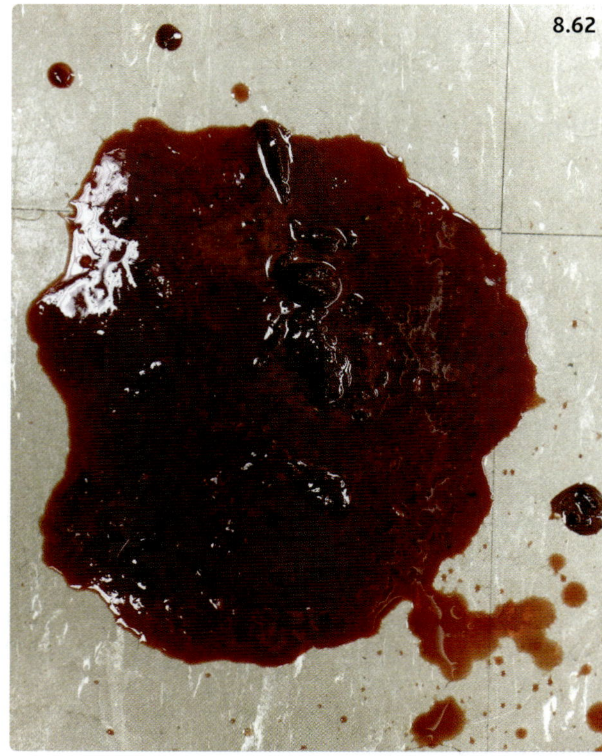

Figure 8.62 Hemorrhagic diarrhea from a dog with acute hemorrhagic diarrhea syndrome.

Differential diagnosis

Parvovirus infection, bacterial infections, salmon poisoning disease, severe parasite infestations, dietary indiscretion, intestinal volvulus or intussusception, acute necrotizing pancreatitis, acute liver disease, hypoadrenocorticism, sepsis, immune-mediated thrombocytopenia, and vitamin K antagonist rodenticide toxicosis.

Diagnosis

Initially, affected dogs typically have a high PCV (often above 65%) and a normal or low serum concentration of total solids (or total proteins, albumin, or globulins). White blood cell counts may be normal, high, or low depending on the severity of disease. Mild thrombocytopenia is common. Other serum biochemistry changes may include prerenal azotemia, increased liver enzymes, hypoglycemia, and electrolyte abnormalities. Metabolic acidosis is often present. Abdominal radiographs usually show an enteritis pattern with fluid- and gas-filled small intestinal loops.

Management

Aggressive fluid therapy. IV boluses of isotonic crystalloid solutions (10–20 ml/kg) should be given to treat hypovolemic shock. Addition of synthetic colloids such as hetastarch may be useful (5–10 ml/kg with 10 ml isotonic crystalloids, continued with CRI of 1 ml/kg/hour). Perfusion and cardiovascular status should be reassessed every 15 minutes, and further boluses administered as required until normal blood pressure is restored. Fluid deficits should be replaced over a 6–12-hour period with crystalloid solutions, adding the maintenance requirements and estimated ongoing losses due to continuing diarrhea. Electrolytes deficits such as hypokalemia should also be corrected. Other treatments include antiemetics and possibly gastric antacids if decreased perfusion of the gastric mucosa is suspected (see **Table 8.6**). The PCV generally normalizes in response to aggressive fluid therapy, and the serum protein concentration usually drops to levels indicative of hypoproteinemia, with both low serum albumin and globulin concentrations (**Figure 8.63**).

Broad-spectrum antibiotics should be administered IV in severe cases with existing or impending sepsis. This is particularly important when mucosal sloughing is present. However, in the absence of these problems, systemic use of antibiotics is not recommended. A recent study showed that cases of mild to moderate severity do not appear to benefit from antimicrobial treatment when endpoints such as time to resolution of diarrhea and length of hospital stay are compared between dogs given amoxicillin and clavulanic acid and those receiving placebo. Probiotics are recommended after resolution of bloody diarrhea (**Box 8.7**)

Dogs with AHDS/HGE should be fasted for 12–24 hours and then offered small quantities of easily digestible food frequently (boiled chicken and rice, adequate commercial prescription diets). Puppies should receive parenteral glucose supplementation.

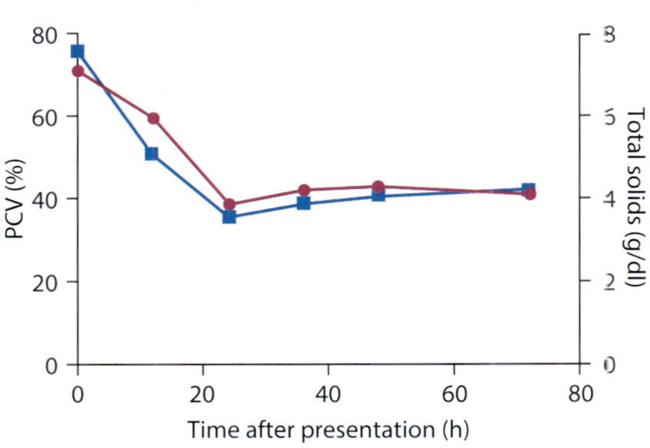

Figure 8.63 Evolution of PCV (red line) and total solids (blue line) with treatment in a 6-year-old Miniature Schnauzer dog with acute hemorrhagic diarrhea syndrome. The initial PCV was 70% (reference range 35–55). The total solids plummeted from 7.5 to 3.5 g/dl within 24 hours with aggressive fluid therapy (reference range 5.8–7.5).

Prognosis

Good when dogs are presented early in the course of the disease. Most dogs can be discharged following 1–7 days of fluid therapy (median 3 days in a recent study). Serious complications may include disseminated intravascular coagulation, sepsis, and aspiration pneumonia in vomiting animals. AHDS/HGE may be fatal if the emergent needs of the patient are addressed too late.

INTESTINAL OBSTRUCTION

Etiology

Small intestinal obstruction most often results from FBs such as peach pits, corn cobs, toys, and fish hooks in dogs and linear foreign bodies in cats. Other differential diagnoses for intestinal obstruction include intussusception and neoplasia. Intussusceptions (**Figure 8.64**) are seen mostly in young animals, particularly in conjunction with severe acute enteritis, such as parvovirus infection or ascarid infestation, but can also be seen in cases of chronic diarrhea, such as IBD, and intestinal neoplasia. Intestinal volvulus (torsion) is a rare disorder in dogs that involves intestinal rotation at the root of the mesentery, with complete occlusion of the cranial mesenteric artery (**Figure 8.65**). This results in bowel necrosis, release of toxins, and life-threatening hypovolemic and septic shock. Most cases have been reported in adult, medium to large breed male dogs.

Pathophysiology

Small intestinal obstruction generally causes an accumulation of intestinal content, fluid, or gas in the loops located craniad to the site of obstruction. Intussusceptions

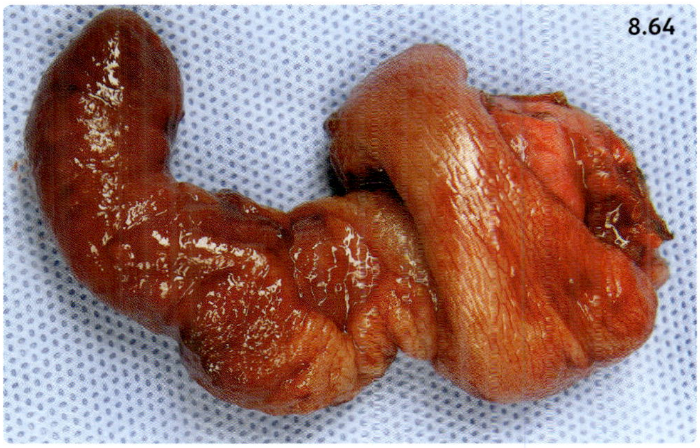

Figure 8.64 An ileocolic intussusception was diagnosed and surgically removed from a 1-year-old male Beagle with chronic diarrhea. Shown is the cecum that was prolapsed into the ascending colon. (Courtesy A. Grooters and K. Saile)

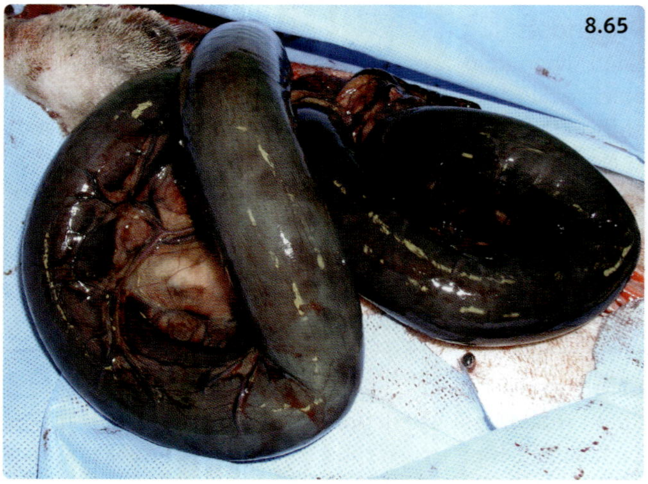

Figure 8.65 Intestinal volvulus in a dog. The small bowel loops are dilated with a hemorrhagic, necrotic wall. (Courtesy R. Husnik)

are thought to occur as a complication of abnormal intestinal motility associated with enteritis or with abnormal intestinal masses.

Clinical presentation

Clinical findings are related to the site, severity, and cause of the obstruction. Complete upper intestinal obstruction results in severe vomiting associated with fluid loss and dehydration and possible hypovolemic shock. Partial obstructions often present with an insidious onset of vomiting and intermittent chronic diarrhea.

Differential diagnosis

Dietary indiscretion or other causes of acute gastroenteritis and acute pancreatitis are the top differentials.

Diagnosis

The history is sometimes helpful for raising suspicion of a FB. A thorough physical examination is important in all cases, including inspection of the base of the tongue for linear foreign bodies, especially in cats (see Chapter 2.4: Vomiting, **Figure 2.6.9**). Abdominal palpation may reveal discomfort or pain, and an FB or intussusception may be identifiable. Abdominal radiographs are essential to document or rule out obstruction (**Box 8.8**). Signs of intestinal obstruction are readily recognizable (**Figures 8.66–8.69**). In severe cases, signs of bowel perforation, such as decreased serosal detail and free abdominal gas, may be present as well. Additionally, abdominal ultrasound may help confirm the diagnosis of intussusceptions and masses. A minimum database consisting of CBC, biochemistry panel, and urinalysis may help characterize the fluid and electrolyte losses and document inflammation or sepsis in complicated cases.

Box 8.8 Practical tip: antiemetics may mask the signs of gastrointestinal foreign bodies.

Several effective antiemetics are currently available to veterinarians:

- Metoclopramide, which can be administered as a CRI to dogs and cats receiving IV fluids (1–2 mg/kg q24h)
- Ondansetron (0.5–1 mg/kg IV or SC q12h) and dolasetron (0.6–1 mg/kg SC or IV q12h)
- Maropitant (1 mg/kg IV or SC q24h)

These antiemetics may suppress vomiting in patients with gastric or small intestinal foreign bodies, and thus delay proper treatment involving foreign body retrieval via exploratory celiotomy or endoscopy (for gastric foreign bodies only). Delayed treatment may make it necessary to resect intestinal tissue (when enterotomy would have been sufficient with early intervention) or even increase the risk of perforation. Consequently, abdominal radiographs should be performed as soon as possible in dogs and cats with history and clinical signs compatible with a GI foreign body in order to rule out obstruction.

Management

Treatment of intestinal obstruction involves surgical removal of the cause of the obstruction (**Figure 8.70**). Broad-spectrum antibiotics should be given IV to patients with signs of intestinal perforation (e.g. amoxicillin, 20 mg/kg q8h; enrofloxacin, 10 mg/kg q24h; and metronidazole, 10–15 mg/kg q12h).

Prognosis

In the absence of complications such as intestinal perforation, the prognosis after surgical extraction of a FB is excellent. The risk of suture dehiscence at the enterotomy or enterectomy site is higher in the presence of peritonitis (i.e. perforation). There is a risk of recurrence for intussusceptions unless the underlying disease is controlled. For intestinal volvulus, the prognosis is usually grave.

CHRONIC ENTERITIS

PARASITIC ENTERITIS

CANINE SCHISTOSOMIASIS

Etiology

Heterobilharzia americana is the agent of canine schistosomiasis, an uncommon disease endemic in the Southeast of the USA and areas bordering the Gulf of Mexico. Raccoons

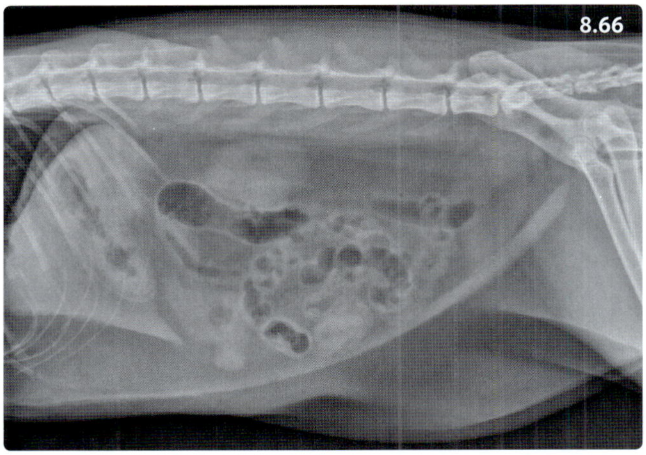

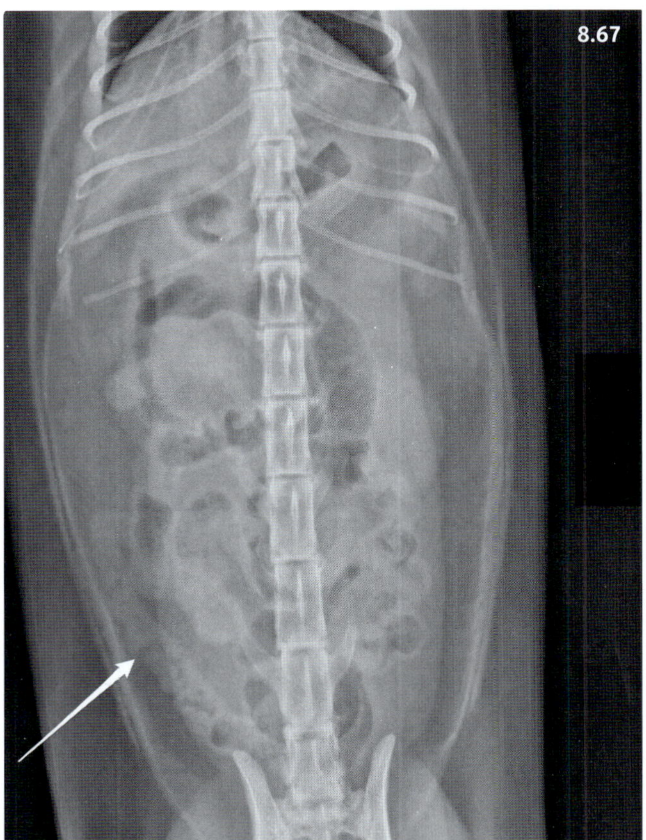

Figures 8.66, 8.67 Cat with a linear foreign body. (8.66) Right lateral abdominal radiograph. All small intestinal loops are located centrally, diffusely plicated, and corrugated in appearance. There are multiple rounded, comma-shaped and paisley-shaped gas opacities of varying size throughout the small bowel. (8.67) Ventrodorsal radiograph of the same cat. The arrow points to a caudally displaced small bowel loop that displays a plicated appearance with content of mixed soft tissue and gas density. (Courtesy L. Gaschen)

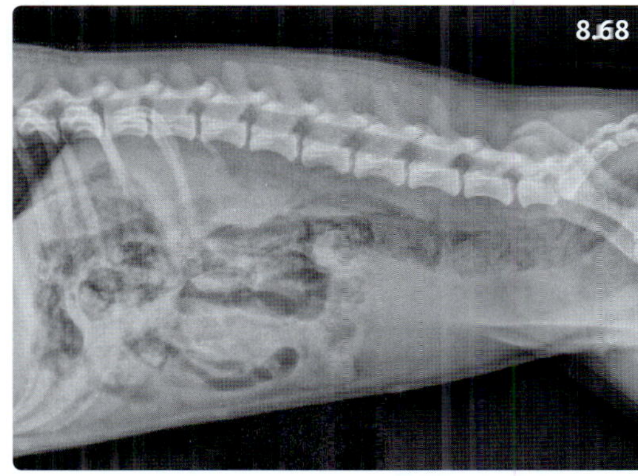

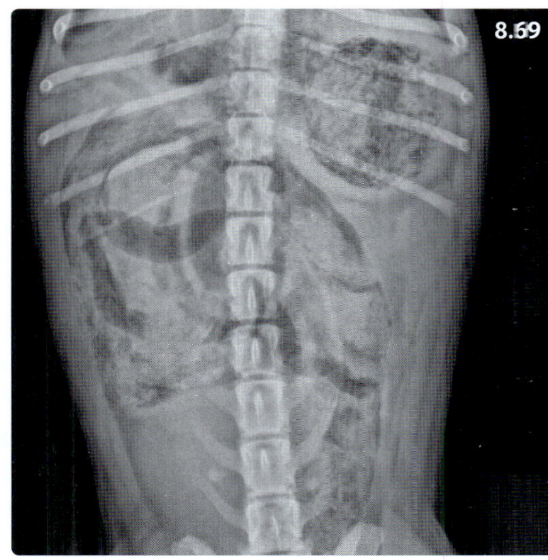

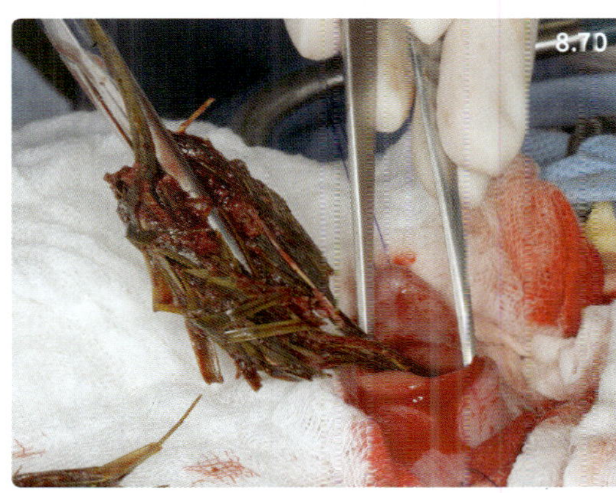

Figures 8.68–8.70 A 2-year-old female Jack Russell Terrier presented with a 4-day history of vomiting. (8.68) Right abdominal radiograph. The serosal detail is decreased throughout the abdomen. The stomach, small intestines, and colon contain a large amount of material with heterogeneous soft tissue and gas density. (8.69) Ventrodorsal radiograph of the same dog. (Courtesy LSU SVM Diagnostic Imaging Service) (8.70) Grass is extracted through a mid-jejunal enterotomy. Large amounts of grass were present throughout the gastrointestinal tract and were impacting the small intestine. (Courtesy A. Grooters and K. Saile)

are the parasite's reservoir host. Freshwater snails are obligatory intermediate hosts.

Pathophysiology

Percutaneous infection occurs through free-swimming cercariae. After migration, adult *Heterobilharzia* produce ova in the terminal branches of the mesenteric veins. The ova are shed through the intestinal mucosa in the feces. Granulomatous inflammation can be found in the intestinal submucosa (**Figure 8.71**) and in other organs as well.

Clinical presentation

Acute to chronic mixed small and large bowel diarrhea. Dysorexia/anorexia, weight loss, often cachexia, lethargy, melena, and/or hematochezia are common.

Differential diagnosis

Includes IBD (including protein-losing enteropathy [PLE]), severe parasitic enteritis, intestinal neoplasia.

Diagnosis

Blood work may reveal anemia, hypoalbuminemia, hyperglobulinemia, and eosinophilia. Hypercalcemia is present in >50% of affected dogs and may cause polyuria/polydipsia. Radiographs may show mineralization of the small intestinal wall. Diagnosis is confirmed with saline sedimentation of feces or a commercially available fecal PCR.

Management

Praziquantel (25 mg/kg q8h for 2–3 days), possibly in combination with fenbendazole (50 mg/kg q24h).

Prognosis

Depends on the severity of lesions at presentation. In a recent retrospective study, the survival rate was 55% after 6–36 months.

GIARDIASIS

Definition/overview

Studies concerning the prevalence of giardiasis in the canine and feline populations report rates of 5–10% in healthy pets and pets presented for veterinary care. The prevalence is greatest in patients that live in high-density group housing, especially when recommended disinfecting protocols are not carried out optimally. In such cases, *Giardia* cysts can easily survive in the environment and continuously infect new animals or reinfect animals after they have been treated.

Etiology

Giardia duodenalis is a flagellated protozoan that exists in two forms: a motile trophozoite of piriform to ellipsoidal shape (**Figure 8.72**) and a cyst form that is highly resistant in the environment. Cysts are absorbed with contaminated food or water, and release trophozoites into the small intestinal lumen. Trophozoites multiply by cell division and become encysted. *Giardia* cysts have four nuclei and a thin envelope. Under favorable conditions they can persist for 3 weeks or even longer in the environment.

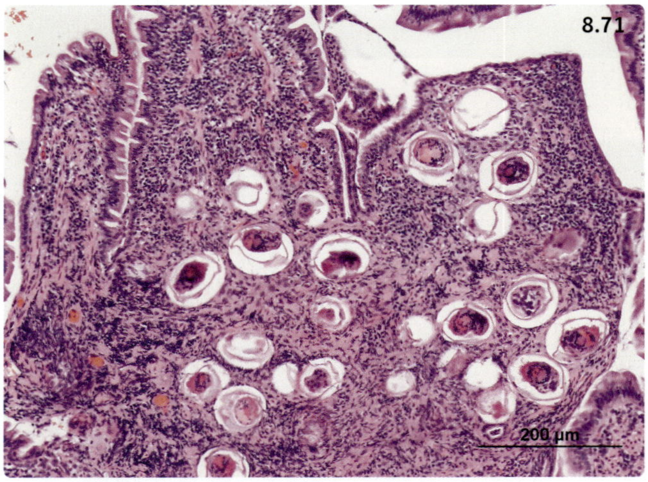

Figure 8.71 Photomicrograph of a duodenal mucosal sample from a dog with canine schistosomiasis. There are numerous eggs present in the mucosa that are associated with granulomatous inflammation. (Courtesy M. Im Hof)

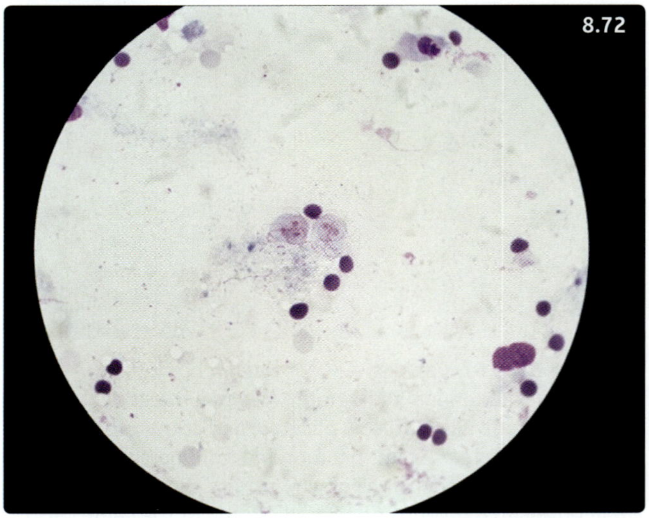

Figure 8.72 Photomicrograph of a fecal smear from a dog with *Giardia* infection. Two trophozoites are visible in the middle of the picture. Wright–Giemsa stain. (Courtesy R. Husnik)

Giardia isolates are further divided into several different genotypes or assemblages with specific host ranges. The zoonotic potential of canine and feline giardiasis is very low. Consumption of water contaminated with *Giardia* cysts is the main origin of infections in people.

Pathophysiology

Trophozoites are found in highest concentration in the duodenum. They attach to the mucosal epithelium and cause disease by affecting epithelial permeability.

Clinical presentation

Diarrhea with watery feces and admixed mucus. In severe and chronic infections, malabsorption and weight loss may occur and the animal may be in poor general condition. Importantly, many infected dogs and cats do not show clinical signs.

Differential diagnosis

Other causes of chronic-intermittent diarrhea and malabsorption, such as other parasite infections, chronic enteropathies (see below), exocrine pancreatic insufficiency, and possibly alimentary lymphoma (cats).

Diagnosis

Several diagnostic tests are available for the diagnosis of *Giardia* infections in dogs and cats (**Table 8.10** and **Figure 8.72**). Confirmation of diagnosis can be complicated by the fact that cysts are shed intermittently.

Table 8.10 Diagnostic tests for *Giardia* in the feces of dogs and cats.

Diagnostic test	Target	Sensitivity
Flotation with zinc sulfate or sugar centrifugation	Cysts	Intermediate, operator-dependent. Can be increased from 70% to 90% if three samples collected at 2–3 day intervals are examined
IFA or ELISA	Specific antigens	Intermediate to good. Diagnostic accuracy of cage-side ELISA test is equivalent to that of antigen tests run in the laboratory
PCR	DNA sequences	Intermediate to high. Only recommended for determination of specific assemblage

Management

The goal of treatment is to stop diarrhea and attempts to fully eliminate *Giardia* infection may not be successful. In dogs, metronidazole (25–30 mg/kg PO q12h for 5–8 days) and fenbendazole (50 mg/kg PO q24h for 3–5 days) are most commonly used. In cats, metronidazole benzoate (25 mg/kg PO q12h for 7 days) is well tolerated and eliminates cyst shedding within 7–10 days of treatment. Fenbendazole can also be used at the same dose as in dogs, although its efficacy may be inferior. Other drugs, including tinidazole (44 mg/kg PO q24h for 3 days), can also be used in cats.

An increased rate of resistance of *Giardia* spp. to metronidazole and other antigiardial agents has been reported in human patients. However, no published data concerning drug resistance of canine or feline giardiasis are currently available.

Dogs kept in group housing should be removed from their runs, shampooed, and rinsed with quaternary ammonium based disinfectants. The runs should be cleaned and disinfected before reuse. Quaternary ammonium containing disinfectants have shown an excellent efficacy for inactivating *Giardia* cysts in a short period of time.

Prognosis

Good

CRYPTOSPORIDIOSIS

Etiology

Cryptosporidium canis (dog) and *C. felis* (cat). The cycle of the parasite is complex and consists of asexual and sexual stages. Sporulated oocysts protected by a wall that is resistant to many environmental factors are passed with the feces and are infectious to appropriate hosts. Prevalence rates between 0% and 38.5% have been reported in different feline populations, while prevalence rates reported in dogs were 0–44.8%. The mode of transmission is via the oral–fecal route.

Pathophysiology

Cryptosporidium spp. are obligate intracellular parasites that infect enterocytes in the small intestine. They damage the epithelial microvilli and enterocytes, and may cause villous atrophy and inflammatory infiltration of the lamina propria.

Clinical presentation

Cryptosporidium infection may be associated with diarrhea, particularly in young animals. In some instances, chronic or intermittent diarrhea, anorexia, and weight loss may occur. However, in many cases, animals do not show clinical signs.

Differential diagnosis

Other causes of chronic small bowel diarrhea such as other parasitoses (e.g. giardiasis), IBD, and alimentary lymphoma (cat).

Diagnosis

The oocysts are small and difficult to see in fecal preparations. Immunoassays for detection of *C. parvum* in human feces have yielded mixed results with feline and canine samples. A fecal PCR test is available to detect *Cryptosporidium* spp. in dogs and cats.

Management

The goal of treatment is to control diarrhea, and underlying diseases such as IBD should be appropriately managed. Feeding a highly digestible diet or an elimination diet may be beneficial as well. There is no drug with documented efficacy against *Cryptosporidium* spp. in small animals. Antibiotics such as azithromycin (10 mg/kg PO q24h) and tylosin (10–15 mg/kg PO q24h) have been used with some success. Nitazoxanide was used in naturally infected laboratory cats (25 mg/kg PO q12–24h) and caused vomiting and foul-smelling dark diarrhea. However, *Cryptosporidium* shedding resolved immediately after the drug was administered. Paromomycin (150 mg/kg PO q12–24 h for 5 days) has also been used in small animals. However, it does not consistently stop oocyst shedding, and is also associated with severe renal failure in cats.

Prognosis

Fair to good. While diarrhea usually resolves with or without therapy in otherwise healthy dogs and cats, treatment may be challenging in the presence of concurrent diseases.

FUNGAL AND OOMYCETAL ENTERITIS

HISTOPLASMOSIS

Etiology

Histoplasma capsulatum is a dimorphic saprophytic fungus that can be found in temperate and subtropical climates. Most cases of canine or feline histoplasmosis described in the literature come from North America, particularly from the Ohio, Missouri, and Mississippi river valleys.

Pathophysiology

Young cats and dogs are predominantly infected by inhalation of microconidia (mycelium). The infection can remain local (respiratory tract). If it propagates, it generally also involves the GI tract.

Clinical presentation

GI signs include chronic small or large bowel diarrhea. Weight loss and poor body condition score are common. Affected animals are sometimes presented with PLE. Other organ systems may be infected and cause additional clinical signs.

Differential diagnosis

Other causes of chronic diarrhea and weight loss such as parasite infections, IBD, and alimentary lymphoma (cat).

Diagnosis

The most reliable diagnosis consists in identifying the organism on cytologic smears from fine needle aspirates of lymph nodes or from rectal scrapings (**Figure 8.73**), or on histologic analysis of intestinal biopsies.

Management

First-line treatment includes itraconazole (10 mg/kg once daily) and must be continued for 4–6 months and at least 2 months beyond clinical remission.

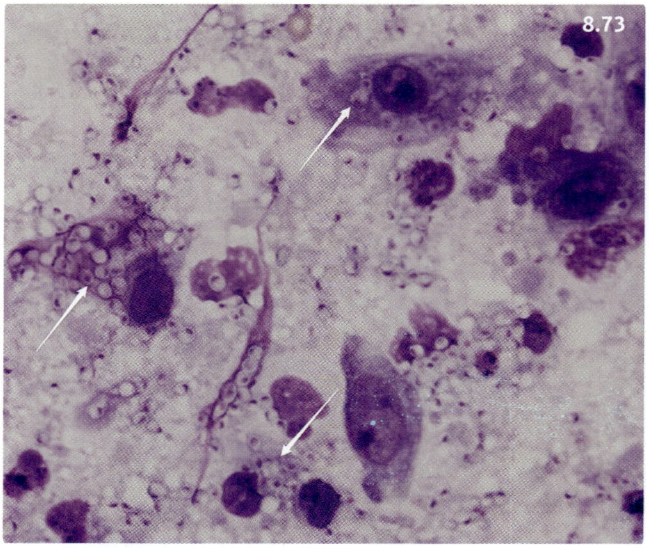

Figure 8.73 Photomicrograph of a fine needle aspirate of a mesenteric lymph node from a dog with intestinal histoplasmosis. The arrows point to macrophages filled with yeast forms of *H. capsulatum*. Wright–Giemsa stain. (Courtesy S. Gaunt)

Prognosis

Guarded to poor in dogs; fair to good in cats.

Pythiosis

Etiology

Pythium insidiosum is a eukaryotic microorganism from the class Oomycota found in subtropical climates (such as the Southeast and Gulf of Mexico regions of the USA) and sporadically in other areas. It causes severe, progressive GI disease. It affects particularly large breed male dogs, probably because of their increased risk of environmental exposure.

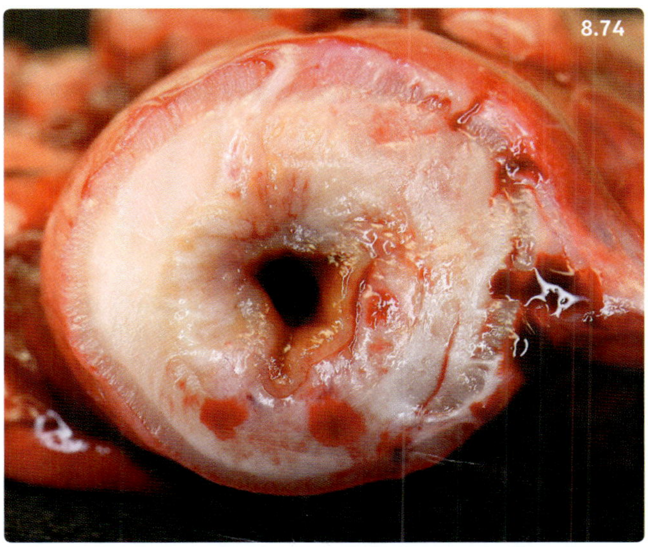

Figure 8.74 Cross-section of a resected jejunal segment from a 2-year-old mixed-breed dog with intestinal pythiosis. The wall is severely thickened and the normal structure is not recognizable. The severe narrowing of the jejunal lumen caused partial intestinal obstruction. (Courtesy A. Grooters)

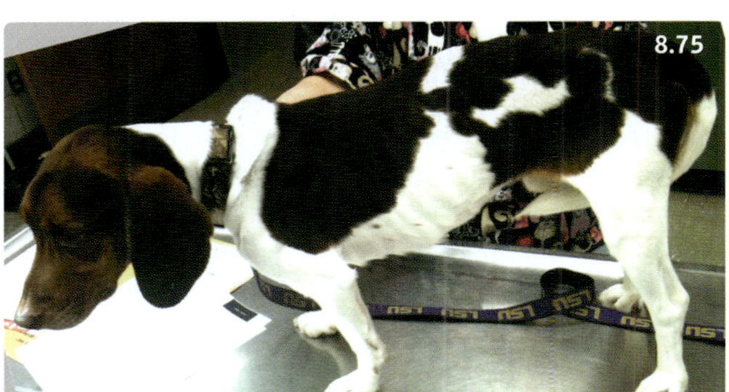

Figure 8.75 Three-year-old male Beagle with a progressive history of chronic-intermittent vomiting. The dog has lost weight and is cachectic. Intestinal pythiosis was diagnosed.

Pathophysiology

Motile *Pythium* zoospores are attracted to and invade damaged GI mucosa. The disease is characterized by transmural inflammation that may affect one or more of the following sites: stomach, small intestine, gastric antrum, colon, and rectum (rarely the esophagus, see above) (**Figure 8.74**). Local lymph nodes are often reactively enlarged.

Clinical presentation

Young, large breed dogs with access to the outdoors are most commonly affected. History commonly indicates a progressive illness. Vomiting, diarrhea, and weight loss (**Figure 8.75**) are also commonly observed, with possible dysorexia. In advanced cases, clinical features are suggestive of obstruction of the proximal GI tract, with vomiting and a palpable intestinal mass. Poor body condition is frequently present. Interestingly, lethargy and other signs of systemic illness are observed only in advanced cases as a consequence of complete GI obstruction or GI perforation.

Differential diagnosis

Intestinal FB, histoplasmosis, parasitic enteritis, IBD, small intestinal neoplasia.

Diagnosis

Peripheral eosinophilia, anemia, hypoalbuminemia, and hyperglobulinemia may be present. Abdominal imaging: radiographs may reveal an abdominal mass with or without obstructive pattern (**Figure 8.76**); ultrasound helps locate the affected segment, which is characterized by transmural thickening with disappearance of the normal small intestinal wall structure (**Figure 8.77**) and lymph node enlargement (**Figure 8.78**). Ultrasound-guided fine needle aspirates can be performed. An ELISA test for detection of serum antibodies is available (locations can be found on the web). Histopathologic diagnosis is granulomatous enteritis affecting mostly the submucosa and muscularis layers (**Figure 8.79**). Oomycetal organisms may be detected with special stains (**Figure 8.80**) or with immunohistochemistry. Fresh infected tissue may also be cultured to confirm the diagnosis.

Management

Aggressive surgical resection of the lesion with 5 cm clean tissue margins on both sides is the preferred treatment for GI pythiosis. Enlarged abdominal lymph nodes

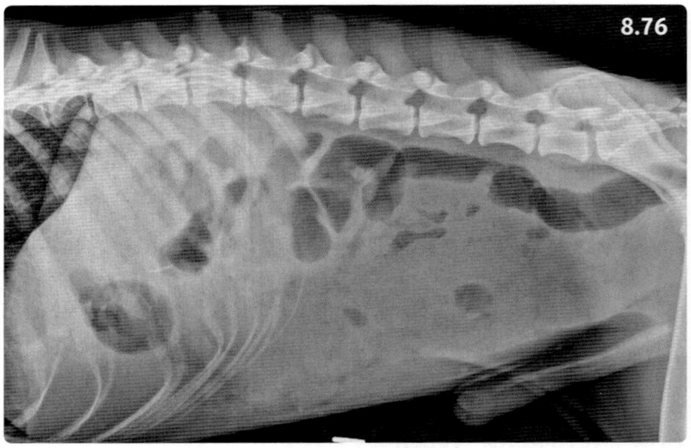

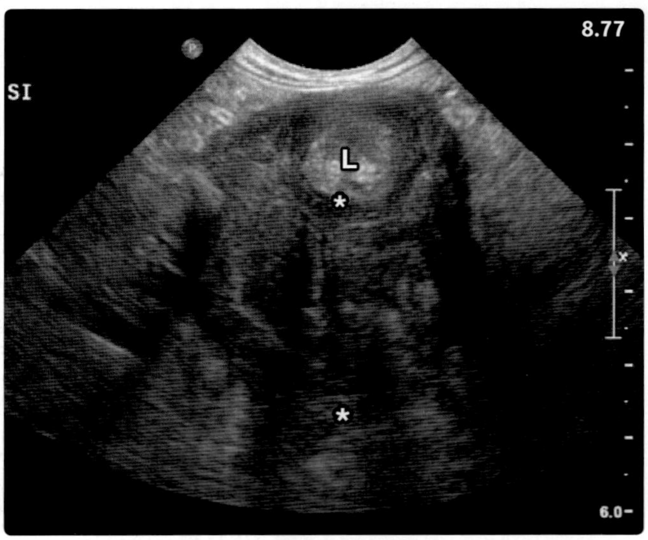

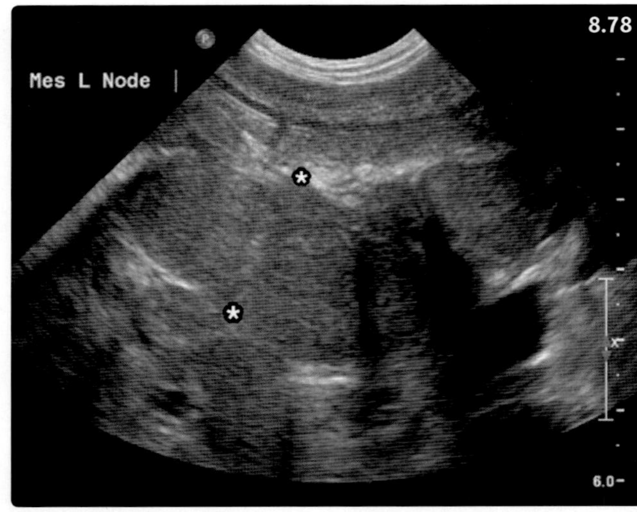

Figure 8.76–8.78 Two-year-old male Catahoula Cur with intestinal pythiosis. (8.76) Left lateral abdominal radiograph. There is an ill-defined central abdominal soft tissue mass that displaces the intestines dorsally and ventrally. (8. 77) Abdominal ultrasound. The cross-section of this small intestinal segment reveals a markedly thickened wall (~3 cm) with abnormal layering (between asterisks). L, intestinal lumen. (8.78) Abdominal ultrasound. Note the very enlarged mesenteric lymph node (between asterisks). The measured size was 2.2 × 6.4 cm. (Courtesy LSU SVM Diagnostic Imaging Service)

should be biopsied, but their resection is not absolutely essential since they are rarely infected. Except in cases where total resection with 5 cm clean margins could be performed (usually mid-jejunal masses), medical treatment with a combination of itraconazole (10 mg/kg PO q24h) and terbinafine (5–10 mg/kg PO q24h) is recommended. Prednisone (1 mg/kg PO q24h) can also be used to decrease local inflammation and to palliate clinical signs in the short term. ELISA serology should be performed at the time of diagnosis and 3 months postoperatively, and medical treatment can be discontinued if the titer decreases by >50%.

Prognosis

Poor, except if complete surgical resection of the GI lesion is possible. Recurrence is common unless full resection with clean margins could be achieved. The disease is fatal if untreated.

CHRONIC CANINE ENTEROPATHIES

Definition/overview

The general term 'chronic enteropathy' (CE) has been used frequently in recent years to describe dogs and cats with chronic intestinal diseases of unknown origin. Diet-responsive diarrhea (DRD), antibiotic-responsive diarrhea (ARD), and IBD are different forms of chronic enteropathy. They may form a continuum, with DRD being the mild form of CE and IBD requiring immunosuppressive treatment representing the severe form of the disease.

Etiology

Based on research in rodent models, people, and dogs, IBD results from a combination of factors that include dysregulation of the immune system and its interactions with

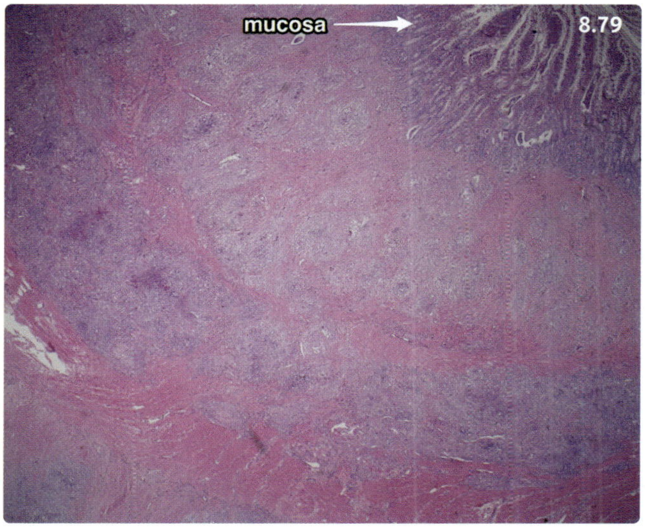

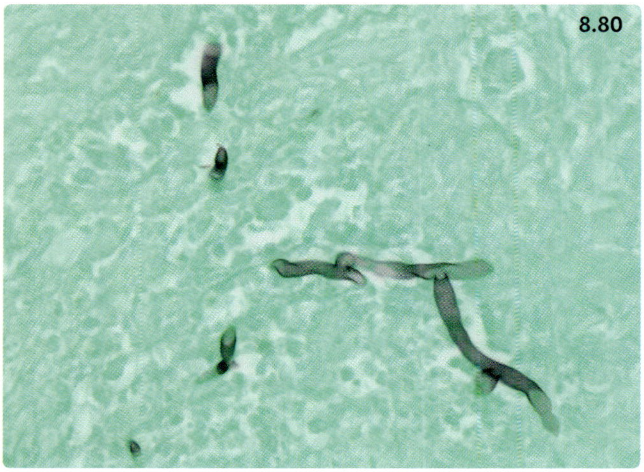

Figure 8.79, 8.80 Dog with pythiosis affecting the jejunum. (8.79) Low-magnification photomicrograph of the intestinal wall. The mucosa is visible at the top right of the image (arrow); the deeper structures (submucosa, muscularis) are obliterated by granulomatous and eosinophilic inflammation. H&E stain. (8.80) High-magnification photomicrograph of an intestinal lesion. Infectious organisms with morphology suggestive of *P. insidiosum* are nonspecifically stained. Grocott's methenamine silver stain. (Courtesy LSU SVM Pathology Service)

intestinal microbiota and/or dietary components, and compromised integrity of the intestinal mucosal barrier.

Specific forms of IBD have been recognized as occurring more frequently in several canine breeds. For instance, in the Southeast UK, Weimaraners, Rottweilers, German Shepherd Dogs, Border Collies, and Boxers were at increased risk of developing IBD. Examples of established breed associations include lymphangiectasia and duodenal crypt inflammation with PLE in Yorkshire Terriers, PLE and protein-losing nephropathy in Soft-Coated Wheaten Terriers, and cobalamin deficiency in Shar Peis. German Shepherd Dogs have a high prevalence of intestinal dysbiosis/ARD and IBD.

Pathophysiology

Recognition of commensal intestinal microbiota by the innate immune system is altered. Toll-like receptors (TLRs) are pattern-recognition receptors located on immune and epithelial cells that are essential for appropriate recognition of intestinal microbiota. Polymorphisms in various TLRs have been identified in the intestinal mucosa of dogs with CE, which may trigger an inflammatory response. In addition, significant changes in the intestinal microbiota were detected using molecular biological approaches that do not rely on microbial culture. In dogs and people, IBD reduces the diversity of the intestinal microbiome. Furthermore, in dogs with IBD, the bacterial taxa Firmicutes (including the Clostridiales), Bacteroidetes, and Fusobacteria are diminished, and Proteobacteria (including Enterobacteriacae) are increased. It is not clear whether these changes are the origin of the intestinal inflammation or if they reflect the altered environment in the chronically inflamed gut, or both.

Clinical presentation

Chronic or chronic-intermittent diarrhea of more than 3 weeks' duration. Mild CE may cause intermittent clinical signs, whereas progressive and severe clinical signs are common in severe IBD. Poor body condition with poor hair coat is frequent with severe disease. Dehydration is possible. Thickened small intestinal loops may occasionally be palpated. Animals may show pain or discomfort on abdominal palpation. Ascites, hydrothorax, and peripheral edema may occur in cases of significant protein loss (see Protein-losing enteropathy). Clinical activity scoring systems have been validated for use in the dog: CIBDAI (Canine Inflammatory Bowel Disease Activity Index) and CCECAI (Canine Chronic enteropathy Clinical Activity Index) (**Table 8.11**). Clinical activity scoring is useful for documenting the severity of clinical signs at presentation and for accurate evaluation of clinical response to treatment.

Differential diagnosis

General differentials include chronic intestinal FB, intestinal parasitoses, bacterial enteritis, fungal enteritis, and diseases originating outside the GI tract such as chronic kidney disease, chronic liver disease, chronic pancreatitis, exocrine pancreatic insufficiency, and atypical hypoadrenocorticism.

Table 8.11 Clinical activity indices used in dogs with chronic enteropathies.

CIBDAI[1]	CCECAI[2]
A: Attitude/activity 0 = normal 1 = slightly decreased 2 = moderate decreased 3 = severely decreased **B: Appetite** 0 = normal 1 = slightly decreased 2 = moderately decreased 3 = severely decreased **C: Vomiting** 0 = no vomiting 1 = mild (1 episode/week) 2 = moderate (2–3 episodes /week) 3 = severe (>3 episodes/week) **D: Stool consistency** 0 = normal 1 = slightly soft feces 2 = very soft feces 3 = watery diarrhea **E: Stool frequency** 0 = normal 1 = slightly increased (2–3 times daily) or fecal blood, mucus or both 2 = moderately increased (4–5 times daily) 3 = severely increased (>5 times daily) **F: Weight loss** 0 = none 1 = mild (<5% body weight) 2 = moderate (5–10% body weight) 3 = severe (>10% body weight) **Evaluation of scores:** CIBDAI 0–3: no clinical significance CIBDAI 4–5: mild IBD CIBDAI 6–8: moderate IBD CIBDAI 9 and above: severe IBD	**A + B + C + D + E + F +** **G: Serum albumin concentration** 0 = >20 g/l 1 = 15–19.9 g/l 2 = 12–14.9 g/l 3 = <12 g/l **H: Ascites and peripheral edema** 0 = none 1 = mild ascites or peripheral edema 2 =moderate amount of ascites or peripheral edema 3 = severe ascites/pleural effusion and peripheral edema **I: Pruritus** 0 = no pruritus 1 = occasional episodes of itching 2 = regular episodes of itching that stop when the dog is asleep 3 = dog regularly wakes up because of itching **Evaluation of scores:** CCECAI 0–3: no clinical significance CCECAI 4–5: mild enteropathy CCECAI 6–8: moderate enteropathy CCECAI 9–11: severe enteropathy CCECAI 12 and above: very severe enteropathy

1 Jergens AE, Schreiner CA, Frank DE *et al.* (2003) A scoring index for disease activity in canine inflammatory bowel disease. *J Vet Intern Med* **17**:291–297.
2 Allenspach K, Wieland B, Gröne A *et al.* (2007) Chronic enteropathies in dogs: evaluation of risk factors for negative outcome. *J Vet Int Med* **21**:700–708.

Diagnosis

Diagnosis of CE consists of an elimination process to rule out other diseases of known etiology that may cause similar clinical signs: fecal flotation and a *Giardia* antigen test should be performed in all dogs. Alternatively, empiric parasiticide treatment can be administered (e.g. fenbendazole, 50 mg/kg q24h for 3–5 days). Subsequently, the diagnostic process is different for dogs with mild clinical signs and no evidence of complications such as hypoproteinemia, and for dogs that are more severely affected.

Mildly affected dogs can undergo a treatment trial with a novel protein or hydrolyzed peptide diet without further diagnostics (see Management, below), while severely affected dogs should be evaluated more thoroughly with collection of a minimal database including

CBC, serum biochemistry, and urinalysis. Presence of hypoalbuminemia, often accompanied by hypoglobulinemia, suggests PLE, particularly if other causes can be ruled out. Sensitivity of abdominal ultrasound is intermediate, and scans may be normal or show focal or diffuse loss of wall layering, presence of mucosal striations or spicules, wall thickening, and enlarged and/or hypoechoic mesenteric lymph nodes. If lesions are present, localization to a specific intestinal segment may be helpful (**Figures 8.81, 8.82**).

Upper GI endoscopy and exploratory celiotomy are both good procedures for collecting intestinal mucosal biopsy samples, and each offers different advantages and drawbacks (**Table 8.12**). Observation of severe mucosal lesions during duodenoscopy is a negative prognostic factor.

Procurement of biopsy samples is necessary to further evaluate disease severity. Biopsy specimens of adequate quality and quantity are required for accurate interpretation by pathologists. The most important justification for histology is to rule out a neoplastic infiltrate. However, it is also useful to evaluate the magnitude of intestinal mucosal inflammation based on the severity and type of the infiltrate and the severity of the architectural mucosal changes. A newly established scoring system takes both architectural and inflammatory mucosal changes into account. Inflammatory infiltration may be of varying severity and consist of lymphocytes and plasma cells (lymphoplasmacytic enteritis), eosinophils, neutrophils or macrophages, or combinations thereof (**Box 8.9**). Examples of small intestinal mucosal architectural changes include villus stunting (**Figure 8.83**), surface epithelial injury, crypt distension (**Figure 8.84**), lacteal dilation (**Figure 8.85**), and mucosal fibrosis. It is noteworthy that in animals responding to treatment, histopathologic lesions do not seem to improve in correlation with clinical signs. This finding may suggest that CE can be controlled clinically, but not healed.

Management

In most instances, the goal of treatment is to manage the clinical signs. Full recovery is possible in mild cases.

The standard approach for a dog with mild to moderate chronic recurrent diarrhea of unknown origin without systemic repercussions is to initiate a food trial with a novel protein or hydrolyzed peptide diet. Many dogs respond at least partially within 10–14 days (**Figure 8.86**). For those who do not, the next step may consist of another treatment trial with another novel protein or hydrolyzed peptide diet and/or antimicrobials.

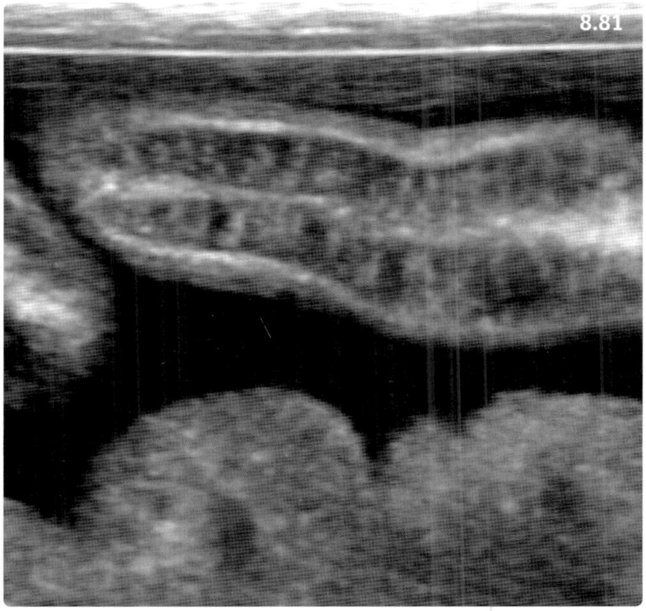

Figure 8.81 Abdominal ultrasound of a dog with inflammatory bowel disease, crypt disease, and protein-losing enteropathy. The normal layers of the intestinal wall are not recognizable in this oblique section of a small intestinal loop. Hyperechogenic striations are present and run from the lumen to the serosa. There is free abdominal fluid. (Courtesy LSU SVM Diagnostic Imaging Service)

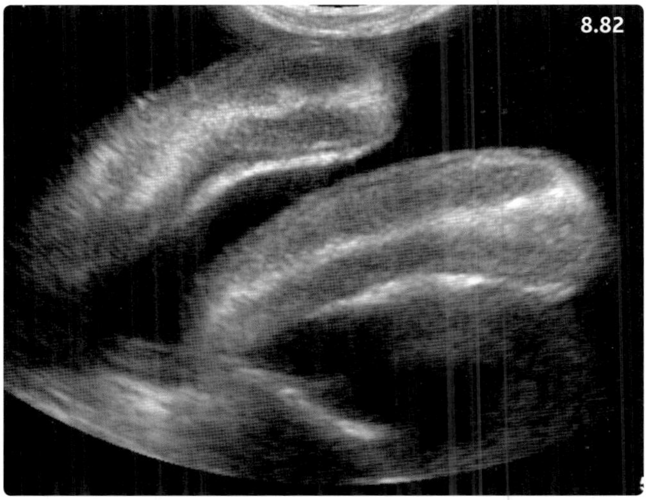

Figure 8.82 Abdominal ultrasound of another dog with severe inflammatory bowel disease and protein-losing enteropathy. The normal layers of the intestinal wall are obliterated by an irregular hyperechogenic pattern. There is free abdominal fluid. (Courtesy LSU SVM Diagnostic Imaging Service)

While dysbiosis (change in the composition of the intestinal microbiota) occurs in most dogs with IBD, a subset of young large breed dogs with CE (particularly

Table 8.12 Advantages and drawbacks of endoscopy and surgery for collecting intestinal mucosal biopsies.

	Endoscopy	Celiotomy
Availabilty of equipment	Limited	Universal
General anesthesia required	Yes	Yes
Rapidity	Depends on endoscopist's experience	Depends on surgeon's experience
Access to gastrointestinal tract	Stomach, duodenum, sometimes proximal jejunum, ileum, colon	Whole GI tract. Full-thickness biopsies of the colon are a more risky procedure
Access to other abdominal organs	No	Yes
Evaluation of intestinal mucosa	Yes	No
Quantity of biopsies	++ to +++	+
Quality of biopsies	+ to +++	+++
Associated risks of complication	Very rare	Minimal, but present, particularly in case of severe panhypoproteinemia
Postinterventional recovery	Rapid	Longer

Box 8.9 Further considerations with different types of intestinal infiltrates.

Lymphoplasmacytic enteritis: most common type of inflammatory infiltrate, nonspecific. A mild to moderate lymphoplasmacytic mucosal infiltrate may be present in the absence of clinical signs.
Eosinophilic enteritis: rule out parasitic enteritis or allergic causes, and in cats eosinophilic syndrome. Idiopathic eosinophilic enteritis may occur in dogs and cats. While it usually responds well to steroids in dogs, this disorder is often steroid resistant in cats.
Neutrophilic (or suppurative) enteritis: bacterial infectious component cannot be ruled out, and treatment with broad-spectrum antibiotic should be considered alone or in association with immunosuppressive drugs.
Granulomatous enteritis: rule out fungal enteritis. Idiopathic transmural granulomatous enteritis usually carries a poor prognosis.

but not exclusively German Shepherd Dogs) respond to prolonged treatment with antimicrobials such as tylosin (20 mg/kg PO q12h) or metronidazole (10–15 mg/kg PO q12h). This may result from an inability of these dogs' immune systems to interact adequately with their intestinal microbiota. Clinical experience accumulated over the past decades indicates that prolonged treatment (4–8 weeks) is necessary, and that relapses are not uncommon.

8.83

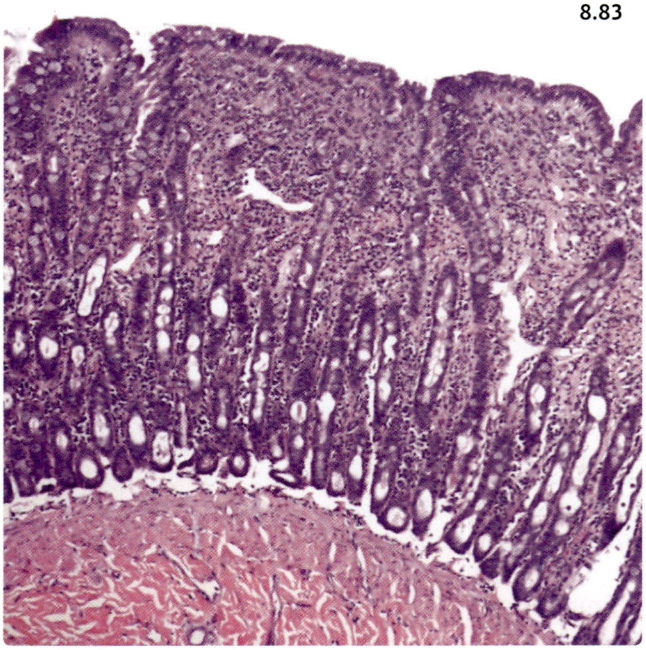

Figure 8.83 Photomicrograph of the duodenal mucosa of a 10-year-old female spayed Domestic Shorthair cat with chronic inflammatory bowel disease. There is marked blunting and fusion of the intestinal villi (compared with Figure 8.52), and a moderate lymphoplasmacytic infiltrate. H&E stain.

In refractory cases, and in dogs with severe disease and evidence of systemic involvement, a more thorough work up with acquisition of a minimal database should be initiated (see Diagnosis, above).

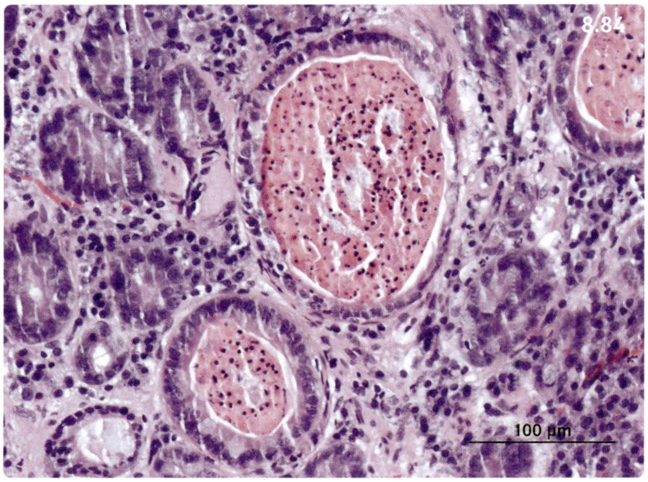

Figure 8.84 Photomicrograph of the duodenal mucosa of a dog with protein-losing enteropathy. Two intestinal crypts are markedly distended and filled with necrotic material. The diagnosis was moderate lymphocytic plasmacytic duodenitis with severe crypt lesions. H&E stain.

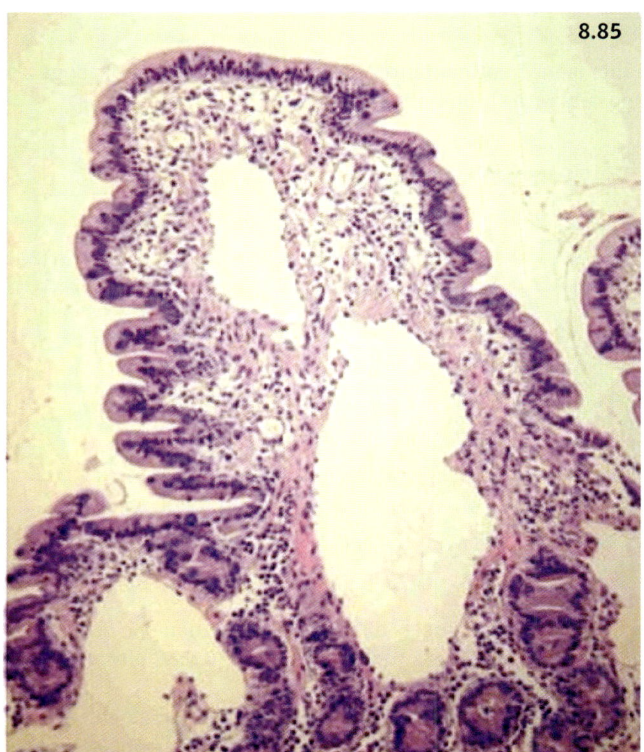

Figure 8.85 Photomicrograph of the duodenal mucosa of a Yorkshire Terrier with protein-losing enteropathy. The villus is markedly distended and dilated lacteals partially filled with eosinophilic material are visible. The diagnosis was moderate idiopathic lymphangiectasia. H&E stain.

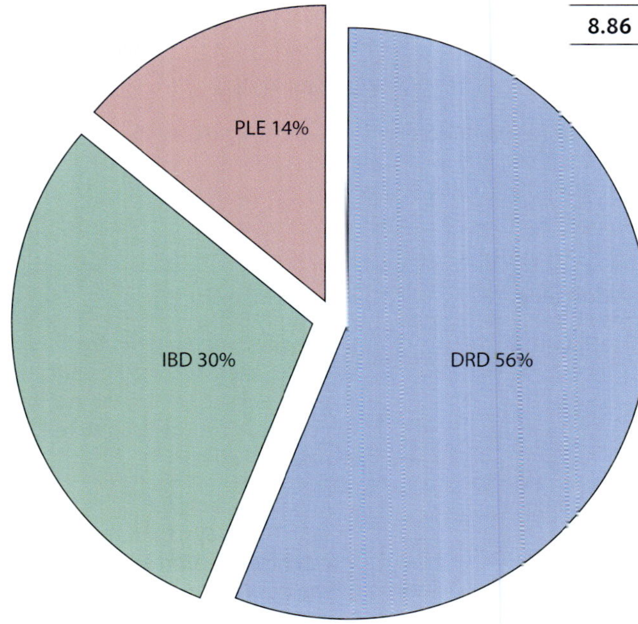

Figure 8.86 Pie chart summarizing the data from a study that included 70 dogs with chronic enteropathy referred to the University of Bern Veterinary Teaching Hospital. 56% of dogs responded within 10 days to a novel protein diet (DRD, diet-responsive diarrhea), while 30% required steroid treatment, and 14% had severe protein-losing enteropathy. (Source: Allenspach K, Wieland B, Gröne A *et al.* (2007) Chronic enteropathies in dogs: evaluation of risk factors for negative outcome. *J Vet Intern Med* **21**:700–708.)

In dogs with histopathologic evidence of IBD, immunosuppressive doses of prednisone or prednisolone (**Table 8.13**) are generally the mainstay of initial treatment. Initially, very high doses (e.g. 2 mg/kg q12h) are recommended for a few days, followed by a regular immunosuppressive dose (2 mg/kg/day, in 1 dose or divided into 2 doses). Dietary treatment consists of hydrolyzed peptide or novel protein diet, which has been shown to be superior to easily digestible low-fat diet for long-term maintenance of remission in moderate to severe canine IBD. A recheck is scheduled after 1–2 weeks to reassess the situation. In cases showing good response, the dose of prednisone should be maintained for another 2 weeks, then slowly decreased in 2–4-week steps.

Treatment failure should prompt the clinician to review the diagnosis and ascertain that no mistakes or erroneous assumptions were made in the diagnostic process. Refractory IBD patients must be examined thoroughly to detect intercurrent diseases that may be contributing to treatment failure. For instance, a significant proportion of dogs with IBD (particularly those with PLE) may develop hypocobalaminemia because of severe involvement of the distal small intestine. Cobalamin

Table 8.13 Dosage of oral immunosuppressive drugs used in the treatment of inflammatory bowel disease in small animals.

Drug	Canine dose	Feline dose	Side-effects
Prednisone, prednisolone	1–2 mg/kg q12–24h	Prednisolone preferred. Same dose as canine	In dogs they include polyuria/polydipsia, panting, alopecia, pot-bellied appearance, calcinosis cutis. Rare in cats, may cause diabetes mellitus
Budesonide	3 mg/m^2 q24h	1 mg/cat q24h	Same as above
Azathioprine	Initially 2 mg/kg q24h for 3 weeks, then 1–2 mg/kg q48h. Up to 3 weeks of treatment may be necessary for the drug to reach maximal effect	Do not use in cats	Hepatotoxicity, pancreatitis, rarely bone marrow suppression
Chlorambucil	Initially 4–6 mg/m^2 q24h for the first 7–21 days, then the dose can be decreased by 25–33%, or the dosage interval increased to every 2–3 days	2 mg/cat 3 times weekly	Rarely bone marrow suppression
Cyclosporine	5 mg/kg q12–24h	Same as canine	Vomiting, nausea, gingival hyperplasia

deficiency may cause a delayed response or lack of response to adequately designed immunosuppressive treatment. Serum cobalamin concentration should be determined. Subcutaneous supplementation is essential in these animals (**Table 8.14**). Relatively frequently, dogs with moderate to severe IBD require treatment with a combination of immunosuppressive agents (**Table 8.13**). In cases with unacceptable corticosteroid side-effects, another immunosuppressive drug may be added in the hope of decreasing the prednisone dose. Alternatively, budesonide can be used. Budesonide is a glucocorticoid that undergoes high first-pass hepatic metabolism after intestinal absorption, but still affects the pituitary–adrenal axis. Budesonide may cause fewer side-effects than prednisone; it has been used in large breed dogs, which tend to be more prone to severe polyuria and polydipsia. There is no documented benefit in using the controlled release formulation compared with the generic substance.

Prognosis

Good in mild cases that respond to dietary trials. Return to a less expensive commercial food may be possible after 2–3 months of dietary treatment; however, some dogs require life-long administration of an elimination diet. Guarded to poor in dogs requiring medical treatment.

Table 8.14 Treatment protocol for hypocobalaminemic dogs and cats with chronic enteropathy.

Dose per SC injection		
Cats:	Any weight	250 µg
Dogs:	<4.5 kg	250 µg
	4.5–9 kg	400 µg
	9–18 kg	600 µg
	18–27 kg	800 µg
	27–36 kg	1,000 µg
	36–45 kg	1,200 µg
	>45 kg	1,500 µg

Schedule:
Administer once weekly dose for 6 weeks, then one dose 30 days later. Recheck serum cobalamin 30 days after the last injection. If it is:

- Above the reference range, and the underlying process has been successfully managed, discontinue cobalamin injections.
- Within the reference range, continue monthly treatment.
- Below the reference range: reassess the patient.

Source: Texas A&M University GI Laboratory website (http://vetmed.tamu.edu/gilab), with permission.

PROTEIN-LOSING ENTEROPATHY

Definition/overview

Intestinal protein loss is a sign of failure of digestive function that may result from severe acute or chronic inflammatory lesions or from a disruption of chyle absorption and intestinal lymph flow.

Etiology/pathophysiology

Primary intestinal lymphangiectasia occurs preferentially in Yorkshire Terriers, Shar Peis, Maltese, Norwegian Lundehunds, and Rottweilers. The pathogenesis of primary intestinal lymphangiectasia is still poorly understood. It results from obstruction to the flow of lymph in the intestinal wall. Secondary intestinal lymphangiectasia is commonly associated with significant intestinal mucosal inflammation (e.g. IBD) and neoplasia (alimentary lymphoma).

IBD may also directly cause PLE. The inflammatory process located in the GI mucosa may lead to protein loss both by preventing absorption of nutrients and by compromising the integrity of the intestinal mucosal barrier, leading to exudation of proteins into the intestinal lumen. PLE of Soft-Coated Wheaten Terriers is a specific form of IBD affecting this breed worldwide. In approximately 50% of these dogs, PLE and protein-losing nephropathy (PLN) occur concurrently, and the pathogenesis includes a hypersensitivity component.

Crypt dilation and necrosis have been frequently associated with PLE. Dogs with small intestinal crypt abscesses have significant hypoalbuminemia and ultrasound changes of their intestinal mucosa, and their clinical presentation is generally severe.

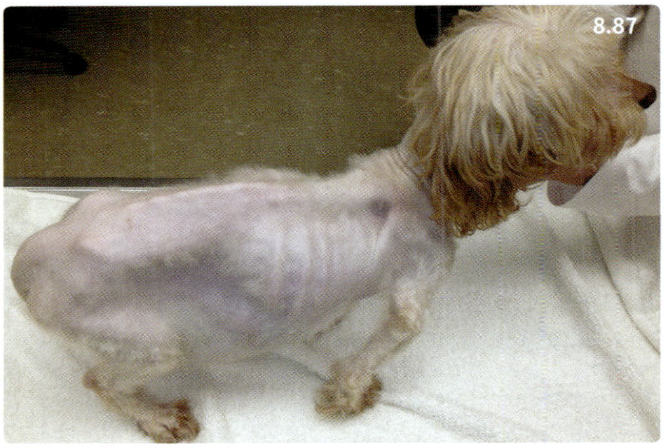

Figure 8.87 Four-year-old male neutered Maltipoo with severe chronic inflammatory bowel disease and protein-losing enteropathy. The dog is cachectic and a pot-bellied abdomen is visible (ascites).

Clinical presentation

Chronic intermittent small intestinal diarrhea with possible vomiting is a common presentation. In severe cases, dysorexia/anorexia and malnutrition with evidence of malabsorption and weight loss may be observed (**Figure 8.87**). Importantly, significant intestinal protein loss and hypoalbuminemia may also occur without obvious diarrheic episodes. In the presence of severe hypoalbuminemia (serum albumin <2.0 g/dl, often ≤1.5 g/dl), the main complaint may relate to significantly decreased oncotic pressure causing cavitary effusion (**Figure 8.88**) and subcutaneous edema (**Figure 8.89**).

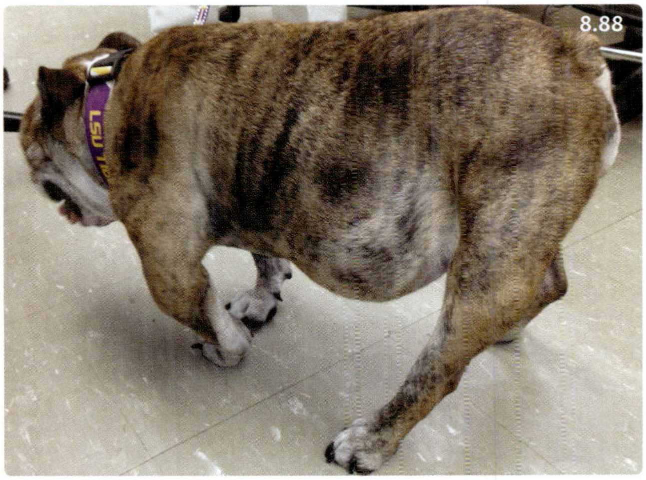

Figure 8.88 Ten-year-old female spayed English Bulldog with chronic inflammatory bowel disease and protein-losing enteropathy. The abdomen is severely distended due to ascites. The dog also had pleural effusion.

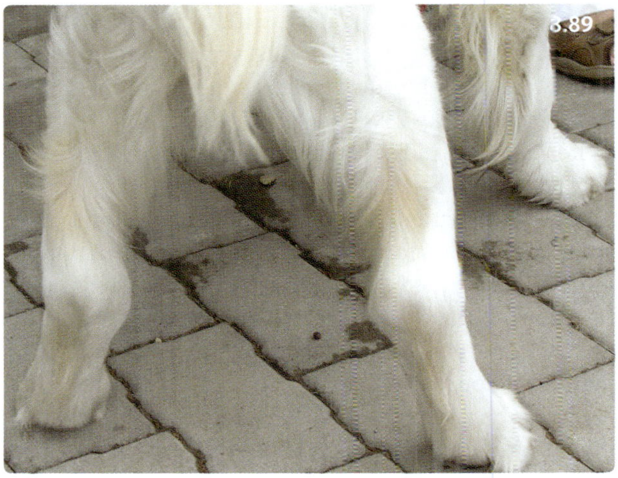

Figure 8.89 One-year-old male Montagne des Pyrenées with inflammatory bowel disease and protein-losing enteropathy. There is subcutaneous edema around both hocks. (Courtesy R. Husnik)

Differential diagnosis

Hypoalbuminemia and associated signs may also occur with liver failure, PLN, third spacing of proteins (vasculitis), or cutaneous loss.

Diagnosis

First, the origin of the protein loss should be established by ruling out other processes. Generally, PLE is associated with panhypoproteinemia due to nonselective protein loss, but exceptions may occur. Other common abnormalities of dogs with PLE include hypocholesterolemia, hypocalcemia (total and ionized), hypomagnesemia, and lymphopenia.

Once the GI tract has been confirmed as the site of protein loss, further work up should include abdominal ultrasound, a technique with acceptable sensitivity that often helps assess the severity and anatomic distribution of intestinal lesions. Hyperechogenic mucosal striations are frequently observed in dogs with PLE, and appear to be quite specific (see **Figure 8.81**).

Endoscopy may reveal a broad range of changes of varying severity (**Figures 8.90, 8.91**). The diagnosis of the cause of PLE requires histopathologic analysis of intestinal biopsies (see **Figures 8.84, 8.85**). In some instances, dogs with severe hypoalbuminemia are poor anesthetic candidates, and it is sometimes preferable to avoid taking excessive risks and postpone endoscopy or surgery. Additionally, many dogs with PLE have bicavitary effusion, and thoracic radiographs are recommended as a screening tool for the presence of thoracic effusion, which may represent an additional anesthetic risk.

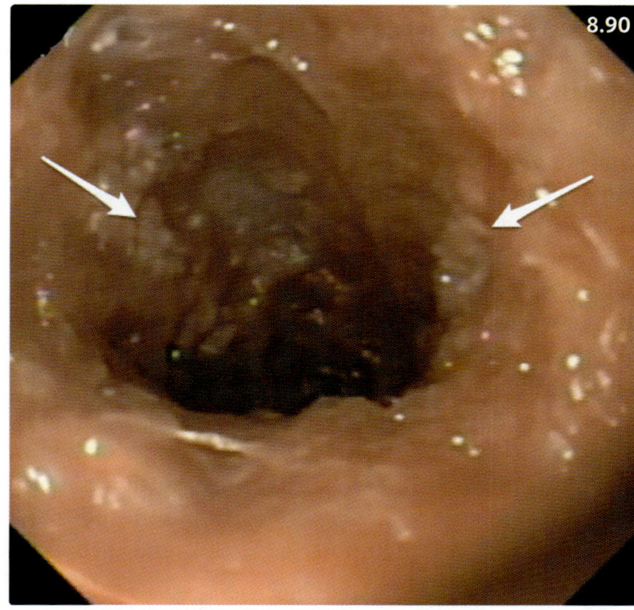

Figure 8.90 Endoscopic picture from the duodenum of the same dog as in Figure 8.81. The surface of the intestinal mucosa is very irregular and abnormal, and patches of recognizable villi are visible (arrows).

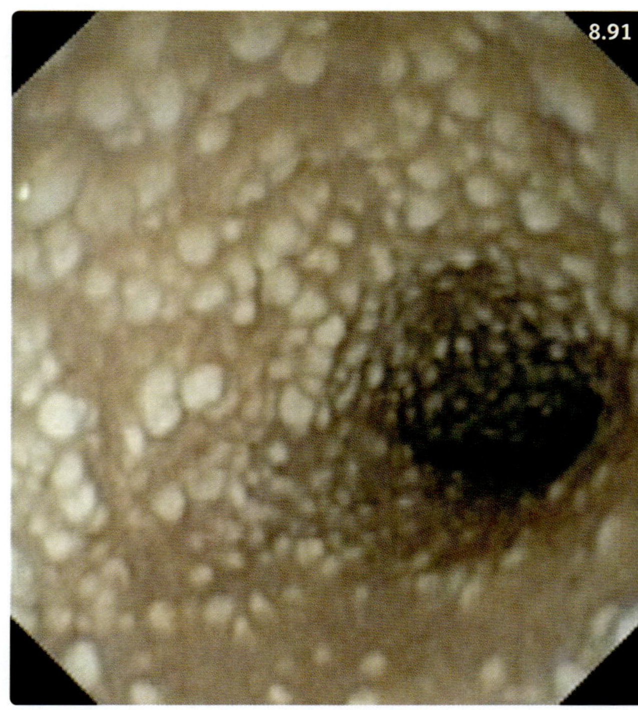

Figure 8.91 Endoscopic view of the duodenum of a 5-year-old Yorkshire Terrier. There are numerous multifocal white spots in the mucosa that represent dilated villi filled with chyme. The histopathologic diagnosis was idiopathic lymphangiectasia.

Management

Dogs with PLE are in a catabolic state, and adequate nutrition is essential. In dogs with primary idiopathic intestinal lymphangiectasia, dietary modification centers on feeding a highly digestible diet with low to very low fat content (10–15% on a dry matter basis) to prevent further dilation and rupture of lacteals. Additionally, the diet should contain highly bioavailable dietary proteins and be low in crude fiber. Dietary therapy should probably be maintained for the length of the dog's life. In dogs with PLE associated with underlying IBD, good success has been reported with exclusive feeding of a diet consisting of hydrolyzed proteins. Novel protein diets are an alternative approach.

In dogs with primary intestinal lymphangiectasia, anti-inflammatory glucocorticoid therapy (e.g. prednisone, 1 mg/kg/day) is useful and often required for proper management of the disease. The main desired effect is to decrease the inflammation associated with lipogranulomas secondary to chyle leakage and therefore help restore an adequate flow in the intestinal lymphatics. In some dogs, anti-inflammatory treatment can be slowly weaned off over 2–3 months or longer.

Immunosuppression is the basis for treatment of severe IBD with PLE (**Table 8.13**).

Complications

Low serum cobalamin concentrations are commonly found in dogs with PLE, especially in the presence of underlying IBD, and may delay proper healing of intestinal inflammation. Treatment consists of weekly SC injections of vitamin B12 (**Table 8.14**).

Recent studies have revealed the high prevalence of hypercoagulability in dogs with PLE, which increases the risk of potentially fatal thromboembolic events. Hypercoagulability does not appear to resolve after successful treatment of PLE. Administration of low doses of aspirin (0.5–1 mg/kg/day) and/or clopidogrel (1–5 mg/kg/day) may be considered in order to prevent thrombosis.

The decrease in serum total calcium is associated with severe hypoalbuminemia. Additionally, low serum ionized calcium concentration occur in association with low 25-hydroxyvitamin D and increased levels of parathyroid hormone in dogs with PLE. In dogs with a moderate to severe decrease in ionized calcium, treatment with calcium and vitamin D is recommended. Concurrent hypomagnesemia may compromise the success of treatment and should be corrected if present.

Prognosis

Generally, hypoalbuminemia (serum albumin <2 g/dl) is associated with a less favorable outcome. A few studies show a high mortality among Yorkshire Terriers with intestinal lymphangiectasia (50–60%). In the author's practice, some Yorkshire Terriers with idiopathic intestinal lymphangiectasia respond well to a strict diet alone or with anti-inflammatory doses of glucocorticoids. There are no known parameters that allow early segregation of dogs likely to be refractory to dietary and steroid treatment. Crypt abscesses in the small intestine are associated with significantly shorter survival.

CHRONIC FELINE ENTEROPATHY

Definiton/overview

While the etiology and pathophysiology are thought to be similar to canine CE, the presentation and approach of cats with CE is partially different.

Clinical presentation

The most commonly observed clinical signs are vomiting, anorexia, diarrhea, and weight loss (**Figure 8.92**). However, some cats may have a normal to increased appetite, and many cats, unlike dogs, will not have diarrhea at

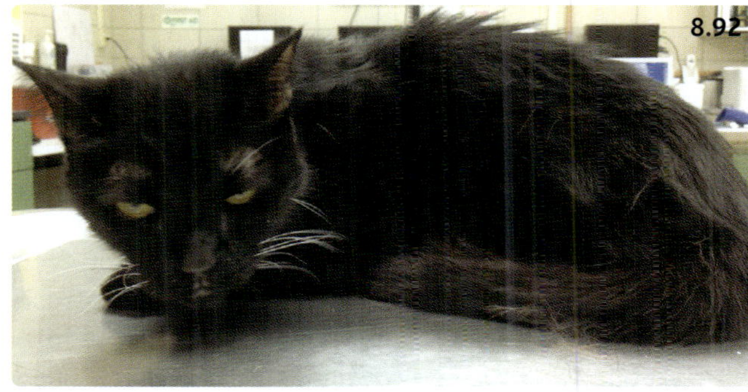

Figure 8.92 Fourteen-year-old male neutered Domestic Longhair cat with chronic diarrhea and occasional vomiting. The cat is lethargic, cachectic, and his hair coat is in poor condition. Inflammatory bowel disease and alimentary lymphoma are among the top differentials.

presentation. Other cats will be presented for dysorexia/anorexia and weight loss. The signs are often waxing and waning, and the owners may seek veterinary attention only late in the course of disease. Abnormal findings on physical examination of cats with CE include loss of body condition, dehydration, palpation of thickened bowel loops, and/or abdominal pain.

Differential diagnosis

Includes diseases originating outside the digestive tract such as hyperthyroidism, diabetes mellitus, chronic kidney disease, and heartworm disease, but also liver disease and pancreatitis. Alimentary lymphoma, particularly diffusely infiltrative low-grade alimentary lymphoma, may be very difficult to differentiate from IBD.

Diagnosis

The clinical signs may be very nonspecific, and the first step is to rule out diseases that may present with a similar clinical picture. A minimal database of CBC, chemistry profile, serum thyroxin concentration, and abdominal imaging (particularly ultrasound) is recommended. Confirmation of diagnosis requires histologic evaluation of intestinal biopsies collected using endoscopy or celiotomy (**Table 8.12**, **Figure 8.83**).

Management

As is the case in dogs, a high proportion of cats with CE may respond to an appropriate diet change (e.g. novel protein or hydrolyzed peptides). Other cats may respond to antimicrobials: metronidazole (10–15 mg/kg PO q12h) is popular, although its therapeutic margin in cats is narrow. Tylosin (20–40 mg/kg PO q12h) is a good alternative. Both drugs also have immunomodulating effects.

Immunosuppressive therapy is the mainstay of IBD treatment. It is best initiated when histologic evidence of intestinal mucosal infiltration is available, but could also be the final option of the empirical treatment sequence started with dietary trial and antimicrobials. Prednisolone (2–4 mg/kg PO q24h or divided into 2 daily doses) is administered for 10–14 days. Once the clinical signs have been controlled for 2 weeks or longer, the dose is reduced by one-half every 10–14 days. The final goal is to maintain the cat on the lowest effective dose, or even to consider discontinuation of steroid treatment if feasible. If the owner is unable to pill the cat, methylprednisolone acetate can be given (10 mg/kg SC q2–4weeks, and tapered to q4–8weeks). Repository steroids may cause more side-effects and do not appear to be very successful in the author's experience. Refractory cases are usually treated with chlorambucil or cyclosporine (**Table 8.13**). Chlorambucil is generally used in combination with prednisolone (2 mg/cat PO every other day [in cats >4 kg body weight] or every 3 days [in cats <4 kg body weight] and then tapered to the lowest effective dose). A CBC should be checked every 2–4 weeks for signs of myelosuppression. Although there are no published reports of cyclosporine use in cats with IBD, the dose generally recommended is approximately 5 mg/kg once daily (25 mg/cat).

Prognosis

In one study, 80% of cats with IBD treated with diet change and prednisone had a positive response to treatment, although clinical signs did not completely resolve. Cats with severe histologic lesions or eosinophilic inflammation may be more difficult to manage. Failure to respond to treatment may indicate refractory IBD or lymphoma. Feline IBD is a disease that is managed but rarely cured.

PARALYTIC ILEUS

Etiology

Primary nonobstructive disorders of intestinal motility are rare. Secondary alterations in motility of the small intestine occur with many diseases. Enteritis is associated with abnormal intestinal motility patterns that resolve with successful treatment of the inflammation. Intestinal hypomotility and ileus may occur after abdominal surgery (postoperative ileus [POI]) or during ischemic or inflammatory conditions affecting abdominal organs, such as peritonitis, pancreatitis, or parvovirus infection. Hyperthyroidism in cats may also alter intestinal transit time and cause diarrhea.

Pathophysiology

POI is thought to be due to inhibition of neural pathways and release of proinflammatory mediators and corticotrophin releasing factor. They may be complicated by the use of opiates for analgesia.

Clinical presentation

Vomiting, bloated abdomen, abdominal discomfort or pain, and/or signs of colic. Hyporexia/anorexia, nausea, increased belching, pica, and/or polydipsia may also be observed.

Differential diagnosis

Differential diagnoses are numerous. Small intestinal obstruction (see above) can result in a very similar presentation, and all necessary steps must be taken to rule it out. Autonomic neuropathy (dysautonomia) is a rare disease, but should also be considered in the appropriate clinical setting.

Diagnosis

Physical signs, abdominal radiographs often show dilated small intestinal segments in the absence of an obstructive pattern (see **Figure 8.61**). Precise evaluation of small intestinal motility is difficult under clinical conditions.

Management

Proper diagnosis and treatment of any underlying disease that might affect gastric motility is an essential premise. Therapy of functional, nonobstructive disorders of gastric motility is based on dietary modification and judicious use of prokinetic drugs. Dietary management is attempted at first: small amounts of a low-fat, low-protein diet given at frequent intervals can help reduce the symptoms of delayed gastric emptying. Medical therapy can be attempted if dietary management alone is unsuccessful (**Table 8.9**).

Prognosis

Generally good if the problem is secondary to an underlying disease that can be treated successfully. Idiopathic disorders of small intestinal motility often represent a therapeutic challenge.

MALIGNANT SMALL INTESTINAL NEOPLASIA

Etiology

In dogs, small intestinal tumors occur relatively frequently (1–8% of all canine cancers). Epithelial tumors include adenocarcinoma, mucinous adenocarcinoma, ring cell carcinoma, and undifferentiated carcinoma and represent 29% of all small intestinal tumors, as does lymphoma. Furthermore, 23% of small bowel neoplasms are leiomyosarcoma. These tumors may metastasize to mesenteric lymph nodes, liver, peritoneum, and lungs (adenocarcinoma metastasis rate is ~50%).

In cats, small intestinal tumors are also relatively common (6–13.5% of all feline cancers), and consist mostly of alimentary lymphoma (74%) and adenocarcinoma (17%). Siamese cats appear to be predisposed. Depending on the source, between one-third and three-quarters of all feline lymphomas are localized in the GI tract. Two main forms are recognized: low-grade alimentary lymphoma (LGAL), which causes a diffuse infiltration of the intestinal wall and consists of T cells; and high-grade alimentary lymphoma (HGAL) which causes focal or segmental disease and consists of B cells.

Pathophysiology

The cause of intestinal neoplasia in dogs and cats is unknown. An association between alimentary lymphoma and chronic inflammation (IBD) has been hypothesized in cats but not demonstrated.

Clinical presentation

Clinical signs develop late in the course of disease. They include chronic progressive vomiting, small bowel diarrhea, hyporexia/anorexia, and melena. An abdominal mass is palpable in 50% of cases with a discrete neoplasm. In diffusely infiltrative tumors, thickening of the small intestinal wall may also be palpable. Enlarged abdominal lymph nodes may also be detected. Clinical features of cats with LGAL may be identical to those of cats with IBD (**Figure 8.92**).

Differential diagnosis

For occlusive tumors, intestinal FB, granulomatous disease (e.g. pythiosis), other cause of vomiting such as pancreatitis, metabolic disease (e.g. chronic kidney disease). Feline IBD is the most common differential diagnosis for cats with LGAL.

Diagnosis

It may be very difficult to differentiate cats with moderate to severe IBD from those with LGAL. Collection of intestinal biopsies of adequate size for histopathologic interpretation is essential but does not guarantee that a final diagnosis will be reached (**Figure 8.93**). There is ongoing debate regarding the value of endoscopy (**Figure 8.94**) versus surgery in obtaining the samples (**Table 8.12**). Special immunohistochemistry stains (**Figure 8.95**) and PCR for antigen receptor rearrangement can be of further help in attempting to confirm a diagnosis of LGAL.

CBC may reveal anemia (chronic disease or blood loss), serum chemistry may show hypoalbuminemia and increased liver enzymes. An obstructive pattern may be seen on abdominal radiographs; thoracic films may reveal metastases. Abdominal ultrasound is the most sensitive imaging method. It allows evaluation of localization, size, and extent of the mass, and can be used to guide fine needle aspiration for cytologic evaluation.

8.93

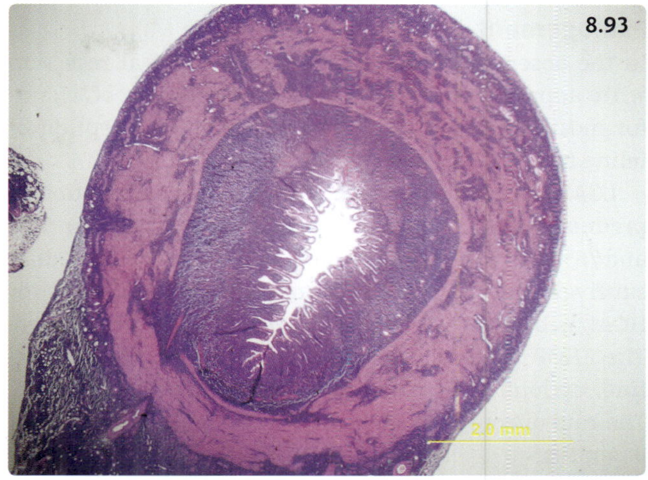

Figure 8.93 Low-power photomicrograph of a resected jejunal segment from a cat with alimentary lymphoma. The very severe infiltration with small lymphocytes extends through all layers of the wall. Inflammatory infiltrates generally do not extend beyond the muscularis mucosae. H&E stain.

8.94

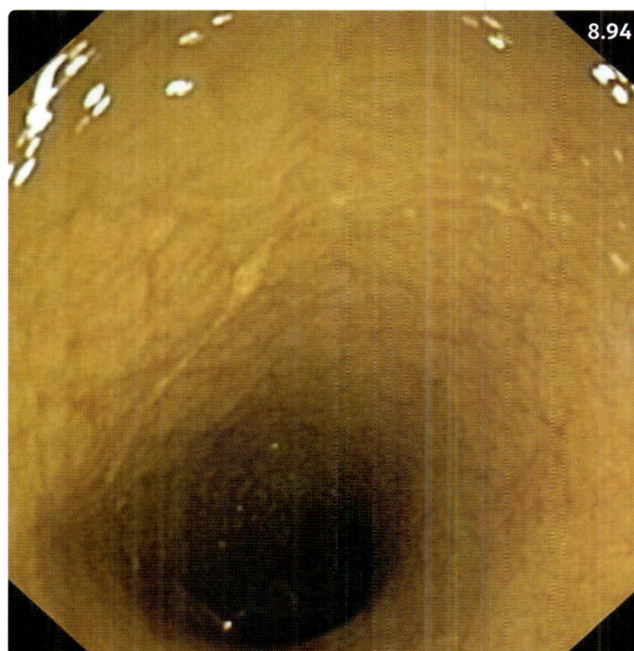

Figure 8.94 Endoscopic view of the duodenal mucosa from a cat with low-grade alimentary lymphoma. The mucosa appears irregular and granular. Changes could be similar in cats with inflammatory bowel disease. (Courtesy R. Husnik)

Management

In the absence of distant metastases, surgical resection with appropriate margins is the treatment of choice for most small intestinal tumors, with the exception of feline LGAL.

LGAL can be treated efficiently with a combination of prednisolone and chlorambucil (**Table 8.13**). Between 55% and 76% of cats achieve complete remission with a median survival time (MST) of 19–29 months. Chemotherapy for HGAL is best initiated after the mass has been resected. The CHOP protocol, consisting of prednisolone, vincristine, cyclophosphamide, and doxorubicin, is preferred. The rate of complete remission is 38–87%, with a MST of 8 months.

Prognosis

Canine adenocarcinoma carries a good prognosis with >2 year survival documented in the absence of metastases and with clean margins, and a MST of 15 months. In cases with metastasis, the MST is usually significantly shorter (3 months). In cats, survival ranges from 5 to 13 months. The benefit of postsurgical chemotherapy has not been scientifically evaluated. MST for canine leiomyosarcoma with or without metastasis ranges from 9 to 22 months.

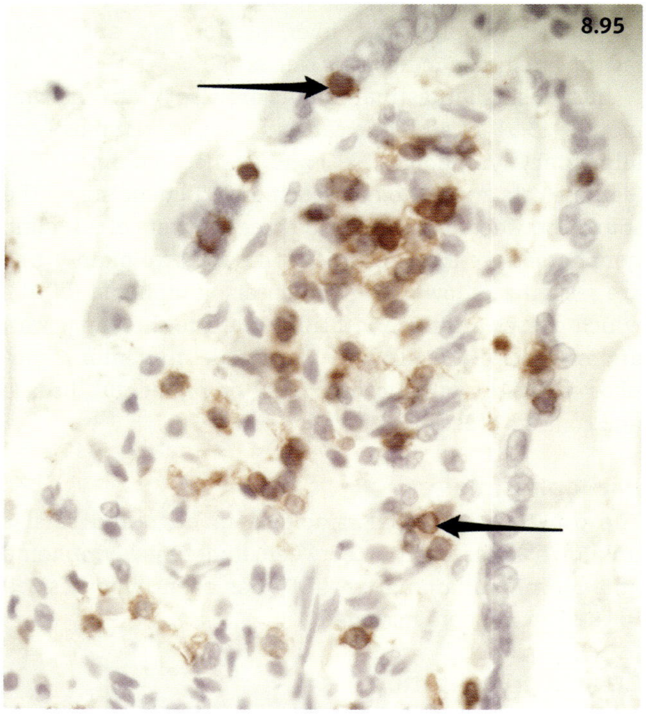

Figure 8.95 Photomicrograph of a small intestinal villus from a cat with low-grade alimentary lymphoma stained with antibodies against CD3, a T-cell marker. There are numerous cells that stain positive. T-cell alimentary lymphoma was diagnosed.

Part 5: Diseases of the large intestine

Overview

Inflammatory diseases of the colon are frequently encountered in dogs and are less common in cats. In many instances, acute nonspecific colitis is self-limiting. Chronic colitis is often associated with a long, sometimes waxing and waning clinical course and specific treatments. Constipation is an uncommon clinical sign usually encountered in older animals, and appears to affect cats more frequently than dogs.

Anatomy and physiology of the large intestine

The large intestine consists of six segments: cecum (a short blind pouch), ascending colon, transverse colon, descending colon, rectum, and anus. The ileocolic valve and its sphincter separate the distal small intestine and the large intestine (**Figure 8.96**). The microscopic structure of the large intestine resembles that of the small intestine. However, the large intestinal mucosa does not form villi, the epithelial cells have fewer microvilli on their apical surface than enterocytes, and numerous goblet cells are interspersed in the epithelial layer (**Figure 8.97**). The colon has two main functions: water absorption, which takes place in the proximal colon, and storage and elimination of feces. Colonic motility includes a few patterns with different functions: stationary contractions mix the content and indirectly promote water absorption and peristaltic contractions move the feces aborally over

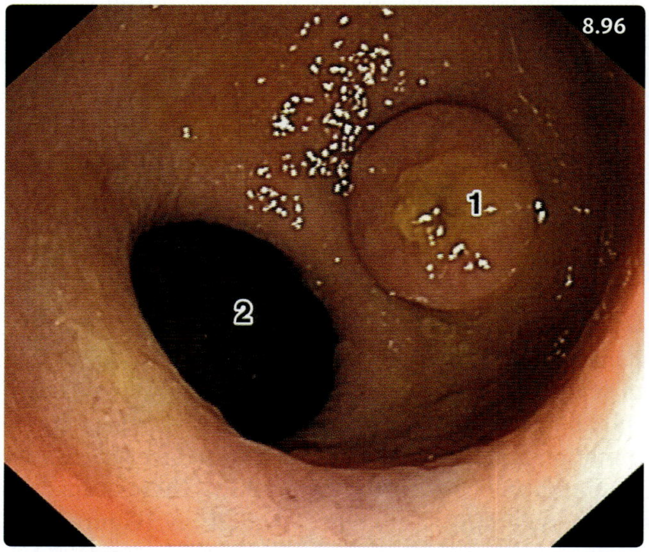

Figure 8.96 Endoscopic view from the ascending colon of a dog. The ileocolic junction (1) and the entrance to the cecum (2) are visible. (Courtesy R. Husnik)

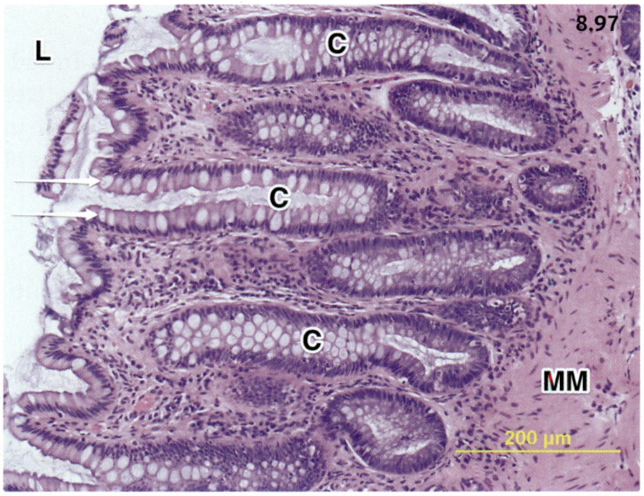

Figure 8.97 Photomicrograph of the canine colonic mucosa. The arrows point to a few of the numerous goblet cells. Mucus can be observed on the surface of the epithelium and in the colonic crypts. There is mild expansion of the lamina propria, with lymphoplasmacytic inflammation. C, colonic crypts; L, lumen; MM, muscularis mucosae.

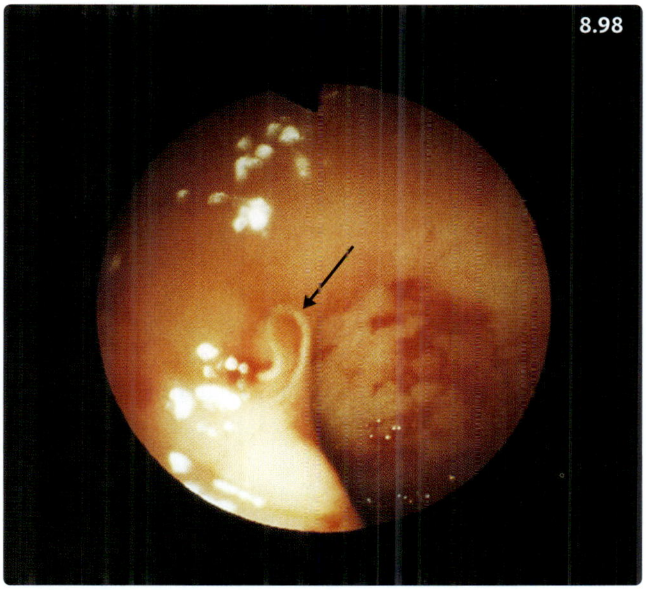

Figure 8.98 Endoscopic view of the colon of a 5-year-old mixed-breed dog with whipworm-induced colitis. The dog had severe bloody mucoid diarrhea for more than a week. Three consecutive fecal examinations were negative for parasitic ova. At endoscopy the mucosa was friable and hemorrhagic, with large numbers of *Trichuris* attached to the mucosa (arrow). The dog was treated with fenbendazole and sulfasalazine and made a good recovery.

small distances. Eventually, giant contractions precede defecation and move feces over longer segments. The gastrocolic reflex is mediated by enteric nerves and enhances colonic motility after a meal, leading to defecation.

CECAL DISEASES

Diseases of the cecum are rarely recognized as a separate entity in cats and dogs. However, the cecum is the preferred place of residence of adult whipworms. Additionally, colonic inflammation can extend to the cecum and cause typhlitis. Clinical signs are characterized by large bowel diarrhea, which cannot be differentiated from colitis.

ACUTE COLITIS

PARASITIC COLITIS (WHIPWORMS)

Definition/overview

As stated earlier, the CAPC maintains a very informative and freely accessible website on intestinal parasites of small animals and this should be consulted for additional information (www.capcvet.org).

Etiology

Trichuris vulpis is a common cause of large bowel diarrhea in dogs. Whipworm infestation in cats is rare, and caused by *T. campanula* and *T. serrata*. The infection mode is fecal-oral. Eggs develop into larvae in the small intestine and larvae ultimately migrate to the cecum and colon, where they develop to adult worms (**Figure 8.98**).

Pathophysiology

Adult whipworms feed on cecal and colonic epithelial cells. Severe typhlitis and colitis may occur with heavy infestations; however, many dogs infested with few whipworms do not show clinical signs.

Clinical presentation

Acute or chronic large bowel diarrhea that may occur in dogs of all ages. Severely affected animals may present with lethargy, hyporexia, and dehydration. Abdominal discomfort or abdominal pain due to accumulation of gas in the large intestinal lumen may also be present. Rarely, whipworm infested dogs may show hyperkalemia and hyponatremia, which is suggestive of hypoadrenocorticism, even though their adrenal glands are fully functional.

Differential diagnosis

Other causes of acute colitis (dietary, idiopathic) or chronic colitis (IBD, granulomatous colitis). In the presence of hyperkalemia and hyponatremia, hypoadrenocorticism.

Diagnosis
Fecal flotation allows identification of the bipolar operculated eggs (**Figure 8.99**). However, fecal shedding of ova may only occur intermittently, particularly if immature worms are involved. Therefore, repeated fecal examinations usually increase the diagnostic yield. Alternatively, empirical treatment may be initiated with a broad-spectrum anthelminthic (see below). Further diagnostic testing is generally not required with the exception of severely dehydrated dogs and animals with pre-existing conditions. In dogs with recurrent episodes of acute diarrhea, a more detailed work up may be indicated.

Management
Fenbendazole (50 mg/kg/day for 3 days) or febantel (25 mg/kg once) are the anthelminthic drugs of choice. Because immature adults and larval stages are less sensitive to the drugs, treatment should be repeated 3 weeks later and again after 3 months. Milbemycin oxime and moxidectin used monthly to prevent heartworm infection are also useful for prevention and treatment of whipworm infestations. Whipworm ova are resistant to unfavorable environmental conditions and may represent a problem in shelter situations.

ACUTE IDIOPATHIC COLITIS

Etiology
Unknown. Some form of dietary indiscretion is usually present.

Pathophysiology
Colonic inflammation is associated with decreased non-propulsive motility and excessive propulsive motility that results in diarrhea with frequent defecation of feces of decreased consistency.

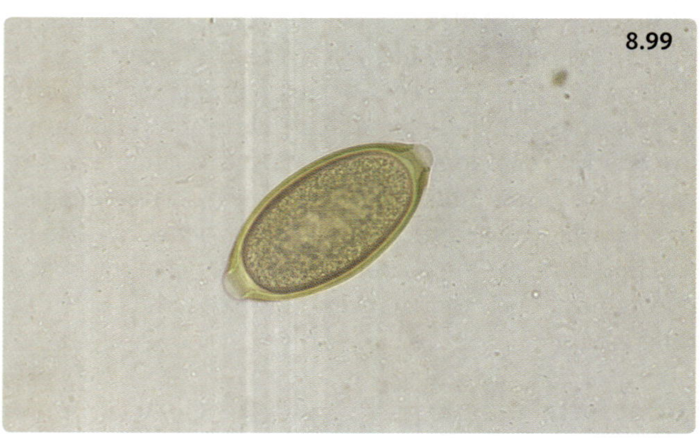

Figure 8.99 *T. vulpis* egg. The egg is lemon-shaped with a plug (operculum) at each pole. (Courtesy B. Delcambre)

Clinical presentation
Large bowel diarrhea with all typical components including hematochezia (see **Figure 2.6.3**), mucoid feces (see **Figure 2.6.5**), and tenesmus (**Figure 8.100**), as listed in **Table 2.6.1**. Acute nonspecific colitis may occur in dogs of any age.

Diagnosis
Elimination of known causes of acute colitis such as whipworm infestation and *C. perfringens* infection.

Management
The disease is usually self-limiting. Mild cases may not require any treatment. Moderate cases respond well to symptomatic treatment that includes dietary manipulations with a 12–24-hour fasting period. An easily digestible low residue diet should be fed for 48–72 hours (small meals several times daily), with progressive return to a good quality commercial diet over the following 48–72 hours. Systematic use of antimicrobials in cases of acute nonspecific colitis is not recommended because increases in the resistance of *C. perfringens* to metronidazole have been reported and are concerning. Metronidazole has been commonly used in the treatment of acute colitis because of its effects on the intestinal microbiome, its properties as a modulator of inflammation, and its spectrum against anaerobic infections. The use of probiotics provides a good alternative to antimicrobials (**Box 8.7**).

In cases with clinical evidence of dehydration, IV fluids should be administered using balanced isotonic crystalloid solutions at appropriate rates in order to

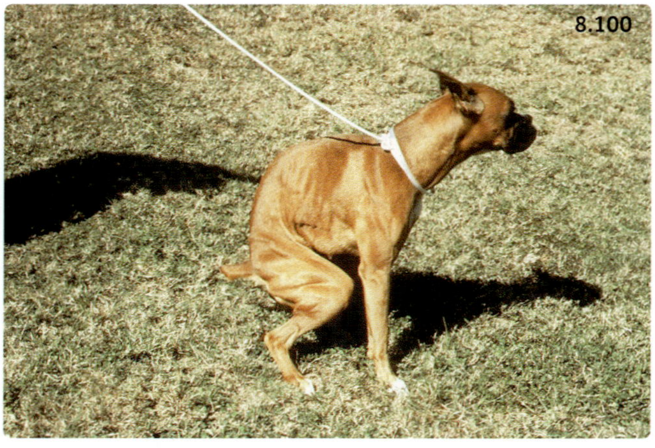

Figure 8.100 Tenesmus in a 2-year-old Boxer with chronic colitis. When walked the dog immediately attempted to defecate. It remained in this position for more than 2 minutes and produced only a small quantity of liquid feces.

rapidly replace fluid deficits and provide maintenance requirements. In dogs with severe acute colitis and consistent abdominal pain, analgesic treatment should be considered.

Prognosis

Good to excellent. The disease is generally self-limiting or it responds well to symptomatic treatment.

CHRONIC COLITIS

FUNGAL AND OOMYCETAL COLITIS

Overview

Animals infected with histoplasmosis may show signs of large bowel diarrhea. Rectal scraping or fine needle aspiration of enlarged abdominal lymph nodes may be diagnostic and reveal large numbers of fungal organisms phagocytized by macrophages (see **Figure 8.73**). Pythiosis is caused by an oomycetal organism and may occasionally diffusely infiltrate the colonic and rectal wall and cause severe clinical signs. The prognosis is generally poor (see **Figure 8.74**).

Further details about histoplasmosis and pythiosis can be found in Part 4: Diseases of the small intestine.

PARASITIC COLITIS

WHIPWORMS

(See Acute colitis.)

TRICHOMONIASIS

Etiology

Tritrichomonas foetus is a protozoal organism associated with chronic, recurring feline colitis in large multi-cat households. Most affected cats come from shelters or belong to breeders, and it is suspected that environmental stress plays a role in their susceptibility to the infection. Co-infections with *Giardia* are common. *T. foetus* is not very resistant in the environment and direct fecal–oral contact is required for transmission (e.g. multi-cat litterbox).

Pathophysiology

T. foetus live in the cecum, descending colon, and ileum, and may cause lymphoplasmacytic and/or neutrophilic inflammation of the mucosa with secondary architectural changes.

Clinical presentation

The disease affects young cats, with onset between birth and 2 years of age. Seventy-five percent or more of affected cats are younger than 1 year of age at the time of diagnosis. Affected cats either live or have lived in a large multi-cat household. Typical clinical signs include waxing and waning large bowel diarrhea, which may contain mucus and blood. The feces are soft and malodorous (**Figure 8.101**). Secondary anal inflammation may be observed.

Differential diagnosis

In shelter or other large multi-cat household situations, other infectious diseases such as infestation with *Giardia* or *Cryptosporidium* (see Chronic enteritis), alone or in combination, may also occur. However, these protozoa more often cause small intestinal or mixed diarrhea. In spite of the young age of cats with suspect *T. foetus* infections, CE should also be considered (DRD, IED).

Diagnosis

Three methods are available for detection of *T. foetus* in the feces. Direct analysis of fresh feces after dilution with saline is an insensitive method (14%), but may yield a positive result in diarrheic feces of severely affected cats (**Figure 8.102**). Feces are best sampled by flushing the colon with saline, and should be analyzed within 2 hours. Under the microscope, *T. foetus* trophozoites may be misdiagnosed as *Giardia*; however, they have a characteristic

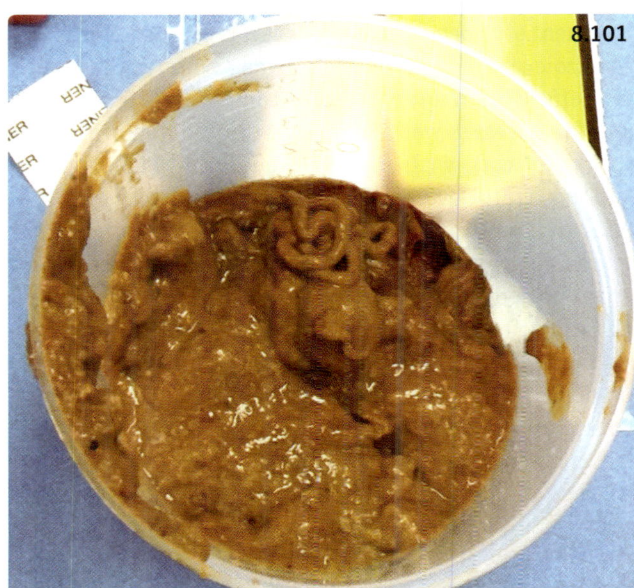

Figure 8.101 Soft and malodorous diarrhea from a cat with *T. foetus* infection. (Courtesy M K. Tolbert)

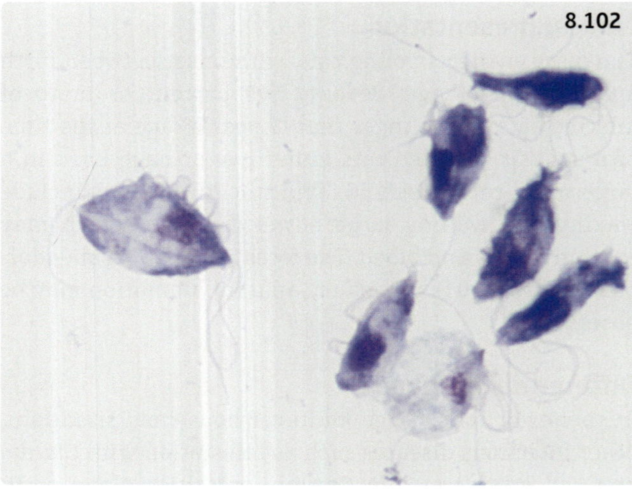

Figure 8.102 Microphotograph of stained *T. foetus* trophozoites. (Courtesy M.K. Tolbert)

forward motion that contrasts with the 'falling leaf' motion of *Giardia* trophozoites. Another method is to inject a small amount of fresh feces into a special culture medium (Feline In Pouch®) and evaluate the medium under the microscope at daily intervals for the presence of *T. foetus* trophozoites. The sensitivity of culture is intermediate (55%). Fecal PCR is the most sensitive method to detect *T. foetus* when the samples are collected adequately. Recommendations to increase the yield of fecal PCR can be found at www.JodyGookin.com.

Management

Treatment of *T. foetus* infection in cats is problematic as fenbendazole and metronidazole, as well as many other drugs, are ineffective. In a recent study, ronidazole (30 mg/kg PO q24h for 2 weeks) was effective at resolving clinical signs in 23 of 27 cats, with most cats becoming PCR negative. Only three cats developed side-effects consisting mostly of lethargy, vomiting, and lack of appetite that resolved after discontinuation of the drug. Ronidazole neurotoxicity has been reported within 3–9 days after initiation of treatment and resolved after discontinuation of the drug. Therefore, ronidazole should be administered only after a definitive diagnosis has been made and only at the dosage listed above. Natural resistance of *T. foetus* to ronidazole has been recently demonstrated in two cats that were refractory to treatment. Ronidazole is not approved for use in cats, and must be compounded in capsules.

Prognosis

Spontaneous resolution of *T. foetus* infection usually occurs within 2 years of onset. However, many cats may remain silent carriers and be able to infect other cats. Ronidazole treatment is most efficacious in animals relocated to single-cat households, as the risk for reinfection is low.

CHRONIC IDIOPATHIC COLITIS

DIET-RESPONSIVE CHRONIC COLITIS

Overview

In a recent study, 56% of 70 dogs with chronic diarrhea responded to an elimination trial with a novel protein diet (see **Figure 8.86**). Of those 39 diet-responsive dogs, 27 (69%) exclusively showed large bowel diarrhea while nine (23%) had mixed large and small bowel signs. Similarly, in another study, 27 (49%) of 55 cats with chronic intestinal disease were diet responsive, while 16 (29%) were diagnosed as food sensitive. Two-thirds of the feline group had abnormal findings on colonic or rectal histopathology.

Based on these data, an elimination trial with hydrolyzed peptide or novel protein diets chosen on the basis of the animal's dietary history should be initiated in all dogs with mild to moderate chronic idiopathic colitis. Clinical signs generally abate within 10–14 days of treatment.

INFLAMMATORY BOWEL DISEASE

Etiology/pathophysiology

The etiology and pathophysiology of IBD are described in Part 4 (Diseases of the small intestine, Chronic enteropathy). While it appears that IBD most often affects the small intestine or both small and large intestine concurrently (especially in cats), colonic IBD is a recognized disease. Synonyms include lymphoplasmacytic colitis, eosinophilic colitis.

Differential diagnosis

Whipworms, diet-responsive colitis, possibly colorectal neoplasia (see below). In cats with compatible signalment and history, *T. foetus* infection.

Diagnosis

The diagnostic approach must be comprehensive in order to rule out all other known causes of colitis (see **Figure 2.6.9**). While a treatment trial with sulfasalazine or olsalazine may be appropriate in dogs with suspect colonic IBD, colonoscopy with collection and histologic evaluation of mucosal biopsies is recommended prior to initiating immunosuppressive treatment. This will confirm the presence and assess the severity of colonic inflammation (**Figures 8.103, 8.104**) and rule out other

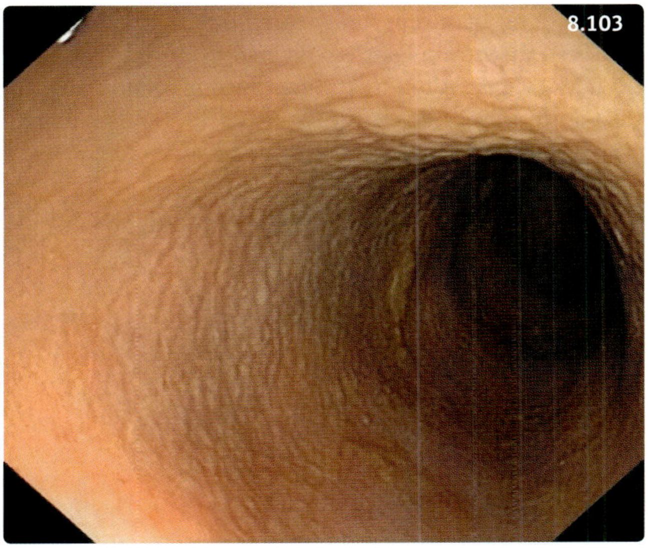

Figure 8.103 Colonoscopy view of a dog with chronic large bowel diarrhea. The inability to see submucosal vessels indicates thickening of the mucosa. The mucosal surface is irregular with a cobblestone pattern. The histopathologic diagnosis was severe lymphoplasmacytic colitis. (Courtesy R. Husnik)

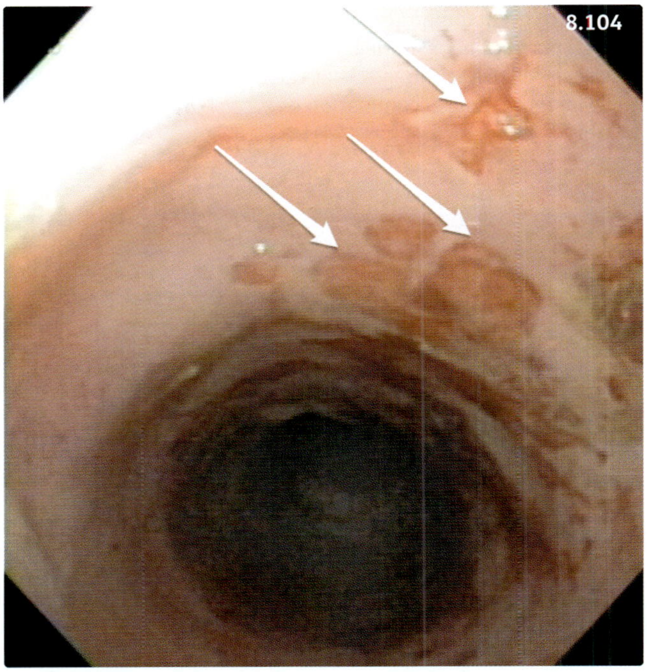

Figure 8.104 Colonoscopy picture of a 6-year-old cat with chronic large bowel diarrhea and hematochezia. There are numerous mucosal ulcerations (arrows). The histopathologic diagnosis was severe, ulcerative lymphoplasmacytic colitis. The cat improved when fed a novel protein diet and treated with immunosuppressive doses of prednisolone.

diseases such as granulomatous colitis (see below) or neoplasia (e.g. lymphoma, especially in cats). Colonoscopy requires appropriate preparation with prolonged fasting (24–48 hours), administration of electrolyte solutions with osmotic laxative effects, and possibly enemas. Rigid proctoscopy can be performed in sedated dogs; however, a full examination of the rectum, colon, and cecum is only possible using flexible endoscopes under general anesthesia.

Management

In dogs with suspect colonic IBD, an anti-inflammatory treatment trial with sulfasalazine may be attempted (10–30 mg/kg [maximum 1 gram total dose] PO q8h for 4–6 weeks). Sulfasalazine liberates 5-aminosalycilic acid in the colon, and is widely used in the treatment of dogs with colitis. After successful completion of the initial treatment regimen, it is best to slowly decrease the dose in stages of 10–14 days. Monitoring tear production regularly during treatment is essential as keratoconjunctivitis sicca is a common complication. Olsalazine (5–15 mg/kg q8–12h) may be used in dogs that do not tolerate sulfasalazine. In addition, dietary fiber supplementation is often helpful (see **Box 8.10**). In cats with colonic IBD and in dogs with confirmed colonic IBD refractory to sulfasalazine or olsalazine, immunosuppressive prednisone should be initiated (**Table 8.13**).

Prognosis

Prognosis for IBD is generally better when only the colon is affected. However, one retrospective study of dogs with IBD did not find any association between localization of disease and outcome. Nevertheless, clinical studies demonstrated that a large number of dogs and cats with colitis respond completely to dietary modification and/or, for dogs only, to sulfasalazine treatment.

Granulomatous colitis

Definition/overview

Granulomatous colitis (GC) is also known as histiocytic ulcerative colitis (HUC). It is a form of IBD that occurs most frequently in young Boxer dogs or, infrequently, in other breeds such as Mastiffs, Alaskan Malamutes, French Bulldogs, and English Bulldogs.

Etiology

Adhesive–invasive *E. coli* or adherent–invasive *E. coli* adhere to and invade intestinal epithelial cells and have been identified as the cause of GC. These *E. coli* are taken up by endosomes and persist in the macrophages instead of being cleared. A genetic predisposition for GC is suspected due to the preponderance of cases in young Boxer dogs. Preliminary results from genetic studies in Boxers with GC and healthy controls point to a defective clearance of *E. coli* in macrophages.

Clinical presentation

The onset of disease generally occurs before 2 years of age. Clinical signs include severe chronic large intestinal inflammation with diarrhea, hematochezia, increased frequency of defecation, tenesmus, and presence of excessive mucus in the feces. Although physical examination findings are most frequently normal, weight loss and inappetence can be seen in severe cases (**Figure 8.105**).

Diagnosis

Signalment, history, and clinical signs are usually very suggestive. While it is tempting to initiate a treatment trial in these dogs, a comprehensive diagnostic work up including endoscopic biopsies is the recommended approach.

Colonoscopy typically reveals sites of severe colonic hemorrhage and ulcerations interspersed with stretches of normal appearing mucosa. Histology may show severe infiltration with neutrophils, macrophages, lymphocytes, plasma cells, and mast cells. Accumulation of large macrophages staining strongly positive with PAS in their cytoplasm is pathognomonic for GC (**Figure 8.106**). Confirmation of the presence of *E. coli* using fluorescent in situ hybridization (FiSH) analysis on formalin-fixed biopsies is now recommended as part of the detailed diagnostic work up of dogs with suspect HUC (**Figure 8.107**).

Management

Treatment of the disease consists of enrofloxacin at 10–20 mg/kg PO q24h for 4–6 weeks. Most affected dogs respond within 10–14 days of initiating therapy. While several dogs were reportedly disease-free after the drug had been discontinued, there is increasing evidence that GC may relapse after treatment. Recent reports suggest that up to 43% of dogs with GC/HUC develop enrofloxacin resistance early in the disease process and may be refractory to treatment if they are treated empirically. Therefore, it is prudent to send colonic biopsies for culture

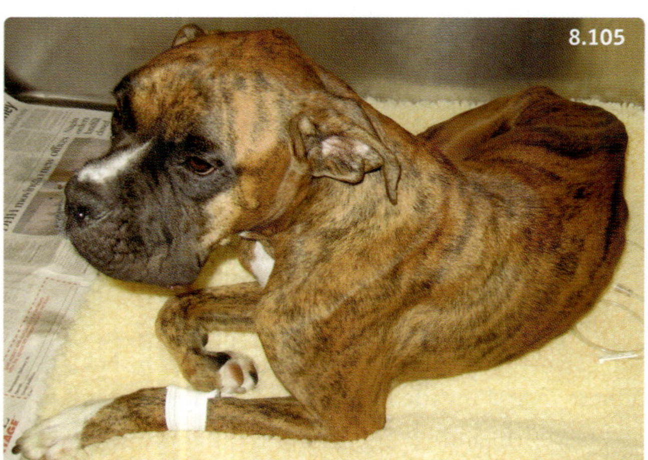

Figure 8.105 Eighteen-month-old Boxer with granulomatous colitis and chronic intermittent large bowel diarrhea, episodes of anorexia, and weight loss.

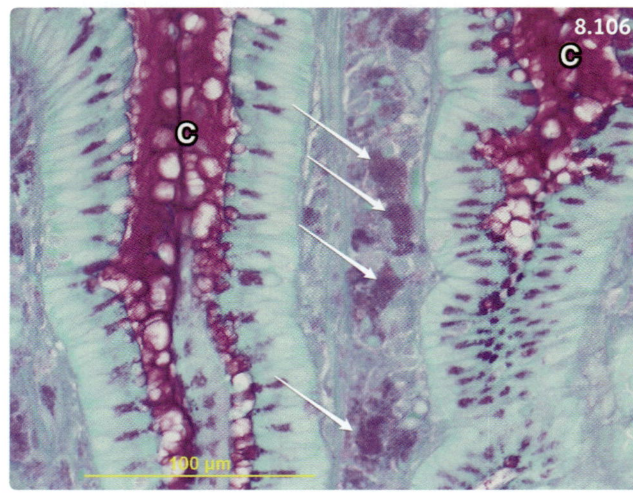

Figure 8.106 Photomicrograph from a colonic biopsy from a Boxer with granulomatous colitis. There are numerous purple-stained macrophages in the lamina propria (arrows point to four such cells). It is thought that the PAS-positive intracellular material represents accumulation of *E. coli*. PAS stain. C, colonic crypts.

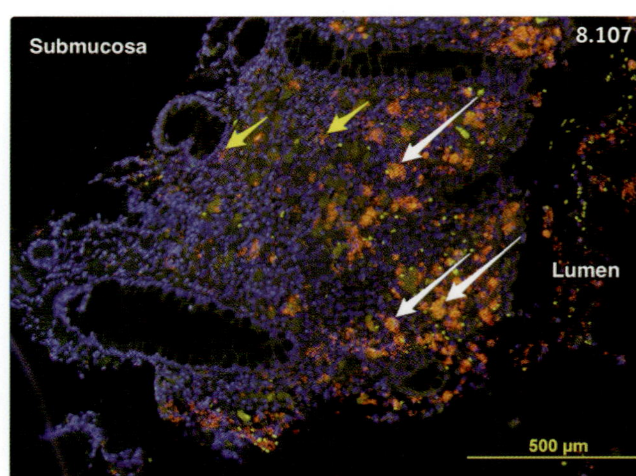

Figure 8.107 Photomicrograph of a colonic biopsy from a dog with granulomatous colitis (fluorescent in situ hybridization or FiSH). Long white arrows show some of the macrophages filled with *E. coli* while short yellow arrows show examples of clusters of *E. coli* within the mucosa. *E. coli*-Cy3 probe stains *E. coli* in red–orange; DAPI stains nuclei in blue. (Courtesy K. Simpson)

and sensitivity before starting treatment, and tailor the choice of antibiotics to the specific sensitivity profile of the cultured *E. coli*.

Prognosis

The long-term prognosis is guarded to poor.

COLORECTAL OBSTRUCTION

Etiology/pathophysiology

Luminal colonic or rectal obstruction may result from a FB or from the presence of hardened feces such as may be the case in constipated or obstipated patients. Alternatively, benign rectal strictures may occur in response to significant trauma of the rectal or distal colonic mucosa (e.g. FB, anorectal surgery). Fibrosis and cellular proliferation are responsible for narrowing of the lumen. Neoplastic masses arising from the colonic wall may also cause an obstruction to the passage of feces in the distal colon and rectum (see below). They may cause malignant strictures. Finally, space-occupying lesions occurring in neighboring organs such as the prostate or sublumbar lymph nodes may also compromise passage of feces through the distal large bowel.

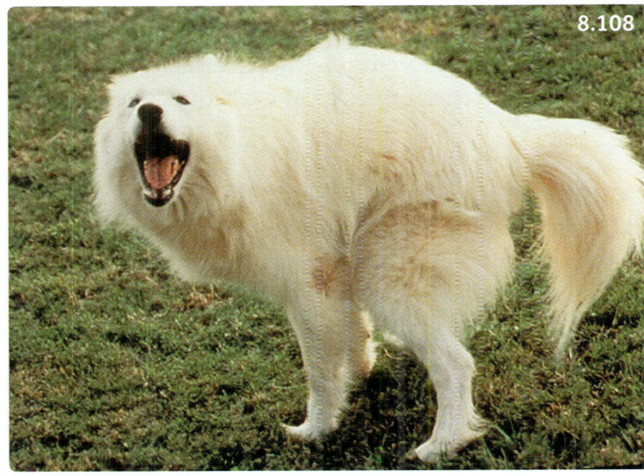

Figure 8.108 Severe tenesmus and dyschezia in a 4-year-old Husky with constipation due to a rectal stricture. The anus was scarred and extremely painful to palpation. The dog vocalized loudly each time it tried to defecate. Eventually, defecation ceased, presumably because it was too painful. Attempts at surgical correction, including anal resection, were unsuccessful and the dog was euthanized.

Clinical presentation

Dyschezia, tenesmus (**Figure 8.108**), passage of ribbon-like feces (**Figure 8.109**), and hematochezia are frequently observed in association with partial or total colorectal obstruction. Severe retention of feces may lead to systemic repercussions such as hyporexia, lethargy, and vomiting.

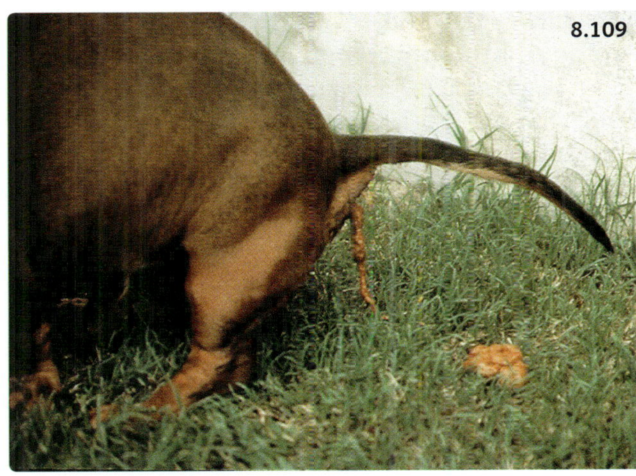

Figure 8.109 This 13-year-old Dachshund was presented with the complaint of tenesmus and 'narrow stools'. The dog strained hard to defecate and passed pencil thin feces. Rectal examination revealed a stricture. Biopsy revealed scar tissue and the dog responded well to balloon dilation and sulfasalazine.

Differential diagnosis

Primary colonic dysmotility, perineal hernia, anal sacculitis, and pseudocoprostasis may all cause dyschezia.

Diagnosis

In animals with a suggestive presentation, abdominal palpation and digital rectal examination often allow confirmation of the presence of partial or total obstruction of the distal large bowel. Sedation may be required for a thorough rectal examination, particularly in animals who are in pain. Radiographs and ultrasound of the abdomen and pelvic canal may be useful to detect a radiopaque FB and/or evaluate the severity of fecal retention and examine the surrounding structures. Endoscopic evaluation can be performed using a rigid proctoscope or a flexible endoscope. This allows visualization of the rectum and distal colon and collection of mucosal biopsies if a neoplastic process is suspected.

Management

Most FBs can be dislodged using repeated warm water enemas with added water-soluble gel. Digital dilation of mild rectal strictures may be successful, although several procedures at intervals of 1 week are generally required. Balloon dilation usually has a higher success rate. In severe cases, or cases refractory to dilatory procedures, surgical removal is required (rectal pull-through if possible or other procedure). The treatment of obstructive neoplasia relies on surgical excision if feasible (see below).

Prognosis

FB, benign polyp – good to excellent. Stricture, other neoplasia – guarded to poor. Anorectal surgery may lead to fecal incontinence or recurrence of stricture.

FUNCTIONAL LARGE BOWEL DISORDERS

CHRONIC IDIOPATHIC LARGE BOWEL DIARRHEA

Definition/overview

Chronic idiopathic large bowel diarrhea (CILBD) affects dogs and is characterized by recurrent large bowel diarrhea in the absence of histopathologic evidence of inflammation. It appears to be comparable to irritable bowel syndrome (IBS), a disease that is relatively common in people. One form of IBS is associated with diarrhea.

Etiology/pathophysiology

The etiology of CILBD is unknown. In people, IBS is associated with visceral hypersensitivity and patients have enhanced perception of visceral events such as contractions and gas throughout their GI tract. Stress, diet, and intestinal and colonic microbiota are all thought to play a role in the pathogenesis. Approximately 40% of dogs with CILBD have abnormal personality traits and/or are exposed to environmental stress factors. Associated behavioral issues may include separation anxiety, submissive urination, noise sensitivity, aggression, or nervous, high-strung dogs. Environmental factors may range from presence of visitors in the household and construction in the house to traveling and moving.

Clinical presentation

Dogs of all ages may be affected (median 6 years old) and exhibit chronic intermittent large bowel diarrhea. Excessive mucus in the feces (**Figure 8.110**), hematochezia, increased number of daily defecations, and/or tenesmus are common. Appetite may be decreased during diarrheic episodes and abdominal pain may be present. Vomiting may occur as well.

Differential diagnosis

Whipworm infestation, diet-responsive colitis, colonic IBD, granulomatous colitis (in Boxer dogs and Bulldogs), colonic neoplasia.

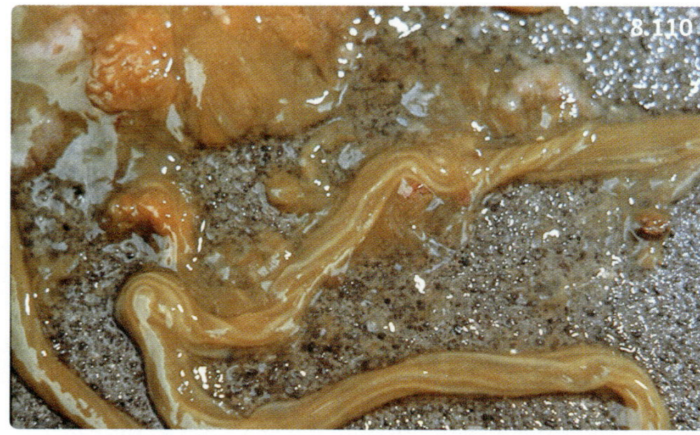

Figure 8.110 Feces from a 13-year-old mixed-breed dog with chronic idiopathic large bowel diarrhea. This dog had intermittent large bowel diarrhea only when the home environment was disturbed. Colonoscopy and mucosal biopsy were normal. The dog responded well to tranquilizers, anticholinergics, and a high-fiber diet.

Diagnosis

CILBD is a diagnosis by exclusion, and all other causes of chronic-intermittent large bowel diarrhea must be ruled out (see **Figure 2.6.9**). Diagnostic criteria for CILBD include chronic or chronic-recurring large bowel diarrhea of at least 4 weeks' duration, absence of or only minimal abnormal findings on physical examination and blood work, no other identifiable cause of diarrhea, and lack (or only minimal) changes observed during colonoscopy. Finally, histopathologic evaluation of the colonic mucosa must be unremarkable.

Management

Between 63% and 96% of dogs with CILBD respond to fiber supplementation alone (**Box 8.10**). In fiber-refractory dogs, a full behavioral assessment should be performed and behavior-modifying drugs prescribed as appropriate. In one study, approximately 60% of dogs requiring drug treatment responded, while 40% did not.

Prognosis

Prognosis is good considering the high response rate to fiber supplementation.

CONSTIPATION

Definition/overview

Constipation is characterized by infrequent or difficult evacuation of feces. Obstipation is the result of recurrent, intractable constipation. Constipation and obstipation may culminate in the syndrome of megacolon. In the cat

Box 8.10 Fiber supplementation in dogs with colitis and chronic idiopathic large bowel diarrhea.

Overall, dietary fibers enhance the structure and function of the intestinal epithelium, and also have beneficial effects on colonic motility. As a trade-off, they may have a negative impact on nutrient digestibility depending on the specific fiber type. Soluble fibers are fermented to short-chain fatty acids (SCFAs) by the colonic flora. SCFAs are an essential source of energy for colonic epithelial cells.

- Psyllium is a soluble fiber derived from the seed of *Plantago ovata.* It has great water holding capacities and forms gels in water, two properties that can contribute to improvement of fecal consistency. Psyllium was very efficient when added to a highly digestible diet in the treatment of chronic idiopathic colitis. The initial daily dosage is 0.5 tablespoon (T) for toy breeds, 1 T for small dogs, 2 T for medium dogs, and 3 T for large dogs. The fiber supplement should be administered with each meal, and the dose adapted to effect. Psyllium is included as an ingredient in a few commercial prescription diets.
- Canned pumpkin is another source of soluble fiber. It is administered with an initial dosage comparable to that of psyllium, and the dose is adapted to effect.

Other sources of SCFAs include fructooligosaccharides and beet pulp, which are included in some high-quality diets.

constipation is a relatively frequent problem while obstipation and megacolon are less common. Constipation and associated problems occur less frequently in the dog.

Etiology

Primary constipation is due to abnormal colonic motility. Neuromuscular dysfunction may occur in animals with lumbosacral disease or in cats with idiopathic megacolon. Dehydration, hypokalemia, and hypocalcemia may all negatively impact colonic motility. Inactivity and obesity may also be a cause of prolonged large bowel transit time. Furthermore, use of opiates and anticholinergics may also lead to constipation.

Secondary constipation is more common and is associated with processes that impair the transit and evacuation of colonic content, such as mechanical obstruction of the colon or rectum. Obstructions can be intraluminal (e.g. fecal impaction, FB, stricture), intramural (neoplasia), or extramural (e.g. narrowing of the pelvic canal, space-occupying lesions impinging on the descending colon or rectum).

Clinical presentation

Typical clinical signs include reduced, absent, or painful defecation, which may be progressive. Other clinical signs associated with a primary underlying disease might be present, such as those associated with hypothyroidism, which is more common in dogs. The onset of distal bowel signs may be insidious and animals may be presented late when the problem is severe. Dyschezia may be observed (**Figure 8.108**). Chronic constipation/obstipation may have systemic repercussions such as anorexia, lethargy, weight loss, and vomiting.

Differential diagnosis

Diseases of the anorectum such as perineal hernia and anal sacculitis may cause painful defecation. Pseudocoprostasis or constipation can be caused by matted hair around the anus, which occasionally occurs in dogs and cats with long hair. Importantly, some cat owners may not be able to differentiate stranguria and dyschezia, and lower urinary tract diseases should always be ruled out.

Diagnosis

A detailed physical examination is required. This may reveal varying degrees of dehydration, weight loss, and abdominal pain. Rectal palpation should be performed and may reveal pelvic canal abnormalities, a rectal FB, a stricture, or presence of a perineal hernia.

A thorough screening of animals presented with recurrent constipation is recommended to identify obstructions and underlying diseases and assess the systemic repercussions of the problem. A minimal database consisting of CBC, biochemistry panel, and urinalysis should be obtained in all cats presented for constipation to rule out metabolic causes and underlying chronic diseases such as chronic kidney disease. Abdominal radiographs help characterize the severity of colonic impaction (**Figures 8.111, 8.112**) and identify predisposing factors such as intraluminal radiopaque foreign material, intraluminal or extraluminal mass lesions, pelvic fractures, and spinal abnormalities. Extraluminal mass lesions may be further evaluated by abdominal ultrasonography and guided biopsy, whereas intraluminal mass lesions are best evaluated by endoscopy.

Management

All identified underlying problems should be treated. If the cause of the obstruction can be addressed in a timely manner, colonic function may be preserved. However, prolonged obstruction is ultimately associated with loss of colonic contractility.

The different methods for treatment of idiopathic, nonobstructive constipation include administration of oral laxatives, enemas (**Table 8.15**), and prokinetic agents such as cisapride (**Table 8.9**).

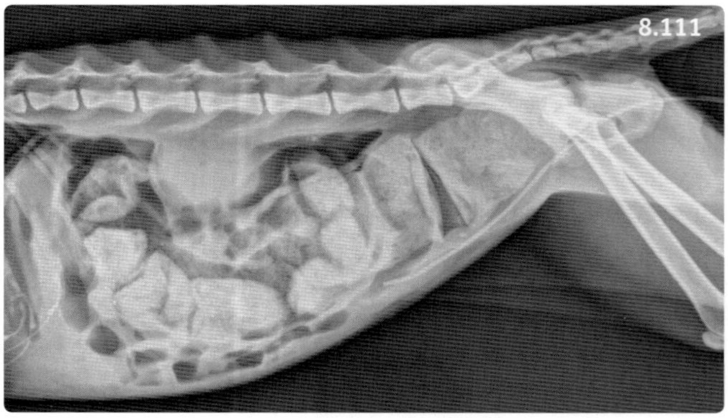

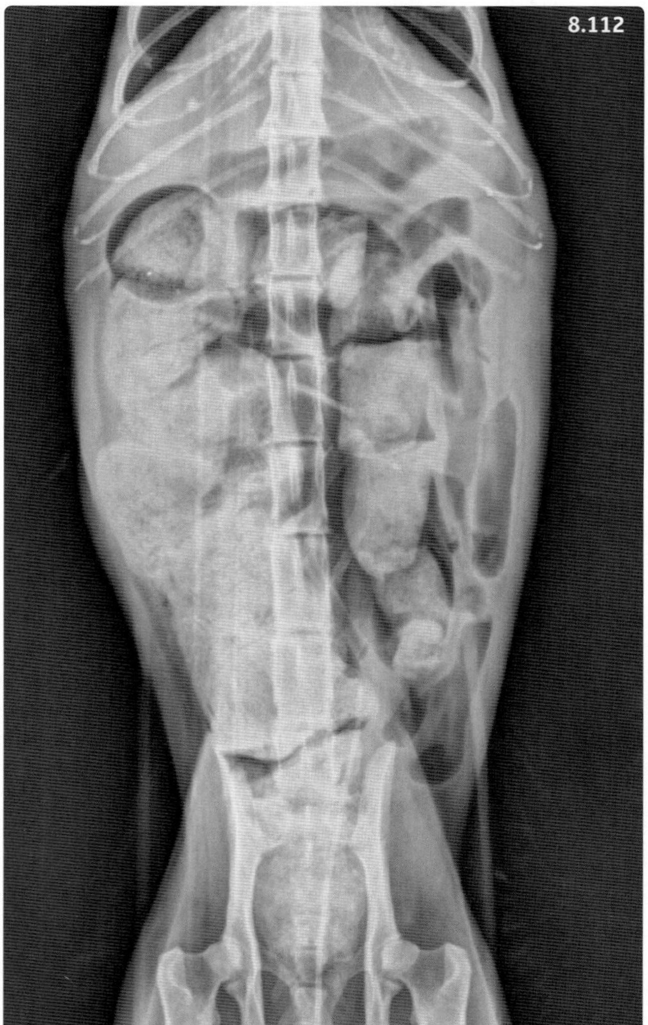

Figures 8.111, 8.112 Ten-year-old female spayed Domestic Shorthair cat. (8.111) Right lateral abdominal radiograph. There is severe dilation of the entire colon from the cecum to the rectum with large amounts of radiopaque fecal material. The cat is in poor body condition. Radiographic diagnosis is megacolon. A urinary catheter is present. (8.112) Ventrodorsal abdominal radiograph. The severely dilated and impacted colon is displaced to the right. (Courtesy L. Gaschen)

In cats with chronic recurrent idiopathic constipation, a stepwise approach has proven useful. Mild to moderate constipation (e.g. first occurrence, recurrence after a long interval with normal defecation) is best treated with an initial enema followed by treatment with laxatives. Maintaining these cats on a psyllium-enriched diet or continuing daily administration of laxatives is recommended. Addition of prokinetics is necessary when management with diet and laxatives fails. Early use of cisapride is likely to prevent the progression of constipation to obstipation and dilated megacolon in these cats. However, some cases become refractory to conservative treatment and slowly progress to obstipation and dilated megacolon.

When treating a constipated cat, enemas should be injected slowly, as rapid administration may cause reflex vomiting and rapid and excessive efflux of the liquid, and may also increase the risk of colonic perforation. If several enemas fail to induce defecation, nasoesophageal administration of PEG 3350 is a relatively noninvasive method with an excellent success rate (**Box 8.11**, **Figure 8.113**). This technique has significantly decreased the number of cases that need to undergo manual extraction of feces, a technique used when all other options have failed. It is best performed on an anesthetized cat with careful transabdominal colonic massage and simultaneous rectal administration of a combination of warm water or physiologic saline with water-soluble lubricants to break down the impacted feces. Some authors recommend administering a low dose of metronidazole

Box 8.11 Conservative treatment of moderate to severe colonic impaction on cats.

Polyethylene glycol (PEG) 3350 is an osmotic laxative that has been shown to be safe and palatable in cats. PEG 3350 can be administered to constipated or obstipated cats through a nasoesophageal tube as a CRI at a rate of between 6 and 10 ml/kg/hour. In a recent study, the mean total dose required was 80 ml/kg (range 40–156), and defecation occurred on average 8 hours after initiation of treatment (range 5–24). The technique has considerably decreased the need for enemas in feline practice (**Figure 8.113**).

Sources: Carr AP, Gaunt MC (2010) Constipation resolution with administration of polyethylene-glycol solution in cats. *J Vet Intern Med* **24:**723 (abstract).

Little S (2014) Personal communication.

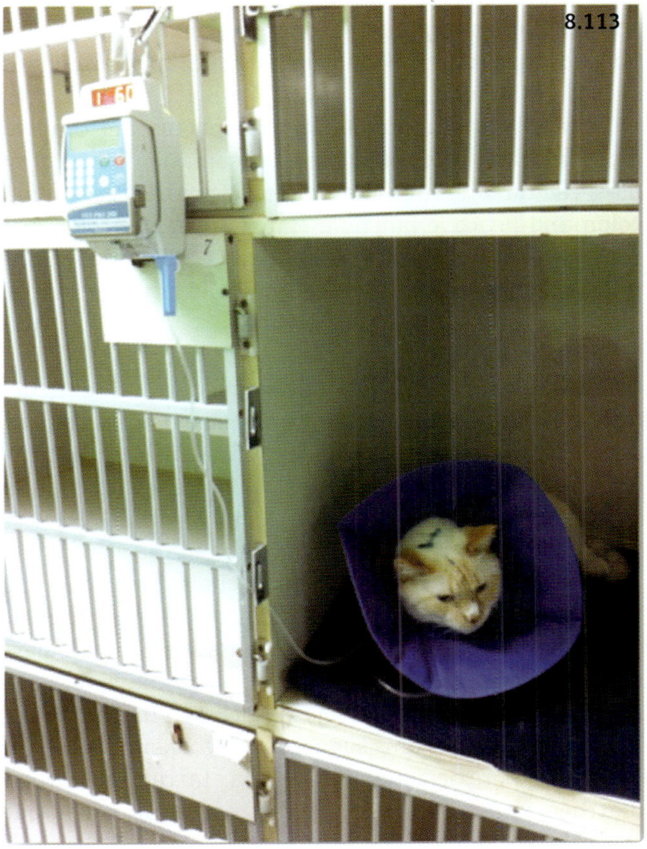

Figure 8.113 Constipated cat receiving PEG 3350 as a constant rate infusion via a nasoesophageal tube. (Courtesy S. Little)

(7.5–15 mg/kg PO q12h) in order to limit the risk of bacterial translocation during or after the procedure.

A surgical approach is the last option for severe cases with obstipation or megacolon that does not respond to conservative treatment options. Different techniques for colectomy have been successful.

Prognosis

Many cats have one or two episodes of constipation without further recurrence, although others may progress to complete colonic failure. When conservative management has failed, colectomy is usually associated with a favorable prognosis, although mild to moderate diarrhea may persist for 4–6 weeks postoperatively in some cases.

RECTAL PROLAPSE

Definition/overview

Prolapse can be partial with protrusion of anal mucosa only (anal prolapse) or complete with protrusion of all layers of the rectum (rectal prolapse).

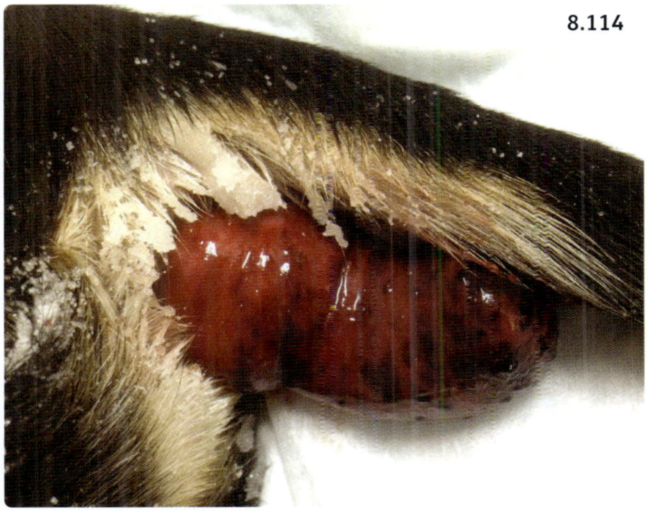

Figure 8.114 Young mixed-breed dog with rectal prolapse. Sugar has been applied to the mucosa to decrease the swelling.

Etiology

Prolapse occurs secondary to tenesmus associated with disorders of the colon, anorectum, or urogenital tract. Prevalence appears to be higher in young animals. Predisposing factors include GI parasitism, typhlitis, colitis, proctitis, colorectal neoplasia, rectal FBs, perineal hernia, diseases of the urinary bladder, prostatic disorders, and dystocia.

Clinical presentation

Anal prolapse is characterized by the presence of red, swollen mucosa protruding from the anus, particularly after defecation. In animals with a rectal prolapse, there is an often round or cylindrical mass protruding from the anus (**Figure 8.114**). The everted rectal mucosa and other wall layers can become ischemic and damaged and necrotic after prolonged exposure.

Diagnosis

A thorough physical examination is necessary to screen for the underlying diseases predisposing to prolapse listed above. If indicated, additional tests, such as fecal parasitologic examination, blood analyses, and abdominal imaging, should be performed.

Management

Reduction under sedation is easiest in animals with anal prolapse using saline and water-soluble lubricant gel. When a significant amount of mucosa is exposed or in rectal prolapse, 50% dextrose can be applied to the mucosa to reduce edema prior to careful repositioning. Corticosteroid cream can also be used to decrease inflammation and straining. A purse-string suture is applied around the anus to narrow the anal orifice while allowing soft feces to pass through, and kept in place for 3–5 days. The animal should be fed a low residue diet; using lactulose (**Table 8.15**) to effect may helpful. If the prolapsed rectal mucosa is traumatized or necrotic, surgical resection is required. Underlying conditions must be addressed to prevent recurrence. Colopexy may be required in animals experiencing recurrent episodes in spite of appropriate treatment.

Prognosis

Generally good if the mucosa is viable and the prolapse can be reduced. Guarded to poor if resection is required because of the risk of stricture.

COLORECTAL NEOPLASIA

Etiology

In dogs, the prevalence of colorectal neoplasia is higher than that of gastric and small intestinal tumors. The sites of predilection are the descending colon and rectum. Adenomas and polyps are relatively common (**Figure 8.115**), and *in-situ* progression to carcinoma has been documented. The most common type of malignant neoplasia is adenocarcinoma, followed by lymphoma and stromal tumors such as leiomyosarcoma. Local tumor invasion appears to be slow, and metastasis to distant sites is uncommon.

In cats, adenocarcinoma and lymphoma are the two most frequent types of colorectal neoplasia, followed by mast cell tumors. Sites of predilection are the descending colon and ileocolic junction. Malignant feline colorectal tumors have a high rate of metastasis. Alimentary lymphoma often involves both the small and large intestines.

Pathophysiology

Colorectal neoplasms may cause mechanical obstruction. Colonic dysfunction with abnormal motility and decreased water reabsorption capacity (with subsequent diarrhea) may also occur.

Clinical presentation

In dogs, common clinical signs include hematochezia, mucoid feces, and dyschezia, with or without concurrent diarrhea. Dyschezia may be associated with passage of feces of a smaller than usual diameter (see **Figure 8.109**). Systemic neoplasia such as lymphoma may be associated with signs suggesting involvement of other organs, hyporexia, and weight loss. In cats, vomiting, diarrhea, and weight loss are common with or without clinical signs of large bowel disease.

Table 8.15 Therapeutic options for conservative management of constipation in cats.

Laxatives (administer in well-hydrated cats only)	**Bulk-forming** (add to moist cat food). More useful in mild cases	Psyllium (1–4 teaspoons per meal); also available incorporated in a proprietary dry extruded diet (Royal Canin Intestinal Fibre Response®)
		Wheat bran (1–2 tablespoons per meal)
	Emollient	Dioctyl sodium succinate (10–15 ml/cat PO)
	Lubricant	Mineral oil (10–15 ml/cat PO); administer with caution due to risk of aspiration
		White petrolatum (1–5 ml/cat PO)
	Osmotic	Lactulose (0.5 ml/kg q8–12h PO)
		PEG 3350 (Colyte®) 1.9 g/cat; dose can be doubled if no results are seen after 48 hours. (See **Box 8.11** for CRI instructions)
	Stimulant	Bisacodyl (5 mg q24h PO)
Removal of feces	**Enemas**	Warm water (5–10 ml/kg)
		Dioctyl sodium succinate or DSS (5–10 ml/cat)
		Mineral oil (5–10 ml/cat)
		Lactulose (5–10 ml/cat)
	Manual extraction	Under anesthesia

Differential diagnosis

Causes of chronic colitis such as IBD, GC, heavy whipworm infestation in dogs, IBD in cats. Also distal colonic or rectal FB or stricture.

Diagnosis

In dogs, rectal palpation can detect up to 80% of rectal tumors. In cats, more than half of colonic masses can be palpated abdominally. Survey radiographs may show an accumulation of feces orad to the neoplasm. Mural masses can be visualized using abdominal ultrasound, and surrounding lymph nodes can also be evaluated. Cytologic evaluation of ultrasound-guided fine needle aspirates can be useful, particularly for diagnosis of lymphoma. However, the diagnosis of most other tumors requires histopathology from a biopsy collected during colonoscopy. Endoscopy also allows a good evaluation of the severity and extent of the tumor (**Figures 8.115, 8.116**). Thoracic radiographs and abdominal ultrasound are used to stage the tumor, looking for pulmonary masses and abnormal abdominal lymph nodes.

Management

Rectal tumors are usually amenable to surgical resection using the rectal pull-through technique. Masses located in the cecum and colon require standard celiotomy for resection. The benefit of chemotherapy has not been established except for alimentary lymphoma. Currently recommended chemotherapy protocols are best found in recent oncology texts.

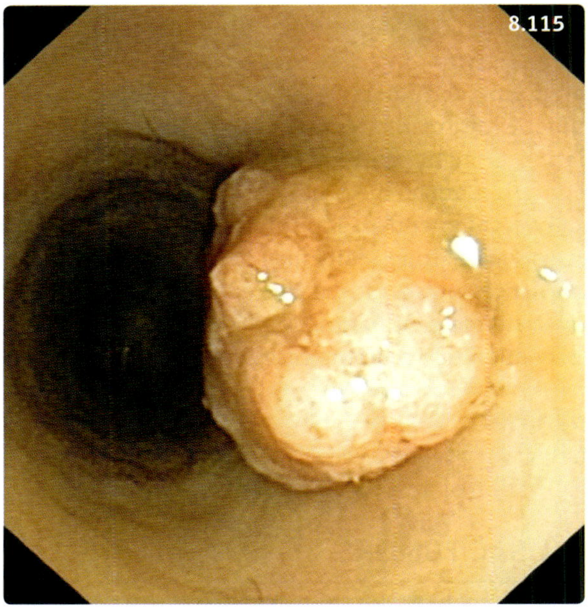

Figure 8.115 Colonoscopic view of an adenoma located in the distal colon of a dog. The parietal mass is pedunculated and could be removed with an electrocautery snare passed through the biopsy channel of the endoscope. (Courtesy R. Husnik)

Prognosis

Surgical excision is generally curative for benign tumors. While the rectal pull-through procedure has few complications, secondary infections may occur after celiotomy and resection of large bowel masses.

Canine carcinomas have been associated with a median survival of 32 months after removal in pedunculated tumors, 12 months for sessile tumors, and less than 2 months for annular tumors. The median survival time for leiomyosarcoma is 9–22 months after resection. Even though feline carcinomas benefit from an aggressive approach (subtotal colectomy), the median survival is only 4–5 months. The approach to alimentary lymphomas in cats is discussed in more detail in Part 4: Diseases of the small intestine.

Part 6: Diseases of the anus and perineum

FECAL INCONTINENCE

Definition/overview

Fecal incontinence is a rare disease that is characterized by involuntary loss of feces. Anal sphincter incontinence may be neurogenic (due to lesions damaging the innervation of the anal sphincter) or primary (in association with direct damage to the sphincter). Reservoir incontinence is uncommon and has been reported with loss of fecal storage capacity after colectomy.

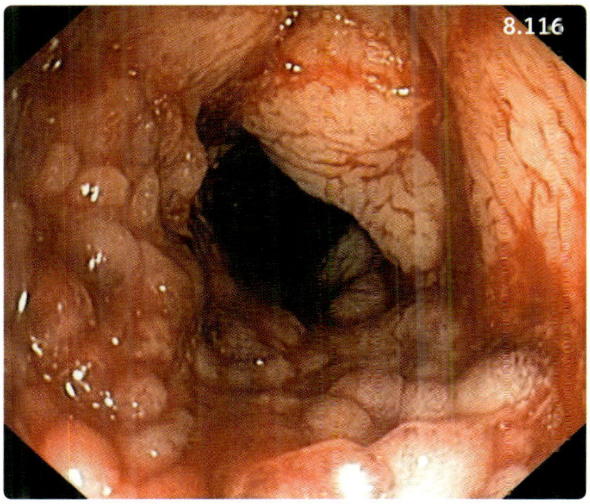

Figure 8.116 Endoscopic view of a dog with a severely abnormal rectal and colonic wall. The histopathologic diagnosis was adenocarcinoma. (Courtesy R. Husnik)

Etiology

Causes of non-neurogenic incontinence include IBD, colitis, colonic, rectal or anal/perianal neoplasia, anorectal trauma or surgery, and perianal fistula. Neurogenic incontinence is associated with sacral spinal cord disorders or peripheral nerve diseases.

Clinical presentation

Affected animals are unable to control defecation, with involuntary elimination of feces, and sometimes continuous fecal dribbling. Concurrent urinary incontinence may be present in animals with neurogenic fecal incontinence. Rectal palpation reveals significantly decreased anal tone. A thorough neurologic examination should be performed to detect other neurologic deficits.

Diagnosis

History and physical examination are usually sufficient. A search for neurologic lesions and their precise location may require cross-sectional imaging.

Management

Mild fecal incontinence may respond to opiates such as loperamide (0.1 mg/kg PO q8h). These drugs increase the tone of the internal sphincter, but are without effect on the external sphincter. Moderate to severe cases are difficult to treat, regardless of their origin.

Prognosis

Guarded to poor in many cases.

DISEASES OF THE ANAL SACS

Definition/overview

Anal sac impaction, anal sacculitis, and abscess formation are common anal sac diseases that may occur in dogs and occasionally in cats. Small breed dogs and some large canine breeds (e.g. German Shepherd Dog) appear to be at higher risk of developing anal sac diseases.

Etiology

The exact cause of anal sac disorders is unknown. Abnormal anal sac emptying may occur with decreased fecal consistency, obesity, and inactivity, or in association with painful perianal processes such as anal furunculosis. Anal sac impaction increases the risk of infection and/or abscessation.

Clinical presentation

Anal sac disease commonly causes anal or perianal pruritus and pain, with excessive licking and/or biting of the area, tail chasing, scooting, and rubbing the anus on the ground. If the perineal area is swollen and painful, the animal may not want to sit. Other frequently associated signs include dyschezia, tenesmus, or even reluctance to defecate. A detailed examination of the perineal area, including rectal palpation, may reveal swelling and pain to the touch.

Differential diagnosis

Anal furunculosis, perianal or anal tumors, and bite wounds (especially in cats).

Diagnosis

History and clinical signs are suggestive. Swelling may be visible in the 4 and 8 o'clock positions ventral to the anus. Rectal palpation confirms the presence of swollen anal sacs, which are often painful. With impaction, pasty thick and malodorous material can be expressed from the swollen sacs. If the expressed material is bloody and/or purulent, anal sacculitis is likely and can be confirmed cytologically by the presence of large amounts of neutrophils with intracellular bacteria. Abscesses often involve the surrounding tissues, and cytology of a fine needle aspirate is diagnostic.

Management

Anal sac impaction is treated with gentle expression of the swollen anal sacs. If digital massage and expression are not successful, flushing the anal sacs with saline is recommended. Instillation of an antibiotic and steroid ointment into the empty sacs is generally recommended. In animals with infected sacs, treatment also consists of emptying and flushing the sacs and instillation of an antibiotic ointment. However, this generally requires sedation or light anesthesia. Systemic antibiotic treatment with a broad-spectrum antibiotic for 10–14 days is usually recommended. Topical treatment with hot compresses several times daily may help reduce swelling and pain. Abscesses should be lanced, flushed, and treated with systemic antibiotics. Anal sacculectomy is a last resort option for recurring cases.

Prognosis

Usually very good. Fecal incontinence is a possible complication of anal sacculectomy.

ANAL SAC TUMORS

Definition/overview

Anal sac tumors are uncommon and very often malignant neoplasms that occur in dogs. They may metastasize to regional lymph nodes and invade surrounding tissues.

Etiology/pathophysiology

The etiology is unknown. Between 50% and 90% of dogs with anal sac adenocarcinomas are hypercalcemic due to production of parathyroid hormone-related peptide by cancerous cells. This malignancy-associated hypercalcemia may ultimately lead to irreversible kidney injury.

Clinical presentation

Anal sac tumors most commonly affect older dogs, with a predilection for females. Dyschezia and perianal swelling may be observed. Up to 40% of dogs may only show clinical signs associated with hypercalcemia of malignancy: polyuria, polydipsia, vomiting, and constipation. A thorough rectal examination is essential to identify nodules associated with the anal sacs. Metastasis to sublumbar lymph nodes is very common at the time of diagnosis, and liver and lungs may be affected as well.

Differential diagnosis

Other perianal tumors, perineal hernia, rectal FB, or stricture. Other causes of hypercalcemia, such as hyperparathyroidism, lymphoma, and other tumors, should also be considered.

Diagnosis

History and physical examination are suggestive. If a mass is present, cytologic evaluation of a fine needle aspirate may be diagnostic. Radiographs and ultrasonography are useful to evaluate the sublumbar area, liver, and lungs for metastasis (**Figure 8.117**). Cross-sectional imaging may also be helpful in complicated cases. A CBC, serum chemistry profile, and urinalysis are essential to detect the presence of hypercalcemia (associated with hypophosphatemia) and possible secondary kidney damage.

Management

Wide surgical excision of the primary tumor and regional lymph node. The benefits of chemotherapy and/or radiation treatment have not been clearly established. Hypercalcemia may need to be addressed prior to surgery in order to avoid additional end organ damage (see Chapter 11: Endocrine disorders).

Prognosis

Poor to fair, with a 40% 1-year survival. Negative prognostic factors include presence of lymph node or distant metastases and tumor size.

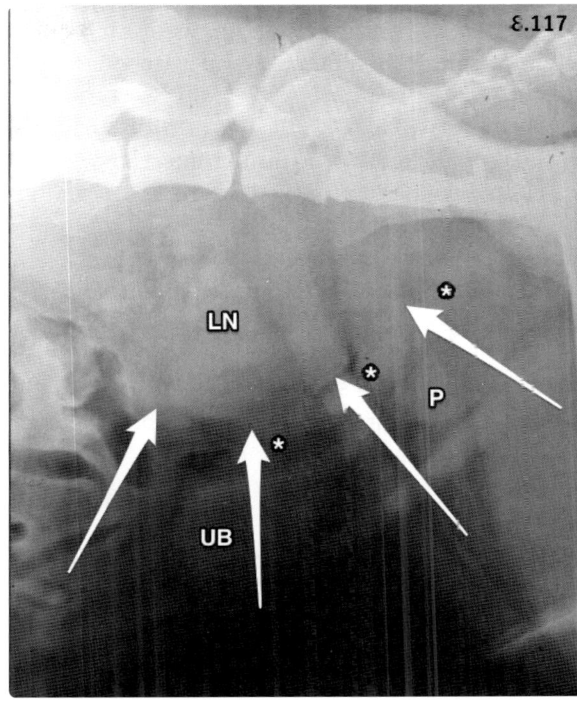

Figure 8.117 Radiograph of the caudal abdomen of a 10 year-old male Akita Inu. The dog was presented with severe hypercalcemia and dyschezia. While the primary anal sac tumor was a few millimeters in diameter, the sublumbar lymph node (LN) was severely enlarged (arrows). Note the ventrally displaced colon (asterisks), urinary bladder (UB), and prostate (P). A metallic plate used to repair a pelvic fracture several years prior to presentation is visible on the ileum.

ANAL FURUNCULOSIS/PERIANAL FISTULAE

Definition/overview

Anal furunculosis is a chronic and painful disease of the canine anorectum that seems to preferentially affect middle aged to old German Shepherd Dogs and German Shepherd Dog mixed breeds, although dogs from other breeds may be also affected. The condition is characterized by inflammation, ulceration, and sinus tracts.

Etiology

The etiology is unknown, but is likely multifactorial

Pathophysiology

The inflammatory process is chronic and consists of a mononuclear to granulomatous infiltrate. It may involve the anal sacs, their excretory ducts, the anal sphincter, and the circumanal glands. Immune dysregulation with aberrant cell-mediated immune response and excessive local production of matrix metalloproteinases has been reported in dogs with anal furunculosis. The lower carriage of the tail in affected dogs may provide the necessary environment for worsening inflammation and infection.

Clinical presentation

Clinical signs include a painfully ulcerated perineal region with perianal discharge (**Figure 8.118**) and associated tenesmus, dyschezia, hematochezia, and/or constipation. In severe cases, anorexia, weight loss, and behavioral changes may be observed. Intensive perianal licking may be an early sign.

Differential diagnosis

Anal sac abscessation, perianal tumor, bite wound, or other traumatic injury.

Diagnosis

Thorough examination of the perianal area may be difficult without sedation. The perineum should be cleaned to appreciate the extent of the disease process. The anus and rectum should be evaluated in detail, as they may be involved as well.

Management

Immunosuppression with cyclosporine (5 mg/kg PO q12–24h for 1–3 months) is effective in 60–98% of cases but can be costly in large dogs. Concurrent use of ketoconazole, an inhibitor of cytochrome P450 enzymes, to increase the half-life of cyclosporine is not recommended because combination therapy results in unpredictable and often subtherapeutic cyclosporine levels. Immunosuppressive doses of prednisone (at least 2 mg/kg PO q24h) only help in one-third of cases. The effect of other immunosuppressive drugs has not been evaluated. Medical treatment followed by surgery (excision of remaining tracts, anal sacculectomy) is associated with a lower risk of recurrence. A significant number of dogs with anal furunculosis have concurrent adverse reaction to food, and feeding an elimination novel-protein or hydrolyzed diet may contribute to decreasing the recurrence rate.

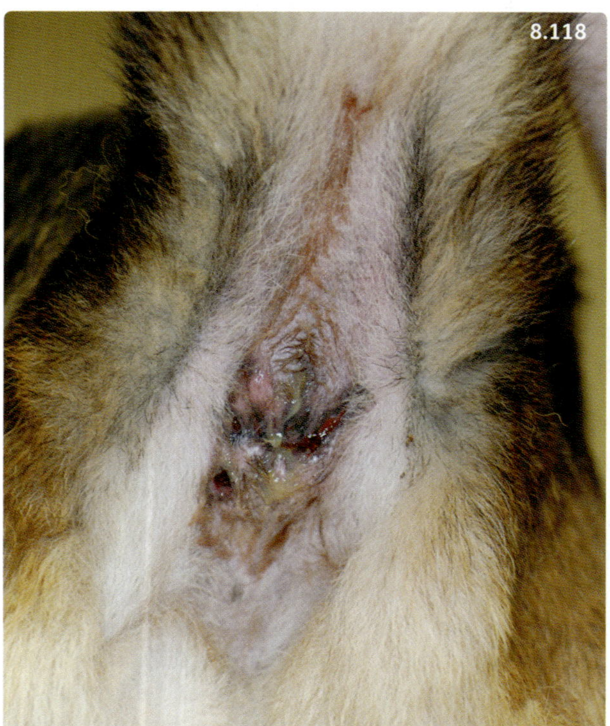

Figure 8.118 View of the cleaned and clipped perianal area of an 8-year-old female spayed German Shepherd Dog with anal furunculosis. Note several fistulous tracts oozing bloody or purulent exudate. (Courtesy LSU SVM Dermatology Service)

Prognosis

Overall guarded. Recurrence is common. Anal sphincter incompetence and fecal incontinence are well known complications of surgery.

PERINEAL HERNIA

Definition/overview

Perineal hernia results from weakness and breakdown of the pelvic diaphragm, with deviation and herniation of the rectum (and, possibly, the urinary bladder, prostate, and small intestine) into the perineum. The pelvic diaphragm consists of the levator ani and coccygeus muscles and the perineal fascia.

Etiology

The condition occurs in middle aged intact male dogs. Predisposed breeds include Pekingese, Boston Terrier, Welsh Corgi, Boxer, Poodle, Bouvier, and Old English Sheepdog. It is occasionally seen in cats as a surgical complication of perineal urethrostomy or colectomy.

Pathophysiology

The exact pathophysiology is unknown, and the disease is most likely multifactorial. The existence of rectal abnormalities (dilation, diverticulum), androgens, gender-related anatomic differences, relaxin (a hormone synthesized in the prostate), prostatic disease, and neurogenic atrophy have all been associated with perineal hernia in dogs.

Clinical presentation

Typical presenting signs include reducible perineal swelling (**Figure 8.119**), tenesmus, dyschezia, and constipation. The disease can be unilateral (if so, the right side is more commonly affected) or bilateral. Rectal examination reveals a defect in the pelvic diaphragm surrounding the rectum. If the bladder is retroflexed, dogs may not be able to void urine and develop postrenal azotemia with associated signs such as vomiting, anorexia, and lethargy.

Differential diagnosis

Perineal tumor.

Diagnosis

History and clinical signs are usually sufficient. Survey and contrast radiographs (**Figures 8.120, 8.121**) or ultrasonography (**Figure 8.122**) are necessary to confirm retroflexion of the urinary bladder or other organs. CBC, serum chemistry, and urinalysis are useful to evaluate kidney function.

Management

Medical management, consisting of maintaining a soft fecal consistency with laxatives such as lactulose (0.5 ml/kg PO q8–12h) or a bulk-forming agent such as psyllium (**Box 8.10**), and occasional enemas, may be successful in the short term with mild cases. However, most cases require surgical treatment. Herniorrhaphy using the internal obturator transposition technique is usually successful. (See surgery textbooks for further details.)

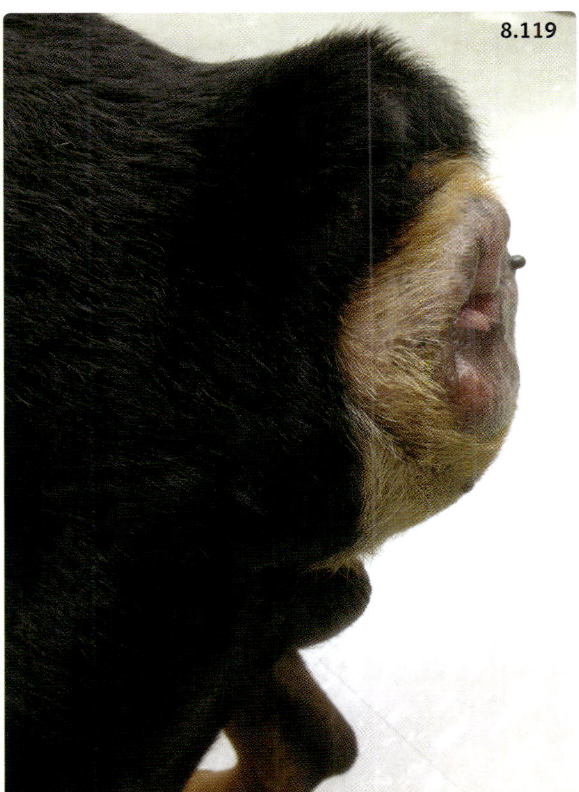

Figure 8.119 Severe bilateral perineal hernia in a 10-year-old intact male Rottweiler.

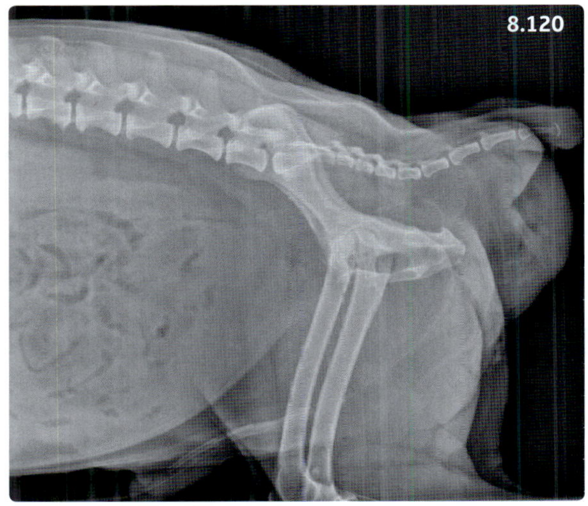

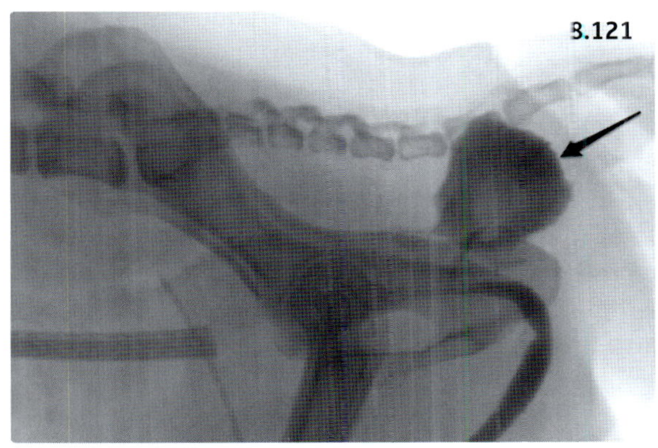

Figures 8.120, 8.121 Another dog with a perineal hernia. (8.120) Caudal abdominal radiograph. A large soft tissue mass representing the hernia can be seen in the perineum. The urinary bladder is not visible in the caudal abdomen. (8.121) Positive contrast retrograde urethrocystography. The bladder is retroflexed in the perineal hernia. (Courtesy L. Gaschen)

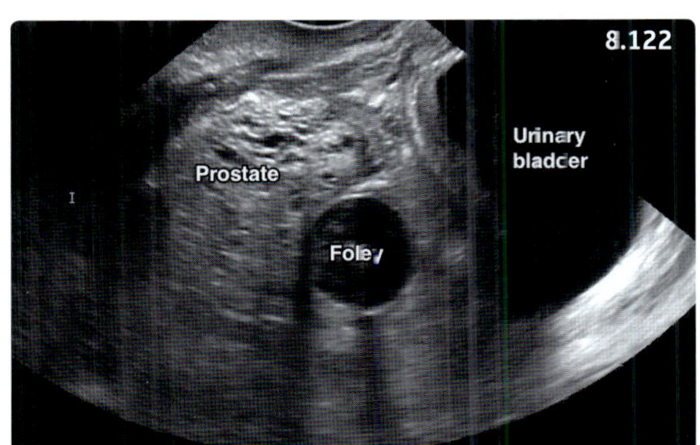

Figure 8.122 Ultrasound image of the dog in Figure 8.119. The prostate and urinary bladder are retroflexed in the retroperitoneal space. The balloon of a Foley catheter passed into the bladder is visible. Orientation: left is cranial; right is caudal.

Surgical complications include seroma, wound infection, fecal incontinence, and sciatic nerve paralysis.

Prognosis

Good if the hernia can be repaired early, guarded in dogs with chronic perineal hernia. In the latter group, recurrence is frequent and repeat surgical intervention is often challenging.

PERINEAL TUMORS

Definition/overview

The perianal region of dogs contains perianal (or circumanal) glands that are located in the dermis in a circular pattern around the anus. Perianal adenomas are the most common perianal tumors, while perianal adenocarcinomas occur considerably less frequently.

Etiology

Perianal adenomas are sex hormone dependent and occur mostly in middle aged to older males. Cocker Spaniels, Beagles, Bulldogs, and Samoyeds may be predisposed. Adenocarcinomas are not influenced by sex hormones and occur in neutered or intact male and female dogs.

Clinical presentation

Adenomas are slow growing, single, multiple or diffuse nonpainful masses located around the anus or on the perineum, and occasionally also on the prepuce, scrotum, and tailhead. Adenocarcinomas grow faster and may be similar to adenomas, but may be more firm, adhere to underlying tissues, and become ulcerated.

Differential diagnosis

Differentiating adenoma from adenocarcinoma is challenging, but important, as more aggressive treatment is required for the malignant perineal tumor. Detection of metastases is strongly indicative of adenocarcinoma.

Diagnosis

Signalment, history, and physical examination are suggestive. Cytologic evaluation of a fine needle aspirate reveals typical sebaceous cells that resemble hepatocytes. However, cytology does not allow reliable differentiation between adenoma and adenocarcinoma.

Management

Adenoma: castration and conservative surgical removal. Adenocarcinoma: wide excision of the primary tumor and affected lymph nodes. Postoperative radiation therapy may be useful. Inoperable cancers may benefit from palliative radiation treatment and chemotherapy.

Prognosis

Adenoma: excellent, low risk of recurrence after excision if the dog is neutered. Adenocarcinoma: removal at an early stage (diameter less than 5 cm) is associated with good survival.

RECOMMENDED FURTHER READING

Ettinger SJ, Feldman EC (2010) (eds) *Textbook of Veterinary Internal Medicine*, 7th edn. Saunders Elsevier, St. Louis.

Little SE (2012) (ed) *The Cat. Clinical Medicine and Management*. Elsevier Saunders, St. Louis.

Nelson RW, Couto CG (2014) (eds) *Small Animal Internal Medicine*, 5th edn. Sauders Elsevier, St. Louis.

Washabau RJ, Day MJ (2013) (eds) *Canine and Feline Gastroenterology*. Elsevier Saunders, St. Louis.

Withrow SJ, Vail DM, Page RL (2013) (eds) *Withrow and MacEwen's Small Animal Clinical Oncology*, 5th edn. Elsevier Saunders, St. Louis.

Chapter 9

Liver disorders

Joseph Taboada

INTRODUCTION

Hepatology (the study of the liver and the diseases that affect it) remains a particularly frustrating area in small animal internal medicine because the liver is involved in hundreds of metabolic processes and can be involved with a variety of pathologic and pathophysiologic changes. Fortunately, the liver has a remarkable functional reserve; in some cases as much as 70–80% of the functional liver mass must be impaired before signs of dysfunction become apparent and, under the right circumstances, the liver is capable of regenerating significant functional capacity over relatively short periods of time.

Alterations in the normal metabolic processes result in many of the clinical findings in animals with liver disease. Some of these important metabolic processes include: normal metabolism of lipids, protein, carbohydrate, vitamins, and minerals; bile acid synthesis and excretion; protein production; detoxification and excretion of many endogenous and exogenous substances; production of urea from ammonia; drug metabolism and excretion; managing translocated bacteria and bacterial products, coagulation, and reticuloendothelial function. Abnormalities of normal protein production and bilirubin metabolism can be especially significant determinants of clinical signs. Impaired albumin synthesis may result in decreased plasma oncotic pressure, therefore edema or ascites and impaired synthesis of procoagulant clotting proteins and anticoagulants may result in bleeding or thrombosis. Cholestasis may result in jaundice.

Despite the importance of the liver in normal metabolism, early diagnosis of liver disease is often impaired by the nonspecific nature of the typical clinical signs and by a paucity of findings at physical examination. Typically, animals with liver disease present with lethargy, anorexia, weight loss, and other nonspecific clinical signs. Signs referable to the gastrointestinal (GI) tract such as vomiting and diarrhea are also common. Vomiting is an important yet nonspecific finding, especially in cats. Either large or small bowel diarrhea may be noted, especially in dogs or in cats with concurrent intestinal or pancreatic disease. Diarrhea is a less common finding than vomiting. Abdominal pain may be noted in animals with acute liver diseases or in patients with concurrent or associated pancreatitis or peritonitis.

Neurologic manifestations of liver disease are common in animals with either congenital or acquired portosystemic shunts (PSSs) or acute fulminating hepatic failure. The signs associated with hepatoencephalopathy are generally those of central nervous system (CNS) depression or overt signs of cerebral and diencephalic dysfunction (**Figure 9.1**). Depression, behavioral changes, ataxia, central blindness, circling, head pressing, pacing, panting, stupor, coma, and seizures may be noted. Seizures are most common in animals with PSSs, especially following attempted surgical correction. Cats with

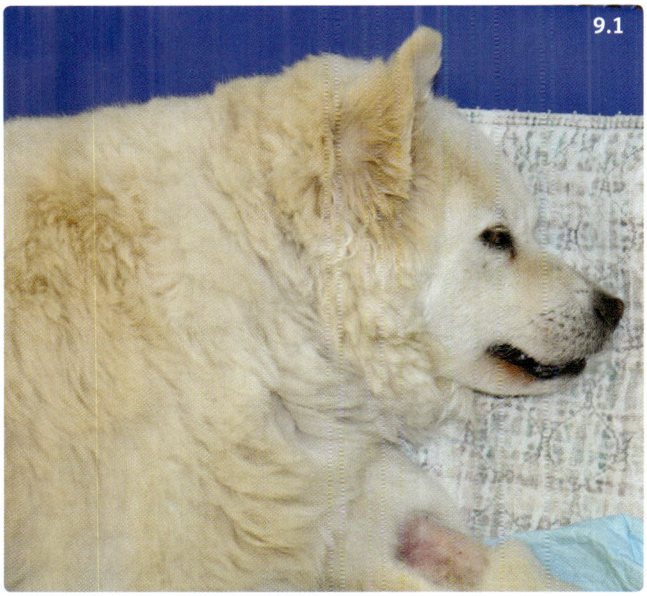

Figure 9.1 A terminally ill dog in an hepatic coma caused by fulminating hepatic lipidosis. Gross pathology and histopathology of this dog's liver showed marked hepatic lipidosis.

hepatoencephalopathy tend to have signs that are more difficult to ascribe to the CNS. Anorexia, CNS depression, and ptyalism are often noted in cats with liver disease and may not be attributed to the influence of hepatotoxins on the CNS, thus leading to underutilization of appropriate medical therapy for hepatoencephalopathy in this species.

Cholestasis resulting in icterus is common in animals with liver disease, but it may not be severe enough to be noted at physical examination early in the disease process. Posthepatic biliary disease, pancreatitis, and hemolytic anemia are also important causes of icterus. Animals with severe liver disease may not produce or normally activate procoagulant clotting factors, resulting in overt bleeding tendencies. GI bleeding is common. Nonspecific signs of anemia may be noted if bleeding is low grade and chronic, or melena may be obvious if bleeding is severe. Ecchymotic hemorrhage may be apparent. Platelet membrane abnormalities associated with changes in lipoprotein metabolism may result in thrombopathia or decrease platelet half-life and thus cause thrombocytopenia with resultant petechia. Changes in anticoagulant protein production may result in thrombosis or thromboembolism. The disrupted balance between bleeding and thrombosis in liver disease can be clinically very confusing.

Unless the patient is jaundiced or exhibits overt signs of encephalopathy or ascites, clinicopathologic abnormalities are frequently the first indicator of liver disease. Increased transaminase activities or increased activities of enzymes indicative of cholestasis are the earliest indicators of liver disease in most cases. Alanine aminotransferase (ALT) and aspartate transaminase (AST) activities are sensitive indicators of liver insult in both dogs and cats, while increased alkaline phosphatase (ALP) and gamma-glutamyltransferase (GGT) activities are indicative of cholestasis. Hypoalbuminemia may indicate decreased hepatic function, as can decreased blood urea nitrogen (BUN) and hypoglycemia. These biochemical indicators are not specific for decreased hepatic function, so more specific tests such as fasting and postprandial bile acids or plasma ammonia concentrations are often evaluated when hepatic dysfunction is suspected. Unfortunately, biochemical recognition of primary hepatic disease is complicated by the fact that disorders that involve the liver secondarily (reactive hepatopathies), as well as certain drugs, can cause abnormal liver test results. In addition to liver tests, radiology, ultrasonography, cross-sectional imaging, and cytologic and histologic examination of liver tissue are employed in the evaluation of the hepatobiliary system.

FELINE HEPATIC LIPIDOSIS

Definition/overview

Feline hepatic lipidosis is a syndrome that can be either a primary idiopathic condition or secondary to a variety of common diseases of cats. Hepatic lipidosis is the most common liver disease of the cat, accounting for approximately 50% of diagnoses. The disorder accounts for approximately 10% of liver related deaths. Other names include feline fatty liver syndrome, steatosis, and fatty liver.

Etiology

A variety of factors have been proposed as potential etiologies, none of which has been confirmed. A multifactoral pathogenesis leading to malnutrition is likely. The major risk factor is obesity and a prolonged reduction of food intake, but obesity is not universally present in affected cats. Anorexia may be caused by concurrent disease, dietary change, or decreased food intake. Environmental stress is potentially an additional important risk factor. Changes in the intestinal microbiome may play an important role.

Pathophysiology

The exact pathogenesis remains to be defined. Decreased caloric intake causes a negative nitrogen balance. Fatty acids are mobilized from tissue stores and transported to the liver. Decreased protein metabolism and amino acid availability means that there is insufficient apoprotein to facilitate removal of fatty acids and fat accumulates in the hepatocytes. Histologically, >80% of hepatocytes will be heavily vacuolated with triglyceride. This decreases the ability of the cell to function and liver function slowly decreases.

Clinical presentation

Most affected animals are 2 years old or older. Cats with secondary hepatic lipidosis tend to be older than cats with idiopathic hepatic lipidosis. There is no apparent breed or gender predisposition, but older females seem to be more at risk. Affected cats are commonly obese and/or have experienced a stressful event of some type (e.g. a change in environment or concurrent disease). This is followed by anorexia and rapid weight loss or muscle wasting. Anorexia persists and the cat is presented for veterinary evaluation usually between 1 and 3 weeks after onset. Jaundice develops in most cats and is usually evident on presentation to a veterinarian.

At examination cats are depressed, dehydrated, and icteric (**Figure 9.2**) and show varying degrees of muscle

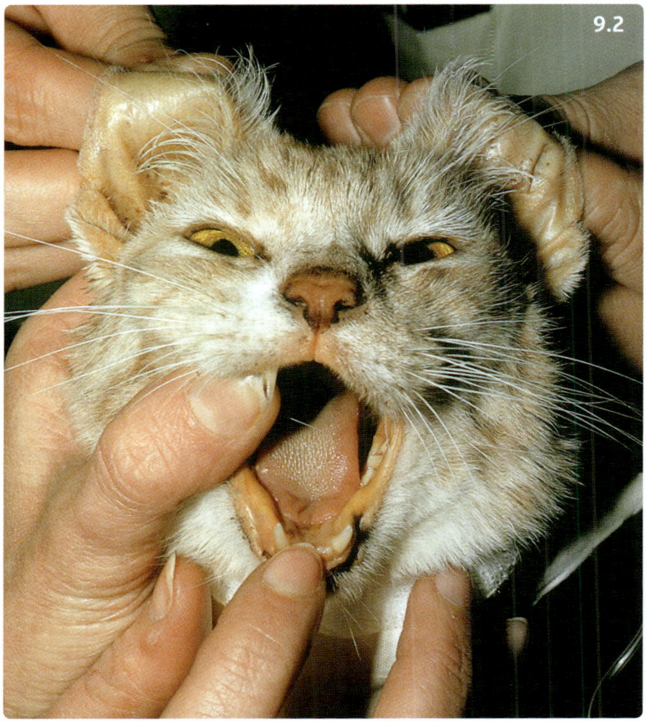

Figure 9.2 Jaundice in a cat with hepatic lipidosis. (Courtesy M. Schaer)

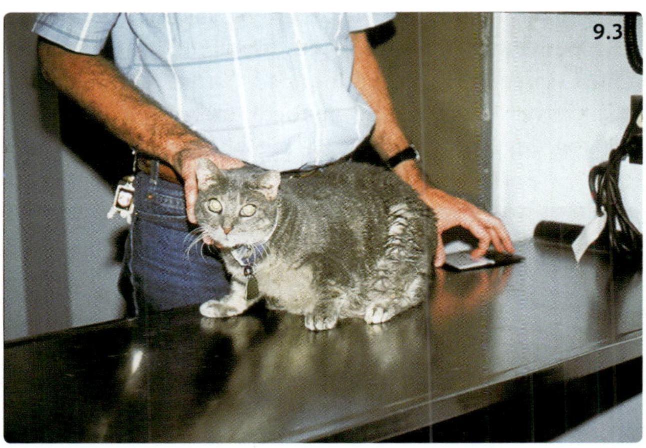

Figure 9.3 Marked subcutaneous fat pads in a cat with hepatic lipidosis. (Courtesy M. Schaer)

wasting. However, fat pads remain intact, reflecting the cat's inability to mobilize fat in this disease and the marked muscle breakdown for gluconeogenesis (**Figures 9.3**, **9.4**). Hepatic encephalopathy (**Figure 9.5**) may be related to severe hepatocellular dysfunction or to a relative deficiency of arginine, to which the anorexic cat is predisposed (cats cannot synthesize arginine and must rely on dietary sources). Abdominal palpation may reveal hepatomegaly that is smooth surfaced.

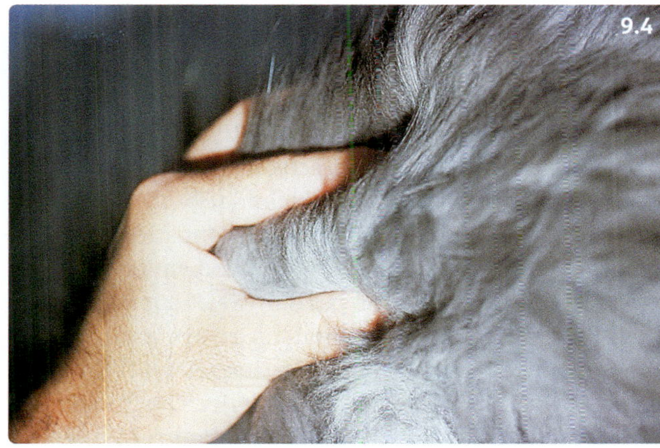

Figure 9.4 Marked muscle wasting along the back of a cat with hepatic lipidosis.

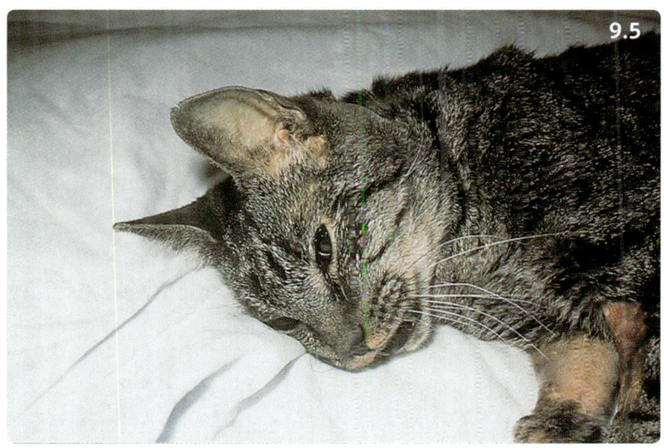

Figure 9.5 A Domestic Shorthair cat with hepatic encephalopathy associated with hepatic lipidosis. (Courtesy M. Schaer)

Differential diagnosis

Idiopathic hepatic lipidosis, secondary hepatic lipidosis, pancreatitis, inflammatory bowel disease (IBD), feline infectious peritonitis (FIP), hepatic lymphoma, cholangitis, liver flukes, biliary neoplasia.

Diagnosis

Diagnosis is based on hepatic cytology or histologic examination of a liver biopsy specimen. Typical laboratory findings are those of cholestasis; total bilirubin values range from normal (5 µmol/l [0.3 mg/dl]) to 256.5 µmol/l (15 mg/dl) or higher. There is usually a mild nonregenerative anemia.

Poikilocytosis is common and target cells may be noted. Liver enzyme activities are increased; ALT is normal or moderately increased (50–450 IU/l), AST is normal or moderately increased (50–450 IU/l), and ALP is occasionally normal but usually moderately to markedly increased (75–1,200 IU/l). Albumin and globulin concentrations are usually normal. Fasting serum bile acid concentrations are above normal (0.75–5.6 µmol/l [0.3–2.3 µg/ml]) in most cats, but it should be noted that measurement of serum bile acids is considered redundant if hyperbilirubinemia is present, as it is in most affected cats. Glucose may be increased due to stress. Hypokalemia is often present. Greater than 50% of cats will have prolongation of PIVKA (proteins induced by vitamin K antagonism or absence), prothrombin time (PT), or partial thromboplastin time (PTT), but overt bleeding tendencies are rare. Of the commonly used coagulation screening tests, PIVKA is the one most likely to detect an abnormality. Coagulopathies associated with hepatic lipidosis are often responsive to vitamin K1.

Abdominal radiographs may reveal hepatomegaly. Ultrasonographic examination of the liver and surrounding structures allows other diseases in the differential diagnosis, such as cholangitis and extrahepatic bile duct obstruction, to be ruled out. The principal ultrasonographic feature of hepatic lipidosis is hyperechogenicity.

Tissue diagnosis can be made by aspiration cytology in some patients, but in others it is achieved by fine needle percutaneous biopsy (**Figure 9.6**), laparoscopy (**Figure 9.7**), or by exploratory laparotomy. Specimens are placed in buffered 10% formalin, in which they usually float.

Management

The mainstay of therapy is complete nutritional support and treatment of known concurrent illness. Protein should not be restricted unless severe signs of hepatoencephalopathy are present and cannot be controlled by other means. Adequate caloric support (80–100 kcal/kg/day) is critical and can rarely be accomplished without enteral support. Food is best administered through an esophagostomy or gastrostomy tube. Nasoesophageal feeding can be used, but the long-term nature of the enteral nutritional support needed makes this a less than ideal delivery method. Feeding tubes should be left in place until the cat is eating on its own. This may take months in some cats. Parenteral treatment with vitamin K1 (0.5–1.5 mg/kg IM) should be administered approximately 12 hours prior to biopsy. Fluids with potassium supplementation are important until an enteral feeding method is established. Serum phosphorus should be monitored closely during the initial 48 hours after starting enteral feeding. Re-feeding-induced hypophosphatemia is common and, if severe, may result in hemolysis or signs of CNS dysfunction that might be confused with hepatoencephalopathy. Careful administration of parenteral phosphate supplementation may be necessary during this period. B vitamins have been recommended in the management of cats with hepatic lipidosis. Soluble multi-B vitamin supplements have been recommended as additives to fluids used in the initial management of cats with hepatic lipidosis. Thiamine and cobalamin have both been implicated in the potential pathogenesis. Serum cobalamin has been noted to be low in cats with hepatic lipidosis, especially those with concurrent pancreatitis or IBD, and supplementation (1 mg IM q1–4weeks) is recommended. Other supplements that have been recommended include L-carnitine (250 mg/day PO), vitamin E (10 mg/kg/day PO), and SAMe

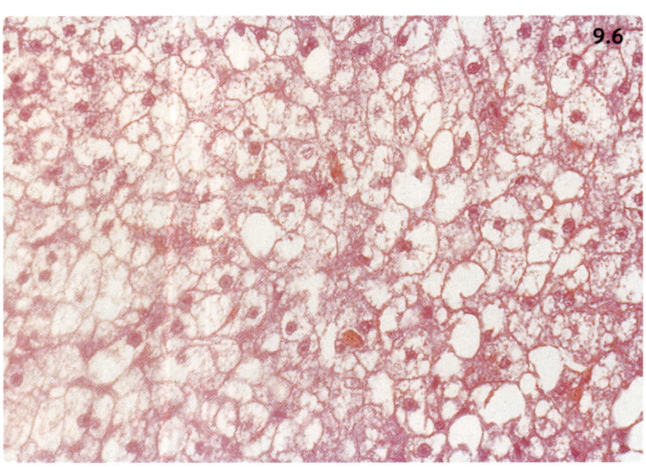

Figure 9.6 Histologic appearance of the liver in feline hepatic lipidosis. Note the empty hepatocytes, which contained fat removed during the fixing process.

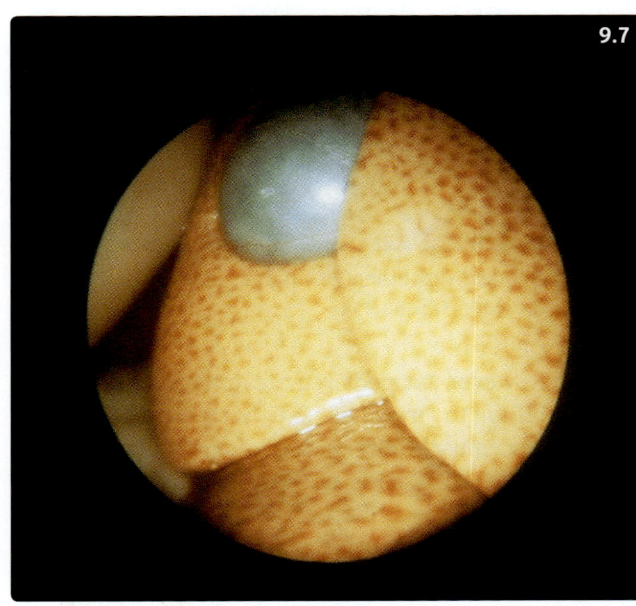

Figure 9.7 Laparoscopic view of the liver of a cat with hepatic lipidosis. Note the fatty liver and distended gallbladder.

(20 mg/kg PO q12h). Efforts should be made to correct any sources of psychological stress that may have triggered the initial anorexia.

The prognosis for cats with idiopathic hepatic lipidosis treated with adequate nutritional support is good. From 75% to >90% of cats will respond completely to therapy. Relapse is rare. If secondary hepatic lipidosis is present, the prognosis is dependent on the underlying disease. Less than 10% of cats with hepatic lipidosis will recover if adequate nutritional support is not maintained.

FELINE INFLAMMATORY LIVER DISEASE

Definition/overview

Chlolangitis is a complex of related inflammatory hepatobiliary disorders that accounts for approximately 25% of the liver diseases in cats. The WSAVA Liver Standardization Group has proposed a nomenclature system that recognizes three distinct forms of cholangitis in cats: neutrophilic, lymphocytic, and cholangitis associated with liver flukes (**Figures 9.8a–c**). The neutrophilic form is subdivided into an acute (neutrophilic infiltrate) and a chronic (mixed infiltrate) form. The term cholangitis has been recommended in preference to cholangiohepatitis.

Etiology

Inflammatory liver diseases are characterized by the predominant inflammatory cell infiltrate seen histopathologically. The inflammation is usually seen in the portal areas and can be characterized as suppurative (neutrophilic) (**Figure 9.9**), nonsuppurative (lymphocytic–plasmacytic) (**Figures 9.10–9.12**), or biliary cirrhosis (fibrosis). Cholangitis is the primary finding, with extension of the inflammation across the limiting plate into the surrounding hepatic parenchyma and periportal necrosis being common. Whether these classifications represent different stages in the progression of one disease, or are separate etiologic entities, is not known, nor is the underlying etiology of inflammatory liver disease in cats.

Pathophysiology

Bacterial, allergic, and immune mechanisms have all been speculated to be involved in the pathogenesis of inflammatory liver disease in cats. Bacterial cholangitis from ascending infection from the duodenum may either initiate the inflammatory process or perpetuate it early in the disease course. Immune mechanisms probably also play a role, especially in lymphocytic cholangitis and chronic mixed cholangitis. Cats with cholangitis, especially those with suppurative disease, may also have

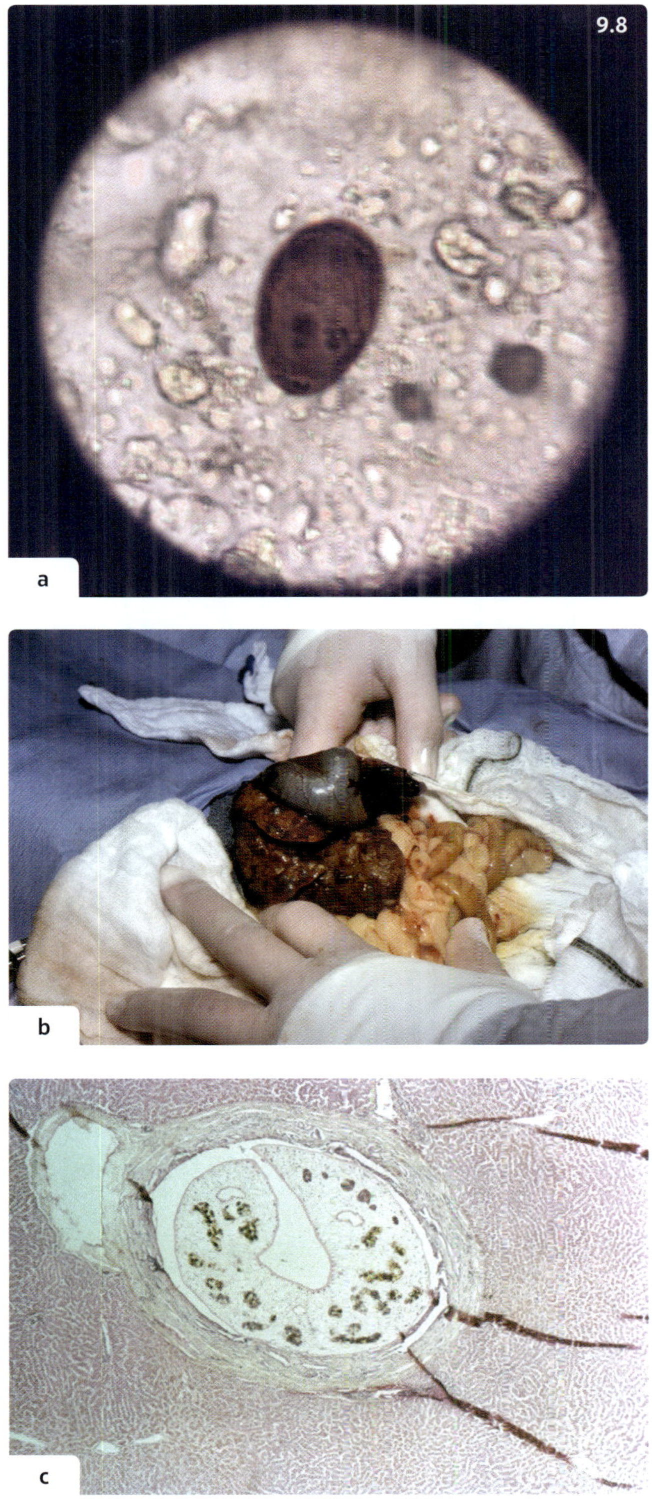

Figures 9.8a–c Liver fluke. (a) Microscopic view of a liver fluke (*Platynosum concinum*) ovum from a cat living in South Florida. (b) Surgical view of liver fluke-induced chronic cholangitis in a cat living in North Central Florida. (c) Histopathology section of liver fluke residing in a bile duct causing inflammation and fibrosis. Taken from the cat in 9.8b. (Courtesy M. Schaer)

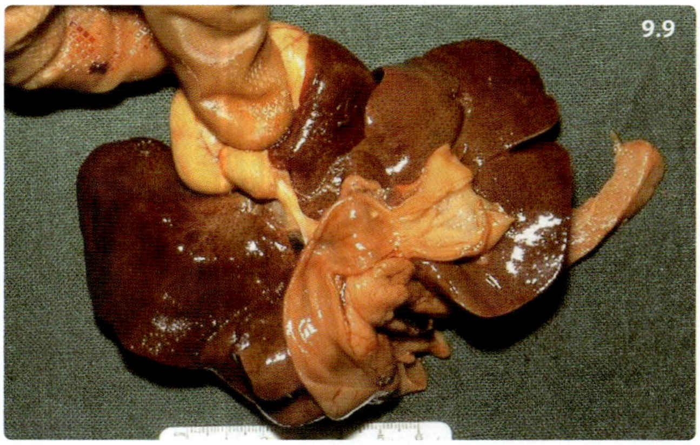

Figure 9.9 Postmortem view of the liver of a cat with suppurative cholangitis and cholecystitis. The cystic duct was obstructed by inspissated bile. (Courtesy M. Schaer)

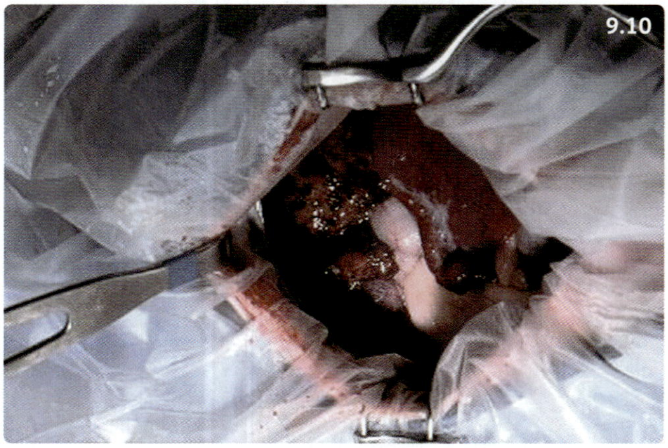

Figure 9.10 Surgical exploratory on a cat with chronic lymphocytic–plasmacytic hepatitis with telangiectasia. (Courtesy M. Schaer)

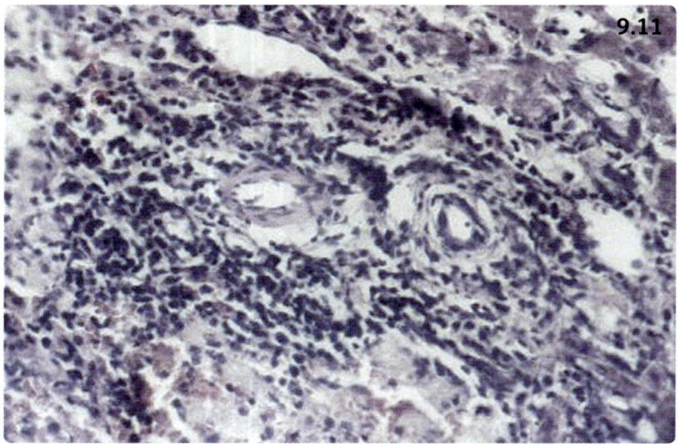

Figure 9.11 Photomicrograph of the specimen in Figure 9.10 showing marked periportal lymphocytic–plasmacytic infiltrates. (Courtesy M. Schaer)

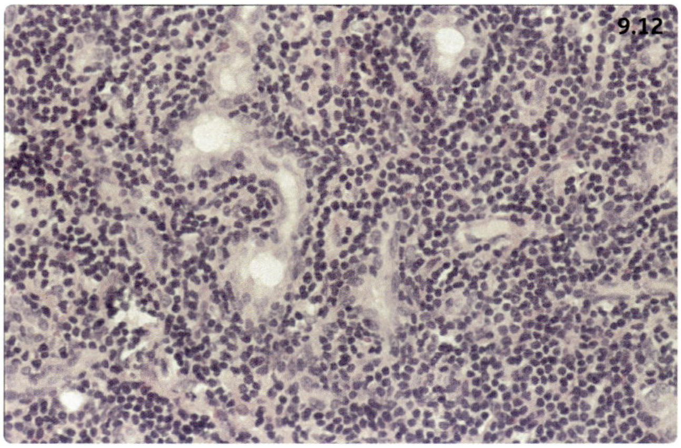

Figure 9.12 High-power photomicrograph of lymphocytic–plasmacytic cholangitis in a cat. (Courtesy M. Schaer)

concurrent cholecystitis, pancreatitis, and IBD. The relationship between these three inflammatory conditions is not well characterized, but it has been speculated that the underlying initiator of the inflammatory process may affect the liver, the pancreas, and the small intestine concurrently. The term 'triaditis' has been coined to describe those situations in which inflammation of the liver, pancreas, and small intestine are seen to occur concurrently.

Clinical presentation

The clinical findings seen in cats with inflammatory liver disease are similar to those seen with hepatic lipidosis and other liver diseases. Vomiting, anorexia, lethargy, and weight loss are typical. Fever is occasionally seen. Diarrhea, while not usual, is more common than in cats with hepatic lipidosis and may represent that subset of cats with concurrent IBD. Affected cats are rarely obese. A mild ascites may be present (**Figure 9.13**). Cats with suppurative cholangitis are more likely to be severely systemically ill when compared with cats with lymphocytic cholangitis. Cats of all ages can be affected. Males predominate in populations of cats with suppurative cholangitis compared with those with lymphocytic cholangitis. Suppurative cholangitis often has an acute course, while disease characterized by lymphocytic–plasmacytic inflammation may be more chronic. In evaluating liver enzymes, ALP tends not to be as elevated as in cats with hepatic lipidosis, while ASDT, ALP, and GGT activities tend to be higher. About 50% of cats will have high serum bilirubin concentrations. Neutrophil counts, transaminase activities, and total bilirubin concentrations tend to be higher in cats with suppurative cholangitis when compared with cats with lymphocytic cholangitis.

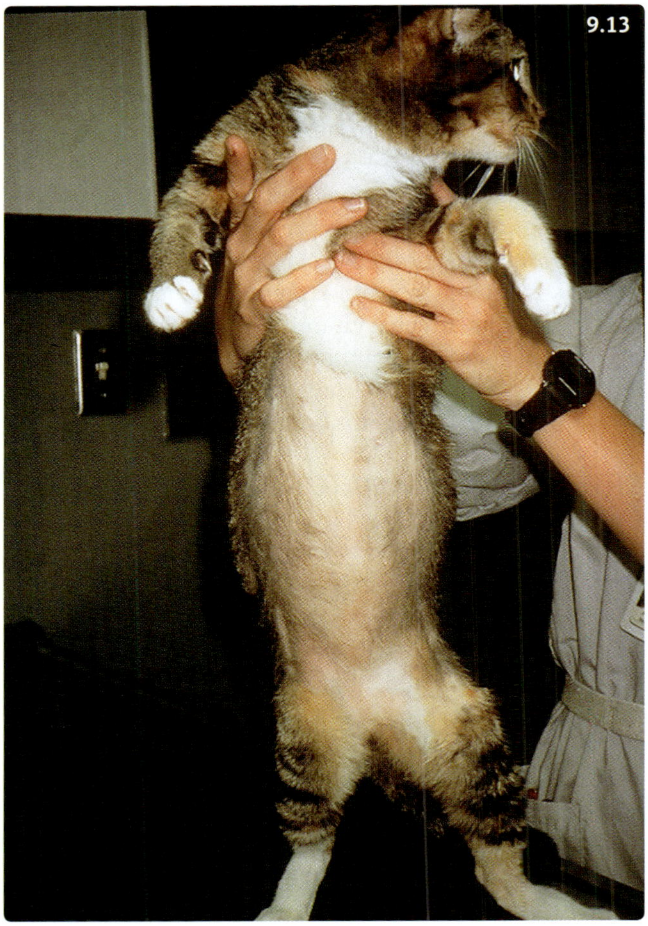

Figure 9.13 Mild abdominal distension caused by a sterile inflammatory exudate in a cat with cholangitis.

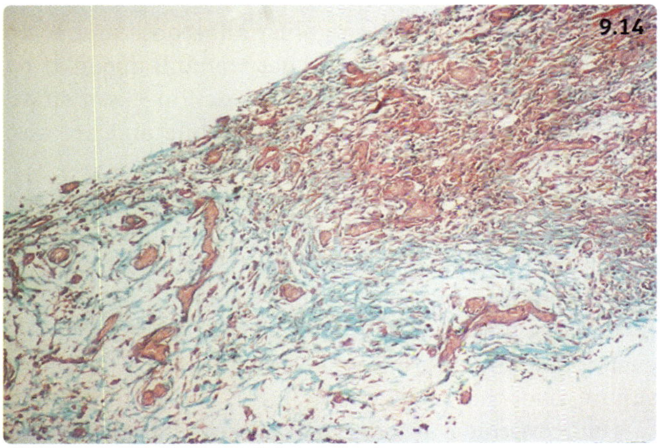

Figure 9.14 Low-power view of a trichrome-stained needle biopsy specimen from the cat in Figure 9.13. There is marked hepatic fibrosis (blue staining) in addition to inflammatory cells.

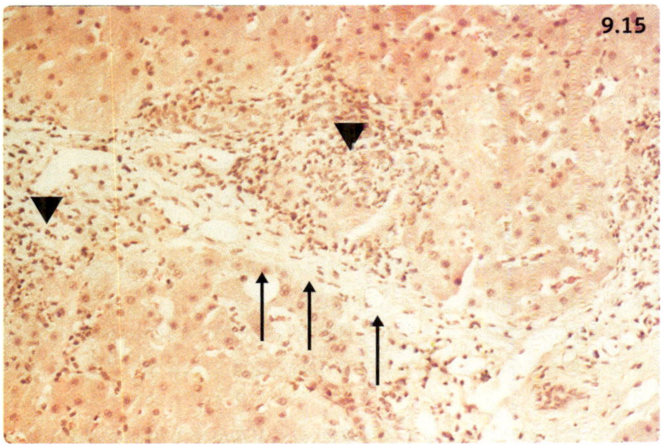

Figure 9.15 Histologic appearance of the liver in a 4-year-old Persian cat with cholangitis. There is marked fibrosis (arrows) and an infiltrate of plasma cells and lymphocytes (arrowheads).

However, all liver enzymes may be normal early in the course of disease.

Differential diagnosis

As for hepatic lipidosis.

Diagnosis

Diagnosis is usually dependent on histopathology, as cytology is often normal or reveals nonspecific changes. Biopsy for both histopathology and culture should be performed if inflammatory liver disease is suspected. The advent of readily available ultrasonography has resulted in needle biopsy becoming the most popular method of obtaining tissue for histopathology (**Figures 9.14**, **9.15**). Ultrasonography can also provide important information pertaining to co-existing cholecystitis. However, the diagnostic accuracy of needle obtained biopsies has been questioned. Laparoscopically or surgically obtained 'wedge' samples should be considered for histopathology and bacterial culture and sensitivity when feasible; the larger samples give the pathologist more tissue to assess (**Figure 9.16**, biopsy comparison). Prior to biopsy, coagulation parameters should be evaluated. As in cats with hepatic lipidosis, PIVKA may be the most sensitive indicator of potential bleeding tendencies. Vitamin K1 (0.5–1.5 mg/kg SC) given 12–24 hours prior to biopsy may decrease the risk of bleeding. Culture of aspirated bile may be a more sensitive indicator of bacterial infection than culture of biopsy specimens.

Management

In addition to the supportive care and nutritional support important in the management of cats with hepatic lipidosis, antibiotics effective against gram-negative and/or anaerobic bacteria should be used when treating cats with inflammatory liver disease. This is probably most important when treating suppurative cholangitis.

Metronidazole is effective against anaerobes and some gram-negative aerobes and it has immune modulating effects. Ampicillin, amoxicillin, amoxicillin–clavulanate, and enrofloxacin are excreted in the bile and are also good choices.

Immunosuppressive agents should be added to the treatment regimen in cats with lymphocytic or mixed inflammatory disease and in cats with suppurative disease that fail to respond to antibiotics alone. Prednisolone (2–4 mg/kg/day initially then slowly tapered to 1 mg/kg every other day) is used most commonly. Other immunosuppressives that may be used in cats responding poorly to glucocorticoids include chlorambucil (approximately 1 mg for cats <3.2 kg, 2 mg for cats >3.2 kg, PO q48h) and oral cyclosporine. Ursodeoxycholic acid (10–15 mg/kg PO q24h) is a safe treatment alternative that can be used in cats with suppurative or nonsuppurative disease. The drug appears to have multiple actions including shifting the bile acid pool to a less toxic hydrophilic population, a choleretic effect, reducing expression of class 2 major histocompatibility complex, and an anti-inflammatory effect. Bile duct patency is required before using ursodeoxycholic acid. Since the drug is commercially available in a 300 mg capsule size in the USA, accurate dosing of ursodeoxycholic acid for a cat can be prepared by a compounding pharmacist.

Antioxidants are important in the management of liver diseases as oxidative damage appears to be an important factor in perpetuation of inflammation and initiation of fibrosis. Vitamin E (aqueous alpha tocopherol, 10–100 IU/kg/day) has been advocated for its antioxidant effects. SAMe (90–180 mg PO q24h) is a precursor of glutathione. Glutathione is an important antioxidant that has been shown to be reduced in dogs and cats with liver disease. The nutraceutical SAMe may help replace glutathione. It also may have hepatoprotective effects in preventing programed cell death (apoptosis), which occurs during inflammatory liver disease. Milk thistle extract (silymarin) is a nutraceutical that is widely used for its hepatoprotective effects. It may be of benefit as an antioxidant, as an antifibrotic agent, or as an aid in hepatic regeneration. The recommended dose is 50–200 mg/kg PO q24h. Two products containing silybin and vitamin E are marketed: Marin®, which is a combination of silybin and vitamin E plus zinc, and Marin® Plus, which contains silybin, vitamin E, zinc, medium chain triglyceride oil, and curcumin. Silybin is one of the active ingredients in milk thistle. Additionally, there is a product (Denamarin®) that contains both silybin and SAMe.

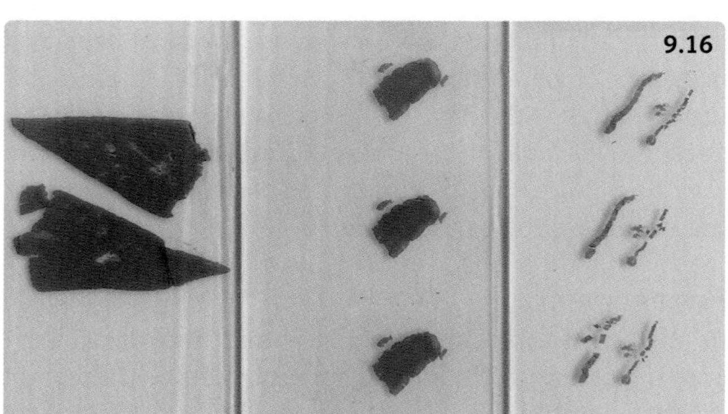

Figure 9.16 Sub-gross views of liver biopsy slides. Laparotomy liver wedge biopsy (left); laparoscopic liver wedge biopsy (middle); ultrasound guided Tru-cut liver biopsy (right). All stained with H&E stain (Courtesy J. Greene and I. Langohr)

CHRONIC INFLAMMATORY LIVER DISEASE IN DOGS

Definition/overview

The dog suffers from a variety of chronic inflammatory liver diseases (e.g. administration of primidone, phenytoin, and phenobarbital; abnormal copper metabolism in the Bedlington Terrier, West Highland White Terrier, Skye Terrier, Dalmatian, and Labrador Retriever; spontaneous and experimentally induced infectious canine hepatitis), often resulting in subsequent cirrhosis (**Table 9.1**). All have similar clinical signs. In the dog, chronic hepatitis (CH) (formerly chronic active hepatitis) has been associated with leptospirosis. A syndrome of CH has also been recognized in the Dobermann, Dalmatian, and American Cocker Spaniel. CH resulting in subsequent cirrhosis is rare in cats.

Etiology

Chronic inflammatory liver diseases have overlapping histologic appearances and are mostly of unknown etiology. Once started, the immune system, oxidative stress, and stellate cell activation with subsequent fibrosis play

Table 9.1 Inflammatory disorders of the canine liver.

- Chronic hepatitis: breed related (e.g. Dobermann, Cocker Spaniel, Labrador Retriever)
- Copper storage hepatopathy: Bedlington Terrier, West Highland White Terrier
- Chronic nonsuppurative hepatitis
- Chronic portal triaditis
- Chronic drug-induced hepatitis
- Chronic cholangiohepatitis
- Chronic cholangitis
- Chronic lobular hepatitis
- Lobular dissecting hepatitis
- Chronic major bile duct obstruction
- Idiopathic hepatic fibrosis

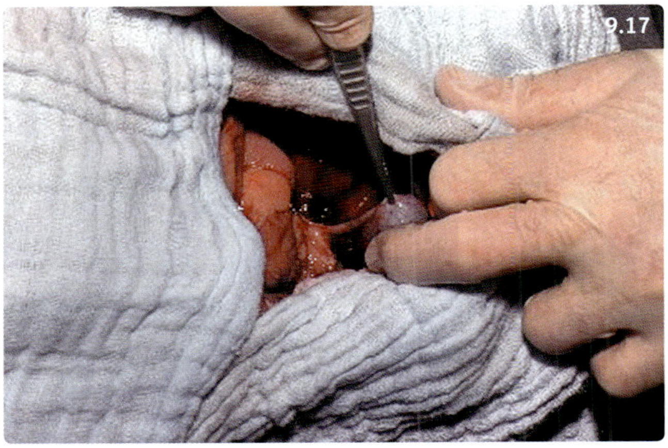

Figure 9.17 Surgical exploratory in a dog showing the gallbladder and parenchymal liver disease that turned out to be chronic lymphocytic–plasmacytic hepatitis on biopsy. (Courtesy M. Schaer)

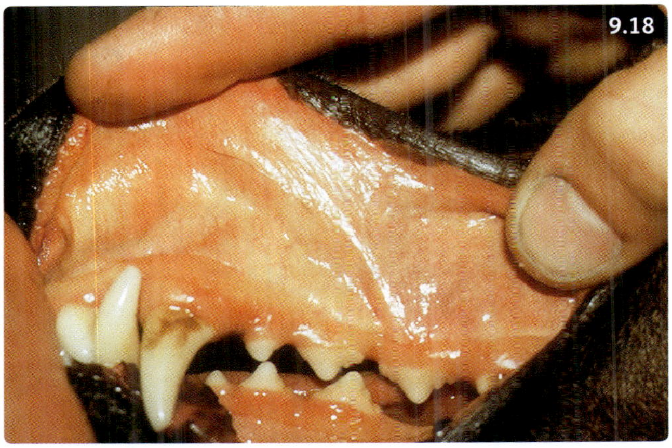

Figure 9.18 Icteric mucous membranes in a 5-year-old female spayed Dobermann with chronic hepatitis.

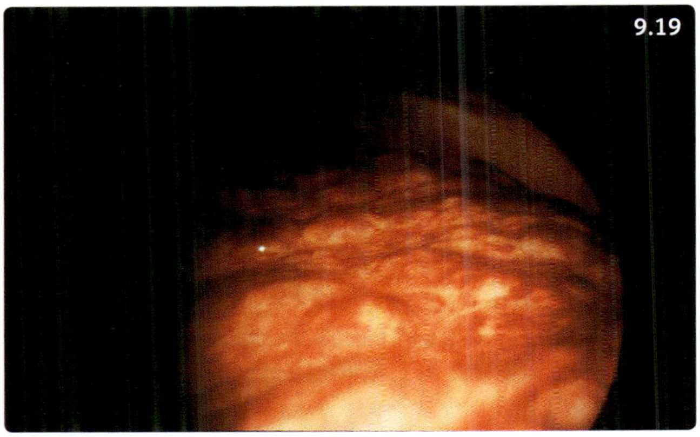

Figure 9.19 Laparoscopic view of regenerative nodules on the liver in a dog with chronic hepatitis

an important role in perpetuation of hepatocellular injury.

Pathophysiology

CH has many potential initiating insults but is often idiopathic. Unless the initiating insult is copper or bacterial infection, the histopathologic description will usually be that of chronic and active inflammation without an obvious etiology. CH (**Figure 9.17**) is characterized by continuing hepatic inflammation, necrosis, apoptosis, fibrosis, and regeneration. The immune system and oxidative injury play an important role in perpetuation of disease.

Clinical presentation

Clinical signs are nonspecific. Inappetence and lethargy are common complaints. Occasional vomiting, diarrhea, and pica may also be reported. Behavioral changes and other signs consistent with hepatoencephalopathy, ascites, and icterus may develop later in the course of disease (**Figure 9.18**). Signs may be chronic or appear acute with the disease often advanced before a diagnosis is made.

Differential diagnosis

Infections; vascular hepatopathy; drug-induced, familial, or lobular dissecting hepatitis.

Diagnosis

Chronic inflammatory liver disease is characterized histologically by hepatocellular apoptosis and necrosis, a variable mononuclear or mixed inflammatory cell infiltrate, regeneration, and fibrosis. More ominous histologic features suggestive of progression are implied when confluent areas of necrosis are identified that form zones of parenchymal collapse that bridge between portal triads and central veins or span lobules between portal triads. Chronic inflammatory liver disease should be suspected when recurrent slight to moderate increases of serum ALT, AST, and ALP activities are observed. Persistence of the chronic inflammatory process for months to years disrupts normal liver architecture (**Figure 9.19**) and the earlier biochemical pattern of 'low-grade' hepatocellular necrosis progresses to one of hepatic insufficiency. The waxing and waning nature of the changes in enzyme activities, as well as the potential for relatively insignificant increases late in the disease course, make chronic inflammatory liver disease sometimes difficult to detect biochemically. However, as the disease progresses, indicators of liver dysfunction, such as hypoalbuminemia, decreased BUN, and prolonged PT, are suggestive of advanced liver disease. Earlier indicators of liver insufficiency are hyperbilirubinemia, hyperammonemia, and increased serum bile acids. Disruption of clotting factor synthesis may result in bleeding, which

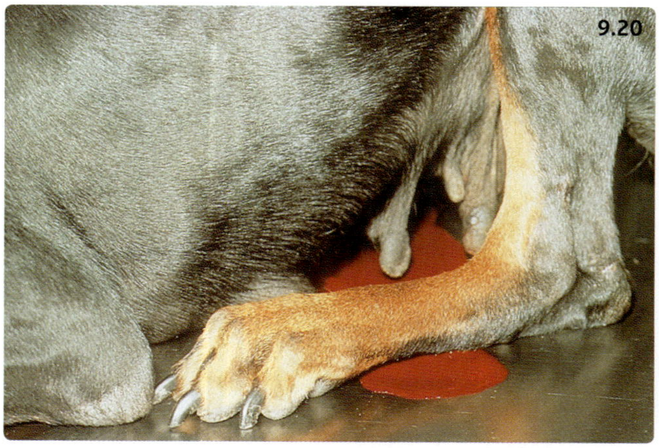

Figure 9.20 Bleeding from the skin after percutaneous liver biopsy in a Dobermann with advanced chronic hepatitis. Prebiopsy clotting studies had been normal.

is most often characterized by GI bleeding, resulting in melena or low-grade anemia (**Figure 9.20**). A hypercoagulable state may also be present, resulting in thrombosis of the portal vasculature. Histologic examination of a liver biopsy sample confirms the diagnosis (**Figures 9.21–9.23**).

Management

Specific treatment is unavailable in most cases and usually depends on the inciting cause. Supportive therapy includes vitamin E, ursodeoxycholic acid, SAMe, and silymarin. Anti-inflammatory or immunosuppressive therapy using prednisolone, cyclosporine, penicillamine, azathioprine, and/or colchicine may be useful.

HEPATIC ABSCESS

Definition/overview

Hepatic abscesses following bacterial infection of the liver occur uncommonly in dogs and cats (**Figures 9.24a–c**).

Etiology

Hematogenous or ascending biliary infection may result in hepatic abscess formation. Gram-negative enteric organisms or gram-positive and gram-negative anaerobic organisms (especially clostridial organisms) may be noted. It may be part of systemic infection. *Bartonella* can cause diffuse hepatic infection and microabscessation.

Pathophysiology

Hepatic abscesses are usually associated with systemic infection or hepatic damage. Bacteria arrive in the liver hematogenously via a systemic arterial or portal venous route (translocation) or via the biliary tree.

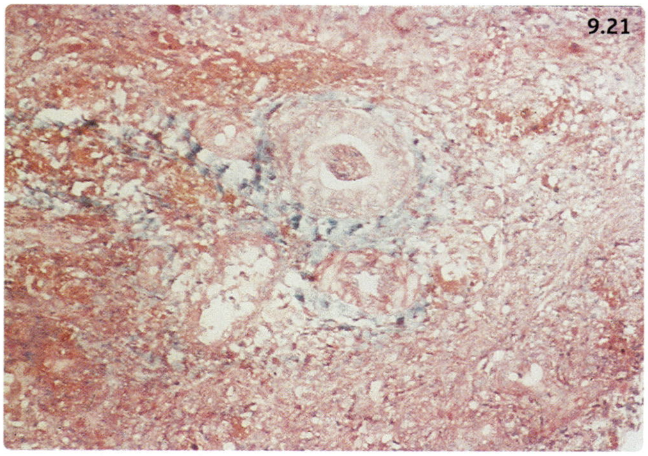

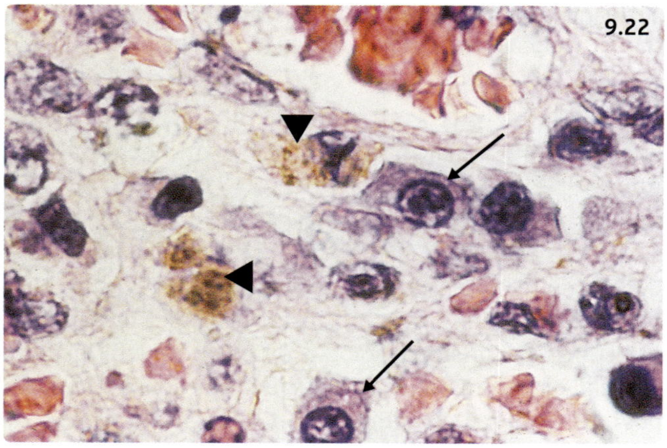

Figures 9.21, 9.22 (9.21) Histologic appearance of the liver in chronic hepatitis. There is widespread hepatocellular degeneration, portal fibrosis (blue staining), and bile stasis. (9.22) Higher-power view in the same patient shows periportal round cells (arrows) and bile stasis (arrowheads).

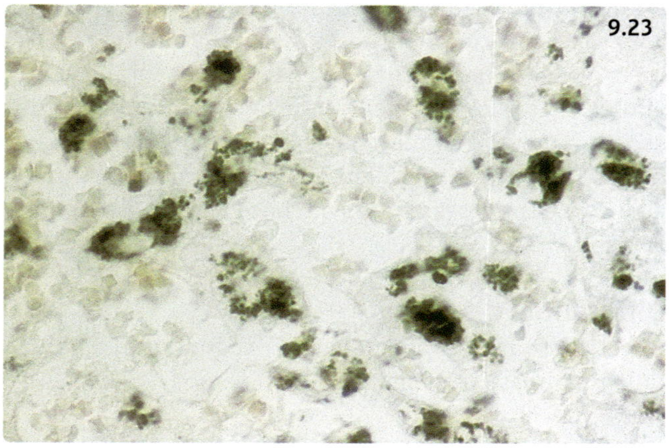

Figure 9.23 Copper stain of the liver in a Dobermann with chronic hepatitis.

Immunosuppression or damaged hepatic parenchyma results in infection and subsequent abscess formation.

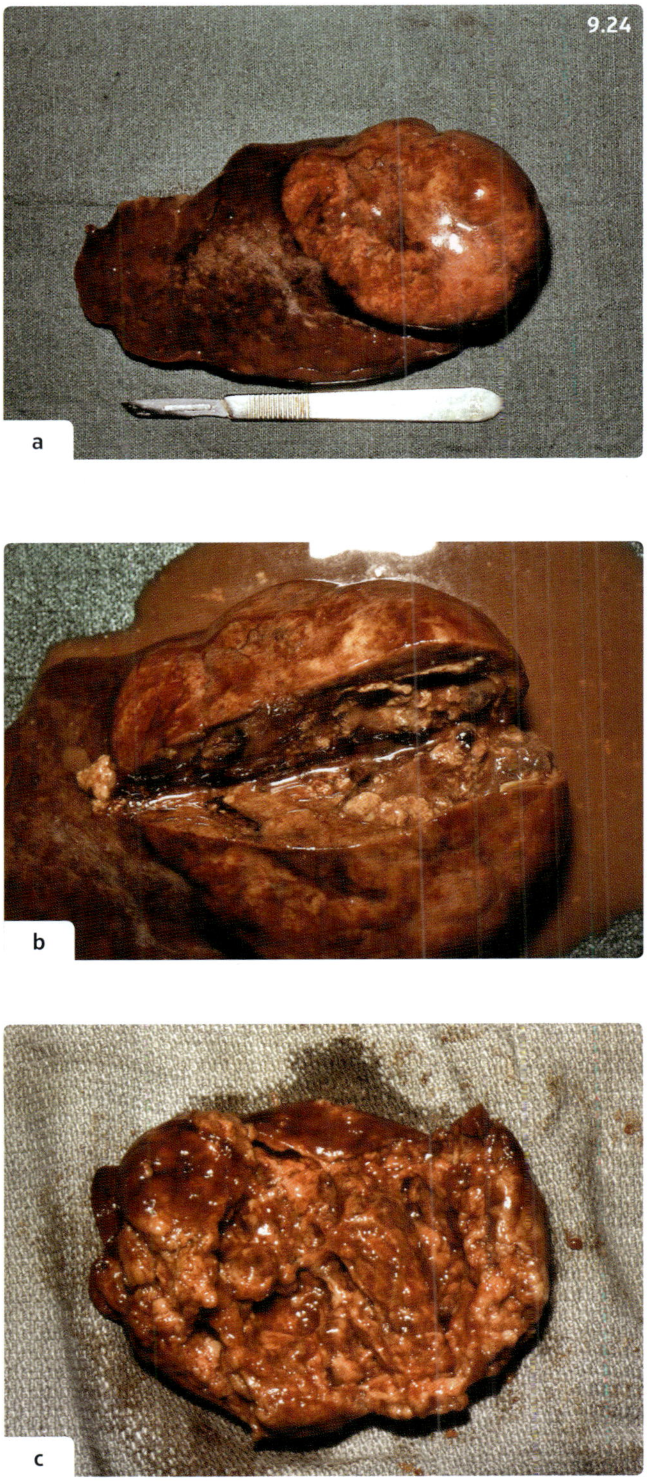

Figures 9.24 a–c Surgical specimen of an abscessed liver lobe showing the intact and necrotic tissue. (Courtesy M. Schaer)

Cats tend to have multiple small abscesses while dogs more often have one or a few larger abscesses.

Clinical presentation

Usually older dogs or cats with nonspecific GI signs or signs of sepsis. Fever may be noted but hypothermia is more likely in cats. Abdominal pain may be noted, especially if rupture of an abscess has occurred resulting in septic peritonitis.

Differential diagnosis

Inflammatory liver diseases, pancreatitis, septic or bile peritonitis, hepatic neoplasia.

Diagnosis

Complete blood count (CBC) findings are consistent with inflammation; septic changes may be noted. ALT and AST activities may be increased but cats may have normal liver enzyme activities. Hypoalbuminemia, hyperglobulinemia, and mild hyperbilirubinemia are common. Hypoglycemia associated with sepsis or decreased hepatic function may be seen. Abdominal ultrasound usually reveals hypo- to anechoic structures with a hyperechoic rim within hepatic parenchyma. Fine needle aspiration for cytology and culture reveals evidence of bacterial infection. Culture and sensitivity are important in directing definitive treatment.

Management

Focal abscesses should be treated with surgical excision or drainage. Percutaneous drainage may be carried out. Antibiotics based on Gram staining and culture and sensitivity should accompany appropriate surgical management. Broad-spectrum coverage with fluoroquinolone and clavulanate-potentiated amoxicillin or sulbactam-potentiated ampicillin, with or without metronidazole for added anaerobic coverage, is appropriate for treatment while waiting for culture results. Definitive antibiotic treatment should be for a minimum of 6–8 weeks with follow-up ultrasound and blood work evaluation. Mortality rates may exceed 50%.

ACUTE HEPATITIS AND ACUTE HEPATOCELLULAR DEGENERATION AND NECROSIS

Definition/overview

Acute hepatitis and acute hepatocellular degeneration are characterized by focal or diffuse damage to the hepatocytes. Hepatocytes may be killed by a spectrum of insults, but death occurs through apoptosis or necrosis. Mild insults may cause apoptosis, while stronger insults will cause necrosis.

Etiology

The causes of hepatocellular disruption are many and varied and are often undetermined. Recognized hepatotoxins include: chemical solvents such as carbon tetrachloride; mycotoxins such as aflatoxin; Cyanophyceae algae; cycasin from cycad plants; drugs such as acetaminophen, azole antifungals, methimazole, and diazepam in the cat; drugs such as mebendazole, oxybendazole, trimethoprim–sulfa antibiotics, immunosuppressives such as cyclosporine, azathioprine, and chlorambucil, nonsteroidal anti-inflammatory drugs (NSAIDs) such as carprofen, azole antifungals, and the artificial sweetener xylitol in some dogs; certain mushrooms (*Amantinum* spp.); viruses including canine adenovirus 1, herpesviruses, FIP virus; bacteria such as *Clostridium piliformis*, *Bartonella*, *Leptospira*, and possibly *Helicobacter*. Clinical signs, biochemical data, and histologic findings do not usually indicate a specific cause, resulting only in a histologic diagnosis of acute hepatic necrosis or 'toxic' hepatitis (**Figure 9.25**).

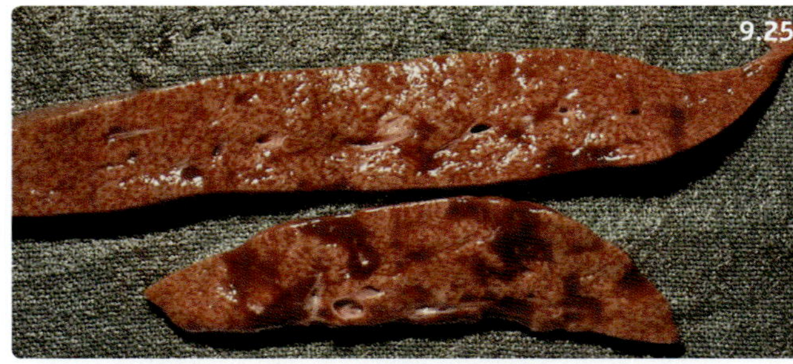

Figure 9.25 Postmortem liver specimen from a dog with fatal peracute hepatic necrosis of unknown etiology. Note the loss of normal parenchymal architecture due to the dark red patches of necrosis. (Courtesy M. Schaer)

Pathophysiology

The predominant lesion of acute hepatitis is multifocal apoptosis and necrosis of individual hepatocytes associated with abnormal liver enzyme activity. The proportion of each cell type varies with time and the host response, as well as with the possible cause.

Clinical presentation

Clinical signs are variable and include inappetence, lethargy, and vomiting. Icterus develops if the hepatocellular insult is extensive. Neurologic signs caused by hepatoencephalopathy may be seen.

Differential diagnosis

Acute pancreatitis, infectious CH, acute gastroenteritis, and some toxicoses.

Diagnosis

The predominant biochemical abnormality is an increase in serum ALT and AST activities, the magnitude of which depends on the severity and extent of the hepatocellular damage. Serum ALP is usually normal or only slightly increased early in the disease process. An increase in serum bilirubin concentration may occur if a sufficient number of hepatocytes have been damaged or destroyed or if there has been sufficient damage to cause cholestasis. The patient will recover if enough functional liver remains to support regeneration.

A liver biopsy is often neither helpful nor essential in the diagnostic evaluation if the history strongly implicates the cause, and it may be contraindicated by liver-associated coagulopathies. Histologic examination can be useful for assessing the severity and extent of the disease process or determining if the acute onset of clinical disease is associated with chronic histologic changes. A liver biopsy is justified if recurrent abnormal ALT/AST values have been documented (see Chronic inflammatory liver disease).

Management

Few hepatotoxins have specific antidotes but silymarin has been shown to be effective at blocking hepatocellular binding sites for some toxins. Successful recovery depends on aggressive supportive therapy and management of oxidative stress. The prognosis is usually good if the inciting cause is removed, permanent loss of functional mass is less than 50%, and the liver has retained the capacity to regenerate.

CIRRHOSIS

Definition/overview

Cirrhosis is the end stage of CH in the dog. It is a diffuse hepatic disease process characterized by fibrosis and by an alteration of normal hepatic architecture by structurally abnormal regenerative nodules. Portocentral vascular anastomoses and acquired PSSs may be present (**Figure 9.26**). The disease occurs in two morphological presentations: (1) micronodular cirrhosis, in which regenerative nodules are less than 3 mm in diameter, and (2) macronodular cirrhosis, in which the nodules are greater than 3 mm and usually up to several centimeters and of different sizes. Lobular dissecting hepatitis is a form of cirrhosis seen in adolescent and young adult dogs.

Etiology

The cause of cirrhosis is varied and is seldom determined.

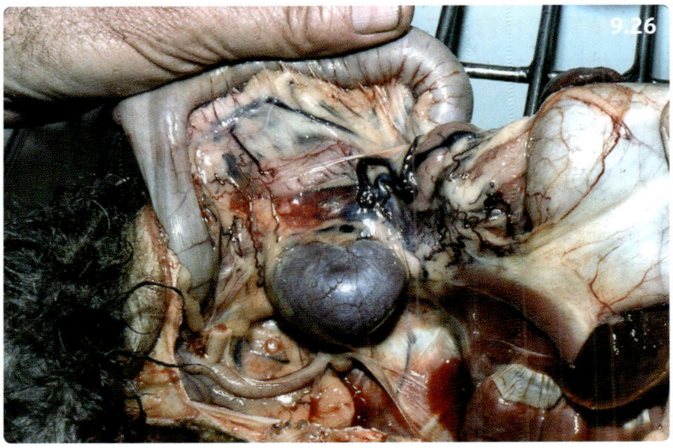

Figure 9.26 Postmortem view showing acquired extrahepatic shunt vessels (dark tortuous vessels) in a Schnauzer that had micronodular cirrhosis. (Courtesy M. Schaer)

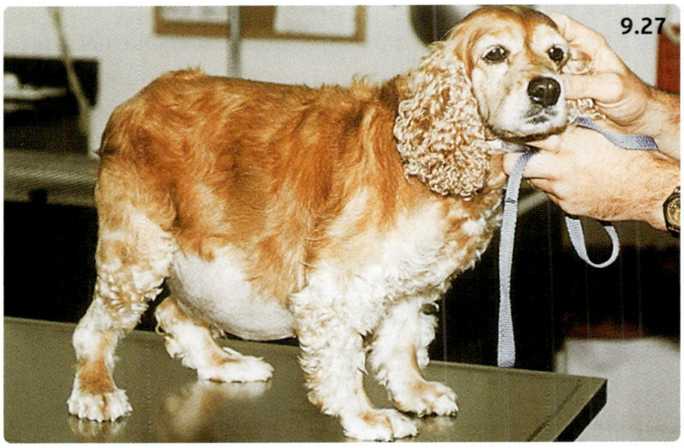

Figure 9.27 Ascites in a Cocker Spaniel secondary to hepatic fibrosis and cirrhosis.

Pathophysiology

Increased hepatic vascular resistance and portal hypertension resulting from the fibrosis and regenerative nodules eventually lead to icterus, ascites, multiple acquired PSSs, and associated hepatoencephalopathy.

Clinical presentation

Cirrhosis is a common presentation in dogs, but is uncommon in cats. Clinical signs most often include lethargy, inappetence, ascites (**Figure 9.27**), and mental depression that can progress to encephalopathy. GI signs such as vomiting and/or diarrhea are occasionally seen. Polyuria and polydipsia are inconsistent findings, but when present may be severe and clinically reminiscent of diabetes insipidus or psychogenic polydipsia. Bleeding, noted as petechiae or ecchymoses, may be seen in more severely affected dogs. GI bleeding is common and may manifest as obvious melena or may be more subtle and contribute to an iron deficiency anemia. Some patients are compensated and show few clinical signs, while others are icteric and show signs of liver failure.

Differential diagnosis

Metastatic disease, nodular regeneration, hepatocutaneous syndrome.

Diagnosis

Biochemical findings may indicate severe liver disease, but they are also often subtle. Serum ALT, AST, and ALP activities may be moderately increased, or they may be normal or only slightly increased because of the decreased hepatic cell mass. Other biochemical abnormalities are more consistent and reflect the reduced functional capacity of the liver and altered hepatic blood flow. Decreased BUN and a decreased serum albumin concentration may be noted. Increased serum bilirubin concentration is a late indicator of liver insufficiency. Persistent bilirubinuria will be detected before jaundice develops. Determination of total serum bile acids and plasma ammonia concentrations are the most reliable tests for detecting hepatic insufficiency. Serum bile acids are appropriately determined in the anicteric patient, but plasma ammonia is a better indicator of hepatic dysfunction in the dog with icterus. Reduced hepatocellular mass, altered portal blood flow and cholestasis result in an increase in serum bile acid concentrations.

Jaundice may develop in the cirrhotic patient without prior clinical evidence of liver disease and may require differentiation from extrahepatic impairment of bile flow. While ultrasound evaluation of the biliary tree is the most effective means of noninvasively determining if extrahepatic bile flow is impaired, the increased total serum bilirubin concentration is often lower (usually <102.6 µmol/l [6 mg/dl]) in the cirrhotic patient than in the patient with extrahepatic biliary obstruction. The absence of a marked increase in serum ALP activity, a decrease in BUN, a decrease in serum albumin concentration, or an increased plasma ammonia concentration supports a diagnosis of cirrhosis.

Histologic confirmation of cirrhosis is important since on gross visual inspection cirrhosis may resemble metastatic disease, nodular regeneration, or hepatocutaneous syndrome (**Figure 9.28, 9.29**).

Management

Supportive measures are aimed at controlling the complications of chronic liver failure (e.g. hepatic encephalopathy, coagulation abnormalities, and infection). Ascites should be managed by reducing the sodium content in the

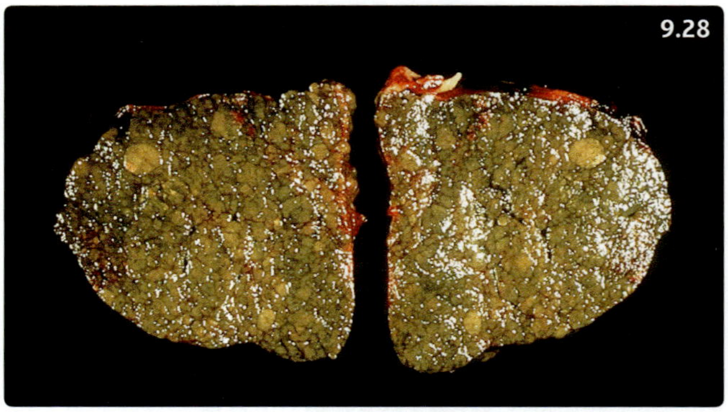

Figure 9.28 Cross-section of the liver of a 4-year-old Spitz with severe cirrhosis. Regenerative nodules are dispersed throughout the parenchyma.

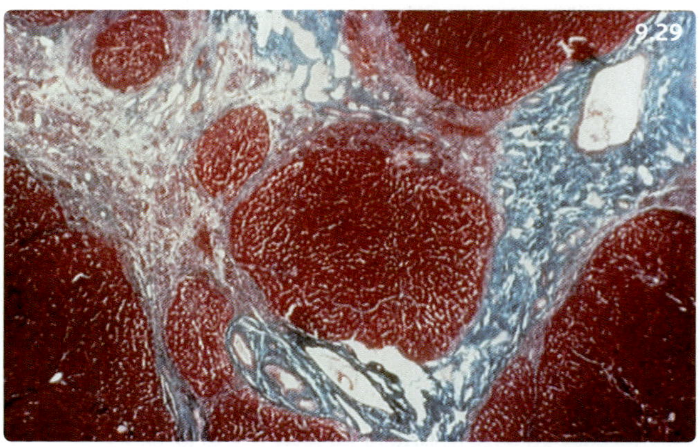

Figure 9.29 Trichrome stain of a section of cirrhotic liver showing fibrosis (blue) and nodules (red).

diet and the judicious use of diuretics. Potassium-sparing diuretics should initially be used as dogs with chronic fibrosis are prone to developing hypokalemia. Any suspected bleeding associated with gastroenteric ulcerations should be treated with anti-ulcer drugs such as sucralfate and proton pump inhibitors. The diet should ideally be one that contains adequate protein and calories to maintain weight. The protein content of the diet should not be reduced until necessitated by evidence of hepatoencephalopathy. When signs of hepatoencephalopathy become apparent it should be managed with lactulose and oral antibiotics such as neomycin or metronidazole. The protein content of the diet should be reduced only to the extent necessary to control the neurologic signs. Management of fibrosis is usually not helpful once a dog is showing signs of liver failure associated with cirrhosis, but prednisone, D-penicillamine, colchicine, and silymarin have all been advocated to reduce fibrosis. Antioxidants and anti-inflammatory drugs, as discussed under chronic inflammatory liver diseases, may also be indicated.

HEPATOCUTANEOUS SYNDROME

Definition/overview

Hepatocutaneous syndrome is a metabolic disease in which a vacuolar hepatopathy is associated with an ulcerative necrolytic dermatitis. Other terms used include superficial necrolytic dermatitis, necrolytic migratory erythema, diabetic dermatopathy, and metabolic epidermal necrosis.

The disease affects primarily middle aged to older dogs, with the average age being about 10 years. Males are more commonly affected than females. No definitive breed predilection has been noted; however, West Highland White Terriers, Shetland Sheepdogs, Cocker Spaniels, German Shepherd Dogs, Scottish Terriers, Lhasa Apsos, and Border Collies may be overrepresented.

Etiology

The cause of the syndrome is unknown. It is characterized by liver disease in which there is extensive hepatocyte vacuolization coupled with parenchymal collapse together with a characteristic superficial necrolytic dermatitis. Diabetes mellitus may also be noted.

Pathophysiology

The consistent finding in dogs is liver disease and skin disease in a patient with severe hypoaminoacidemia. The cause of either set of lesions is not understood, but it is speculated that a metabolic derangement that results in increased catabolism or loss of amino acids is present, and this sets up an environment that has a detrimental effect on the skin, resulting in striking inter- and intracellular edema and marked parakeratosis, with resulting ulceration, exudation, and crusting. The footpads are often affected. Whether the changes in the liver are a cause or an effect of the hypoaminoacidemia is not known. In humans, this syndrome is most often seen as a paraneoplastic condition associated with glucagonomas. This has been documented in dogs, but in most cases a glucagonoma or evidence of a pancreatic mass is not seen. In addition to the characteristic vacuolar hepatopathy, this syndrome has been seen with phenobarbital and primidone-associated liver disease and intestinal malabsorption.

Clinical presentation

The most common presentation is the development of skin lesions that include erythema, crusting, exudation, ulceration, and alopecia involving the footpads, pressure points on the trunk and limbs, perineum, muzzle, and periocular areas **(Figures 9.30–9.34)**. Lameness due

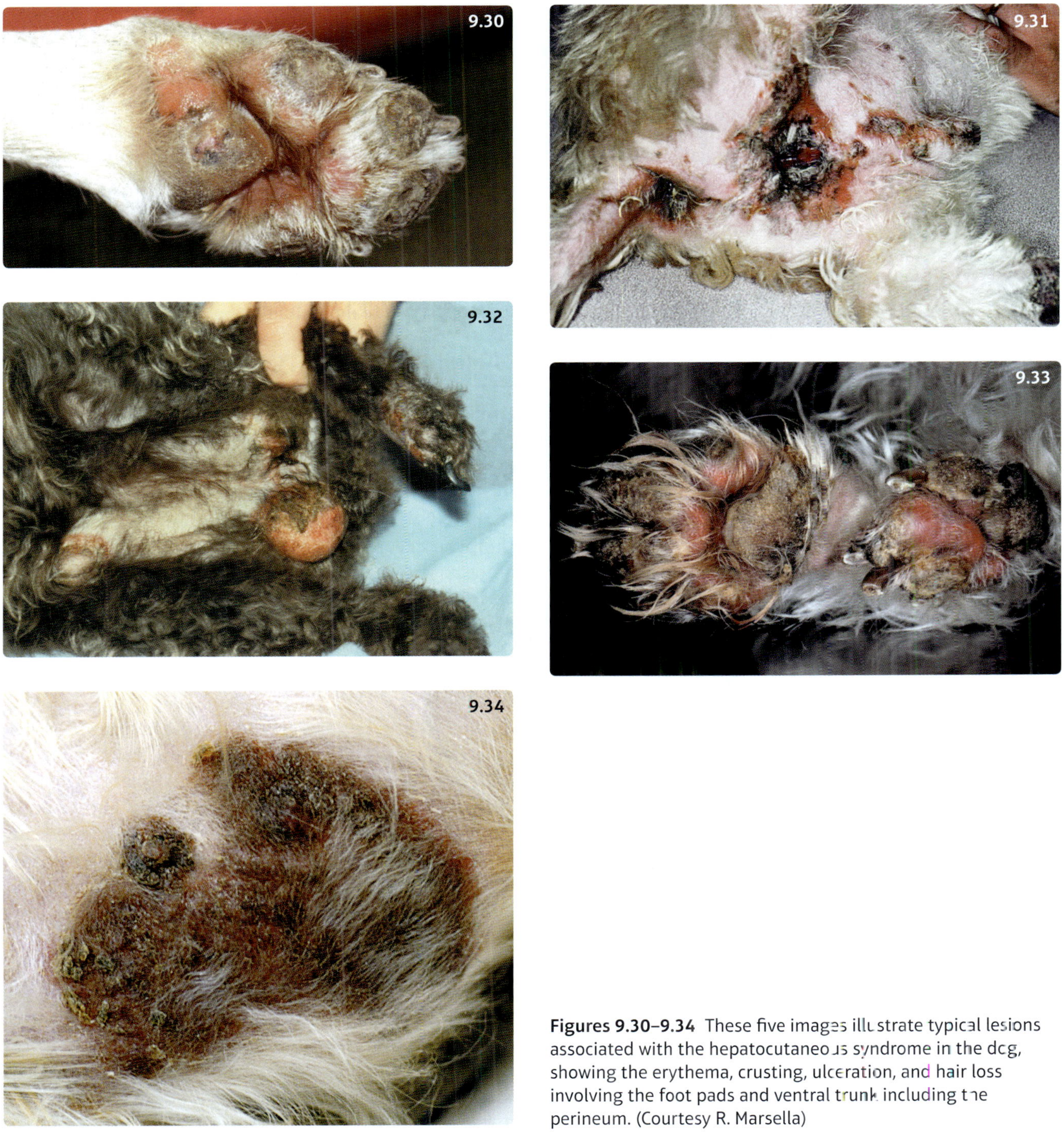

Figures 9.30–9.34 These five images illustrate typical lesions associated with the hepatocutaneous syndrome in the dog, showing the erythema, crusting, ulceration, and hair loss involving the foot pads and ventral trunk including the perineum. (Courtesy R. Marsella)

to footpad ulceration is often an initial presenting complaint. Some dogs may present only for liver disease and typically show lethargy and anorexia. Most of these dogs either will have subtle skin lesions at the initial presentation or will develop the skin lesions within weeks of the initial presentation.

Differential diagnosis
Macronodular cirrhosis, metastatic neoplasia, glucagonoma.

Diagnosis
Serologic abnormalities seen in affected dogs include: increased ALT, AST, and ALP activities; variable glucagon concentrations (increased in only some patients with glucagonoma, diabetes mellitus, pancreatitis, and chronic hepatic insufficiency); fluctuating hyperglycemia without ketoacidosis; nonregenerative to mildly regenerative anemia; abnormalities in red cell morphology (polychromasia, anisocytosis, poikilocytosis, target cells); hypoalbuminemia; and severe hypoaminoacidemia. Liver function test results can range from normal to severely abnormal. Results of liver cytology are consistent with severe, vacuolar degeneration of hepatocytes.

Ultrasonographic imaging of the liver in dogs with hepatocutaneous syndrome can be very striking. A unique 'honeycomb' pattern is found and this has been reported as being pathognomonic. This pattern consists of variably sized hypoechoic regions measuring 0.5–1.5 cm in diameter surrounded by highly echogenic borders.

Skin biopsy is the most consistent means of definitively diagnosing hepatocutaneous syndrome. Skin biopsy specimens should be taken from multiple sites; include the footpad when lesions are present. The dermatohistopathology of the disease is unique and striking, with changes consisting of marked inter- and intracellular edema, which is localized to the upper half of the epidermis. Severe edema produces loss of cellular structure and resultant intraepidermal clefts and vesicles. Basal cell hyperplasia is also seen. Irregular epidermal hyperplasia is overlaid by marked diffuse parakeratotic hyperkeratosis.

The liver lesions reflect chronic hepatocellular degeneration with severe intracellular fat accumulation. Severe lobular collapse and nodular regeneration are residual evidence of ongoing hepatocellular regeneration and degeneration, with resultant parenchymal loss.

Management
Amino acid supplementation has been the primary approach to treatment either by increasing protein in the diet or by parenteral administration of amino acid mixtures. Amino acid solution (Aminosyn™ 10%; a crystalline amino acid solution) can be administered at a dose of 24 ml/kg slowly over about 8–12 hours into a large central vein (jugular), initially weekly, then less often as the lesions improve. Oral protein supplements used by body builders can supplement the IV administration of amino acids. Consideration should be given to measuring blood ammonia concentrations before initiating this treatment because it is possible to worsen hepatoencephalopathy with the therapy; however, hepatoencephalopathy is rarely seen in patients with hepatocutaneous syndrome. Measuring blood ammonia concentrations can be done daily or weekly until improvement is noted. Some dogs may require monthly IV amino acid infusions, but many dogs can go several months between infusions. The prognosis is guarded, but some dogs will respond well, with long-term survival possible.

FAMILIAL COPPER TOXICITY

Definition/overview
A hereditary metabolic disturbance resulting in excessive hepatic copper accumulation is seen in breeds such as the Bedlington Terrier, Labrador Retriever, Skye Terrier, West Highland White Terrier, and Dalmatian. The defect is best characterized in Bedlington Terriers where there is an autosomal recessive pattern of inheritance and is similar to hepatolenticular degeneration in humans (Wilson's disease). The disease is one form of chronic liver disease that progresses to cirrhosis.

Etiology
In the Bedlington Terrier, the disease is caused by an inherited metabolic defect caused by a deletion in the COMMD1 gene leading to an abnormal metallothionein copper-binding protein. The abnormal protein, or other derangements in copper metabolism in other breeds, leads to a defect in copper transport, which causes an accumulation of copper in hepatocytes resulting in inflammation or necrosis.

Pathophysiology
Accumulation of copper leads to major hepatic injury as the hepatic mitochondria become damaged by oxidants. Acute release of copper from the necrotic hepatocytes may cause hemolytic anemia. With progressive disease, the liver diminishes in size and a mixture of micro- and macronodular cirrhosis develops.

Clinical presentation
Young adults may present for signs of acute hepatic failure or the clinical signs and biochemical findings may be similar to those described for CH.

Differential diagnosis
Infections; drug-induced, familial, or lobular dissecting hepatitis; idiopathic CH.

Diagnosis

Diagnosis is suggested by increased ALT/AST activities and confirmed by measurement of the copper concentration of fresh liver tissue. Hepatic copper concentrations tend to increase slowly until middle age, but the concentration is often high enough at 1 year of age to suggest the presence of a defect.

Management

Dogs are best treated before clinical signs become severe. Asymptomatic animals may be helped by treating with zinc supplements and restriction of dietary copper. Treatment with D-penicillamine (10–15 mg/kg PO q12h) or another chelator such as trientine hydrochloride (10–15 mg/kg PO q12h) prevents progression of the disease in many dogs and will slowly result in decreased hepatic copper concentrations. Affected dogs and carriers of the gene should be identified and removed from breeding programs.

DRUG-INDUCED LIVER DISEASE

Definition/overview

Drugs can cause liver injury ranging from a transient asymptomatic increase in serum transaminase activity to clinically overt acute or chronic liver disease.

Etiology

Drugs can induce liver injury either by a direct toxic action, the formation of toxic metabolites, or indirectly via a hypersensitivity reaction.

Pathophysiology

Direct-acting hepatotoxins usually cause acute necrosis when the drug or a metabolite interacts chemically with an essential structural component or metabolic enzyme system of the hepatocyte (e.g. acetaminophen). A drug or its metabolite may induce liver injury either by altering the regulatory system of the immune response so that reactions to self-antigens are no longer suppressed, or by altering hepatocyte antigens so that they are no longer recognized as self-components.

Clinical presentation

Animals may present with several signs depending on the inciting cause and include depression, ataxia, weight loss, anorexia, vomiting, behavioral changes, coagulopathy, jaundice, and ascites.

Differential diagnosis

Infections; familial, lobular, or dissecting hepatitis; idiopathic CH.

Diagnosis

A hypersensitivity response is very difficult to prove, since challenge exposes the patient to unnecessary risk. Sulfa-containing drugs, anticonvulsants anthelmintics, NSAIDs, halothane, azole antifungals, xylitol artificial sweeteners, cyclophosphamide, methimazole, and others have been implicated in veterinary medicine (**Figures 9.35, 9.36**).

Management

It is prudent to discontinue the inciting drug. If the drug is essential, then the dose should be modified as much as possible. Fasting and postprandial bile acid concentrations (assuming there is no increase in serum bilirubin) should be determined, as major hepatic damage is less likely if the concentrations are normal.

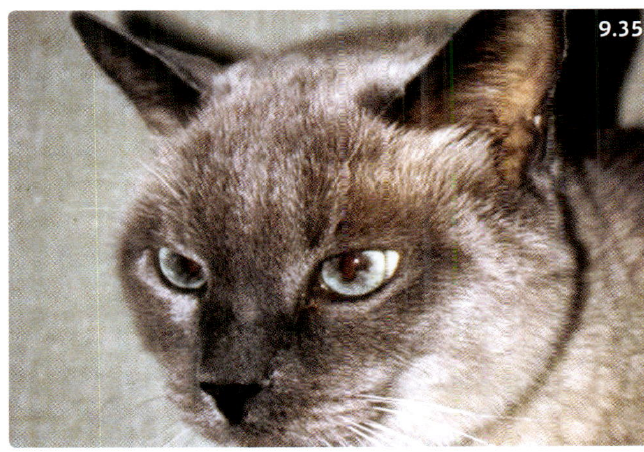

9.36

HEMATOLOGY	
PCV	0.35 l/l (35%)
Total WBCs	7.68 × 10^9/l (7.68 × 10^3/μl)
Platelets	Normal
URINALYSIS	
SG	1.025
pH	6.5
Bilirubin	>68 μmol/l (>4 mg/dl)
CHEMISTRIES	
AP	424 U/l
AST	320 U/l
ALT	835 U/l
Total bilirubin	195 μmol/l (11.4 mg/dl)
Total protein	86 g/l (8.6 g/dl)
Creatinine	212 μmol/l (2.4 mg/dl)
BUN	4.6 mmol/l (28 mg/dl)

Figures 9.35, 9.36 This 11-year-old hyperthyroid male Siamese cat had methimazole hepatotoxicosis. He had icterus (9.35) and elevated liver enzyme levels (9.36) (Courtesy M. Schaer)

EXTRAHEPATOBILIARY OBSTRUCTION (EXTRAHEPATIC IMPAIRMENT OF BILE FLOW)

Definition/overview

Extrahepatic biliary obstruction refers to the impairment of bile flow in the biliary system between the liver and the duodenum. Acute, total extrahepatic impairment of bile flow is rare.

Etiology

Neoplasia (**Figure 9.37**), infection, and trauma should be considered. Chronic pancreatitis and tumors of the pancreas and the bile duct epithelia are the most common causes, although cholelithiasis and choledocholithiasis have been reported in both the cat and the dog. Inspissated bile (most often associated with an underlying liver disorder), liver flukes, duodenal or pyloric neoplasia, diaphragmatic hernia, congenital abnormalities, and mucinous cystic hyperplasia are additional causes.

Pathophysiology

Neoplasia or pancreatitis in the dog and cat may result in a mass effect or sufficient inflammation/fibrosis/fat necrosis to cause an extraluminal anatomic obstruction involving the common bile duct (**Figure 9.38**). Scars usually form around or within the bile ducts. No matter the cause, obstruction causes leakage of bile from the ducts into the connective tissue of portal areas. This causes inflammation and fibrosis of the portal areas, with bile duct proliferation and an inflammatory infiltrate of pigment-laden macrophages, lymphocytes, neutrophils, and plasma cells.

Clinical presentation

Signs include inappetence, icterus, and repeated vomiting (especially if the pancreas is involved). Both cats and dogs may be presented with a chronic history of anorexia, lethargy, and jaundice. Physical findings are usually unremarkable except for icterus. If a patient with suspected pancreatic pathology (see Chapter 10: Pancreatic disorders) remains icteric beyond 10–14 days of symptomatic medical management, an extrahepatic component should be suspected and managed accordingly.

Differential diagnosis

Liver flukes, neoplasia, cholelithiasis, traumatic gallbladder or bile duct lesion.

Diagnosis

Extrahepatic cholestasis causes a marked increase in the hepatic expression of ALP, resulting in a concomitant increase in serum activity. Increased serum cholesterol concentrations can also occur. Retained bile acids also cause hepatocellular damage, with an associated mild to moderate increase in ALT activity. Severe cholestasis results in decreased bile acid excretion into the small intestine with subsequent fat, and therefore fat soluble vitamin, malabsorption. Clotting studies reveal increased PT and PTT, which should revert to normal with parenteral vitamin K1 therapy. Bilirubinuria will be noted on urine dipsticks as strongly positive. Ultrasonography is a valuable, noninvasive diagnostic tool since it allows visualization of a dilated extrahepatic bile duct and may reveal the cause of obstruction (**Figure 9.39**).

Acute pancreatitis occasionally causes a mild to moderate increase in ALT activity, a marked increase in ALP activity, and increased total serum bilirubin

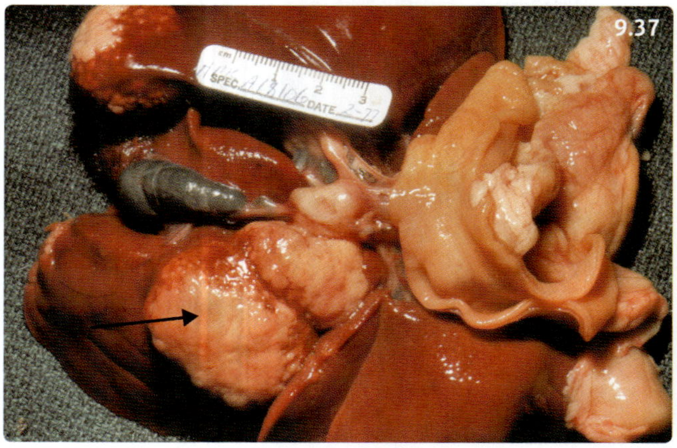

Figure 9.37 Postmortem image of a cat that had a cystadenocarcinoma (arrow) of the common bile duct. (Courtesy M. Schaer)

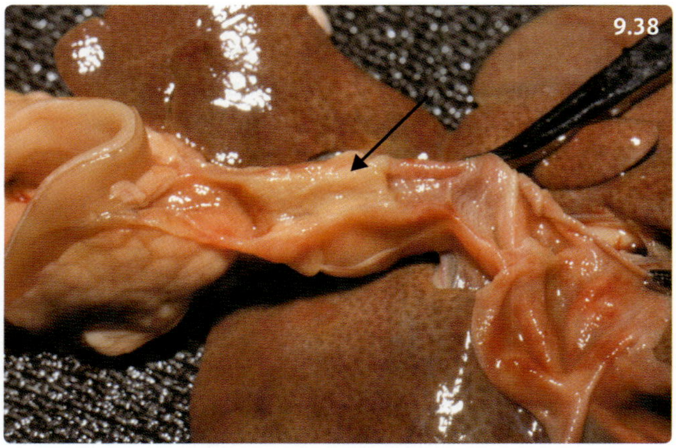

Figure 9.38 Postmortem image of a cat that had a common bile duct occlusion (arrow) caused by metastatic pancreatic adenocarcinoma. (Courtesy M. Schaer)

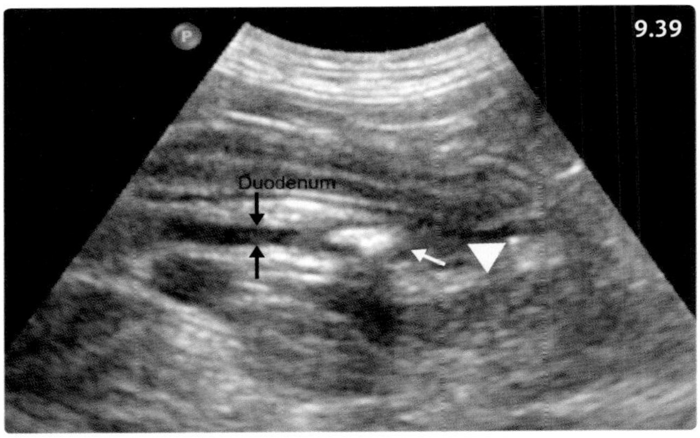

Figure 9.39 Ultrasound image of a cat with a cholelith located in the distal portion of the common bile duct (white arrow). The common bile duct is dilated above the obstruction (black arrows). The duodenal papilla is visible (white arrowhead). (Courtesy L. Gaschen)

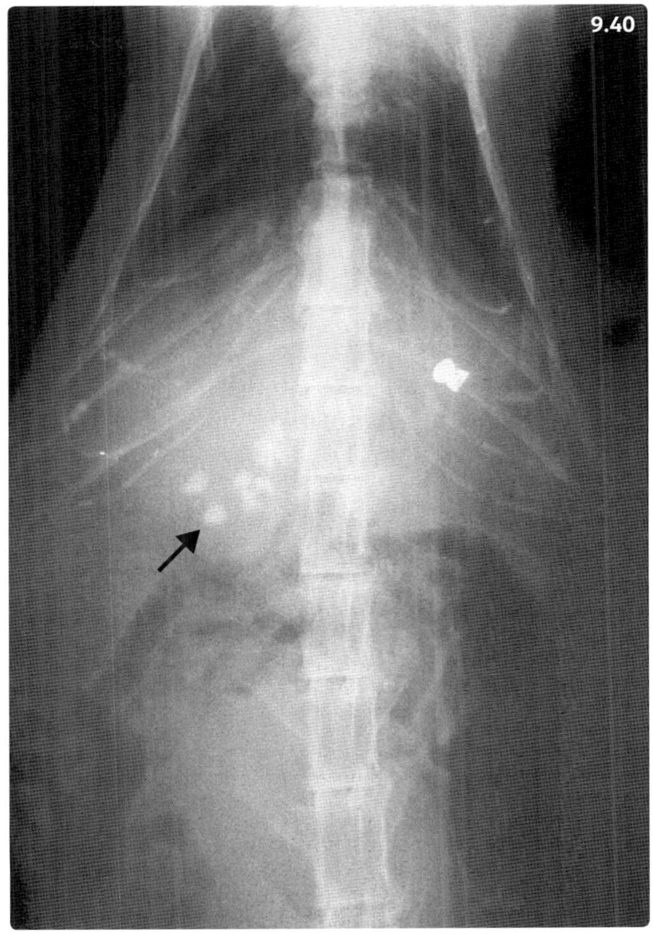

Figure 9.40 Survey abdominal radiograph in a cat showing a collection of gallstones (arrow). This was an incidental finding (as was the airgun pellet). (Courtesy B. Jones)

concentration. The biochemical pattern may appear similar to that of extrahepatic biliary obstruction or CH with intrahepatic cholestasis. An acute onset of repeated vomiting preceding the development of jaundice suggests acute pancreatitis. Marked increases in serum pancreatic lipase immunoreactivity (cPLI, fPLI) may be noted. Suggested causes for the transient increase in the liver enzymes and bilirubin associated with acute pancreatitis include inflammation of the peripancreatic tissue, which compresses the bile duct, the release of proteases into the portal blood, which damage hepatobiliary tissue, and oxidative stress, which damages hepatocellular membranes and results in proinflammatory cytokine release.

Management

Surgical correction is the treatment of choice. If no obstruction is found at laparotomy, the liver should be biopsied and the patient managed accordingly. Treatment with ursodeoxycholic acid and antioxidants such as acetylcysteine, SAMe/silybin combinations, or vitamin E is also helpful.

CHOLETHIASIS (GALLSTONES)

Definition/overview

Cholelithiasis occasionally occurs in dogs and cats. Most are incidental findings on abdominal radiographs or at necropsy (**Figure 9.40**). On rare occasions, choleliths can cause obstruction of the common bile duct, but simply finding them on radiographs in patients with evidence of liver disease is not justification for removal.

Etiology

Dogs and cats typically develop mixed choleliths composed of calcium salts, bilirubin, and occasionally cholesterol. This is different from humans where choleliths are typically dietary-induced cholesterol-containing stones.

Pathophysiology

Gallstones in dogs usually contain mucin, calcium, and bilirubin. In cats they are more often calcium carbonate and mixed choleliths composed of calcium carbonate, calcium bilirubinate, and cholesterol.

Clinical presentation

Dogs and cats with cholelithiasis are often asymptomatic. If signs are apparent, they may include vomiting, icterus (the stones move into the common bile duct and cause obstruction), anorexia, fever, and abdominal pain. Middle aged small breed dogs and cats are predisposed.

Occasionally, perforation of the gallbladder or common bile duct is seen.

Differential diagnosis

Parasitism, neoplasia, nonbiliary tract disorders, gallbladder mucocele.

Diagnosis

While seldom radiopaque, choleliths are typically easily diagnosed by abdominal ultrasonography (**Figures 9.41, 9.42**). They appear as hyperechoic foci with acoustic shadowing originating from the gallbladder or common bile duct. Dilation of the common bile ducts and/or intrahepatic ducts may be noted.

Management

In cases with evidence of bile flow obstruction, exploratory laparotomy for surgical removal of stones should be performed and the patency of the common bile duct assessed. Follow-up therapy with ursodeoxycholic acid, antioxidants, and antimicrobials is recommended.

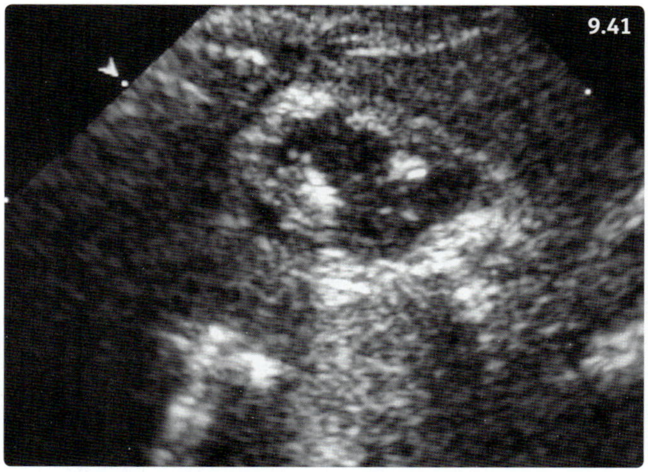

9.41

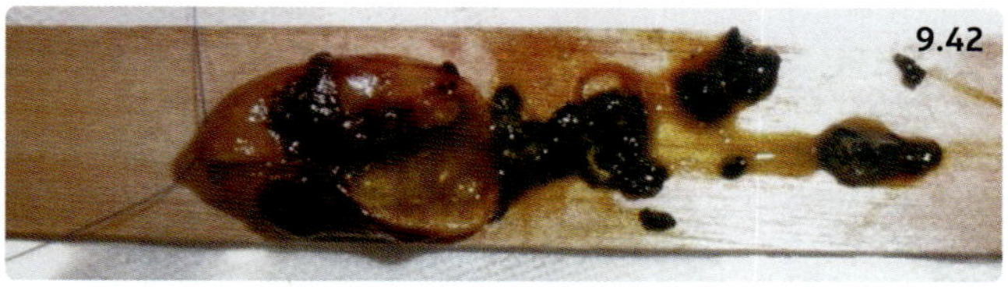

9.42

Figures 9.41, 9.42 Dog with cholecystitis and bilirubin gallstones. (9.41) Ultrasound image. (9.42) The surgically removed gallbladder, which was diagnosed as cholecystitis. Gallstones are also present. (Courtesy M. Schaer)

BILE DUCT RUPTURE

Definition/overview

Obstruction or trauma may result in perforation or rupture of the structures of the biliary tract. The common bile duct, distal to the opening of the last hepatic duct, seems to be the most common site of ductal rupture.

Etiology

Blunt trauma, penetrating wounds, pathology associated with a tumor or infection, and liver biopsies have been associated with rupture of the biliary system.

Pathophysiology

Extravasation of bile elicits a strong inflammatory response and causes transudation of lymph from serosal surfaces (**Figure 9.43**).

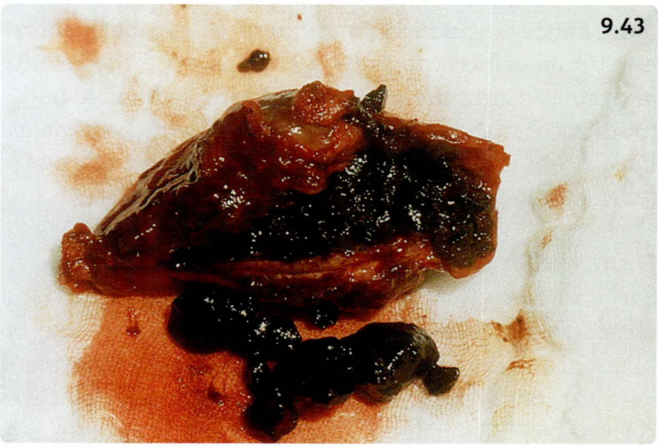

9.43

Figure 9.43 Cholecystitis in a 4-year-old German Shepherd Dog. The inflamed gallbladder had ruptured, causing a bile peritonitis. Note the inspissated bile in the gallbladder. A pure culture of *E. coli* was grown from the purulent abdominal fluid.

Clinical presentation

The clinical course is usually protracted. There is acute abdominal pain for the first 48 hours followed by anorexia, depression, fever, slow abdominal distension, and icterus. Hepatobiliary sepsis is life-threatening.

Differential diagnosis

Hepatic tumors, acute pancreatitis, FIP.

Diagnosis

An exudative, yellow–green-colored abdominal effusion is found at abdominocentesis. Macrophages containing bile pigment may be noted in a smear of the fluid (**Figure 9.44**).

Management

Exploratory surgery is always indicated.

GALLBLADDER MUCOCELES

Definition/overview

Gallbladder mucoceles are an increasingly common finding in dogs; they appear as dilation or distension of the gallbladder with accumulated mucus. Marked distension

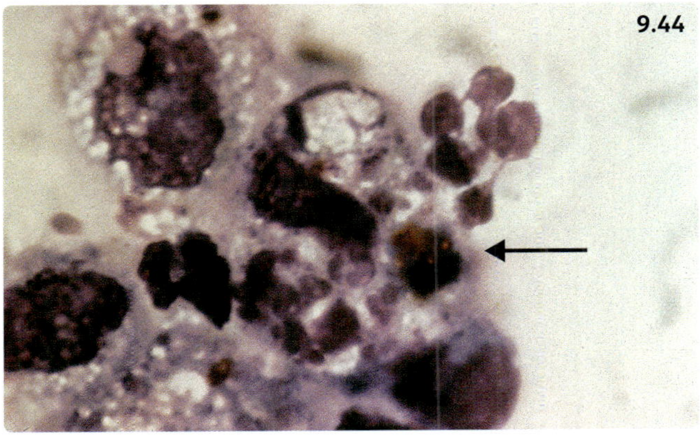

Figure 9.44 Cellular appearance of the fluid in bile peritonitis. Note the neutrophils and macrophages containing bile (arrow). (Courtesy D. Meyer)

may eventually result in rupture of the gallbladder and subsequent peritonitis.

Etiology

The cause is not known, but it is suspected that gallbladder mucoceles result from dysfunction of mucus-secreting cells within the gallbladder mucosa and altered wall contractility.

Pathophysiology

Mucus hypersecretion and formation of a biliary sludge result in the formation of a semi-solid mass of gallbladder contents that cannot pass from the gallbladder to the common bile duct. Over time the gallbladder distends and secondary cholecystitis may result. Rupture of the gallbladder and resultant peritonitis is possible, but is not seen in all cases. An association with hyperadrenocorticism and hypothyroidism has been postulated.

Clinical presentation

Nonspecific clinical signs such as vomiting, anorexia, and lethargy are usually the presenting complaint, but the finding of a gallbladder mucocele can be an incidental finding on ultrasound examination of the abdomen for another reason (**Figure 9.45**). Physical examination findings can include abdominal pain, jaundice, and fever if there is inflammation of the hepatobiliary tree.

Differential diagnosis

Pancreatitis, bile duct obstruction.

Diagnosis

Ultrasonography is a highly reliable means of identifying gallbladder mucocele and gallbladder rupture. The gallbladder may have a 'kiwi fruit' appearance.

Management

The management of dogs that are not showing clinical signs is controversial, as it is unknown what percentage of dogs with gallbladder mucoceles will progress to a gallbladder rupture. Asymptomatic dogs should be treated with ursodeoxycholic acid, antioxidants, and antimicrobials and monitored via abdominal ultrasound. Dogs showing clinical signs should have a cholecystectomy (**Figure 9.46**).

LIVER TUMORS

Definition/overview

Primary and metastatic tumors occur in the liver. Metastatic tumors are reportedly twice as frequent as primary tumors. Primary tumors include bile duct

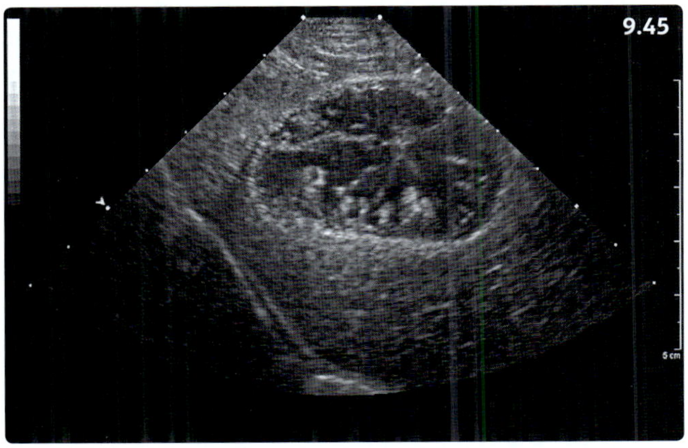

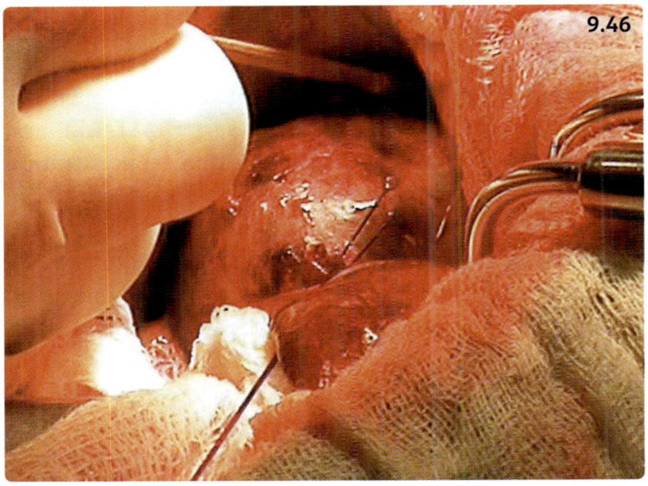

Figures 9.45, 9.46 Dog with a mucocele. (9.45) Ultrasound image. (9.46) Different dog at surgery, showing a severely inflamed gallbladder with several foci of necrosis. These would have perforated if surgery had not been done immediately. (Courtesy M. Schaer)

carcinoma, hepatocellular adenoma and carcinoma (hepatoma), and lymphoma. Hepatocellular carcinomas have been associated with a paraneoplastic hypoglycemia in the dog. Lymphosarcoma is the most common liver tumor, especially in cats.

Etiology

The cause of primary tumors is not usually determined. Metastatic tumors in the dog often arise from the pancreas, mammary glands, adrenals, bone, lungs, thyroid, GI tract, and spleen, whereas in the cat they usually arise from the kidney, pancreas, and GI tract. Malignant transformation of cystadenomas is possible.

Pathophysiology

Biliary and hepatocellular cancer occur as multifocal nodular or diffuse infiltrations of large areas of liver or as solitary masses.

Clinical presentation

Clinical signs are vague and nonspecific in most patients. They include inappetence progressing to anorexia, weight loss, vomiting, abdominal distension, and terminal jaundice in some patients (**Figure 9.47**).

Differential diagnosis

Parasitism, hepatobiliary cysts, cirrhosis.

Diagnosis

Those tumors that do not cause extrahepatic biliary obstruction may cause increases in serum AST, ALT, and ALP activities and total serum bilirubin concentration that may appear similar to the pattern associated with CH.

Abdominal radiographs are often read as normal, but they may reveal hepatomegaly (**Figure 9.48**). Hepatocellular carcinomas may be very large and noted on palpation or abdominal radiographs. Ultrasound-guided biopsy or laparotomy and biopsy are essential for diagnosis of neoplastic disease. The gross appearance of neoplastic lesions may appear similar to nodules associated with cirrhosis (**Figure 9.49**). Histologic evaluation can differentiate between the two lesions. Microscopic examination of a hepatic aspirate can help diagnose hepatic lymphoma (**Figure 9.50**).

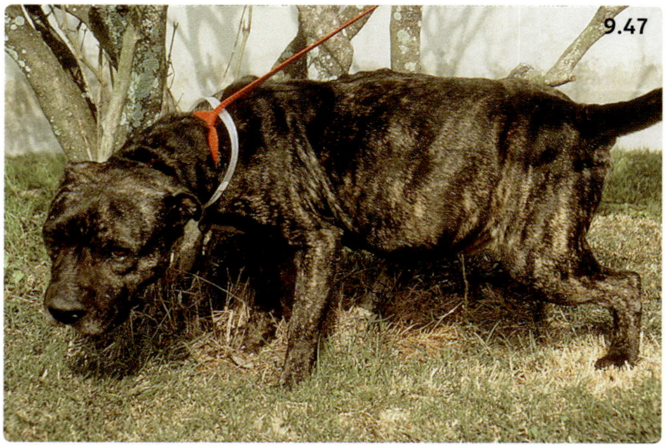

Figure 9.47 Abdominal distension and loss of muscle mass in a Bull Terrier suffering from advanced hepatocellular carcinoma.

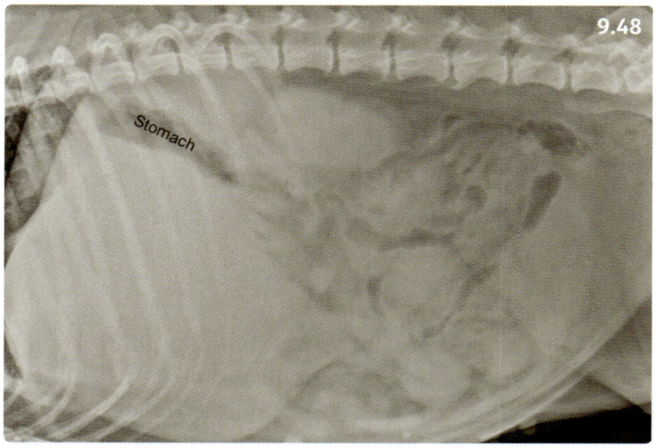

Figure 9.48 Lateral abdominal radiograph showing marked hepatomegaly and dorsal displacement of the stomach in an older dog with hepatic carcinoma. (Courtesy L. Gaschen)

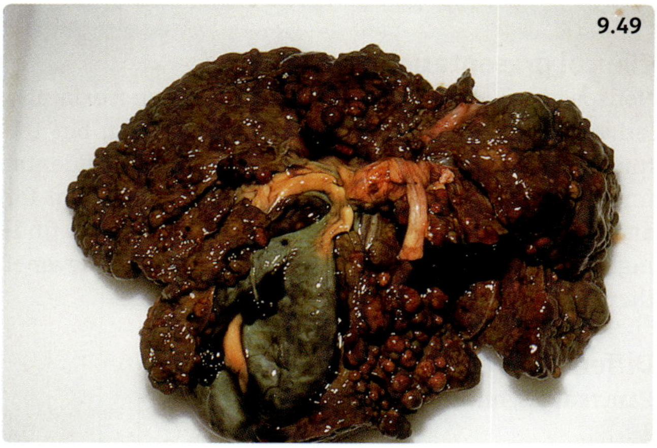

Figure 9.49 Postmortem specimen from a dog with macronodular cirrhosis. (Courtesy M. Schaer)

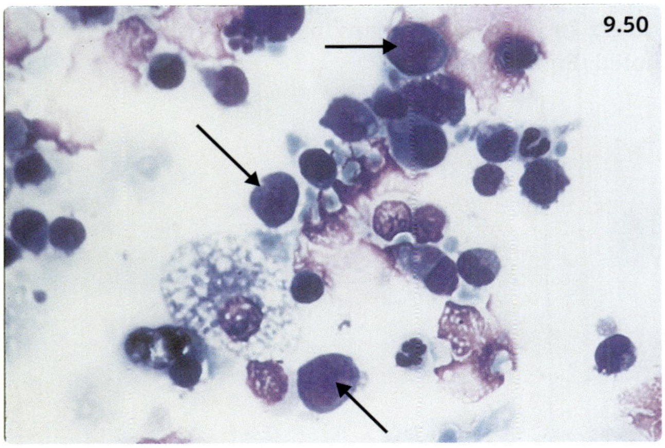

Figure 9.50 Microscopic examination of an hepatic aspirate can help differentiate between hepatic lymphoma and lipidosis in cats with jaundice and hepatomegaly. This aspirate from the liver of a 13-year-old Siamese confirmed a diagnosis of lymphoma (arrows).

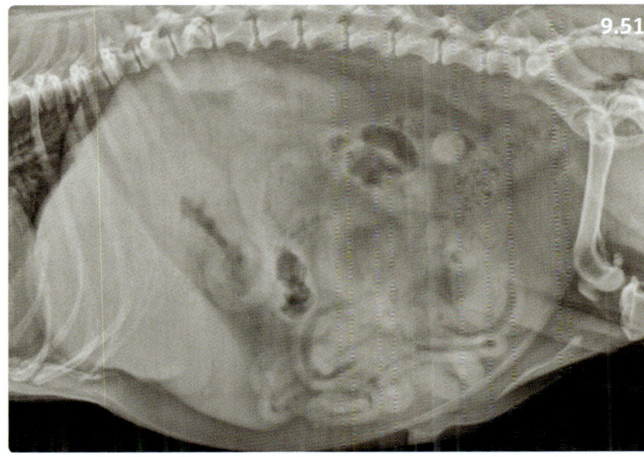

Figure 9.51 Lateral abdominal radiograph showing the typical cushingoid pendulous abdomen with liver enlargement. (Courtesy L. Gaschen)

Management

Primary tumors confined to a single lobe may be resected surgically. The abdominal cavity should be evaluated for metastatic spread and biopsy specimens of hepatic lymph nodes should be obtained. Chemotherapy may be appropriate in selected patients.

VACUOLAR AND STEROID HEPATOPATHY

Definition/overview

This is a unique and idiosyncratic response of the canine liver to either exogenous administration or endogenous overproduction of corticosteroids and perhaps adrenal sex hormones. The disorder is characterized by hepatocellular glycogen accumulation, with associated hepatomegaly and a variety of clinical and laboratory signs, most often associated with the steroids themselves. Scottish Terriers are reported to have a breed-specific syndrome associated with a vacuolar hepatopathy and elevated serum ALP.

Etiology

Exogenous administration of glucocorticoids and naturally occurring hyperadrenocorticism can induce morphologic changes in hepatocytes and abnormal clinicopathologic test results in the dog. Other steroid hormones and adrenal sex hormones may cause similar changes. Some dogs can acquire vacuolated hepatopathy without any specific etiology. Steroid hepatopathy is not typically seen in cats.

Pathophysiology

While most dogs receiving glucocorticoids accumulate hepatocellular glycogen, not all develop the same degree of change. Some dogs develop focal necrosis and severe hepatomegaly, whereas others exhibit almost no response. The reason for this individual variation is unknown. Scottish Terriers with vacuolar hepatopathy typically do not have clinical signs. Increased ALP activity is often dramatic. Adrenal steroids are thought to play a role in the development of the vacuolar hepatopathy in most cases. Progression to inflammation and fibrosis is more likely in Scottish Terriers than other dogs with steroid hepatopathy.

Clinical presentation

Dogs present with clinical signs associated with corticosteroid use – a history of polydipsia/polyuria, polyphagia, nocturnal restlessness, panting, and weight gain. Later there may be a history of ventral and lateral abdominal hairlessness, thin skin, pendulous abdomen (**Figure 9.51**), and muscle wasting. There may be palpable hepatomegaly. Icterus is absent. There may be a history of oral, otic, or ophthalmic administration of corticosteroids. Failing this, endogenous overproduction of glucocorticoids should be suspected.

Differential diagnosis

Includes all causes of hepatomegaly including hepatic neoplasia, other causes of vacuolar hepatopathy, and hepatic amyloidosis.

Diagnosis

Increased ALP activity is the most consistent finding. The increased ALP activity is predominantly due to an isoenzyme of ALP produced by the canine liver in response to glucocorticoids. ALP activity may be dramatically increased, similar to the increases associated with extrahepatic biliary obstruction and cholangitis. In contrast, serum bilirubin concentration remains normal in most dogs with steroid hepatopathy. Also, while ALT may show a mild to moderate increase, the AST usually remains close to normal (**Figure 9.52**). The serum bile acid concentration may be mildly increased (usually <25 µmol/l in the fasted state [10.25 µg/ml]).

Microscopic examination of a hepatic aspirate or biopsy specimen reveals a characteristic vacuolar degeneration as glycogen is lost during tissue fixation and staining (**Figure 9.53**).

Management

Withdrawal of steroid therapy or treatment of endogenous adrenal production is usually all that is required. Treatment with ursodeoxycholic acid and SAMe may hasten recovery.

CANINE HEPATIC LIPIDOSIS

Definition/overview

Accumulation of small (microvesicular) lipid-containing vacuoles within the cytoplasm of hepatocytes is seen rarely in dogs. Accompanying hepatic failure may be noted (**Figures 9.54a, b**).

9.52

Glucose	5.2 mmol/l (93 mg/dl)
BUN	6.1 mmol/l (17 mg/dl)
Creatinine	61.9 µmol/l (0.7 mg/dl)
Cholesterol	**15.6 mmol/l (607 mg/dl)**
Total bilirubin	5.1 µmol/l (0.3 mg/dl)
Total protein	65 g/l (6.5 g/dl)
Albumin	34 g/l (3.4 g/dl)
AP	**2,519 U/l**
Calcium	2.5 mmol/l (10.1 mg/dl)
Phosphorus	0.6 mmol/l (2.0 mg/dl)
AST	88 U/l
ALT	**239 U/l**
Globulin	31 g/l (3.1 g/dl)
Chloride	107 mmol/l (107 mEq/l)
Sodium	146 mmol/l (146 mEq/l)
Potassium	3.9 mmol/l (3.9 mEq/l)
Total CO_2	22 mmol/l (22 mEq/l)

Figure 9.52 Serum chemistry profile showing some of the commonly elevated parameters (in bold) caused by glucocorticoid hepatopathy in the dog.

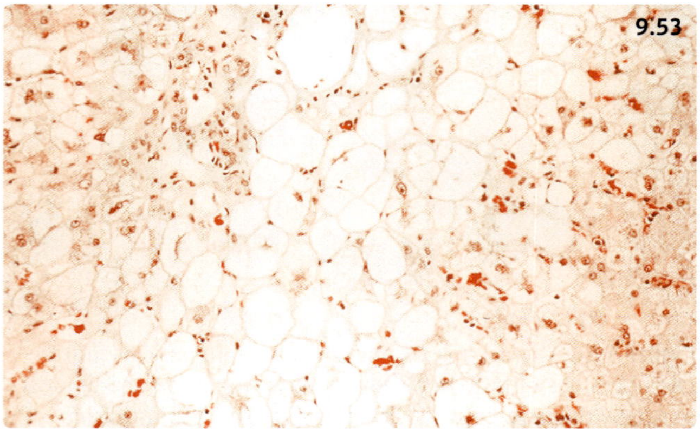

Figure 9.53 Histologic appearance of canine glucocorticoid hepatopathy. Note the vacuolated cells that contained glycogen prior to fixation.

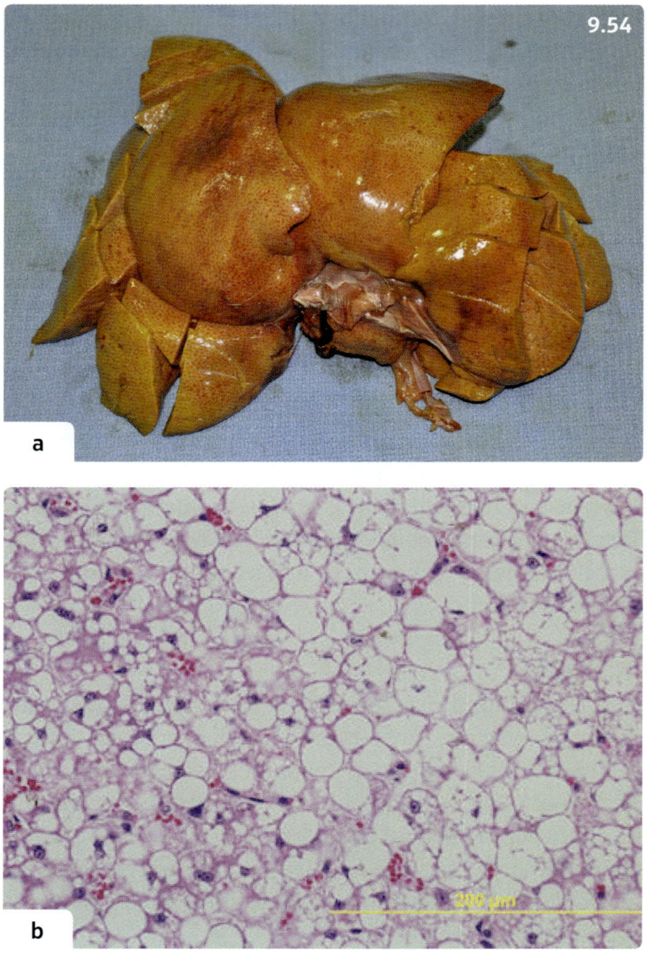

Figures 9.54a, b Postmortem specimen and histopathology from a diabetic ketoacidotic dog dying from fuminating hepatic lipidosis. (Courtesy M. Schaer)

Etiology

Hepatic lipidosis in dogs is usually associated with ketoacidotic diabetes mellitus or juvenile hypoglycemia of small breed dogs.

Pathophysiology

Excessive transport of fatty acids into the liver from mobilization of fat stores associated with insulin resistance, decreased hepatocyte and mitochondrial oxidation of fatty acids, and decreased transport of lipoproteins from the liver. Severe lipid accumulation may result in severe hepatic failure.

Clinical presentation

Clinical signs are usually due to ketoacidotic diabetes mellitus or associated with starvation and hypoglycemia in toy breed neonates.

Diagnosis

Hepatic cytology or biopsy.

Management

Glucose supplementation, nutritional support, and treatment of any underlying disease should be attempted in neonatal toy breed puppies with hepatic lipidosis. Dogs with diabetes mellitus should be treated for ketoacidosis. Because liver failure and hepatoencephalopathy may be contributing to clinical signs, appropriate treatment of fulminant hepatic failure and hepatoencephalopathy is important.

CONGENITAL PORTOSYSTEMIC VASCULAR ANOMALIES (PORTOSYSTEMIC SHUNTS)

Definition/overview

Congenital anomalies of the portal vascular system (PSSs) occur commonly in the dog and are being recognized with increasing frequency in the cat. The anomalous vascular development can involve one or more vessels of the hepatic portal circulation. Single intrahepatic shunts are more common in large breed dogs and single extrahepatic shunts are more common in cats and small breed dogs. Other intrahepatic vascular anomalies are being identified.

Etiology

The reason, or reasons, congenital PSSs develop is not known, but there appears to be a genetic basis in certain lines of Miniature Schnauzers, Irish Wolfhounds, Old English Sheepdogs, and Cairn Terriers. A proposed microvascular dysplasia within the liver has been reported for the latter breed as well as in other small breeds and in cats. Yorkshire Terriers and Miniature Schnauzers are breeds that appear to be at increased risk. Mixed breed cats are most commonly affected and of the purebreds, Himalayans and Persians appear to be at increased risk. Affected male dogs and cats are often cryptorchid. Most animals develop signs by 10 months of age, but they may be subtle and adequately compensated (or accepted by the owner) until they become more prominent later in life (up to 10 years of age).

Pathophysiology

Pathologic changes are secondary to decreased portal venous blood flow with subsequent increased hepatic arteriolar flow. Portal blood shunts past sinusoidal flow and hepatocellular contact, resulting in systemic delivery of materials absorbed from the GI tract including products of the intestinal microbiome. The liver appears grossly small and often mottled, and there is typically atrophy of the hepatocytes, with arteriolar hyperplasia and small or absent portal veins. Other features include sinusoidal congestion, biliary hyperplasia, lipogranulomas, increased periportal connective tissue, and periportal vacuolization.

Clinical presentation

The signalment and history provide important clues to the diagnosis. Affected animals may be normal in stature or may be small for their age, less active than their littermates, and may be labeled 'poor-doers'. Neurologic signs are common in the dog and include seizures and personality changes (**Figures 9.55**, **9.56**). Intermittent depression, disorientation, aggression, head pressing, blindness, mydriasis, and seizures have also been observed. Cats often show depression and anorexia. Polydipsia/polyuria, ptyalism (**Figure 9.57**), and recurrent formation of

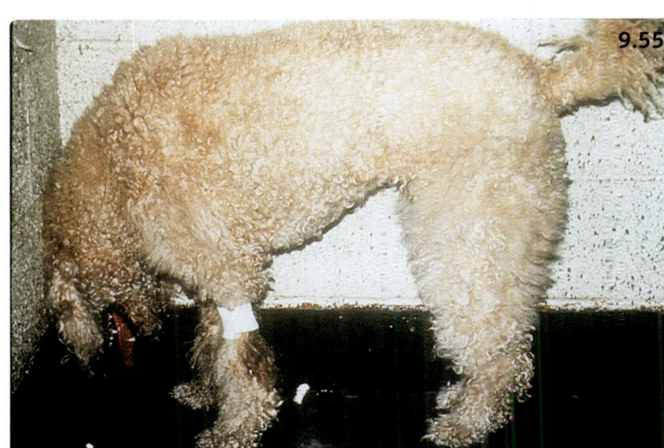

Figures 9.55 A Poodle with hepatic encephalopathy demonstrating behavioral changes such as head pressing and 'getting lost' in corners.

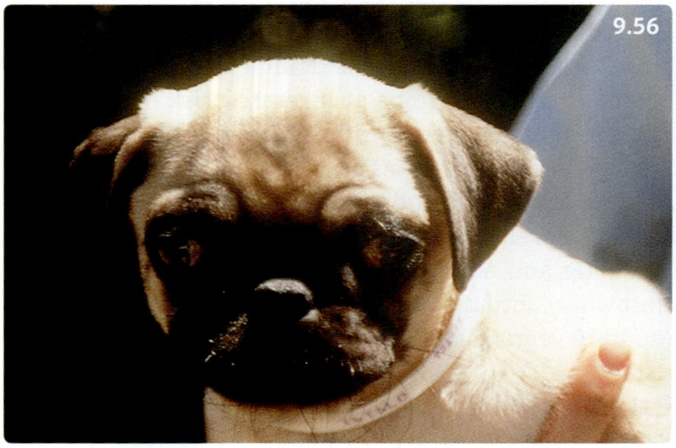

Figure 9.56 An abrasion on the head of a Pug as a result of head pressing. The animal was diagnosed with a portosystemic shunt and the signs disappeared after corrective surgery.

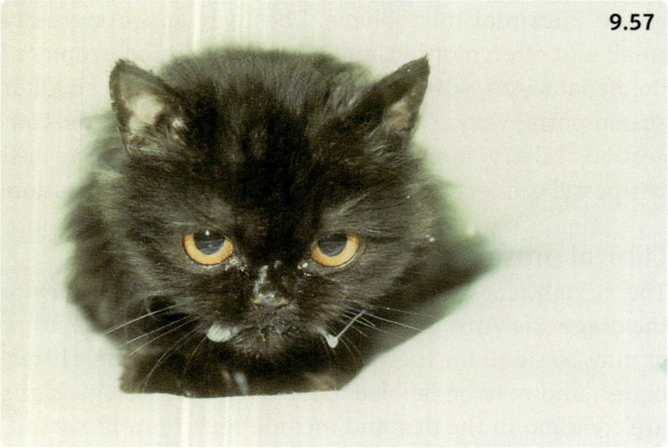

Figure 9.57 Ptyalism in a Himalayan kitten with hepatic encephalopathy as a result of a portosystemic shunt.

urinary calculi are also common findings. Renal, cystic, and urethral calculi may be the first clinical indication of an underlying congenital PSS in some dogs. Urate urolithiasis develops commonly. Signs may or may not be associated with eating. Unexpected prolonged recovery from general anesthesia or an exaggerated response to tranquilizers has been noted.

Findings on physical examination are often unremarkable. Occasionally, an inappropriately small body stature is present (**Figure 9.58**). Slightly enlarged kidneys have been palpated in some cats or small dogs, but this is more often detected radiographically.

Differential diagnosis

Portal vein hypoplasia, congenital enzyme deficiency of the urea cycle, infectious diseases (canine distemper, FIP, diseases related to feline leukemia virus and feline immunodeficiency virus, toxoplasmosis), idiopathic epilepsy, metabolic disorders (e.g. hypoglycemia, thiamine deficiency), hydrocephalus, toxicity.

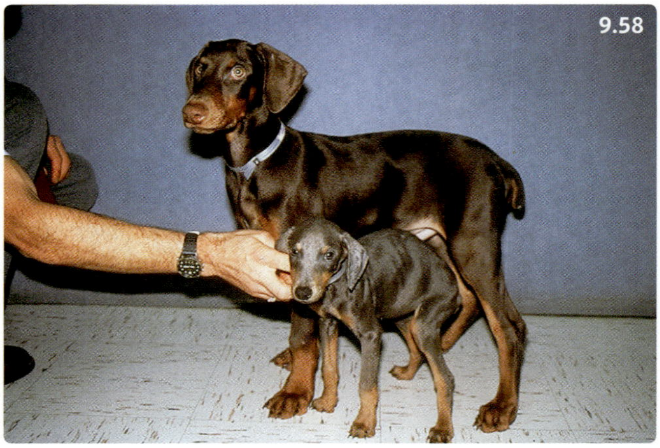

Figure 9.58 Dobermann littermates. The smaller dog has a portosystemic shunt with associated stunted growth.

Diagnosis

ALT and ALP activities may be normal or only slightly increased. Serum albumin and BUN concentrations are decreased in many patients with a PSS. Decreased concentrations occur because of hepatic atrophy and insufficient portal blood flow. These two parameters are valuable indicators of liver insufficiency on the biochemical profile.

A mild hypoglycemia may also be detected. The combination of a compatible history and biochemical abnormalities indicates the need for a function test such as serum bile acids or blood ammonia. Ammonium biurate crystals may be observed in the urine sediment (**Figure 9.59**) and evaluation of the hemogram may reveal a slightly decreased MCV. Serum iron is decreased in over 50% of dogs with confirmed PPS.

Imaging may reveal microhepatica in some patients (**Figure 9.60**). Visual confirmation of the portal vascular anomaly requires ultrasonography, CT angiography, scintigraphy, a cranial mesenteric angiogram, splenoportography, or jejunal vein portography (**Figure 9.61**).

Histologically, the liver may appear normal architecturally or there may be subtle changes of hepatic cord atrophy, small or absent portal veins, and an increase in arteriolar structures. Other nonspecific findings that may be reported include periportal or midzonal vacuolization, mild to moderate biliary hyperplasia, mild periportal fibrosis, and foci of iron-rich fatty macrophages (lipogranulomas). The latter finding is rare in normal dogs under the age of 6 years and should raise the suspicion of an underlying congenital portosystemic shunt.

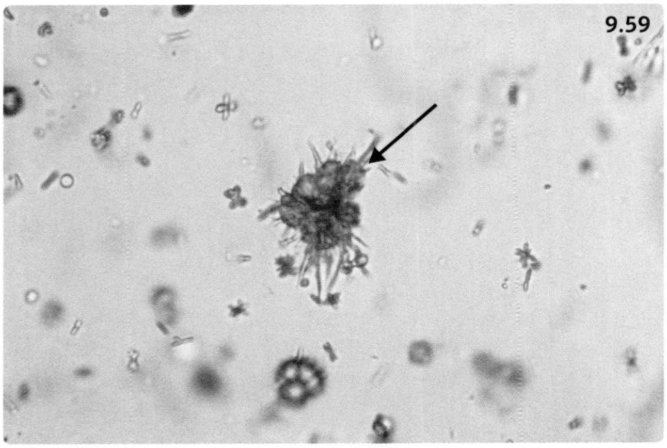

Figure 9.59 Ammonium biurate crystal (arrow) in the urine sediment in a dog with a portacaval shunt.

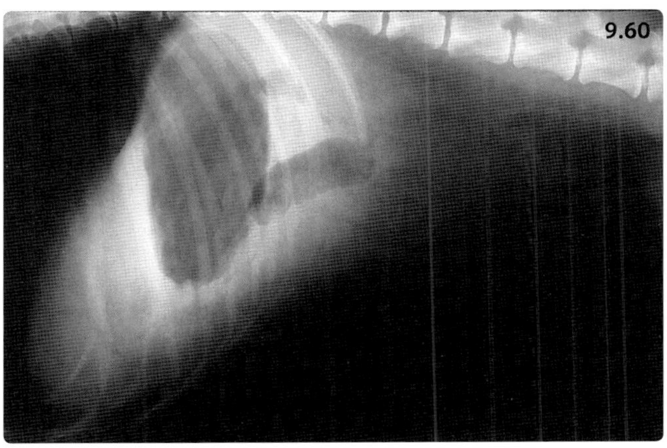

Figure 9.60 Lateral radiograph showing microhepatica, as evidenced by the vertical gastric axis, in a Dalmatian with a portosystemic shunt.

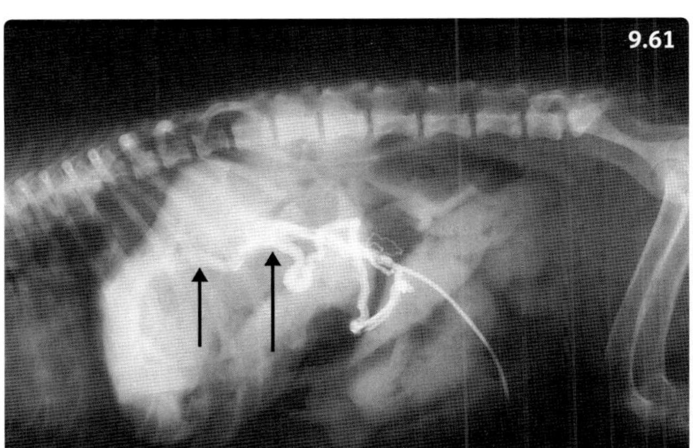

Figure 9.61 Mesenteric venous portography confirmed a shunt (arrows) in this 2-year-old Lhasa Apso.

Management

Surgical ligation or compression of the anomalous vessel is the treatment of choice in the dog and cat, but some shunts are now being treated by the implantation of coils under fluoroscopic guidance. If surgery is not an option, medical management with a low-quantity, high-quality protein diet, plus lactulose and neomycin or metronidazole to ameliorate signs of encephalopathy, may provide satisfactory results for months to several years depending on the severity of the vascular insufficiency.

FURTHER READING

Ettinger SJ, Feldman EC (2010) *Textbook of Veterinary Internal Medicine*, 7th edn. Elsevier Saunders, St. Louis.

Nelson RW, Couto CG (2014) *Small Animal Internal Medicine*, 5th edn. Elsevier Mosby, St. Louis.

Rothuizen J, Bunch SE, Charles JA *et al.* (2006) *WSAVA Standards for Clinical and Histological Diagnosis of Canine and Feline Liver Disease – WSAVA Liver Standardization Group*. Elsevier Saunders, St. Louis.

Washabau RJ, Day MJ (2013) *Canine & Feline Gastroenterology*. Elsevier Saunders, St. Louis.

Chapter 10

Pancreatic disorders

Michael Schaer

INTRODUCTION

Disorders of the digestive tract occur commonly in dogs and cats. The clinical signs involving diseases of the liver, pancreas, and bowel can show considerable overlap. This makes an accurate diagnosis a formidable challenge to the small animal practitioner.

Most experienced internists will attest that there is seldom anything pathognomonic about acute pancreatitis. Therefore, if a diagnosis is to be made, a thorough review of all the available clinical findings is necessary.

ACUTE PANCREATITIS

Definition/overview

Of the various clinical disorders treated by the small animal practitioner, there is probably none more difficult and frustrating to treat than acute pancreatitis. Despite the continuing acquisition of new knowledge regarding pancreatic physiology and pathophysiology, there is still no miracle treatment that can directly counteract the ravages of acute necrotizing pancreatitis. However, the optimal therapeutic outcome depends to a great extent on the clinician's working knowledge of the physiology, pathophysiology, clinical features, and medical and surgical treatments for this disorder in the dog and cat.

Etiology

Fortunately, the dog and cat are spared from many of the causes of pancreatitis that affect humans (**Table 10.1**). However, there are several general mechanisms that should be considered such as obstruction to the pancreatic duct, dietary factors, infectious agents, trauma, toxic drug reactions, metabolic abnormalities, and vascular alterations.

Table 10.1 Some causes of acute pancreatitis in humans.

Causes
* Biliary tract disease
Ethanol abuse
Infectious agents (viral, bacterial, toxoplasmosis)
Peptic ulcer
Methanol
* Trauma, surgery
Scorpion bites (Trinidad)
* Vascular factors – ischemia, thrombosis
* Carcinoma of the pancreas
* Hyperlipoproteinemias (type , IV, and V in humans)
* Hypotensive shock
* Hypercalcemia
* Ductal obstruction by tumors
* Drugs
* High-fat diet – dogs only
Hereditary pancreatitis, pancreas divisum

* Causes that have been implicated in dogs and cats

Pathophysiology

At the cellular level the calcium-dependent intra-acinar cell activation of pancreatic digestive zymogens, particularly proteases, is an early event in the initiation of acute pancreatitis. Activation of transcription factor NF-κB also occurs early in experimental pancreatitis. Early pathologic Ca^{2+} mobilization into acinar cells has a central role in the pathogenesis of acute pancreatitis. Another early acinar cell event is thought to be a decrease in compartmental pH. Other contributing factors to pathogenesis include neurally mediated inflammation and the production of large amounts of reactive oxygen species along with the simultaneous depletion of antioxidants.

The neutrophil migration that takes place is a result of the activation of trypsin, chymotrypsin, and oxygen radicals. The cytokines that are subsequently produced go on to cause the systemic inflammatory response syndrome. Other factors that augment the inflammatory response include altered pancreatic microcirculation, a shift from acinar cell apoptosis to necrosis, and the activation of other vasogenic pathways.

Prostaglandins are thought to have a key role in the pathogenesis of acute pancreatitis (**Figure 10.1**). Suspected mechanisms for these cyclo-oxygenase-2 effects include regulating heat shock protein 70 expression, inducible nitric oxide synthase activity, release of substance P,

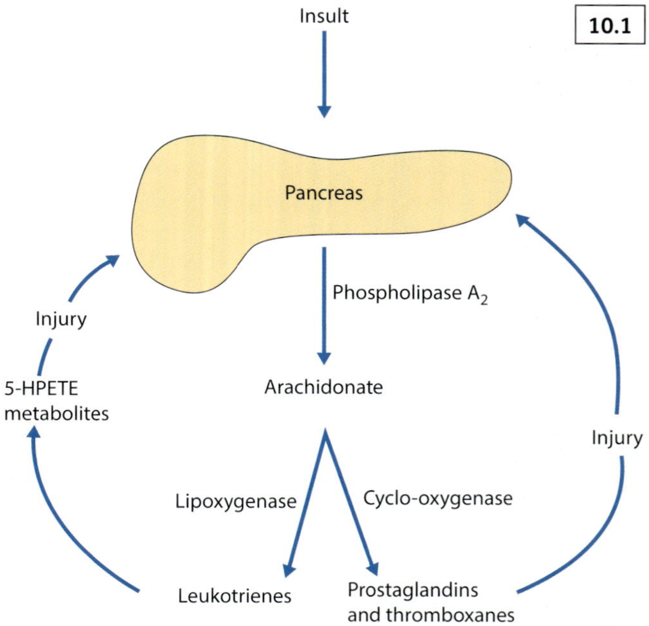

Figure 10.1 The role of prostaglandins in acute pancreatitis. Arachidonic acid metabolites are important mediators of inflammation in acute pancreatitis. 5-HPETE, 5-hydroperoxyeicosatetraenoic acid. (Source: Nager AB, Gorelick FS (2004) Acute pancreatitis. *Current Opinions in Gastroenterology* **20(5)**:439–443.)

and neutrophil function. A number of factors that can cause the described disturbances of cellular metabolism will cause increased permeability of cellular lipoprotein membranes surrounding the lysosomal hydrolases in the acinar cells, with resultant inappropriate proenzyme activation and autodigestion. At first the antiproteases will attempt to counteract the released proteases, but eventually the activation of the pancreatic proteolytic enzyme cascade will prevail and cause clinical acute pancreatitis. The characteristics of activated pancreatic enzymes and their effects on the pancreas and other tissues are shown in **Table 10.2** and illustrated pathologically in **Figures 10.2–10.22**.

Marked hypotension can be observed in dogs and cats with acute pancreatitis, and it is probably the main contributing factor to their demise. Studies of the hemodynamic consequences of severe pancreatitis in humans demonstrate that the cardiac index is increased and the systemic vascular resistance is decreased; these findings are similar to those in patients with sepsis. The mechanisms responsible for these effects involve various inflammatory mediators including interleukin (IL)-1, IL-2, IL-6, IL-8, tumor necrosis factor (TNF), platelet activating factor, and interferon gamma. Circulating vasoactive

Table 10.2 Characteristics of the pancreatic enzymes.*

Enzyme	Substrate	Effects
Lipase	Triglyceride	Fat necrosis Hypocalcemia Cell membrane damage
Phospholipase A_2	Cell membranes Phosphatides	Lysophosphatide formation Membrane destruction Vascular leakage Acute respiratory distress syndrome
Trypsin	Other proenzymes Kallikreinogen Scleroproteins	Coagulation necrosis Vascular leakage, shock Proteolysis Coagulopathy Kinin release
Chymotrypsin/ carboxypeptidase	Scleroproteins	Coagulation necrosis Proteolysis Vascular leakage
Elastase	Scleroproteins Elastic/collagen fibers of blood vessels	Coagulation necrosis Elastocollagenolysis Proteolysis Vascular leakage Hemorrhage
Kallikrein	Kinins	Kinin release

Modified from Büchler MW, Uhl W, Malfertheiner P *et al.* (2004) (eds.) *Diseases of the Pancreas*. Karger, Basel.

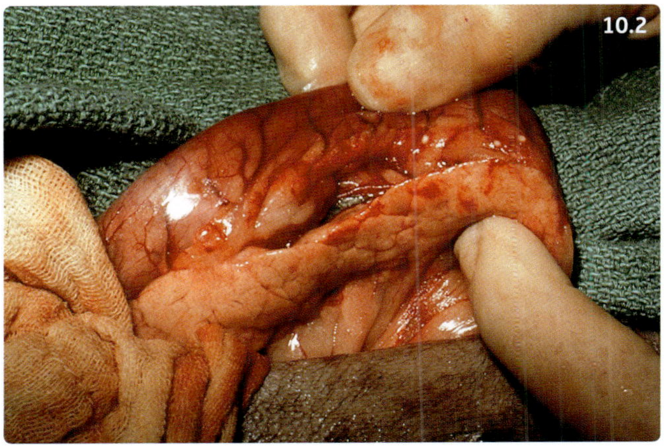

Figure 10.2 This 7-year-old male Poodle was taken to surgery after a 5–7-day period of medical treatment accompanied by persistent vomiting. Shown is edematous pancreatitis.

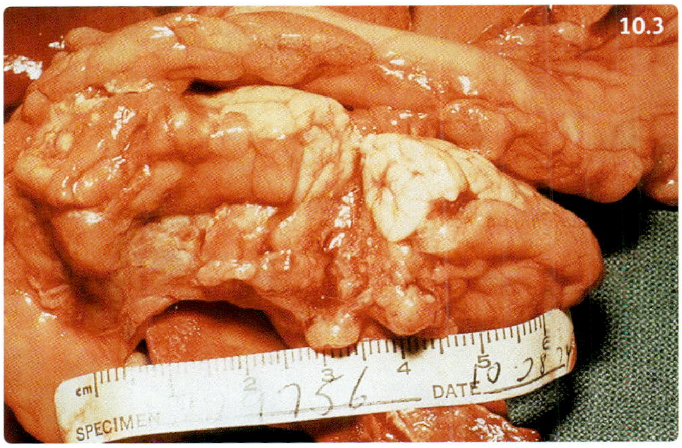

Figure 10.3 Postmortem specimen illustrating edematous pancreatitis and extensive peripancreatic fat necrosis. This patient was a 4-year-old female Yorkshire Terrier that also had diabetic ketoacidosis and renal failure.

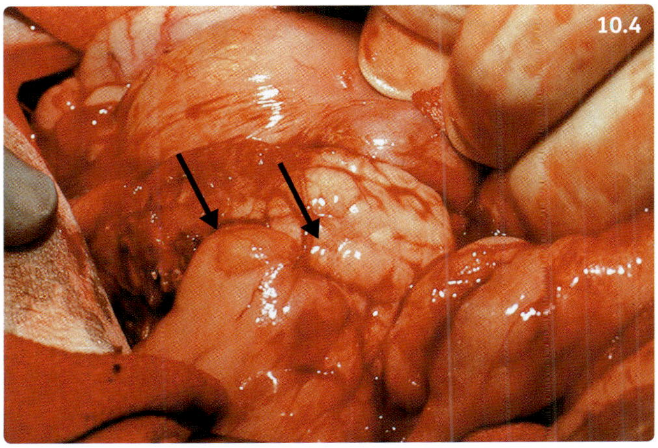

Figure 10.4 Surgical view of hemorrhagic necrotic pancreatitis in a 10-year-old male Wirehaired Fox Terrier. Note how one half of the pancreas is hemorrhagic and the other half is edematous (arrows).

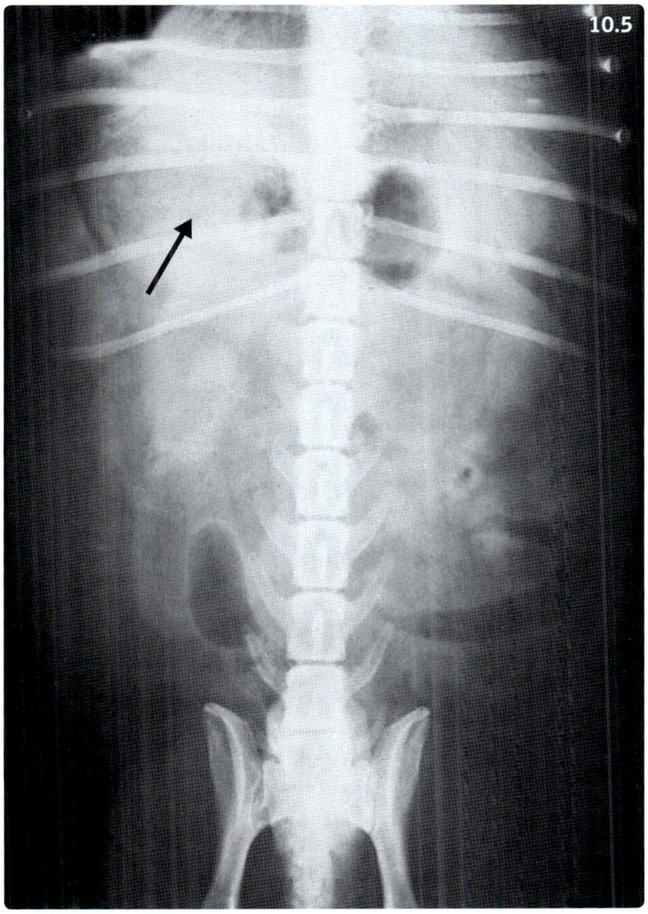

Figure 10.5 Radiograph, taken from the dog in Figure 10.4, typical of acute pancreatitis, showing increased fluid density in the right upper abdominal quadrant (arrow) and lateral displacement of the duodenum.

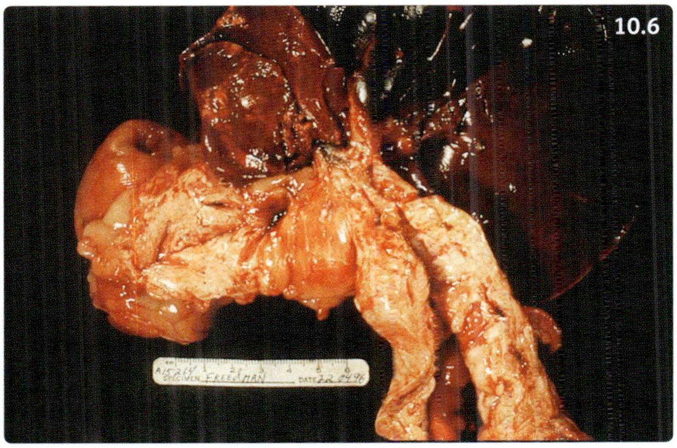

Figure 10.6 Over the ensuing year, the dog in Figures 10.4 and 10.5 had several episodes of relapsing pancreatitis that eventually terminated with renal shutdown. This postmortem specimen shows chronic pancreatic scarring along with recent necrotic changes.

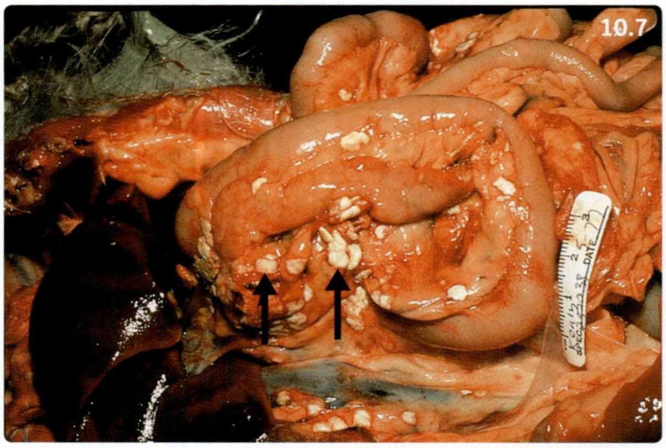

Figure 10.7 Postmortem view of the abdomen of a 13-year-old female Lhasa Apso showing diffuse edematous pancreatitis accompanied by diffuse calcium soap deposition (arrows) throughout the mesentery and omentum.

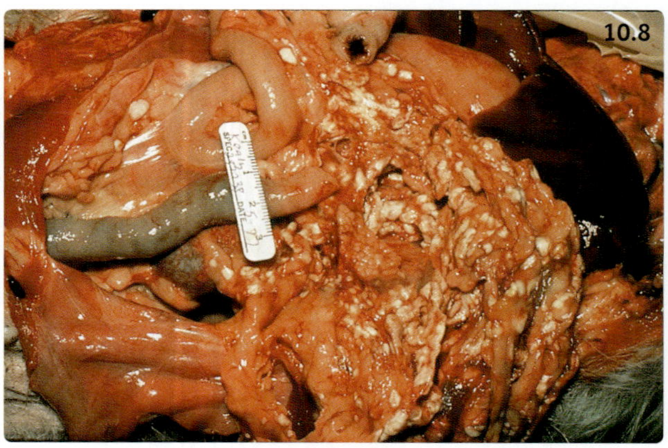

Figure 10.8 Another view of the specimen shown in Figure 10.7. This calcium soap formation is one of the accepted explanations for the lowered serum calcium level that can accompany acute pancreatitis.

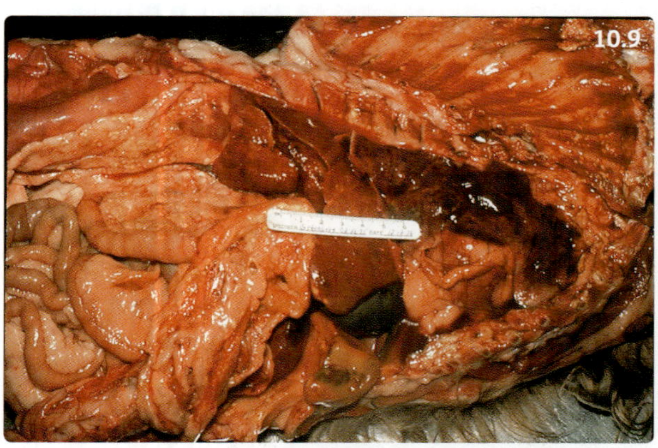

Figure 10.9 This 14-year-old male Dachshund had pleural effusion along with acute pancreatitis. Shown is the serosanguineous pleural effusion that is accompanied by calcium soap deposits on the pleural membranes underlying the thoracic viscera.

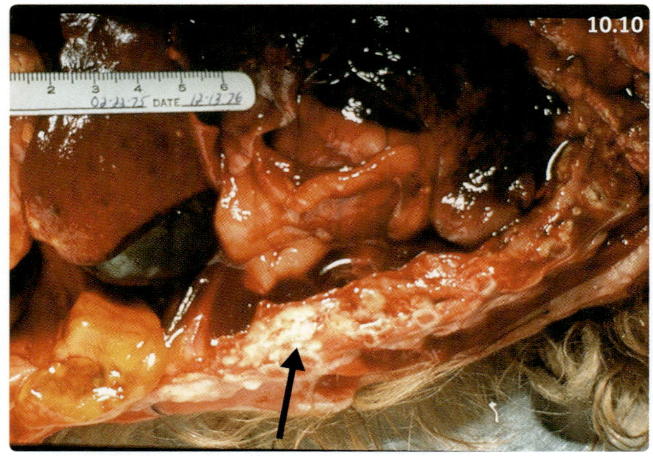

Figure 10.10 The same dog as in Figure 10.9, showing the intercostal muscles with calcium soap deposits (arrow).

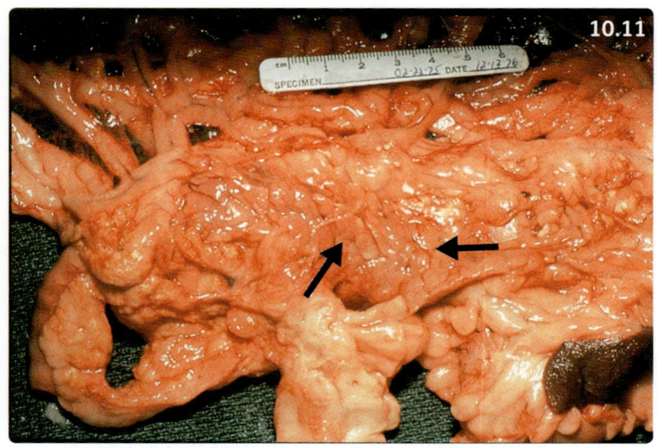

Figure 10.11 The dog in Figures 10.9 and 10.10 had edematous pancreatitis (arrows).

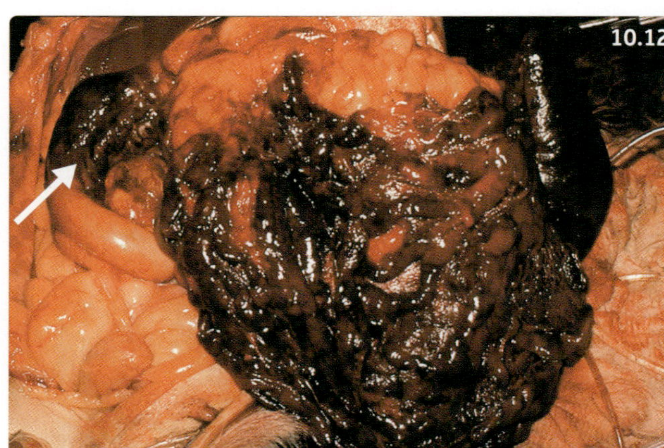

Figure 10.12 Postmortem findings of severe hemorrhagic pancreatitis complicated by pathologic coagulation causing infarction to the duodenum (arrow) and omentum.

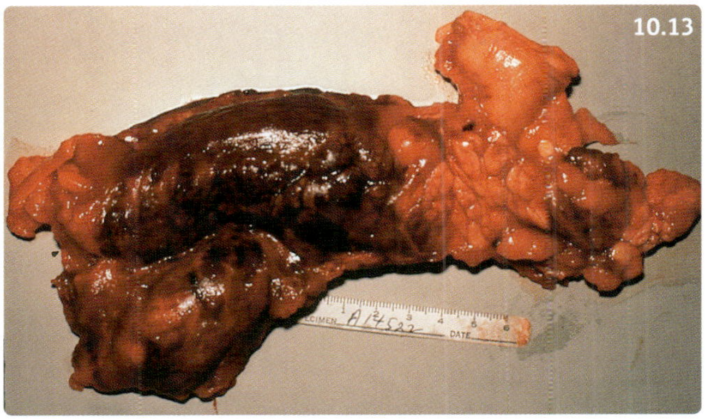

Figure 10.13 Marked pancreatic necrosis in the specimen shown in Figure 10.12. The peripancreatic lymph node is markedly enlarged from hemorrhagic necrosis.

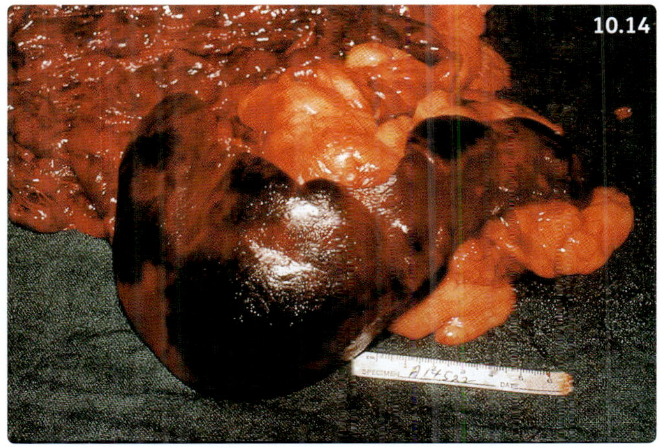

Figure 10.14 Multiple splenic infarcts in the 9-year-old dog in Figures 10.12 and 10.13. It was taken to surgery where it expired. Disseminated intravascular coagulation was the cause of the hypercoagulable state.

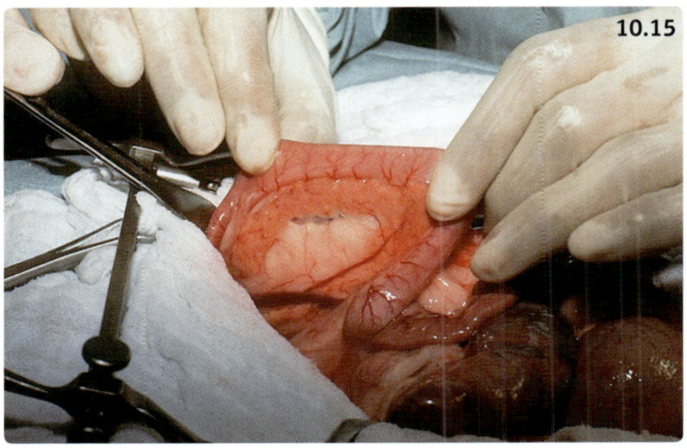

Figure 10.15 Surgical view of a 16-year-old cat with chronic active pancreatitis. This cat had been hospitalized 3 years earlier with acute pancreatitis, which responded well to conservative treatment.

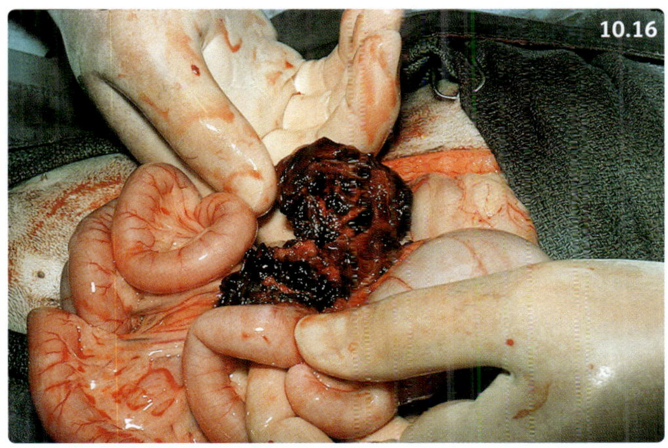

Figure 10.16 This 10-year-old cat was taken to surgery for the primary problems of vomiting, depression, and a hemorrhagic abdominal effusion. Shown is hemorrhagic pancreatitis. Copious surgical lavage and the insertion of abdominal drains until 2–3 days postoperatively would be the usual surgical measures for this type of pathology.

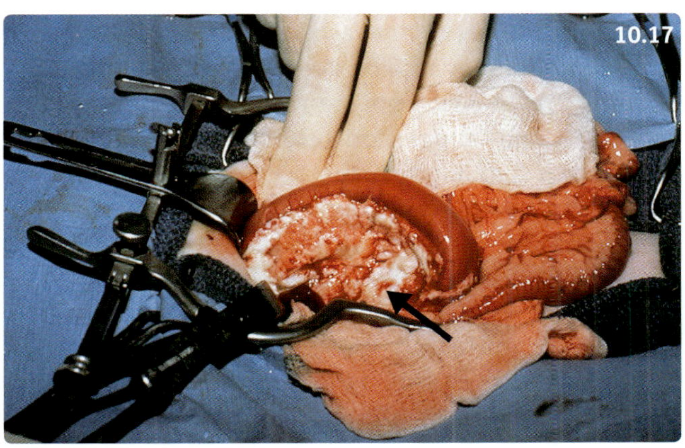

Figure 10.17 After 7 days of medical therapy, this 12-year-old female cat was taken to surgery because it showed no signs of improvement. Shown is hemorrhagic pancreatitis accompanied by extensive peripancreatitic and mesenteric calcium soap formation (arrow). Postoperatively, nutrition was provided through a jejunostomy tube that was inserted at the time of surgery. This cat survived after 3 weeks of illness.

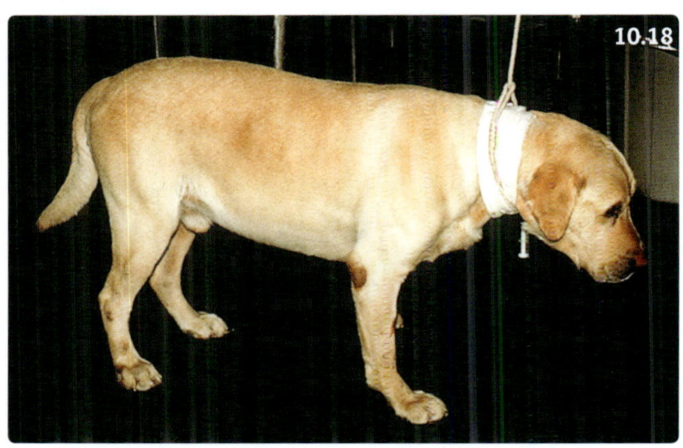

Figure 10.18 This 5-year-old male Labrador Retriever had vomiting, fever, depression, and abdominal pain.

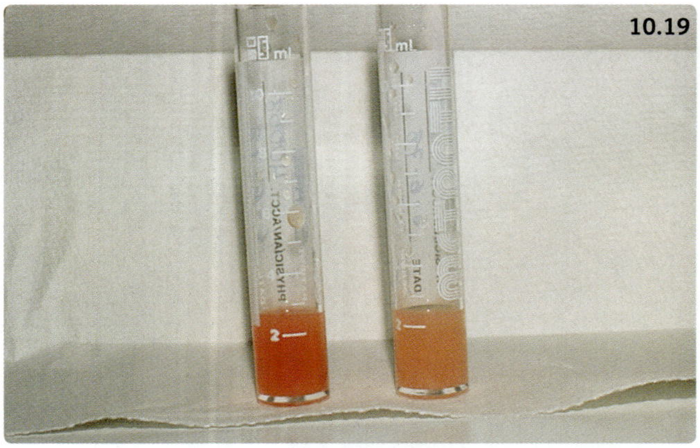

Figure 10.19 Blood samples taken from the dog shown in Figure 10.18 were markedly lipemic. The patient died despite intensive medical efforts.

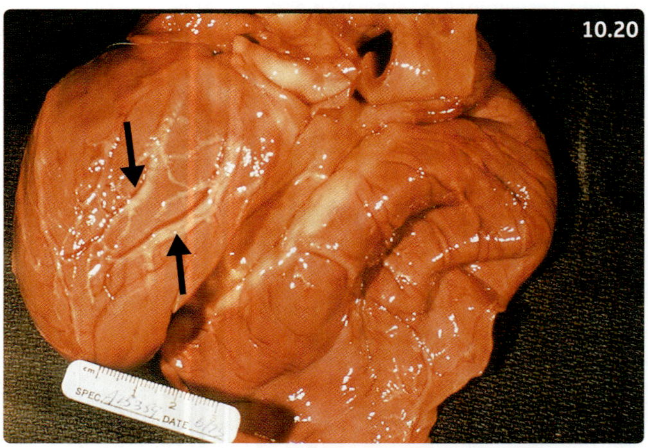

Figure 10.20 Postmortem examination of the dog in Figure 10.18 showed diffuse thyroid atrophy. The severe atherosclerotic vascular lesions shown here involved the coronary arteries (arrows).

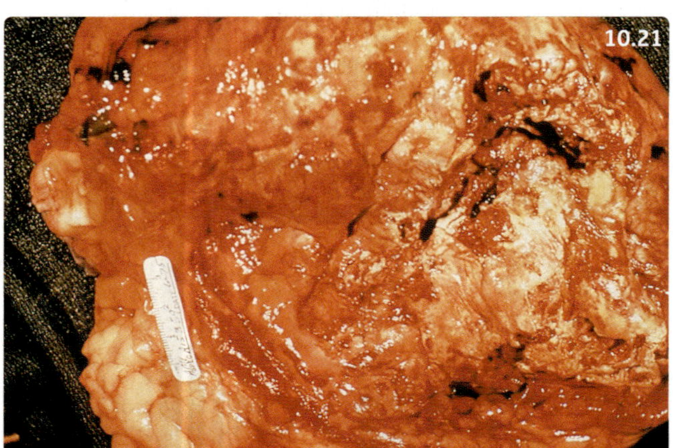

Figure 10.21 There was also extensive pancreatic phlegmon formation in the dog shown in Figure 10.18. The primary cause of this dog's pancreatitis was hypothyroidism, which caused marked hyperlipidemia; this, in turn, could have triggered the acute pancreatitis. Hyperlipidemia is a well-known common cause of acute pancreatitis in humans.

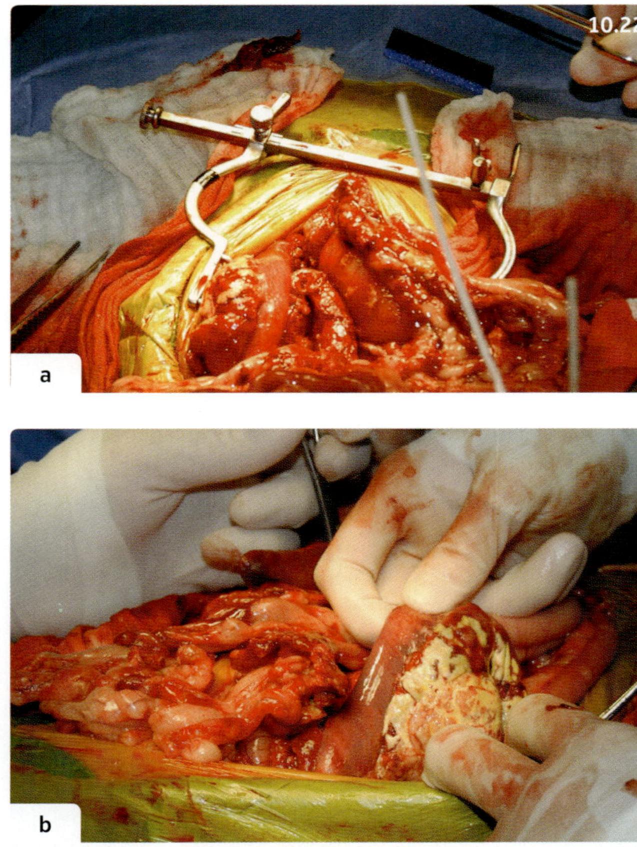

Figures 10.22a, b (a) Pancreatic phlegmon is illustrated in this surgical view showing extensive parapancreatic soft tissue adhesions. (b) The pancreas from the same dog showing extensive saponification.

com-pounds, such as bradykinin and myocardial depressant factor (in the dog), resulting from pancreatic necrosis, also contribute to the vasomotor instability. The low blood pressure may also be due to sequestration of fluid from the plasma space into the 'third spaces' of the peritoneal cavity and retroperitoneum. Experiments in the dog have shown that approximately 35% of the total plasma volume can be lost from the circulation 4 hours after the induction of acute pancreatitis. The local and systemic effects of acute pancreatitis are shown in **Figure 10.23**.

Clinical presentation

Most occurrences of acute pancreatitis in the dog involve middle aged, obese females; however, dogs with normal weight and male dogs can also be affected. The most common historical signs involve a sudden onset of vomiting, anorexia, and mental depression. Some occurrences reportedly follow the ingestion of a fatty meal, although this might not be a consistent finding. Initially, the vomitus might contain partially undigested food and this may be followed subsequently by vomitus consisting of bile and

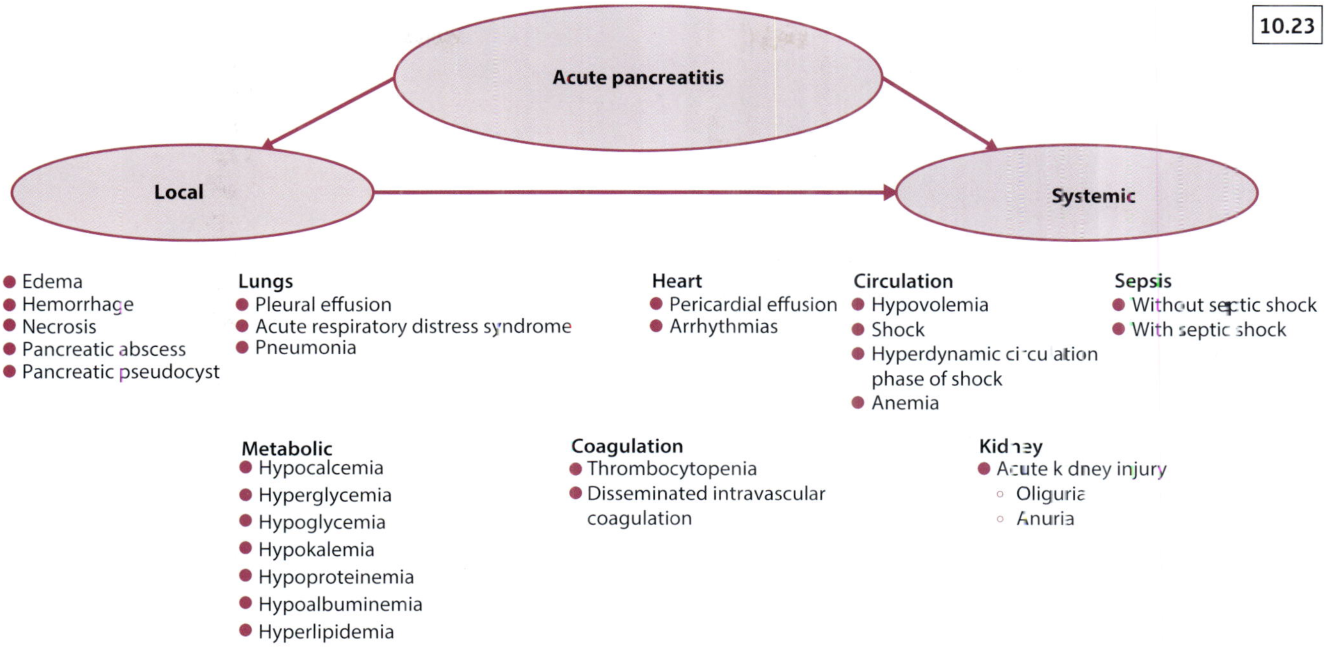

Figure 10.23 Pathophysiologic consequences of acute pancreatitis. The adverse effects of acute pancreatitis are far reaching, with involvement of several organ systems. In many cases this can lead to multiple organ dysfunction and the patient's demise. (Modified from Büchler MW, Uhl W, Malfertheiner P *et al.* (2004) *Diseases of the Pancreas*. Karger, Basel.)

watery mucus. After the initial vomiting, the dog might show regurgitant movements only because of nausea. Its attitude will vary from mild to marked depression, and its posture will either be normal, upright with abdominal tucking, or lateral recumbency depending on the degree of pain and hypovolemia (**Figures 10.24–10.28**). Diarrhea might occasionally occur, but scant or absent feces is more common due to the peritonitis-induced ileus.

The age of cats affected with acute pancreatitis can range from young to old, although in one study the majority of the cats were older than 8 years. Many have normal body weight. The clinical signs are similar to those in the dog, although vomiting might be occasionally absent and the clinical presentation much more subtle (**Figures 10.29, 10.30**).

The physical examination findings vary with the severity of the problem. Dogs and cats with mild pancreatitis might only show mild mental depression, normal vital signs, and equivocal palpable abdominal tenderness. Signs associated with the hemorrhagic necrotic form include: marked mental depression; fever; hypotension with accompanying tachypnea, tachycardia, and weak femoral pulse; a painful abdomen; and a moderate to marked degree of dehydration. Abdominal palpation in the cat can sometimes detect bowel adhesions (**Figure 10.31**). One retrospective study involving 40 cats reported the most common signs being severe lethargy, anorexia, and dehydration. Histopathology identified

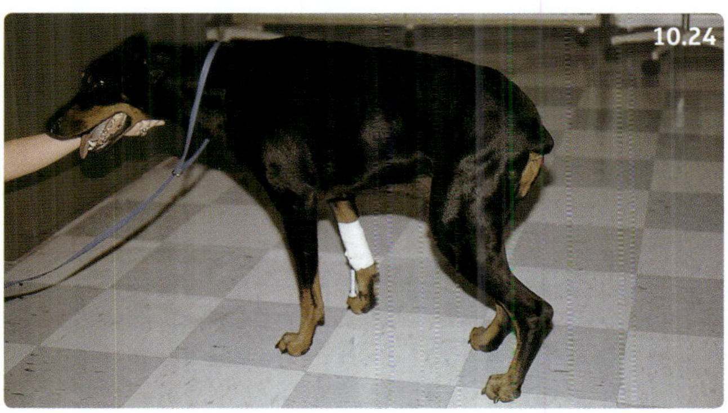

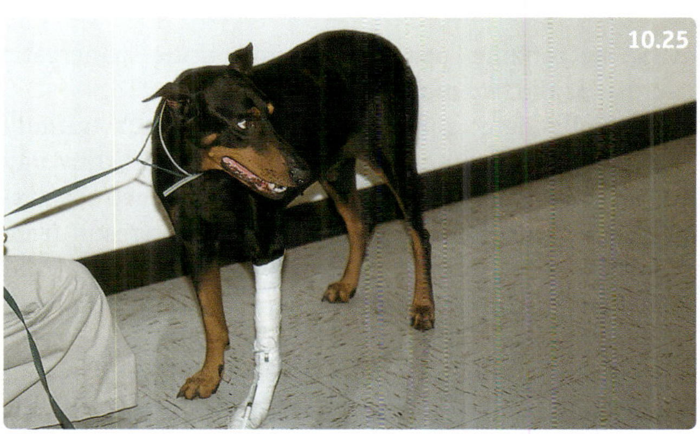

Figures 10.24, 10.25 This 5-year-old male Dobermann displays an abnormal posture from abdominal pain caused by acute pancreatitis. After 3 days of treatment the dog was pain free and its posture was normal.

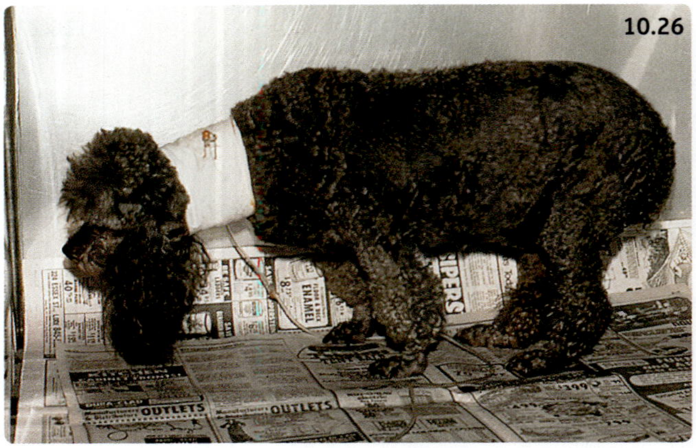

Figure 10.26 The clinical signs of acute pancreatitis can vary from mild to marked. This 13-year-old female Poodle had acute vomiting, mental depression, and marked abdominal pain peracutely immediately after dinner. Despite the use of intensive fluid therapy, the dog died from hemorrhagic necrotic pancreatitis.

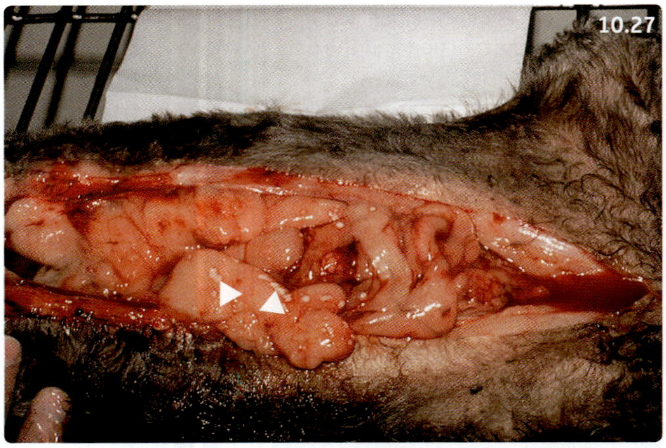

Figure 10.27 Postmortem examination of the dog in Figure 10.26. Shown here are calcium soap deposits (arrowheads) on the abdominal fat and pancreatic ascites.

acute necrotizing pancreatitis and acute pancreatic necrosis as the two main types.

Clinically detectable icterus will not occur initially with pancreatitis, but it might be evident by the third day and usually results from cholestasis; bile duct obstruction occurs rarely. Abdominal distension can result from paralytic ileus. A reddish-brown colored ascitic fluid (pancreatic ascites) can sometimes accumulate with hemorrhagic necrotic pancreatitis. A guarded to grave prognosis should always be given to pancreatitis patients that assume a lateral recumbent posture and have mental dullness, oliguria/anuria, and hypotension that is resistant to treatment. A more detailed and practical severity scoring system is provided in **Table 10.3**.

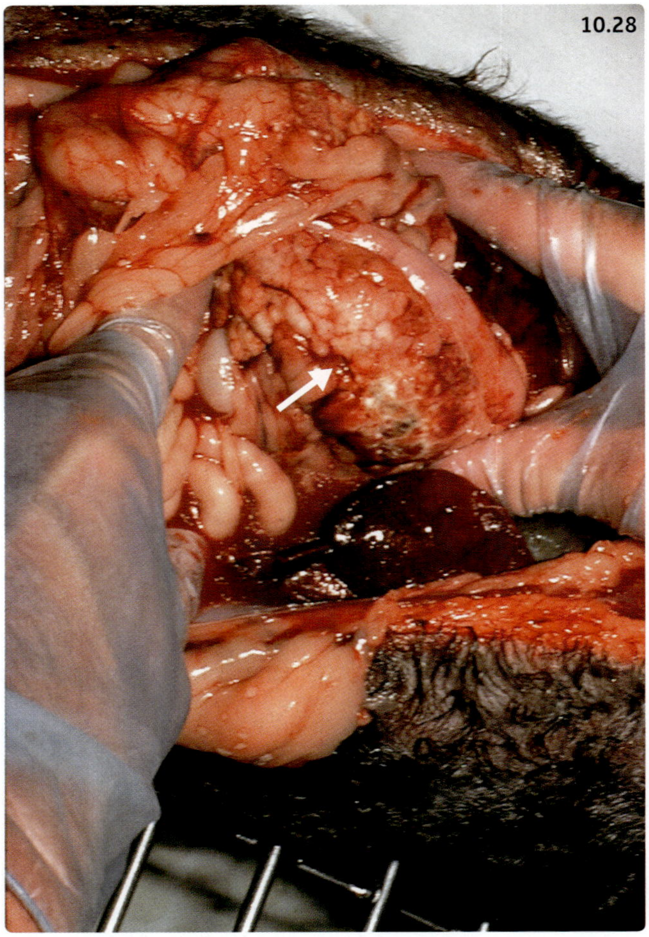

Figure 10.28 Severe hemorrhagic pancreatic necrosis (arrow) in the postmortem examination of the dog shown in Figure 10.26.

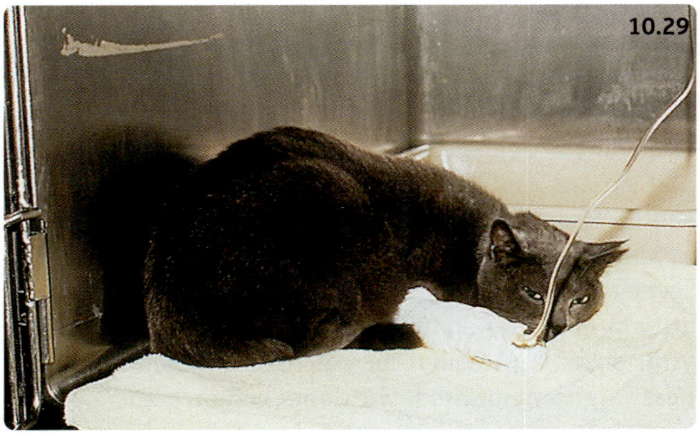

Figure 10.29 Pancreatitis in cats is typically accompanied by anorexia, mental depression, and marked inactivity. Although many cats will vomit, there are those who will not. Most cats with pancreatitis will show abdominal tenderness and varying degrees of radiographic pathology. A definitive diagnosis can only be obtained by visualizing the pancreas grossly with or without biopsy and histopathology.

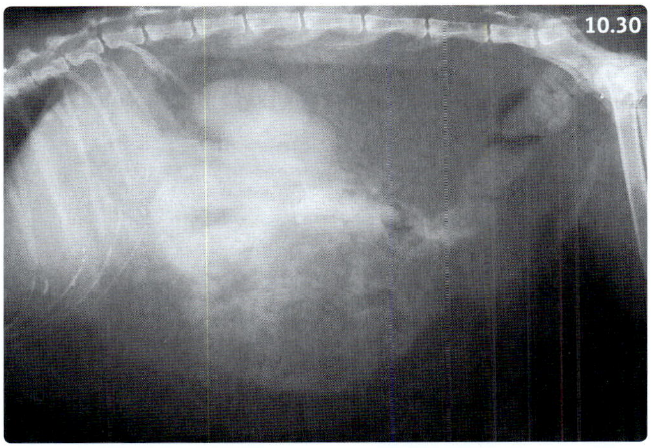

Figure 10.30 Lateral abdominal radiograph of the cat in Figure 10.29, which presented with acute pancreatitis, showing a diffuse abdominal effusion and a 'gathering effect' of the small bowel. These lesions were evident at surgery (see Figure 10.31). The abundant amount of retroperitoneal fat causes ventral depression of the descending colon.

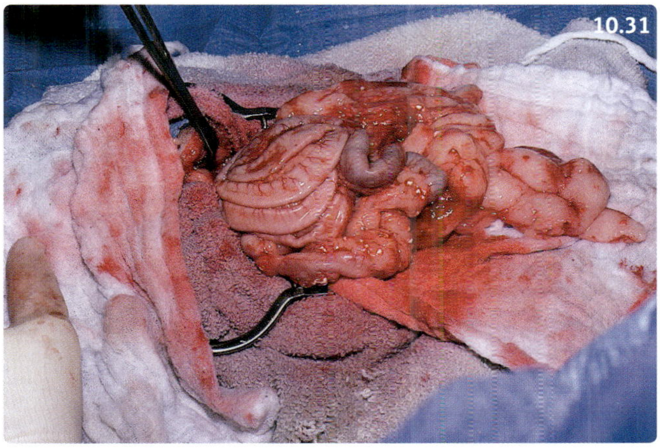

Figure 10.31 This surgical view of a 16-year-old female Domestic Shorthair cat shows small bowel adhesions, which were detectable on abdominal palpation. Also shown are diffuse calcium soap deposits on the parietal and visceral peritoneal surfaces. These deposits are pathognomonic of acute pancreatitis.

Table 10.3 Practical severity scoring in dogs.

Disease severity	Score*	Prognosis	Clinical presentation and typical therapy
Mild	0	Excellent	Often resolves spontaneously. Recovery is uncomplicated. Managed as an outpatient, if hydration status is good. Intravenous fluids can be given if necessary. Pancreatic rest (no food for 1–2 days if vomiting or nauseous) and/or pain control is usually all that is required. Maropitant will help the vomiting and nausea
Moderate	1	Good to fair	Usually dehydrated – the renal system is most often compromised (prerenal azotemia). Treatment involves the administration of crystalloids at twice the maintenance rate together with electrolytes. Nothing by mouth until vomiting stops, with analgesia and maropitant as appropriate. Recovery is usually uncomplicated provided adequate fluid therapy is given. If anorexia lasts for more than 2 days, consider additional nutritional support
	2	Fair to poor	Dehydrated, hypovolemic, often prerenal azotemia and degenerative left shift leukocytosis. Animals usually recover with intensive therapy, but may have to be euthanized for financial reasons. Intravenous crystalloids (initially administered as per treatment for shock) followed by colloids, with or without plasma, in many cases. Monitor urine output, renal function, and lung sounds. Control pain and consider special nutritional support. Monitor coagulation status carefully and intervene early with fresh frozen plasma and heparin, if necessary. May need referral if there is a poor response to initial therapy
Severe	3	Poor	Extensive therapy and life support is required with constant monitoring. Early referral is advised. Surgical intervention and peritoneal lavage may be necessary. Ventilatory support, central venous pressure monitoring, and high volume fluid therapy are usually needed. Jejunostomy feeding or total parenteral nutrition is often required. Most patients die and euthanasia may have to be considered. The pathology in these patients can include extensive pancreatic necrosis, pancreatic abscess, phlegmon formation, and macroscopic vascular compromise caused by regional infarction
	4	Grave	

Modified from Ruaux and Atwell (1998) and Ruaux (2000).
*The severity scoring system is based on the number of organ systems, apart from the pancreas, that show evidence of failure or compromise at initial presentation.

Table 10.4 Differential diagnosis of acute pancreatitis in the dog and cat.

Acute gastroenteritis
Intoxications
Blunt abdominal trauma
Gastrointestinal obstruction
Gastrointestinal perforation
Intestinal volvulus
Intestinal ischemia and infarction
Emphysematous cholecystitis
Ruptured organs (e.g. uterus, urinary bladder, gallbladder)
Acute kidney injury
Acute hepatopathy

Differential diagnosis

The initial differential diagnosis of acute pancreatitis includes a variety of clinical disorders (**Table 10.4**). The list is extensive because the signs mimic any number of acute abdominal syndromes. Several are surgical emergencies that require rapid diagnosis and treatment.

Diagnosis

Imaging findings

The two most commonly used modalities are radiology and ultrasonography. Abdominal radiographs of dogs and cats with acute pancreatitis can show several abnormalities. In the mild edematous form the findings can range from normal to mild ileus involving the stomach and duodenum. The more severe forms cause the following changes as a result of the peritonitis: increased fluid density with loss of visceral detail in the anterior abdomen, right-sided lateral displacement of a gas-distended duodenum, and gastric distension (**Figures 10.32–10.34**). In the dog, visualization of the right kidney becomes apparent on the ventral dorsal projection of the abdominal radiograph (**Figures 10.35a, b, 10.36).** This finding has been demonstrated in many dogs in the author's experience and the results corroborated at surgery or at necropsy. The exact mechanism for this phenomenum has not been thoroughly explained, but local adhesions associated with the regional peritonitis might be major factors. In addition to these classic findings, acute pancreatitis can also cause radiographically demonstrable pleural effusion and pulmonary fluid accumulations, as shown in the pathologic illustrations (see **Figures 10.9, 10.10**). In the most advanced stages of this disease, the acute respiratory distress syndrome can occur as a result of the systemic inflammatory response syndrome. The outcome associated with this syndrome is usually ominous (**Figures 10.37a–c**). In cats, pleural and pericardial effusions have been described.

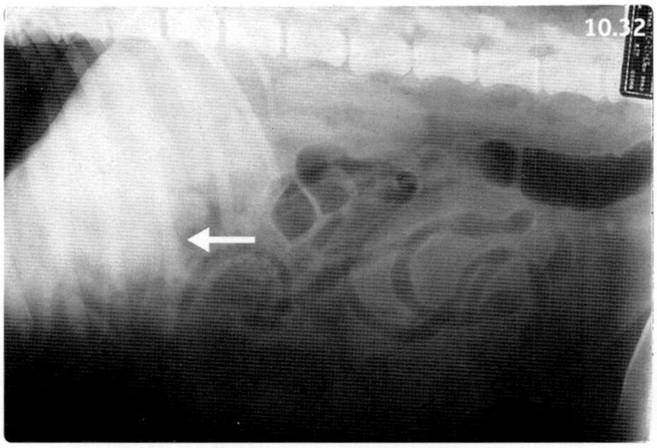

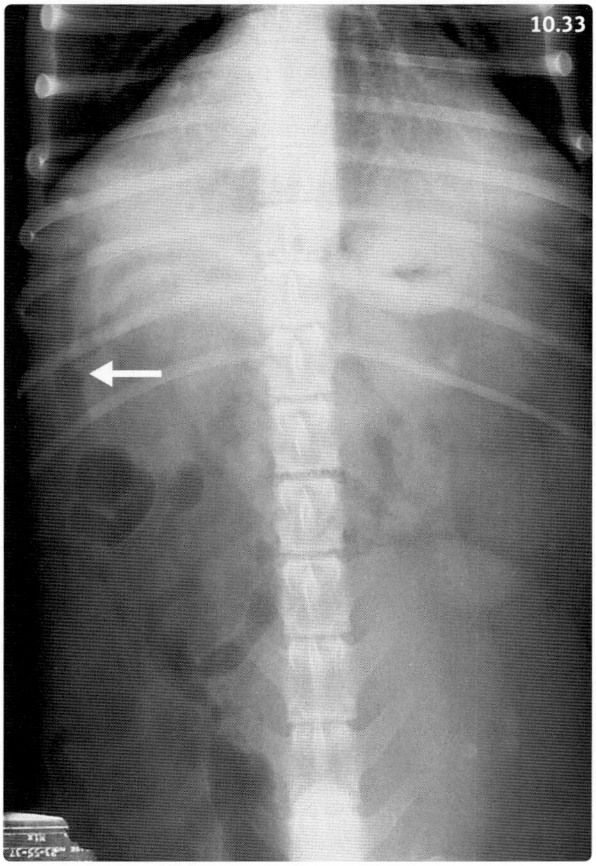

Figures 10.32, 10.33 Lateral and ventrodorsal abdominal radiographs of a dog illustrating several abnormalities indicative of acute pancreatitis. The lateral projection shows a loss of detail in the anterior mid abdomen and an increased fluid density in the anterior abdomen just caudal to the liver (arrow). The ventrodorsal view shows an increased right upper abdominal fluid density along with duodenal ileus and lateralization (arrow).

Ultrasonography is very useful in detecting pathology associated with pancreatitis in the dog and cat. While the normal pancreas is seldom visualized, the inflamed organ in the dog acquires an increased hypoechogenicity.

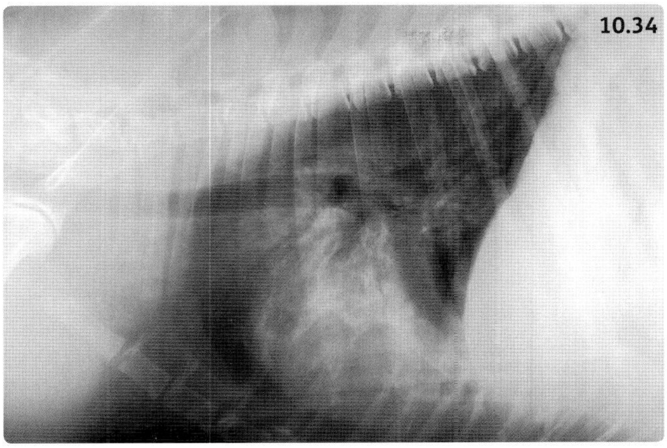

Figure 10.34 Lateral thoracic radiograph from an adult Labrador Retriever showing a pleural effusion as well as pulmonary infiltrate. The dog had hemorrhagic necrotic pancreatitis and secondary acute respiratory distress syndrome.

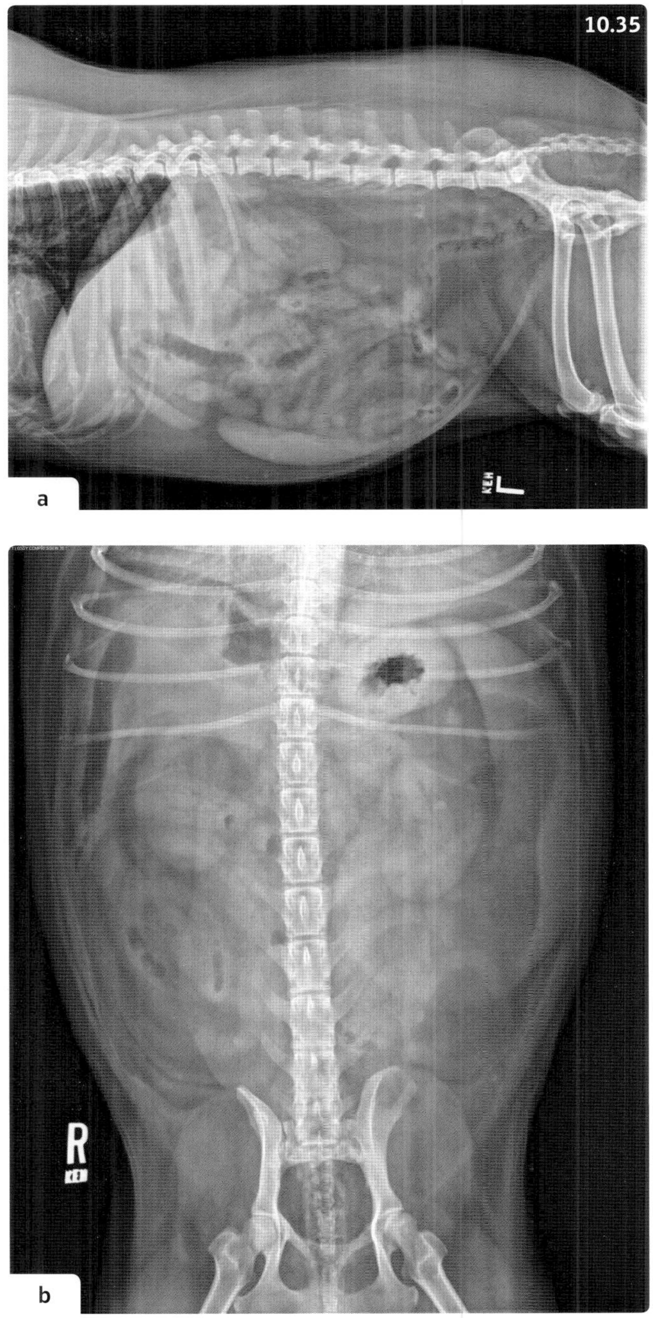

Figures 10.35a, b Lateral and ventrodorsal radiographs of a dog with acute pancreatitis showing a summation soft tissue fluid effect in the cranial abdomen on the lateral view. The ventrodorsal view clearly shows the right kidney.

In the presence of peripancreatic fat inflammation, the perimeter of the pancreas becomes hyperechogenic. Additional findings in the dog include pancreatic enlargement and irregularity, peritoneal effusion, and evidence of extrahepatic biliary obstruction. Inflammation of the right pancreatic limb can cause the duodenum to appear thickened. One study describing the ultrasonographic findings of acute pancreatitis in cats included hypoechogenic pancreas, hyperechoic peripancreatic mesentery, peritoneal effusion, pancreatic enlargement, hyperechoic hepatomegaly, and mixed pancreatic hypo- and hyperechogenicity. Pancreatic anechoic pseudocyst and abscess formation and pancreatic ascites can also be detected with ultrasonography (**Figures 10.38, 10.39, 10.40a–d**). Overlying distended bowel loops are the major limitation to this imaging technique, but in most instances abdominal ultrasonography is a helpful diagnostic modality (**Figures 10.41–10.44**).

Clinicopathologic findings

The characteristic laboratory test abnormalities of acute pancreatitis in dogs and cats have been described. These are listed in **Table 10.5** and illustrated in **Figure 10.45**. In cats the serum biochemical profile is variable, ranging from normal to abnormalities involving renal, liver, glucose, protein, and electrolyte parameters. The hemogram often indicates an inflammatory response. One study of 46 cats with pancreatitis suggests that low plasma ionized calcium concentration is common and is associated with a guarded to grave prognosis, especially when ionized calcium concentrations are ≤1.0 mmol/l (4.0 mg/dl).

Choosing between amylase or lipase as a diagnostic test has been a subject of controversy for several years, because both enzyme levels can be normal or elevated from other conditions despite the presence of acute pancreatitis, thus causing them to lack both sensitivity and specificity. Increases in serum amylase levels to 3–5 times normal are strongly suspicious of acute pancreatitis in the appropriate clinical setting.

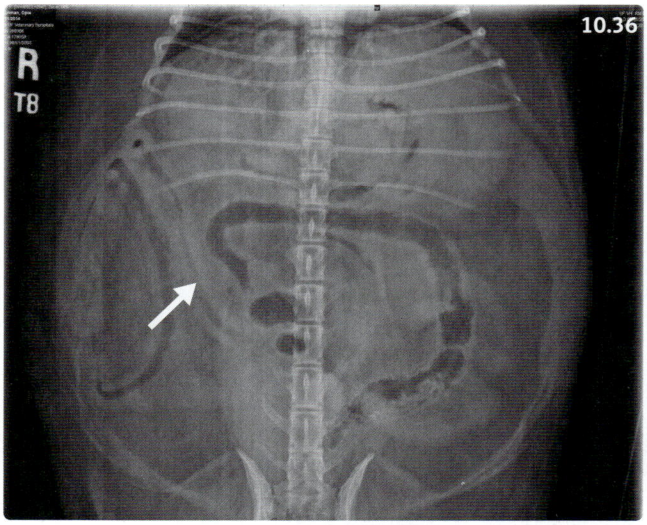

Figure 10.36 Ventrodorsal radiograph of another dog with acute pancreatitis showing a highly visible right kidney outline (arrow).

Serum lipase level has been reported to be more reliable than amylase for diagnosing acute pancreatitis in the dog. However, lipase as well as amylase may be elevated in patients with serious abdominal illnesses such as hepatopathies and renal and neoplastic disease. Serum amylase and lipase activities can be normal or even decreased despite the presence of serious pancreatic damage because of rapid renal clearance and diminished quantity after the initial elevation. The interpretation of serum amylase and lipase results should always be made solely within the context of the patient's other ongoing clinical findings.

In feline pancreatitis the appearance of abnormally elevated serum amylase and lipase levels is typically variable and should never be the sole criteria for diagnosis. Normal levels of both enzymes commonly occur in the cat despite the presence of acute pancreatitis. A two-fold or more increase in serum amylase and lipase activity in the presence of normal renal function is suggestive of acute pancreatitis when used with other supportive clinical findings.

When the feline trypsin-like immunoreactivity (TLI) concentration test first became available, there was a false dependence on its supposed accuracy. It is no longer recommended as a diagnostic test for acute pancreatitis in cats.

In dogs the canine pancreatic lipase immunoreactivity (PLI) test is supposed to be fairly sensitive for diagnosing acute pancreatitis. The diagnostic cut-off value is 200 μg/l. This test can now be done in-house with a commercially available kit in addition to it being done in commercial laboratories. A recent (2012) multi-institutional study evaluating the canine pancreatic lipase immunoassay and the point of care (SNAP®) assay, showed that the tests

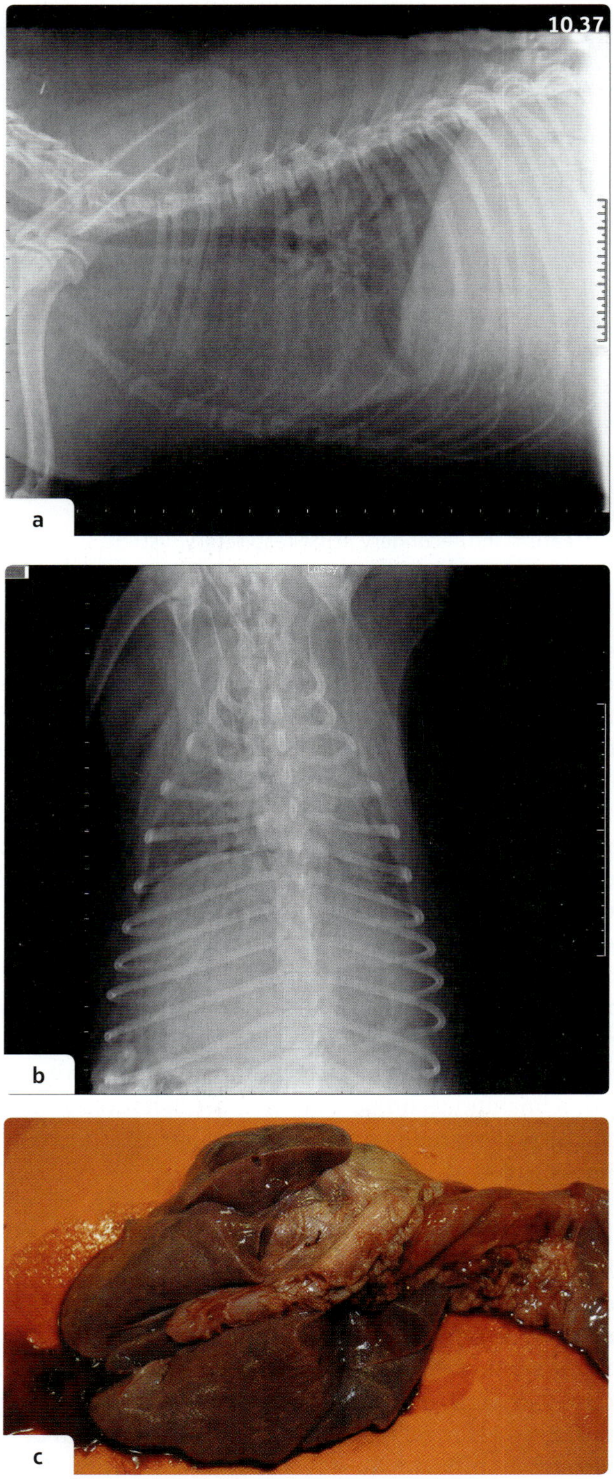

Figures 10.37a–c Thoracic radiographic images (a, b) from a dog that has severe acute pancreatitis with a pancreatic abscess. The dog acquired acute respiratory distress syndrome (ARDS) and was eventually euthanized. The radiographs, taken during the final days, show diffuse pulmonary infiltrate and some pleural effusion. The lungs as seen at necropsy (c) were consolidated and the histopathology features confirmed ARDS.

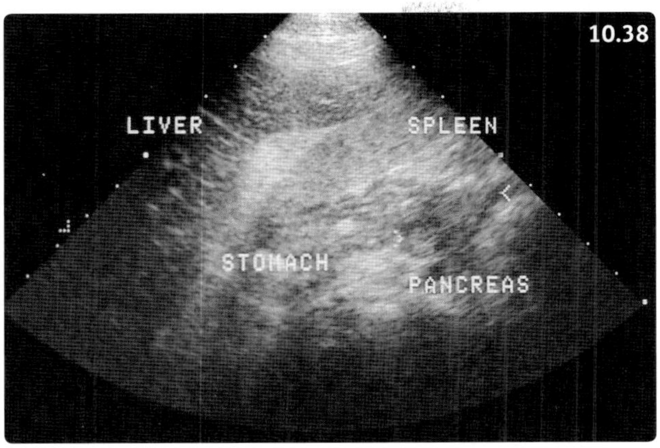

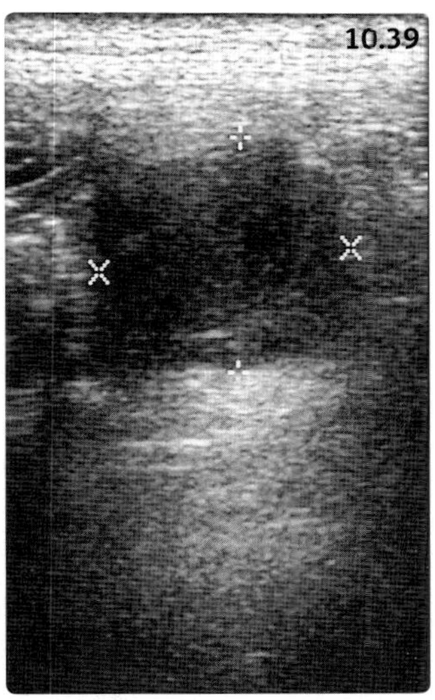

Figures 10.38, 10.39 Abdominal ultrasonograms from a 5-year-old male Irish Setter taken 2 weeks after a bout of acute pancreatitis. (10.38) General orientation of the dog's upper abdomen showing an anechoic area in the pancreas. (10.39) More detailed view of the pancreatic cavitation. The transabdominal fine needle aspiration yielded a dark colored fluid that was composed of sterile amorphous debris. All of the 'cystic' fluid was removed by aspiration and the dog recovered well.

have higher sensitivities and specificities than the serum amylase and lipase tests. However false-positive test results are still possible with both of these tests and their results should be interpreted along with other diagnostic modalities such as imaging.

There is also a feline PLI test that adds to the clinician's diagnostic acumen for acute pancreatitis in the cat. This feline pancreatic lipase test (fPLI) has been shown to have greater diagnostic accuracy than the feline TLI test. The same caution regarding interpretation of this test in the dog should be used when using this test in the cat. It is essential to realize that there is no one laboratory test that is 100% accurate in diagnosing acute pancreatitis in the dog and cat and that the newly available PLI tests are simply another diagnostic tool that can help lead to a diagnosis. The gold standard test for diagnosing acute pancreatitis in veterinary patients is gross observation of the pancreas with or without biopsy and histopathology.

Management

Medical therapy

Therapy entails the restriction of oral intake (nothing by mouth) if the animal is vomiting profusely, while providing fluid and electrolyte needs by parenteral means. The steps listed in **Table 10.6** provide guidelines for treating the more severe form of pancreatitis.

Patients who have suspicious yet mild historical and physical signs with unremarkable laboratory test results can often be treated conservatively with small feedings for 1–2 days, if they will eat voluntarily, and periodic offerings of water.

Esophageal, gastric, or jejunal feeding tubes can be placed early in the course of treatment and low-volume frequent feedings can be given through the tubes.

Initially, the most important component of treatment of severe pancreatitis is the provision of adequate parenteral fluids. Marked hypotension in the dog should be treated with rapid volume expansion with lactated or acetated Ringer's at an initial dosage of 20 ml/kg (for cats give 7–10 ml/kg) over the first 15 minutes of treatment and repeated at 15-minute intervals until the blood pressure is normalized. Normal saline (0.9%) is no longer a preferred fluid because of its tendency to cause hyperchloremic metabolic acidosis. Saline will be indicated if the patient is hyponatremic. Close patient monitoring is essential in order to prevent intravascular fluid overload. This can be done crudely by observing breathing quality and listening to lung sounds. After the vital signs are stabilized and urine output is noted as adequate, a maintenance fluid rate of 60–120 ml/kg can be given gradually over the remaining 20–22-hour period. The amount of maintenance fluid depends on the patient's vasomotor stability, the degree of abdominal effusion accumulation ('third spacing'), and the presence of ongoing losses through vomiting and diarrhea. The intravenous maintenance solution can consist of 2.5–5% dextrose in 0.45% saline solution supplemented with potassium chloride (3–5 mmol/kg/day [3–5 mEq/kg/day]) and soluble vitamin B complex. Any acid–base abnormalities should be recognized and treated appropriately. Severely hypoproteinemic animals (serum albumin <20 g/l [2.0 g/dl]) should receive fresh plasma (5–20 ml/kg per day IV). This will temporarily increase the plasma oncotic pressure

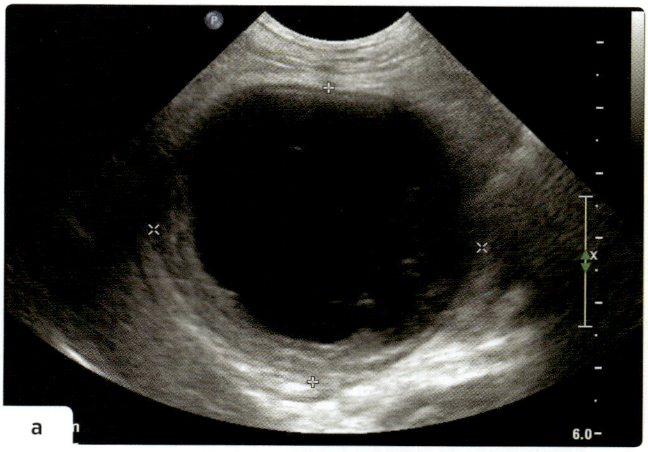

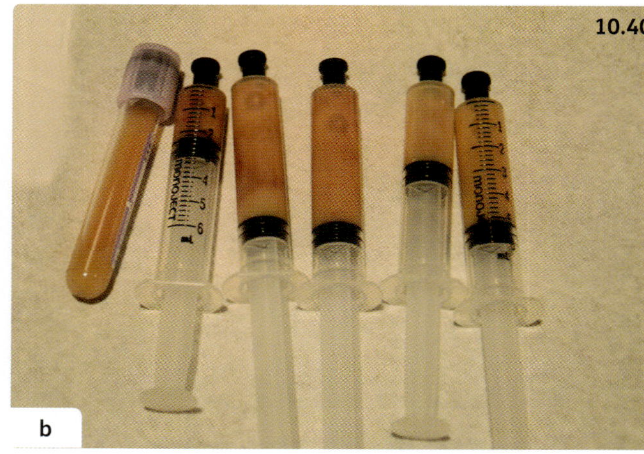

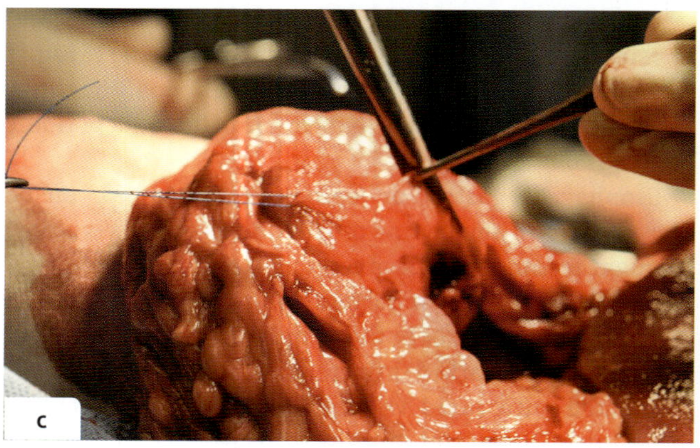

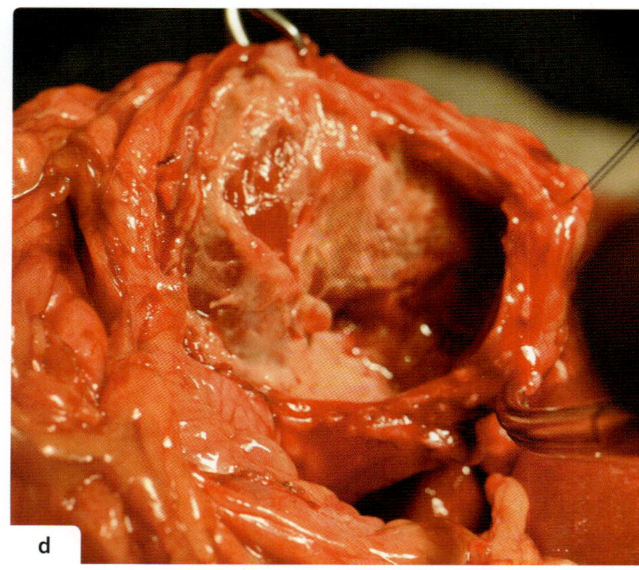

Figures 10.40a–d Images of a large pancreatic pseudocyst in a dog showing its ultrasonographic appearance, the cyst contents from a fine needle aspiration procedure, and the cyst at surgery (intact and after resection).

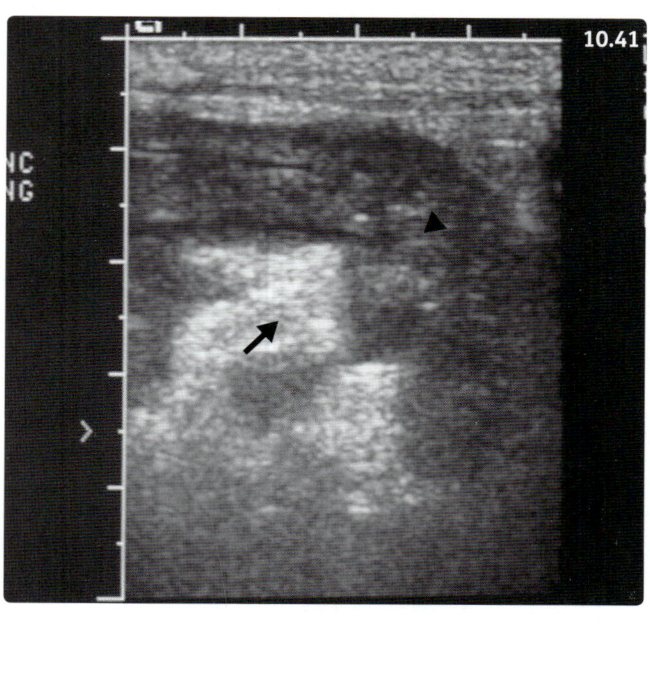

Figure 10.41 Abdominal ultrasound examination of a 7-year-old male English Cocker Spaniel showing lesions typical of acute pancreatitis, including hypoechogenicity of the pancreatic parenchyma (arrowhead) and prominent hyperechogenicity of the inflamed peripancreatic fat, which contained ample calcium soap deposits (arrow). This dog was also in an addisonian crisis. He became anuric and was subsequently euthanized. The postmortem findings included acute necrotizing pancreatitis (similar to that shown in Figure 10.27), bilateral adrenocortical atrophy, and thyroid atrophy. It was thought that the untreated hypothyroidism caused hyperlipidemia, which could have predisposed the dog to acute pancreatitis. The adrenal and thyroid conditions could have been associated with an autoimmune polyhypoendocrinopathy condition.

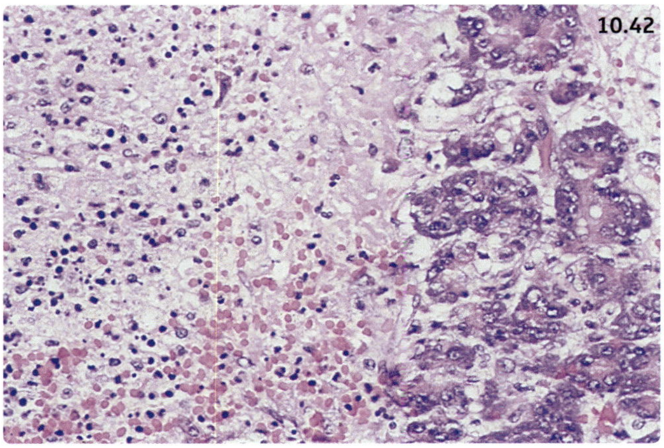

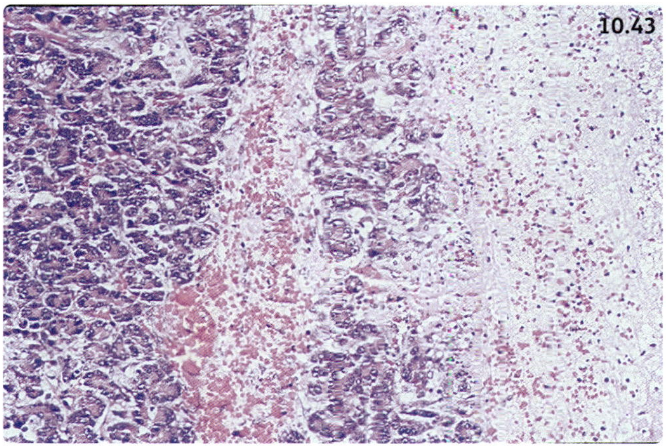

Figures 10.42, 10.43 Histopathology of the pancreas of the dog in Figure 10.36 showing glandular necrosis, hemorrhage, edema, and inflammatory infiltrate consisting of neutrophils and macrophages. (H&E) (Courtesy P. Ginn)

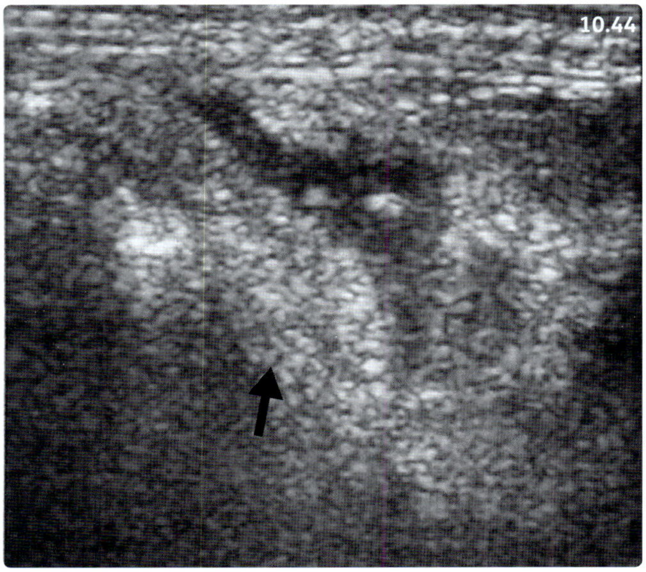

Figure 10.44 Cats can also have typical ultrasonographic signs of acute pancreatitis, as evidenced by the parenchymal hypoechogenicity and a 'rim' of hyperechogenicity (arrow). This 7-year-old male cat was also a ketoacidotic diabetic who gradually improved with 3 weeks of intensive medical treatment alone. He eventually became cured of both diseases.

and help prevent edema formation, pleural effusion, pulmonary edema, and renal failure. Note that the actual volume of plasma needed and the usual prohibitive cost per unit will usually limit the actual amounts administered. Plasma (10 ml/kg IV over a 3–6-hour period) is also a source of pancreatic protease inhibitors, but studies in humans have shown no clinical benefit from this antiprotease activity in transfused plasma. Other colloidal solutions, such as hydroxyethyl starch (20 ml/kg IV over 24 hours) or dextrans (10–20 ml/kg IV over 24 hours), were formerly used as plasma substitutes, but they are no longer recommended because of the potential complications they can cause in the patient (acute kidney injury and bleeding, respectively).

Urine output should be closely monitored after the volume of the patient's plasma space is adequately expanded. Oliguria or anuria should prompt a furosemide-induced diuresis after rehydration is completed, even though it will not reverse acute kidney injury. Potassium supplementation should be discontinued if hyperkalemia develops. The induction of osmotic diuresis should be avoided if the animal's plasma is already hyperosmotic (usually from hyperglycemia). During oliguria the maintenance parenteral fluid volumes should be equal to the volume of urine produced plus any insensible fluid losses (10–15 ml/kg/day). During anuria any unsuccessful forced IV fluid diuresis attempts can cause potentially fatal pulmonary edema.

Drugs used to treat gastrointestinal disorders (e.g. atropine and propantheline) were commonly used in the past to help stop vomiting. However, their adverse parasympatholytic side-effects often exceeded any benefits. The current recommendation is to administer maropitant (1.0 mg/kg SC), which functions as a neurokinin (NK1) receptor antagonist antiemetic. If vomiting persists, metoclopramide can be used without the parasympatholytic effects of the early-generation antiemetics. The recommended dosage is 0.2–0.4 mg/kg SC q6–8h or 1 mg/kg/q24h by continuous IV infusion. Ondansetron is a centrally acting antiemetic that can be given to dogs and cats at a dosage of 0.15 mg/kg IV over a 6–12-hour period and repeated every 6–12 hours.

Famotidine, an H2 blocker, and gastric acid inhibitors, such as the proton pump blockers

Table 10.5 Clinicopathologic abnormalities accompanying acute pancreatitis in the dog and cat.

Abnormality	Proposed mechanism(s)
Leukocytosis	Inflammation, stress, hemoconcentration, secondary infection
Leukopenia	Mobilization to inflamed site, bone marrow suppression from endotoxemia
Hemoconcentration	Dehydration, translocation of plasma into abdominal cavity
Hypoalbuminemia	Intestinal loss, translocation into the abdominal cavity and peripancreatic tissues
Thrombocytopenia	Consumption from thrombus formation
Anemia	Hemorrhagic abdominal effusion, iatrogenic crystalloid fluid infusion
Azotemia	Prerenal from dehydration, renal from hypovolemia or disseminated intravascular coagulation, idiopathic renal failure
Liver enzyme and bilirubin elevations	Focal hepatic necrosis, hepatic lipidosis, cholangitis, cholangiostasis
Hyperglycemia	Elevated 'stress' hormones (growth hormone, glucocorticoids, glucagon, epinephrine), hypoinsulinemia, destruction of islet β-cells
Hypoglycemia	Sepsis with impaired gluconeogenesis
Hypocalcemia	Calcium soap formation is most widely accepted mechanism
Hyperlipidemia	Might pre-exist as separate entity; can occur with pancreatitis, but exact mechanism unknown, possibly related to 'stress' hormone release
Hypernatremia	Dehydration
Hyponatremia	Vomiting, pseudohyponatremia from hyperlipidemia
Hypokalemia	Vomiting, failure to supplement parenteral fluids, osmotic diuresis from hyperglycemia
Hyperamylasemia and hyperlipasemia	Direct venous absorption of enzymes from the inflamed pancreas and absorption via transperitoneal lymphatics, and lymphatic drainage from the pancreas and peripancreatic tissues
Prolonged prothrombin and partial thromboplastin times, hypofibrinogenemia, thrombocytopenia	Disseminated intravascular coagulation

10.45

Glucose	48.6 mmol/l (884 mg/dl)
BUN	35.7 mmol/l (100 mg/dl)
Creatinine	424 µmol/l (4.8 mg/dl)
Cholesterol	7.8 mmol/l (300 mg/dl)
Total bilirubin	61.5 µmol/l (3.6 mg/dl)
Total protein	74 g/l (7.4 g/dl)
Albumin	26 g/l (2.6 g/dl)
AP	492 U/l
Calcium	2.2 mmol/l (8.8 mg/dl)
Phosphorus	1.5 mmol/l (4.7 mg/dl)
AST	110 U/l
ALT	46 U/l
Globulin	48 g/l (4.8 g/dl)
Chloride	103 mmol/l (103 mEq/l)
Sodium	130 mmol/l (130 mEq/l)
Potassium	4.4 mmol/l (4.4 mEq/l)
Total CO_2	12 mmol/l (12 mEq/l)
Amylase	3,000 U/l
Lipase	2.0 U/l
Osmolality	360 mOsmol/kg

Figure 10.45 Example of marked serum biochemical abnormalities taken from the dog in Figure 10.3. These results support the additional clinical diagnoses of hyperosmolar diabetic ketoacidosis and acute kidney injury. The serum amylase and lipase exceeded the upper limits of normal by two-fold, thus supporting the main clinical diagnosis of acute pancreatitis. The lowered serum calcium level is attributed to calcium soap formation. The elevated liver enzymes are likely due to hepatic lipidosis and cholangiostasis, while the hyponatremia could have been due to losses from impaired renal tubular sodium reabsorption, osmotic diuresis, and vomiting. Pseudohyponatremia could have also been present from hyperlipidemia or marked hyperglycemia. The low total CO_2 reflects metabolic acidosis, and the hyperosmolality is due to the marked hyperglycemia.

Table 10.6 Basic principles for treating severe pancreatitis in the dog.

Admit to intensive care and insert an indwelling intravenous catheter
Nothing by mouth if vomiting is profuse
Small amounts of oral nutrition can be given in the absence of severe vomiting
Pain relief
Antibiotics
Parenteral fluid replacement
Insulin (where appropriate)
Nutrition support eventually by total parenteral nutrition or enteral nutrition using jejunostomy tube if oral intake is not possible
Surgical débridement and drainage – if infected or not responsive to medical treatment

omeprazole (0.5–1.0 mg/kg q24h) and pantoprazole (0.7–1.0 mg/kg IV over 15 minutes q24h) have been recommended because of their effective anti-ulcer effects. Although there are theoretical justifications for their use, there are no well-controlled clinical trials that substantiate any proven benefit in the treatment of acute pancreatitis.

Antibiotics are usually reserved for moderately and severely ill patients. Such animals are prone to various complications including septicemia, urinary tract infection (especially when an indwelling urethral catheter is used), pneumonia, and pancreatic abscess formation. Since some of these infections are polymicrobial, broad-spectrum antimicrobial coverage for both aerobic and anaerobic bacteria is recommended. Bacterial infection of the pancreas can be due to the spread of bacteria from the portal lymph nodes, biliary tree, colon, or from other body sites. Ampicillin, quinolones, and first-generation cephalosporin antimicrobials can be used safely. Aminoglycoside antibiotics should be used with caution due to their potential nephrotoxicity in a clinical setting where renal function might already be impaired. The literature currently does not recommend antimicrobial use in the absence of a documented infection.

Glucocorticoids are not routinely used in acute pancreatitis. Although they might be helpful because of their anti-inflammatory activity, they can predispose the patient to infections that can be very detrimental.

Providing adequate nourishment is essential. Although 5% dextrose solution provides the small amount of calories that might suffice for the first few days of treatment, it falls far short of providing the patient's caloric and protein needs over the 1–2-week period of inappetence caused by the animal's abdominal discomfort and persistent vomiting. Many patients will be able to resume the intake of liquids and then solids after the first 5–7 days following cessation of vomiting. A low-fat diet is recommended during this recovery period and for the long term thereafter. In cats, the introduction of food is also gradual, but without any apparent need for fat restriction.

Intravenous parenteral nutrition or enteral tube feeding should be considered if the patient will not voluntarily eat. The former is somewhat controversial because there is evidence that intravenous infusion of amino acid and lipid solutions can stimulate pancreatic secretion in the dog. Problems associated with intravenous hyperalimentation include catheter-associated phlebitis and septicemia and plasma hyperosmolarity. Meticulous preparation is required. There is a need for multiple cannulae, and expense must be taken into consideration. Intravenous hyperalimentation is therefore usually reserved for tertiary medical facilities where the logistics are conducive to this particular treatment modality. Enteral tube feeding is an alternative way of nourishing an animal that has protracted acute pancreatitis. J-tube feeding is the preferred choice for extended nutritional support in postoperative patients because of its ease of maintenance and the advantages it provides to the small bowel mucosa.

Analgesic treatment using opioids should be reserved for animals that have severe and intractable pain. Phenothiazine drugs are contraindicated initially because they might worsen hypotension (see **Table 10.7** for specific drugs and dosages). Epidural analgesia can also be used for pain control (**Figures 10.46, 10.47**).

Table 10.7 Analgesia for the dog and cat with acute pancreatitis.

Species	Drug	Dose
Small dogs and cats	Fentanyl transdermal	25 μg/hour
Dogs 5–10 kg	Fentanyl transdermal	25 μg/hour
Dogs 10–20 kg	Fentanyl transdermal	50 μg/hour
Dogs 20–30 kg	Fentanyl transdermal	75 μg/hour
Dogs >30 kg	Fentanyl transdermal	100 μg/hour
Cats and dogs	Butorphanol	0.1–1.0 mg/kg IM, IV, or SC q1–3h
Cats and dogs	Buprenorphine	0.01–0.02 mg/kg IM, IV, or SC q6–12h

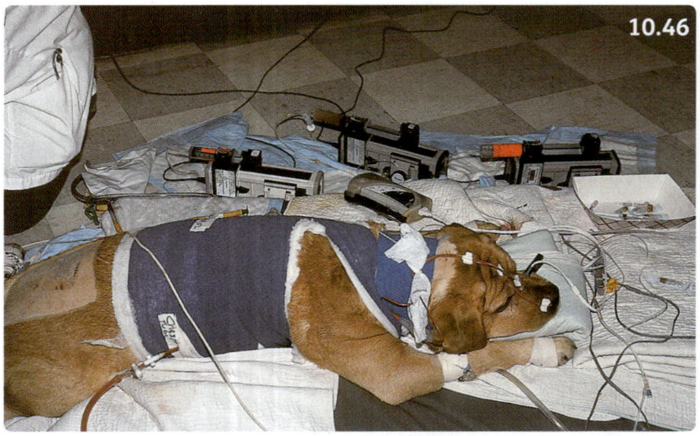

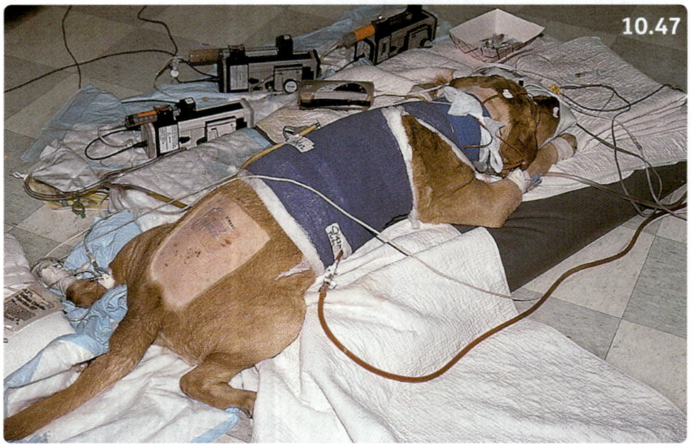

Figures 10.46, 10.47 This 5-year-old male Labrador Retriever was referred to surgery because of severe hemorrhagic pancreatitis. He required critical care, which included epidural analgesia, intensive patient monitoring, and the need for multiple intravenous and intra-arterial cannula sites. The dog died despite all the intensive care provided.

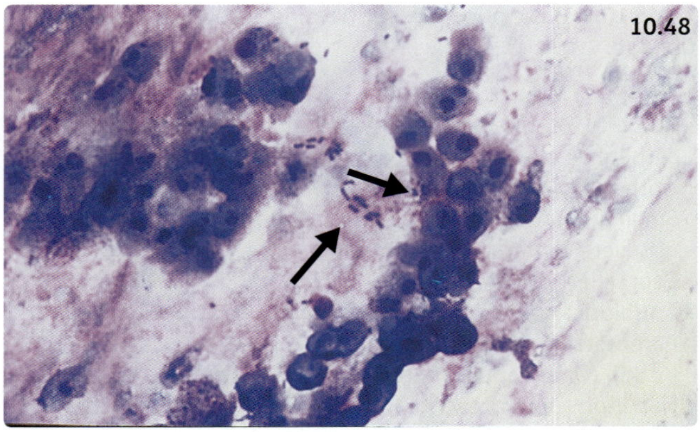

Figure 10.48 One of the indications for surgery in acute pancreatitis patients is the formation of pancreatic phlegmon and the onset of secondary bacterial infection. This cytology sample, from abdominal fluid in a dog with marked pancreatic necrosis with phlegmon and abscess formation, shows toxic neutrophils containing bacteria as well as free bacteria (arrows). Gram-negative bacteria are the most common organisms present on culture if infection occurs. (Courtesy D.J. Meyer)

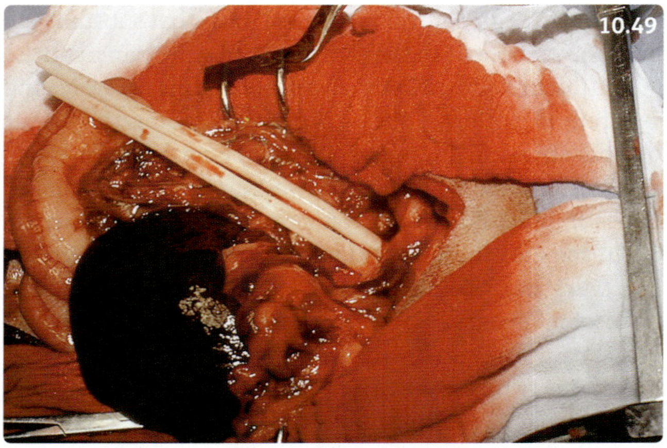

Figure 10.49 Surgery for pancreatitis in a 3-year-old female Schnauzer that was refractory to medical therapy alone. Shown here is peritonitis and an isolated mesenteric abscess containing drains that were surgically implanted and remained in place for 3 days postoperatively. This dog required two separate surgical procedures for débridement and drainage. She required intensive care for 5 weeks and went on to do well.

Insulin treatment is indicated when the blood glucose level exceeds 16.7 mmol/l (300 mg/dl). Regular crystalline zinc insulin (initial SC injection of 0.5 U/kg body weight) is preferred because of its short duration of action, especially if the hyperglycemia is transient. If the patient shows a continued need for insulin, it should be managed according to current protocol. Regular insulin should be given by slow constant IV infusion (0.05–0.1 U/kg/hour) if the patient is hypotensive, during which time subcutaneous absorption is impaired and undependable.

Surgical therapy

There are several major indications for surgery in patients with acute pancreatitis: to treat potentially correctable disease such as pancreatic pseudocyst or abscess; to eliminate diseases initiating pancreatic inflammation; to remove necrotic or infected foci during the septic phase of hemorrhagic necrotizing pancreatitis; and to correct complicating problems such as bile duct obstruction (**Figures 10.48–10.53**). Laparotomy also allows for the insertion of a J-tube and the commencement of enteral feeding. Although some might prefer earlier surgical intervention, the current recommendation in human medicine calls for delays of as long as 2 weeks in order to allow time for diffuse inflammation to subside and for any pancreatic abscess or pseudocyst to assume the form of a discrete mass.

Laparotomy and peritoneal lavage are recommended for moderately to severely sick animals that fail to

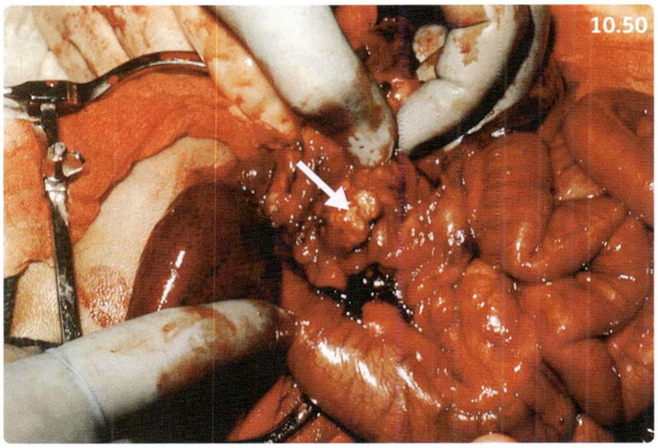

Figure 10.50 Surgery on a 10-year-old Yorkshire Terrier showing caseous debris (arrow) and peritonitis associated with acute hemorrhagic necrotic pancreatitis. Débridement and abdominal drains were used to treat this dog.

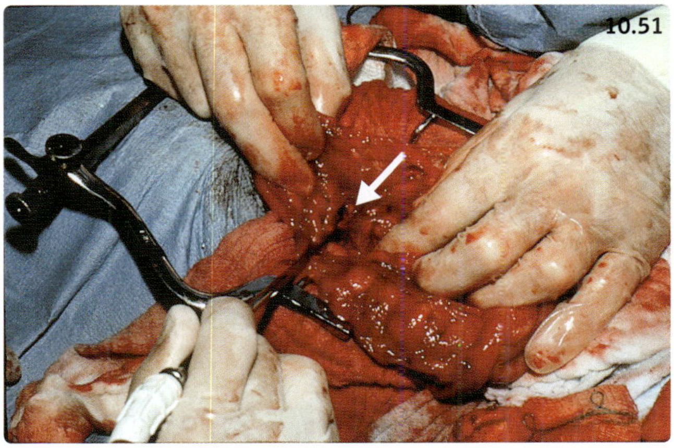

Figure 10.51 This 7-year-old male Wirehaired Fox Terrier had hemorrhagic pancreatitis that could barely be identified at surgery among the inflamed abdominal tissues. Shown is a large abscess cavity (arrow) that was located at the root of the mesentery.

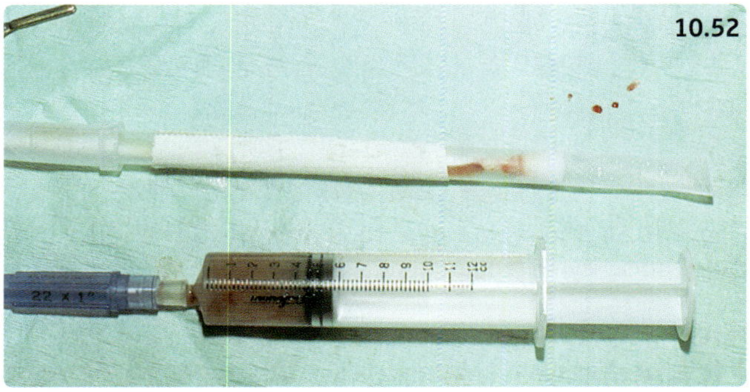

Figure 10.52 The cavity shown in Figure 10.51 contained a remarkable amount of pus from which *E. coli* was isolated.

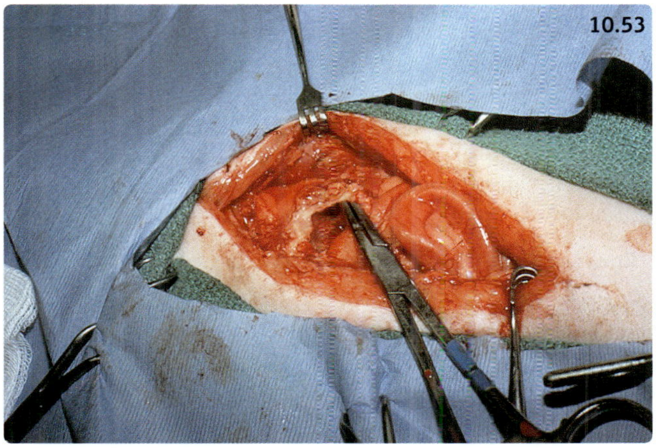

Figure 10.53 Acute pancreatitis in cats can cause similar pathology to that seen in dogs. Shown here is a phlegmon with cavitation that was found during an abdominal ultrasound examination preoperatively. Abdominal drains were inserted after the necrotic debris was removed. This 6-year-old male Siamese cat required two abdominal surgeries before recovery was attainable.

respond to medical treatment after the first 5–7 days or for those in the early stages of severe hemorrhagic necrotic pancreatitis. In many of these cases, the optimal time for surgery is left to the discretion of the clinician. Cases of infected pancreatitis should also be treated surgically as soon as possible, much in the same light as a septic abdomen would be treated. This condition is frequently associated with a guarded to grave prognosis. The diagnosis of infected pancreatitis is made by the cytologic demonstration of bacteria obtained from abdominal fluid or tissue via ultrasound-guided fine needle aspiration or through surgical exploration. Microbial isolation for identification and sensitivity should also be done, ideally prior to antibiotic administration. Lavage-induced hypoproteinemia and serum electrolyte deficiencies should be corrected with plasma and appropriately adjusted electrolyte solutions, respectively.

Complications and long-term management

Table 10.8 outlines the several complications that can occur during the acute or chronic (beyond 2 weeks) phase of pancreatitis. Long-term medical management for the dog includes a low-fat diet that is divided into two or three feedings per day. Diabetes mellitus and exocrine pancreatic insufficiency (EPI) should be treated according to established protocols. The diabetic condition can be either temporary or permanent and is the result of substantial beta-cell destruction (70–90%) as a result of the pancreatitis.

Table 10.8 Complications of acute or chronic pancreatitis.

Complication	Phase of disease
Diabetes mellitus	Acute or chronic
Pancreatic abscess and pseudocyst	Acute
Bowel infarction	Acute
Bowel obstruction	Acute
Bile duct obstruction and/or cholangiostasis	Acute
Renal failure	Acute
Septicemia	Acute
Consumption coagulopathy	Acute
Pulmonary edema (acute respiratory distress syndrome)	Acute
Pleural effusion	Acute
Relapsing pancreatitis	Chronic
Pancreatic exocrine insufficiency	Chronic

Note: 'Acute' refers to first 14 days; 'chronic' extends beyond 14 days.

EXOCRINE PANCREATIC INSUFFICIENCY

Definition/overview

EPI is a malnutrition disorder caused by a deficiency of pancreatic digestive enzymes. It is much more common in dogs than in cats.

Etiology

In the dog, where it is most commonly seen in German Shepherd Dogs and Rough-coated Collies, EPI is usually caused by an atrophy of the zymogen-containing acinar cells. The atrophy was once thought to be idiopathic, but recent studies show that an immune-mediated lymphocytic inflammatory process leads to the atrophy in the aforementioned breeds. The typical age of onset is between 1 and 5 years. EPI can also be caused by recurrent pancreatitis and the associated loss of acinar cells. It rarely occurs with pancreatic adenocarcinoma because the malignancy will often lead to the patient's demise long before it destroys the majority of the exocrine pancreatic cells. EPI occurs rarely in cats (**Figures 10.54–10.56**), where the signs are similar to those in the dog; chronic pancreatitis is thought to be the cause.

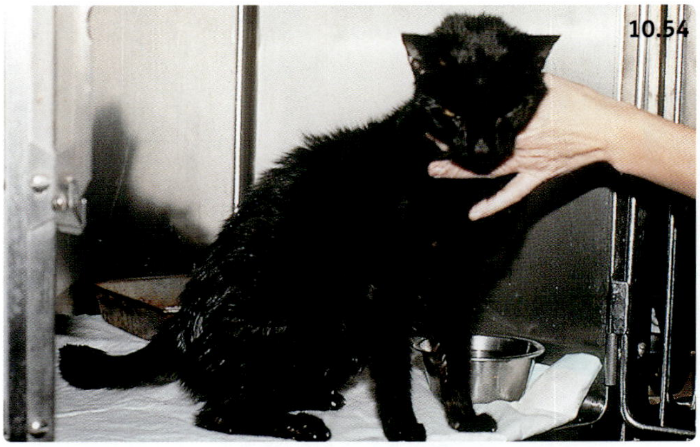

Figure 10.54 Exocrine pancreatic insufficiency is rare in the cat. This emaciated 13-year-old female Domestic Shorthair cat showed typical signs of weight loss and polyphagia in the absence of hyperthyroidism.

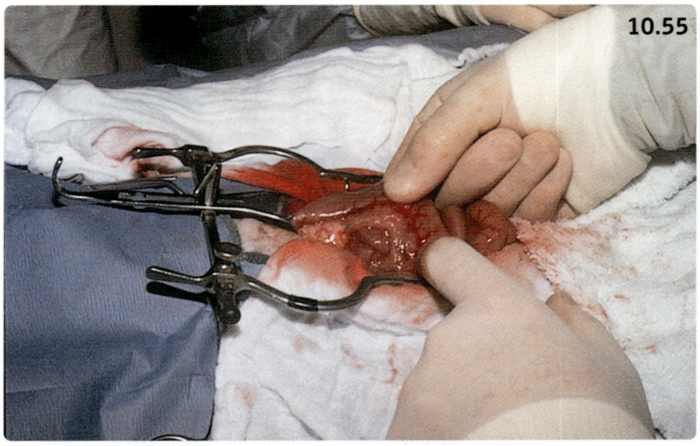

Figure 10.55 The fibrotic and atrophic pancreas of the cat in Figure 10.54 was evident at laparotomy.

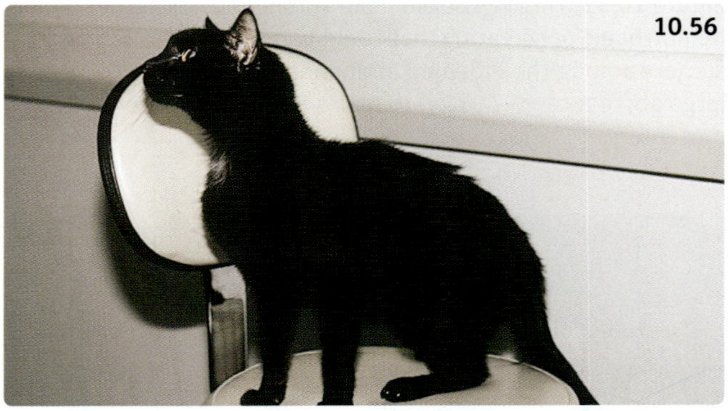

Figure 10.56 The cat in Figure 10.54 after treatment with pancreatic enzyme replacement.

Pathophysiology

A lack of digestive enzymes resulting in poor intraluminal digestion is the main cause of the malabsorption in this syndrome. This is furthered by changes in the small intestinal mucosa including abnormal intestinal enzyme activity, impaired transport function, villous atrophy, and inflammatory cell infiltration. Bacterial overgrowth is a frequent complication of EPI and may contribute to some of the pathology.

Clinical presentation

The classic signs include polyphagia, weight loss, and hyperdefecation. Pica and coprophagia, flatulence, and borborygmus can also occur. The stool quality ranges from diarrhea to semi-formed, while the color varies from brown to yellow (**Figure 10.57**). Polydipsia and polyuria can be present if diabetes mellitus coexists.

EPI patients are typically thin and have dull dry haircoats reflecting their chronic malnourished condition (**Figures 10.58–10.60**). Examination of the stool and, sometimes, the perineum often shows a greasy texture caused by steatorrhea. The feces can give off a very foul odor. In cats, EPI must be differentiated from hyperthyroidism, and the physical examination should

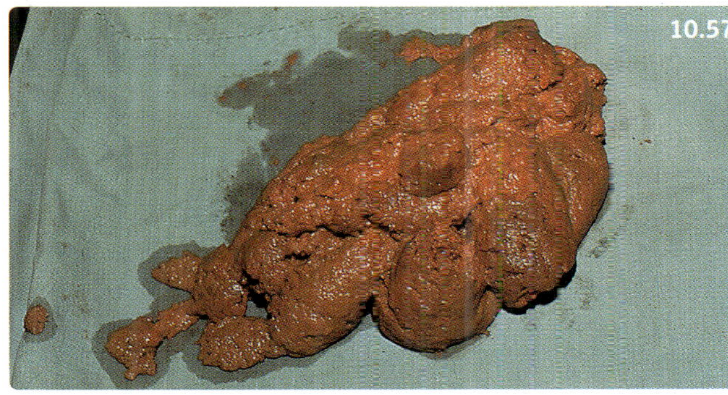

Figure 10.57 Fecal sample from a dog with exocrine pancreatic insufficiency and steatorrhea showing the typical yellow color and greasy texture.

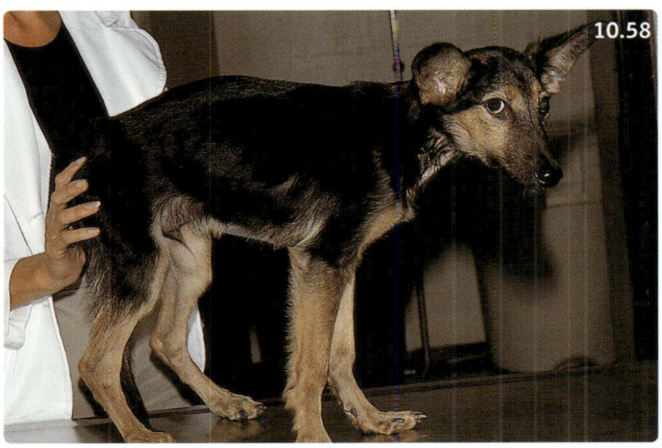

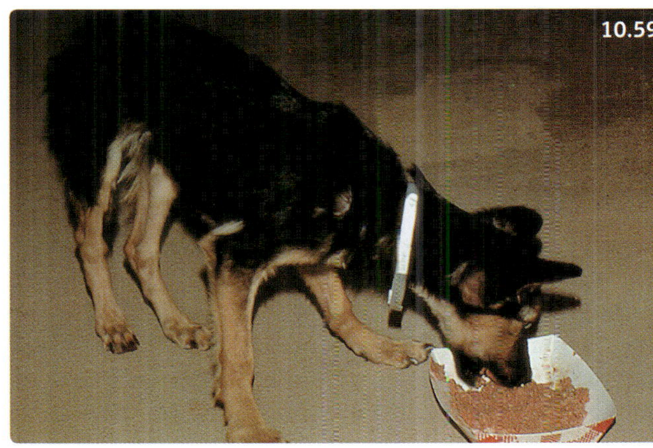

Figures 10.58, 10.59 A 10-month-old male German Shepherd Dog showing its frail body and stunted growth (10.58) and its voracious appetite (10.59).

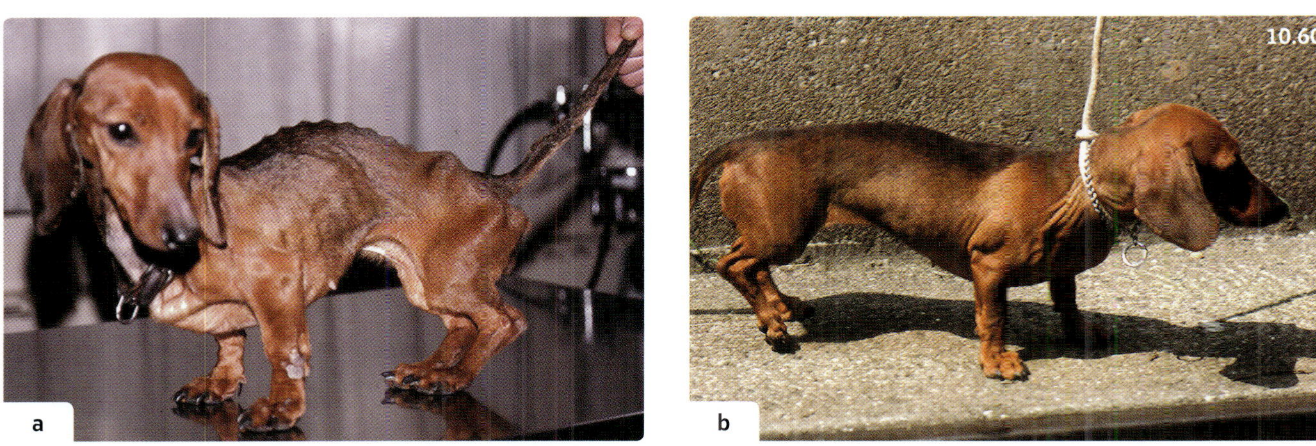

Figures 10.60a, b This young female Dachshund suffered severe emaciation from exocrine pancreatic insufficiency. The same dog is shown approximately 4 months after pancreatic enzyme replacement treatment.

include a thorough palpation of the neck in search of goiters, which will lend support to this diagnosis.

Differential diagnosis

Small intestinal malabsorption, pancreatic duct obstruction, primary small intestinal disease, parasitism, hyperthyroidism.

Diagnosis

The hemogram will be normal or show a mild normochromic normocytic anemia from the malnutrition. Serum chemistry levels are usually normal; however, hypoproteinemia can occur in some patients as a result of the faulty digestion and impaired assimilation of ingested proteins. Hyperglycemia can occur if most of the pancreatic beta cells have been destroyed by earlier pancreatitis.

Examination of feces for the presence of fat, carbohydrate, and trypsin activity (film digestion) is an empirical test and frequently yields inaccurate results (**Figures 10.61, 10.62**). However, a fecal proteolytic enzyme test has been found to be useful in cats. The serum TLI assay is a sensitive and accurate quantitative test for diagnosing EPI in the dog and cat. A value of <2.5 µg/l is diagnostic. In German Shepherd Dogs and Rough-coated Collies, serum TLI values ranging between 2.5 and 5 µg/l suggests subclinical EPI and partial atrophy.

Management

Once the diagnosis is made, treatment is simple, entailing the provision of a powdered ox- or pig-derived commercial pancreatic enzyme product. The powdered form is preferred over tablets. It should be thoroughly mixed in a moist, nutritionally balanced ration (one teaspoonful per 0.5 kg of food) at each feeding. Providing a balanced vitamin–mineral tablet will also be helpful. Some dogs with coexisting intestinal bacterial overgrowth will require antimicrobial treatment (tetracycline, 15 mg/kg q8h) in order to enhance the effectiveness of treatment. Gradually increased amounts of food should be provided until the patient's normal body weight is reached.

The outlook for the majority of these patients is excellent so long as they are maintained on their required amount of pancreatic enzyme therapy (**Figure 10.63**). In most cases, where regeneration of pancreatic exocrine tissue rarely occurs, treatment will be life-long (**Figures 10.64, 10.65**). Insulin-dependent diabetes mellitus might also require life-long insulin treatment if the EPI is the result of acute pancreatitis.

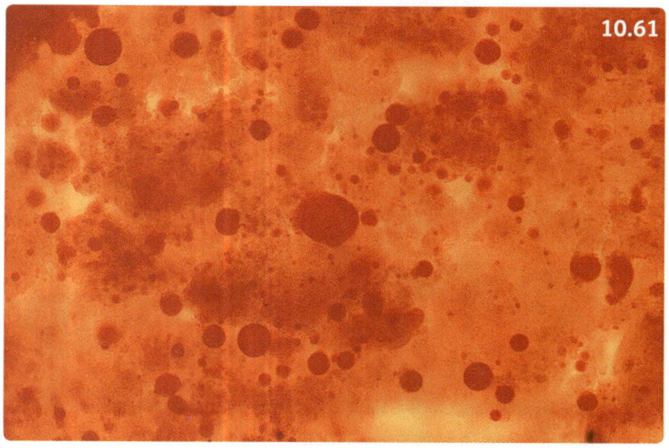

Figure 10.61 A microscopic view of steatorrheic stool stained with Oil Red O showing the large sized red-colored fat globules reflecting undigested fat (×100).

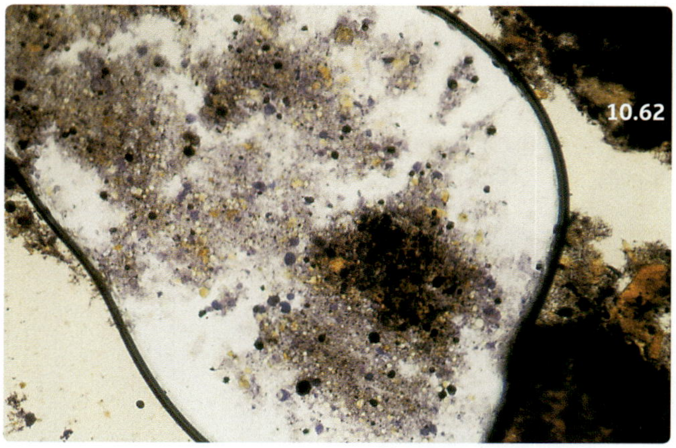

Figure 10.62 Lugol solution will stain starch a dark purple color, as shown on this microscopic view of a stool smear taken from a dog with exocrine pancreatic insufficiency (×100).

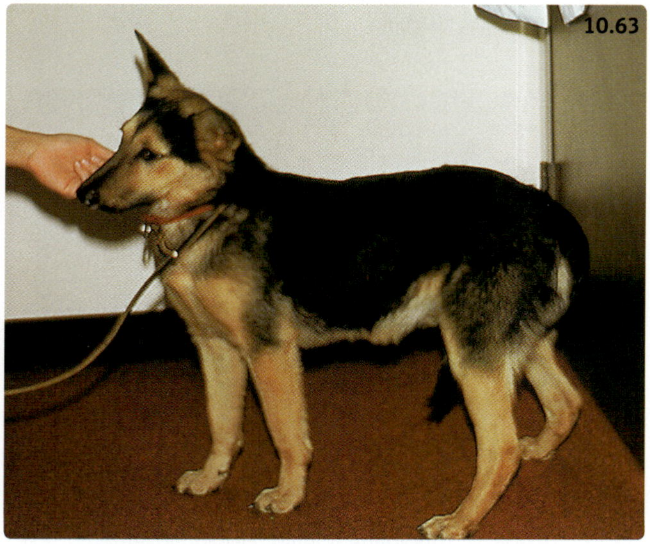

Figure 10.63 The dog in Figures 10.58 and 10.59 after 4 months of treatment with pancreatic enzyme replacement, showing marked improvement in stature.

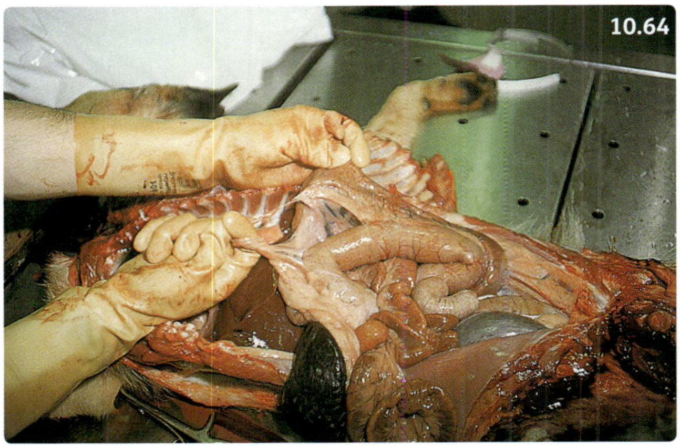

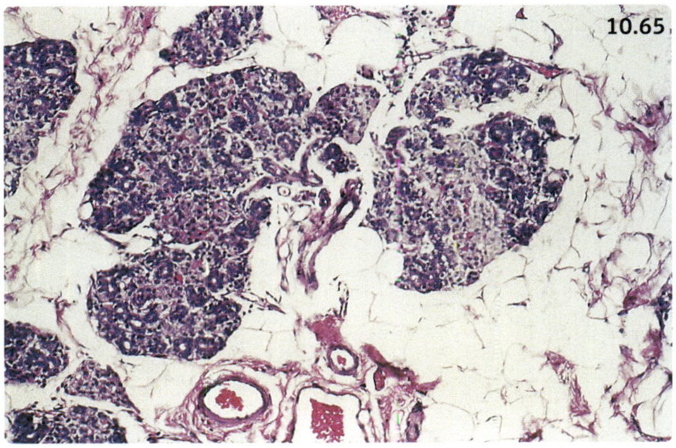

Figures 10.64, 10.65 (10.64) A postmortem examination of a dog with exocrine pancreatic insufficiency showing marked pancreatic atrophy. (10.65) A microscopic view of the pancreas showing diminished numbers of acinar epithelial cells (H&E. ×40).

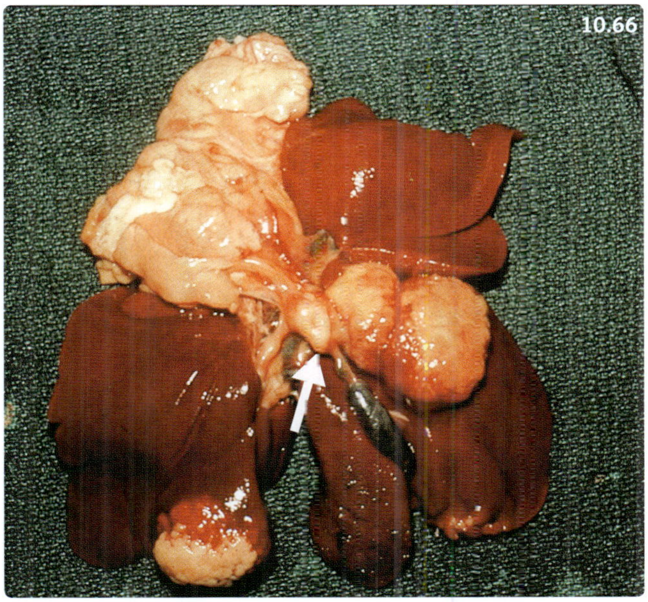

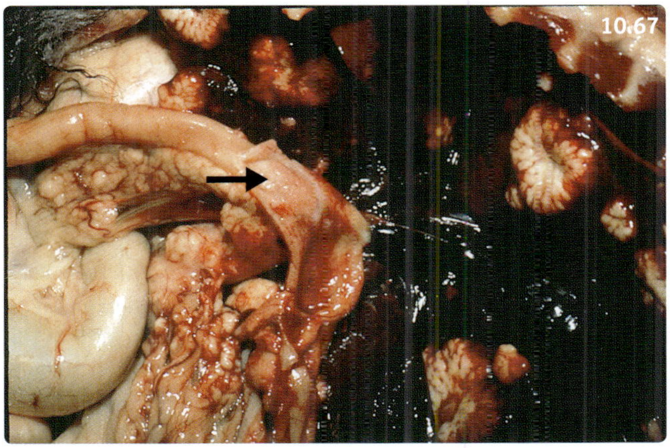

Figures 10.66, 10.67 Pancreatic adenocarcinoma in the cat usually involves the older age group. The usual signs include anorexia and weight loss. Icterus commonly occurs and is associated with obstructed bile flow. Shown here are postmortem findings on two aged cats illustrating rather large metastatic lesions involving the liver. One cat (10.66) had obstructed bile flow due to obstruction along the common bile duct (arrow), while the other cat's icterus was due to carcinoma involving the duodenal papilla (10.67) (arrow).

PANCREATIC TUMORS

Definition/overview

Exocrine cancer of the pancreas is rare in the dog and cat. The majority of the tumors are epithelial and most are adenocarcinomas of ductular or acinar origin. These tumors often have an aggressive behavior, with implantation on the peritoneum and metastasis to the liver common. The liver nodules can be small or quite large (**Figures 10.66–10.71**).

Etiology

There are no known causes of pancreatic adenocarcinoma in either the dog or the cat.

Pathophysiology

The exact stimulus for this particular tumor formation in the dog and cat is unknown.

Clinical presentation

The most common clinical signs are weight loss and anorexia. Vomiting is sporadic. Ascites from peritoneal implants and icterus from common bile duct obstruction can also occur (**Figures 10.72, 10.73**).

Differential diagnosis

Chronic pancreatitis, any malignant tumor, chronic gastroenteric disease, chronic liver disease.

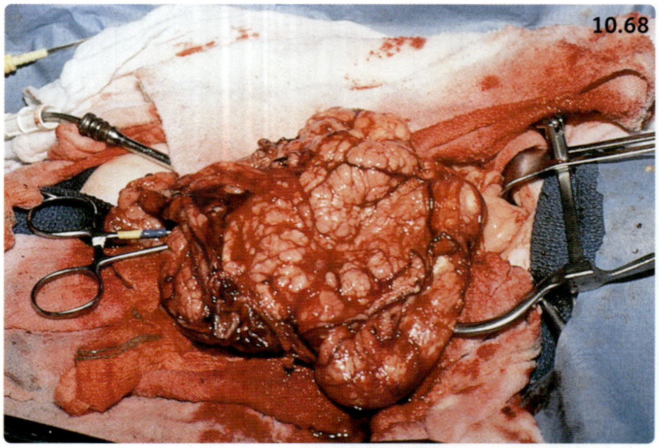

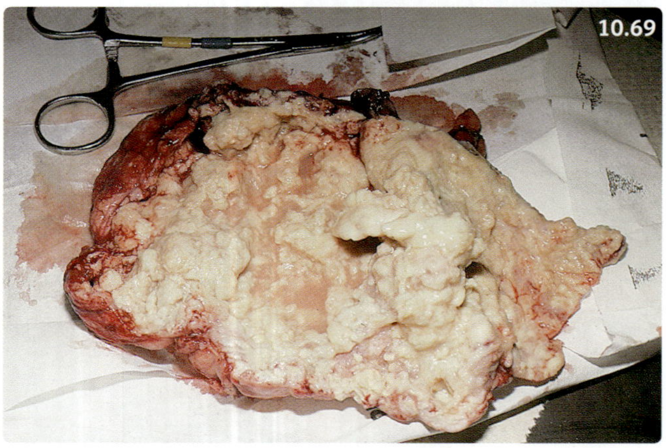

Figures 10.68, 10.69 This large pancreatic adenocarcinoma was found in a 12-year-old Siamese cat that was examined for the primary complaints of anorexia, weight loss, lethargy, and gradual abdominal enlargement. Physical examination revealed a large (>5 cm) anterior mid-abdominal mass. The only clinicopathologic abnormalities included a leukocytosis and a mildly elevated total bilirubin. Shown is the tumor at surgery (10.68) and its necrotic interior in the extirpated specimen (10.69).

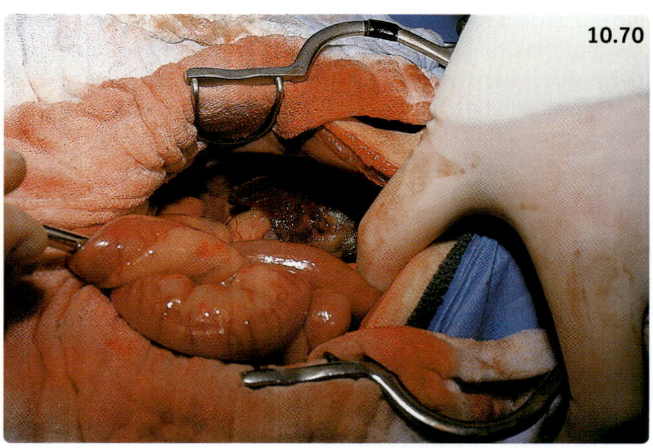

Figure 10.70 Surgical view of pancreatic adenocarcinoma in a 13-year-old male Poodle showing the metastatic lesions to the liver.

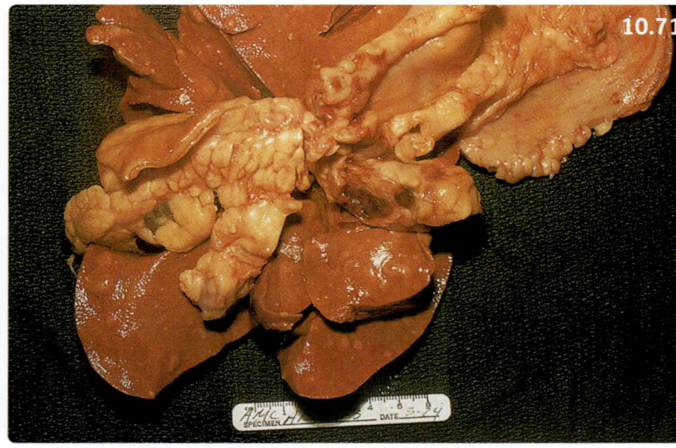

Figure 10.71 Postmortem view of a 15-year-old dog with pancreatic carcinoma with diffuse liver metastasis.

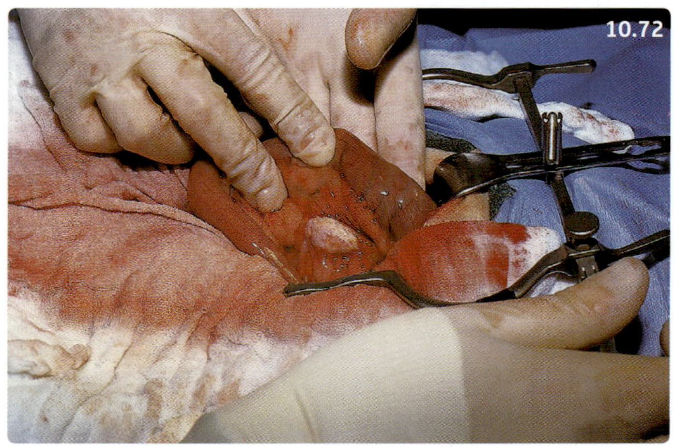

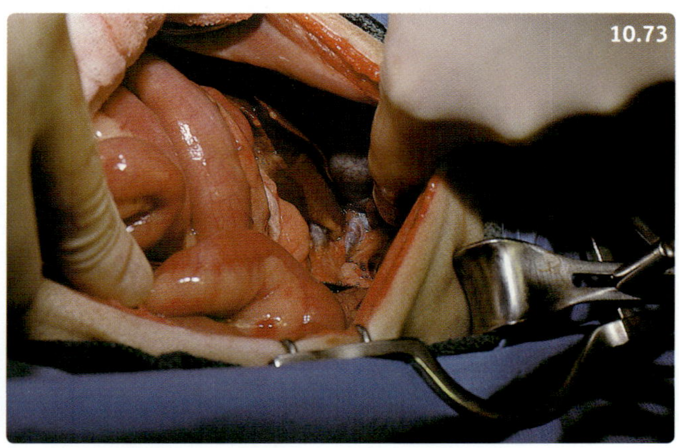

Figures 10.72, 10.73 Surgical views of a pancreatic adenocarcinoma in a 13-year-old male Poodle that has signs of anorexia and icterus. 10.72 shows the primary neoplasm and 10.73 shows metastatic lesions obstructing the bile duct. The pertinent serum chemistry abnormalities were: cholesterol 9.64 mmol/l (371 mg/dl), total bilirubin 117.9 mmol/l (6.9 mg/dl), ALP 28,240 U/l, AST 271 U/l, ALT 380 U/l. The serum amylase and lipase concentrations were normal at 1,332 and 0.6 U/l, respectively, as was the CBC.

Diagnosis

There are no specific diagnostic tests for pancreatic cancer. The hemogram and serum chemistry panel might reflect the effect of the disease, as seen with the cholangiostasis associated with metastasis involving the hepatobiliary tree. Pancreatic lipase assays will give varying results. One of the author's canine patients had markedly elevated levels of cPLI associated with lymphoma infiltrating the pancreas. Abdominal ultrasound can demonstrate abnormal pancreatic parenchyma and metastatic lesions involving the liver. The definitive diagnosis is obtained through a diagnostic laparotomy and histopathology on biopsied tissue specimens.

Management

Optimal treatment would be complete surgical extirpation of the tumor. However, a diagnosis is hardly ever made early enough before the malignancy has had a chance to spread. The prognosis is always grave.

RECOMMENDED FURTHER READING

Büchler MW, Uhl W, Malfertheiner P *et al.* (2004) (eds.) *Diseases of the Pancreas*. Karger, Basel.

Freeman LM, Labato MA, Rush JE *et al.* (1995) Nutritional support in pancreatitis: a retrospective study. *J Emerg Med Crit Care* **5(1):**32–41.

Gerhardt A, Steiner JM, William DA *et al.* (2001) Comparison of the sensitivity of different diagnostic tests for pancreatitis in cats. *J Vet Intern Med* **15:**329–333.

Hess RS, Sanders M, VanWinkle TJ *et al.* (1998) Clinical, clinicopathologic, radiographic, and ultrasonographic abnormalities in dogs with fatal acute pancreatitis: 70 cases (1986–1995). *J Am Vet Med Assoc* **213(5):**665–670.

Hill RC, Van Winkle TJ (1993) Acute necrotizing pancreatitis and acute suppurative pancreatitis in the cat: a retrospective review of 40 cases (1976–1989). *J Vet Intern Med* **7:**25–33.

Kimmel SE, Washabau RJ, Drobatz KJ (2001) Incidence and prognostic value of low plasma ionized calcium concentration in cats with acute pancreatitis: 46 cases (1996–1998). *J Am Vet Med Assoc* **219(8):**1105–1109.

Mansfield C (2012) Pathophysiology of acute pancreatitis: potential application from experimental models and human medicine to dogs. *J Vet Intern Med* **26:**875–887.

McCord K, Morley PS, Armstrong J *et al.* (2012) A multi-institutional study evaluating the diagnostic utility of spec cPL™ and SNAP™ in clinical acute pancreatitis in dogs. *J Vet Intern Med* **26:**888–896.

Nagar AB, Gorelick FS (2004) Acute pancreatitis. *Curr Opin Gastroenterol* **20(5):**439–443.

Ruaux CG (2000) Pathophysiology of organ failure in severe pancreatitis in dogs. *Compend Contin Educ Pract Vet* **22:**531–542.

Ruaux CG, Atwell RB (1998) A severity score for spontaneous canine acute pancreatitis. *Aust Vet J* **76:**804–808.

Saunders HM, Van Winkle TJ, Drobatz K *et al.* (2002) Ultrasonographic findings in cats with clinical, gross pathologic, and histologic evidence of acute pancreatic necrosis: 20 cases (1994–2001). *J Am Vet Med Assoc* **221(12):**1724–1730.

Steiner JM, Williams DA (2000) Serum feline trypsin-like immunoreactivity in cats with exocrine pancreatic insufficiency. *J Vet Intern Med* **14:**627–629.

Swift NC, Marks SL, MacLachlan NJ *et al.* (2000) Evaluation of serum feline trypsin-like immunoreactivity for the diagnosis of pancreatitis in cats. *J Am Vet Med Assoc* **217(1):**37–42.

Tenner, S, Baillie J, DeWitt J *et al.* (2013) American College of Gastroenteritis Guideline: management of acute pancreatitis. *Am J Gastroenterol* **108:**1400–1415.

Watson P (2004) Pancreatitis in the dog: dealing with a spectrum of disease. *In Practice* **26(2):**64–77.

Wiberg ME, Westermarck E (2002) Subclinical exocrine pancreatic insufficiency in dogs. *J Am Vet Med Assoc* **220(8):**1183–1187.

Chapter 11

Endocrine disorders

Michael E. Herrtage

INTRODUCTION

The presentations of endocrine diseases are diverse and the findings in the history and physical examination reflect this diversity. Some of the more common presentations are listed in **Table 11.1**. Although multiple endocrine disorders can occur in the same animal (for example, autoimmune polyendocrine syndromes or multiple endocrine neoplasia), most abnormalities affect a single hormone system. A working knowledge of endocrine physiology is essential not only for a good understanding of the pathophysiology of endocrine disease, but also for understanding the rationale and limitations of endocrine function tests.

Advances in our knowledge of endocrine diseases have been made possible by the widespread availability of sensitive methods for measuring hormone concentrations and improved diagnostic imaging techniques. The release of some hormones shows marked diurnal variation, making single determinations difficult to interpret. The pattern of release may also vary with age, sex, stress, diet, or concurrent disease or medication.

In order to overcome some of these problems of interpretation, dynamic tests have been developed that determine the response of a gland to stimulation or suppression. Stimulation tests assess the functional reserve of an endocrine gland by its ability to increase its hormonal output. The response may be exaggerated in conditions where there is excessive function or reduced if the gland is structurally or functionally damaged. Suppression tests use the administration of a pure hormone to test the negative feedback mechanism. Hormonal production is normally suppressed in these tests, but production persists where the gland is hyperplastic or if a functional endocrine tumor is present.

This chapter has been structured to provide a practical guide for veterinarians in the diagnosis and management of the more common endocrine disorders.

Table 11.1 Common presentations of endocrine disease.

Polyuria–polydipsia
Weight gain/obesity
Weight loss
Poor growth or stunting
Symmetrical alopecia
Episodic weakness and collapse
Hypertension

DISORDERS OF THE PITUITARY

The pituitary gland is a small ovoid structure that lies in a distinct fossa, the sella turcica, just ventral to the hypothalamus and caudal to the optic chiasma. The pituitary consists of two distinct parts, an anterior and a posterior lobe, each of which has separate functions. The hypothalamus and pituitary form a complex functional unit that controls much of the endocrine system, and any space-occupying lesions arising in this area can therefore cause a wide range of effects.

The hypothalamus is important in the regulation of anterior and posterior pituitary function. The release of hormones from the anterior lobe of the pituitary is controlled by hypothalamic peptides, which are transported to the anterior pituitary by the capillaries of the hypothalamic–hypophyseal portal circulation (**Figure 11.1**). The hypothalamus contains a number of autonomic centers that control thirst, satiety, body temperature, emotional reactions, and sympathetic responses, and it serves as an important link between the brain and the endocrine system.

The posterior pituitary releases stored vasopressin (antidiuretic hormone [ADH]) and oxytocin, which have been synthesized in the supraoptic and paraventricular nuclei of the hypothalamus.

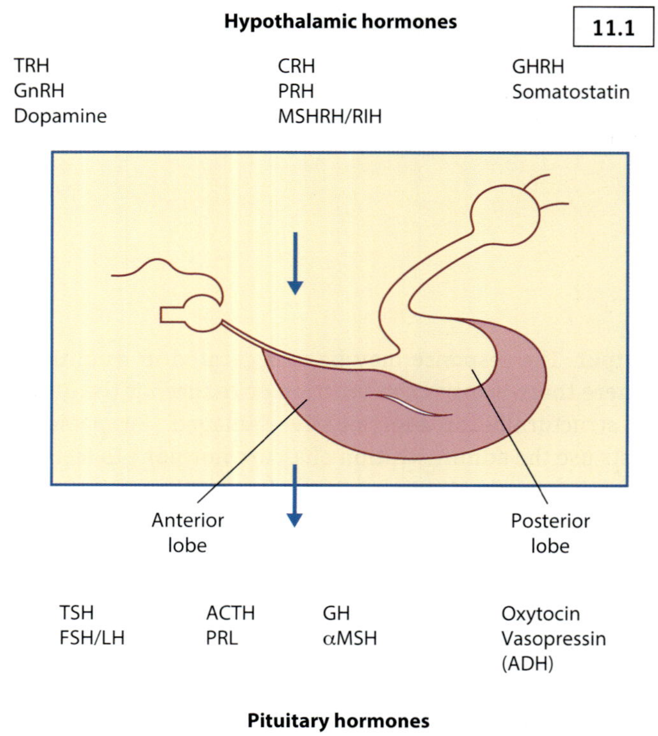

Figure 11.1 Physiology of hypothalamic–pituitary function.

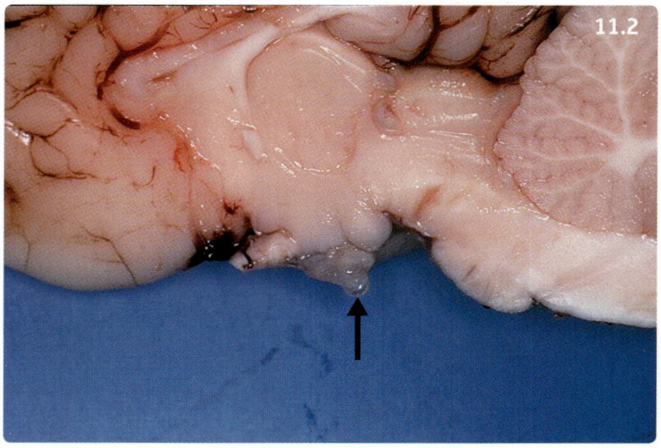

Figure 11.2 Cystic dilatation of Rathke's pouch (arrow) in a German Shepherd Dog with hypopituitarism.

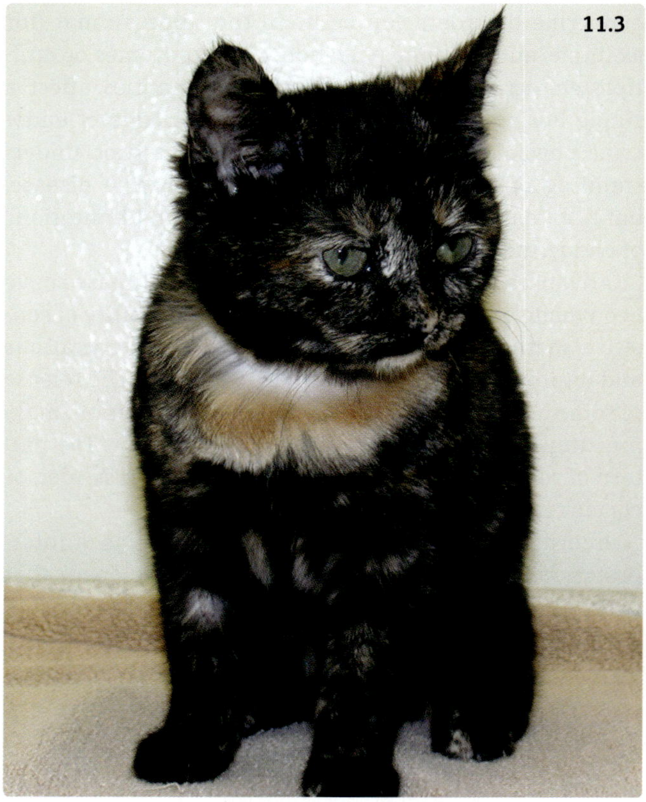

Figure 11.3 A 5-month-old kitten with congenital hypopituitarism.

CONGENITAL HYPOPITUITARISM

Definition/overview

Congenital hypopituitarism results from inadequate secretion of growth hormone (GH) and resultant retardation of growth (pituitary dwarfism).

Etiology

The condition is rare, but it has been reported in a number of breeds of dog. It is most commonly seen in German Shepherd Dogs, where it has been shown to be inherited as an autosomal recessive trait. In the dog, pituitary dwarfism is most commonly associated with cystic dilatation of Rathke's pouch, which arises as a result of the failure of the anterior lobe of the pituitary to develop normally and results in reduced secretion of anterior pituitary hormones (**Figure 11.2**). Hypoplasia of the pituitary has been reported in the cat but also appears to be rare (**Figure 11.3**).

Pathophysiology

In many affected animals a cystic vestigial adenohypophysis is present, although some animals have either a hypoplastic pituitary or one that appears grossly normal. Pituitary dwarfism is not usually caused by an isolated GH deficiency, but is due to a combined pituitary hormone deficiency affecting anterior lobe function.

Clinical presentation

Affected animals appear normal at birth, but growth retardation is usually evident by weaning (**Figure 11.4**). A deficiency of GH produces proportionate dwarfism (**Figure 11.5**). The degree of stunting is variable and probably depends on the extent of pituitary damage. Delayed growth plate closure and dental eruption have been reported in some cases.

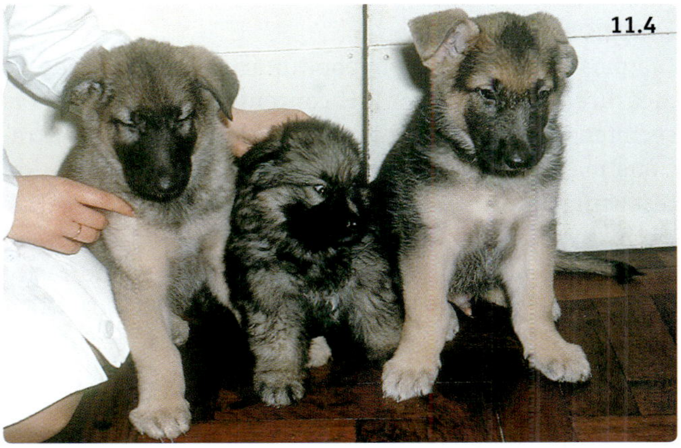

Figure 11.4 Three 6-week-old German Shepherd Dog puppies. The middle puppy is affected with congenital hypopituitarism and shows growth retardation.

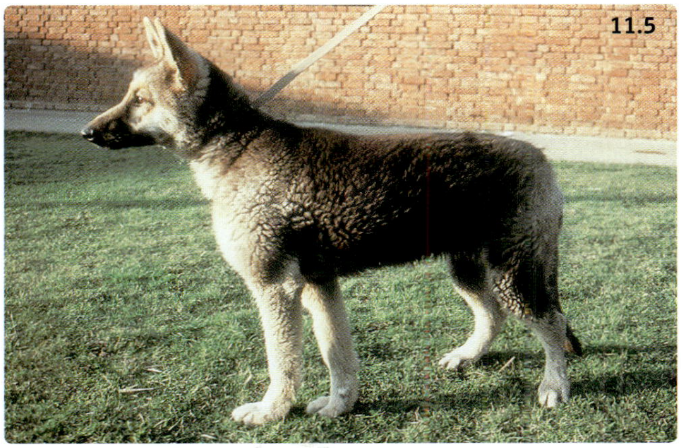

Figure 11.5 An 8-month-old German Shepherd Dog with congenital hypopituitarism demonstrating proportionate dwarfism and a woolly coat.

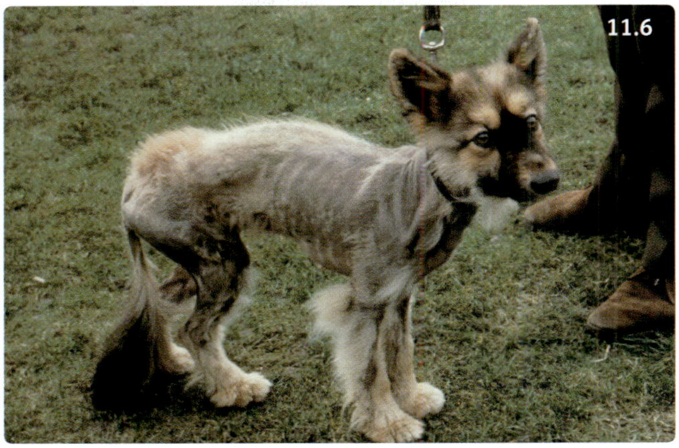

Figure 11.6 An 18-month-old German Shepherd Dog with congenital hypopituitarism showing bilaterally symmetrical alopecia. The hair loss is mainly from areas of friction, such as the flanks, neck, and ventral abdomen, and where hair is lost, the skin usually becomes hyperpigmented.

GH is required to produce a normal adult hair coat in the dog. In pituitary dwarfism the fine puppy coat is retained and becomes matted and woolly in appearance (**Figure 11.5**). The hair coat is slowly lost from the trunk, leading to the development of bilaterally symmetrical, nonpruritic alopecia by 1 year of age (**Figure 11.6**). Other areas, such as the head and feet, are generally spared and affected dogs retain the facial characteristics of a puppy (**Figure 11.7**). Hair loss does not appear to be a feature of congenital hypopituitarism in the cat.

The function of other endocrine systems controlled by the anterior pituitary is also often affected. In German Shepherd Dogs with congenital hypopituitarism, there is usually a combined deficiency of GH, thyroid-stimulating hormone (TSH), and prolactin together with impaired release of gonadotropins. While clinical signs of secondary hypothyroidism may develop, signs of secondary hypoadrenocorticism are not seen in the German Shepherd Dog because adrenocorticotropic hormone (ACTH) secretion is preserved. Gonadal involvement may result in testicular atrophy in the male and abnormal estrous cycles in the bitch.

Differential diagnosis

(See **Table 11.2**)

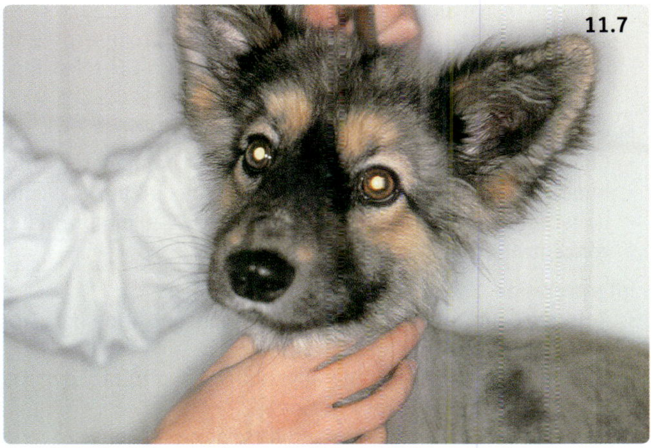

Figure 11.7 The same dog as in Figure 11.6 showing the retention of puppy-like facial features.

Table 11.2 Differential diagnosis of poor growth or stunting.

Endocrine causes:
- Congenital hypopituitarism (pituitary dwarf)
- Congenital hypothyroidism (disproportionate dwarf)
- Juvenile-onset diabetes mellitus
- Hyperadrenocorticism
- Hypoadrenocorticism
- Diabetes mellitus

(continued)

Table 11.2 Differential diagnosis of poor growth or stunting. (*continued*)

Nonendocrine causes:

• Malnutrition
• Maldigestion (e.g. exocrine pancreatic insufficiency)
• Malabsorption (e.g. villous atrophy)
• Severe intestinal parasitism
• Severe metabolic disorders associated with major organ dysfunction, for example:
  ◦ Portosystemic shunting
  ◦ Congenital renal dysplasia
  ◦ Congenital heart defects (e.g. tetralogy of Fallot)
  ◦ Mucopolysaccharidoses
• Skeletal dysplasias causing disproportionate dwarfism, for example:
  ◦ Enchondrodystrophy in the English Pointer
  ◦ Chondrodysplasia of the Alaskan Malamute

Diagnosis

Diagnosis of congenital hypopituitarism can be made by measurement of plasma GH concentrations. Since GH is secreted in pulsatile fashion, basal plasma GH concentrations may be low in healthy animals and a stimulation test using GH-releasing hormone or an alpha2-adrenergic agonist, such as clonidine or xylazine, should be performed (**Table 11.3**). GH concentration can be assessed indirectly by measuring insulin-like growth factor-1 (IGF-1). IGF-1 has the advantage of a long half-life and its secretion is not episodic. Pituitary dwarfs also have abnormally low serum IGF-1 concentrations. Thyroid function tests and, if necessary, adrenal function tests should be performed to assess thyroidal and adrenal function (see **Tables 11.8** and **11.15**).

Table 11.3 Protocols for testing growth hormones.

GH stimulation test Indication: • Used to diagnose pituitary dwarfism (congenital hypopituitarism) and acromegaly and to evaluate patients with adult-onset GH-responsive alopecia • Basal concentrations of GH are often difficult to interpret due to the overlap between normal dogs and those with GH deficiency. Therefore, provocative testing with GH-releasing hormone (GHRH) or an alpha2-adrenergic agonist (such as clonidine or xylazine) is recommended
Method: • Collect 5 ml of blood into EDTA, centrifuge immediately, and store plasma frozen (<–20°C) for basal GH concentration • Inject either GHRH (1 µg/kg IV) or clonidine (10 µg/kg IV, maximum dose 300 µg) or xylazine (100 µg/kg IV) • Collect second 5 ml blood sample into EDTA 20 minutes later, centrifuge immediately, and store plasma frozen (<–20°C) for GH concentration
Interpretation: • Reference range in dogs for basal GH concentration is 1–4 ng/ml (µg/l) and peak post-stimulation value is 10–58 ng/ml (µg/l), but check laboratory reference range • GH concentrations are generally reduced in pituitary dwarfism (<1 ng/ml [µg/l]) and show little or no response to stimulation with GHRH, clonidine, or xylazine • Reduced GH concentrations and little or no response to stimulation may be found in adult-onset GH-responsive alopecia. However, reduced responses may be found in dogs with hypothyroidism or hyperadrenocorticism and these more common disorders must be excluded as possible diagnoses first • Basal GH concentrations are generally elevated in acromegaly (>100 ng/ml [µg/l]) and are not usually further stimulated by GHRH, clonidine, or xylazine
Basal serum insulin-like growth factor-1 Indication: Used in the diagnosis of pituitary dwarfism and acromegaly. IGF-1 concentration is regulated by GH and nutritional status and is less subject to fluctuation than GH. This makes a single determination more meaningful. The assay is more readily available
Interpretation: • Reference range for IGF-1 in normal adults is >200 ng/ml and for animals up to 1 year of age is >500 ng/ml • Serum IGF-1 concentrations are decreased in pituitary dwarfs (<50 ng/ml). The sensitivity can be increased by comparing IGF-1 concentrations with those of normal littermates. IGF-1 concentrations may also be depressed in chronic debilitating disease • Elevated IGF-1 concentrations are seen in dogs and cats with acromegaly (>1,000 ng/ml)

A genetic test is available for German Shepherd Dogs with pituitary dwarfism, which have a mutation of the gene encoding the transcription factor LHX3. The genetic test not only identifies affected individuals, but also identifies carriers of the mutation.

Management

Canine GH is not available for therapeutic use, but bovine, porcine, and human GH preparations have been used for treatment. The diagnosis of hypopituitarism is usually made too late in development to influence growth significantly and affected animals remain permanent dwarfs. However, GH administration (0.1 IU/kg SC 3 times a week for 4–6 weeks) has been shown to be effective in some cases in producing regrowth of hair. Treatment with exogenous GH can be associated with the development of antibodies, which could interfere with its subsequent action. GH is expensive and its repeated use may result in the development of diabetes mellitus.

More recently, progestogens, principally proligesterone and medroxyprogesterone acetate, have been used to stimulate endogenous GH from the mammary gland in both male and female pituitary dwarfs with some success. This treatment avoids the development of autoantibodies to GH. Proligesterone given subcutaneously at a dose of 10 mg/kg every 3 weeks until the serum IGF-1 concentration has normalized has been recommended. Adverse effects such as cystic endometrial hyperplasia and acromegaly have been reported in some cases.

Thyroid hormone replacement should be used in cases of secondary hypothyroidism (see Hypothyroidism). Thyroid hormone therapy has been used, with variable success, in an attempt to stimulate hair growth in pituitary dwarfs with normal thyroid function. Half the normal replacement dose of thyroxine is administered for several months to assess the response to treatment.

ACROMEGALY

Definition/overview

The excessive secretion of GH in adult animals results in acromegaly, an insidious condition associated with overgrowth of connective tissue and bone.

Etiology

In the dog, acromegaly is mainly caused by progestogen therapy or by endogenous progesterone produced during the diestrous phase of the estrous cycle, which induces GH secretion. Progesterone-induced GH excess originates from hyperplastic ductular epithelium in the mammary gland and not from the pituitary.

In the cat, acromegaly is caused by a pituitary tumor that secretes excess GH. This cause has been reported in one dog.

Pathophysiology

GH antagonizes the effects of insulin. In acromegaly, mild glucose intolerance or overt diabetes mellitus develops, which can lead to polyuria and polydipsia. Diabetes mellitus induced by GH may be reversible or permanent depending on the duration and degree of the excessive GH secretion. Initially, hyperglycemia is associated with increased insulin concentrations, but as the disease progresses, beta-cell exhaustion will result in lowered insulin secretion. Most cases of acromegaly present with insulin-resistant diabetes mellitus, and patients usually require abnormally high doses of exogenous insulin to control blood glucose concentrations.

Clinical presentation

Clinical signs of acromegaly develop slowly and insidiously in middle aged to older cats and bitches. The bitches are entire and are either cycling normally or being given regular treatment with progestogens to prevent estrus.

Initially, there is increased soft tissue swelling, particularly around the head and neck and this may result in excessive panting, inspiratory stridor, and exercise intolerance (**Figure 11.8**). There may be excessive skin folds and thickened skin around the head, neck, and distal extremities (**Figures 11.9, 11.10**), and separation of the teeth with increased interdental spacing, particularly of the incisor teeth (**Figure 11.11**).

Differential diagnosis

Hyperadrenocorticism, hypothyroidism, diabetes mellitus.

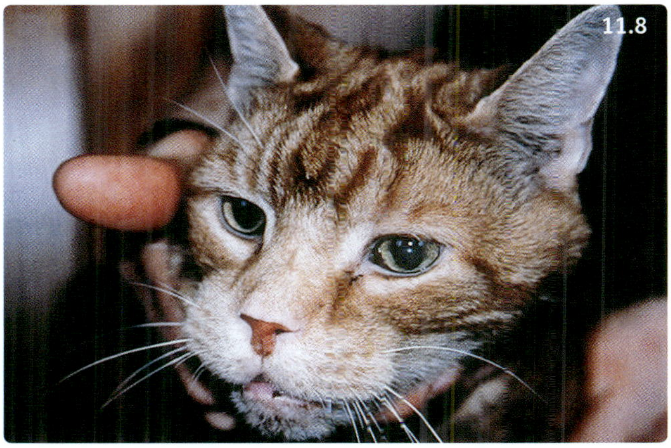

Figure 11.8 A 14-year-old Domestic Shorthair cat with acromegaly. Note the broad muzzle.

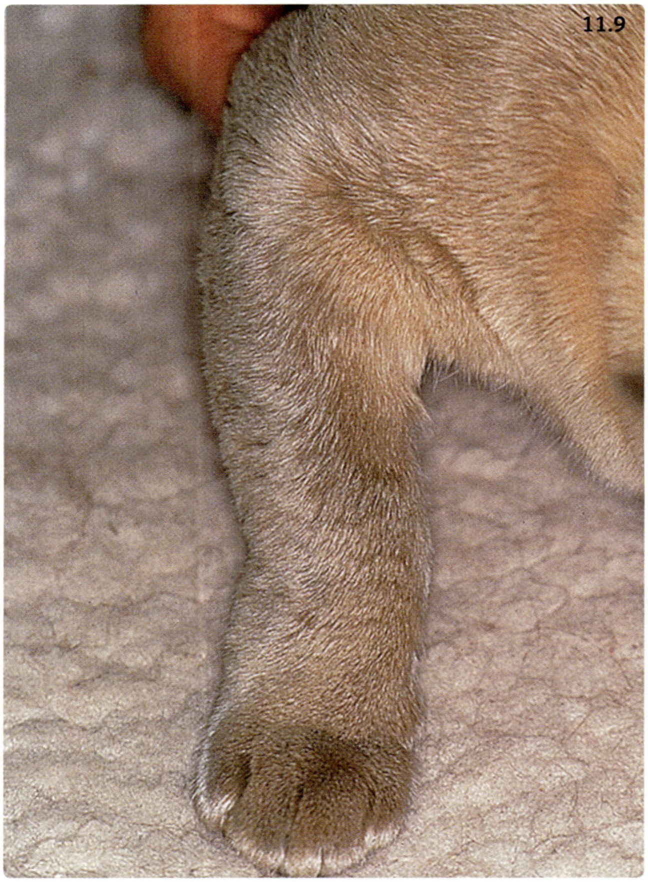

Figure 11.9 A nine-year-old Burmese cat with acromegaly showing enlargement of the paw.

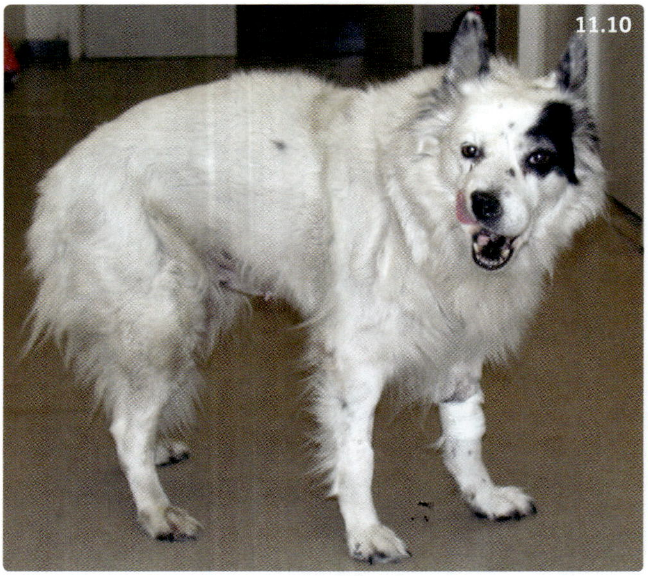

Figures 11.10 A 12-year-old Collie-cross dog with acromegaly showing increased soft tissue around the head and neck.

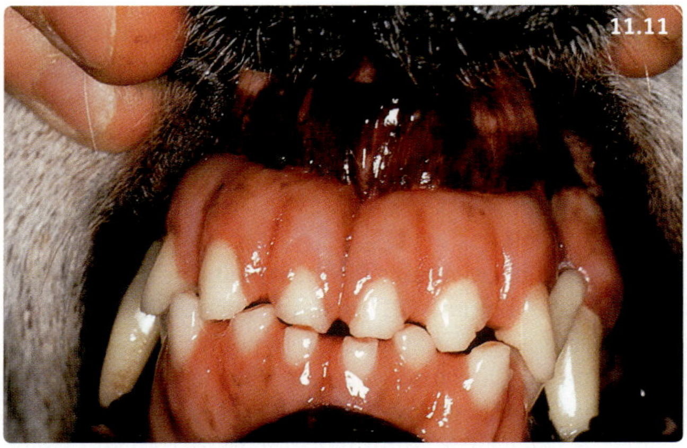

Figure 11.11 A 12-year-old Labrador Retriever with acromegaly showing separation of incisor teeth with increased interdental spacing.

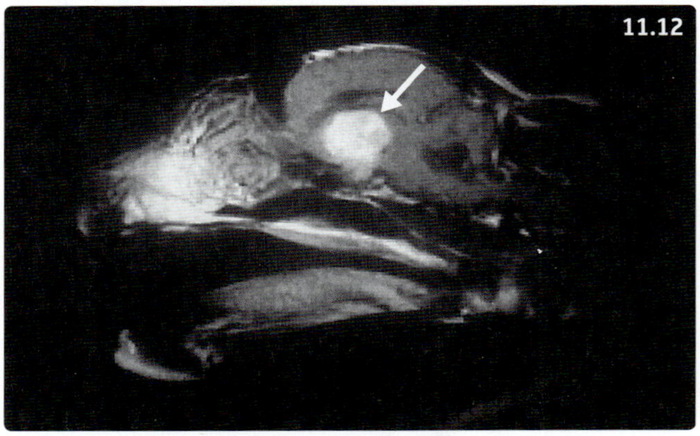

Figure 11.12 An MR image of the brain of a Domestic Shorthair cat with acromegaly showing a large pituitary mass (arrow).

Diagnosis

Laboratory findings of uncontrolled or poorly regulated diabetes mellitus with hyperglycemia and glycosuria are found in most cases. A definitive diagnosis of acromegaly can be made by demonstrating elevated serum concentrations of GH or IGF-1.

CT or MRI of the cranium is required in the cat to demonstrate the size and position of the pituitary tumor (**Figure 11.12**).

Management

Successful treatment of acromegaly in the bitch involves the withdrawal of progestogen therapy and ovariohysterectomy for estrus control. Insulin requirements may decrease dramatically or even cease completely following the withdrawal of progestogen therapy or after ovariohysterectomy. Patients should therefore be monitored very closely to avoid insulin overdosage and the development of hypoglycemia.

In the cat, pituitary irradiation using a linear accelerator or cobalt-60 source has been successful in reducing the GH secretion and allowing resolution or improved control of the diabetes mellitus. Successful treatment following transsphenoidal hypophysectomy has been described in a limited number of cats, but further evaluation and long-term follow-up are required before the treatment can be confidently recommended.

PITUITARY TUMORS

Definition/overview

Primary and secondary tumors can involve the pituitary. Primary tumors may be functional or non-functional. Adenomas of the anterior lobe of the pituitary are the most common tumor and many of these will secrete ACTH, resulting in pituitary-dependent hyperadrenocorticism.

Pathophysiology

Functional pituitary tumors may produce signs associated with excess hormone production by the tropic endocrine glands. The space-occupying effects of large tumors may cause compression and destruction of surrounding pituitary tissue (**Figure 11.13**, arrows), leading to a reduction in the secretion of tropic hormones, which may result in clinical signs of hormone deficiency.

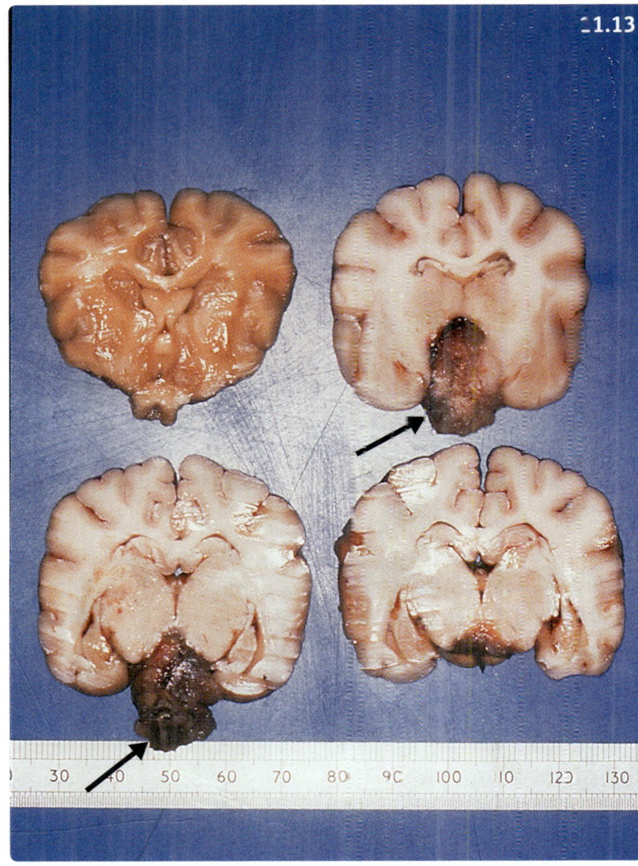

Figure 11.13 Postmortem specimen showing the effects of a large pituitary tumor (arrows).

Clinical presentation

Clinical signs may include those associated with endocrine upset such as polyuria and polydipsia due to excess secretion of ACTH by a functional corticotroph adenoma or impaired vasopressin synthesis or release by compression of the posterior pituitary, lethargy and weight gain due to secondary hypothyroidism, or atrophy of the sex organs due to reduced gonadotropin release.

Space-occupying effects of a pituitary tumor include listlessness, depression, anorexia, vomiting, adipsia, aimless wandering, head pressing, staring, apparent blindness, ataxia, incoordination, head tilt, circling, and seizures (**Figure 11.14**).

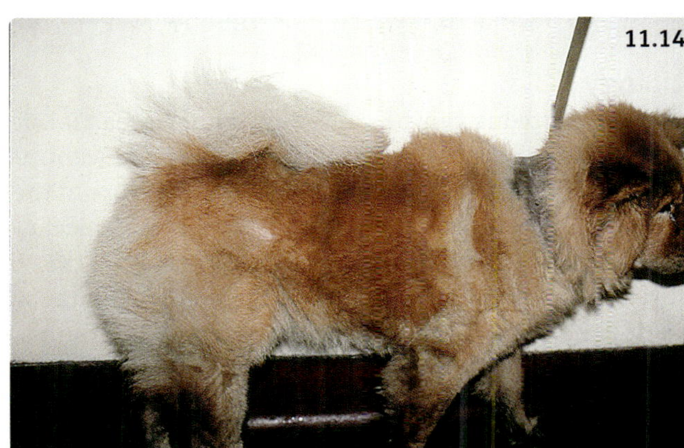

Figure 11.14 A 5-year-old Chow Chow with signs of depression and circling due to a pituitary tumor.

Differential diagnosis

Hyperadrenocorticism, acromegaly, hypothyroidism, diabetes insipidus, neurologic conditions.

Diagnosis

Diagnosis of a pituitary mass can be confirmed by CT or MRI (**Figure 11.15**). Endocrine function tests will help demonstrate if the tumor is functional or not, or if hypopituitarism is present.

Management

If neurologic signs are present, radiotherapy using megavoltage radiation is the treatment of choice and has proved successful in reducing the size of the pituitary mass. Pituitary-dependent hyperadrenocorticism can be

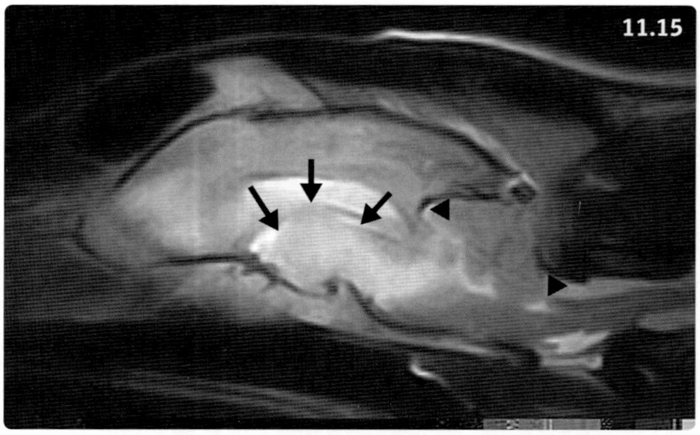

Figure 11.15 Sagittal T2-weighted MR image of a 12-year-old Dalmatian with a large pituitary mass (arrows) causing both caudal transtentorial and foramen magnum herniation (arrowheads).

treated with trilostane or mitotane (see p. 430). Secondary hypothyroidism can be treated by replacement thyroxine (see p. 402).

DIABETES INSIPIDUS

Definition/overview

Vasopressin (ADH) released from the posterior lobe of the pituitary increases the permeability of the distal convoluted tubules and collecting ducts of the kidney and thus controls water excretion. Diabetes insipidus results from a deficiency of vasopressin and is characterized by severe and uncontrolled polyuria, with resultant polydipsia.

Etiology

Diabetes insipidus can be caused by either a partial or total failure to synthesize or release vasopressin (central diabetes insipidus [CDI]) or a partial or total failure of the renal tubules to respond to vasopressin (nephrogenic diabetes insipidus [NDI]).

Both forms of diabetes insipidus may be congenital or acquired. CDI may result from neoplasia or head trauma, but is usually idiopathic in the dog and cat. Rarely, inflammatory and parasitic lesions have been associated with CDI. NDI may be secondary to various drugs, a variety of renal and metabolic disorders including chronic kidney disease, renal medullary fibrosis, tubular necrosis, hyperadrenocorticism, pyometra, and hypercalcemia, or it may be idiopathic.

Pathophysiology

Plasma osmolality is the major determinant of vasopressin release, but hypovolemia and hypotension can also stimulate ADH production. In total CDI there is little increase in urine osmolality with increasing plasma osmolality. In partial CDI, vasopressin is released with increasing plasma osmolality, but concentrations are subnormal.

Clinical presentation

Clinical signs of diabetes insipidus include marked polyuria, frequently with nocturia and incontinence, and severe polydipsia, with the animal often drinking more than 100 ml/kg/24 hours. In acquired cases the onset of clinical signs is usually sudden. Affected dogs and cats start searching for water and may become anorexic and lose weight as a result. Despite their increased thirst, affected animals remain mildly to moderately dehydrated. Affected animals generally show no other clinical signs, although neurologic signs may be noted, particularly if diabetes insipidus is associated with a space-occupying mass such as a pituitary tumor or if the animal becomes severely hypernatremic when deprived of water.

Differential diagnosis

The differential diagnosis of polyuria and polydipsia is given in **Table 11.4**. Diabetes insipidus must be differentiated from primary polydipsia with resultant polyuria, so-called psychogenic polydipsia (PP), where there is a relative lack of vasopressin due to overhydration and,

Table 11.4 Differential diagnosis of polydipsia–polyuria.

Polyuria with compensatory polydipsia Osmotic diuresis: • Diabetes mellitus • Primary renal glycosuria/Fanconi's syndrome • Polyuric renal failure/postobstructive diuresis
Interference with ADH release and/or renal response to ADH Chronic kidney disease Glomerulopathy/nephrotic syndrome Pyelonephritis Pyometra Hyperadrenocorticism Chronic liver disease Hypercalcemia Hypoadrenocorticism Central diabetes insipidus Nephrogenic diabetes insipidus Hypokalemia Hyperthyroidism Drugs/diet
Primary polydipsia Psychogenic polydipsia

frequently, reduced renal concentrating power due to a decrease in medullary hypertonicity from the wash-out effect of handling large quantities of fluid.

Diagnosis

Hematologic, biochemical, and electrolyte profiles are generally unremarkable in animals with CDI or idiopathic NDI. When abnormalities are noted they are usually secondary to dehydration. The most significant finding is very dilute urine of low specific gravity (SG), usually between 1.001 and 1.005. The urine SG is almost invariably less than that of glomerular filtrate (i.e. <1.010), indicating good renal tubular function with resorption of solute in excess of water.

Urine osmolality is low and typically below that of plasma, which is often mildly or moderately elevated due to the concomitant dehydration (**Table 11.5**). In PP the plasma osmolality is usually decreased due to the overhydration.

A carefully monitored water deprivation test (**Table 11.6**) will confirm the animal's inability to concentrate its urine in diabetes insipidus, despite becoming dehydrated. Renal function must be assessed before undertaking this test and the test must always be discontinued if the patient loses more than 5% of its body weight. Urine and plasma osmolality measurements provide more definitive information than urine SG alone (**Figure 11.16**).

The ADH response test (**Table 11.6**) is used to distinguish CDI from NDI. Dogs and cats with CDI will concentrate their urine in response to the administration of exogenous ADH, whereas dogs with NDI will show no response.

Management

Successful treatment of CDI requires long-term replacement therapy using desmopressin, a vasopressin analog. Desmopressin is available in the form of an injection, nasal drops, or tablets. It can provide antidiuretic activity for about 8 hours. One to four drops of the nasal preparation placed in the conjunctival sac twice daily will control the polydipsia and polyuria in most dogs and cats with CDI. Oral therapy (200 µg 1–3 times daily) has proved effective in some cases, but generally the tablets appear to be less effective.

Chlorpropamide, an oral sulfonylurea hypoglycemic agent, potentiates the effects of vasopressin on the renal tubules and, therefore, requires at least the presence of

Table 11.5 Differentiation of central diabetes insipidus, nephrogenic diabetes insipidus, and psychogenic polydipsia.

Parameter	Before water deprivation	After water deprivation		
		CDI	NDI	PP
Urine				
Specific gravity	<1.010	<1.010	<1.010	<1.025
Osmolality	<300	<300	<300	<700
Plasma				
Osmolality	>300 CDI or NDI	>310	>310	±310
	<295 PP			
U:P osmolality	<1.0	<1.0	<1.0	2–3
ADH response test				
Urine specific gravity	<1.010	>1.015	<1.010	<1.025
U:P osmolality	<1.0	>1.0	<1.0	>1.0

Note: Osmolality measured in mOsm/kg.

Table 11.6 Protocol for water deprivation and antidiuretic hormone response testing.

Water deprivation test Indication: • Used in the diagnosis of diabetes insipidus. Does not differentiate between the central and nephrogenic forms of the disease The test should only be performed in animals with normal blood urea and creatinine concentrations
Method: • Collect 5 ml of urine and plasma if osmolality is being measured. If specific gravity is to be measured, only urine is required • Weigh patient • Withhold all fluids and food • Collect urine and plasma after 8 hours and then at 2-hour intervals until the test is complete. It is rarely safe or necessary to continue this test for 24 hours • Weigh patient each time urine and plasma is collected • Stop test if patient demonstrates adequate concentrating ability (specific gravity >1.020) or if patient becomes dehydrated and loses 5% of its body weight or more
Interpretation: • Cases of central or nephrogenic diabetes insipidus fail to concentrate urine (specific gravity <1.010) and urine osmolality remains low and does not exceed that of plasma • This test does not always give conclusive results, especially if plasma and urine osmolality are not measured
Vasopressin (ADH) response test Indication: • Used to differentiate between central and nephrogenic diabetes insipidus
Method: • Collect 5 ml of urine and plasma if osmolality is being measured. Only urine is required if specific gravity is to be measured • Inject desmopressin intramuscularly. Use 2 μg for dogs <15 kg and 4 μg for dogs >15 kg • Collect urine and plasma samples every 2 hours
Interpretation: • Dogs with nephrogenic diabetes insipidus will show very little or no response to exogenous vasopressin and the urine specific gravity and osmolality will remain low • Dogs with central diabetes insipidus will concentrate their urine, usually within 6 hours (specific gravity >1.015); the urine osmolality will rise by 50% or more and will exceed the plasma osmolality

11.16

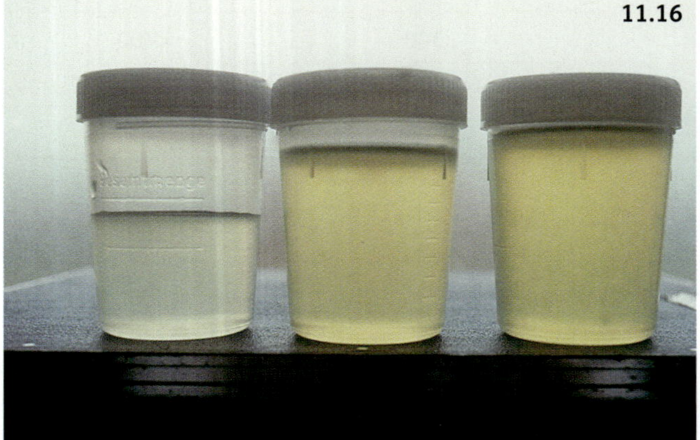

Figure 11.16 Urine samples from a dog with central diabetes insipidus taken during a water deprivation test. The specific gravity never increased above 1.008 despite the dog losing 5% of its body weight during the test.

some endogenous vasopressin in order to be effective. Chlorpropamide has been shown to be effective in partial CDI in humans; however, the results in dogs with CDI have been inconsistent. In some cases it may take several weeks to obtain an effect. Hypoglycemia is a potential adverse effect. A dose of 10–40 mg/kg PO q24h has been suggested in dogs. Chlorpropamide is not recommended for use in cats.

Thiazide diuretics such as hydrochlorothiazide and chlorothiazide have a paradoxical effect in both CDI and NDI. Urine output may be decreased by up to 50%, although the urine is still dilute. The suggested doses for hydrochlorothiazide and chlorothiazide are 2–4 mg/kg q12h and 20–40 mg/kg q12h, respectively. The precise dose should be tailored to each patient and the effect may be enhanced by concurrent use of a sodium-restricted diet. Patients should be monitored periodically for electrolyte disturbances, particularly hypokalemia.

Idiopathic CDI has a favorable prognosis with treatment. Animals with an expanding hypothalamic or pituitary tumor have a more guarded prognosis, especially if neurologic signs are present. CDI following head trauma carries a variable prognosis; spontaneous recovery may occur within a few days or weeks in some cases, but in others the damage is permanent. NDI tends to have a more guarded prognosis and a search for a primary cause should be undertaken in order to provide more appropriate therapy.

DISORDERS OF THE THYROID GLAND

The thyroid gland consists of two lobes, which are not normally palpable in healthy dogs or cats. Palpable enlargement of the thyroid from any cause is referred to as goiter. Two parathyroid glands are associated with each thyroid lobe. The internal parathyroids usually lie within the thyroid capsule at the caudal pole of each lobe.

The thyroid gland actively takes up inorganic iodide, resulting in concentrations that are 10–200 times that of serum. The inorganic iodide enters the thyroid follicular cells and is transformed into the metabolically active thyroid hormones thyroxine (T4) and triiodothyronine (T3). The synthesis and secretion of T4 and T3 are controlled by TSH secreted by the thyrotroph cells of the anterior pituitary. Secretion of TSH is stimulated by thyrotropin releasing hormone (TRH), a hypothalamic tripeptide. A classic negative feedback system operates to maintain the plasma concentrations of T4 and T3 within close limits (**Figure 11.17**).

In plasma, more than 99% of T4 and T3 is bound to plasma proteins, mainly albumin and globulins. It is the free (unbound) hormones that are metabolically active. Although T4 is the major secretory product of the thyroid gland, the metabolic activity of T3 is much greater. About 80% of the plasma T3 concentration is produced by deiodination of T4 in peripheral tissues, mainly the liver, muscle, and kidneys. In catabolic states, such as those produced by starvation, anorexia, or debilitating disease, T4 is deiodinated to reverse T3 (rT3), an inactive metabolite, at the expense of T3 production.

Thyroid hormones play a dominant role in controlling metabolism. They increase basal metabolic rate, stimulate cellular oxygen consumption, promote carbohydrate absorption from the intestine, and regulate lipid metabolism. Thyroid hormones are also essential for normal growth and development and they activate the anagen (growth) phase of the hair cycle. Some effects of thyroid

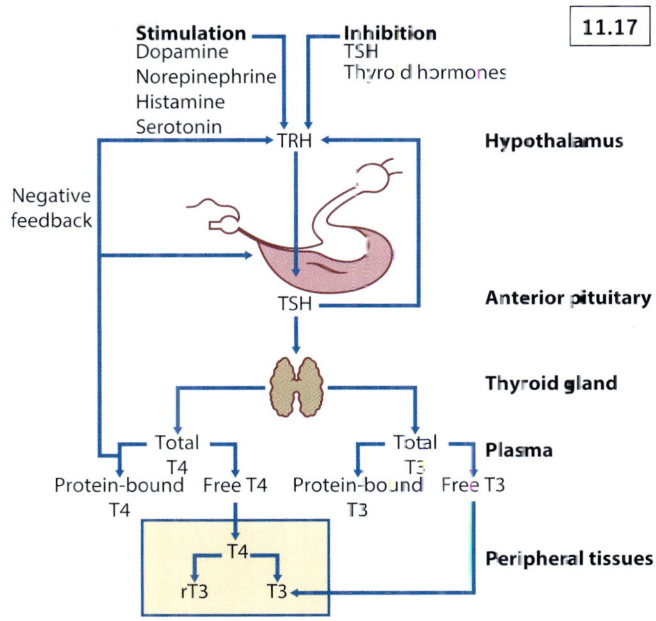

Figure 11.17 Physiology of thyroid function.

hormones, such as stimulation of the nervous and cardiovascular systems, are mediated by increased sensitivity to catecholamines.

HYPOTHYROIDISM

Definition/overview

Hypothyroidism is a multisystemic disorder resulting from inadequate circulating thyroid hormone concentrations. It is considered a common endocrinopathy in the dog and estimates of incidence range from 1 in 156 to 1 in 500 depending on the criteria for diagnosis. However, in the past hypothyroidism may have been overdiagnosed, as the clinical signs are vague and nonspecific and diagnostic tests frequently give false positive results in euthyroid dogs.

Naturally occurring hypothyroidism is a rare clinical disorder in cats.

Etiology

Primary hypothyroidism is caused by an intrinsic disorder of the thyroid gland and is the most common type of hypothyroidism in the dog. Hypothyroidism usually results from lymphocytic thyroiditis or thyroid atrophy. Thyroid atrophy may be the end-stage of lymphocytic thyroiditis (**Figures 11.18a, b**). Thyroid neoplasia can occasionally be associated with hypothyroidism, although most dogs with thyroid tumors have normal thyroid function. Congenital hypothyroidism (cretinism) is rare and may be caused by thyroid agenesis, dysgenesis, or dyshormonogenesis. Secondary hypothyroidism is usually associated with pituitary neoplasia, but it may also occur with congenital panhypopituitarism. Hypothalamic dysfunction, iodine deficiency, and serum transport defects are rare causes of hypothyroidism.

The most common cause of feline hypothyroidism is iatrogenic destruction or removal of the thyroid gland following radioactive iodine therapy or surgery for the treatment of hyperthyroidism. Spontaneous acquired hypothyroidism has been reported in a cat with lymphocytic thyroiditis. Congenital hypothyroidism has been reported in the cat and may be associated with goiter.

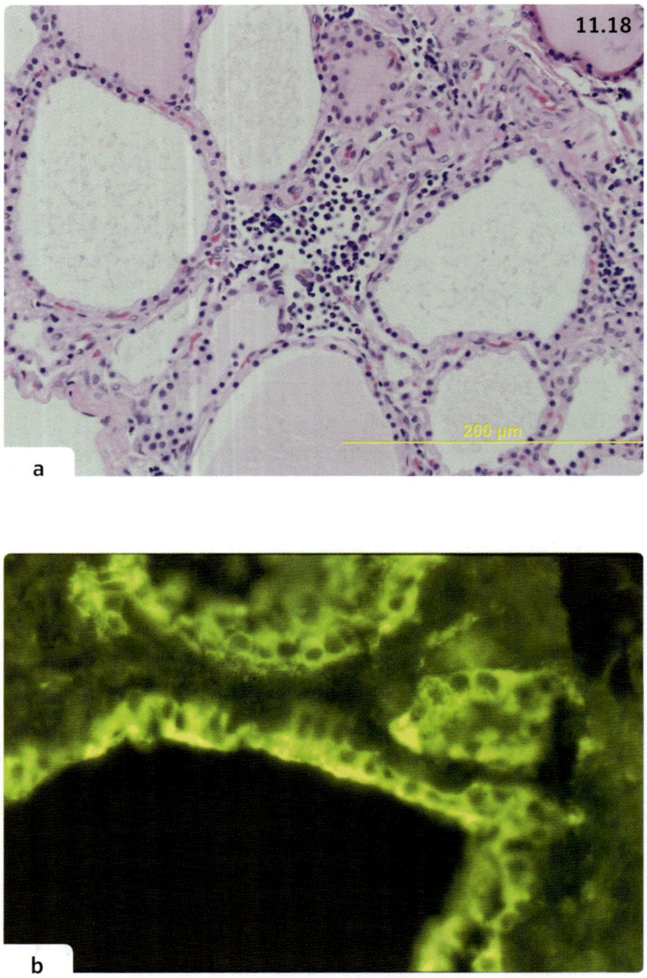

Figures 11.18a, b Hypothyroidism. (a) Histopathologic microscopic view of lymphocytic thyroiditis in a dog showing the infiltrating lymphocytes. (H&E stain). (b) Histopathologic indirect immunofluorescent demonstration of autoimmune thyroiditis. The immunofluorescence represents antibodies that are bound to the thyroid epithelial cells. (Courtesy M. Schaer)

Pathophysiology

Hypothyroidism may result from dysfunction of any part of the hypothalamic–pituitary–thyroid axis. In lymphocytic thyroiditis there is infiltration of the thyroid gland by lymphocytes, macrophages, and plasma cells. Leukocytes and degenerate follicular cells may be found within vacuolated colloid. The parenchyma becomes progressively destroyed and replaced by fibrous connective tissue. In follicular atrophy the parenchyma is replaced by adipose connective tissue. In secondary hypothyroidism the follicular epithelial cells become flattened and the follicles become distended with colloid.

Clinical presentation

The clinical signs of hypothyroidism are very variable and often vague. Some cases present with a classic combination of clinical signs, whereas others may exhibit only one sign. Hypothyroidism usually affects young to middle aged dogs of the larger breeds. Golden Retrievers, Dobermanns, Boxers, Great Danes, and Irish Setters appear to be overrepresented.

Lethargy, mental dullness, bradycardia, poor exercise tolerance, weight gain without an increase in food intake, intolerance to cold, and hypothermia are the most common clinical signs associated with hypothyroidism. Bilaterally symmetrical, nonpruritic alopecia affecting the flanks, thorax, ventral trunk, and neck is associated with inhibition of the hair cycle (**Figure 11.19**). The remaining hair coat is dry and dull. The skin is often thickened (myxedematous) and hyperpigmented. Myxedema of the skin is most evident on the head, resulting in a 'tragic' facial expression (**Figure 11.20**). The skin, particularly on the ventral abdomen, may be cold and clammy to the touch. Comedones, seborrhea, and recurrent pyoderma may also be noted. Intact females often have abnormal estrous cycles and reduced fertility. Constipation and corneal lipidosis (**Figure 11.21**) may occasionally be noted.

Neurologic signs may be seen in some dogs with hypothyroidism and include neuromuscular dysfunction with cranial nerve abnormalities, laryngeal paralysis, megaesophagus, lower motor neuron disease, and encephalopathy (**Figures 11.22, 11.23**). Clinical signs of lameness, dragging of the feet, quadriparesis, hearing impairment, and nystagmus have also been reported. Electromyography may reveal fibrillation potentials and positive sharp waves. Motor nerve conduction velocities may be decreased and tendon reflexes appear sluggish.

Congenital hypothyroidism has been reported in a number of breeds including the Boxer and the Giant Schnauzer. Clinical signs of congenital hypothyroidism

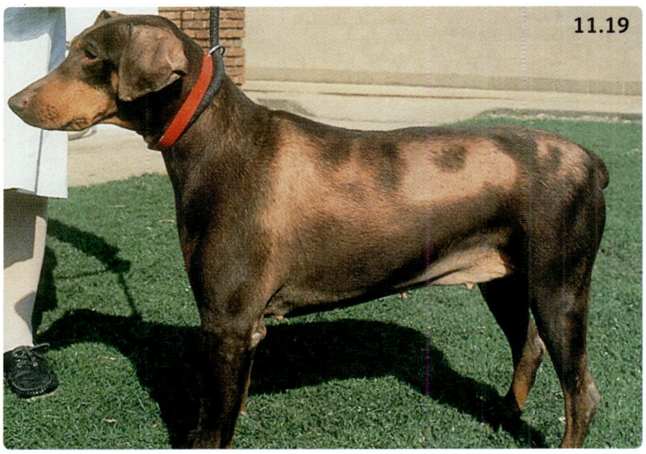

Figure 11.19 A 6-year-old Dobermann with bilaterally symmetrical alopecia due to hypothyroidism.

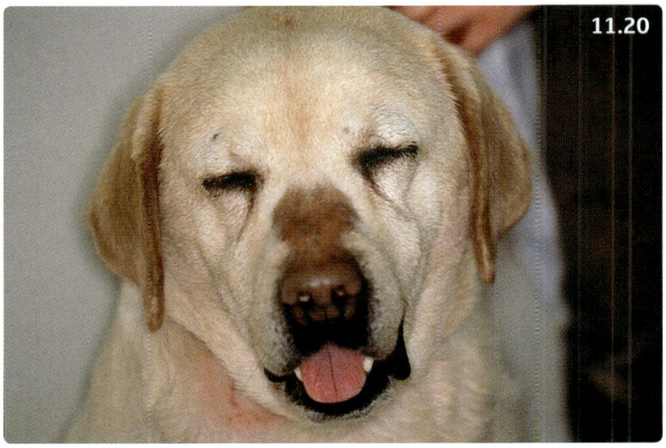

Figure 11.20 A 7-year-old Labrador Retriever with hypothyroidism showing a 'tragic' expression.

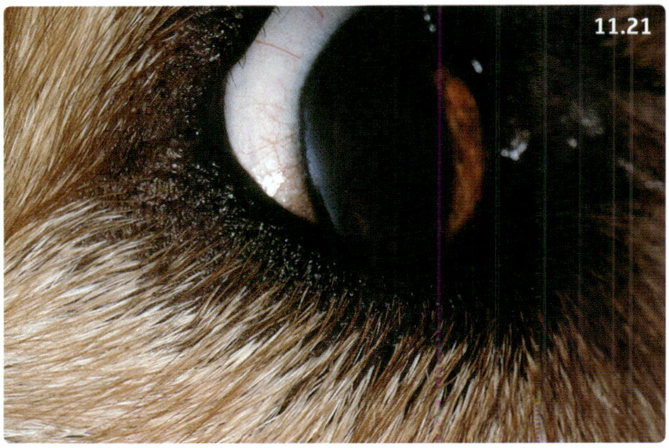

Figure 11.21 An 8-year-old Golden Retriever with hypothyroidism showing corneal lipidosis around the limbal margin.

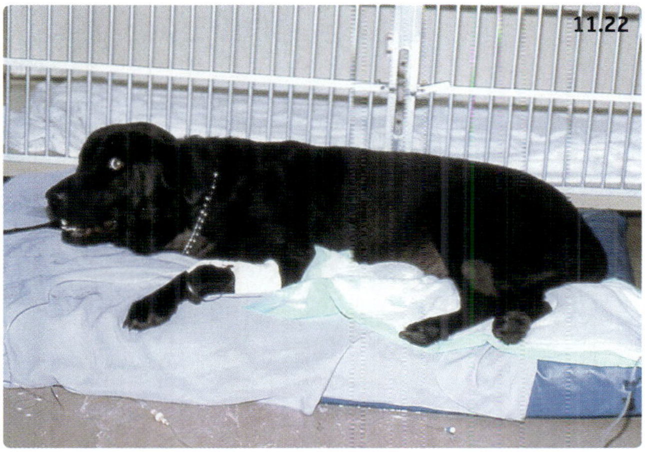

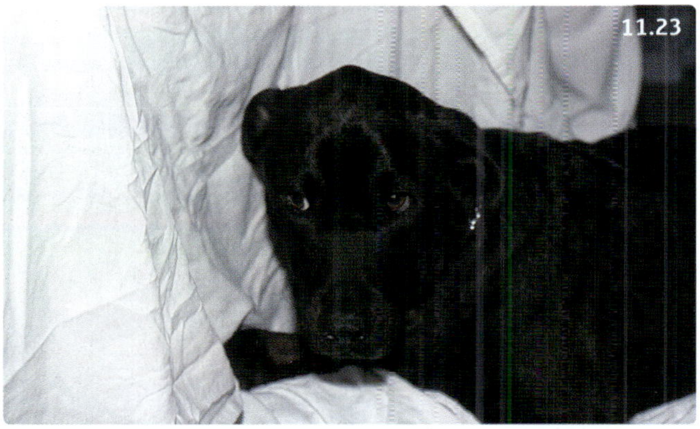

Figures 11.22, 11.23 This young Labrador Retriever was referred to neurology for signs of tetraparesis and abnormal cranial nerve function (note the dysconjugate eye positioning). The diagnosis was hypothyroid neuropathy. The dog made a complete recovery with levothyroxine replacement treatment. (Courtesy M. Schaer)

include hypothermia, lethargy, disproportionate dwarfism with a short, broad skull, short thick limbs and kyphosis, delayed dental eruption, thickened skin, and a dry hair coat (**Figure 11.24**). Radiographic changes include delayed epiphyseal ossification and epiphyseal dysgenesis (**Figure 11.25**). Congenital hypothyroidism has also been seen in the cat (**Figure 11.26**).

Differential diagnosis

Pituitary tumor or cyst, surgery (thyroidectomy or hypophysectomy), drugs (particularly antithyroid drugs and glucocorticoids), diet/obesity, hyperadrenocorticism.

Diagnosis

Laboratory findings

Hypercholesterolemia is found in about 70% of hypothyroid dogs. Thyroid hormones stimulate biliary excretion of cholesterol and a deficiency of these

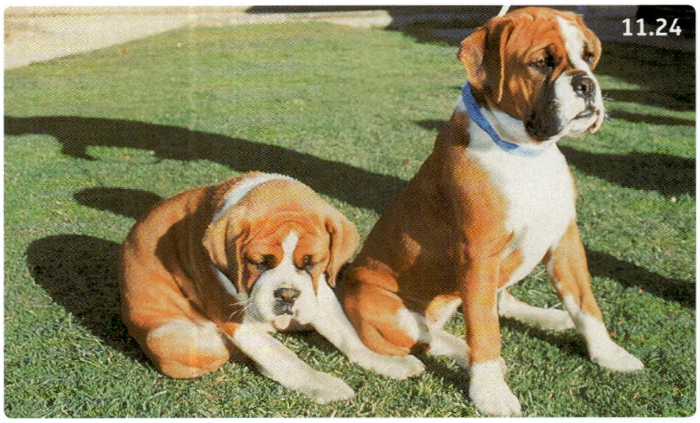

Figure 11.24 Two 7-month-old Boxer littermates. The puppy on the left has congenital hypothyroidism.

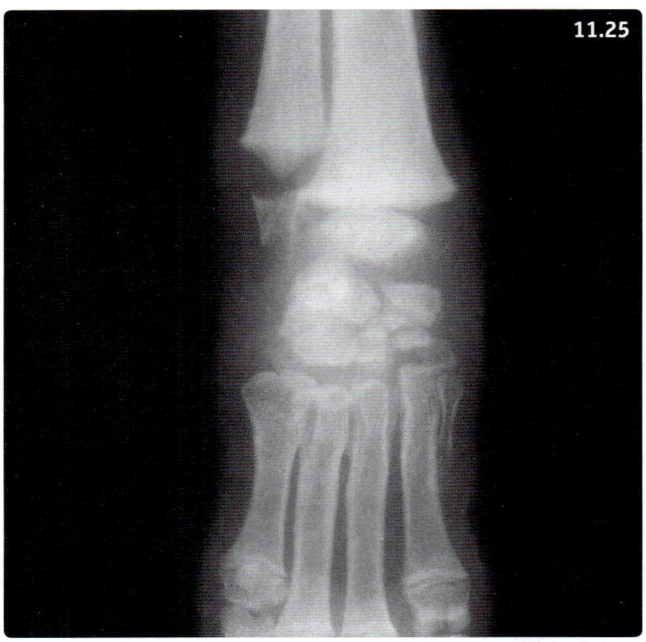

Figure 11.25 Craniocaudal radiograph of the carpus of a 10-month-old Boxer with congenital hypothyroidism showing delayed ossification and epiphyseal dysgenesis.

hormones results in an increase in the cholesterol content of the liver. To prevent overloading the liver with cholesterol, the low-density lipoprotein receptors are downregulated to limit low-density and high-density lipoprotein uptake from the circulation. Plasma concentrations of these lipoproteins rise, causing hypercholesterolemia. Causes of hypercholesterolemia are listed in **Table 11.7**.

Mild normocytic, normochromic, nonregenerative anemia occurs in about 30% of hypothyroid dogs and represents a physiologic response to the lowered basal metabolic rate.

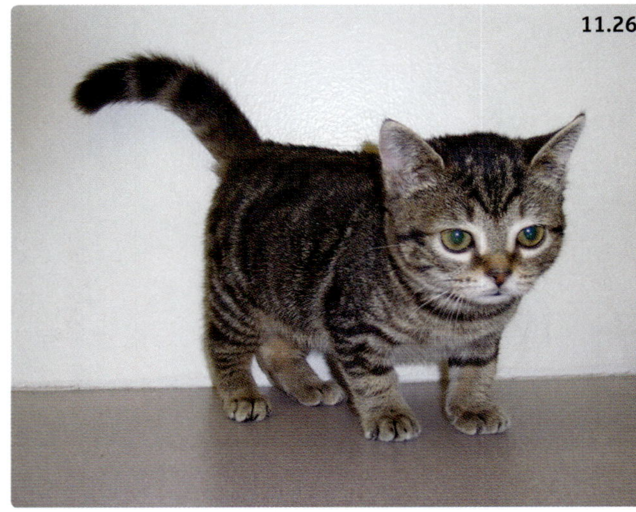

Figure 11.26 This approximately 6-month-old kitten was the runt of the litter due to its congenital hypothyroid condition. (Courtesy A. Specht)

Table 11.7 Causes of hypercholesterolemia.

Causes
Postprandial hyperlipidemia
Secondary hyperlipidemia: • Hypothyroidism • Hyperadrenocorticism • Diabetes mellitus • Cholestatic liver disease • Nephrotic syndrome
Primary (idiopathic) hyperlipidemia

Mild to moderate increases in serum activity of ALT, AST, ALP, and CK may be noted. Increased CK activity is particularly associated with myopathy in cases of hypothyroidism.

Thyroid function tests

The dynamic thyroid function tests and their protocols are listed in **Table 11.8**.

Serum total and free T4

Baseline serum T4 concentration using a validated assay is more accurate than serum T3 in assessing the status of thyroid gland function and is recommended for initial evaluation of the thyroid gland. Random fluctuations in serum T4 concentrations occur, but a true circadian rhythm has not been identified.

Serum T4 concentrations can be affected by breed, age, illness, and drug administration. Certain breeds, particularly sighthounds, have lower serum T4 concentrations than other breeds and this is important when interpreting results from Greyhounds or Afghan

Table 11.8 Protocol and interpretation of the TSH and TRH stimulation tests.

TSH stimulation test Protocol: • Collect plasma or serum sample for basal T4 concentration • Administer 50–75 µg/dog recombinant human TSH intravenously • Collect second sample for T4 concentration 6 hours later
Interpretation: • A diagnosis of primary hypothyroidism can be confirmed if both the pre- and post-T4 samples are below the reference range for basal T4 concentration • In normal animals the T4 concentration should be stimulated to well within or above the normal reference range for T4. In most animals the T4 concentration should increase by at least 1.5 times the basal concentration • Interpretation of intermediate results is more difficult and may occur in association with nonthyroid illness, treatment with certain drugs, secondary hypothyroidism, or possibly in the early stages of primary hypothyroidism
TRH stimulation test Protocol: • Collect plasma or serum sample for basal T4 concentration • Administer 200 µg/dog protirelin (TRH-[Cambridge Laboratories, UK]) intravenously. Injection may cause salivation, vomiting, and tachycardia • Collect second sample for T4 concentration 4 hours later
Interpretation: • Similar to TSH stimulation test, although stimulation of T4 concentrations is less than with TSH and the response to TRH shows greater individual variation

Hounds, for example. Serum T4 concentrations tend to be higher in young growing puppies and lower in old dogs when compared with normal adult concentrations. Concurrent illness can suppress serum thyroid hormone concentrations (sick euthyroid syndrome). The degree of suppression is dependent on the severity of the illness or catabolic state rather than the specific disorder. Various drugs can alter thyroid hormone metabolism and serum binding, particularly glucocorticoids, anticonvulsants, NSAIDs, potentiated sulfonamides, furosemide, and anesthetic agents.

Serum free T4 concentrations measure metabolically active T4 and should not be influenced by the effects of serum binding. However, measurement of serum free T4 by most assays, which do not employ equilibrium dialysis, has not proved to be any more reliable than total T4 concentrations in the diagnosis of hypothyroidism. Serum free T4 measured by equilibrium dialysis can prove useful in differentiating genuine hypothyroidism when the total T4 concentration is in the reference range.

A low basal serum T4 concentration, with a history and clinical signs compatible with hypothyroidism, may be sufficient evidence to warrant a therapeutic trial. In one study the predictive value of a positive test result was 0.75 and of a negative test result was 0.87 when using T4 concentrations to diagnose hypothyroidism. Serum T4 concentrations in the low normal or nondiagnostic range should have further tests performed (e.g. a canine TSH concentration and/or a TSH or TRH stimulation test) provided the index of suspicion is still high for hypothyroidism.

Serum T4 concentrations in the normal range are unlikely to be associated with hypothyroidism. However, antibodies to thyroid hormone can cause discordance between measured thyroid hormone concentrations and the clinical status of the dog. Depending on their concentration, binding affinity, and the assay method employed, thyroid antibodies can result in either falsely elevated or falsely low thyroid hormone concentrations. Autoantibodies to T4 and T3 can be measured in these cases.

Serum total T3 and free T3

Baseline serum T3 concentrations are less accurate for predicting hypothyroidism than serum T4. Random fluctuations in serum T3 concentrations are greater than with serum T4 and have a greater tendency to be misleading with respect to the status of thyroid gland function. Possible explanations for this discrepancy include the normal thyroid gland's preference for secreting T4, the intracellular formation and location of most T3, the preferential secretion of T3 compared with T4 as thyroid function progressively fails, and the development of anti-T3 antibodies. The diagnostic value of serum T3 concentrations in hypothyroidism is therefore inferior to serum T4.

Endogenous canine TSH

Measurement of canine TSH (c-TSH) has revolutionized the testing for hypothyroidism, particularly in primary hypothyroidism where the concentrations should be high because of loss of the negative feedback effect of thyroid hormones. A validated c-TSH assay is now widely available, but unfortunately it has been shown that not all cases of primary hypothyroidism exhibit elevated c-TSH concentrations and that some euthyroid dogs as well as some dogs with nonthyroidal illness may have elevated TSH concentrations. The general conclusions are that c-TSH measurements are useful when measured together with serum total T4 concentrations in the diagnosis of cases of suspected hypothyroidism; however, the sensitivity and specificity of the assay, particularly at lower concentrations, are insufficient to obviate the need for a dynamic test (TSH or TRH stimulation test) to confirm the diagnosis in some cases of hypothyroidism.

TSH stimulation test

The administration of exogenous TSH to measure thyroid secretory reserve is the most definitive method currently available for the diagnosis of hypothyroidism. Unfortunately, pharmaceutical grade bovine TSH has limited availability, but more recently recombinant human TSH has become available. The protocol and interpretation criteria are given in **Table 11.8**. The use of this test is limited by the expense of the TSH injection.

Peak serum T4 responses are decreased by nonthyroidal illness and drug administration in the same way as basal T4 concentrations. Thyroid function testing is thus best performed after resolution of nonthyroidal illness and, if possible, with the patient off all medication.

TRH stimulation test

TRH is readily available and less expensive than TSH. However, the T4 response to TRH is less predictable and peak concentrations tend to be lower than with TSH stimulation. Increasing the dose of TRH increases the duration but not the magnitude of the T4 response. TRH administration may cause cholinergic signs such as salivation, vomiting, and defecation. Responses are also affected by nonthyroidal illness and drug administration.

Reverse T3 (rT3)

Measurement of serum rT3 concentration can be useful in identifying cases with significant nonthyroidal illness and should be reserved for those cases with discordant or equivocal T4 concentrations. If the serum rT3 concentration is high in a dog with low or low-normal T4, hypothyroidism is unlikely to be the cause of the animal's clinical signs.

Thyroglobulin autoantibodies (TgAA)

Lymphocytic thyroiditis is a major cause of canine hypothyroidism and, as part of the inflammatory process, antibodies to thyroid antigens are released into the circulation. Thyroglobulin is the principal antigen for which measurable serum antibodies are present. Therefore, measurement of TgAA provides evidence of an active inflammatory process in the the thyroid gland. However, the presence of TgAA does not provide information about thyroid function, since at least 60–70% of the gland has to be destroyed before thyroid dysfunction occurs. Consequently, both lymphocytic thyroiditis and TgAA can be found in dogs that are not hypothyroid and, in dogs where hypothyroidism is caused by thyroid atrophy, circulating TgAA may not be present at all.

Thyroid biopsy

Although not commonly performed, histologic examination of a thyroid gland biopsy provides an accurate method of differentiating between primary and secondary hypothyroidism. In primary hypothyroidism there is loss of thyroid follicles resulting from either lymphocytic thyroiditis or thyroid atrophy. In secondary hypothyroidism the thyroid follicles become distended with colloid and the follicular epithelial cells are flattened. Testing thyroid function is still required to make a diagnosis of hypothyroidism, since the degree of histologic change does not always relate to reduced hormone production and release.

Management

Thyroid hormone replacement is required for the treatment of hypothyroidism. Synthetic forms of T4 and T3 are available. Sodium levothyroxine (L-thyroxine) is the treatment of choice because it most closely resembles the preferential secretion of T4 by the normal thyroid gland. Synthetic T4 is readily deiodinated to T3 in peripheral tissues and therefore does not bypass the normal cellular regulatory processes that control the production of the more potent T3 in those tissues.

An initial replacement dose of L-thyroxine is 20–40 µg/kg daily in divided doses. Although it has been suggested that once daily dosing is sufficient in many cases, the author has documented a number of cases where once daily administration has failed to maintain adequate serum concentrations throughout the day, with a consequent failure of the clinical signs to resolve fully. Poor absorption and a shorter half-life for T4 explain why dogs require higher doses and more frequent administration than human patients with hypothyroidism.

Therapy should always be continued for a minimum of 3 months. Improved activity and mental alertness are usually seen within 2 weeks, but skin and hair coat changes may take up to 6 months to resolve.

The effect of treatment can be monitored by measurement of post-pill serum T4 concentrations. Sampling 4–6 hours after dosing will give a peak serum T4 concentration and a sample taken just prior to dosing will give the lowest serum T4 concentration. The dose and frequency of administration should be adjusted to maintain the serum T4 concentration in the high end of the reference range throughout the day. Underdosage may lead to treatment failure and overdosage can lead to iatrogenic hyperthyroidism. Replacement therapy is required for life.

Possible causes for cases failing to respond to replacement therapy include misdiagnosis, inadequate dose or frequency of administration, poor gastrointestinal (GI) absorption, and peripheral tissue resistance.

Congenital hypothyroidism should be treated as early as possible to achieve normal growth and development. The dose will require adjustment as the patient grows and becomes older, so post-pill assessments are required at monthly intervals during the first year of life.

HYPOTHYROID MYXEDEMA

Definition/overview

Myxedema coma is an extreme form of hypothyroidism with an acute presentation that can prove life-threatening. It is considered to be a complication of chronic hypothyroidism and is manifest by impaired mental status, thermoregulation, respiratory and cardiovascular function.

Clinical presentation

Affected dogs, mostly Dobermanns, are profoundly dull and present stuporous or comatose with hypothermia in the absence of shivering (**Figures 11.27a–c**). The skin can

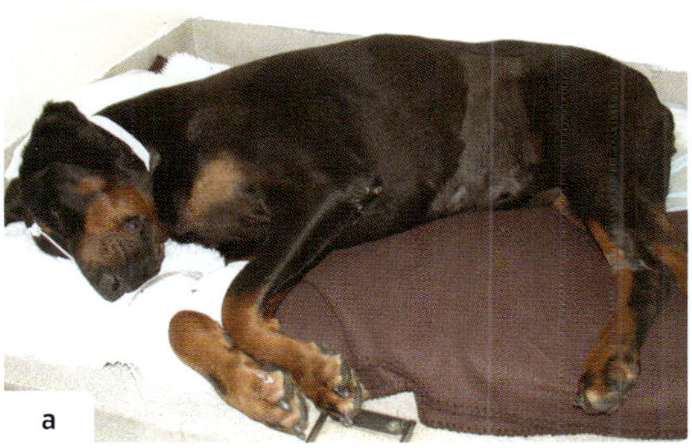
a

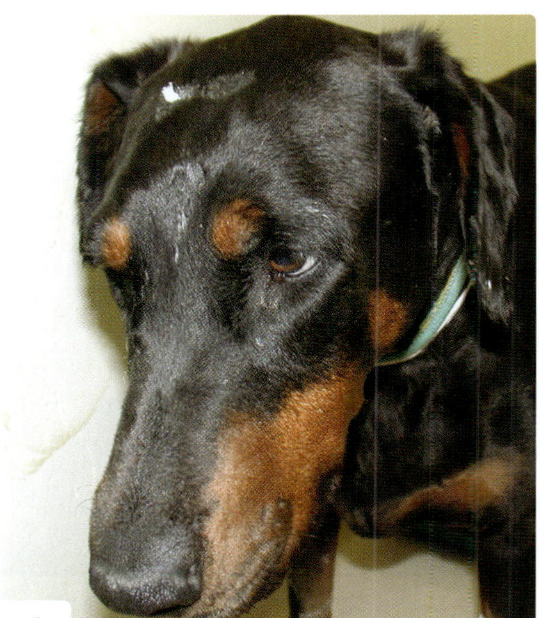
c

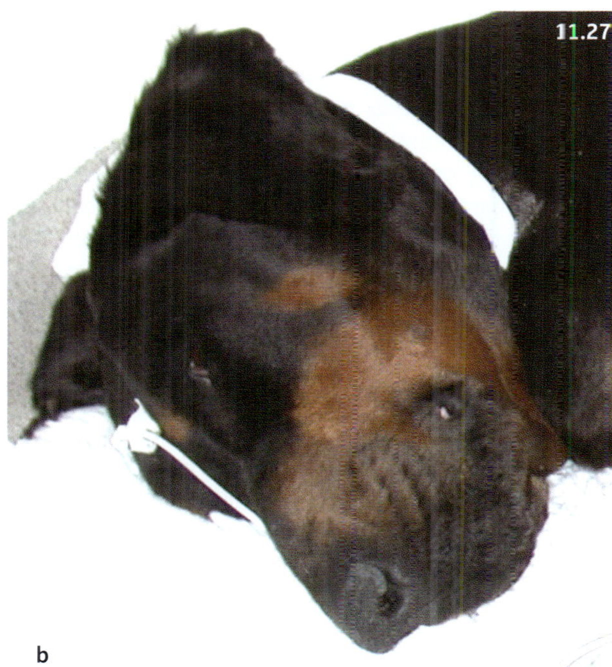

b

Figures 11.27a–c This Dobermann was referred to the neurology service to evaluate generalized weakness. The dog was profoundly mentally depressed and recumbent. Shown is the dog initially (a, b) and subsequently improved with treatment (c).

be myxedematous due to the accumulation of mucopolysaccharides and hyaluronic acid. Bradycardia, hypotension, and hypoventilation are also evident.

Diagnosis

Laboratory test results are characteristic of hypothyroidism.

Management

Treatment entails gradual warming, avoiding overhydration from IV fluids, monitoring ventilation and providing support if needed, and administration of glucocorticoids and L-thyroxine.

HYPERTHYROIDISM

Definition/overview

Hyperthyroidism (thyrotoxicosis) is a multisystemic disorder resulting from excessive circulating concentrations of T4 and/or T3. Hyperthyroidism is the most common endocrine disorder of the domestic cat, but is rare in the dog.

Etiology

Functional adenomatous hyperplasia (adenoma) affecting one or, more commonly, both thyroid lobes is the most common cause of feline hyperthyroidism. Iatrogenic hyperthyroidism caused by excessive thyroid hormone supplementation is recognized occasionally. Thyroid carcinoma is a rare cause of hyperthyroidism in the cat. In the dog, although thyroid carcinoma is the most common thyroid tumor, it is rarely functional.

Pathophysiology

The pathogenesis is unknown, but the frequent involvement of both thyroid lobes would suggest a circulating factor may be involved. Recent epidemiologic studies suggest there is an increased risk of developing feline hyperthyroidism associated with indoor living and consumption of canned cat food, in particular fish flavors.

Clinical presentation

Hyperthyroidism is a disease of middle aged to older cats, with a mean age of 13 years and a range of 6–21 years. Only about 6% of hyperthyroid cats are younger than 10 years of age at the time of diagnosis. There is no breed or sex predisposition.

The clinical signs of hyperthyroidism relate to the excessive secretion of thyroid hormones and their general stimulatory effect on different body systems. The frequency and severity of the clinical signs are highly variable in cats with hyperthyroidism and are influenced by the duration of hyperthyroidism, the ability of the body systems to cope with the demands imposed by thyroid hormone excess, and the presence of concomitant disease in the older animal. In most cases the clinical signs of hyperthyroidism are slowly progressive, with an insidious onset.

The major presenting sign, therefore, is progressive weight loss frequently accompanied by polyphagia (**Figure 11.28**). Since most cats maintain a good appetite and remain active for their age, owners frequently feel the cat is in good health until weight loss or other signs develop. Affected cats are often hyperactive and become irritable or aggressive, which can make clinical examination difficult (**Figure 11.29**). Polydipsia and polyuria are common. Intermittent GI signs such as vomiting, diarrhea, and the passage of voluminous fatty feces

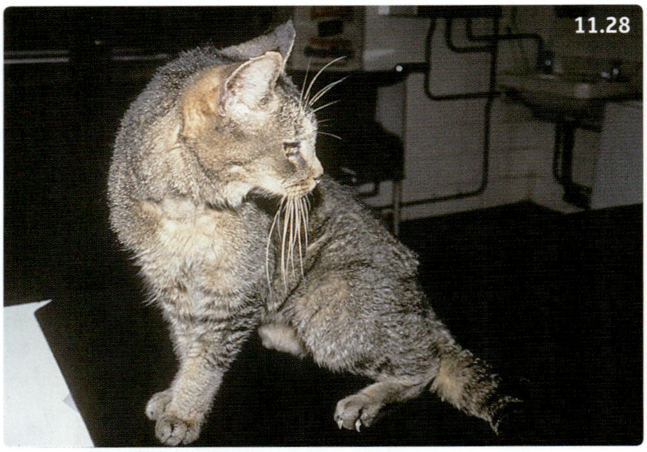

Figure 11.28 A 13-year-old Domestic Shorthair cat with hyperthyroidism.

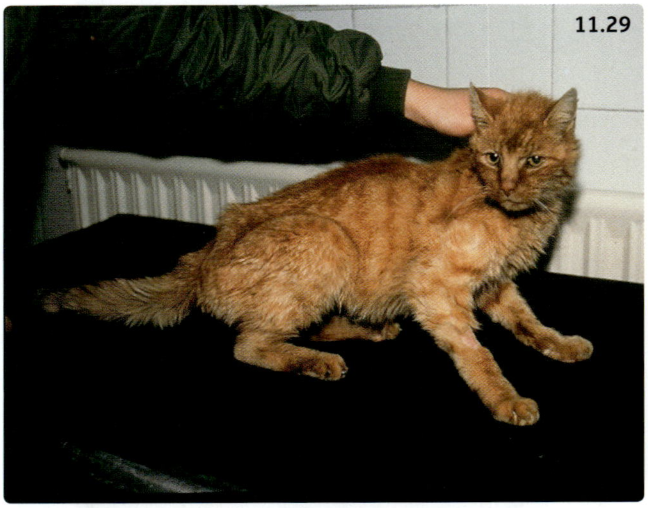

Figure 11.29 A 15-year-old Domestic Shorthair cat with hyperthyroidism showing irritation.

are also frequent clinical signs. Occasionally, systemic hypertension with retinal hemorrhages and/or detachment may occur, but generally, hypertension, if present, is only mild to moderate in severity.

Cardiac abnormalities are frequently recognized in hyperthyroid cats. There is usually a tachycardia with a heart rate in excess of 240 bpm. Systolic murmurs, gallop rhythms, or dysrhythmias are frequently detected on auscultation. In severe cases, clinical signs of congestive heart failure (CHF) may develop and these may include dyspnea resulting from pulmonary edema or accumulation of pleural fluid and ascites. The cardiac signs are associated with cardiomyopathy, usually the hypertrophic form, which develops secondarily to excessive thyroid hormone secretion. Electrocardiographic abnormalities may include tachycardia, increased R wave amplitude, particularly in lead II, and various atrial and ventricular dysrhythmias and conduction disturbances (**Figure 11.30**).

Although there are no specific skin lesions, the coat of cats with hyperthyroidism is often matted and unkempt (**Figure 11.31**). Affected cats may also develop heat intolerance with panting and dysphonia. Although most hyperthyroid cats are polyphagic and hyperactive, about 10% of cases are presented with severe depression and muscle weakness, which may result in ventroflexion of the neck. Weight loss remains a feature, but is usually associated with anorexia rather than increased appetite. Cardiac abnormalities are also common. This clinical presentation is referred to as 'apathetic' hyperthyroidism.

In most cases there is palpable enlargement of one or both thyroid lobes (**Figure 11.32**). Thyroid palpation requires both skill and practice. The thyroid gland is not usually palpable in the normal cat. Enlarged lobes of the thyroid are usually located just distal to the larynx, but they can be quite mobile and descend down the neck and occasionally pass into the thoracic inlet. Ectopic thyroid tissue located anywhere from the base of tongue to the base of the heart is occasionally involved in the pathogenesis of the condition.

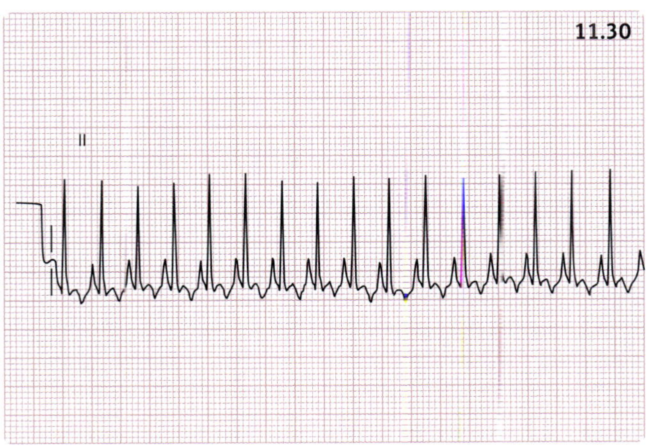

Figure 11.30 ECG from a 13-year-old Domestic Shorthair cat with hyperthyroidism showing sinus tachycardia. The heart rate is approximately 260 bpm.

Differential diagnosis

Chronic kidney disease, intestinal disorders (e.g. inflammatory bowel disease), lymphoma, diabetes mellitus, chronic liver disease.

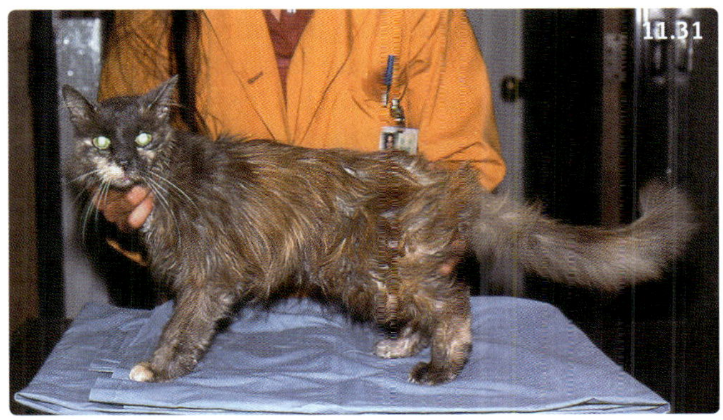

Figure 11.31 Hyperthyroid cat showing its unkempt hair coat. (Courtesy M. Schaer)

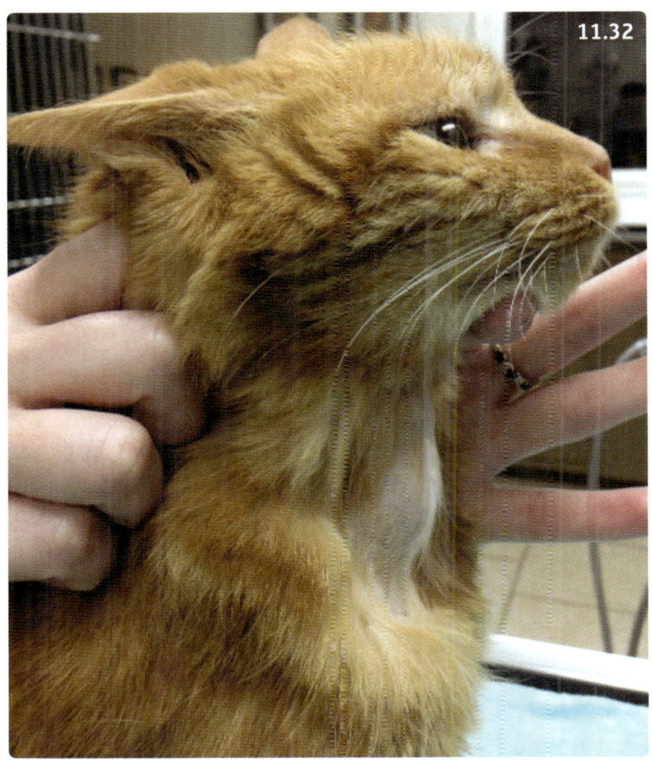

Figure 11.32 Hyperthyroid cat showing a large goiter. (Courtesy M. Schaer)

Diagnosis

Laboratory findings

Routine hematologic and biochemical screening tests are useful not only because results may show alterations that support a diagnosis of hyperthyroidism, but because they may also indicate evidence of concurrent disease in the older cat. The most frequent hematologic change is a relative polycythemia with a mild to moderate increase in red cell parameters (red blood cell count, PCV, and Hgb concentration). A mature neutrophilia with lymphopenia and eosinopenia is also common and probably reflects a stress response. However, eosinophilia and lymphocytosis are found in some cats with hyperthyroidism.

A mild to moderate increase in serum activity of the enzymes ALT, AST, ALP, and LDH is a frequent but nonspecific finding. The reason for the increase is not clear, but in some cases it might be related to a relative hypoxemia in the portal circulation. Evidence of concurrent renal dysfunction in hyperthyroidism is common, with mild to moderate elevations in serum creatinine and urea. These increases may be related to increased protein catabolism and prerenal azotemia. Careful consideration should be given to the method of treatment selected for hyperthyroid cats with concomitant azotemia, since some of these cats may develop clinical signs of renal failure caused by a deterioration in renal function when the hyperthyroid state is corrected.

Thyroid function tests

Increased serum basal thyroid hormone concentrations are diagnostic of hyperthyroidism. In the majority of cases both serum T4 and T3 concentrations are increased, often markedly; however, in a few cases serum T3 concentrations are in the normal range despite obvious elevation of the serum T4 concentration. There is, therefore, usually no advantage in determining serum T3 concentrations and serum total or free T4 concentrations provide a reliable indication of hyperthyroidism.

About 5% of cases of hyperthyroidism have serum thyroid hormone concentrations within reference intervals at the time of examination and this may be due to an early stage of the disease, significant daily fluctuations of thyroid hormone concentrations, or the effect of concurrent nonthyroidal illness. In cases where hyperthyroidism is still suspected on clinical grounds, a diagnostic T4 concentration may be obtained by re-testing the animal in 3–6 weeks. Alternative diagnostic tests for equivocal cases of hyperthyroidism include the TRH stimulation test and the T3 suppression test.

Diagnostic imaging

Hyperthyroid cats with secondary cardiomyopathy usually show cardiac enlargement, which is evident on both radiographic and echocardiographic examinations. However, it is important to recognize that significant concentric hypertrophy can occur without affecting the appearance of the cardiac silhouette on thoracic radiographs (**Figure 11.33**), and the diagnosis of cardiomyopathy in these cases can only be made on echocardiographic findings (**Figure 11.34**).

Thyroid imaging using radioactive iodine or technetium-99m is a useful diagnostic technique if gamma camera facilities are available. The technique determines whether there is unilateral or bilateral lobe involvement, which is valuable if surgical thyroidectomy is to be performed (**Figure 11.35**). The technique also determines

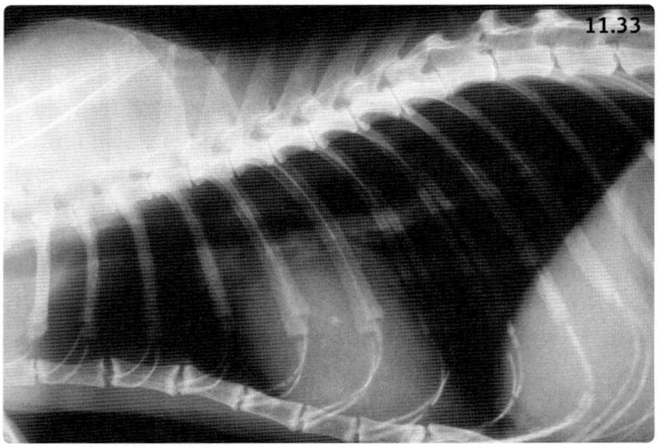

Figure 11.33 Lateral thoracic radiograph of a 12-year-old Domestic Shorthair cat with hyperthyroidism and hypertrophic cardiomyopathy. Note the cardiac silhouette is not enlarged.

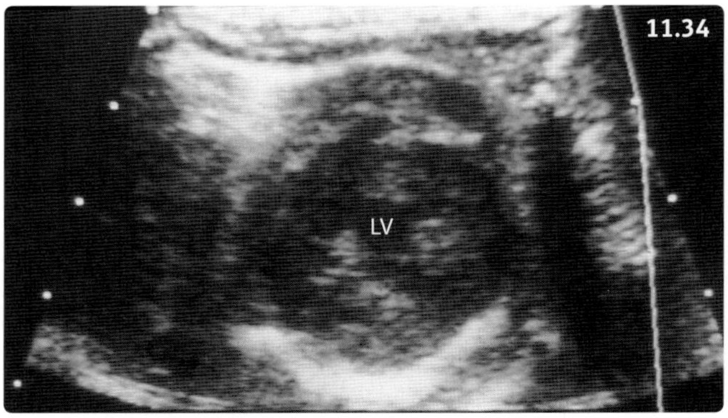

Figure 11.34 Short-axis 2D echocardiogram from the cat in Figure 11.33 showing the degree of concentric hypertrophy and the reduction in the size of the left ventricular lumen (LV).

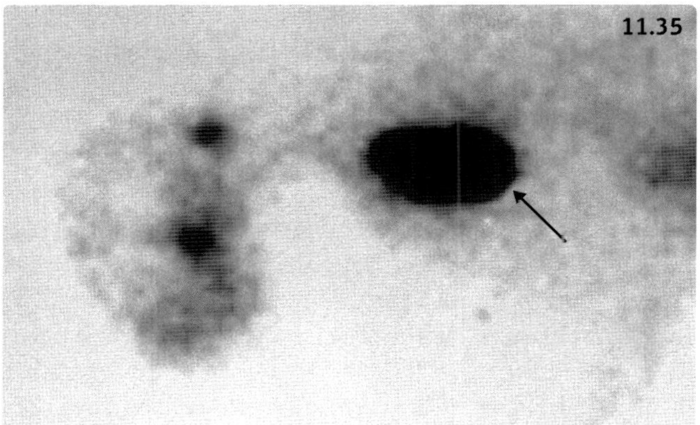

Figure 11.35 Thyroid scan using technetium-99m of a cat with hyperthyroidism. The head is seen to the left, with uptake in the salivary glands. The greatest uptake of technetium is by the thyroid adenoma (arrow).

any alteration in the position of the thyroid gland, the rare case of abnormal ectopic thyroid tissue within the thorax, or the presence of distant metastases from a functioning thyroid carcinoma.

Management

There are four options for treatment of hyperthyroidism: dietary management, medical management (antithyroid medication), surgical thyroidectomy, and radioactive iodine.

Dietary management

The release of a prescription diet with very low-iodine content (Hills y/d) in 2011 marked a new development in the management of feline hyperthyroidism; however, long-term, independent studies are required to fully appreciate its advantages and limitations. The diet must be used as the sole food source for the affected cat, as even small quantities of other foods (including milk) are likely to make the diet ineffective. The diet must not be used as the sole food source for healthy cats, which may restrict its use in multicat households. In addition, the diet must not be used at the same time as antithyroid medication or radio-iodine as hypothyroidism may result. The diet needs up to 14 weeks to work, so for cats that are seriously ill with hyperthyroidism, conventional management would be preferred.

The diet does not treat the underlying adenoma, which will get bigger and more able to produce thyroid hormone. Ultimately, the adenoma is likely to 'break through' and conventional medical, surgical, or radioactive iodine treatment will be needed. However, for mildly affected animals this may to be an effective treatment. Monitoring serum total T4 concentrations is essential to judge the effect of therapy.

Medical management

Medical management of hyperthyroidism using antithyroid drugs is indicated when preparing hyperthyroid cats for surgical thyroidectomy in order to improve their general condition and reduce the risk of complications arising during or following surgery. Antithyroid drugs are also recommended for the initial treatment of hyperthyroid cats with concurrent azotemia in order to ascertain whether significant deterioration in renal function is likely to occur after medical control of the hyperthyroid state. If there is no deterioration in renal function after 3–4 weeks of treatment, surgical thyroidectomy or radioactive iodine therapy for hyperthyroidism can be considered. Antithyroid drugs can also be used for long-term management of hyperthyroidism, particularly in cases where owners refuse surgical treatment.

Carbimazole and methimazole inhibit thyroid hormone synthesis. Carbimazole is the antithyroid drug most widely used in Europe and methimazole is the most widely used antithyroid drug in the USA and elsewhere. They are a safe and effective form of treatment and are undoubtedly the treatment of choice for aged cats and those with concurrent disease. Carbimazole is rapidly converted to methimazole after oral administration.

Carbimazole is initially administered at a dose of 5 mg PO q8h, whereas methimazole is given at a dose of 2.5 mg PO q12h and subsequently titrated to effect. Serum total thyroxine concentrations decrease to within the reference range after 3–15 days. Within 2 weeks the dose of carbimazole can be reduced in most cats to 5 mg PO q12h and for methimazole to 2.5 mg PO q24h. These doses can usually be continued for the remainder of the cat's life. Periodic assessment of thyroid hormone is necessary to confirm that the hyperthyroid state is being adequately controlled. Adjustment of the dosage is required in some cases to maintain the euthyroid state. A slow-release form of carbimazole, which only requires once daily administration, is available in some countries.

Adverse reactions to carbimazole and methimazole include anorexia, vomiting, and lethargy, which are usually transient, but more serious reactions such as pruritus, self-induced excoriation, hepatopathy, jaundice, and bleeding diatheses have been reported and necessitate withdrawal of these drugs.

Surgical management

The aim of surgical thyroidectomy is to remove all of the abnormally functioning thyroid tissue. Surgical thyroidectomy is a highly effective treatment for feline hyperthyroidism, but it can be associated with significant morbidity and mortality if cats are not carefully assessed and stabilized prior to surgery. Preoperative treatment with carbimazole or methimazole and propranolol (2.5–5 mg PO q8h for 7–14 days before surgery) will control the excessive thyroid hormone production and protect the heart against the effects of excess thyroid hormone.

The anesthetic protocol for the hyperthyroid cat should be carefully considered, using agents that have the minimum effect on cardiac rhythm. Techniques for unilateral and bilateral thyroidectomy have been reported for cats with hyperthyroidism. Both intracapsular and extracapsular techniques have been designed to preserve parathyroid function after removal of the abnormal thyroid tissue.

The potential complications associated with thyroidectomy include hypoparathyroidism, Horner's syndrome, and laryngeal paralysis. The most serious complication is hypocalcemia associated with damage to, or removal of, the parathyroid glands. Since only one parathyroid gland is required for maintenance of normocalcemia, hypoparathyroidism is mostly identified in cats treated by bilateral thyroidectomy. Hypocalcemia is usually transient and may be manifested by clinical signs including anorexia, vocalization, lethargy, muscular tremors, tetany, and convulsions. The treatment of postoperative hypocalcemia is outlined in **Table 11.9**.

Radioactive iodine therapy

Radioactive iodine therapy is a safe and effective method of treating hyperthyroidism; however, it does require the cat to be housed in licensed premises with restricted access until the radiation dose rate has decreased to an acceptable level. This usually requires hospitalization for around 4 weeks, depending on local laws on the use of radioisotopes. The radioisotope used most commonly is iodine-131 (^{131}I), which has a half-life of 8 days and emits both beta-particles and gamma-radiation. The beta-particles cause most of the required tissue damage. Radioactive iodine can be administered subcutaneously and has not been associated with any adverse reactions.

DISORDERS OF THE PARATHYROID GLAND

The normal dog or cat usually has four small parathyroid glands. One pair of glands is generally found in the fascia cranial to each of the thyroid lobes. The caudal pair of parathyroid glands is embedded in the parenchyma of each thyroid lobe. The location and number of the parathyroid glands can vary. Each parathyroid gland contains chief cells, which synthesize and secrete parathyroid hormone (PTH).

PTH secretion is controlled by the serum-ionized calcium concentration in order to maintain the serum-ionized calcium within narrow limits. If the serum-ionized calcium concentration falls below the set point (reference range: dog, 1.2–1.5 mmol/l [4.8–6.0 mg/dl]; cat, 1.1–1.4 mmol/l [4.4–5.6 mg/dl]), PTH release is enhanced. Concentrations of serum-ionized calcium above the set point inhibit PTH secretion. Total serum calcium consists of ionized and protein-bound calcium. Although serum protein-bound calcium is affected by several factors, including the circulating albumin concentration and the acid–base status, it is only the ionized calcium that is physiologically active. It is important to appreciate this, since most laboratories only measure total serum calcium.

PTH tends to increase serum-ionized calcium concentrations through a number of integrated actions. In the kidney, PTH increases tubular reabsorption of calcium and enhances renal excretion of phosphate. PTH also activates 1-alpha-hydroxylase, the renal enzyme that converts 25-hydroxy-cholecalciferol to the active form of vitamin D, 1,25-dihydroxy-cholecalciferol (calcitriol). Increased circulating 1,25-dihydroxycholecalciferol

Table 11.9 Management of postoperative hypocalcemia.

Immediate therapy
• Administer 1.0–1.5 ml/kg of 10% calcium gluconate or calcium glubionate by slow intravenous injection • Stop injection if bradycardia develops. Repeat as necessary
Maintenance therapy
• Begin oral supplementation as soon as possible using 50–75 mg/kg/day of calcium equivalent in three or four divided doses (equivalent to 500–750 mg/kg/day of calcium gluconate or 400–600 mg/kg/day of calcium lactate) and 0.03 mg/kg/day of dihydrotachysterol or 0.05 μg/kg/day of alfacalcidol (calcitrol) • Monitor the serum calcium concentration and decrease the dihydrotachysterol by 0.01 mg/kg every other day or alfacalcidol by 0.01 μg/kg every other day once serum calcium is within the reference range. Adjust doses of dihydrotachysterol or alfacalcidol and calcium supplementation according to subsequent serum calcium concentrations. In most cases, hypocalcemia is temporary

enhances calcium and phosphate absorption by the intestine. In bone, PTH promotes the release of calcium and phosphate into the extracellular fluid by stimulating osteoclast and osteocyte activity and by suppressing osteoblastic activity. The combination of calcium mobilization from bone and retention of calcium by the kidneys causes the serum-ionized calcium concentration to rise.

Calcium plays an important role in neuromuscular excitability, membrane permeability, muscle contraction, enzyme activity, hormone release, and blood coagulation, as well as acting as an essential structural component of the skeleton.

HYPOPARATHYROIDISM

Definition/overview

Hypoparathyroidism is caused by inadequate production and secretion of PTH (primary hypoparathyroidism) or, more rarely, by deficient end-organ responsiveness to circulating PTH (pseudohypoparathyroidism).

Etiology

The two most common causes of primary hypoparathyroidism are iatrogenic injury or removal of the parathyroid glands during thyroidectomy (see p. 407) and idiopathic hypoparathyroidism due to destruction and atrophy of the parathyroid glands. Idiopathic hypoparathyroidism probably results from immune-mediated destruction of the parathyroid glands, and this is supported by the diffuse lymphocytic infiltration found in the parathyroid glands of some affected animals.

Pathophysiology

Cessation of gland activity results in increased plasma phosphate concentrations and decreased serum calcium concentrations. Loss of PTH leads to changes in calcium and phosphate mobilization from bone, increased intestinal absorption of calcium and phosphate, and retention of calcium and enhanced renal excretion of phosphate. Neuronal membrane permeability is increased when extracellular calcium ion concentrations are below normal and the nervous system becomes more excitable. Spontaneous discharge of nerve fibers initiates impulses to peripheral skeletal muscles, causing tetanic contractions.

Clinical presentation

Idiopathic hypoparathyroidism is rare, but it has been reported in the dog and cat. The disease affects young to middle aged animals of various breeds. A female bias has been reported in dogs. The clinical signs relate to neuromuscular abnormalities that develop secondary to hypocalcemia and include seizures, focal trembling or twitching, generalized muscle fasciculations, ataxia, stiff gait, weakness, panting, anorexia, and lethargy. The fact that the clinical signs tend to be intermittent, often precipitated by exercise, excitement, or stress, suggests a physiologic adaptation to severe hypocalcemia. Posterior lenticular cataract formation can occur secondary to hypocalcemia in dogs and cats (**Figure 11.36**). Electrocardiography may show prolongation of QT interval in some cases of hypoparathyroidism.

Differential diagnosis

(See **Table 11.10**.)

Diagnosis

Profound hypocalcemia (serum total calcium <2 mmol/l [<8 mg/dl]) and severe hyperphosphatemia (serum phosphate >1.3 mmol/l [>4 mg/dl]) with normal renal function (blood urea and serum creatinine) are found in cases of primary hypoparathyroidism.

PTH assays are available and have been validated for use in the dog and cat. Inappropriately low plasma PTH concentration in a hypocalcemic animal is diagnostic of primary hypoparathyroidism. Careful sample handling is essential to avoid erroneous results, since PTH is heat labile. Simultaneous measurement of serum calcium and PTH is essential in order to be able to interpret the PTH result.

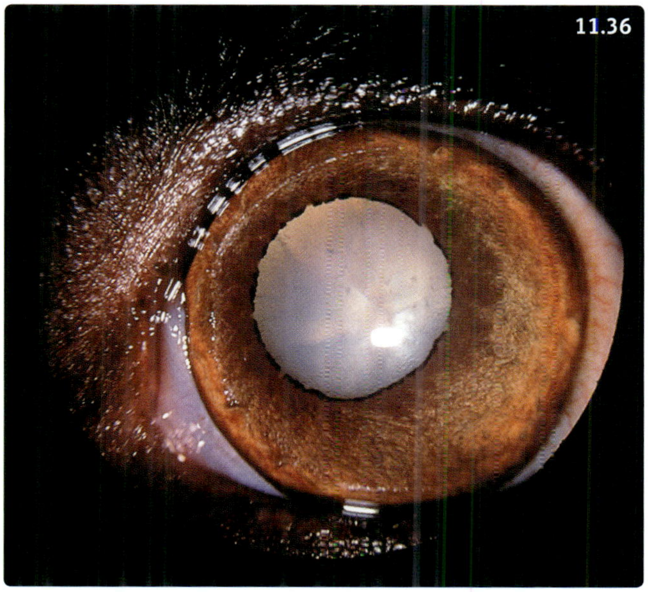

Figure 11.36 Lenticular cataracts in a Springer Spaniel with primary hypoparathyroidism.

Table 11.10 Differential diagnosis of hypocalcemia.

Primary hypoparathyroidism
Chronic kidney disease*
Hypoalbuminemia*
Intestinal malabsorption*
Acute pancreatitis*
Eclampsia
Acute kidney injury
Ethylene glycol toxicity
Phosphate-containing enemas

* Not usually associated with clinical signs of tetany

Management

The treatment protocol for hypocalcemia is outlined in **Table 11.9**; similar principles are used when treating dogs and cats. Parenteral calcium preparations should be used as emergency therapy to correct hypocalcemic tetany. Maintenance therapy using calcium and vitamin D supplementation must be tailored to the individual patient and the dose adjusted according to the serum calcium concentration. Dihydrotachysterol (commercial availability varies) supplementation can prove expensive in larger dogs. Vitamin D2 (1,000–6,000 IU/kg/day), alfacalcidol (0.05 µg/kg/day), or calcitriol (0.03–0.06 µg/kg/day) may be used as alternatives. These starting doses may need to be exceeded to bring the serum calcium into the reference range.

With adequate monitoring of the serum calcium concentration, the prognosis in cases of primary hypoparathyroidism is usually excellent, but supplementation is usually required for life.

HYPERPARATHYROIDISM

Definition/overview

Hyperparathyroidism is caused by excess production and secretion of PTH, which can be primary or secondary. Primary hyperparathyroidism is an uncommon disease of older dogs and cats. There is no sex predisposition, but there is a breed predilection as the Keeshond is overrepresented.

Etiology

Primary hyperparathyroidism is a disorder resulting from autonomous and excessive secretion of PTH by one or more of the parathyroid glands. Secondary hyperparathyroidism is an adaptive increase in PTH secretion as a result of chronic stimulation from conditions that tend to reduce the concentration of ionized calcium in plasma. Secondary hyperparathyroidism may occur as a result of chronic kidney disease (see Chapter 12: Nephrology/urology) and calcium deficiency during growth (see Chapter 14: Disorders of the nervous system and muscle).

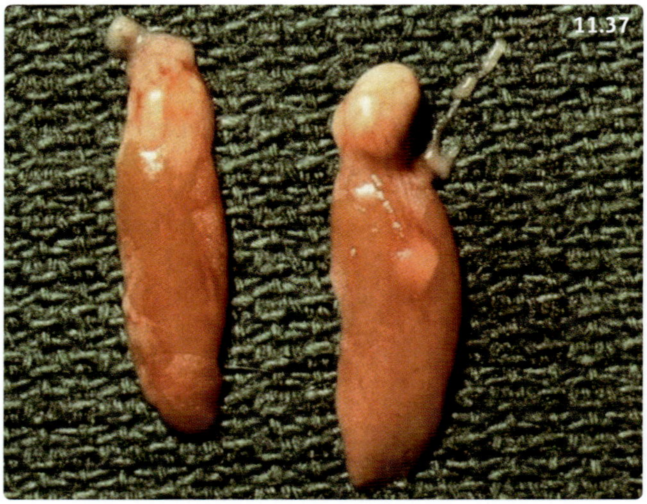

Figure 11.37 Necropsy specimen from a Dachshund that had several endocrinopathies. Shown are both thyroid glands, with one containing a parathyroid adenoma. (Courtesy M. Schaer)

Primary hyperparathyroidism is most commonly caused by a small solitary parathyroid adenoma (**Figure 11.37**). PTH excess may also be caused by nodular hyperplasia in one or more parathyroid glands. Very rarely the disease is caused by a parathyroid carcinoma. The Keeshond has an autosomal dominant form of primary hyperparathyroidism that has partial age-dependent penetrance.

Pathophysiology

The normal negative feedback control regulating calcium concentration is lost by the entry of excess calcium into the extracellular fluid. The kidneys lose their ability to excrete the excess calcium and are unable efficiently to reabsorb sodium and water.

Clinical presentation

The clinical signs in hyperparathyroidism are variable. The disease may be asymptomatic or may result in mild to severe systemic illness. The clinical signs relate to hypercalcemia and include polyuria, polydipsia, anorexia, vomiting, depression, muscle weakness, constipation, and weight loss. Urinary calculi can occur. Clinical examination may reveal bradycardia. The small size of the parathyroid lesions means that the nodules are rarely palpable.

Differential diagnosis

(See **Table 11.11**.)

Diagnosis

Laboratory findings

Hypercalcemia (serum total calcium >3 mmol/l [>12 mg/dl]) and hypophosphatemia (serum phosphate concentration <1.3 mmol/l [<4 mg/dl]) are found in cases of primary hyperparathyroidism provided that renal function is normal. Prolonged increases in the circulating calcium concentration will facilitate calcium deposition in the kidneys, causing renal function to deteriorate and serum phosphate concentrations to rise. If renal failure develops, primary hyperparathyroidism is difficult to differentiate from secondary renal hyperparathyroidism.

Circulating PTH concentrations are inappropriately increased in animals with primary hyperparathyroidism. A PTH assay provides a useful differentiation in hypercalcemic patients because plasma PTH concentrations are low in dogs with cancer-associated hypercalcemia. Careful handling of the sample is essential to avoid erroneous results, since PTH is heat labile. Plasma PTH-related protein (PTH-rp) concentrations are elevated in most cases of cancer-associated hypercalcemia, but are low in primary hyperparathyroidism.

Diagnostic imaging

Ultrasonographic examination of the parathyroid glands is useful in the evaluation of hypercalcemic dogs and can be used to identify hyperplastic parathyroid glands and parathyroid adenomas (**Figures 11.38–11.40**). Ultrasound examination of the kidneys in the dog may also reveal the hyperechoic medullary band characteristic of nephrocalcinosis (**Figure 11.41**). This medullary band may be seen in normal cats.

Management

Treatment of the hypercalcemic crisis

The hypercalcemic crisis should be treated by aggressive IV fluid therapy using 0.9% sodium chloride solution. Saline will restore the circulating fluid volume and promote calcium excretion. Furosemide (2–4 mg/kg IV q12h) may also be administered to enhance calcium excretion. Bisphosphonates are osteoclast inhibitors and have also been used in dogs to control hypercalcemia. Clodronate, etidronate, alendronate, and pamidronate have been used; disodium etidronate (5 mg/kg PO q24h) has been used most frequently in the dog and alendronate (5–10 mg/cat/week) in the cat.

Table 11.11 Differential diagnosis of hypercalcemia.

Cancer-associated hypercalcemia: • Lymphoproliferative disease • Apocrine cell adenocarcinoma of the anal sac • Multiple myeloma • Other solid tumors
Hypoadrenocorticism
Chronic kidney disease
Primary hyperparathyroidism
Granulomatous diseases (e.g. the systemic mycoses)
Vitamin D intoxication

Surgical treatment

Primary hyperparathyroidism should be resolved following parathyroidectomy. Parathyroid adenomas are usually easily identified and removed (**Figure 11.42**). Postoperative complications include hypocalcemia, since the remaining parathyroid glands may be atrophic and require a period of adaptation before control of circulating calcium is regained. For this reason, it is advisable to begin supplementation with vitamin D (dihydrotachysterol or alfacalcidol) and calcium gluconate 24 hours before surgery in those patients with calcium concentrations >3.75 mmol/l (>15 mg/dl).

DISORDERS OF THE ADRENAL GLANDS

The adrenal glands are located craniomedially to each kidney in retroperitoneal fat. Each gland consists of a cortex and a medulla. The cortex completely surrounds the medulla and consists of three distinct zones: the outer zona glomerulosa, the middle zona fasciculata, and the inner zona reticularis.

The adrenal cortex produces about 30 different hormones, many of which have little or no clinical significance. The hormones can be divided into three groups

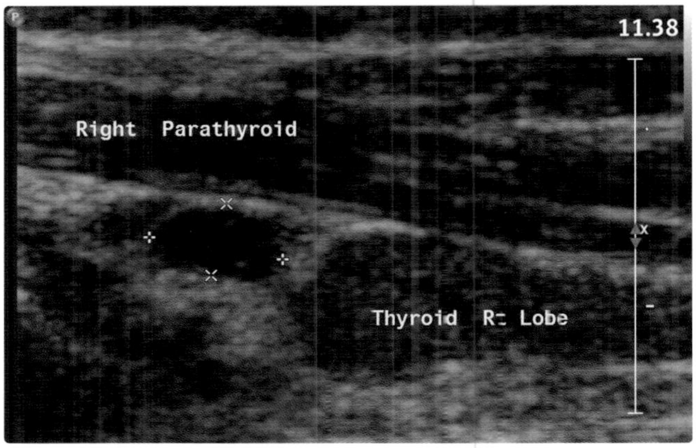

Figure 11.38 This ultrasound image shows a large parathyroid adenoma at the cranial aspect of the right thyroid gland. (Courtesy M. Schaer)

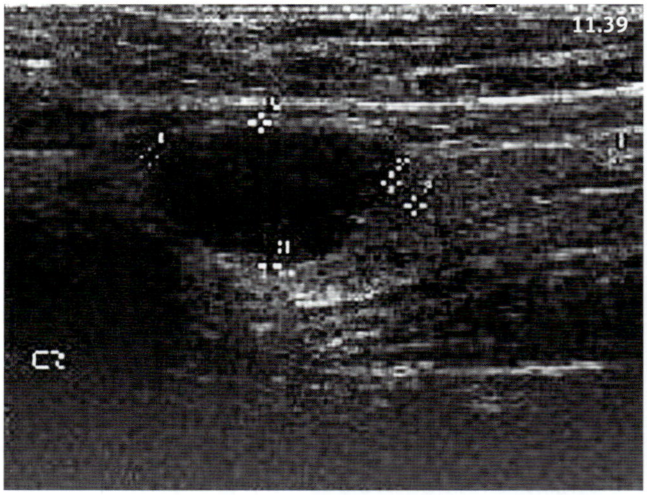

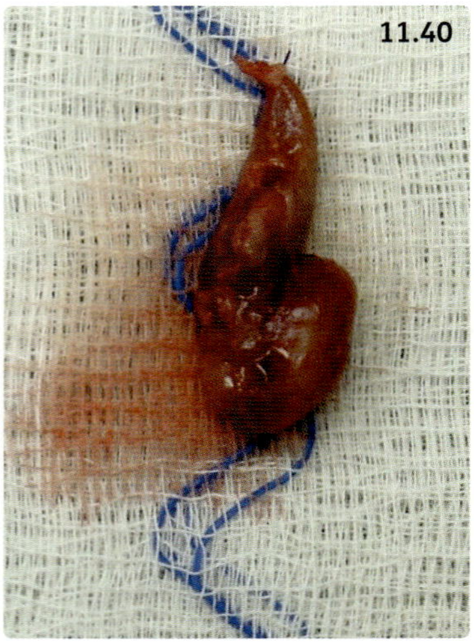

Figures 11.39, 11.40 (11.39) Ultrasonogram of the cervical region showing a large cystic parathyroid adenoma at the cranial pole of a thyroid lobe. (11.40) Surgical specimen showing the similarity to the image. (Courtesy M. Schaer)

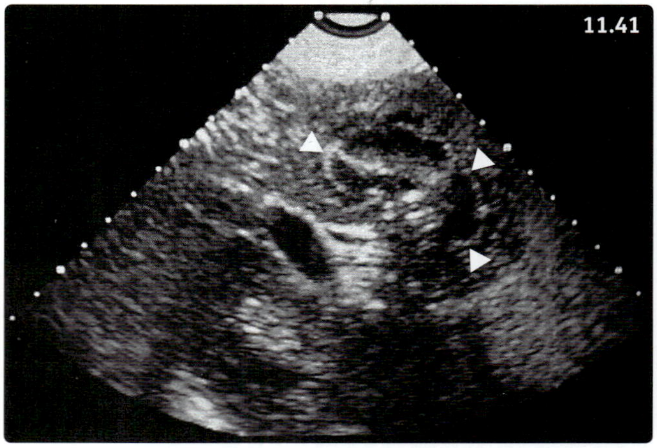

Figure 11.41 Ultrasonogram of the kidney of a Labrador Retriever with hypercalcemic nephropathy. Note the echogenic rim in the medulla (arrowheads).

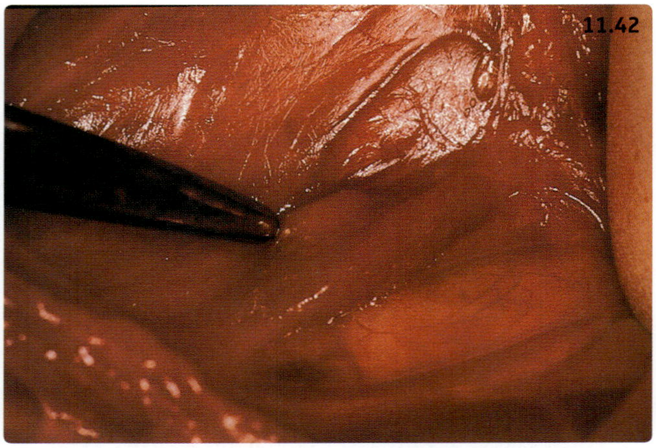

Figure 11.42 Parathyroid adenoma adjacent to the thyroid gland being pointed out at surgery.

based on their predominant actions: mineralocorticoids, which are important in electrolyte and water homeostasis; glucocorticoids, which promote gluconeogenesis; and small quantities of sex hormones, particularly male hormones that have weak androgenic activity. Aldosterone is the most important mineralocorticoid and is produced by the zona glomerulosa. The principal glucocorticoid (cortisol) and the sex hormones are produced in the zonae fasciculata and reticularis.

Glucocorticoid and mineralocorticoid release are controlled by different mechanisms. Glucocorticoid release is controlled almost entirely by ACTH secreted by the anterior lobe of the pituitary, which in turn is regulated by corticotropin-releasing hormone (CRH) from the hypothalamus (**Figure 11.43**). CRH is secreted by the neurons in the anterior portion of the paraventricular nuclei within the hypothalamus, and it is transported to the anterior pituitary by the portal circulation, where it stimulates ACTH release. There is probably an internal or 'short loop' negative feedback control by ACTH on CRH. ACTH secreted into the systemic circulation causes cortisol release, with concentrations rising almost immediately. Cortisol has direct negative feedback effects on the hypothalamus (decreases formation of CRH) and on the anterior lobe of the pituitary (decreases the formation of ACTH). These feedback mechanisms help regulate the plasma concentration of cortisol.

Secretion of CRH and ACTH is normally episodic and pulsatile, which results in fluctuating cortisol concentrations during the day. Diurnal variation is superimposed on this type of release. It is usually stated that in the dog, CRH and ACTH, and thus cortisol concentrations, are highest in the early hours of the morning and that in the cat they are greatest in the evening. However, a true circadian rhythm of cortisol concentrations has been difficult to confirm in the dog and cat. The episodic release of CRH and ACTH is perpetuated by the reciprocal effect of cortisol acting through negative feedback control. This reciprocal arrangement does not hold during periods of stress when both ACTH and cortisol are maintained at high concentrations, because the effects of stress tend to override the normal negative feedback control.

Aldosterone release is influenced primarily by the renin–angiotensin system and by plasma potassium concentrations (**Figure 11.44**). Renin is secreted into the blood by the cells of the juxtaglomerular apparatus, which consists of specialized cells in the wall of the afferent arteriole immediately proximal to the glomerulus and the specialized epithelial cells of the distal convoluted tubule adjacent to that arteriole, the macula densa. Renin release may be stimulated by stretch receptors in the juxtaglomerular apparatus in response to hypotension or reduced renal blood flow, or by sodium and chloride receptors in the macula densa. Renin is also released by sympathetic nerve stimulation and is inhibited by angiotensin II, ADH, hypertension, and increased reabsorption of sodium by the renal tubules.

Renin is an enzyme that splits circulating angiotensinogen, produced by the liver, into angiotensin I. Angiotensin I is converted to angiotensin II by angiotensin-converting enzyme, which is located almost entirely in the pulmonary capillary endothelium. Angiotensin II is a powerful vasoconstrictor and it stimulates aldosterone secretion from the zona glomerulosa. Through its action on the distal convoluted tubule, aldosterone has a negative feedback effect on the juxtaglomerular apparatus.

Potassium has a direct stimulatory effect on the zona glomerulosa cells to release aldosterone. ACTH and sodium play a less significant role in aldosterone secretion. ACTH is necessary to maintain normal aldosterone output. In the absence of ACTH the zona glomerulosa partially atrophies, causing mild to moderate aldosterone deficiency, whereas there is almost total loss of glucocorticoid synthesis and release.

The main function of aldosterone is to protect against hypotension and potassium intoxication. Aldosterone promotes sodium, chloride, and water reabsorption, as well as potassium excretion, in many epithelial tissues including the intestinal mucosa, salivary glands, sweat glands, and kidneys. Its main site of action is the renal tubule, where it promotes sodium and chloride reabsorption in the proximal convoluted tubule and sodium reabsorption by exchange with potassium in the distal convoluted tubule. It is one of the complex regulatory systems for the regulation of extracellular fluid electrolyte concentrations, extracellular fluid volume, blood volume, and arterial pressure.

11.43

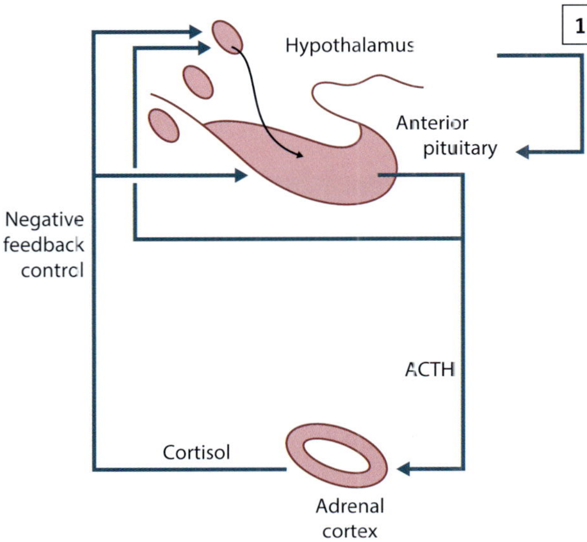

Figure 11.43 Physiology of the hypothalamic–pituitary–adrenal axis.

11.44

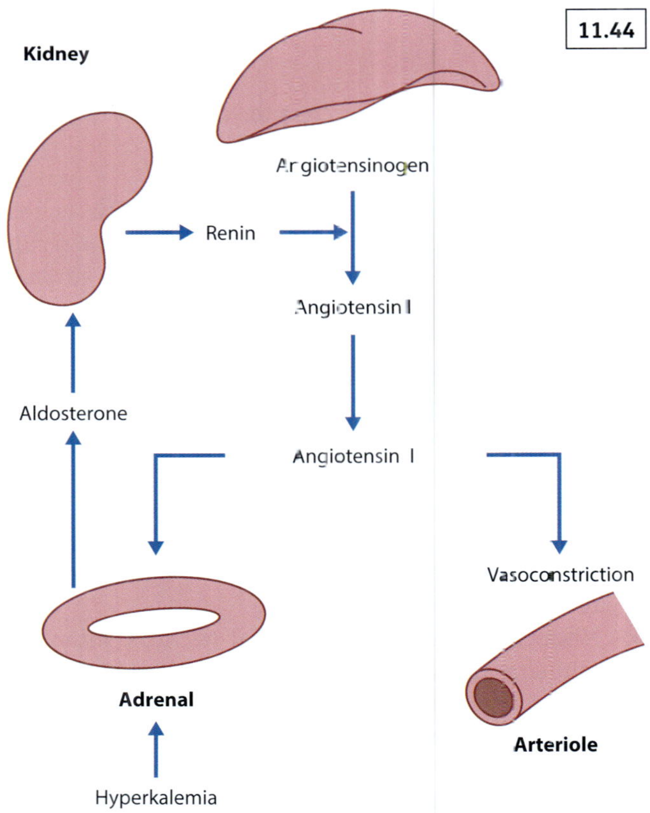

Figure 11.44 Physiology of the renin–angiotensin system.

HYPOADRENOCORTICISM

Hypoadrenocorticism is a syndrome that results from a deficiency of both glucocorticoid and mineralocorticoid secretion from the adrenal cortices. Destruction of more than 95% of both adrenal cortices causes a clinical deficiency of all adrenocortical hormones and is termed primary hypoadrenocorticism (Addison's disease). Secondary hypoadrenocorticism is caused by a deficiency in ACTH, which leads to atrophy of the adrenal cortices and impaired secretion of glucocorticoids. The production of mineralocorticoids, however, usually remains sufficient to maintain normal electrolyte concentrations.

PRIMARY HYPOADRENOCORTICISM (ADDISON'S DISEASE)

Definition/overview

Primary hypoadrenocorticism is caused by the destruction or loss of the adrenal cortices. Addison's disease occurs more frequently in the dog than is recognized, but it is much less common than hyperadrenocorticism (Cushing's disease). Hypoadrenocorticism is rare in the cat. The clinical signs, diagnosis, and treatment of hypoadrenocorticism in the dog and cat are similar.

Etiology

Primary hypoadrenocorticism in the dog has been associated with the following conditions:

- Idiopathic adrenocortical insufficiency. This is the most common cause in the dog and is thought to result from immune-mediated destruction of the adrenal cortex. The presence of antiadrenal antibodies in two dogs and characteristic histopathologic findings in another support this hypothesis (**Figures 11.45-11.47**). In humans, hypoadrenocorticism has been found to be associated with other immune-mediated endocrine disorders such as lymphocytic thyroiditis, diabetes mellitus, hypoparathyroidism, primary gonadal failure, and atrophic gastritis. A similar autoimmune polyglandular disease has also been recognized in dogs.
- Mitotane-induced adrenocortical necrosis. Although mitotane usually spares the zona glomerulosa and, therefore, mineralocorticoid secretion, cases of complete adrenocortical failure can occasionally occur (**Figures 11.48**) (see Hyperadrenocorticism).
- Trilostane-associated adrenocortical necrosis. Although trilostane is a competitive inhibitor of steroid synthesis, it can cause acute adrenal necrosis, which can lead occasionally to complete adrenocortical failure (see Hyperadrenocorticism).
- Other causes. Bilateral adrenalectomy, hemorrhage or infarction of the adrenal cortex, or mycotic or neoplastic involvement of the adrenal glands can also lead to adrenal insufficiency, but these are rare causes.

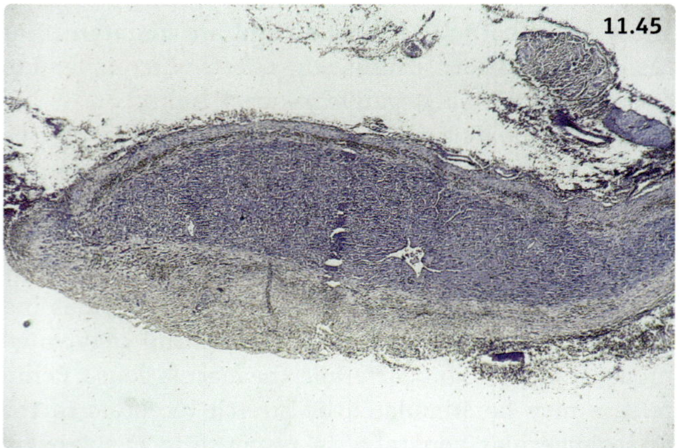

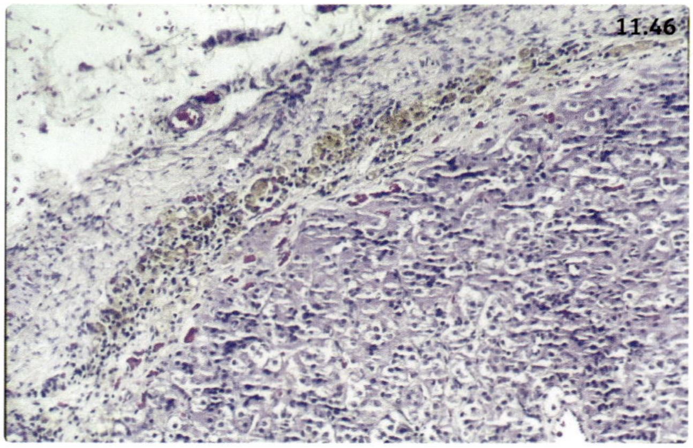

Figures 11.45, 11.46 These histopathologic specimens are from a dog that had Addison's disease. They show adrenocortical atrophy and lymphocytic and plasmacytic infiltrates within the cortex. (Courtesy M. Schaer)

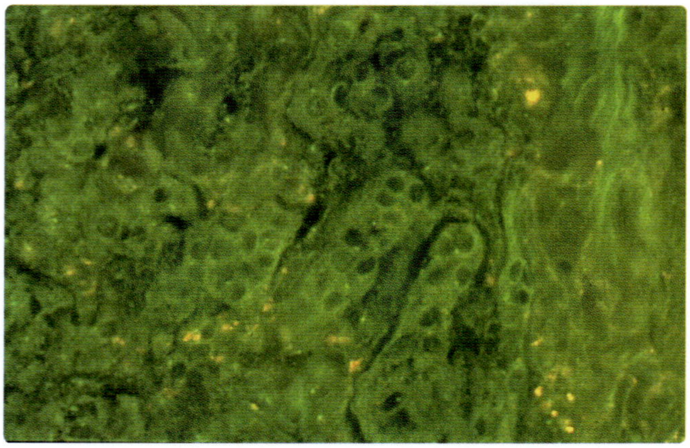

Figure 11.47 Indirect immunofluorescence stain of an adrenal cortex template showing the positive reaction for antiadrenal antibodies as illustrated with the bright yellow iridescence. (Courtesy M. Schaer)

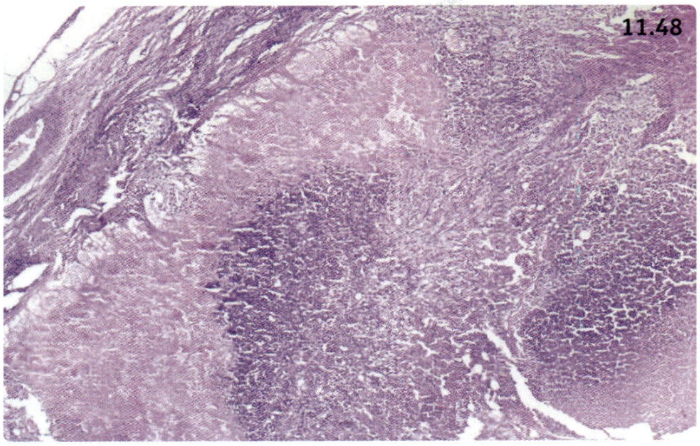

Figure 11.48 This histopathologic specimen is from a cushingoid dog that became toxic from mitotane therapy. Shown is widespread adrenocortical necrosis. (Courtesy M. Schaer)

Pathophysiology

Loss of or damage to the adrenal cortex leads to mineralocorticoid and glucocorticoid deficiency. Aldosterone is the major mineralocorticoid and deficiency causes impaired ability to conserve sodium and water and failure to excrete potassium, leading to hyponatremia and hyperkalemia. Hyponatremia induces lethargy, depression, and nausea and leads to the development of hypovolemia, hypotension, reduced cardiac output, and decreased renal perfusion. Hyperkalemia causes muscle weakness, hyporeflexia, and impaired cardiac conduction. Glucocorticoid deficiency causes decreased tolerance to stress, loss of appetite, and a mild normocytic normochromic anemia.

Clinical presentation

There are no breed predilections, but the possibility of a hereditary factor has been suggested in some breeds, for example Standard Poodles, Bearded Collies, Portuguese Water Dogs, Nova Scotia Duck Tolling Retrievers, and Leonbergers. Hypoadrenocorticism appears to be a disease of the young and middle aged dog, with an age range of 3 months to 14 years and a median age of 4–5 years. Approximately 70% of reported cases are female. The progression of adrenocortical insufficiency may be acute or chronic. Chronic hypoadrenocorticism is far more common than the acute disease in the dog.

Acute primary hypoadrenocorticism

The clinical appearance of the acute form is that of hypovolemic shock (adrenocortical crisis). The animal is usually found in a state of collapse or collapses when stressed. Other signs include a weak pulse, profound bradycardia, abdominal pain, vomiting, diarrhea, dehydration, and hypothermia. The condition is rapidly progressive and life-threatening. Aggressive fluid therapy will help most patients and allow more time to make a diagnosis.

Chronic primary hypoadrenocorticism

The clinical signs in the chronic form are often vague and nonspecific (**Table 11.12**). The diagnosis should be considered in any dog with a waxing and waning type of illness or who shows episodic weakness and collapse. The most consistent clinical signs include anorexia, vomiting, lethargy, depression, and/or weakness. The severity of each sign can vary during the course of the disease and may be interspersed with periods of apparent good health, often following nonspecific veterinary therapy, usually consisting of corticosteroid medication and/or fluid administration. Other common clinical signs include dehydration, bradycardia and weak femoral pulses. In a few cases, severe GI hemorrhage can occur resulting in profound anemia.

Differential diagnosis

Chronic renal insufficiency, primary neuromuscular disorders, diseases that cause weight loss, weakness, anorexia, vomiting, and diarrhea.

Diagnosis

Laboratory findings

The most common laboratory findings are listed in **Table 11.13**. Hematologic changes may include lymphocytosis, eosinophilia, and mild normocytic, normochromic nonregenerative anemia. However, these findings are not as consistent as those changes seen in hyperadrenocorticism. Normal or elevated eosinophil and

Table 11.12 Clinical signs of primary hypoadrenocorticism (in approximate decreasing order of frequency).

Anorexia
Lethargy/depression
Vomiting
Weakness
Weight loss
Waxing/waning course
Dehydration
Diarrhea
Previous response to therapy
Collapse
Hypothermia
Slow capillary refill time
Shaking
Polyuria/polydipsia
Melena
Weak pulse
Bradycardia (<60 bpm)

Table 11.13 Laboratory findings in primary hypoadrenocorticism.

Hematology Lymphocytosis Eosinophilia Relative neutropenia Anemia (usually a normocytic, normochromic, nonregenerative anemia, but can be blood loss anemia associated with GI hemorrhage)
Biochemistry Azotemia Hyponatremia (<135 mmol/l [<135 mEq/l]) Hyperkalemia (>5.5 mmol/l [5.5 mEq/l]) Reduced sodium:potassium ratio (<25:1) Reduced bicarbonate and total CO_2 concentrations Hypochloremia Hypercalcemia Hypoglycemia
Urinalysis Specific gravity variable (usually 1.015–1.030)
Endocrine testing Low basal serum cortisol concentration with a failure to stimulate in response to ACTH administration Raised plasma ACTH concentration

lymphocyte counts in an ill animal with signs compatible with hypoadrenocorticism are significant, because the expected response to stress is eosinopenia and lymphopenia. The mild anemia may not be obvious until the dog has been rehydrated, since dehydration may mask the anemia.

The most consistent laboratory findings in hypoadrenocorticism are prerenal azotemia, hypocholesterolemia, hyponatremia, and hyperkalemia. Blood urea and serum creatinine and phosphate concentrations are increased as a result of reduced renal perfusion and decreased glomerular filtration rate. Reduced renal perfusion results from hypovolemia, reduced cardiac output, and hypotension, which in turn result from chronic fluid loss through the kidneys, acute fluid loss through vomiting and/or diarrhea, and inadequate fluid intake.

Prerenal azotemia is usually associated with concentrated urine (SG >1.030), whereas the urine in primary renal failure is often isosthenuric or only mildly concentrated (1.008–1.025). However, some severe cases of hypoadrenocorticism may develop impaired concentrating ability because the chronic sodium loss reduces the renal medullary concentration gradient. Therefore, the laboratory findings may resemble those of chronic kidney disease. With adequate fluid therapy the blood urea will return to normal in cases of hypoadrenocorticism.

Sodium concentration is usually <135 mmol/l (<135 mEq/l) and potassium concentration >5.5 mmol/l (>5.5 mEq/l). The ratio of sodium to potassium may be more reliable than the absolute values. The normal ratio of sodium to potassium varies between 27:1 and 40:1, whereas in patients with hypoadrenocorticism the ratio is commonly less than 25:1 and may be below 20:1, however, there are other medical disorders that can produce a similar serum electrolyte pattern. Blood samples must be collected before IV fluids are administered, otherwise the electrolyte concentrations can quickly return to normal. Despite this, approximately 10% of cases may have normal electrolyte concentrations (referred to by some authors as atypical) at the time of presentation and these are usually thought to be early cases of hypoadrenocorticism.

Mild to moderate hypercalcemia is seen in about one-third of cases of hypoadrenocorticism, usually those dogs that are most severely affected by the disease. Hypercalcemia is caused by hemoconcentration, increased renal tubular reabsorption, and decreased glomerular filtration.

Cases of hypoadrenocorticism have a tendency to develop hypoglycemia because glucocorticoid deficiency reduces glucose production by the liver and peripheral cell receptors become more sensitive to insulin. Severe hypoglycemia is uncommon, but the potential should remain a concern for the clinician.

Electrocardiographic findings

Hyperkalemia impairs cardiac excitation and conduction, which can be assessed by an ECG examination (**Figure 11.49**). Although the ECG changes do not correlate directly with serum potassium levels, the guidelines shown in **Table 11.14** have proved helpful. Changes in the ECG can also be used for monitoring the patient during treatment.

Radiographic findings

Dogs with hypoadrenocorticism may show radiographic signs of hypovolemia, which include microcardia, decreased size of pulmonary vessels, and reduced size of the caudal vena cava (**Figure 11.50**). The changes are not specific and only represent changes associated with hypovolemia and dehydration, irrespective of the cause. A few dogs with hypoadrenocorticism develop esophageal dilatation as a result of generalized muscle weakness and this can be seen on thoracic radiographs (**Figure 11.51**).

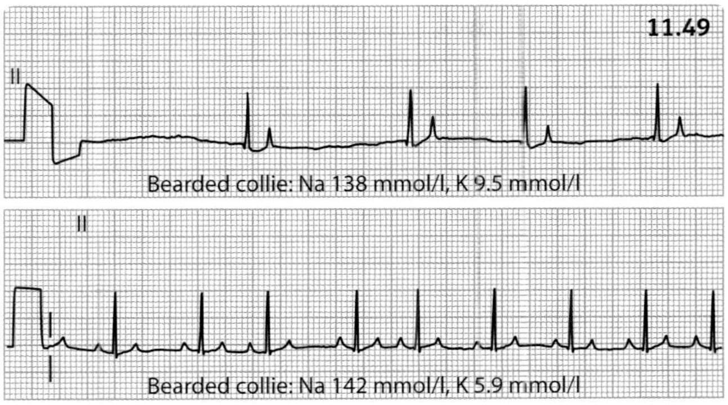

Figure 11.49 Electrocardiogram of an addisonian crisis. Note the slow ventricular rate and absence of P waves. The serum potassium was 9.5 mmol/l (9.5 mEq/l). Shown are the pre- and post-treatment electrocardiograms.

Table 11.14 ECG changes with hyperkalemia

>5.5 mmol/l (>5.5 mEq/l) – peaking of the T wave, shortening of the Q-T interval
>6.5 mmol/l (>6.5 mEql/l) – increased QRS duration
>7.0 mmol/l (>7.0 mEq/l) – P wave amplitude decreased, P-R interval prolonged
>8.5 mmol/l (>8.5 mEq/l) – P wave absent, severe bradycardia (sinoventricular rhythm)

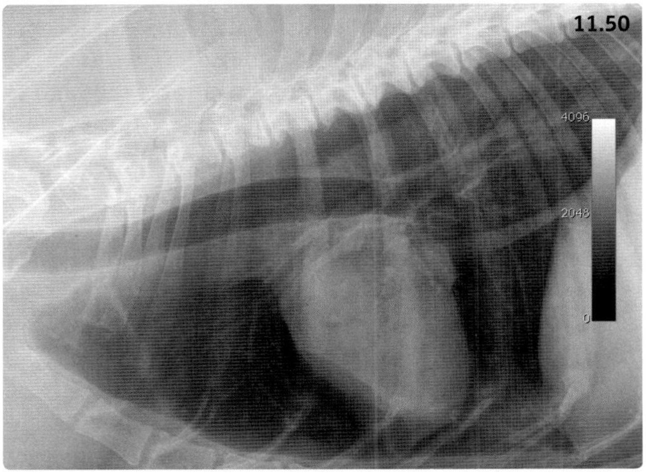

Figure 11.50 Lateral thoracic radiograph of a Bearded Collie with hypoadrenocorticism showing microcardia due to dehydration and hypovolemia.

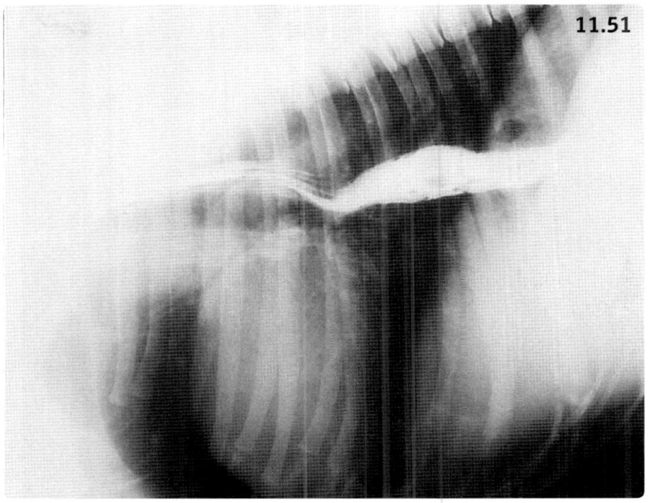

Figure 11.51 Lateral thoracic radiograph of a Dobermann with hypoadrenocorticism. A barium swallow has been performed to show a megaesophagus, which resolved following treatment of the hypoadrenocorticism.

Endocrine testing

The ACTH stimulation test (**Figure 11.52**) is commonly used to confirm the presence of hypoadrenocorticism; the protocol is described in **Table 11.15**. The IV preparation of ACTH (tetracosactin [cosyntropin in the USA]) should be used, as absorption by other routes cannot be relied on if the patient is collapsed or dehydrated. The ACTH stimulation test, however, does not distinguish between primary and secondary hypoadrenocorticism. While aldosterone concentrations pre- and post-ACTH are not routinely measured, they may be useful in addition to cortisol concentrations in those cases with normal electrolyte concentrations (so-called atypical hypoadrenocorticism) to determine whether mineralocorticoid supplementation is likely to be indicated.

Plasma ACTH concentrations are required to differentiate primary and secondary hypoadrenocorticism. Plasma ACTH concentrations are low in secondary hypoadrenocorticism and markedly raised in primary hypoadrenocorticism.

Management

Acute primary hypoadrenocorticism

Aggressive IV fluid therapy using 0.9% saline should be used in the acute crisis to treat the hyperkalemia, which is life-threatening. Once stabilized, 0.45% saline may be used since the serum sodium should not be increased by more than 8–12 mmol/l (8–12 mEq/l) per 24 hours in order to avoid causing central pontine myelinosis (osmotic demyelination). This is particularly important when the

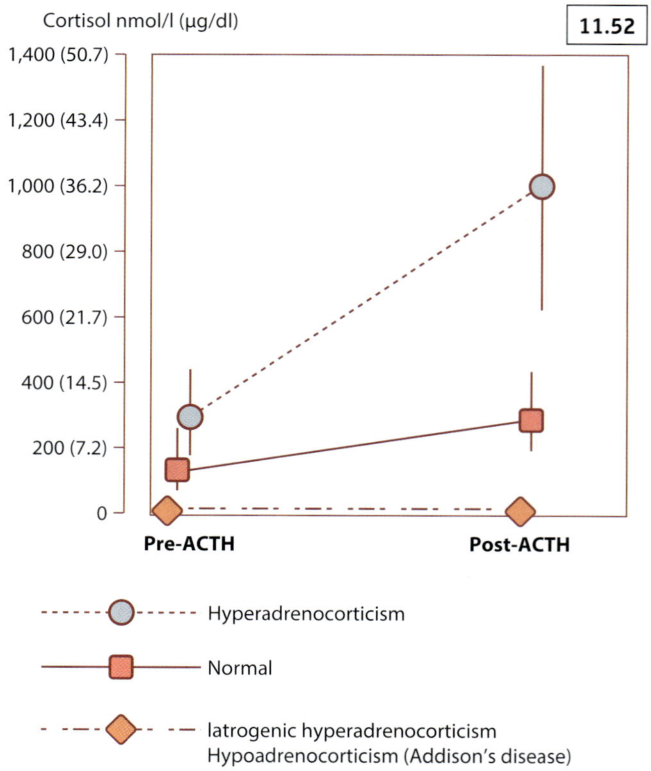

Figure 11.52 ACTH stimulation test.

Table 11.15 Protocol for endocrine testing for hypoadrenocorticism.

ACTH stimulation test Protocol: • Collect 3 ml plasma or serum sample for basal cortisol concentration* • Inject 0.25 mg of synthetic ACTH (tetracosactrin; Synacthen, Ciba) IV in dogs >5 kg. Use only 0.125 mg in dogs <5 kg • Collect a second sample for cortisol concentration 30–60 minutes later *The recent administration of glucocorticoids, such as hydrocortisone, prednisolone, or prednisone, may result in elevated cortisol concentrations due to cross-reactivity in many cortisol assays. For this reason these glucocorticoids should be withheld for at least 24 hours before testing. There is no cross-reactivity with dexamethasone, although dexamethasone will suppress cortisol concentrations in patients with an intact hypothalamic–pituitary–adrenal axis
Interpretation: • In normal dogs, pre-ACTH cortisol concentrations are usually between 20 and 250 nmol/l (0.7 and 9.1 µg/dl), with post-ACTH cortisol concentrations between 200 and 450 nmol/l (7.2 and 16.3 µg/dl) • Reduced responses to ACTH are also seen in primary hypoadrenocorticism (Addison's disease). Usually both pre- and post-ACTH cortisol concentrations are <20 nmol/l (<0.7 µg/dl)

serum sodium level is <120 mmol/l (<120 mEq/l). The response to treatment is predictable and often dramatic, while acute kidney injury will slow down the improvement process. Glucose and insulin therapy or calcium administration are therefore not usually required for the treatment of hyperkalemia due to hypoadrenocorticism, unless there are life-threatening ECG abnormalities such as atrial standstill or the appearance of sine waves. The serum potassium falls because of the dilution effect of the saline and the improvement in renal perfusion. The increased renal blood flow allows further excretion of potassium into the urine.

Glucocorticoid therapy should be used early in the treatment of the acute crisis. Once the animal has improved with saline and glucocorticoids, maintenance therapy with mineralocorticoids can be instigated (see below). Glucocorticoids of choice in the acute crisis include:

- Hydrocortisone sodium succinate (10 mg/kg IV repeated every 3–6 hours or a CRI of 0.5 mg/kg/hour).
- Prednisolone sodium succinate (5 mg/kg IV repeated every 3–6 hours).
- Dexamethasone sodium phosphate (0.5–1.0 mg/kg IV given once).

If plasma cortisol concentrations are to be measured for the diagnosis of hypoadrenocorticism, dexamethasone should be used, as the other preparations cross-react with cortisol in the assay.

Chronic primary hypoadrenocorticism (maintenance therapy)

Fludrocortisone acetate is an oral synthetic adrenocortical steroid with mineralocorticoid effects. It is the treatment of choice for maintenance therapy in the dog. An initial dose of 15 µg/kg/day of fludrocortisone is given and serum electrolytes measured after 5–7 days. The dose rate should then be adjusted until the sodium and potassium concentrations are within the reference range. The daily maintenance dose required is usually between 15 and 30 µg/kg. The dose often has to be increased during the first 6–18 months of therapy and the drug may need to be administered twice daily in some cases. Desoxycorticosterone pivalate, a long-acting ester of desoxycorticosterone, can be used as an alternative. The dose is 2 mg/kg IM or SC q25days (lower doses and longer treatment intervals can be efficacious in some dogs).

Daily glucocorticoid supplementation is not required after initial treatment with fludrocortisone acetate in the majority of cases, as fludrocorticosone has some glucocorticoid activity. However, the owners of animals with hypoadrenocorticism should be given a supply of prednisolone tablets to be administered if the patient appears unwell. Prednisolone at a dose of 0.1–0.2 mg/kg daily should be sufficient as a physiologic replacement for those cases that do require glucocorticoid medication.

Salt supplementation using salt tablets or salting the food should be instigated initially to help correct hyponatremia, but this can be gradually reduced and phased out as it is not usually required long term. However, dogs requiring unusually high doses of fludrocortisone may respond to oral salt and fewer fludrocortisone tablets.

The prognosis for primary hypoadrenocorticism is generally excellent providing owner education is adequate. Hypoadrenocorticism can occur in conjunction with other endocrine deficiencies, such as hypothyroidism, diabetes mellitus and hypoparathyroidism, or with other immune-mediated diseases, such as immune-mediated hemolytic anemia or thrombocytopenia.

Secondary hypoadrenocorticism

Definition/overview

Secondary hypoadrenocorticism is associated with a deficiency of glucocorticoids caused by a deficiency in ACTH production and/or release. The production of mineralocorticoids, although reduced, generally remains adequate. Secondary hypoadrenocorticism occurs in both dogs and cats.

Etiology

Secondary hypoadrenocorticism can be associated with destructive lesions (e.g. nonfunctional tumors) in the hypothalamus or anterior pituitary. More commonly, however, the condition is iatrogenic, with clinical signs occurring after the cessation of glucocorticoid therapy. In these cases, secondary hypoadrenocorticism is caused by prolonged suppression of ACTH secretion from glucocorticoid therapy. In the cat, secondary hypoadrenocorticism is also seen following prolonged megestrol acetate therapy.

Pathophysiology

Destructive lesions in the pituitary or hypothalamus may result in deficiencies of several pituitary hormones, including ACTH. Alternatively, exogenous glucocorticoid administration may suppress ACTH production and release. Both situations result in atrophy of the adrenal cortices and decreased glucocorticoid synthesis and release.

Clinical presentation

The clinical signs are variable and may include depression, anorexia, occasional vomiting or diarrhea, a weak pulse, and sudden collapse when stressed. If the secondary hypoadrenocorticism is associated with cessation of glucocorticoid therapy, clinical signs of iatrogenic hyperadrenocorticism (Cushing's disease) are usually present.

Differential diagnosis

Diabetic ketoacidosis, septic peritonitis, acute necrotizing pancreatitis.

Diagnosis

Diagnosis is based on a failure of the animal's cortisol levels to respond to ACTH stimulation.

Management

Glucocorticoid replacement using prednisolone (0.1–0.2 mg/kg q24h) is indicated for immediate correction of the clinical signs. Further treatment and the prognosis depend on the cause and whether glucocorticoid therapy can be eliminated.

HYPERADRENOCORTICISM (CUSHING'S DISEASE)

Definition/overview

Hyperadrenocorticism is associated with excessive production or administration of glucocorticoids and is one of the most commonly diagnosed endocrinopathies in the dog. Hyperadrenocorticism is rare in the cat.

Etiology

Hyperadrenocorticism can be spontaneous or iatrogenic. Spontaneously occurring hyperadrenocorticism may be associated with inappropriate secretion of ACTH by the pituitary (pituitary-dependent hyperadrenocorticism [PDH]) or with a primary adrenal disorder (adrenal-dependent hyperadrenocorticism) (**Figure 11.53**).

Pathophysiology

Pituitary-dependent hyperadrenocorticism

PDH accounts for 80–85% of dogs and the majority of cats with naturally occurring hyperadrenocorticism. Excessive ACTH secretion results in bilateral adrenocortical hyperplasia and increased cortisol secretion. There is a failure of the negative feedback mechanism of cortisol on ACTH. However, episodic secretion of ACTH results in

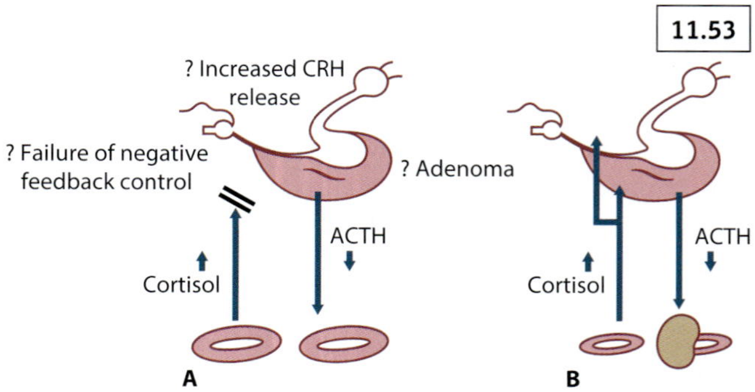

Figure 11.53 Pituitary-dependent hyperadrenocorticism (A); adrenal-dependent hyperadrenocorticism (B).

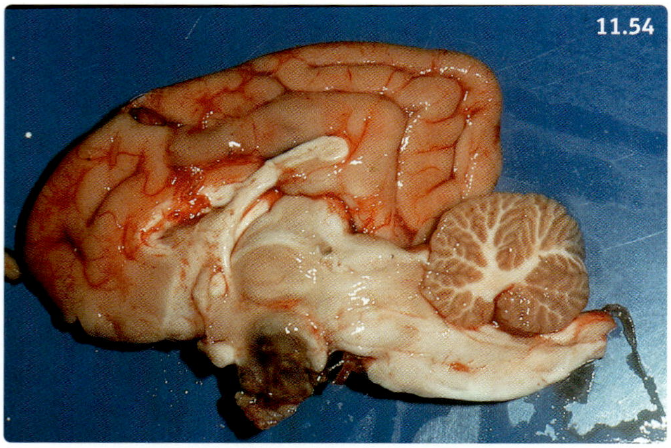

Figure 11.54 A large corticotroph adenoma associated with pituitary-dependent hyperadrenocorticism. The dog was successfully treated for 5 years while the tumor was gradually enlarging.

fluctuating cortisol concentrations that may at times be within the normal range. The presence of excessive cortisol secretion can be confirmed by measuring urine cortisol excretion over a 24-hour period.

Pathologic changes in PDH include microadenomas and macroadenomas of the corticotroph cells and a primary failure of the negative feedback response. Microadenomas are <1 cm in diameter. The incidence of corticotroph adenomas associated with PDH varies widely, probably because detection of small tumors requires careful microdissection, experience, and special stains. In one study using immunocytochemical staining, more than 80% of dogs with PDH were positive for pituitary adenomas. Macroadenomas are >1 cm in diameter and only a small percentage of dogs have large corticotroph adenomas (**Figure 11.54**). These may compress the remaining pituitary and extend dorsally into the hypothalamus. However, they are generally slow growing and do not always produce neurologic signs. Malignant pituitary tumors are rare.

The defect responsible for PDH unassociated with pituitary neoplasia is unknown. A primary failure of the negative feedback response by cortisol has been proposed. Others suspect an overproduction of CRH from the hypothalamus, which may cause diffuse hyperplasia of ACTH-producing cells in the anterior pituitary. From a clinical point of view the precise pituitary pathology is not of great importance unless neurologic signs are present at the time of diagnosis or become apparent during the initial treatment.

Adrenal-dependent hyperadrenocorticism

The remaining 15–20% of spontaneous cases of hyperadrenocorticism in dogs and cats are caused by unilateral or, occasionally, bilateral adrenal tumors, which can be benign or malignant. Adrenocortical adenomas are small (usually <4 cm in diameter), well-circumscribed tumors that do not metastasize and are not locally invasive. Approximately 50% are partially calcified. Adrenocortical carcinomas are usually larger, locally invasive, hemorrhagic, and necrotic. Tumor calcification also occurs in about 50% of dogs. The tumors frequently invade the phrenicoabdominal vein and caudal vena cava and metastasize to the liver, lung, and kidney.

In dogs, adrenocortical adenomas and carcinomas occur in approximately equal proportions. The cortex contiguous to the tumor and that of the contralateral gland will tend to become atrophied in the presence of functional adenomas and carcinomas (**Figure 11.55**). This is important if the tumor is removed surgically, as postoperatively the animal may not be able to secrete sufficient glucocorticoids. Function of the zona glomerulosa should not be affected.

Clinical presentation

Any breed of dog can develop hyperadrenocorticism, but Poodles, Dachshunds, Spaniels, and small terriers (e.g. Yorkshire Terrier, Jack Russell Terrier, and Staffordshire Bull Terrier) appear more at risk of developing PDH. Adrenocortical tumors occur more frequently in larger breeds of dog. No breed predisposition has been recorded in cats.

PDH is usually a disease of the middle aged to older dog, with an age range of 2–16 years and a median age of 7–9 years. Dogs with adrenal-dependent hyperadrenocorticism tend to be older, with a range of 6–16 years and a median age of 10–11 years. There is no significant difference in sex distribution in PDH; however, female dogs are three times more likely to develop adrenal tumors than males. Affected dogs usually develop a classic combination of clinical signs associated with increased glucocorticoid levels. These are listed in **Table 11.16** in approximate decreasing order of frequency. Some dogs, however, and particularly those of the larger breeds, may not show all the classic signs.

Hyperadrenocorticism has an insidious onset and is slowly progressive over many months or even years. Many owners consider the early signs as part of the normal aging process of their dog. In a few cases, clinical signs may be intermittent, with periods of remission and relapse, and in other cases there may be rapid onset and progression of clinical signs.

Polydipsia, defined as water intake in excess of 100 ml/kg body weight/day, and polyuria, defined as urine production in excess of 50 ml/kg body weight/day, are seen in virtually all cases of hyperadrenocorticism.

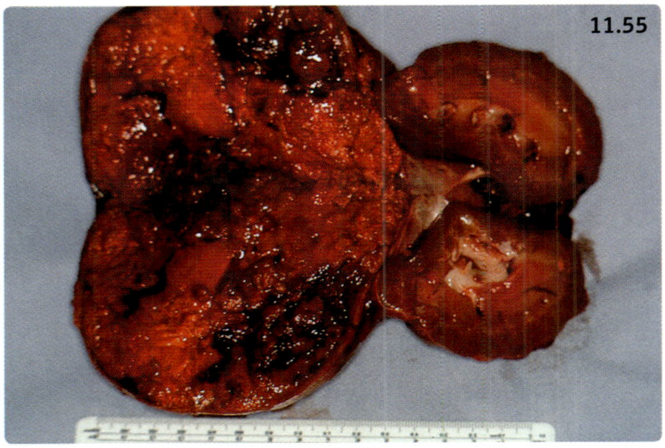

Figure 11.55 A large adrenal tumor invading the kidney from a dog with adrenal-dependent hyperadrenocorticism.

Table 11.16 Clinical signs of hyperadrenocorticism (in approximate decreasing order of frequency).

Polydipsia and polyuria
Polyphagia
Abdominal distension
Liver enlargement
Muscle wasting/weakness
Lethargy, poor exercise tolerance
Skin changes
Alopecia
Hypertension
Persistent anestrus or testicular atrophy
Calcinosis cutis
Myotonia
Neurologic signs

Excessive thirst, nocturia, and/or urination in the house are usually noted by owners. The polydipsia occurs secondary to the polyuria, which is only partially responsive to water deprivation.

Increased appetite is common, but most owners often assess this as a sign of good health. However, a voracious appetite and scavenging or stealing food may give rise to concern, especially if the dog previously had a poor appetite. Polyphagia is assumed to be a direct effect of glucocorticoids.

A pot-bellied appearance is very common in hyperadrenocorticism, but it may be so gradual that owners fail to recognize its significance (**Figure 11.56**). The abdominal distension is associated with redistribution of fat to the abdomen, liver enlargement, and abdominal muscle wasting and weakness.

The gradual onset of lethargy and poor exercise tolerance are usually considered by most owners to be compatible with aging. Only when muscle weakness is severe, as reflected by an inability to climb stairs or jump into the car, does the owner become concerned. Lethargy, excessive panting, and poor exercise tolerance are probably an expression of muscle wasting and weakness. Apart from the development of a pendulous abdomen, decreased muscle mass may be noted around the limbs, over the spine, or over the temporal region. Muscle weakness is the result of muscle wasting caused by protein catabolism.

Occasionally, dogs with hyperadrenocorticism develop myotonia, characterized by persistent active muscle contractions that continue after voluntary or involuntary stimuli (**Figure 11.57**). All limbs may be affected, but the signs are usually more severe in the hindlimbs. Animals with myotonia walk with a stiff stilted gait. The affected limbs are rigid and rapidly return to extension after

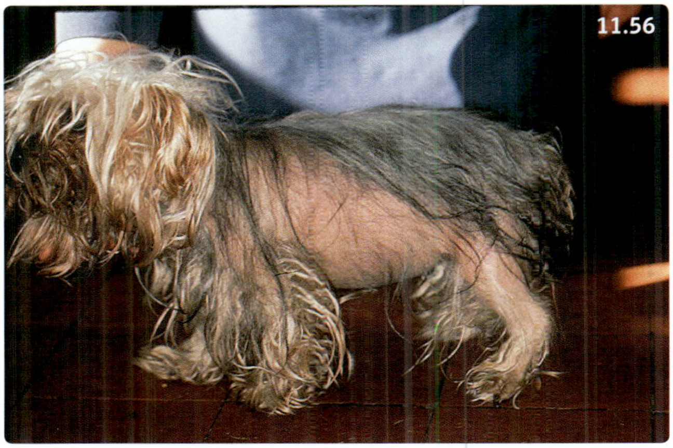

Figure 11.56 A 10-year-old Yorkshire Terrier with hyperadrenocorticism showing a pot-bellied appearance and bilaterally symmetrical alopecia.

being passively flexed. Spinal reflexes are difficult to elicit because of the rigidity, but pain sensation is normal. The muscles are usually slightly hypertrophied rather than being atrophied, and a myotonic dimple can be elicited by percussion of the affected muscle. Bizarre high-frequency discharges are noted on electromyography.

The skin, particularly over the ventral abdomen, becomes thin and inelastic (**Figure 11.58**). Elasticity can be assessed clinically by tenting the skin between the thumb and forefinger. In the normal dog the skin will flow back to a smooth contour, but in hyperadrenocorticism it remains tented. Striae can form as a result of this inelasticity. The abdominal veins are prominent and easily visible through the thin skin. There is often excessive surface scale and comedones, caused by follicular plugging, are seen, especially around the nipples (**Figure 11.59**). Hyperpigmentation of the skin is rare in canine hyperadrenocorticism.

Protein catabolism, causing atrophic collagen, also leads to excessive bruising following either venepuncture or other minor trauma. Wound healing is extraordinarily slow, presumably because of inhibition of fibroblast proliferation and collagen synthesis. Healing wounds often undergo dehiscence and even old scars may start to break down (**Figure 11.60**).

Calcinosis cutis is a frequent finding in biopsy material from the skin; however, clinical evidence of calcinosis cutis is less common. The gross appearance can vary, but the predilection sites are the neck, axilla, ventral abdomen, and inguinal areas (**Figure 11.61**). Calcinosis cutis usually appears as a firm, slightly elevated, white or cream plaque surrounded by a ring of erythema. Large plaques tend to crack, become secondarily infected, and develop a crust containing white powdery material. The exact pathogenesis is unknown, but plasma calcium and phosphorus concentrations are usually normal. Mineralization of the

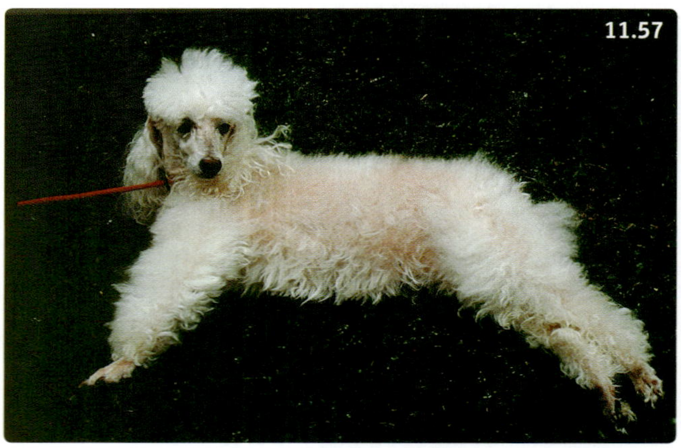

Figure 11.57 An 11-year-old Poodle with hyperadrenocorticism showing rigidity associated with myotonia.

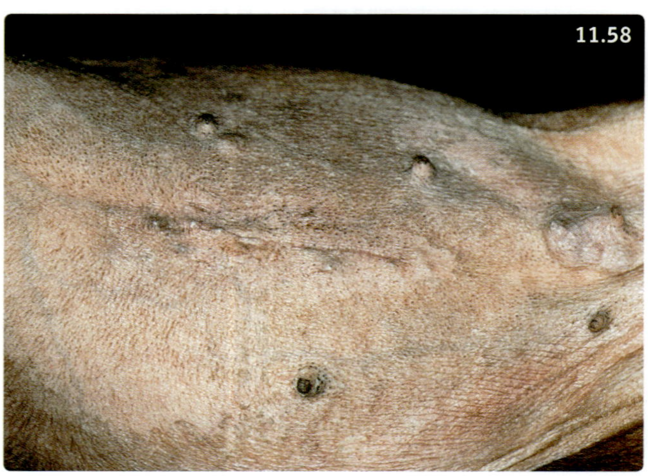

Figure 11.58 Thin, inelastic skin on the ventral abdomen of a Dachshund with hyperadrenocorticism.

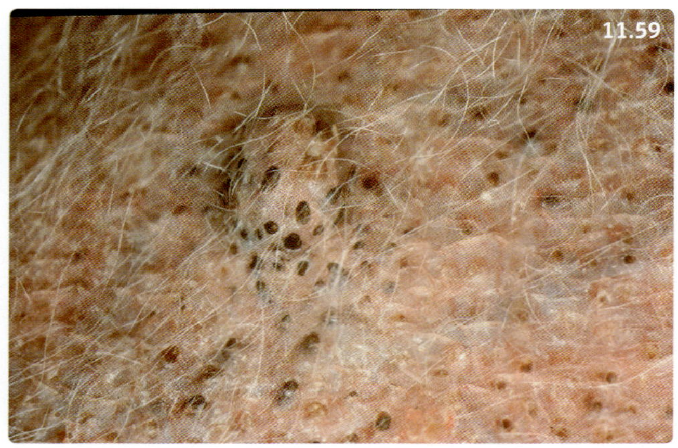

Figure 11.59 A close up of comedones around the nipple of a Poodle with hyperadrenocorticism.

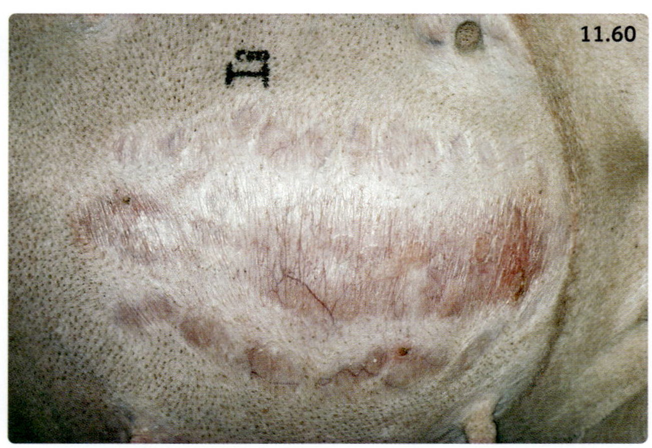

Figure 11.60 Stretching of an abdominal scar and striae on the ventral abdomen of a Boxer with hyperadrenocorticism.

soft tissues may be seen at other sites (e.g. the bronchial walls and kidneys) on radiographic examination.

Thinning of the hair coat, leading to bilaterally symmetrical alopecia, is frequently seen with hyperadrenocorticism and occurs because of the inhibitory effect of cortisol on the anagen or growth phase of the hair cycle. The remaining hair is dull and dry because it is in the telogen or resting phase of the hair cycle. The alopecia is nonpruritic and affects mainly the flanks, ventral abdomen and chest, perineum, and neck. The head, feet, and tail are usually the last areas to be affected (**Figure 11.62**). The coat color is often lighter than normal.

Systemic hypertension and associated proteinuria may be found in cases of hyperadrenocorticism. In the majority of cases, the degree of hypertension is moderate and not associated with clinical signs; however, hypertension-induced blindness due to intraocular hemorrhage and retinal detachment has occasionally been reported.

Entire bitches with hyperadrenocorticism usually cease to cycle. The length of anestrus (often years) indicates the duration of the disease process. In the intact male both testes become soft and flabby. Anestrus and testicular atrophy occur due to the negative feedback effect of high concentrations of cortisol on the pituitary, which also suppresses secretion of gonadotropic hormones.

Although uncommon at the time of presentation, a few cases develop neurologic signs associated with large expanding functional pituitary tumors. The most common clinical signs are dullness, depression, loss of learned behavior, anorexia, aimless wandering, head pressing, circling, ataxia, blindness, anisocoria, and seizures. More often, however, neurologic signs develop during initial treatment of PDH with mitotane or trilostane. This is thought to involve removal of the negative feedback of cortisol, which can cause some pituitary tumors to enlarge rapidly.

Differential diagnosis

Causes of polydipsia/polyuria (**Table 11.4**), liver disease, hypothyroidism, Sertoli cell tumor, ovarian imbalance.

Diagnosis

Laboratory findings

The main hematologic, biochemical, and urinalysis findings are listed in **Table 11.17**. The most consistent hematologic finding is a stress leukogram with a relative and absolute lymphopenia (<1.5 × 10^9/l [<1.5 × 10^3/µl]) and eosinopenia (<0.2 × 10^9/l [<0.2 × 10^3/µl]). Lymphopenia is most likely the result of steroid lymphocytolysis and/or redistribution of T cells to lymphoid tissues, and the eosinopenia results from bone marrow sequestration of eosinophils. A mild to moderate neutrophilia and monocytosis may be present, and it is thought that excessive glucocorticoids result in decreased capillary margination and diapedesis and increased release from the bone marrow. The red cell count is usually normal, although mild polycythemia may occasionally be noted. Platelet counts may also be elevated. These findings are thought to result from stimulatory effects of glucocorticoids on the bone marrow.

Glucocorticoids, both endogenous and exogenous, induce a specific hepatic isoenzyme of ALP in the dog. The increase in serum ALP is commonly 5–40 times the normal level and is perhaps one of the most reliable indicators of hyperadrenocorticism. Measurement of the specific steroid-induced isoenzyme of ALP has been used for more accurate assessment of elevated serum ALP activity. A marked increase in serum ALP is rarely seen in cats

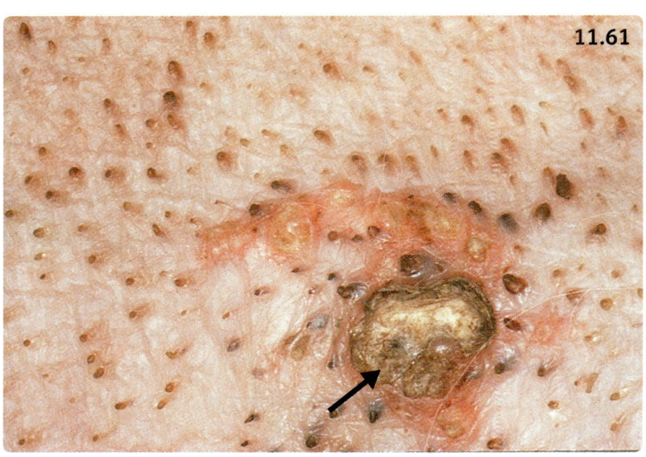

Figure 11.61 Calcinosis cutis (arrow) and comedones on the ventral abdomen of a Poodle with hyperadrenocorticism.

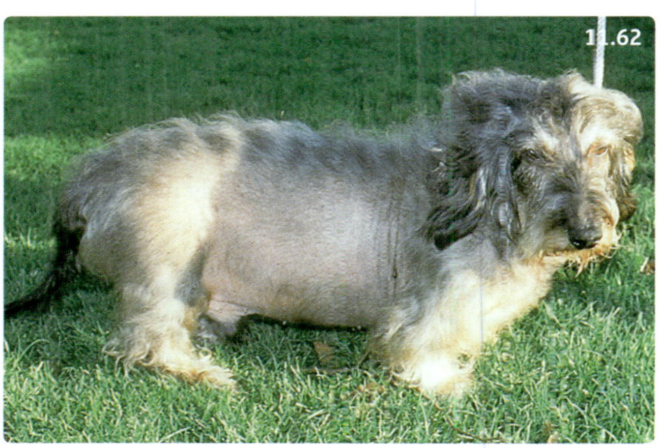

Figure 11.62 Bilaterally symmetrical alopecia in a Wirehaired Dachshund with hyperadrenocorticism.

Table 11.17 Laboratory findings in hyperadrenocorticism.

Hematology
Lymphopenia (<1.5 × 10^9/l [<1.5 × 10^3/μl])
Eosinopenia (<0.2 × 10^9/l [<0.2 × 10^3/μl])
Neutrophilia
Monocytosis
Erythrocytosis
Biochemistry
Increased ALP (often markedly elevated); dog only
Increased ALT
High normal fasting blood glucose; rarely diabetic except for the cat
Decreased blood urea
Increased cholesterol (>8 mmol/l [>309 mg/dl])
Lipemia
Increased bile acid
Urinalysis
Urine SG <1.015
Glycosuria (<10% of canine cases)
Urinary tract infection
Other findings
Low T4 concentrations
Subnormal T4 response to TSH or TRH stimulation

with hyperadrenocorticism because they do not possess a steroid-induced isoenzyme and have the ability to clear serum of excess ALP. ALT is commonly elevated in hyperadrenocorticism, but the increase is usually only mild and is believed to result from liver damage caused by swollen hepatocytes due to glycogen storage. Blood glucose is usually in the high normal range, but about 10% of canine cases will develop overt diabetes mellitus. The gluconeogenic effect of glucocorticoids results in insulin antagonism and subsequent development of pancreatic islet cell exhaustion. Cats appear to be more prone to developing hyperglycemia and overt diabetes. In contrast to the dog, where polydipsia and polyuria are amongst the earliest clinical signs of hyperadrenocorticism, the onset of polydipsia and polyuria is delayed in the cat and coincides with the development of moderate to severe hyperglycemia and glycosuria. Hyperadrenocorticism should be suspected in any cat that requires high daily insulin doses to control the hyperglycemia and glycosuria.

Blood urea is usually below normal due to the continual urinary loss associated with glucocorticoid-induced diuresis. Serum creatinine concentrations also tend to be in the low to normal range. Cholesterol and lipid concentrations are usually increased due to glucocorticoid stimulation of lipolysis. Cholesterol is usually >8 mmol/l (>309 mg/dl) but this is not a specific finding as cholesterol is also raised in hypothyroidism, diabetes mellitus, chronic liver disease, and chronic renal disease, all of which may be differential diagnoses. Lipemia is important as it can interfere with the accurate assessment of a number of laboratory parameters. Resting and postprandial bile acid concentrations may show a mild to moderate increase in some cases of hyperadrencorticism due to steroid hepatopathy.

The SG of the urine is usually <1.015 and is often hyposthenuric (<1.010) provided water has not been withheld. Dogs with hyperadrenocorticism can concentrate their urine if deprived of water, but their concentrating ability is usually reduced. Urinary tract infection is common and occurs in about half the cases of hyperadrenocorticism; however, it does not result in typical signs of cystitis due to the anti-inflammatory effects of excess glucocorticoids. Proteinuria, defined as a urine protein:creatinine ratio of equal to or greater than 1.0, is present in over 40% of untreated cases of hyperadrenocorticism. Glycosuria is present in the 10% of cases with diabetes mellitus.

Basal thyroxine concentrations are decreased in about 70% of dogs with hyperadrenocorticism. This is, in part, due to inhibition of TRH and reduced pituitary secretion of TSH. Excess cortisol, however, may also alter thyroid hormone binding to plasma proteins and enhance the metabolism of thyroid hormone. The response to stimulation by TSH usually parallels that of normal dogs, but thyroxine concentrations both before and after stimulation with TSH are subnormal. Endogenous canine TSH concentrations are usually low, but may be increased in some cases, mimicking the changes seen in hypothyroidism.

Diagnostic imaging

Radiography

Radiographic examination of the thorax and abdomen is advisable in all cases of suspected or proven hyperadrenocorticism. Although positive diagnostic information is only obtained in the small number of cases in which adrenal enlargement can be detected, the number and frequency of radiologic changes consistent with hyperadrenocorticism provide a useful aid to diagnosis. In addition, survey radiographs may reveal significant concurrent disease. The most common radiologic signs of hyperadrenocorticism are listed in **Table 11.18**.

Hepatomegaly is the most consistent radiographic finding in hyperadrenocorticism. Good radiographic contrast permits easy identification of the abdominal structures because of the large deposits of intra-abdominal fat. Hepatomegaly may be mild to severe and the ventral lobe borders vary in shape between distinctly rounded

Table 11.18 Radiologic signs of hyperadrenocorticism.

Abdominal radiographs
Liver enlargement
Good radiographic contrast
Pot-bellied appearance
Calcinosis cutis/soft tissue mineralization
Distended bladder
Cystic or renal calculi
Adrenal enlargement/calcification
Osteopenia
Thoracic radiographs
Tracheal and bronchial wall calcification
Pulmonary metastasis from adrenocortical carcinoma
Osteopenia
Pulmonary interstitial mineralization (rare)
Congestive heart failure (rare)
Pulmonary thromboembolism (rare)

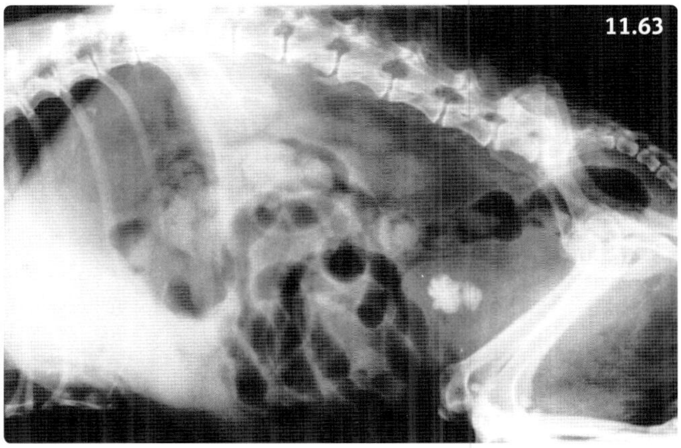

Figure 11.63 Lateral abdominal radiograph of a case of hyperadrenocorticism. Cystic calculi are also present.

and sharply wedge shaped. The pot-bellied appearance is usually very obvious on the recumbent lateral projection (**Figure 11.63**). Hepatomegaly and a pendulous abdomen are the most consistent radiographic findings in cats with hyperadrenocorticism.

Adrenal enlargement is the least common finding on abdominal radiographs. Gross enlargement is suggestive, although not diagnostic, of an adrenocortical carcinoma. Unilateral mineralization in the region of an adrenal gland suggests the possibility of an adrenal tumor (**Figure 11.64**). Both adrenocortical adenomas and carcinomas can become calcified. Radiography of the abdomen not infrequently demonstrates calcification of the adrenal glands in normal older cats and is not associated with any functional abnormality.

Calcinosis cutis tends to have a nodular mineralization pattern, whereas calcification in the fascial planes (e.g. just dorsal to the thoracolumbar spine) tends to be linear. Mineralization may also be seen in the renal pelvis, liver, gastric mucosa, and abdominal aorta.

A grossly distended urinary bladder may be seen radiographically even when the animal has been allowed to urinate prior to the radiographic examination. Cystic calculi may also be present and are usually associated with urinary tract infection. Occasionally, the impression of osteopenia is gained from a distinct reduction in radiographic density of the lumbar vertebral bodies relative to the vertebral end plates. Tracheal and bronchial wall calcification is frequently seen radiographically in cases of hyperadrenocorticism. However, calcification of these structures can be seen in animals as part of the normal aging process and is not considered to be a highly significant finding.

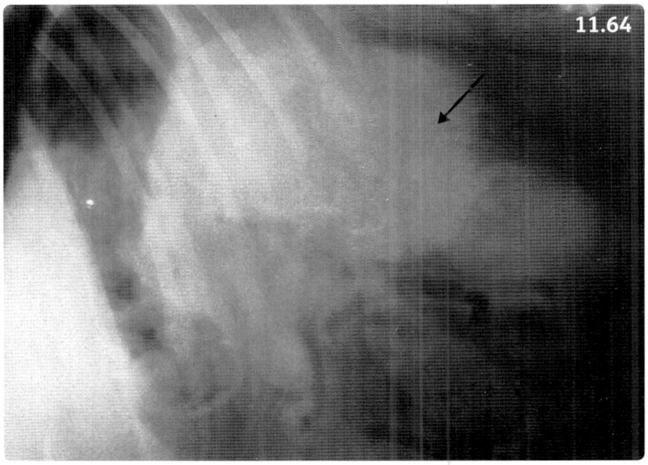

Figure 11.64 Lateral abdominal radiograph of a 9-year-old German Shepherd Dog with a right adrenal tumor (arrow).

The thoracic radiographs should also be examined for evidence of pulmonary metastases from an adrenocortical carcinoma, CHF, osteoporosis of the thoracic spine, or pulmonary thromboembolism. The latter is a rare complication of hyperadrenocorticism and may be suspected when the radiographic signs include pleural effusion, increased diameter and blunting of pulmonary arteries, decreased vascularity of the affected lobes, and overperfusion of the unobstructed pulmonary vasculature. However, in some cases of pulmonary thromboembolism the radiographs may reveal no abnormalities.

Ultrasonography

Abdominal ultrasonography is frequently used to examine the adrenal glands. It is a challenge for the ultrasonographer to distinguish consistently between normal and hyperplastic adrenal glands, since the diagnosis of adrenal hyperplasia is somewhat subjective. Measurement of the thickness (ventrodorsal dimension) of the adrenal gland has been shown to be more sensitive than either the length or width of the gland. A thickness of >7.5 mm for the left adrenal gland would be suggestive of adrenal hyperplasia (**Figures 11.65, 11.66**). If both adrenal glands are of similar size and normal shape in a dog or cat with hyperadrenocorticism, it confirms the disease is PDH.

Abdominal ultrasonography can also detect adrenocortical tumors (**Figure 11.67**). Adrenal masses are diagnosed by the location of the mass and the clinical signs exhibited by the animal. There is a propensity for adrenal tumors to invade nearby vessels and surrounding tissues, therefore a thorough ultrasonographic examination of adjacent vessels and tissues should be performed (**Figures 11.68, 11.69a, b**). Mineralization is frequently associated with benign and malignant adrenocortical tumors in the dog, and acoustic shadowing may aid in localizing the adrenal tumor. If an adrenal mass is identified, the liver should also be examined ultrasonographically for evidence of hepatic metastases.

CT and MR imaging

CT and MR imaging have proved helpful in the diagnosis of adrenal tumors, adrenal hyperplasia, and large pituitary tumors (**Figure 11.70**), but these techniques are more expensive.

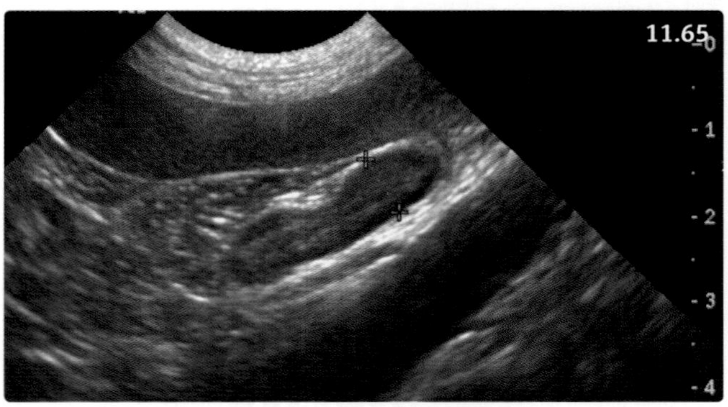

Figure 11.65 Ultrasonogram of a Boxer with adrenal hyperplasia due to PDH.

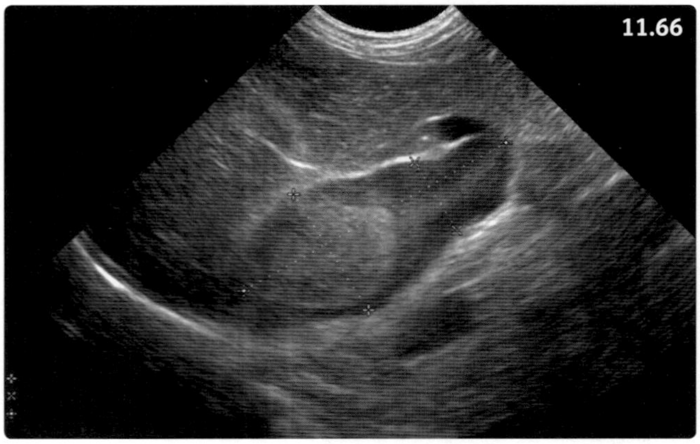

Figure 11.66 Ultrasonogram showing right-sided adrenal enlargement with nodular hyperplasia. The dog was being treated with trilostane, which can cause treatment-associated adrenomegaly.

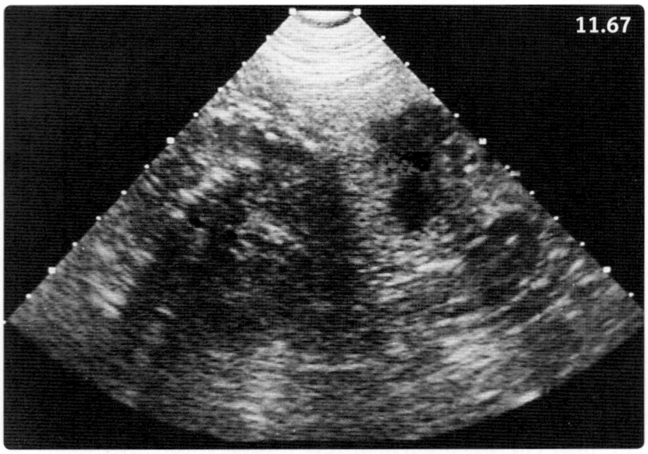

Figure 11.67 Ultrasonogram of a large adrenal tumor adjacent to the left kidney in a Rottweiler with adrenal-dependent hyperadrenocorticism.

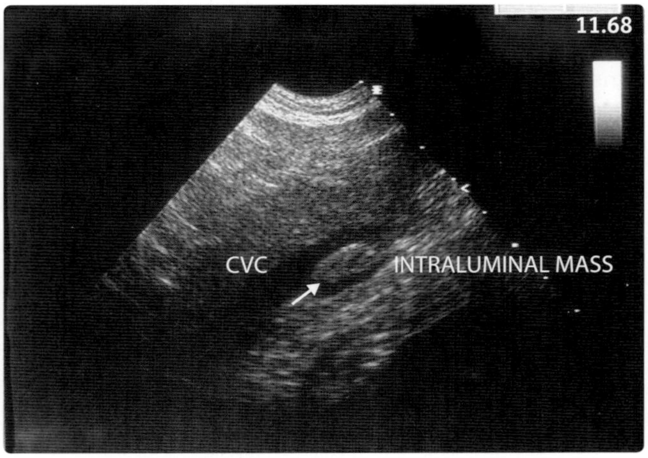

Figure 11.68 Ultrasonogram of an adrenal tumor (arrow) invading the caudal vena cava in a Labrador Retriever with adrenal-dependent hyperadrenocorticism.

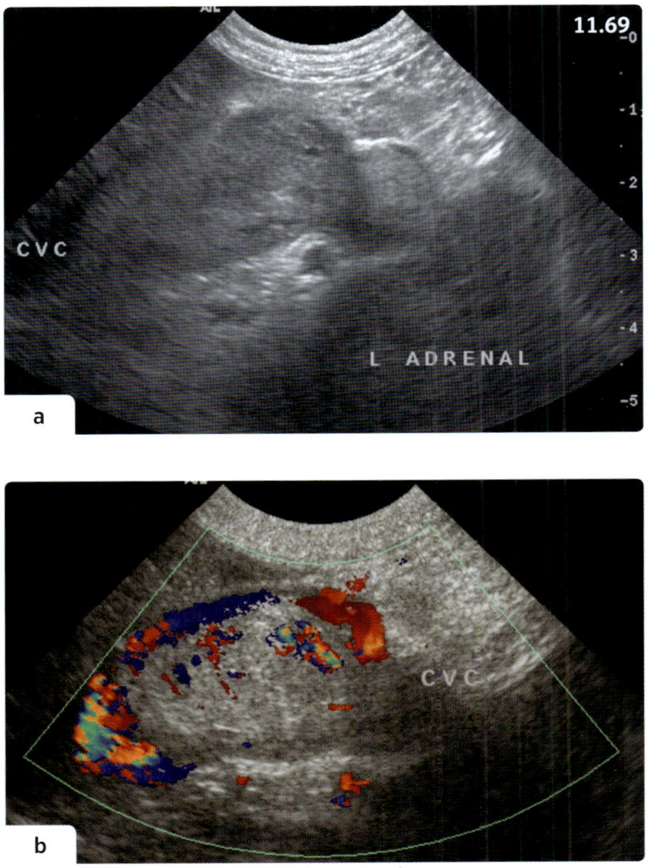

Figure 11.69a, b A plain abdominal ultrasound examination (a) and a flow Doppler evaluation (b) showing invasion of the caudal vena cava by a malignant adrenocortical carcinoma.

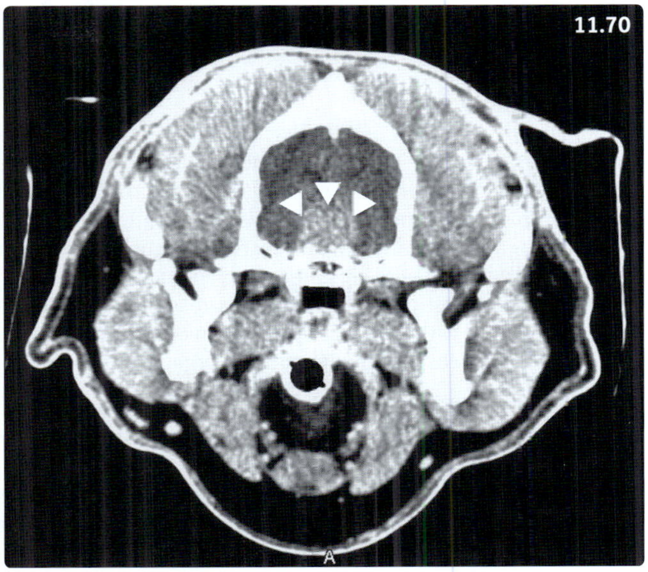

Figure 11.70 A contrast CT scan of a cushingoid dog showing a large pituitary macroadenoma (arrowheads) expanding deep into the diencephalon. (Courtesy M. Schaer)

Endocrine screening tests

A presumptive diagnosis of hyperadrenocorticism can be made from clinical signs, physical examination, routine laboratory tests, and diagnostic imaging findings, but the diagnosis must be confirmed by either an ACTH stimulation test or a low-dose dexamethasone suppression test (LDDST) (see **Table 11.19**).

ACTH stimulation test

The ACTH stimulation test (see **Figure 11.52**) is the best screening test for distinguishing spontaneous from iatrogenic hyperadrenocorticism. It reliably identifies about 85% of dogs with PDH, but only about 50% of those dogs with adrenal-dependent hyperadrenocorticism. It is a simple test to perform and the only one that directly documents excessive production of glucocorticoids by the adrenal cortex. The information gained also provides a baseline for monitoring trilostane or mitotane therapy. However, the ACTH stimulation test does not reliably differentiate adrenal-dependent hyperadrenocorticism from PDH. A diagnosis of hyperadrenocorticism should not be excluded on the basis of a normal ACTH response if the clinical signs are compatible with the disease. Occasionally, an animal under chronic stress may develop some degree of adrenal hyperplasia, which produces an abnormal or equivocal ACTH response result. The author has seen this in a number of severe systemic diseases (e.g. uncontrolled diabetes mellitus and pyometra) and has documented a normal ACTH response after treatment in each case. The ACTH response test is not as reliable for diagnosing this disorder in the cat.

Low-dose dexamethasone suppression test

The LDDST (**Figure 11.71**) is more reliable than the ACTH stimulation test in confirming hyperadrenocorticism, since the results are diagnostic in most adrenal-dependent cases and in 90% of dogs with PDH. However, it is not as useful as the ACTH stimulation test for the detection of iatrogenic hyperadrenocorticism. It is also affected by more variables, takes 8 hours to complete, and does not provide pretreatment information that may aid in monitoring the effects of trilostane or mitotane therapy. The LDDST, like the ACTH stimulation test, does not reliably differentiate PDH from adrenal-dependent hyperadrenocorticism.

Interpretation of the results of a LDDST must be based on the laboratory's normal range of cortisol values for the dose and preparation of dexamethasone administered. If the dose of dexamethasone fails to suppress adequately

Table 11.19 Protocols for endocrine screening tests for hyperadrenocorticism.

ACTH stimulation test Protocol: • Collect 3 ml plasma or serum sample for basal cortisol concentration* • Inject 0.25 mg of synthetic ACTH** (tetracosactrin; Synacthen, Alliance) IV in dogs >5 kg. Use only 0.125 mg in dogs <5 kg • Collect a second sample for cortisol concentration 30–60 minutes later *The recent administration of glucocorticoids, such as hydrocortisone, prednisolone, or prednisone, may result in elevated cortisol concentrations due to cross-reactivity in many cortisol assays. For this reason glucocorticoids should be withheld for at least 24 hours before testing. There is no cross-reactivity with dexamethasone, but dexamethasone will suppress cortisol concentrations in patients with an intact hypothalamic–pituitary–adrenal axis **Sold in USA as cosyntropin (Cortrosyn, Organon)
Interpretation: • In normal dogs, pre-ACTH cortisol concentrations are usually between 20 and 250 nmol/l (0.7 and 9.1 µg/dl), with post-ACTH cortisol concentrations between 200 and 450 nmol/l (7.2 and 16.3 µg/dl) • An exaggerated response (post-ACTH cortisol concentrations >600 nmol/l [>21.7 µg/dl]) is expected in dogs and cats with hyperadrenocorticism. The ACTH stimulation test reliably identifies more than 50% of dogs with adrenal-dependent hyperadrenocorticism and about 85% of dogs with PDH. Exaggerated responses to ACTH may also be seen in chronic illness (e.g. uncontrolled diabetes mellitus) • The ACTH stimulation test is the best screening test for distinguishing spontaneous hyperadrenocorticism from iatrogenic Cushing's disease where reduced responses to ACTH are recorded due to adrenocortical suppression as a result of long-term or high-dose glucocorticoid administration
Low-dose dexamethasone suppression test (LDDST) Protocol: • Collect 3 ml plasma or serum sample for cortisol determination • Inject 0.01 mg/kg of dexamethasone IV • Collect a second sample for cortisol concentration 4 hours later and a third sample 8 hours after dexamethasone administration
Interpretation: • A plasma or serum cortisol concentration exceeding 40 nmol/l (1.5 µg/dl) at 8 hours is regarded as diagnostic for hyperadrenocorticism. The LDDST reliably identifies all dogs with adrenal-dependent hyperadrenocorticism and about 90% of PDH. However, stress during therapy may cause animals without hyperadrenocorticism to break the suppressive effect of dexamethasone • Cortisol concentrations at 0 and 4 hours are not required for the diagnosis of hyperadrenocorticism, but may be informative in the differential diagnosis. Suppression of the cortisol concentration to <30 nmol/l (<1.1 µg/dl) at 4 hours with a rebound escape of suppression at 8 hours would be suggestive of PDH. Cases of adrenal-dependent hyperadrenocorticism do not show significant suppression of cortisol at 4 hours; however, up to 40% of dogs with PDH will not show suppression at 4 hours either
Urine cortisol:creatinine ratio Protocol: • Urine (5 ml) is collected in the morning for cortisol and creatinine measurements. It is preferable for the dog to be at home for this test so that it is as little stressed as possible. The urine cortisol:creatinine ratio is determined by dividing the urine cortisol concentration (in nmol/l) by the urine creatinine concentration (in µmol/l)
Interpretation: • The reference ratio for normal dogs is less than 10×10^6. The urine cortisol:creatinine ratio is increased above the normal ($>10 \times 10^6$) in dogs with hyperadrenocorticism. However, the ratio is also increased in many dogs with nonadrenal illness. Therefore, while this simple test appears highly sensitive in detecting hyperadrenocorticism in dogs, it is not specific. The test does provide a good screening test for hyperadrenocorticism and values in the normal range make a diagnosis of hyperadrenocorticism highly unlikely

circulating cortisol concentrations in a dog with compatible clinical signs, a diagnosis of hyperadrenocorticism is confirmed. While basal and 8-hour post-dexamethasone samples are most important for interpretation of the test, one or more samples taken at intermediate times (for example, 2, 4, or 6 hours) during the test period may also prove helpful. If a plasma cortisol concentration determined 2–6 hours after dexamethasone injection is

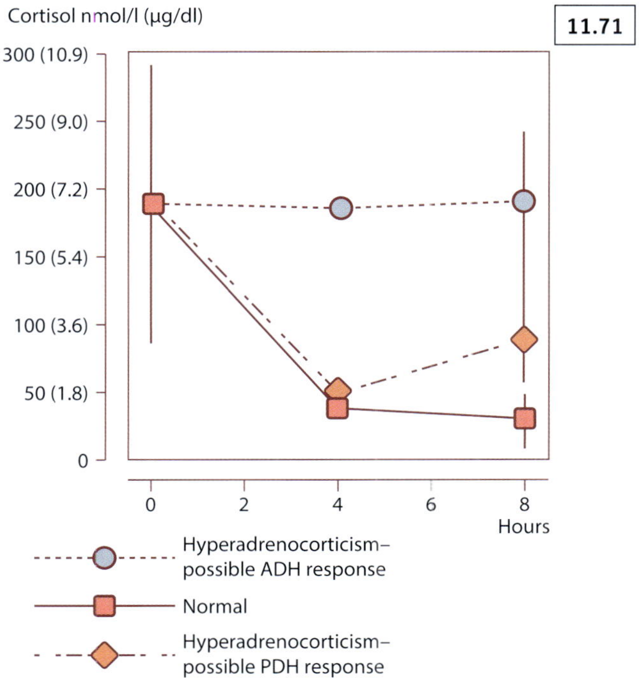

Figure 11.71 Low-dose dexamethasone suppression test.

suppressed to <40 nmol/l (<1.5 µg/dl), while the 8-hour sample shows escape from cortisol suppression, then a diagnosis of PDH can be made. While some cases of PDH will not suppress at any stage during a LDDST, any suppression during the 8-hour period essentially rules out a diagnosis of adrenal-dependent hyperadrenocorticism. This test is variable and thus not always reliable for diagnosing hyperadrenocorticism in the cat.

Other screening tests

Evaluation of urinary corticoid:creatinine ratio rather than the more laborious 24-hour urinary corticoid excretion has been shown to be a simple and valuable screening test that is highly sensitive in detecting hyperadrenocorticism; however, it lacks specificity and is affected by many variables. The test does provide useful information in that values within the reference range make a diagnosis of hyperadrenorcorticism highly unlikely.

Endocrine tests to differentiate the cause of hyperadrenocorticism

The ability to differentiate between PDH and adrenal-dependent hyperadrenocorticism is important in order to provide a better prognosis and the most effective method of management for the disease. An accurate test is therefore required to differentiate pituitary from adrenal causes of hyperadrenocorticism. The protocols for such tests are listed in **Table 11.20**.

Table 11.20 Protocols for endocrine tests to differentiate the cause of hyperadrenocorticism.

High-dose dexamethasone suppression test • Collect 3 ml serum or plasma sample for cortisol determination • Inject 0.1 mg/kg (although some authors recommend 1.0 mg/kg) of dexamethasone IV • Collect two post-dexamethasone samples, one at 4 hours and a second at 8 hours after the dexamethasone
Plasma endogenous ACTH concentration • Blood (5 ml) is collected into a cooled plastic EDTA tube and centrifuged at 4°C immediately • The plasma should then be harvested and stored frozen (at <– 20°C) in a plastic tube • Samples must be transported to the laboratory frozen and kept frozen until assayed • Stringent and meticulous sample handling is crucial since hormone activity in the plasma will reduce rapidly, resulting in falsely low values and incorrect interpretation • The endogenous ACTH assay must be validated for use in dogs, otherwise the test may provide spurious results that could be misleading

Plasma ACTH concentration

The determination of plasma ACTH concentrations in the dog provides a reliable test for differentiating pituitary and adrenal causes of hyperadrenocorticism providing sample handling is meticulous. Dogs with adrenal tumors have undetectably low endogenous ACTH concentrations, whereas cases of PDH have normal or high concentrations.

High-dose dexamethasone suppression test

The high-dose dexamethasone suppression test was the most commonly used test for differentiating the cause of hyperadrenocorticism, but it is less accurate than abdominal ultrasonography or plasma ACTH measurements. This test may be indicated in cases where the diagnosis of hyperadrenocorticism has been established by a screening test, but the differentiation between adrenal-dependent hyperadrenocorticism and PDH has not been determined. The high dose of dexamethasone inhibits pituitary ACTH secretion through negative feedback in PDH, thus suppressing serum cortisol concentrations by 50% or more by 4 hours. Adrenocortical tumors are autonomous, therefore serum cortisol is not suppressed at 4 hours if an adrenocortical tumor is present. However, approximately 20–30% of PDH cases will not suppress with this test, and the test does not differentiate adrenocortical adenomas from adrenocortical carcinomas. This test has been recommended for diagnosing hyperadrenocorticism in the cat, but the high dose of dexamethasone can cause or worsen concurrent diabetes mellitus.

Management

Treatment of pituitary-dependent hyperadrenocorticism

Trilostane therapy

Trilostane is a short-acting, synthetic steroid analog that competitively inhibits 3 beta-hydroxysteroid dehydrogenase, thus interfering with adrenal steroid biosynthesis. It has been successfully used to treat hyperadrenocorticism in dogs with relatively few adverse effects.

Treatment is initiated at 2–6 mg/kg once daily with food and the dosage adjusted on the results of the ACTH stimulation test carried out 4 hours after the administration of trilostane. Following the introduction of trilostane therapy, patients should be re-examined and an ACTH stimulation performed at 7–14 days and then at 30 and 90 days, or more frequently if problems occur. If the post-ACTH cortisol concentration is <20 nmol/l (<0.7 µg/dl), trilostane should be stopped for 5–7 days and then re-started at a lower dose. If the post-ACTH cortisol concentration is >120 nmol/l (>4.3 µg/dl), the dose of trilostane should be increased. If the post-ACTH cortisol concentration is between 20 and 120 nmol/l (0.7 and 4.3 µg/dl) and the patient appears clinically well controlled, the dose should remain unchanged. If, however, the patient's clinical signs appear poorly or only partially controlled, trilostane may need to be given twice daily.

Minor adverse effects such as mild lethargy, diarrhea, or decreased appetite may occur soon after starting therapy and are usually transient and respond to a reduction in dose. If more serious adverse effects such as vomiting, severe or hemorrhagic diarrhea, or severe depression develop, trilostane should be stopped and prednisolone replacement therapy instigated. Acute adrenal necrosis has been associated with death in a few cases. Hypoadrenocorticism has also been associated with trilostane therapy. The median survival time for dogs with PDH treated with trilostane is 22 months. Trilostane is effective for treating cats with PDH. The starting dose for cats is 1.0 mg/kg per day and this is subsequently titrated to effect.

Mitotane therapy

Mitotane (o'p'DDD; Lysodren, Bristol Laboratories) was formerly the treatment of choice for PDH, but many clinicians have since switched to trilostane as their preferred treatment. During its evaluation as an insecticide, mitotane was discovered to have adrenocorticolytic effects. It selectively destroys the zona fasciculata and zona reticularis while tending to preserve the zona glomerulosa.

Mitotane therapy should only be considered once the diagnosis of hyperadrenocorticism has been confirmed. Because of its powerful effects, it should never be used empirically. Before treatment is instigated, the patient's daily water consumption should be measured over at least two consecutive 24-hour periods. If the water intake and appetite are not increased, baseline lymphocyte and eosinophil counts and an ACTH stimulation test are required to monitor the response to therapy.

The author prefers to hospitalize the patient for the initial course of treatment, although many clinicians have dogs treated by their owners at home, with the owners doing the necessary monitoring. Mitotane is given orally with food at a dose rate of 50 mg/kg/day. Concomitant glucocorticoid treatment is not advised, although if the dog is being treated at home, the owner should be given a small supply of prednisolone tablets. Daily mitotane therapy should be continued until any of the following changes are noted:

- The water intake of a polydipsic dog drops to below 60 ml/kg/day.
- The dog takes longer to consume its meal than before treatment or stops eating completely.
- The dog vomits or has diarrhea.
- The dog becomes listless and depressed.

The initial course of mitotane is then stopped and the dog put on maintenance therapy (see below). The importance of close monitoring of the patient during this period cannot be overemphasized.

Mitotane therapy is comparatively safe and the side-effects that commonly occur (e.g. anorexia, vomiting, or diarrhea) are rarely serious providing they are noticed early so that the mitotane can be withheld. Some of the problems occasionally encountered during treatment are summarized in **Table 11.21**, together with their suggested management. Mitotane is ineffective in dogs being treated with phenobarbital because the latter drug will enhance mitotane hepatic metabolism.

The majority of dogs with PDH require between 7 and 14 days of treatment, with an average of 10 days, before water consumption drops to below 60 ml/kg/day. If the dog is not polydipsic or polyphagic, treatment should continue until the lymphocyte count is above 1.0×10^9 cells/l or the eosinophil count is above 0.3×10^9 cells/l. However, the best method of evaluating treatment is by use of the ACTH stimulation test. In adequately treated cases the basal and ACTH stimulated serum cortisol concentrations

Table 11.21 Possible problems arising from mitotane therapy and their management.

Problem	Management
Vomiting or anorexia within the first 3 days of treatment (gastric irritation)	Discontinue mitotane and reassess patient. Divide dose and give 2–4 times per day
Profound weakness, depression, and anorexia usually around 4th or 5th day of treatment	Discontinue mitotane and reassess patient. Check sodium and potassium levels and institute prednisolone (0.2 mg/kg/day). Reassess ACTH stimulation test. Start maintenance therapy with mitotane
Acute onset of neurologic signs (due to sudden expansion of the pituitary tumor)	Reassess patient. Continue mitotane unless the dog is anorexic, vomiting, or depressed. Give prednisolone (2.0 mg/kg/day) or dexamethasone (0.1 mg/kg/day) and decrease dose slowly once neurologic signs have resolved
Failure to resume normal water intake	Recheck urinalysis and blood urea. Reassess ACTH stimulation test. Increase mitotane by 50% if post-ACTH cortisol level is >200 nmol/l (>7.2 µg/dl)
Failure to regrow hair	Reassess ACTH stimulation test. Determine baseline T4. Increase mitotane by 50% if post-ACTH cortisol level is >200 nmol/l (>7.2 µg/dl). (If <120 nmol/l [<4.3 µg/dl], perform a TRH/TSH stimulation test)
Excessive depression or weakness related to weekly maintenance therapy	Reassess patient. Check sodium and potassium levels. Repeat ACTH stimulation test. If cortisol level post-ACTH is <15 nmol/l (<0.5 µg/dl), reduce maintenance dose or give every other week

should be <120 nmol/l (<4.3 µg/dl). If the serum cortisol concentrations exceed 200 nmol/l (7.2 µg/dl) with ACTH stimulation, further mitotane should be administered until the cortisol concentrations are adequately suppressed. A few dogs respond in 2–3 days and occasionally others require more than 60 consecutive days of treatment. It is important to emphasize that each dog must be treated as an individual if treatment is to be successful.

Having produced sufficient adrenocortical damage with daily mitotane treatment, it is important to continue therapy, albeit at a lower dose, otherwise the zona glomerulosa will regenerate a hyperplastic zona fasciculata and zona reticularis and the clinical signs will recur. Mitotane is given at a dose of 50 mg/kg/week with food. Cases that are well controlled may sleep for a few hours after the weekly dose and for that reason it is often recommended that the treatment is given in the evening. More profound depression or weakness requires re-evaluation and possibly a reduction of the maintenance dose. Failure to control the polydipsia may require an increased dose of mitotane (**Table 11.21**).

Treated dogs should be re-examined 6–8 weeks after completion of the initial therapy, unless there are any problems. Marked improvement should be noted at this time. The most obvious response is a rapid reduction in water intake, urine output, and appetite, and this is usually obvious at the end of the initial course of therapy. Muscle strength and exercise tolerance improve over the first 3–4 weeks. Skin and hair coat changes take longer and the progress is variable. The skin and alopecia may deteriorate markedly before improving; alternatively, there may be a gradual and noticeable resolution of the dermatologic signs. Although improvement should be noted at 8 weeks, the skin and hair coat may not return to normal for 3–6 months (**Figures 11.72, 11.73**). A few dogs have dramatic changes in coat color following successful therapy.

Re-examination every 3–6 months is recommended for the remainder of the animal's life. Relapses and episodes of overdosage do occur and reassessment of adrenal reserve by ACTH stimulation testing is indicated. Relapses may require a short course of daily mitotane therapy or an increase in the maintenance dosage. Overdosage requires reassessment by an ACTH stimulation test and a reduction of the maintenance dose. The median survival time of treated dogs is 30 months with a range of a few days to over 7 years.

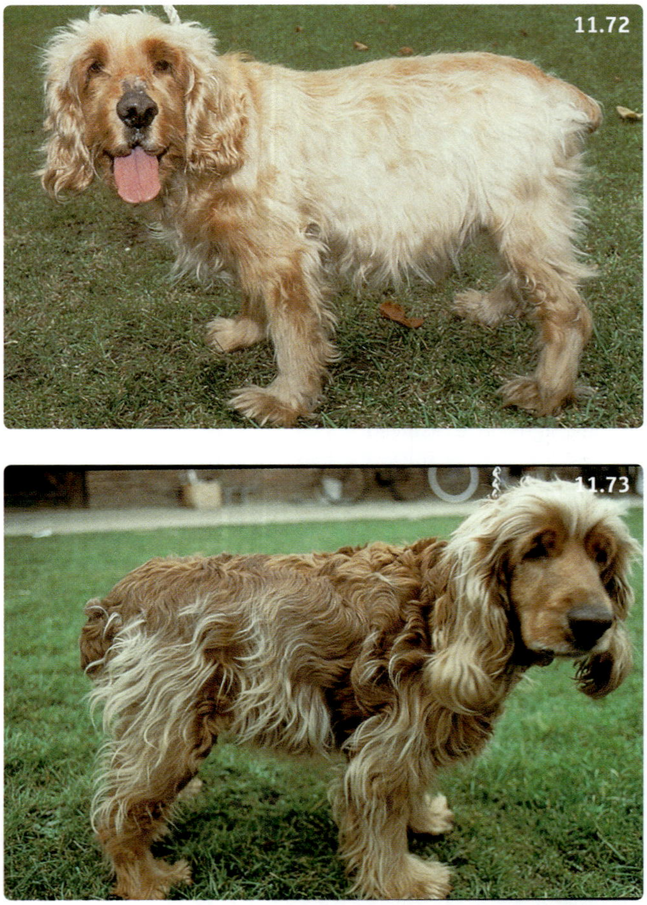

Figures 11.72, 11.73 Response to mitotane therapy. An 8-year-old Cocker Spaniel before treatment (11.72) and 4 months after treatment (11.73).

Mitotane has been shown to be ineffective in the cat because of its rapid hepatic metabolism.

Other therapeutic options for pituitary-dependent adrenocorticism

- L-deprenyl (selegiline hydrochloride) is a monoamine oxidase inhibitor that inhibits ACTH secretion by increasing dopaminergic tone to the hypothalamic–pituitary axis. The use of L-deprenyl for treatment of hyperadrenocorticism has been evaluated in dogs. Although the effectiveness of treatment is variable, one major advantage of L-deprenyl is the lack of any severe adverse effects, including iatrogenic hypoadrenocorticism. Treatment is initiated at a dosage of 1 mg/kg daily. If an inadequate response is seen after 2 months, the dosage is increased to 2 mg/kg/day. If this dosage also proves ineffective, alternative treatment is required. However, if the treatment with L-deprenyl is effective, daily treatment should be continued for the remainder of the dog's life. Response to treatment is evaluated by the resolution of clinical signs, since there is minimal measurable endocrinological improvement. More than 50% of dogs fail to respond adequately to L-deprenyl.
- Ketoconazole has a reversible inhibitory effect on glucocorticoid synthesis while having minimal effects on mineralocorticoid production. Ketoconazole has been used effectively to control hyperadrenocorticism in dogs, but it is not effective in cats. However, ketoconazole is not uniformly efficacious in dogs and between one-third and one-half of all dogs treated fail to respond adequately. The initial recommended dosage of ketoconazole is 10 mg/kg q12h for 14 days. Alternatively, treatment is initiated at 5 mg/kg q12h for the first 7 days to assess drug tolerance, then increased to 10 mg/kg. The efficacy of the initial 14-day course of treatment is determined by an ACTH stimulation test. To ensure adequate control of hyperadrenocorticism, both the pre- and post-ACTH serum cortisol concentrations must be lowered into the basal reference range. If the serum cortisol concentrations remain above this range, the dosage is increased to 15 mg/kg q12h and an ACTH response test repeated in 14 days.
- Bilateral adrenalectomy has been employed successfully, but it involves the risk of putting an ill animal with a compromised immune system and poor wound healing through a difficult surgical procedure. Bilateral adrenalectomy used to be the recommended treatment for feline hyperadrenocorticism despite its accompanying postoperative morbidity. Patients treated by this approach require lifelong treatment for hypoadrenocorticism. More recently, trilostane has been found to be an effective treatment option for treating PDH in the cat.
- Hypophysectomy has been successfully performed in the dog for the treatment of PDH, but the operation is technically difficult.

Treatment of adrenal-dependent hyperadrenocorticism

Dogs diagnosed as having adrenal-dependent hyperadrenocorticism carry the best prognosis if the tumor can be completely removed surgically, although mitotane (for dogs) or trilostane (for dogs and cats) therapy is also recommended.

Unilateral adrenalectomy

This procedure requires considerable expertise because of the complex anatomy. Preoperative staging using ultrasonography and radiography or CT is essential. Adrenalectomy is best performed via a ventral midline

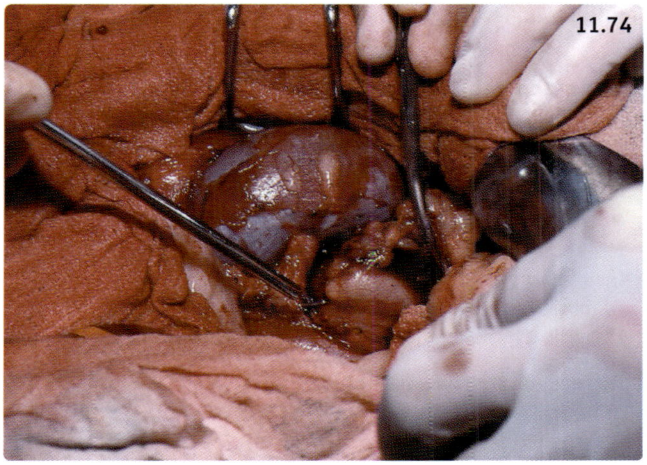

Figure 11.74 Surgical view of an adrenocortical carcinoma that had a spontaneous bleed into the retroperitoneal space. (Courtesy M. Schaer)

laparotomy (**Figure 11.74**). It should only be performed by experienced surgeons as perioperative mortality is high. Postoperative support is important, as the contralateral adrenal cortex will be atrophic and unable to respond to the stress. Replacement glucocorticoid and mineralocorticoid therapy may therefore be required for 7–10 days postoperatively. Even with experienced surgeons, there is a high morbidity and mortality rate and perioperative mortality can be as high as 30%. The median survival time is around 2 years, with some dogs surviving for longer than 4 years. Heparin has been recommended for some dogs in the perioperative period because of hypercoagulability.

Mitotane therapy

Mitotane is effective and relatively safe in dogs with adrenal-dependent hyperadrenocorticism. Dogs with adrenal tumors, however, tend to be more resistant to mitotane than dogs with PDH. Generally, dogs with adrenal-dependent hyperadrenocorticism require higher daily induction doses (50–75 mg/kg/day) and a longer period of induction (>14 days) than dogs with PDH. Frequent monitoring of treatment by ACTH stimulation testing is important to ensure adequate control of the hyperadrenocorticism. Maintenance doses are also generally higher (75–100 mg/kg/week) and, again, frequent monitoring of the cortisol response to ACTH stimulation is required to maintain optimal control of the disease. Adverse effects of treatment are similar to those described for PDH. Those dogs requiring higher dose rates tend to be more prone to adverse effects. The adrenal tumor and metastatic mass will often reduce in size due to the cytotoxic effects of mitotane, but in other cases the tumor will continue to grow despite increasing doses of mitotane. The median survival time is 11 months, with a range from a few weeks to more than 5 years.

Trilostane therapy

Trilostane is also effective and relatively safe in dogs and cats with adrenal-dependent hyperadrenocorticism. The dose of trilostane needs to be tailored to the individual patient with an adrenal tumor on the basis of the results of regular ACTH stimulation testing. There is a tendency for the dose to increase as the tumor continues to grow. Survival times similar to mitotane therapy (in dogs) for adrenal tumors have been reported.

PRIMARY HYPERALDOSTERONISM

Definition/overview

Primary hyperaldosteronism is characterized by excessive autonomous secretion of aldosterone from one or both adrenal glands resulting in clinical signs relating to hypertension and/or hypokalemia. It is a disease of middle aged to old aged cats, with a mean age of 13 years. There is no breed or sex predisposition. The condition is rare in dogs.

Etiology

Adrenocortical tumors are the most common cause of primary hyperaldosteronism in cats. There is an approximately equal incidence of adenomas and carcinomas with the right and left adrenal glands being affected with almost equal frequency. Rarely, bilateral tumors have been reported. More recently, primary hyperaldosteronism has been recognized in association with adrenocortical hyperplasia.

Pathophysiology

Increased autonomous secretion of aldosterone leads to excessive sodium and water retention, with resultant hypertension, and excessive potassium secretion leading to hypokalemia. The elevated plasma aldosterone and increased circulating blood volume have a negative feedback effect on renin release, resulting in reduced plasma renin activity.

Clinical presentation

The most common presenting sign is muscular weakness due to the hypokalemia. This can range from mild weakness and lethargy to severe generalized weakness, ataxia, depressed spinal reflexes, and flaccidity. Ventroflexion of the neck may be noted (**Figure 11.75**). Blindness, which may be sudden or gradual in onset, is due to systemic hypertension and usually results from retinal detachment and intraocular hemorrhage. Systemic hypertension can

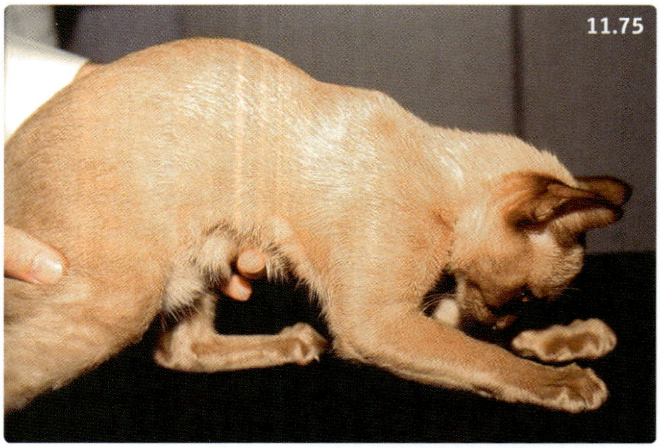

Figure 11.75 A Burmese cat showing ventroflexion of the neck due to hypokalemia.

also lead to left ventricular hypertrophy and cardiac murmurs. Impaired renal function is common and many cats also exhibit polydipsia and polyuria.

Differential diagnosis

The differential diagnoses of hypokalemia and hypertension are given in **Tables 11.22** and **11.23**, respectively.

Diagnosis

The diagnosis of primary hyperaldosteronism is based on demonstrating the presence of an adrenal tumor, together with an elevated plasma aldosterone concentration.

Adrenal tumors can usually be identified using ultrasonography (**Figure 11.76**). Abdominal ultrasonography can also be used to identify metastases and evidence of invasion of surrounding structures, particularly the caudal vena cava. CT and MRI have also been used.

Plasma aldosterone concentrations are usually raised to between 2 and 30 times the reference range. Although ACTH stimulation has been described when measuring plasma aldosterone, there is no clear evidence of improved diagnostic performance following ACTH stimulation. It should be noted, however, that raised aldosterone concentrations are not pathognomonic for primary hyperaldosteronism and that diseases that activate the renin–angiotensin–aldosterone system (RAAS), especially chronic kidney disease and CHF, will cause secondary hyperaldosteronism.

Adrenal hyperplasia can only be diagnosed by demonstrating a raised plasma aldosterone:plasma renin activity ratio. In primary hyperaldosteronism, plasma aldosterone is raised, which exerts a negative feedback effect on renin, resulting in reduced plasma renin activity, as distinct from secondary hyperaldosteronism where the RAAS has been activated. When renin

Table 11.22 Differential diagnosis of feline hypokalemia.

Differential diagnosis
Decreased intake Anorexia Potassium-deficient intravenous fluids Potassium-deficient diet
Potassium translocation Metabolic alkalosis Insulin administration Diabetic ketoacidosis Periodic hypokalemia (Burmese cats)
Increased gastrointestinal loss Vomiting Diarrhea
Increased renal loss Polyuria Chronic kidney disease Acute kidney injury (polyuric phase) Diuretic administration (loop or thiazide diuretics) Renal tubular acidosis Primary hyperaldosteronism Liver failure Congestive heart failure
Note: Hypokalemia in some diseases may have more than one mechanism.

Table 11.23 Differential diagnosis of feline hypertension.

Differential diagnosis
Chronic kidney disease
Hyperthyroidism
Diabetes mellitus
Hyperaldosteronism
Hyperadrenocorticism
Chronic anemia
Liver disease

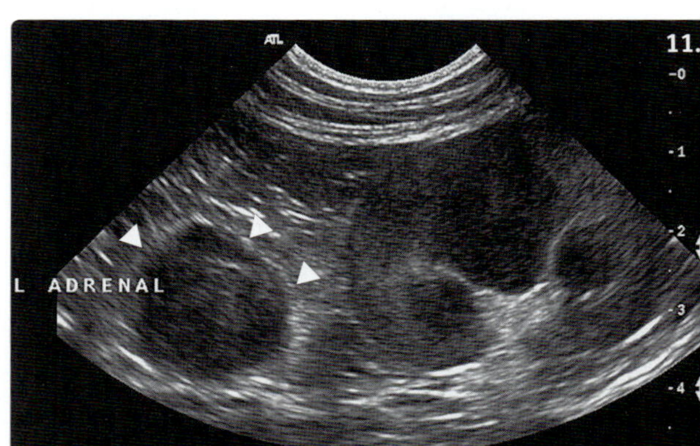

Figure 11.76 Ultrasonogram of an adrenal tumor (arrowheads) in a Domestic Longhair cat with primary hyperaldosteronism.

assays are unavailable, the combination of clinical signs and elevated serum aldosterone levels in the absence of any demonstrable adrenal mass is highly suggestive of adrenocortical hyperplasia as the cause of the hyperaldostonism.

Management

Initial therapy should be aimed at controlling hypokalemia and hypertension. Hypokalemia can be treated with potassium supplementation and the competitive aldosterone antagonist spironolactone. Hypertension can usually be controlled with amlodipine and beta-blockers. Treatment with these drugs can be continued for life and survival times from 4 months to 2.5 years have been reported. Medical management is the recommended treatment for cases associated with adrenal hyperplasia.

Although unilateral adrenalectomy is the treatment of choice for adrenal tumors, perioperative mortality is relatively high, with intra- and postoperative hemorrhage the most common cause of death. However, those patients who survive surgery frequently live for more than a year.

PHEOCHROMOCYTOMA

Definition/overview

Tumors of the adrenal medulla (pheochromocytomas) are rare in dogs and have only been reported rarely in cats. They are usually unilateral, benign, slow growing tumors that may reach a considerable size. Rarely, they are malignant and may invade the caudal vena cava or metastasize to lung, liver, or bone. Pheochromocytomas may secrete excessive amounts of catecholamines.

Pathophysiology

The physiologic effects of catecholamines secreted by pheochromocytomas account for many of the diverse clinical signs. The presence of the tumor mass may also contribute to the clinical presentation.

Clinical presentation

Clinical signs of a pheochromocytoma may relate to an abdominal mass compressing adjacent structures or to the secretion of catecholamines. Clinical signs related to tumor size might include a palpable abdominal mass, ascites, and hindlimb weakness. Secretion of catecholamines may be intermittent or persistent and can cause hypotension or hypertension, tachycardia, tachyarrhythmias with episodic weakness and trembling, head pressing, or seizures. Epistaxis and retinal hemorrhages may also be noted. The clinical signs vary depending on whether an excess of epinephrine or norepinephrine is predominant. In some cases, there may be no reported clinical signs and an adrenal mass is found incidentally, usually during abdominal ultrasonography.

Differential diagnosis

Causes of episodic weakness (**Table 11.24**).

Table 11.24 Differential diagnosis of episodic weakness.

Cardiovascular disorders Bradyarrhythmia Tachyarrhythmia Congenital heart disease (e.g. aortic or pulmonic stenosis, tetralogy of Fallot, reverse shunting PDA) Acquired heart disease (e.g. valvular, myocardial, pericardial) Heartworm disease (dirofilariasis, angiostrongylosis) Vasovagal syncope Vasodilation (Aortic) thromboembolism
Respiratory disorders Laryngeal paralysis Brachycephalic airway disease Tracheal collapse Severe coughing *Filaroides osleri* Pulmonary disease Pleural effusions Thoracic masses Hematologic disorders
Anemia Myeloproliferative disorders Polycythemia Hyperviscosity syndrome Hemoglobinopathies Pyrexia of unknown origin Orthopedic disorders
Degenerative joint disease, particularly hips or stifles Polyarthritis – various types
Neuromuscular disorders Myasthenia gravis Polymyositis Hereditary myopathy of Labrador Retrievers Sex-linked muscular dystrophy – Irish Terriers, Golden Retrievers Myotonia in Chow Chows, Staffordshire Terriers Malignant hyperthermia Mitochondrial myopathies Exertional myopathy (rhabdomyolysis)

(continued)

Table 11.24 Differential diagnosis of episodic weakness. (*continued*)

Neurologic disorders
Congenital or acquired spinal disorders including wobbler syndrome
Epilepsy (various causes)
Vestibular disease
Cerebellar disorders
Thiamine deficiency
Congenital disorders (e.g. hydrocephalus)
Acquired disorders (e.g. old dog encephalitis, cerebral vascular accident, tumors)
Lysosomal storage diseases
Giant axonal neuropathy
Progressive axonopathy – Boxer
Tetanus
Botulism
Narcolepsy/cataplexy – Dobermann, Poodle, Labrador Retriever
Generalized tremor
Jack Russell Terrier ataxia
Scottie cramp – also in the Norwich and Jack Russell Terrier, Dalmatian
Episodic falling in the Cavalier King Charles Spaniel
Metabolic disorders
Hepatic encephalopathy
Uremic encephalopathy
Hyperglycemia
Hypoglycemia
Hyponatremia
Hyperkalemia
Hypokalemia
Hypercalcemia
Hypocalcemia
Hypermagnesemia
Hypomagnesemia
Acidosis
Hyperthermia (heatstroke)
Hypoxia
Shock
Endocrine disorders
Insulinoma
Hyperadrenocorticism – myotonia
Hypoadrenocorticism
Hypoparathyroidism
Hypothyroidism
Pheochromocytoma
Diabetic ketoacidosis

Diagnosis

A diagnosis of pheochromocytoma should be suspected in any unexplained case of episodic weakness. Radiographic and ultrasonographic examinations will often reveal a mass in the adrenal area (**Figures 11.77–11.79**). However, confirmation requires quantification of

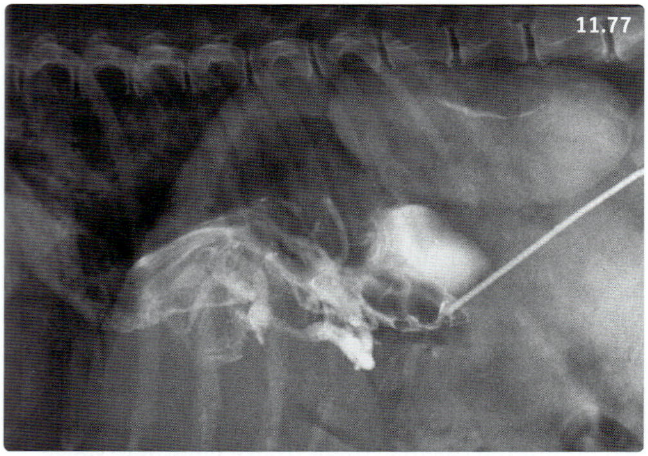

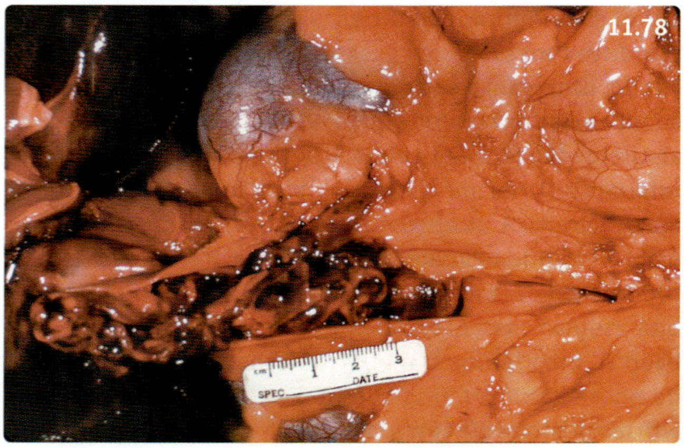

Figures 11.77, 11.78 (11.77) Contrast venogram radiographic study showing abnormal dispersion of the contrast medium in the posterior vena cava. This was caused by a pheochromocytoma invading the vessel. (11.78) The pathology at postmortem is shown. (Courtesy M. Schaer)

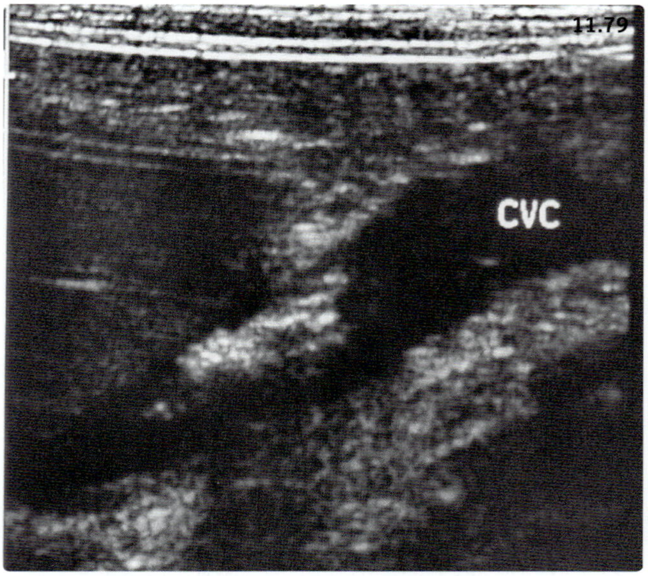

Figure 11.79 Ultrasonogram of a dog with a pheochromocytoma invading the postcava. (Courtesy M. Schaer)

plasma catecholamines and their metabolites or urinary excretion of catecholamines and their metabolites, but these tests are not widely available and the results are not always reliable.

Management

Surgical removal (**Figures 11.80, 11.81**) is the treatment of choice, but this should only be performed by experienced surgeons since excessive handling of the tumor during surgery may provoke massive secretion of catecholamines and the tumors tend to be invasive. Phentolamine, an alpha-adrenergic antagonist for IV use, can be used at a dose of 0.02–0.1 mg/kg to lower blood pressure while manipulating the tumor. However, phenoxybenzamine (0.2–1.5 mg/kg PO q12h) may be the drug of choice due to its long duration of action. Improved surgical survival has been associated with the use of oral phenoxybenzamine treatment for 2 weeks prior to surgery. Lidocaine or propranolol can be administered intravenously as necessary during surgery to control tachycardia or tachyarrhythmias.

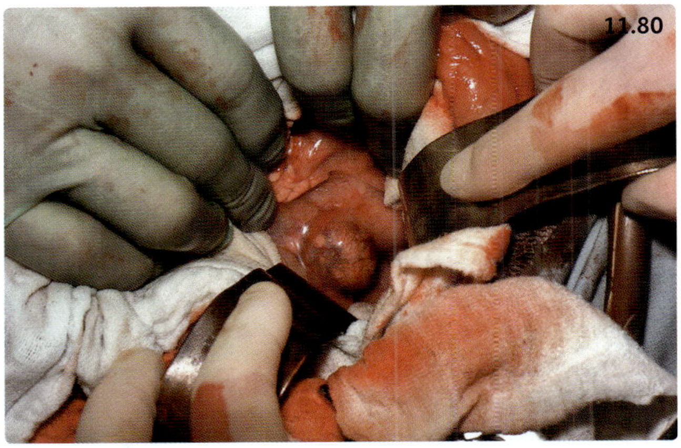

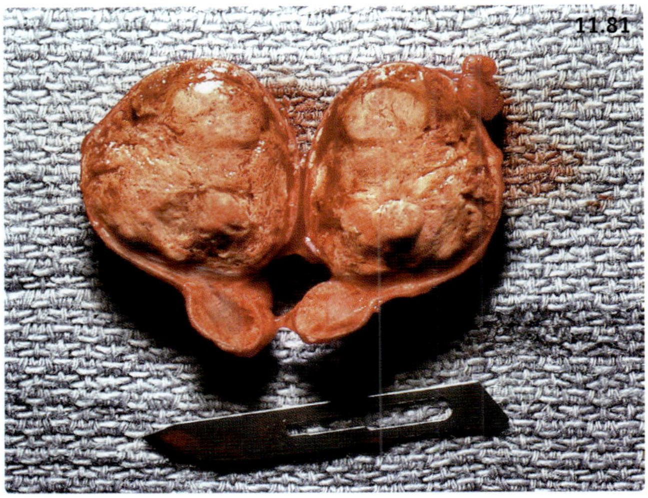

Figures 11.80, 11.81 Surgical view (11.80) and resected specimen (11.81) of a well-localized and noninvasive pheochromocytoma. (Courtesy M. Schaer)

DIABETES MELLITUS

Definition/overview

Diabetes mellitus is a heterogeneous syndrome in the dog and cat rather than a single disease entity. It is characterized by a relative or absolute deficiency of insulin secretion by the beta cells of the islets of Langerhans in the pancreas.

Etiology

Carbohydrate metabolism, and in particular blood glucose concentration, is controlled by the balance between the action of catabolic hormones (e.g. glucagon, cortisol, catecholamines, and GH) on the one hand and the principal anabolic hormone, insulin, on the other.

Pathophysiology

A relative or absolute deficiency of insulin results in decreased utilization of glucose, amino acids, and fatty acids by peripheral tissues, particularly liver, muscle, and adipose tissue. Failure of glucose uptake by these cells leads to hyperglycemia. Once the renal threshold for glucose reabsorption is exceeded, an osmotic diuresis ensues with loss of glucose, electrolytes, and water in the urine. A compensatory polydipsia prevents the animal becoming dehydrated. The loss of glucose leads to catabolism of the body's reserves, especially of fats. Excessive fat catabolism leads to the production and accumulation of ketone bodies and the onset of diabetic ketoacidosis (**Figure 11.82**). In diabetic ketoacidosis the patient is unable to maintain an adequate fluid intake and becomes rapidly dehydrated due to the uncontrolled osmotic diuresis. The

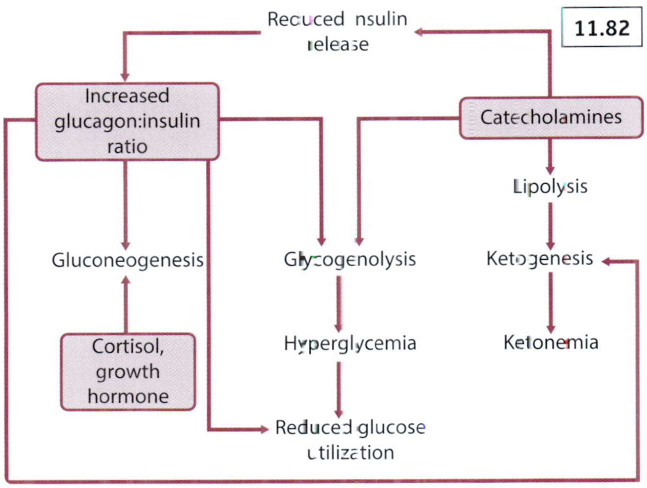

Figure 11.82 Etiology of diabetic ketoacidosis.

dehydration and acidosis require emergency care if the animal is to survive.

In humans diabetes is classified as type I insulin-dependent diabetes mellitus and type II noninsulin-dependent diabetes mellitus. This classification has not proved very useful in veterinary medicine, since nearly all dogs with diabetes mellitus require insulin therapy regardless of the underlying etiology. However, in cats, type II diabetes mellitus is the most common form of the disease and is characterized by variable loss of insulin secretory capacity and insulin resistance. Classifying diabetes mellitus into primary and secondary causes is of more use clinically in the dog (**Table 11.25**). In secondary diabetes, which is caused by peripheral insulin resistance, there is initially a compensatory increase in insulin secretion, but after a period of time the islet cells become exhausted, the beta cells are destroyed, and their function is permanently lost.

Clinical presentation

Diabetes mellitus is a disease of middle aged dogs with a peak incidence around 8 years of age. Genetic predisposition to diabetes has been found in Keeshonds and Samoyeds. Cairn Terriers, Tibetan Terriers, Poodles, and Dachshunds may also be overrepresented. Entire bitches are more frequently affected than male dogs and this is due mainly to the induction of GH by progesterone or progestogens.

Diabetes mellitus is the second most common endocrine disorder in cats after hyperthyroidism. Its incidence appears to be increasing, probably due to an increase in obesity in the cat population. Several risk factors have been identified including age, obesity, neutering, and sex. The disease is seen in middle aged to older cats and appears to be more common in males than females and in neutered cats rather than entire cats.

Table 11.25 Etiology of diabetes mellitus in the dog and cat.

Primary islet cell degeneration
Islet cell destruction (?autoimmune) Chronic pancreatitis Amyloidosis
Secondary diabetes mellitus
Obesity – causing downregulation of insulin receptors Antagonism to insulin by counterregulatory hormones: • Hyperadrenocorticism • Progesterone-induced GH excess (dogs only) • Acromegaly Antagonism to insulin by drug therapy: • Glucocorticoids • Progestogens

Polyuria, polydipsia, increased appetite, and weight loss develop over a few weeks in uncomplicated cases (**Figure 11.83**). In entire bitches this usually occurs in the diestrus phase of the estrous cycle. Hepatomegaly, muscle wasting, and infections of the urinary or respiratory tract may be noted on clinical examination. Ulcerative skin lesions and cutaneous xanthomata have occasionally been reported. If the diabetes remains uncontrolled, an accumulation of ketone bodies may occur, which causes metabolic acidosis and leads to depression, anorexia, vomiting, and rapid dehydration (**Figure 11.84**). Coma and death may result from severe hypovolemia and circulatory collapse.

Differential diagnosis

Primary renal glycosuria, stress, hyperadrenocorticism, pancreatitis, renal insufficiency, exocrine pancreatic neoplasia, acromegaly, diestrus, pheochromocytoma, postprandial hyperglycemia.

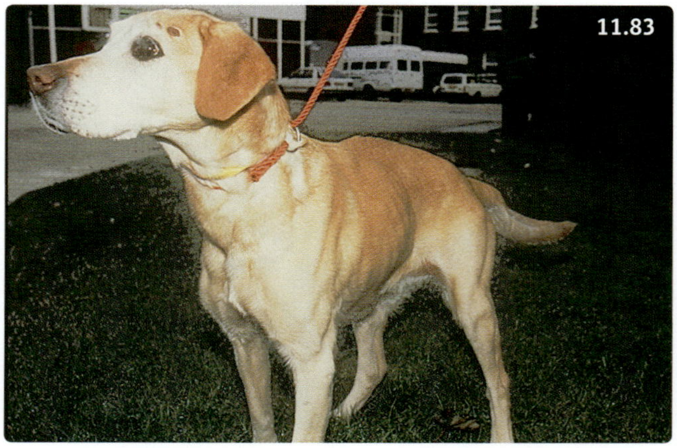

Figure 11.83 A 12-year-old Labrador Retriever with diabetes mellitus. Note the weight loss.

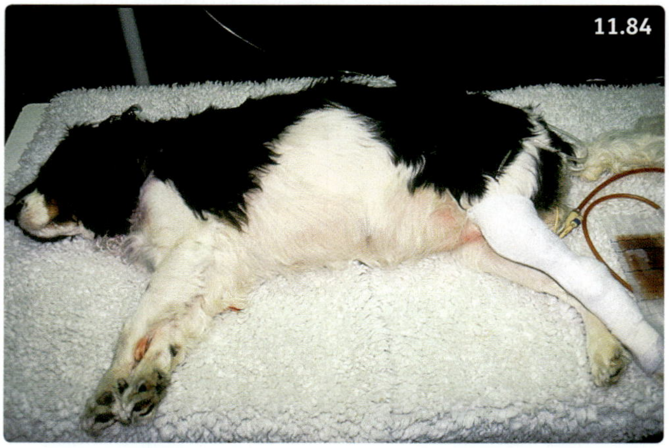

Figure 11.84 A 3-year-old Cavalier King Charles Spaniel in a diabetic ketoacidotic coma.

Diagnosis

Urinalysis reveals persistent glycosuria and often ketonuria. Despite the high solute load in the urine, which would tend to increase the SG of the urine, many older dogs and cats may have impaired renal concentrating power and thus the SG of the urine is variable, typically between 1.015 and 1.045. Bacterial cystitis is common and occasionally may involve gas-producing organisms, which can cause emphysematous cystitis (**Figure 11.85**).

Plasma biochemistry reveals hyperglycemia (>9 mmol/l [>162 mg/dl]) and hyperlipidemia. In some patients the blood will be lactescent due to lipemia. Liver enzymes are usually raised and liver function tests such as bile acid concentrations may be abnormal. In cases where diabetes is associated with pancreatitis, canine or feline-specific pancreatic lipase immunoreactivity may be elevated.

Diabetic ketoacidosis is often triggered by an underlying condition such as systemic inflammatory disease (pancreatitis, urinary tract infection, pyometra, or pneumonia) or a condition that causes dehydration. In diabetic ketoacidosis there are serious derangements in fluid, electrolyte, and acid–base status. The most frequent abnormalities are prerenal azotemia, hyponatremia, hypokalemia, and acidosis.

Management

Treatment can be divided into the acute management of diabetic ketoacidosis and the stabilization of the uncomplicated diabetic. The ketoacidotic dog can be stabilized as for the uncomplicated case, once it has started to feed normally.

Acute management of diabetic ketoacidosis

Although the healthy (still eating and drinking) ketotic diabetic can usually be managed conservatively without fluid therapy or intensive care, diabetic ketoacidosis characterized by hyperglycemia, ketonemia, metabolic acidosis, dehydration, and electrolyte imbalance is a medical emergency that is associated with a high mortality. Treatment should consist of replacement of fluid and electrolytes, reduction of blood glucose concentrations, correction of acidosis, and identification of precipitating causes. A treatment protocol is given in **Table 11.26**, but diagnosis and treatment of the underlying trigger is also important.

Fluid therapy

IV replacement of fluid and electrolytes is essential for the successful management of diabetic ketoacidosis. Unless serum electrolytes suggest otherwise, 0.9% sodium chloride or lactated Ringer's solution is the initial fluid of choice. The fluid deficit is usually about 10% of body weight and this should be replaced over a period of 24–48 hours. Sodium chloride may be alternated with lactated Ringer's solution or, if the blood glucose falls below 10 mmol/l (180 mg/dl), a solution containing 0.18% sodium chloride and 4% glucose (or some other comparable isotonic crystalloid–glucose solution). Urine output should be measured and, if possible, a central venous catheter used so that central venous pressure can be monitored during fluid therapy.

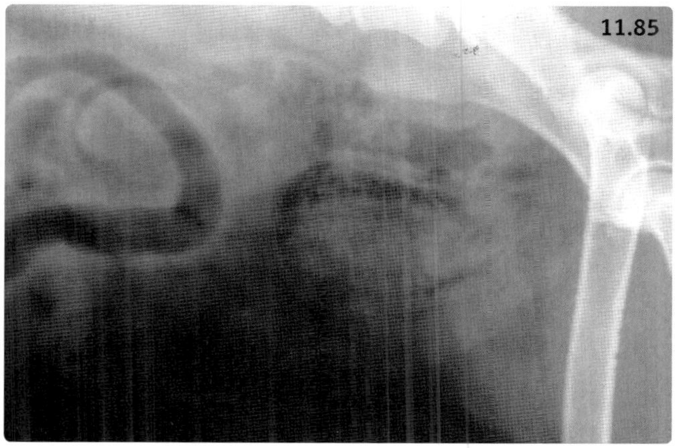

11.85

Figure 11.85 Abdominal radiograph of a diabetic dog showing emphysematous cystitis. (Courtesy M. Schaer)

Insulin therapy

Soluble insulin ('regular') should be used in the treatment of diabetic ketoacidosis. Although intermittent administration using the IV and IM routes has been used, low-dose IV insulin infusion (0.1 U/kg/hour) is effective and appears to be associated with fewer side-effects, such as hypokalemia and hypoglycemia. Low-dose IV insulin infusion provides a steady, gradual reduction in blood glucose and ketone concentrations and is less likely to cause the increases in glucagon, cortisol, and GH that can occur with intermittent bolus administration of insulin.

Blood glucose should be monitored every 2 hours. Glucose-containing fluids should be introduced when the blood glucose concentration falls below 10 mmol/l (180 mg/dl) and the insulin infusion should be stopped when the blood glucose reaches 6 mmol/l (108 mg/dl). Once the insulin infusion is halted, blood glucose concentrations will increase, so that further infusion of insulin may be required if the patient is not eating or a longer-acting insulin preparation may be introduced if its appetite has returned.

Table 11.26 Treatment protocol for diabetic ketoacidosis in the dog.

Intravenous fluid and electrolyte replacement • 0.9% sodium chloride initially then alternate with lactated Ringer's solution. Monitor urine output and, if possible, central venous pressure
Insulin therapy • Low-dose insulin infusion. Add 25 units soluble (Regular) insulin to 500 ml 0.9% sodium chloride solution or 2.5 units in a 50 ml syringe (0.05 U/ml) and infuse at a rate of 0.1 U/kg/hour through a separate IV catheter. Use of an infusion pump, syringe driver or pediatric burette is helpful in controlling the rate of infusion. Monitor blood glucose concentration every 2 hours • Soluble insulin injection. A dose of 1 U/kg is divided and one-quarter of the dose given IV and three-quarters IM. The dose is repeated every 4–6 hours. Monitor blood glucose concentration every 2 hours
Continue intravenous fluid and electrolyte replacement • Continue alternating 0.9% sodium chloride with lactated Ringer's solution while blood glucose remains >10 mmol/l (>180 mg/dl). Use 0.18% sodium chloride with 4% glucose solution when blood glucose falls to <10 mmol/l (<180 mg/dl)
Potassium supplementation • Ideally, supplementation with potassium should be based on serum potassium concentrations. In the absence of serum potassium measurements, add 20 mmol/l (20 mEq/l) of potassium chloride to each 500 ml bag of IV fluid solution. Two to three times more potassium will be necessary with potassium concentrations <3.0 mmol/l. The rate of administration should not exceed 0.5 mmol/kg/hour, although in dire circumstances (potassium <2.0 mmol/l), the rate can be increased to 1.5 mmol/kg/hour with simultaneous ECG monitoring. This treatment will be safe providing the patient has adequate urine production
Phosphate supplementation • Phosphate shifts in the same way as potassium. Hypophosphatemia is only likely to occur in severe diabetic ketoacidosis, but can be severe (<0.5 mmol/l [0.5 mEq/l]). Dose of 0.01–0.03 mmol/kg/hour of potassium phosphate in calcium-free fluid (e.g. normal saline) is required if hypophosphatemia is detected. In cases of severe hypophosphatemia, the dose may be increased to 0.12 mmol/kg/hour
Correction of acidosis • Bicarbonate therapy is not necessary provided renal function has been re-established. It is only indicated in life-threatening (pH <7.0) acidosis and only one-third of the calculated replacement dose should be used to prevent excessive blood HCO_3^- concentrations
Antibiotic therapy • If indicated

Potassium supplementation

A deficit in total body potassium is usually masked by the acidosis, which sometimes causes potassium to move extracellularly. Serum potassium concentration can decrease rapidly as renal function improves and insulin therapy causes potassium to move back into the cells. Although hypokalemia is less likely to occur with low-dose insulin infusion, replacement therapy should be started within a few hours of instigating fluid and insulin therapy. In the absence of serum potassium measurements, 20 mmol of potassium chloride should be added to every 500 ml of IV fluid solution. Insulin treatment is best delayed for several hours if the patient is initially hypokalemic in order to avoid a further lowering of the serum potassium concentration (see **Table 11.26**).

Phosphate supplementation

Phosphate moves between the intracellular and extracellular compartments in the same way as potassium. Hypophosphatemia can cause hemolytic anemia, weakness, ataxia, and seizures. Phosphate supplementation is only usually required in dogs and cats with severe diabetic ketoacidosis. Potassium phosphate (0.01–0.03 mmol/kg/hour IV) is recommended to correct hypophosphatemia.

Bicarbonate therapy

The use of sodium bicarbonate to correct the acidosis in diabetic ketoacidosis is controversial. Rapid correction of the acidosis with bicarbonate can lead to metabolic alkalosis, tissue anoxia due to a shift to the left of the hemoglobin–oxygen dissociation curve, and paradoxical cerebral acidosis because carbon dioxide crosses the blood–brain barrier more rapidly than bicarbonate ions. For these reasons, bicarbonate should be used only in life-threatening acidosis (arterial pH <7.0). Provided normal renal function is restored and adequate fluid therapy is given, the acidosis will resolve without bicarbonate administration.

Antibiotic therapy

Initially, broad-spectrum antibiotic therapy might be preferred by some clinicians because bacterial infection is a common precipitating factor for diabetic ketoacidosis and the use of IV and urinary catheters may predispose the patient to infection.

Concurrent problems

Other common concurrent illnesses in the dog and cat with diabetic ketoacidosis include pancreatitis, renal failure, CHF, hyperadrenocorticism, and pyometra. Entire bitches may be resistant to insulin therapy during the diestrus phase of their estrous cycle, thus requiring ovario-hysterectomy as soon as the patient is physiologically stable during the first 2–3 days of hospitalization.

Stabilization of uncomplicated diabetes mellitus

The primary goal of diabetes therapy is to maintain normoglycemia and thereby control the signs that occur secondary to hyperglycemia and glycosuria and result in the development of complications (**Table 11.27**). The essentials of good stabilization of diabetes mellitus require understanding by the owner and adherence to a regular daily routine that involves diet, insulin administration, and regular controlled exercise. Stabilization can be carried out satisfactorily at home but, particularly if the patient is ketotic, it may be preferable to hospitalize the animal during stabilization, since it is easier to monitor blood glucose more closely.

Most diabetic dogs are presented with complete islet cell degeneration and atrophy. Therefore, diabetes mellitus in dogs is insulin dependent. Rarely, bitches may be presented during the diestrus phase of the estrous cycle before islet cell exhaustion has occurred. If ovario-hysterectomy is performed in these patients immediately the signs of diabetes become apparent, there can be complete resolution of the disease. However, in the majority of bitches this opportunity is missed or goes unnoticed and permanent damage to the islet cells occurs.

Table 11.27 Complications associated with diabetes mellitus.

Hypoglycemia
Ketoacidosis
Cataract formation
Hepatic lipidosis
Pancreatitis
Infections
Retinopathy
Diabetic neuropathy
Diabetic nephropathy
Skin disease

While a small percentage of cats may respond to diet and oral hypoglycemic agents, principally glipizide (a sulfonylurea), it is generally considered that insulin provides better glycemic control and, therefore, more chance of attaining diabetic remission. Remission of diabetes in cats usually occurs within 1 month of beginning insulin therapy, but can occur as late as 6–8 months after the start of treatment.

Dietary therapy

Appropriate dietary therapy is an essential part of the management of diabetes. The diet must be well-balanced and constant in both composition and the amount fed at each meal. It is therefore most convenient to use a commercial diet. Canned or dry foods that contain digestible complex carbohydrates should be fed, as slow digestion minimizes the fluctuations in postprandial blood glucose concentrations. Semi-moist foods containing a predominance of easily assimilated carbohydrates in the form of disaccharides and propylene glycol should be avoided because of marked postprandial hyperglycemia. There is evidence that diets with a high-fiber content improve glycemic control by delaying starch hydrolysis and glucose absorption, thereby reducing postprandial fluctuations in blood glucose. High-fiber diets are also beneficial in correcting obesity. However, there may be disadvantages in using high-fiber diets (e.g. reduced palatability and the fact that the low caloric density may cause patients to lose excessive weight or fail to gain weight if already below ideal body weight). The author tends to reserve high-fiber diets for those patients that are difficult to stabilize and/or are obese.

Correction of obesity and minimizing the impact of the diet on postprandial blood glucose concentrations are also important dietary considerations in diabetic cats. Following weight reduction, glycemic control often improves and, in some cats, remission of diabetes may occur. Although high-fiber diets have been used in cats with diabetes, palatability can prove a problem. More recently, high-protein, low-carbohydrate diets have been used in the management of feline diabetes. Since cats are strict carnivores and maintain their blood glucose mainly through gluconeogenesis from amino acids, these diets produce a more stable blood glucose level and insulin requirements are reduced.

Finally, the feeding schedule should be designed to enhance the action of insulin and minimize postprandial hyperglycemia. The daily caloric intake should occur when insulin is present in the circulation and capable of handling glucose absorbed from the intestine. Several small meals are preferable to one large feed, as these will help minimize postprandial hyperglycemia and thus help to control fluctuations in blood glucose. The author routinely recommends two equal meals fed at times to coincide with insulin activity. In cases that prove difficult to stabilize, 3–4 smaller meals are fed during the day. Titbits and scavenging must be avoided as they tend to destabilize diabetic patients.

Insulin therapy

For routine stabilization in the dog, insulin zinc suspension (lente), which contains a mixture of 30% insulin zinc suspension (amorphous) and 70% insulin zinc suspension (crystalline), is the preparation of choice in the UK. When given by subcutaneous injection it is an intermediate-acting insulin with an onset of activity at 1–2 hours, peak activity around 6–12 hours, and a duration of action of between 18 and 26 hours in the dog. The times for peak activity and duration of action vary with the individual, but in some dogs once daily administration is adequate, although in the majority of cases twice daily administation is required to maintain good glycemic control. In the USA, most clinicians use NPH insulin, which has a shorter duration of action, and administer it to diabetic dogs in a divided twice daily dosage.

Cats tend to metabolize insulin more quickly than dogs; therefore, a long-acting insulin such as protamine zinc insulin is often recommended if once daily dosing is to be tried, although PZI is often administered twice daily as with other intermediate to long-acting insulins. However many clinicians use twice daily dosing with lente insulin to gain good glycemic control. Insulin glargine, a long-acting insulin analog, has been used in cats with encouraging results (a dose of 0.25–0.5 U/kg q24h or q12h has been recommended). Insulin glargine forms microprecipitates at the site of injection from which small amounts of insulin are slowly released.

Lente insulin can be given as a single morning injection at the same time as or just before the first meal, with the second meal given 6–8 hours later to coincide with peak insulin activity. However, because of the frequency of hypoglycemia associated with once daily treatment, the lente insulin can also be given in a divided twice daily treatment protocol (see below). An initial dose of between 0.5 and 1.0 U/kg is used. Insulin is probably best dosed on body surface area rather than a simple weight basis. Thus, small dogs (<15 kg) tend to require 1.0 U/kg and larger dogs (>25 kg) receive 0.5 U/kg. Although the subcutaneous route is ideal for long-term use, the intramuscular route may be used initially, especially in dehydrated or 'healthy' ketotic animals, because absorption from subcutaneous depots in these patients may be slow and erratic. Regular insulin can also be given by the intramuscular or intravenous route.

Insulin should be administered using specific 0.3, 0.5, or 1.0 ml syringes calibrated in units (100 U/ml or 40 U/ml depending on the concentration of the preparation). Insulin preparations should be stored in a refrigerator at 2–8°C (35.6–46.4°F) because they are adversely affected by heat or freezing. Preparations should be rolled gently to resuspend the particles before use. A diabetic patient will usually take 2–4 days to respond fully to a dose of insulin or a change in preparation. It is important to avoid increasing the dose too quickly before equilibration has occurred, as this can lead to a sudden and precipitous fall in blood glucose due to overdosage with insulin. In most cases, adjustments in the insulin dose should be made in small changes of 1–4 units per injection, depending on the size of the patient and the severity of the hyperglycemia. The type of preparation and frequency of administration may require alteration in those patients that prove difficult to stabilize with this standard routine. However, it is good for the clinician to become familiar with one type of insulin preparation and only change from that preparation if the insulin is the cause of the instability.

The standard routine for a dog would be:

8.00 am	Give lente insulin injection SC
8.30 am	Feed half of the measured daily ration
2.30 pm	Feed second half of the daily ration

for once daily treatment (although administering the insulin in divided doses SC is recommended) and:

8.00 am	Give lente insulin injection subcutaneously
8.30 am	Feed half of the measured daily ration
8.00 pm	Give lente insulin injection subcutaneously
8.30 pm	Feed second half of the measured daily ration for twice daily treatment.

Keep the daily routine constant, including exercise; avoid titbits and scavenging.

Monitoring therapy

Ideally, monitoring should consist of serial blood glucose concentrations, as tighter diabetic control can be gained than with urine glucose estimations. Initially, at least two blood glucose estimations should be made, one before insulin is administered and the second just before the second feed. Once the patient appears fairly stable, more frequent blood samples should be taken throughout the day to assess the degree of stabilization. An assessment of daily water intake can also provide useful information about the degree of diabetic control.

Blood glucose concentrations should ideally be maintained at between 5 and 9 mmol/l (90 and 162 mg/dl) (**Figure 11.86**). The blood glucose concentration will usually be highest in the morning before insulin is administered and lowest just before the second feed. A trace of glucose in the morning urine sample may be acceptable, but the urine should be negative at other times in the day. However, it is important to remember that urine glucose may not reflect the blood glucose concentration at the same point in time and, if the urine glucose is negative, the blood glucose concentration could be hypoglycemic (<3.0 mmol/l [<54 mg/dl]), normoglycemic, or hyperglycemic (>5.5 mmol/l [>99 mg/dl]). Although the author's clients monitor urine for glucose and ketones regularly, he does not advocate adjusting daily insulin dosages on the basis of morning urine glucose measurements. Instead, he prefers to continue with a fixed insulin dosage unless the patient remains unstable for more than several days.

Measurement of glycated proteins such as fructosamine and glycosylated Hgb are used increasingly in the dog and cat to monitor the response to treatment. The irreversible, nonenzymatic glycation process occurs throughout the life span of the protein, mainly albumin in the case of fructosamine, and is proportional to the glucose concentration over that time. These measurements reflect the average blood glucose concentration over the preceding 1–2 weeks in the case of serum fructosamine and 2–3 months in the case of glycosylated Hgb. Fructosamine concentrations <400 mmol/l indicate good glycemic control, whereas concentrations >500 mmol/l are found in newly diagnosed or poorly controlled diabetics. Glycosylated Hgb is less routinely available as an assay. Well-controlled diabetic dogs have between 4% and 6% glycosylated Hgb, whereas poorly controlled diabetics have concentrations >7%.

Diabetic records (**Figure 11.87**) should be kept by the owner for each patient, as alterations to stability can be assessed more easily over a period of time. Insulin requirements will be increased by infection, estrus (particularly the metestrus phase of the cycle), pregnancy, and ketoacidosis. It is therefore recommended that entire bitches should undergo ovariohysterectomy in order to avoid insulin resistance at subsequent seasons.

Investigation of instability

If a patient appears to be poorly stabilized at home despite repeated attempts to provide adequate glycemic control, the diabetic record should be checked and the patient examined for signs of disease that could cause insulin resistance (e.g. infection, estrus, pregnancy, ketoacidosis, hyperadrenocorticism, or acromegaly). The daily routine should be discussed with the owner to make sure that the diet is constant and measured and that there is no access to titbits or scavenging. The insulin preparation should be checked for type, expiry date, and storage, as should the ability of the owner to administer the insulin (adequate mixing, correct dosage, and injection technique).

If an obvious cause cannot be determined, the patient should be hospitalized on its daily routine and serial blood glucose determinations made every 1–2 hours throughout the day. Determinations made with glucose

11.86

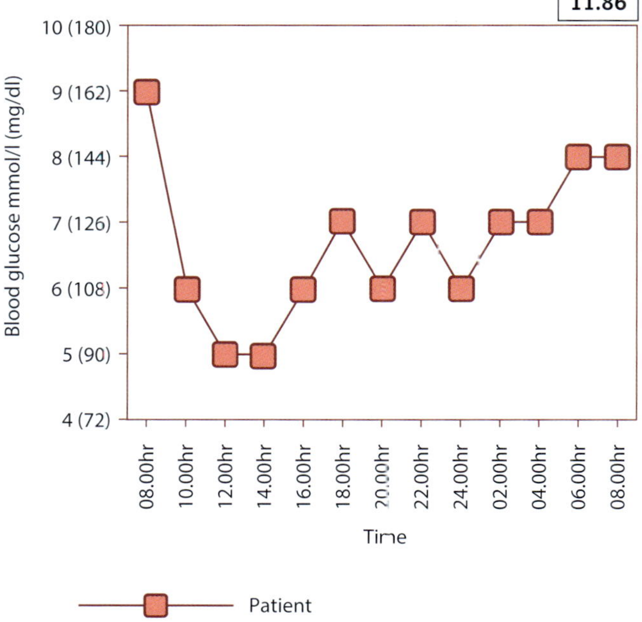

Figure 11.86 Ideal blood glucose curve.

11.87

Date	Urine exam	Insulin dose & time of injection	Food	Drink	Body weight	Blood results	Note
15 March	am glucose-ve ketones-ve	18 units lente insulin s.c. 8.00 am	3/4 tin Dogga 8.30 am 2.30 pm	0.9 L	24 kg	2.00 pm blood glucose 4.6 mmol/l	Bright and alert

Figure 11.87 Diabetic record.

reagent strips and a glucose meter are simple, fast, and sufficiently accurate for this purpose. Some owners are prepared to record these measurements at home environment, which is useful as it provides a more realistic assessment of the patient in its own home environment. The use of a continuous glucose monitoring system has proved useful but is more expensive. The results should then be plotted on a graph against time, although it is important to realize that precise glucose curves may vary from day to day in any diabetic patient.

Three major causes of instability can be deduced from the graph of serial blood glucose determinations:

- The first is insulin-induced hyperglycemia, also called the Somogyi overswing, where excessive insulin dosage leads to paradoxical hyperglycemia (**Figure 11.88**). The blood glucose concentration is high in the morning before insulin is given, but falls sharply to hypoglycemic concentrations (<3.5 mmol/l [<63.1 mg/dl]) after insulin administration. The hypoglycemic period is short in duration and is not associated with signs of hypoglycemia. In fact, the nadir can easily be missed if frequent sampling is not performed. The low blood glucose concentration stimulates the release of hormones antagonistic to insulin (e.g. glucagon, cortisol, and catecholamines), and these cause the glucose concentration to rebound quickly to high levels. If blood glucose and/or urine glucose concentrations were measured only before insulin and before the second feed, the concentrations would be high and this could easily be misinterpreted as a reason for increasing the daily insulin dose, when in fact the patient is already being overdosed. The treatment for insulin-induced hyperglycemia is to reduce the daily dose of insulin in order to prevent the hypoglycemia that causes the dramatic swing in blood glucose concentrations.
- The second cause of instability is due to rapid metabolism of insulin, which means that an intermediate-acting insulin preparation does not last for a full 24 hours (**Figure 11.89**). In such cases the blood glucose concentration is high in the morning before insulin is given, but falls to normal levels for much of the day. However, after the second feed the blood glucose concentration rises and remains high for the remainder of the day. This leads to a considerable period of hyperglycemia and results in glycosuria in the morning and often nocturnal polydipsia and polyuria. The treatment for rapid insulin metabolism is either to try a longer-acting insulin preparation (e.g. protamine zinc insulin or insulin glargine [**Note:** Ultralente is no longer available in the USA]) or to administer two doses of lente insulin 12 hours apart, with two meals

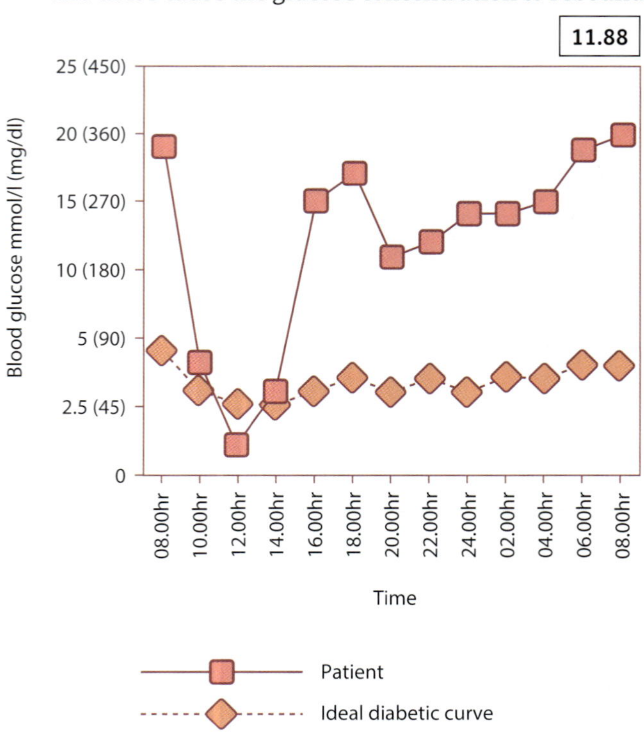

Figure 11.88 Insulin-induced hyperglycemia (Somogyi overswing).

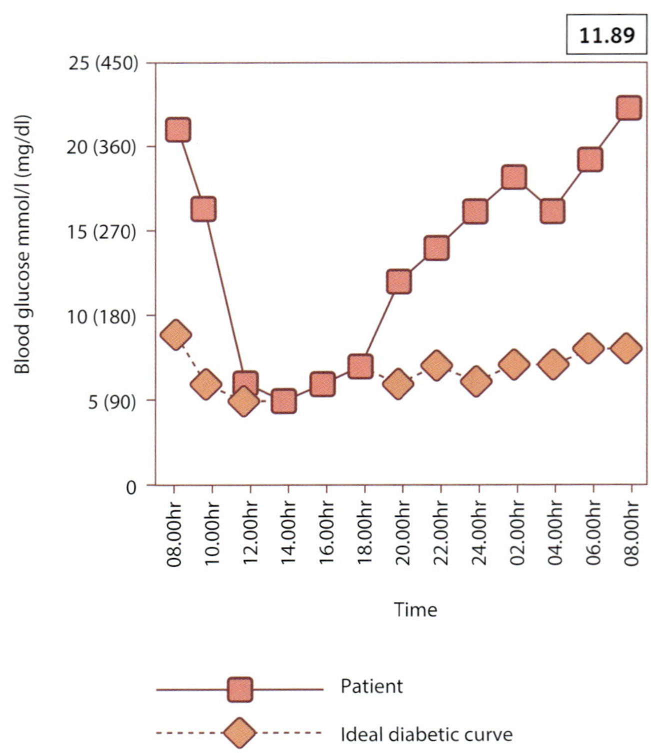

Figure 11.89 Rapid metabolism of insulin.

at the time of injection or four small meals given at approximately 6-hour intervals.

- The third cause of instability is associated with insulin resistance. In these cases the animal remains persistently hyperglycemic despite an insulin dosage of more than 2.2 U/kg/day (**Figure 11.90**). Although some patients can be stabilized satisfactorily at doses higher than this, peripheral antagonism to insulin activity is likely to be present. In cases where adequate stabilization is not possible, a thorough investigation of the patient is required to try and identify the precise cause of the insulin resistance. Some of the causes of insulin resistance are listed in **Table 11.28**. Correction or treatment of the underlying cause will usually enable the patient to be stabilized at a lower dose of insulin with improved glycemic control.

INSULINOMA

Definition/overview

Functional islet cell tumors (insulinomas) are the most frequently occurring tumors of the endocrine pancreas in dogs. Most insulin-secreting tumors are malignant islet cell carcinomas that metastasize to regional lymph nodes and/or the liver. Early diagnosis is important, as dogs with metastases have significantly reduced survival times.

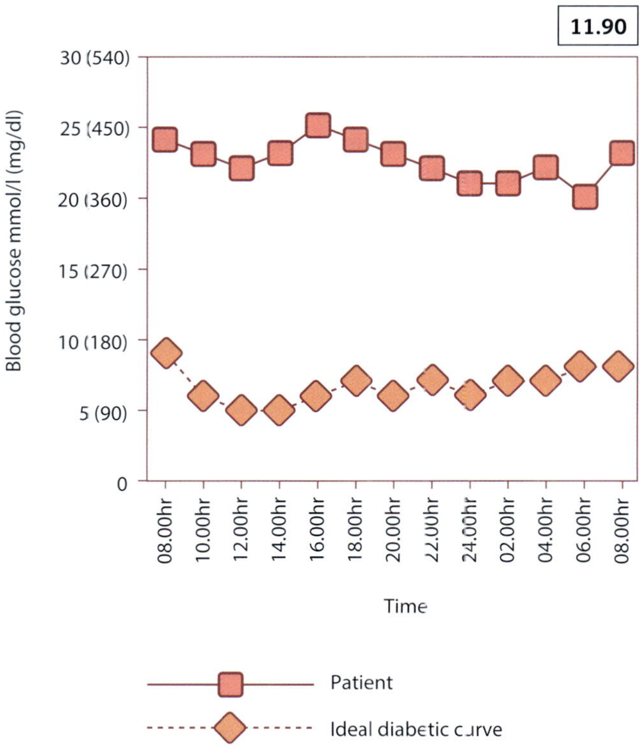

Figure 11.90 Insulin resistance.

Etiology

Causes of episodic weakness (**Table 11.24**), causes of hypoglycemia in adults (**Table 11.29**).

Pathophysiology

Insulinomas release insulin despite the presence of hypoglycemia. Hypoglycemia is normally the major inhibitory stimulus for insulin secretion. As a result of hyperinsulinism, tissue utilization of glucose continues, the hypoglycemia worsens, and ultimately clinical signs develop. The onset and severity of clinical signs are determined by the degree of hypoglycemia and the rate at which the plasma concentration of glucose falls. A rapid decline in plasma glucose concentration may occur with fasting, exercise, or excitement in dogs with insulinomas. The brain is an obligate consumer of glucose. Cerebral cells have limited stores of glycogen and a limited ability to utilize protein and amino acids for energy. These cells will be the first

Table 11.28 Causes of insulin resistance.

Obesity
Hyperadrenocorticism
Exogenous glucocorticoid administration
Metestrus phase of the estrous cycle
Exogenous progestogen administration
Acromegaly
Hypothyroidism
Hyperthyroidism
Impaired absorption of insulin
Excessive insulin antibody formation
Pheochromocytoma
Glucagonoma

Table 11.29 Differential diagnosis of hypoglycemia in dogs.

Incorrect anticoagulant/delayed separation of serum from red blood cells
Functional islet cell tumor (insulinoma)
Excessive insulin administration
Extrapancreatic tumors, particularly hepatic tumors
Liver disease
Septicemic or endotoxic shock
Hypoadrenocorticism
Idiopathic hypoglycemia in working dogs
Severe polycythemia

affected by hypoglycemia. Prolonged and profound hypoglycemia causes ischemic neuronal cell damage.

Hypoglycemia is a potent stimulus for the release of hormones that have an antagonistic action to insulin. These include glucagon, GH, glucocorticoids, catecholamines, and possibly thyroid hormones. These hormones act in concert to raise the plasma glucose concentration. Some of the clinical manifestations of hypoglycemia, such as muscle tremors, nervousness, restlessness, and hunger, may in fact result from stimulation of the sympathetic nervous system and increased levels of circulating catecholamines.

Clinical presentation

Insulinomas usually occur in middle aged to older dogs (mean age of 9 years) of any breed, although medium to large breeds appear to be predisposed. No sex predisposition has been reported. Insulinomas appear to be very rare in cats. A tentative diagnosis of hyperinsulinism is generally based on fulfilment of the criteria from Whipple's triad:

1. The presence of neurologic signs typical of hypoglycemia, which may be precipitated by exercise or excitement.
2. Hypoglycemia (plasma glucose <3 mmol/l [<54 mg/dl]) at the time of the clinical signs.
3. Resolution of clinical signs following feeding or administration of intravenous glucose.

Clinical signs associated with hypoglycemia include fatigue, generalized weakness, collapse, muscle tremors, altered behavior, confusion/disorientation, apparent blindness, ataxia, incoordination, stupor, and seizures. These signs are usually episodic in nature and may occur with fasting, exercise, or excitement in dogs with insulinomas. Provocative stimuli, such as IV administration of glucagon or glucose, result in excessive secretion of insulin from neoplastic beta cells. This response may be even greater if glucose is administered orally, as numerous intestinal hormones (glucagon, secretin, cholecystokinin, gastrin, and gastric inhibitory peptide) are secreted in response to oral glucose and these in turn increase insulin secretion. It is by this mechanism that feeding has been reported to initiate clinical signs in dogs with insulinomas.

Seizure activity is one of the most common clinical manifestations of hypoglycemia. The seizures may be grand mal or focal in nature and are normally self-limiting, lasting between 30 seconds and 5 minutes. Peripheral neuropathy with nerve degeneration and demyelination has also been associated with canine insulinoma in a few cases. Insulinomas are generally small tumors and do not lead to malignant cachexia. Thus weight loss is not a feature of this disease.

Diagnosis

Laboratory findings

A presumptive diagnosis of insulinoma is based on the presence of typical clinical signs in association with persistent hypoglycemia and an inappropriately high plasma insulin concentration. A fasting plasma glucose concentration of 3 mmol/l (54 mg/dl) or less is found in most cases. Some dogs with insulinoma show no clinical signs despite having extremely low blood glucose concentrations (<2 mmol/l [<36 mg/dl]) because they are able to adapt to these low concentrations over a prolonged period of time. Serum fructosamine concentrations are also reduced (<250 µmol/l), supporting substantial periods of hypoglycemia even in those patients with normal or low-normal fasting blood glucose concentrations.

Plasma insulin concentrations greater than 20 mU/l in association with hypoglycemia are inappropriate and an insulin:glucose ratio >4.2 is considered diagnostic.

In borderline cases an IV glucose tolerance test using 0.5 g glucose/kg body weight has proved useful. Insulin-secreting tumors retain a degree of responsiveness to the glucose challenge; a glucose half-life of <20 minutes and/or a fractional clearance rate of more than 3%/minute is highly suggestive of insulinoma in the dog.

Although hypoalbuminemia, hypokalemia, and increases in serum ALP concentrations have occasionally been reported, these findings are not specific or helpful in achieving a definitive diagnosis.

Ultrasonography

Abdominal ultrasonography using a high-quality diagnostic ultrasound machine has been used to examine the pancreas of dogs with suspected insulinomas. Most insulinomas are quite small (<4 cm) and are isoechoic when compared with the surrounding pancreatic tissue. In one study a pancreatic mass was identified as a spherical or lobular hypoechoic nodule in 75% of dogs with insulinomas (**Figure 11.91**). Tumors as small as 7 mm have been identified in the pancreas. However, ultrasonography has proved less sensitive compared with CT for the detection of hepatic or lymphatic metastases from insulinomas.

Management

Management of insulinomas should be directed at specific treatment of the tumor, reduction of insulin secretion, and correction of hypoglycemia. Sometimes, IV glucagon is needed to increase the blood glucose to desirably safe levels. The initial glucagon dose is 50.0 ng/kg as an IV bolus followed with a maintenance dose of 5–10 ng/kg/minute.

Surgical management

Surgical resection of the pancreatic tumor and metastatic tumor masses should be the first approach to therapy (**Figure 11.92–11.94**). Most insulinomas are located in the left lobe of the pancreas, with masses in the right lobe or body occurring less frequently. Tumors are usually solitary, but multiple masses may occur. Rarely, there is a diffuse islet cell tumor with no discrete nodule. There does not appear to be a difference in survival in relation to tumor location within the pancreas, but there is a suggestion that tumors with a high mitotic count carry a worse prognosis.

Postoperative recovery is routine in many cases, but complications including pancreatitis, hyperglycemia, overt diabetes mellitus, and hypoglycemia occur. In nearly all cases, hypoglycemia will recur eventually due to metastasis.

Medical management

Medical management should be used if widespread metastasis is present or if hypoglycemia recurs after surgery. This should consist of dietary control (frequent small meals of a diet high in proteins, fats, and complex carbohydrates) and the use of prednisolone, which inhibits insulin and stimulates glycogenolysis, and diazoxide,

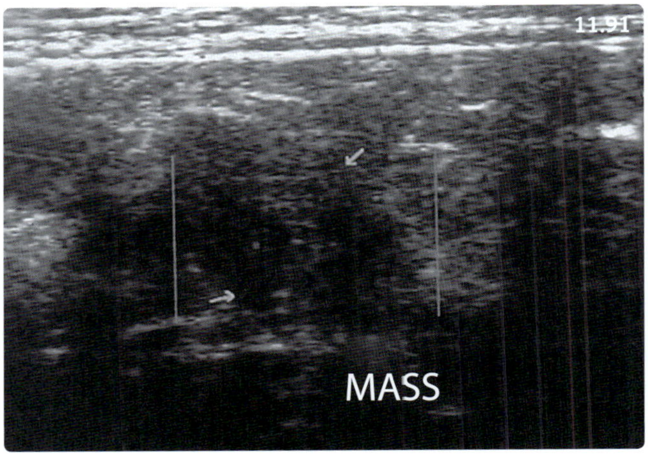

Figure 11.91 Ultrasonogram of the pancreas of a crossbred dog showing a hypoechoic mass, which proved to be an insulinoma on histology.

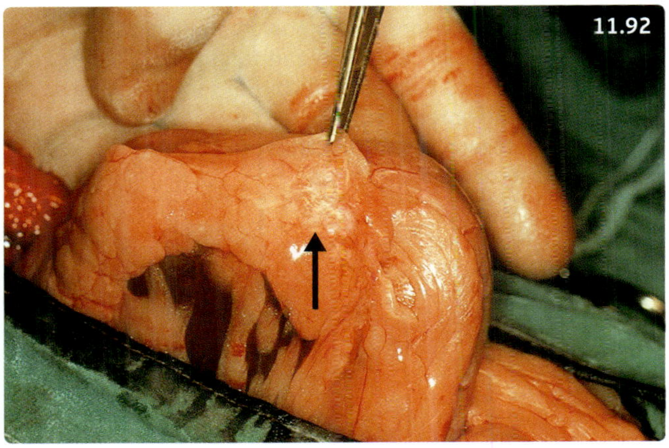

Figure 11.92 An insulinoma being pointed out at surgery (arrow).

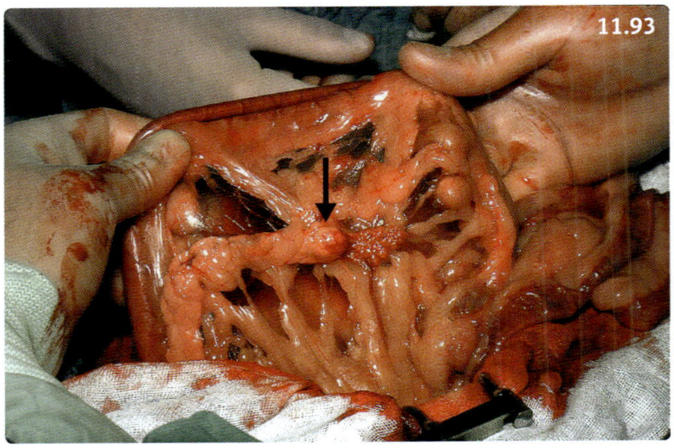

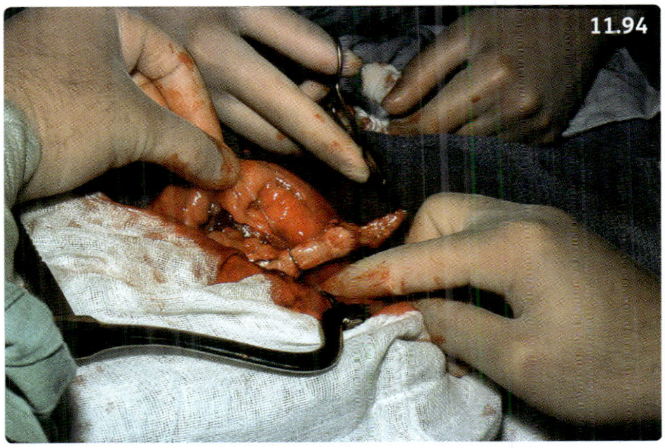

Figure 11.93, 11.94 Surgical view of an insulinoma before (arrow) and during its ligation for removal. (Courtesy M. Schaer)

Table 11.30 Management of hypoglycemia.

- In acute hypoglycemic crisis, give 1 ml/kg of a 40–50% glucose solution by slow IV injection or, if the animal is still conscious, provide a meal containing glucose. Glucose administration is an emergency treatment and cannot be used for long-term control
- Management of chronic hypoglycemia requires a combination of therapies:
  - Diet: feed small meals high in protein and low in simple sugars 5–6 times daily
  - Exercise should be restricted
  - Diabetogenic drugs:
    - Glucocorticoids: prednisolone (0.5–1 mg/kg daily in divided doses)
    - Diazoxide, a nondiuretic benzothiadiazine antihypertensive drug that acts by suppressing insulin secretion (10 mg/kg in divided doses increasing up to 60 mg/kg daily if necessary)
    - Octreotide, a long-acting somatostatin analog that inhibits insulin synthesis and secretion (10–20 µg SC q12h or q8h). Only effective in some dogs. Close monitoring required
    - Streptozotocin and alloxan are nephrotoxic and not recommended

a nondiuretic, benzothiadiazine antihypertensive drug that inhibits insulin secretion (**Table 11.30**). Octreotide, a somatostatin analog that inhibits insulin synthesis and secretion, has also been used and has been shown to be effective in some cases.

The prognosis is guarded due to the malignant nature of the disease. However, many dogs do well with medical and surgical management. The median time to recurrence of clinical signs after surgery is 12 months (range 4–16 months) and the median postoperative survival time is 14 months (range 10–33 months).

RECOMMENDED FURTHER READING

Ettinger SJ, Feldman EC (2010) (eds.) *Textbook of Veterinary Internal Medicine*, 7th edn. Elsevier Saunders, St Louis.

Feldman EC, Nelson RW, Reusch C *et al.* (2015) (eds.) *Canine and Feline Endocrinology and Reproduction*, 4th edn. Elsevier, St Louis.

Mooney CT, Peterson ME (2012) (eds.) *BSAVA Manual of Endocrinology*, 4th edn. British Small Animal Veterinary Association, Gloucester.

Rijnberk A, Kooistra HS (2010) (eds.) *Clinical Endocrinology of Dogs and Cats*, 2nd edn. Schluetersche, Germany.

Chapter 12

Nephrology/urology

Mark J. Acierno

INTRODUCTION

The kidneys are responsible for maintaining the body's fluid and electrolyte balance, filtering metabolic waste, and performing several hormonal functions. Reduced renal function manifests itself in several ways including increased blood levels of blood urea nitrogen (BUN) and creatinine. The increase in these nitrogenous compounds is referred to as azotemia. Uremia refers to the constellation of clinical signs that results from azotemia and includes vomiting, lethargy, anorexia, diarrhea, oral ulcerations, and uremic breath.

Azotemia is categorized by its underlying cause. This is clinically important because not all azotemia is the result of actual renal disease. Prerenal and postrenal factors can result in increased levels of nitrogenous compounds despite otherwise healthy kidneys.

- **Prerenal azotemia** is the result of decreased kidney perfusion in the absence of existing renal disease or injury. Decreased renal blood flow leads to a reduction in glomerular filtration and a compensatory activation of the renin–angiotensin–aldosterone system. The ensuing increase in tubular sodium reabsorption and antidiuretic hormone-induced water reabsorption leads to production of low sodium concentrated urine. Clinically, this is important, as the hallmark of prerenal azotemia is mild to moderate azotemia with an increased urine specific gravity (USG). Treatment of the underlying condition (**Table 12.1**) will often lead to resolution of clinical signs with no residual renal compromise.
- **Postrenal azotemia** can result from either an obstruction in urine outflow or leakage of urine into the abdomen. With a urinary obstruction, the blockage causes increased pressure proximal to the impasse. This results in increased hydrostatic pressure in Bowman's capsule and decreased glomerular filtration rate (GFR). This is most commonly observed in urethral obstructions since single ureteral obstructions leave one kidney functioning normally; however, azotemia can occur with unilateral ureteral obstructions if a patient has pre-existing kidney disease. A rupture of the urinary tract results in the accumulation of fluid in the abdomen. Because urea is highly diffusible, it is quickly resorbed back into circulation while creatinine, which is not diffusible, becomes trapped in the fluid. Patients who experience a rupture of the urinary tract develop an accumulation of fluid that has a BUN comparable to serum plasma but a creatinine that is elevated.
- **Renal azotemia** is a direct result of renal parenchymal disease.

Table 12.1 Causes of prerenal azotemia.

Hypotension	Anesthesia Dehydration Hypoadrenocorticism (Addison's disease) Hemorrhage
Hypoperfusion	Cardiac disease
Thrombosis	Renal artery or vein obstruction

Because of differing etiology, prognosis, and treatment, primary renal disease is classified clinically into acute kidney injury (AKI) or chronic kidney disease (CKD) and histologically as glomerular or tubular disease.

Differentiation between AKI and CKD is important in determining etiology, prognosis, and treatment options (**Table 12.2**). Immediate intervention and aggressive therapy are more likely to produce clinical recovery in AKI since underlying causes may be identified and treated. In addition, if significant numbers of nephrons are unaffected, these will undergo hypertrophy and compensate for the damaged ones. Lastly, damaged nephrons are capable of recovering from some insults if given sufficient time.

It is unlikely that a treatable cause of kidney disease will be identified in the CKD patient. Also, it is doubtful

Table 12.2 Differentiation of acute kidney injury (AKI) and chronic kidney disease (CKD).

	AKI	CKD
History	Exposure to toxins or drugs Acute illness Ischemic episode	PU/PD for some time Anorexia Weight loss over extended period
Body condition	Normal	Thin/emaciated
Renal size (radiography/ ultrasound)	Normal/increased	Small and irregular
Packed cell volume	Normal/increased	Anemia
Acidosis	Moderate/severe	Moderate
Serum potassium	Normal/increased	Normal/ decreased
Osteodystrophy	None	Some cases (rubber jaw)

that remaining nephrons have additional compensatory capacity and there is little hope for nephron repair. Treatment in the CKD patient is more directed toward supportive care. Although differentiation between the two conditions is essential, there is no single test to discriminate between the two. Diagnosis is made based on a combination of history, clinical signs, physical examination findings, and diagnostic tests.

ACUTE KIDNEY INJURY

Definition/overview

AKI is a condition characterized by a rapidly progressive impairment in the kidney's ability to filter metabolic waste, as well as maintain the body's fluid and electrolyte balance.

Etiology

AKI is the result of damage that can be caused by ischemia, nephrotoxins, infectious agents, or systemic disease (**Table 12.3**). In companion animal medicine, AKI is most commonly the result of exposure to toxins and infectious agents.

Pathophysiology

There are many specific mechanisms by which the kidney can be injured. The pathophysiology of the most common causes of renal failure can be found in **Table 12.4**.

Table 12.3 Common causes of acute kidney injury.

Nephrotoxins	Ethylene glycol Toxic plants (e.g. lilies [cats]; grapes [dogs]) Melamine Jerky treats (cause undetermined) NSAIDs Aminoglycosides Amphotericin B Cisplatin and carboplatin Cyclosporin
Infectious agents	Leptospirosis Rocky Mountain spotted fever Ehrlichiosis Babesiosis Leishmaniasis Pyelonephritis
Systemic disease	Heat stroke
Ischemia	Hypotension (e.g. anesthetic induced)

Development of azotemia after an insult to the kidney is dependent on a combination of four features:

1. Injury decreases glomerular permeability (**Figure 12.1**) and causes vasoconstriction (**Figure 12.2**). This directly reduces GFR and ultrafiltrate production. Filtration of the blood significantly decreases.
2. As a result of the injury, dead epithelial cells, cellular debris, and proteins are discarded into the tubular lumen and form obstructive casts (**Figure 12.3**). Ethylene glycol exposure results in calcium oxalate crystals precipitating and causing tubular obstruction. Lastly, acute swelling and inflammation of the damaged renal parenchyma externally compresses renal tubules. These obstructive forces increase hydrostatic pressure within Bowman's capsule and arrest glomerular filtration.
3. The death of tubular epithelial cells leaves areas of the tubules with no barrier to prevent diffusion of electrolytes and fluids (**Figure 12.4**). Thus, up to 50% of glomerular filtrate can be lost to 'back leak', and urea, creatinine, electrolytes, and fluids undergoing glomerular filtration fail to be excreted.
4. For reasons that are not entirely clear, toxic and ischemic insults are often followed by a period of intrarenal vasoconstriction. This decreases the blood flow delivered to the glomerulus, leading to a decrease in GFR, and affects blood supply to the entire kidney. The resulting hypoxia is most profound in the S3

Table 12.4 Mechanism for common causes of acute kidney injury.

Ethylene glycol	Used as an anti-freeze in cars (prohibited in some countries) Toxic dose: 1.4 ml/kg in cats; 4.4 ml/kg in dogs Ethylene glycol is broken down in the liver by a series of oxidative steps. Several of the ethylene glycol metabolites are directly toxic to renal epithelial cells. One of the metabolites, oxalate, leads to the formation of calcium oxalate crystals within the tubules
Leptospirosis	Zoonotic disease. Caused by a number of antigenically distinct serovars of the bacteria *Leptospira* Maintained in the wild by asymptomatic wild animals (hosts), which shed the bacteria in urine. Infection occurs when leptospires penetrate mucous membranes or broken skin. Renal tubular epithelial cells become colonized resulting in interstitial lymphoplasmacytic inflammation
NSAIDs	Block the cyclo-oxygenase pathway preventing the formation of locally protective prostaglandins in the kidney. Activation of the renin–angiotensin system leads to vasoconstriction in the glomerular capillary bed. As the arterioles constrict, blood flow out of the glomerulus and into peritubular capillaries decreases. If left unchecked, the resulting decreased blood flow to the medulla of the kidney leads to ischemic injury. Suppression of the renin–angiotensin system by IV fluid therapy can help prevent this vasoconstriction
Cholecalciferol-based rodenticides	Cholecalciferol is metabolized to calcitriol, the active form of vitamin D. Calcitriol increases intestinal absorption, stimulates bone resorption, and encourages renal tubular reabsorption of calcium. This can lead to soft tissue (e.g. kidney) mineralization
Lilium and *Hemerocallis* (true lilies)	Lilies of the genera *Lilium* and *Hemerocallis* (e.g. Easter lilies, tiger lilies) are extraordinarily nephrotoxic; however, the mechanism of toxicity is not known. It is important to note that not all 'lilies' are members of this group. Peruvian and peace lilies are examples of plants that are not toxic
Grapes/raisins	The mechanism of toxicity is not known; however, it does not appear to be related to heavy metals, pesticides, or mycotoxins. Ingestion has been shown to cause acute tubular necrosis of the proximal tubule

(straight) segment of the proximal convoluted tubule (PCT) and the ascending loop of Henle, where metabolic activity is quite high and blood supply is limited. This can lead to further permanent nephron loss.

Clinical presentation

General

Clinical signs of AKI are somewhat dependent on the underlying cause, severity of the azotemia, and electrolyte imbalances. Clinical signs that are often noted include depression, weakness, dehydration, anorexia, vomiting, diarrhea, uremic breath, oral ulcers (**Figures 12.5, 12.6**), and hypothermia.

Ethylene glycol specific

Ethylene glycol is an alcohol that does not become toxic until metabolized by the liver. Early clinical signs are due to the alcohol's effect on the central nervous system (CNS) and include ataxia, proprioceptive deficits, muscle tremors, nausea, vomiting, and seizures. Polyuria and polydipsia are common because ethylene glycol and its metabolites have a diuretic effect. Since it is potentially treatable in the early stages, ethylene glycol exposure should be considered in every dog with acute unexplained neurologic signs.

Differential diagnosis

Prerenal azotemia, postrenal azotemia, CKD.

Diagnosis

Determining the likely underlying cause of the kidney injury is critical in accessing prognosis as well as for developing an appropriate treatment plan. The importance of the client interview cannot be overemphasized. Questions should focus on possible exposure to environmental nephrotoxins (e.g. ethylene glycol, cholecalciferol-based rodenticides), household toxins (lilies, grape products), current medications (both human and pet), and recent travel history. Often, travel will expose a patient to diseases not commonly encountered in the local environment.

Once the presence of azotemia (increased BUN, creatinine, and phosphorus) is confirmed, possible differential diagnoses (prerenal azotemia, postrenal azotemia, and CKD) must be eliminated from consideration.

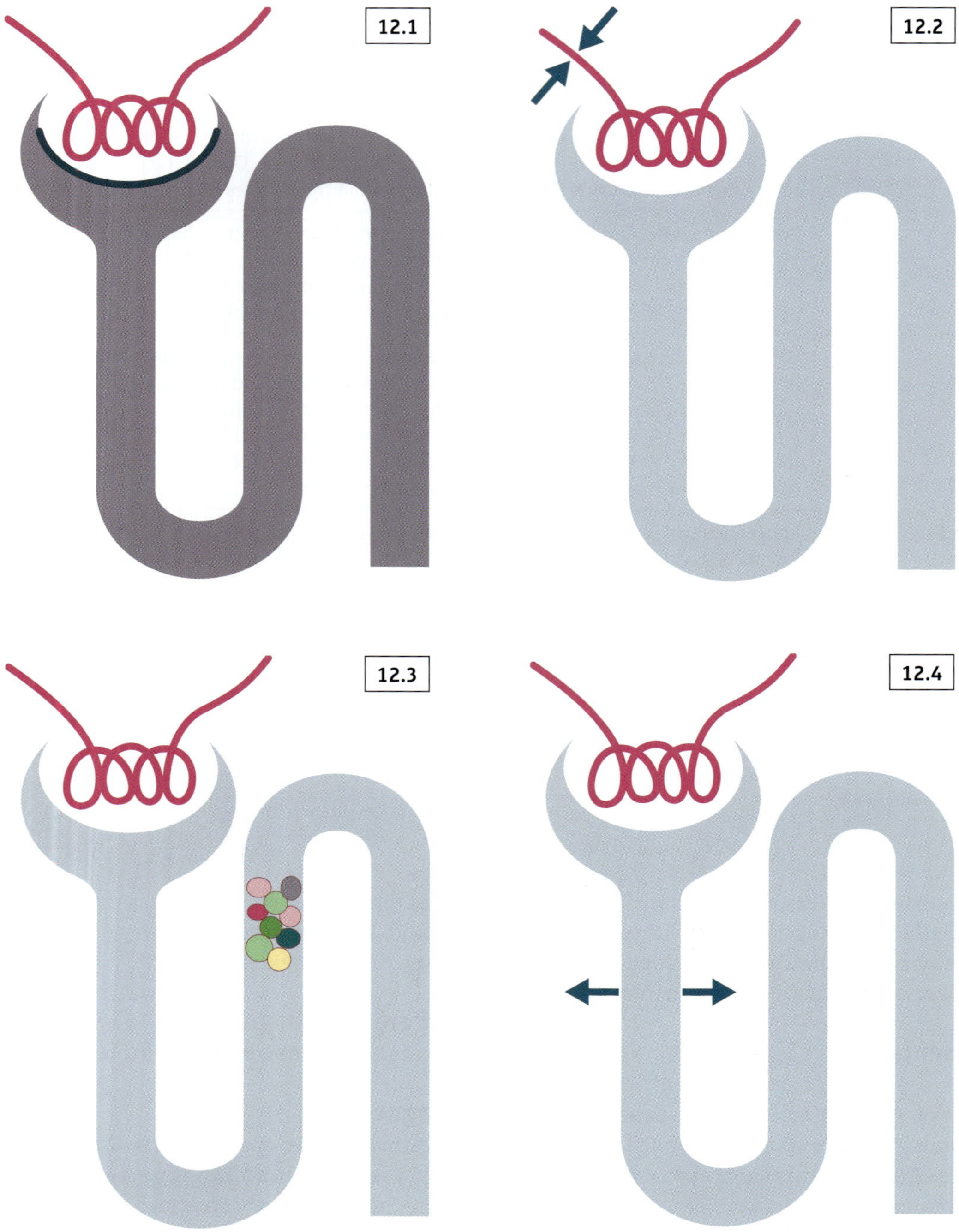

Figures 12.1–12.4 Hypothesized causes of oliguria in acute kidney injury. (12.1) Reduced glomerular permeability; (12.2) vasoconstriction; (12.3) tubular obstruction; (12.4) back leak.

The hallmark of prerenal azotemia is a moderate elevation in BUN and creatinine with an increase in USG. Postrenal azotemia should be suspected in animals with elevations in BUN and creatinine that present with a distended bladder or free fluid in the abdomen. If this fluid is from the urinary tract, it will have a BUN that is similar to the patient's serum but a creatinine concentration that is higher. Once a diagnosis of AKI is suspected, a complete blood count (CBC), serum chemistry, urinalysis, aerobic urine culture, ultrasound, and serology testing should be performed.

Urinalysis

Urinalysis can be used to quickly differentiate between prerenal and renal azotemia. Isosthenuria is typical of AKI while a USG of >1.025 in the dog and >1.035 in the cat is typically associated with prerenal azotemia. The presence of glucosuria in the absence of hyperglycemia is suggestive of acute proximal tubule dysfunction, but is also seen with Fanconi syndrome. The discovery of protein, in the absence of bacteria, red blood cells (RBCs), white blood cells, or casts may be suggestive of glomerular disease (see Protein-losing nephropathy). Only a urine protein:creatinine (UPC) ratio can provide a quantitative assessment of urine protein concentration and should be performed on every proteinuric patient. Microscopic examination of the urine sediment allows detection of calcium oxalate monohydrate crystals, which are associated with ethylene glycol toxicity (**Figure 12.7**). The presence of casts can provide important diagnostic information (**Figure 12.8**). Bacteria may be seen in cases of pyelonephritis; however, the absence of bacteria and/or inflammatory cells does not eliminate pyelonephritis as a cause of AKI. Casts, often observed in AKI, can help determine the underlying cause (**Figure 12.8**; **Table 12.5**).

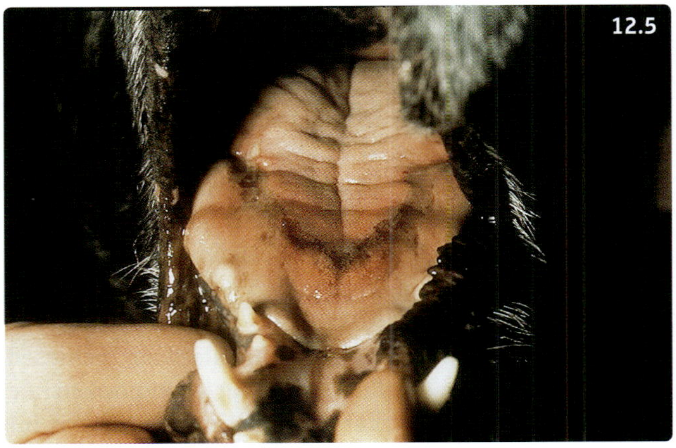

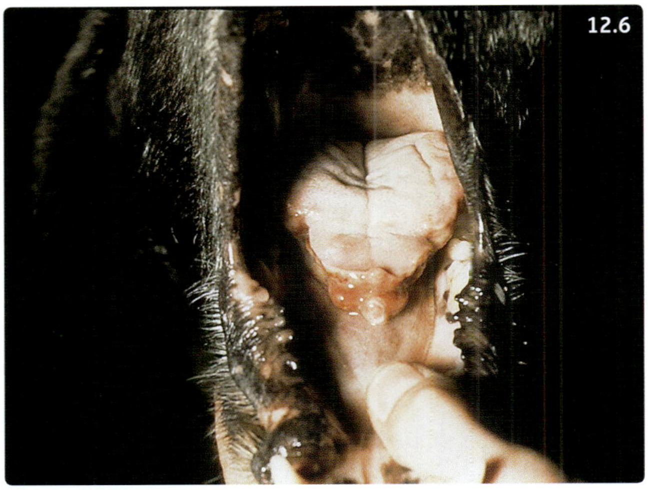

Figures 12.5, 12.6 Lingual necrosis in a dog with acute kidney injury. (12.5) The necrotic tip of the tongue shows discoloration. (12.6) Appearance of the tongue after the necrotic area has sloughed. (Courtesy D.F. Senior)

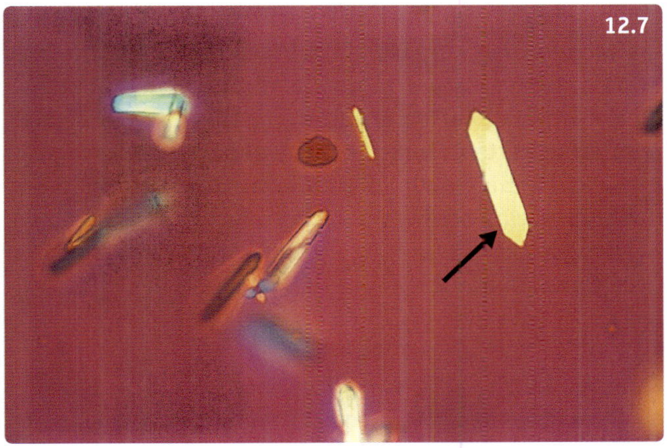

Figure 12.7 Calcium oxalate monohydrate crystals (arrow) typical of those observed in the urine sediment of animals with ethylene glycol intoxication. (Courtesy C.A. Osborne)

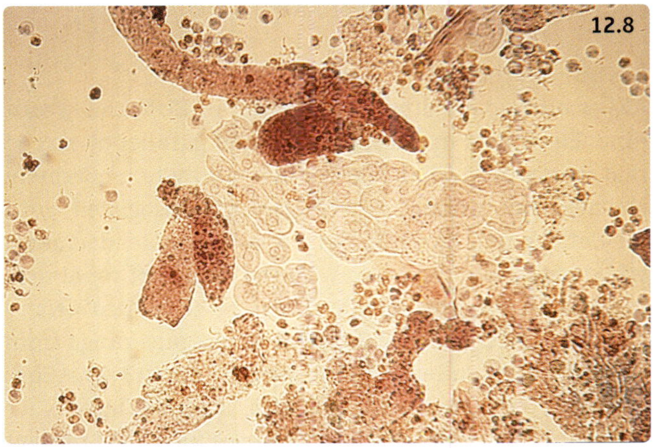

Figure 12.8 Granular casts in the urine sediment of a dog with acute kidney injury. (Courtesy D.F. Senior)

Table 12.5 Types of casts and associated conditions.

Hyaline casts	Proteinuria: glomerulonephritis and amyloidosis
Granular casts	Degeneration of cells or precipitation of proteins Ischemic or toxic tubular injury
Fatty casts	Granular casts containing lipid Nephrotic syndrome & diabetes
White cell casts	Pyelonephritis
Waxy casts	Final degeneration of granular casts Intrarenal stasis

Urine culture

Urine culture should be performed regardless of the appearance of the urine sediment. Microscopic examination of urine sediment is not highly sensitive for detection of bacteria. Kidneys may only shed a small number of bacteria into the urine and these microorganisms can be missed when examining dilute urine. At one time, the presence of white blood cells was used to gauge the need for a urine culture; however, this too has proven to be unreliable.

Complete blood count

Changes in the CBC are often non-specific. However, elevations in the white blood cell count can be associated with pyelonephritis and systemic infectious diseases. The absence of a stress leukogram (neutrophilia, lymphopenia, and eosinopenia) in a sick patient should raise the suspicion that the patient could have hypoadrenocorticism (Addison's disease), not AKI.

Serum chemistry

AKI is accompanied by an elevation in BUN and creatinine. Elevations in phosphate usually parallel or exceed that of creatinine. Calcium is often mildly to moderately elevated but dramatic decreases are associated with ethylene glycol toxicity. Serum bicarbonate decreases while potassium increases with the degree of renal dysfunction. Anion gap should always be calculated ($[Na^+ + K^+] - [Cl^- + HCO_3^-]$). Normal canine anion gaps range from 12 to 24 mEq/l, while normal feline values are 13–27 mEq/l. Increases can be associated with ketones, lactate, or uremia; however, significant increases in an AKI patient are suggestive of toxin ingestion. In veterinary medicine, the most common nephrotoxin is ethylene glycol, although methanol, ethanol, and salicylic acid should be considered.

Radiography and ultrasound

When available, ultrasound is the preferred imaging modality (**Figure 12.9**). Ultrasound can provide information about the renal architecture and outflow tract, and allows interrogation of the renal blood flow. In addition, ultrasound can be used to obtain renal biopsies in a minimally invasive fashion. Patients with AKI usually present with kidneys of normal to increased size while small, irregular shaped kidneys are suggestive of chronic disease.

Infectious disease serology

In areas where leptospirosis is endemic, titers for the prevalent serovars should be submitted in all patients where the cause of the AKI is not immediately identified. Generally, a microscopic agglutination titer of >1:800 in the absence of recent vaccination suggests exposure, while a four-fold increase in paired titers 14 days apart indicates an active infection. There are PCR assays for leptospirosis. They may be positive in early infection before a rise in specific antibody detected by MAT or ELISA is present. There are some questions as to the sensitivity and specificity of the test. Other serologic tests (e.g. leishmaniasis, rickettsia, babesiosis) should be considered based on the location of the patient and the relevant travel history.

Ethylene glycol blood test

Any patient with a severe metabolic acidosis, increased anion gap, calcium oxalate crystalluria, hypocalcemia, or any combination of these signs should be tested for ethylene glycol exposure. This should be done regardless of the compatibility of the history with exposure. It is important to note that some of the commercially available test kits may not be sensitive enough to detect

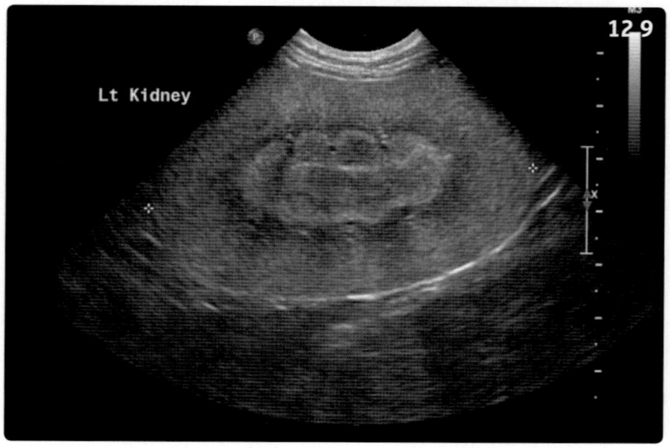

Figure 12.9 Ultrasound of a kidney from a dog with ethylene glycol intoxication. Note the dramatically increased echogenicity of the renal cortex consistent with, but not diagnostic, for this toxin. (Courtesy L. Gaschen)

ethylene glycol exposure in cats, as the lethal serum concentration may be below the threshold of the test.

Management

Successful treatment of AKI is dependent on determining an underlying cause, correcting dehydration, establishing a brisk diuresis, and correcting life-threatening electrolyte imbalances. Often, treatment must begin before the cause can be established; however, the importance of accurate fluid therapy cannot be overemphasized. Studies in people and animal models clearly demonstrate that even small amounts of excessive fluid administration can be fatal in AKI patients.

Due to inappetence, vomiting, and an impaired ability to concentrate urine, dehydration is common in AKI patients. Initial fluid therapy must account for three factors: patient dehydration, maintenance fluids, and insensible losses. A balanced electrolyte solution can be used (LRS, Normosol); however, if hyperkalemia exists, 0.9% saline should be substituted.

First, the patient's degree of dehydration must be estimated (**Table 12.6**) and then the total volume of fluids needed to correct dehydration can be calculated using the equation:

$$\text{deficit in liters} = \%\ \text{dehydration} \times \text{kg body weight}$$

So that fluids have time to equilibrate between the vascular, interstitial, and cellular compartments, this deficit must be divided and administered over 8–12 hours. Commonly available formulae for calculating 'maintenance' fluids assume normally functioning kidneys and are of little utility in formulating fluid therapy

Table 12.6 Signs used to determine degree of dehydration.

% dehydration	Clinical signs
<5%	Not detectable
5–6%	Subtle loss of skin elasticity
6–8%	Delay in return of skin to normal position Slight increase in CRT Dry mucous membranes
10–12%	Skin stands in place when tented Increase in CRT Eyes sunken Dry mucous membranes Shock: tachycardia, cold extremities, weak pulses
12–15%	Death imminent

plans for AKI patients; rather, an indwelling urinary catheter should be aseptically placed to measure urine output. Hourly urine output is then used as the surrogate 'maintenance' fluid rate. Finally, insensible losses can be estimated as 20 ml/kg/day plus any fluids lost to vomiting or diarrhea. For example:

A 10 kg dog presenting for AKI is found to be 10% dehydrated and is producing 5 ml/hour urine. Total dehydration is determined to be 1 liter (10 kg × 0.10), to be given over 8–12 hours. Thus, the dehydration component of the hourly fluid therapy is 83 ml/hour (1,000 ml/12 hours). The patient is producing 5 ml/hour and this represents the maintenance fluids. There has been no vomiting or diarrhea reported so the insensible losses are 8 ml/hour ([20 ml/kg × 10]/24). Therefore, the hourly fluid rate for the next 12 hours should be 96 ml/hour (83 ml/hour + 5 ml/hour + 8 ml/hour). Urine output per hour is monitored regularly and the maintenance fluid component of the formula adjusted.

Once dehydration has been corrected, fluid therapy should account only for maintenance fluids and insensible losses. To determine maintenance fluids, urine should be collected and quantified at a regular interval (e.g. every 4 hours) and the hourly urine production rate can be used as the 'maintenance' rate. Insensible losses can be estimated as 20 ml/kg/day plus any fluids lost to vomiting or diarrhea. For example:

The 10 kg dog is now well hydrated. The patient is producing 9 ml/hour and this represents the maintenance fluids. There has been no vomiting or diarrhea reported so the insensible losses are 8 ml/hour (20 ml/kg × 10/24). Therefore, the hourly fluid rate for the next 12 hours should be 17 ml/hour (9 ml/hour + 8 ml/hour). Urine output is monitored regularly (e.g. every 4 hours) and the maintenance component of the formula adjusted.

AKI patients are at high risk for fluid overload and death; therefore, whenever possible, central venous pressure (CVP) should be monitored in addition to urine output (**Figure 12.10**). An increase in CVP of >5 cm H_2O above baseline, or an absolute value of >9 cm H_2O, suggests an excessive fluid administration rate. Although patient weight can provide information on the patient's hydration status, it is too insensitive an indicator to be useful as the sole method of monitoring.

The goal should be a brisk diuresis of at least 1 ml/kg/hour. Well-hydrated animals that produce <0.25 ml/kg/hour of urine are considered to be in oliguric renal failure, while anuric renal failure patients fail to produce any urine. These conditions necessitate aggressive treatment. Occasionally, AKI patients will produce large volumes of urine once dehydration is corrected. Polyuric patients

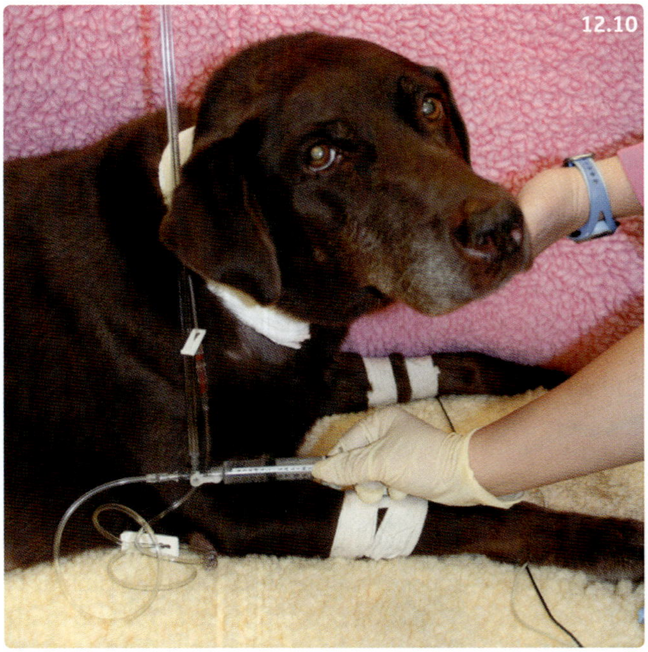

Figure 12.10 Central venous pressure measurement in a dog. (Courtesy K. Ryan)

are probably either less severely affected or represent a later course of the disease process. Polyuric patients are generally easier to manage clinically, as they are less likely to develop life-threatening electrolyte abnormalities and fluid overload; however, they still require careful monitoring. Urine production needs to be quantitated regularly and adjusted as previously described or dehydration can occur rapidly. Significant azotemia and uremia can persist during this polyuric phase and should not be considered a negative prognostic indication.

In oliguric and anuric animals that are not fluid overloaded and are well hydrated, mannitol is considered to be the initial treatment of choice. Experimental models of renal failure have shown mannitol to increase renal blood flow, shrink swollen tubular cells, dislodge tubular obstructions, and scavenge free radicals. It is given as a 0.25–1.0 g/kg IV bolus over 30 minutes. If urine production improves, a CRI of 1–2 mg/kg/minute can be started. Mannitol is contraindicated in patients with ethylene glycol intoxication because it can further exacerbate hyperosmolality, thus exacerbating the neurologic signs. If there is no response to therapy or in an overhydrated animal, therapy with furosemide should be attempted.

Furosemide is a loop diuretic that as been associated with the induction of diuresis and resolution of tubular obstructions under experimental conditions. Furosemide is typically given as a bolus (2 mg/kg) and if urine production increases, it is continued as a CRI (0.25–1.0 mg/kg/hour). (**Note:** Aminoglycoside toxicity should not be treated with furosemide as it can potentiate further renal injury.) Studies in people have failed to demonstrate improved survival in AKI patients who received furosemide or mannitol; however, widespread access to advanced therapies such as dialysis makes it unclear if these studies are directly applicable to animals. At one time, furosemide was given with dopamine for alleged synergistic effects; however, the use of dopamine is not supported.

Small retrospective studies had suggested that fenoldopam, a peripheral dopamine D1 receptor agonist, and diltiazem, a calcium channel blocker, might be helpful in the treatment of AKI. More recent prospective studies have failed to demonstrate a benefit of either drug. Some research suggests that use of diltiazem may actually be contraindicated depending on the inciting cause of the AKI; therefore, use of these drugs cannot be recommended at this time.

Patients that produce significant amounts of urine in response to rehydration or mannitol/furosemide therapy are less likely to require specific treatment for electrolyte and acid–base imbalances. Oliguric and anuric renal failure patients that do not respond to medical management can quickly develop fatal hyperkalemia and metabolic acidosis.

Hyperkalemia

The most common life-threatening electrolyte imbalance encountered in AKI is hyperkalemia. Restoring urine production is critical for long-term survival. Elevation in serum potassium causes a reduction of the transmembrane electrochemical gradient and changes nerve and muscle cell excitability. Clinically, signs of hyperkalemia include muscle weakness, reduced cardiac contractility, arrhythmias, and neurologic abnormalities. Classic ECG findings include bradycardia, disappearance of the P wave, spiking of the T wave, and widened QRS complexes (**Figure 12.11**). These changes begin to appear when potassium approaches 6.5 mEq/l. Cardiac arrest can occur at any time.

In the absence of adequate urine production, only dialysis can provide a long-term solution to hyperkalemia; however, there are several strategies for short-term management of this condition (**Table 12.7**).

Metabolic acidosis

Metabolic acidosis is also common in AKI, as the renal tubules are responsible for recapturing filtered bicarbonate as well as manufacturing new buffer. Generally, metabolic acidosis is not treated unless

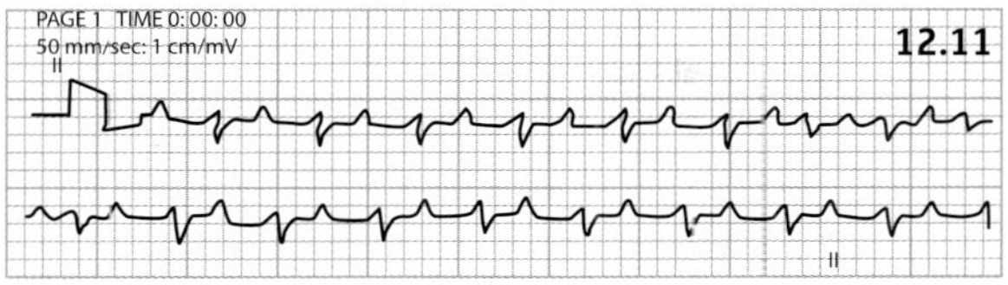

Figure 12.11 Example of an ECG of a patient with hyperkalemia (lead II).

Table 12.7 Management of hyperkalemia.

- Calcium gluconate (10% solution): 0.5–1.0 ml/kg given IV over 10–15 minutes. Protects against cardiac toxicity for approximately 30 minutes
- Regular insulin (0.1–0.25 units/kg) and glucose (1–2 g/unit of insulin). Potassium transported into cells with glucose. Provides short-term correction
- Sodium bicarbonate (1–2 mEq/kg over 20 minutes). Corrects for acidosis, allowing potassium back into cells. Effects can last 1–2 hours

Table 12.8 Protocols used to control emesis in acute kidney injury patients.

Antiemetic protocols	Metoclopramide (Reglan): dopamine inhibition (1.0–2.0 mg/kg IV or CRI q24h)
	Maropitant citrate (Cerenia): NK1 inhibition (1.0 mg/kg SC q24h [dogs]; 0.5–1.0 mg/kg SC q24h [cats])
	Ondansetron (Zofran): 5HT3 inhibitor (0.1–0.2 mg/kg IV [slow push] q6–12h)
	Dolasetron (Anzemet): 5HT3 inhibitor (0.4–0.6 mg/kg IV q24h)
Gastric irritation	Omeprazole (Prilosec): proton pump inhibitor (0.7–1.0 mg/kg PO q12–24h)
	Sucralfate (Carafate): gastric coating (0.5–1.0 mg/kg PO [dog]; 0.25 mg/kg [cat])
	Famotidine (Pepcid): H2 receptor antagonist (0.5 mg/kg PO, SQ, or IV q24h)

serum bicarbonate is <12 mEq/l and pH <7.2. A dose for bicarbonate can be calculated as (body weight in kg × 0.3) × (16 minus measured bicarbonate [mEq/l]). Typically, only two-thirds of the dose is given, with one-third given IV over 30 minutes while another one-third can be given with IV fluids over 4 hours. Acid–base status should be re-evaluated before additional bicarbonate is administered.

Emesis

Quite commonly, AKI patients experience significant vomiting that can complicate treatment, worsen electrolyte abnormalities, and contribute to dehydration. The vomiting is likely due to both stimulation of the chemoreceptor trigger zone by uremic toxins and gastric irritation. These should be addressed with a combination of antiemetic and gastric protectant medications (**Table 12.8**). Until emesis is controlled, these medications should only be given IV.

Drug dosage

Many drugs are excreted by the kidneys. In AKI, dosages of these drugs must be adjusted to reflect the reduced clearance. One method is to monitor serum drug levels and adjust dosages accordingly. This is rarely performed in veterinary or human medicine due to the cost and test availability. A more commonly used method is to reduce dosages by multiplying them by 1/serum creatinine. This is based on the principle that increases in serum creatinine are inversely proportionate to the fall in GFR. Thus, as serum creatinine increases, GFR and drug clearance decreases by a proportionate amount; however, this approximation is valid only until serum creatinine approaches 4 mg/dl (354 μmol/l). Many will reduce the dosages based on serum creatinine until it rises above 4 mg/dl, and then use the calculation as a guide while empirically adjusting the dosage. Unless serum levels are being measured or GFR calculated, nephrotoxic drugs and those drugs that are cleared by the kidney and have a narrow therapeutic range must be avoided.

Leptospirosis

Patients should be treated as outlined above with special attention paid to fluid therapy. Patients who are oliguric or anuric benefit from advanced renal therapies such as dialysis, and referral should be considered. Whenever possible, doxycycline should be used as the initial antimicrobial therapy as it both treats the leptospiremia and clears the carrier state; however, doxycycline is metabolized by the liver and excreted in the bile. Supraphysiologic serum concentrations can occur in patients with liver impairment, which is common in leptospirosis patients. In patients with evidence of liver involvement, antibiotics in the beta-lactam category (penicillin, ampicillin) should be used for 2 weeks to clear the leptospiremia. This is then followed with 2 weeks of doxycycline to clear the carrier state.

Specific toxin ingestion

Ethylene glycol

Exposure is always a medical emergency. Several cage-side tests are now available for the detection of this toxin. These tests differ in their sensitivity as well as the complexity of the testing procedure. In the absence of an in-hospital diagnostic test, the treatment of ethylene glycol should begin whenever a combination of compatible laboratory findings (severe metabolic acidosis, increased anion gap, hypocalcemia, calcium oxalate crystalluria) is seen in an animal demonstrating appropriate clinical signs. If ingestion is discovered in the first hour, vomiting should be induced and activated charcoal administered. Initial serum chemistry should be obtained and repeated at 24 and 48 hours. Methylpyrazole, an antidote, should be administered at once (**Table 12.9**). The first step in ethylene glycol's metabolism into toxic intermediaries takes place in the liver by alcohol dehydrogenase. Methylpyrazole binds to and inactivates alcohol dehydrogenase so that the ethylene glycol can leave the body unchanged through the kidneys. Although ethanol can be administered IV as an antidote, methylpyrazole is far safer and more efficacious. IV fluids should be started at a rate of 4 ml/kg/hour and urine output monitored for at least 48 hours. If urine output decreases, follow AKI fluid therapy recommendations outlined above.

In dogs, the greatest benefit of medical management is seen in the first 5–8 hours and cats within 3 hours of ingestion. In one study, those cats treated 3 hours or less after exposure with 4-methylpyrazole (4-MP), had 100% survival while those treated with ethanol had 25% survival; however, 4 hours after ethylene glycol ingestion, there was 100% mortality regardless of the treatment.

Table 12.9 Treatment of ethylene glycol toxicity.

Canine	4-MP (methylpyrazole 50 mg/ml): 20 mg/kg IV first dose; 15 mg/kg at 12 hours; 15 mg/kg at 24 hours; 5 mg/kg at 36 hours
Feline	4-MP (methylpyrazole 50 mg/ml): 126 mg/kg slow IV initial dose; 31.25 mg/kg IV at 12 hours; 31.25 mg/kg IV at 24 hours; 31.25 mg/kg IV at 36 hours
Alternative treatment	A 7% ethanol solution is made by removing 175 ml from a 1 L bag of saline and adding 175 ml of an 80 proof vodka, or by removing 74 ml from a 1 L bag of saline and adding 74 ml of 190 proof alcohol. For both cats and dogs, give a loading dose of 8.6 ml/kg 7% ethanol (slow IV), then continue with a CRI of 1.43 ml/kg/hour. Remember to use only 'clear' alcohols

It has been reported that cats treated with hemodialysis after the onset of renal failure secondary to ethylene glycol had a significantly better survival rate. (**Note:** The 4-MP dose for cats is approximately six times the dose used for dogs.)

NSAID toxicity

Because of its rapid absorption and depressive effect on the CNS, vomiting should be induced only if ingestion is immediately detected. Initial serum chemistry should be obtained and repeated at 24 and 48 hours. IV fluids should be started at a rate of 4 ml/kg/hour and urine output monitored for at least 48 hours. If urine output decreases, follow the AKI fluid therapy recommendations outlined above. Misoprostol, a synthetic prostaglandin E1 analog, can be given to dogs at a dose of 2.0–5.0 µg/kg q8h. Due to its long half-life, naproxen toxicity should be treated for at least 72 hours.

Cholecalciferol-based rodenticides

If ingestion is discovered in the first 24 hours, vomiting should be induced and activated charcoal administered. Because of enterohepatic recirculation, activated charcoal administration should be repeated. Initial serum chemistry should be obtained and then repeated every 12 hours for 4 days. Intravenous fluids (0.9% sodium chloride) should be started at a rate of 4 ml/kg/hour and urine output monitored for at least 48 hours. Sodium chloride is preferred as it increases calcium excretion. If urine output decreases, the AKI fluid therapy recommendations outlined above should be followed. A combination of furosemide (2 mg/kg q6h) and prednisone (2–3 mg/kg q12h) should be administered to reduce calcium resorption and increase its excretion. If oral intake is possible, oral phosphate binders (e.g. aluminum hydroxide) can be used as needed. If calcium and phosphorus levels remain elevated, a single dose of pamidronate 1.3–2.0 mg/kg given IV over 2 hours may be effective. Often one dose is needed for the entire treatment. Calcium and phosphorus levels should be monitored for 6 weeks. Due to their prolonged half-life, treatment of these toxicities can be prolonged and expensive.

Grapes, raisins, lily ingestion

If ingestion is discovered in the first 4 hours, vomiting should be induced and activated charcoal administered. Initial serum chemistry should be obtained and then repeated at 24 hours. IV fluids should be started at a rate of 4 ml/kg/hour and urine output monitored for at least 48 hours. If urine output decreases, the AKI fluid therapy recommendations outlined above should be followed. Prognosis for cats presenting for lily ingestion is guarded. In one small study, 50% of cats that presented for ingestion of lily plants died despite aggressive therapy. Dogs suffering AKI secondary to grape ingestion also have a guarded prognosis. In one study, more than half of affected patients survived; 65% of those that survived had complete resolution of signs. Since grape toxicity appears to be idiosyncratic, all exposures should be considered potentially lethal. It is important to realize that raisin containing products such as breads, cakes, and 'trail mix' are also potentially toxic.

Advanced renal therapies

In recent years, the increasing availability of veterinary dialysis centers has made this modality a viable option. Indications for extracorporeal blood purification include significant uremia, anuria, oliguria, hyperkalemia, and exposure to dialyzable drugs/toxins. The removal of toxins by dialysis is dependent on several characteristics of the drug (size, protein binding, volume of distribution, water solubility) as well as the dialysis equipment available. Dialysis centers maintain lists of dialyzable drugs. Many centers can also perform therapeutic plasma exchange, which has the potential for removing some toxins that cannot be dialyzed.

Until recently, veterinary patients requiring dialysis universally received intermittent dialysis (**Figure 12.12**), which is performed at set intervals, often several times a week for 6–8 hours. Continuous renal replacement therapy (**Figure 12.13**) is a newer modality that differs from intermittent dialysis in several aspects. The most obvious difference is that this modality is administered on a slow, continuous basis rather than intermittently. It is not clear which modality, if any, is associated with better outcomes.

If an owner is interested in dialysis, a center should be consulted as soon as possible. The chance of a successful treatment increases with early intervention. In addition, if there is any chance that a client may be interested in dialysis, the jugular veins should not be disturbed. In many patients, these are the only veins in which a dialysis catheter can be placed and even a single blood draw can render a vein unusable. An up-to-date list of dialysis centers around the world can be found at http://www.queenofthenephron.com

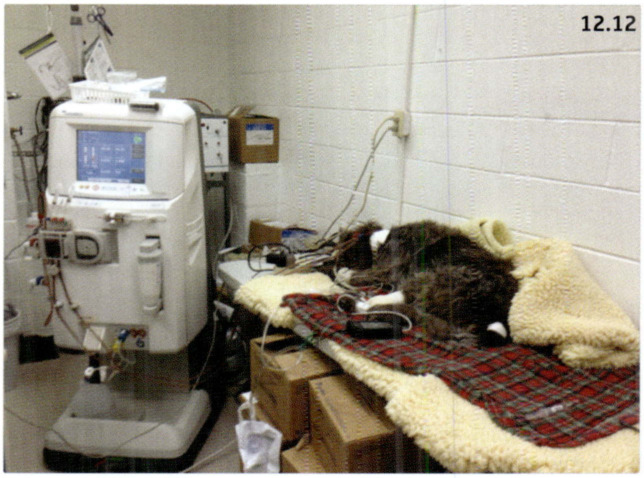

12.12

Figure 12.12 Patient receiving intermittent hemodialysis.

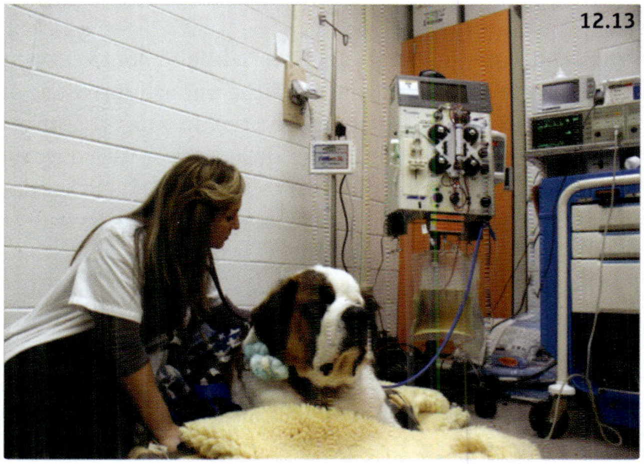

12.13

Figure 12.13 Patient receiving continuous renal replacement therapy.

CHRONIC KIDNEY DISEASE

Definition/overview

CKD is characterized by a progressive decrease in the kidney's ability to concentrate urine, excrete nitrogenous waste, produce hormones, and maintain electrolyte balance. This deterioration in renal function is due to a gradual, irreversible loss of nephrons and is the most common type of renal disease in companion animals. CKD is often divided into two categories based on the underlying etiology: congenital and acquired.

In congenital renal disease, the animal is either born with lesions present in the kidneys (e.g. aplasia) or born with a condition that will lead to renal disease in the future (e.g. polycystic kidney disease). While most cases of congenital renal disease are thought to be inherited, the mode of genetic transmission and pathogenesis is often unknown. The patient's condition usually becomes apparent early in life, often in the first year, and is progressive (**Table 12.10**).

Acquired CKD is the result of an insult to the renal parenchyma that causes nephron loss and precipitates a

Table 12.10 Congenital causes of chronic kidney disease in the dog and cat.

Condition	Breed
Amyloidosis	Shar Pei, Beagle, Abyssinian, Oriental Shorthair
Renal dysplasia	Shi Tzu, Lhasa Apso, Golden Retriever, Soft-coated Wheaten Terrier, others
Glomerulopathy	Soft-coated Wheaten Terrier, Cocker Spaniel
Fanconi syndrome	Basenji
Polycystic kidney disease	Cairn Terrier, Persian
Glomerulonephritis	Bernese Mountain Dog

gradual decline in renal function. While in some cases it is possible to determine and treat the underlying cause of the renal disease (e.g. pyelonephritis), in most instances the nature of the initial insult is never discovered. Regardless of the etiology, most cases of CKD have a similar clinical presentation, course, and treatment.

Pathophysiology

Although the exact pathophysiology of CKD is not known, it is now believed that an initial insult reduces the number of functioning nephrons (**Figure 12.14**). This could be a sequela of AKI, a congenital defect, or the result of a chronic disease process (e.g. hypertension). Remaining nephrons compensate by dilation of the glomerular arterioles, increased intraglomerular capillary pressure, increased renal plasma flow, and increased single nephron GFR in a phenomenon that has been called hyperfiltration. Hyperfiltration increases the clearance of nitrogenous wastes in each surviving nephron, but elevated intraglomerular capillary pressure eventually leads to mechanical disruption of the capillaries and protein loss through the glomerulus. Excess filtered protein is reabsorbed by the epithelial cells of the PCT, broken down by cellular lysosomal mechanisms and re-enters the blood as amino acids. The process of breaking down proteins releases oxygen free radicals, which stimulate the release of inflammatory cytokines. The resulting inflammation damages epithelial cells. Increased intraglomerular capillary pressure also results in scarring and eventual occlusion of the glomerular capillaries. Continued damage to tubular epithelial cells, combined with glomerular capillary injury, leads to tubulointerstitial fibrosis, which is the hallmark of CKD (**Figures 12.15, 12.16**). Thus, what starts as a compensatory mechanism eventually perpetuates additional renal damage.

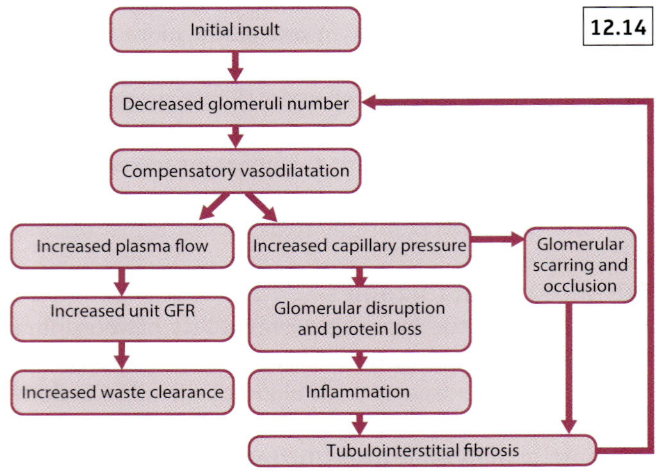

Figure 12.14 Pathophysiology of chronic kidney disease.

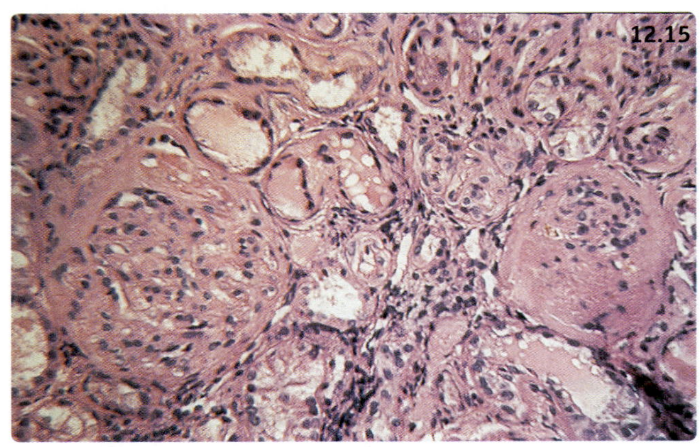

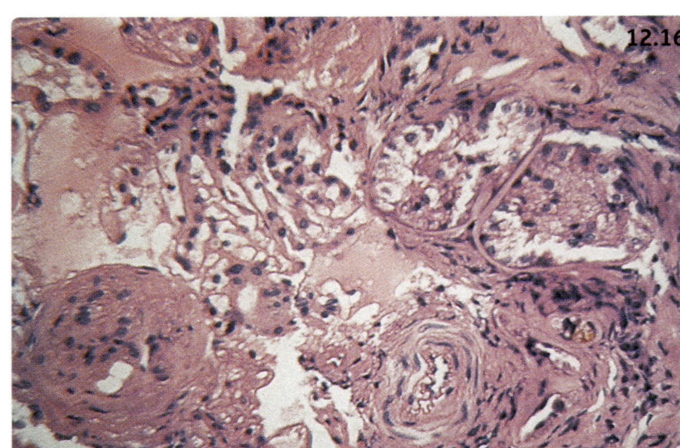

Figures 12.15, 12.16 Histopathology of the kidney from a dog with chronic kidney disease. (12.15) Glomerulosclerosis and a mononuclear interstitial infiltrate. (12.16) Tubular atrophy and interstitial fibrosis. (Courtesy D.F. Senior)

Differential diagnosis

Prerenal, primary renal, or postrenal azotemia, AKI.

Clinical presentation

Common clinical features of CKD include polyuria/polydipsia, weight loss, lethargy, anorexia, vomiting, dehydration, oral ulcers, and uremic breath. In cats, blindness secondary to hypertension is not uncommon and is often the primary reason that owners seek veterinary care.

Diagnosis

The diagnosis of CKD is made on the basis of history, physical examination, and laboratory blood work. Once the presence of azotemia is confirmed, possible differential diagnoses (prerenal azotemia, postrenal azotemia, and AKI) must be eliminated from consideration. A CBC, serum chemistry, urine analysis, aerobic urine culture, and ultrasound should be performed on all CKD patients.

Serum chemistry

CKD is accompanied by an elevation in BUN and creatinine; however, as advanced CKD patients are often severely muscle wasted, creatinine may not be as elevated as one would expect. Elevations in serum phosphate often exceed those of serum creatinine. Calcium is often mildly to moderately elevated as a result of secondary hyperparathyroidism. Serum bicarbonate decreases with the degree of renal dysfunction and significant decreases may be associated with a worse long-term prognosis. Potassium levels are usually maintained in the normal range, but hypokalemia can be observed in cats. Recently, a new blood test, symmetric dimethylarginine (SDMA), has become available. Preliminary studies have shown that SDMA is an accurate predictor of CKD and may become elevated 9 months before creatinine in dogs and 17 months earlier in cats. At the time of writing, the best way to utilize this information in developing a treatment regimen is not known.

Complete blood count

A normochromic, normocytic, nonregenerative anemia is the most common hematologic finding in patients with CKD. Elevations in the white blood cell count can be associated with chronic pyelonephritis or a systemic infectious disease; however, the white blood cell counts are usually unremarkable.

Urinalysis

The most common urinalysis finding in CKD is isosthenuria (SG = 1.007–1.015); however, some cats may still be able to concentrate urine in the early phases of CKD. Mild azotemia in the presence of highly concentrated urine is the hallmark of prerenal azotemia. The finding of large amounts of glucose is suggestive of proximal tubular dysfunction and can be seen in dogs with Fanconi syndrome (**Figure 12.17**). The detection of large amounts of protein, in the absence of hematuria, bacteria, or white blood cells in the urine sediment, may be the result of glomerular damage. A quantitative assessment of urine protein concentration requires that a UPC ratio be performed (see Glomerular disease). In cats, the UPC ratio may be prognostic even in the absence of overt proteinuria. Research suggests that cats with CKD and a UPC ratio of <0.43 lived approximately 2 years from the time of diagnosis. Those with a UPC ratio of >0.43 lived only about 9 months. Even if no bacteria are microscopically detected in the urine, an aerobic urine culture should always be performed to help rule out chronic pyelonephritis as a contributing factor to the progression of CKD.

Blood pressure measurement

Arterial hypertension is a common complication of CKD that eventually affects the majority of cats and dogs. Not only can hypertension have negative consequences for the eyes, heart, and nervous system, it can also potentiate further kidney damage; therefore, identifying and treating these patients is essential. Since hypertension may develop at any point in the disease process, all CKD patients should have their blood pressure checked

	12.17
Fanconi facts	• Failure of proximal tubule transport • Sodium, bicarbonate, potassium, glucose, amino acids not resorbed • 10–16% of Basenjis affected, documented in other breeds
Diagnosis	• Signs of CKD and glucosuria with normal blood glucose are suggestive • Aminoaciduria is diagnostic
Treatment	• Oral supplementation: bicarbonate goal (serum >12 mmol/l [12 mEq/l]); potassium goal (serum 4–6 mmol/l [4–6 mEq/l]); calcium goal (serum 2.25–2.5 mmol/l [9–10 mg/dl]) • Renal failure diet
Prognosis	• Good with proper treatment

Figure 12.17 Fanconi syndrome characteristics.

regularly. Specific guidelines for measuring and treating arterial hypertension can be found later in this chapter (see Hypertension).

Radiography and ultrasound

When available, ultrasound is the preferred imaging modality. Not only does it provide an unparalleled view of the renal architecture and outflow tract, but it can also be utilized to obtain renal biopsies when indicated. Typically, CKD is characterized as bilateral loss of renal mass; however, certain disease processes, such as polycystic kidney disease, have a characteristic ultrasound appearance. Enlarged kidneys are suggestive of an underlying disease process with secondary renal involvement (e.g. lymphoma, feline infectious peritonitis [FIP], hydronephrosis), primary renal neoplasia, or AKI. Mild dilatation of the renal pelvis (pyelectasia) is often seen with chronic renal infections. Congenital renal dysplasia and aplasia are characterized by an abnormal renal architecture with loss of the delineation between the cortex and medulla.

Management

Staging

Patients with CKD should be staged according to the guidelines developed by the International Renal Interest Society (IRIS). These guidelines, which have been accepted by the both the American and European Societies of Veterinary Nephrology and Urology, classify patients on the basis of renal function, proteinuria, and blood pressure (**Tables 12.11–12.13**). For example, using these criteria, a 15-year-old cat with a creatinine of 3.0 mg/dl (265 µmol/l), a UPC of 2.0, and a blood pressure of 170 mmHg would be classified as a stage 3 proteinuric, stage II hypertensive patient. Using this staging system not only allows for a common nomenclature for describing and discussing patients, but allows for the development and application of appropriate guidelines for the prognosis and treatment of CKD.

Table 12.11 IRIS stages of CKD based on serum creatinine values (mg/dl [µmol/l]).

	Dog	Cat
Stage 1	<1.4 [<125]	<1.6 [<140]
Stage 2	1.4–2.0 [125–179]	1.6–2.8 [140–249]
Stage 3	2.1–5.0 [180–439]	2.9–5.0 [250–439]
Stage 4	>5.0 [>440]	>5.0 [>440]

Table 12.12 IRIS classification of proteinuria based on the urine protein:creatinine ratio.

	Dog	Cat
Proteinuric	>0.5	>0.4
Borderline proteinuric	0.2–0.5	0.2–0.4
Nonproteinuric	<0.2	<0.2

Table 12.13 IRIS classification of arterial hypertension.

	Systolic blood pressure
Stage 0	<150 mmHg
Stage I	150–159 mmHg
Stage II	160–179 mmHg
Stage III	>180 mmHg

Fluid therapy

Many patients with CKD present with some degree of dehydration. This can complicate management of CKD as dehydration leads to hypoperfusion and prerenal azotemia. Proper rehydration often causes significant reductions in azotemia. Therefore, the degree of dehydration should be estimated and, if significant, a regimen of replacement fluids should be calculated and administered IV over 12–24 hours. In mildly dehydrated patients, SC fluids can be administered during the clinic visit. In either case, when patients have difficulty maintaining proper hydration, the daily administration of SC fluids at home can help prevent dehydration, reduce azotemia, and significantly improve the patient's quality of life (**Figures 12.18a, b**). In cases where the patient is uncooperative or the owner is unwilling to give SC fluids, a SC fluid port (GIF-Tube®) can be inserted (**Figures 12.19a, b**). This port provides easy access for fluid administration and avoids the need for needles; however, some cats will not tolerate these tubes. Alternatively, an esophagostomy tube can be placed (**Figures 12.20a–h**). These are easily inserted, can remain in position for extended periods of time, and can be used to provide the patient's fluid and nutritional needs.

Control of acidosis

One of the primary functions of the kidney is to maintain acid–base balance. The renal tubules reabsorb filtered bicarbonate, generate new bicarbonate, and excrete acids. As CKD progresses, the ability of the kidneys to perform this function fails. Even when mild, chronic

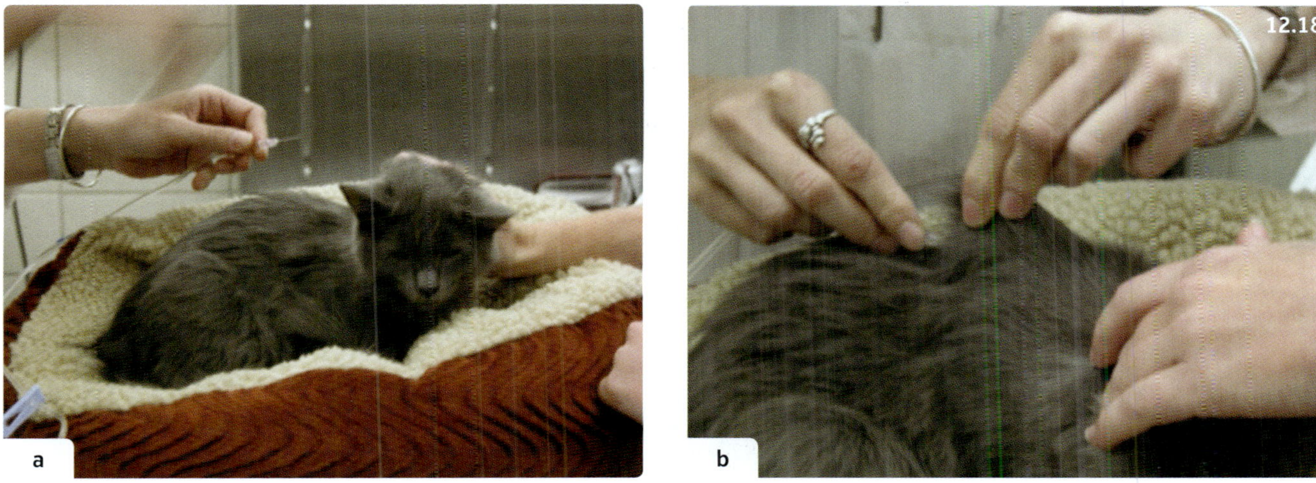

Figures 12.18a, b Cat with chronic kidney disease receiving subcutaneous fluids.

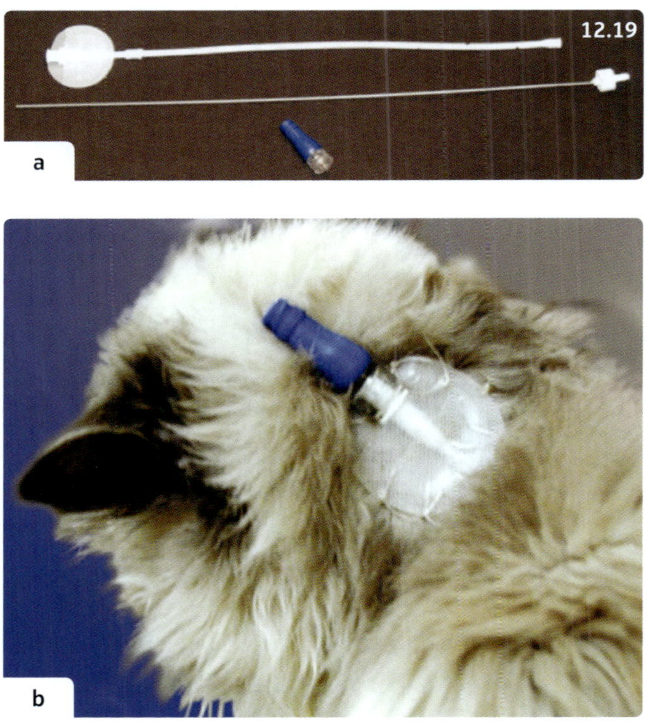

Figures 12.19a, b Gif-Tube (a) and a patient with a Gif-Tube inserted (b). (Courtesy Practivet)

acidosis enhances protein catabolism, promotes bone demineralization, and contributes to the array of clinical signs experienced by the renal failure patient. Because most feline maintenance diets are acidified, changing the patient to an appropriately buffered renal failure diet helps prevent and correct metabolic acidosis. When the patient is being fed an appropriate diet additional oral alkalization therapy is only indicated when total CO_2 is <18 mEq/l or serum bicarbonate is <17 mEq/l. Initially, sodium bicarbonate at a dose of 5–10 mg/kg q8–12h or potassium citrate at 40–60 mg/kg q8–12h can be given. The exact dose, which initially requires frequent monitoring, needs to be tailored to the individual patient.

Potassium

Hypokalemia is a common finding in cats with CKD and is associated with muscle weakness, muscle mass loss, ileus, and potentially fatal cardiac arrhythmias; however, the most commonly observed manifestation is anorexia. This condition is not recognized in dogs. The mechanism by which cats develop hypokalemia is unknown; however, it is generally believed to be a combination of malnutrition and excessive renal losses. In one study, one-third of healthy cats fed a potassium restricted diet developed interstitial nephritis and fibrosis. This suggests that low potassium is not only an effect of renal failure but can contribute to its progression. For this reason, most feline renal failure diets are potassium supplemented and, in most cases, will prevent hypokalemia. In patients that do not respond to diet therapy, oral supplementation with potassium citrate (20–30 mg/kg PO q24h) or potassium gluconate (2–6 mEq/cat q24h) can be given.

Hyperphosphatemia

Because of its role in muscle and nerve conduction, calcium is highly regulated within the body. Parathyroid hormone (PTH) is released by the parathyroid gland in response to small decreases in circulating calcium (**Figure 12.21**). PTH causes the release of stored calcium and stimulates an enzyme in the renal tissue, alpha-1 hydroxylase, to convert calcidiol to calcitriol. Calcitriol, the active form of vitamin D, stimulates absorption of calcium from the intestinal tract and also provides the

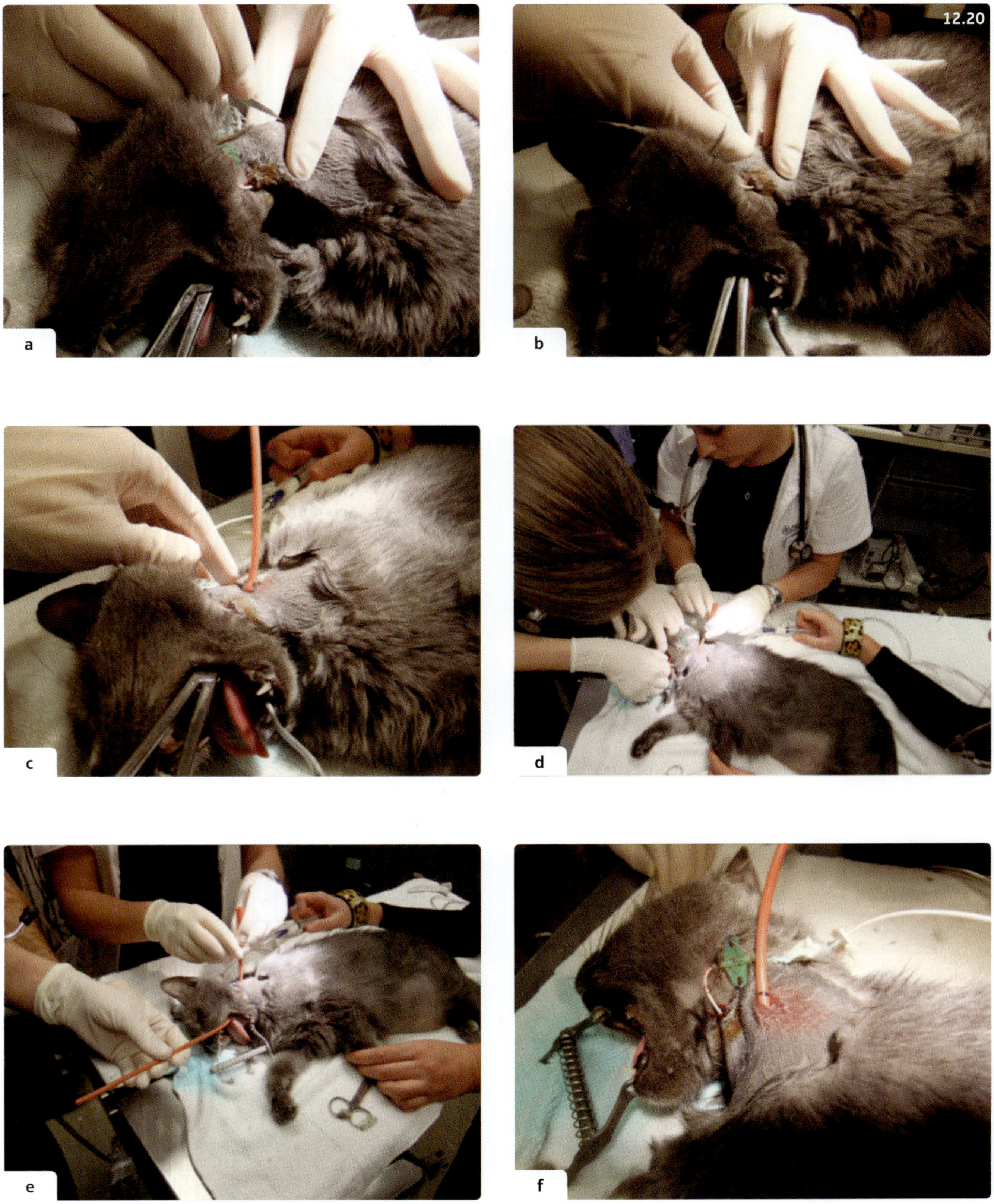
12.20
a
b
c
d
e
f

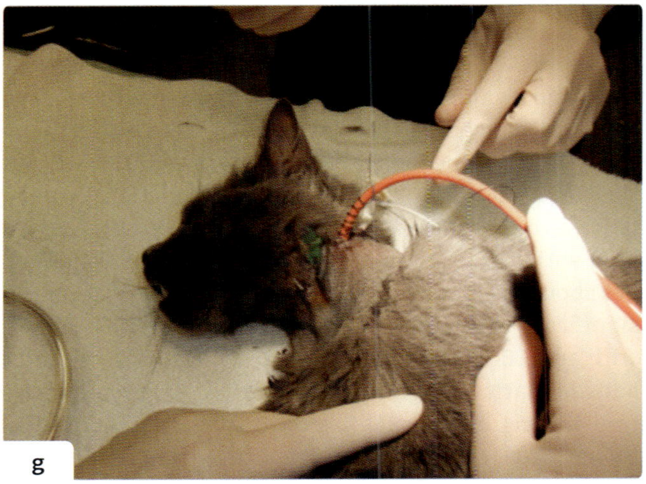

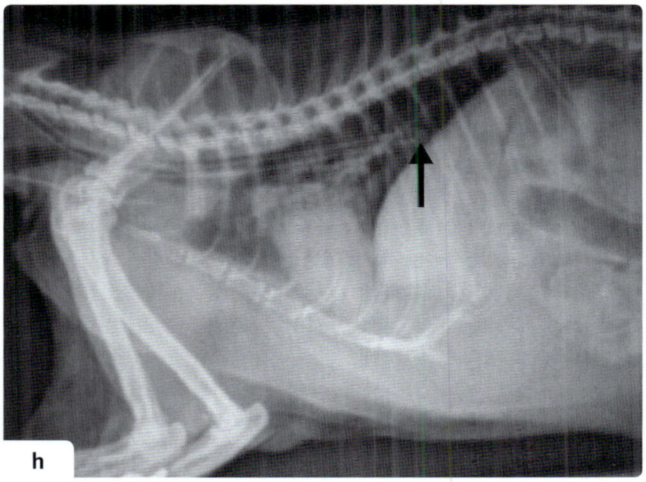

Figures 12.20a–h Esophagostomy tube placement. The patient is anesthetized and monitored. Although most tubes are placed on the left lateral cervical area, the right can be used as well. A red rubber or silicone tube is selected and marked so that the end of the tube will be located in the esophagus between the 6th and 9th intercostal spaces. The left lateral cervical area is clipped and scrubbed. The jugular vein is identified and isolated. (a) A pair of Mixter hemostats (tip forms a right angle) is inserted into the mouth and a small stab incision is made through the skin just over the tip of the hemostat. (b) The hemostat is seen poking through the skin. (c) A feeding tube is inserted into the open jaws of the hemostat. (d) The feeding tube is pulled into the esophagus and out of the mouth. (e, f) The tube is fed back into the mouth and down the esophagus. (g) A purse-string suture and a finger trap are placed to hold the tube in place. (h) Radiography confirms correct placement. Note the end of the tube is caudal to the heart and cranial to the lower esophageal sphincter (arrow).

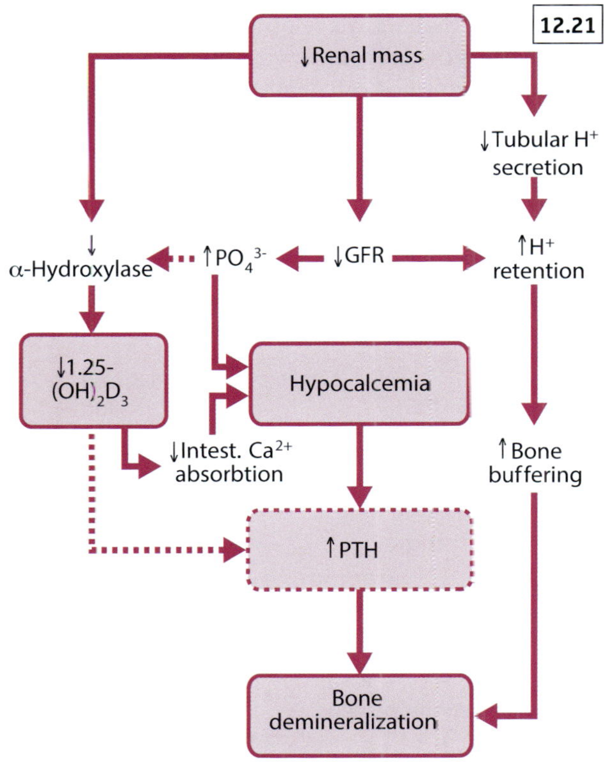

Figure 12.21 Pathogenesis of renal secondary hyperparathyroidism in chronic kidney disease. Renal production of calcitriol normally inhibits parathyroid hormone production and release by the parathyroid gland. Broken arrows indicate an inhibitory action.

negative feedback for PTH release. Phosphate is normally absorbed from the diet, used for metabolic processes, and subsequently undergoes renal excretion. As renal mass decreases and GFR falls, excessive levels of phosphate accumulate in the blood. Phosphate acts to inhibit alpha-1 hydroxylase, thus preventing the formation of calcitriol and removing the negative feedback on PTH release. Thus, hyperphosphatemia leads to loss of calcitriol, unabated PTH release from the parathyroid, and release of calcium and phosphorus from bone. Soft tissue mineralization becomes a concern when the product of serum calcium (mg/dl) and phosphorus (mg/dl) approaches 70. This is often seen in advanced CKD patients. In addition to its role in calcium regulation, calcitriol may also play a role in slowing the progression of renal disease. Therefore, controlling hyperphosphatemia is essential.

Other than hemodialysis there is no treatment that will rapidly decrease serum phosphorus levels, although fluid therapy can help in dehydrated patients. Since the primary source of serum phosphorus is dietary the first step is to change the patient's diet to a low phosphorus diet. In many cases, this will adequately control serum phosphorus levels. If after 2–3 weeks, hyperphosphatemia has not resolved, a phosphate-binding agent should be added to the diet. Aluminum hydroxide and aluminum carbonate (30–80 mg/kg q24h divided and given with meals) are commonly used and are effective in binding phosphorus in the intestine. Cats may find aluminum-based liquid phosphate binders to be unpalatable. Lanthanum carbonate (Fosrenol®) (30 mg/kg divided and given with meals) is an excellent alternative. It should be crushed and mixed well with food. Recently, a veterinary specific lanthanum-based phosphate binding product has been introduced (Renalzin®). Although it is both palatable and effective, it is not available in all countries. Calcium acetate (60–90 mg/kg q24h divided with meals) may also be effective in binding phosphate but increases calcium absorption in the intestine and may contribute to hypercalcemia; therefore, monitoring of serum calcium is essential. Regardless of the binder selected, the medication should be started at the lowest dose and then adjusted as needed based on serum phosphorus levels. Two weeks should be given between rechecks. Recently, several new phosphate binders have been introduced for use by human renal disease patients. These drugs were produced in response to concerns that small amounts of aluminum absorbed over long periods of time could lead to health problems. These new drugs are expensive and have not been shown to be more effective or safer in cats and dogs.

Since elevated PTH levels result from inhibition of calcitriol synthesis, supplementation with exogenous calcitriol has been proposed as a treatment for secondary hyperparathyroidism. Also, studies suggest that calcitriol therapy slows progression of CKD and improves survival in CKD dogs; however, similar results have not been documented in cats. Therefore, dogs with CKD should receive calcitriol therapy. Prior to calcitriol use, calcium and phosphate serum levels should be within normal range. Calcitriol (2.0–2.5 ng/kg/day) has been effective in normalizing serum PTH levels; however, required dosages vary widely and must be tailored to each patient. Ionized calcium and PTH must be monitored. The goal is to minimize PTH without inducing hypercalcemia. Since calcitriol can significantly increase intestinal calcium and phosphorus absorption, it must not be given with food. Use of calcium containing phosphate binders should be avoided. The primary complication associated with calcitriol treatment is hypercalcemia, which can occur at any time. Therefore, it is recommended that calcium and phosphate levels be monitored 1 week after starting therapy and then once monthly.

Proteinuria

Proteinuria can accelerate the progression of CKD and steps to mitigate protein loss should be taken when the UPC ratio exceeds 0.4 in the cat and 0.5 in the dog. Therapy usually involves feeding a renal failure diet and administration of an angiotensin-converting enzyme inhibitor (ACEI). The goal of the therapy is to reduce the UPC ratio by at least 50%, and preferably into the normal range. Although enalapril can be used, it is cleared exclusively through the kidney, while benazepril (0.25–0.5 mg/kg PO q12–24h), which has renal and hepatic clearance, is preferred. In some patients, ACEIs have been associated with a worsening of azotemia; therefore, renal values should be checked 7–14 days after starting therapy. If significant reductions in proteinuria cannot be achieved with an ACEI alone, angiotensin receptor blockers can be added. Pharmacologic data are sparse; however, irbesartan (1–5 mg/kg PO q24) has been suggested. Additional information can be found later this chapter (Protein-losing nephropathy).

Treatment of anemia

The cause of anemia in CKD is multifactorial and includes decreased RBC life span due to uremic toxins, nutritional deficiencies impairing RBC production, and intestinal bleeding; however, the most important cause of anemia is the loss of erythropoietin production by renal interstitial cells (**Figure 12.22**). Erythropoietin is a glycoprotein that increases the number of committed stem cells in the bone marrow that will develop into erythrocytes. In the absence of erythropoietin, erythroid stem cells undergo apoptosis (programed cell death). Release of erythropoietin depends on oxygen sensors located on renal interstitial cell membranes. These sensors upregulate production of erythropoietin during hypoxia and downregulate production when blood oxygen levels are normal.

12.22

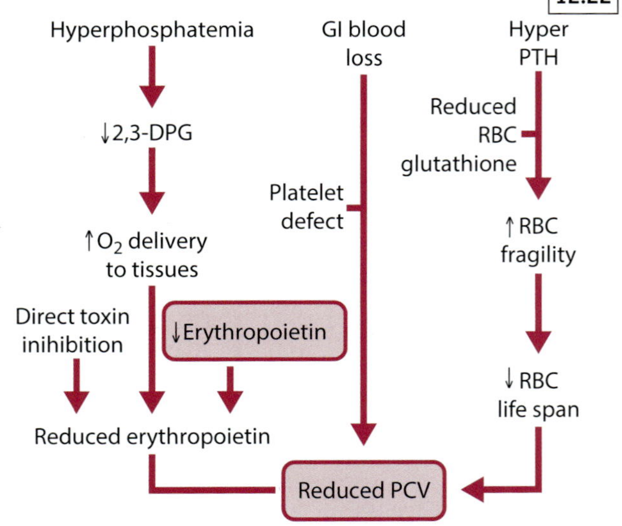

Figure 12.22 Pathogenesis of anemia in chronic kidney disease. The major cause of anemia is reduced renal production of erythropoietin.

Patients who are symptomatic for their anemia or have a dangerously low packed cell volume (PCV <20%) should immediately receive a compatible transfusion. Patients with a low PCV that are not symptomatic or critical should be started on a recombinant erythropoietin replacement therapy. Two alternatives exist: epoetin alfa (Epogen®) and darbepoetin alfa (Aranesp®). Epoetin alfa is more widely used because it is less expensive and there is more veterinary experience with this drug. Because it is a human recombinant protein, epoetin alfa can stimulate an immune response that can inactivate endogenous erythropoietin as well as the exogenous hormone. Some patients may become transfusion dependent. For this reason, it should be reserved for patients with significant anemia. The induction dose is 44–120 units/kg SC three times a week. Response time is variable but increases in PCV are usually seen in 1–2 weeks and target PCV should be obtained within a month. Once PCV has returned to 24–28%, the dose is tapered down to the minimum needed to maintain efficacy. Often, 44–88 units/kg SC 1–2 times a week is sufficient. The PCV should be rechecked every 2 weeks during induction and then monthly. Failure of the PCV to rise despite increasing dosages of epoetin alfa is strongly suggestive of an immune response. The drug should be discontinued at once and its use can be re-attempted in 3–4 weeks. As the immune response is likely to persist, these patients may never again respond appropriately to therapy. In addition, once an immune response develops to epoetin alfa, darbepoetin alfa is unlikely to be effective. Use of epoetin alfa has also been associated with hypertension and, therefore, blood pressure should be checked regularly.

Darbepoetin alfa is newer and more costly, but experience suggests that it is much less likely to stimulate an immune response. The induction dose is 1.5 units/kg SC once a week. This is continued until the patient's PCV reaches the low end of the normal range. At this point, the patient is changed to every other week dosing. Initially, PCV should be checked weekly to avoid overdosing. Eventually, the PCV can be checked monthly. Due to the high demand for iron needed for erythropoiesis, it is recommended that patients receiving either epoetin alfa or darbepoetin alfa receive iron supplementation (10 mg/kg IM every 3–4 weeks).

Diet

The mainstay of CKD treatment has been the correction of dehydration and nutritional support. Dietary formulations for patients with CKD have traditionally focused on protein restriction in the hope of slowing the progression of renal failure. While protein restriction does help reduce uremia and can significantly improve the patient's quality of life, it is not clear that controlling dietary protein alone can significantly change the disease course. Nevertheless, it is clear that patients with CKD who are fed a renal failure diet live longer than those fed a maintenance formulation. Certainly, control of acidosis, hyperphosphotemia, and hypokalemia are helpful in treating these patients. Studies demonstrate that proper regulation of serum phosphorus alone can improve survival of patients with CKD. However, it is now believed that the ratio of omega-3 to omega-6 fatty acids may also play an important role in slowing the progression of renal disease. All major commercially available renal failure diets are generously supplemented with omega-3 fatty acids.

Anorexia

Patients with CKD often suffer from anorexia. While the exact cause of inappetence is unknown, it is probably related to uremic toxins combined with irritation of the gastrointestinal tract. Due to their low protein, restricted phosphorus, and reduced sodium, renal failure diets can be unpalatable to even healthy pets. Owners should try several different brands and formulations in order to find one that their pet will eat. Some owners report good success with rotating several different diets. Many CKD pets will eat frequent small meals rather than one or two large ones; therefore, feeding schedules and amounts may need to be adjusted. Warming of wet food can make a renal diet more palatable, especially to cats; however, when utilizing a microwave oven, care must be taken as nonuniform heating can lead to oral burns. Mirtazapine, a tetracyclic antidepressant, may help improve appetite in anorexic cats (1–3 mg/cat PO q72h). Because hypergastrinemia can occur with CKD, many patients respond to H2-histamine receptor blockers such as famotidine (0.5 mg/kg IV or PO q24h). When present, nausea can usually be relieved with either dopamine or serotonin (5HT) inhibitors (**Table 12.8**).

Advanced renal therapies.

Renal transplantation for cats with CKD is now being performed at referral centers around the world. In order to be a candidate, a patient must be documented to be free of infectious diseases such as feline leukemia virus, feline immunodeficiency virus, and toxoplasmosis. Recent thoracic radiographs and an abdominal ultrasound are required to show the absence of a malignancy. In addition, an echocardiogram may be required to demonstrate that the patient does not have significant cardiac disease. A good candidate would be a middle aged cat that is suffering from increasing azotemia despite appropriate therapy and yet is still in good body condition. Six-month survival approaches 60% while 3-year survival is >40%. While renal transplantation has been performed in dogs, the success rates have not been encouraging due to problems with tissue rejection. Centers performing renal transplantation can be found on line at: www.queenofthenephron.com

Hemodialysis for the CKD patient is available at select centers. While technically feasible, cost and the need for treatments several times a week have made this option impractical for most pet owners.

PROTEIN-LOSING NEPHROPATHY

Definition/overview

Normally, the glomerulus provides an effective barrier against the loss of albumin and other large proteins into the urine. In protein-losing nephropathy (PLN), the barrier is disrupted and excessive amounts of protein cross the glomerular filtration barrier into the tubules. As a result, tubules become damaged by inflammation and fibrosis. Thus, what starts as a localized disruption of the glomerulus leads to a generalized disease of the nephron.

Pathophysiology

The glomerular capillary bed is unique in that it can filter molecules based on the size and charge of a molecule. The wall of the glomerular capillary is composed of three distinct layers: endothelial cells, glomerular basement membrane, and epithelial cells (**Figure 12.23**). The endothelial cells form the inner lining of the capillary tube. While the endothelial cells do not provide a significant filtration barrier, they do serve other important functions such as inhibition of clot formation. The basement membrane, which provides the structural scaffold of the glomerulus, possesses a negative change that helps establish glomerular charge selectivity. It is composed of type IV collagen, laminin, and heparan sulfate. Collagen is primarily responsible for the structural support, laminin is involved with cell adhesion, and heparan sulfate provides the basement membrane with its negative charge. Epithelial cells, called podocytes, freely float in Bowman's space. These cells give rise to an array of parallel projections called foot processes, which are attached to the basement membrane. The projections interdigitate to form slit pores. Proteins, such as nephrin, bridge slit pores and limit the size of molecules that can pass through.

The degree to which a protein can pass across the glomerular capillary wall is a function of molecular size and charge (**Figure 12.24**). Size selectivity is based primarily on podocyte slit pores while charge selectivity is a function of the negative charge generated by all three layers.

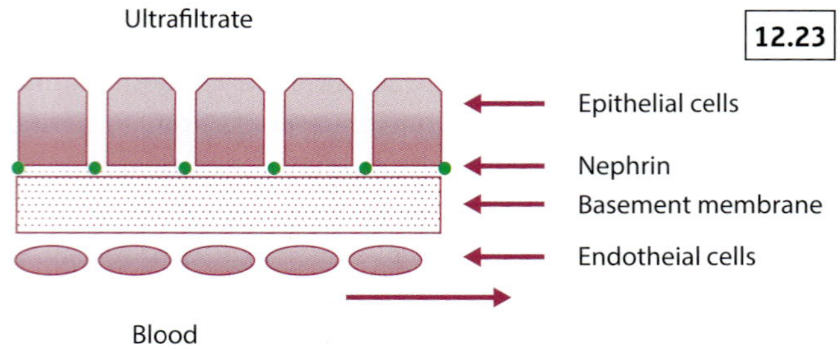

Figure 12.23 The components of the glomerular membrane.

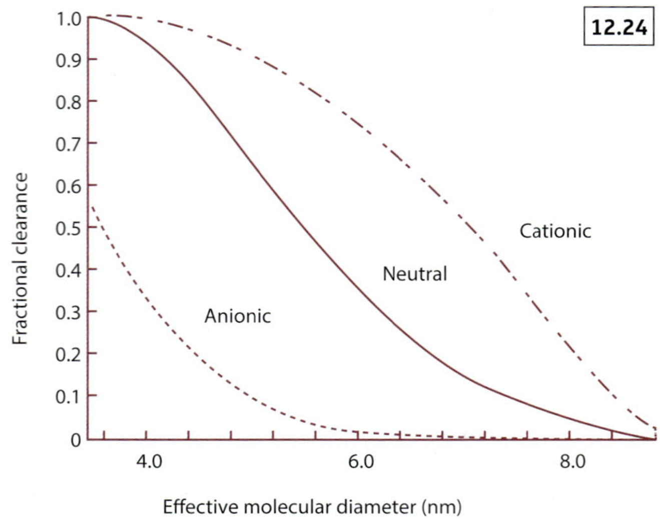

Figure 12.24 Charge selectivity of glomerulus demonstrated by fractional clearance of anionic and neutral molecules. The neutral molecule is more freely filtered because it is not repelled by the membrane's charge.

Typically, small negatively charged proteins, such as inulin (5,200 MW) are freely filtered, larger ones such as myoglobin (17,000 MW) are partially filtered, and albumin (69,000 MW) is only slightly filtered. Under normal circumstances, all filtered proteins are reabsorbed in the PCT. Large proteins are taken into the tubular epithelial cells by carrier-mediated endocytosis and then catabolized in the lysosomes where they are broken down into amino acids. The process of breaking down large amounts of proteins into amino acids is thought to release oxygen free radicals and leads to the release of inflammatory cytokines. The resulting inflammation causes fibrosis and scarring of the tubules.

There are two disease processes associated with disruption of the normal filtration barrier of the glomerulus and the development of PLN: amyloidosis and glomerulonephritis (GN). These cannot be distinguished from each other on the basis of clinical signs or laboratory data. Only a renal biopsy can be used to differentiate the two conditions.

Amyloidosis

Amyloidosis is caused by an inappropriate deposition of fibrils into the glomerulus. These fibrils are formed by the polymerization of protein subunits, which have a specific tertiary structure called the beta-pleated sheet. These subunits, such as serum amyloid A (SAA), are produced in the liver and are one of a number of acute-phase reactants manufactured in response to inflammation. The exact function of these proteins is unknown, but production appears to be simulated by interleukin (IL)-2, IL-6, and tumor necrosis factor, which are released by macrophages in response to tissue injury. Once polymerized, the amyloid fibrils cannot be degraded because the beta-pleated sheet conformation prevents enzymatic degradation. When deposited in the glomerulus, the fibrils act to disrupt normal function.

Glomerulonephritis

GN results from the deposition of preformed circulating immune complexes or *in-situ* reaction of circulating antibodies with exogenous or endogenous antigens on the glomerular basement membrane. The presence of immune complexes leads to activation of complement, neutrophil chemotaxis, platelet aggregation, and activation of the coagulation system. This leads to protein spilling across the glomerulus and into the proximal tubules. Eventually, the glomerulus responds to the immune response with cellular proliferation, thickening of the basement membrane, and eventually sclerosis.

GN can be divided into three categories based on histologic appearance: membranoproliferative glomerulonephritis (MPGN), membranous nephropathy (MN), and proliferative glomerulonephritis.

- Membranoproliferative glomerulonephritis (MPGN) is the most common type of GN seen in the dog and accounts for up to 60% of all cases. While a familial form of the disease is seen with Bernese Mountain Dogs and a rapidly progressive form has been associated with *Borrelia burgdorferi* infection, the underlying cause of many cases is unknown. The classic histopathologic appearance is that of thickened capillary loops and mesangial hypercellularity (**Figures 12.25–12.28**).
- Membranous nephropathy (MN) is the second most common type of GN lesions seen in the dog and the most common type in the cat (GN2). In this condition, the glomerular basement membrane becomes thickened due to the deposition of immune complexes in the subepithelial spaces and the resulting proliferation of the basement membrane (**Figures 12.29–12.32**).
- Proliferative glomerulonephritis accounts for as little as 2% of GN cases and is characterized by endocapillary or mesangial proliferation.

Clinical presentation

Generally, PLN is a disease of middle aged to older dogs. Clinical features of PLN are somewhat dependent on the underlying cause and degree of azotemia. Some cases are detected on routine urine analysis in otherwise healthy patients. Lethargy, anorexia, vomiting, and weight loss are among the most common clinical signs in patients with overt renal disease. Less commonly noted are polyuria, polydipsia, and ataxia.

Diagnosis

Urinalysis

The hallmark of PLN is the finding of inappropriate amounts of urine protein in the absence of bacteria, casts, or blood cells. It is impossible to determine the significance of proteinuria detected on routine urinalysis or a urine dipstick; therefore, the finding of proteinuria always warrants further investigation.

Normal renal protein excretion in dogs and cats is <20 mg/kg/day. A 24-hour urine collection is the gold standard for quantifying the magnitude of protein excretion; however, this is neither convenient nor practical in the clinical setting. Because the UPC ratio has been shown to closely correlate with 24-hour protein excretion, this value is most commonly used in clinical applications. Healthy dogs and cats have been shown to have a UPC ratio of <0.5 and <0.4, respectively. It is important to note that the presence of white blood cells, bacteria, epithelial cells, and casts can significantly increase the UPC ratio. Therefore, UPC ratio should only be performed in tandem with a full urinalysis and sediment examination. In addition, studies suggest that the UPC ratio can have significant day-to-day variability associated with actual protein loss fluctuations. One strategy to minimize this variability is to have the owner collect three samples of urine at home and store them at 40°F (4.4°C). In the clinic, equal volumes of these samples are pooled and submitted for analysis.

Serum chemistry

Kidney injury is usually accompanied by elevations in BUN, creatinine, and phosphorus and a decrease in bicarbonate. Proteinuria may be detected prior to onset of azotemia; however, in most cases, serum albumin will be decreased.

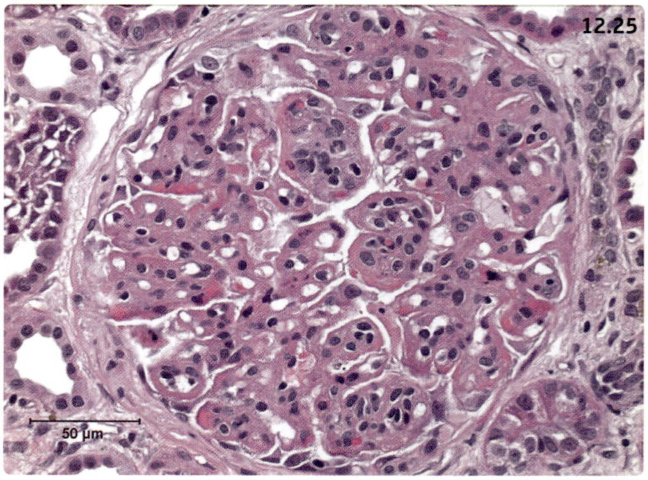

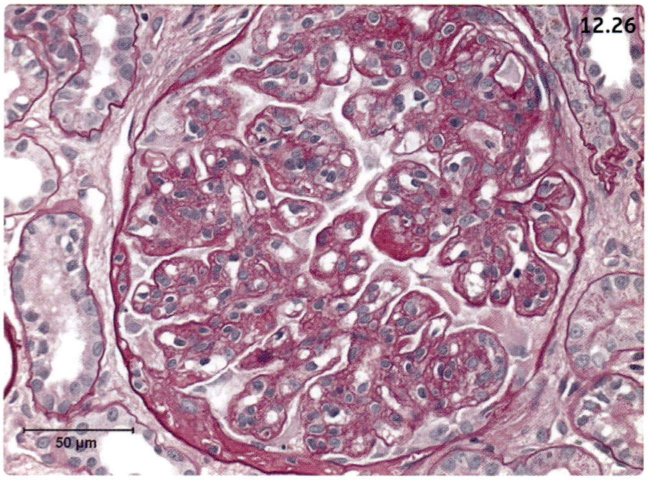

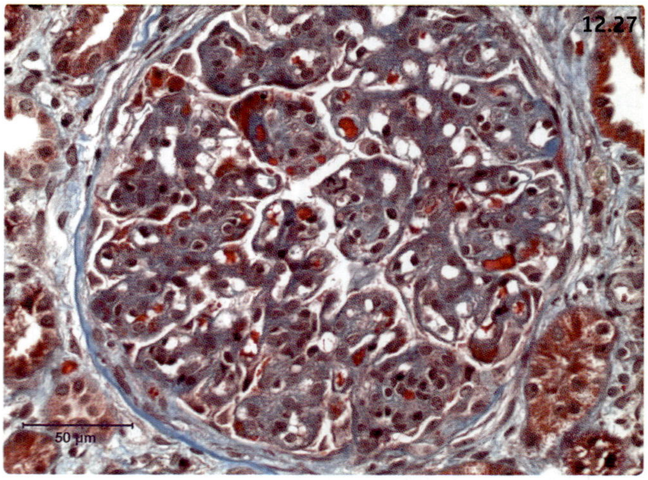

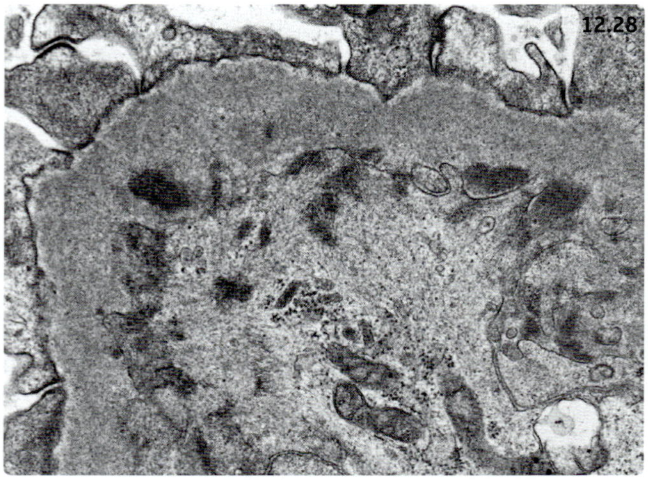

Figures 12.25–12.28 Illustrations of the histologic and ultrastructural features of membranoproliferative gomerulonephritis in a dog. The light microscopic appearance of a single glomerulus is shown stained with with H&E (12.25), PAS (12.26), and Masson's trichrome (12.27). The transmission electron micrograph (12.28) shows subendothelial electron-dense immune deposits in the capillary wall. (Courtesy R.P. Groman, G.E. Lees, B.R. Berridge, and F.J. Clubb Jr.)

Complete blood count

Anemia is by far the most common CBC finding in PLN patients. The cause of anemia is probably multifactorial and involves decreased RBC life span, decreased erythropoietin production, and the anemia of chronic disease. Changes in the white blood count are often nonspecific, although elevations are suggestive of an infectious disease process.

Management

Underlying cause

As GN is often secondary to an identifiable underlying disease (**Table 12.14**) and amyloidosis is associated with chronic inflammation, a thorough search for an inciting cause is essential. Infectious, neoplastic, endocrine, inflammatory, and drug-related causes must be considered.

Infectious disease serology

Serologic tests should be selected on the basis of the patient's geographic location and relevant travel history. Infectious diseases associated with PLN include Rocky Mountain spotted fever, ehrlichiosis, borreliosis, leishmaniasis, babesiosis, and heartworm infection.

Radiography and ultrasound

Imaging plays an important role in the diagnostic plan for PLN. PLN can be secondary to a neoplastic process and ultrasound and radiographic studies, in combination with

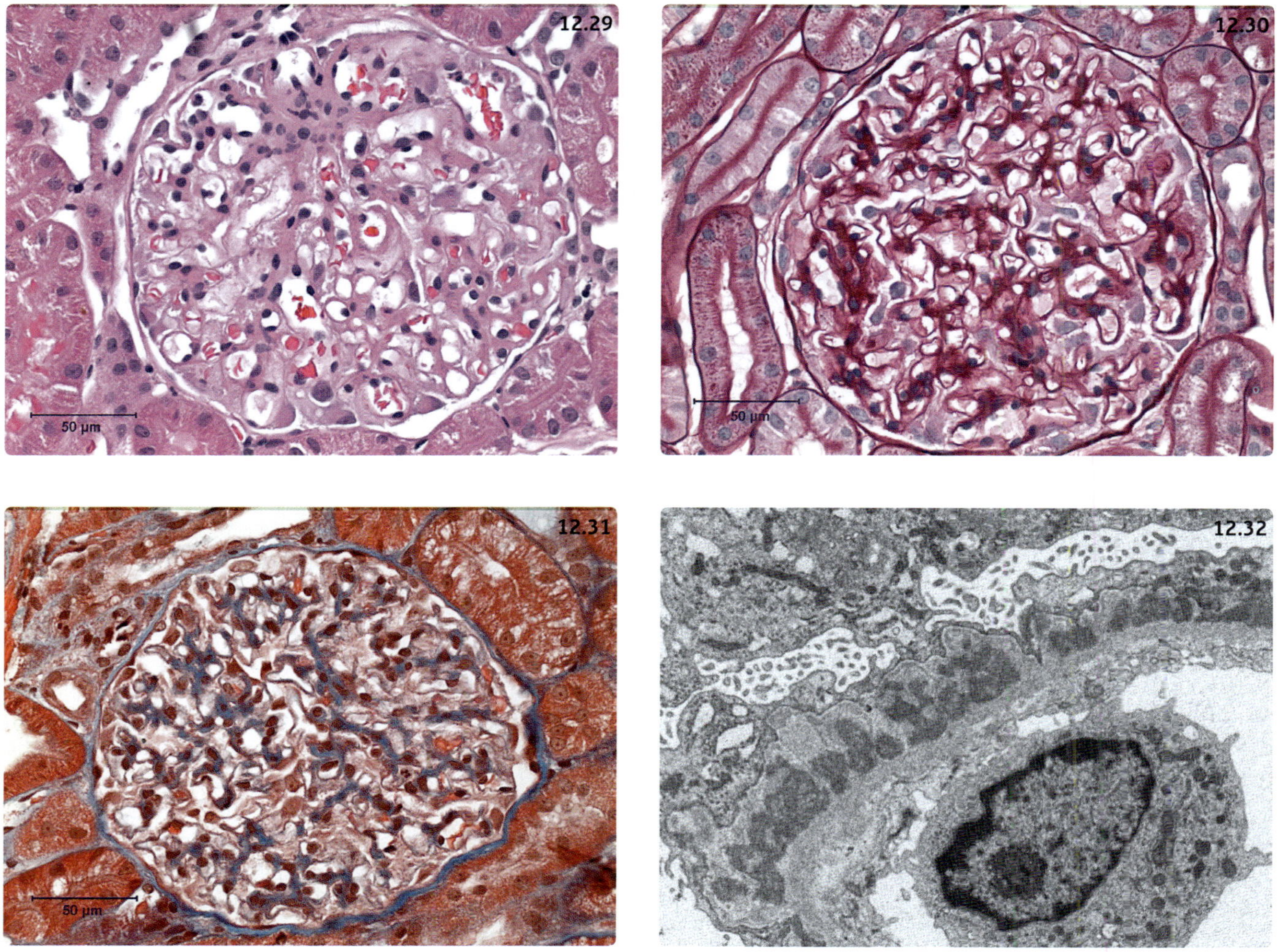

Figures 12.29–12.32 Illustrations of the histologic and ultrastructural features of membranous glomerulonephritis in a dog. The light microscopic appearance of representative glomeruli is shown stained with H&E (12.29), PAS (12.30), and Masson's trichrome (12.31). The transmission electron micrograph (12.32) shows intramembranous electron-dense immune deposits in the capillary wall. (Courtesy R.P. Groman, G.E. Lees, B.R. Berridge, and F.J. Clubb Jr.)

a thorough physical examination, are essential in eliminating this as a possible underlying cause. Ultrasound can also provide information about the renal architecture and outflow tract, and it can be used to obtain renal biopsies in a minimally invasive fashion.

If an underlying disease process is found, then therapy aimed at treating the primary condition should be initiated; otherwise, the condition is labeled as idiopathic. Prognosis may be better if the cause can be identified and treated.

Amyloidosis vs. glomerulonephritis

The only way to differentiate amyloidosis from GN is by renal biopsy. There is no meaningful difference between the clinical pathology and physical examination findings in these two conditions. In addition, several forms of GN are now recognized and can only be differentiated on analysis of a renal biopsy sample examined by light, electron, and immunofluorescence microscopy (GN and GN2). At a minimum, examination by light microscopy should be performed on all cases. Tissue samples should be stained with periodic acid–Schiff (PAS), methenamine silver, trichrome, and Congo red: PAS allows inspection of the glomerular basement membrane for evidence of scarring; methenamine silver allows for examination of the basement membrane of the tubules, glomeruli, and Bowman's capsule; trichrome allows for visualization of immunoglobulin deposits; Congo red, when viewed with polarized light, will confirm or rule out the presence of amyloid (**Figure 12.33**). There are two collaborating

Table 12.14 The various causes of protein-losing glomerulonephritis in the dog and cat.

	Canine	Feline
Infectious	Canine hepatitis	Feline leukemia virus
	Bacterial endocarditis	Feline infectious peritonitis
	Brucellosis	Mycoplasmal polyarthritis
	Dirofilariasis	
	Ehrlichiosis	
	Leishmaniasis	
	Pyometra	
	Borreliosis	
	Rocky Mountain spotted fever	
	Trypanosomiasis	
Neoplasia	Leukemia	Leukemia
	Lymphoma	Lymphoma
	Systemic histocytosis	Others
	Others	
Inflammatory	Pancreatitis	Pancreatitis
	Systemic lupus erythematosus	Systemic lupus erythematosus
	Polyarthritis	Polyarthritis
	Prostatitis	Cholangiohepatitis
	Immune-mediated hemolytic anemia	
Other	Hyperadrenocorticism	Familial
	Steroid administration	Idiopathic
	Familial	
	Idiopathic	

centers, one in North America (International Veterinary Renal Pathology Service) and one in Europe (Utrecht Veterinary Nephrology Service), with extensive experience analyzing renal biopsy specimens. Since different

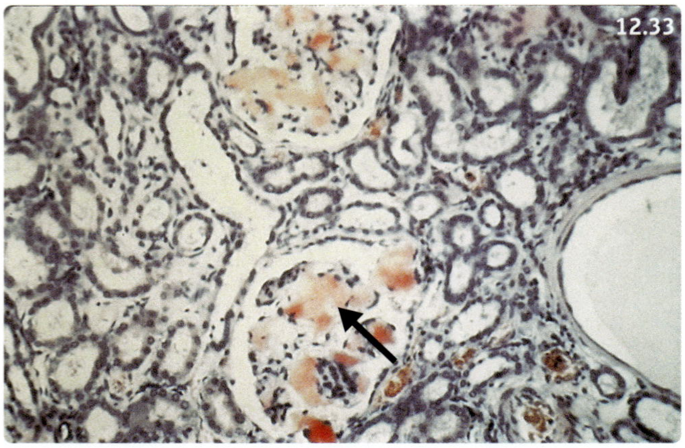

Figure 12.33 Histopathology of the kidney of a dog with amyloidosis. Red-staining amorphous amyloid is evident in the glomeruli (arrow). (Courtesy D.F. Senior)

forms of GN have different treatment options and prognosis, these pathology services should be utilized whenever possible.

Amyloid-specific treatment

Colchicine, an inhibitor of microtubule assembly, has been shown to inhibit release of SAA from hepatocytes and may be of benefit before signs of renal failure develop. It has been used in humans with familial Mediterranean fever to prevent onset of renal amyloidosis. The efficacy of this drug in the treatment of renal amyloidosis in animals is not established. Colchicine has significant side-effects including vomiting, diarrhea, and nausea. In addition, there is no known benefit to starting treatment after renal failure develops. The currently recommended canine dose is 0.02–0.04 mg/kg PO q24h.

Dimethyl sulfoxide (DMSO) has been advocated for the treatment of amyloidosis. Theoretical benefits include solubilization of amyloid fibrils and reduced serum concentration of SAA as well as reduced renal inflammation. There are no controlled clinical studies to determine if DMSO is beneficial for small animals suffering from amyloidosis, but an individual case report suggested a positive response. The canine dose is 80 mg/kg diluted 1:4 with sterile saline given SC three times a week. Methylsulfonylmethane (MSM) is a derivative of DMSO that can be given orally. Theoretical benefits are the same as for DMSO but it is considered more convenient since it can be given at home. It should be noted that there are no clinical data to support the use of MSM. The currently recommended canine dose is 88 mg/kg q8h.

Glomerulonephritis-specific treatment

Angiotensin-converting enzyme inhibition

In a blinded multicenter study of dogs with biopsy confirmed GN, the ACEI enalapril (0.5 mg/kg q12–24h) decreased the UPC ratio, lowered blood pressure, and improved clinical outcome. Some of the effect is likely due to decreased glomerular hypertension secondary to dilation of the efferent arterioles. There is also evidence that ACEIs may inhibit cytokine production, thereby decreasing interstitial fibrosis. The goal of the therapy is to reduce the UPC ratio by at least 50%, and preferably into the normal range. Although enalapril can be used, it is cleared exclusively through the kidney, while benazepril (0.25–0.5 mg/kg PO q12–24h), which has renal and hepatic clearance, is preferred. If significant reductions in proteinuria cannot be achieved with ACE inhibition alone, angiotensin receptor blockers can be added. Pharmacologic data are sparse; however, irbesartan (1–5 mg/kg PO q24h) and telmisartan (1.0–2.0 mg/kg PO q24h) have been suggested.

Immunosuppression

The role of immunosuppressive drugs in the treatment of dogs with GN has changed dramatically in recent years. When histopathologic evidence of an active immunologic basis for the PLN exists, immunosuppressive therapy is strongly recommended. Such evidence would include electron-dense deposits detected on electron microscopy and immunoglobulin or complement-associated immune complexes detected by immunofluorescent microscopy. Therefore, renal biopsies are strongly recommended in all cases of PLN. In cases where the PLN is progressive and histopathology is unavailable, the use of immunosuppressive drugs could be considered providing the owner is aware of potential risks. In cases of peracute or rapidly progressive GN, mycophenolate (10 mg/kg PO q12h) has been recommended with or without cyclophosphamide (200–250 mg/m^2 every 3 weeks). Response to treatment can be measured by changes to the UPC ratio. A complete response is defined as a UPC ratio of <0.5, while a partial response is defined as a reduction of the UPC ratio by 50% of the pretreatment value. In dogs that demonstrate no response to immunosuppressive therapy after 8 weeks, an alternative therapy can be considered (**Table 12.15**). If after 3–4 months there is no clinically significant response, therapy should be discontinued. In patients that do have a response to therapy, immunosuppressive therapy should be continued for 12–16 weeks, after which the dose may be tapered while monitoring the UPC ratio and degree of azotemia.

Common amyloidosis and glomerulonephritis therapies

Diet

Patients with PLN should be fed a properly formulated renal failure diet that is low in protein, high in omega-3 polyunsaturated fatty acids, and low in sodium. Although initially counterintuitive, PLN patients should be fed a moderately protein-restricted diet. Studies in people with PLN have shown that feeding a high protein diet is associated with increased glomerular protein loss, additional renal pathology, and higher mortality. Conversely, patients fed a low protein diet lose less protein in their urine, have less renal pathology, and live longer. The

Table 12.15 Immunosuppressive drugs used in glomerulonephritis.

Agent	Mechanism	Dose
Azathioprine	Antagonizes purine metabolism. Interferes with DNA and RNA synthesis. Cytotoxic to lymphocytes	2 mg/kg PO q24h for 1–2 weeks, then 1–2 mg/kg q48h
Chlorambucil	Alkylating agent. Interferes with DNA replication and RNA transcription	0.2 mg/kg PO q24–48h
Cyclophosphamide	Alkylating agent. Interferes with DNA replication and RNA transcription	Pulse therapy 200–250 mg/m^2 every 3 weeks
Cyclosporine	Calcineurin inhibitor. Prevents activation of T cells	5–20 mg/kg PO q12h, taper dose upward from low to high
Mycophenolate	Antagonizes guanosine metabolism. Suppresses T- and B-cell proliferation	10 mg/kg PO q12h

reason for this paradox is unclear but may involve the damage caused to the tubule by the increased protein available for loss into the urine.

Thromboembolism

Thromboembolism is the cause of death for a significant number of dogs with glomerular disease. Much of the blame has been placed on antithrombin III which, because of its size, is lost through the damaged glomerulus at a rate comparable to albumin (**Figures 12.34, 12.35**). However, not all animals with low albumin experience thromboembolic events and therefore other factors are likely involved. Risk of thromboembolism is greatest when antithrombin III is less than 75% of normal. This correlates with a serum albumin of approximately 2.0 g/dl. There are few studies on which to base anticoagulation recommendations. A low dose of aspirin has been recommended to inhibit platelet aggregation and clot formation; however, one recent study suggests that the previously recommended dose of 0.5 mg/kg may be too low to be efficacious. A dose of 1.0–5.0 mg/kg q24h has now been suggested. Another option is clopidogrel (1.1 mg/kg q24h). Clopidogrel is a platelet aggregation inhibitor, which may be used in conjunction with or in place of aspirin. Clopidogrel should not be given simultaneously with proton pump inhibitor antacid drugs because the latter will delay the metabolism of the clopidogrel and predispose to bleeding problems associated with platelet dysfunction.

Blood pressure

The vast majority of dogs with glomerular disease develop significant hypertension during the course of their disease. Hypertension can lead to ocular, cardiac, and cerebral damage and potentiate further kidney injury. Therefore, blood pressure should be checked periodically and antihypertensive therapy administered as needed (see Hypertension, below, for more information).

Fluid therapy

While fluid therapy is a cornerstone in the treatment of AKI and CKD, it should be used with great caution in PLN patients. These patients are extremely vulnerable to fluid overload and edema. In addition, studies in people and animal models suggest that colloids should not be used to prevent or treat edema as they can further potentiate renal damage. When necessary, only enough fluids to correct dehydration should be administered. This should be done over relatively long periods of time (~24 hours) and under close supervision. In patients where edema has already occurred, fluid therapy should be stopped and diuretic therapy with furosemide or spironolactone should be considered.

HYPERTENSION

Definition/overview

Historically, the definition of 'normal' canine and feline blood pressure has been the subject of debate. While there is no clear definition, it is generally accepted that a single blood pressure estimation of >150/95 mmHg in a patient with clinical signs attributed to hypertension or a blood pressure >150/95 mmHg on three separate visits in a patient who demonstrates no clinical signs is compatible with hypertension.

Etiology

Clinically, hypertension is divided into two categories based on the underlying etiology: primary and secondary. Primary hypertension is the result of an imbalance

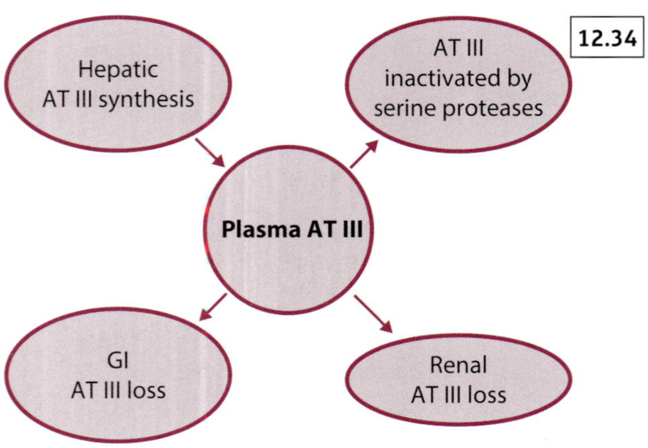

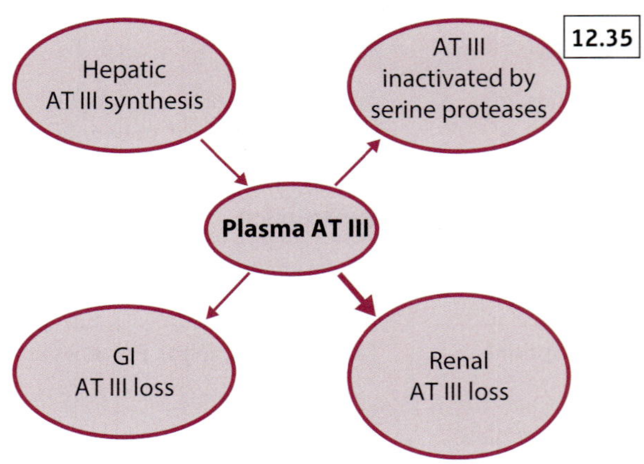

Figures 12.34, 12.35 Antithrombin III (AT III) balance in normal dogs (12.34) and in dogs with glomerulonephropathy (12.35). Loss of glomerular sieve selectivity leads to massive renal excretion with subsequent reduced serum levels.

between cardiac output, systemic vascular resistance, and the autonomic nervous system. Although primary hypertension accounts for more than 90% of all cases of elevated blood pressure in human patients, it is thought to be uncommon in dogs and cats. Secondary hypertension occurs as a consequence of another disease or medical treatment and accounts for the majority of small animal cases. Renal disease, hyperadrenocorticism, thyroid disease, diabetes mellitus, liver disease, pheochromocytoma, chronic anemia, and drugs including erythropoietin and glucocorticoids have all been associated with hypertension in dogs and cats. Clinically, this is important because it allows clinicians to focus their blood pressure screening efforts on specific 'at-risk' populations.

Pathophysiology

Normal blood pressure is the result of a complex interaction between the heart, the kidneys, the autonomic nervous system, and the endothelial signaling mechanisms (**Figure 12.36**). These factors determine cardiac output and systemic vascular resistance, which are the ultimate blood pressure determinants (BP = CO × SVR). Although the relationship between renal disease and hypertension has been studied extensively, the connection between the two remains elusive. Recent data suggest that the cause of hypertension in renal failure patients is multifactorial.

Clinical presentation

When increases in blood pressure are mild the patient usually demonstrates no clinical signs directly attributable to hypertension. As the elevations in systolic pressure approach 200 mmHg, the eyes, heart, brain, and kidneys are organs in which clinical signs of hypertension become apparent. Choroidopathy and retinopathy are so common in cats with CKD that loss of vision and not the underlying renal disease often initiates the clinic visit. Retinal edema, tortuous vessels, and hemorrhage characterize hypertensive retinopathy (**Figures 12.37a, b**) while choroidopathy results in ischemic necrosis of the choriocapillaries and the retinal pigmented epithelium. This presents clinically as blindness due to retinal detachment.

As the pressure against which the heart must pump increases, changes occur in the cardiac muscle. Dogs

12.36

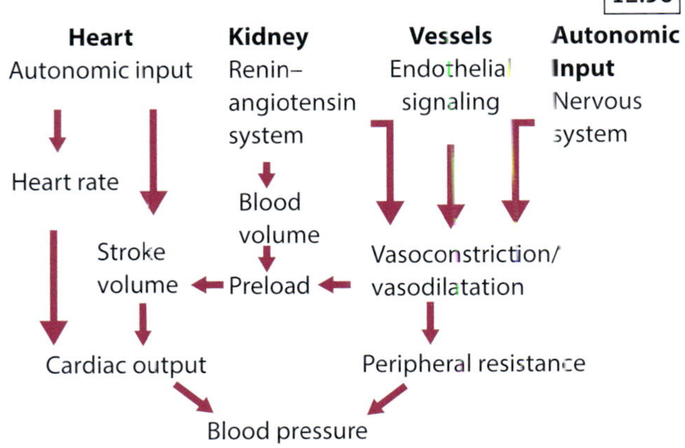

Figure 12.36 Complex interactions between heart, kidneys, vessels, nervous system, and endothelial signaling system, which determine blood pressure.

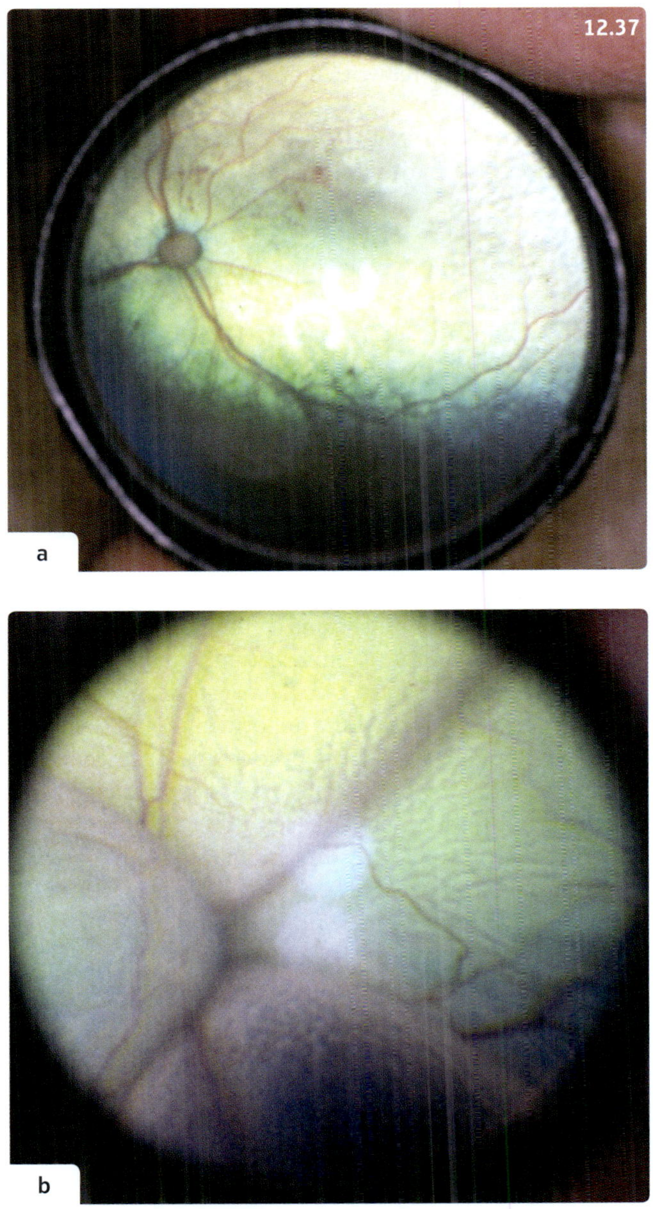

Figures 12.37a, b (a) Ocular changes consistent with hypertension. Note the tortuous vessels, hemorrhage, and edema. (b) Retinal detachment secondary to hypertension. (Courtesy P. Miller)

develop left ventricular hypertrophy and commensurate mitral valve insufficiency. Typically, cats develop thickening of the interventricular septum, hypertrophy of the left ventricular free wall, reduced diastolic ventricular internal diameter, and dilation of the proximal aorta. Clinically, these changes can be detected as a murmur, an arrhythmia, or a gallop rhythm.

As systolic blood pressure exceeds the capacity of the autoregulatory mechanisms of the cerebral vasculature, hypertensive encephalopathy becomes apparent. This is characterized by a head tilt, ataxia, depression, disorientation, and seizures. This condition constitutes an emergency and is associated with a guarded prognosis.

Differential diagnosis

White coat effect, error in measurement.

Diagnosis

Systolic and diastolic blood pressure can be measured directly by placing a catheter in a suitable artery and connecting it to a transducer (**Figures 12.38a, b**). While this is the most accurate way to measure blood pressure, it is invasive, painful, and neither convenient nor practical in the clinical setting. Indirect measurements of blood pressure using Doppler and oscillometric techniques are most useful in the clinic.

Oscillometric devices work by inflating a cuff around a distal extremity until arterial blood flow is occluded (**Figure 12.39**). The unit then slowly deflates the cuff while monitoring for pulsations created by arterial blood flow. Interestingly, these units actually measure mean arterial pressure and then calculate systolic and diastolic pressures using proprietary algorithms. Oscillometric units are popular in clinical practice because they are automated and provide systolic, diastolic, and mean arterial pressure. Nevertheless, these units can significantly underestimate blood pressure when used on cats and small dogs (<10 kg). Recently, new devices have been produced that claim to have been optimized for veterinary use. The accuracy of these devices is not clear at this time.

Doppler flow detectors are less expensive, easy to use, and suitable for dogs and cats of all sizes (**Figure 12.40**). These devices work by emitting an ultrasound wave and then comparing the frequency of the initial signal to the one that is reflected back to the probe. If the wave is reflected off of the surface of a moving object, such as blood cells coursing through an artery, the frequency is shifted. The Doppler unit makes this change in frequency audible and the operator hears this as a characteristic 'swoosh' sound.

The first step in measuring blood pressure with a Doppler unit is to palpate an artery in the distal portion of an extremity (**Figures 12.41–12.45**). The hair over the artery is clipped and a cuff with a width 30–40% of the circumference of the limb is placed proximal to the clipped area. To ensure conduction, ultrasound gel is placed on the Doppler probe and the probe is placed over the clipped area. The probe is then adjusted until the sound of arterial blood pulsations can be clearly heard. The cuff is inflated approximately 10–20 mmHg past the point at which blood flow can no longer be detected. Then, the cuff is gradually deflated while the operator observes the sphygmomanometer's display. The pressure at which the sound of blood flow first returns is the systolic pressure. Sometimes, a second sound, which represents the diastolic pressure, can be heard as cuff

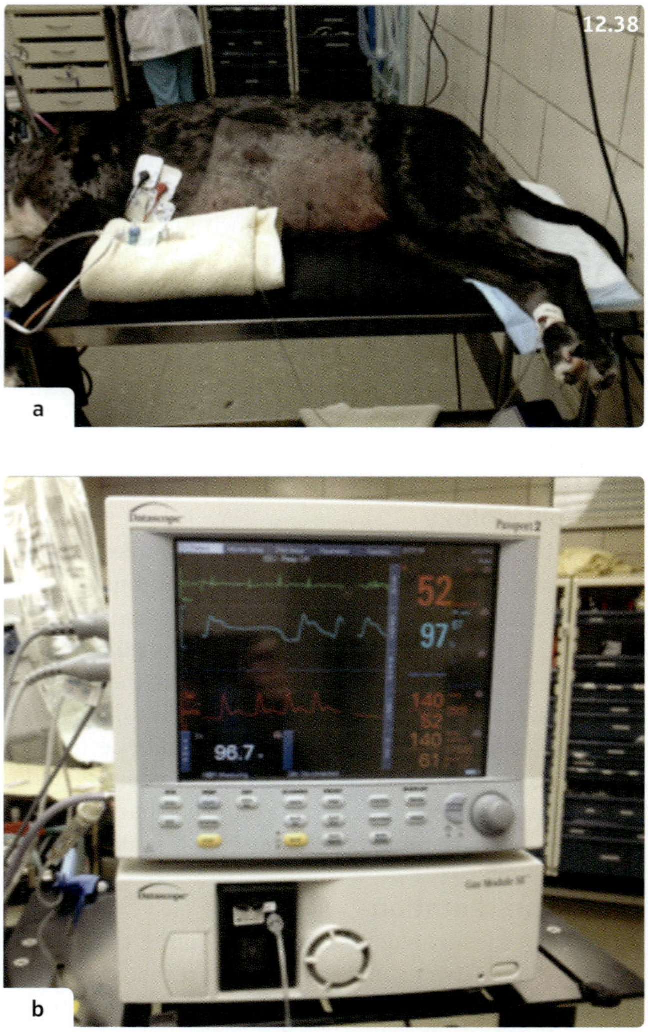

Figures 12.38a, b Direct blood pressure measurements are made by placing a catheter in an artery, connecting the catheter to a transducer, and displaying the blood pressure on a monitor. (a) Patient with arterial catheter in a hindlimb and the transducer at the level of the heart. (b) Multifunction monitor displaying blood pressure.

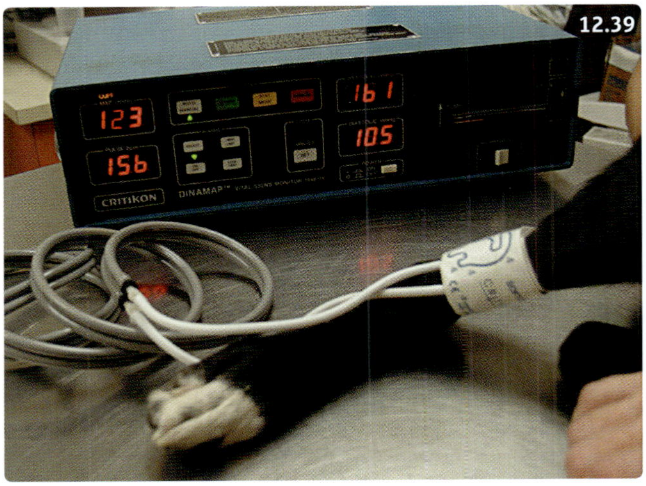

Figure 12.39 Oscillometric blood pressure measuring device.

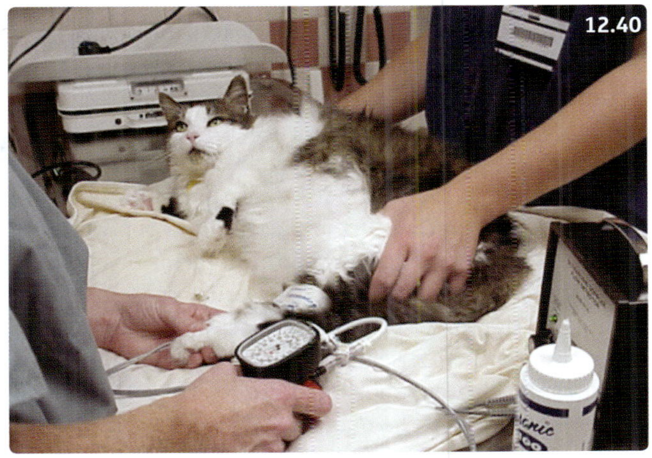

Figure 12.40 Feline patient having blood pressure measured with a Doppler device.

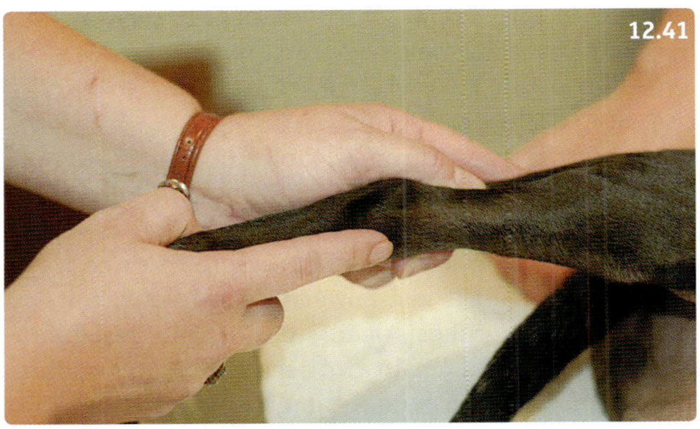

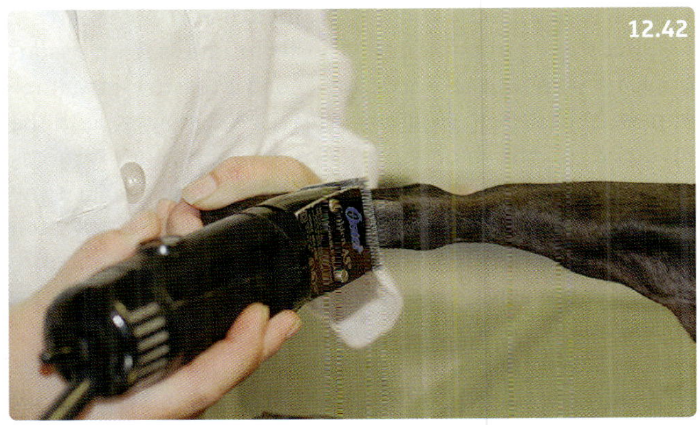

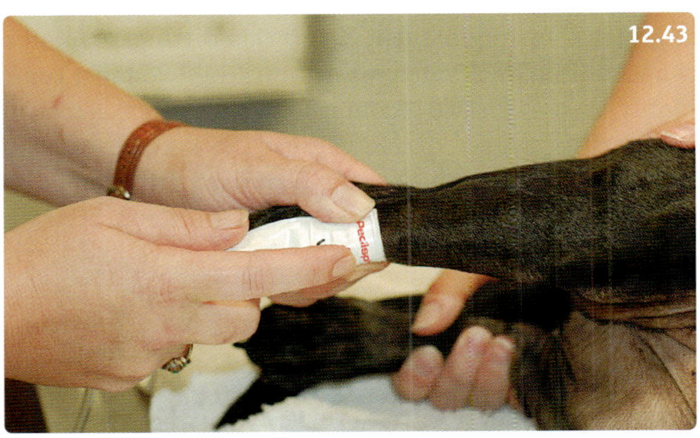

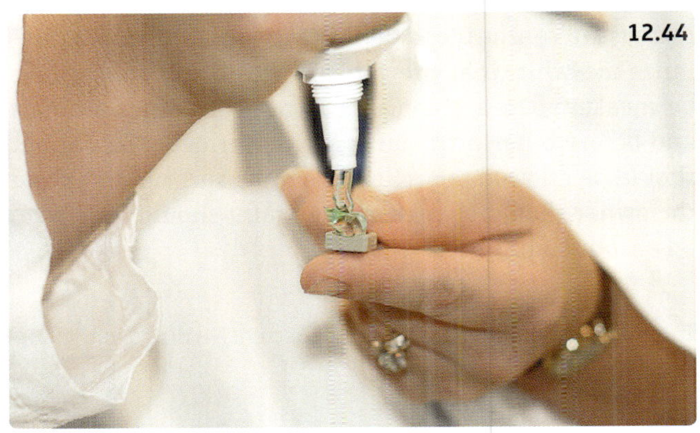

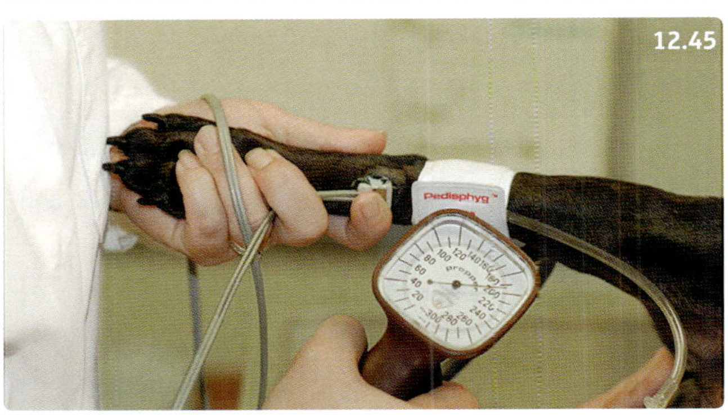

Figures 12.41–12.45 Measuring blood pressure using the Doppler method. The artery is palpated (12.41) and an area over the artery is clipped (12.42). A cuff, whose width is 30–40% the circumference of the limb, is selected (12.43). Ultrasound gel is placed on the probe to improve conduction (12.44). The probe is placed over the artery and the sound of blood flowing is heard. The cuff is inflated to 20 mmHg greater than needed to occlude the blood flow and then the cuff is slowly deflated until the sound of blood flowing is heard again (12.45). This sound represents systolic blood pressure

deflation continues. Although the systolic blood pressure is easily obtained, determining diastolic pressure can be technically challenging.

Regardless of which blood pressure measuring technology is used, four principles help to ensure accurate measurements: proper cuff size selection, consistency of personnel, acclimation of the patient, and repeatability of results. Perhaps the most important factor in attaining accurate and repeatable blood pressure measurements is the selection of a correctly sized cuff. Although some veterinary oscillometric devices come with an integrated cuff selection system, most blood pressure measurement devices require that the operator select an appropriately sized cuff. The width of the cuff should be 30–40% of the circumference of the extremity. A cuff that is too wide will underestimate blood pressure, while a cuff that is too small will artificially increase values.

Consistency of personnel and technique are an essential part of obtaining accurate blood pressure measurements. Whenever possible, the same team should be involved in the blood pressure measurement process and they should utilize the same technique each time blood pressure is measured. The phenomenon by which this produces more accurate measurements is probably related to operator experience.

The 'white coat effect' refers to the stress created by a visit to the veterinarian and the effect that this can have on blood pressure. While cats may be somewhat more susceptible, nervousness or excitement can induce an increase in canine blood pressure as well. In order to minimize the 'white coat effect', blood pressure should always be measured in a quiet area away from other animals and before other procedures are performed. The patient should be allowed to acclimatize to its surroundings and the owner should be present. Restraint should be kept to an absolute minimum.

Individual blood pressure measurements can be inaccurate for a variety of reasons. Blood pressure measurements should be repeated four or five times and the individual measurements compared. If there is a significant variation (>10%) between the measurements, the readings should be discarded and the process repeated. A diagnosis of hypertension in an asymptomatic patient should be confirmed by repeating the blood pressure measurements on three different office visits.

Management

As most small animals with elevated blood pressure suffer from secondary hypertension, the first step should be to identify and, when possible, treat the underlying condition. Often, this will decrease systolic blood pressure and make the hypertension more amenable to therapy; however, in some conditions, such as CKD, therapy may have minimal effect on blood pressure.

Dog-specific therapy

ACEIs are the initial drug of choice in treating canine hypertension (**Table 12.16**). ACEIs exert their effect by blocking the conversion of angiotensin I to angiotensin II and help lower blood pressure in three ways. First, angiotensin II is a powerful vasoconstrictor and inhibiting its synthesis leads to systemic vasodilatation. Second, angiotensin II directly promotes sodium absorption in the proximal tubule; this leads to intravascular volume expansion. Last, aldosterone release is stimulated by angiotensin II and this further promotes renal sodium and water resorption. The two most commonly used ACEIs are enalapril and benazepril. Because enalapril is cleared exclusively by the kidneys and its half-life can be significantly increased by renal disease, its use should be avoided in CKD patients. Instead, benazepril, which is cleared by the kidneys and liver,

Table 12.16 Commonly used antihypertensive drugs in the dog and cat.

Drug	Class	Canine dose	Feline dose
Enalapril	ACE inhibitor	0.5–1.0 mg/kg PO q12–24h	0.25–0.5 mg/kg PO q12–24h
Benazepril	ACE inhibitor	0.25–0.5 mg/kg PO q12–24h	0.25–0.5 mg/kg PO q12–24h
Amlodipine	Ca^{++} channel blocker	0.05–0.1 mg/kg PO q24h	0.625–1.25 mg/cat PO q24h
Atenolol	Beta-1 blocker	0.25–1.0 mg/kg PO q12–24h	6.25–12.5 mg/cat PO q12–24h
Propranolol	Beta blocker	2.5–10 mg/dog PO q8–12h	2.5–5 mg/cat PO q8–12h
Prazosin	Alpha blocker	0.5–2.0 mg/dog q12h	Not recommended
Spironolactone	Aldosterone inhibitor	1.0–2.0 mg/kg PO q12h	1.0–2.0 mg/kg PO q12h

is preferred. In some CKD patients, ACEIs have been associated with a worsening of azotemia; therefore, renal values should be checked 7–14 days after starting therapy in these patients.

Often, ACEIs fail to produce the desired decrease in blood pressure as sole agent therapy. In these hypertensive patients, a calcium channel blocker can be added to the ACEI therapy. These agents exert their effects by blocking the influx of calcium needed to cause smooth muscle contraction and act to decrease systemic vascular resistance. Amlodipine besylate (**Table 12.16**) is the most widely used calcium channel blocker. Channel blockers have the potential to worsen renal disease when used as a monotherapy agent in dogs. This effect is thought to be due to the calcium channel blocker's preferential dilation of the glomerular afferent arteriole resulting in glomerular hypertension. ACEIs preferentially dilate the efferent arteriole, normalizing glomerular pressures and preventing renal damage; therefore, calcium channel blockers should be used in conjunction with ACEIs when treating canine hypertension.

Cat-specific therapy

ACEIs are less effective in treating feline hypertension. Studies have shown that as many as 50% of hypertensive cats fail to respond to enalapril. While benazepril has been shown to produce a statistically significant decrease in feline blood pressure, the actual reduction is relatively modest. For this reason, calcium channel blockers have become the drug of choice in controlling feline hypertension. Amlodipine besylate (**Table 12.16**) is the most widely utilized calcium channel blocker for controlling feline hypertension. As in the dog, it is long acting and gradual in effect. Although use of amlodipine as a monotherapy agent is discouraged in the dog, using calcium channel blockers alone does not appear to cause glomerular injury in cats; therefore, they are considered safe as a single agent therapy. In cases where amlodipine fails to produce the desired decrease in blood pressure, an ACEI can be added to the treatment protocol (**Table 12.16**).

Adjunctive therapy

Beta blockers are useful adjunctive therapy in dogs or cats where the initial antihypertensive agent has failed to produce the desired effect. Beta-adrenergic receptors are found in both the heart (beta-1) and lungs (beta-2). Blockade of the beta-1 receptors slows the heart and lowers blood pressure while blockade of the beta-2 receptors can trigger bronchial constriction. Therefore, only selective beta-1 antagonists (**Table 12.16**) should be utilized.

Alpha blockers decrease blood pressure by selectively antagonizing adrenergic receptors on the systemic vasculature, resulting in a decrease in systemic vascular resistance. Prazosin, a potent alpha inhibitor, has successfully been used as primary and adjunctive treatment for hypertension in the dog (**Table 12.16**). The use of prazosin in cats as an antihypertensive agent has not been fully evaluated and is therefore not recommended.

It has long been known that aldosterone contributes to hyptertension by stimulating sodium and water reabsorption in the kidney and thereby increasing intravascular volume. Aldosterone antagonists such as spironolactone have been used to counteract these hypertensive effects. More recently, it has become apparent that aldosterone plays a role in the inflammation, fibrosis, and necrosis seen in hypertension-induced end organ damage. Inhibiting aldosterone appears to protect the heart, brain, and kidneys from the deleterious effects of hypertension. Although this information is preliminary and more research is needed, hypertensive patients may benefit from the use of aldosterone antagonists such as spironolactone (**Table 12.16**)

Goals and monitoring

The goal of treating hypertensive patients is to gradually lower systolic pressure to <160 mmHg. It is important in the initial stages of treatment to monitor the patient regularly and avoid making rapid adjustments in medication. Changes in antihypertensive therapy should only be made every 2 weeks. Once the patient's blood pressure has been regulated, it should be rechecked every 3 months. CBC and serum chemistry should be checked twice a year.

INCONTINENCE

Definition/overview

Incontinence refers to involuntary escape of urine during the storage phase of the urinary cycle. This can present in different ways; however, the most common presentation is an intermittent or continuous dribbling of urine combined with episodes of normal voiding.

Etiology

Causes of incontinence include urethral sphincter incompetence, anatomic abnormality in the termination of the ureters, an inability of the bladder to dilate, spasms of the bladder, or damage to the nerves controlling micturition (**Table 12.17**); however, urethral sphincter incompetence and ectopic ureters (EUs) account for 85% of all incontinence cases.

Table 12.17 Causes of incontinence in dogs.

Cause	Typical signalment	Clinical signs	Relative frequency
Urethral incompetence	Post-spay female	Dribbling of urine when resting. Previously normal urination	Frequent
Ectopic ureters	Young female	Continual urine dribbling. Noted from early age	Common
Detrusor instability: • Urge incontinence • Idiopathic instability	Middle aged female	Nocturia, pollakiuria, urgency, incontinence	Less common
Neurologic disease	None	Upper motor: erratic reflexive bladder emptying with a difficult to express bladder. Lower motor: no attempts to urinate, easily expressed bladder	Less common
Pelvic entrapment of bladder	Adult large breed female	Continual urine dribbling	Less common
Urovaginal fistula	Incontinence following spaying	Continual urine dribbling	Uncommon
Urorectal fistula	Young dog or post trauma	Chronic urinary tract infection, with passage of urine from rectum	Uncommon

Pathophysiology

The urinary cycle is divided into two phases: the filling phase, and the emptying phase (**Figure 12.46**). During the filling phase, the hypogastric nerve provides sympathetic stimulation of beta receptors in the body of the bladder, resulting in relaxation and stretching, while stimulation of alpha receptors in the bladder's trigone region and proximal urethra causes constriction (**Figure 12.47**). Thus, the sympathetic branch of the autonomic nervous system dominates the filling phase of micturition by constricting the outflow of the bladder while allowing the body of the bladder to distend. Additionally, sympathetic stimulation blocks parasympathetic transmission thereby inhibiting urination.

As the bladder fills, sensory receptors embedded in the wall of the bladder become active and signals travel via the pelvic nerve to the spinal cord. This information is relayed to the brainstem where afferent impulses are integrated with information from the forebrain. Once it is an appropriate time to void, the impulse to empty the bladder is carried down the spinal cord. Parasympathetic neurons located in the pelvic nerve transmit impulses to the parasympathetic ganglia in the bladder wall. Nerve fibers leave this nucleus and innervate smooth muscle fibers of the detrusor muscle causing contraction of the bladder body and relaxation of the bladder neck. At the same time, reflex contraction of the striated muscle of the urethra, mediated by the pudendal nerve, is inhibited.

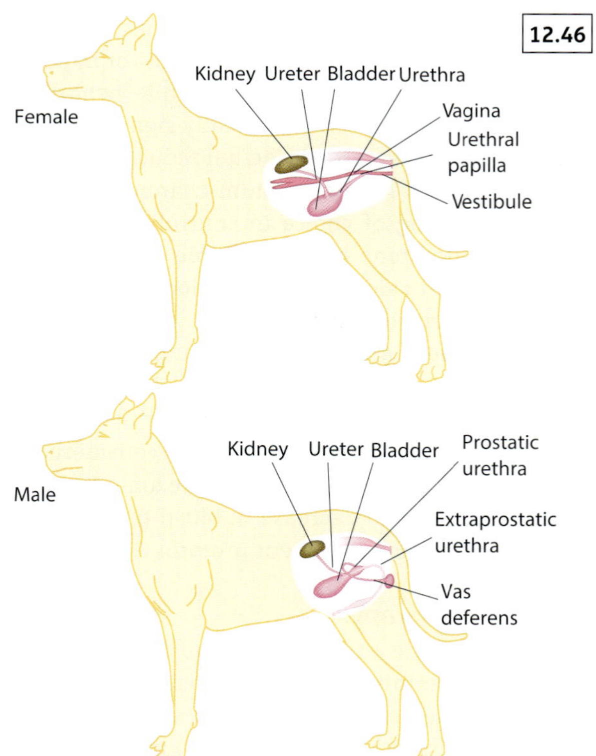

Figure 12.46 Functional components of the urinary tract. Urine is produced in the kidney, travels to the bladder via the ureter, and is stored in the bladder. The urethra acts as a valve and prevents the dribbling of urine and, when appropriate, directs urine out of the body.

12.47

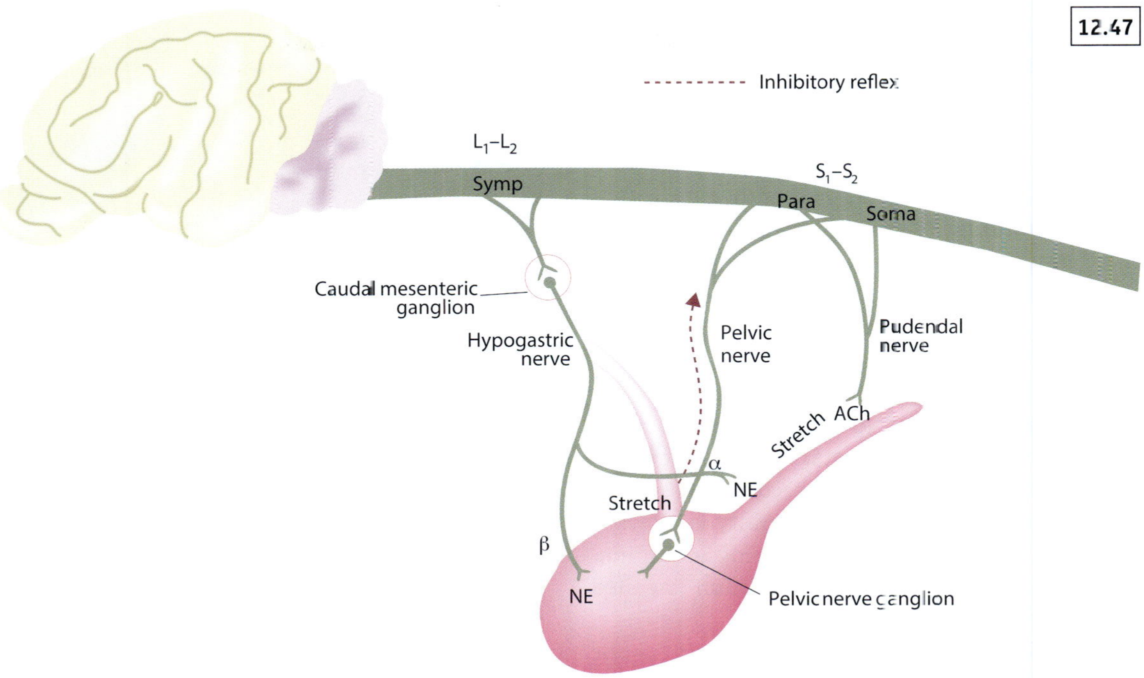

Figure 12.47 Schematic diagram representing the autonomic and somatic innervation of the bladder and urethra. Sympathetic nerve fibers responsible for the storage phase of urination travel in the hypogastric nerve and stimulate receptors in the body and neck of the bladder. Beta receptors in the body of the bladder allow the detrusor muscle to relax and fill. Alpha receptors in the neck of the bladder and proximal urethra result in contraction and continence. Parasympathetic nerve fibers responsible for the voiding phase of the urinary cycle travel in the pelvic nerve. Sensory information travels from the bladder to the spinal cord via the pelvic nerve. Somatic control of the external urethral sphincter travels in the pudendal nerve.

The parasympathetic nervous system dominates the emptying phase of the urinary cycle by coordinating the contraction of the bladder as well as relaxation of the bladder neck, proximal urethra, and external sphincter.

Urethral sphincter incompetence is the most common cause of canine urinary incontinence. Although it has been reported in males, it is much more common in females and affects approximately 10% of all spayed females. The incidence in large breed dogs approaches 12.5%. The onset of incontinence is usually seen 2–3 years after an uneventful ovariohysterectomy but can occur any time after the procedure. In dogs with severe abnormalities, incontinence can occur before ovariectomy and the condition is worsened after the spay operation. Owners typically describe a dribbling of urine that is most noticeable when the animal is asleep. The exact mechanism by which removal of the ovaries leads to incontinence is unknown. Estrogen increases both the number and sensitivity of the alpha-adrenergic receptors of the smooth muscle internal urethral sphincter, so decreased estrogen stimulation tends to reduce the contractile responsive of the urethral smooth muscle to sympathetic stimulation. However, a number of dogs with spay-related urinary incontinence do not respond to estrogen supplementation and dogs in which estrogen secretion has been suppressed with progesterone do not appear to develop urethral incompetence.

12.48

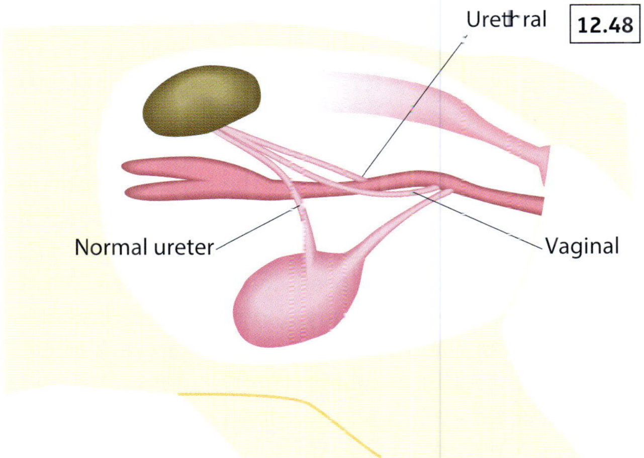

Figure 12.48 Normal termination of the ureter contrasted with extramural ectopic ureters.

EUs are a congenital abnormality characterized by termination of one or both ureters at a point distal to the neck of the bladder (**Figure 12.48**). Thus, the flow of urine bypasses the neck of the bladder and affected animals typically leak urine from birth. EUs are categorized as extramural and intramural based on their point of attachment and behavior. An extramural EU attaches and empties directly into the urethra or, in rare cases, the vagina or uterus. Intramural EUs attach to the bladder and tunnel below the submucosa and into the urethra or vagina. In cases of unilateral EU, normal urine voiding is reported as one ureter is properly emptying into the bladder. Normal urination may or may not occur in bilateral cases. Almost 90% of canine EUs occur in females and 25% of these are bilateral. Although EUs have been reported in cats, they are less common than in dogs.

Detrusor instability is characterized by sudden urgency to urinate and an involuntary bladder contraction (**Figure 12.49**). When this occurs secondary to infection, neoplasia, or urolithiasis, this instability is referred to as urge incontinence. When an underlying inflammatory condition is not diagnosed, the condition is called idiopathic detrusor instability.

Caudal location of the bladder within the pelvis ('pelvic bladder') has also been associated with urinary incontinence. Although this condition is most often seen in large breed female dogs, it has also been reported in males. In normal patients, the bladder is positioned in the abdomen while in affected dogs the bladder neck and some portion of the body are located in the pelvic canal. It is not clear why 50% of dogs with this condition are incontinent while the others are unaffected. It has been proposed that 'pelvic bladder' is part of a syndrome characterized by shortened urethra, dysfunctional detrusor, and abnormal urethral musculature.

Urovaginal and urethrorectal fistulas are both uncommon causes of incontinence in the dog. Urethrorectal fistulas typically present with persistent urinary tract infections (UTIs) and passage of urine from the anus. Urovaginal fistulas have been documented as a complication of ovariohysterectomy and develop secondary to entrapment of the distal ureter by a ligature. Typically, these present for incontinence shortly after an otherwise uneventful spay and are unresponsive to medical management. Urethrorectal fistulas may be congenital or be the result of trauma. Although English Bulldogs are thought to have a genetic predisposition to developing a congenital form of this condition, it has been described in other breeds.

Clinical presentation

The most common presentation is an intermittent or continuous dribbling of urine combined with episodes of normal voiding.

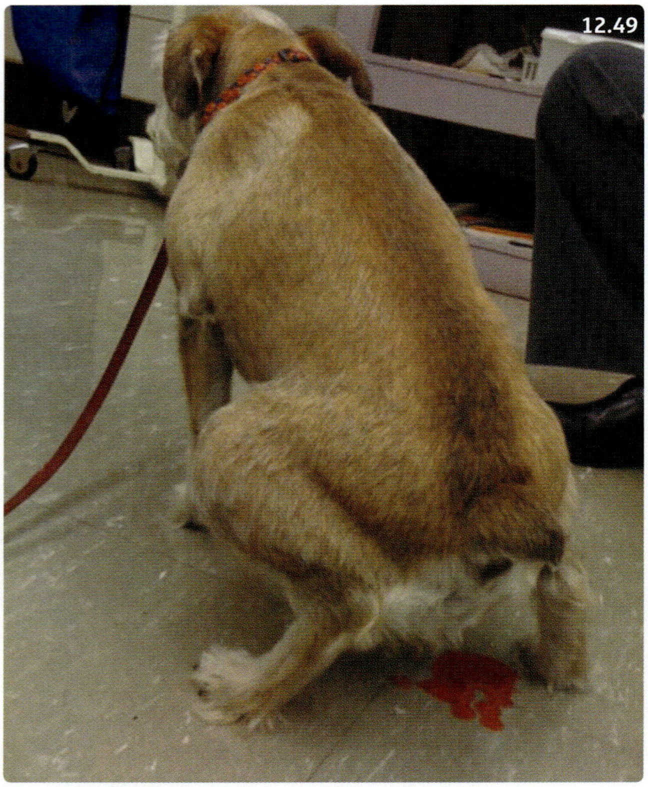

Figure 12.49 Dog with urge incontinence. The patient was later found to have a bladder mass.

Differential diagnosis

Nocturia, pollakiuria, and urgency.

Diagnosis

A detailed history that focuses on the timing, volume, events surrounding the leakage of urine (e.g. sleeping, excitement), and spinal trauma are essential. In addition, determining the quality and quantity of the purposeful urinations is important. Nocturia, pollakiuria, and urgency, which can all be confused with incontinence, can be eliminated on the basis of a thorough history.

A detailed inspection of the genitals should be performed. The area around the genitals should be checked for moisture, urine staining of the fur, and skin scalding. The external genitalia should be examined to be sure they are anatomically correct. Observing the animal urinate can be helpful in confirming normal micturition.

Laboratory data should include a CBC, serum chemistry panel, and urinalysis with aerobic culture. The CBC and chemistry panel help rule out systemic disease while the urinalysis may implicate cystitis as a cause of the incontinence. Urine culture results can be difficult to interpret.

Although UTIs can lead to urge incontinence, infection can also be the result of anatomic abnormalities.

A thorough neurologic examination is a critical part of the incontinence work up. Disorders affecting the spinal cord above the fifth lumbar vertebra (upper motor neuron lesions) produce an involuntary, erratic, reflexive emptying of the bladder with increased resistance of the external urethral sphincter. Clinically, these animals present with significant neurologic abnormalities that are relatively easy to detect, including paresis, paralysis, hyperreflexia, decreased proprioception, and decreased pain perception. Lesions of the sacral spinal cord (lower motor neuron lesions) prevent bladder sensation from traveling up the spinal cord and as a result, the patient makes no attempts to urinate even as the bladder becomes overdistended. Sacral lesions also affect the pudendal nerve and result in the loss of external sphincter resistance. Typically, patients with sacral lesions have an easily expressed overdistended bladder and they dribble urine. Lower motor neuron lesions can be more difficult to detect as they present with no obvious signs of neurologic dysfunction. In cases where the function of the pudendal nerve is in question, squeezing the distal portion of the penis or edge of the vulva and observing the anus for a reflexive contraction can help evaluate afferent and efferent pudendal nerve function.

Spay-related incontinence

Due to the prevalence of urethral incompetence in middle aged spayed dogs, the typical clinical presentation, and the relative safety of the drugs used to treat this condition, the diagnosis is often made empirically (**Table 12.17**). Definitive diagnosis requires a urethral pressure profile. In this test, a special multilumen catheter is pulled through the length of the urethra (**Figure 12.50**). The catheter is designed so that while one lumen measures the pressure generated by the urethra, another at the tip of the catheter measures the pressure in the bladder. At the end of the procedure a computer calculates the pressure generated by the urethra that is in excess of that which is generated by the bladder (urethral closure pressure). It also determines the functional length of the bladder. Using this information, the clinician can determine if the force exerted and the length of the urethra are normal. The cost and availability of this procedure limit its use to atypical cases and those that fail to respond to medical management.

Ectopic ureters

Typically, EUs are suspected in young female dogs that have a history of dribbling urine since they were very young. Interestingly, because of the small volume of urine produced and the expectation that young puppies will have 'accidents', this condition is often overlooked until the patient is several months old. The diagnosis of EUs has historically been made on the basis of excretory urography, retrograde vaginourethrography, or some combination of these procedures. Collectively, these tests have a sensitivity of only 70–80%. More recently, the use of rigid cystoscopy has been shown to be 100% sensitive and has become the method of choice for diagnosing this condition (**Figure 12.51**).

12.50

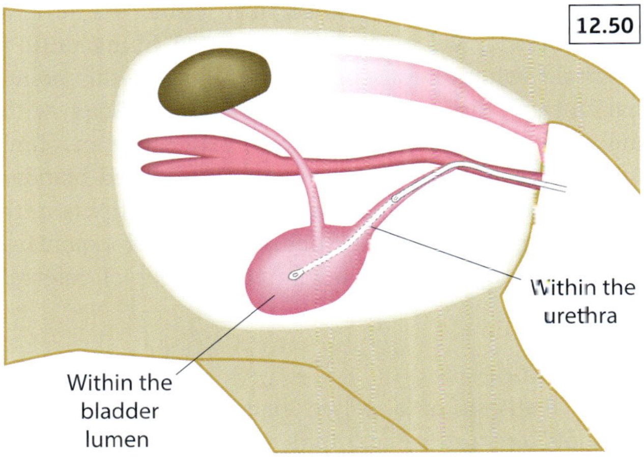

Figure 12.50 Urethra pressure profile.

12.51

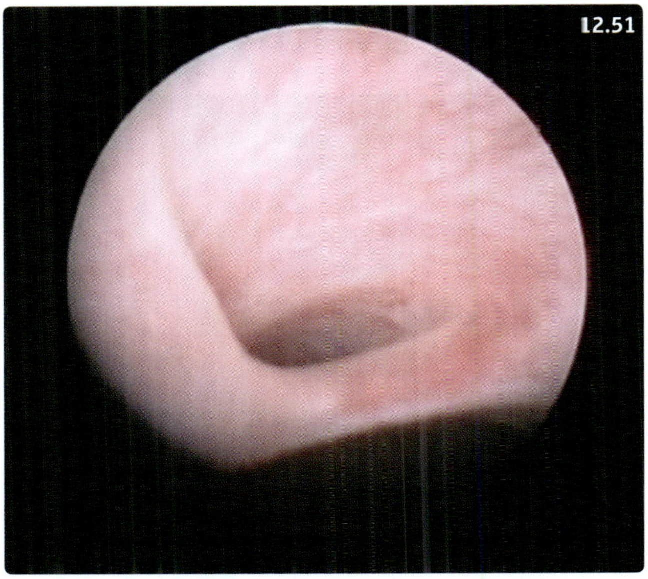

Figure 12.51 Example of an ectopic ureter opening into the urethra as seen with a rigid cystoscope.

Urge incontinence/idiopathic detrusor instability

The diagnosis of urge incontinence is made on the basis of finding an underlying cause for the bladder instability. As in all cases of incontinence, a thorough physical examination, neurologic examination, history, and urinalysis with microscopic examination of the sediment and culture are essential. Radiography and ultrasound of the lower urinary tract are also important to look for neoplasia, urolithiasis, or structural abnormalities (**Figure 12.52**). Diagnosis of idiopathic detrusor instability is made first by ruling out all possible causes of urge incontinence and then on the results of a cystometrogram. During this test, a catheter is placed in the bladder and is slowly filled with saline. The normal canine bladder will allow uninterrupted filling until a threshold volume of 22 ml/kg is reached. At this point, involuntary bladder contractions begin. Dogs with idiopathic detrusor instability will experience involuntary bladder contractions at a greatly reduced bladder volume. While simple in principle, the equipment to perform this test is quite sophisticated and expensive and is only available at a limited number of referral institutions.

Pelvic bladder

Initial diagnosis of a pelvic bladder is made on the basis of contrast radiographs (**Figures 12.53, 12.54**). Contrast radiographs show an abnormally shaped, caudally displaced bladder that fails to taper at the junction with the urethra. Since dogs with pelvic bladder syndrome will demonstrate a dysfunctional detrusor and an abnormal urethral musculature, a urethra pressure profile is indicated.

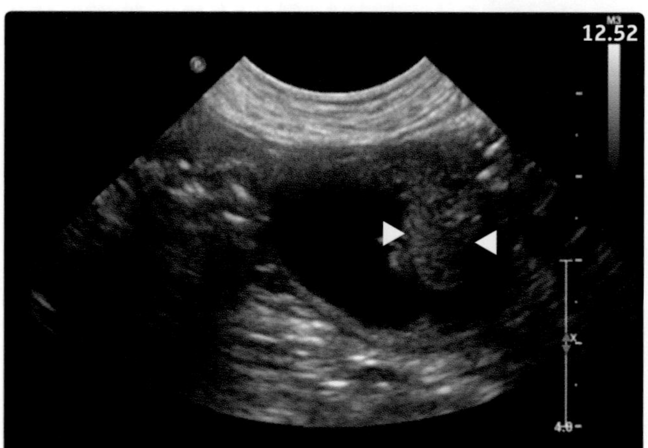

Figure 12.52 Ultrasound of a bladder reveals a mass (between arrowheads). The mass was eventually determined to be a tissue reaction to suture material used in a previous cystotomy.

Urovaginal/urethrorectal fistulas

Diagnosis of urovaginal and urethrorectal fistulas requires specialized radiographic procedures. Urovaginal fistulas are often visualized with IV urography but may require more invasive techniques such as antegrade ureterography. Urethrorectal fistulas can be diagnosed with

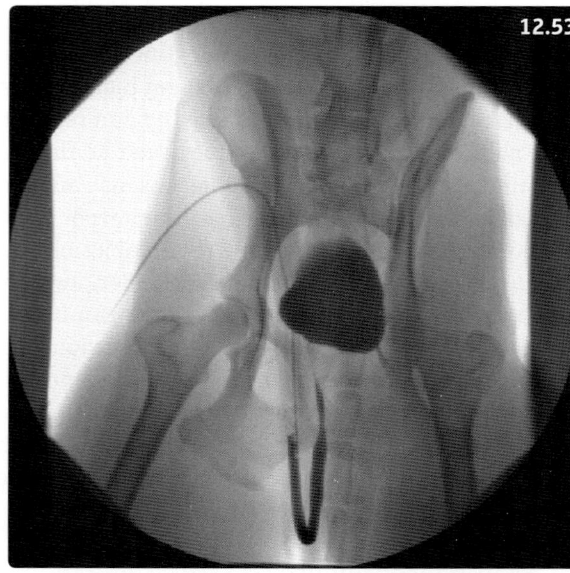

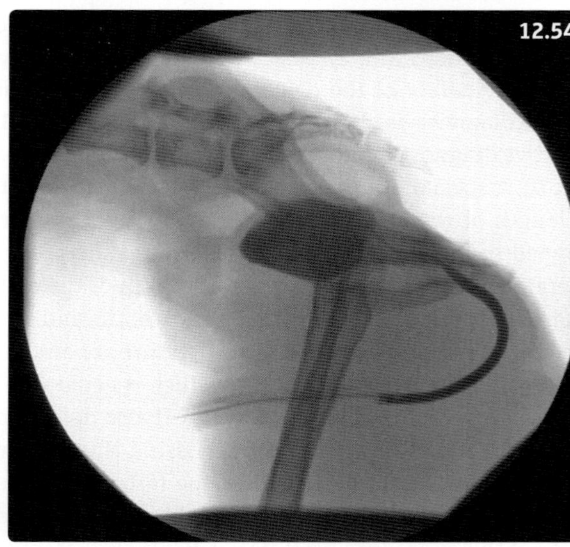

Figures 12.53, 12.54 Pelvic bladders are usually seen in female dogs; however, this example is in a 2-year-old male Greyhound. Note the position of the bladder and its failure to taper at the junction with the urethra. A urethral pressure profile and cystometrogram revealed a nonresponsive detrusor muscle and incompetent urethra.

either a cystogram or retrograde urethrogram performed under fluoroscopy.

Management

Spay-related incontinence

For many years, alpha-adrenergic agonists such as phenylpropanolamine have been the mainstay for the treatment of spay-related urethral incompetence (**Table 12.18**). Total resolution of urinary incontinence can be expected in 85% of cases, while a significant improvement in clinical signs occurs in most dogs. Since the side-effects of phenylpropanolamine include hypertension, tachycardia, increased intraocular pressure, and hepatic glycogenolysis, this drug should be avoided in patients with hypertension, glaucoma, or diabetes mellitus. Recently, the United States Food and Drug Administration has approved estriol (Incurin™), a synthetic estrogen, for urethral sphincter incompetence. This medication, which is now available in many countries, has proven to be efficacious when used alone or in combination with phenylpropanolamine. Common side-effects include loss of appetite, vomiting, excessive water drinking, and a swollen vulva. For most patients, these seem to resolve fairly quickly. Unlike previously available estrogen formulations, estriol does not appear to cause bone marrow suppression, alopecia, behavioral change, or signs consistent with estrus.

For the small percentage of urethral incompetence patients that do not adequately respond to medical management, several procedural options exist. The first, urethral collagen injection, involves the endoscopic placement of collagen or extracellular matrix into the urethral submucosa. In one study, 68% of dogs treated with this method attained full urinary continence, and an additional 25% of owners reported a significant decrease in their pet's urine dribbling. These endoscopically placed injections result in bulging of the urethra into the lumen and significantly improved urethral closure pressure. The primary limitation of this procedure seems to be its temporary nature, as many dogs return to incontinence over time. While many of the dogs that relapse will respond to medical management, most will eventually require additional urethral injections.

Another option is the surgical placement of a hydraulic urethral occluder, which is an inflatable silicone cuff that is surgically placed around the proximal urethra (**Figures 12.55a–d**). The cuff is attached to an inflation port, which is secured subcutaneously to the abdominal wall. The occluder works by providing resistance to the proximal urethra. When the patient urinates, pressure in the bladder overcomes the resistance and normal micturition occurs. Interestingly, the resistance provided by the occluder can be adjusted through the injection port.

Ectopic ureters

Since extramural EUs attach and directly empty into the urethra, the vagina, or the uterus, they must be surgically reimplanted. Intramural EUs, however, attach to the bladder correctly and then tunnel below the submucosa and into the urethra or vagina. These are amenable to correction by laser ablation, which is less invasive, more effective, and associated with fewer complications than currently performed surgical techniques (**Figures 12.56a, b**).

Many dogs will experience some degree of incontinence after EU correction. Although the reason for the sphincter incompetence is not clear, a urethral pressure profile may help identify which animals will be continent, continent with medication, or incontinent after surgery. Unfortunately, this procedure is not definitive, is expensive, and is available at a limited number of referral institutions.

Table 12.18 Commonly used drugs for treating incontinence.

Drug	Class	Dose
Phenylpropanolamine	Alpha-agonist	1.0–4.0 mg/kg q8–12h
Estriol (Incurin™)	Synthetic estrogen	2.0 mg/dog q24h for 14 days then decrease to lowest possible dose. Allow 7 days between adjustments
Flavoxate	Anticholinergic	100–200 mg/dog q6–8h
Oxybutinin	Anticholinergic	5.0 mg/dog q6–8h
Dicyclomine	Anticholinergic	10.0 mg/dog q6–8h

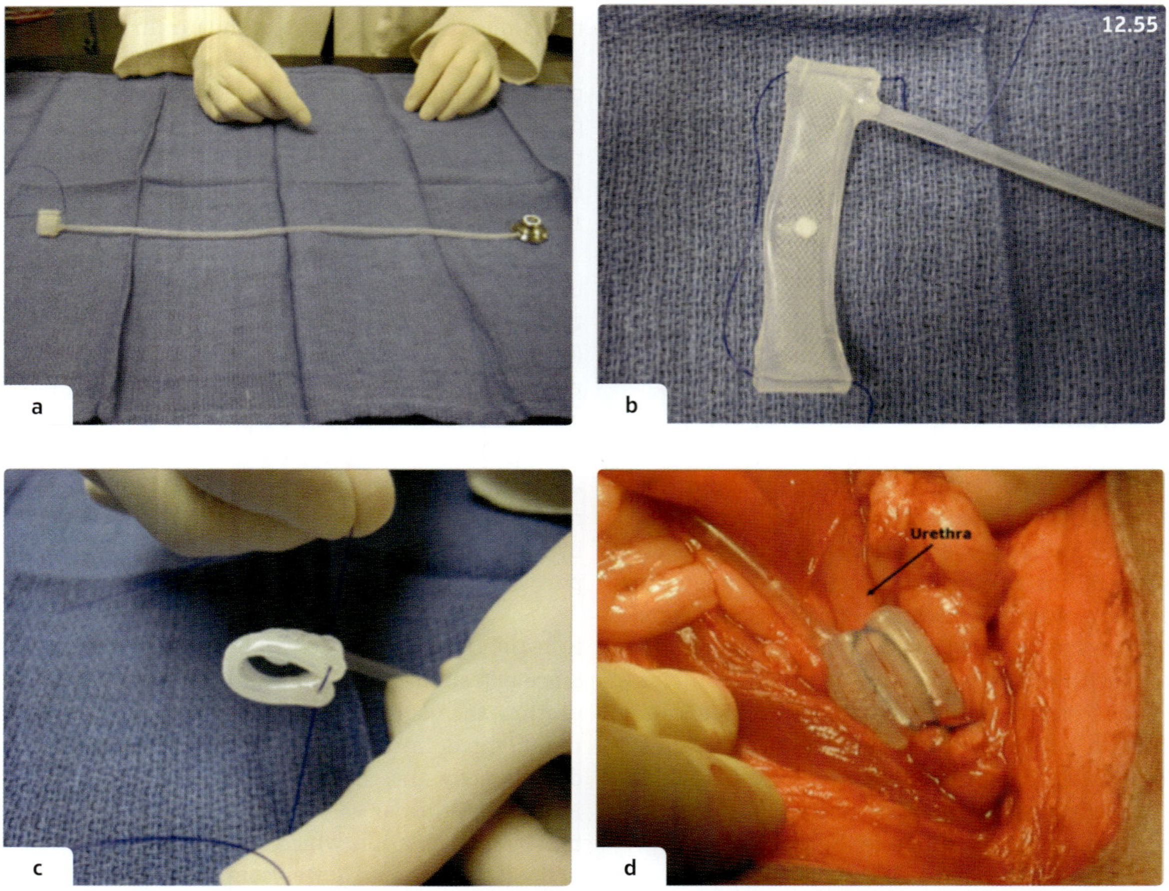

Figures 12.55a–d (a) Hydraulic urethral occlusion device. Note the cuff, which will be surgically placed around the urethra, and the inflation port, which will be secured subcutaneously to the abdominal wall. (b, c) Close-up of a cuff that will be placed around the neck of the bladder. (d) Cuff placed around the urethra. (Courtesy A. Berent)

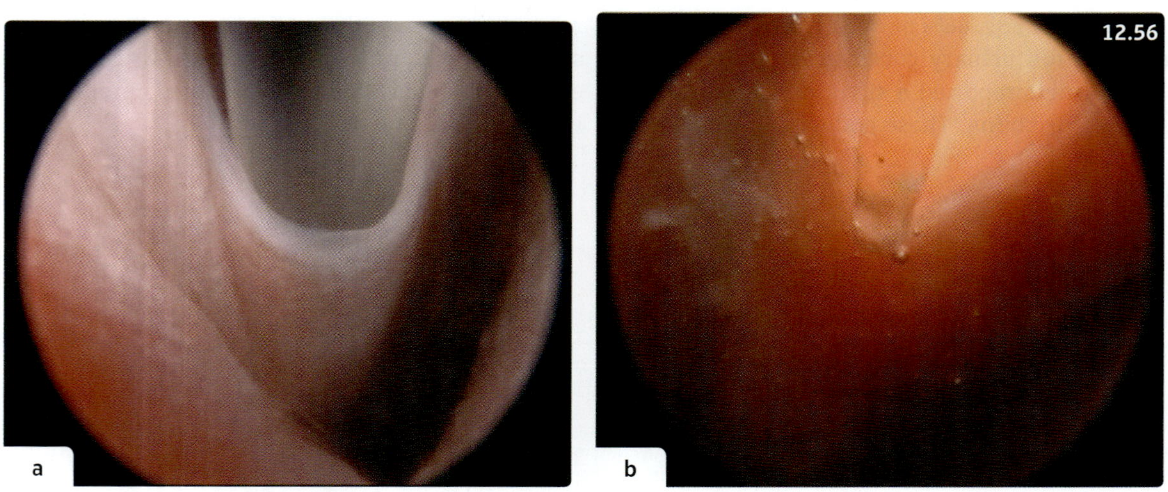

Figures 12.56a, b Example of an intramural ectopic ureter corrected by laser ablation. (a) An endoscope has been used to place a guide wire in an ectopic ureter. Note that the ectopic ureter tunnels alongside and opens into the urethra near the opening into the vestibule. (b) Endoscopically directed holmium YAG laser fiber being used to oblate the ectopic ureter. This procedure continues until the ureter opens into the bladder.

Hydronephrosis is common in dogs born with EUs. Abdominal ultrasound should be performed to examine the architecture of the kidney and determine the need for additional renal function testing. A hydronephrotic functionless kidney should be removed.

Urge incontinence/idiopathic detrusor instability

Treatment of urge incontinence is based on successful resolution of the underlying condition. Usually, no additional therapy is needed. Treatment for idiopathic detrusor instability relies on anticholinergic drugs that interfere with the parasympathetic nervous system's stimulatory effect on the detrusor muscle. Commonly used drugs include flavoxate, oxybutynin, and dicyclomine (**Table 12.18**).

Pelvic bladder

Treatment of pelvic bladder syndrome is often unrewarding. Treatment with phenylpropanolamine is thought to be helpful but unlikely to resolve incontinence (**Table 12.18**). Some have recommended colposuspension, a surgery where the bladder is repositioned in the abdomen in cases where medical management is unrewarding. At this time, there is little evidence to support the use of this procedure.

Urovaginal and urethrorectal fistulas

Surgical correction of these abnormalities has been described. Generally, a good outcome is expected.

FELINE LOWER URINARY TRACT DISEASE

Definition/overview

Feline lower urinary tract disease (FLUTD) is a term given to cats that present exhibiting certain clinical signs including straining to urinate, hematuria, pollakiuria, and periuria. FLUTD accounts for nearly 5% of all cats presenting for veterinary care. The condition can be divided into two groups: cats that present with a urethral obstruction, and cats that are not obstructed but are displaying clinical signs. While the former group is almost always male, the latter can be male or female. A cat with an obstructed urethra is always a medical emergency.

Etiology

The most common cause of all cases of FLUTD is idiopathic cystitis. This is a diagnosis of exclusion and accounts for almost 70% of affected cats. Only about 15% of cats with lower urinary tract signs have uroliths. UTIs are extremely uncommon and make up less than 2% of these patients.

Pathophysiology

Most obstructions are the result of urethral spasms and/or plugs. Urethral spasms are thought to be the result of inflammation and irritation of the urethral musculature. The origin of the 'urethral plug' is unknown, although they are often a mix of a proteinaceous matrix and struvite crystals (**Figure 12.57**). It is thought that inflammation of the urinary tract leads to leakage of plasma, including albumin and bicarbonate, into the urine. This provides the protein needed for matrix formation and increases the urine pH, promoting the formation of struvite crystals. The protein matrix forms a web-like structure in the urethra that traps the struvite crystals, thus leading to the plug.

In the nonobstructed patient, periuria (urinating around) is the clinical sign that most often initiates the visit to a veterinarian. The clinician must differentiate cats with FLUTD from those with behavioral issues. Other potential considerations include uroliths, UTIs, and neoplasia. Urine osmolality in young healthy cats is so high that it acts to inhibit bacterial growth. This, combined with host defense mechanisms make UTIs extremely rare in these patients; therefore, empirical treatment with antibiotics is unlikely to be efficacious. Urinary tract neoplasia is also uncommon. Despite extensive diagnostics, no specific underlying cause (e.g. stones, UTI) can be determined in more than 70% of FLUTD cats, and these are categorized as feline idiopathic cystitis (FIC).

When normal cats are subjected to stressful events, (e.g. change in the environment), there is an initial catecholamine release followed by a period of acclimation and a return to baseline levels. Cats with FIC may have an exaggerated and extended catecholamine response that may be similar to anxiety disorders seen in some people.

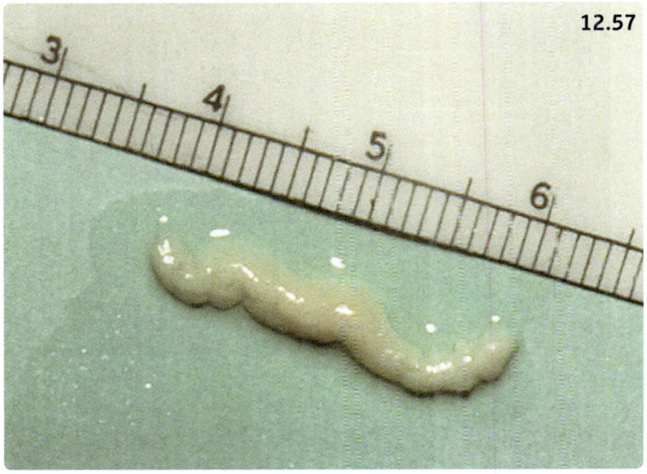

Figure 12.57 Urethral plug from a cat with urethral obstruction. (Courtesy M. Schaer)

This suggests that cats with FIC may have an inappropriate response to stress.

Besides generalized anxiety, this catecholamine release can also have an effect on specific organs. For example, in the bladder, sensory neurons are activated and perpetuate bladder wall inflammation.

Cats with FIC also have abnormalities in the mucus covering of the uroendothelium, histologic changes in the endothelium of the bladder wall, and abnormalities of the hypothalamic–pituitary–adrenal axis. How these findings fit together to produce the constellation of clinical signs seen with FIC is not clear. Glycosaminoglycans (GAGs) are an important part of the protective mucus layer that covers the urinary tract. Cats with FIC produce smaller amounts of GAGs (particularly GAG GP-51) than normal felines. Without this protective layer, irritants (e.g. hydrogen, calcium, potassium) found in urine come in contact with the bladder wall. Sensory neurons (C fibers) relay information through the spinal cord, causing the brain to sense pain. Locally, the noxious stimuli cause neurogenic inflammation (substance P release resulting in vascular leakage and histamine release) (**Figure 12.58**).

Clinical presentation

Obstructive

Urethral obstruction typically occurs in male cats between 1 and 6 years of age. Obstructed cats strain unproductively to urinate and may cry out during the attempt. Owners often mistake these attempts for constipation.

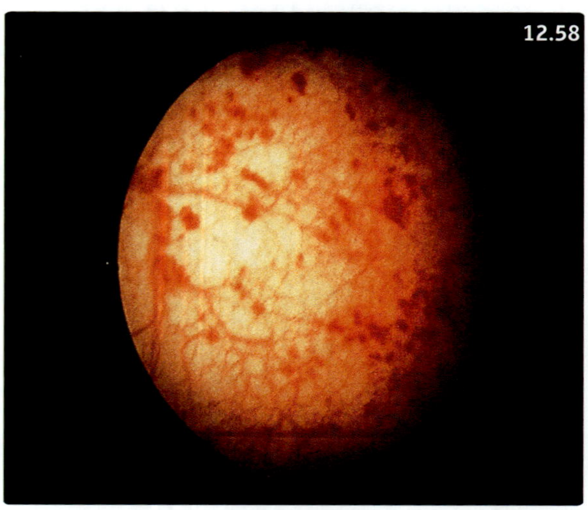

Figure 12.58 Cystoscopic view of submucosal hemorrhages, called glomerulations, in a cat with idiopathic feline lower urinary tract disease. This lesion is seen when the bladder is distended to about 80 cm of water pressure. The finding is nonspecific but does not appear in normal cats. (Courtesy D.F. Senior)

Licking of the genital region is also frequently observed. Patients often hide in a secluded area. Patients examined soon after obstruction may be fractious and resist examination. After more prolonged obstruction, patients become progressively more depressed. An enlarged firm bladder is felt on abdominal palpation.

Nonobstructive

Signs of nonobstructive FLUTD are variable but usually include stranguria, pollakiuria, hematuria, and dysuria. Affected cats may vocalize during urination and urinate in inappropriate places. The bladder of cats with nonobstructed FLUTD is usually small with a thickened wall. Attempts at collecting urine through cystocentesis are often unrewarding due to the frequent attempts at urination that occur, especially when the patient is handled.

Differential diagnosis

Inappropriate urination (behavorial), uroliths, UTI, neoplasia, anatomic defects.

Diagnosis

All cats presenting for FLUTD should have diagnostic imaging performed. This will allow for inspection of the urinary tract for uroliths, anatomic malformations, and neoplasia. As for many urinary tract conditions, ultrasound in the hands of a skilled operator is likely to yield more information than radiography. Nevertheless, treatment of an unstable obstructed patient should not be delayed. In these cases, imaging studies should be performed once the obstruction is relieved.

Obstructive

Obstructive FLUTD is identified by palpation of an enlarged, firm bladder. Urinalysis and urine culture can be performed on urine collected by cystocentesis before urethral catheterization or via the catheter after relief of the obstruction. Serum creatinine and BUN allow assessment of the degree of azotemia; however, these are likely to resolve quickly once the obstruction is relieved. Serum potassium levels and an ECG tracing should always be performed in depressed cats to assess cardiotoxicity associated with hyperkalemia.

Nonobstructive

Along with diagnostic imaging, laboratory data should include a CBC, serum chemistry panel, and urinalysis with aerobic culture. The CBC and chemistry panel help rule out systemic disease. Crystalluria is not an uncommon urinalysis finding and is unlikely to be the cause of the condition; rather, it is most likely a result of the inflammation. For this reason, the crystalluria is not usually considered a therapeutic target. The presence of white cells is not unexpected with inflammation and should not be associated with UTIs.

Management

The first step in assessing a cat that presents with FLUTD is to quickly recognize patients that are obstructed. These cats are almost always male and can be identified by palpation of an enlarged, firm bladder. Affected cats may be azotemic, hyperkalemic, acidotic, or bradycardic, and have an ECG consistent with atrial standstill secondary to hyperkalemia (e.g. absence of P waves, prolonged QRS, spiked T waves) (**Figure 12.59**). Patients should have an IV catheter placed and be sedated (e.g. ketamine and valium). A treatment algorithm is shown in **Figure 12.60**.

Once a urinary catheter is placed (**Figures 12.61a, b**), urine output should be monitored for at least 24–48 hours for evidence of postobstructive diuresis. This is a high rate of urine output that occurs when an obstruction is relieved. The cause is unknown; however, significant amounts of dilute urine can be produced, leading to hypovolemia. Recommendations are to measure urine output every 2–4 hours and set an IV fluid rate such that IV fluids given match those lost to excessive urination. Fortunately, postobstructive diuresis is self-limiting and usually resolves in 24–48 hours. It is not clear if there is an optimal amount of time to leave the urinary catheter in place; however, it seems prudent to wait for postobstructive diuresis (if any) to resolve and the urine to seem clear.

A wide variety of empirical treatments have been claimed to be successful in the treatment of idiopathic FLUTD. The waxing–waning nature of the clinical signs makes evaluation of treatment modalities difficult. Compounding the problem is a lack of well-controlled clinical trials. Nevertheless, a multifaceted approach involving environmental enrichment, diet, pheromones, and drugs seems to alleviate signs and decrease recurrence in many cats.

Environmental enrichment

FIC may actually be a clinical manifestation of a physiologically inappropriate response to stress. This is similar to the colitis that some dogs experience when subjected to a stressful event such as boarding. As such, it is important to look for possible stressors in the cat's environment and ways to reduce them. FLUTD surveys that require the owner to answer questions about the home environment have been developed. These surveys are helpful in extracting information from the owner in a systematic and concise way, which may be difficult in a time limited clinic interaction (**Figure 12.62**).

In multi-cat households the 'cats +1' rule should be applied to all shared resources. If there are two cats in the household, there should be three litter boxes, three

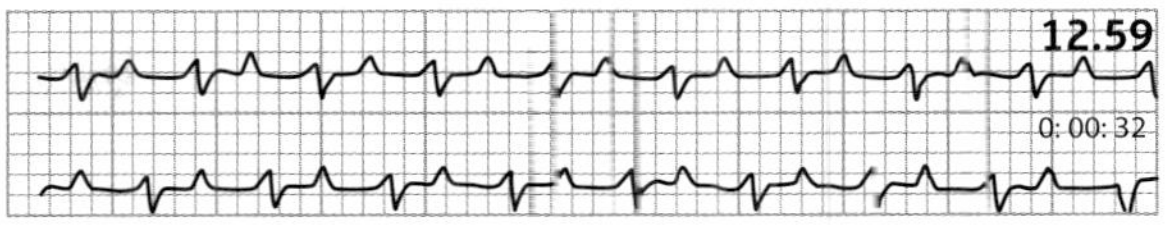

Figure 12.59 An ECG example of hyperkalemia causing atrial standstill. Note the characteristic absence of P waves, prolonged QRS, and spiked T waves.

12.60

Obstructive algorithm:

- Draw blood for possible serum chemistry and electrolytes.
- Place IV catheter and begin fluids.
- Monitor ECG and treat hyperkalemia as needed (**Table 12.7**).
- Carefully attempt to catheterize with a sterile Slippery Sam™ or 3.5-French open-end tomcat catheter (**Figures 12.61a, b**).
- If obstruction cannot be relieved, attempt to dislodge by flushing urethra with sterile saline or lactated Ringer's solution.
- If bladder is extremely firm, remove urine by cystocentesis. This decreases back-pressure and allows for aseptic collection of urine for analysis and culture.
- If obstruction will not dislodge, use retropulsion with the urethral orifice pinched off.
- A small amount of lidocaine gel may be infused into the catheter to decrease urethral spasm.

Once urethral patency is established:

- If a 'Slippery Sam' catheter was used to relieve obstruction, the catheter can be sutured in place.
- If a tomcat catheter was used:
  - Measure distance from prepuce to neck of bladder.
  - Note distance on a sterile 5-French polyvinyl catheter (soft red rubber) and insert into the urethra up to that point.
  - Place tape on external part of tube (as close to prepuce as possible) and suture tape to prepuce with two sutures.
  - Tape free end of tube to tail.
  - Attach extension set to urinary catheter and place sterile collection bag on the other end of the extension set.
- Place e-collar before the patient awakens.

Figure 12.60 Algorithm for treating obstructed cats.

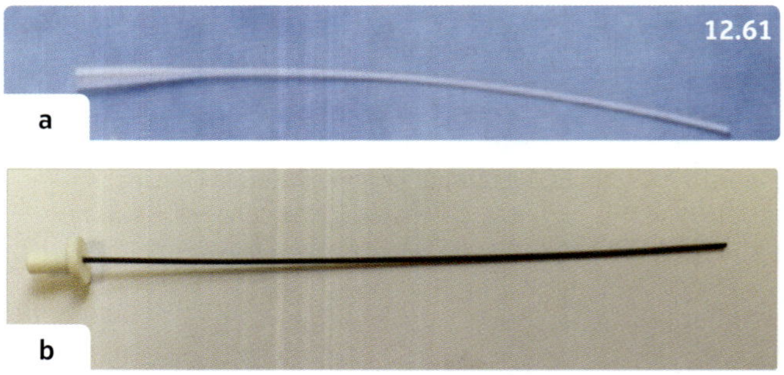

Figures 12.61a, b Examples of a tomcat catheter (a) and a Slippery Sam™ catheter (b).

food bowls, three water bowls, three scratching posts, etc. Litter boxes should be kept very clean and away from other pets. Having a dog interrupting private time in the box or rummage through the litter looking for 'treats' can be very stressful. Water bowls need to be kept clean and filled. Some cats seem reluctant to drink if their whiskers can touch the sides of the bowl; therefore, an extra wide drinking bowl may be helpful. As with litter boxes, bowls should be out of the reach of curious children and hungry dogs. Cats seem to prefer surveying the environment from elevated vantage points. This gives

12.62

Household Resource Checklist

The following questions ask about your cat's resources so we can learn more about the environment your cat(s) live in. Please ✓ **DK** if you don't know, **NA** if it does not apply, or **Yes** or **No** after each question. If you have more than one cat, please answer for **all** cats. Resources (food, water, litter, and resting areas) for each cat are assumed to be out of (cat) sight of each other, such as around a corner or in another room. If they are in sight of each other, please answer **No**.

Space		**DK**	**NA**	**Yes**	**No**
1	Each cat has its own resting area in a convenient location that provides some privacy.	☐	☐	☐	☐
2	Resting areas are located such that another animal cannot sneak up on the cat while it rests.	☐	☐	☐	☐
3	Resting areas are located away from appliances or air ducts that could come on unexpectedly (machinery) while the cat rests.	☐	☐	☐	☐
4	Perches are provided so each cat can look down on its surroundings.	☐	☐	☐	☐
5	Each cat can move about freely, explore, climb, stretch, and play if it chooses to.	☐	☐	☐	☐
6	Each cat has the opportunity to move to a warmer or cooler area if it chooses to.	☐	☐	☐	☐
7	A radio or TV is left playing when the cat is home alone.	☐	☐	☐	☐
Food and water					
8	Each cat has its own food bowl.	☐	☐	☐	☐
9	Each cat has its own water bowl	☐	☐	☐	☐
10	Bowls are located in a convenient location to provide privacy while the cat eats or drinks.	☐	☐	☐	☐
11	Bowls are located such that other animals cannot sneak up on the cat while it eats or drinks	☐	☐	☐	☐
12	Bowls are washed regularly (at least weekly) with a mild detergent.	☐	☐	☐	☐
13	Bowls are located away from machinery.	☐	☐	☐	☐
Litter boxes					
14	Each cat has its own box (one box per cat, plus 1).	☐	☐	☐	☐
15	Boxes are located in convenient, well-ventilated locations that still give each cat some privacy while using it.	☐	☐	☐	☐

16	Boxes are located on more than one level in multi-level houses.	☐	☐	☐	☐
17	Boxes are located so another animal cannot sneak up on the cat during use.	☐	☐	☐	☐
18	Boxes are located away from machinery that could come on unexpectedly during use.	☐	☐	☐	☐
19	The litter is scooped daily.	☐	☐	☐	☐
20	The litter is completely replaced weekly.	☐	☐	☐	☐
21	Boxes are washed regularly (at least monthly) with a mild detergent (like dishwashing liquid), rather than strongly scented cleaners.	☐	☐	☐	☐
22	Unscented clumping litter is used.	☐	☐	☐	☐
23	A different brand or type of litter is purchased infrequently (less than monthly).	☐	☐	☐	☐
24	If a different type of litter is provided, it is put in a separate box so the cat can choose to use it (or not) if it wants to	☐	☐	☐	☐
Social contact					
25	Each cat has the opportunity to play with other animals or the owner if it chooses to on a daily basis.	☐	☐	☐	☐
26	Each cat has the option to disengage from other animals or people in the household at all times.	☐	☐	☐	☐
27	Do any cats interact with outdoor cats through windows?	☐	☐	☐	☐
Body care and activity					
28	Horizontal scratching posts are provided.	☐	☐	☐	☐
29	Vertical scratching posts are provided.	☐	☐	☐	☐
31	Chew items (e.g. cat-safe grasses) are provided.	☐	☐	☐	☐
32	Toys to chase that mimic quickly moving prey are provided.	☐	☐	☐	☐
33	Toys that can be picked up, carried, and tossed in the air are provided.	☐	☐	☐	☐
34	Toys are rotated on a regular basis (at least weekly) to provide novelty.	☐	☐	☐	☐

If you have additional comments on any of the questions, please write them below, including the question #.

Please help us understand what your cat does around the house by placing a check (✓) in the box next to each behavior that best describes how commonly your cat does each of the behaviors described below.

Does your cat	All of the time	Most of the time	A good bit of the time	Some of the time	A little bit of the time	None of the time	Does not apply
Leave household articles (furniture, drapes, clothing, plants, etc.) alone.	☐	☐	☐	☐	☐	☐	☐
Eat small amounts calmly at intervals throughout the day.	☐	☐	☐	☐	☐	☐	☐
Drink small amounts calmly at intervals throughout the day.	☐	☐	☐	☐	☐	☐	☐
Use the litterbox.	☐	☐	☐	☐	☐	☐	☐

Get along with people in the home.	☐	☐	☐	☐	☐	☐	☐
Get along with other pets in the home.	☐	☐	☐	☐	☐	☐	☐
Remain calm when left alone.	☐	☐	☐	☐	☐	☐	☐
Stay relaxed during normal, everyday handling (grooming, petting).	☐	☐	☐	☐	☐	☐	☐
Calm down quickly if startled or excited.	☐	☐	☐	☐	☐	☐	☐
React calmly to everyday events (telephone or doorbell ringing).	☐	☐	☐	☐	☐	☐	☐
Play well with people.	☐	☐	☐	☐	☐	☐	☐
Play well with other family cats.	☐	☐	☐	☐	☐	☐	☐
Show affection without acting clingy or annoying.	☐	☐	☐	☐	☐	☐	☐
Tolerate confinement in a carrier (including travel).	☐	☐	☐	☐	☐	☐	☐
Groom entire body calmly.	☐	☐	☐	☐	☐	☐	☐
Use scratching posts.	☐	☐	☐	☐	☐	☐	☐
Play with toys.	☐	☐	☐	☐	☐	☐	☐

Comments: anything else your cat regularly does or does not do that you think might be helpful for us to know about?

Figure 12.62 Example of a Household Resource questionnaire that can be used to collect information about the pet's environment. (Courtesy C.A. Buffington)

cats a place where they can feel safe cat-napping. Cat hammocks and window perches can provide them with the necessary comfort. When there is conflict between pets, steps must be taken to mitigate adverse interactions, even if it requires physical separation of the pets. Toys that encourage interaction between owners and their pets should be encouraged.

Diet

The role of diet in controlling FIC is somewhat controversial. Although many feline diets have been acidified and, in some cases, magnesium restricted 'for urinary tract health', there is no proven benefit of this practice. Struvite crystals do not damage normal urinary tract epithelium and their presence does not appear to be the cause of FIC. Nevertheless, the feeding of canned moist diet has been shown to lower the incidence and recurrence of FIC. It is important, however, not to 'switch' diets, especially in cats accustomed to a dry kibble food. The stress associated with an abrupt diet change has the potential to trigger further episodes of cystitis or, worse, anorexia and hepatic lipidosis. Rather, the new diet should be offered alongside the cat's usual food, and the pet should be allowed to choose between them. Most cats will eventually choose the wet food. If the cat will only eat dry food, a change should not be instituted.

While it is clear that ingestion of a wet food diet decreases urine osmolality and, therefore, concentration of noxious substances, other factors may be involved. The feeding of a wet food involves a different type of interaction between the owner and pet. Bowls need to be washed, cans opened, food scooped and prepared and, finally, the cat is presented with its meal. This can be contrasted with scooping and 'dumping' of a dry kibble. Whether it is the moisture content of the food, the ritual involved, or both, the feeding of a wet food diet should be encouraged. A recent study suggests that a specific diet (Hill's® c/d® Multicare), which is high in omega-3 fatty acids, may decrease recurrence of FLUTD.

The eating environment should be analyzed for potential stress. Many cats prefer to eat alone where they will not be disturbed by other animals, sudden movement, or unexpected noises. Other cats seem to be more social and may enjoy human companionship during their meals. The goal is to minimize stress and maximize the pleasure of the dining experience.

Pheromones

Pheromones are chemical messengers that convey information between members of the same species. Cats release several pheromones from facial scent glands, and they deposit these pheromones by rubbing their heads on objects, including their human companions, when they feel safe. A synthetic analog (Feliway®, Ceva Santé Animale) is available as both a room diffuser and spray. The proposed effect of this product is to decrease anxiety-related behavior. While studies examining the use of this product in cats with FIC are lacking, there is evidence that this product may decrease marking and scratching behavior in multi-cat households, as well as increase grooming and eating in hospitalized patients. It has been suggested that the spray can be applied to the area in which the cat is inappropriately urinating or that an entire room can be treated with a plug-in diffuser.

Drugs

Amitriptyline is a tricyclic antidepressant drug with anti-anxiety, analgesic, and anti-inflammatory properties. Although some small studies have shown no benefit from the use of amitriptyline for the treatment of FLUTD, one large study in 2003 found a significant benefit from its use. Not only does amitriptyline decrease anxiety and provide analgesia both peripherally and in the CNS, it has been shown to be a potent relaxer of urethral tissue. The recommended dosage is 1 mg/kg PO q24h.

Prazosin (0.5mg/cat PO q24h) is an alpha-blocker that may decrease urethral spasms. There is some empirical evidence to support its use.

Other

While the exact cause of FLUTD is unknown, a multifaceted approach combining environmental enrichment, diet, pheromones, and drugs appears to give many patients relief. In cases in which symptoms cannot be controlled, a perineal urethrostomy may be required. Because of the risk of incontinence, the required anatomic modification, and high lifelong risk of infection, this should only be considered when other possible alternatives have been exhausted.

UROLITHIASIS

Definition/overview

The most common uroliths in dogs and cats are composed of struvite and calcium oxalate, while uroliths composed of ammonium urate and cystine are less common (**Tables 12.19, 12.20**).

Table 12.19 Uroliths in dogs.

	Struvite	Calcium oxalate	Urate	Cystine
Age	2–9 years*	5–12 years	1–5 years	1–7 years
Breed	Min. Schnauzer, Min. Poodle, Bichon Frise, Cocker Spaniel	Min. Schnauzer, Std. Schnauzer, Lhaso Apso, Yorkshire Terrier, Min. Poodle, Shi Tzu, Bichon Frise	Dalmatian, English Bulldog, Min. Schnauzer, Yorkshire Terrier, Shi Tzu	English Bulldog, Dachshund, Bassett Hound, Newfoundland
Sex:				
Female	>80%			
Male		>5 years**	>6 years**	Majority
Urinalysis:				
PH	≥7.0	≤7.0	≤7.0	≤7.0
Crystals	Struvite	Calcium oxalate	Urate	Cystine
Culture	*Staph. intermedius*			
Serum		↑ Ca^{2+}[†]	↓ Albumin[††] ↓ BUN (urea)[†]	
Radiography	Large, >2 cm smooth surface	Medium size spiked surface	Small rounded	Small rounded
Opacity	2+–4+	4+	0–2+	1+–2+

* If less than 1 year old, very high chance of struvite.
** Higher probability if in this age category.
[†] Only rarely found.
[††] In portosystemic shunts.

Etiology

Urine is a complex solution made up of dissolved substances, some of which have a tendency to precipitate out of solution while others actively inhibit precipitation by increasing solubility. For example, as the concentration of calcium in urine increases, there is an increased risk of it binding to oxalate and forming crystals and stones; however, citrate, which is also present in urine, binds to calcium and makes it unavailable for binding. In **Figure 12.63**, there is a region on the chart called the solubility product. If urine were only made up of substances that have a tendency to precipitate out of solution, this would be the maximum saturation that could be achieved. However, the presence of substances that actively inhibit precipitation allows urine to achieve a metastable supersaturation state. Under normal circumstances, there is a balance between precipitators and inhibitors and urine exists in this metastable state; however, in the presence of an excess of precipitators or a shortage of inhibitors, crystals and uroliths can form. In some cases, urine pH can also directly impact the solubility of these solutes.

Table 12.20 Uroliths in cats.

	Struvite	Calcium oxalate	Urate
Age:* 1–4 years >10 years	 79% 60%	 21% 40%	 Rare
Breed	Any	Burmese, Himalayan, Persian	
Sex: Male Female	 65% 75%	 35% 25%	
Urinalysis: PH Crystals Culture Serum	 ≥7.0 Struvite *Staph. intermedius*	 ≤7.0 Calcium oxalate ↑ Ca^{2+}††	 ≤7.0 Ammonium urate ↓ Albumin†† ↓ BUN
Radiograph	Discoid‡ Ovoid/smooth‡‡	Spiked surface	Rounded
Opacity	2+–4+	4+	0–2+

* If less than 1 year old, usually due to urease-producing infection.
† Only rarely found.
†† In portosystemic shunts.
‡ Usually sterile.
‡‡ Associated with urease-producing infection.

Pathophysiology

Struvite

In dogs, the most common urolith is struvite (magnesium ammonium phosphate). These stones, once called triple phosphate, are associated with urease-producing bacteria (*Staphylococcus intermedius, Proteus mirabilis, Pseudomonas* spp., *Klebsiella* spp.). Urea is plentiful in the urine and urease splits it to form ammonium and bicarbonate **(Figure 12.64)**. Ammonium combines with magnesium and phosphate while the bicarbonate raises the urine pH. The change in pH decreases the solubility of the ammonium–magnesium–phosphate complex, leading to the formation of struvite crystals and stones. The anatomic configuration of the female makes urease-producing infections more common than in males.

In contrast to those in dogs and people, struvite uroliths found in young healthy cats are usually not associated with UTIs. Although the exact pathophysiology is not well understood, diet, breed, sex, and urine pH all seem to play a role.

Calcium oxalate

The second most common canine urolith is calcium oxalate. The formation of these stones can be the result of excessive calcium/oxalate excretion or an absence of urolith inhibitors. Although most cases are idiopathic, possible causes of excessive calcium excretion into urine should be investigated. Increased calcium excretion can

12.63

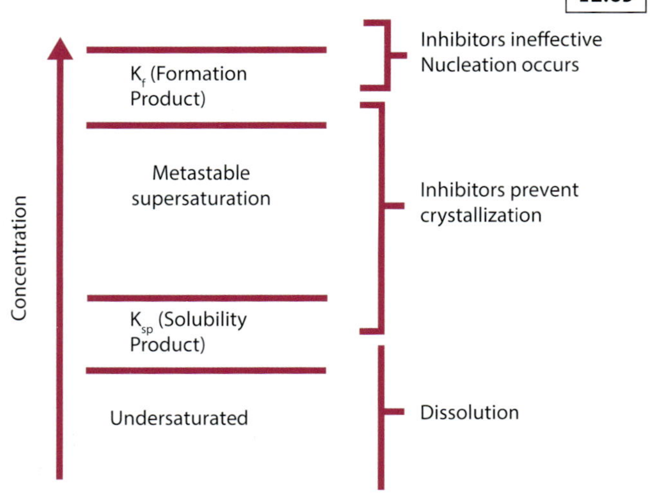

Figure 12.63 Factors that increase urine concentration above the supersaturation point or decrease the formation product (e.g. loss of precipitation inhibitors) will lead to crystal and stone formation.

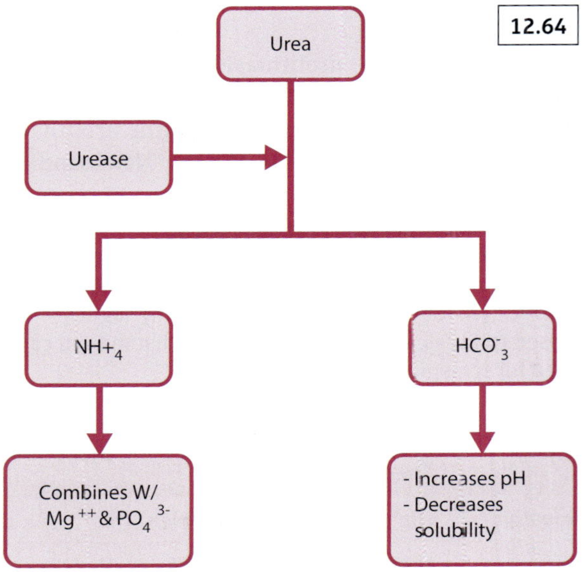

Figure 12.64 Bacterial urease splits urea, which is plentiful in urine, to form ammonium and bicarbonate. Ammonium combines with magnesium and phosphate while the bicarbonate raises the urine pH. The change in pH decreases the solubility of the ammonium–magnesium–phosphate complex, leading to the formation of struvite crystals and stones.

be the result of kidney leakage (failure to reabsorb), or excessive renal excretion due to elevated blood levels. Elevated blood levels can be secondary to abnormal intestinal absorption, hyperparathyroidism, paraneoplastic syndromes, granulomatous disease, or calcitriol toxicosis. Although excessive loss of oxalate into the urine (hyperoxaluria) plays a role in urolith formation in people, it is not believed to be important in dogs. In addition, while it was once thought that urine pH had a great effect on calcium oxalate formation, it is now generally accepted that urine acidity plays only a minor role.

Serum calcium levels should be measured in all patients who present with calcium oxalate uroliths or crystals. This information, when combined with calcitriol, PTH, and PTH-related peptide (PTHrP), can be helpful in determining the underlying cause of calcium oxalate formation (**Table 12.21**). For example, dogs with excessive intestinal calcium absorption have mildly increased serum calcium, which suppresses the release of PTH. In the kidney, increased amounts of calcium are passed through the glomerulus; however, the absence of PTH prevents tubular reabsorption. This results in hypercalciuria and stone formation. Dogs with this condition will often have calcium levels still within the upper limits of 'normal range' with suppression of both PTH and calcitriol. Since no tumor is involved, PTHrP will be undetectable.

Calcium oxalate uroliths have been reported in dogs secondary to hyperparathyroidism. In these patients, excessive PTH results in osteoclastic reclamation of bone and excessive formation of calcitriol (1,25-hydroxyvitamin D) by the kidney. Calcitriol increases intestinal absorption of calcium. These two actions result in elevations in blood calcium levels. In the kidney, excessive amounts of calcium are passed through the glomerulus. Although PTH simulates renal calcium reabsorption, the filtered amount overwhelms the kidney's capacity, resulting in hypercalciuria and stone formation.

Although uroliths have been reported secondary to paraneoplastic hypercalcemia in people, it is not clear if this occurs in dogs. In these patients, PTHrP, a PTH analog that is produced by the tumor, is elevated and stimulates osteoclastic reclamation of bone. In addition, PTHrP stimulates conversion of calcidiol to calcitriol. The resulting elevation in serum calcium levels overwhelms the kidney's resorptive abilities, resulting in hypercalciuria.

Leakage hypercalciuria is a failure of the renal tubules to resorb filtered calcium despite the presence of adequate PTH. As calcium is lost, PTH is released from the parathyroid gland, mobilizing calcium from bone and stimulating the conversion of calcidiol to calcitriol. Although large amounts of calcium can be lost into the urine, serum levels are normal due to the actions of PTH and calcitriol. For reasons that are not entirely clear, hyperadrenocorticism (Cushing's disease) can promote tubular calcium loss.

Although many cases of feline calcium oxalate uroliths are idiopathic, all patients should be screened for idiopathic hypercalcemia, malignancy hypercalcemia, and primary hyperparathyroidism. Since increases in total calcium can be unimpressive with some of these conditions, ionized calcium should be measured in all feline patients with calcium oxalate crystals and/or uroliths. If high, PTH and PTHrP levels should be measured. Based

Table 12.21 Causes of canine hypercalcemia can often be determined by measuring calcium, parathyroid hormone (PTH), calcitriol, and parathyroid hormone-related peptide (PTHrP).

	Ca^{++}	PTH	Calcitriol	PTHrP
Intestinal	E	L	L	O
Leakage	N	N	N	O
Hyperparathyroid	E	E	E	O
Paraneoplastic	E	L	E	E
Granulomatous	E	L	E	O
Calcipotriol	E	L	E	O

E, elevated; L, low; N, normal; O, zero.

on these three parameters, the likely cause of the hypercalcemia can be determined (**Table 12.22**).

Cats with idiopathic hypercalcemia may have only slight elevations in total calcium, while ionized calcium can be dramatically affected. While at least half of affected cats will have no clinical signs, others will experience weight loss, anorexia, and/or oxalate stones. Besides removing the calcium oxalate stones, these patients should be fed a high-fiber alkaline urine forming diet. Many will respond to high dose prednisone (10 mg/cat q24h), others may require a bisphosphonate such as alendronate (10 mg/cat q7days).

Urate

Urate stones are the third most common urolith in dogs and account for 8% of canine urinary calculi. A genetic predisposition (autosomal recessive) has been documented in Dalmatians and is suspected in English Bulldogs. Urate stone formation has also been associated with hepatic dysfunction, especially hepatic portal shunts. Interestingly, a significant number of dogs that are not Dalmatians or English Bulldogs and have no evidence of liver disease develop urate uroliths. While the mechanism of urate stone formation in these dogs is unclear, Yorkshire Terriers, Shih Tzus, and Miniature Schnauzers appear to be overrepresented.

In most dogs, dietary purines are metabolized in a series of steps to the highly soluble allantoin (**Figure 12.65**). This process, which takes place in the liver, involves converting purines to hypoxanthine. Through the action of xanthine oxidase, hypoxanthine is converted to xanthine and then uric acid. Uric acid, which is poorly soluble, is then converted to the highly soluble allantoin through the enzymatic action of uricase.

Although Dalmatians possess all the necessary enzymes to convert purines to allantoin, it appears that a defective cell membrane transport system decreases hepatic metabolism of uric acid and large amounts of uric acid are then presented to the kidney. The resulting hyperuricosuria may not completely explain the urolith formation, as not all Dalmatians with increased urate excretion are affected. It is likely that other factors including urine pH and a decrease in the production of crystallization inhibitors play a role. The fact that most Dalmatians that present for urate stones are male is probably due to anatomic differences (e.g. decreased urethral diameter) between the sexes.

Urate uroliths have been observed in cats. There does not appear to be a breed predilection. Most urate uroliths occur in younger cats and may be secondary to liver disease or portal vascular anomaly; however, many appear to be idiopathic.

Cystine

In the USA, cystine urolithiasis is uncommon and accounts for only 1–2% of all uroliths; the incidence may be higher in parts of Europe. While cystine uroliths have been reported in many breeds of dogs, Newfoundlands,

Table 12.22 Causes of feline hypercalcemia can often be determined by measuring ionized calcium, parathyroid hormone, and parathyroid hormone-related peptide. Since idiopathic hypercalcemia can present with only slightly increased total calcium, it is recommended that ionized calcium be used for screening.

	Ionized Ca++	PTH	PTHrP
Idiopathic	High	Normal/high	0
Cancer	High	Low	High
Primary	High	High	0

12.65

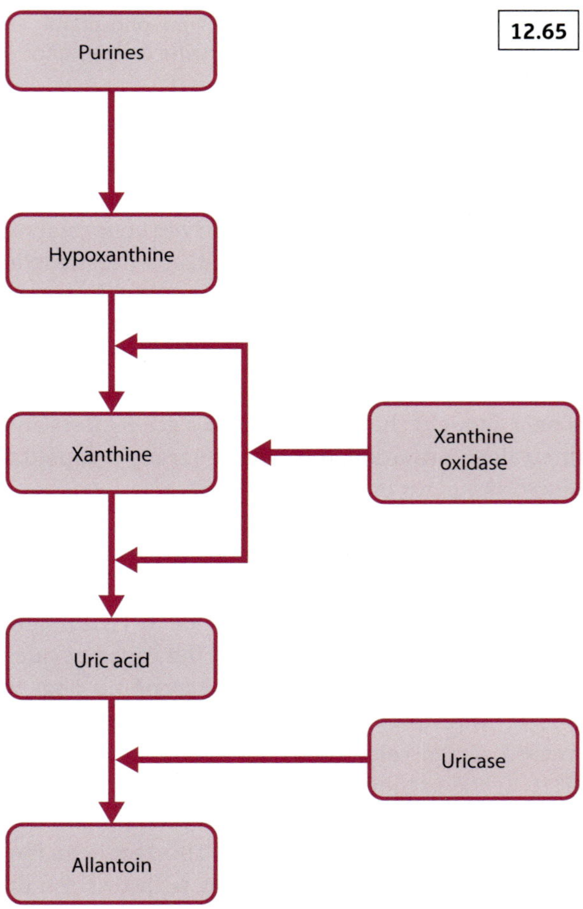

Figure 12.65 Dietary purines are metabolized in a series of oxidative steps to the highly water soluble allantoin. In some patients, the process is interrupted, leaving large amounts of the poorly soluble uric acid.

Pit Bull Terriers, Dachshunds, and Chihuahuas appear to be overrepresented.

In the kidney, cystine is freely filtered by the glomerulus and then reabsorbed in the PCT. In affected dogs, there is a defect in the proteins needed for cystine reabsorption and excessive amounts of the poorly soluble amino acid are excreted in the urine. In Newfoundlands, the condition is inherited as an autosomal recessive condition; however, this has not been demonstrated in other breeds. There is now a genetic test specifically for Newfoundlands (University of Pennsylvania).

Clinical presentation

Clinical signs vary with the location of the uroliths. Nephroliths may cause sublumbar pain and hematuria but they often cause no clinical signs. Bladder uroliths cause signs of lower urinary tract inflammation with hematuria, pollakiuria, and stranguria. Urethral uroliths in male dogs cause stranguria and intermittent incontinence with a full bladder. They can cause complete urethral obstruction in both dogs and cats.

Differential diagnosis

Lower urinary tract inflammation (hematuria and proteinuria), trauma, neoplasia, UTI, idiopathic cystitis (cats).

Diagnosis

Presence, number, size, and location of uroliths are usually determined by radiographic and/or ultrasound examination (**Tables 12.19, 12.20**). As size and radiolucency can vary substantially, ultrasound has proved to be more diagnostically useful than radiographs

The likely mineral composition of uroliths can be predicted on the basis of clinical data including the age, breed, and sex, and the radiographic density and shape of the uroliths (**Figure 12.66a, b**), the mineral composition of crystals in the urine sediment (**Figures 12.67–12.70**), urine pH, and bacterial culture of the urine; however, actual mineral composition can only be determined by quantitative analysis of recovered uroliths. These tests, which include optical crystallography, x-ray diffraction, and infrared spectroscopy, are only performed at specialty laboratories.

Management

Uroliths can be treated in several different ways depending on their location in the urinary tract. Stones located in the kidney are usually left untreated unless they obstruct the ureter, at which point they would be surgically managed. Stones that become lodged in the ureter represent a surgical emergency because in a matter of days they can lead to hydronephrosis and irreversible kidney damage. Traditionally, these have been surgically removed; however, today, options such as ureteral stents (**Figure 12.71**) and subcutaneous ureteral bypass devices have become possible.

Struvite, urate, and cystine uroliths are all amenable to being dissolved (**Figure 12.72**); however, in male patients, this is associated with a high risk of urethral obstruction. Removal of tiny stones can be attempted

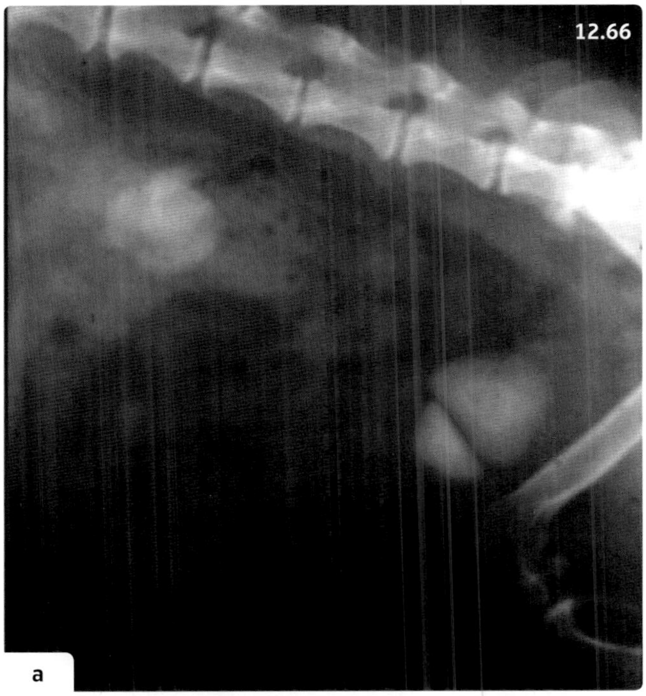

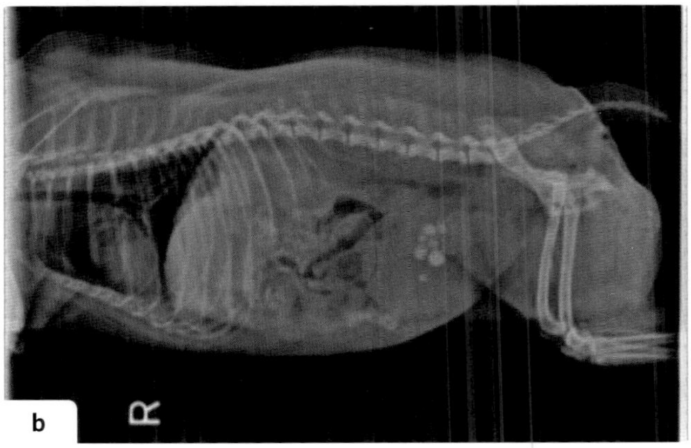

Figures 12.66a, b Although struvite uroliths are classically described as being large with flattened edges between the stones (a), they can appear as many small stones (b), making predicting the composition of the uroliths based on clinical data challenging. In addition, uroliths of a mixed composition are not uncommon; therefore, whenever possible, uroliths should be submitted for analysis.

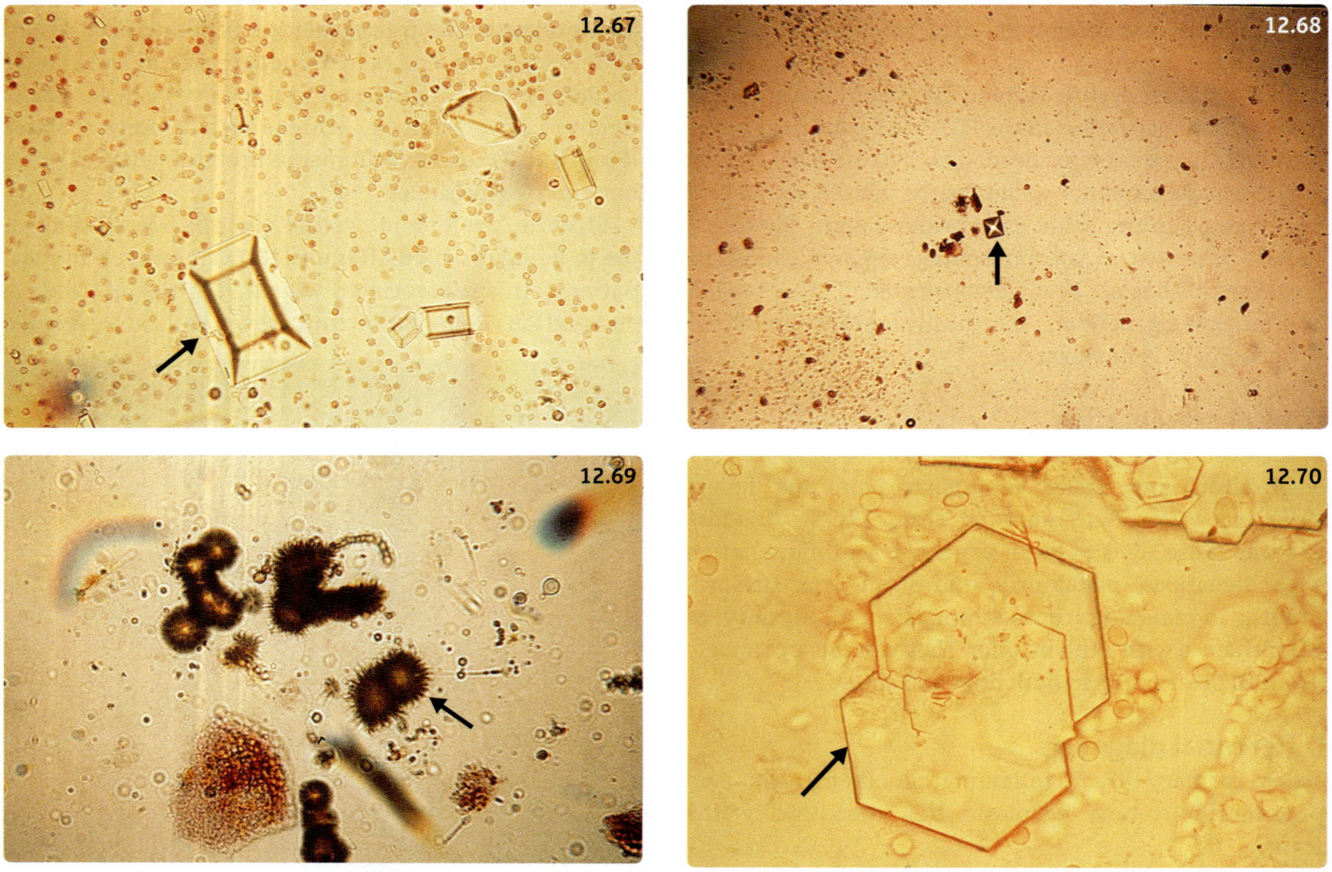

Figures 12.67–12.70 Appearance of crystals in urine corresponding to the common uroliths (arrows): (12.67) struvite; (12.68) calcium oxalate dihydrate; (12.69) ammonium urate; (12.70) cystine. (Courtesy D.F. Senior)

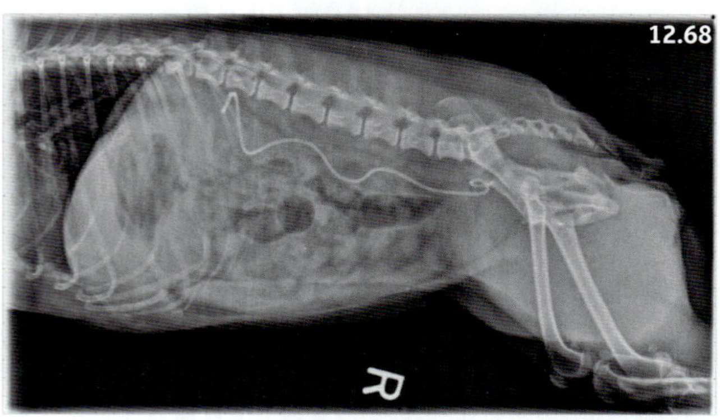

Figure 12.71 Example of a ureteral stent in a patient with ureteral obstruction. (Courtesy M. Ellison)

12.72

Preliminary: Urine obtained by cystocentesis submitted for culture and sensitivity.
Initiate therapy: Start oral antimicrobial drugs based on urine culture and sensitivity results and begin feeding commercially available struvite dissolving diet. Antimicrobial therapy must continue for duration of dissolution therapy.
Every 30 days: Physical examination, urinalysis, abdominal radiographs. If pH is >7.0, suspect resistant infection and submit urine for culture and sensitivity. Adjust antimicrobial as indicated.
Continue protocol: Continue therapy for 30 days after the first follow-up radiographic examination that shows no evidence of uroliths.

Figure 12.72 Canine struvite uroliths dissolution flowchart.

with catheter-assisted retrieval. Small stones may be removed with urohydropropulsion or an endoscope utilizing a stone basket (**Figure 12.73**). Larger stones can be removed via surgery or fragmented and removed by lithotripsy. Once removed, all stones should be submitted for analysis. While diagnostic imaging and urine analysis can provide information about the likely composition of the stone (**Tables 12.19 and 12.20;** see **Figures 12.67–12.70**), only a proper stone analysis can provide definitive information regarding stone composition.

Canine struvite uroliths

Struvite uroliths can be dissolved over time; however, this carries the risk of urethral obstruction. In males, the long narrow urethra and the potential for stones to become lodged in the area of the os penis makes this is especially concerning. A discussion with the owner about the relative risks and benefits of medical and surgical management should occur before deciding on a therapy. The owner should be made aware that in dogs, the dissolving process takes many months.

Dissolution of struvite uroliths involves a combination of antimicrobial and dietary therapy (see **Figure 12.72**). Appropriate antimicrobial selection can only be made on the basis of a urine culture and sensitivity. The urine must be obtained by cystocentesis and examined in a timely fashion. Since bacteria are often sequestered and protected in the layers of the stone, antibiotic therapy must be continued throughout the entire dissolution process. There are several commercially available struvite-dissolving diets. These diets tend to be low in protein and acidify the urine. Every month, the patient's progress should be evaluated by performing abdominal radiography and a urine analysis. If the pH is >7.0, a resistant UTI should be suspected and a urine sample, obtained by cystocentesis, submitted for culture.

Inhibition of struvite formation requires prevention of alkaline urine; therefore, the urinary tract must be free of infections. At-home monitoring can be performed by measuring urine pH on a regular basis. This can be accomplished using urine dipsticks or with an inexpensive pH meter. The presence of alkaline urine indicates that a urine culture is necessary. Dogs with recurrent UTIs despite the resolution of uroliths should be evaluated for structural abnormalities that may predispose the patient to UTI. The author has found that most of these cases are related to an involuted vulva (**Figures 12.74a, b**). Some patients benefit from long-term, low-dose antibiotic

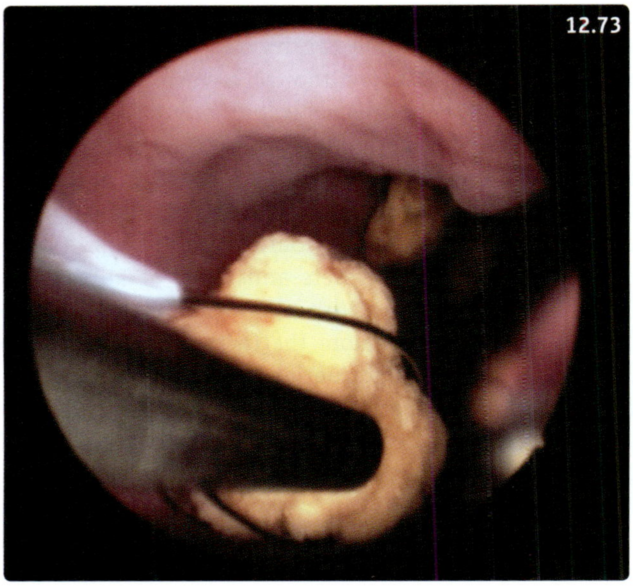

Figure 12.73 Urolith removed with a urethroscope and retrieval basket.

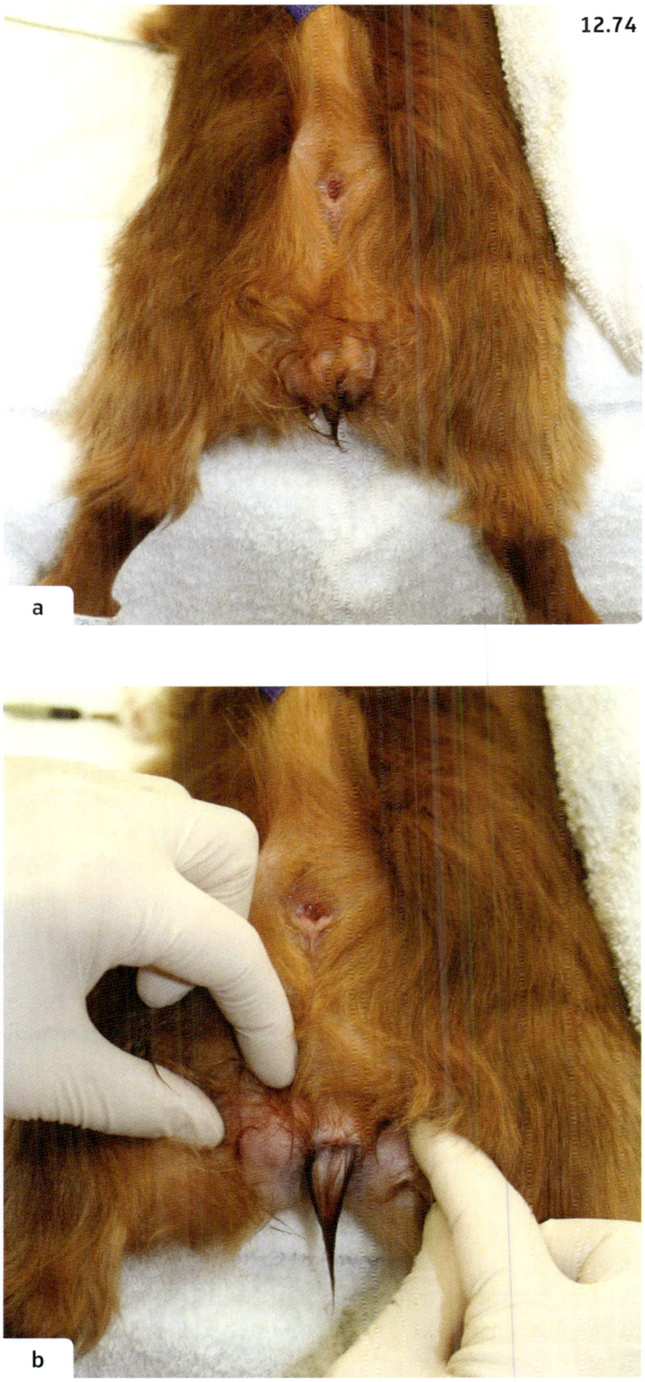

Figures 12.74a, b Dog with an involuted vulva. Note how the extent of the involution is not apparent until a complete genital examination is performed.

therapy: ampicillin (10 mg/kg PO q24h) or amoxicillin (5 mg/kg PO q24h) administered at bedtime.

Feline struvite uroliths

Sterile struvite uroliths can be dissolved by feeding a diet that is both restricted in magnesium, phosphorus, and protein and induces aciduria. There are several commercial diets formulated to accomplish struvite dissolution is cats; however, male cats may be at risk of obstruction. Compared with dogs, in which the process can take many months, complete dissolution of stones can be often accomplished in days to weeks.

Canine calcium oxalate

Calcium oxalate uroliths cannot be dissolved and must be removed using urohydropropulsion, a stone basket (see **Figure 12.73**), surgery, or lithotripsy.

Dogs with elevations in blood calcium levels should be treated appropriately for any underlying condition. One of the most important steps in preventing calcium oxalate crystals and uroliths in otherwise healthy dogs is to increase water intake, which can be partially accomplished by feeding a canned diet. The optimum diet composition to prevent calcium oxalate urolith formation is unknown. Previously, it had been recommended that diets be low in protein and sodium restricted; however, recent epidemiologic studies have challenged this approach. Currently recommended diets include Royal Canin S/O, Hill's u/d, and Hills w/d. Despite appropriate diet therapy, as many as 50% of dogs will have recurrence within 3 years.

The owner should purchase a refractometer and urine dipsticks. Urine should be checked regularly (at least weekly) to be certain the USG remains <1.020 and pH is 7.0–7.5. Radiographs should be taken every 2–4 months so that stones can be detected while they are small enough to be removed by stone basket, catheter-assisted retrieval, or urohydropropulsion.

Thiazide diuretics have been shown to decrease urinary calcium excretion and should be considered in dogs with persistent calcium oxalate crystalluria or recurrence of uroliths despite appropriate diet therapy (hydrochlorothiazide, 2 mg/kg PO q12h). Citrate is a urolith inhibitor that is thought to form complexes with calcium and increases its solubility. In people, oral potassium citrate ingestion increases urine pH and increases the amount of citrate in the urine; however, supplementation in dogs does not result in a significant change in urine citrate concentration. Therefore, the benefit of potassium citrate supplementation is not clear. Nevertheless, some experts recommend potassium citrate supplementation (25–50 mg/kg PO q12h).

Feline calcium oxalate

Cats with elevations in ionized calcium should be treated appropriately for any underlying condition. Once the hypercalcemia is addressed the amount of calcium spilling into the urine will abate and they should not continue to form uroliths. For patients with idiopathic calcium oxalate uroliths, there are two diets that are formulated for the prevention of these stones. These diets contain potassium citrate (as an alkalinizing agent and as a source of citrate) and induce a urine pH of approximately 7.0. Neither has been evaluated in actual calcium oxalate-forming cats; nevertheless, cats consuming c/d multicare (Hill's Pet Nutrition) and S/O (Royal Canin) do demonstrate a decreased urine calcium oxalate saturation.

Urate

Although urate uroliths in dogs that do not have liver disease can be medically dissolved, there is a risk of urethral obstruction in male dogs. A discussion with the owner about the relative risks and benefits of medical and surgical management should occur before selecting a therapy. Dissolution should not be attempted in dogs with known liver disease.

The dissolution of urate uroliths involves dietary changes, medical intervention, and urine modification. Reduction of urate excretion can be achieved by restricting total protein and by offering low purine content proteins (e.g. eggs) instead of high purine content proteins (e.g. fish). Feeding a protein-restricted diet can dilute urine by decreasing the urea available for the medullary concentration gradient of the kidney. Feeding a canned diet in order to increase water intake can further dilute urine.

Allopurinol, a xanthine oxidase inhibitor, prevents the conversion of soluble xanthine to the insoluble uric acid (see **Figure 12.65**). Although a variety of adverse reactions have been reported in humans, the most commonly reported adverse effect in dogs is the formation of xanthine uroliths. This is usually seen when protein intake is not properly restricted. Prevention of urate urolith recurrence is best accomplished through a combination of low-protein diets and urine alkalinization. Prophylactic treatment with allopurinol is not recommended as it may promote the formation of xanthine uroliths. Urate urolith formation is inhibited in alkaline urine as the concentration of ammonium ions needed for stone formation decreases. The target pH range is 7.0–7.4. Low-protein diets favor an alkaline pH; however, sometimes further urine alkalinization is needed. Potassium citrate (40–90 mg/kg PO q12h) can be given. A urine pH of 7.5 or higher should be avoided, as this may favor the formation of calcium phosphate and struvite uroliths.

Response to medical therapy can be evaluated by periodic monitoring of urine pH (7.0–7.4), USG (<1.015), and serum BUN (<10 mg/dl).

Cystine

Although cystine uroliths can be medically dissolved (1–3 months), there is a significant risk of urethral obstruction, as these occur predominantly in male dogs (98%). A discussion with the owner about the relative risks and benefits of medical and surgical management should occur before selecting a therapy.

Dissolution of cystine uroliths involves dietary changes, medical intervention, and urine modification. Reduction of cystine excretion can be achieved by restricting total protein. Furthermore, feeding a protein-restricted diet can dilute urine by decreasing the urea available for the renal medulla. Increasing urine volume and thereby further diluting cystine concentration can be achieved by feeding a canned diet. Thiol-containing drugs catalyze the conversion of the poorly soluble cystine to more soluble compounds. N-(2-mercaptopropionyl) glycine (Thiola®) (20 mg/kg PO q12h) can be used for this purpose. Side-effects, including aggression, myopathy, proteinuria, anemia, and thrombocytopenia, may limit its use. Cystine urolith formation is inhibited in alkaline urine. The target pH range is 7.0–7.4. Low-protein diets favor an alkaline pH; however, sometimes further urine alkalinization is needed. Potassium citrate (40–90 mg/kg PO q12h) can be given. A urine pH of 7.5 or higher should be avoided, as this may favor the formation of calcium phosphate and struvite uroliths. Response to medical therapy can be evaluated by periodic at-home checking of urine pH (7.0–7.4) and USG (<1.015).

TUMORS OF THE LOWER URINARY TRACT

Definition/overview

Tumors of the lower urinary tract are relatively rare, representing less than 2% of all canine neoplasms and an even lower percentage of feline neoplasms. Most are malignant and the common histologic types include transitional cell carcinoma, squamous cell carcinoma, adenocarcinoma, undifferentiated carcinoma, rhabdomysarcoma, and fibroma. In both dogs and cats, transitional cell carcinoma is the most common neoplasm of the urethra and bladder. Other malignant mesenchymal tumors, lymphoma, and benign masses have been reported.

Etiology

A relationship between dipping dogs with parasiticides and the use of certain lawn products and the appearance of transitional cell carcinoma has been suggested. Scottish Terriers have an 18-fold increased risk of developing transitional cell carcinoma, while Shetland Sheepdogs and Beagles have a 4-fold increased risk. In cats, the tumor types are much more varied, with many different primary cell types involved. As many as 20% of bladder tumors in cats are benign mesenchymal masses.

Pathophysiology

Transitional cell carcinomas spread by direct extension through the wall of the bladder or urethra to adjacent tissue and to draining lymph nodes. At diagnosis about 40% have undergone metastasis, most commonly to the local lymph nodes, the lungs, the urethra, and the ventral lumbar vertebrae. Secondary UTIs are common, a development that can intensify clinical signs.

Clinical presentation

Affected animals present with signs of lower urinary tract inflammation including pollakiuria, dysuria, stranguria, and hematuria. Urethral obstruction may be evident in patients with urethral tumors. On physical examination, the bladder wall may be thickened and a mass may be palpable. With urethral tumors in dogs, a portion or all of the urethra may be thickened on rectal examination.

Differential diagnosis

Abnormal micturition: UTI, urolithiasis, behavioral disturbances, urethral stricture, granulomatous urethritis, neurologic disorders, cystitis

Diagnosis

Urinalysis can fail to detect neoplastic cells on microscopic examination of the urine sediment; cytospin examination of saline flushes of the bladder may be much more reliable. When the neoplasm is in the urethra, a suction biopsy can also be obtained for accurate cytologic evaluation (**Figure 12.75**). This is performed by placing a side-hole catheter in the urethra while using rectal palpation to guide the catheter tip into the affected area. Suction is then applied using a syringe so that the catheter adheres to the urethral wall and abnormal tissue is drawn inside the lumen of the side-hole. Then the catheter is forcibly removed while continuing to apply suction. The diagnostic sample is flushed out of the catheter using a syringe filled with saline.

Plain radiographs are usually unrewarding, but contrast studies including a retrograde urethrogram can reveal filling defects and defects in the normally smooth contrast agent–mucosal interface (**Figure 12.76**).

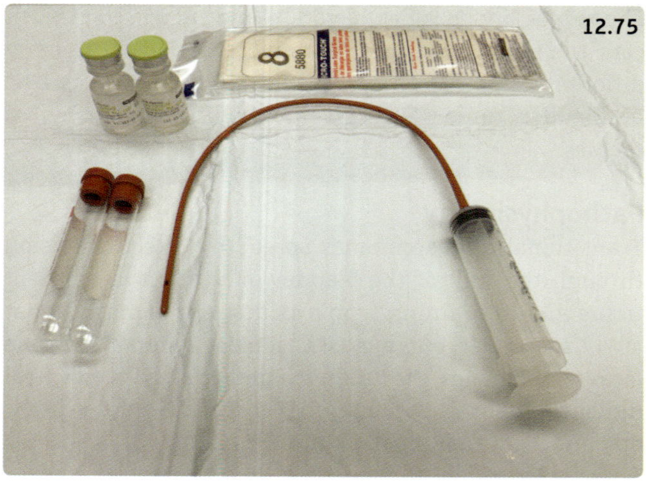

Figure 12.75 Example of simple equipment needed for effective urethral suction biopsy. The patient is sedated and a catheter inserted into the urethra using rectal palpation to guide the catheter tip into the affected area. Suction is applied using the syringe and the catheter is forcibly removed.

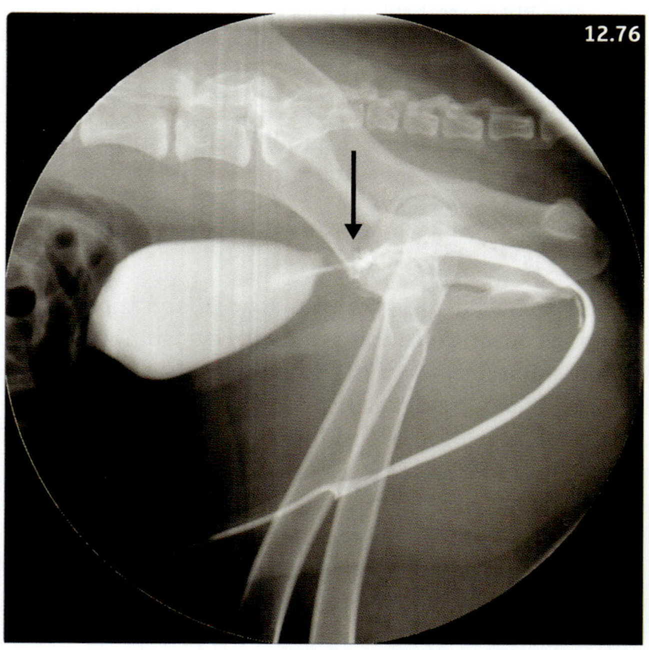

Figure 12.76 Example of a retrograde urethrogram in a patient with urethral obstruction due to transitional cell carcinoma. The arrow indicates an area of filling defect.

Ultrasound can be supportive. Because of the risk of spreading the neoplasm into the abdomen, fine needle aspirates should not be attempted. When avaliable, urethroscopy and cystoscopy are the most rewarding procedures (**Figure 12.77**). Not only do they allow visual inspection of the urethra and bladder, they also facilitate tissue biopsies.

Management

The success of surgical intervention is limited by the late stage at which the diagnosis of tumors of the lower urinary tract is generally made. Urethral stenting can provide palliative relief of obstructed urethras (**Figure 12.78**). The most effective chemotherapeutic agent for dogs with transitional cell carcinoma of the bladder is piroxicam (0.3 mg/kg PO q24h). In one study of 34 dogs, 14.7% went into partial or complete remission; median survival was 155 days and 1-year survival rate was 20.6%. Cisplatin (50 mg/m^2 body surface area every 4 weeks for two or more treatments) provided a partial response in some patients. Some success has been reported with both intraoperative and postoperative radiation. Control of concurrent UTI and treatment with an anticholinergic agent such as propantheline (7.5–15 mg PO q8–12h) to reduce bladder spasm can alleviate some of the urge incontinence experienced by affected dogs.

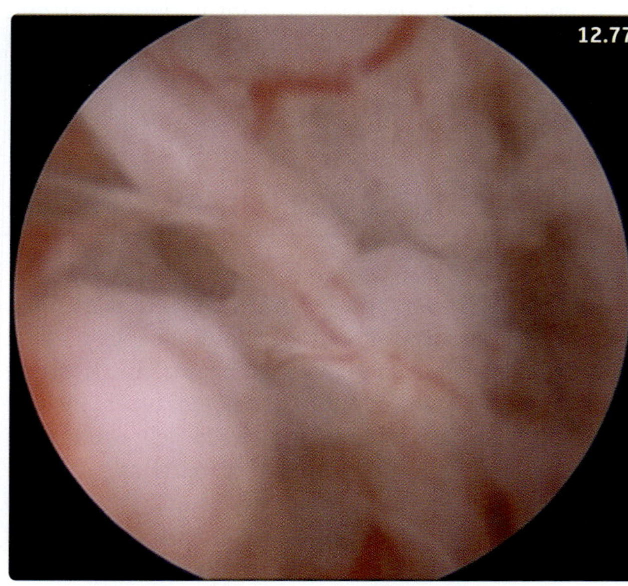

Figures 12.77 Example of a urethra affected by transitional cell carcinoma as seen during cystoscopy.

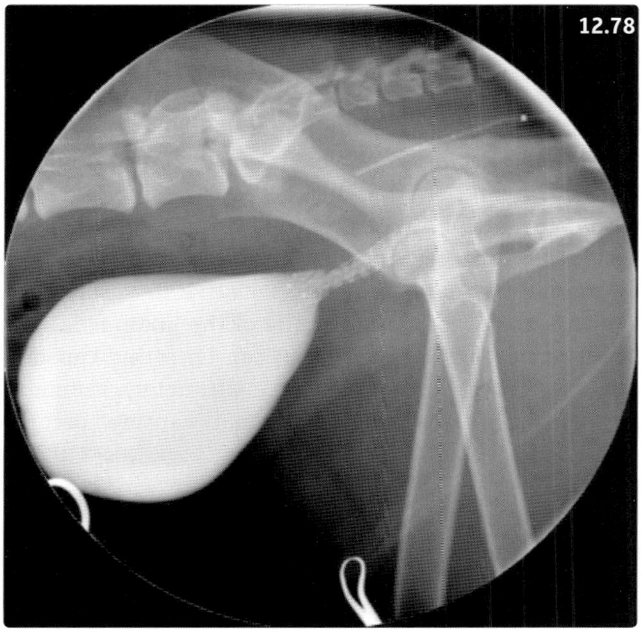

Figure 12.78 The same patient as in Figure 12.77 after placement of a urethral stent.

CYSTIC DISEASE

Definition/overview

Polycystic kidney disease (PKD) is a bilateral condition that has been reported in Persian cats, Cairn Terriers, and West Highland White Terriers. Rare solitary renal cysts can be seen in dogs and cats. Cats occasionally develop unilateral or bilateral perirenal pseudocysts.

Etiology

PKD has a genetic basis with autosomal dominant inheritance in Persian cats and autosomal recessive inheritance in Cairn Terriers and West Highland White Terriers.

Pathophysiology

The precise changes in the nephron wall that lead to PKD are not known. A weakening of the tubular basement membrane and support structures could be a possibility. Hyperplasia of tubular epithelial cells with consequent occlusion and obstruction of the tubule has also been theorized. A combination of the above factors may be present. Persian cats can appear normal as kittens and only develop pronounced renomegaly and renal failure as adults. In the single report of PKD in Cairn Terriers, the dogs developed renal failure as very young puppies. The cysts of PKD can become infected. The cause of perirenal pseudocysts in cats is unknown and most affected animals present with CKD.

Clinical presentation

Animals with PKD or perirenal pseudocyst develop extreme bilateral renomegaly with concurrent signs of CKD. Affected Persian cats can be any age on initial presentation but in Cairn Terriers and West Highland White Terriers, affected animals are usually very young. Solitary renal cysts are most often diagnosed as an incidental finding.

Differential diagnosis

Renomegaly, neoplasia, hydronephrosis, amyloidosis, FIP.

Diagnosis

In Persian cats, an ultrasound performed at 16 weeks has been reported to have a sensitivity of 75% and a specificity of 100%, while an ultrasound performed at 36 weeks of age has a sensitivity of 91% and a specificity of 100%. Cairn Terrier PKD is characterized by the presence of cysts in the liver and kidney, while West Highland White Terriers develop PKD as puppies.

Once bilateral renomegaly is recognized on physical examination, ultrasound examination can differentiate between PKD, solitary cysts, and perirenal pseudocysts. In PKD the cysts are multiple, of variable size, and throughout the parenchyma of the kidney (**Figures 12.79a, b**), whereas in perirenal pseudocysts the renal capsule is extremely distended, completely surrounding the kidney with fluid (**Figure 12.80**).

Management

No specific treatment is available to manage cats with PKD or perirenal pseudocyst other than support for their concurrent CKD. Antibiotics to control secondary pyelonephritis may prevent some of the malaise suffered by cats with PKD.

HYDRONEPHROSIS

Definition/overview

Hydronephrosis is caused by pressure atrophy of renal tissue due to partial or complete urine outflow obstruction. The renal papilla and renal medulla are affected first. Hydronephrosis is a relatively uncommon condition that often goes unrecognized if only one kidney is affected.

Etiology

Hydronephrosis is caused by obstruction to urine flow. Cancers in the trigone of the bladder, of the ureter, and in the renal pelvis can all induce hydronephrosis. Uroliths, ureteroliths, congenital and acquired strictures, EUs, and misplaced sutures (usually in association with ovariohysterectomy) are also reported.

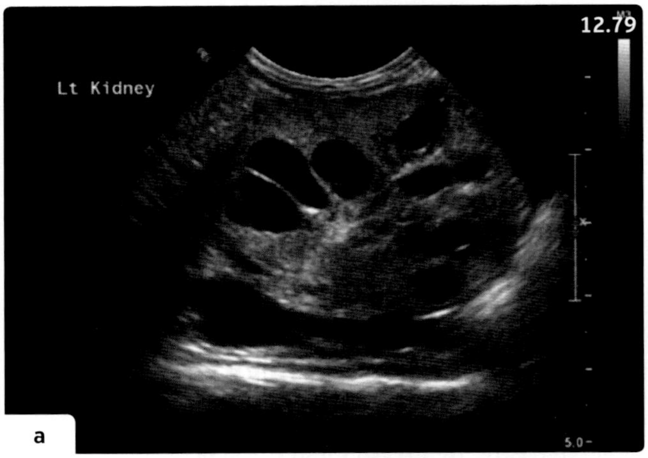

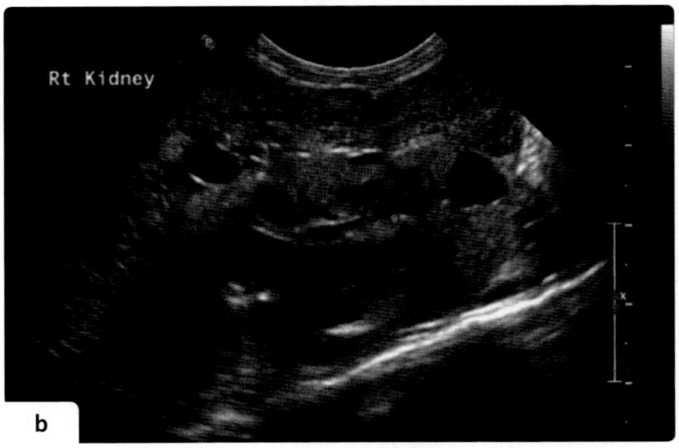

Figures 12.79a, b Ultrasonograms of a Persian cat (age unknown) with polycystic kidney disease. (Courtesy R. Baumruck)

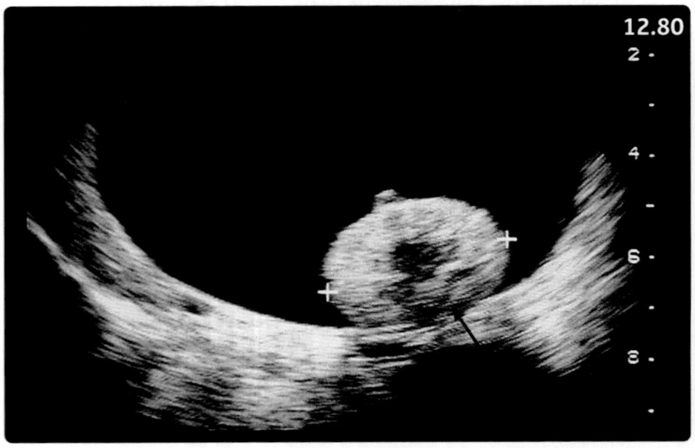

Figure 12.80 Ultrasonographic appearance of the kidney (arrow) and the surrounding cystic structure in a cat with a perirenal pseudocyst. (Courtesy AM Grooters; from *Compendium on Continuing Education for the Practicing Veterinarian*, 1997, **9:**1226, with permission.)

Pathophysiology

When urine cannot flow freely from the renal pelvis, increased pressure is reflected back up into the nephron via the collecting duct. The back pressure eventually becomes sufficiently high to stop glomerular filtration both by direct pressure and a reflex vasomotor action. When partial ureteral obstruction exists, increased hydrostatic pressure in the collecting tubules renders them less sensitive to vasopressin and this, combined with atrophy of the juxtamedullary nephrons, causes reduced renal concentrating capacity and increased urine volume. Ultimately, remaining cortical tissue and the renal capsule become distended.

Clinical presentation

Unilateral hydronephrosis is often clinically silent and signs are induced by the underlying condition causing the hydronephrosis (e.g. bladder cancer in the trigone region of the bladder). Acute obstruction can lead to sensitivity often thought to be 'back pain'. Partial obstruction can lead to increased urine volume with polydipsia. Bilateral partial ureteral obstruction leads to renal failure.

Differential diagnosis

Renomegaly: neoplasia, amyloidosis, FIP, cystic disease.

Diagnosis

An enlarged kidney may be apparent on abdominal palpation or on radiographs. The presence of hydronephrosis can be confirmed on ultrasound (**Figure 12.81**), but the

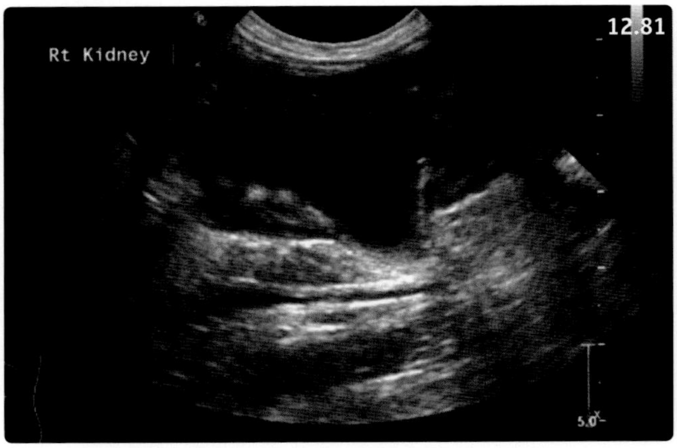

Figure 12.81 Middle aged female Shih Tzu with a ureterolith causing hydronephrosis of the right kidney. (Courtesy R. Baumruck)

cause of obstruction may only become apparent with further imaging studies and exploratory surgery.

Management

Expeditious surgical correction of outflow obstruction is essential, as significant kidney function can be lost in just days. Extreme hydronephrosis is managed by surgical excision of the affected kidney.

RENAL TUMORS

Definition/overview

Primary kidney tumors are rare and account for less than 2% of all canine cancer. Most are tumors that have metastasized from a remote site. The most common histologic types in dogs include renal tubular cell carcinoma, transitional cell carcinoma, and renal cell papilloma. Carcinoma, sarcoma, fibroma, hemangiosarcoma, lymphoma, and nephroblastoma have also been reported. In cats, lymphoma is the predominant renal neoplasia.

Etiology

The large renal blood supply results in the kidney being the site of distant metastases from primary tumors elsewhere in the body.

Pathophysiology

Tumors cause pain, hematuria, hydronephrosis (if they obstruct urine outflow), and displacement of normal renal tissue, which can lead to CKD. Early metastasis by the time of initial presentation is usual. Paraneoplastic syndromes have been described including polycythemia and hypertrophic osteopathy. In German Shepherd Dogs, a hereditary multifocal renal cystadenocarcinoma is accompanied by cutaneous nodules (dermatofibrosis).

Clinical presentation

At presentation, affected animals usually exhibit anorexia and weight loss. Dogs and cats with nonlymphomatous renal tumors often present with red–brown urine that appears the same color both at the beginning and at the end of urination. In addition, pollakiuria, stranguria, and urgency are not usually observed. Unilateral renal enlargement and pain may be evident on abdominal palpation. Unilateral tumors do not cause signs of kidney disease.

In dogs with renal lymphoma, renal involvement can be diffuse, so both kidneys can be enlarged. Gross hematuria is not common and evidence of the tumor can usually be detected involving other organs. In cats, lymphoma usually causes lumpy bilateral renomegaly. In both dogs and cats, the diffuse bilateral nature of renal lymphoma generally leads to CKD and renal failure.

Differential diagnosis

Renomegaly: hydronephrosis, amyloidosis, FIP, cystic disease.

Diagnosis

Radiographs of the abdomen show an irregularly enlarged kidney and areas of mineralization may be visible. While an IV urogram can be used to find abnormal blood perfusion or distortion of the collection system, ultrasonic imaging can readily detect the abnormal tissue (**Figure 12.82**). Cytologic evaluation of the urine has proven unreliable, so only a fine needle aspirate or biopsy of the mass can provide a definitive diagnosis. Chest radiographs and an abdominal ultrasound should be taken to rule out metastasis of a renal tumor or a primary tumor in another organ.

Management

Treatment of discrete renal tumors is by surgical resection (**Figure 12.83**). Prognosis is poor because of the late stage at which these tumors are generally diagnosed; however, nephroblastoma is less metastatic than other tumors and nephrectomy can be curative. Usual treatments for

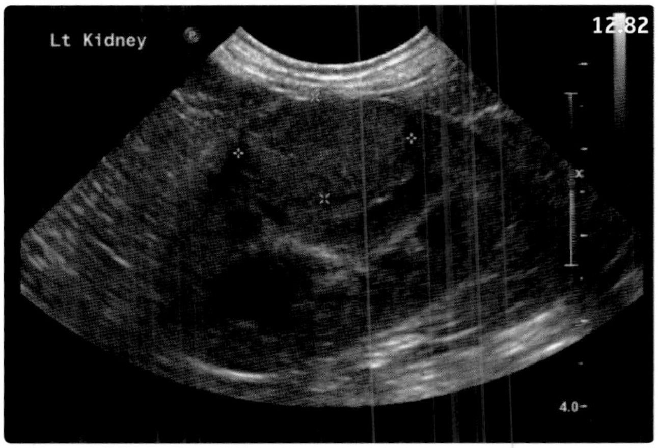

Figure 12.82 Renal mass in the right kidney later confirmed to be anaplastic carcinoma.

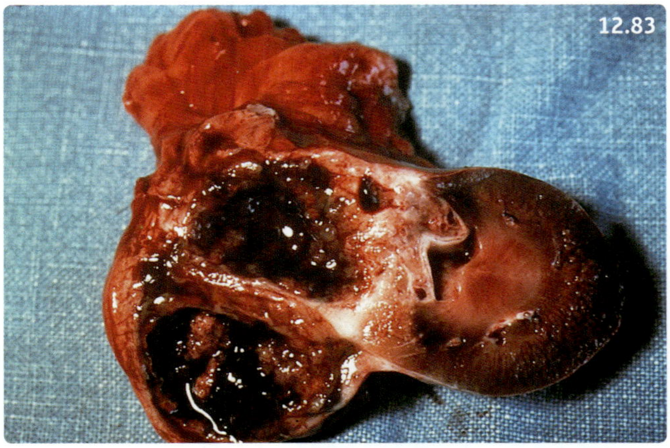

Figure 12.83 Gross specimen showing a unilateral renal carcinoma following surgical resection. (Courtesy D.F. Senior)

lymphoma are indicated and renal function can show some improvement if remission is achieved.

URINARY TRACT INFECTION

Definition/overview

UTI is common in dogs, but uncommon in young and middle aged cats.

Etiology

Infection of both the upper and lower urinary tract is almost always the result of bacteria ascending through the urethra. Direct hematologic spread to the kidneys is thought to be relatively rare. UTIs develop when bacterial number and virulence are sufficient to overcome host defenses.

Pathophysiology

The normal healthy urinary tract has a number of defense mechanisms that prevent bacterial colonization. These include: a tight sphincter; frequent forceful voiding; a long urethra; a glycosaminoglycan coating; regular shedding of epithelial cells; urinary secretion of immunoglobulin; and high urine osmolality (especially in the cat). When there is loss of normal defense mechanisms or an overwhelming inoculation of pathogenic bacteria, the normally sterile urinary tract can become infected. The resulting inflammation results in the commonly seen clinical signs. Rectal and genital bacteria are thought to serve as a reservoir for infection. Although more than 20 different species of bacteria can be found colonizing this area, only seven account for the vast majority of UTIs (**Table 12.23**).

Table 12.23 Frequency of bacterial isolates from urinary tract infection in dogs (%).

Microorganism	**%**
Escherichia coli	26–67
Staphylococcus spp.	11–19
Proteus mirabilis	3–32
Enterococcus/Streptococcus spp.	3–22
Klebsiella pneumoniae	2–8
Pseudomonas aeruginosa	2–4
Enterobacter cloacae	2–6

Clinical presentation

Clinical signs are dependent on whether the upper urinary tract, the lower urinary tract, or both, are affected. Lower UTIs can be completely asymptomatic or have any combination of pollakiuria, stranguria, dysuria, hematuria, or urge incontinence. Most of these signs are due to inflammation of the bladder and/or urethra. It is important to note that infections involving only the lower urinary tract cannot cause polyuria, which is the result of bacterial lipopolysaccharide inhibition of vasopressin. When the upper urinary tract is involved, signs consistent with AKI and septicemia may predominate.

Although a mucopurulent or bloody discharge is sometimes seen at the distal end of the penis or vulva, physical examination findings in UTI patients with lower urinary tract involvement are usually unremarkable. Intact male dogs may exhibit pain on rectal palpation, suggesting prostatic involvement. Patients with upper UTIs (pyelonephritis) may exhibit signs of back pain.

Differential diagnosis

Lower urinary tract inflammation (hematuria and proteinuria): trauma, neoplasia, urolithiasis, idiopathic detrusor instability.

Diagnosis

Diagnostic work up for UTI should include a thorough physical examination, diagnostic imaging, a CBC, serum chemistry, urine analysis, and culture. While radiographs are commonly performed, ultrasound has more diagnostic value. Ultrasound is more sensitive and specific for finding uroliths, discovering structural abnormalities, and detecting pyelectasia, which supports the diagnosis of pyelonephritis. Patients with UTIs that are confined to the lower urinary tract should have no CBC or serum chemistry abnormalities. White blood cell counts in patients with pyelonephritis can range from normal to leukocytosis, while serum chemistry analysis can be normal or demonstrate signs of azotemia depending on the degree of kidney involvement. The presence or absence of white blood cells on microscopic analysis of urine sediment does not help in the diagnosis of a UTI. The presence of white blood cells simply suggests inflammation, which can have many causes. In addition, UTIs can be diagnosed in animals in which few white blood cells are found in urine sediment. While the finding of bacteria on urine microscopic analysis is diagnostic for a UTI, in some cases the number of bacteria shed into the urine is low enough to avoid detection.

The cornerstone of diagnosing and treating UTIs is a urine culture. The fact that more than half of all urine samples submitted to veterinary diagnostic laboratories fail to grow bacteria suggests that clinical signs are not specific for UTIs. In addition, widespread antibiotic resistance makes antimicrobial susceptibility testing essential.

Urine should be collected aseptically by cystocentesis. Often, patients with a UTI will experience pollakiuria, resulting in a small bladder and making cystocentesis difficult. In these cases, ultrasound can be helpful in sample collection. When cystocentesis is not possible, urine may be collected by catheterization, although in cats and female dogs, sedation would be required. Although a midstream urine collection can be attempted, the potential for sample contamination makes this option the least desirable.

There are several options for processing collected samples. The first, and most cost effective, is to plate and incubate samples 'in-house'. A calibrated loop is used to streak urine on blood and MacConkey agar plates, which are then incubated at 37°C (**Figure 12.84**). Blood agar will support the growth of urinary bacterial pathogens, while MacConkey agar prevents *Proteus* spp. from swarming. If after 48 hours no bacterial growth is noted, the plates can be discarded and the patient assumed to be free of a UTI; however, if growth occurs, the agar plates are submitted to a commercial laboratory for bacterial identification and antimicrobial susceptibility testing. A second option is to refrigerate urine for a limited period of time (e.g. 12 hours) before it is plated at a commercial laboratory. Refrigerating samples has the potential for affecting colony counts and time between collection and plating should be minimized. Specialized tubes, designed to protect urine pathogens while refrigerated, are available but not widely used. Samples should never be left at room temperature, as bacterial count can double in less than 1 hour, amplifying potential contaminates and eventually leading to bacterial death.

12.84

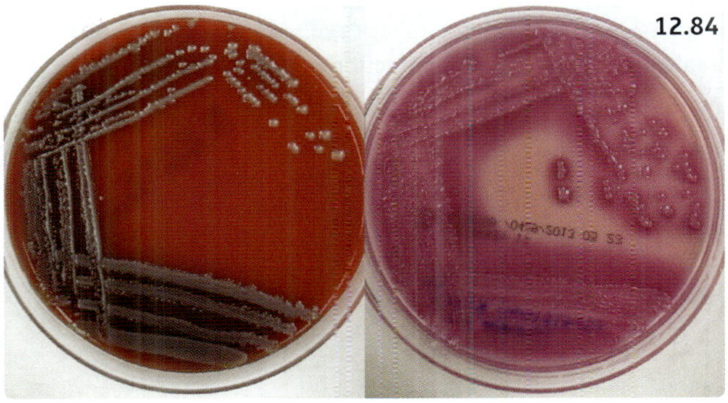

Figure 12.84 Examples of blood agar and blood and MacConkey agar plates from a patient suspected of having a urinary tract infection.

Antimicrobial susceptibility testing provides essential information for selecting an appropriate antibiotic therapy. Results are often reported as (S)ensitive, (I)ntermediate, and (R)esistant on the basis of the Kirby–Bauer disk diffusion technique. With this method, the uropathogen that was isolated from the patient's urine is grown on a specialized agar plate in which disks impregnated with commonly used antibiotics are placed. The antibiotics diffuse out from the disks and their ability to inhibit bacterial growth determines the susceptibility of the bacteria. While this method is quite effective, the results are based on typical serum concentrations for the antibiotic being tested. Because many drugs are excreted into the urine at higher concentrations, some antibiotics reported as (I)ntermediate may be quite effective in treating UTIs.

In the minimum inhibitory concentration (MIC) test, isolates of the patient's uropathogen are incubated with different dilutions of an antibiotic. The minimum concentration of the antibiotic that will inhibit the growth of the bacteria represents the bacteriostatic dose. If the achievable urine concentration of the antibiotic can be expected to be four or more times the MIC, then this drug would be an acceptable choice even if the antimicrobial susceptibility testing suggests the antibiotic would be (I)ntermediate (**Table 12.24**).

Management

UTIs can be divided into two general categories: uncomplicated and complicated. Uncomplicated cases are those first-time UTIs in which no underlying predisposing

Table 12.24 Dose, minimum inhibitory concentration (MIC), and mean urinary concentration (MUC) of antimicrobials used in the treatment of urinary tract infection in dogs. (Data developed by GV Ling, University of California.)

	Dose	MIC break-point (µg/ml)	MUC (µg/ml)
Amoxicillin	11 mg/kg PO q8h	50	201 ± 93
Amoxicillin/clavulanate	11 mg/kg PO q8h	50	201 ± 93
Ampicillin	25 mg/kg PO q8h	77	309 ± 55
Cephalexin	25 mg/kg PO q8h	56	225
Chloramphenicol	33 mg/kg PO q8h	32	124 ± 40
Enrofloxacin	5 mg/kg PO q12h	0.5	25
Nitrofurantoin	4 mg/kg PO q8h	25	100
Penicillin G	36,600 U/kg PO q8h	74 (U/ml)	294 ± 210 (U/ml)
Penicillin V	26.4 mg/kg PO q8h	32	148 ± 98
Sulfisoxazole	11 mg/kg PO q8h	360	1,466 ± 832
Tetracycline	18 mg/kg PO q8h	34	138 ± 65
Trimethoprim–sulfadiazine	13 mg/kg PO q8h	8/20	26/79
Amikacin	5 mg/kg SC q18h	85	342 ± 153
Gentamicin	2.2 mg/kg SC q8h	25	107 ± 33
Kanamycin	5.5 mg/kg SC q12h	132	530 ± 151
Tobramycin	1 mg/kg SC q8h	16	66 ± 39

Note: Bacteria with MIC levels above the break-point are unlikely to be effective. Values assume normal urine concentration; polyuria decreases urine antimicrobial concentration.

condition can be identified. Complicated cases include those with a predisposing condition, a history of recurrent UTIs, and all intact male dogs. Predisposing conditions include systemic diseases (e.g. renal disease, hyperadrenocorticism, diabetes mellitus, hyperthyroidism), structural abnormalities (e.g. vulvar malformations, uroliths, tumors), and immunosuppressive medications.

In uncomplicated cases, treatment with amoxicillin, cephalexin, or trimethoprim–sulfamethoxazole can be started while waiting for the results of susceptibility testing. Antibiotic therapy should be re-evaluated once the results of antimicrobial susceptibility testing become available. An effective therapy should be continued for 10–14 days.

In complicated cases, it is important to attempt to correct any underlying condition. Endocrine disorders such as hyperadrenocorticism, diabetes mellitus, and hyperthyroidism must to be regulated in order for UTIs to be adequately controlled. A recessed vulva (see **Figures 12.74a, b**) is a common malformation that contributes to many UTIs in female dogs. Many female dogs with recurrent UTIs have a recessed vulva, which allows for trapping and pooling of urine. Although urine is sterile when produced, it is a rich medium for bacterial growth. This allows normal defense mechanisms to be overwhelmed. This problem is easily corrected with surgery. This is easily corrected with surgery. Immunosuppressive medications should be reduced to the lowest effect dose. Repeated courses of antibiotics without correcting the underlying problem are likely to result in multidrug resistant infections.

In intact male dogs, UTIs often involve the prostate and only certain antibiotics can penetrate this organ. If appropriate antibiotic therapy is not selected, the urinary tract can be repeatedly reinfected by sheltered bacteria. Antibiotic selection needs to be guided by the results of antimicrobial susceptibility testing as well as by considering which drugs are likely to penetrate the prostate. Macrolides, lincosamides, sulfonamides, chloramphenicol, and fluoroquinolones all seem to be reasonable choices.

Despite appropriate therapy and a failure to diagnosis a predisposing underlying cause, persistent and recurrent UTIs occur. One strategy to prevent reinfection is oral administration of methenamine hippurate (500 mg PO q12h [dog]; 250mg PO q12h [cat]). Methenamine is converted to formaldehyde in the presence of acidic urine (pH <5.5). Ammonium chloride can be used to acidify the urine (65 mg/kg PO q8h in dogs;

20 mg/kg PO q12h in cats). Long-term low-dose antimicrobial treatment can also be used in the treatment of recurrent UTIs. Patients are given a full course of antimicrobial based on sensitivity test results for 3–4 weeks. Treatment is then continued for at least 6 months by giving 50% of the regular daily dose at night after the patient has voided.

RECOMMENDED FURTHER READING

Acierno MJ, Labato MA (2011) Kidney diseases and renal replacement therapies. *Vet Clin North Am Small Anim Pract* **41(1)**.

Bartges J, Polzin DJ (2011) *Nephrology and Urology of Small Animals*. Wiley-Blackwell, Ames.

Ettinger SJ, Feldman EC (2010) *Textbook of Veterinary Internal Medicine*, 7th edn, Vol 2. Elsevier Saunders, St. Louis.

Chapter 13

Approach to abdominal radiographs

L. Abbigail Granger

BASICS OF ABDOMINAL RADIOGRAPHY

To properly interpret abdominal radiographs, the basics of lesion description using the six Roentgen signs (size, shape, margination, opacity, location, and number) must be performed in order to reliably research differential diagnoses; the goal is to translate an image to text. Additionally, the five radiographic opacities must be known to avoid misinterpretation of findings, such as falciform fat being mistaken for fluid. The five radiographic opacities in order from most lucent to most opaque are: air, fat, soft tissue/fluid, bone/mineral, and metal. The abdomen is primarily composed of soft tissue opaque structures that are surrounded by fat. Organs are visible because fat is decreased in opacity when compared with soft tissue/fluid. It must be understood that soft tissue and fluid are of identical radiographic opacity, therefore thickness of gastrointestinal (GI) walls and the urinary bladder wall cannot be determined on radiographs without the use of contrast.

Technique and positioning

Positioning

An abdominal study should include the entire diaphragm as the cranial boundary and the coxofemoral joints as the caudal boundary. The right and left lateral views are named according to the recumbency of the animal. The ventrodorsal view is obtained with the animal in dorsal recumbency and is the primary orthogonal view obtained in abdominal imaging. A dorsoventral view with the animal positioned in sternal recumbency is rarely obtained. With each view, the hindlimbs should be extended caudally to limit crowding of abdominal organs.

Choosing the abdominal views

Like any radiographic study, at least two views must be obtained of the abdomen in order to properly evaluate the study and reconstruct a 3-D description from a set of 2-D images. Most commonly, right lateral and ventrodorsal views are obtained. In the right lateral view, the tail of the spleen is more commonly visible and the kidneys are better distinguished as separate structures when compared with the left lateral view. Gravity, mobility of organs, and the changes in distribution of gas and fluid with recumbency can be used to optimize the diagnostic capability of radiographic studies in many common clinical scenarios. Because of this, many radiologists advocate the use of right and left lateral views in addition to an orthogonal view as standard practice for imaging the thorax and the abdomen.

The variation in abdominal organ appearance with recumbency is most notable in the GI tract. Luminal contents within the stomach and small intestine often contain some degree of fluid and gas. Because patients are positioned in recumbency (rather than standing) and views are obtained with a vertical beam (rather than horizontal beam), the classic appearance of a combination of contents in the GI tract is a summation of opacities created by both gas and fluid that changes with positioning (**Figure 13.1**). The redistribution of gas within the GI tract (without administration of additional contrast agents) by obtaining a left lateral view has been used to diagnose pyloric outflow obstructions, locate obstructions within small intestines, highlight intussusceptions, distinguish colon from dilated small intestine, rule out gastric malpositioning, and definitively locate the pylorus, among other applications.

Special views

Depending on the clinical circumstances, an additional view outside the standard protocol may provide vital diagnostic information. For example, a flexed hindlimb view of the caudal abdomen can be obtained to evaluate the entire penile urethra for calculi in a male dog while avoiding superimposition of the femurs. Simple additional techniques include positional radiography (left lateral abdominal projection and horizontal beam radiography), compression radiography, and simple negative contrast radiography (pneumocolon and

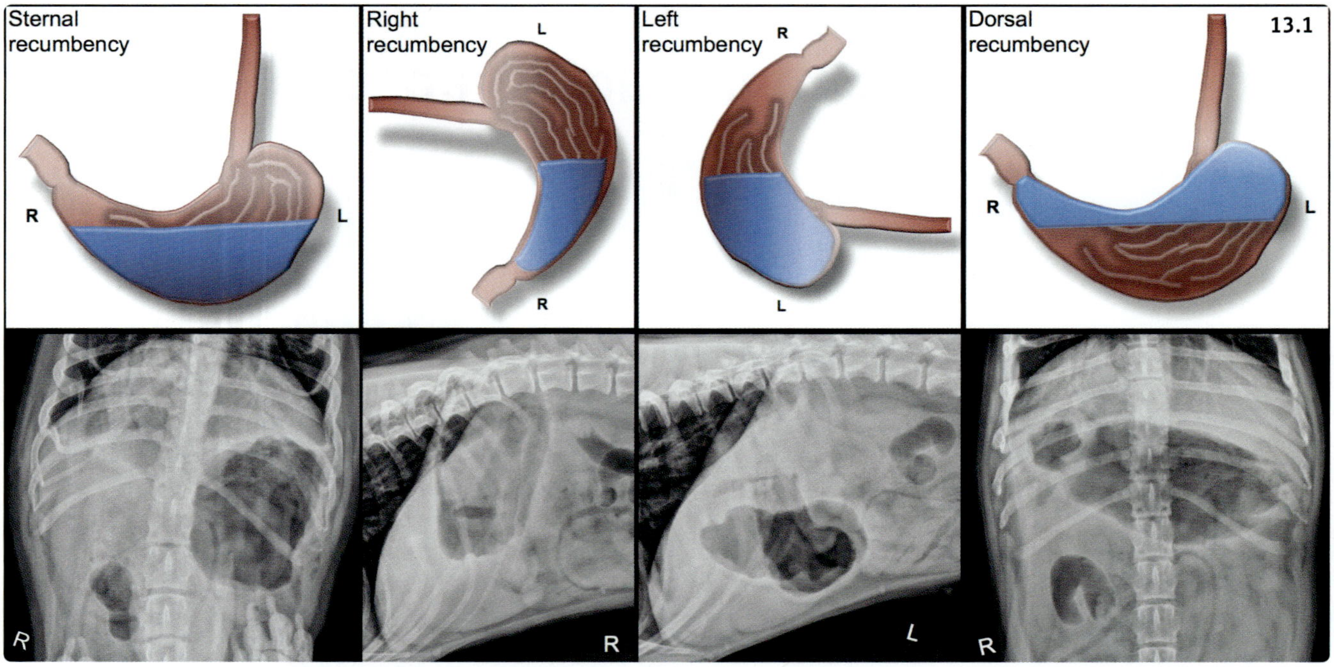

Figure 13.1 Diagram showing the distribution of gravity-dependent stomach contents with recumbency. An accompanying radiographic appearance is shown below each diagram. When the animal is positioned in sternal recumbency (dorsoventral view), gas tends to rise to the most dorsal part of the stomach, the fundus, and fluid will fall to the most ventral part, the gastric body. As a result, the gastric fundus is more apparent because luminal gas creates more contrast. In the right lateral view, mobile fluid falls to the most gravity-dependent part of the stomach, the pylorus, while gas rises to the fundus, the largest gastric compartment. As a result, the gastric fundus is most visible on right lateral view. On the left lateral recumbent view, gas rises to the nongravity-dependent pylorus, while fluid falls to the fundus, making the region of the pylorus more radiographically evident. Finally, when animals are positioned in dorsal recumbency (ventrodorsal view), gas rises to the most ventral part of the stomach, the gastric body, while fluid falls to the gastric fundus and pylorus. This results in increased visibility of the gastric body.

pneumogastrogram). These views will be addressed in appropriate sections throughout the chapter.

READING ABDOMINAL RADIOGRAPHS

The reading of abdominal radiographs must be done systematically. An organ approach can be used to ensure that each structure is evaluated on each view (**Box 13.1**). Evaluating each organ on every study regardless of clinical signs increases the comfort level in recognizing normal from abnormal structures. The familiarity gained from a systematic approach will prevent newly recognized organs or organs better seen in one patient versus another from being automatically or inappropriately deemed abnormal. Also, many structures within the abdomen are not seen in normal animals on radiographs. The location of these structures should be kept in mind so that when radiographically evident abnormalities do occur, they will be considered by interpreter.

INTERPRETATION OF ABDOMINAL ABNORMALITIES

Extra-abdominal structures

Extra-abdominal structures must be reviewed early in the interpretation process. On some occasions, structures associated with the abdominal wall can give the false impression of intra-abdominal abnormalities, such as wet hair mimicking peritoneal effusion, therefore early recognition will prevent misinterpretation.

Abdominal wall, skeleton, and visible thorax

Initially, the ventral abdominal wall should be characterized as tucked, pendulous, or normal. This will assist with differentiating potential causes of decreased detail, if it exists, and gives an overall clue as to the body habitus of the animal. An animal with a tucked abdominal contour may have decreased abdominal detail because of thin body condition, whereas an animal with a pendulous contour and decreased peritoneal detail may have

Box 13.1 Systematic evaluation of the abdomen.

- Extra-abdominal structures:
  - Abdominal wall, including soft tissues and axial skeleton
  - Visible thorax
  - Visible hindlimbs
- Peritoneal space:
  - Peritoneum*
  - Mesentery, omentum, falciform fat
  - Mesenteric lymph nodes*
- Liver:
  - Gallbladder*
- Spleen
- Retroperitoneal space:
  - Retroperitoneal fat
  - Medial iliac and other sublumbar lymph nodes*
- Upper urinary tract:
  - Kidneys
  - Ureters*
- Adrenal glands*
- Reproductive tract:
  - Ovary/uterus*
  - Prostate*
- Lower urinary tract:
  - Urinary bladder
  - Urethra*
- Gastrointestinal tract:
  - Stomach
  - Small intestine
  - Colon
- Pancreas*

*Organs not normally seen radiographically

peritoneal effusion or large volumes of peritoneal fat deposition causing increased scatter. Young animals also tend to have a pendulous contour and decreased detail.

Abnormalities within the visible thorax and skeleton may not be responsible for clinical signs but can assist with appropriate ranking of differential diagnoses if intra-abdominal abnormalities are seen.

Peritoneal space

Peritoneal effusion

The influence of fluid within the peritoneal space can range from a mild decrease in detail to a total border effacement of abdominal organs (**Figures 13.2a, b**). Smaller volumes of peritoneal effusion may cause soft tissue opaque streaking within the falciform and mesenteric fat, making serosal margins less distinct. In some cases, fluid is so severe that the only indication of organ position is the gas within small intestinal loops An asymmetric distribution of small intestine may indicate mass effect or may simply be due to an absence of gas-filled intestine in a particular region. When differentiating various causes of abdominal effusion, a fluid composition approach is most inclusive. Fluid may be due to transudates, exudate, hemorrhage, urine, bile, or chyle. The causes of each fluid type can then be considered as potential differential diagnoses. Clinical history is also very useful in differentiating causes of effusion. In many instances, fluid sampling and subsequent analysis is the next step when peritoneal effusion is suspected.

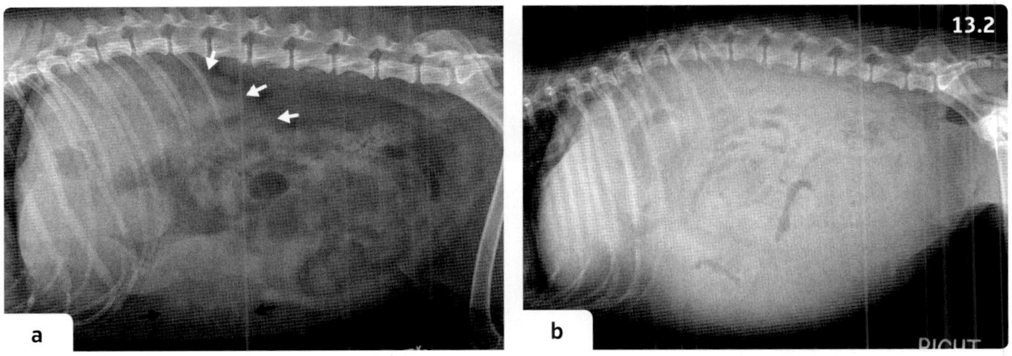

Figures 13.2a, b Lateral abdominal radiographs in a dog with a small volume of peritoneal effusion (a) and a dog with marked peritoneal effusion (b). In the dog with the smaller volume of peritoneal effusion, soft tissue opaque streaking can be seen within the ventral abdominal fat (a, between black arrows). The margins of the liver, spleen, intestines, and urinary bladder are somewhat visible, but are less distinct than in a normal animal. The splenic tail, although it is less distinct, can be recognized as having a nodular appearance. In this case, the margins of the kidneys remain sharp because they are retroperitoneal in location and effusion is not concurrently present in the retroperitoneal space (white arrows). In the dog with a large volume of peritoneal effusion (b), the serosal margins of the peritoneal structures are completely obscured. The only indication of organ location is the distribution of intestines containing gas. Abdominal ultrasound and/or fluid analysis are the next logical steps in evaluating cases with this volume of effusion.

Decreased serosal detail (**Box 13.2**) can include the entire abdomen or can have a clear regional distribution indicating disease limited to local organs. Focal or global regions of decreased detail may also be due to peritonitis, which appears similar to small volumes of effusion. In such cases, attempts to sample may be unrewarding and ultrasound is recommended to determine the underlying cause.

Horizontal beam radiography

Abnormalities within the peritoneal space may manifest as excess lucency rather than increased opacity. Free gas within the abdomen can highlight serosal margins, making them apparent when they otherwise would not be visible. Potential causes of free peritoneal gas are listed in **Box 13.3**. Additionally, most causes of free peritoneal gas also cause some degree of abdominal effusion, resulting in a mixed gray opacity that can be difficult to differentiate from GI contents if care is not taken to avoid misinterpretation. In such cases, horizontal beam radiography can be immensely helpful in confirming suspicion of free gas; however, suspicion of free gas must be present in order to consider use of horizontal beam radiographs.

Horizontal beam views of the abdomen can be obtained by placing the animal in left lateral or dorsal recumbency (**Figures 13.3a–d**). The basis of these views is to force gas

Box 13.2 Potential causes of reduced peritoneal detail.

- Underexposure
- Wet air artifact
- Young animal (typically pendulous contour)
- Abdominal effusion (pendulous contour)
- Mass effect (pendulous contour)
- Obesity (pendulous contour)
- Emaciation or thin body condition (tucked contour)
- Peritonitis
- Carcinomatosis or neoplastic seeding (typically pendulous contour)

Box 13.3 Causes of free peritoneal gas.

- Perforated hollow viscus:
  - Stomach
  - Small intestine
  - Colon
  - Uterus
  - Urinary bladder (gas rarely present)
- Penetrating or perforating injury
  - Bite wound
  - Gunshot
- Ruptured abscess (gas-producing bacteria)
- Recent abdominal surgery (within about 3 weeks)

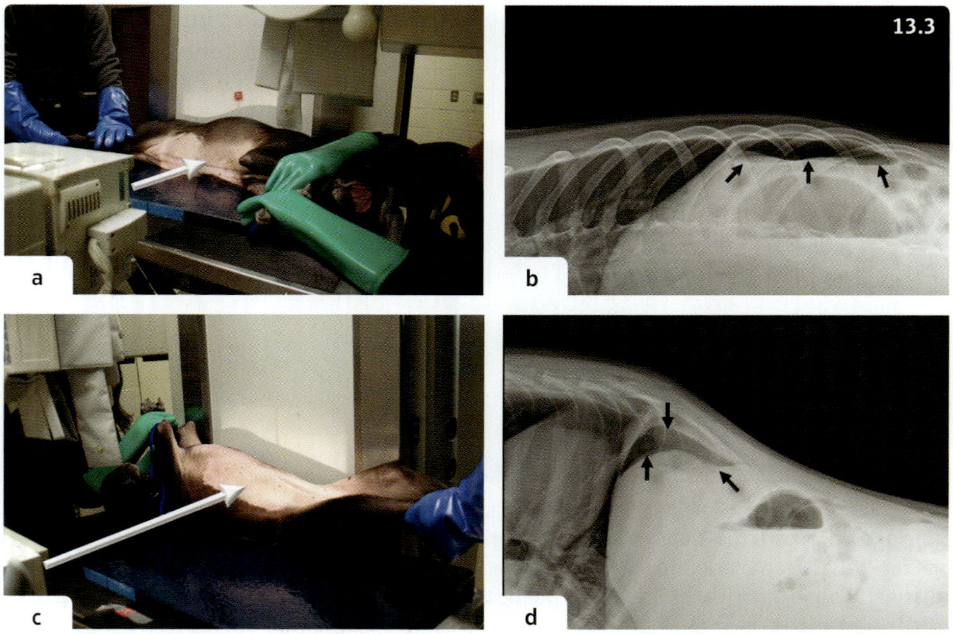

Figures 13.3a–d Horizontal beam radiography of the abdomen. Positioning (a) to obtain a horizontal beam radiograph with the patient in left lateral recumbency; arrow denotes direction of the x-ray beam. Resultant horizontal beam ventrodorsal view (b) showing free peritoneal gas accumulated caudal to the diaphragm on the right side (arrows). Positioning (c) to obtain horizontal beam radiograph with the patient in dorsal recumbency; arrow denotes direction of the x-ray beam. Resultant horizontal beam lateral view (d) showing free peritoneal gas accumulated caudal to the diaphragm, ventrally (arrows).

to accumulate in a predictable location (i.e. non-gravity dependent) and radiograph this location.

Pneumoperitoneum is most often caused by a penetrating/perforating wound or a perforated hollow viscus, usually the GI tract. Unless the cause of the pneumoperitoneum is iatrogenic (i.e. previous abdominal surgery within about 3 weeks), the diagnosis of pneumoperitoneum often indicates septic peritonitis and surgical intervention is required.

Compression radiography

The purpose of compression radiography is to isolate a specific region of interest or remove superimposition of peritoneal structures by use of a radiolucent compression device. The most typically used device is a radiolucent wooden spoon or spatula; however, any rigid radiolucent device with a handle can be used. The indications for this study include isolation of specific organs of interest that are otherwise obscured by superimposition or to better delineate margins of a normal or abnormal structure seen on survey radiographs. This technique has been used to better delineate palpable or radiographically visible abdominal masses, isolate the urinary bladder to prove presence or absence of calculi, remove superimposition of the GI tract on kidneys, separate small intestines from each other, and confirm the presence of uterine enlargement, among other potential applications.

Patient positioning depends on the region of interest to be evaluated. Often, standard abdominal views are used to assist in determining the region of interest and positioning for the compression study. Palpation may also dictate a specific region of interest. The specific location should be isolated with a hand, then the hand replaced by the wooden spoon or other compression device. The device should be similar in size to or 1.5 times larger than the specific organ or regions of interest being isolated. The act of compressing reduces the thickness in the region of interest; therefore, the radiographic technique should be reduced to avoid overexposure (decrease kVp by 10%). Collimating is advisable to avoid personnel exposure and optimize the image (**Figures 13.4a–c**).

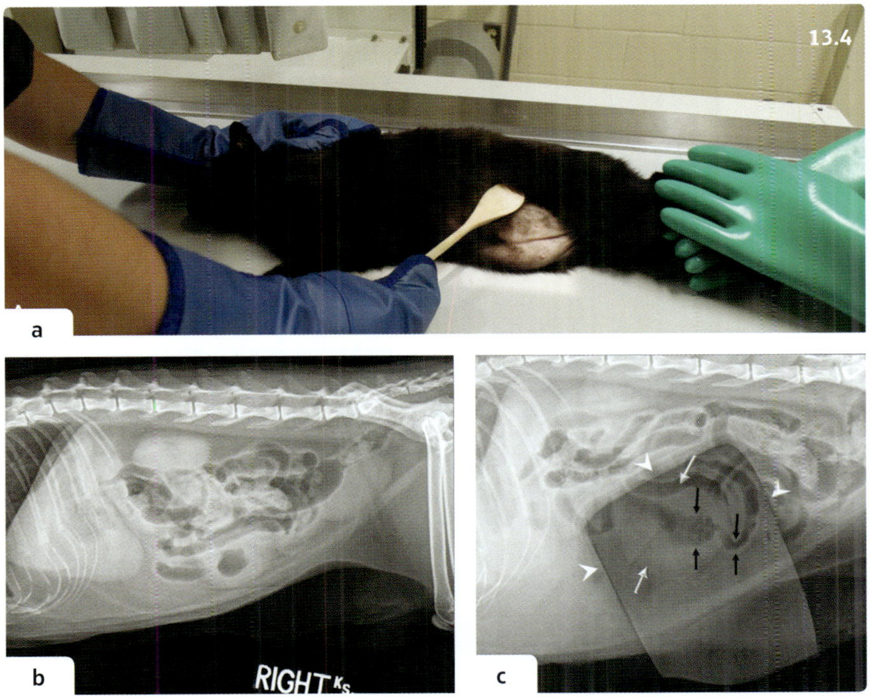

Figures 13.4a–c Positioning for obtaining a compression view, and lateral abdominal survey and compression radiographs in an 11-year-old female spayed Domestic Shorthair cat presenting with a year-long history of intermittent vomiting. Typical positioning for a palpable abdominal mass is shown in (a). A ventrally located soft tissue opacity having an indistinct dorsal margin is seen on the survey radiograph (b). A lateral radiograph was obtained after using a radiolucent wooden spatula to isolate the mass (c). The wooden spatula decreases the thickness of tissues in the region of the mass, which results in an increase in overall apparent exposure in the location of the spatula (c, white arrowheads). The soft tissue opacity is better defined on the compression view (white arrows). Also, a gas-containing small intestinal loop leads into the mass, which has an irregular tubular gas center (black arrows) consistent with a small intestinal organ of origin.

Compression should be avoided in cases where rupture is a potential concern, such as a severely enlarged uterus or splenic mass, or in cases of diaphragmatic hernia where organs may be further displaced into the pleural space.

Mass effect

The visibility of serosal margins can be diminished when organ crowding occurs. Mass effect is the altered distribution of organs within the peritoneal space. A mass is the object that causes the altered distribution of organs. The description of mass effect is the biggest clue as to the most likely organ of origin for an abdominal mass. For the sake of description of mass effect, the abdomen can be considered to have defined compartments on the lateral and ventrodorsal views. Potential organs of origin for visible masses correspond to the location of the mass effect related to these compartments, as shown in **Table 13.1**. Description of the organ displacement is the key to determining the most likely compartment for a mass effect

Table 13.1 Potential organs of origin for masses located in regions of the peritoneal space. Separate regions are numbered and delineated with black lines.

Lateral view

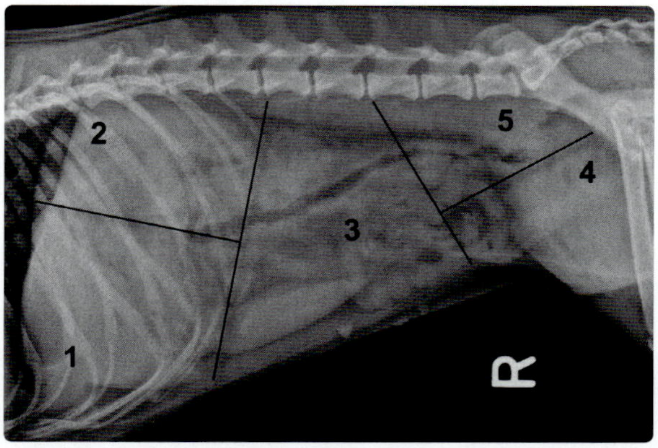

Location of mass effect	Potential organ of origin
1. Cranioventral	• Liver • Spleen • Gastric body and pylorus • Right pancreatic limb • Gallbladder and biliary system • Hepatic and gastric lymph nodes
2. Craniodorsal	• Liver • Splenic head • Gastric fundus • Kidneys • Adrenal glands • Ovary • Left pancreatic limb • Splenic lymph nodes
3. Central	• Spleen • Mesenteric lymph nodes • Mesentery • Uterus • Intestine • Ovary • Retained testicle • Left kidney

(Continued)

Location of mass effect	Potential organ of origin
4. Caudoventral	• Urinary bladder • Prostate • Uterus • Retained testicle
5. Caudodorsal	• Sublumbar lymph nodes • Distal descending colon • Ureters
Ventrodorsal view	
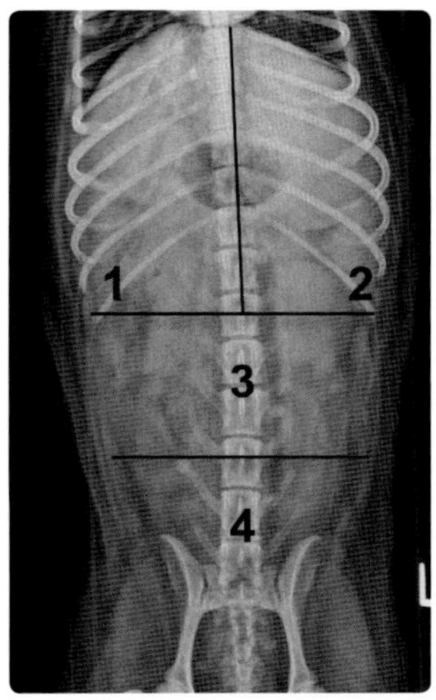	
Location of mass effect	**Potential organ of origin**
1. Right cranial	• Liver • Gallbladder and biliary system • Pancreas • Right kidney • Right adrenal • Pylorus and proximal duodenum • Gastric and hepatic lymph nodes
2. Left cranial	• Spleen • Liver • Gastric fundus • Left pancreatic limb • Left adrenal
3. Central	• Spleen • Mesenteric lymph nodes • Intestine • Left kidney • Uterus • Ovary • Retained testicle
4. Caudal	• Urinary bladder • Uterus • Prostate • Sublumbar lymph nodes • Distal descending colon

and, therefore, the most likely organ of origin and the most likely differential diagnoses for the mass. Location of the mass effect needs to be considered on orthogonal views in order to assign the most likely organ of origin. Keep in mind that a mass effect can be identified without a well-defined mass being visible; however, displacement of organs such as the small intestines indicates the presence of an abnormality. Very few differential diagnoses exist for abdominal masses and they are highlighted in **Box 13.4**.

Liver

Hepatic size is a subjective determination based on its shape and the position of the stomach. The axis of the stomach is a line drawn from the gastric fundus to the ventral aspect of the gastric body/pylorus. The gastric axis should be roughly parallel to the ribs or perpendicular to the spine. When the axis of the stomach is angled cranially, causes of microhepatia should be considered; when the axis is angled caudally, causes of hepatomegaly should be considered. The majority of the liver is within the confines of the costal arch; however, it can extend caudal to the arch in normal animals. Increased caudal extension of the caudoventral liver margin indicates hepatic enlargement. Additionally, in some cases of hepatic enlargement, the caudoventral liver margin will appear rounded, rather than sharp and triangular.

Box 13.4 Differential diagnoses for abdominal masses.

- Cyst
- Hematoma
- Abscess
- Neoplasia
- Granuloma
- Nodular regeneration, hyperplasia, extramedullary hematopoiesis (liver and spleen)
- Physiologic enlargement (e.g. renal hypertrophy or splenomegaly due to tranquilization)
- Distension of a hollow viscus (gastrointestinal tract, urinary bladder, uterus)
- Organ torsion/congestion

Increased liver size

Hepatomegaly can be categorized as focal, generalized, or nodular. The distinction is important because differential diagnoses are based on the categorization (**Table 13.2**). Generalized hepatomegaly will most often appear as a rounded caudoventral margin with increased extension beyond the costal arch and caudal displacement of the gastric axis (**Figure 13.5**). The pylorus tends to be dorsally displaced and the right kidney is often caudally displaced. With generalized hepatomegaly, often the right stomach (pylorus) is more caudally displaced than the left. Severe asymmetric displacement, however, indicates focal hepatomegaly.

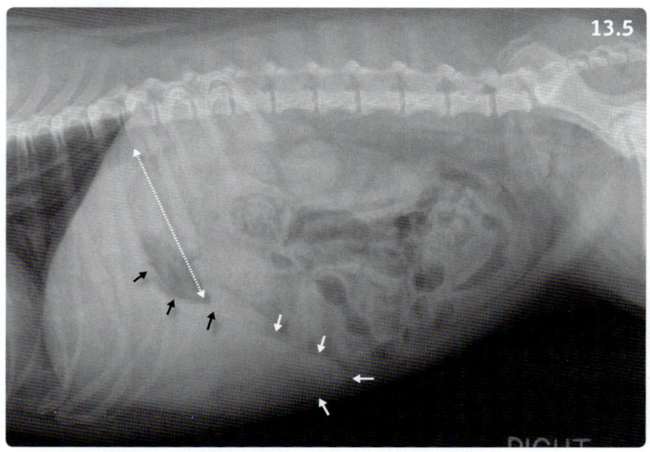

Figure 13.5 Lateral abdominal radiograph of a dog with generalized hepatomegaly due to vacuolar hepatopathy associated with hyperadrenocorticism. There is caudal extension of the caudoventral liver margin, which is rounded (white arrows). The gastric axis is caudally displaced (dotted white line) due to caudal and dorsal displacement of the gastric body and pylorus relative to the gastric fundus (black arrows).

Table 13.2 Classification of hepatomegaly with respective differential diagnoses.

Generalized hepatomegaly	Focal hepatomegaly	Nodular liver
• Vacuolar hepatopathy (e.g. steroid hepatopathy, hepatic lipidosis) • Passive congestion • Hepatitis • Infiltrative neoplasia (e.g. lymphoma, mast cell tumor) • Amyloidosis	• Primary hepatic neoplasia (e.g. hepatocellular carcinoma in dogs, biliary cystadenoma in cats) • Regenerative changes • Cyst • Abscess • Hematoma • Granuloma • Liver lobe torsion	• Metastatic neoplasia (with hepatomegaly) • Nodular regeneration (with hepatomegaly) • Hepatocutaneous syndrome (with hepatomegaly) • Cirrhosis/fibrosis (with microhepatia)

Nodular hepatomegaly will appear as a generalized enlargement; however, margination is very irregular, rather than the smooth margins maintained by true generalized hepatomegaly. Differential diagnoses are ranked differently with metastatic neoplasia, nodular regeneration, and hepatocutaneous syndrome being most likely.

Focal hepatomegaly is caused by a mass. Differential diagnoses for masses are listed in **Box 13.4**. However, once it is determined that the organ of origin is most likely to be liver, the ranking can be organized to include neoplasia, regenerative changes, cyst, and abscess at the top of the list. Focal hepatomegaly causes focal caudal displacement of the stomach to the right or left side, depending on its location. The margin of the liver at the location of the mass tends to be rounded rather than sharp. Most liver masses appear ventral in location, but dorsal masses can occur. Masses cranial to the stomach are typically hepatic in origin; however, in some cases, hepatic masses can extend caudal to the stomach (called a pedunculated liver mass), appearing in the location of the splenic tail on lateral views (**Figures 13.6a, b**). The most common cause of liver masses in dogs and cats is neoplasia. The most common mass-like neoplasm in the canine liver is hepatocellular carcinoma; in cats it is biliary cystadenoma.

Reduced liver size

Microhepatia is diagnosed when the liver size is small, as denoted by a cranially positioned gastric axis. The causes of microhepatia are shown in **Box 13.5**. Shape can sometimes be used to distinguish the causes of microhepatia. In cases of cirrhosis/fibrosis the liver margin may be irregular in shape, giving it a nodular appearance. This abnormal shape is not always radiographically apparent, however. Additionally, ascites is uncommonly present in dogs with a congenital portosystemic shunt, so the presence of peritoneal effusion makes cirrhosis, fibrosis, or noncirrhotic portal hypertension more likely.

Alterations in hepatic opacity

Radiographic abnormalities within the liver can sometimes appear as an alteration in opacity. Hepatic mineralization is most commonly due to mineralization within

Box 13.5 Causes of microhepatia.

- Congenital portosystemic shunt
- Cirrhosis
- Fibrosis
- Microvascular dysplasia
- Noncirrhotic portal hypertension (portal vein hypoplasia)

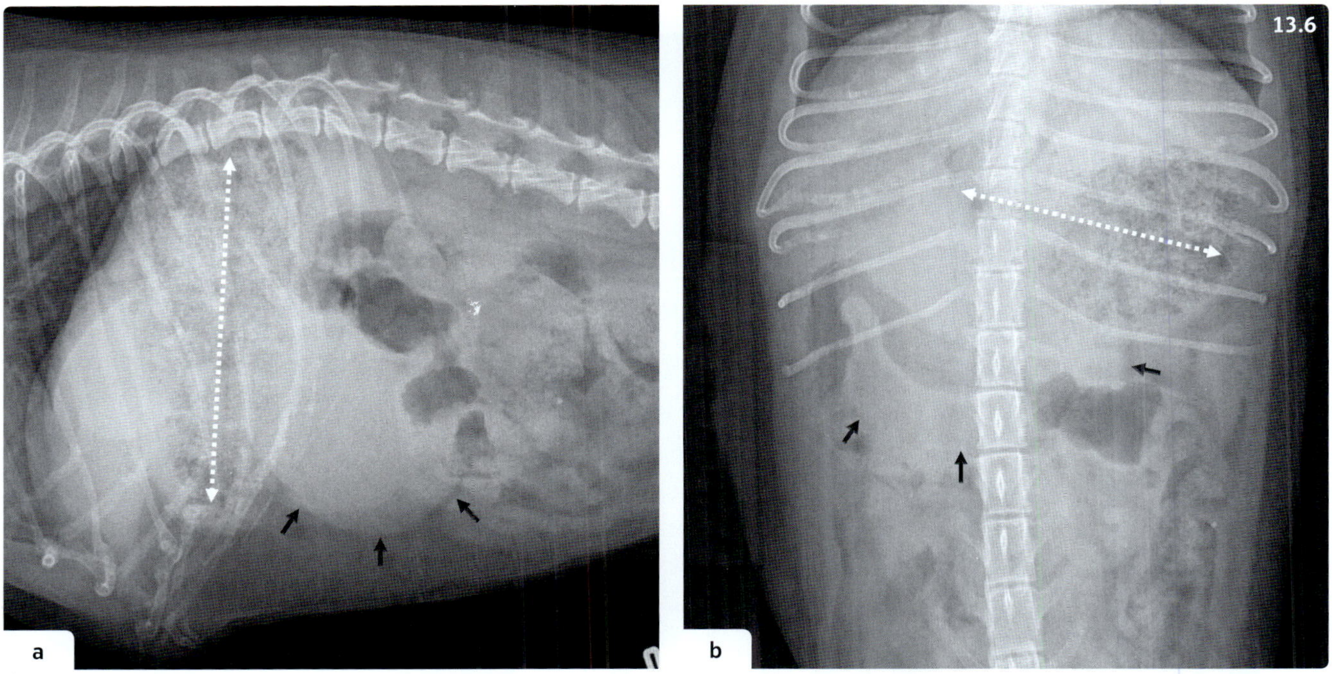

Figures 13.6a, b Lateral (a) and ventrodorsal (b) abdominal radiographs in a dog with a pedunculated liver mass. A soft tissue opaque mass with a well-defined rounded ventral and caudal margin (black arrows) is located caudal to the gastric axis (dotted white line). The mass in located on the right side, causing the stomach to be displaced to the left. Right-sided small intestines are caudally displaced. A single pedunculated hepatic mass was found on ultrasound examination. A hepatocellular adenoma was subsequently diagnosed with aspirates.

the intrahepatic biliary system rather than within the hepatic parenchyma itself.

This causes linear branching mineral opacities that are most commonly accumulated in the right liver. This finding is often incidental; however, previous biliary disease or active disease cannot be ruled out. Mineralized calculi can also accumulate within the gallbladder. These choleliths can be incidental findings or can result in obstruction of the common bile duct. They appear as single, rounded mineral opacities or as an accumulation of mineral opacities within the right ventral liver in the region of the gallbladder. When multiple smaller calculi are present, the ventral margin of the accumulated choleliths tends to be rounded. Finally, the gallbladder wall itself can mineralize due to chronic cholecystitis or cystic mucinous hyperplasia. This appears as a well-defined, rounded, thin mineral-rimmed structure in the right cranial liver in the region of the gallbladder.

Hepatic gas accumulations occasionally occur within the liver parenchyma. Parenchymal hepatic gas is most often associated with a mass due to abscessation. Hepatic abscesses are uncommon, typically exist as a single mass lesion, and most often do not contain gas. On occasions where gas is present, it will accumulate within the margins of the mass (**Figures 13.7a, b**). Concurrent peritoneal effusion is commonly present. Most often, gas located within the abscess does not extend to the peritoneal space.

Spleen

After the liver, the spleen should be located and evaluated. The spleen can be divided into a cranial head, body, and caudal tail. It can be variable in position due to the mobility of the splenic tail. On the lateral view in dogs, the tail of the spleen, when visible, is typically in the cranioventral abdomen caudal to the margin of the liver and stomach. This is most reliably seen on the right lateral projection. In normal cats, the splenic tail is typically not visible on the lateral view of the abdomen. The head of the spleen is sometimes visible on the lateral view in the craniodorsal abdomen near the plane of the right kidney. The head of the spleen is in a more predictable, stable position due to the presence of the gastrosplenic ligament. On the ventrodorsal view, the head of the spleen is the portion that is most consistently visible, caudal to the gastric fundus and cranial to the left kidney, as a triangular soft tissue opacity that is formed where the spleen appears end-on near the junction of the splenic head and body. The overall apparent size of the spleen is smaller in cats than in dogs. Abnormalities within the spleen

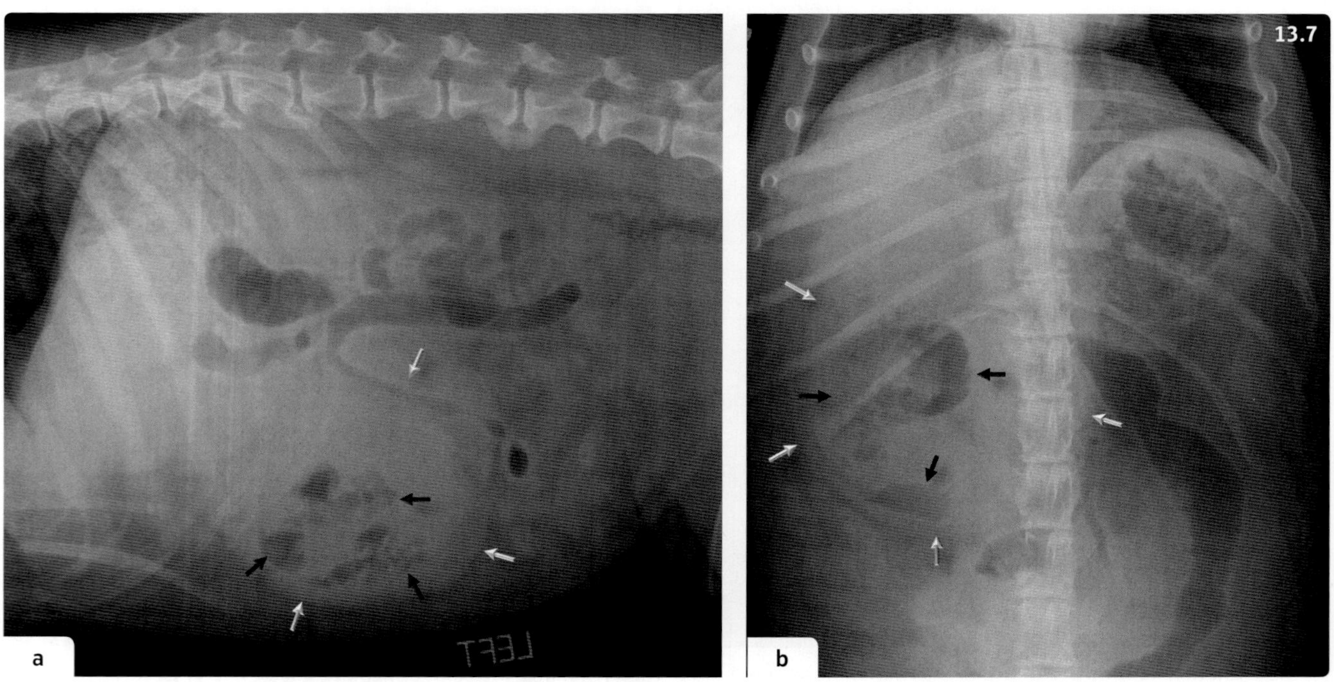

Figures 13.7a, b Lateral (a) and ventrodorsal (b) abdominal radiographs in a dog with a hepatic abscess. A large, well-defined, rounded soft tissue opacity is present in the right cranioventral abdomen (white arrows). The mass causes caudal and dorsal deviation of small intestines and leftward deviation of the stomach. Multiple, well-defined, variably sized and shaped gas opacities are located within the mass (black arrows).

will typically manifest as an alteration in size, shape, location/orientation, and rarely, opacity.

Splenomegaly

Splenic size can be subjectively assessed. Generalized splenic enlargement will appear as a subjective increase in thickness of the splenic tail or head. The margins of the spleen will be rounded and may or may not be irregular, indicating nodular changes. Mass effect associated with generalized splenic enlargement will typically cause rightward displacement of small intestines on the ventrodorsal view and dorsal displacement of intestines on the lateral view (**Figures 13.8a, b**). Generalized splenomegaly can cause cranial and ventral displacement of the gastric fundus. In cats, if the splenic tail is visible on the lateral view, it is considered to be enlarged. Focal splenomegaly occurs when mass lesions are present within the spleen. Given the focal nature of many splenic masses, unaffected sections of the spleen can appear radiographically normal. Masses associated with the splenic head will be located in the craniodorsal abdomen and on the left side. Masses associated with the splenic body or tail are typically more ventral in location and can be right or left sided. Masses are more commonly seen within the splenic tail and body, therefore most splenic masses are located in the ventral cranial to mid abdomen. As a general rule, masses within the splenic body or tail can appear identical to pedunculated liver masses (**Figures 13.9a, b**). Distinction between generalized and focal splenomegaly is important, as differential diagnoses differ (**Table 13.3**).

Alterations in splenic location

Splenic malpositioning due to torsion can occur as a single event (isolated splenic torsion) or, more commonly, in association with gastric dilatation and volvulus (GDV). Splenic torsion is often accompanied by peritoneal effusion, making the margins of the spleen somewhat indistinct. Indications of splenic torsion include a mass effect in the cranial to mid-ventral abdomen, a loss of visibility of the normal splenic head and body in the left cranial abdomen on the ventrodorsal view, visibility of overt splenomegaly, or gas accumulations within the spleen or within the mass effect associated with the ventral abdomen. Finally, in cases where splenic margins are readily identified, the position of the spleen may appear as a reverse 'C' shape in the ventral mid-abdomen on the lateral view.

Alterations in splenic opacity

Splenic mineralization occurs, most often, secondary to metabolic diseases such as hyperadrenocorticism; however, it is uncommonly detectable on radiographs. Gas opacity within the splenic parenchyma rarely occurs, but can be a sequela to necrotizing splenitis or gas-producing bacteria within the spleen. This most commonly occurs secondary to splenic torsion and creates a classic mass (**Figures 13.10a, b**).

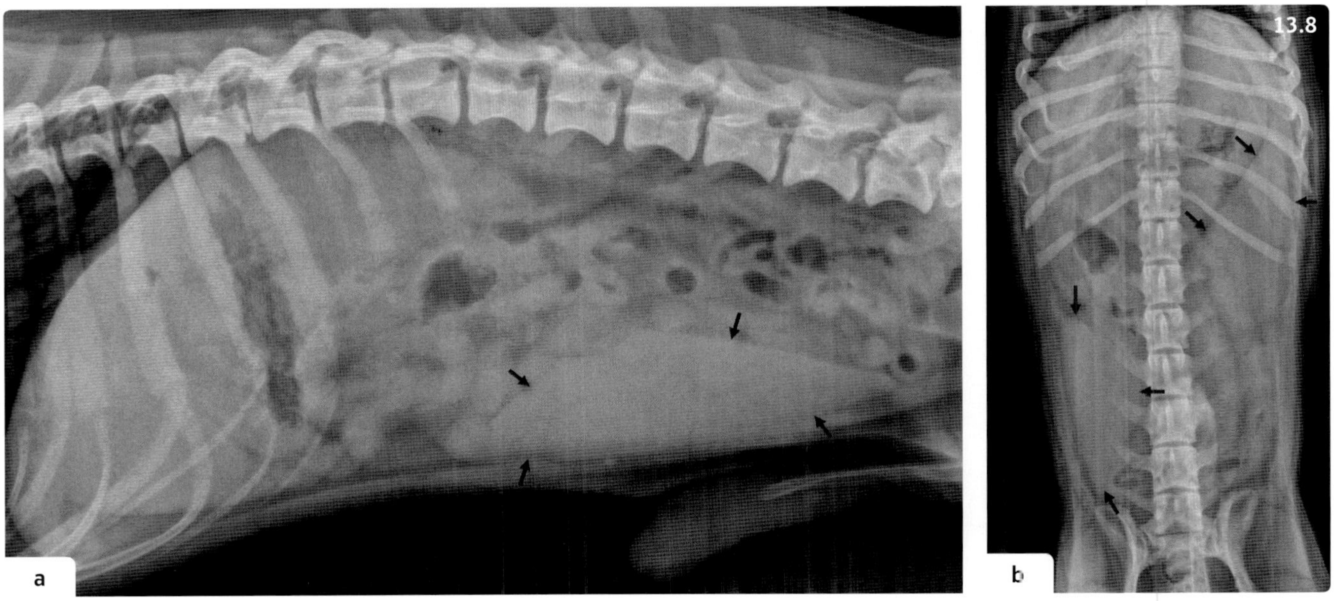

Figures 13.8a, b Lateral (a) and ventrodorsal (b) abdominal radiographs in an anemic dog with marked generalized splenomegaly due to benign extramedullary hematopoiesis. The margins of the spleen are rounded and there is subjectively increased thickness of the spleen on both views (arrows). The spleen extends excessively caudally approaching the pelvic inlet. Additionally, the spleen extends to the caudal abdomen on the right side, as seen on the ventrodorsal view.

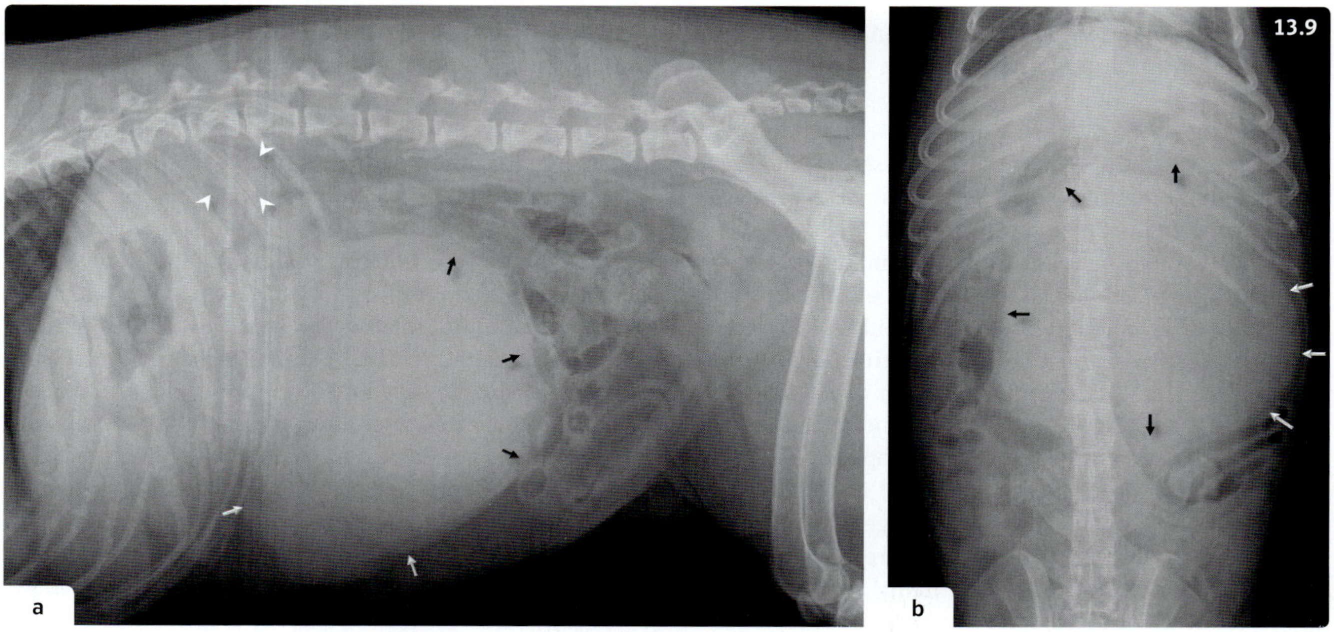

Figures 13.9a, b Lateral (a) and ventrodorsal (b) abdominal radiographs in a dog with a splenic mass. In the lateral view, a normal splenic head is seen in the craniodorsal abdomen (white arrowheads). A large, predominantly round, well-defined soft tissue opacity is present in the left cranial to mid-ventral abdomen (white arrows). The mass causes marked caudal, dorsal, and rightward displacement of the small intestines and cranial displacement of the gastric fundus (black arrows). Other than spleen, the main differential for the organ of origin is a pedunculated liver mass.

Table 13.3 Classification of splenomegaly with respective differential diagnoses.

Generalized splenomegaly	Focal splenomegaly (mass)
• Inflammatory splenomegaly (splenitis): ∘ Systemic or peritoneal bacterial infection ∘ Chronic systemic infection • Hyperplastic splenomegaly: ∘ Chronic infection ∘ Hemolytic disorders • Extramedullary hematopoiesis • Congestion: ∘ Tranquilization ∘ Right heart failure ∘ Portal hypertension (rare) ∘ Splenic torsion • Infiltrative neoplasia: ∘ Lymphoma ∘ Mast cell tumor ∘ Multiple myeloma ∘ Acute and chronic leukemia ∘ Malignant histiocytosis • Amyloidosis	• Non-neoplastic: ∘ Hematoma ∘ Abscess ∘ Nodular hyperplasia ∘ Infarction ∘ Cyst ∘ Granuloma • Neoplastic: ∘ Hemangiosarcoma ∘ Hemangioma ∘ Leiomyosarcoma ∘ Leiomyoma ∘ Myelolipoma ∘ Lymphoma

Retroperitoneal space

The retroperitoneal space should be the next area evaluated. This space, being physically divided from the peritoneal space, can serve as a comparison for detail of organ visibility, where effusion causing reduced detail in the peritoneal space often spares the retroperitoneal space, and vice versa. Causes of retroperitoneal effusion or mass effect must be considered, with knowledge of organs that

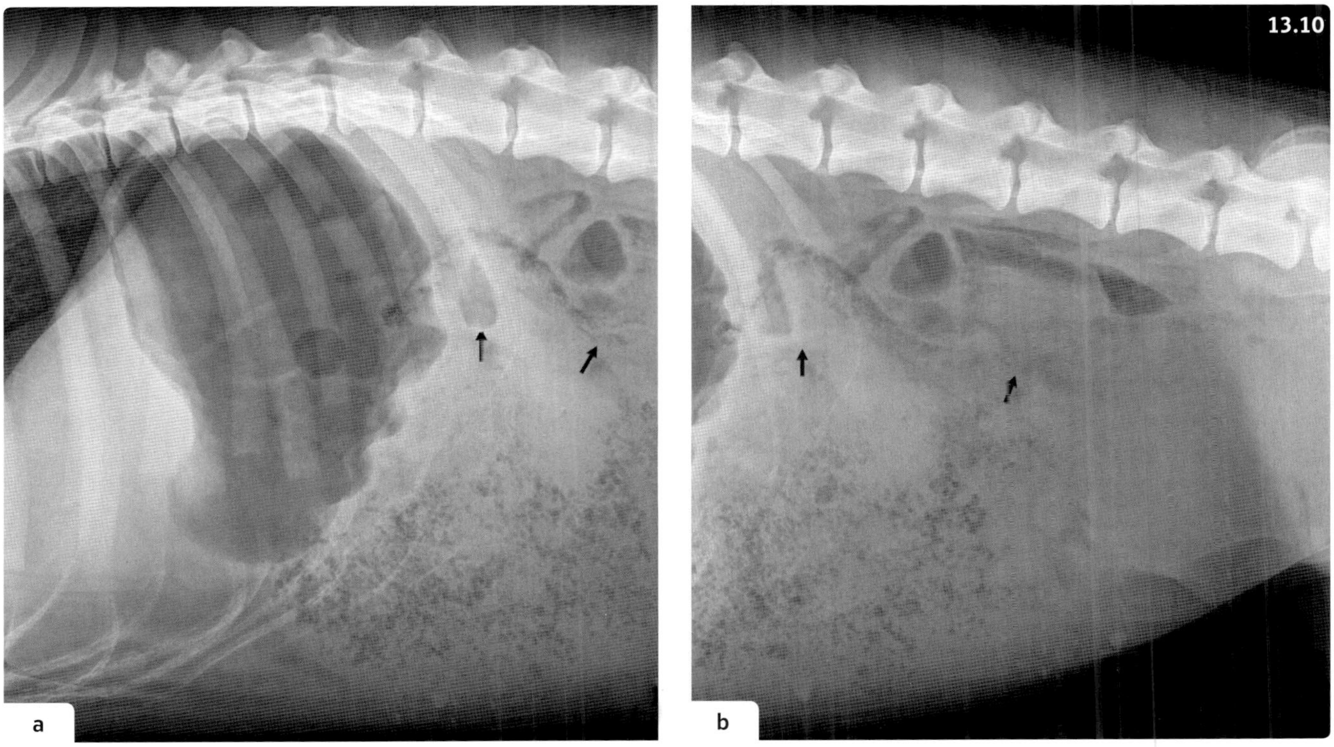

Figures 13.10a, b Lateral cranial (a) and caudal (b) abdominal radiographs in a dog with splenic torsion and secondary splenitis. Peritoneal detail is reduced due to effusion. A large mass effect is present in the ventral abdomen, which is causing dorsal displacement of small intestines (arrows). A mass with indistinct margins is located in the ventral abdomen, which is soft tissue opaque and contains numerous, well-defined, contained gas bubbles. The location and opacity of the mass are classic for splenic torsion and splenitis.

exist in this space, such as the kidneys, adrenal glands, and ureters.

Retroperitoneal effusion and mass effect

Poor retroperitoneal detail is most often caused by effusion and/or mass. Retroperitoneal effusion causes a decrease in delineation of the renal margins. This may be unilateral or extend across the right and left peritoneal spaces. A large volume of fluid can cause a mass effect within the peritoneum where the colon and small intestines are pushed ventrally. When retroperitoneal detail is poor, the concurrent presence of a mass may not be readily visible. The masses themselves can cause similar border effacement of retroperitoneal structures. Causes of retroperitoneal effusion are shown in **Box 13.6** and are best distinguished by considering fluid types. Causes of effusion must be considered together with history and clinical signs. For example, a history of trauma makes urine or hemorrhage the most likely cause of retroperitoneal hemorrhage, whereas a renal neoplasm is more likely if the animal has a history of hematuria.

Box 13.6 Causes of retroperitoneal effusion.

- Urine:
  - Kidney rupture
  - Ureteral rupture
- Hemorrhage:
  - Kidney rupture
  - Rodenticide/coagulopathy
  - Neoplasia (renal, adrenal gland, retroperitoneal sarcoma)
- Exudate:
  - Renal abscessation
  - Retroperitoneal abscess (including migrating foreign body)
- Transudate/modified transudate:
  - Urinary obstruction
  - Severe acute interstitial nephritis

Neoplastic effusion

Sublumbar lymph nodes

The medial iliac lymph nodes are located lateral to the aorta near the location of its trifurcation where the external iliac arteries branch from the abdominal aorta. Caudal to this, the internal iliac lymph nodes are located where the internal arteries branch. These lymph nodes combined are often called the sublumbar lymph nodes. They are radiographically invisible in normal cats and dogs. With severe enlargement, the sublumbar lymph nodes can cause a mass effect, displacing the distal descending colon ventrally near the pelvic inlet (**Figure 13.11**). When sublumbar lymphadenopathy is present, urogenital/perineal neoplasms or multicentric lymphoma should be considered first.

Upper urinary tract

Both kidneys and the ureters are retroperitoneal. The normal renal size in dogs is within 2.5–3.5 times the length of the L2 vertebral body as measured on the ventrodorsal view. In cats, the size of normal kidneys is within 2.0–3.0 times the length of the L2 vertebral body on the ventrodorsal view. Also, both kidneys should be similar in size. Normal ureters are never seen radiographically; excretory urography is the only imaging modality that will allow assessment of the ureters.

Kidneys

Abnormalities associated with the kidneys will appear as an alteration in size, shape, opacity, and, rarely, number. Abnormal renal size must always be considered in combination with renal shape. Additionally, differential diagnoses are often ranked according to whether the radiographic abnormalities are unilateral or bilateral. An algorithmic approach can be used to determine differential diagnoses for the appearance of the kidneys, while taking clinical abnormalities into consideration (**Box 13.7**). Compression radiographs should be obtained in cases where the kidneys are not easily seen due to a superimposed GI tract and when clinical evidence suggests renal disease.

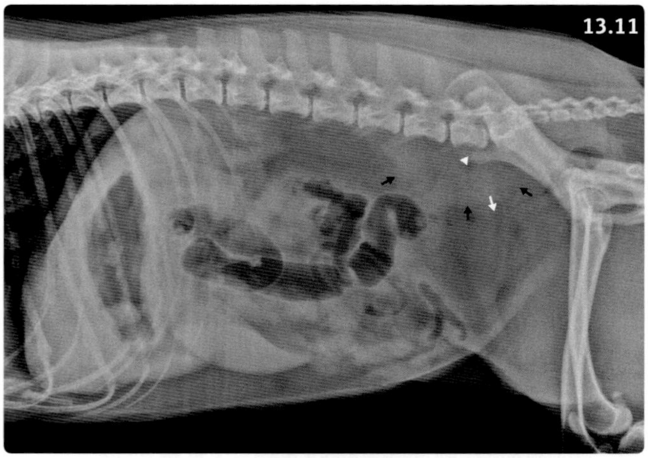

Figure 13.11 Lateral abdominal radiograph in a dog with transitional cell carcinoma of the urinary bladder. A moderately well-defined soft tissue opaque mass is present in the caudal dorsal abdomen (black arrows). The mass is causing ventral displacement of the distal descending colon (white arrow). Additionally, there is a very indistinct, irregular periosteal reaction associated with the ventral L7 vertebral body consistent with an aggressive bone lesion and metastatic disease (arrowhead).

Small kidneys

Small irregular kidneys (**Figures 13.12a, b**) are most often secondary to chronic renal disease or chronic obstructive uropathy. Renal dysplasia must also be considered in young animals having small irregular kidneys, as the two causes can appear identical.

Renomegaly

Enlarged kidneys can cause a mass effect in the dorsal abdomen that can be right sided, left sided, or both, depending on the laterality of the diseased kidney(s). Ventral displacement of the intestines can be seen with renal masses or retroperitoneal effusion. Enlarged kidneys that are smoothly marginated or irregular have numerous causes that often require more advanced imaging, such as excretory urography or ultrasonography, to differentiate them. Determination of the presence of unilateral or bilateral disease can assist with likely diagnoses, as some diseases such as acute kidney injury (AKI), pyelonephritis, lymphoma, feline infectious peritonitis, and amyloid deposition tend to be bilateral, while hydronephrosis and pyonephrosis tend to be unilateral. Renal carcinoma can be unilateral or bilateral and is often accompanied by retroperitoneal effusion due to hemorrhage. Peritoneal effusion is also occasionally seen because of invasion through the peritoneal lining. Subcapsular fluid accumulations due to perinephric pseudocyst occur in cats and dogs, but are more commonly reported in cats where subcapsular edema can accompany AKI and urinary obstruction. Renomegaly can be severe and may be bilateral **(Figures 13.13a, b)** or unilateral. Polycystic kidneys are most commonly seen in Persian cats where they have an autosomal dominant mode of inheritance, but the condition has been reported in Bull Terriers, which also have an autosomal dominant mode of inheritance.

Renal mineralization and nephroliths

Nephroliths associated with the kidneys are typically located in the region of the renal pelvices and can be variable in size. Nephroliths may persist indefinitely in the renal pelvis or they may migrate into the ureter, increasing the risk of urinary obstruction.

Box 13.7 Algorithmic approach to differentiating causes of abnormal kidneys.

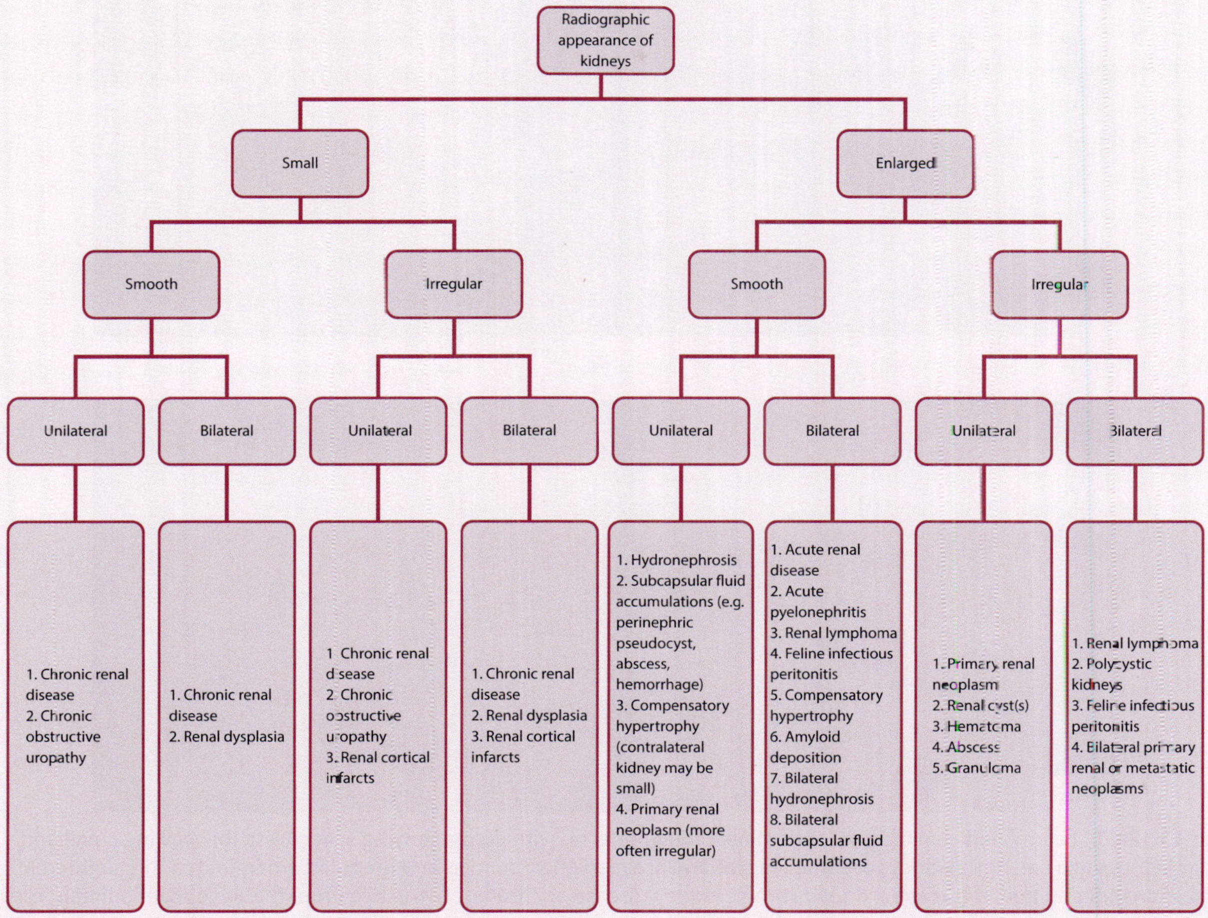

Nephrocalcinosis because of parenchymal mineralization may be dystrophic due to chronic disease or metastatic due to diseases resulting in altered calcium and phosphorus metabolism. Classic nephrocalcinosis appears as parallel linear mineralization located in the region of the renal diverticula. Parenchymal mineralization can accompany oxalate crystal deposition in ethylene glycol intoxication; however, this is generally not visible radiographically. When the presence of nephroliths or nephrocalcinosis is unclear because of superimposition, compression of the kidneys could be performed to confirm suspicion (**Figures 13.14a, b**).

Emphysematous pyelonephritis

On rare occasions, gas can accumulate within the kidneys, most often within the renal pelvis, due to the presence of gas-forming bacteria or reflux of gas from the urinary bladder. Emphysematous pyelonephritis most often occurs in combination with emphysematous cystitis in diabetic animals (see Lower urinary tract).

Ureters

As previously mentioned, ureters should never be seen radiographically without contrast in normal animals. The most common cause of ureteral visibility is due to ureterolithiasis. Ureteroliths appear as mineral opacities that are superimposed in the presumed location of a ureter (**Figures 13.15a, b**). In many instances, excretory urography or abdominal ultrasound is needed to confirm the presumed location of the calculus within the ureter.

Adrenal glands

Both adrenal glands are retroperitoneal in location. They are paired and located medial to the cranial poles of each kidney. The aorta borders the left adrenal gland

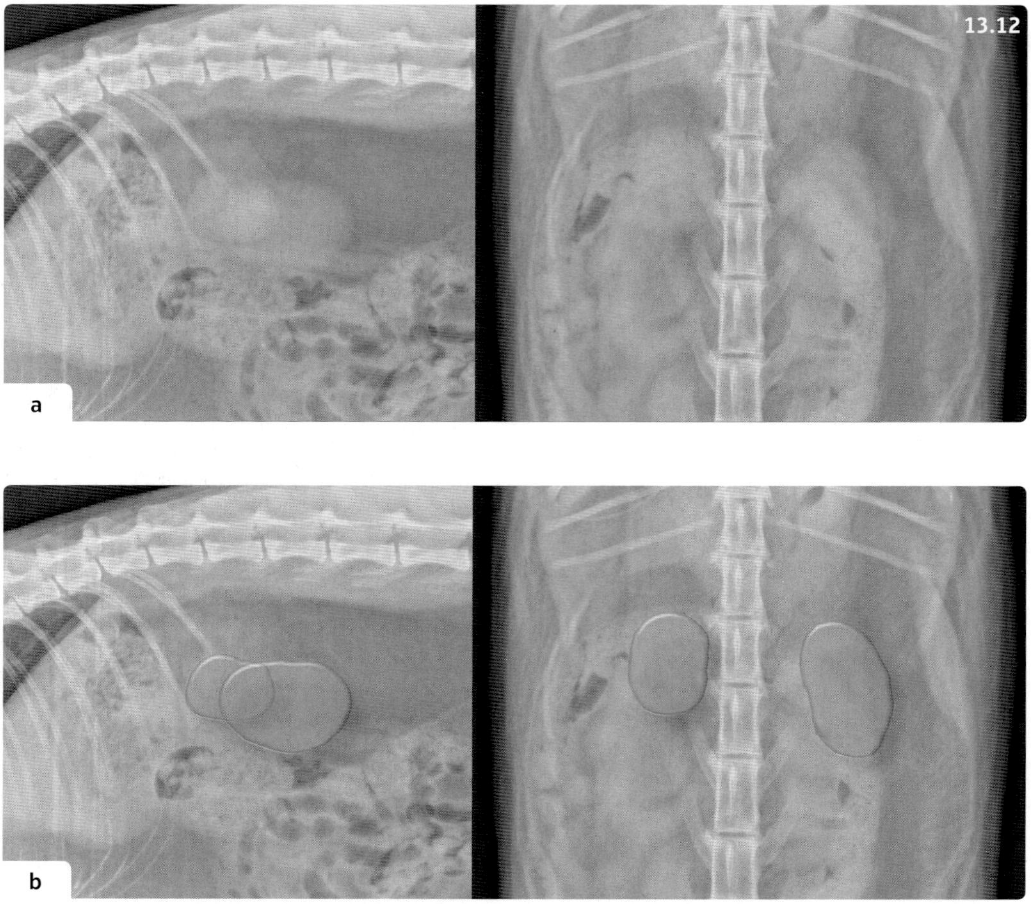

Figures 13.12a, b Lateral and ventrodorsal abdominal radiographs (a) with accompanying schematics (b) showing small and irregular kidneys in a cat. Both kidneys are small in size and are markedly rounded and irregularly marginated (highlighted in 13.12b). In an older animal, this may be due to chronic kidney disease or chronic obstructive uropathy. In younger animals, renal dysplasia must also be considered.

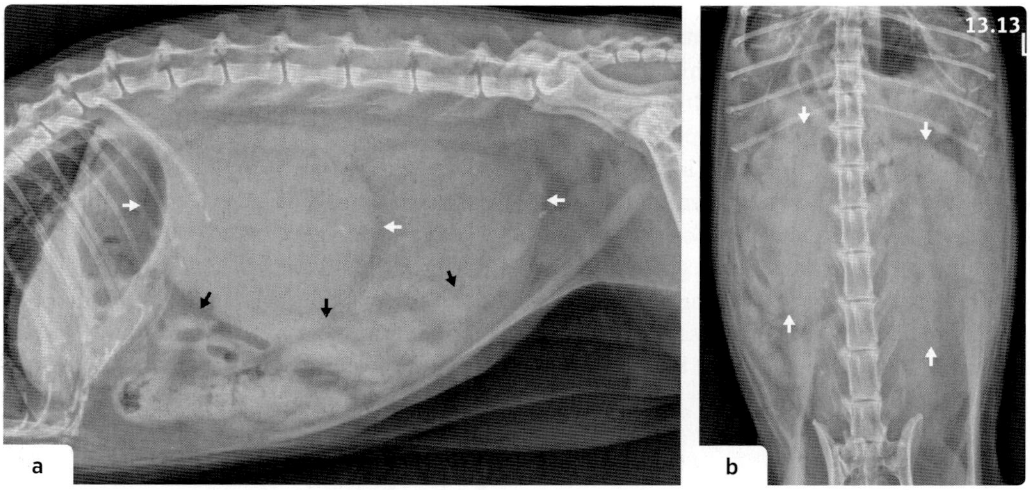

Figures 13.13a, b Lateral (a) and ventrodorsal (b) radiographs in a cat with a history of chronic kidney disease and an increasingly distended abdomen due to bilateral perinephric pseudocysts. A marked mass effect is seen causing ventral displacement of the colon and small intestines (black arrows), indicating a retroperitoneal organ of origin. The kidneys are markedly enlarged, but remain smoothly marginated (white arrows).

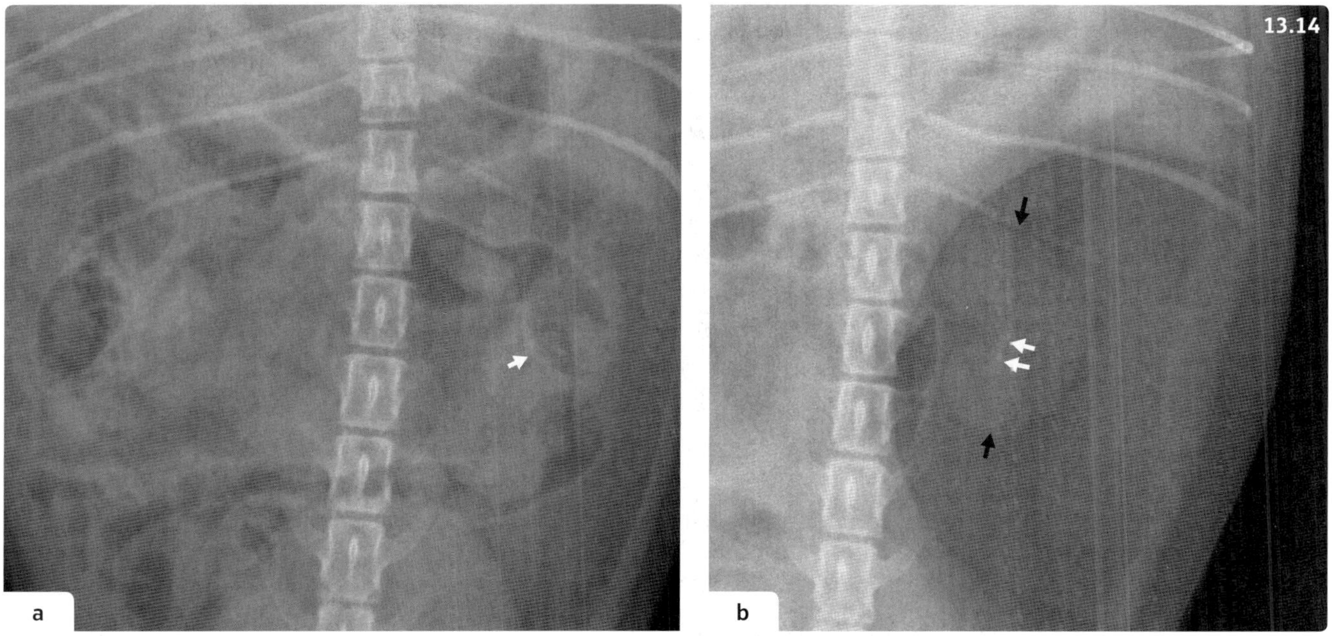

Figures 13.14a, b Ventrodorsal (a) and compression ventrodorsal (b) abdominal radiographs in a dog with small nephroliths. The kidneys were poorly seen on the survey study due to superimposed colon and small intestines. Superimposed over the left kidney, a small mineral opacity appeared to extend beyond the margins of the colon (a, white arrow). On the compression view, the margins of the left kidney are better identified (b, black arrows) and small calculi can be seen in the region of the renal pelvis (b, white arrows).

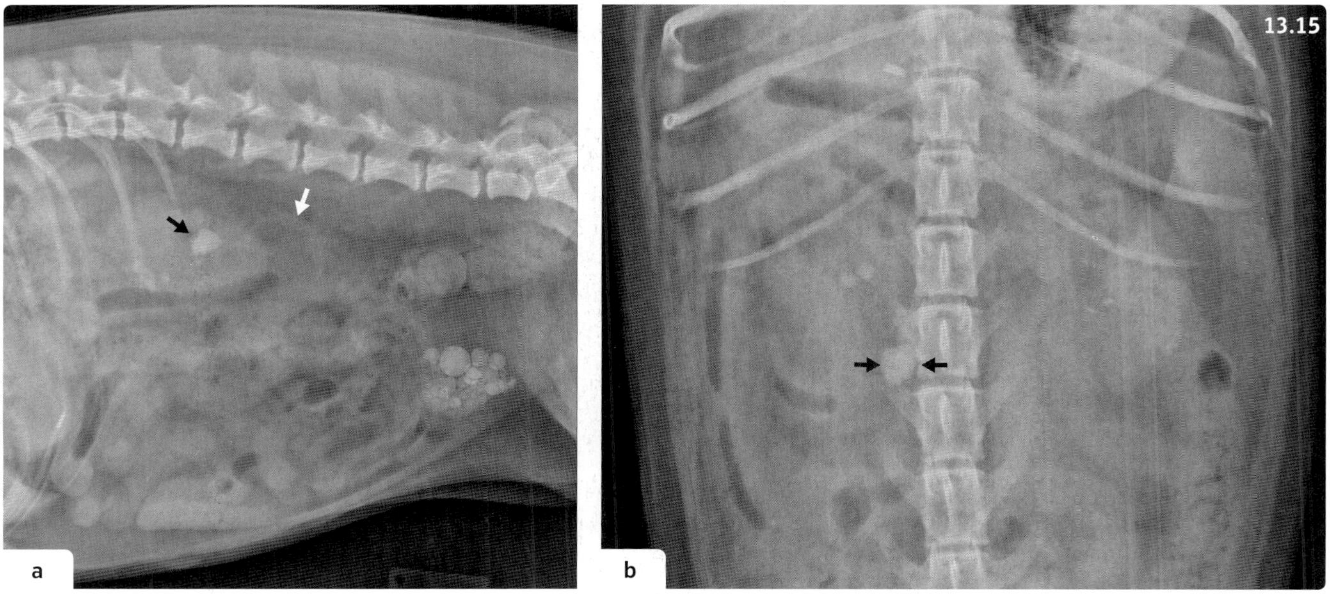

Figures 13.15a, b Lateral (a) and ventrodorsal (b) abdominal radiographs in a dog with azotemia and lethargy. Multiple mineral opaque calculi are superimposed over the kidneys. The largest calculus (black arrows), however, is superimposed medial to the margin of the right kidney in the expected location of a ureter. A small amount of soft tissue opaque streaking is present in the retroperitoneal space (white arrow). Urinary obstruction due to ureterolithiasis was confirmed on ultrasound examination. Numerous, round, well-defined calculi are also present within the urinary bladder.

medially. The right adrenal gland is bordered by the caudal vena cava medially. Adrenal glands are not identified radiographically in normal animals. However, their position relative to the kidneys creates a unique appearance when they are enlarged and a mass effect is created. When an adrenal gland creates a mass effect, it can cause lateral displacement of the cranial pole of its adjacent kidney. When severely enlarged, adrenal masses cause caudal displacement of the adjacent kidney and, often, the cranial pole of the kidney is dorsally displaced (**Figures 13.16a, b**). Masses associated with the adrenal glands are most commonly neoplastic. Animals with adenomas or adenomatous hyperplasia due to pituitary-dependent Cushing's disease do not usually have radiographically visible adrenal glands. Bilateral adrenal mineralization can occur as a normal aging process in cats.

Reproductive tract

Female reproductive tract

The uterine body is a tube located between the urinary bladder and the descending colon; its horns extend to each ovary. The uterus is typically not radiographically visible in normal animals. Visibility of the uterus is considered abnormal and indicates enlargement. The uterus is not expected to be larger in diameter than the small intestines in the normal animal.

Uterine enlargement results in a mass effect that causes dorsal, cranial, and medial displacement of small intestines. Various degrees of uterine enlargement can be seen ranging from mild to severe (**Figures 13.17a, b**). Differential diagnoses for generalized uterine enlargement include pregnancy, pyometra, mucometra, and hydrometra. Incorporation of clinical signs and history are needed to distinguish these causes. Mass lesions due to neoplasia, abscess, granuloma, hematoma, or cyst can also occur and create a mass effect with similar displacement of organs. Concurrent peritoneal effusion is often present with pyometra, stump pyometra, or inflammatory uterine diseases.

Uterine enlargement is readily detectable in pregnant cats and dogs prior to fetal mineralization. In dogs, the uterus is visible at 30 days post luteinizing hormone (LH) surge. In cats, uterine swelling can be seen at 17–21 days. Mineralization of the fetal skeleton initiates in the axial skeleton, beginning at 45 days after the LH surge in dogs and

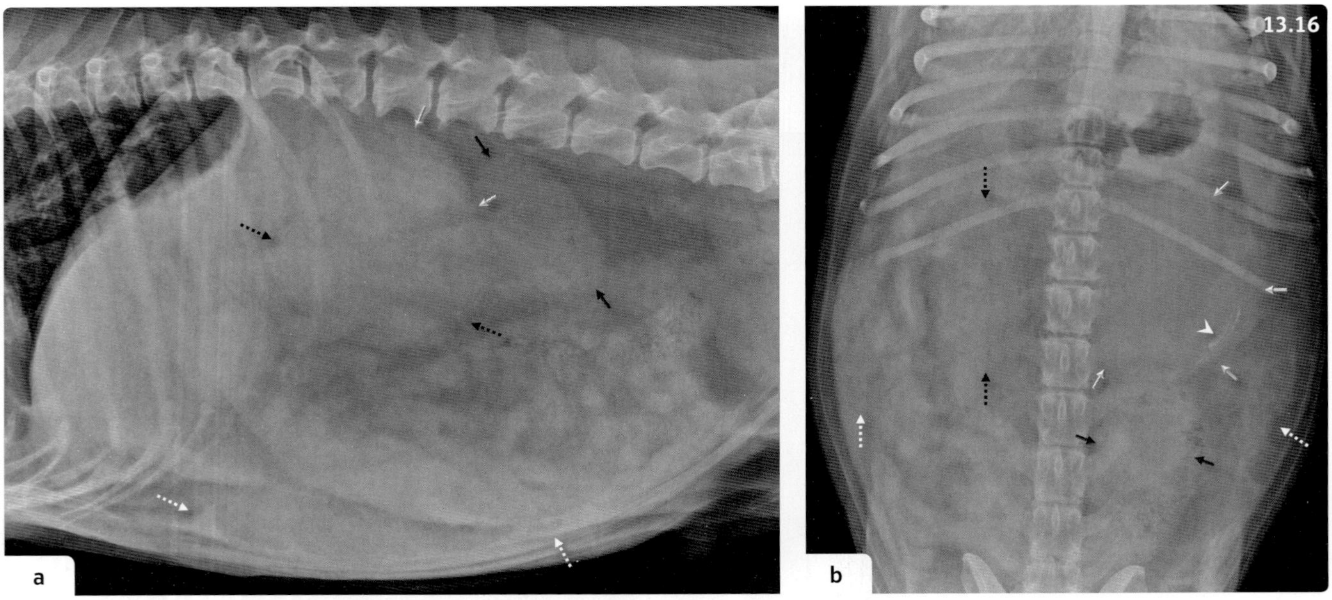

Figures 13.16a, b Lateral (a) and ventrodorsal (b) abdominal radiographs in a dog presenting for acute vomiting and a suspected foreign body. A retroperitoneal mass effect is present (white arrows), causing ventral and rightward displacement of cranial abdominal small intestines. Normal shaped right (dotted black arrows) and left (black arrows) kidneys are visible. An additional, large, round, soft tissue opacity having a well-defined dorsal and lateral margin is visible in the left craniodorsal abdomen. This structure is causing marked caudal displacement and altered orientation of the left kidney, causing its cranial pole to be dorsally displaced. A rim of mineral is present at the lateral caudal periphery of the mass (white arrowhead). A mild amount of soft tissue opaque streaking is present in the peritoneal space (dotted white arrows), which is causing mild decreased detail.

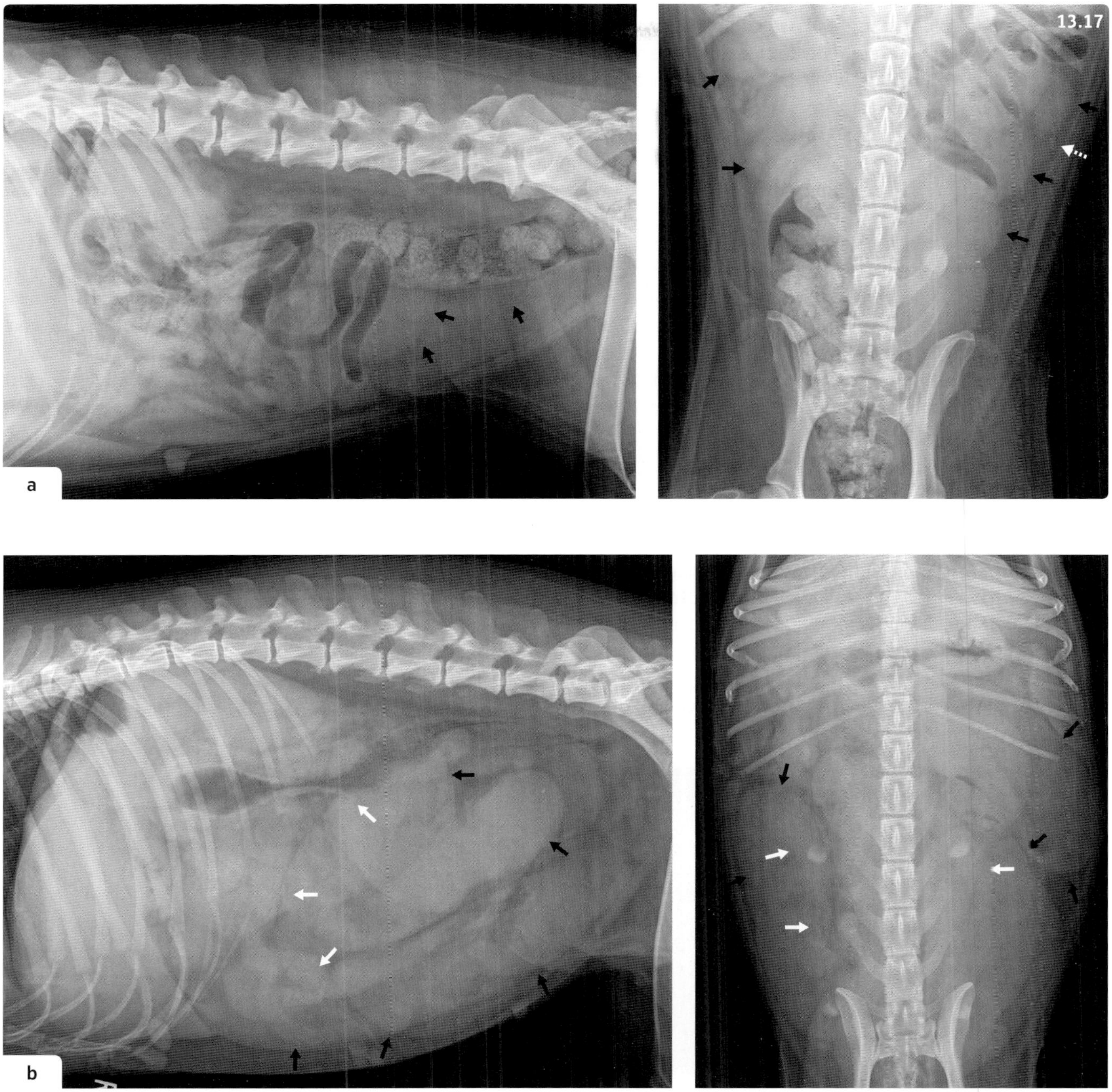

Figures 13.17a, b Lateral and ventrodorsal abdominal radiographs in two dogs with different degrees of uterine enlargement due to pyometra. In 13.17a, there is moderate uterine enlargement with a soft tissue opaque tube visible bordering the dorsal aspect of the urinary bladder and located at the periphery of the right and left abdomen (a, black arrows). A small amount of soft tissue opaque streaking is present within abdominal fat near the left body wall (dotted white arrow), denoting a small volume of regional effusion. Marked uterine enlargement is shown in 13.17b. Tubular-shaped soft tissue opacities are located in the caudal ventral to mid abdomen (b, black arrows). The typical mass effect for uterine enlargement is cranial and dorsal displacement of intestines, which are often pushed medially (b, white arrows).

at 36–45 days after breeding in cats. Mineralization of the skeleton can be used to roughly estimate the stage of pregnancy and the likelihood of imminent parturition. In dogs and cats, the final skeletal structures to mineralize are the distal limbs (metatarsi, metacarpi, and phalanges) and the teeth. Once these are radiographically mineralized and visible, parturition can be expected within 0–5 days in dogs and 0–6 days in cats.

Radiography is insensitive to fetal distress compared with ultrasound. If fetuses have been dead for >24 hours, signs of death may be visible as emphysematous changes within the uterus or fetus (**Figures 13.18a, b**) or collapse of the axial skeleton. Additionally, some causes of fetal dystocia are radiographically visible, such as fetal malposition, extreme maternofetal disproportion, or narrowed pelvic canal due to previous trauma.

Male reproductive tract

The prostate gland encircles the proximal urethra. The prostate gland in cats is not visible. To the author's knowledge, abnormalities causing a radiographically visible prostate in cats have never been reported. In neutered dogs, the prostate gland is typically not identified, but is occasionally seen when the colon is empty or when compression radiography is used. When an enlarged prostate is present, the most reliable indicator of a prostatic organ of origin is the fat opaque triangle located between the urinary bladder and the prostate gland.

In intact males, the prostate gland most often becomes radiographically visible because of benign hypertrophy, which is the most common cause of prostatic enlargement (**Figure 13.19**). The prostate usually encompasses <50% of the diameter of the pelvic inlet from the sacrum to the pubis on the lateral view. The prostate will be intrapelvic in young dogs and will become intra-abdominal as the prostate enlarges in older intact males. Scottish Terrier dogs are reported to have increased severity of prostatomegaly due to benign hypertrophy. Prostatitis can cause radiographically visible enlargement and is more commonly diagnosed in intact dogs. Occasionally, regional peritoneal effusion and peritonitis is present when prostatitis is severe. Regardless, prostatic disease should be considered in male dogs having a ventral caudal abdominal mass effect.

The incidence of prostatic neoplasia is similar in intact and neutered males; however prostatic neoplasia is highly likely in neutered males having a radiographically visible prostate and signs associated with prostatic disease. Mineralization is a common feature of prostatic neoplasia, but it is also less commonly found in benign prostatic enlargements. Generally, mineralization that occurs with benign prostatic diseases is not radiographically visible,

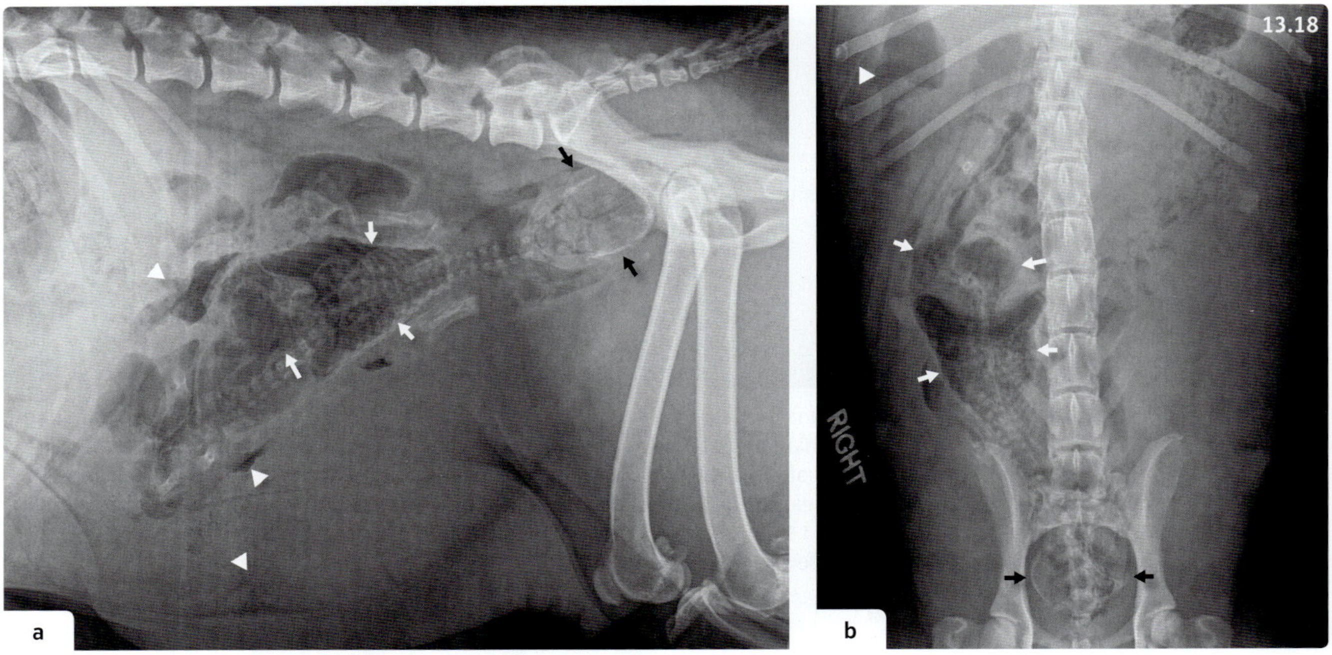

Figures 13.18a, b Lateral (a) and ventrodorsdal (b) abdominal radiographs in a dog having dystocia of unknown duration. A single full-term fetus is present. Dystocia likely occurred due to maternofetal disproportion where the skull (black arrows) was unable to pass through the pelvic canal. Emphysematous metritis is present (white arrowheads), evidenced by gas accumulations within the uterus and surrounding the fetus. Gas is also present within the fetal thorax and abdomen (white arrows).

but can be more readily identified on ultrasound examination. Prostatic neoplasms commonly metastasize to the sublumbar lymph nodes, caudal lumbar spine, and pelvis. In male dogs with visible sublumbar lymphadenopathy or aggressive bone lesions of the caudal lumbar spine or pelvis, prostatic neoplasia should be ruled out as an underlying cause, regardless of whether prostatic enlargement or mineralization is radiographically visible or not (**Figure 13.20**).

Prostatic mass effects due to abscessation, cyst, or paraprostatic cyst occur less commonly. Prostatic abscesses and intraprostatic cysts will have a similar radiographic appearance to benign hypertrophy or prostatitis. However, inflammatory prostatic lesions due to abscessation are more likely to have regional peritoneal effusion. Paraprostatic cysts occur peripheral to the prostate and have a radiographic appearance that is distinct from prostatomegaly alone. In most cases, the paraprostatic cyst is located to the right or the left of the urinary bladder, thus overlapping the urinary bladder on the lateral view, rather than being located caudal to the urinary bladder. Therefore, the typical fat opaque triangle associated with prostatic enlargement may not be a feature of paraprostatic cyst unless concurrent radiographically visible prostatomegaly is present. The appearance of paraprostatic cysts mimics that of a supernumerary urinary bladder.

Lower urinary tract

Urinary bladder

The urinary bladder is almost always visible on the lateral view in cats and dogs regardless of its size. It must be moderately distended before becoming visible on the ventrodorsal view. Bladder size can be variable, therefore its position is inconsistent. Abnormalities associated with the urinary bladder are typically seen as an alteration in opacity or an abnormally large size in an animal showing clinical signs associated with urinary obstruction. Urinary bladder position can also be abnormal, but this is less commonly encountered.

Mineral opacity associated with the urinary bladder is most commonly due to radiopaque urocystic calculi. Calculi are radiopaque because of the presence of calcium in their composition. This includes mainly calcium phosphate and calcium oxalate stones or combinations of stone that are mixed (e.g. magnesium ammonium phosphate, also called struvite, which often contains calcium phosphate). Urate and cystine urocalculi are often radiolucent, but may contain some degree of calcification, making them faintly visible. In general, the determination of urocystic calculus composition cannot be definitively made radiographically. Urinary calculi can be variable in size and shape. Urocystic calculi should be mobile, therefore they will most often be superimposed over the body of the urinary bladder centrally

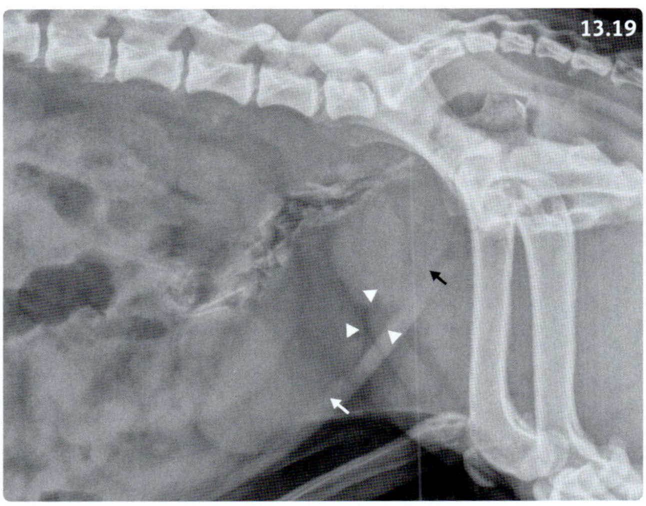

Figure 13.19 Lateral abdominal radiograph in a dog with prostatomegaly due to benign hypertrophy. The fat triangle (between white arrowheads) located between the prostate and the urinary bladder indicates a prostatic organ of origin for the rounded soft tissue opacity at the pelvic inlet. The prostate is enlarged (black arrow), encompassing less than 50% of the dorsoventral diameter of the pelvic inlet. The urinary bladder is cranially positioned (white arrow) likely due to prostatomegaly.

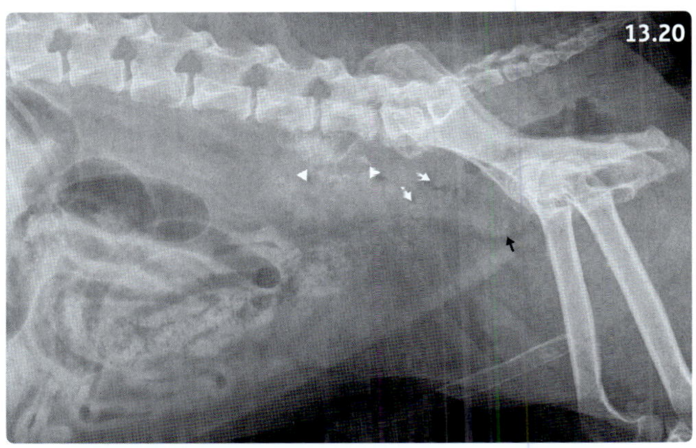

Figure 13.20 Lateral abdominal radiograph in a dog with prostatic neoplasia. The prostate is radiographically visible (black arrow) and contains a small amount of pinpoint mineral near its ventral margin. There is mass effect in the caudal dorsal abdomen, which is causing mild ventral displacement of the distal descending colon (white arrows) consistent with sublumbar lymphadenopathy. Indistinct mineral is superimposed ventral to the caudal lumbar spine (white arrowheads). The ventral margin of these vertebrae is indistinct, indicating an aggressive bone lesion. This is due to metastatic disease from prostatic neoplasia.

on orthogonal views. Mineral that is superimposed in a noncentral location over the urinary bladder indicates a lack of mobility and may be due to adherent luminal calculi or sediment, mineralization of the urinary bladder wall, or mineralized neoplasia.

Gas opacity is occasionally identified within the urinary bladder associated with the lumen or the urinary bladder wall. Most commonly, gas is found in the lumen and is iatrogenic due to catheterization or cystocentesis. In these cases, the gas bubble is mobile and will locate in the most nongravity-dependent part of the urinary bladder as the animal is positioned in lateral or ventrodorsal recumbency. As a result, the bubble will be located at the level of the urinary bladder body on both views. Rarely, gas can be located within the urinary bladder due to gas-forming bacteria, most commonly in diabetic animals with glucose-fermenting infections. Emphysematous cystitis can result in luminal gas or mural gas within the urinary bladder wall. When gas is located within the urinary bladder wall, it will remain superimposed over the same portion of the urinary bladder regardless of the view or the position of the animal and is curvilinear in shape, following the margin of the urinary bladder wall (**Figures 13.21a, b**). Reflux of gas through the ureters or presence of concurrent emphysematous pyelonephritis will cause gas to be located within the region of the renal pelvis.

Urethra

In male dogs, the urethra can be divided into the prostatic urethra, the membranous urethra, and the penile urethra. As its name implies, the prostatic urethra is located in the prostate; the membranous urethra is located caudal to the prostate. The landmark for the junction between the membranous urethra and the penile urethra is the ischial arch. The penile urethra distal to the ischial arch is the longest portion in dogs. The male feline urethra is divided into pelvic and penile parts, where the ischial arch is the landmark for the junction between the two sections. The pelvic part is the longest portion of the urethra in the male cat and includes preprostatic, prostatic, and postprostatic parts. The female urethra in cats and dogs has a pelvic and postpelvic part. When the urinary bladder is distended, the pelvic urethra is more cranially positioned and can be radiographically visible within the abdomen, especially in cats. Otherwise, the urethra is not identified as a separate structure radiographically.

When assessing male dogs for suspected urinary calculi, especially if evidence of urinary obstruction is present or the urinary bladder is distended, a flexed hip view centered at the pelvis and including the perineal region should be incorporated into the protocol so that the entire urethra is visible without superimposition by the femurs (**Figures 13.22a, b**). Evaluation of the urethra on both lateral and flexed lateral views will also prevent mistaking the

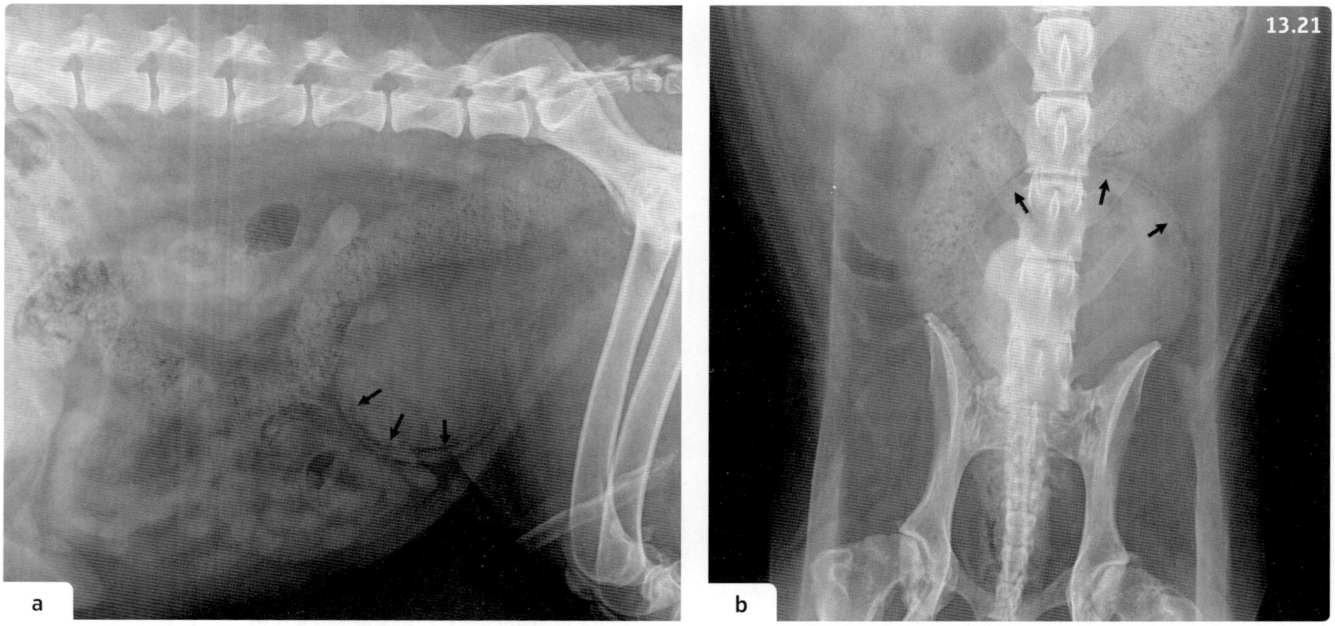

Figures 13.21a, b Lateral (a) and ventrodorsal (b) abdominal radiographs in a dog with emphysematous cystitis. Rather than gas being superimposed over the body of the urinary bladder, as would be expected with mobile luminal gas, a curvilinear rim of gas is present at the bladder apex, consistent with its presence within the urinary bladder wall (arrows).

fabellae for penile urethral calculi, as the fabellae will move with the femur with each view. Keep in mind that, in male dogs, urethral calculi tend to obstruct at the level of the os penis (**Figures 13.22a, b**). The flexed hip view is not necessary in cats or in female dogs; however, the views should include the entire perineal region. The pelvic urethra is another location common for obstruction, especially in female dogs. The portion of the urethra within the pelvis must be closely evaluated on both views to ensure that a calculus is not overlooked as a normal part of the bony pelvis (**Figures 13.23a, b**). The size of a urinary calculus that can pass through the entire urethra is not reliably predictable.

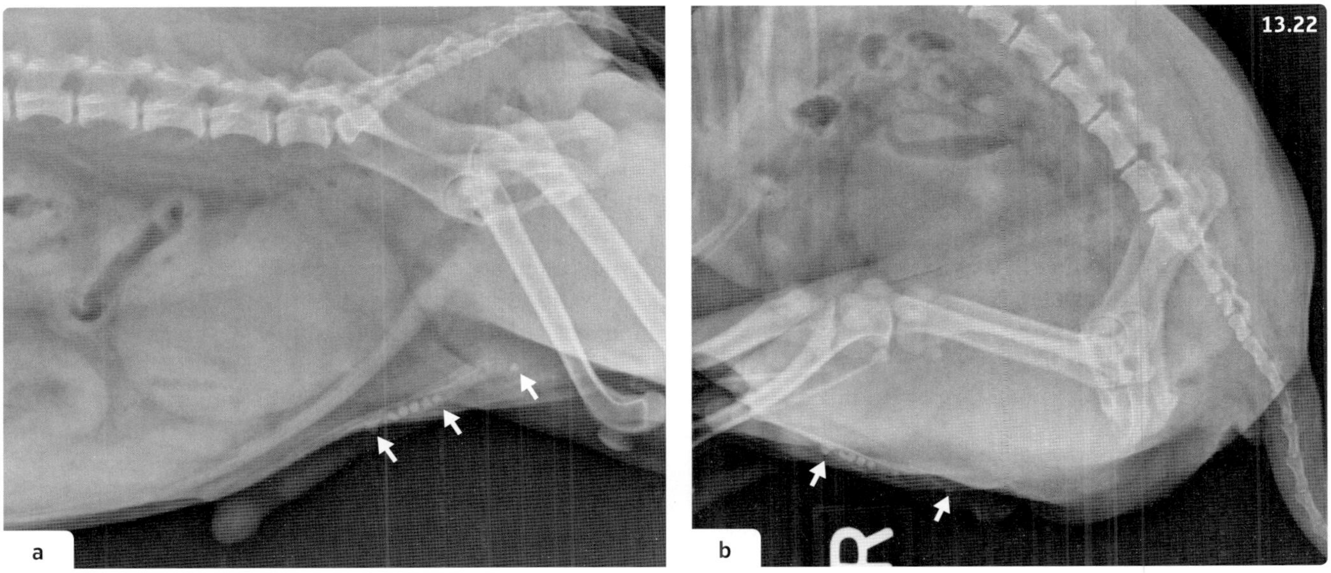

Figures 13.22a, b Standard lateral (a) and flexed hindlimb lateral (b) abdominal radiographs in a male dog with clinical signs consistent with urinary obstruction. Multiple, round, well-defined calculi are present within the penile urethra (arrows). To confirm the correct number of calculi, a flexed hindlimb view (b) is needed to view the entire urethra and remove superimposition of the femurs over the urethra.

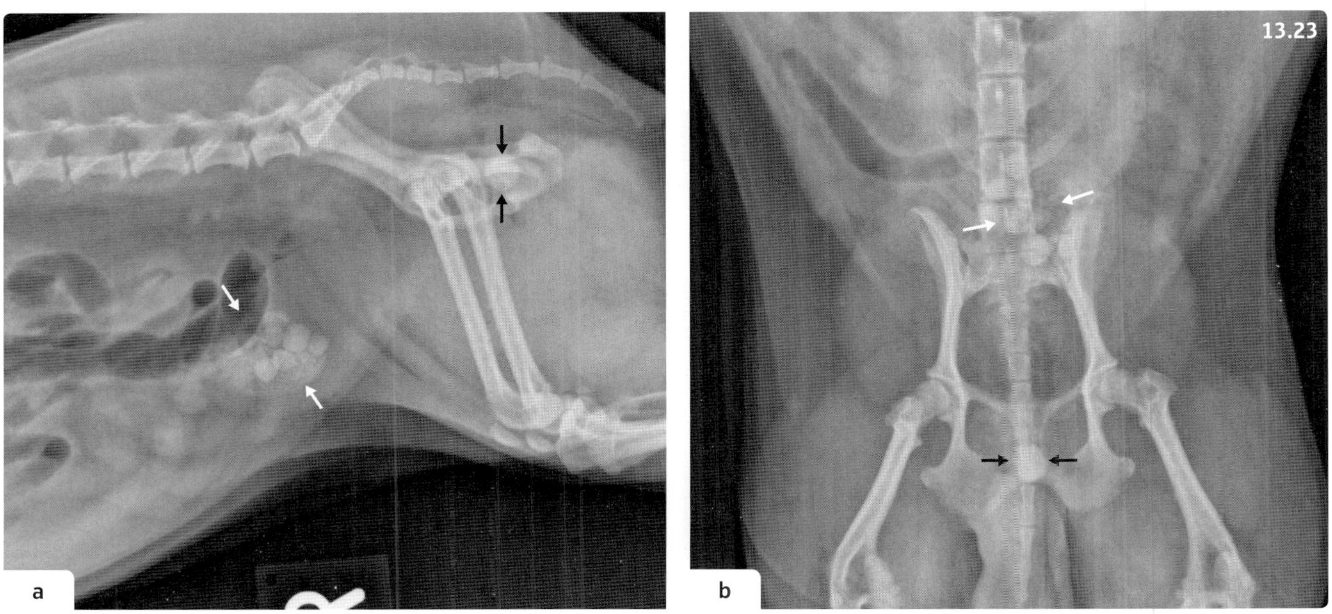

Figures 13.23a, b Lateral (a) and ventrodorsal (b) abdominal radiographs in a female dog with clinical signs associated with urinary obstruction. Numerous calculi are readily visible within the urinary bladder (white arrows). A single, large calculus is present within the pelvic urethra, which is superimposed over the bony pelvis on both views (between black arrows). This calculus was not initially identified prior to removal of the bladder calculi and was removed on a subsequent cystotomy.

Gastrointestinal tract

When evaluating the intestines, the colon should be identified first because it is in a more predictable location and is easier to recognize. Next, any remaining intestine that is distended or has abnormal contents is probably within small intestine, making it more likely to be of clinical significance. It is common for beginner interpreters to only recognize portions of the GI tract containing gas and ignore portions that are empty or contain only fluid opacity. Attempts must be made to evaluate portions that are soft tissue/fluid opaque as they may be abnormal and the gas-filled loops more normal. Also, many beginner interpreters assume a decrease in peritoneal detail when evaluating the abdomen of an animal having little to no luminal gas within the intestines. Evaluation of serosal margins to determine their visibility will confirm or reject the presence of decreased serosal detail.

Stomach

A normal size measurement for the stomach does not exist; therefore, distension is a subjective determination. An empty stomach is typically intercostal in location. With increasing distension, the stomach extends caudally and ventrally, as commonly seen in cats and especially dogs that have recently eaten large volumes. The fundus is always the largest portion of the stomach regardless of the degree of distension (this is useful when evaluating the stomach for malpositioning). The fundus should be located on the left side of the abdomen and is dorsal. In dogs, the gastric body crosses from left to right and is the most ventral portion of the stomach. The pyloric antrum and pylorus are slightly more dorsal in location than the gastric body and are located on the right side. In cats, the stomach is 'J' shaped and is primarily located on the left side, with the pylorus being close to midline. Alterations in stomach size, position, and opacity can occur.

Gastric distension

A distended stomach causes caudal displacement of small intestines and the head and tail of the spleen. Gastric dilatation can be caused by mechanical or functional ileus. Several considerations should be made when evaluating a distended stomach. The clinical signs, history, and description of the luminal content alter the ranking of differential diagnoses associated with a distended stomach. In the case of recent ingestion, the luminal content of the stomach is usually an inhomogeneous mixture of gas, soft tissue, and, sometimes, granular or faint mineral opaque material. The content of the stomach can rarely be definitively distinguished as food or foreign material. Foreign materials, such as tough, expansile glues containing diphenylmethane diisocyanate, and indigestible materials, such as fabric or grass, can have an inhomogeneous appearance similar to that of recently ingested food. When it is unclear whether or not the stomach is filled with food or foreign material, repeat radiographs should be obtained 6–8 hours after fasting to see if gastric emptying is occurring. If the stomach is identical after this period of time, foreign or indigestible material (**Figures 13.24a, b**) should be considered.

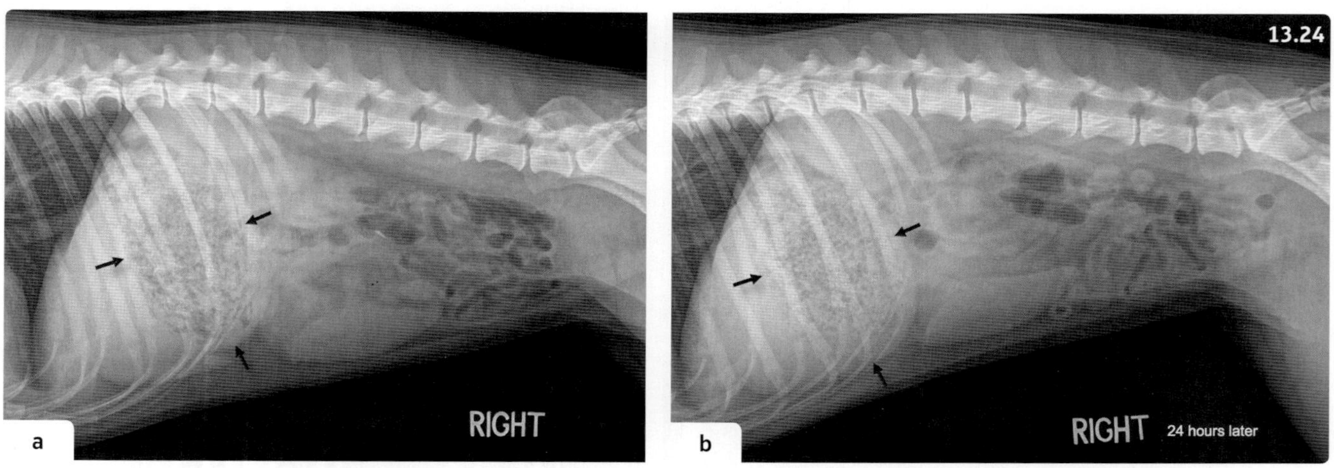

Figures 13.24a, b Lateral abdominal radiographs in an anorexic dog that vomited once prior to presentation. The stomach is moderately distended with inhomogeneous gas and soft tissue opaque material (a, arrows). This could be due to recent ingestion of food or to indigestible foreign material. The dog was fasted for 24 hours and the study repeated (b). The stomach is almost identical in appearance (arrows), consistent with a lack of movement of content from the stomach and the presence of indigestible material. A large volume of hay was removed endoscopically.

In an animal with a functional ileus or a pyloric outflow obstruction, the stomach may or may not be distended, depending on the effectiveness of vomiting. Gastric contents in an animal that is concurrently anorexic often appear as a homogeneous shade of gray consistent with a combination of gas and fluid (**Figures 13.25a, b**) rather than the inhomogeneous opacity seen with recent ingestion of food or a stomach filled with nondigestible material. Pyloric outflow obstructions can occur due to luminal foreign material that is nonmobile and lodged within the pylorus/proximal duodenum or can be due to mural thickening or a mass at the same level. The most common causes of a functional gastric ileus are acute gastritis or pancreatitis.

When a stomach containing homogeneous gas and fluid is encountered, the next step is to obtain a left lateral view. The left lateral view will allow luminal fluid to fall to the gravity-dependent gastric fundus on the left side, while gas rises to the nongravity-dependent pyloric antrum on the right side. This recumbency will allow gas to highlight materials that may be obstructing the pylorus and are not mobile, given that these materials are often soft tissue opaque (**Figures 13.26a, b**). Mobile soft tissue opaque materials (food or foreign) will follow luminal fluid with recumbency, being similarly gravity dependent, and may remain effaced by any fluid present, depending on the volume of gas versus fluid present in the stomach. Therefore, mobile foreign objects are not readily identified unless they are mineral or metal opaque or are surrounded, at least in part by gas, allowing their structure to be revealed. Effort should be made to determine the degree to which foreign material extends into the small intestinal tract, as lengthy or linear foreign bodies must be removed surgically rather than endoscopically. The left lateral projection can be used to highlight some mural gastric wall or pyloric abnormalities if they are large enough to extend into the lumen or create an irregular gas pattern in the pyloric antrum (**Figures 13.27a–c**).

In cases where the left lateral view does not reveal a luminal foreign object, a mural abnormality or luminal obstruction not highlighted by gas cannot totally be ruled out; however, causes of functional ileus such as gastritis and pancreatitis are considered higher on the differential diagnosis list, especially if acute vomiting is the predominant clinical sign. The left lateral projection can also be used to prove that a cranioventral mass is a distended stomach rather than a liver or splenic mass.

Gastric wall masses are not usually diagnosed on radiographs alone because it can be difficult to differentiate a mass typically effaced by surrounding organs and luminal content unless a luminal abnormality can be highlighted by gas. A stomach wall mass can cause a similar mass

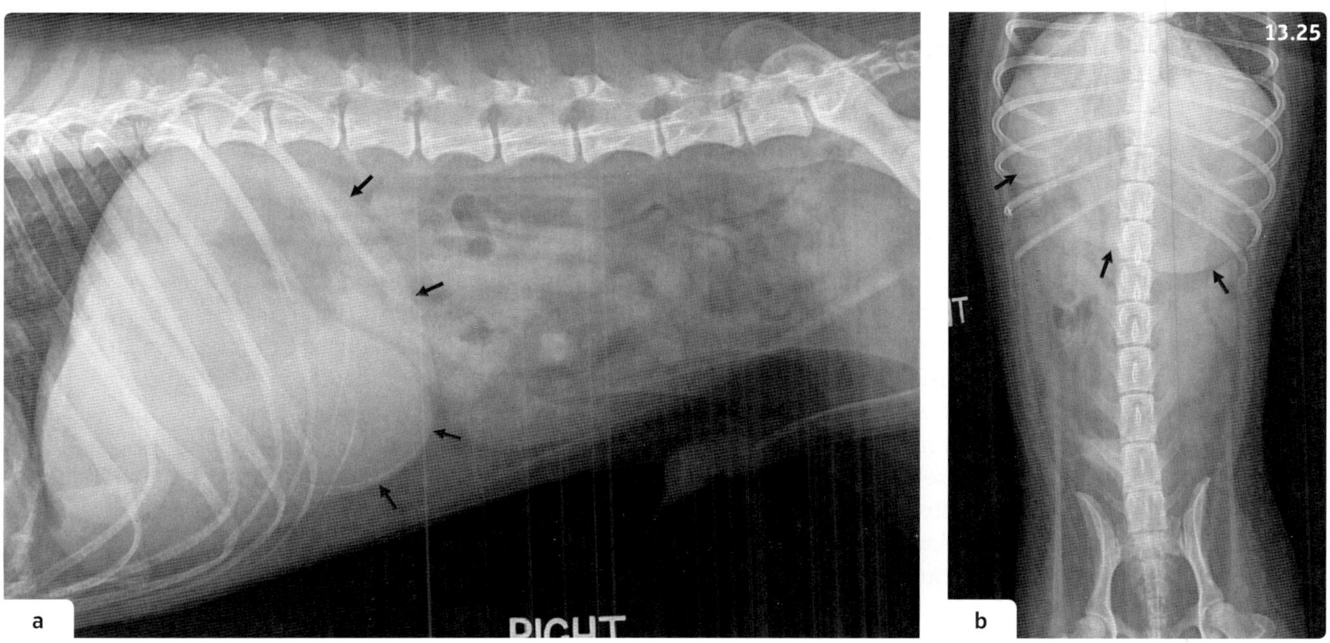

Figures 13.25a, b Lateral (a) and ventrodorsal (b) abdominal radiographs in a dog presenting for vomiting. The stomach is distended (arrows), causing caudal displacement of the small intestines and the spleen. The stomach is a homogeneous shade of gray created by a combination of luminal gas and fluid. This appearance is not typical for an animal that has recently eaten. It is more typical for a functional ileus or a pyloric outflow obstruction.

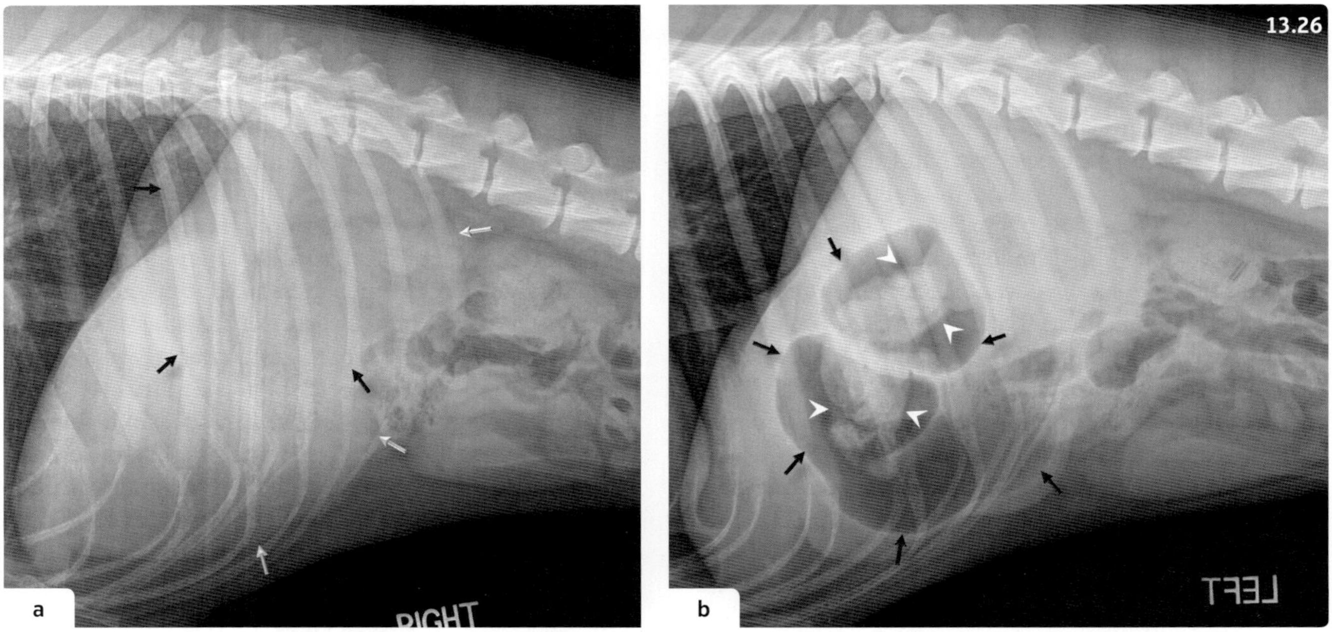

Figures 13.26a, b Right (a) and left (b) lateral radiographs in a dog presenting for acute and frequent vomiting. On the right lateral view, a distended stomach is seen (a, white arrows) which contained a shade of gray consistent with gas and fluid content. Due to recumbency in the right lateral view, gas is located in the gastric fundus (a, black arrows) and fluid is located at the level of the pylorus. Because of the clinical signs and appearance of the stomach, a left lateral projection was obtained. On this view, gas fills the nongravity-dependent pyloric antrum (b, black arrows) while fluid falls to the gastric fundus. Gas within the pylorus highlights a well-defined, tubular, soft tissue opacity (b, white arrowheads). This opacity is pyloric in location and must be nonmobile because it did not fall with luminal fluid to the gravity-dependent gastric fundus in the left lateral view, indicating positive evidence for obstruction. A rope toy and plastic pieces were removed surgically.

effect to that seen with luminal gastric distension (i.e. caudal displacement of small intestines and the spleen). In many cases a positive (barium sulfate, most commonly) or negative (room air, most commonly) contrast upper GI study or an abdominal ultrasound is ultimately required to determine the presence of a gastric wall mass.

Gastric malpositioning

Alterations in stomach positioning can occur due to mass effect from surrounding organs or to volvulus. If the diaphragm is ruptured, the stomach can be cranially displaced within the pleural space or in the location of the liver, and may be difficult to locate unless distended or contrast is administered. A small liver can cause a cranially positioned stomach. Conversely, hepatomegaly can cause caudal displacement of the stomach.

Volvulus occurs when the stomach axis rotates, typically clockwise when viewing the animal from caudal to cranial, altering the relative positions of the gastric fundus and pylorus. The pylorus rotates cranially, dorsally, and to the left while the fundus rotates to the right and ventrally. Often, the stomach is massively dilated concurrent with volvulus, hence the term GDV. In most cases the stomach contains a large volume of gas; however, fluid or inhomogeneous ingesta may be the most notable luminal contents. The motion of gas and fluid within the normal stomach must be understood in order to appreciate the radiographic abnormalities that occur with GDV. The right lateral recumbent view is often the only view needed to evaluate for the presence of gastric malpositioning; however, additional views can be performed, if necessary. Due to gastric malpositioning with GDV, instead of fluid falling to the pylorus in the right lateral view, gas will rise to the pylorus, which is abnormally located on the left side. Therefore, having gas present in the pylorus on the right lateral view is a positive indication of gastric malpositioning (**Figure 13.28**). The volvulus combined with the severe distension creates a compartmentalized appearance to the stomach, which appears to be divided by a soft tissue band. This descriptive configuration of gastric malpositioning occurs with a 180-degree torsion, which is the most common torsion. In the case of a 360-degree torsion, gas and fluid will behave as expected in a normal animal, except that massive gastric distension will be seen, making this degree of volvulus more easily overlooked.

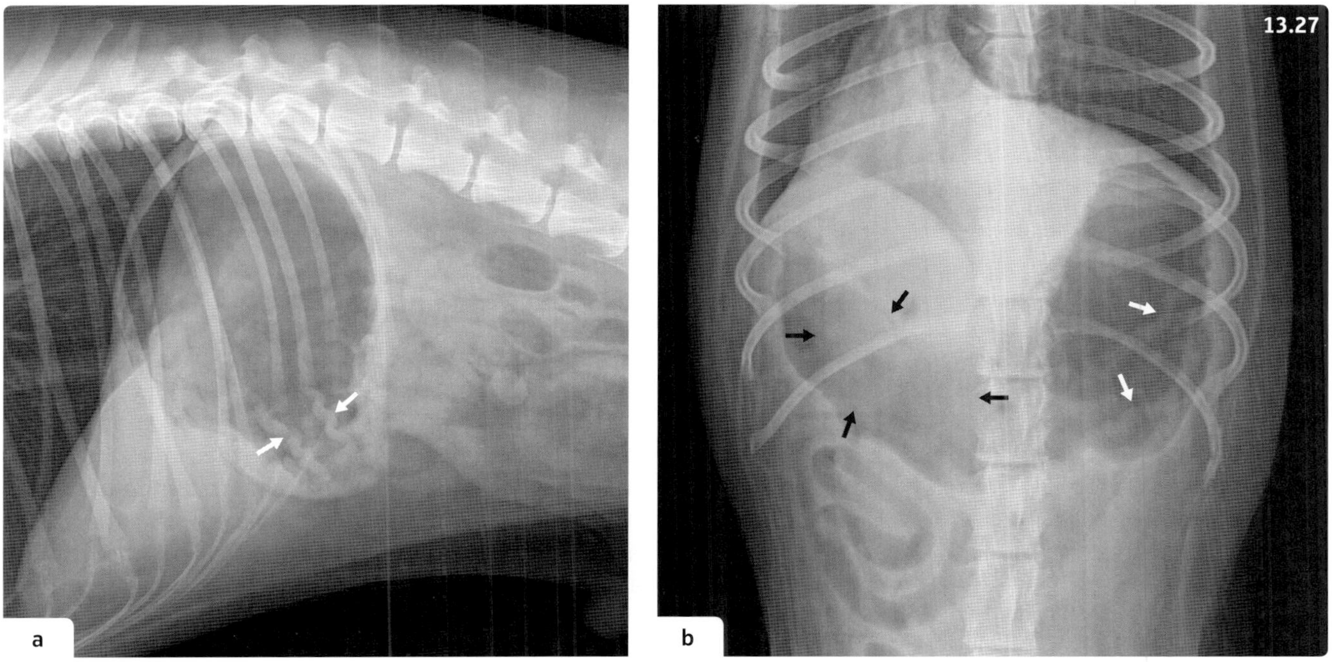

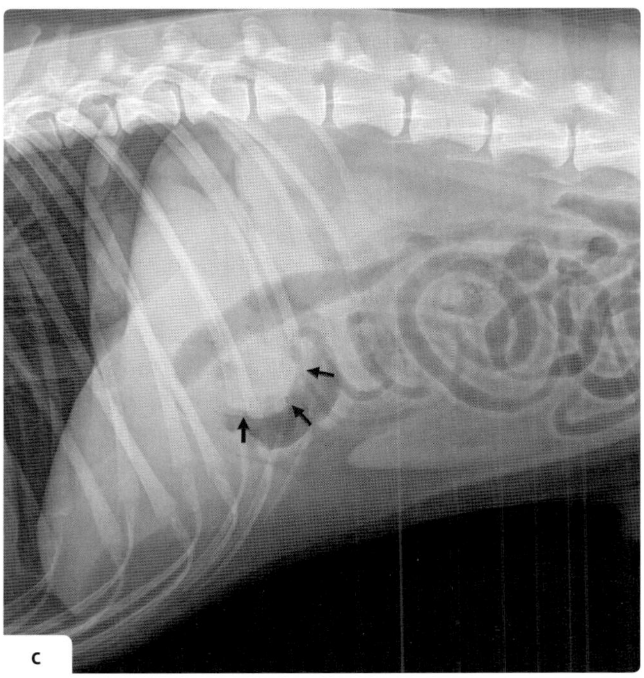

Figures 13.27a–c Right lateral (a), ventrodorsal (b), and left lateral (c) abdominal radiographs in a dog presenting for increasing episodes of vomiting over several weeks. The stomach is moderately distended and contains a large amount of gas, causing a darker gray opacity; however, some fluid is also present, which makes the gravity-dependent part of the stomach difficult to evaluate. In the right lateral projection (a), gas is present in the fundus, while luminal fluid falls to the gravity-dependent part of the stomach, the pylorus. Rugal folds located within the gastric body and fundus are highlighted by gas on the right lateral and ventrodorsal views (a and b, white arrows). Additionally, an indistinct soft tissue opacity is seen at the right gastric body and pyloric antrum on the ventrodorsal view (b, black arrows). This may be mobile luminal fluid or ingested content. On the left lateral view (c), gas has risen to the nongravity-dependent pyloric antrum and highlights a soft tissue mass that is partially surrounded by gas, has an irregular luminal margin (black arrows), and provides a more convincing view of a mural abnormality. Gastric adenocarcinoma was diagnosed via endoscopic samples.

Several secondary changes are commonly encountered in conjunction with a GDV. Microcardia, small pulmonary vasculature, and a small caudal vena cava occur secondary to poor cardiovascular return of volume and shock. An obstructive megaesophagus and small intestinal paralytic ileus also commonly occur. Due to the gastrosplenic ligament, rotation of the stomach can result in concurrent splenic torsion. Finally, necrosis of the gastric wall, although not commonly evident on radiographs, can manifest as pneumatosis or gas within the stomach wall (**Figure 13.28**).

An alteration in stomach opacity occurs most commonly due to radiopaque luminal material that may

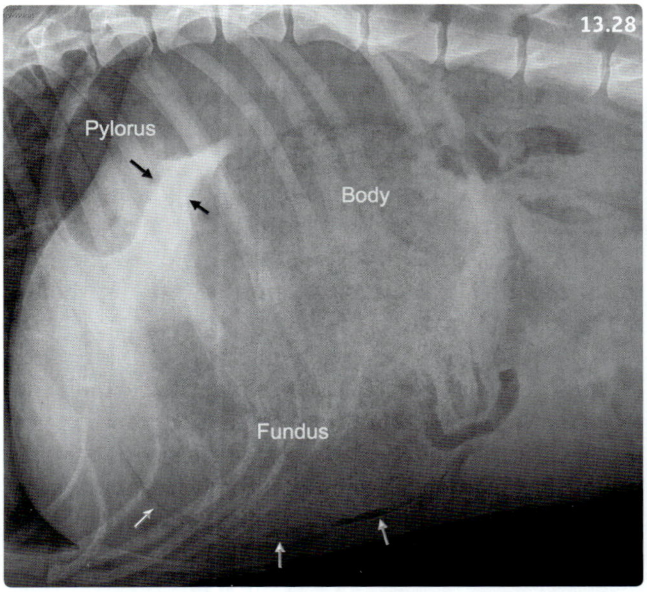

Figure 13.28 Right lateral abdominal radiograph in a dog with gastric dilatation and volvulus. Each portion of the stomach is labeled. On a right lateral view, the pylorus should contain fluid. In this case, the pylorus (identified as being the smallest gastric compartment) contains gas and is located dorsally and cranially. The fact that the pylorus contains gas in right lateral recumbency indicates that it is located on the left side of the dog. A thick soft tissue opaque band (between black arrows) is present between the gastric body and pylorus, typical for the compartmentalization seen with massive distension and volvulus. Additionally, an irregular line of gas borders the ventral aspect of the gastric fundus, indicating intramural gas (gastric pneumatosis) and wall necrosis (white arrows).

be mineral or metal opaque and can be obstructive, or benign. True alterations in stomach opacity can occur due to mural gas (gastric pneumatosis) or mucosal mineralization as reported with uremic gastritis. In cats, fat within the submucosal layer of the stomach is sometimes radiographically visible as a lucent line paralleling the gastric wall and is a normal finding. This fat layer is not present in dogs and its identification in cats must not be mistaken for pneumatosis. Mineralization associated with uremic gastritis occurs in the mucosal layer and can result in a faint mineral line that follows the rugal folds, likely due to metastatic mineralization and formation of whitlockite crystals.

Small intestines

Inexperienced interpreters often rely solely on small intestinal diameter as an indication of abnormality. Several other descriptors exist that should be evaluated when interpreting small intestine and are summarized in **Box 13.8**. With regard to small intestinal diameter,

Box 13.8 Descriptors for evaluation of small intestines.

- Location
- Luminal content
- Serosal margin shape and margination
- Path of small intestinal loops
- Apparent number of small intestinal loops
- Diameter

multiple measurements have been published for normal small intestine diameter. In dogs, the normal small intestinal diameter should be less than two rib widths. Also, an increase in diameter of a small intestinal segment >50% of the diameter of the remaining small intestinal loops is considered abnormal. Small intestinal dilation >1.6 times the dorsoventral diameter of the narrowest point of the L5 vertebral body is significantly associated with mechanical obstruction. Small intestines in cats should measure <12 mm in diameter. Small intestine must be distinguished from colon. The diameter of the colon can vary greatly, being quite large and often containing inhomogeneous fecal material in normal animals. Finding similar luminal material within small intestines to that normally seen within the colon is often of significance.

The luminal content in small intestines should be homogeneous in appearance. The small intestines normally contain gas or fluid, or are empty, producing a shade of gray depending on the volume of gas located within the segment. Additionally, normal luminal gas forms well-defined tubes or ovals without causing distension. Dogs tend to have more luminal gas than cats; however, great variation exists depending on the degree of aerophagia. Because they tend to be more evident, loops containing gas are often evaluated more closely by beginner interpreters than uniformly soft tissue opaque loops; attempts must be made to evaluate loops that are empty or have homogeneous soft tissue opaque content. Inhomogeneous small intestinal content, having either a definable structure or more descriptively matching luminal feces located within the large intestine, should raise suspicion of foreign material, especially when associated clinical signs are present. Obtaining right and left lateral recumbent views redistributes luminal gas and fluid within the small intestines and can make the presence of an abnormality more visible.

The serosal margin of small intestinal loops should be linear, smooth, and well defined. A roughened serosal margin most commonly occurs with fine plication due to the typically thin thread-like material, which causes linear foreign bodies in cats. Mural small intestinal masses can also cause an irregular serosal surface to small intestinal loops.

Normal intestinal loops have a path comprised of multiple broad turns. The presence of a tortuous path consisting of tight turns should raise suspicion for plication due to linear foreign material. Plication also tends to create a reduction in the apparent number of small intestinal loops. With severe small intestinal dilation, the small intestinal path can have extremely tight turns (so-called hairpin turns) giving the loops a stacked appearance with squared-off ends, indicating small intestinal crowding due to increased luminal volume (**Figure 13.29**).

The diameter of the small intestines should be uniform across all segments and should be within measurements previously discussed. When considering causes of dilated small intestines, segmental distribution of dilation is probably the most useful descriptor in determining the presence of obstruction; uniform dilation is more often associated with a functional ileus and the presence of dilated small intestinal loops in combination with loops that are normal in diameter is more characteristic of mechanical obstruction.

Small intestinal mechanical obstruction

Small intestinal mechanical obstruction falls into two main categories, focal discrete obstruction and linear obstruction, and these have important differences in radiographic appearance. The typical radiographic appearance for a discrete obstruction is small intestinal dilation that is segmental in nature. In other words, some distended loops are identified and, importantly, some loops that are normal in diameter are also identified. With more distal obstructions, an increase in the number of dilated small intestinal loops relative to normal ones is often identified because distension occurs orad to the obstruction. Potential causes for a discrete obstruction include luminal foreign material, a mural mass, or an intussusception. Close evaluation of small intestinal content may reveal the presence of focal structured or inhomogeneous material, further raising suspicion of mechanical obstruction due to foreign material. Sometimes, the discrete obstruction can have a characteristic appearance, such as a corncob having a lucent grid at regular intervals (**Figure 13.29**) or a textile having linear gas and soft tissue opaque striations (**Figure 13.30**). Additionally, luminal intestinal gas can highlight a foreign object, creating a gas–soft tissue interface that is inconsistent with a normal luminal gas bubble (**Figure 13.31**). Redistribution of gas using both lateral recumbencies can assist with foreign body diagnosis by potentially highlighting such interfaces. The lack of identification of the obstructing material should not preclude a diagnosis of obstruction when remaining descriptors indicate mechanical ileus.

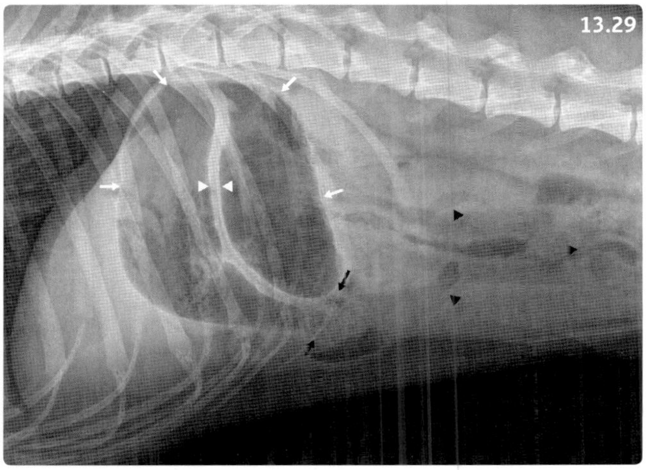

Figure 13.29 Lateral abdominal radiograph in a dog presenting for acute, frequent vomiting. A massively distended loop of small intestine containing mostly gas is present in the cranial abdomen (between white arrows). Due to the extreme distension, the loop of intestine is stacked upon itself and takes a hairpin turn, creating a squared-off end in the dorsal abdomen. The stacked intestinal walls create an apparent soft tissue opaque band (between white arrowheads) separating the luminal gas within each segment. Ventrally, a structured inhomogeneous opacity composed of gas and soft tissue is present, which is partially surrounded by gas (between black arrows). Multiple small intestinal loops are normal in diameter (black arrowheads). Mechanical obstruction due to a corncob foreign body was diagnosed.

Small intestinal masses can cause a focal, discrete obstruction. Small intestinal masses are most commonly neoplastic due to adenocarcinoma, lymphoma, or leiomyosarcoma. Focal masses can be circumferential surrounding the entire lumen (more typical of adenocarcinoma) or eccentric involving one side of the intestine (more typical of leiomyosarcoma). Diffuse or multifocal neoplasms such as lymphoma also occur. Focal, discrete, circumferential masses are most likely to cause mechanical obstruction. An accumulation of granular mineral material at a location within the intestinal tract (called a gravel sign) indicates a partial chronic obstruction, most likely due to a focal mural small intestinal mass where mineral opaque or desiccated material accumulates at the site of obstruction. The absence of small intestinal dilation does not rule a mechanical obstruction out. Especially with proximal small intestinal mechanical obstructions, frequent and effective vomiting can limit visible distension. In general, the small intestinal dilation seen with focal, discrete mechanical obstruction is often greater than the dilation seen with a paralytic or functional ileus.

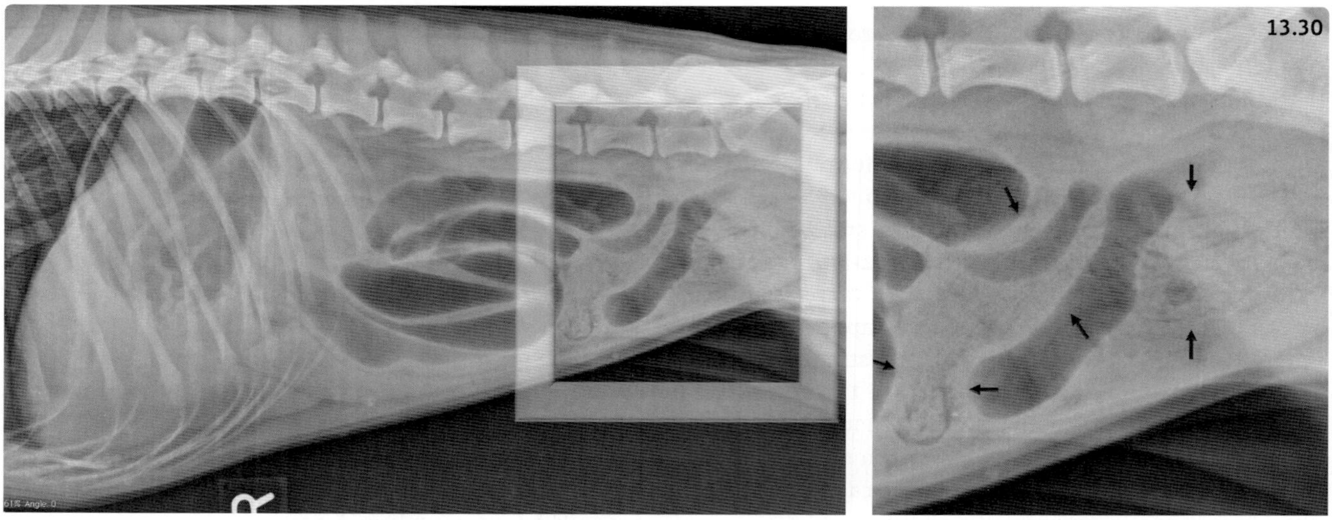

Figure 13.30 Lateral abdominal radiograph in a dog presenting with acute, frequent vomiting. Multiple gas-filled small intestinal loops are dilated. Too many visible dilated loops are present to be due to colon alone. In the caudoventral abdomen, a loop containing inhomogeneous luminal material having linear gas and soft tissue opaque striations is present (in boxed inset and between arrows), which is typical for textile material. A hand towel was surgically removed.

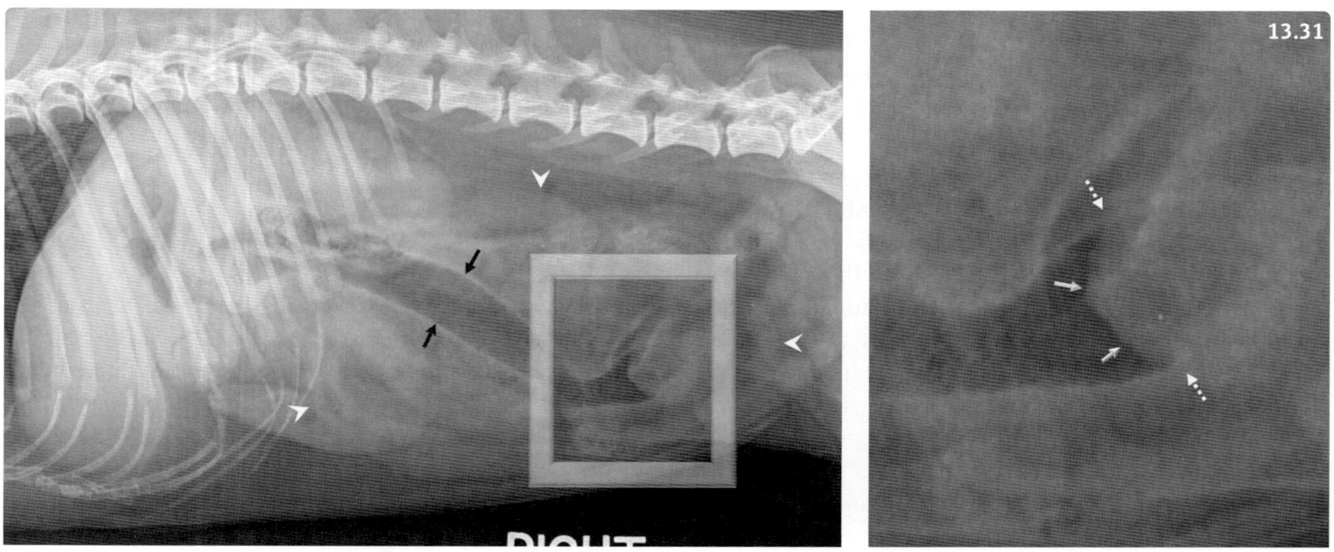

Figure 13.31 Lateral abdominal radiograph of a dog that had been vomiting for 1 week. A gas-distended small intestinal loop is present (between black arrows). Several normal diameter loops are also present (white arrowheads). At the caudal aspect of the gas-distended loop, an irregularly marginated interface between the gas and a soft tissue opacity is seen (boxed inset, white arrows). The small intestinal loop visibly dilates at the level of this soft tissue opacity (dotted white arrows). A plastic toy nose was removed surgically.

Linear foreign material tends to span large portions of the GI tract, causing small intestinal plication but not necessarily dilation. A tortuous path of small intestine or the presence of visible plication creating an irregular serosal margin is the most reliable evidence of a linear foreign body. Plication occurs because the material is fixed in one position while one end travels distally through the GI tract, where continual peristalsis causes the intestine to gather around the material like pleats in a drape. Two main features distinguish linear foreign bodies in cats from those in dogs. First, in cats, linear foreign material is usually very thin, such as thread or floss. Because of this, the plication that occurs with linear foreign material tends to be fine, appearing as an irregular serosal margin with little to no measurable small intestinal distension **(Figures 13.32a, b)**. The small intestines can appear decreased in number and aggregated in a focal location (usually the right abdomen); however, these are often the least useful features for identification of linear foreign bodies and can be confused with the intestinal appearance in normal animals, especially obese cats. Some small intestinal loops may have small, irregular gas bubbles that are piriform in shape as gas becomes trapped in the pleats. Also, in cats, the material often becomes anchored at the base of the tongue, so examination of the mouth may confirm suspicion of linear foreign material. Linear foreign material in dogs tends to be thick textile material, such as socks, rope toys, and towels. This material tends to anchor at the level of the pylorus, causing an outflow obstruction. Because of the size of the linear material, small intestinal dilation is commonly seen with linear foreign body obstructions in dogs **(Figures 13.33a, b)**. Also, due to the location of the obstruction at the pylorus, a left lateral view of a stomach containing adequate gas often reveals the origin of the linear object. Due to the thick nature of the textile causing most obstructions, the plication seen in a dog is characterized by frequent changes in direction of the small intestinal loop rather than the fine pleating that occurs with linear foreign material in cats.

Functional ileus

Functional ileus results in visible dilation of small intestines that is often diffuse, but on some occasions can be focal. Focal narrowing of small intestine due to segmental peristaltic contractions is not seen radiographically when paralytic ileus is the cause of small intestinal dilation. Peritonitis, pancreatitis, enteritis, and infiltrative bowel neoplasms (e.g. lymphoma and mast cell tumor) are the most common causes of functional ileus. The distension that occurs with functional ileus is not usually as great as that seen with mechanical obstruction. Regardless, functional ileus cannot always be distinguished from a distal mechanical obstruction without ultrasound examination or a positive contrast GI study. Less common causes of functional ileus, such as bowel ischemia and thrombosis or dysautonomia, can cause a profound small intestinal dilation that may be segmental rather than diffuse.

Colon

The colon is in a relatively predictable location and often contains luminal gas or feces, making it readily identifiable in most cases Locating the colon should be the first step in evaluating the intestinal tract. The cecum is rarely identified in cats. The normal colon is typically larger in diameter than the small intestines and, as previously mentioned, is the only intestinal segment whose contents should be inhomogeneous, appearing as a mixture of gas, soft tissue, and granular mineral in locations where fecal material is present. Material of this characterization located in small intestines would be considered abnormal. Normal large intestinal diameter is difficult to characterize because it is so variable; however, the colon diameter should not exceed the length of the L7 vertebral body.

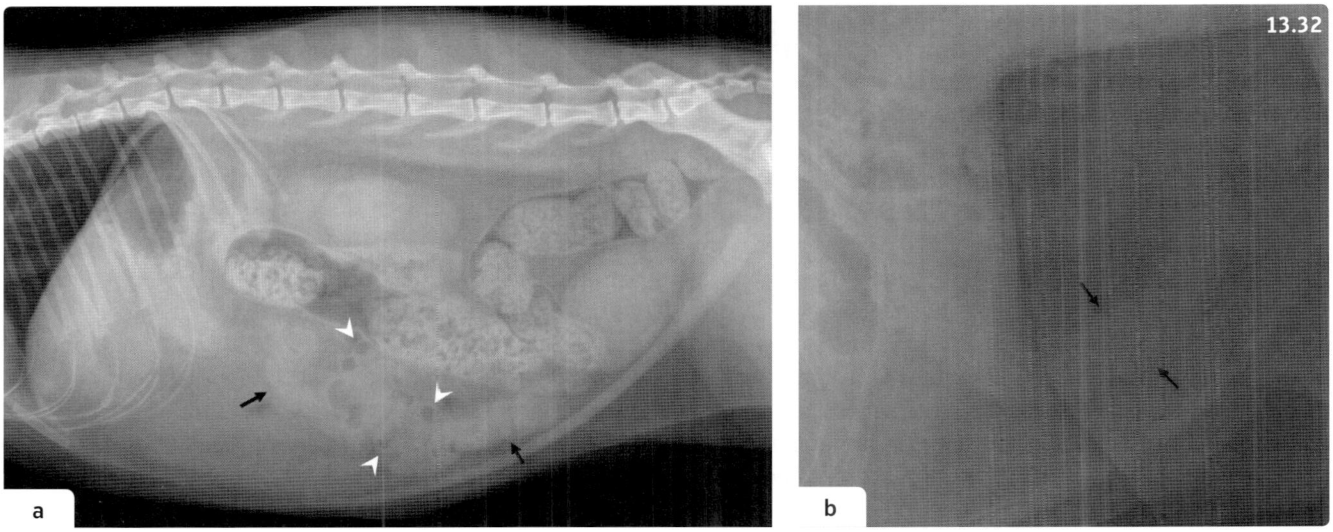

Figures 13.32a, b Lateral abdominal radiograph (a) and magnified compression view (b) in a cat presenting for acute vomiting. The serosal margins of the loops are irregular with a tortuous path (a and b, black arrows). Several, small gas bubbles are trapped within the pleats of the plicated intestinal loops (a, white arrowheads). The plication of small intestines causes an apparent reduction in the number of intestinal loops.

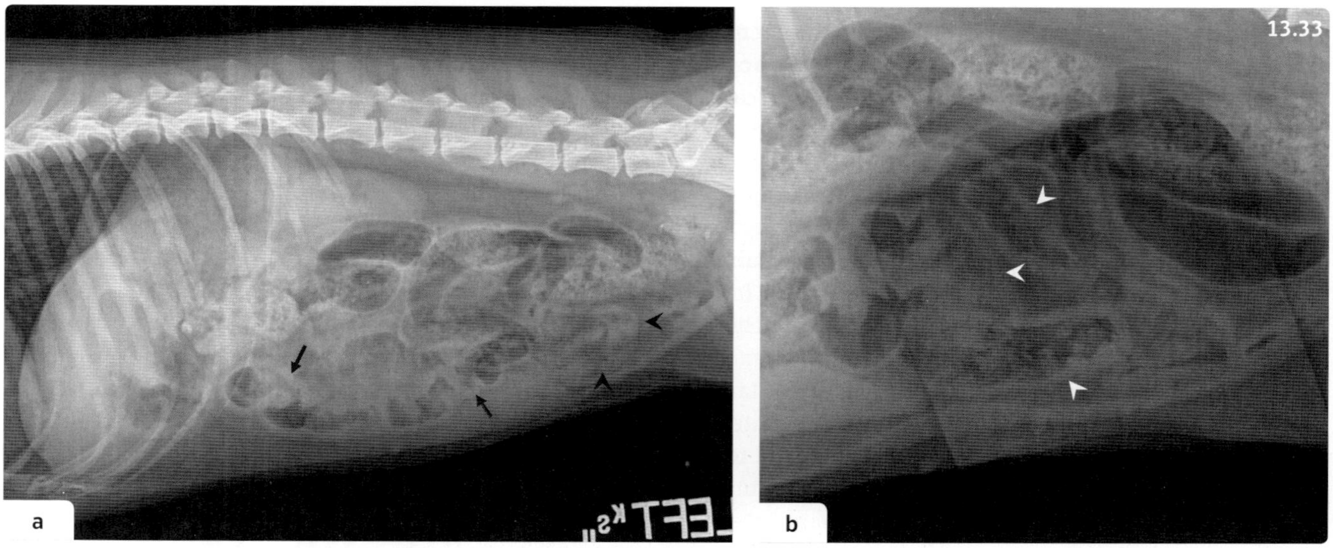

Figures 13.33a, b Lateral abdominal radiograph (a) and magnified compression view (b) in a dog presenting with acute, frequent vomiting. Multiple ventrally located small intestinal loops have a tortuous path (a, black arrows). The loops are also increased in diameter when compared with more normal loops (a, black arrowheads). The luminal content within the tortuous loops is nonhomogeneous (b, white arrowheads), indicating foreign material. An unraveled carpet was removed surgically.

Alterations in colon location, size, and opacity can occur in diseased animals. Colon displacement occurs most commonly due to the abdominal mass effects previously discussed. Mass effects causing concurrent colon displacement and compression with subsequent extramural obstruction occur near the pelvic inlet, usually due to sublumbar lymph node or prostatic enlargement. Abnormal luminal distension is either due to functional or mechanical obstruction. Functional causes of colon enlargement due to nutritional, metabolic, neurologic, or chronic obstructive causes will result in a generalized enlargement of the colon (called megacolon). Mechanical causes of colon dilation result in enlargement orad to the obstruction and can be due to extramural, mural, or luminal causes. The most common location for a mechanical colon obstruction is at the level of the pelvic inlet, therefore generalized megacolon tends to occur with functional or mechanical causes. Alterations in opacity of the colon most typically occur due to changes in luminal content. In animals having diarrhea, the colon will be characterized by a homogeneous gas or fluid opaque lumen rather than the inhomogeneous mixture typically seen with formed feces, making its contents similar in appearance to small intestinal content. Of course, an empty colon will appear soft tissue opaque and will be small in diameter. Colon masses or intussusceptions appear homogeneously soft tissue opaque. In many cases, an interface will occur where the homogeneously opaque obstructive mass or intussusceptum contacts inhomogeneous feces in a dilated colon (**Figure 13.34**). In most cases, when foreign material is positively located within the colon, surgical intervention is not required. Therefore, the interpreter must ascertain the origin of any radiopaque foreign objects or structured appearing materials prior to deciding on a treatment plan. In some cases, contrast procedures are needed to confirm the exact location of suspicious material or a distended loop of intestine (pneumocolonography using room air is very useful to delineate the true location of the colon).

Pancreas

The right pancreatic limb borders the duodenum, the pancreatic body is located near the cranial duodenal flexure, and the left pancreatic limb borders the greater curvature of the stomach. The pancreas is never identified radiographically in the normal dog. Occasionally, in fat cats, the pancreas can be seen as an indistinct soft tissue opacity located between the gastric fundus, left kidney, and the spleen. Pancreatic diseases most often produce clinical GI signs. Rarely, radiographically visible changes are seen with pancreatic disease; however, radiographs are still recommended to assist with ruling out other potential causes of clinical signs. On occasions where radiographic changes of pancreatic disease are present, it will typically manifest as a loss in peritoneal detail (focal

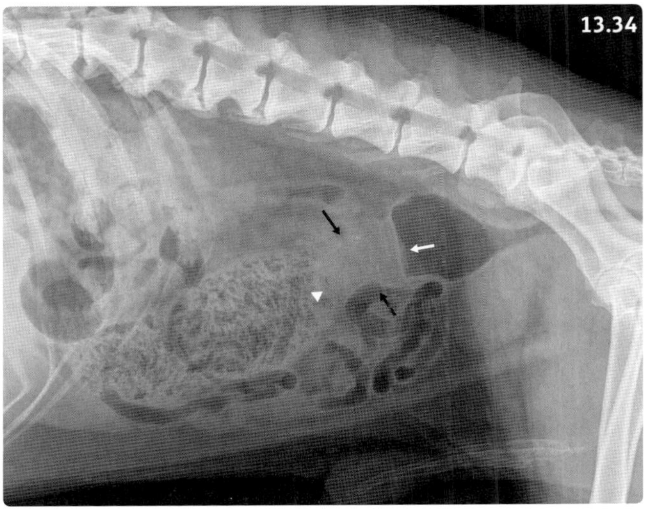

Figure 13.34 Lateral abdominal radiograph in a dog straining to defecate. The descending colon is markedly distended, causing it to be ventrally located in the abdomen. A portion of the colon is nearly homogeneously soft tissue opaque (between black arrows). Homogeneous soft tissue opacity is unexpected in a colon that is distended with fecal material. The cranial aspect of the soft tissue opacity interfaces with more typical inhomogeneous soft tissue and gas opaque fecal content (white arrowhead). The caudal aspect of the soft tissue opacity has a well-defined, flat interface with gas (white arrow). This configuration indicates gas highlighting a luminal structure. A circumferential colonic wall mass was found on abdominal ultrasound. Colonic adenocarcinoma was diagnosed on aspiration.

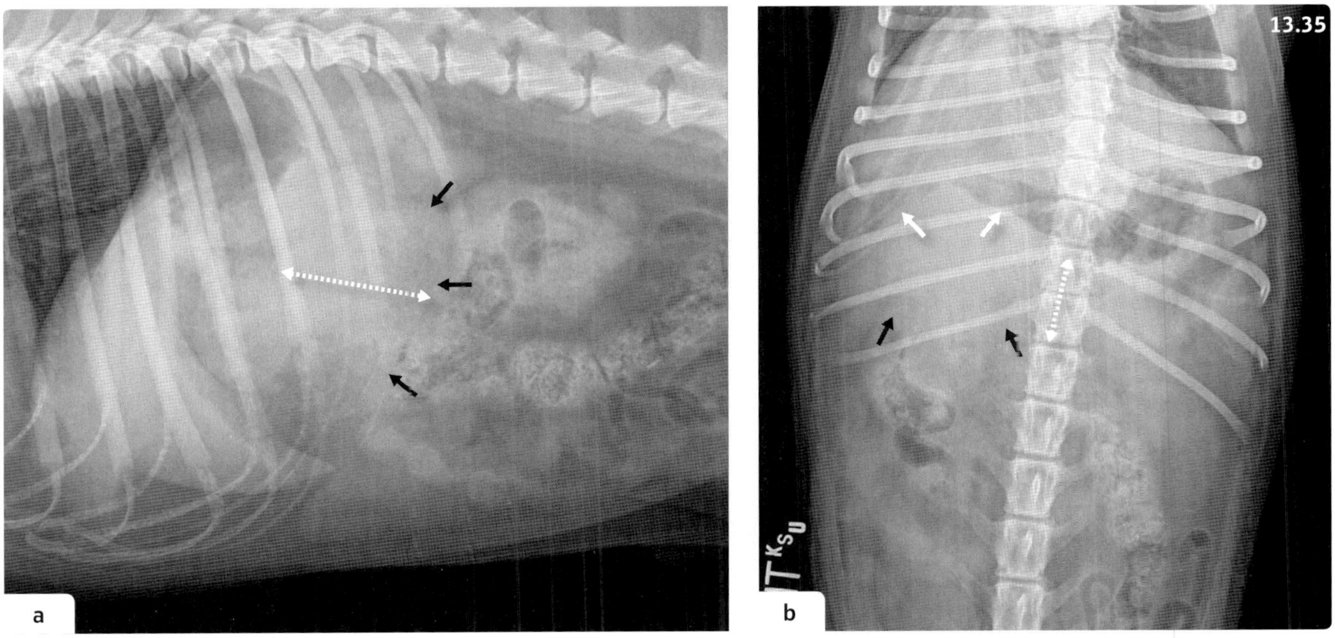

Figures 13.35a, b Lateral (a) and ventrodorsal (b) abdominal radiographs in a dog with acute pancreatitis. A focal loss of detail is present in the cranial abdomen, with an indistinct increase in soft tissue opacity in the right cranial abdomen (black arrows). The gastric body and pyloric antrum are cranially displaced and compressed with increased left-sided positioning of the stomach (white arrows). There is increased distance between the stomach and the transverse colon (dotted white line).

or diffuse), a right cranial abdominal mass effect, separation of the stomach from the transverse colon, and/or dilation of the stomach and the duodenum due to functional ileus (**Figures 13.35a, b**). The right cranial abdominal mass effect classically causes leftward displacement of the gastric body with rightward displacement of the duodenum towards the body wall. Additionally, the intestines are pushed caudally. Acute pancreatitis is the most common cause of a mass effect associated with the pancreas; however, pancreatic abscesses, pseudocysts, and neoplasms can have a similar appearance. Additionally, other organs of origin for a right cranial abdominal mass, such as liver, gallbladder, and duodenum, must be considered.

SUMMARY

When beginning a review of each study, the focus should be on systematic evaluation of each organ, keeping in mind those organs not normally seen radiographically. Also, an attempt should be made to increase the diagnostic usefulness of abdominal radiography with compression and positional views, and contrast procedures as warranted. When radiographs fail to diagnose or definitively rule out disease in a clinical patient, referral for abdominal ultrasound or computed tomography may be warranted.

RECOMMENDED FURTHER READING

Dennis R, Kirkberger RM, Wrigley RH *et al.* (2001) *Handbook of Small Animal Radiological Differential Diagnosis*. WB Saunders, London.

Kealy JK, McAllister H, Graham JP (2011) *Diagnostic Radiology and Ultrasonography of the Dog and Cat*. WB Saunders, St. Louis.

O'Brien TR (1978) *Radiographic Diagnosis of Abdominal Disorders in the Dog and Cat: Radiographic Interpretation, Clinical Signs, Pathophysiology*. WB Saunders, Philadelphia.

Thrall DE (2013) *Textbook of Veterinary Diagnostic Radiology*, 6th edn. WB Saunders, St. Louis.

Chapter 14

Disorders of the nervous system and muscle

Simon R. Platt

DISORDERS OF THE BRAIN

Introduction

Diseases of the forebrain (cerebrum and thalamus) are very complex and may affect the whole of the central nervous system (CNS). In veterinary medicine, the clinical symptoms of brain dysfunction can be relatively mild despite being often associated with a severe lesion. Dogs and cats with forebrain dysfunction may exhibit clinical signs that include altered mental status (obtundation more likely than stupor or coma), behavioral changes, circling in a wide arc, head-pressing, visual impairment, focal and/or generalized seizure activity, and hemi-inattention (unilateral hemineglect) syndrome. Conscious proprioceptive deficits with a normal to near-normal gait are characteristic of forebrain dysfunction. Neck pain may be appreciable in some patients with structural brain lesions. Lesions from the midbrain (mesencephalon) through the medulla (myelencephalon) may lead to altered mental status (stupor or coma more likely than with forebrain lesions), proprioceptive and gait abnormalities, deficits in cranial nerves (CNs) III–XII, and central vestibular dysfunction.

Neurodiagnostic investigation

Depending on the localization of the disease, appropriate diagnostic tests should be performed to rule in or out each disease on the differential diagnosis list. Sometimes, the underlying disorder is evident, such as with cranial trauma; however, all too often animals with brain disease can present a diagnostic challenge. If the animal presents in a coma, emergency evaluation of airway patency and vital signs including cardiac function and respiration should be undertaken, as for animals with head trauma. The important aspects of the evaluation of animals with brain disease include:

- Response to noxious stimulation.
- The presence of voluntary motor movement.
- Posture (i.e. decerebrate rigidity).
- Pupillary reactivity to light.
- Eye movements (physiologic nystagmus).
- Segmental spinal reflexes.

This evaluation is very similar to that of the patient with severe head trauma and in some respects the Modified Glasgow Coma Scale (GCS) system may be useful, although it has not been universally utilized or validated. Unless the diagnosis is established from the history (e.g. toxin ingestion), further testing is usually necessary:

- Routine laboratory analysis is essential – the minimal acceptable information should include packed cell volume (PCV), total protein concentration, blood urea nitrogen (BUN), electrolytes, and glucose concentrations.
- Urinalysis and urine production rate should be assessed, which may necessitate urethral catheterization.
- Liver function tests.
- Thoracic and abdominal radiographs may be useful to supplement physical examination findings.
- Cerebrospinal fluid (CSF) analysis is indicated primarily to confirm an inflammatory lesion. Although such analysis is rarely specific, when it is assessed in conjunction with the patient's signalment, history, neurologic signs, and the results of other diagnostic tests (such as serologic assays) it can help to better define the underlying etiology. If there is evidence or even a suspicion of increased intracranial pressure (ICP) (anisocoria, lack of pupil response to light, reduced or absent physiologic nystagmus, decreased or absent response to noxious stimulation), diagnostic imaging should be performed prior to cisterna magna or lumbar puncture, which risks promoting further herniation. In these cases, reducing the ICP using mannitol (0.5–2.0 g/kg IV) should be considered.
- Advanced imaging studies such as computed tomography (CT) and magnetic resonance imaging (MRI) are strongly indicated to assess the integrity of the intracranial structures.
- An electroencephalogram (EEG) records the electrical activity associated with forebrain structures. An EEG is rarely specific and with certain cerebral conditions it also lacks sensitivity. Although rarely used as a diagnostic tool, electroencephalography can provide

confirmation of brain death (flat or isoelectric EEG). However, other factors, such as patient body temperature, concurrent drug administration, and cardiac function, must be considered before brain death is diagnosed.

VASCULAR DISEASE

Definition/overview

Cerebrovascular disease refers to any abnormality of the brain caused by a pathologic process compromising blood supply. Pathologic processes that may result in cerebrovascular disease include occlusion of the lumen by a thrombus or embolus, rupture of a blood vessel wall, a lesion or altered permeability of the vessel wall, and increased viscosity or other changes in the quality of the blood. Stroke or cerebrovascular accident is the most common clinical presentation of cerebrovascular disease and is defined as a sudden onset of nonprogressive focal brain signs secondary to cerebrovascular disease.

Etiology

Vascular disturbances of the nervous system can arise due to a loss of adequate blood supply (ischemia/infarct) or hemorrhage into the nervous tissue. The initial process is focal in the majority of cases. However, it is possible with a disturbance in systemic perfusion that there is a multifocal, diffuse hemorrhagic process in the brain with a subsequent multifocal course. Vascular damage to the nervous system can be due to various different causes such as neoplasia, endocrine diseases, CNS infections, atherosclerosis, carcinogenic emboli, vasospasm, hematologic disturbances, vasculitis, hyperviscosity syndrome, hypertension, coagulopathy, disseminated intravascular coagulation, or sepsis.

Pathophysiology

Ischemia means the reduction of the blood flow to a level that is not compatible with normal function. An infarct is a large and continual reduction in the blood flow resulting in tissue necrosis. Hypoxia/ischemia initially particularly affects the most sensitive elements of the tissue and then subsequently disturbs all the tissue components. The main mechanism of cell damage found in an infarct is a reduced energy metabolism.

Spontaneous intracranial hemorrhage is caused by a bleed within the brain or in its immediate surroundings without accompanying trauma. A brain hemorrhage can be epidural, subarachnoidal, intraparenchymal, or intraventricular. Epi- or subdural hemorrhages are always associated with cranial trauma. Although not well documented, hypertension appears to play a role in the development of primary intraparenchymal hemorrhage in the dog and cat. Secondary intraparenchymal hemorrhages are associated with reperfusion disturbances after infarcts, congenital arteriovenous malformations, intracranial tumors, and coagulopathies. The damage to the brain is the result of compression or destruction of the surrounding brain tissue. In addition, reduced blood flow to the brain, increased ICP, and obstructive hydrocephalus can be the consequence of an intracranial hemorrhage.

Clinical presentation

Generally, cerebrovascular diseases start suddenly and have a nonprogressive course. The brain dysfunction due to an infarct is usually focal. The neurologic deficits depend on the size of the lesion and are usually asymmetrical. The forebrain symptoms are mainly seizures, possibly in clusters, with contralateral visual and proprioceptive deficits. Behavioral changes are common and involve compulsive pacing, disorientation, and sudden attacks of anxiety or aggression. Ipsilateral circling or head tilt can often be seen.

Differential diagnosis

Head trauma, neoplasia, CNS inflammation.

Diagnosis

Complete blood count (CBC), biochemistry profile, coagulation tests, and a urinalysis are helpful in excluding renal disease, sepsis, hyperviscosity syndrome, or coagulopathy. Assessment of systemic blood pressure at several time points is vital. Endocrine evaluations may be necessary if an endocrine association is suspected based on clinical evaluation of the patient. Thoracic and abdominal imaging is important to consider to rule out cavity neoplasia. Electrocardiography and an ultrasonographic investigation of the heart may be necessary to diagnose heart disease, although this is a rare association in veterinary medicine.

The most useful specific diagnostic methods are imaging techniques such as CT or MRI. Abnormal changes in patients with brain infarcts can be visualized with CT within a few hours. These changes depend on the age of the lesion and are normally shown as a slightly hypodense region. An increase in contrast can occur after a few days in the periphery of the lesion and reflects the capillary proliferation. CT is a sensitive method of imaging acute hemorrhages. These appear as hyperdense regions, which become more demarcated over the next 72 hours and attain a constant pattern after roughly 4 weeks.

In MRI, an infarct is hypointense in T1-weighted sequences and hyperintense in T2-weighted sequences (**Figures 14.1a–e**). These changes can already be seen an

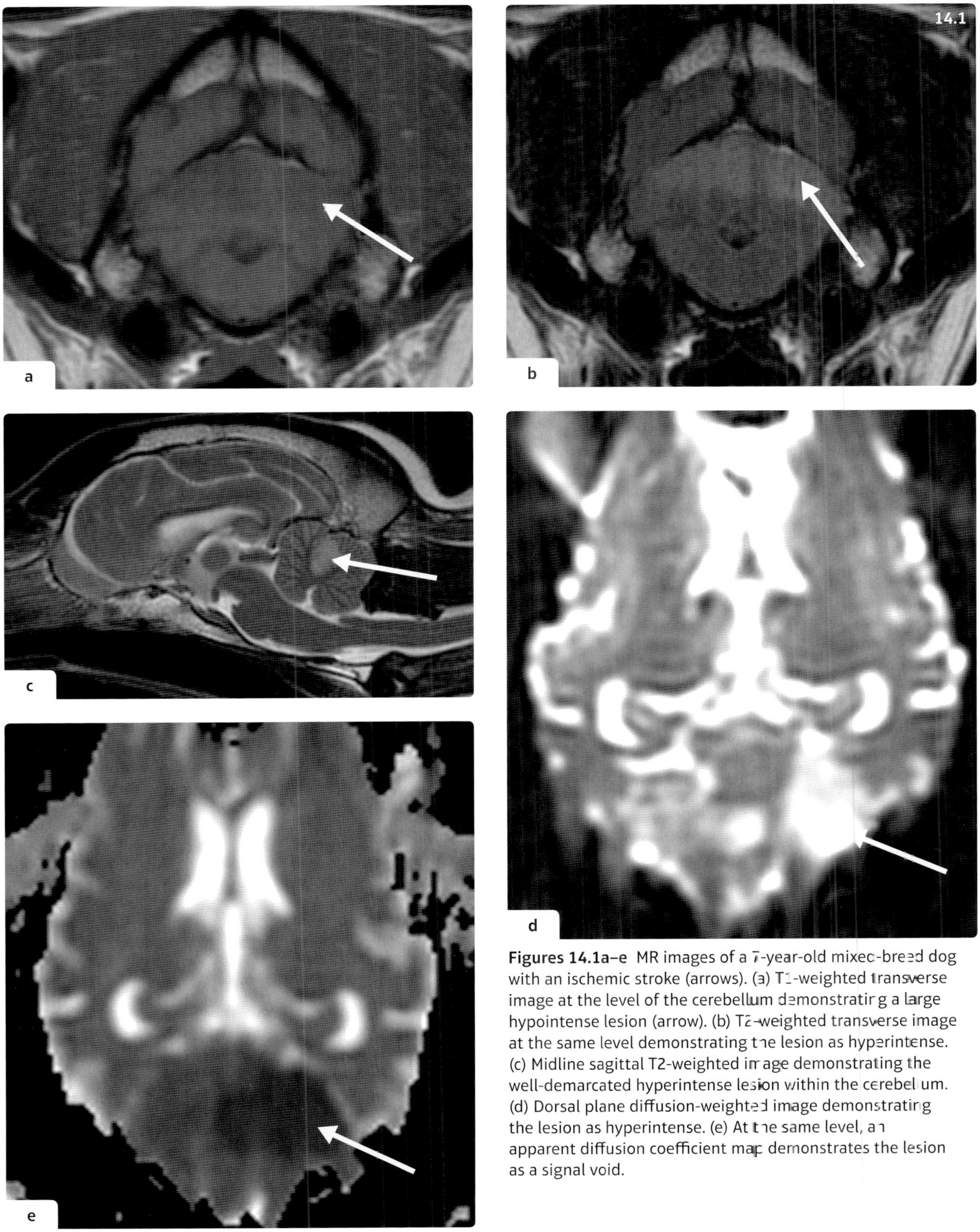

Figures 14.1a–e MR images of a 7-year-old mixed-breed dog with an ischemic stroke (arrows). (a) T1-weighted transverse image at the level of the cerebellum demonstrating a large hypointense lesion (arrow). (b) T2-weighted transverse image at the same level demonstrating the lesion as hyperintense. (c) Midline sagittal T2-weighted image demonstrating the well-demarcated hyperintense lesion within the cerebellum. (d) Dorsal plane diffusion-weighted image demonstrating the lesion as hyperintense. (e) At the same level, an apparent diffusion coefficient map demonstrates the lesion as a signal void.

hour after the start of the infarct, meaning that MRI is more sensitive for the visualization of an infarct than CT. In comparison, the depiction of a hemorrhage with MRI is more complicated and depends on the age of the lesion. As infarct and hemorrhage can occur at the same time, CT is often preferred in the acute stages to differentiate between these two different types of disease.

Management

Treatment of dogs with ischemic events to the brain is largely supportive. The aim of the treatment is to ensure an adequate oxygen supply to the tissue, to treat neurological problems and the causative disease.

Oxygen supplementation is often enough in many cases. Hypovolemia should be treated with fluids, although administration of large volumes of crystalloids should be avoided as this causes a worsening of cerebral edema and can increase the ICP. Diazepam (0.5–1.0 mg/kg IV) and barbiturates (phenobarbital 2–5 mg/kg PO q12h) can be used to control seizure activity and reduce the brain metabolism.

The prognosis for dogs with focal brain infarcts is variable, but most have a guarded to fair prognosis for recovery of partial or full function.

ANOMALOUS/DEVELOPMENTAL DISORDERS

CONGENITAL HYDROCEPHALUS

Definition/overview

Hydrocephalus is the term used to describe a condition of abnormal dilatation of the ventricular system within the brain. It can be further subdivided into obstructive and nonobstructive types. Ventricular dilatation occurs with some frequency in dogs and cats due to a variety of intracranial disease processes. Some breeds are predisposed to congenital hydrocephalus, including Chihuahuas, Pomeranians, Yorkshire Terriers, English Bulldogs, Lhasa Apsos, Toy Poodles, Cairn Terriers, Boston Terriers, Pugs, Pekingese, and Maltese.

Etiology

Hydrocephalus can result from:

- Obstruction (intraventricular or extraventricular) of the ventricular system (e.g. brain tumor).
- Increased size of the ventricles due to loss of brain parenchyma (hydrocephalus *ex vacuo*).
- No obvious cause (congenital).
- The overproduction of CSF associated with a choroid plexus tumor (rare).
- Obstruction of CSF flow in cats as a result of ependymitis and vasculitis associated with CNS infection with feline coronavirus (which causes feline infectious peritonitis [FIP]).

Pathophysiology

Diffuse ventricular enlargement suggests congenital ventricular dilatation or obstruction at the level of the lateral apertures or foramen magnum. Focal ventricular enlargement suggests focal obstruction or loss of parenchymal cells. It is not uncommon to have asymmetrical bilateral lateral ventricle enlargement. Animals with an asymmetrical appearance of the ventricles should be critically evaluated for focal obstruction of, or impingement on, the ventricular system due to mass effect. Elevation of ICP associated with hydrocephalus can occur in cases of acute severe obstruction to CSF flow or chronically enlarged ventricles with little cortical mantle remaining to absorb pressure.

Initial pathologic changes are found in the ependyma at the angles of the lateral ventricles. Loss of integrity of the ependymal surface allows water to leak into the periventricular white matter, causing edema. Further enlargement of the ventricles causes direct damage to the white matter due to compression. Treatment needs to be considered prior to damage affecting the cerebral cortex.

Clinical presentation

Hydrocephalus can result in clinical signs due to loss of neurons or neuronal function and/or alterations in ICP and all of its consequences. Clinical signs of hydrocephalus can reflect the anatomic level of disease involvement or can represent a diffuse disease process. The severity of the clinical signs is not necessarily dependent on the degree of ventricular dilatation, but rather on a host of concurrent abnormalities including the underlying disease process, associated ICP changes, intraventricular hemorrhage, and the acuity of ventricular obstruction. In animals with severe hydrocephalus, the compressed layer of cortex is prone to tearing either spontaneously or with minor trauma, causing a sudden onset of focal signs of forebrain disease.

In young dogs prior to ossification of the cranial sutures, hydrocephalus may contribute to abnormalities of skull development such as a thinning of the bone structure, a dome-shaped or bossed appearance to the head (**Figure 14.2**), or a persistent fontanelle.

A ventral and/or lateral strabismus has been noted in humans and animals with hydrocephalus. This is sometimes referred to as the 'setting sun sign'. Confusion remains as to the underlying reason for this clinical finding. It has been suggested that this appearance is associated with skull deformity and distortion of the orbits. Others suggest that because this abnormality can be improved with shunting of the lateral and third ventricles, the strabismus is associated with pressure on the mesencephalic tegmentum.

As a result of the involvement of the forebrain and brainstem structures in hydrocephalus, alterations in awareness and cognition are common. Many congenitally affected animals may appear less intelligent than normal and be difficult to house train. In addition to alterations in consciousness, aggression, circling, paresis, and seizures may also be seen. Central visual dysfunction can occur with compression of the optic radiations and occipital cortex.

Occasionally, when hydrocephalus is associated with fourth ventricle enlargement, there may be pronounced vestibular dysfunction.

Differential diagnosis

Lissencephaly, hepatic (metabolic) encephalopathy.

Diagnosis

The diagnosis of hydrocephalus is aided by information obtained from a variety of imaging and electrophysiologic studies. Historical invasive techniques (such as pneumoventriculography and contrast ventriculography) have been replaced by noninvasive evaluations

Ultrasonography can be used to diagnose hydrocephalus (**Figure 14.3**). This is most readily accomplished when a fontanelle is present, as it provides an acoustic window (ultrasound waves do not adequately penetrate the skull). In general, correlation between the degree of ventricular enlargement and clinical signs is poor. CT is often useful for defining ventricular size. The ventricular system is usually readily identifiable due to its relatively dark signal in comparison with the parenchyma. CT evaluation also affords the ability to examine the majority of the ventricular system as well as additional intracranial structures. MRI also affords evaluation of the ventricular system (**Figure 14.4**). It is now recognized that many toy breeds that are predisposed to hydrocephalus also have anomalies such as Chiari-like malformations, which can potentially complicate their management and are only detected on MRI.

Management

Although the prognosis for resolution of hydrocephalus is uncertain, there are several medical and surgical options that may be beneficial. The choice of treatment

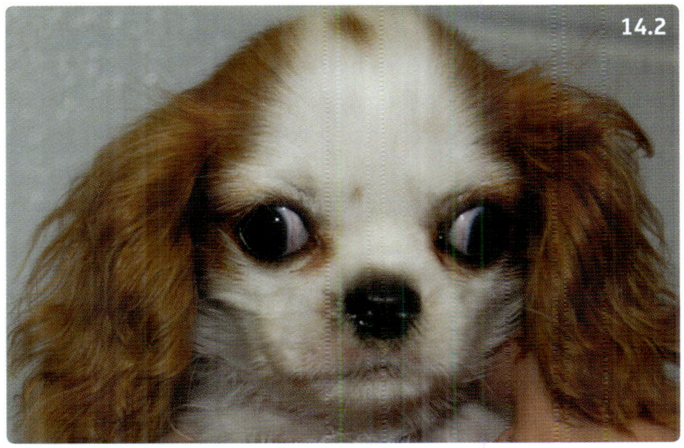

Figure 14.2 A 2-year-old Cavalier King Charles Spaniel with a domed skull due to its underlying hydrocephalus.

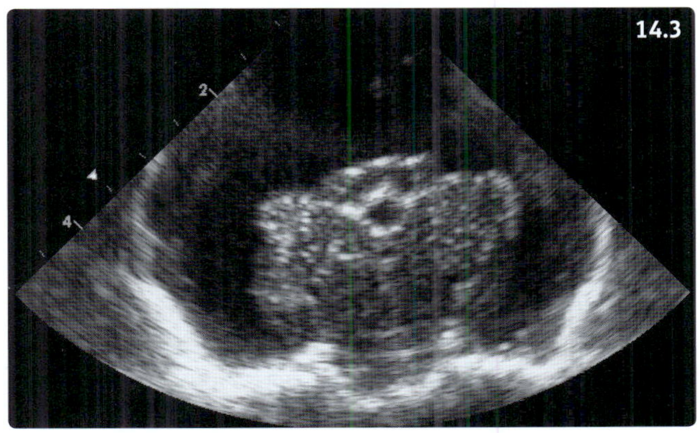

Figure 14.3 Ultrasound of the cerebral cavity reveals extensive ventricular volume as a hypoechoic (dark) signal within the more hyperechoic parenchyma.

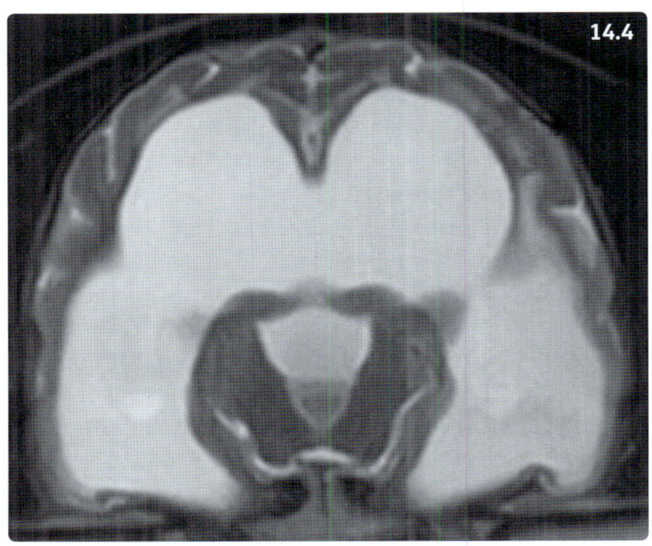

Figure 14.4 T2-weighted transverse MR image at the level of the brainstem depicts large lateral ventricles hyperintense to the surrounding parenchyma.

is generally dictated by physical status, age of the animal, and cause of the hydrocephalus. Medical treatment may include general supportive care and drugs to limit CSF production and reduce ICP. Surgical treatment is designed to provide drainage of CSF from the brain to another site for absorption. Glucocorticoids are often used for medical treatment. Prednisone may be given (0.25–0.5 mg/kg PO q12h, then gradually reduced at weekly intervals to 0.1 mg/kg PO q48h). This dose is continued for at least 1 month, after which time it is discontinued, if possible. Some animals can be adequately managed with long-term glucocorticoid administration at low doses. If no clinical benefits are observed within 2 weeks, or if side-effects develop, other forms of therapy should be tried. Acetazolamide (a carbonic anhydrase inhibitor) is thought to reduce CSF pressure by decreasing CSF production. Its effectiveness in treating hydrocephalus is inconsistent. Omeprazole has also been administered for the treatment of clinical signs related to hydrocephalus; however, positive outcomes are also inconsistent.

Surgery is generally required for those animals that do not improve within 2 weeks, if deterioration occurs during corticosteroid therapy, or if there is an obstructive cause such as a tumor that cannot be resected. As a successful outcome may be more likely in animals that have minimal clinical signs, surgery may be appropriate in animals with a VB (height of ventricle to height of brain) ratio >60%, although, few owners are willing to undergo the expense and risk of shunt placement if their dog appears healthy. Ventriculoperitoneal shunts are most commonly used in small animals. Complications of shunt placement occur in approximately 20% of cases.

CHIARI-LIKE MALFORMATION SYNDROME

Definition/overview

Chiari-like malformation syndrome (CLMS) is the canine analog of Chiari type I malformation of people. Although only recently described in dogs, CLMS appears to be a very common neurologic disorder in this species. This disease is almost exclusive to small breed dogs, with the Cavalier King Charles Spaniel (CKCS) being the most overrepresented. Other breeds commonly encountered with CLMS include Brussels Griffon, Miniature/Toy Poodle, Yorkshire Terrier, Maltese, Pug, Pomeranian, and Pekingese.

Etiology

The disorder is a congenital malformation of the suboccipital bone, leading to overcrowding of the caudal fossa and compression of the cervicomedullary junction at the level of the foramen magnum. There is convincing evidence in the CKCS breed that CLMS is a heritable disease, although the exact mode of inheritance has not been determined.

Pathophysiology

Progressive alterations in pressure dynamics between the intracranial and spinal compartments are believed to be responsible for the development of clinical signs of CLMS. Although aberrant pressure dynamics due to obstruction of CSF pathways at the level of the foramen magnum are generally agreed to cause syringomyelia in CLMS, the exact mechanism of this development is unknown and there are multiple theories proposed to explain it. Newer theories suggest that the syringomyelia fluid is actually derived from extracellular fluid from the cord itself, either driven into the central canal via a pulse pressure wave from behind the foramen magnum obstruction and/or drawn into the central canal via a centrifugally directed hydrostatic pressure force within the spinal cord. Common to all theories of syrinx development in CLMS is the causative factor of obstruction of normal CSF flow at the foramen magnum.

The clinical sign of scratching activity is believed to be due to the syrinx interfering with spinothalamic tracts and/or dorsal horn neurons, resulting in abnormal sensations (dysesthesia/paresthesia). Scoliosis (torticollis) is most likely due to asymmetric syrinx damage to sensory proprioceptive neurons innervating cervical musculature; an alternative, less likely, hypothesis is syrinx damage to lower motor neurons (LMNs) innervating cervical musculature.

Clinical presentation

Most dogs with CLMS are presented for evaluation as young adults, between 3 and 6 years of age. However, the age range for this disorder is very broad, ranging from less than 6 months to more than 12 years of age. Dogs that are presented at <2 years of age often have more severe clinical signs than older dogs. There is a wide spectrum of possible neurologic presentations for dogs with CLMS, including cervical myelopathy, cerebellovestibular dysfunction, and forebrain dysfunction (e.g. seizure activity). Cervical dysfunction and cerebellovestibular dysfunction are the most common and are often both present (e.g. multifocal CNS disease). Some specific clinical findings in dogs with CLMS include cervical and cranial hyperesthesia, forelimb weakness, hindlimb ataxia, persistent scratching (at the head, neck, and shoulder region, often without making skin contact), scoliosis, and facial nerve paresis/paralysis (unilateral or bilateral).

Scratching activity and neck discomfort often are exacerbated by stress or excitement, and physical contact with the neck/shoulder region (e.g. collar).

Diagnosis

Consistent findings on MR imaging indicative of CLMS are attenuation/obliteration of the dorsal subarachnoid space at the cervicomedullary junction and rostral displacement of the caudal cerebellum by the suboccipital bone (**Figure 14.5**). Other common MRI findings in CLMS include syringomyelia (usually C2 level caudally), herniation of the caudal cerebellum through the foramen magnum, and a 'kinked' appearance of the caudal medulla. In the absence of concurrent disease processes, CSF analysis is usually normal; occasionally, a mild mononuclear pleocytosis may be apparent.

Management

Treatment of CLMS can be divided into medical and surgical therapy. Medical therapy generally falls into three categories: analgesic drugs (implies relief of dysesthesia/paresthesia also), drugs that decrease CSF production, and corticosteroid therapy. By far the most useful drug available for relief of the scratching activity associated with syringomyelia is gabapentin (10 mg/kg PO q8h). Orally administered opioid drugs are sometimes helpful in alleviating neck and head pain in CLMS dogs. A number of drugs aimed at decreasing CSF production have been used in CLMS patients in an effort to diminish the CSF pulse pressure. They include omeprazole (a proton pump inhibitor), acetazolamide (a carbonic anhydrase inhibitor), and furosemide (a loop diuretic). Corticosteroids are often used in medical management of CLMS. An initial anti-inflammatory prednisone dose of 0.5 mg/kg PO q12h is often effective in controlling clinical signs. In most cases of CLMS, medical therapy will diminish the severity of clinical signs, but resolution is unlikely. The preferred surgical procedure for treatment of CLMS in dogs is foramen magnum decompression.

INTRACRANIAL ARACHNOID CYST (DIVERTICULUM)

Definition and overview

Intracranial arachnoid cyst (IAC) (also termed intra-arachnoid cyst) is a developmental brain disorder in which CSF is thought to accumulate within a split of the arachnoid membrane. All reported canine cases have been in the caudal fossa. Because IAC is typically associated with the quadrigeminal cistern in dogs, these accumulations of fluid are often called quadrigeminal cysts in this species. The vast majority of reported IAC cases in dogs have been small breeds, with a predominance of brachycephalic dogs.

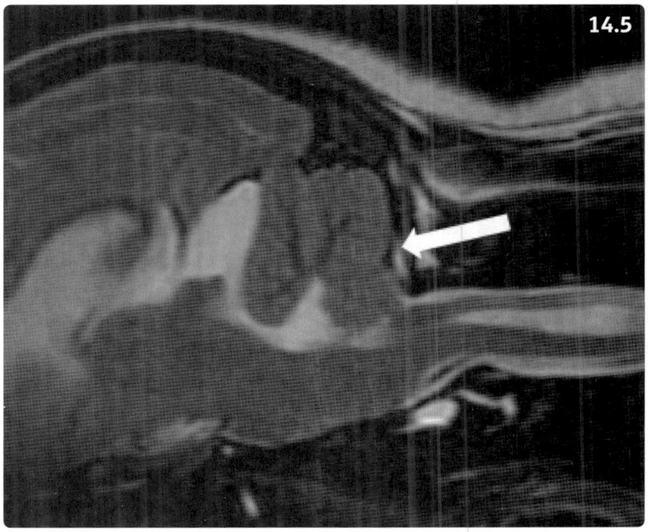

Figure 14.5 T2-weighted sagittal MR image of the brain and skull of a Brussels Griffon dog; the arrow points to a hypoplastic occipital bone, which is causing compression and herniation of the cerebellum through the foramen magnum classic for Chiari-like malformation in dogs.

Etiology

The cause of this developmental anomaly is unknown.

Pathophysiology

It is believed that some aberration of CSF flow from the choroid plexuses during development forces a separation within the forming arachnoid layer, eventually leading to the creation of an IAC. The mechanisms by which an IAC continues to expand with fluid are unknown. Fluid may be secreted by the arachnoid cells lining the cyst cavity.

Clinical presentation

There is a wide age range at clinical presentation for dogs with IAC (2 months to 10 years), with an approximate average age of 4 years. The most common clinical signs seen with IAC are forebrain (including seizure activity) and/or central vestibular (cerebellovestibular) dysfunction. Dogs may also present with a primary complaint of neck pain. They can be incidental findings.

Differential diagnosis

Hydrocephalus, congenital portosystemic shunt, hepatic encephalopathy, infectious CNS disease, toxicities.

Diagnosis

Diagnosis is typically made via CT or (preferably) MRI (**Figure 14.6**). IACs can also be visualized using ultrasound imaging (via foramen magnum, temporal window, and/or persistent bregmatic fontanelle), especially in younger dogs. The characteristic appearance of an IAC is a large, well-demarcated, fluid-filled structure, isointense with the CSF spaces and located between the caudal cerebrum and rostral cerebellum. Because IAC may be an incidental finding, it is important to rule out concurrent inflammatory disease (i.e. by using CSF examination).

Management

Medical treatment for IAC is identical to that described for congenital hydrocephalus (see above) (e.g. corticosteroids, diuretics, anticonvulsants if indicated). Dogs with an IAC tend to respond initially to medical therapy, but the response is often temporary. Surgical management of IACs is typically either achieved via cyst fenestration or cystoperitoneal shunt placement.

DEGENERATIVE DISEASES

INHERITED NEURODEGENERATIVE DISEASES

Definition/overview

Neurodegenerative diseases can affect any part of the nervous system and commonly result in dysfunction of the brain. Examples include multisystem neuronal degeneration of Cocker Spaniels, spongiform degenerations in Labrador Retrievers, Samoyeds, Silky Terriers, Dalmatians (cavitating leukodystrophy), mixed-breed dogs and Egyptian Mau kittens, and multisystemic chromatolytic neuronal degeneration in Cairn Terriers.

Etiology

The likely etiology for many of these diseases is genetic, although it has not been elucidated in most of them.

Pathophysiology

Storage diseases are due to an inborn error of metabolism and the absence of a vital enzyme necessary to break down endogenous body substances. These substances then accumulate within the neuron or other cells associated with the nervous system and eventually cause cellular dysfunction (**Figure 14.7**). The numerous storage diseases of small animals have been reviewed in detail in other publications (see Recommended further reading).

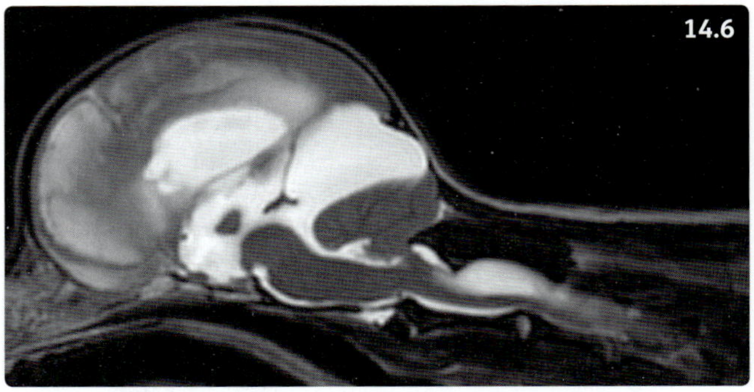

Figure 14.6 Sagittal T2-weighted midline brain MR image of a 2-year-old toy breed dog with a large cyst dorsal to and compressing the cerebellum and brainstem.

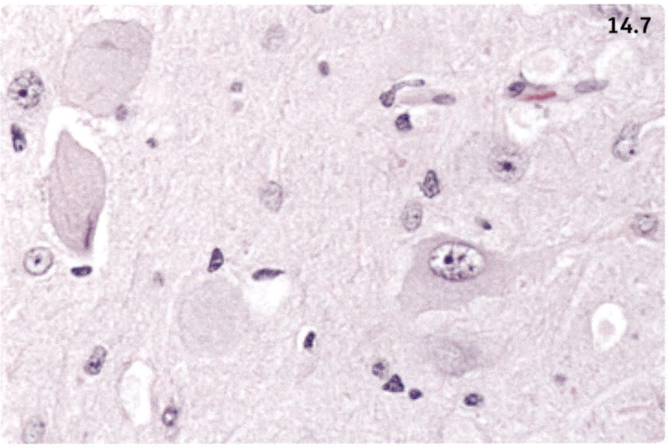

Figure 14.7 Intracytoplasmic storage material in the majority of the neurons of the trigeminal ganglion of a dog with GM2 storage disease. The tissue is stained with hematoxylin and eosin.

Clinical presentation

The majority of degenerative diseases involving the nervous system result in clinical signs early in life, usually with an onset at <1 year of age. Many are breed related and presumed inherited. Clinical signs are slowly progressive with severe alterations in consciousness occurring relatively late in the disease course. Most diseases cause multifocal neurologic signs and many affect the cerebellum.

Differential diagnosis

Hydrocephalus, congenital portosystemic shunt, hepatic encephalopathy, infectious CNS disease, toxicities.

Diagnosis

Antemortem diagnosis requires biopsy of the affected tissue. Determination of the lysosomal enzyme activity within the brain and other cells may be helpful, but is not universally clinically available.

Screening blood and urine for accumulation products indicative of inborn errors of metabolism may suggest the presence of a lysosomal storage disease, and in some cases can be diagnostic. Depending on the disease, abnormal accumulations may be evident within cells (particularly macrophages) on buffy coat blood smears and in biopsy samples from the liver, spleen, lymph nodes, bone marrow, or nerves. Screening tests performed on fresh urine samples should include evaluation for the following analytes:

- Urinary organic acids. The accumulation of organic acids within the body fluids (particularly urine) is indicative of inborn errors of metabolism such as L-2-hydroxyglutaric aciduria in Staffordshire Bull Terriers.
- Urinary oligosaccharides. The accumulation of mannose-containing oligosaccharides in cats is indicative of mannosidosis. The accumulation of high molecular weight oligosaccharides in dogs and cats is indicative of GM1 and GM2 gangliosidosis, and of fucosidosis in English Springer Spaniels.
- Urinary glycosaminoglycans. The accumulation of dermatan sulfate is indicative of mucopolysaccharidosis (MPS) I, II, VI, and VII. The accumulation of heparin sulfate is indicative of MPS IIIA and IIIB.

Where the signalment and neurologic signs are suggestive of one or more lysosomal storage diseases, and where the underlying enzyme defect is known for those diseases, then an enzyme analysis can be performed against known normal control animals. A reduction in the level of enzyme activity is indicative of that particular lysosomal storage disease. Washed white blood cells or cultured skin fibroblasts are usually the most appropriate cell source and can be assayed either fresh or fresh-frozen.

Characteristic MRI changes may be apparent with some canine and feline genetic diseases, although the changes are rarely specific for a single disease. The lesions usually appear bilaterally symmetrical (e.g. as seen with L-2-hydroxyglutaric aciduria in Staffordshire Bull Terriers) and often result in a decrease in the apparent size of the cerebellum. Fucosidosis in English Springer Spaniels and some of the gangliosidoses can also result in notable MRI abnormalities.

Management

Currently, there is no effective treatment for degenerative diseases of the CNS. Symptomatic therapy, such as anticonvulsants and anti-anxiety drugs, can help alleviate clinical signs, but these diseases are inevitably progressive. Often, helping the owner decide when to elect euthanasia for a dog affected by a slowly progressive brain disease is the most challenging aspect of these diseases.

COGNITIVE DISORDER

Definition/overview

This neurodegenerative syndrome affects older dogs and cats. The frequency of this condition is unknown but it does not seem to affect a specific breed of animal more commonly.

Etiology

There is no specific etiology identified for this condition.

Pathophysiology

The normal aging brain progressively accumulates oxidative damage and other types of neuropathology that ultimately result in neuronal dysfunction and cognitive decline. This syndrome has been likened to the early stages of Alzheimer's disease in humans. In fact, diffuse beta-amyloid plaques may develop in the cerebral cortex in dogs, but the neurofibrillary tangles seen in humans have not been reported in dogs.

Clinical presentation

Affected animals show chronic progressive behavioral abnormalities such as loss of learned behavior, failure to recognize their owners, and disturbed sleep cycles.

Differential diagnosis

Brain tumor, cerebrovascular disease, metabolic encephalopathy, hypertensive encephalopathy.

Diagnosis

Cognitive disorder is diagnosed by excluding other causes of the behavioral abnormalities. However, due to the nonspecific clinical signs associated with this clinical syndrome, it is difficult to make a definitive diagnosis. An extensive evaluation for other causes of intracranial signs in older dogs should be undertaken. Measurement of the interthalamic adhesion thickness using MRI has been suggested as a criterion for the confirmation of brain atrophy in dogs, as it is significantly smaller in older dogs with cognitive dysfunction.

Management

Diets rich in antioxidants have been useful in slowing age-related behavioral changes in experimental colonies of dogs. The use of L-deprenyl has also been advocated. Antidepressant and anti-anxiety medications may be beneficial in the symptomatic management of some animals.

METABOLIC DISEASES

Numerous metabolic abnormalities may alter cerebrocortical and brainstem function. Liver disease (hepatic encephalopathy), renal disease (renal encephalopathy), pancreatic disease (pancreatic encephalopathy), glucose abnormalities (hyperglycemia or hypoglycemia), electrolyte abnormalities (sodium, potassium, chloride, calcium, magnesium), cardiovascular diseases (resulting in ischemia and hypoxia), and acid–base abnormalities are examples of metabolic diseases. Endocrine abnormalities (thyroid hormones and cortisol) may also affect consciousness.

HEPATIC ENCEPHALOPATHY

Definition/overview

When liver function is compromised due to organ failure, hepatic microvascular dysplasia, or portosystemic shunting, CNS signs quickly ensue.

Pathophysiology

Hepatic encephalopathy occurs when numerous putative neurotoxins reach the brain without being metabolized as a result of passing through an abnormally functioning liver. Suspected toxins include neurotransmitters (e.g. gamma-aminobutyric acid [GABA] and glutamate), aromatic amino acids, and ammonia.

Clinical presentation

Animals with hepatic encephalopathy are most often admitted for seizures, ptyalism (especially in cats), and mentation changes, which range from behavioral abnormalities to coma. Signs of hepatic dysfunction, such as weight loss, polydipsia, anorexia, and vomiting, may be present. These animals are often sensitive to the administration of benzodiazepines and barbiturates, as both these types of drug are metabolized by the liver. Overzealous administration of these drugs may result in stupor and coma due to CNS depression.

Differential diagnosis

Hydrocephalus, inflammatory CNS diseases, toxicity, other metabolic encephalopathies.

Diagnosis

The diagnosis of hepatic encephalopathy is supported by abnormal liver function studies such as bile acid testing and resting ammonia levels. Other associated abnormalities may include microcytic red blood cells, low albumin, cholesterol, glucose, and urea concentrations, and elevated liver enzymes if there is parenchymal damage. The preferred imaging studies to confirm a diagnosis of portosystemic shunt include mesenteric portography, abdominal ultrasonography, and per rectal scintigraphy. Transcranial color-coded duplex ultrasonography and MRI have also been used to characterize the brain tissue of animals with hepatic encephalopathy.

Management

Treatment of hepatic encephalopathy aims to:

- Treat the underlying liver disease.
- Treat any associated seizures.
- Reduce the level of hematogenous neurotoxins (e.g. ammonia) or factors that can increase ammonia production (e.g. metabolic alkalosis, hypokalemia, gastrointestinal [GI] bleeding).

A diet of high-quality, low-quantity protein can help to minimize ammonia production in the gut. Lactulose (0.5–1.0 ml/kg PO q8h) is frequently used to assist with this aim as it reduces the amount of colonic ammonia produced and 'traps' ammonia by creating an acidic environment within the gut. Lactulose can also be administered as an enema to comatose patients (1–2 ml/kg q4–6h until loose stool is seen). In addition, neomycin (20 mg/kg PO q8h), ampicillin (22 mg/kg PO q8h), or metronidazole (7.5 mg/kg PO q8h) can be given to reduce the number of urea-splitting bacteria in the colon. Potassium bromide can be used in these cases, but requires load-dosing to rapidly attain steady-state levels. The ideal anticonvulsant to use is levetiracetam (PO, IM or IV). Seizures following surgical ligation of portosystemic shunts can be especially severe and difficult to effectively treat. Cautious use of a constant rate infusion of diazepam or midazolam may be used for status epilepticus in this situation; however, it can be difficult to dose due to the underlying alterations in liver function. Reduced dosages titrated to effect can be helpful but require vigilant patient monitoring and assessment.

HYPOGLYCEMIA

Definition/overview

The neurons in the brain require glucose for energy metabolism. A decrease in the availability of glucose to the brain neurons can cause a constellation of clinical abnormalities.

Etiology

Decreases in the blood glucose level alter intracranial neuronal function.

Pathophysiology

Hypoglycemia can occur secondary to insulinoma, liver disease, hypoadrenocorticism, glycogen storage diseases, insulin overdose in diabetic animals, toxicity (e.g. xylitol), infectious diseases, and extrapancreatic neoplasia. Toy breeds and neonates may become hypoglycemic during times of stress. Some dogs that undertake significant exercise (e.g. hunting dogs) and young animals with metabolic stresses (such as caused by a parasitic infestation) are also at risk of developing hypoglycemia.

Clinical presentation

Hypoglycemia can cause a variety of neurologic signs including anxiety, a ravenous appetite, lethargy or depression, tremors, seizures, and coma. Exercise or fasting may precipitate signs. The speed with which the glucose concentration changes influences signs to a certain extent. A sudden drop in the blood glucose level causes a sympathetic discharge, hence anxiety and hunger, whereas a chronically low glucose concentration causes lethargy. Central blindness is a frequent finding in animals that present with hypoglycemic seizures. This can be a permanent residual deficit if severe damage has occurred.

Differential diagnosis

Hydrocephalus, inflammatory CNS diseases, toxicity, other metabolic encephalopathies.

Diagnosis

Serum glucose concentrations <3.3 mmol/l (<60 mg/dl) accompanied by consistent neurologic signs are suggestive of significant hypoglycemia. If the glucose level decreases slowly, some animals can tolerate a lower concentration (<2 mmol/l; <35 mg/dl) without serious clinical problems. Imaging can be used to demonstrate the presence of a pancreatic mass, which may be one of several types of pathology including insulinoma (beta cell carcinoma).

Management

Treatment depends on the underlying cause. Feeding multiple small meals can help dogs with insulinomas. Direct correction of hypoglycemia is indicated in emergency situations. Syrup can be applied to the gums when IV access is not available (e.g. by owners). It should be noted that if the suspected diagnosis is insulinoma, giving large amounts of glucose, either in the form of a large meal or IV, can sometimes cause a further increase in insulin release into the circulation and exacerbate the problem.

ELECTROLYTE DISTURBANCES

SODIUM ABNORMALITIES

Definition/overview

Both hypernatremia and hyponatremia may affect the CNS and result in abnormalities of mentation.

Etiology

Any cause of an abnormal sodium concentration will result in neurologic dysfunction. Hypernatremia is most extreme in animals with abnormalities of thirst and drinking, which may also be associated with hypothalamic disease.

HYPERNATREMIA

Pathophysiology

Hypernatremia is synonymous with hyperosmolality and can lead to shrinkage of the brain parenchymal cells, which in turn can cause stretching of the small intracranial blood vessels and hemorrhage. After 2–3 days, the brain attempts to compensate for the altered extracellular sodium level by producing osmotically active intracellular substances (idiogenic osmoles). Thus, overly rapid correction of chronic hypernatremia can cause sudden swelling of the brain parenchyma and ultimately be fatal.

Clinical presentation

The clinical signs of hypernatremia include lethargy and irritability progressing to ataxia, tremors, myoclonus, seizures, blindness, coma, and death.

Differential diagnosis

Hydrocephalus, inflammatory CNS diseases, toxicity, other metabolic encephalopathies.

Diagnosis

Demonstration of an abnormal electrolyte level in the presence of an encephalopathy, which improves with appropriate correction, confirms the diagnosis.

Management

Guidelines for the treatment of sodium abnormalities have been suggested but are crude. Appropriate therapy is based on replacement of the water deficit (calculated using the following equation) in conjunction with addressing the underlying cause:

Water deficit (l) = 0.6 × bodyweight (kg) × (patient's sodium concentration/normal sodium concentration -1)

However, calculations such as this are only used as a guide to begin therapy. With chronic serum sodium abnormalities, cautious fluid therapy with frequent monitoring for neurologic deterioration is imperative. In an animal with established hypernatremia, the water deficit should be corrected either orally or by fluid therapy administered conservatively over 2–3 days. An isotonic maintenance fluid (such as lactated Ringer's solution) should be used, initially at 1.5 times the normal maintenance rate. Serum sodium concentrations should be monitored every 4–6 hours and the rate of fluid therapy administration adjusted up or down accordingly. If the serum sodium concentration is lowered too rapidly, cerebral edema may result, with a clinical deterioration in consciousness. With slow onset hypernatremia (occurs over 48 hours or more), the maximal daily decrease with treatment should not exceed 0.5 mEq/hour or 8–12 mEq/l per 24 hours.

HYPONATREMIA

Pathophysiology
Hyponatremia is synonymous with hypo-osmolality and can result in swelling of the brain parenchymal cells with subsequent edema. After 2–3 days the brain tries to compensate for this by actively extruding osmotically active intracellular components. As with hypernatremia, rapid correction of hyponatremia can be fatal.

Clinical presentation
The clinical signs of hyponatremia include lethargy, nausea, and vomiting progressing to seizures, coma, and death.

Differential diagnosis
Hydrocephalus, inflammatory CNS diseases, toxicity, other metabolic encephalopathies.

Diagnosis
Demonstration of an abnormal electrolyte level in the presence of an encephalopathy, which improves with appropriate correction, confirms the diagnosis. T2-weighted and fluid-attenuated inversion recovery (FLAIR) MR images of the thalamic area of the brain reveal characteristic bilateral hyperintense abnormalities. These abnormalities are often focal and oval.

Management
Appropriate therapy is based on correction of the sodium deficit (calculated using the following equation) in conjunction with addressing the underlying cause:

Sodium deficit (mEq/l) = 0.6 × bodyweight (kg) × (normal sodium concentration – patient's sodium concentration)

As for hypernatremia, cautious fluid therapy and frequent monitoring are paramount. Too rapid correction of established hyponatremia can result in thalamic lesions. When hyponatremia has occurred over a period of >24 hours, treatment is adjusted so that the maximal increase does not exceed 0.5 mEq/l/hour or 8–12 mEq/l per 24 hours.

NEOPLASTIC DISEASES

Definition/overview
Brain tumors most commonly affect older dogs and cats. Brain tumors may arise primarily from the brain or surrounding tissues, extend into the brain from adjacent structures, or metastasize to the brain from another location in the body. Tumors result in clinical signs either through primary mechanical damage or as a consequence of secondary pathophysiologic events such as edema and hemorrhage.

The median age of dogs diagnosed with a brain tumor is reported to be 9 years (range: 4–13 years). The most commonly affected breeds include Golden Retrievers, Labrador Retrievers, Boxers, Collies, Bulldogs, and Boston Terriers. The median age at the time of diagnosis of brain tumors in cats is reported to be 11.3 years (± 3.8 years).

Pathophysiology
Tumors of the intracranial space may be primary (arising from tissues in the intracranial space) or secondary (arising from tissues adjacent to the intracranial space or from metastasis). Primary intracranial tumors include:

- Meningiomas. The most common brain tumors in dogs and cats. These tumors arise from the arachnoid layer of the meninges, originating at the periphery of the brain parenchyma and expanding inwards.
- Gliomas. Arise from the supporting cells of the brain parenchyma. These include astrocytes and oligodendrocytes forming astrocytomas, oligodendrogliomas, and the extremely malignant glioblastoma multiforme. Brachycephalic breeds such as Boxers and Boston Terriers may be more often affected with these tumors.
- Ependymomas. Arise from the ependymal lining of the ventricular system.
- Choroid plexus tumors. Arise from areas where the choroid plexus is concentrated (the lateral, third, and fourth ventricles).

- Pituitary gland tumors. Macroadenomas may enlarge dorsally from the sella and compress the diencephalon. Neurologic impairment can be surprisingly minimal. The relative size of the tumor cannot be predicted from the endocrine test result.

Secondary intracranial lesions arise as a result of metastasis or direct extension from extraneural sites. Numerous tumors in older animals metastasize to the brain including hemangiosarcomas, lymphomas, and mammary gland and other carcinomas.

Clinical presentation

Most canine brain tumors affect the forebrain. The most common presenting complaint in these cases is seizures. Seizures are sometimes the only sign of a structural intracranial abnormality, with the remainder of the neurologic examination findings being normal. This is particularly true with more rostral and olfactory lobe lesions. Otherwise, the clinical signs associated with tumors affecting the brain depend on the location within the brain, brainstem, or cerebellum. Disorientation, circling, ataxia, depression, and CN signs can variably be seen.

Most feline intracranial neoplasia affects the forebrain. The most common neurologic signs include altered consciousness (depression, stupor, or coma), circling, seizures, ataxia, and behavioral changes.

Differential diagnosis

CNS inflammatory diseases such as granulomatous meningoencephalomyelitis (GME) and those due to infections.

Diagnosis

Advanced imaging modalities, such as CT and MRI, are most commonly used to investigate cases of suspected neoplasia (**Figures 14.8a–h**). CT-guided, freehand needle biopsy of brain tumors has been reported in dogs with intracranial lesions to obtain a histologic diagnosis prior to treatment. Although CT-guided, freehand needle biopsy is a relatively safe procedure, the diagnostic yield can be variable.

An MRI-compatible stereotactic brain biopsy system has recently been validated for use in dogs. This modified frameless stereotactic system has been shown to have acceptable precision for obtaining biopsy samples and has been used successfully in a clinical setting.

CSF analysis is often not helpful for the definitive diagnosis of a brain tumor, and in some instances can even be misleading. Typically, CSF in dogs with a brain tumor contains an increased level of protein without a concurrent pleocytosis (albuminocytologic dissociation). However, in a significant proportion of these cases cellular changes consistent with inflammation are present and, interpreted alone, may falsely suggest a primary inflammatory disease. Occasionally, CSF in a dog with a brain tumor is normal. The presence of neoplastic cells in the CSF is specific; however, it is a very rare finding.

Management

Treatment for brain tumors in dogs depends on tumor type, location, natural history of the tumor, associated morbidity/mortality with the treatment modality, and cost. While studies of brain tumor treatment in dogs and cats exist in the veterinary literature, many have incomplete diagnoses, nonstandardized treatment protocols, lack of a control population, and different tumor types being grouped together to increase overall case numbers. These problems make it difficult to make definitive statements regarding treatment efficacy.

Glucocorticoid therapy provides minimal supportive care for patients with brain tumors, although its use can often be necessary and helpful. The aims of glucocorticoid treatment are to control the secondary conditions of acquired hydrocephalus and peritumoral edema, and to reduce ICP. Clinical signs in many patients improve following the initiation of steroid treatment, which may give some indication of tumor invasion and what could be achieved with surgery.

Surgery is ideal for superficially located, encapsulated, relatively small benign tumors, of which meningiomas are the most common example (**Figure 14.9**). Median survival times reported in dogs following surgery for all types of brain tumor vary, but tend to cluster around 140–150 days. For meningiomas, median survival times may be slightly longer (240 days) and there is evidence that improving surgical excision using ultrasonic aspiration or endoscopy does improve survival times. Surgical excision is more readily accomplished in cats, as meningiomas in this species tend to be well encapsulated and easily delineated from normal brain tissue. Studies have determined the median survival time in cats following meningioma resection to be between 22 and 27 months.

Conventional radiation therapy has been shown to be effective for brain tumors in dogs. The main goal of treatment is to administer the highest possible dose to the tumor while minimizing the dose to the surrounding normal tissue. Median survival time in dogs is around 150 to 350 days.

Chemotherapy is used as a primary therapy or as an adjunct to surgery in selected instances in animals with brain tumors. Carmustine and lomustine are alkylating

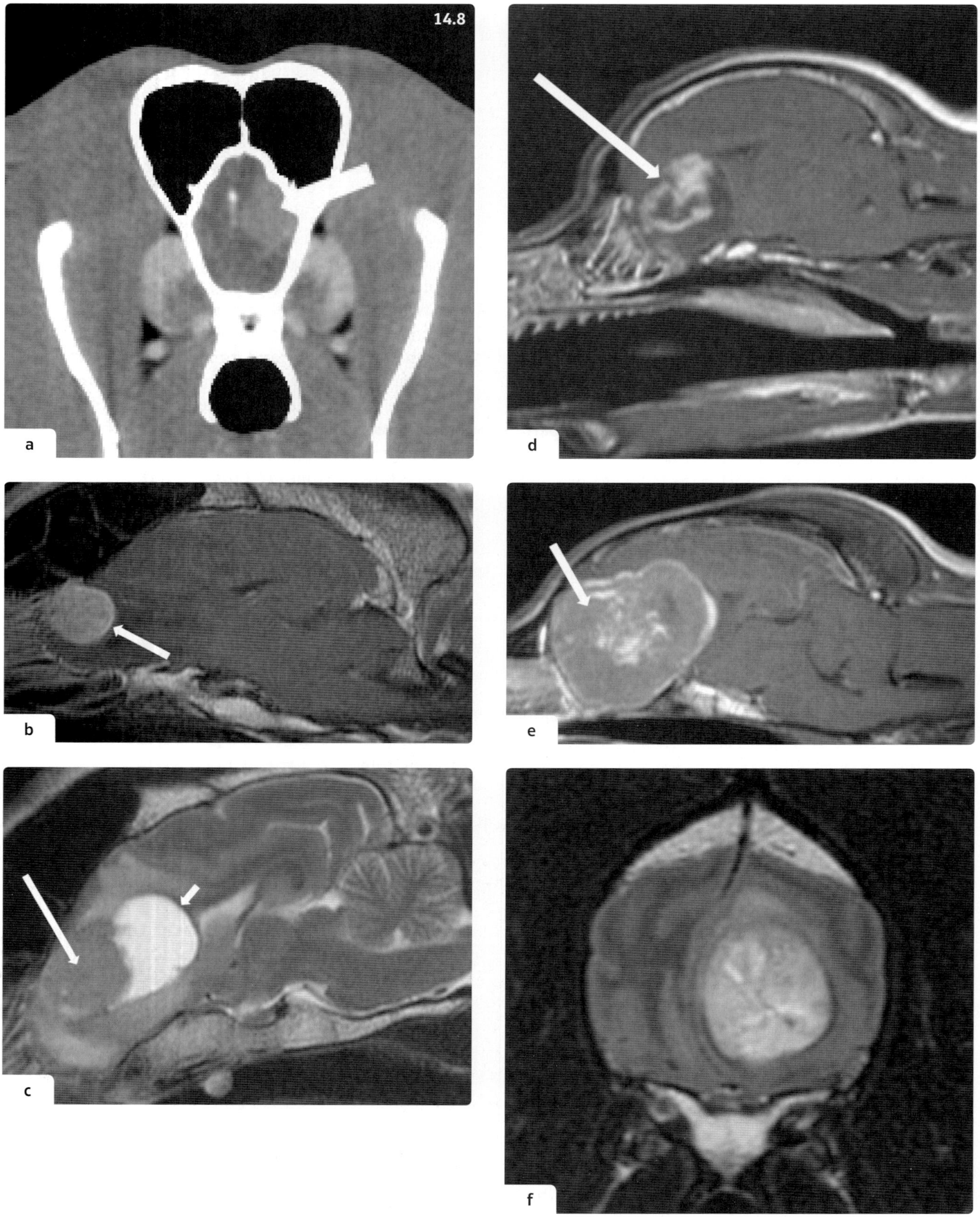
14.8
a
b
c
d
e
f

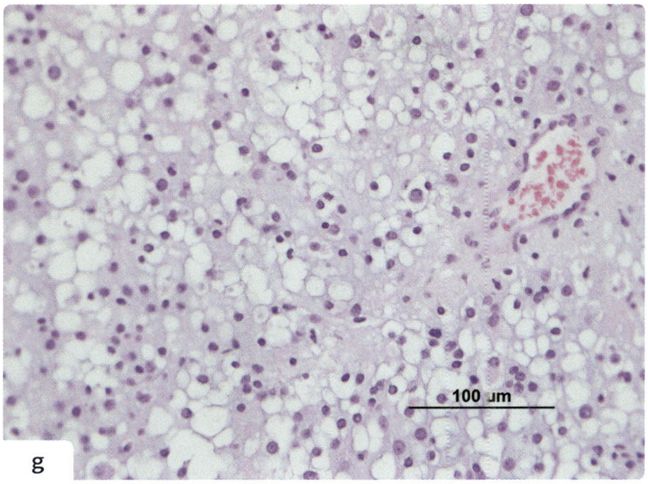

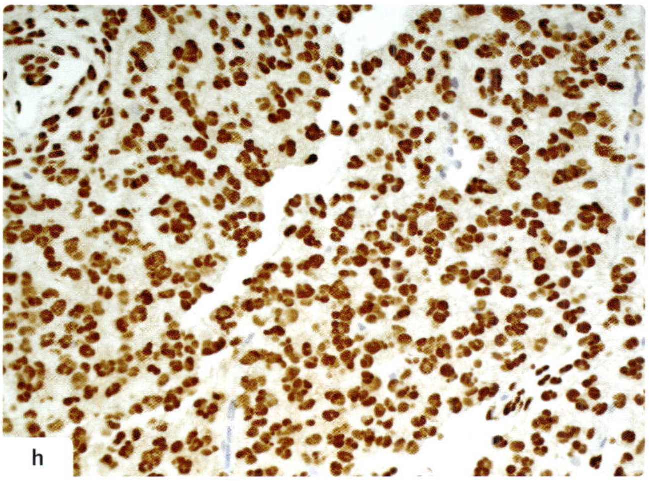

Figures 14.8a–h (a) Post-contrast transverse CT brain scan at the level of the olfactory bulbs and frontal sinuses. A well-defined contrast-enhanced lesion can be identified (arrow), which was confirmed to be meningioma on histopathology following resection. (b) T1-weighted post-contrast midline sagittal brain MR image depicting a homogeneously enhancing lesion in the olfactory bulb (arrow), characteristic for a meningioma. (c) T2-weighted midline sagittal brain MR image depicting an iso- to hyperintense lesion in the olfactory bulb (long arrow), which is accompanied by a cystic component (short arrow), which is well described for meningiomas. (d) T1-weighted post-contrast midline sagittal brain image depicting a heterogeneously enhancing lesion in the frontal lobe characteristic for a glioma, which in this case was an astrocytoma. (e) T1-weighted post-contrast midline sagittal brain MR image depicting a heterogeneously enhancing lesion in the olfactory bulb and the frontal lobe. The lesion was a nasal adenocarcinoma extending caudally from the nasal cavity. (f) T2-weighted transverse brain MR image clearly showing a large well-demarcated heterogeneously hyperintense lesion causing mass effect (midline shift of the brain). The lesion was confirmed as an oligodendroglioma. (g) The oligodendroglioma shown in 14.8f is stained with hematoxylin and eosin. (h) The oligodendroglioma shown in 14.8f stains positively immunohistochemically with Olig2.

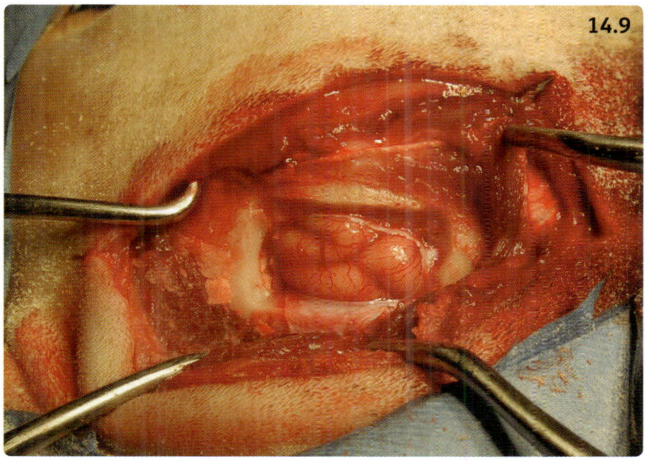

Figure 14.9 A lateral rostrotentorial craniectomy is used to approach the parietal lobe of the brain for the purposes of tumor resection.

agents that have some effectiveness against gliomas. Hydroxyurea (30–45 mg/kg PO three times a week, with monitoring of the blood cell count for evidence of myelosuppression) is gaining popularity for treatment of meningiomas. There is little to no data available on the effectiveness of chemotherapy for canine or feline brain tumors.

INFLAMMATORY INFECTIOUS CNS DISEASES

Definition/overview

Encephalitis and infectious diseases often exist concurrently in dogs and cats.

Etiology

Numerous infectious agents have been implicated:

- Viral: distemper, parvovirus, parainfluenza, herpesvirus, feline coronavirus (which causes FIP), West Nile virus, pseudorabies, and rabies.
- Bacterial.
- Rickettsial: Rocky Mountain spotted fever and *Ehrlichia*.
- Fungal: blastomycosis, histoplasmosis, cryptococcosis, coccidioidomycosis, and aspergillosis.
- Protozoal: toxoplasmosis and neosporosis.
- Unclassified organisms: protothecosis.

Pathophysiology

The specific pathophysiology of the above mentioned infectious diseases in the CNS is discussed below. Inflammation of the structures of the brain (encephalitis) can co-exist with inflammation of the meninges (meningitis) and, occasionally, with inflammation of the spinal cord (myelitis).

Clinical presentation

As a general rule, inflammatory diseases tend to be acute in onset and progressive, with a multifocal or diffuse, often asymmetrical, distribution within the CNS. Neurologic manifestations are quite variable and reflect the location of the inflammatory foci within the nervous system. Central vestibular signs are commonly encountered and can be seen alone or in combination with other neurologic signs. Neck pain can also be present as a manifestation of meningeal inflammation. Animals with CNS infections frequently do not have evidence of systemic involvement. Therefore, the absence of fever, anorexia, and depression and the presence of a normal hemogram cannot be used to exclude the possibility of an infectious etiology in an animal with neurologic signs.

Differential diagnosis

Sterile causes of CNS inflammatory disease, brain tumor, metabolic and toxic encephalopathies.

Diagnosis

A thorough ophthalmologic examination should be performed in every neurologic case to look for evidence of fundic changes or uveitis compatible with inflammatory disease. Definitive diagnosis of CNS inflammatory disease is typically based on finding an increased total nucleated cell count or an abnormal cell type distribution, with a concomitant increase in protein concentrations, on CSF analysis. In rare instances, normal CSF can be obtained from an animal with confirmed CNS inflammatory disease. This can occur if the inflammation does not involve the meninges or the ependymal lining of the ventricular system, or if the animal has been treated with corticosteroids prior to CSF collection. Elevations in protein concentration can result from breakdown of the blood–brain barrier or intrathecal antibody production. It is likely that both of these mechanisms contribute toward the elevated protein levels recognized with most CNS inflammatory disease. Cytologic evaluation of the fluid provides additional information as to possible causes (**Figure 14.10**).

Additional testing, based on the cytologic evaluation, is performed in an attempt to identify the infectious cause of the inflammation. These tests can include:

- CSF culture for bacterial or fungal organisms.
- Serum and CSF antibody or antigen titers.
- CSF polymerase chain reaction (PCR) analysis.

However, despite extensive testing, an underlying cause for the inflammation is not determined in most cases.

14.10

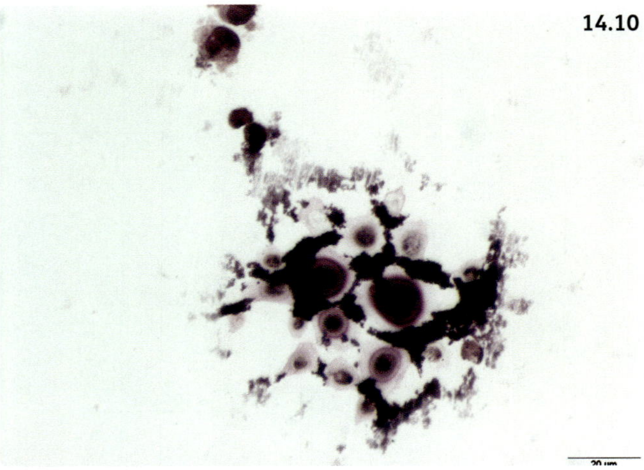

Figure 14.10 *Cryptococcus* organisms can be seen in this cytologic analysis from CSF of a dog with seizure episodes. (Courtesy R. Di Terlizzi)

Management

Treatment is aimed at the primary disease process. Treatment with clindamycin (10–15 mg/kg PO q12h) and/or trimethoprim/sulfonamide (15 mg/kg PO q12h) for potential protozoal infections can be initiated once a diagnosis of encephalomyelitis has been made based on CSF results, while additional test results are pending. If no infectious cause is discovered on additional testing, or the animal does not respond to initial antimicrobial therapy, treatment with corticosteroids should be initiated. Anti-inflammatory doses are often effective at alleviating the clinical signs, but higher immunosuppressive doses may be required in some instances to appropriately manage the immune-mediated disease. Prognosis is variable and depends on both the cause of the inflammation and the extent and severity of associated neurologic deficits. Some infections, especially those caused by protozoal and fungal agents, are difficult to eradicate and relapses are common. In addition, residual neurologic deficits can persist despite successful treatment of an infection due to irreversible damage caused by the inciting agent.

RABIES

Definition/overview

Rabies is caused by an enveloped RNA neurotropic virus of the genus *Lyssavirus* in the family Rhabdoviridae. All warm-blooded animals are vulnerable to infection with rabies, but species susceptibility varies tremendously. Foxes, coyotes, jackals, and wolves are amongst the most susceptible animals with skunks, raccoons, bats, and cattle also having a high susceptibility.

Pathophysiology

Infection most often occurs as a result of being bitten by an infected animal with rabies virus in its saliva. The incubation period is influenced by multiple factors, including patient age, bite site, the variant, and the amount of virus inoculated. After IM inoculation, the virus enters the neuromuscular junctions following a variable period (from days to 6 months) of replication in the local tissues. The virus rapidly spreads up the peripheral nerves and then the spinal cord to the forebrain, causing damage to the nervous tissue *en route* and resulting in progressive nervous system signs.

Clinical presentation

There are several overlapping phases during the progression of the disease. In dogs there is usually a prodromal phase (lasts for 2–3 days) during which clinical signs such as apprehension, nervousness, anxiety, and variable fever may be seen. Overall, a significant change in the normal behavior of the animal is noted by the owner. Affected animals can be seen to constantly lick the site of viral inoculation. Cats may also exhibit this prodromal phase, but it more commonly consists of erratic behaviour for 1–2 days.

The furious or psychotic form of rabies usually lasts up to a week in dogs and is manifest by cerebral dysfunction with exaggerated responses to sound and touch. Affected animals can bite at imaginary objects or their cage and become extremely irritable. At this stage they frequently exhibit generalized tonic–clonic seizure activity, during which they can die. Occasionally, dogs can exhibit a pre-death paralyzed state. Cats typically develop the furious stage, resulting in unprovoked attacks and appearing 'disconnected' from the environment.

The paralytic or dumb form of rabies is often seen within 2–4 days following the onset of clinical signs and is manifest by flaccid paralysis. In both dogs and cats, a bite to the neck or head may more commonly result in CN dysfunction. Dysphonia, dysphagia, excessive salivation, and a dropped jaw may be seen, and these clinical signs are also classed as part of the paralytic form. Coma and death usually follow these signs within 2–4 days.

Differential diagnosis

Other infectious and sterile causes of CNS inflammatory disease, brain tumor, metabolic and toxic encephalopathies.

Diagnosis

Rabies should always be suspected in any animal presenting with neurologic dysfunction and living in an area known to have a virus reservoir in the local wildlife. Particular concern should be raised for animals that are known to be unvaccinated and that have exhibited clinical signs for <5 days.

There are no antemortem tests sensitive enough to be consistently reliable for confirming a diagnosis of rabies, and there are no hematologic or serum biochemical changes characteristic of the disease. CSF analysis may reveal elevated protein levels and white blood cell count with a lymphocytic predominance. Serologic tests are rarely performed because of the low percentage of animals that have time to develop antibodies. However, a serologic assay can be used to assess vaccine efficacy.

A direct fluorescent antibody assay test of the nervous tissue can be performed on thin touch impression smears and is rapid and sensitive for a definitive diagnosis. The most commonly affected areas on examination are the brainstem, hippocampus, cerebrum, and cerebellum (**Figure 14.11**). Reverse transcriptase PCR (RT-PCR) is a relatively new method for rabies diagnosis and is very useful when the sample size is small (e.g. CSF sample).

Management

There is no specific treatment for this fatal disease. A dog or cat suspected of contracting the disease should be quarantined as recommended by the local heath authorities or euthanized and the brain submitted for examination. Exposure of all healthcare providers to the animal and/or its tissues should be restricted.

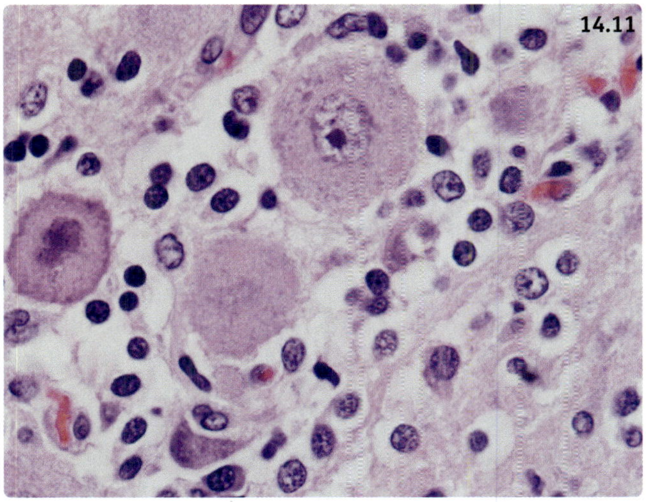

Figure 14.11 Intracytoplasmic inclusion bodies can be seen within the neuronal cells of a dog with rabies virus infection.

BACTERIAL MENINGOENCEPHALITIS

Definition/overview

Bacterial infection is a relatively rare cause of encephalitis in dogs and cats when compared with other species.

Etiology

Bacterial infection of the CNS.

Pathophysiology

Bacterial infection of the brain is usually a consequence of direct extension of infection from the middle ear or sinuses or a penetrating injury to the skull (surgical or traumatic). Hematogenous spread can occur less commonly. Both aerobic and anaerobic infections have been reported. It is possible for the infection to be limited to the extradural or subarachnoid space, especially following bite wounds, in which case the infection can remain localized (intracranial empyema or abscess) and signs might not be so rapidly progressive. Clinical signs are largely the result of the inflammatory reaction that bacteria incite.

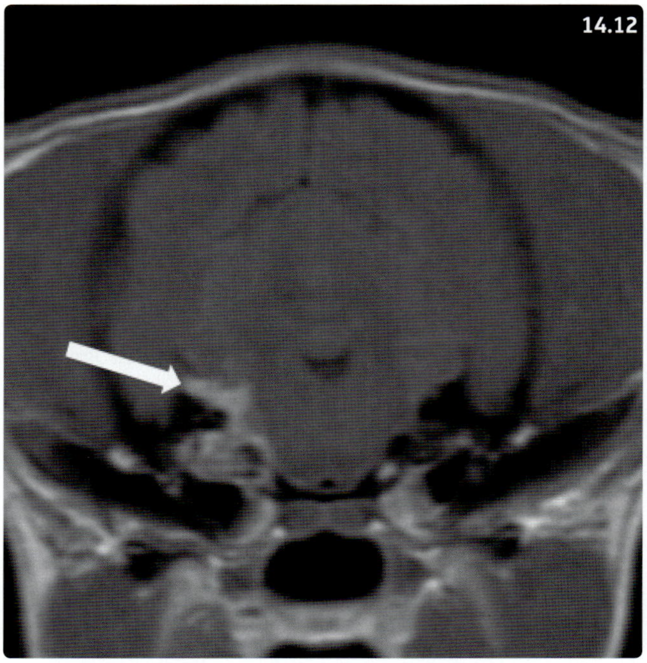

Figure 14.12 T1-weighted post-contrast transverse brain MR image at the level of the bullae reveals extension of otitis media/interna into the central nervous system (arrow) in an 8-year-old Yorkshire Terrier.

Clinical presentation

Animals can exhibit a variety of signs including vestibular dysfunction, seizures, cerebellar signs, paresis, cervical hyperesthesia, and coma. Fever is present in approximately 50% of cases at presentation. The signs are usually rapidly progressive and frequently fatal.

Differential diagnosis

Other infectious and sterile causes of CNS inflammatory disease, brain tumor, metabolic and toxic encephalopathies.

Diagnosis

Routine blood work usually reflects an inflammatory process, but can be normal. A urine sample should be cultured if bacterial encephalitis is suspected and blood cultures are indicated in animals in which there is no obvious source of infection. Imaging of the brain (CT or MRI) is helpful to identify defects in the skull and otitis media/interna (OMI) and can be suggestive of an inflammatory process (**Figure 14.12**). CSF analysis is the most useful test. Typically, there is a marked elevation in the protein level and total nucleated cell count and the majority of cells are degenerate neutrophils. Bacteria may be visible in the spinal fluid. However, CSF analysis can be unremarkable or show more nonspecific inflammatory changes. CSF should be cultured if it contains degenerate neutrophils, although it is common for the cultures to be negative.

Management

Treatment with an antibacterial drug that penetrates the CNS should be initiated while waiting for culture results. The most common bacterial isolates are *Escherichia coli*, *Streptococcus* and *Klebsiella*, but anaerobic infections can also occur. Appropriate drugs include fluoroquinolones and third-generation cephalosporins. Many patients are in a critical condition and need IV fluids and anti-inflammatory drugs. Mechanical ventilation might be necessary in comatose patients. Prognosis is poor in animals with rapidly progressing severe signs. Early appropriate treatment is vital to obtain a good outcome.

CANINE DISTEMPER VIRUS INFECTION

Definition/overview

Canine distemper is a multisystemic viral disease that causes multifocal CNS dysfunction. It most commonly affects unvaccinated dogs.

Etiology

Canine distemper virus (CDV) is a paramyxovirus that commonly infects the CNS of dogs.

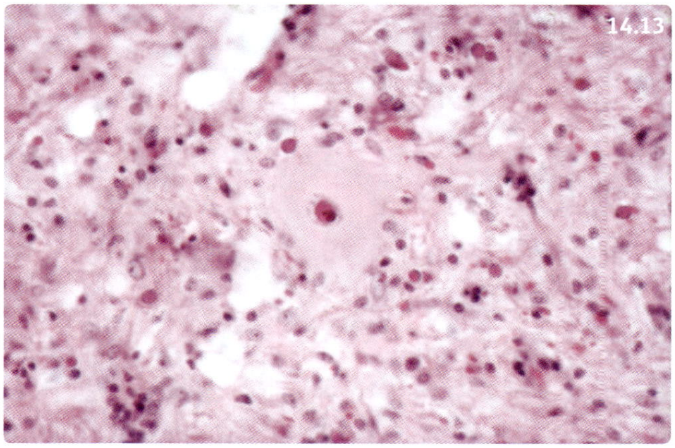

Figure 14.13 Intranuclear inclusion material in a neuron of a dog with distemper virus infection. The tissue is stained with hematoxylin and eosin.

Pathophysiology

The presence and severity of the neurologic signs depend on factors such as the age and immunocompetence of the host and the neurovirulence of the virus strain. Many dogs probably develop transient CNS infections without concurrent clinical signs. In the CNS, CDV initially replicates in the neurons and glial cells (**Figure 14.13**), and can cause both gray and white matter lesions, with one usually predominating. These early degenerative lesions are not characteristically inflammatory. A chronic course of CNS infection results from a late or insufficient immune response to CDV, with characteristic inflammatory demyelinating lesions. Polioencephalomyelopathy has been reported most frequently in immature dogs, while leucoencephalomyelopathy or a combination of both is more common in mature animals.

Clinical presentation

Seizures, visual deficits, vestibular dysfunction, cerebellar signs, paresis, and myoclonus. The presence of myoclonus is most commonly associated with CDV infection but is not pathognomonic, as it has been described with other inflammatory CNS disorders. Neurologic disease associated with CDV infection tends to have a progressive course. Disease can develop in well-vaccinated animals, so previous vaccination history does not exclude the possibility of CDV-associated disease. Systemic signs, such as respiratory and GI involvement, are reported to precede the neurologic signs by 2–3 weeks. However, many dogs have no previous history of disease prior to the onset of neurologic signs. Extraneural signs include conjunctivitis, rhinitis, fever, respiratory signs, GI signs, tonsillitis, cachexia, enamel hypoplasia, and hyperkeratosis of the footpads or nose. These signs are frequently mild. Fundic examination is recommended in all suspected cases, as many dogs have evidence of chorioretinitis.

Differential diagnosis

Other infectious and sterile causes of CNS inflammatory disease, brain tumor, metabolic and toxic encephalopathies.

Diagnosis

An indirect fluorescent antibody test for viral antigen in conjunctival smears can be positive in many dogs with CNS distemper, regardless of whether the disease is acute or chronic. Viral antigen can also be demonstrated in tracheal washings and urine sediment. Results of CSF analysis are variable. During the acute stage of the disease, an inflammatory response is lacking and thus the cell count and protein levels can be normal. In the chronic stage of the disease, lymphocytic pleocytosis is more frequently identified. An elevated CSF titer of antibody against CDV relative to the serum titer is supportive of a diagnosis. Biopsy samples of haired skin from the dorsal neck can be used antemortem for immunohistochemical testing for acute CDV infection. PCR analysis of urine and CSF samples for CDV has proven most useful in the antemortem diagnosis of distemper-associated neurologic disease.

Management

There is no specific treatment for CDV-associated neurologic disease. Overall, the prognosis is poor, especially in cases with rapidly progressive signs. However, some dogs can survive with residual neurologic deficits. Seizures are reported to be an unfavorable prognostic sign as they are often difficult to control with antiepileptic drugs. Consequently, in cases where the neurologic signs are not severe, it is recommended that the animal is provided with supportive care and the disease progression monitored over 1–2 weeks before considering euthanasia.

FELINE INFECTIOUS PERITONITIS

Definition /overview

FIP is a multisystemic viral disease that causes multifocal CNS dysfunction.

Etiology

Feline coronavirus is the causative agent of FIP, which is the most common cause of meningoencephalomyelitis in cats.

Pathophysiology

The disease occurs most commonly in cats <3 years old and from multiple cat households; however, cats as old as 15 years have been diagnosed with the disease. Neurologic involvement is most common with the noneffusive or 'dry' form of the disease. Up to one-third of cats with the non-effusive form of the disease have been reported to have either primary neurologic FIP or neurologic signs as part of the overall disease presentation. FIP induces a pyogranulomatous and immune complex-mediated vasculitis involving the meninges, ependymal lining, periventricular brain tissue, and choroid plexus of the CNS. Secondary hydrocephalus can be seen due to obstruction of the ventricular system by the inflammation.

Clinical presentation

Neurologic signs include seizures, cerebellar signs, vestibular dysfunction, and paresis. The disease often has an insidious onset and can lack distinct clinical signs. Affected cats may have concurrent systemic signs, including anorexia and weight loss. Ocular lesions have also been identified, including anterior uveitis, iritis, keratic precipitates (**Figure 14.14**), retinitis, and anisocoria.

Differential diagnosis

Other infectious and sterile causes of CNS inflammatory disease, brain tumor, metabolic and toxic encephalopathies.

Diagnosis

Hematological findings can include anemia, leukocytosis, and hyperglobulinemia; however, in some affected cats no abnormalities are present. Serum tests for anti-coronavirus antibodies are often positive, but they have low specificity. In addition, a negative serum titer (i.e. a complete absence of antibody) does not exclude the possibility of FIP-associated neurologic disease because soluble antibodies can form immune complexes and escape detection by standard tests. Advanced imaging of the brain often reveals the presence of ventricular dilatation and periventricular contrast enhancement can be visible with MRI (**Figure 14.15**). Results of CSF analysis are variable. The characteristic finding is a marked neutrophilic to pyogranulomatous pleocytosis, with cell counts often in the hundreds, and an associated increase in protein concentration to >200 mg/dl. However, the CSF can be normal, show a mild mononuclear pleocytosis, or have a normal cell count with an elevated protein concentration. Positive CSF titers can be a useful antemortem indicator of neurologic disease. However, positive antibody titers must be interpreted with respect to the integrity of the blood–brain barrier. PCR assays performed on CSF samples have not been shown to be reliable for confirming disease.

Management

Prognosis for cats with CNS FIP is poor. Definitive treatment is not available. The use of immunosuppressive drugs can slow the progression of disease. Affected animals should be isolated from other cats to prevent the spread of infection.

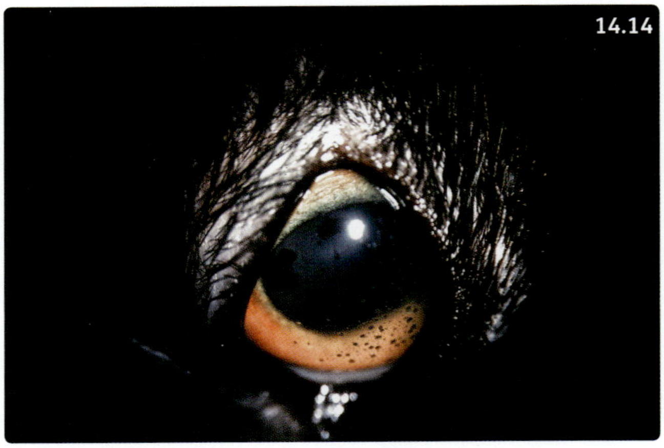

Figure 14.14 Ocular feline infectious peritonitis in a cat, showing keratic precipitates. (Courtesy Ophthalmology Service, University of Florida)

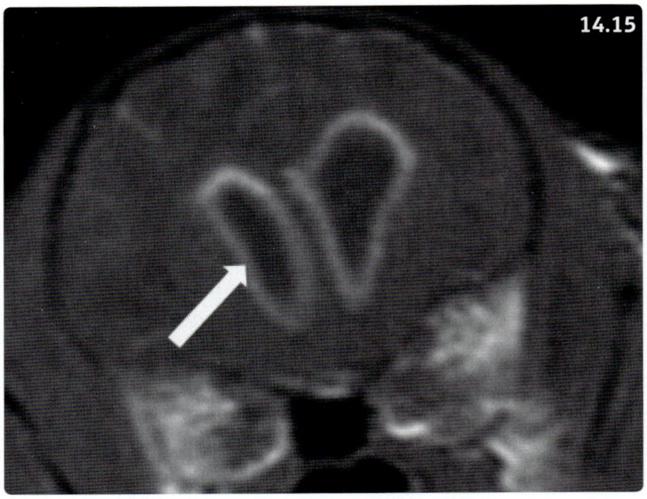

Figure 14.15 T1-weighted transverse brain MR image of a 3-year-old Domestic Shorthair cat with feline infectious peritonitis; marked enhancement of the lateral ventricular lining (arrow) is associated with the infection in this cat.

TOXOPLASMOSIS AND NEOSPOROSIS

Definition/overview

Toxoplasmosis and neosporosis are multifocal CNS diseases that are relatively uncommon following systemic infection with *Toxoplasma* or *Neospora*.

Etiology

Toxoplasma gondii is an intracellular protozoan parasite of humans and animals that can cause encephalitis in infected dogs and cats. *Neospora caninum* is a protozoan parasite that is known to cause neurologic disease in dogs but not cats.

Pathophysiology

Ingestion of tissue from infected intermediate hosts is the most common cause of *T. gondii* infection in dogs and cats. In the case of *N. caninum* infection, dogs are commonly infected *in utero*, although they can also be infected by ingestion of intermediate host tissue.

Clinical presentation

Signs of disease are seen most frequently in young or immunocompromised animals, and can occur with concurrent CDV infection or FIP. Neurologic signs include seizures, behavioral changes, CN deficits, cerebellar signs, and diffuse neuromuscular disease. A progressive cerebellar ataxia has been described in adult dogs with neosporosis. A characteristic early sign of disease is progressive rigidity of one or more limbs as a result of myositis and neuritis. Concurrent ocular abnormalities can be identified on fundoscopic examination.

Differential diagnosis

Other infectious and sterile causes of CNS inflammatory disease, brain tumor, metabolic and toxic encephalopathies.

Diagnosis

Imaging can reveal the presence of either solitary or multiple mass lesions in the brain of affected animals. CSF analysis typically demonstrates pleocytosis with a mixed population of neutrophils and the presence of small and large mononuclear cells. Eosinophils can also be seen. With toxoplasmosis, a presumptive diagnosis is based on positive antibody titers in the CSF. However, a positive titer can be seen in animals previously exposed to the organism following nonspecific immune stimulation and therefore is not definitive evidence of active disease. Serum and CSF anti-*Neospora* antibody titers are more reliable than serum titers alone. However, for both infections, evidence of a rising titer should be obtained. PCR assays performed on CSF samples can aid in the antemortem diagnosis of these protozoal infections.

Management

Clindamycin and/or trimethoprim/sulfonamide therapy for 3–4 weeks is recommended in animals with CNS protozoal infections. Trimethoprim/sulfonamide can be combined with pyrimethamine (0.5–1.0 mg/kg PO q24h for 2 days, then 0.25 mg/kg PO q24h for 2 weeks) and a folic acid supplement (5 mg/day PO) once the diagnosis has been confirmed. Neurologic signs typically improve with treatment but might not resolve because of permanent damage caused by the organism. In addition relapses are possible.

CRYPTOCOCCOSIS

Definition/overview

Cryptococcus neoformans is the most common fungal organism that affects the CNS. It occurs more commonly in cats than in dogs and causes multifocal signs.

Etiology

Cryptococcus is a saprophytic yeast with a worldwide distribution. The organism can be isolated from several sources, although its main reservoir is pigeon droppings.

Clinical presentation

Nonspecific signs include anorexia, weight loss, lethargy, lymphadenopathy, and pyrexia. Respiratory signs include nasal discharge, sneezing, and coughing. Ocular disease (including anterior uveitis, chorioretinitis, and retinal detachment) can be seen in association with neurologic signs. Neurologic signs often reflect a diffuse or multifocal localization and frequently include altered mentation, CN deficits, and gait abnormalities.

Pathophysiology

Dogs and cats most frequently become infected following inhalation of the organism. Neurologic involvement results from hematogenous spread or local extension of an infection through the cribriform plate.

Differential diagnosis

Other infectious and sterile causes of CNS inflammatory disease, brain tumor, metabolic and toxic encephalopathies.

Diagnosis

MRI findings are variable and include multifocal or solitary lesions with uniform or peripheral contrast enhancement (**Figures 14.16a, b**). Meningeal enhancement can also be observed. A hemogram can reveal the presence of monocytosis. In animals with extraneural disease, a definitive diagnosis can often be made based on cytology and/or culture of urine, nasal discharge, lymph node aspirates, or cutaneous masses. In addition, these animals often have positive CSF or serum titers for cryptococcal capsular antigen. Diagnosis of CNS cryptococcosis can often be made by cytologic evaluation of the CSF. Neutrophilic, mononuclear, or mixed pleocytosis can be seen, with neutrophilic pleocytosis most common in cats. Eosinophils are frequently present. The encapsulated organism can be seen in cytologic preparations in the majority of cases. The use of India ink, new methylene blue, or Gram stain allows the organisms to be identified more readily (**Figure 14.17**). In cases in which the organism is not observed on cytology, diagnosis can be made

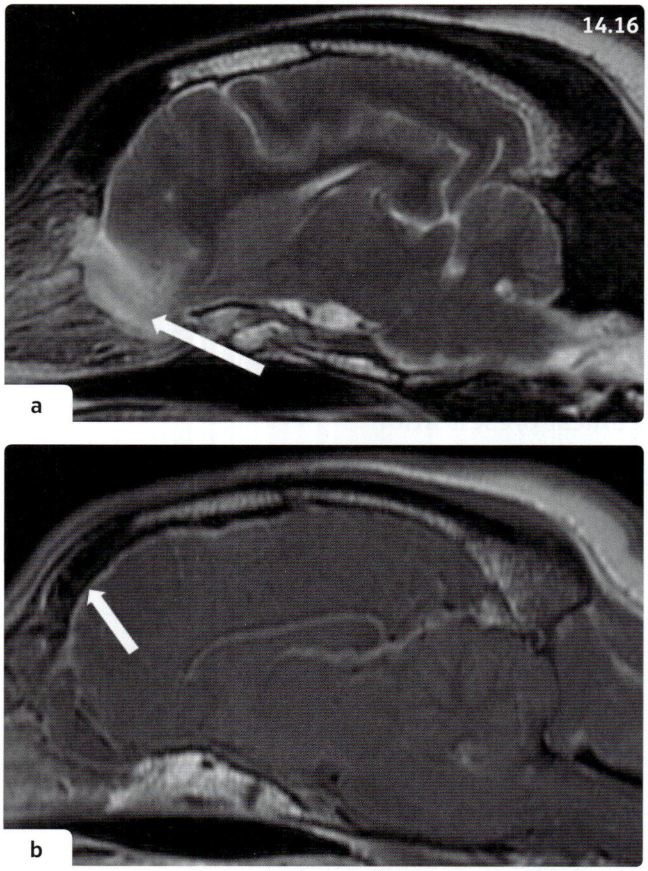

Figures 14.16a, b (a) Midline sagittal T2-weighted MR image of a dog's brain with *Cryptococcus* infection showing a granuloma adjacent to the cribriform plate in the olfactory bulb (arrow). (b) Midline sagittal T1-weighted MR image of the same dog reveals marked meningeal contrast enhancement (arrow) compatible with inflammation associated with the fungal infection.

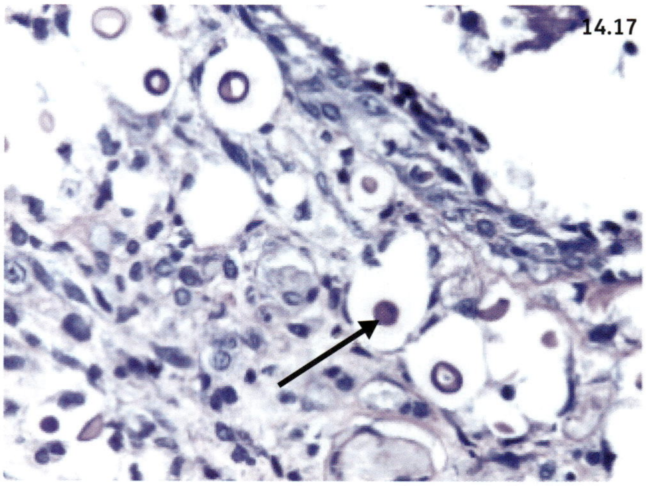

Figure 14.17 Brain tissue stained with periodic acid–Schiff to highlight the fungal bodies in purple (arrow) with the capsular area shown in white.

either by detecting cryptococcal capsular antigen in the CSF or by culturing CSF samples.

Management

Treatment with amphotericin, fluconazole, or itraconazole is recommended, although overall prognosis is fair to poor. Nonsteroidal anti-inflammatory drugs (NSAIDs) should be administered when antifungal therapy is initiated, to counteract the intense inflammatory reaction that accompanies the killing of *Cryptococcus*. Long-term treatment is required, ranging from several months to years. It is difficult to completely rid the body of the organism and relapses are common. Treatment should be continued until serum cryptococcal titers are negative or for 2 months beyond the resolution of clinical signs.

INFLAMMATORY NONINFECTIOUS CNS DISEASES

Inflammatory, noninfectious causes of CNS dysfunction in dogs include such diseases as GME and necrotizing encephalitis. These diseases are often grouped together antemortem within the term meningoencephalitis of undetermined etiology.

GRANULOMATOUS MENINGOENCEPHALOMYELITIS

Definition/overview

GME is an inflammatory disease of unknown etiology that affects the CNS of dogs and, rarely, cats.

Etiology

The etiology is unknown, although infectious, autoimmune, and neoplastic causes have been proposed.

Pathophysiology

Although the cause of GME is unknown, characteristics of the lesion suggest a possible immunologic basis for the disease and an immune-mediated pathogenesis is suspected

Clinical presentation

The disease is most common in middle aged toy and small breed dogs, with a possible breed predisposition in Poodles and Terriers. Three clinicopathologic forms of the disease are described: (1) an ocular form, which manifests with acute onset of dilated, unresponsive pupils due to optic neuritis; (2) a focal form, which presents with clinical signs suggestive of a single space-occupying mass, with areas of predilection in the pontomedullary region and forebrain; and (3) a diffuse form, which presents with clinical signs suggestive of a multifocal CNS disorder, with the cerebrum, brainstem, cerebellum, and cervical spinal cord most commonly involved. Clinical signs are usually acute in onset and progressive.

Differential diagnosis

Other infectious and sterile causes of CNS inflammatory disease, brain tumor, metabolic and toxic encephalopathies.

Diagnosis

CSF analysis typically reveals a mononuclear pleocytosis with an associated increase in protein concentration. However, both neutrophilic pleocytosis and normal CSF analysis have been reported. A mass lesion may be evident on imaging with the focal form of the disease, while the brain parenchyma can have a patchy, heterogeneous appearance with the diffuse form (**Figure 14.18**). A definitive diagnosis can only be made histologically on postmortem examination or by biopsy. Antemortem diagnosis is usually presumptive, by exclusion of infectious etiologies.

Management

The most commonly prescribed treatment for GME consists of immunosuppressive doses of corticosteroids. Other immunomodulatory drugs are frequently used in combination with corticosteroids and include cytosine arabinoside, cyclosporine, mycophenolate procarbazine, lomustine, and azathioprine. Radiation therapy has also been recommended as a treatment for dogs with the focal form of the disease. Overall, prognosis is poor, but survival times range from weeks to years. The diffuse form of the disease carries the worst prognosis, with a survival time of weeks to months.

NECROTIZING MENINGO(LEUKO)ENCEPHALITIS

Definition/overview

Necrotizing meningo(leuko)encephalitis is a chronic progressive neurologic disorder reported in Pugs (Pug encephalitis), Yorkshire Terriers, Chihuahuas, and Maltese. There are also sporadic reports of similar findings in other small breed dogs, such as the Chihuahua, Pekingese, and Shih Tzu.

Etiology

The etiology of the disease is unknown.

Pathophysiology

Infection with an alpha-type herpesvirus has been suggested based on histologic similarities with this type of infection in humans. However, attempts at viral isolation have been unsuccessful. The disease is associated with necrosis and a nonsuppurative meningoencephalitis, predominantly in the cortex. The subcortical white matter is frequently involved (**Figure 14.19**). Areas of necrosis can also be seen in the brainstem. Recent research suggests that genetics may play a role in disease susceptibility in Pugs.

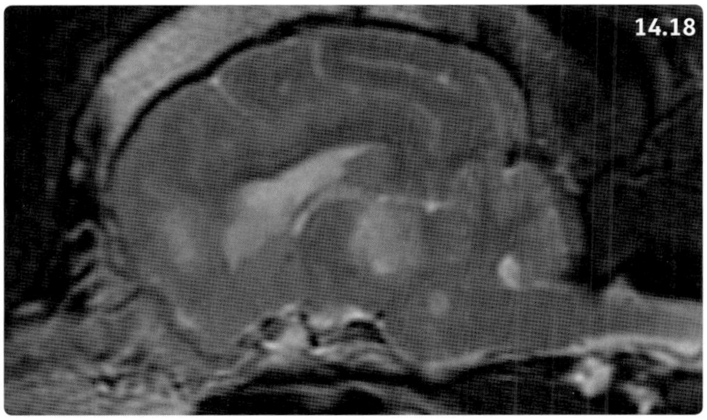

Figure 14.18 Sagittal paramedian T2-weighted brain MR image of a 2-year-old French Bulldog demonstrating multifocal hyperintensities confirmed to be GME on histopathology.

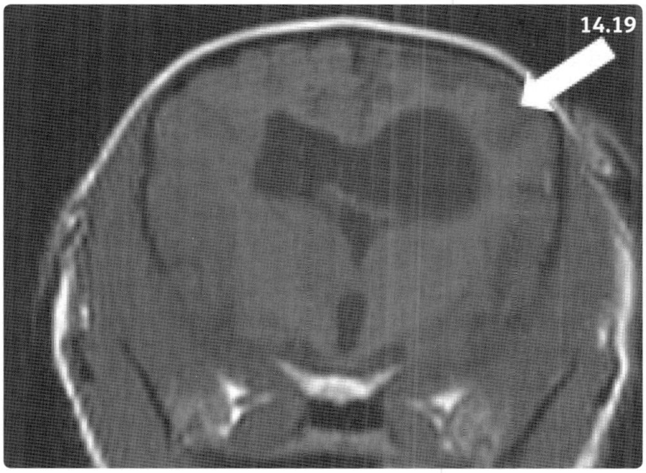

Figure 14.19 Transverse T1-weighted brain MR image depicting a loss of subcortical parenchyma (arrow) associated with necrotizing meningoencephalitis in a dog.

Clinical presentation

Pug encephalitis is most commonly seen in juvenile to young adults, and causes seizures and other signs of forebrain dysfunction. The disease described in Maltese also has a predilection for the forebrain. The disease in Yorkshire Terriers causes signs of forebrain and brainstem involvement. Chihuahuas with necrotizing meningoencephalitis present with neurologic signs, which include seizures, blindness, mentation changes, and postural deficits. Multifocal loss or collapse of cortical gray/white matter demarcation is identified on MRI. Multifocal asymmetrical areas of necrosis or collapse in both gray and white matter of the cerebral hemispheres is seen on post mortem.

Differential diagnosis

Other infectious and sterile causes of CNS inflammatory disease, brain tumor, metabolic and toxic encephalopathies.

Diagnosis

CT may reveal a focal hypodense area within the brain parenchyma relating to the area of necrosis. Multifocal, asymmetrical areas of high signal intensity in the brain can be seen on T2-weighted MR images, with variable contrast enhancement of the parenchyma and meninges visible on T1-weighted images. A lymphocytic pleocytosis is most frequently recognized on CSF analysis. A definitive diagnosis is based on histopathology.

Management

Prognosis is poor and the disease is typically fatal. Combined immunosuppressive protocols similar to those utilized for the treatment of GME are recommended. As with GME, there is limited information on the efficacy of such treatments in cases of histologically confirmed disease.

NUTRITIONAL DISEASES (THIAMINE DEFICIENCY)

Definition/overview

Thiamine deficiency is a rare problem in dogs and cats that results in an acute progressive multifocal disease of the brain.

Etiology

Thiamine must be provided in the diet, as dogs and cats are unable to produce it endogenously. Fish is high in thiaminase, and feeding an all-fish diet to cats can lead to thiamine deficiency. Overcooking canned food or meat, causing heat destruction of thiamine, has led to thiamine deficiency in dogs. Feeding meat preserved with sulfur dioxide to dogs and cats may also result in thiamine deficiency.

Pathophysiology

Thiamine (vitamin B1) is a necessary cofactor for normal carbohydrate oxidation, and its deficiency results in insufficient ATP production in the brain with subsequent neuronal dysfunction and death (if not treated).

Clinical presentation

Neurologic dysfunction due to thiamine deficiency tends to be acute and rapidly progressive. In both dogs and cats, signs of neurologic dysfunction due to thiamine deficiency typically include vestibular ataxia, decreased mentation (obtundation leading to coma, if not treated), ventroflexion of the head and neck, seizure activity, pupillary dilation with absent menace responses, and head tremors (**Figures 14.20a, b**). Left untreated, affected animals progress to a comatose state with opisthotonus (decerebrate posture) and ultimately death.

Differential diagnosis

CNS inflammatory disease, cerebrovascular disease, toxicity.

Diagnosis

Antemortem diagnosis of thiamine deficiency is typically based on characteristic clinical signs of thiamine deficiency in a dog or cat receiving a thiamine-deficient diet. A positive response to thiamine administration also supports the diagnosis. Elevated blood pyruvate and lactate levels and decreased erythrocyte transketolase activity are supportive of the diagnosis, but these tests are rarely done. There are reports of MR imaging in dogs with thiamine deficiency; similar to other metabolic encephalopathies, bilaterally symmetric brain lesions (hyperintense on T2-weighted images) were evident. In animals that die because of thiamine deficiency, characteristic bilaterally symmetric lesions (petechial hemorrhages) are appreciable throughout the brain at necropsy, especially in the caudal colliculi of the midbrain.

Management

Treatment of suspected thiamine deficiency is with IM or SC thiamine hydrochloride. Rapid IV injection of thiamine can cause an acute anaphylactoid reaction, therefore this route of administration is contraindicated. Anaphylactoid reactions are still possible, albeit more unlikely, with the IM and SC routes. The dosage is

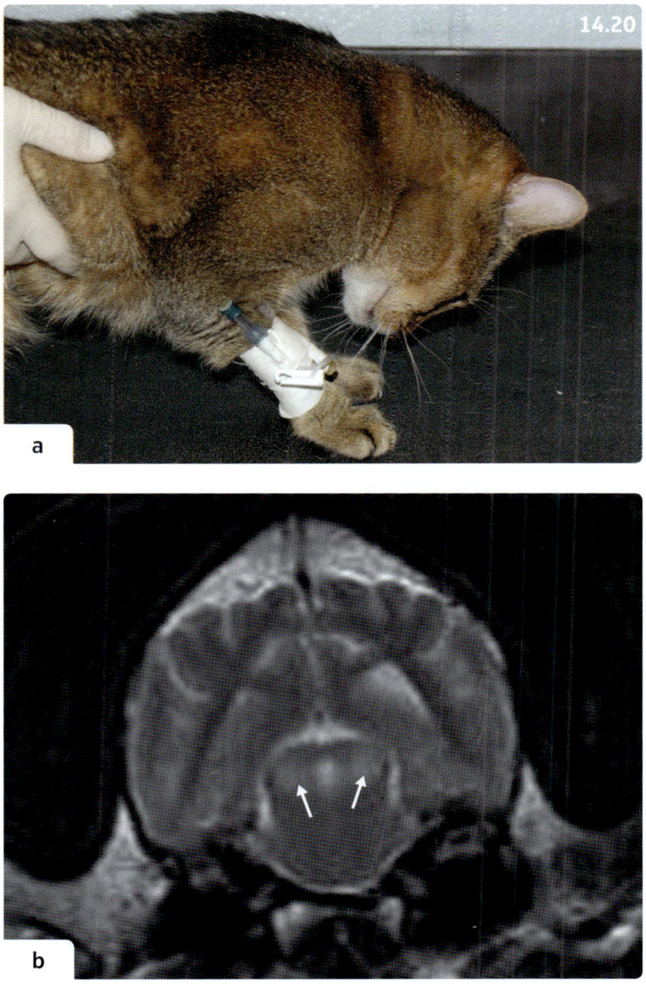

Figures 14.20a, b (a) A 7-year-old Domestic Shorthair cat exhibiting ventroflexion associated with its thiamine deficiency. (b) Transverse T2-weighted brain MR image of a dog with thiamine deficiency depicting bilateral hyperintensities associated with the colliculi (arrows).

5–50 mg/day for dogs and 1–20 mg/day for cats. If recognized and treated early, prognosis for survival of thiamine deficiency is good. If not treated rapidly in the early period of neurologic dysfunction, prognosis for survival is guarded to poor.

HEAD TRAUMA

Definition/overview

Severe head trauma is associated with high mortality in animals. The appropriate therapy for head trauma patients remains controversial in veterinary medicine due to a lack of objective information on the treatment of dogs and cats with head injuries. Treatment of affected animals must be immediate if the animal is to recover to a level that is both functional and acceptable to the owner. Many dogs and cats can recover from severe brain injuries if systemic and neurologic abnormalities that can be treated are identified early enough.

Etiology

Common causes of head injuries in cats and dogs include road traffic accidents, falls, kicks, gunshot or pellet wounds, and bites from larger animals. Traumatic injuries to the brain may result from blunt or penetrating insults; most canine head trauma results from blunt vehicular trauma, while most feline head trauma is associated with crush injury.

Pathophysiology

Head trauma pathophysiology can be divided into primary and secondary injury. Primary injury to the brain cannot be reversed, occurs immediately, and describes the physical disruption of brain tissue; this includes contusions, hematomas, lacerations, and diffuse axonal injury leading to vasogenic edema. The underlying vascular and cellular pathophysiology of head trauma is similar to that described for spinal cord trauma, but is complicated by elevations in ICP. This secondary injury is delayed and progressive, potentially providing targets for treatment. In addition to excitatory neurotransmitter release, ATP depletion resulting in cytotoxic edema, intracellular calcium accumulation causing activation of intracellular enzyme systems, and oxygen radical production resulting in lipid peroxidation occur. Traumatic brain injury is associated with a marked inflammatory response. The secondary injury 'cascade' is exacerbated by systemic abnormalities present in the patient, which include hypotension, hypoxia, hypo- or hyperglycemia, hypo- or hypercapnia, and hyperthermia.

After head trauma, the volume of the brain tissue compartment increases, usually due to edema or hemorrhage. As the brain tissue compartment increases, the CSF and the blood compartments must decrease or ICP will increase. Compensation for increased brain tissue volume initially involves the translocation of CSF out of the skull; this is followed by decreased production of CSF and, eventually, decreased cerebral blood flow. These compensatory mechanisms prevent increases in ICP for an undetermined period. Once the ability for compensation is exhausted, a further small increase in intracranial volume will result in dramatic elevations of ICP, with the immediate onset of clinical signs. Increases in ICP are often responsible for clinical decline after head trauma. Marked increases in ICP lead to an elevation of mean arterial blood pressure (MABP) and reflex bradycardia (Cushing reflex). In addition to a drop in heart rate coupled with an elevated MABP, other clinical manifestations of ICP elevation include anisocoria, miosis, mydriasis, altered mentation, and loss of motor function with the development of vertical nystagmus and extensor rigidity toward the end stages.

Differential diagnosis

Cerebrovascular disease, toxicities.

Diagnosis

Imaging of the patient's head is often indicated, especially in animals that fail to respond to aggressive medical therapy or deteriorate after initially responding. Skull radiographs are unlikely to reveal clinically useful information about brain injury but may occasionally reveal evidence of calvarial fractures (**Figures 14.21a–f**). CT is the preferred modality for imaging the head in cases of severe head injury associated with fractures. Even patients with 'mild' head trauma can exhibit abnormalities on the CT scan and so the initial decision to image the patient's head should not be based on the neurologic examination alone. CT image acquisition time is faster and often less expensive than MRI, and CT also demonstrates bone detail better than MRI. However, MRI has been shown to provide key information relevant to the prognosis based on its ability to detect subtle parenchymal damage not evident on CT imaging. The detection of midline parenchymal shift and ventricular obliteration on MR images is associated with a poor prognosis for survival, based on a recent canine study. Furthermore, lesions of the intracranial structures that may benefit from surgical therapy, such as hematomas and pneumocephalus, can be accurately identified using advanced imaging. Cervical spinal radiographs are also advised at the time of any skull imaging to rule out concurrent spinal lesions. As for spinal trauma (see below), thoracic radiographs will help to evaluate for evidence of thoracic and cardiac trauma.

Management

A detailed assessment is important for determining the way in which treatment is tailored to the individual patient. Systemic and neurologic assessment must be undertaken rapidly and continually reassessed. In humans, traumatic brain injury is graded as mild, moderate, or severe on the basis of an objective scoring system (e.g. GCS). A modification of the GCS has been proposed for use in veterinary medicine. The modified scoring system incorporates three categories of the examination (level of consciousness; motor activity; brainstem reflexes), which are assigned a score from 1 to 6, providing a total score of 3 to 18, with the best prognosis being the higher score.

The most important consideration in head injury is maintenance of cerebral perfusion by treatment of hypotension and elevated ICP.

The basic goal of fluid management of head trauma cases is to maintain a normovolemic to slightly hypervolemic state to ensure an adequate cerebral perfusion pressure. Initial resuscitation usually involves IV administration of hypertonic saline and/or synthetic colloids. Use of these solutions allows rapid restoration of blood volume and pressure while limiting the volume of fluid administered. In contrast, crystalloids will extravasate into the interstitium within an hour of administration and thus larger volumes are required for restoration of blood volume. If isotonic crystalloids are chosen for administration (appropriate in mild head trauma), an aliquot of the shock dose (90 ml/kg in the dog and 60 ml/kg in the cat) can be given rapidly and repeated until improved tissue perfusion is achieved. Hypertonic saline administration (4–5 ml/kg over 2–5 minutes; 4 ml/kg of 7.5% or 5.3 ml/kg of 3%) draws fluid from the interstitial and intracellular spaces into the intravascular space, which improves blood pressure and cerebral blood pressure and flow, with a subsequent decrease in ICP. Colloid solutions can be administered after hypertonic saline is used to maintain the intravascular volume, possibly due to retention of fluids in the intravascular compartments, maintaining an intravascular oncotic gradient. The co-administration of hypertonic solutions and colloids is more effective at restoring blood volume than either alone. A dose of 4 ml/kg total of a 1:2 combination of 23.4% hypertonic saline with 6% hydroxyethyl starch (Hetastarch) has been recommended.

Osmotic diuretics are very useful in the treatment of intracranial hypertension. Use of mannitol is recommended once vascular volume has been stabilized. Mannitol has an immediate plasma-expanding effect, which reduces blood viscosity, increasing cerebral blood flow and oxygen delivery. This results in vasoconstriction within a few minutes, causing an almost immediate decrease in ICP. The better known osmotic effect of mannitol reverses the blood–brain osmotic gradient, thereby reducing extracellular fluid volume in both normal and damaged brain. Mannitol should be administered as a bolus over a 15-minute period, rather than as an infusion, in order to obtain the plasma-expanding effect; its effect on decreasing brain edema takes approximately 15–30 minutes to establish and lasts between 2 and 8 hours. Doses of 0.5–2.0 g/kg appear to be equally

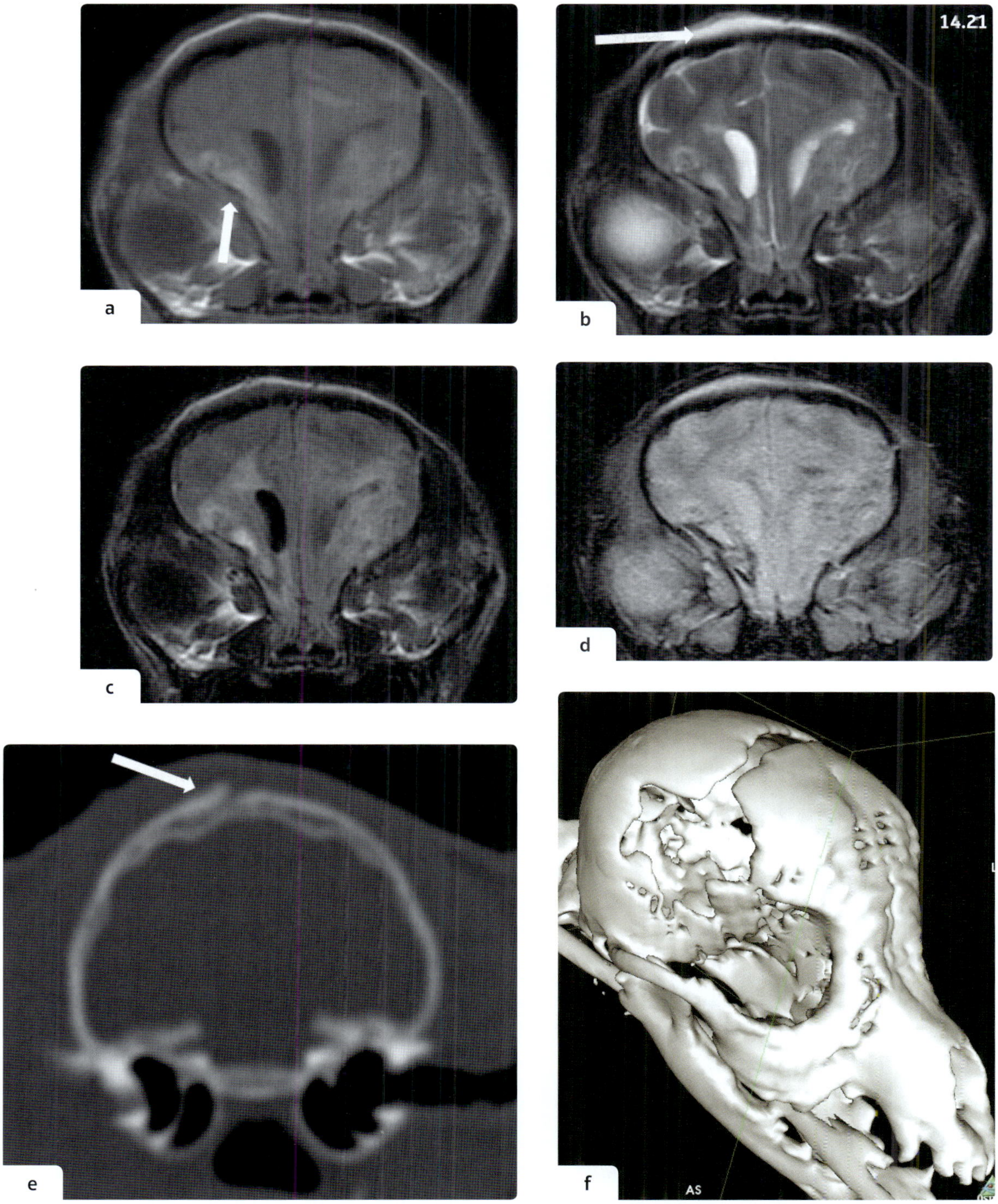

Figures 14.21a–f (a) T1-weighted transverse MR image of a dog 24 hours following a head trauma. A linear fracture of the skull associated with the orbit (arrow) can be seen. Multifocal areas of parenchymal damage can be identified within the frontal lobes. (b) T2-weighted transverse MR image of the dog in 14.21a. In addition to the parenchymal damage, a focal area of soft tissue damage can be seen on the dorsum of the head as a hyperintensity (arrow). (c) T2-weighted FLAIR MR image suppressing free fluid seen on the T2-weighted image and highlighting pathologic hyperintensities alone. (d) Transverse gradient echo MR image detailing hemorrhage and bone as black, making both easier to determine in comparison with the other sequences. (e) Transverse skull CT scan of a cat following a bite on the head. A small nondepressed fracture of the skull can be made out (arrow) with this modality, although underlying parenchymal damage is difficult to discern. (f) 3-D reconstruction of a dog with a depressed skull fracture.

effective in lowering ICP, but the duration of effect is shorter with the lower doses.

Oxygen supplementation is recommended for most acutely brain injured animals. Supplemental oxygen should be administered initially via flow by, as oxygen cages are usually ineffective because constant monitoring of the patient does not allow for a closed system. As soon as possible, nasal oxygen catheters or transtracheal oxygen catheters should be used to supply a 40% inspired oxygen concentration with flow rates of 100 ml/kg/minute and 50 ml/kg/minute, respectively.

CRANIAL NERVE DISEASES

HEAD TILT AND NYSTAGMUS

Definition/overview

Head tilt and nystagmus are relatively common presentations typically associated with vestibular disease (**Figure 14.22**). A thorough neurologic evaluation is critical to successful management. By determining the location of the disturbance within the vestibular system, a list of differential diagnoses and a diagnostic plan can be formulated.

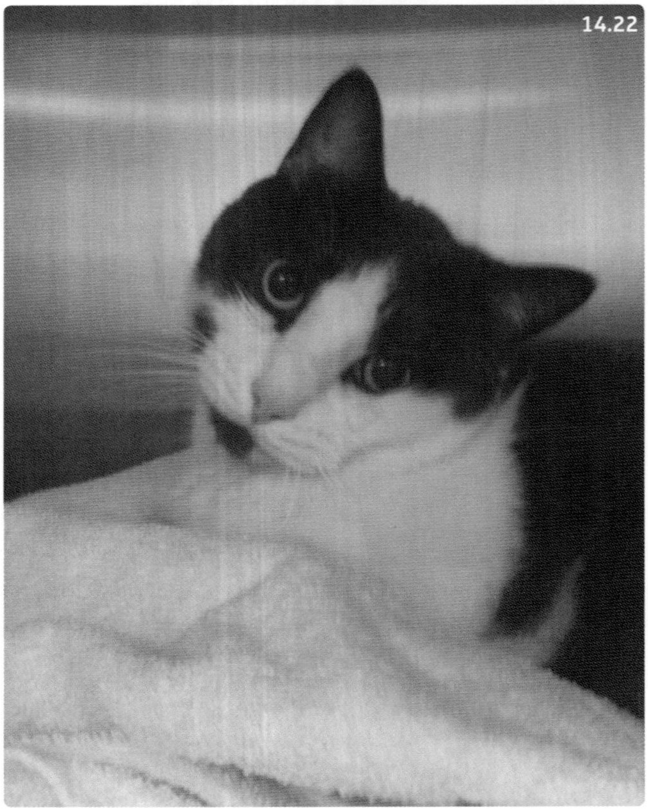

Figure 14.22 An 8-year-old Domestic Shorthair cat with a left-sided head tilt.

Etiology

For peripheral vestibular disease, OMI, idiopathic vestibular disease, hypothyroidism, toxicity, trauma, and neoplasia should be considered. For central vestibular disease, CNS inflammation, cerebrovascular accident, neoplasia, hydrocephalus, trauma, metronidazole toxicity, thiamine deficiency, and lysosomal storage diseases should be considered.

Pathophysiology

The vestibular system functions to maintain an animal's balance and orientation with respect to gravity. The system detects linear acceleration and rotational movement of the head, and is responsible for maintaining the position of the eyes, trunk, and limbs in reference to the position of the head. The sensory receptors for vestibular input are located in the membranous labyrinth of the inner ear. Input from the receptors enters the brain via the vestibular portion of CN VIII, where the majority of fibers terminate in one of four vestibular nuclei. The remaining axons terminate in the cerebellum. Pathways from the vestibular nuclei project to the nuclei of CNs III (oculomotor), IV (trochlear), and VI (abducent) to control eye movements, as well as to other brainstem centers and the cerebellum, cerebral cortex, and spinal cord. A head tilt results from the loss of anti-gravity muscle tone on one side of the neck. Jerk nystagmus develops from the dysfunction of the pathways responsible for integrating vestibular input with the extraocular eye muscles.

Clinical presentation

Head tilt is described as a rotation of the head about the first cervical vertebra such that one of the ears is held lower than the other. Head tilt is indicative of vestibular disease and is the most consistent sign of a unilateral vestibular deficit. Nystagmus is a term used to denote the involuntary rhythmic oscillation of the eyeballs; the eye movements have a slow phase in one direction and a rapid recovery in the opposite direction, which can be horizontal, rotary, or vertical in character. Other clinical signs of vestibular dysfunction include ataxia, a wide-based stance, circling, leaning, falling or rolling toward the side of the head tilt, and positional strabismus, where the eye on the affected side deviates ventrally or ventrolaterally when the head is elevated. Animals with acute vestibular disease can present with anorexia or vomiting associated with the disequilibrium.

Differential diagnosis

The differential diagnoses for an animal with vestibular disease vary considerably depending on whether the vestibular deficits are determined to be central or peripheral in origin. The two most common disease processes that cause central vestibular signs are neoplasia and infection/inflammation, while the two most common diagnoses in animals with peripheral vestibular signs are OMI and idiopathic vestibular disease.

Diagnosis

A CBC, blood chemistry, thyroid panel, and urinalysis should be performed in all animals presenting with vestibular signs. This can be useful for identifying potential inflammatory or metabolic disturbances that might be responsible for the clinical signs, in addition to serving as a general health screen, because further diagnostic testing usually requires anesthesia. Blood pressure measurements should also be obtained, as hypertension can manifest as vestibular dysfunction. An animal found to have peripheral vestibular disease should undergo a thorough otoscopic examination, performed under anesthesia, along with radiographs of the tympanic bullae to assess for OMI. It should be noted that normal radiographs do not rule out OMI. If there is evidence of OMI, a sample of fluid should be obtained via myringotomy and submitted for cytology and bacterial culture. CT and MRI of the tympanic bullae are the most sensitive means of identifying fluid within the middle ear, and can be considered in cases posing a diagnostic challenge (**Figures 14.23a–c**). If the equipment is available, hearing can be assessed using a brainstem auditory evoked response to evaluate for involvement of the cochlear branch of CN VIII. Cats should undergo a thorough pharyngeal examination to check for possible inflammatory polyps. Diagnostic testing in an animal found to have central vestibular disease should include advanced imaging of the brain (preferably MRI) to identify any structural abnormalities. Analysis of

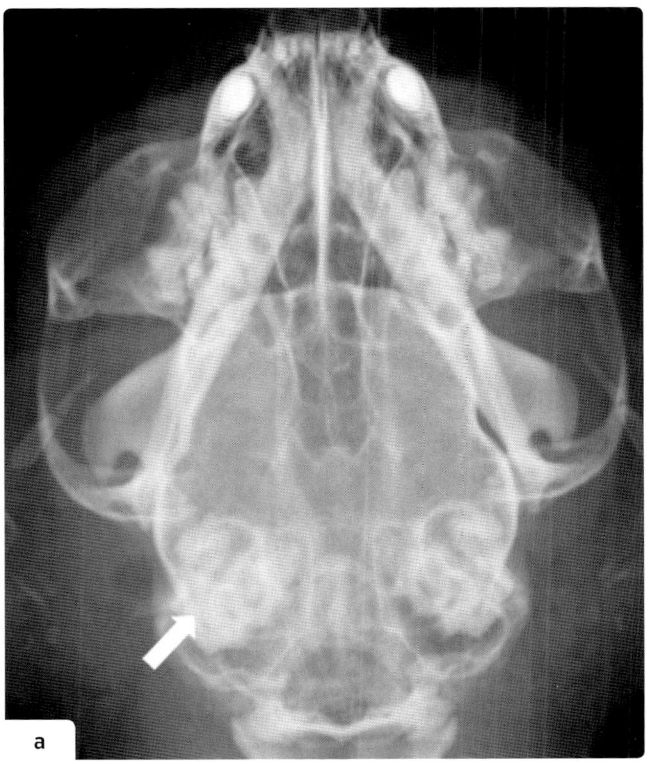

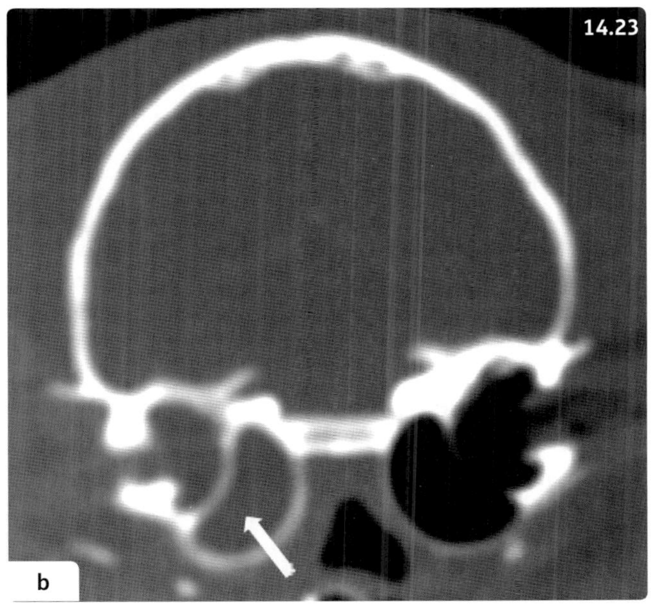

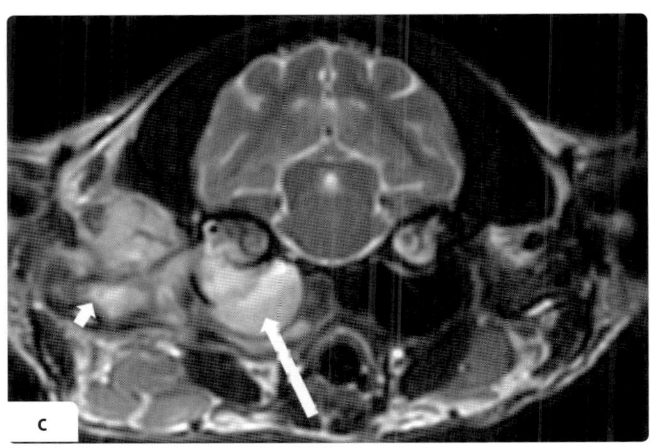

Figures 14.23a–c (a) Ventrodorsal radiograph of a cat with a right-sided head tilt. There is increased bone density associated with the osseous bulla on the right side (arrow), compatible with middle ear disease. (b) Transverse CT scan of the cat in 14.23a at the level of the osseous bullae. Soft tissue opacity (arrow) can be seen within both of the cat's middle ear cavities on the right side, accompanied by increased bone density. (c) Transverse T2-weighted MR image of the same cat at the level of the bullae confirming abnormal signal within the middle (arrow) and external ear cavities. The cat had a severe otitis media/interna, which had extended from the external ear canal and resulted in peripheral vestibular signs.

CSF collected from the cerebellomedullary cistern can also be helpful. Serologic ± CSF testing for potential infectious agents is indicated where CSF testing shows inflammation.

Management

Treatment options for vestibular dysfunction are determined by the underlying etiology. Supportive care should consist of administering IV fluids to animals that are vomiting and confining the animal to a well-padded area in order to minimize self-trauma secondary to disorientation. Meclizine or maropitant can be given to treat nausea.

PERIPHERAL VESTIBULAR DISEASES

IDIOPATHIC VESTIBULAR DISEASE

Definition/overview

Idiopathic vestibular disease is a common cause of vestibular disturbance in both dogs and cats.

Etiology

The cause of idiopathic vestibular disease is unknown.

Pathophysiology

Idiopathic vestibular disease is characterized by the acute or even peracute onset of nonprogressive peripheral vestibular signs, which has been associated with inflammation of the membranous labyrinth of the semicircular canals.

Clinical presentation

The clinical signs most commonly reflect unilateral involvement of the peripheral vestibular system and can be quite severe and acute at onset. Occasionally, bilateral disease is seen, especially in cats. In contrast with many of the other diseases that affect the peripheral vestibular system, facial paresis and Horner's syndrome are not features of idiopathic vestibular disease.

Differential diagnosis

OMI, ototoxicity, trauma, aural neoplasia, hypothyroidism, nasopharyngeal polyps.

Diagnosis

Diagnosis is based on the presence of a compatible history and physical examination findings and by the exclusion of other causes of peripheral vestibular disease, particularly OMI. Typically, improvement in clinical signs is seen within 2–3 days without specific treatment, and this can be used to help confirm the diagnosis.

Management

No treatment is recommended aside from supportive care, which consists of administering IV fluids to animals that are vomiting and confining the animal to a well-padded area in order to minimize self-trauma secondary to disorientation. Meclizine or maropitant can be given to treat nausea. Prognosis is good as the condition resolves on its own within 2–4 weeks in dogs and 4–6 weeks in cats. A mild residual head tilt or ataxia can persist in some animals.

OTITIS MEDIA/INTERNA

Definition/overview

OMI is one of the more commonly recognized causes of peripheral vestibular disease in both dogs and cats.

Etiology

OMI is caused by bacterial infection of the middle and inner ear.

Pathophysiology

OMI typically develops as an extension of otitis externa (OE), with common bacterial isolates including *Staphylococcus intermedius* and *Pseudomonas* spp. OMI can occur in the absence of OE, in which case it is believed to be due to ascent of bacteria from the oral cavity through the auditory tube or hematogenous spread.

Clinical presentation

Evidence of OE can be apparent on general physical examination. Facial nerve paralysis, neurogenic keratoconjunctivitis sicca, and/or Horner's syndrome can be seen in association with the vestibular signs, due to the close association of CN VII and the sympathetic supply with the petrous temporal bone. Disease is most frequently unilateral, but bilateral disease can also occur.

Differential diagnosis

Idiopathic vestibular disease, ototoxicity, trauma, aural neoplasia, hypothyroidism, nasopharyngeal polyps.

Diagnosis

Diagnosis is based on a thorough otoscopic examination and imaging of the tympanic bullae. Radiography of the tympanic bullae can reveal evidence of fluid density within, and sclerosis of, the bulla. However, radiographs can be normal in some cases, particularly early in the course of disease, and thus additional imaging techniques such as CT or MRI might be required to provide more sensitive imaging of the bone and soft tissue in the affected area. Any exudate noted in the external ear canal should be removed by gentle saline irrigation to visualize the tympanic membrane. The tympanic membrane is frequently ruptured; if it is intact, it can appear to be bulging into the external ear canal. If fluid is visualized within the middle ear, an attempt should be made to obtain a sample via myringotomy. This can be performed under general anesthesia by inserting a 22-gauge spinal needle or tomcat catheter through the ventral aspect of the tympanic membrane, using an otoscope for guidance. The fluid present can then be gently aspirated into a syringe and submitted for cytology and bacterial culture.

Management

The treatment for bacterial OMI consists of a 4–6-week (at least) course of systemic antibacterial drugs. The choice of drugs should be based on the results of culture and sensitivity testing (if samples are successfully obtained via myringotomy). Otherwise, a drug that is effective against the most common causative organisms and penetrates the tympanic bullae (e.g. amoxicillin/clavulanate, a cephalosporin, or a fluoroquinolone) should be chosen. Otic cleansing products should not be used, particularly if the tympanic membrane initially cannot be visualized. If cleansing products escape into the middle ear, they can worsen the vestibular signs and cause deafness. Prognosis is good for resolution of the infection, although neurologic deficits can persist after effective medical therapy due to irreversible damage to the neural structures. Cases that are unresponsive to medical therapy might require surgical drainage and débridement via bulla osteotomy. Occasionally, an infection can extend into the cranial vault, causing central rather than peripheral vestibular signs to predominate. Aggressive management, including surgical drainage of the tympanic bulla and cranial vault via a bulla osteotomy and appropriate drug therapy, can result in a favorable outcome in such cases.

NASOPHARYNGEAL POLYPS

Definition/overview

Nasopharyngeal (inflammatory) polyps comprise well-vascularized fibrous tissue lined by epithelium. Disease is identified most frequently in cats from 1 to 5 years of age but has been reported in dogs.

Etiology

These benign polyps are usually secondary to inflammation of the Eustachian tube.

Pathophysiology

Nasopharyngeal polyps originate in the auditory tube or the lining of the tympanic cavity and grow passively into the nasopharynx or middle ear of cats and, very rarely, dogs. OMI can be a complication of auditory tube obstruction by the polyp.

Clinical presentation

Polyps can cause signs of upper respiratory disease and dysphagia in addition to peripheral vestibular dysfunction. Evidence of otitis externa is often present.

Differential diagnosis

Idiopathic vestibular disease, CMI, ototoxicity, trauma, aural neoplasia, hypothyroidism.

Diagnosis

Diagnosis is based on visualizing the polyp in the nasopharynx or external ear canal during a thorough pharyngeal and otoscopic examination performed under anesthesia. Radiography can reveal occlusion of the nasopharynx or sclerosis and soft tissue opacity within the tympanic bulla. Advanced imaging can provide additional information on the extent of soft tissue involvement associated with the polyp.

Management

Treatment involves removal of the polyp. Many polyps are attached to the auditory tube by a narrow stalk of tissue and this can be successfully removed with simple traction. More extensive polyps may require surgical removal via ventral bulla osteotomy. Horner's syndrome is a common postoperative complication following ventral bulla osteotomy, but tends to be transient. Overall, the prognosis is good. However, recurrence is possible, especially for polyps removed non-surgically.

OTOTOXICITY

Definition/overview

Peripheral vestibular dysfunction can occur secondary to administration of several systemic or topical medications.

Etiology

Systemic administration of aminoglycosides is most commonly associated with ototoxicity.

Pathophysiology

Prolonged therapy for >2 weeks with high doses of the drug are necessary to induce changes in normal animals; however, animals with renal impairment are more susceptible to developing toxicity. Of the aminoglycosides, streptomycin is most often associated with damage to the vestibular system. Due to the potential for ototoxicity, topical otic preparations should never be introduced into the ear when the tympanic membrane cannot be visualized or is found to be ruptured.

Clinical presentation

Ototoxic agents can affect vestibular function, hearing, or both. Other agents can induce ototoxicity when used topically, the most notable of which are the iodophors and chlorhexidine.

Differential diagnosis

Idiopathic vestibular disease, OMI, nasopharyngeal polyps, trauma, aural neoplasia, hypothyroidism.

Diagnosis

Diagnosis is based on the acute onset of compatible clinical signs in an animal that has recently been administered an ototoxic agent, in addition to the exclusion of other causes. Deafness can be confirmed with brainstem auditory evoked response testing.

Management

No definitive treatment is possible. Vestibular signs usually improve over time due to resolution of the damage or compensatory mechanisms, but deafness tends to be permanent.

CENTRAL VESTIBULAR DISEASES (SEE ALSO OTHER CAUSES OF BRAIN DISEASE)

METRONIDAZOLE TOXICITY

Definition/overview

Central vestibular signs have been reported in dogs (and rarely in cats) following administration of metronidazole.

Etiology

Dogs reported to have developed metronidazole toxicity were typically treated with an oral dose of >60 mg/kg/day, although doses as low as 30 mg/kg/day have been incriminated. Metronidazole toxicity has also been reported in cats, but affected animals display signs of forebrain and cerebellar involvement rather than vestibular signs. Toxicity can be seen with lower doses than those reported for dogs.

Pathophysiology

The pathogenesis is poorly understood, but it is hypothesized to be related to the interaction of metronidazole with GABA receptors in the cerebellum and vestibular nuclei.

Clinical presentation

Initial clinical signs include anorexia and vomiting, and can progress rapidly to include bilateral central vestibular signs with either a symmetrical or asymmetrical generalized ataxia and a positional vertical nystagmus. Head tilt and seizures are observed less frequently. The onset of clinical signs can occur as soon as 3 days after initiating treatment but can also be seen following chronic therapy.

Diagnosis

A history of metronidazole administration and compatible clinical signs should lead to a high suspicion for this disorder.

Management

Treatment consists of discontinuation of the drug and provision of nursing care. In addition, administration of diazepam (0.5 mg/kg IV followed by 0.5 mg/kg PO q8h for 3 days has been recommended) has been shown to shorten recovery times in dogs. Recovery is typically seen within 1–3 days in dogs treated with diazepam and within 2–3 weeks in dogs for which treatment only consists of drug discontinuation and supportive care. As with dogs, clinical signs in cats are reversible with discontinuation of the drug.

DROPPED JAW

Definition/overview

Weakness of the jaw muscles may manifest as a reduction in voluntary movement of the jaw causing dysphagia or a complete loss of jaw muscle tone and inability to close the mouth (**Figure 14.24**).

Etiology

The cause of dropped jaw is a bilateral lesion affecting the motor component of CN V (trigeminal nerve). Most commonly this is due to idiopathic trigeminal nerve palsy, which is thought to be a neuritis of unknown cause. Lymphoma and immune-mediated inflammatory diseases are less common differentials that should be considered.

Pathophysiology

The inability to close the mouth implies a bilateral lesion affecting the motor component of CN V, since a unilateral lesion does not cause sufficient weakness to prevent mouth closure. The bilateral nature of the trigeminal lesion strongly implies that it involves the peripheral nerves rather than the brainstem (since a lesion in the brainstem large enough to affect both trigeminal nuclei would likely be fatal). The motor neurons of CN V are located in the pons near the rostral cerebellar peduncles and their axons are distributed to the muscles of mastication by the mandibular branch of CN V.

It is important to differentiate a lesion affecting only CN V from one affecting multiple CNs since both may cause an animal to drool. This can be achieved by examining the animal's ability to use its tongue and swallow food when its mouth is held partially closed; these functions are mediated by CN XII (hypoglossal nerve) and CN IX (glossopharyngeal nerve), respectively, which are not affected by an isolated motor trigeminal neuropathy. Apparent inability to close the mouth must also be distinguished from an unwillingness to close the mouth, which can be caused by painful conditions of the head, such as masticatory muscle myositis, retrobulbar lesions, temporomandibular joint disease, or craniomandibular osteopathy.

Diagnosis

Diagnosis of idiopathic trigeminal neuritis is made largely through recognition of the typical pattern of clinical signs, absence of any other neurologic disease, and allowing a period of time to elapse in which recovery can occur. MRI and CSF can be helpful to rule out other causes.

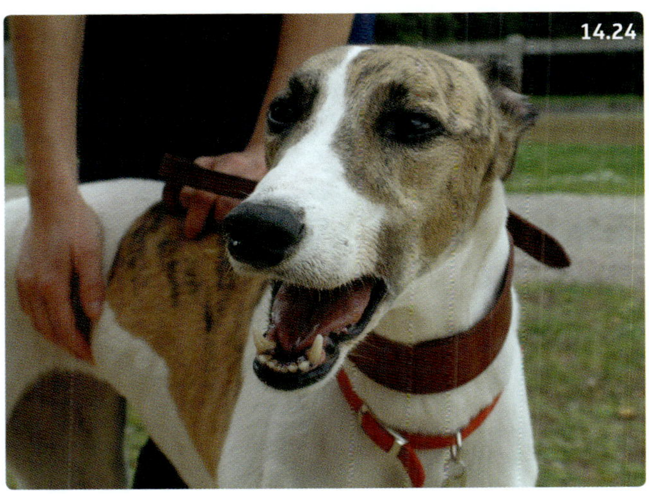

Figure 14.24 A 7-year-old Greyhound with an acute onset of dropped jaw.

Management

Treatment of idiopathic trigeminal neuritis is supportive: helping the animal to eat by offering boluses of soft food and assisting with drinking, or the placement of a temporary feeding tube. It has been suggested that holding the mouth partially closed with a muzzle facilitates eating and drinking during recovery. Most animals recover rapidly and are able to eat unassisted within 3 weeks.

ATROPHY OF THE MASTICATORY MUSCLES

Definition/overview

Masticatory muscle atrophy can occur bilaterally or unilaterally (**Figure 14.25**). In spite of dramatic muscle atrophy, the ability to close the mouth usually appears unimpaired. However, opening the mouth may be very limited in cases in which there has been muscle inflammation and subsequent fibrosis.

Etiology

Masticatory muscle atrophy can result from impaired muscle innervation due to lesions of the motor branch of CN V, diseases of the muscles themselves, or systemic

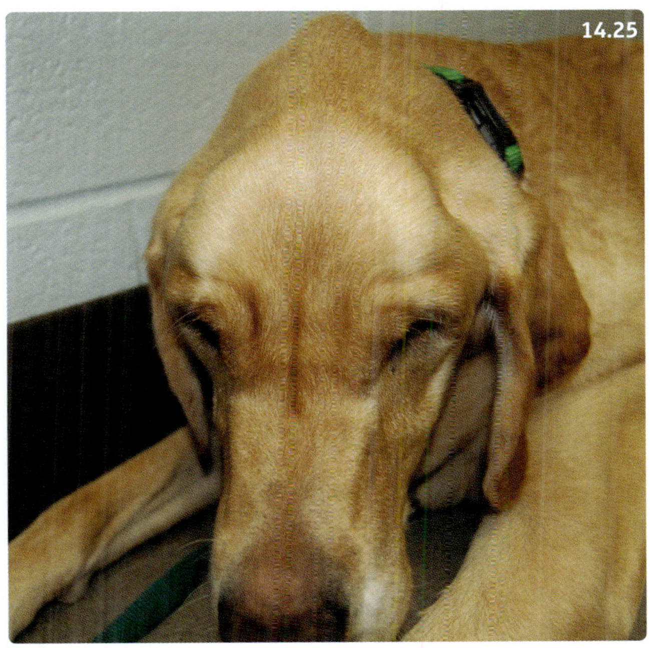

Figure 14.25 Bilateral temporal muscle atrophy is seen in this dog with generalized masticatory muscle atrophy.

disorders such as cachexia or hyperadrenocorticism (or exogenous steroid administration). Unilateral loss of temporal muscle mass can occur in the absence of any sensory signs; it is recognized that nerve sheath tumors may be responsible.

Pathophysiology

Bilateral atrophy can be caused by many systemic diseases, most notably cachexia (associated with cancer) and hyperadrenocorticism (associated with exogenous or endogenous corticosteroids). However, bilateral atrophy most commonly occurs as a consequence of masticatory myositis due to the destruction of muscle fibers and scarring, which can occur rapidly. This is an immune-mediated disorder in which antibody-directed inflammation is targeted at the muscles of mastication, including the masseter, temporalis, and pterygoid muscles. The specific antigen is part of the unique myofiber (type 2M) contained within these muscles. There is no gender predisposition documented for masticatory myositis and breeds noted to have a predisposition include the German Shepherd Dog, Hungarian Vizsla, and Cavalier King Charles Spaniel. Most affected dogs are of large breeds and are often young adults; cats are infrequently affected.

Clinical presentation

Atrophy of the masticatory muscles can occur unilaterally or bilaterally. Bilateral atrophy is not associated with failure to close the mouth, but some individuals exhibit limited mouth opening (trismus). Third eyelid protrusion may follow severe temporal and masseter muscle atrophy, resulting in enophthalmos (due to loss of muscle support to the orbit), which may be sufficiently severe to impair vision. Swelling of the muscles of mastication can occur in the acute phase of masticatory myositis with trismus and exophthalmos. Palpation of the muscles or attempting to open the jaws may cause pain, and occasionally a 'locked jaw' syndrome can result, in which animals are unable to either open or close their mouth. Exophthalmos in the absence of masticatory muscle swelling can result from myositis of the extraocular muscles. Young Golden Retrievers may be predisposed to this unusual disease.

Diagnosis

Detection of a significant concentration of anti-type 2M muscle fiber antibodies confirms masticatory myositis, although by the time the chronic phase is reached, the antibody response may well have subsided. Serum creatine kinase (CK) levels may also be elevated. Muscle biopsy may reveal an inflammatory infiltrate, myofiber necrosis, and phagocytosis. It may also specifically identify antibody localization to the type 2M myofibers. Electromyography often identifies spontaneous abnormalities and should always be performed to evaluate the rest of the musculature in cases where a more generalized myopathy is suspected. CT or MRI is required to diagnose nerve sheath tumors in cases with unilateral masticatory muscle atrophy (**Figure 14.26**).

Management

Masticatory muscle atrophy as a result of systemic disease does not appear to be reversible but does not often cause significant deficits. Masticatory myositis is treated with immunosuppressive doses of corticosteroids, but some cases of atrophy are too far advanced for this therapy to be effective. The recommended dose of prednisolone is 1–2 mg/kg PO q12h for 3–4 weeks, after which the dosage is tapered slowly to achieve the lowest dosage q48h that eliminates the clinical signs. Most dogs treated aggressively in the early stages show a good response to therapy, but relapses are possible. Some cases require the addition of a further immunosuppressive medication, such as azathioprine. While cases that respond rapidly often have a favorable prognosis, chronic loss of muscle may lead to trismus and permanent dysphagia. Feeding regimens should be discussed with the owner, as even in the early stages of a responsive condition feeding tubes

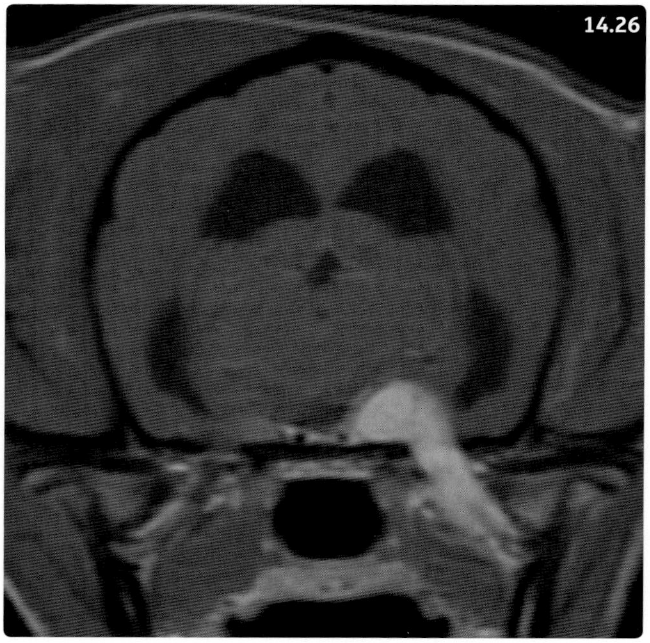

Figure 14.26 Transverse T1-weighted post-contrast brain MR image at the level of the brainstem; the hyperintense lesion compressing the brainstem and seen to exit the skull was confirmed to be a trigeminal nerve sheath tumor.

may be necessary, if only to reduce the potential for aspiration pneumonia. Additional therapy such as vigorous physiotherapy of the jaw muscles (by encouraging the dog to chew rawhides or play with tennis balls) is advisable.

FACIAL PARALYSIS

Definition/overview

Dogs and less commonly cats can present with a drooping of the face due to reduced innervation of the muscles of facial expression. This is most commonly seen as a drooping lip but can also affect the eyelids (**Figure 14.27**).

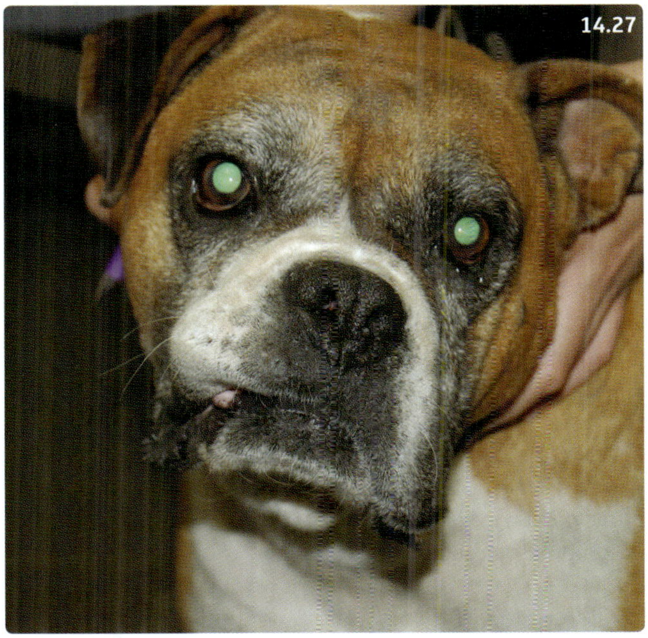

Figure 14.27 A 6-year-old female Boxer with left-sided facial paresis.

Etiology

Facial nerve dysfunction may be due to disease of the peripheral facial nerve caused by OMI, trauma, hypothyroidism, neoplasia of the middle/inner ear, or polyneuropathies. Disease of the facial nerve nucleus in the medulla of the brainstem can result from any disease affecting the CNS. The most common cause of peripheral facial nerve paralysis has been reported to be idiopathic (75% of dogs and 25% of cats with facial paralysis). In addition, facial nerve palsy is sometimes observed in animals with more generalized peripheral neuropathies (e.g. those affecting multiple limbs).

Pathophysiology

Muscles that control facial expression and maintain the normal appearance of the palpebral fissures and mouth are innervated by the facial nerve. The neuron cell bodies are located in the facial nuclei of the rostral medulla and axons leave the ventrolateral surface of the medulla ventral to CN VIII (vestibulocochlear nerve). CN VII (facial nerve) enters the petrosal bone through the internal acoustic meatus on the dorsal aspect of CN VIII and emerges from the skull through the stylomastoid foramen. Any disease affecting CN VII along its path can result in facial paresis, which is often seen as an acute-onset disease.

Clinical presentation

Facial nerve paralysis or palsy may be unilateral or bilateral. Widening of the palpebral fissure and laxity of the facial muscles of expression may be seen. The lip may droop on the affected side and food or saliva may fall from that side of the mouth. The nasal philtrum can be deviated to the normal side in the early stages and drooping of the ears may be apparent in some breeds. There are some signs of CN VII dysfunction, for which pet owners may seek veterinary attention, that do not immediately suggest a facial nerve lesion. Owners may observe the third eyelid flicking over the eye. In these cases, the animal substitutes globe retraction (with concomitant third eyelid protrusion) for blinking with the paralyzed lids. Additionally, accumulation of food in cheeks that have poor muscle tone may lead to halitosis.

Loss of the palpebral and corneal reflexes predisposes the animal to exposure keratitis, which can occur subsequent to improper lubrication of the cornea, despite normal tear production. Clinical signs are usually maximal within 7 days and recovery can take 3–6 weeks if it occurs at all. With chronicity, muscle contracture can lead to narrowing of the palpebral fissure, widening of the mouth and, in unilateral cases, deviation of the nostrils towards the affected side.

Diagnosis

All possible causes of facial paresis and/or paralysis should be excluded before this specific diagnosis of idiopathic facial paresis can be made. A thorough investigation for ear disease should be undertaken in addition to blood tests for hypothyroidism and electromyography to rule out polyneuropathies. MRI may reveal contrast enhancement of the intratemporal facial nerve, which may suggest a poorer prognosis.

Management

There is no effective treatment for the underlying disease but it is important to ensure that the cornea is adequately lubricated (either by endogenous production or eye drops). The prognosis for idiopathic facial palsy varies; many animals make a gradual recovery (weeks to months) but some are left with permanent deficits. These deficits may progress to muscle contracture and deform the facial expression permanently. This can be mistakenly interpreted as hemifacial spasm, an uncommon syndrome in dogs and cats.

SPINAL DISORDERS

Clinical signs of spinal cord dysfunction

The clinical signs associated with spinal cord dysfunction depend on the location, size, and rate of development of the lesion. A small lesion on one side of the spinal cord without a great deal of associated cord swelling (e.g. a slowly growing tumor) will likely cause signs predominantly on the side of the lesion. However, a large lesion or a lesion associated with substantial cord swelling (e.g. an acute disk herniation in the thoracolumbar region) will likely result in bilateral signs of dysfunction. In most spinal cord disorders, bilateral deficits will be observed, but the deficits are often more pronounced on the side of the lesion. Proprioceptive and nociceptive information traveling toward the brain, as well as voluntary motor impulses traveling from the brain, can be affected with spinal cord disease. With progressive spinal cord disease, proprioception is usually the first deficit observed, followed by deficits in voluntary motor ability and finally deficits in the ability to perceive painful stimuli (nociception).

The clinical signs listed below for each of the anatomic subdivisions of the spinal cord represent all of the possible abnormalities that may be encountered with lesions in these respective areas. The clinician may, for example, encounter cases of cervical myelopathy in which severe neck pain is the only clinically detectable abnormality. Alternatively, cases may be encountered with more extensive lesions in the same anatomic location in which the patient is tetraplegic with minimal pain perception to the limbs and having respiratory difficulty. There is a spectrum of possible clinical presentations between these two extreme examples. A topic that is sometimes confusing to clinicians is that of upper motor neuron (UMN) fecal incontinence. Although it is apparently less common than with cauda equina lesions, fecal incontinence may result from cervical or thoracolumbar spinal cord lesions (particularly dorsal lesions, commonly of a cystic nature). This may be due to interruption of ascending information from the rectum to brainstem and cerebral centers responsible for a normal, coordinated defecation reflex, interruption of descending inhibitory influence from such centers on the local spinal cord sacral defecation reflex, or a combination of the two. Since fecal incontinence in these cases does not directly involve the LMNs innervating the anal sphincter musculature or the sensory neurons or nerves innervating the perineum, perineal sensation (in patients with intact pain sensation), as well as anal sphincter tone and perineal reflexes (e.g. anal reflex), are typically normal. The clinical information regarding UMN fecal incontinence in veterinary patients is limited, but it suggests that it may be more responsive to surgical intervention than LMN fecal incontinence. The cauda equina is defined as the nerve roots derived from the cord segments L7 and caudally. Damage to the spinal cord segments supplying the cauda equina will produce the same clinical signs of dysfunction as disruption of the respective nerve roots.

Clinical signs related to disease of C1–C5 spinal cord segments

- Cervical pain (hyperesthesia).
- Proprioceptive deficits ipsilateral to the lesion (forelimb and hindlimb) or all four limbs.
- Voluntary motor deficits ipsilateral to the lesion (forelimb and hindlimb) or all four limbs, varying from paresis to plegia. The paresis or plegia (hemiparesis, hemiplegia, tetraparesis, tetraplegia) is UMN in nature, with normal to hyperactive reflex activity in all limbs.
- Horner's syndrome ipsilateral to the lesion or bilaterally.
- Respiratory difficulty (severe lesions) involving both chest excursions and diaphragmatic movements.
- UMN bladder dysfunction.
- UMN fecal incontinence is possible.
- Nociceptive (pain perception) deficits are possible in all four limbs.

Clinical signs related to disease of C6–T2 spinal cord segments

- Cervical pain (hyperesthesia).
- Proprioceptive deficits ipsilateral to the lesion (forelimb and hindlimb) or all four limbs.
- Voluntary motor deficits ipsilateral to the lesion (forelimb and hindlimb) or all four limbs, varying from paresis to plegia. The paresis or plegia is classically LMN in nature in the forelimbs (involvement of the gray matter of C6–T2 or the efferent axonal processes from that gray matter) and UMN in nature in the hindlimbs. In some instances (e.g. caudal cervical spondylomyelopathy), caudal cervical lesions may result in obvious signs of UMN paraparesis, with subtle or clinically inapparent forelimb deficits.

- Horner's syndrome ipsilateral to the lesion or bilaterally.
- Decreased or absent cutaneous trunci (panniculus) reflex ipsilateral to the lesion or bilaterally. The deficit is due to impairment of the efferent arm of the reflex arc.
- Respiratory difficulty with severe lesions. The respiratory pattern often differs from that seen with C1–C5 spinal cord lesions. Since the phrenic nerve arises from spinal cord segments C5–C7, there is usually enough phrenic nerve function to provide diaphragmatic movement, but impulses from the medullary respiratory centers cannot effectively traverse the damaged cord segments to stimulate the cell bodies of the intercostal nerves. This is the reason for the 'abdominal breathing' pattern seen with severe caudal cervical myelopathies. The thoracic cage moves minimally, if at all, and the exaggerated activity of the diaphragm causes the abdominal contents to move passively.
- UMN bladder dysfunction.
- UMN fecal incontinence is possible.
- Nociceptive deficits are possible in all four limbs.

Clinical signs related to disease of T3–L3 spinal cord segments

- Thoracolumbar pain (hyperesthesia).
- Proprioceptive deficits in the hindlimb ipsilateral to the lesion or both hindlimbs.
- Voluntary motor deficits in the hindlimb ipsilateral to the lesion or both hindlimbs. The paresis or plegia (monoparesis, monoplegia, paraparesis, paraplegia) is UMN in nature, with normal to hyperactive reflex activity in the hindlimbs.
- The forelimbs are neurologically normal (normal proprioception, normal voluntary motor activity). Schiff–Sherrington posture may be seen in the forelimbs and should not be confused with a cervical spinal cord problem. Schiff–Sherrington posture is an anatomic phenomenon, not a prognostic indicator. Depending on the nature of the injury, spinal shock is also a possibility.
- Horner's syndrome is possible with very cranial lesions (T3 spinal cord level), but less likely in comparison with cervical lesions.
- Decreased or absent cutaneous trunci (panniculus) reflex, approximately one to four vertebral levels caudal to the spinal cord lesion. The deficit is due to impairment of the afferent arm of the reflex arc.
- UMN bladder dysfunction.
- UMN fecal incontinence is possible.
- Nociceptive deficits are possible in both hindlimbs.

Clinical signs related to disease of L4–S3 spinal cord segments

- Lumbar pain (hyperesthesia).
- Proprioceptive deficits in the hindlimb ipsilateral to the lesion or in both hindlimbs.
- Voluntary motor deficits in the hindlimb ipsilateral to the lesion or both hindlimbs. The paresis or plegia (monoparesis, monoplegia, paraparesis, paraplegia) is LMN in nature, with a decreased to absent patellar reflex ipsilateral to the lesion or bilaterally. The withdrawal and gastrocnemius reflexes may be normal or decreased, depending on the extent of damage to the L6 spinal segment (L6 contributes to the sciatic nerve).
- A decreased or absent panniculus (cutaneous trunci) reflex may or may not be appreciable one to four vertebral levels caudal to the lesion, because the last three or four lumbar spinal nerves do not give off dorsal cutaneous branches.
- LMN bladder dysfunction.
- LMN fecal incontinence is possible. Decreased anal tone is possible.
- Nociceptive deficits are possible in both hindlimbs and the tail.

Neurodiagnostic investigation

History and findings of physical and neurologic examinations will identify a neurologic problem and assist with neuroanatomic localization and consideration of differentials. The onset (acute or chronic), rate of progression (rapid or gradual), and temporal relation (intermittent and/or episodic, stable or insidious) can be established. A recommended diagnostic approach to spinal cord diseases is as follows:

- CBC, serum biochemistry profile, and urinalysis.
- Thoracic radiographs in animals >5 years of age and after trauma.
- Survey spinal radiographs can assist with recognition of obvious abnormalities such as diskospondylitis, luxations, and bone neoplasia. If an abnormality is not seen, advanced imaging and CSF analysis are indicated.
- CSF collection, preferably from the cerebellomedullary cistern and caudal lumbar region (**Figures 14.28a, b**).

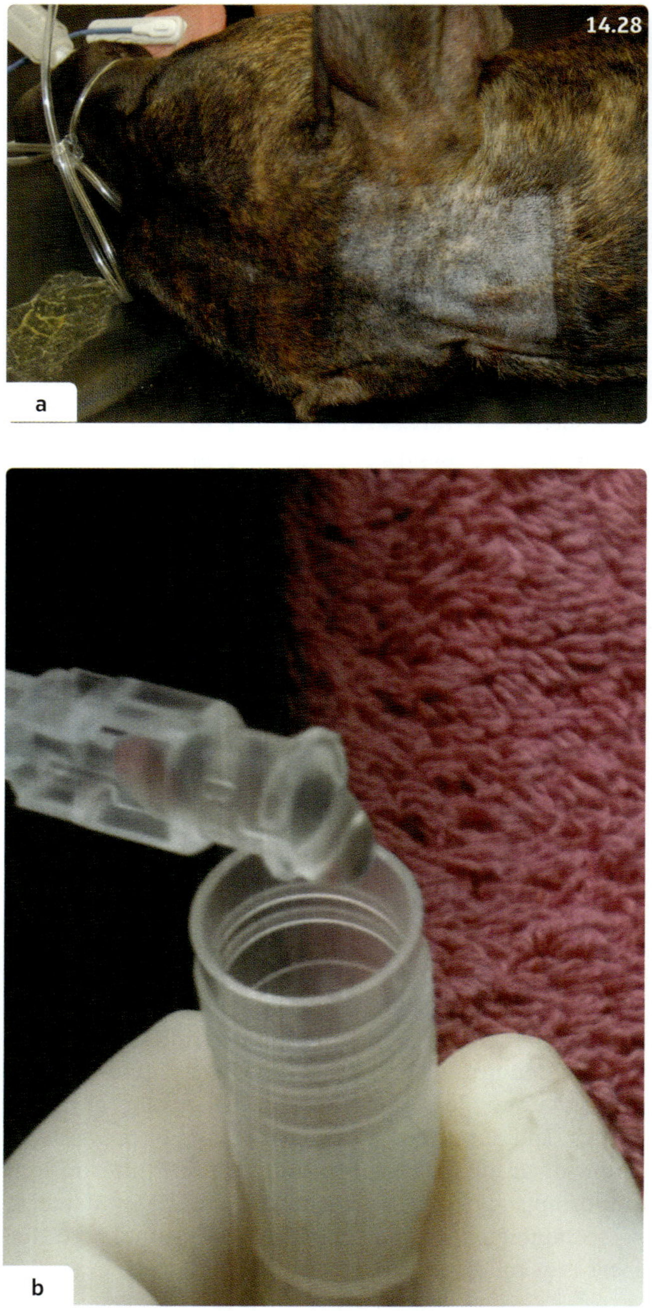

Figures 14.28a, b (a) The skin over the caudal skull and cranial cervical column is shaved and prepared in a sterile fashion for a CSF tap at the cerebellomedullary cistern. (b) A spinal needle with a translucent hub is used to obtain CSF and it is allowed to drip into a sterile polypropylene tube.

- Myelography and epidurography are useful for the detection and characterization of compressive spinal cord lesions (extradural, intradural, and intramedullary) and for determining the extent of the compression (**Figure 14.29**).

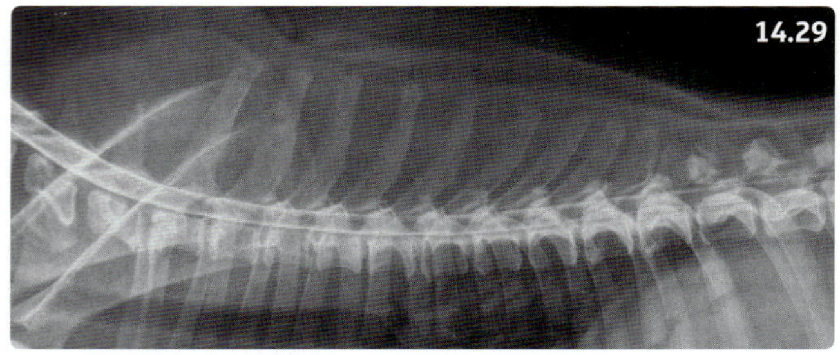

Figure 14.29 A lateral cervicothoracic myelogram.

- CT is used as a primary method to evaluate the spine or assist with determining lesion extent after myelography.
- MRI is becoming more available to veterinarians in general and specialty practice and is considered the standard of care in the detection of lesions within the spinal cord.

Additional diagnostic procedures include electrodiagnostic evaluation (electromyography and nerve conduction studies), nerve and muscle biopsy, CSF protein electrophoresis, serology, PCR, and exploratory surgery.

VASCULAR DISEASE

FIBROCARTILAGINOUS EMBOLIC MYELOPATHY

Definition/overview

Fibrocartilaginous embolic myelopathy (FCEM) is characterized by acute spinal cord infarction caused by embolism of fibrocartilage identical to that of the nucleus pulposus of the intervertebral disk. Acute tetra-, para-, or monoparesis or monoplegia can be seen based on the location of the ischemic injury to the cord. Most commonly this affects large breed dogs. FCEM rarely affects cats.

Etiology

FCEM is caused by embolism of fibrocartilage identical to that of the nucleus pulposus of the intervertebral disk (IVD).

Pathophysiology

Many theories exist as to the pathophysiology for embolization. Entry of disk material into the vascular system and embolization from the point of entry to the arteries and veins of the spinal cord has yet to be elucidated. The gray matter is more severely affected because of its higher metabolic demand. Nonchondrodystrophoid breeds are predisposed, which may relate to the disk being more gelatinous and prone to cause microextrusion. FCEM is frequently recognized in large and giant breed dogs but also affects small- to medium-sized dogs. Purebred dogs that have been documented with FCEM include Miniature Schnauzers, German Shepherd Dogs, and Irish Wolfhounds. FCEM is rare in cats. In dogs the male-to-female ratio varies in different studies and the median age in most studies is 5 or 6 years with a wide age range. In cats, males and females are equally represented with most cats older than 7 years.

Clinical presentation

Neuroanatomic localization often is associated with the spinal cord intumescences, but other spinal cord regions can be involved. Thoracolumbar signs are more common than cervicothoracic signs. Clinical signs usually are associated with trauma or exercise. Asymmetrical lesion distribution is a clinical feature due to the distribution of the blood vessels to the spinal cord parenchyma; however, the lesion can be symmetrical. Symmetrical lesions more often are associated with loss of nociception. Spinal hyperesthesia can be present initially but is absent after the onset of ischemia. Maximal neurologic deficits usually occur within the first 24 hours. Dogs with lumbosacral intumescent involvement more often have loss of deep pain perception.

Diagnosis

Diagnosis is based on history, signalment, and clinical signs. Intramedullary spinal cord swelling provides early myelographic evidence of FCEM. MRI is the preferred diagnostic imaging modality for detection of intramedullary lesions and a presumptive diagnosis of FCEM. MRI findings include a focal, sharply demarcated, and often asymmetric intramedullary lesion, which predominantly affects the gray matter (**Figure 14.30**). CSF analysis may reveal abnormalities in severe cases. Dogs that are ambulatory on presentation are more likely to have normal MRI. The severity of neurologic signs has been associated with the extent of longitudinal and transverse lesions on MRI. Diagnosis of FCEM is confirmed by histopathology and documentation of nucleus pulposus in the spinal cord vasculature.

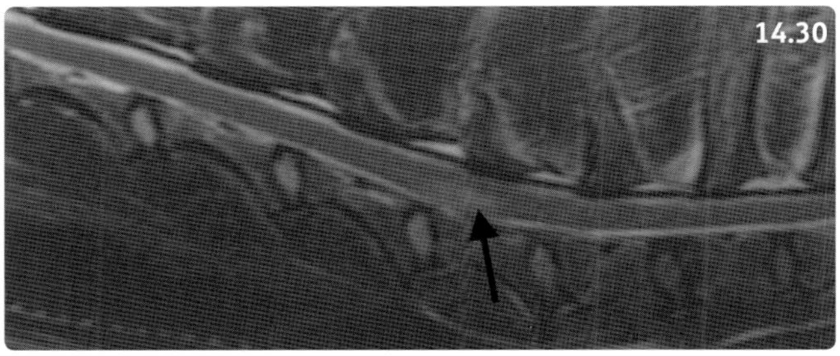

Figure 14.30 Sagittal T2-weighted cervical spinal MR image of a 6-year-old Labrador Retriever with a hyperintense lesion within the parenchyma of the spinal cord (arrow), confirmed histopathologically to be associated with a fibrocartilaginous embolus.

Management

Treatment is with supportive care. As for all spinal cord injuries, physical rehabilitation is important in the process of recovery.

Depending on inclusion criteria, recovery rates have ranged from 54% to 84%. Partial or complete recovery is dependent on the extent of spinal cord damage. Negative indicators of prognosis have been correlated with involvement of the intumescences, symmetry of signs, severe neurologic dysfunction, lack of improvement within 14 days, and decreased deep pain sensation Outcome also has been associated with the longitudinal and transverse extent of the ischemic intramedullary lesion on MRI. However, no associations have been identified between recovery times and clinical or MRI variables. Dog size and severity of clinical signs contribute to owners electing for euthanasia. Animals with functional recovery within 2 weeks have a better prognosis; however recovery may not be complete.

AORTIC THROMBOSIS

Definition/overview

Aortic thromboembolism, also known as saddle thrombus, often causes acute neurologic dysfunction affecting the hindlimbs in addition to clinical signs of poor peripheral perfusion, such as nail bed cyanosis. Cats with systemic thromboembolic disease have a thrombus that obstructs the terminal aorta. The disease can occasionally affect dogs and may present more chronically as lameness or exercise intolerance affecting the hindlimbs.

Etiology

Cats with systemic thromboembolic disease have a thrombus that obstructs the terminal aorta. The most frequent underlying disease in cats with thromboembolism is hypertrophic cardiomyopathy, but also other unclassified cardiomyopathies. In dogs, the disease is more commonly associated with steroid use, hyperadrenocorticism, and neoplasia.

Pathophysiology

Aortic thromboembolism is also known as saddle thrombus. Thrombi form in the left atrium and dilation of the left atrium is one of the greatest risk factors for aortic thromboembolism. The three conditions that favor thrombus formation include blood stasis, hypercoagulability, and endothelial damage (Virchow's triad). Once the thrombus forms, it usually follows a path of least resistance and eventually lodges at the aortic trifurcation. Restriction of blood flow by the embolus and release of vasoactive substances cause ischemic injury to the nerves and muscles of the hindlimbs.

Clinical presentation
Clinical signs consist of acute onset of an asymmetrical hindlimb paresis and/or paralysis. Abyssinian, Birman, Ragdoll, and male cats were overrepresented in one study. The femoral pulse is weak or absent. The limbs are cold and the nail beds are cyanotic and fail to bleed when cut. The hindlimbs are stiff and the muscles are hard and painful on palpation. Typically, there is loss of hindlimb nociception distally. Tachypnea and hypothermia are frequently seen. Congestive heart failure and arrhythmias can each be seen in over 40% of cats.

Diagnosis
Aortic thromboembolism is suspected based on clinical signs. Common biochemical abnormalities in these cats include hyperglycemia, hyperkalemia, azotemia, and a markedly elevated CK concentration soon after the embolic episode. Evidence of cardiac disease is further supported by physical examination findings, thoracic radiographs, and echocardiography. Doppler ultrasonography and/or CT of the aorta and its trifurcation can sometimes identify thrombotic disease (**Figure 14.31**).

Management
Initially, therapy involves management of the cardiac disease and supportive care. Cats benefit from administration of appropriate fluid therapy, acepromazine maleate (ACP), thromboembolism treatment, and pain management. Use of ACP is controversial; although it may improve collateral blood flow and decrease anxiety, it may cause hypotension and current advice is to avoid its use. Specific therapies for the clot include surgical removal, anticoagulants, and thrombolytic agents; but risks versus benefits need to be considered because in time the clot may undergo spontaneous thrombolysis. The use of agents to prevent more clot formation is controversial. Therapies include use of warfarin, heparin, aspirin, and thienopyridine derivatives. Low-dose aspirin (5 mg/cat q72h) has been shown to produce similar survival time and recurrence rates to high-dose aspirin (>25 mg/cat q72h) but with fewer side-effects. Long-term prognosis for cats with aortic thromoboembolism is guarded in the early recovery phase but may improve if cats live to discharge. Studies have shown rates of survival to discharge to range between 27% and 35% using various treatments. Median survival times of cats surviving after discharge range from 117 to 345 days. Cats with congestive heart failure tend to have a significantly shorter survival time than cats without this problem.

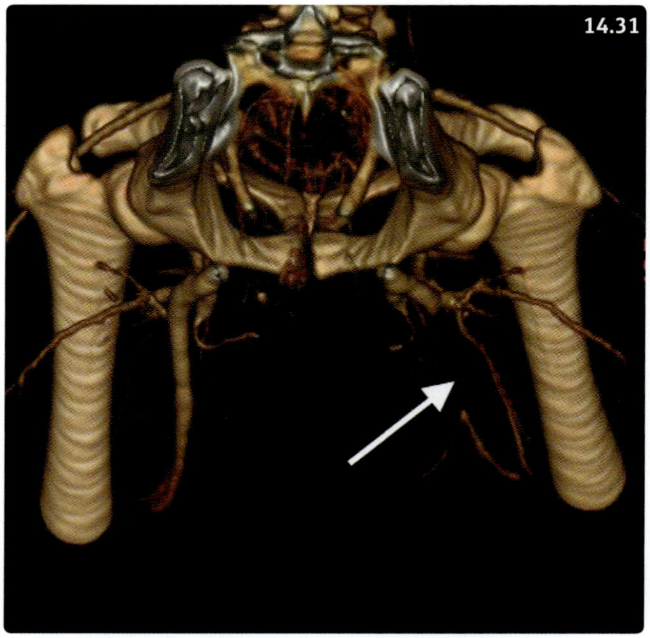

Figure 14.31 3-D reconstructed CT scan of the pelvis and hindlimbs identifying a lack of vascular perfusion in the left femoral artery (arrow) secondary to an intravascular thrombus. (Courtesy Davies Veterinary Specialists)

TRAUMATIC DISEASES

FRACTURES AND LUXATIONS

Definition/overview
Spinal fracture and luxation in dogs and cats are most commonly associated with severe external trauma, occurring in approximately 6% of cases as the cause of spinal cord dysfunction. The resulting clinical signs can vary from pain to paralysis with loss of nociception.

Etiology
Automobile-related injury is the most common cause of exogenous trauma to the spine.

Pathophysiology
The thoracolumbar junction is the most commonly injured site in dogs and cats. Fractures occur between T11 and L6 in 50–60% of patients after blunt trauma. Fractures in the thoracic spine may have little displacement because of

the protection provided by the ribs, ligamentous support, and epaxial musculature. Fractures and luxations of the thoracolumbar spine are often associated with other systemic injuries (e.g. pneumothorax, pulmonary contusions, orthopedic injuries, urogenital injuries, and diaphragmatic hernia). Approximately 20% of patients with thoracolumbar fractures have a second spinal column fracture. In the neck, the atlantoaxial junction is relatively unstable and therefore particularly at risk. The axis is the most commonly fractured cervical vertebra because it acts as a fulcrum between the caudal cervical spine and the so-called cervicocranium (the skull, atlas, dens, and body of the axis) (**Figures 14.32a–c**).

Primary mechanical injury to neural tissue can subsequently lead to secondary biochemical injury. The amount of neural tissue injury is related to the rapidity and severity of insult and the amount and duration of compression.

Clinical presentation

The neurologic signs are determined by the level of any associated spinal cord damage. Schiff–Sherrington posture is a common finding associated with acute thoracolumbar injury but is not a prognostic indicator (**Figure 14.33**). Pain perception is carefully assessed in paraplegic animals to assist with determination of prognosis. Respiratory crises may be noted with acute cervical spinal cord injury.

Diagnosis

Results of the neurologic examination are used to determine neuroanatomic localization and severity of the spinal cord injury. It is important to perform the neurologic examination with care to prevent further injury and displacement of the spine. The neurologic examination findings are most important in establishing the prognosis, irrespective of radiographic

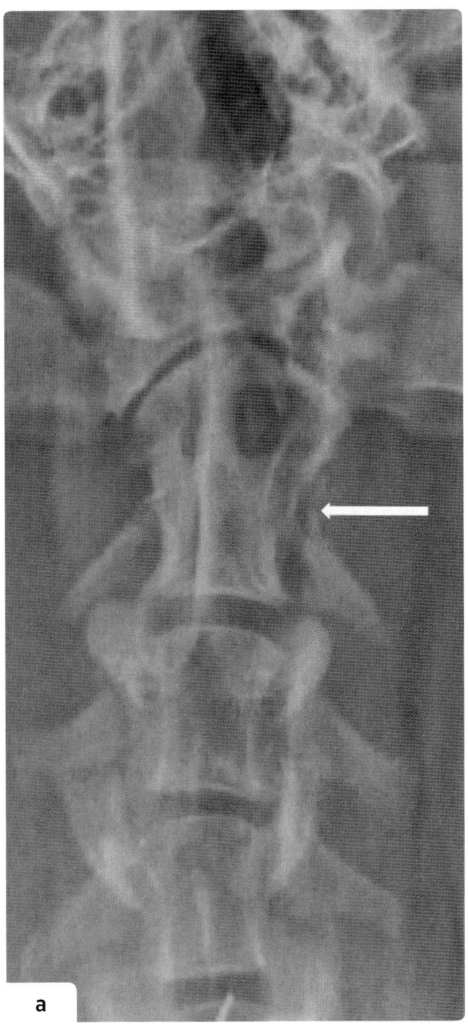
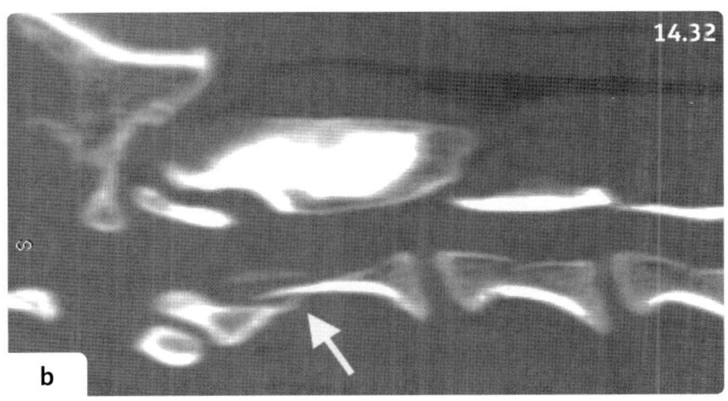
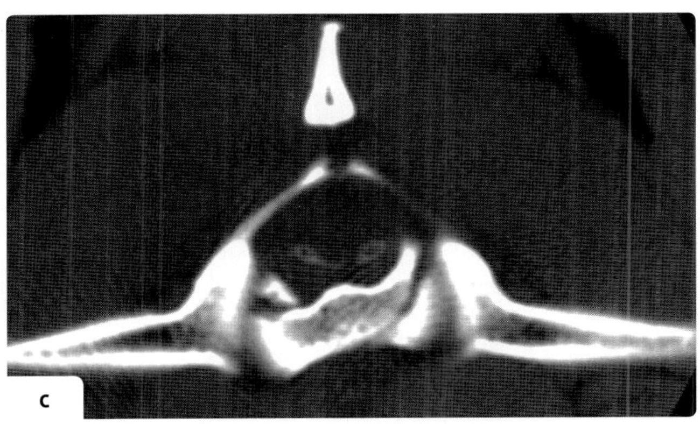

Figures 14.32a–c (a) Ventrodorsal radiograph of the cranial cervical spinal column. A fracture of the cranial aspect of the body of C2 (arrow) can be identified. (b) Sagittal CT scan of the cranial cervical spinal column of the same dog as in 14.32a showing the linear fracture (arrow). (c) Transverse reconstruction through the C2 vertebra showing displacement of the body fracture.

findings. Plain radiography of the entire spine should be performed. Two views are used while minimizing patient movement by obtaining the ventrodorsal view using horizontal beam. Results of survey radiography are used to determine the precise lesion location(s) and extent, demonstrate multiple lesions, and guide appropriate management (**Figure 14.34**). Myelography or cross-sectional imaging is used when the radiographic findings do not correlate with the neurologic examination, to evaluate spinal cord swelling in concussive injuries and to further assess severity of spinal cord compression. CT or MRI is useful for further evaluating bone and spinal cord tissues, respectively, and provide a 3-D configuration of the fracture/luxation extent for assessment of spinal stability (**Figures 14.35a–d**).

Management

The critical factor in determining whether conservative or surgical management of spinal fracture and luxation is appropriate depends on the presence of instability. Spinal stability is assessed using a three-compartment theory (**Figure 14.36**). Priority is placed on treatment of extraneural injuries, beginning with management of shock and hemorrhage. Management of an animal with spinal trauma focuses on the prevention of secondary injury to the spinal cord parenchyma. Indications for nonsurgical management include minimal neurologic deficits, minimal vertebral displacement, and lack of myelographic evidence of spinal cord compression. Principles of conservative management are appropriate confinement for 6–8 weeks and use of external coaptation. The aim of external support is to provide immobilization of the vertebral segments cranial and caudal to the damaged area. It is important to follow principles of bandage care when using methods of external support. The patient will need to be turned regularly and kept clean and dry to prevent urine scalding.

Surgical management often provides a better chance for more rapid and complete neurologic recovery. However, the role of surgery for spinal trauma remains unclear. Indications include severe neurologic deficits and deteriorating neurologic status, imaging evidence of compression, and damage of two or more vertebral compartments. Timely surgical intervention is important to allow for maximal recovery. The objectives for surgical management of spinal trauma are decompression, realignment, and stabilization. The decompressive procedure should be conservative so as not to disrupt further the integrity of the vertebrae, but large enough to allow for removal of compressive material. Successful outcome after surgical fixation depends on the type and strength of fixation, the surgeon's skill and knowledge of the spinal anatomy, and the accuracy of vertebral column alignment (**Figure 14.37**).

Careful attention to postoperative care is imperative for the wellbeing of the patient. Potential complications include urinary tract infections, decubital ulcers (**Figures 14.38a, b**), and implant failure. Physical rehabilitation is important in the recovery process.

The prognosis for animals with acute spinal injury is dependent on the results of the neurologic examination. The prognosis for recovery from a spinal fracture or luxation that results in paraplegia with loss of deep pain perception is considered poor. Patients that maintain pain perception may still require months to recover and have residual neurologic deficits including urinary and/or fecal incontinence. Studies of thoracolumbar fracture and luxation have summarized a 70–95% recovery rate for conservative management on selected cases. Although displacement can vary, results of spinal stabilization tend to be good if pain perception remains intact.

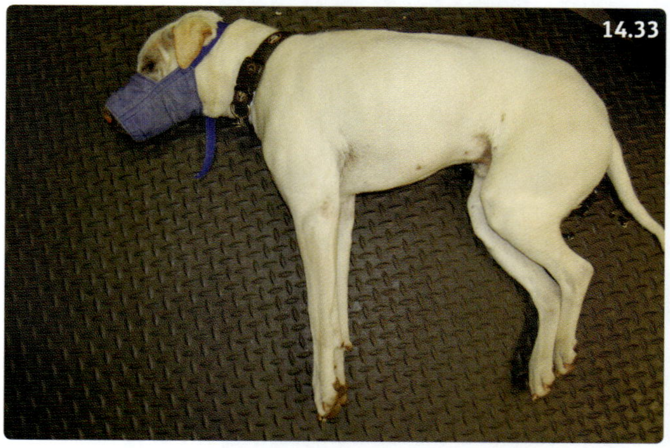

Figure 14.33 A 4-year-old mixed-breed dog exhibits Schiff–Sherrington posture secondary to an acute thoracolumbar spinal trauma.

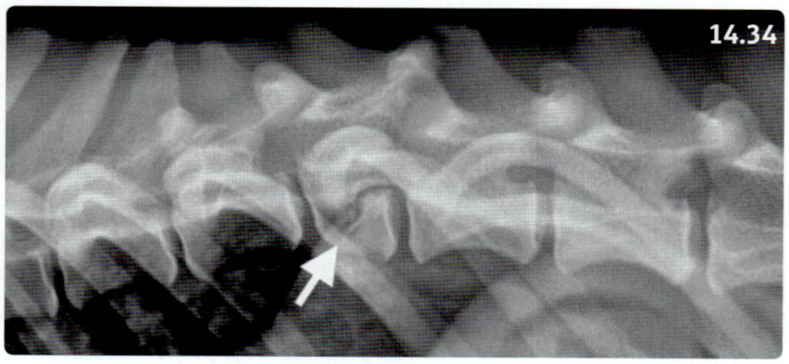

Figure 14.34 Lateral radiograph of a canine thoracic vertebral column, showing a T12 compressed body fracture (arrow).

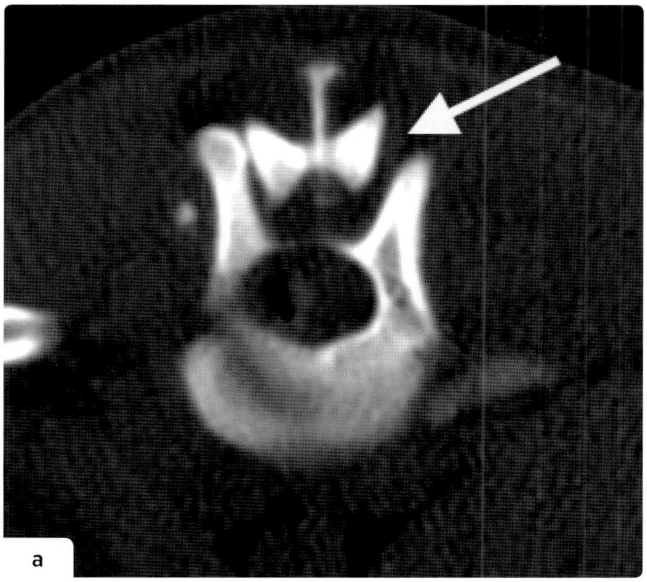

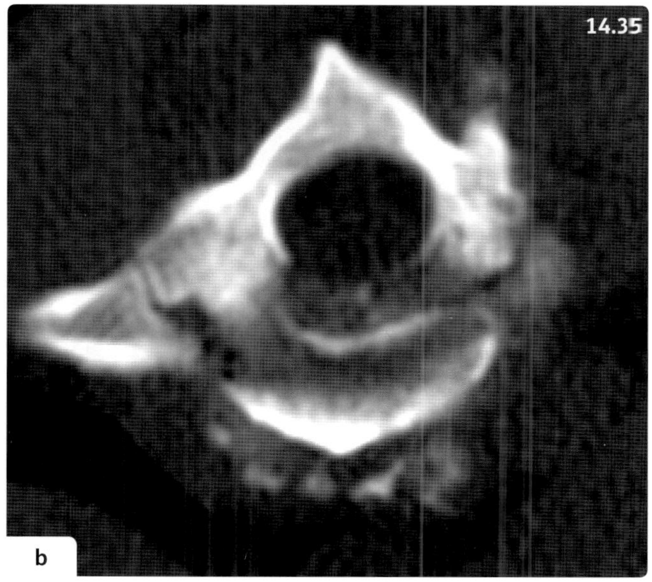

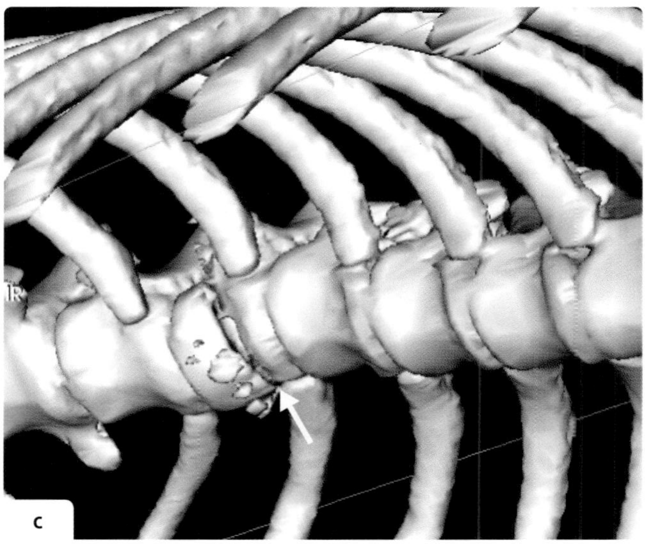

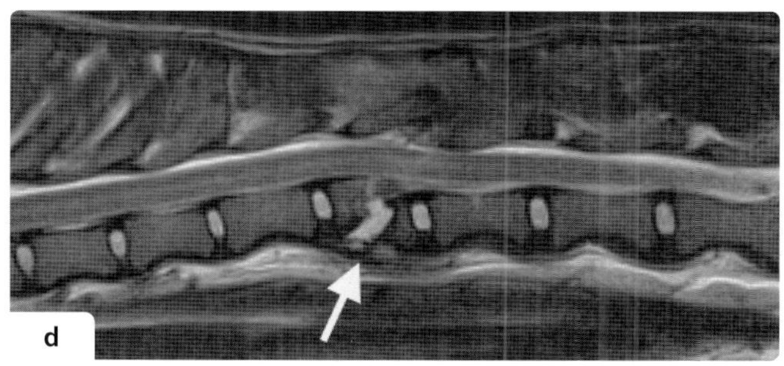

Figures 14.35a–d (a) Transverse T12 and T13 vertebrae CT scan of the fracture depicted in Figure 14.34. Note the subluxation of the articular processes (arrow). (b) Transverse T12 vertebral body CT scan showing the fracture depicted in Figure 14.34. (c) 3-D reconstructed CT scan of the thoracic vertebrae helps identify the ventral aspect of the T12 body fracture (arrow). (d) Sagittal T2-weighted MR image of the thoracic vertebrae is useful to visualize the effect of the T12 fracture (arrow) on the spinal cord.

BRACHIAL PLEXUS AVULSION

Definition/overview

Traumatic injuries causing avulsion of the nerve roots of the brachial plexus are the most common cause of acute forelimb monoparesis or monoplegia in small animals.

Etiology

These injuries are usually a result of abduction and simultaneous caudal displacement of the forelimbs caused by road traffic accidents or falls from a height.

Pathophysiology

The site of root avulsion is usually intradural where the nerve roots arise from the spinal cord. At this point, nerve roots lack a well-defined perineurium and constitute the weakest structure between the spinal cord and the peripheral nervous system. If the avulsion is severe enough, it may place traction over the spinal cord and damage spinal cord pathways, causing ipsilateral hindlimb neurologic deficits. Both dorsal and ventral nerve roots can be affected, but the motor roots appear to be more susceptible to this type of trauma.

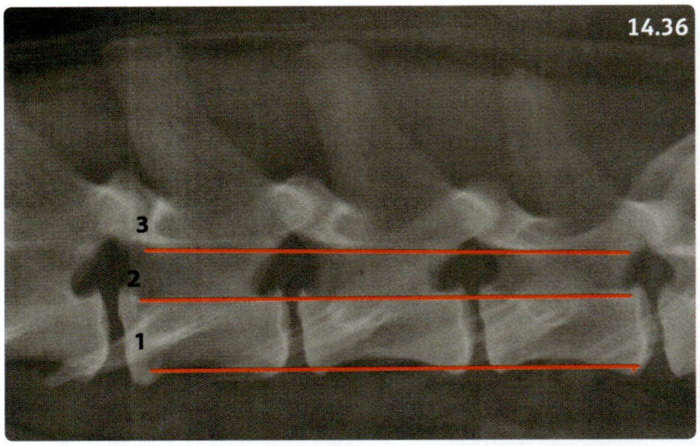

Figure 14.36 Three-compartment model of vertebral instability. Compartment one contains the ventral three-quarters of the vertebral body and disk and the ventral longitudinal ligament. The second compartment consists of the dorsal one-quarter of the vertebral body, the disk, and the dorsal longitudinal ligament. The third compartment includes the articular processes, lateral pedicles, dorsal laminae, interarcuate ligaments, and dorsal spinous processes.

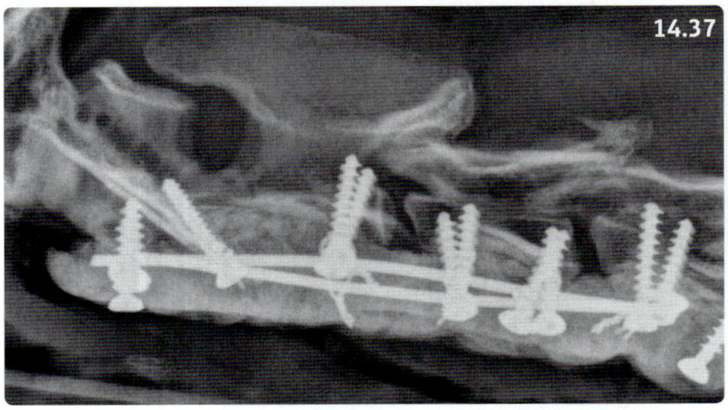

Figure 14.37 Lateral post-spinal fixation radiograph of the dog with a C2 vertebral fracture illustrated in Figure 14.33.

Clinical presentation

Signs are peracute in onset following the traumatic incident. Depending on which nerve roots are affected, avulsions are divided into three types:

- Cranial avulsions (C6–C7 nerve roots).
- Caudal avulsions (C8–T2 nerve roots).
- Complete avulsions (C6–T2 nerve roots).

Cranial avulsions are rare and result in few clinical signs. The elbow extensor muscles are not affected, so the animal can bear weight on the affected limb. There is loss of shoulder movement and elbow flexion, and atrophy of supraspinatus and infraspinatus muscles usually develops.

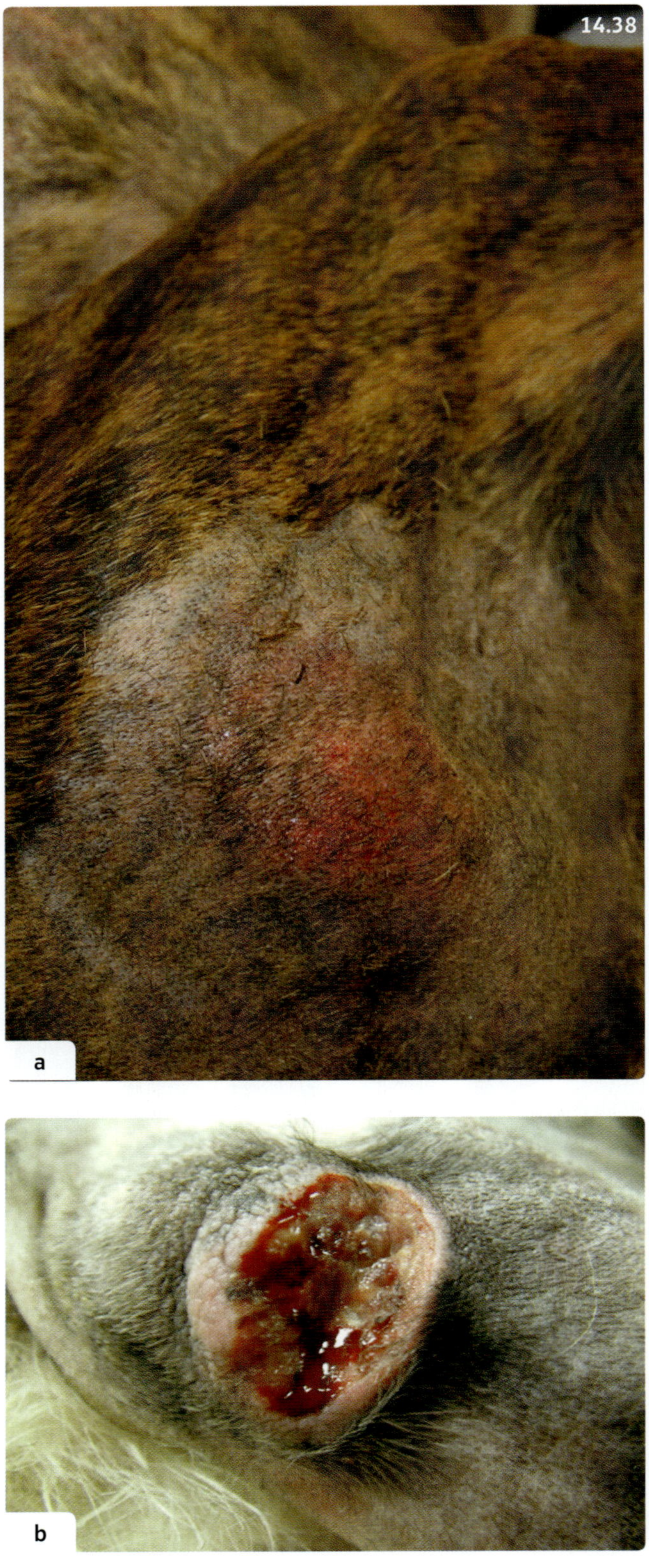

Figures 14.38a, b (a) An early stage decubital ulcer appearing over the ischium following a short period of recumbency in a paralyzed dog. (b) A later stage, open and granulating decubital ulcer.

Caudal and complete avulsions are more common and cause more severe clinical signs. They both cause paralysis of the triceps brachii muscle, so the animal cannot extend the elbow or bear weight on the affected limb. Affected animals drag the limb knuckled over (**Figure 14.39**). Forelimb muscles are hypotonic and severe neurogenic atrophy starts about 1 week after the injury. Spinal reflexes and postural reactions are reduced. If the elbow flexor muscles are spared (caudal avulsions), the animal can carry the limb flexed at this level, avoiding contact with the floor.

Sensory signs are also common. The pattern of decreased or absent sensation in the affected limb allows better determination of the type of avulsion. Cutaneous sensation should be checked in the entire limb, but particular attention should be paid to nociception in the medial (radial and musculocutaneous) and lateral (radial and ulnar) digits, since it is essential in determining a prognosis.

A high percentage of patients with brachial plexus avulsions show partial Horner's syndrome and/or loss of cutaneous trunci reflex ipsilateral to the side of the avulsion. Avulsion of the T1 ventral nerve root causes injury to the preganglionic sympathetic nerve fibers to the eye, causing ipsilateral miosis (partial Horner's syndrome). Loss of the cutaneous trunci reflex is caused by damage to the C8–T1 ventral spinal nerve roots that form the lateral thoracic nerve and innervate the cutaneous trunci muscle. The contralateral reflex is usually present after ipsilateral stimulation.

Diagnosis

A history of forelimb monoparesis after a traumatic incident should raise a high suspicion of brachial plexus avulsion. Every animal unable to use one forelimb after trauma should be examined carefully to detect orthopedic as well as neurologic abnormalities. MRI of the affected plexus may provide information on the degree of nerve and associated soft tissue trauma. Electromyography allows detection of spontaneous electrical activity in the denervated muscles 7–10 days after the injury. Nerve conduction velocity studies of the radial and ulnar nerves allow determination of the degree of injury. Since the radial nerve is commonly injured in brachial plexus avulsions, serial electrodiagnostic evaluations of this nerve may provide useful diagnostic and prognostic information.

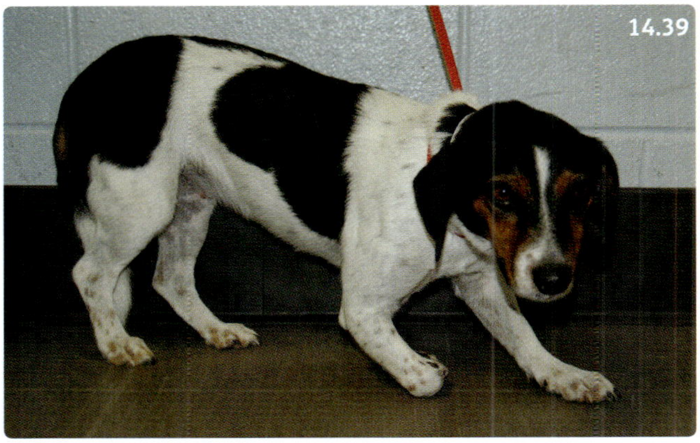

Figure 14.39 Forelimb monoplegia and moderate proximal limb muscle atrophy are evident in this dog with a right-sided brachial plexus avulsion following a traumatic insult.

Management

Unfortunately, there is no routinely effective treatment for this type of injury. The degree of recovery depends only on the severity of the nerve lesion at the time of injury.

If nociception is present in the medial and lateral digits, prognosis for recovery is good and aggressive physiotherapy should be recommended to the owner. If nociception is absent, prognosis will depend on the severity of the axonal injury, being good for neurapraxic lesions but guarded to poor for axonotmetic (nerve injury to axon while sparing the myelin) and neurotmetic (disruption of axon, myelin sheaths, and connective tissue) lesions. Pure axonotmesis occurs rarely, so the potential for recovery, although present, is low and prognosis poor.

When the proximal branches of the radial and musculocutaneous nerves are spared – so that the elbow flexor and extensor muscles are not denervated – corrective surgery can be used to provide carpal extension and prevent the distal part of the limb from collapsing. Tendon transplantation or carpal arthrodesis procedures can be performed.

Animals with caudal and complete brachial plexus avulsions have a poor to guarded prognosis if neurotmesis has occurred. Only those with neurapraxic (temporary loss of sensory and motor function due to nerve injury) injuries show improvement and recover completely. However, most animals do not improve but go on to show severe limb atrophy, eventually developing serious complications such as trophic ulcers, joint contractures or self-mutilations from paresthesia, or abnormal sensation in the affected areas produced by regeneration of sensory nerves. In these cases, amputation of the limb is necessary. The best predictor of complete recovery seems to be nociception. Preservation of nociception is an indicator of a milder type of injury and should prompt the clinician to recommend supportive therapy while waiting for motor function to recover. However, if no improvement is seen during the first 2 months, recovery is unlikely to occur.

DEGENERATIVE DISEASES

DEGENERATIVE MYELOPATHY

Definition/overview

Degenerative myelopathy (DM) is a slowly progressive nonpainful paresis and ataxia usually affecting large breed dogs (especially the German Shepherd Dog).

Etiology

For many years the etiology of DM remained unknown. A mutation in the superoxide dismutase 1 (*SOD1*) gene is now associated with this disease.

Pathophysiology

The uniformity of clinical signs, histopathology, age, and breed predilections suggested an inherited basis for DM. Segregation of DM in families has been reported in the Siberian Husky, Pembroke Welsh Corgi, and Chesapeake Bay Retriever. Dogs testing homozygous for the mutation are at risk for developing DM. Some dogs are homozygous for the mutation but remain free of clinical signs, which suggests age-related incomplete penetrance. A progressive degeneration of the spinal cord, predominantly in the T3–L3 region, is responsible for the clinical signs.

Clinical presentation

Dogs with DM show an insidious, progressive ataxia and paresis of the hindlimbs ultimately leading to paraplegia and euthanasia. If hindlimb hyporeflexia is observed, reflecting nerve root involvement, the disease is sometimes termed canine degenerative radiculomyelopathy. Although the German Shepherd Dog is the most commonly affected breed, DM has been reported in many other pure and mixed breeds. There is no sex predilection. In most breeds, the mean age of onset of neurologic signs is 9 years.

Progressive, asymmetric UMN paraparesis, hindlimb ataxia, and lack of paraspinal hyperesthesia are key clinical features of DM. The clinical course of DM can vary after the presumptive diagnosis. Pet owners usually elect euthanasia when dogs can no longer support weight in their hindlimbs and need walking assistance (**Figures 14.40a, b**). Smaller breed dogs can be cared for by the pet owner over a longer time. The median disease duration in the Pembroke Welsh Corgi is 19 months. As a result of a longer survival time, affected Pembroke Welsh Corgis often have signs of forelimb paresis at the time of euthanasia. The earliest clinical signs of DM are general proprioceptive ataxia and mild paresis in the hindlimbs. Worn nails and asymmetric hindlimb weakness are apparent on physical examination. Asymmetry of signs at disease onset is frequently reported. At disease onset, spinal reflex abnormalities are consistent with UMN paresis localized in the T3–L3 spinal cord segments. Patellar reflexes may be normal or exaggerated;

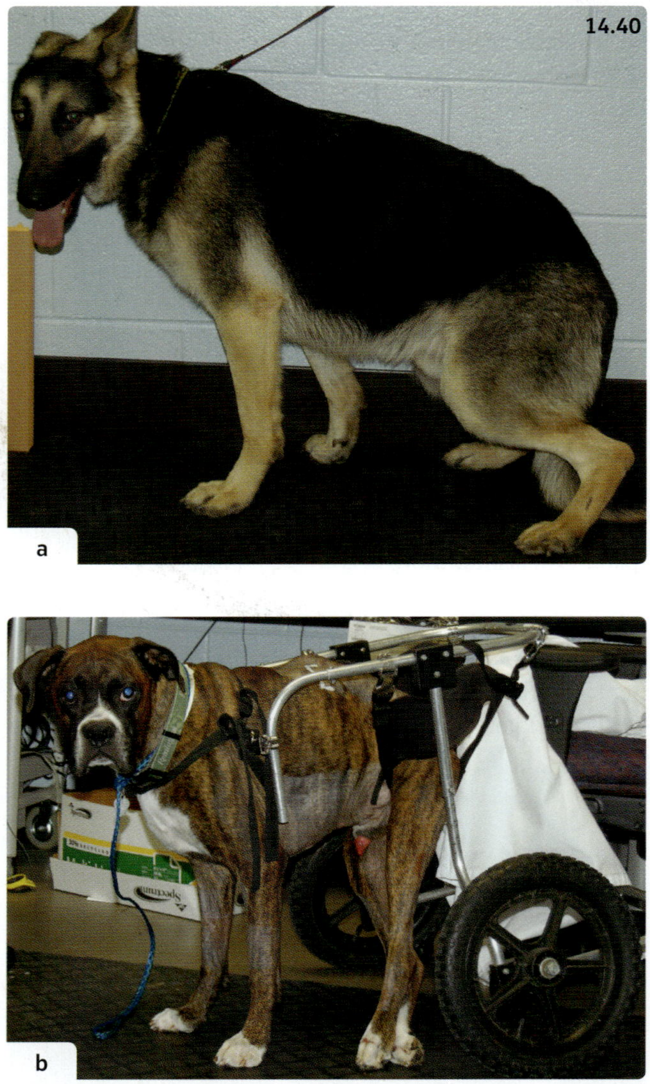

Figures 14.40a, b (a) A 9-year-old German Shepherd Dog with degenerative myelopathy demonstrates profound weakness of the hindlimbs. (b) Severe motor dysfunction of the hindlimbs can be assisted with the use of canine support carts, as shown in this photo.

however, hyporeflexia of the patellar reflex has also been described in dogs at a similar disease stage. Flexor reflexes may also be normal or show crossed extension (suggestive of chronic UMN dysfunction). Most large breed dogs progress to nonambulatory paraparesis within 6–9 months from onset of clinical signs and are euthanized during this disease stage. If the dog is not euthanized early, clinical signs will progress to LMN paraplegia and ascend to affect the forelimbs. Flaccid tetraplegia ultimately occurs in dogs with advanced disease. The paresis becomes more symmetrical as the disease progresses. LMN signs emerge as hyporeflexia of the patellar and withdrawal reflexes, flaccid paralysis, and widespread muscle atrophy beginning in the hindlimbs as the dogs become nonambulatory. Widespread and severe loss of muscle mass occurs in the appendicular muscles in the late stage of DM.

Diagnosis

Tentative antemortem diagnosis is presently based on ruling out other diseases causing progressive myelopathy. Common differentials include intervertebral disk disease (IVDD), inflammatory disease, and spinal cord neoplasia. Hip dysplasia and degenerative lumbosacral stenosis often can be confused with the diagnosis of DM, although the neurologic findings are different if a careful examination is performed. It is not uncommon for DM affected dogs to have coexisting neurological and orthopedic diseases. Diagnostic testing is typically performed in the early disease stage. The lack of abnormal findings of electrodiagnostic testing and myelography or cross-sectional imaging (MRI, CT), along with characteristic disease pattern for progression of neurologic signs, support a presumptive diagnosis of DM. Definitive diagnosis of DM is determined postmortem by histopathologic examination of the spinal cord. A blood test is available to identify SOD1 mutations but the results can only suggest the disease or help rule it out rather than confirm it.

Management

Treatment regimens have been empiric, with lack of evidence-based medicine approaches. Moreover, there exists no prophylactic or curative treatment for human DM. Aminocaproic acid, an antiprotease agent, has been advocated for long-term management of DM; however, there have been no published clinical data to support drug efficacy. While treatment of vitamin deficiencies can resolve neurologic disease in some animals, therapy with parenteral cyanocobalamin or oral alpha-tocopherol did not affect neurologic progression in a study of DM affected dogs. Physical rehabilitation regimens have been advocated for management of DM. Overall, long-term prognosis is considered poor.

HANSEN TYPE I INTERVERTEBRAL DISK DISEASE

(See also Chapter 15: Musculoskeletal disorders)

Definition/overview

Herniation of degenerate nucleus pulposus can result in sudden onset of clinical signs ranging from spinal pain to the loss of motor function and pain sensation. This is most common in the thoracolumbar spinal column but can affect the cervical spinal cord as well.

Etiology

Herniation of the nucleus pulposus through the annulus of the disk and extrusion of nuclear material into the spinal canal, resulting in concussion of the spinal cord and concurrent compression.

Pathophysiology

Hansen type I IVDD is herniation of the nucleus pulposus through the annular fibers and extrusion of nuclear material into the spinal canal. The condition is typically associated with chondroid disk degeneration. The disk extrudes through the dorsal annulus, causing ventral, ventrolateral, or circumferential compression of the spinal cord. Acute disk extrusion is characterized by the presence of soft disk material within the vertebral canal and extradural hemorrhage. Chronic disk extrusion is characterized by extradural fibrous adhesions around the herniated disk material, which has often become a hard mineralized mass. Hansen type I IVDD typically affects chondrodystrophic breeds and has an acute onset. However, large nonchondrodystrophic breeds of dog such as the Dobermann and Labrador Retriever may also be affected. The Dachshund has the highest incidence followed in succession by the Pekingese, Welsh Corgi, Beagle, Lhasa Apso, and Miniature Poodle. In Dachshunds, severe disk degeneration denoted by presence of mineralization on spinal radiography is highly heritable. Hansen type I IVDD most commonly occurs within the thoracolumbar region of chondrodystrophic breeds. The thoracolumbar junction (T12–T13 to L1–L2) accounts for the highest incidence of all disk lesions. The incidence of thoracolumbar IVDD progressively decreases from T12–T13 caudally. The most common site for Hansen type I IVDD in large, nonchondrodystrophic breeds is the interspace between L1 and L2.

Clinical presentation

Onset of neurologic signs may be peracute (<1 hour), acute (<24 hours), or gradual (>24 hours). Dogs presented with peracute or acute thoracolumbar disk extrusions may manifest clinical signs of spinal shock or Schiff–Sherrington postures. These indicate acute and severe spinal cord injury but do not determine prognosis. The degree of neurologic dysfunction is variable and affects prognosis. Clinical signs vary from spinal hyperesthesia only to paraplegia with or without nociception. Dogs with pain only are usually reluctant to walk and may show kyphosis (**Figure 14.41**); these dogs often have myelographic, CT, and MRI evidence of substantial spinal cord compression. Dogs with paraplegia and lack of nociception usually have undergone acute and severe disk extrusions (**Figure 14.42**).

Diagnosis

The initial diagnosis of IVDD is obtained from the signalment, history, and neurologic examination. Differential diagnoses to be considered include trauma, fibrocartilaginous embolism, diskospondylitis, neoplasia, and (meningo)myelitis. Diagnosis of thoracolumbar disk extrusion and/or protrusion is confirmed by cross-sectional imaging and surgery.

Survey spinal radiography can help to determine the diagnosis and site of a thoracolumbar disk extrusion if radiographic signs are well defined and consistent with neuroanatomic localization. Radiographic findings signifying suspected IVD extrusion include the following (**Figure 14.43**):

- Narrowing of the IVD space.
- Wedging of the disk space.
- Narrowing of the intervertebral foramen.
- Mineralized material in the spinal canal or superimposed over the intervertebral foramen.

As survey radiographs identify the correct site of disk extrusion in only about 70% of cases, further imaging, such as myelography or cross-sectional imaging (CT, MRI), is strongly recommended prior to surgery.

CT or MRI is used alone or as an adjunct to myelography to more completely delineate lateralization of extruded disk material and lesion extent. CT alone has been shown to be more accurate than myelography at identifying the major site of disk herniation and has the advantage of being a more rapid test with fewer side-effects than myelography. Mineralized disk material and acute hemorrhage can be identified in the vertebral canal using noncontrast-enhanced CT (**Figure 14.44**). Acutely extruded disk material typically is recognized as

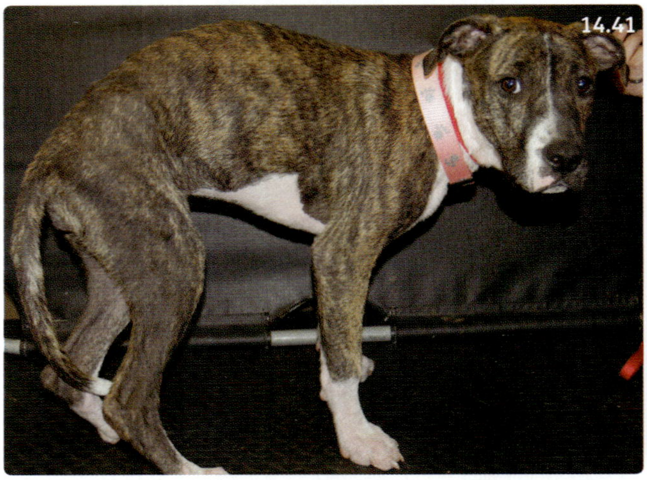

Figure 14.41 An arched back (kyphosis) is often indicative of thoracolumbar pain.

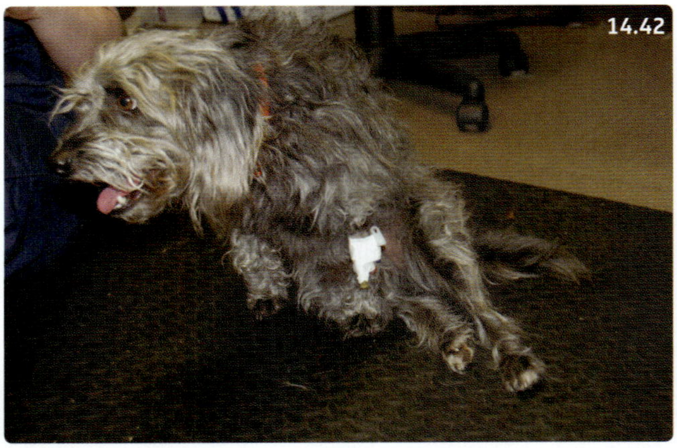

Figure 14.42 Typical posture adopted by dogs with paraplegia.

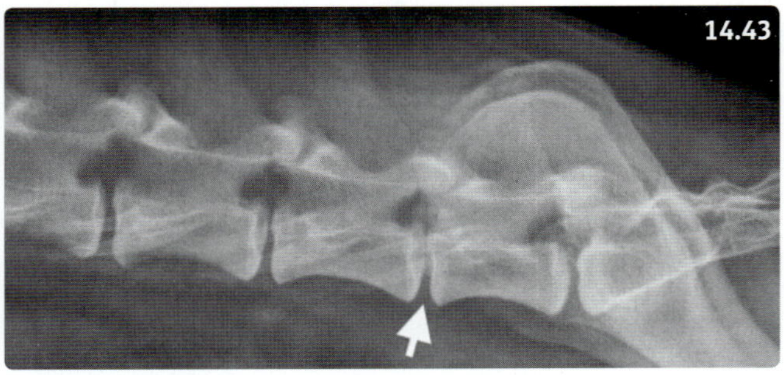

Figure 14.43 The radiographic characteristics of intervertebral disk disease are highlighted in this radiograph at L6/L7 (arrow).

a heterogeneous hyperattenuating extradural mass. The attenuation of the disk material increases with the degree of mineralization. Chronically extruded disk material has a more homogeneous hyperattenuating appearance.

MRI provides a more sensitive technique in recognition of spinal cord pathology (e.g. edema and hemorrhage) and 3-D delineation of the spinal cord compression, allowing for an accurate surgical approach and determining the extent of surgical decompression required. MRI is considered the best method for early recognition of *in-situ* disk degeneration and for determining localization and extent of extruded disk material within the epidural space (**Figure 14.45**). MRI may have diagnostic value in detecting myelomalacia. Findings from a recent study in dogs with IVD extrusion and lack of nociception suggested that an area of hyperintensity >6 times the length of L2 on T2-weighted sagittal images may allow for a presumptive diagnosis of myelomalacia.

Management

Indications for nonsurgical treatment of thoracolumbar IVDD include a first-time incident of spinal pain only, mild to moderate paraparesis, and the financial constraints of the client. The last is the only reason for nonsurgical treatment of a recumbent patient, which should always be considered a surgical candidate, if possible. Dogs can be managed with strict cage rest for 4–6 weeks combined with pain relief using anti-inflammatory drugs, opioids, and muscle relaxants. GI protectants also may be necessary with use of anti-inflammatory therapies. Never use NSAIDs in combination with corticosteroids, as gastric ulcers can result and in some cases these may lead to the death of the animal. Acupuncture also has been advocated as a treatment for pain management. Dogs should be monitored closely for deterioration of neurologic status. If pain persists or the neurologic status worsens, surgical management is recommended. Studies have shown that recovery rates in nonambulatory dogs are lower and recurrence rates higher following conservative rather than surgical treatment. Success rates for conservative management of ambulatory dogs with pain only or mild paresis range from 82% to 100%. More recent retrospective studies of conservatively managed dogs with thoracolumbar disk disease documented 30–50% recurrence rates in dogs with minimally affected ambulatory status. Recurrence of spinal pain in dogs with thoracolumbar IVDD that are conservatively managed usually occurs within 6 months to 1 year from onset of the initial clinical signs. Methylprednisolone sodium succinate is not recommended for the treatment of this disease due to the lack of demonstrated efficacy and the side-effects.

Indications for surgical management of thoracolumbar IVDD include spinal pain or paresis unresponsive to medical therapy, recurrence or progression of clinical signs, nonambulatory paraparesis or paraplegia with intact nociception, and paraplegia without nociception for <24–48 hours. Prolonged loss of nociception (>48 hours) carries a poor prognosis and owners should be made aware of this prior to surgery. However, it is often difficult to know when nociception was lost; in addition, recovery has been observed in dogs that had surgery >5 days after the onset of paraplegia. Surgery includes

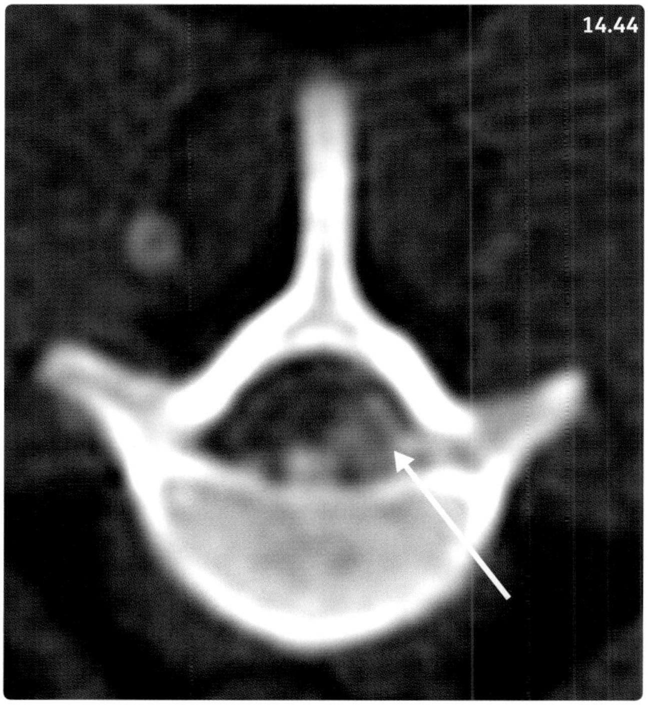

Figure 14.44 Transverse CT scan of the lumbar spinal column at the site of an acute mineralized intervertebral disk extrusion (arrow).

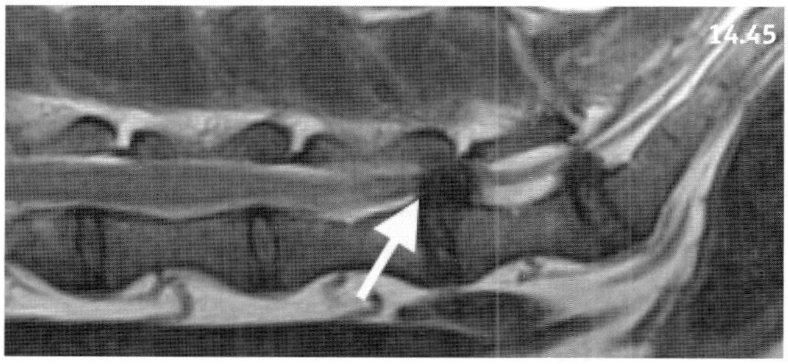

Figure 14.45 Sagittal T2-weighted MR image of the lumbar spine of the dog in Figure 14.43. An acute mineralized disk extrusion (arrow) is seen to compress neural tissue at L6/7.

spinal cord decompression by removal of extruded disk material. Chronicity of disk extrusion at the time of surgery may influence the ease with which extruded disk material can be removed.

HANSEN TYPE II INTERVERTEBRAL DISK DISEASE

Definition/overview

Herniation of the annulus fibrosus can result in slow progressive clinical signs ranging from intermittent spinal pain, through ataxia and paresis to the loss of motor function in the later stages. This is most common in the thoracolumbar spinal column but can affect the cervical and lumbosacral spinal cord as well, where it can be accompanied by degenerative changes of the vertebrae creating a more dynamic/position-associated disease. (See cervical spondylomyelopathy and degenerative lumbosacral syndrome.)

Etiology

Herniation of the annulus of the disk (protrusion) into the spinal canal resulting in spinal cord compression.

Pathophysiology

Hansen type II IVDD is annular protrusion caused by shifting of central nuclear material and is commonly associated with fibroid disk degeneration. The annulus fibrosus slowly protrudes into the spinal canal to cause spinal cord compression. The chronic compression can lead to focal ischemia and other microvascular derangements of the spinal cord. Type II IVDD usually occurs at the mobile points of the spinal column and is more common in older, nonchondrodystrophic breeds of dog. It is not uncommon to identify multiple affected disk spaces. Chronic spinal instability may be an underlying predisposition to type II IVDD.

Clinical presentation

The clinical signs of Hansen type II IVDD include slowly progressive hindlimb ataxia, weakness, reluctance to rise or jump on furniture, and difficulty climbing stairs. Onset of clinical signs is considered chronic and progressive, although acute exacerbations of signs are not uncommon. Localization is focal with asymmetrical or symmetrical weakness. Paraspinal hyperesthesia may or may not be present.

Diagnosis

Diagnosis may be suspected on routine spinal radiographs that show the presence of degenerative changes in the spinal column, such as spondylosis. Myelography, CT myelography, or MRI is necessary to locate the spinal cord compression (**Figure 14.46**).

Management

Medical therapy is indicated in animals with early onset type II IVDD and mild deficits. It also is indicated in those animals that are concurrently afflicted with suspected DM. Medical therapy involves administration of NSAIDs or corticosteroids. The use of a muscle relaxant such as diazepam or methocarbamol should be considered in patients with spinal hyperesthesia. Clinical signs do not always respond to medical therapy and often return after discontinuation of these therapies. Surgical decompression may offer a better long-term outcome.

The type of surgical decompression depends on the location of the lesion. A hemilaminectomy is performed for lesions in the thoracic spine and lumbar spine cranial to L5 (**Figures 14.47a, b**). A dorsal laminectomy is performed if the lesion is located in the lumbosacral area (**Figure 14.48**). Typically, type II disk protrusions require more spinal cord manipulation to relieve the compression from the annulus. The protrusion is usually excised; however, decompression by laminectomy alone may also be adequate in cases where the disk material is irretrievable. Lateral corpectomy is an alternative method for decompression of ventral and lateroventral thoracolumbar disk disease. Often the neurologic status of the animal is worse after surgery but this is usually temporary. Often dogs with chronic clinical signs have multiple IVDD herniations, which complicate surgical decision making.

If surgery is instituted early, prognosis is usually fair to good when patients are considered refractory to medical therapy. If the disease has coursed for several months and is associated with severe neurologic signs (i.e. paraplegia), the prognosis is considered guarded.

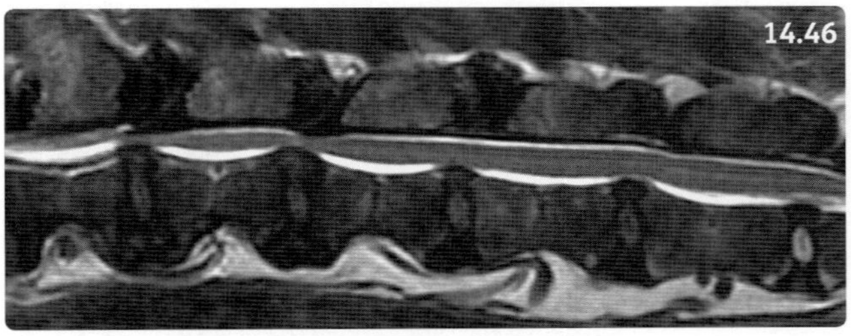

Figure 14.46 Sagittal T2-weighted MR image of the thoracolumbar spinal column in a dog with multiple type II intervertebral disk herniations.

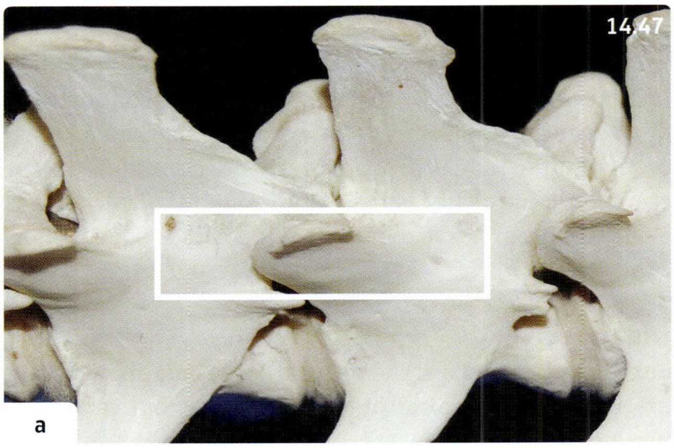

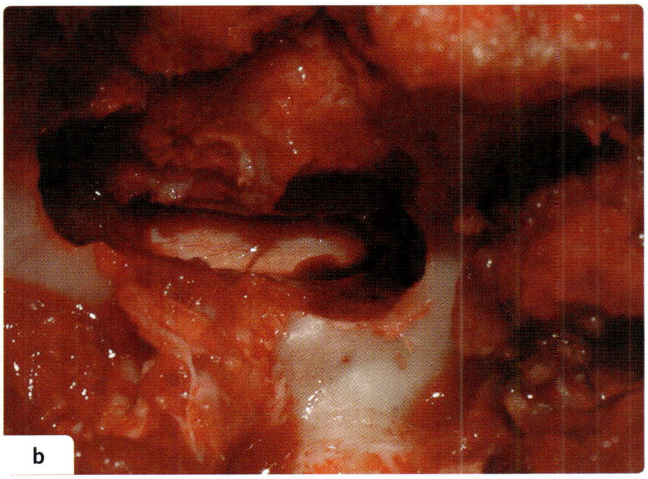

Figures 14.47a, b (a) The surgical 'window' for a hemilaminectomy is illustrated on a spinal column model. (b) The spinal cord is visible through the hemilaminectomy window made in the vertebrae.

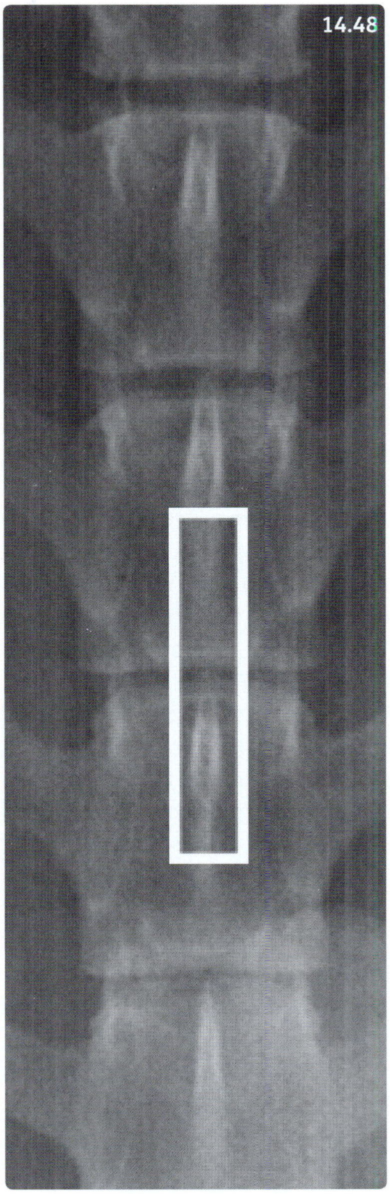

Figure 14.48 The surgical 'window' for a dorsal laminectomy is illustrated in this lumbar vertebral radiograph.

CERVICAL SPONDYLOMYELOPATHY (WOBBLER SYNDROME)

Definition/overview

Cervical spondylomyelopathy describes a syndrome of compression of the cervical spinal cord as a result of degenerative and congenital changes in the cervical spine. There are many names for this syndrome including wobbler syndrome, caudal cervical stenotic myelopathy, cervical malformation/malarticulation, and disk-associated wobbler syndrome (DAWS). Classically, this is thought of as a disease of large (e.g. Dobermann, Dalmatian) and giant breed (e.g. Great Dane, Mastiff breeds, Bernese Mountain Dog) dogs, although identical changes also occur in toy and small breed dogs such as Chihuahuas and Yorkshire Terriers.

Etiology

The etiology of these changes is most likely multifactorial. Genetic factors probably play a role as the disease is seen in specific breeds of dog, although a pattern of inheritance has not been established in commonly affected breeds. Overnutrition and excess calcium supplementation in the first year of life has been implicated in Great Danes, but correction of these feeding patterns has not prevented occurrence of the disease in this breed. It has also been postulated that conformation of the head and neck influences the development of lesions. However, a study on Dobermanns failed to find a correlation between various body dimensions and radiographic or neurologic signs. It is believed by many that the degenerative changes seen in this syndrome ultimately result from relative instability of the cervical spinal column.

Pathophysiology

Progressive spinal cord compression results from both congenital stenosis and degenerative changes in the vertebral column. The changes can be listed as:

- Hypertrophy and protrusion of the annulus fibrosus, often associated with 'tipping' of vertebrae. This change is classically associated with DAWS in Dobermanns.
- Hypertrophy of the ligamentum flavum and dorsal longitudinal ligament. These changes are also common in DAWS.
- Hypertrophy of synovial membrane and formation of synovial cysts at the articular facets, occurring in giant breed stenotic myelopathy and associated with remodeling of the facets.
- Stenosis of the vertebral canal; historically this has been described in giant breed stenotic myelopathy. However, there is evidence that Dobermanns also have a relative stenosis of their cervical vertebral canal.
- Degenerative joint disease and remodeling of the articular processes, commonly found in giant breed stenotic myelopathy.

Clinical presentation

Clinical signs include progressive ataxia, tetraparesis, and, sometimes, neck pain (**Figure 14.49**). Signs in the hindlimbs are more severe than the forelimbs. Dogs with caudal cervical compression frequently have a short stilted forelimb gait with a dysmetric, disconnected hindlimb gait. Nerve root entrapment can cause forelimb lameness and muscle atrophy; in particular, compression of the suprascapular nerve can produce marked atrophy of the supra- and infraspinatous muscles, making the scapular spine easily palpable. Although typically this is a chronic progressive disease, acute onset of severe signs can occur.

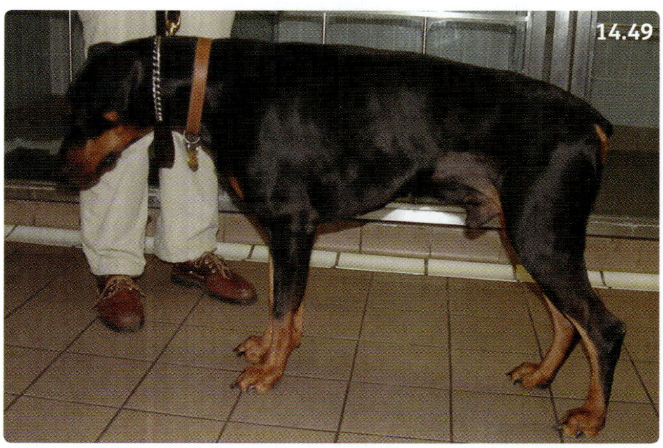

Figure 14.49 An 8-year-old Dobermann with cervical vertebral spondylomyelopathy (wobbler syndrome) presenting with neck pain.

Diagnosis

Survey radiographs of the cervical spine may show degenerative changes typical of this syndrome, but cannot be used to identify sites of spinal cord compression. Stressed views should not be taken as compression of the spinal cord can be exacerbated. Myelography combined with CT used to be the gold standard for diagnosis of cervical spondylomyopathy and for surgical planning. Linear traction views of the myelogram are used to determine whether compression can be addressed by distraction and fusion of vertebrae (i.e. a dynamic lesion). However, MRI has largely replaced CT and myelography. The advantages of MRI include greater accuracy at detecting spinal cord compression and parenchymal disease in addition to decreased morbidity associated with this imaging modality (**Figures 14.50a–d**).

Management

Dogs with neurologic deficits should be treated surgically, as this is a chronic progressive disease. However, many owners cannot afford, or do not wish, to have surgery performed; medical therapy can be considered in such cases and in dogs with mild deficits. Medical management includes treatment of pain with anti-inflammatory drugs and muscle relaxants, and restriction of unmonitored activity combined with controlled exercise and physical therapy. Anti-inflammatory doses of corticosteroids have been used to reduce vasogenic edema but do not appear to influence the outcome. Acupuncture can be useful to control chronic pain in some dogs. Dogs managed in this way should be monitored weekly to biweekly to allow early recognition of deterioration and recommendation for surgical intervention.

The aims of surgery are to decompress and/or stabilize the cervical spine. Surgical strategies include the ventral slot (to remove disk material from the canal), distraction/stabilization techniques (to treat lesions responsive to traction) (**Figure 14.51**), and dorsal laminectomy (to remove dorsal compression or address multiple disk protrusions). Postoperative rehabilitation of patients is critical to their recovery and owners need to be fully informed about the implications of rehabilitating a nonambulatory

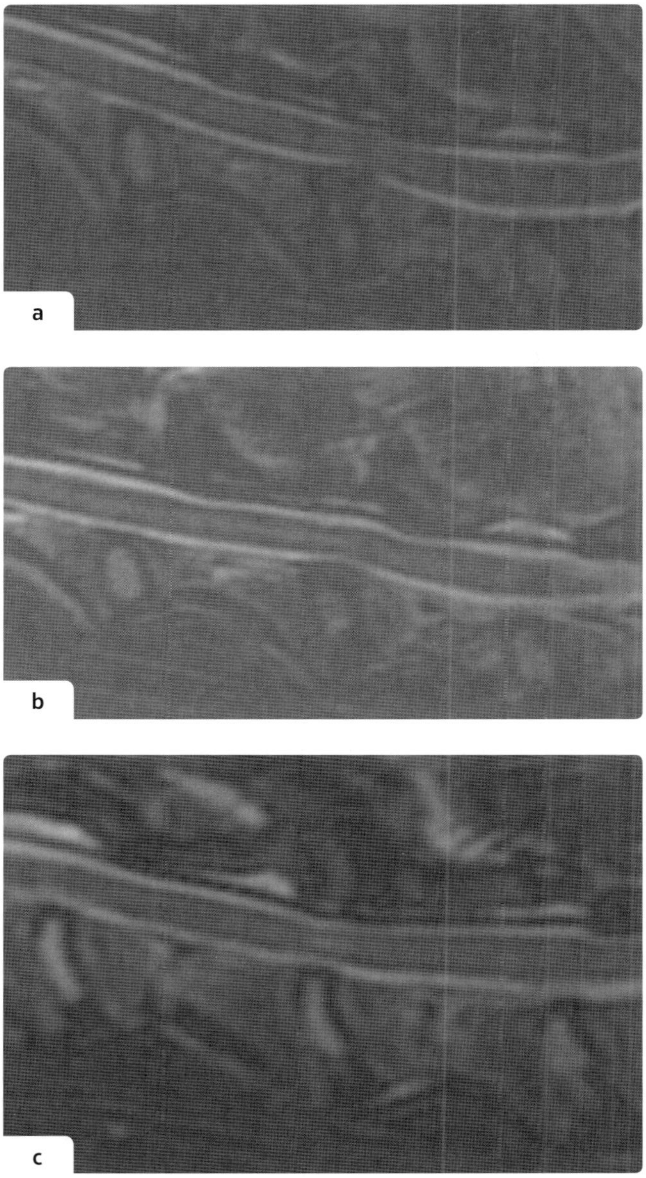

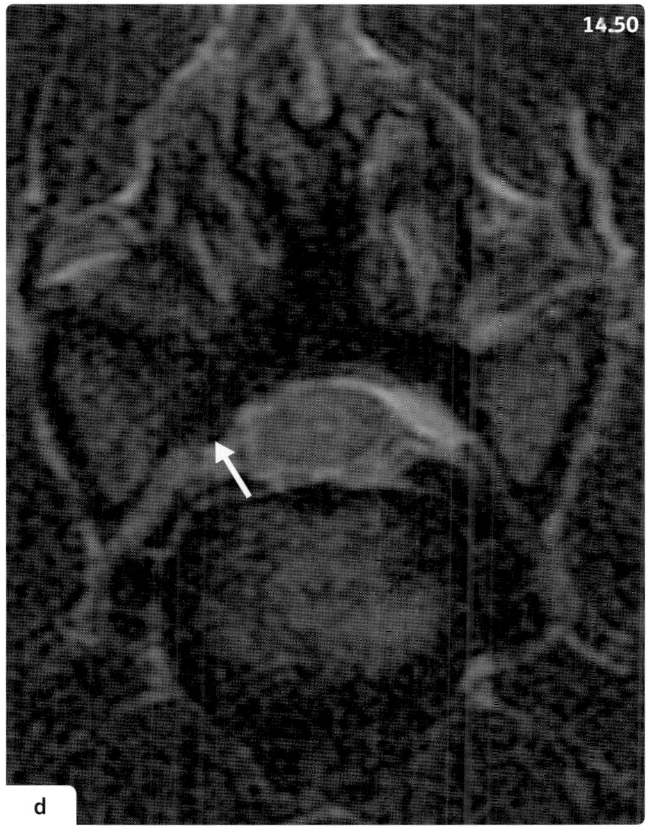

Figures 14.50a–d (a) T2-weighted sagittal caudal cervical MR image of the Dobermann in Figure 14.49. A ventrally compressive lesion is seen over the disk space of C6/C7. (b) Following mild traction applied to the neck, the MRI is repeated and shows a concurrent mild reduction in the degree of ventral compression, indicating a traction-responsive lesion. (c) T2-weighted sagittal caudal cervical MR image of a 1-year-old Great Dane with chronic progressive tetraparesis. Mild compression of the cord can be seen, as can central cord hyperintensity related to the chronic compression. (d) T2-weighted transverse MR image at the level of the compression seen in 14.50c confirming that the compression is due to articular process malformation (arrow) and concurrent stenosis of the spinal canal.

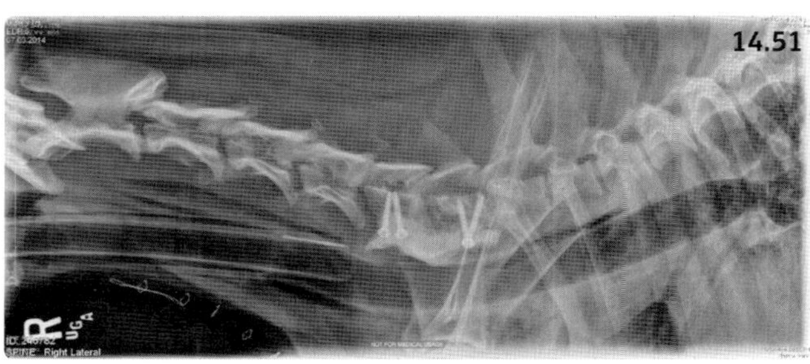

Figure 14.51 Lateral postoperative radiograph of the cervical spine of the dog with the traction-responsive compression in Figure 14.50. A distraction fusion surgery has been performed using cancellous screws and polymethylmethacrylate cement.

large or giant breed dog. Rehabilitation includes passive range of motion exercises and massage in the recumbent dog, hydrotherapy, and controlled exercise. Recovery of these dogs can be prolonged (6–12 weeks or more) due to the chronic nature of the disease.

DEGENERATIVE LUMBOSACRAL STENOSIS

Definition/overview

Lumbosacral stenosis (cauda equina syndrome, lumbosacral malarticulation and malformation, lumbosacral instability, lumbosacral spondylopathy) is common in middle to old aged, large breed dogs and represents a plethora of orthopedic abnormalities associated with the lumbosacral anatomy. Degenerative lumbosacral stenosis is also being recognized with increasing frequency in the cat.

Etiology

Neurologic abnormalities occur coincident with tissue (joint capsule, interarcuate ligament, disk, bone, fibrous adhesions) impingement on the cauda equina, the nerve roots at the level of the foramina, or the vascular supply. Transitional vertebrae have been identified as a predisposing cause of cauda equina syndrome in German Shepherd Dogs and other breeds.

Pathophysiology

The pathologic process begins with Hansen type II IVD degeneration followed by osteophyte formation of the L7–S1 endplates and articular processes. The syndrome is characterized by stenosis of the spinal canal from vertebral subluxation and/or stenotic intervertebral foramina. Concurrent with compressive disease, underlying instability may further accentuate the clinical signs, especially in active dogs.

Clinical presentation

Neuroanatomic localization to the lumbosacral region is determined by the neurologic examination based on signs related to sensory, motor, and autonomic dysfunction. Nonspecific observations include reluctance to rise and hindlimb lameness. Neurologic signs commonly include pain and motor dysfunction as a result of LMN weakness (sciatic, pudendal, caudal nerves). Pain is the most consistent clinical sign and reflective of compressive or inflammatory processes affecting pain-sensitive structures (nerve root, meninges, periosteum, and joints). It is the opinion of the author that the pain primarily originates from nerve root (radicular pain) compression (particularly L7). The affected patient often stands with the hindlimbs tucked under the caudal abdomen to flex the spine and lessen the nerve root compression (**Figure 14.52**). Motor dysfunction varies in severity. The patient may have mild to severe gait and postural reaction deficits. The gait is frequently short strided or shuffled. Postural reaction deficits are often asymmetrical, depending on the degree of cauda equina involvement. Reflex dysfunction of the limbs commonly involves those muscles innervated by the sciatic nerve (L6–S1 nerve roots but L7 and S1 provide the major contribution), particularly the flexor and extensor muscles of the hock. The patellar reflex may appear hyperreflexic due to loss of antagonism from the flexor muscles (pseudohyperreflexia). The cranial tibial and gastrocnemius reflexes may be hyporeflexic. The withdrawal reflexes are reduced in the stifle and hock joints. Less commonly, the pudendal and caudal nerves may be involved. The pudendal nerve (S1, S2, and S3) innervates the perineal region, including the external anal and urethral sphincters. The caudal nerves innervate the tail. Decreased tail tone is assessed on palpation and inability to wag. Other less common clinical signs include fecal and urinary incontinence. If micturition dysfunction is suspected, it is important to closely evaluate sensory perception of the perineal region and the anal reflex.

Diagnosis

A diagnosis of lumbosacral syndrome is suspected from the neurologic examination. Definitive diagnosis of degenerative lumbosacral stenosis is difficult because no one test has 100% specificity and sensitivity, leading to false-positive and false-negative results. Dynamic imaging is important to investigate mobility of the joint and concurrent changes

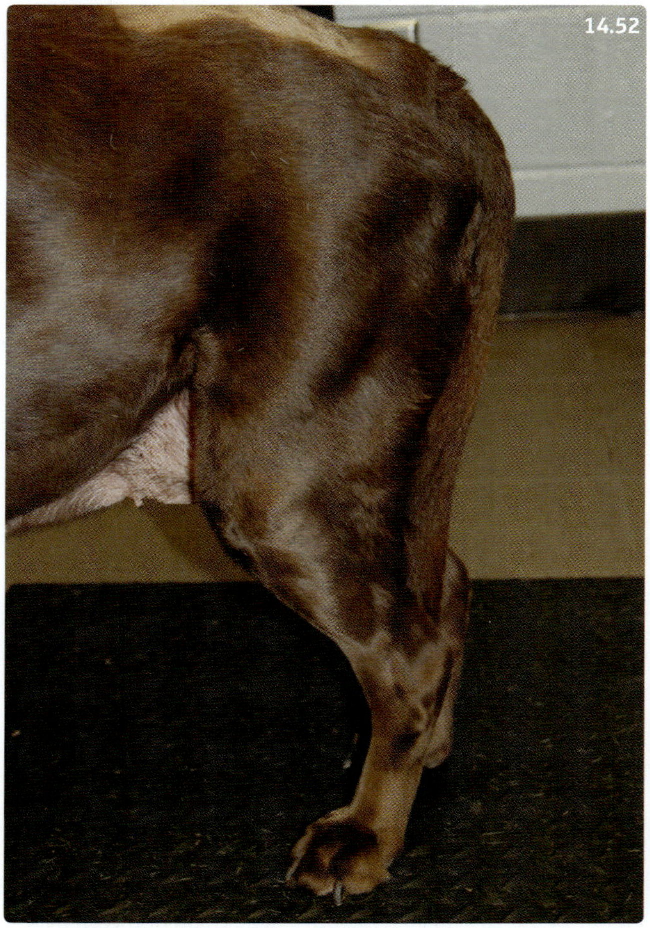

Figure 14.52 A Labrador Retriever with degenerative lumbosacral disease exhibiting reduced tail tone, hindlimb muscle atrophy, and a weak stance.

in nervous tissue compression. Diagnostic procedures to test for degenerative lumbosacral stenosis include electrophysiology, survey and contrast radiography, CT, and MRI. Survey radiography is useful to rule out other causes of cauda equina syndrome. Abnormal findings associated with degenerative lumbosacral stenosis include: osteochondrosis of the sacral endplate; transitional vertebrae; spondylosis; subluxation; sclerosis of the endplates; and bony proliferation of the articular processes.

Stress radiography (extension and flexion views) has been used to identify underlying 'instability' of the lumbosacral junction; however, normal dogs might also have evidence of such 'instability'. MRI is superior to radiography for demonstrating dynamic compression of the neural tissues.

CT has the advantage of better soft tissue and bone resolution. Cross-sectional, dorsal, and sagittal images allow determination of lesion extent. The articular processes, IVDs, and foraminae can be evaluated. CT imaging studies should be performed prior to injecting contrast medium into the vertebral canal or subarachnoid space. Abnormalities detected by CT include loss of epidural fat, increased soft tissue opacity in the intervertebral foramen, bulging of the IVD, thecal sac displacement, spondylosis, narrowed vertebral canal, thickened articular processes, and osteophyte formation on the articular processes in the intervertebral foramen.

MRI is superior to CT with regard to soft tissue definition (**Figure 14.53**). The spinal cord, CSF, IVDs, ligaments, and nerve roots can be directly visualized. MRI may allow early recognition of IVD degeneration and a more accurate assessment of epidural fat displacement, although this is open to overinterpretation. Parasagittal and transverse views can provide evidence of stenosis within the L7–S1 intervertebral foramina. As with radiography, extension and flexion views of the lumbosacral spine can provide evidence of dynamic disease. Importantly, CT and MRI imaging findings may not correlate with the severity of the clinical signs, and thus should not be used to predict surgical outcomes or determine the prognosis.

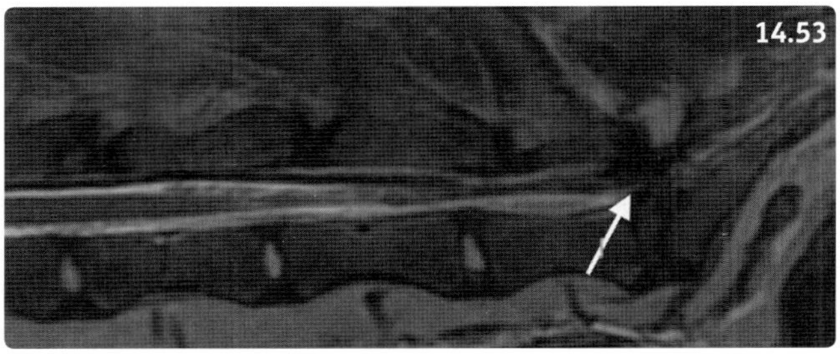

Figure 14.53 Sagittal T2-weighted caudal lumbar spinal MR image of the dog in Figure 14.52 confirming marked neural tissue compression at the L7/S1 intervertebral disk space (arrow).

Management

Indications for medical management include the first episode of clinical signs or intermittent pain. Management consists of strict confinement for 8–14 weeks, anti-inflammatory medication using low-dose prednisolone or NSAIDs, and weight loss. The recovery rate with medical management is between 24% and 50%. A recent report described the use of methylprednisolone sodium acetate (40 mg/ml) injections into the lumbosacral epidural space at a dose of 1 mg/kg. The treatment resulted in clinical improvement in 79% and complete resolution of clinical signs in 53% of dogs mildly affected by degenerative lumbosacral stenosis. The protocol included injections at 0, 2, and 6 weeks, with additional injections as needed.

Indications for surgical management include failure of medical management, severe pain, and moderate to severe neurologic deficits (in particular incontinence). Surgical techniques include decompression and excision of the proliferative tissue, and fixation and fusion of the lumbosacral junction. Surgical decompression is the most common treatment, although distraction–fusion techniques may also be used if indicated. The most crucial aspect of postoperative care is strict cage confinement for 8–12 weeks and a gradual return to fitness. It is important to institute controlled exercise as part of the physical rehabilitation program. In addition, bladder management involves proper monitoring of bladder emptying to avoid urinary tract infections. If the clinical signs resolve with surgery, then the prognosis is fair to good. Dogs with severe neurologic deficits and urinary and fecal incontinence for more than a few weeks prior to surgery have a guarded to poor prognosis. Rates of postoperative improvement range from 41% to 95%.

SPONDYLOSIS DEFORMANS

Definition/overview

Degenerative change associated with the vertebrae, most often the vertebral bodies, easily seen on radiographs but rarely a cause of clinical disease.

Etiology

Degenerative, often age-related change.

Pathophysiology

Spondylosis deformans is characterized by formation of bony growths and bridges at the intervertebral spaces. The condition is a common radiographic finding in older dogs along the thoracic and lumbar spine. Most likely spondylosis is associated with degeneration of the annulus fibrosus of the IVD. Presence of spondylosis deformans has been associated with type II IVDD and degenerative lumbosacral stenosis; however, these diagnoses are often made independent of the presence of spondylosis.

Clinical presentation

Spondylosis rarely causes neurologic signs, but is occasionally associated with back pain.

Diagnosis

The lesion is radiographically identifiable (**Figure 14.54**). The osteophyte formation usually does not compress the neural tissue or encroach within the vertebral canal.

Management

NSAIDs or steroids have been reported to lessen spinal discomfort in animals with severe ankylosing spondylosis. Spondylosis deformans is usually an incidental finding and is rarely associated with clinical signs, therefore the prognosis is good.

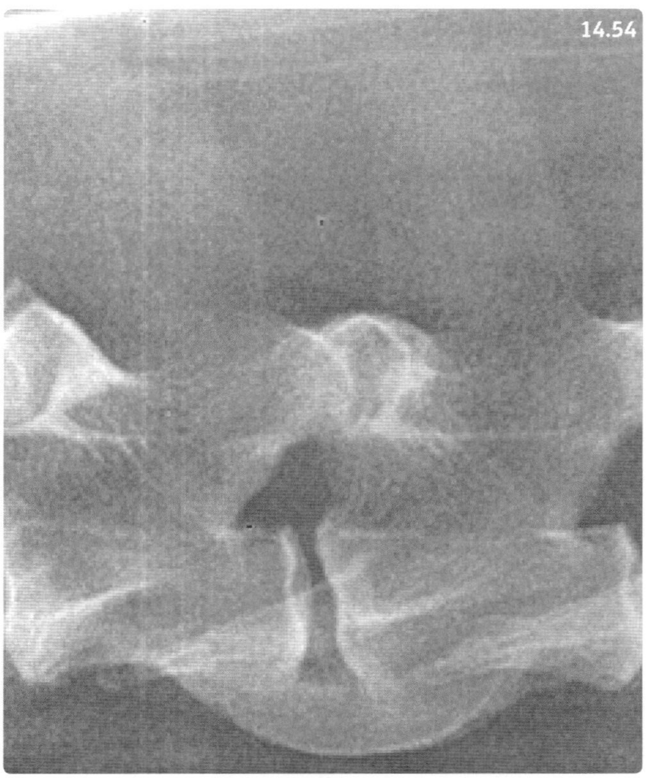

Figure 14.54 Lateral radiograph of the lumbar vertebrae demonstrating ventral bridging spondylosis.

SPINAL SYNOVIAL CYSTS

Definition/overview

Spinal synovial cysts occur in the cervical spine of young large breed dogs but more commonly involve the thoracolumbar region in older large breed dogs.

Etiology

Cysts originate from synovial joint lining of vertebral joints.

Pathophysiology

Spinal extradural synovial cysts and ganglion cysts arise from the articular facets. Some authors have referred to both structures as intraspinal cysts due to the confusion of tissue origination. Pathogenesis of synovial cysts has been associated with degenerative disease and trauma. Increased mechanical stress and joint motion may predispose the thoracolumbar junction to osteoarthritis and synovial cyst formation. Histopathology of the cyst reveals fibrous connective tissue with a synovial cell lining.

Clinical presentation

Clinical signs are consistent with a progressive myelopathy and include paraspinal hyperesthesia.

Diagnosis

Radiographic findings include degenerative changes and remodeling of the articular processes. Myelography demonstrates spinal cord compression, especially on the ventrodorsal view, with attenuation of the contrast column medial to the articular processes. Attenuation of the ventral and dorsal columns (giving an hourglass appearance) is also present on lateral projections. The lesion is better defined using CT myelography and MRI. Cysts will appear as hyperintense lesions on both T2-weighted and STIR images (**Figure 14.55**). Albuminocytologic dissociation is a consistent finding on lumbar CSF analysis.

Management

The treatment often involves surgical decompression and excision of the cyst. Surgical intervention is indicated with severe neurologic deficits and refractory pain. A hemilaminectomy is often performed if one side is affected. The cyst and any protruding disk material are removed. Marked improvements in gait and neurologic deficits occur post surgically.

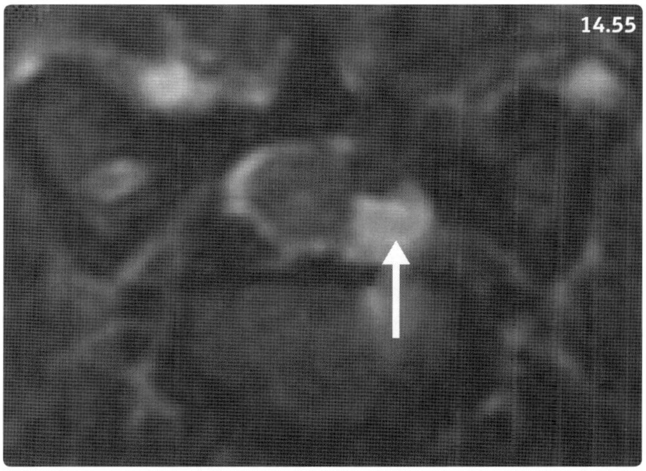

Figure 14.55 T2-weighted transverse spinal MR image showing compression of the spinal cord by a laterally situated fluid-filled synovial cyst (arrow).

ANOMALOUS DISEASES

CHIARI-LIKE MALFORMATION SYNDROME AND SYRINGOMYELIA (SEE ALSO BRAIN DISEASE SECTION)

Overview/definition

CLMS, also known as caudal occipital malformation syndrome, and syringomyelia (SM) often occur together, although both may occur independently of the other. SM is a condition characterized by the presence of a fluid-filled cavity (syrinx) or cavities within the parenchyma of the spinal cord. CLMS and SM are most common in toy and small breed dogs, best described in the CKCS and the Brussels Griffon.

Etiology

In CKCSs, CLMS/SM is a hereditary condition, possibly autosomal recessive with incomplete penetrance. CLMS is caused by congenital hypoplasia of the supraoccipital bone resulting in overcrowding of the structures within the caudal fossa; this finding is in line with human studies. SM is secondary to abnormal CSF flow and is usually associated with CLMS, although it may be associated with other trauma, inflammation, and neoplasia.

Pathophysiology

The CSF, which normally moves through the foramen magnum during systole of the cardiac cycle, becomes turbulent as laminar flow is interrupted by obstruction at the craniocervical junction due to the CLMS. The altered fluid flow in the subarachnoid space leads to fluid accumulation within the spinal cord. The pathogenesis of SM appears to be multifactorial, as its dorsoventral size and sagittal extent do not correlate well with a single morphologic abnormality. The location of the syrinx within the dorsal aspect of the spinal cord affecting the dorsal horn is thought to be one mechanism behind the development of pain, specifically neuropathic pain. Neuropathic pain is secondary to disordered processing of sensory information within the nervous system and results in spontaneous pain, paresthesia, dysthesia, allodynia, or hyperpathia.

Clinical presentation

Onset of signs may be acute or chronic in dogs ranging from 6 months to 10 years of age, but no sex predisposition has been identified. Clinical signs can be seen in dogs with CLMS alone and are usually related to neuropathic pain syndromes. In the presence of SM, neuropathic pain syndromes and neurologic deficits related to spinal cord destruction can present variably. The most common sign of CLMS/SM is pain, predominately isolated to the cervical region, occurring in 35% of affected dogs and 80% of people with the similar condition. Dogs may vocalize spontaneously without apparent stimulation or when the neck or shoulders are touched. Sensory abnormalities, including rubbing of the face, chewing the feet, and intolerance to neck collars or touch, have been described in some dogs, especially evident during times of stress or excitement. 'Phantom scratching', where the dogs will attempt to scratch often without making contact with their skin, is the most notable manifestation of these neuropathic pain abnormalities and has been described in affected dogs, ranging from an infrequent to a near constant problem. Other clinical signs include scoliosis and neurologic deficits relating to cervical spinal cord dysfunction; tetraparesis, sensory ataxia, and abnormal proprioceptive positioning in all limbs have been noted in dogs with CLMS/SM. Intracranial signs, such as facial paresis and vestibular dysfunction, have also been reported. However, dogs may be completely asymptomatic for CLMS and/or SM. SM can be present in up to 44% of clinically normal CKCSs and in 24% of clinically normal Brussels Griffons.

Diagnosis

These structural abnormalities are best diagnosed with MRI, but they may be clinically silent; therefore, their significance must be carefully considered when such abnormalities are discovered. SM is seen as hyperintensity on T2-weighted MR images and as hypointensity on T1-weighted images; a prominent or dilated central canal can be seen in some dogs. The extent of SM is very variable, with some cases exhibiting a focal cyst-like structure most commonly in the dorsal cervical cord (predominantly gray matter) and others exhibiting multifocal, multiloculated lesions throughout the entire spinal cord (holocord syringomyelia) (**Figure 14.56**). Suggestive of a 'pre-syrinx' is a local area of T2-weighted FLAIR hyperintensity associated with the central canal. It is important to rule out other concurrent diseases as being the cause of clinical signs, which can be difficult, but performing CSF analysis is important. As CLMS/SM occurs in toy breed and small dogs, it is essential to consider a CSF tap to investigate the possibility of an inflammatory disease and imaging to rule out disk disease. Evaluating the clinical significance of CLMS or SM MRI findings is difficult. In addition to the 2-D measurements of skull and cerebellar sizes, it has become apparent that volumetric ratios of the caudal fossa size can be useful in supporting an association with clinical signs.

Management

Treatment may not be necessary in asymptomatic dogs or dogs with mild nonprogressive signs. Dogs exhibiting pain, more severe neurologic deficits, or progressive signs can be treated either medically or surgically. Typically, medical therapy is pursued initially, involving the use of analgesics and drugs that reduce CSF formation. Furosemide (1–2 mg/kg PO q12h) and prednisone (0.5–1.0 mg/kg PO q24h, tapering dose) are frequently used. Other treatments used in an attempt to decrease CSF production include acetozolamide and omeprazole. Treatment of neuropathic pain with a drug such as gabapentin (10–20 mg/kg PO q8h) is also an important aspect of therapy; pregabalin may be a useful alternative to gabapentin.

Approximately 70% of patients show some improvement, but it is rarely complete and it does not prevent disease progression. If medical therapy does not alleviate the clinical signs, surgical decompression of the foramen magnum has been suggested (suboccipital craniectomy) and is the treatment of choice in people. Foramen magnum decompression has been performed in dogs with success rates reported at about 80%; however, recurrence is common in nearly half of cases in the long term and neuropathic pain and the accompanying signs of scratching may persist, requiring continued medical therapy. Additionally, multiple surgeries may be necessary if scar tissue develops at the surgical site, obstructing CSF flow, although cranioplasty may reduce the likelihood of this complication. Improvement may not result in the reduction of syrinx size, which usually persists.

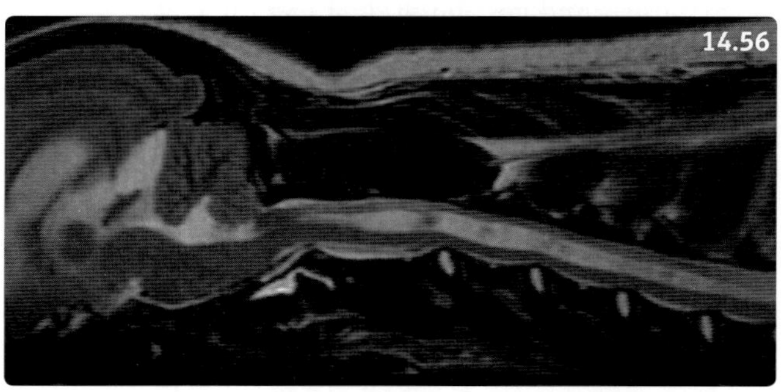

Figure 14.56 T2-weighted sagittal cervical spinal MR image. A large centrally located fluid-filled cavity can be seen within the spinal cord, representing syringomyelia.

ARACHNOID DIVERTICULA (SUBARACHNOID CYSTS)

Definition/overview

Arachnoid diverticula (also known as subarachnoid cysts, meningeal cysts, intra-arachnoid cysts, and leptomeningeal cysts) can cause compression of the cervical or thoracolumbar spinal cord.

Etiology

Congenital, traumatic.

Pathophysiology

Arachnoid diverticula occur in the intradural–extramedullary space. Thoracolumbar arachnoid diverticula more commonly occur over the caudal thoracic vertebrae (T11–T13) and may expand over two vertebrae. Age of onset in dogs with thoracolumbar cysts is older than in dogs with cervical diverticula. Congenital forms may be associated with other neural tube defects and syringohydromyelia. Spinal arachnoid diverticula also occur in cats.

Clinical presentation

Clinical signs reflect a progressive spinal cord disease based on the segmental location of the cyst; the condition usually lacks paraspinal hyperesthesia. Incontinence may be a prominent clinical feature.

Diagnosis

Myelography is useful for detecting the diverticula within the intradural space. On MRI the diverticula appear as focal, well-circumscribed lesions that are isointense to CSF on both T1-weighted and T2-weighted images (**Figure 14.57**). MRI is more sensitive than CT in detecting associated intramedullary lesions such as SM.

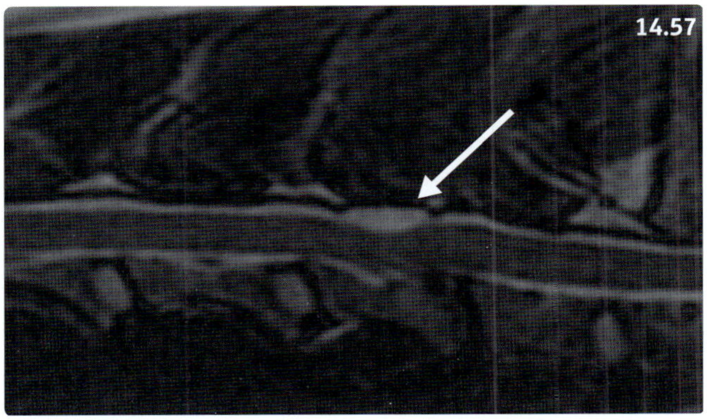

Figure 14.57 T2-weighted caudal cervical spinal MR image depicting a dorsal fluid-filled lesion (arrow) associated with the spinal cord and subarachnoid space. This is often referred to as a subarachnoid cyst or diverticulum.

Management

Surgical decompression of the spinal cord is the recommended treatment. Various surgical procedures involve spinal cord decompression and removal or drainage of the fluid-filled structure with fenestration or marsupialization of the dura mater. Dogs that have the cyst marsupialized may have a better long-term outcome than if the cyst is fenestrated. Conservative management is indicated in dogs with mild neurologic deficits and includes anti-inflammatory doses of prednisolone and controlled exercise. The prognosis is good for young dogs if treated soon after development of clinical signs. Dogs older than 3 years of age and those with clinical signs for a duration of >4 months have a poor long-term outcome when treated with only fenestration of the cyst.

VERTEBRAL COLUMN MALFORMATIONS

ATLANTOAXIAL INSTABILITY

Definition/overview

Subluxation of the atlantoaxial junction is a relatively common problem in toy breed dogs and causes acute to chronic tetraparesis, ataxia, and pain.

Etiology

Trauma, congenital malformation.

Pathophysiology

The atlas (first cervical vertebra) and axis (second cervical vertebra) are held together by ligaments that run from the dens of the axis to the atlas and the skull, over the dens binding it to the floor of the atlas (the transverse ligament), and between the dorsal lamina of the atlas and the dorsal spinous process of the axis. The dens is a bony projection from the cranial aspect of the body of the axis and develops from a separate growth plate. The atlanto-axial and atlanto-occipital region is prone to congenital defects, which can predispose to this luxation:

- Aplasia, hypoplasia, or dorsal angulation of the dens (toy and small breeds of dog are predisposed to this condition).
- Congenital absence of the transverse ligament.
- Incomplete ossification of the atlas.

Clinical presentation

Onset of signs in dogs with the congenital form of the disease usually occurs in young dogs (<2 years of age), although problems can develop at any age. Signs can develop acutely or gradually, and waxing and waning of signs is often reported, presumably a reflection of instability at the atlantoaxial junction causing repeated injury to the spinal cord. Signs include neck pain (variably present), ataxia, tetraparesis, and postural reaction and conscious proprioceptive deficits with normal to increased muscle tone and myotatic reflexes in all four legs. In severe cases, animals can present with tetraplegia and difficulty breathing and they may die acutely as a result of respiratory failure. Some animals present with seizure-like episodes that involve sudden onset of opisthotonus and vocalization, presumably reflecting intermittent compression of the spinal cord and nerve roots, causing severe but transient pain and paresis.

Diagnosis

Atlantoaxial subluxation can be diagnosed from survey radiographs of the cervical spine, although extreme care must be taken when restraining and moving dogs in which this disease is suspected. If the animal is sedated or anesthetized, the head and neck should be supported in slight extension to avoid further spinal cord injury. On lateral radiographs an increased space can be seen between the dorsal lamina of the atlas and the dorsal spinous process of the axis. In severe cases, malalignment of the bodies of the atlas and axis is clearly visible. The presence and size of the dens can be evaluated most accurately on ventrodorsal views. If there is no evidence of subluxation on the lateral views, the neck can be carefully flexed to see if there is instability (the space between the dorsal lamina of the atlas and the dorsal spinous process of the axis should be evaluated). It is preferable to do this with fluoroscopy so that the movement can be monitored to prevent accidental iatrogenic subluxation. Advanced imaging is commonly performed to aid in decision making for surgery. CT allows clear identification of the bony components of the atlantoaxial region, facilitating surgical planning for implant placement. MRI highlights the spinal cord and brainstem parenchyma, allowing diagnosis of concurrent abnormalities such as CLMS or hydrocephalus, which might complicate recovery from surgery (**Figure 14.58**).

Management

Dogs with mild signs can be treated conservatively by placing an external splint for at least 6 weeks. The splint must immobilize the atlantoaxial junction and so must come over the head cranial to the ears and go back to the level of the chest. The aim is to stabilize the junction while the ligamentous structures heal. The dog and splint should be checked daily by the owner for signs of decubital ulcers and checked weekly by the veterinarian, with regular bandage changes if necessary (**Figure 14.59**). Splint placement addresses instability and can produce an immediate improvement, although severe displacement of the atlantoaxial junction may not be adequately addressed. In one study, six of 16 dogs failed to improve following splint placement and were euthanized, while the remaining 10 dogs responded well and maintained a good outcome 1 year after splint removal. Surgery is recommended in dogs with neurologic deficits, although it can be associated with high perioperative morbidity and mortality (**Figure 14.60**). Dorsal and ventral approaches to the atlantoaxial junction have been described, but dorsal approaches, although requiring less dissection and

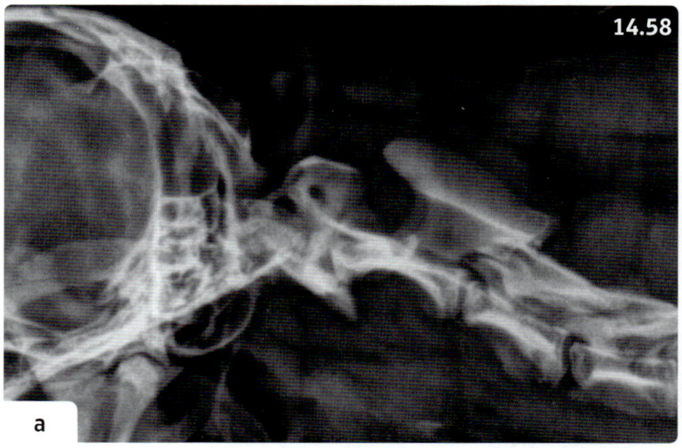

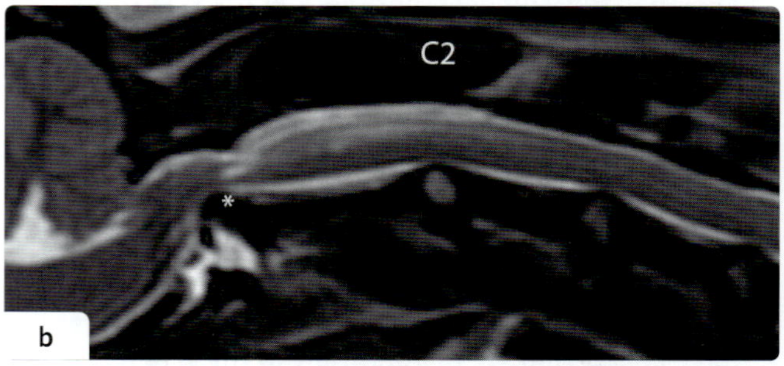

Figures 14.58a, b (a) Lateral radiograph of a Yorkshire Terrier with acute-onset neck pain. There is a notable space present between the dorsum of C1 and the dorsal arch of C2 compatible with atlantoaxial subluxation. (b) Sagittal T2-weighted MR image of the cranial cervical spine of the dog shown in 14.58a. Marked cord compression can be seen associated with a subluxation of the dens (*).

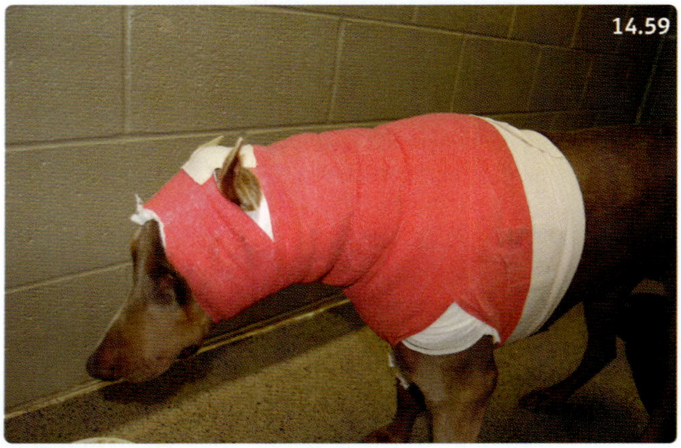

Figure 14.59 External stabilization of the neck requires a ventral splint and bandaging, which needs to extend from the mandible to the mid-thorax.

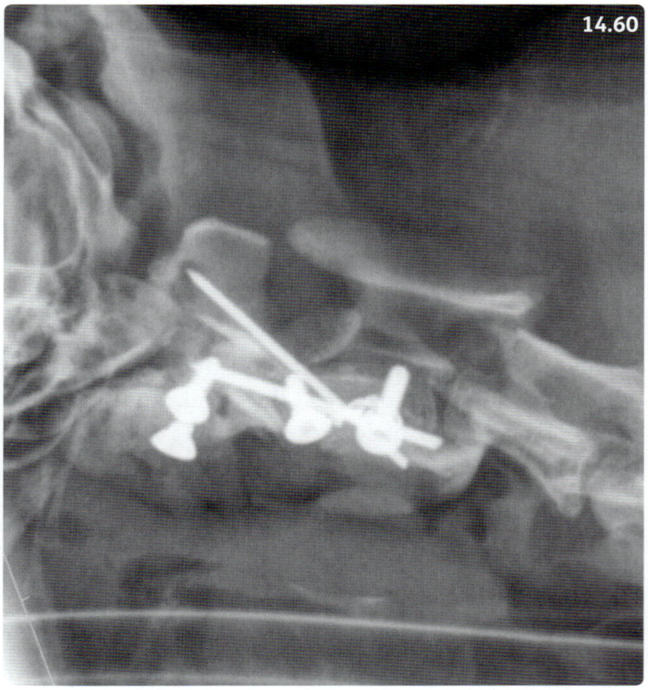

Figure 14.60 Lateral postoperative radiograph of the dog in Figure 14.58. A ventral fixation approach using transarticular pins, screws, and polymethylmethacrylate cement has been used.

retraction of important soft tissue structures such as the esophagus, pharynx, and larynx, are associated with a greater risk of causing spinal cord injury during surgery and a higher incidence of implant failure. A neck splint may be placed postoperatively while fusion occurs if transarticular screws alone are used. This is a problematic area to repair surgically; bone quality is often poor, the bones are small, movement of the vertebrae may cause additional injury to the spinal cord, and the pharynx and larynx can be damaged during retraction. There is a risk of respiratory arrest and death in the perioperative period as a result of additional spinal cord injury or inflammation of the upper airways secondary to retraction. While this is a serious disease, dogs treated surgically have an excellent prognosis if they survive the 48-hour perioperative period. Although reported surgical success rates range from 50% to 90%, the majority report a mortality rate in the region of 20%, with the majority of deaths occurring either during or immediately after surgery. As with all spinal cord diseases, prognosis is worse in animals with severe and chronic neurologic deficits. It has also been shown that prognosis is better in young dogs (<24 months).

Vertebral anomalies

Definition/overview

Vertebral anomalies (e.g. hemivertebra, butterfly vertebra, block vertebra, spina bifida) involve defects in formation of the vertebra and segmentation defects. Congenital anomalies of the vertebral column may be associated also with anomalies of the spinal cord (dysraphism) and/or other organ systems (e.g. cardiovascular and urogenital). Spina bifida is considered a form of spinal dysraphism and is characterized by failure of the vertebral arches to fuse, with or without protrusion of the spinal cord and meninges.

Etiology

Congenital.

Pathophysiology

Vertebral anomalies are common in the brachycephalic and 'screw-tailed' breeds of dog such as Bulldogs and Boston Terriers, and the 'tail-less' cat, the Manx. If they are associated with clinical signs, it can be due to associated osseous compression, disk disease, or associated soft tissue abnormalities (subarachnoid diverticula).

Clinical presentation

Vertebral anomalies are often an incidental finding and usually cause no clinical signs. Malformations involving the spinal cord are more likely to cause neurologic deficits, the nature of which is determined by the location of the abnormality.

Diagnosis

Diagnosis is suspected based on clinical signs, signalment, and survey radiographic findings. Myelography and cross-sectional imaging are useful for determining the extent of compression, stenosis, or other possible spinal cord and spinal column deformities. MRI is more sensitive for determining spinal cord involvement and associated defects of altered CSF flow (cyst, syrinx, edema).

Management

If clinical signs are nonprogressive, conservative management is recommended. Decompressive surgery is recommended with clinical signs of compressive myelopathy. Likewise, spinal instability and malalignment require vertebral stabilization techniques. The prognosis is good for most vertebral anomalies because the majority of cases do not produce clinical signs. The prognosis is considered guarded if signs of spinal cord dysfunction are present. Multiple anomalies may exist concurrently.

Spinal stenosis

Definition/overview

Spinal stenosis indicates a malformation of the spine present at birth and occurs as a primary lesion or in association with other anomalies that predispose to stenosis.

Etiology

Congenital.

Pathophysiology

Relative stenosis refers to canal narrowing that does not cause compression of neural tissue, whereas absolute stenosis refers to a stenosis causing spinal cord compression. Dobermanns have a relative stenosis that most commonly involves the cranial thoracic vertebrae (T3–T6). There have also been reports of thoracic vertebral stenosis in Bull Mastiffs, Great Danes, Basset Hounds, Dogues de Bordeaux, and English Bulldogs.

Clinical presentation

Neurologic signs reflect the neuroanatomic localization of the stenosis. Onset is usually insidious and progressive.

Diagnosis

Diagnosis is based on survey radiography that defines associated vertebral anomalies but requires myelography and/or cross-sectional imaging to determine the presence of stenosis. MRI of the spinal cord is recommended to further delineate associated neural tissue anomalies or abnormalities.

Management

Surgical decompression may relieve the compression; however, associated vertebral and spinal cord anomalies need to be taken into account. The prognosis is considered guarded due to chronicity and presence of other anomalies. The lack of information available with regard to surgical follow-up makes it difficult to give an accurate prognosis.

NEOPLASTIC DISEASES

SPINAL MENINGIOMAS

Definition/overview

Tumors affecting the spinal cord are described based on their location as extradural, intradural–extramedullary, or intramedullary. Intradural–extramedullary tumors include meningioma and nerve sheath tumors. Meningiomas affecting the spinal cord are most common in the neck.

Etiology

Unknown.

Pathophysiology

Spinal meningiomas are the most common primary spinal cord tumor in cats older than 8 years of age. The mean age for spinal meningiomas in dogs is 9 years. Spinal meningiomas in dogs are most common in the cervical spinal cord, but can occur in any region of the spinal cord.

Clinical presentation

Meningiomas of the spinal cord in dogs and cats tend to present with a progressive paraparesis. The clinical signs represent the spinal cord region involved. Paraspinal pain may or may not be present.

Diagnosis

Myelography typically shows an intradural–extramedullary compressive lesion. With MRI, these tumors are iso- to hypointense on T1-weighted images, hyperintense on T2-weighted images, and demonstrate strong, uniform contrast enhancement (**Figure 14.61**).

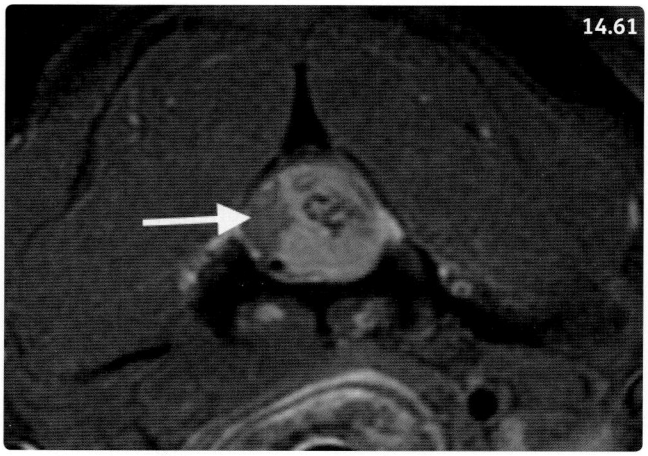

Figure 14.61 Transverse post-contrast T1-weighted MR image at the level of C2 showing a strongly enhancing lesion markedly compressing the cord (arrow) to a fraction of its normal size. Surgical resection of the lesion was performed and confirmed a meningioma.

Management

These lesions should be surgically explored because many meningiomas can be completely or partially removed and therefore may be associated with prolonged survival after surgery. Postoperative radiation therapy may be used adjunctively to prolong survival in dogs with incompletely excised tumors. Treatment with surgery and radiation therapy can result in an improved outcome and prevent recurrence. Surgical results are guarded when meningiomas are associated with an intumescence, a ventral location, and invasion of the neural parenchyma.

NERVE SHEATH TUMORS

Definition/overview

Peripheral nerve sheath tumors (PNSTs) are neoplasms that arise from cells surrounding the axons in peripheral nerves or nerve roots, and they are divided into benign and malignant variants. Most PNSTs in dogs are anaplastic, have a high mitotic index, and an aggressive biological behavior, so they are designated as malignant PNSTs. Malignant nerve sheath tumors are common in dogs, but rare in cats. No sex or breed predilection has been demonstrated for PNSTs in dogs. Most affected animals are adults over 7 years of age, but younger animals may also be affected.

Etiology

Unknown.

Pathophysiology

Malignant PNSTs in dogs most commonly affect the caudal cervical (C6–C8) and the cranial thoracic (T1–T2) nerve roots, although nerve sheath tumors have also been described affecting the sciatic nerve and femoral nerve. These tumors may have their origin in the nerve roots or the brachial or lumbosacral plexi, or they may arise from more peripheral locations in the nerves. Usually, the tumor spreads slowly, both distally and proximally, and may invade the vertebral canal, causing spinal cord compression and associated neurologic deficits. As the tumors grow proximally they spread to neighboring nerves in the plexus bundle, with a high percentage of dogs showing evidence of multiple nerve involvement at the time of diagnosis. PNSTs are highly invasive locally, but they rarely metastasize, although pulmonary metastasis in advanced cases has been described.

Clinical presentation

Malignant PNSTs typically affect older dogs and have been described occasionally in cats. Slowly progressive forelimb lameness or paresis and muscle atrophy are the predominant clinical signs of malignant PNSTs (**Figure 14.62**). In addition, pain on palpation of the limb or axillary region may be encountered. A palpable axillary mass may be present in some cases, but it is not common. Enlargement of the affected limb has been described in one case. Clinical signs progress slowly and orthopedic disease is often suspected before a definitive diagnosis is made. As the PNST spreads proximally and compresses the spinal cord, neurologic deficits may develop in the ipsilateral hindlimb, progressing to all four limbs. If the dorsal cervical nerve roots are affected, animals may also show cervical pain.

Unilateral, partial, or complete Horner's syndrome may appear if the cranial thoracic nerve roots are affected by the tumor itself or if there is cord compression at this point (**Figure 14.63**). Similarly, the ipsilateral cutaneous trunci reflex may be absent due to invasion of the C8–T1 ventral nerve roots or compression of these spinal cord segments.

Diagnosis

Orthopedic disease must be excluded by careful orthopedic examination and radiographs of the appropriate joints. Complete blood work (CBC, serum biochemistry panel), thoracic radiographs, and abdominal ultrasonography should be performed in any dog suspected of having a malignant PNST in order to rule out metastatic disease and assess general health status. Survey radiographs of the spine are often normal. Oblique views may reveal enlargement of the affected intervertebral foramen due to pressure atrophy, caused by the thickened nerve root. Occasionally, lysis of the affected vertebral bodies may be observed. CT imaging allows visualization of some malignant PNSTs, and masses as small as 1.0 cm can be identified on contrast-enhanced CT scans. Enhancement of the mass with iodinated contrast medium provides excellent views, helps differentiate vascular structures, and allows subtle differences in soft tissue opacity created by tumor vasculature to be seen. MRI evaluation of the brachial plexus or peripheral nerves provides excellent diagnostic images but again, not all PNSTs can be detected using this imaging modality early in the course of the disease (**Figure 14.64**).

Ultrasound examination of the affected limb may allow visualization of large, hypoechogenic tubular masses that displace vessels and destroy normal architecture, and ultrasound-guided fine needle aspirates of the masses may be useful to reach a final diagnosis in some

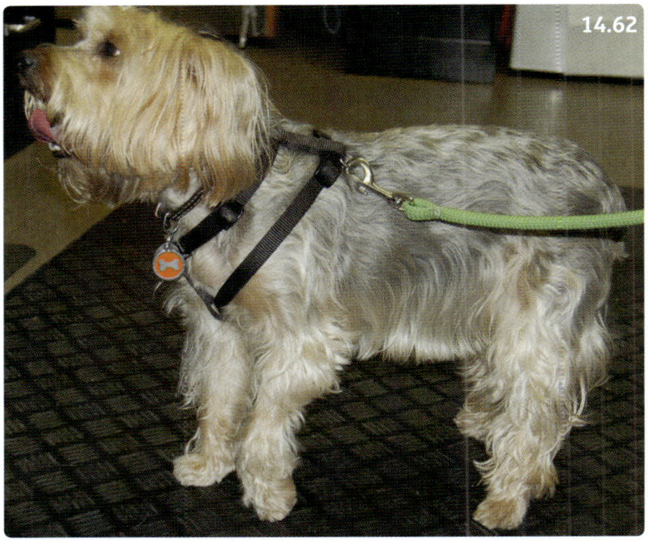

Figure 14.62 A Yorkshire Terrier demonstrating left forelimb root signature associated with a peripheral nerve sheath tumor.

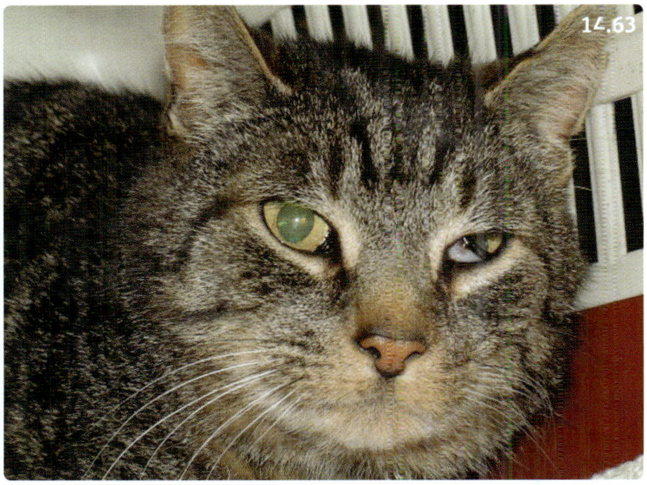

Figure 14.63 Left-sided Horner's syndrome comprising ptosis, miosis, and third eyelid protrusion is seen in this adult cat.

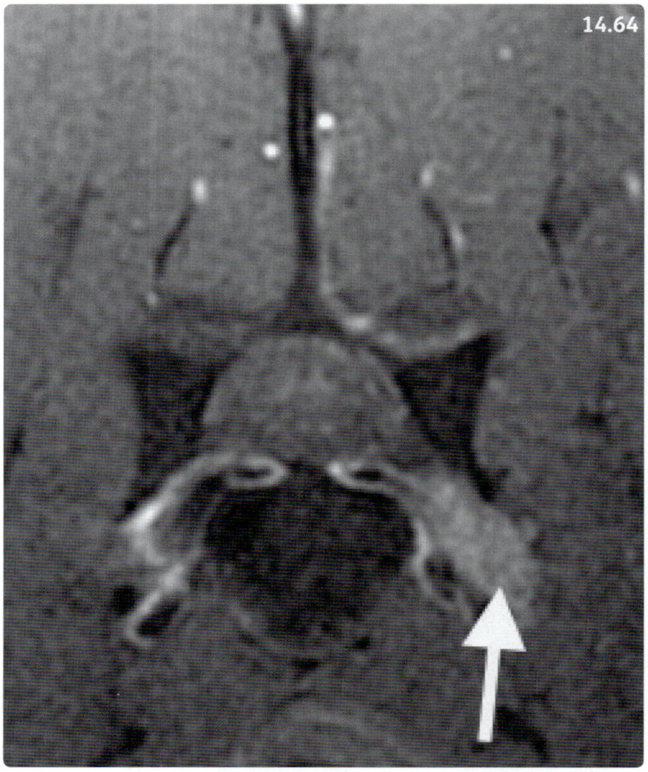

Figure 14.64 Nerve root enhancement (arrow) associated with a nerve sheath tumor is depicted on this transverse post-contrast T1-weighted MR image at the level of C7.

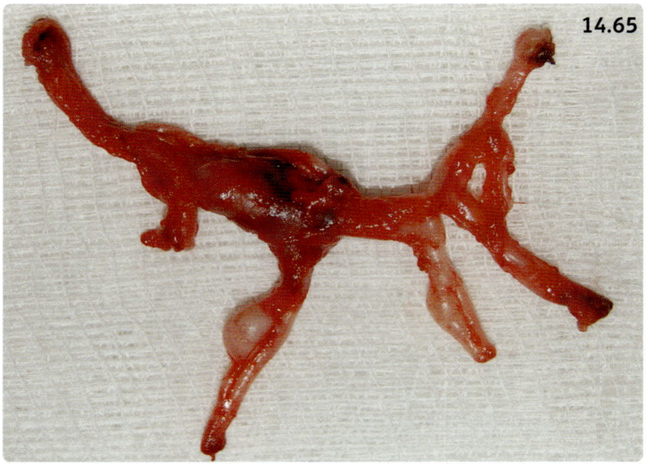

Figure 14.65 The lumbar plexus of a dog affected with an extensive malignant peripheral nerve sheath tumor.

cases. Electromyography reveals abnormal, spontaneous electrical activity in the affected limb muscles and is of great assistance in differentiating neurologic from orthopedic disease.

Managment

Unfortunately, there is usually no curative treatment for PNSTs. Complete surgical resection may be difficult due to the invasive behavior of these tumors and the late detection of the disease in most cases. Tumors within the brachial plexus or peripheral nerves are treated with local excision or amputation of the affected limb. Repeated surgeries may be needed as recurrences are common. In many instances, amputation of the limb is the only option. Early diagnosis and aggressive surgical intervention are recommended to maximize the possibility of complete tumor resection. Aggressive surgical resection at an early stage, if the tumor is peripheral, can be curative (**Figure 14.65**). Amputation is only advisable when the tumor is distal and there is no invasion of the spinal canal. In addition, amputation is performed in some cases just to prevent or avoid self-mutilation and injuries to the limb in cases of loss of sensation or paresthesias. Surgery can be followed by a course of radiation therapy, but it is unclear whether this positively affects the prognosis, since these tumors are poorly responsive to radiation. Despite aggressive management, the overall prognosis is poor for most cases of malignant PNSTs. Recurrence rate after surgery is high. There is a tendency for dogs with more proximally located tumors to respond less favorably to surgery and to relapse earlier (1 month for nerve root tumors and 7.5 months for plexus tumors) than those with peripherally located tumors (>9 months after surgery). Incomplete resection is common, indicating that grossly visible margins at the time of surgery are frequently inaccurate indicators of tumor excision.

VERTEBRAL BODY TUMORS

Definition/overview

Tumors affecting the spinal cord are described based on their location as extradural, intradural–extramedullary, or intramedullary. Extramedullary tumors are the most frequent and most commonly are primary vertebral tumors.

Etiology

Unknown.

Pathophysiology

Vertebral body tumors are primary or metastatic tumors most frequently reported in large and giant breed dogs. Commonly described tumors in dogs include osteosarcoma, fibrosarcoma, chondrosarcoma, hemangiosarcoma, plasma cell tumor, carcinoma, lymphoma, and liposarcoma. Small breed dogs have a higher rate of vertebral metastasis than large breed dogs. In cats, the most commonly described vertebral body tumor is osteosarcoma.

Primary vertebral body tumors will cause a secondary myelopathy by compression or direct spinal cord invasion.

Clinical presentation

Clinical signs may be focal or multifocal depending on the extension of the tumor. Signs include pain and paraparesis or paralysis. Pathologic fractures of the vertebral body result in an acute onset of neurologic deficits.

Diagnosis

Dagnosis is often based on survey radiographic findings, such as lysis and pathologic fractures secondary to tumor destruction of the bone. Other supportive diagnostic techniques, such as CT, MRI, and myelography, are used to determine lesion extent (**Figure 14.66**). MRI and scintigraphy can be used to detect multiple metastases. Fluoroscopic-guided needle aspiration or surgical biopsy can be used to obtain a definitive diagnosis.

Management

Palliative treatment options include surgery, radiation therapy, chemotherapy, or various combinations of the three. A vertebrectomy with a bone allograft fusion has been used for the treatment of a primary vertebral neoplasm in a dog. Decompression or stabilization techniques are used in patients that are rapidly deteriorating. The overall prognosis is considered guarded for dogs and cats with vertebral neoplasia. Survival is not impacted greatly by various treatments but is often determined by the neurologic deficits at the time of diagnosis.

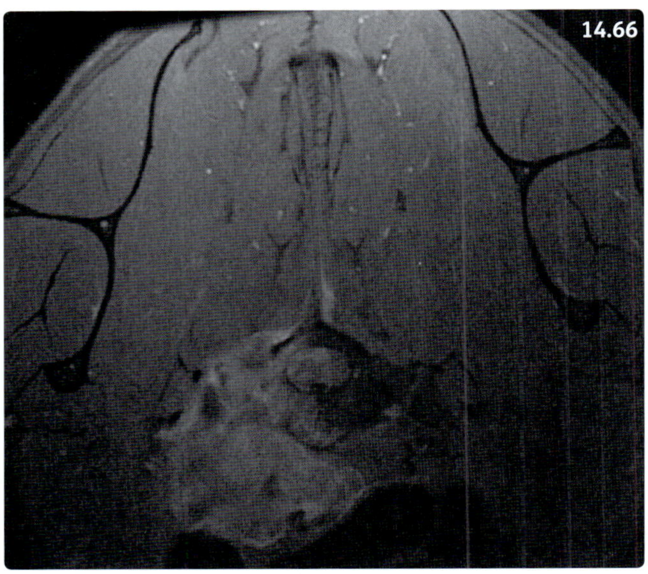

Figure 14.66 Transverse post-contrast T1-weighted MR image at the level of the T2 vertebra clearly demonstrating a large irregular lesion associated with the vertebral body and compressing the spinal cord. The lesion was confirmed to be a chondrosarcoma.

THORACOLUMBAR SPINAL TUMOR OF YOUNG DOGS (SPINAL NEPHROBLASTOMA)

Definition/overview

Canine nephroblastoma is an intradural–extramedullary neoplasm in young dogs located between T10 and L2 in the spinal cord. Occasionally, this tumor is extradural or intramedullary.

Etiology

The origin of the tumor is unknown but descriptions have included medulloepithelioma, embryonal nephroma, nephroblastoma, and Wilm's tumor (**Figure 14.67**).

Pathophysiology

Primary spinal nephroblastoma is thought to arise from embryonic tissue trapped within the dura during fetal development. Histologic appearance may vary. Usually, neuroepithelioma involves one kidney or the spinal cord, but not both. Rarely, renal neuroepithelioma will secondarily metastasize to the spinal cord, bone marrow, and spinal canal.

Clinical presentation

Clinical signs of spinal nephroblastoma are dependent on tumor location. The most common neurologic findings include progressive paraparesis and ataxia. Clinical signs of spinal neuroepitheliomas consist of a progressive asymmetrical T3–L3 myelopathy.

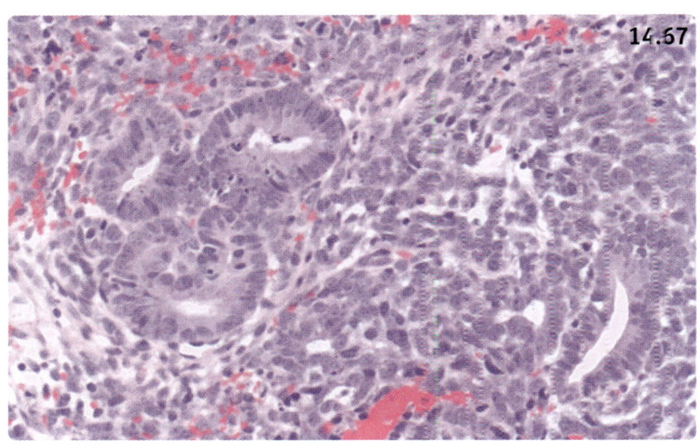

Figure 14.67 Histopathologic section of a nephroblastoma stained with hematoxylin and eosin.

Diagnosis

Survey radiography of the spine shows no abnormalities. Myelography is useful for determining location and lesion extent. CT or MRI of the spine can better assess vertebral and spinal cord involvement (**Figures 14.68a, b**). Abdominal radiography and ultrasonography can assess for primary renal involvement if present. Immunohistochemistry is used to identify the mesenchymal or epithelial components of neuroepithelioma. Staining with Wilm's tumour 1 (WT-1) antibody can support a diagnosis of nephroblastoma.

Management

If detected early, surgical excision can lead to long-term survival with limited morbidity. Adjunct irradiation is considered when total surgical resection is not possible, and may provide a good functional outcome. Overall prognosis is uncertain because of the limited number of cases reported. Prognosis is considered guarded to poor because spinal cord involvement is often extensive by the time of diagnosis. Long-term prognosis is poor because of tumor recurrence.

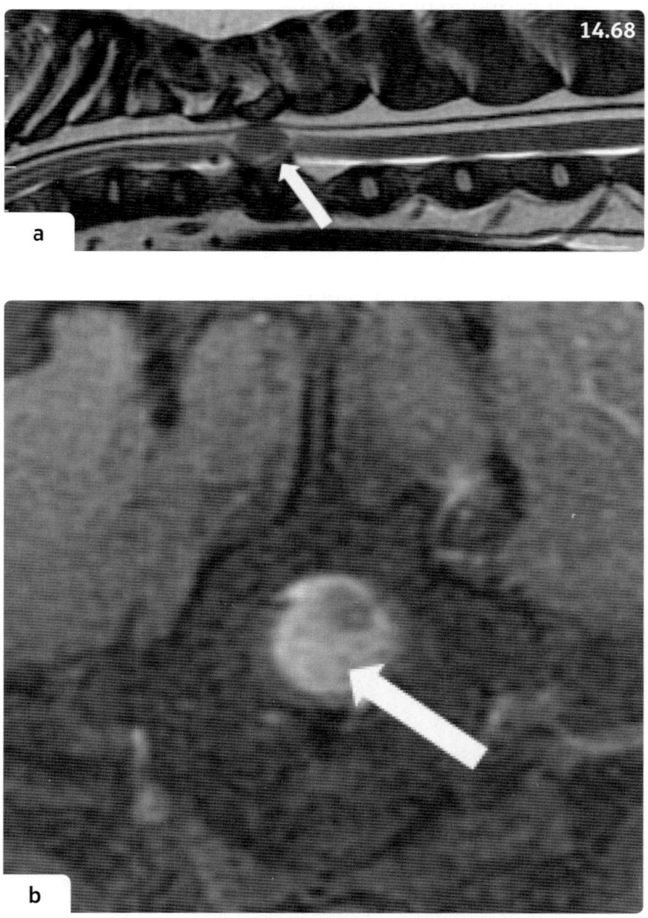

Figures 14.68a, b (a) Sagittal T2-weighted and (b) transverse post-contrast T1-weighted MR images of a nephroblastoma (arrows) compressing the spinal cord in the thoracic spine.

SPINAL LYMPHOMA

Definition/overview

Extradural lymphoma is the most common tumor to induce spinal cord dysfunction in cats and occurs less commonly in dogs.

Etiology

Unknown.

Pathophysiology

Feline leukemia virus has been implicated and is an important factor associated with lymphoma in young cats. Feline spinal lymphoma has a predilection for the thoracic and lumbar spinal cord. Most affected cats are <2 years of age but older animals may also be affected. Lymphoma in cats commonly is found in extraneural sites. Renal lymphoma is likely to relapse in the CNS. Lymphoma is the most commonly diagnosed malignant tumor in dogs, but involvement of the nervous system is relatively unusual. Involvement of the CNS is more common than the peripheral nervous system in both dogs and cats.

Clinical presentation

Neurologic signs are related to the location of the lymphoma and are often insidious but there can be an acute exacerbation with rapid deterioration. Often, cats with lymphoma have multifocal signs reflective of multiple lesions in the CNS. The most common initial clinical sign in cats is paraparesis, with pain and other nonspecific abnormalities such as anorexia, lethargy, weight loss, and respiratory tract infection.

Diagnosis

The safest and most reliable method of obtaining a diagnosis of lymphoma in the CNS may be by confirming the presence of lymphoma in other organ systems. The abdominal organs and bone marrow are commonly aspirated but may not be affected. CSF analysis may detect the presence of malignant lymphocytes, but lack of this finding cannot rule out CNS involvement (**Figure 14.69**). Survey spinal radiography may detect bone involvement. Myelography is useful for determining lesion extent and determining extradural, intradural–extramedullary, or intramedullary involvement. Spinal lymphoma is detected most commonly as an extradural lesion. MRI may detect intramedullary lesions (**Figure 14.70**). A definitive diagnosis can be determined from cytologic

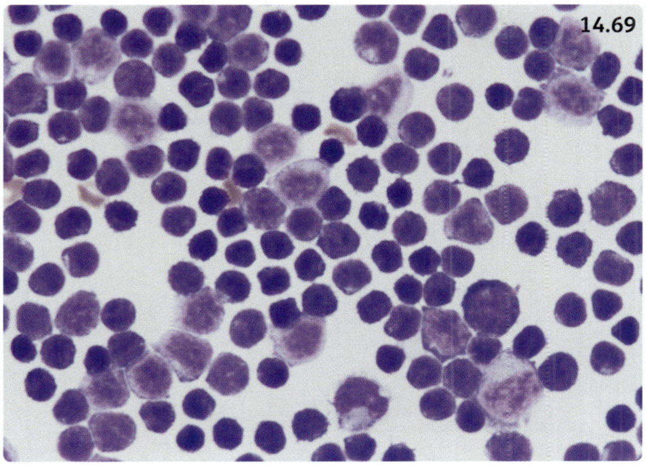

Figure 14.69 Cytologic analysis of CSF from a dog with a CNS lymphoma.

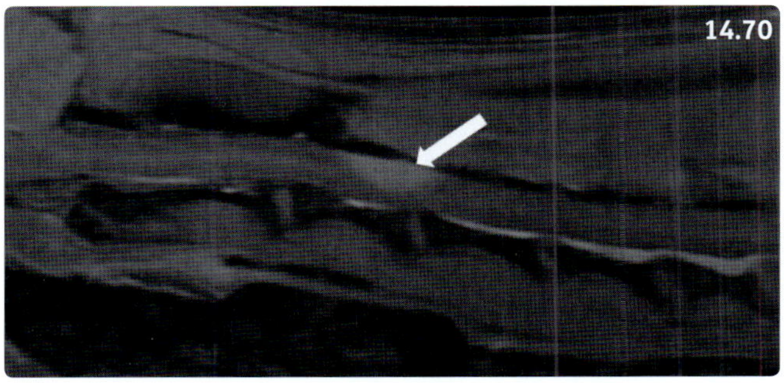

Figure 14.70 Sagittal post-contrast T1-weighted cervical spinal cord MR image of a dog with a spinal cord lymphoma (arrow).

examination of the contents of fluoroscopic-guided fine needle aspirations or a surgical biopsy.

Management

Therapies used in combination or alone include surgical resection, focal irradiation, and systemic chemotherapy (e.g. cytarabine or methotrexate and corticosteroids). A laminectomy procedure provides an accurate histologic diagnosis and adequate decompression. Surgical treatment is necessary for cats that fail to respond rapidly to chemotherapy. Duration and remission times vary among studies. Intramedullary lymphoma is difficult to treat because of poor penetration across the blood–brain barrier of some chemotherapeutic agents. Effectiveness of chemotherapy for lymphoma with neural involvement still remains to be determined. In general, the prognosis for hindlimb paresis or paralysis in cats is guarded to poor. The median duration of complete or partial remission in six cats with spinal lymphoma and severe neurologic deficits, treated with vincristine sulfate, cyclophosphamide, and prednisolone, has been reported as 14 weeks (range 5–28 weeks) and 6 weeks (range 4–10 weeks), respectively.

INFLAMMATORY DISEASES

DISKOSPONDYLITIS/OSTEOMYELITIS

Definition/overview

Diskospondylitis is due to infection of the intervertebral disk and adjacent vertebral endplates; if the infection is confined to the vertebral body, it is called vertebral osteomyelitis or spondylitis. The sites most commonly affected are L7–S1, caudal cervical, midthoracic, and thoracolumbar spine. The infection is usually slowly progressive but can result in acute signs due to secondary pathologic vertebral fractures and IVDD. Its most common clinical sign is that of spinal pain but neurologic signs are seen and related to the localization. An association with empyema has been documented in several dogs, which may represent an extension of the disease and should be considered when considering diagnostic tests and/or when dealing with a refractory case.

Etiology

Coagulase-positive *Staphylococcus* spp. (*S. intermedius* or *S. aureus*) are the most common etiologic agents associated with canine diskospondylitis; other less commonly identified organisms include *Streptococcus* spp., *Escherichia coli*, *Actinomyces* spp., and *Brucella canis*, as well as *Aspergillus* spp. Young German Shepherd Dog bitches seem to be predisposed to aspergillosis, whereas young Basset Hounds contract diskospondylitis due to systemic tuberculosis.

Pathophysiology

Hematogenous spread from distant foci of infection (urogenital tract, skin, dental disease), penetrating wounds, surgery, or plant material migration can cause direct infection of the disk space or vertebrae, the latter of which is usually seen at the level of L2–4 at the insertion of the diaphragmatic crus. Immunosuppression due to factors such as hyperadrenocorticism is considered a predisposing cause. Infection causes osseous lysis, proliferation, and soft tissue reaction, which can cause neural compression.

Clinical presentation

Spinal pain is the most common initial clinical sign in this disease, which is most frequently seen in large intact male young to middle aged dogs. With proliferation of inflammatory tissue, compression of neural tissue can lead to ataxia, paresis, and occasionally paralysis dependent on where the lesion is located. Although it can occur in any animal, the condition is less common in toy and chondrodystrophoid breeds of dog, and rare in cats. Purebred dogs seem more commonly affected than mixed breeds. Approximately 30% of dogs have signs of systemic illness such as fever and weight loss.

Diagnosis

Hematological changes are usually not present unless there are concurrent conditions such as endocarditis. Urine cytology may reveal bacterial or fungal agents. Blood and urine cultures should be performed in all suspected cases and are positive in up to 75% and 50% of cases, respectively. Ideally, these should be performed prior to initiating antibiotic therapy. Serology for brucellosis should also be performed, especially in view of its zoonotic potential; this has been reported to be positive in up to 10% of cases.

Definitive diagnosis is usually made with spinal radiographs, although radiographic change may not be evident in the first 2–4 weeks of infection (**Figures 14.71a–c**). The most commonly affected site is L7–S1, but other frequently affected sites include the caudal cervical/cranial thoracic vertebrae and the thoracolumbar junction. As this can be a multifocal disease, the entire spine should be radiographed. Radiographic evidence of disease includes narrowing of the disk space, accompanied by subtle irregularity of both endplates, through to gross lysis and osseous proliferation of the adjacent vertebral bone, and even fractures. Radiography can also be used to monitor the response to treatment or the progression of the disease, although clinical progression is equally important, as radiographic change can lag behind clinical improvement.

CT can identify subtle endplate erosion and paravertebral soft tissue swelling more readily than radiography. Post-myelogram CT clearly defines compression of the neural tissues by infected tissues, as does MRI. Diskospondylitis appears to have increased signal intensity on T2-weighted images and decreased signal intensity on T1-weighted images, changes also seen in the paravertebral tissues in all cases. MRI can also highlight the inflammation in the surrounding muscles (**Figures 14.71b, c**).

If urine and blood culture and brucellosis serology have not identified an etiologic agent in cases of diskospondylitis, percutaneous needle aspiration of the disk space can be a safe procedure to obtain tissue for bacterial and fungal cultures and cytology. However, this procedure requires general anesthesia, sterile surgical preparation, and fluoroscopic or CT guidance of the needle, and is usually only performed in patients unresponsive to initial broad-spectrum antibiotics. The procedure has been documented to be up to 75% sensitive; open biopsy

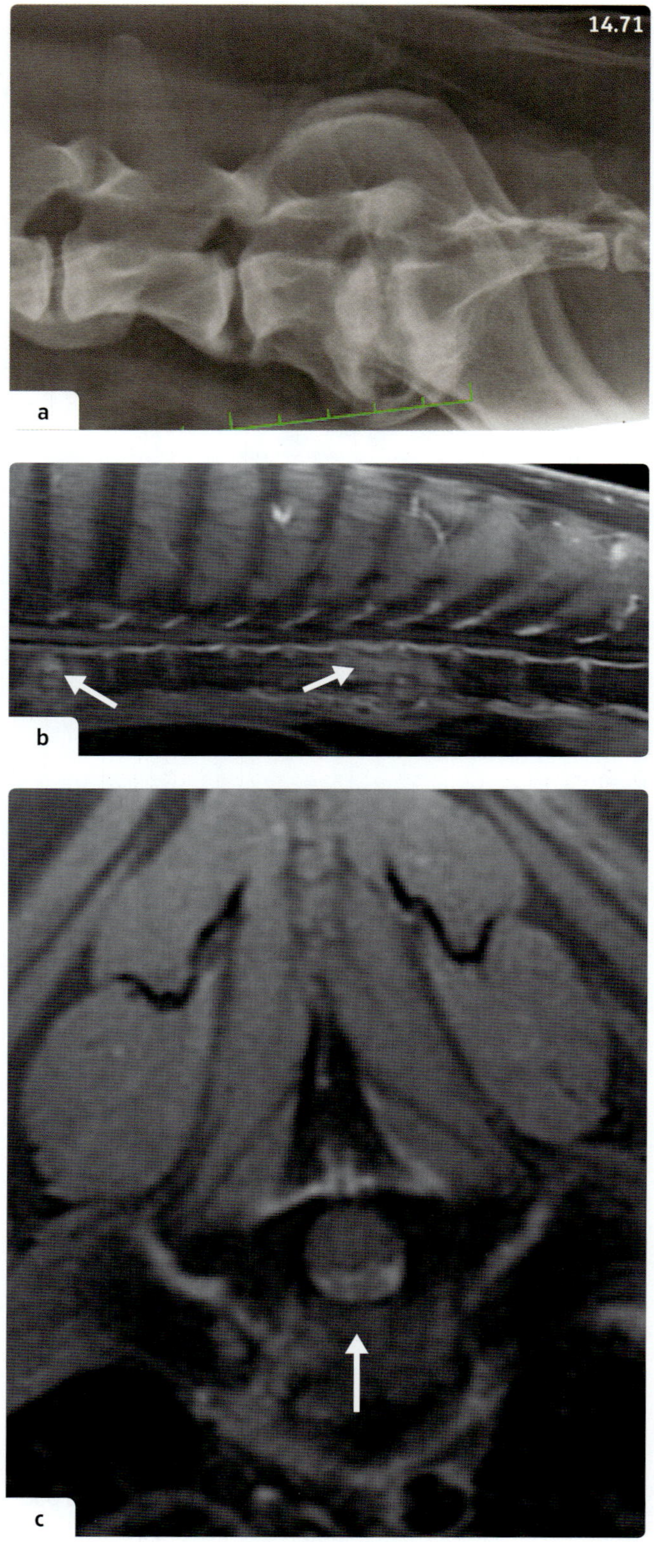

Figures 14.71a–c (a) Lateral radiograph of the lumbosacral joint of a dog with diskospondylitis. Note the endplate sclerosis and lysis. (b) Sagittal and (c) transverse post-contrast T1-weighted MR images of the thoracic spinal column of a dog with multifocal diskospondylitis illustrating the marked vertebral body uptake of contrast (arrows).

of the vertebrae may be considered if needle aspiration is unrewarding. This has yielded positive cultures in approximately 80% of patients. In all cases, diagnostic investigation of potential systemic infectious foci should be considered. This should include abdominal ultrasonography for prostatic or renal disease, thoracic radiographs for pulmonary disease, and cardiac ultrasonography for endocardial disease.

Management

Once radiographic evidence of diskospondylitis is present, treatment for the common potential pathogen *S. intermedius* infection may be started. Initial treatment of diskospondylitis consists of antibiotics (potentiated amoxicillin or cephalexin), cage rest, and analgesics. Results of cultures may require alteration of this choice.

IV antibiotics should be considered if severe neurologic compromise or signs of sepsis are present; otherwise, oral antibiotics are acceptable. However quickly the patient improves, continuation of the antibiotics for 8–16 weeks is recommended. Resolution of clinical signs, such as pain and fever, should be expected within 5 days of initiating therapy; however, complete neurologic resolution may take 2–3 months. Residual deficits may remain, but persistent pain indicates an active disease, and these patients should be treated with an additional antibiotic and considered for further diagnostics, as they may have a potential fungal infection or surgical lesion. Diskospondylitis associated with *Aspergillus* spp. has been treated with itraconazole (5 mg/kg of body weight PO q24h), although long-term reports of success are lacking, with the belief being that chronic recurrence and progression are likely.

Surgical decompression is rarely needed, and should only be considered in refractory cases or those with severe neurologic deficits that show no sign of improvement within 3–5 days. Although internal fixation can be acceptable even at the site of an infection, it may be more appropriate to consider external skeletal fixation, as has been successfully described in dogs with lumbosacral diskospondylitis.

The prognosis for this disease is generally very good unless the etiology is fungal, there are multiple lesions, vertebral fracture or subluxation occurs, or there is endocarditis. The potential for recurrence should be considered, especially if brucellosis has been diagnosed or an underlying immunosuppressive condition is present. Residual neurologic deficits are possible, and in those cases that have severe neurologic deficits associated with the infection, the prognosis should initially be guarded.

STEROID-RESPONSIVE MENINGITIS–ARTERITIS

Definition/overview

Steroid-responsive meningitis–arteritis (SRMA), also termed necrotizing vasculitis, juvenile polyarteritis syndrome, corticosteroid-responsive meningitis/meningomyelitis, aseptic suppurative meningitis, panarteritis, and pain syndrome, is a noninfectious inflammatory condition reported in Beagles, Bernese Mountain Dogs, Boxers, German Short-haired Pointers, and Nova Scotia Duck Tolling Retrievers, but is noted and probably occurs in other medium to large dog breeds.

Etiology

An immunologic cause of this disease is suspected, resulting in a vasculitis. The etiopathogenesis is unknown but an infectious cause has been suggested, although none as yet identified.

Pathophysiology

Notably increased levels of CSF and serum IgA, increased CSF and blood B-cell/T-cell ratios, and CSF IL-8 levels are all thought to be compatible with immune system stimulation. High CD11a expression on polymorphonuclear cells appears to be an important factor in the pathogenesis of SRMA and may be involved in the enhanced passage of neutrophils into the subarachnoid space leading to meningitis and clinical signs. Matrix metalloproteinase-2 seems to also be involved in the neutrophilic invasion into the subarachnoid space. Involvement of such molecular markers provides a potential therapeutic target. Subsequent to neutrophilic invasion of the subarachnoid space, there is development of a fibrinoid arteritis and leptomeningeal inflammation in the spinal cord and, to a lesser degree, the brain. With chronic progression of the lesions, rupture and hemorrhage of the weakened vasculature may be present, accompanied by thickened leptomeninges with less severe inflammation.

Clinical presentation

Affected dogs are often young adults (8–18 months old) but may be of any age, and are usually febrile and hyperesthetic, with cervical rigidity and anorexia (**Figure 14.72**). Neurologic deficits can be seen in the chronic form of this disease and, rarely, severe motor dysfunction may result from spontaneous bleeding into the subarachnoid space. Some dogs (up to 46%) with immune-mediated polyarthritis, especially Bernese Mountain Dogs, Boxers, and Akitas, may show similar clinical signs to dogs with SRMA and have concurrent meningitis. Some dogs may have concurrent glomerulonephritis.

Diagnosis

A marked peripheral neutrophilia with a left shift may be seen at the time of the clinical signs. CSF often reveals a marked neutrophilic pleocytosis and protein elevation; cell counts of >100 cells/μl are common. Neutrophils are nondegenerative, unlike bacterial meningitis. In the majority of dogs with either acute or chronic disease, there are elevations of IgA levels in the CSF and the serum, although this is not specific for this disease. IgA CSF concentrations are significantly higher in dogs with SRMA compared with other disease categories, with the exception of inflammatory CNS disease, and so are considered nonspecific.

Management

The prognosis can be good if dogs are treated early and aggressively with immunosuppressive doses of corticosteroids, with up to 80% of cases going into long-term remission. Infectious diseases should be ruled out before this treatment is initiated. The treatment is long term, and has been reported to be required for over 2 years in some dogs; however, after this time, serum and CSF IgA levels were still elevated in some dogs, so are not considered valuable for disease monitoring. Monitoring of CSF cell count in dogs with this condition is a sensitive indicator of success of treatment. In refractory cases or in patients having steroid-related side-effects, alternative immunomodulation therapy should be considered, such as azathioprine.

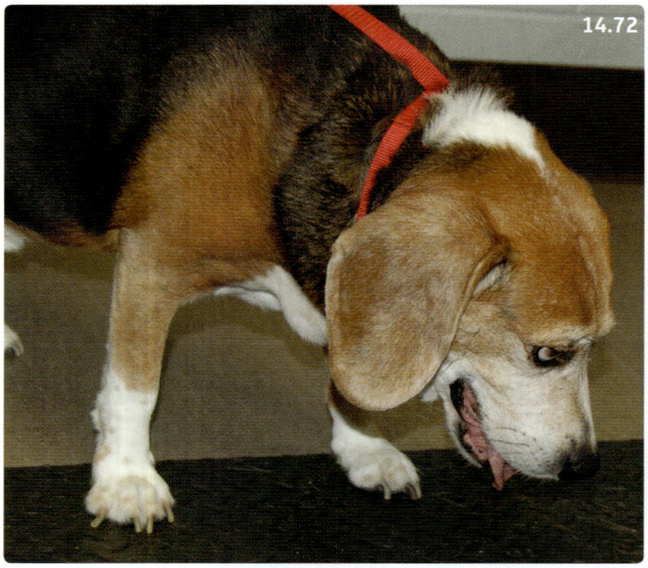

Figure 14.72 A Beagle with severe neck pain associated with its sterile meningitis.

SPINAL EMPYEMA

Definition/overview

Spinal empyema is defined as an extensive accumulation of purulent material in the epidural space of the vertebral canal. This is an uncommon condition.

Etiology

Direct extension of osteomyelitis or diskospondylitis is the main cause of the infection in veterinary medicine. Infection could also be subsequent to surgery, foreign bodies, and trauma.

Pathophysiology

Extension or introduction of an infectious agent into the spinal canal can cause a purulent accumulation, which can result in compression of the spinal cord and systemic signs of an infectious disease.

Clinical presentation

Characteristic clinical signs are a high fever, acute progressive spinal hyperesthesia, and progressive myelopathy.

Diagnosis

Hematology reveals an inflammatory leukogram. Blood cultures can be positive. *Staphylococcus* and *Streptococcus* spp. are commonly isolated. Radiography may reveal vertebral physitis or diskospondylitis. Diagnosis is aided by myelography, CT, or MRI with identification of extradural compression that extends over multiple spinal cord segments. MRI is most sensitive for assessment of severity and extent of changes associated with infection of the paraspinal muscle and other soft tissue structures (**Figure 14.73**). Cross-sectional imaging can further help guide surgical therapy.

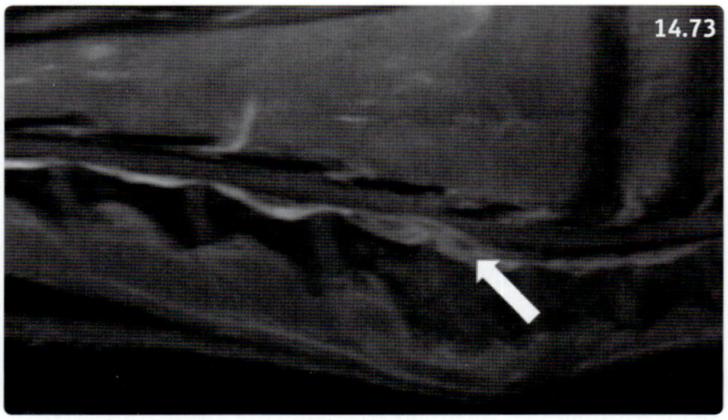

Figure 14.73 Epidural soft tissue material compressing the cord (arrow) and confirmed to be empyema can be seen on this sagittal post-contrast T1-weighted MR image of the caudal cervical spine.

Management

Effective treatment is rapid institution of an appropriate antibiotic therapy and surgical drainage of the epidural fluid. Surgery is the treatment of choice because it allows for spinal cord decompression, drainage of the infected material, and direct culture of the organism. Dogs with spinal empyema have a good outcome when treated with surgery and the appropriate long-term antibiotic therapy based on culture and sensitivity.

INFLAMMATORY SPINAL CORD DISEASES

CANINE DISTEMPER VIRAL MYELITIS

Definition/overview

CDV is a *Morbillivirus* within the family Paramyxoviridae that can cause focal or diffuse lesions in both the gray and white matter of the CNS. Focal or diffuse demyelination can occur in the white matter of the spinal cord. Neurologic forms often occur as the only clinical manifestation in dogs with intermediate levels of viral immunity.

Etiology

CDV.

Pathophysiology

The type of lesion produced in the CNS depends on host immunity and the age and duration of infection. The type of lesion ranges from acute polioencephalomyelopathy with glial and neuronal necrosis in immature or immunodeficient dogs to more chronic leukoencephalomyelopathy with demyelination in older or immunosuppressed dogs. Demyelination is therefore a more prominent feature in the chronic stages of disease.

Clinical presentation

Respiratory, enteric, neurologic, and ocular manifestations have been described in naturally occurring disease. Respiratory and enteric forms of the disease are more common in puppies or severely immunosuppressed adult dogs. Neurologic signs, whether acute or chronic, are usually progressive. Neurologic signs vary with the area of the CNS infected but spinal cord signs can predominate. Clinical signs of CDV myelitis are focal or diffuse, with the T3–L3 spinal region more frequently involved. Paraspinal hyperesthesia can occur as a result of meningeal inflammation. Myoclonus (involuntary twitching of muscles) can present without other neurologic signs, but as the spinal cord disease progresses there may be UMN signs in the affected limbs.

Diagnosis

Diagnosis of CDV infection is based on history and clinical signs. A definitive antemortem diagnosis of CDV is difficult to obtain. MRI may provide evidence of white matter involvement in the brain and spinal cord. Clinical laboratory findings and CSF analysis are often nonspecific. Immunofluorescent techniques for CDV antigen on conjunctival tissue, CSF, urine, skin, or blood can facilitate diagnosis but lack sensitivity. Multiple methods of detection increase diagnostic suspicion of CDV. PCR and analysis of CSF-specific IgG levels and determining the CSF:serum ratio can be used to detect chronic CDV infections.

Management

The treatment of CDV myelitis is often unsuccessful. Corticosteroid therapy of short duration may provide some remedy. Clinical signs typically wax and wane over time followed by a more rapid progression. The prognosis is considered poor for recovery.

FELINE INFECTIOUS PERITONITIS, MYELITIS, AND MENINGITIS

Definition/overview

FIP is a common viral disease in cats caused by the ubiquitous feline enteric coronavirus. FIP is an immune complex forming disease involving virus, antibodies, and complement, which results in multifocal inflammatory lesions affecting the nervous system.

Etiology

Mutated feline coronavirus.

Pathophysiology

Histologic findings include granulomatous inflammation of the meninges, ependymal cells, and choroid plexus. FIP occurs in two forms: non-effusive (dry) and effusive (wet). CNS involvement is seen most commonly with the dry form.

Clinical presentation

Most cats infected are <2 years of age but cats of any age can be infected. Clinical signs are often insidious and present with focal, diffuse, or multifocal distribution. Signs often are vague and reflect multiple organ system involvement. Keratic precipitates can be present on the corneas (see **Figure 14.14**). Systemic signs include pyrexia, weight loss, dullness, and anorexia. Commonly recognized spinal signs are hindlimb or generalized ataxia and paraspinal hyperesthesia. When the virus affects the spinal cord, the resulting pathology includes hydromyelia and myelitis. Other areas of the CNS such as the spinal cord can be involved, but not as commonly as intracranial signs.

Diagnosis

Confirmation of FIP antemortem is very difficult. Biopsy confirmation of infected tissue is the only method to definitively diagnose FIP. CSF analysis is abnormal with an elevated total nucleated cell count and protein levels. The white blood cell differential often reflects a neutrophilic pleocytosis but cellular distribution can be variable. CSF protein concentration can be extremely elevated (1,000–2,000 mg/dl). Results of serologic testing are difficult to interpret reliably. The most useful antemortem indicators of disease are a positive anti-coronavirus titer in CSF, a high serum total protein concentration, and findings on imaging that include periventricular enhancement, ventricular dilatation, and hydrocephalus.

Management

FIP is an incurable disease and clinical management involves supportive and palliative care. Use of corticosteroids and other immunosuppressive drugs may slow the progression of the disease. Various other drugs such as antiviral and immunomodulating (interferon) drugs have been used but none have been shown to be effective. The prognosis for cats with FIP is poor.

PROTOZOAL MYELITIS

Definition/overview

Protozoal infection can cause a focal or disseminated myelopathy in dogs and cats, respectively. Meningoencephalomyelitis and myositis are common lesions associated with *Neospora caninum* infection. Rapid ascending myelitis is more common with *N. caninum* infection. Many previously reported cases of *Toxoplasma gondii* are now thought to be due to *N. caninum*.

Etiology

N. caninum and *T. gondii*.

Pathophysiology

Infection can occur *in utero*, by ingestion of oocysts (due to fecal contamination), or by ingestion of bradyzoites (in muscle). Although subclinical infection is common, clinically significant protozoal infections tend to occur in immunocompromised or young animals, and can affect muscle, peripheral nerves, and the CNS.

Clinical presentation

The neurologic signs of protozoal infection reflect disseminated or progressive multifocal disease. Dogs as young as 4 weeks of age may develop a progressive asymmetrical or symmetrical paraparesis from *T. gondii* or *N. caninum* infection. The organism infects the lumbosacral nerve roots and muscles and often causes a myelitis and/or meningitis. These dogs may have a 'bunny-hopping' gait or present with severe rigid extension of the hindlimbs (**Figure 14.74**). The limbs are rigid because of muscle fibrosis and tendon contracture. The patellar and withdrawal reflexes are lost and severe muscle atrophy often ensues. Rarely, the disease progresses rapidly to tetraparesis and respiratory paralysis.

Diagnosis

Diagnosis is suspected based on history and clinical signs. Electromyography shows diffuse fibrillation potentials and sharp waves in the lumbar paravertebral and hindlimb musculature. CSF analysis shows a mixed cell or mononuclear pleocytosis and an elevated protein concentration, occasionally positive for organisms (**Figure 14.75**). Histology of the muscle and identification of the organism confirms the diagnosis. Serology for *T. gondii* and *N. caninum* is often positive, and PCR analysis of the CSF can confirm the diagnosis.

Management

Early treatment for 2–4 weeks with combinations of trimethoprim–sulfadiazine or ormetoprim sulfadimethoxine and clindamycin may improve clinical signs.

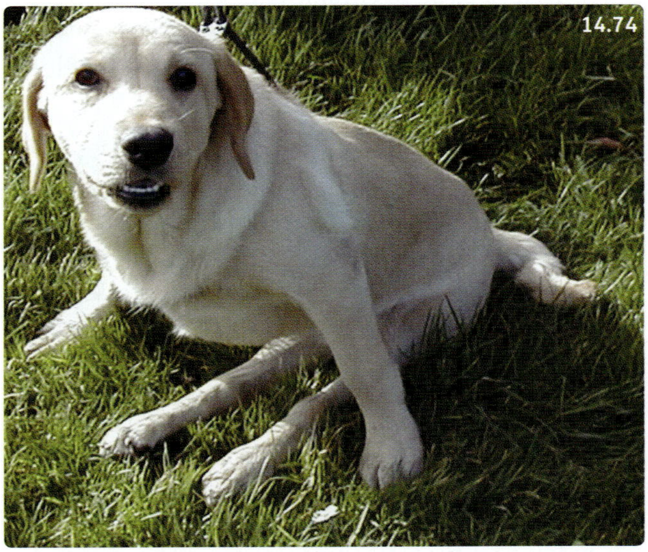

Figure 14.74 A Labrador Retriever puppy exhibiting hindlimb hyperextension associated with a *Toxoplasma* infection of the local nerves and muscles.

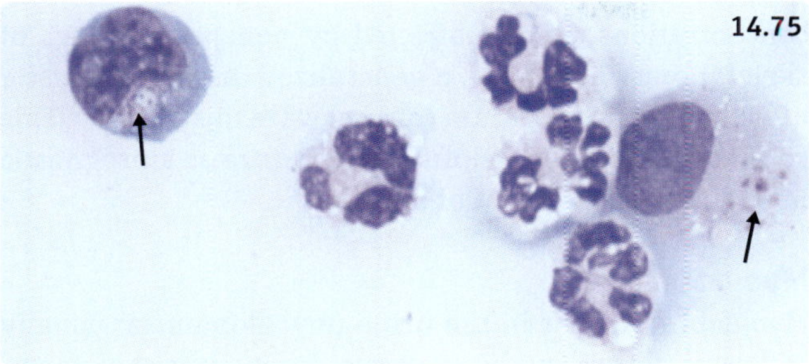

Figure 14.75 Cytologic analysis of CSF from a dog with *Toxoplasma gondii* infection revealed intracytoplasmic organisms in many cells (arrows).

Pyrimethamine may be added to the regimen but can cause bone marrow suppression in young animals. Early antibiotic treatment may improve clinical signs but recovery is often incomplete. Poor prognostic indicators for resolution of clinical signs include rapidly progressive disease, signs of multifocal CNS disease, hindlimb hyperextension, and a long time interval between onset of clinical disease and treatment.

NEUROMUSCULAR DISORDERS

Clinical signs

The classical clinical sign of neuromuscular disease is weakness. A paretic gait is usually manifested as a stilted stride that becomes progressively shorter with accompanying ventroflexion of the neck, reluctance to walk or run, lying down, and collapse. If ataxia is present, this suggests a UMN disorder or a sensory neuropathy. Following rest, muscle strength may greatly improve, but such a finding is not consistent. In between episodes, animals may be completely normal or clinical signs of weakness may persist.

Lesion localization

A thorough history and physical and neurologic examination are essential to determine if weakness is a result of a neuromuscular disease or other systemic disorder. Metabolic and systemic diseases, cardiorespiratory disease, orthopedic, and central neurologic causes of weakness should be ruled out. It is important to approach the patient in a thorough and logical manner, excluding diseases by utilizing the least complex and least invasive tests first.

It is best to perform a standardized clinical examination so that a full physical and neurologic examination is consistently performed. A practical format used for the general examination includes inspection and palpation of muscles and nerves, passive motion of joints, percussion of muscles and tendons, sensory testing, and gait analysis.

Muscle atrophy or hypertrophy can be readily observed at rest, as can spontaneous muscle activity such as fasciculations or tremors. Weakness can often be observed at rest; however, it is easier to detect with moderate walking activity. Weakness of the paraspinal muscles can result in abnormal postures including thoracic kyphosis and scoliosis. Extraocular, laryngeal, and pharyngeal muscles should also be examined at this time, particularly if the history is suggestive of dyspnea or dysphagia. A complete neurologic examination should be performed in all patients with a history of weakness, exercise intolerance, or collapse.

Gait disturbances can require close observation. An abnormal gait will result from weakness of any of the principle flexor or extensor muscles of the limbs, in addition to any structural abnormalities of the articular surfaces, joint capsules, or ligaments. A normal gait also requires coordination by the CNS, which stimulates or inhibits flexors, extensors, adductors, and abductors for counteracting gravity. In general, gait abnormalities result from (1) pain, (2) muscle weakness, (3) reduced range of joint motion, (4) weakness of UMN or LMN origin, (5) spasticity, (6) dystonia, (7) rigidity, and (8) ataxia. The gait should be observed from both sides as well as from front and back, with ample ambulating space. There are four phases of the gait that should be inspected: palmar or plantar strike (as the foot meets the floor), midstance, push off, and mid-swing. The examiner should note the rhythm, symmetry, and strength of strides, the base width of the gait, and the duration of the phases. The base width is the distance between the feet during the strides; assessment is subjective but a base width larger than the width of the trunk can suggest sensory deficits causing the ataxia.

Exercise testing in muscle disorders provides the means to assess exercise capacity quantitatively, to reproduce exercise-induced symptoms, and to investigate the pathophysiology of exercise limitations. Exercise is a powerful tool for evaluating the integrity of the metabolic pathways that power muscular work and for assessing the physiologic responses that are linked to the state of muscle energy metabolism. Thus, exercise testing is particularly useful in the investigation of disorders of muscle energy metabolism. In addition, exercise can be utilized to assess objectively the effectiveness of treatment in metabolic myopathies.

Neurodiagnostic investigation

The diagnostic plan is dependent on the localization of signs, as well as their suspected underlying mechanism. As some of these problems are episodic, their frequency must be taken into account and it should be recognized that many of the tests will need to be performed at the time of an 'episode'. Most neuromuscular disorders, however, will result in continual signs, which may vary in severity based on the level of activity.

The following tests should be considered for all cases with weakness or collapse, particularly if a neuromuscular disorder is suspected.

Video footage

If the episodes are so infrequent that they are not observed by the clinician, the owners should attempt to capture the event on videotape. Observation of the event is critical to the diagnosis. Without observation, the nature of the event must be surmised by listening to the 'eye-witness' description offered by the owner.

Minimum database

Comprehensive hematology, serum biochemistry (including CK, lactate, and electrolytes), urine analysis, a fecal examination, and a resting electrocardiogram, as well as thoracic and abdominal radiographs, should be considered the minimum essential database. A thyroid panel and an adrenocorticotropic hormone (ACTH) stimulation test should also be considered, as neuromuscular disease may be the first and only manifestation of endocrine disorders. Resting blood pressure assessments should also be performed if there is any concern about a cardiorespiratory disease and peripheral vascular pulses should always be palpated to evaluate the potential of peripheral vascular compromise.

Serum creatine kinase

CK is a specific enzyme marker of myofiber damage and the one most frequently used in the diagnosis of muscle diseases. CK is often increased in necrotizing, inflammatory, and dystrophic myopathies and is usually normal in muscle diseases in which necrosis is not a feature (e.g. myotonia). The enzyme is very labile and so is nonspecific. As the half-life is only about 2 hours, the magnitude and persistence of increased CK activity is an indication of severity and activity of an underlying muscle disease. However, this enzyme can be elevated following IM injections, surgery, prolonged recumbancy, and even anorexia in cats. Conversely, muscle disease should never be ruled out based on a normal CK level.

Cardiac troponin I

Troponin is located in myofibrils and is the regulatory protein of contractile skeletal and cardiac muscle. Cardiac muscle can be affected by generalized myopathies including muscular dystrophy, mitochondrial myopathies, and necrotizing myopathies. Although cardiac troponin concentrations are not affected by nonspecific types of skeletal muscle damage, a generalized disease of muscle affecting the myocardium could elevate this enzyme. This could be potentially helpful in the future as a prognostic marker based on extent of disease.

Myoglobin

Myoglobin present in the urine (myoglobinuria) usually indicates severe muscle damage, frequently rhabdomyolysis following trauma, toxins, infections, and malignant hyperthermia. However, a correlation does not exist between serum CK and myoglobinuria and so it is considered an insensitive test. Recurrent myoglobinuria may be detected in inherited metabolic myopathies and in muscular dystrophy. Myoglobin is toxic to the renal tubules and can cause acute kidney injury.

Serology and PCR

Investigations of infectious diseases may require extensive serologic tests and their interpretation may be difficult but, depending on the potential for exposure, serology should be performed on all possible infectious candidates (particularly *Toxoplasma gondii*, *Neospora caninum*, *Hepatozoon* spp. and *Leishmania* spp.) depending on geographic locale and travel history. Serology for autoimmune conditions such as rheumatoid arthritis, systemic lupus, and myasthenia gravis may be warranted if suspected. Antibodies against the acetylcholine receptor (AChR) should be measured in all dogs with acquired megaesophagus and dysphagia. Testing blood with PCR methods for these infections is likely to be more sensitive and specific, if it is available.

Electrophysiology

Extensive electrophysiologic testing may be required to confirm the precise lesion localization of the disease if a neuromuscular abnormality is suspected. An abbreviated needle electromyography (EMG) test may be worthwhile in the initial investigations, as it can quickly aid identification of an axonal or muscular disease. This is particularly helpful in cases with obvious muscle hypertrophy or atrophy. Repetitive nerve stimulation and single fiber EMG should be considered for neuromuscular junction assessment (**Figure 14.76**).

Advanced imaging

Unless a CNS abnormality is suspected, it may not be necessary to consider spinal radiographs, CT, or MRI studies. Thoracic radiographs can assist with the diagnosis of megaesophagus and associated aspiration pneumonia. Fluoroscopy or contrast-enhanced radiography may

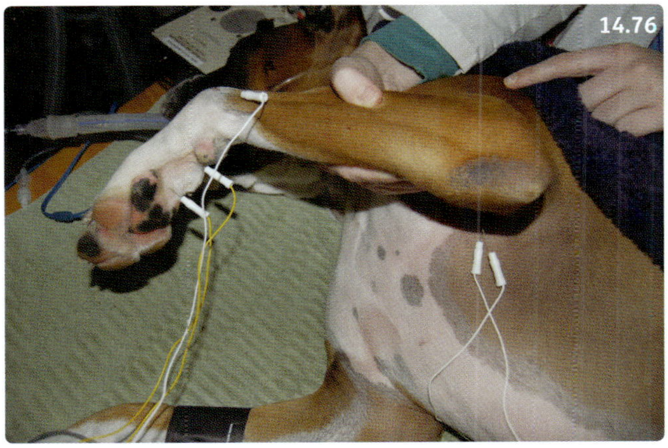

Figure 14.76 Electrophysiologic assessment of the nerves in the forelimb. Stimulating needles are placed proximally in close association to a specific nerve and recording electrodes are placed distally in the interosseous muscles to detect the resultant action potentials.

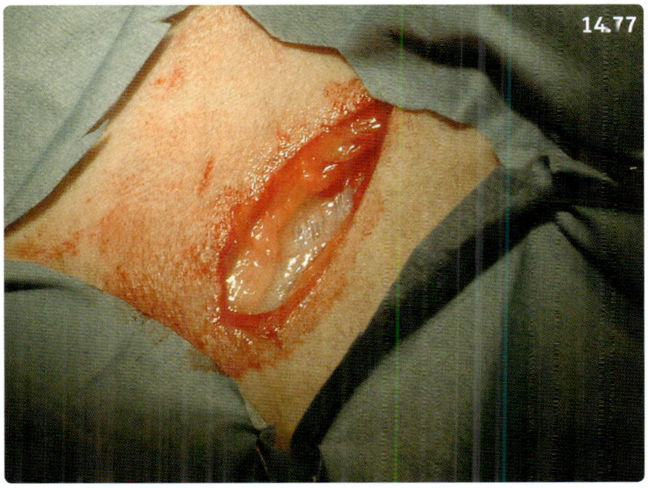

Figure 14.77 A linear skin incision exposes subcutaneous fat and shiny underlying muscle fascia. The fascia needs to be incised, which will allow a small piece of muscle to be sampled for histopathologic assessment.

be helpful to evaluate the function of the esophagus if enlargement is not obvious on plain survey radiographs and swallowing if dysphagia is present. Cardiac ultrasonography may be required if a cardiorespiratory condition is suspected.

MRI and CT scans have recently been utilized to document the presence of muscle pathology, particularly on post-contrast images. The location of the contrast uptake within the muscles detected on MRI or CT can assist with choosing suitable areas for a more high-yield biopsy, which is important in early onset, localized, or patchy myopathies.

Cerebrospinal fluid analysis

A CSF tap may help to rule out CNS diseases as well as diffuse inflammatory conditions of the nerve roots, but rarely is it a specific test and rarely will it be helpful in cases of neuromuscular collapse. Evaluation for infectious diseases can be achieved with serologic techniques or with PCR analysis of the CSF.

Muscle and nerve biopsy

If a neuromuscular disease is suspected, a muscle or nerve biopsy can provide a specific diagnosis of the underlying cause (**Figure 14.77**). Since a peripheral nerve can react in only a limited number of ways to a variety of insults, the biopsy in most instances just confirms the presence of axonal degeneration, demyelination, abnormalities of supporting structures, inflammation, or infiltrative neoplasia. However, a nerve biopsy can provide information on regeneration, remyelination, and degree of fiber depletion and fibrosis, which are important for prognosis. The muscle biopsy is of utmost importance in the diagnosis of most muscle diseases, particularly the inherited diseases.

NEUROPATHIES

BREED-RELATED NEUROPATHY

Definition/overview

Inherited and breed-related neuropathies are rare diseases that usually affect young animals and can produce generalized motor, mixed motor and sensory, pure sensory, and/or autonomic deficits.

Etiology

Unknown, suspected genetic in many breeds.

Pathophysiology

Progressive, usually chronic, degeneration of the myelin and/or the axons of sensory and/or motor fibers.

Clinical presentation

Typically, progressive LMN paresis develops, often affecting the hindlimbs first, but eventually involving the forelimbs. The concurrent development of laryngeal paralysis and megaesophagus is recognized as a syndrome called laryngeal paralysis polyneuropathy complex. This syndrome has been reported in young Rottweilers, Dalmatians, Leonbergers, white coated German Shepherd Dogs, and Pyrenean Mountain Dogs amongst others; it is now recognized that older dogs with idiopathic laryngeal paralysis, in particular Labrador

Retrievers, also suffer from a more generalized neuropathy that is likely hereditary. Several different breeds of cat are also reported to have hereditary neuropathies.

Familial sensory neuropathies are particularly unusual but have been reported in English Pointers, English Springer Spaniels, French Spaniels, and Longhaired Dachshunds, with sporadic reports in other breeds of dog. Dachshunds present with nociceptive deficits, mild ataxia, and loss of conscious proprioception. These dogs have been reported to self-mutilate their penis and dribble urine. The disease in English Pointers and French and English Spaniels is more severe and more specific to nociception. They lose nociception in their distal limbs around 3–8 months of age and as a result lick, chew, and even autoamputate their digits. These dogs do not have conscious proprioceptive deficits.

Diagnosis

Diagnosis is by recognition of typical breed, age of onset, and presentation and ruling out other disorders by electrophysiologic evaluation of nerve function and nerve biopsy.

Management

Therapy is limited to symptomatic management of signs in most diseases. This includes laryngeal tie back in dogs with upper airway obstruction secondary to laryngeal paresis/paralysis and physical therapy to maintain range of motion and muscle mass. One exception is hyperchylomicronemia in cats, which can be treated successfully by feeding a low-fat, high-fiber diet. It is important to recognize problems and diagnose the cause of signs in animals used for breeding.

ENDOCRINE NEUROPATHY

Definition/overview

Endocrine diseases that are known or suspected to cause a peripheral neuropathy include diabetes mellitus, hypoglycemia (most commonly as a result of insulinoma in dogs), hypothyroidism, and hyperadrenocorticism. These diseases are associated with chronic progressive diffuse weakness with or without systemic signs of the specific endocrine disease.

Etiology

Diabetes mellitus, hypoglycemia (most commonly as a result of insulinoma in dogs), hypothyroidism, and hyperadrenocorticism.

Pathophysiology

Poorly controlled diabetes mellitus causes distal axonal degeneration, with the longest peripheral nerves affected first.

Clinical presentation

The most common manifestation of diabetes mellitus is a sciatic neuropathy in cats causing a plantigrade stance in the hindlimbs at rest and when walking. Affected cats retain the ability to ambulate but hock flexion is absent when the withdrawal reflex is tested. As the signs progress, they also develop a palmigrade stance. Although pathologic changes and sporadic cases of neuropathy have been detected in diabetic dogs, it is usually a subclinical problem in this species. However, when it does occur, it resembles a degenerative myelopathy, which will reverse with improved diabetic regulation. Hypothyroidism has been reported to be a cause of weakness in dogs as a result of a generalized peripheral neuropathy. In addition, idiopathic neuropathies such as facial or laryngeal paralysis, peripheral vestibular syndrome, and megaesophagus have been linked to hypothyroidism.

Diagnosis

Diagnosis of diabetic neuropathy is strongly suspected in animals with poorly controlled diabetes and classic neurologic findings. Definitive diagnosis is made by electrophysiologic studies and nerve biopsy. Although axonal degeneration can be present in severely affected animals, the most common findings are abnormalities in Schwann cells and myelin. Diagnosis of hypothyroidism is made by measurement of serum total and free T4 and thyroid-stimulating hormone levels.

Management

Prognosis for full recovery of peripheral nerve function associated with diabetes mellitus is good in most cases. Restoring normoglycemia prevents progression and in most cases may result in complete resolution of neurologic signs. Supplementation with thyroxine may reverse the signs of generalized peripheral neuropathy associated with hypothyroidism over 2–3 months, but laryngeal and esophageal abnormalities usually persist.

INSULINOMA

Definition/overview

Chronic, severe hypoglycemia (<3 mmol/l [54 mg/dl]) is almost invariably associated with insulinomas in dogs and can result in a generalized neuropathy.

Etiology
Pancreatic beta cell tumor.

Clinical presentation
The most common neurologic signs result from the effects of hypoglycemia on the CNS (seizures, weakness, exercise intolerance, and collapse). However, persistent hypoglycemia may also cause a distal peripheral neuropathy that manifests initially as a stiff gait, particularly in the hindlimbs, but progresses to more obvious signs of a generalized peripheral neuropathy with prominent sciatic deficits.

Diagnosis
Diagnosis is based on documention of hypoglycemia with concurrent inappropriate hyperinsulinemia in the presence of the clinical signs and associated with a pancreatic mass, documented with ultrasound or MRI or surgical exploration (**Figure 14.78**) and histopathology following resection.

Management
Treatment of the insulinoma may improve the gait depending on the extent of the underlying disease.

INFLAMMATORY DISEASES

CHRONIC INFLAMMATORY DEMYELINATING POLYNEUROPATHY

Definition/overview
Chronic inflammatory demyelinating polyneuropathy (CIDP) causes slowly progressive LMN tetraparesis in adult dogs and cats with no gender or breed bias.

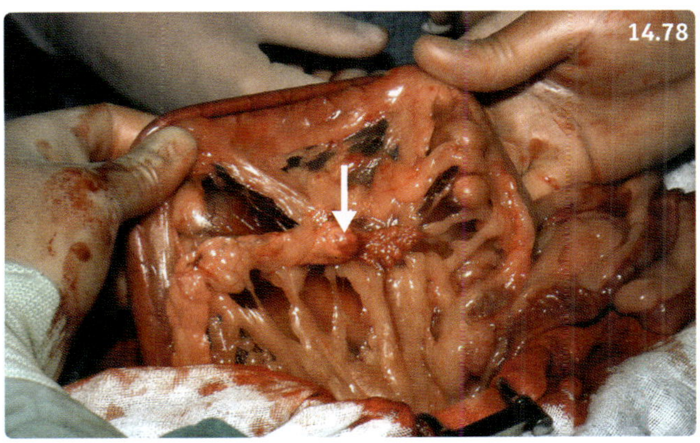

Figure 14.78 Insulinoma (arrow) as viewed at surgery in a dog. (Courtesy M. Schaer)

Etiology
The etiology of CIDP is unknown but it appears to be similar to chronic inflammatory demyelinating polyneuropathy in humans.

Pathophysiology
CIDP is an apparently immune-mediated disease in which the inflammatory reaction is focused on peripheral nerve myelin.

Clinical presentation
Signs can relapse intermittently and can progress from paraparesis to tetraplegia. Shifting lameness, a plantigrade stance, and ventroflexion of the neck have been described in cats, along with megaesophagus and regurgitation. Leg tremors and laryngeal and facial paralysis have been noted in dogs.

Diagnosis
Diagnosis is reached by a combination of electrophysiologic studies and nerve biopsy. Typically, motor nerve conduction velocity is reduced. There is multifocal paranodal demyelination in teased nerve fiber preparations, and thinly myelinated fibers are visible on semithin sections. Electron microscopy reveals macrophages stripping myelin, and the presence of demyelinated and remyelinated fibers. There is also a mononuclear infiltrate.

Management
Treatment consists of immunosuppression with prednisone (initial dose of 2 mg/kg PO divided q12h for 1–2 weeks followed by gradual tapering over a period of weeks). Most cases respond favorably to this regimen, although some eventually relapse and become steroid resistant.

POLYRADICULONEURITIS

Definition/overview
Polyradiculoneuritis (inflammation of peripheral nerves and nerve roots) is probably the most common peripheral neuropathy of dogs and cats.

Etiology
The disease can be subclassified according to cause as Coonhound paralysis, (seen in North America, with onset of signs 7–10 days after raccoon bites), idiopathic polyradiculoneuritis, and post-vaccinal polyradiculoneuritis (extremely rare). An important association in

man is concurrent infection with a specific serotype of *Campylobacter jejuni*, but a variety of other infectious agents can also trigger the disease in humans, including *Toxoplasma gondii*. Recently, it was shown that dogs with idiopathic acute polyradiculoneuritis are more likely to have positive titers for *T. gondii* than control dogs.

Pathophysiology

Signs are caused by an inflammatory reaction to axons and myelin sheaths, which is most intense at the level of the ventral nerve root. Electrophysiologic findings in dogs suggest that it is primarily a motor axonopathy.

Clinical presentation

Affected dogs suffer from an acute ascending paralysis that progresses over 2–4 days to LMN tetraparesis or plegia. Spinal hyperesthesia has been noted in some dogs and CNs can become involved, leading to dysphonia and facial weakness. Severe cases may suffer respiratory failure.

Diagnosis

The number of diseases that cause acute onset of LMN tetraparesis/tetraplegia is limited and polyradiculoneuritis should always be suspected when this clinical picture occurs. Other diseases to consider include botulism and, in the USA and Australia, tick paralysis. EMG reveals spontaneous electrical activity consistent with denervation (fibrillation potentials and positive sharp waves); nerve conduction velocities are dispersed and reduced, with nerve roots more severely affected than the distal nerve. Definitive diagnosis is established with a nerve biopsy.

Management

Treatment is focused on supportive care and rehabilitation. Corticosteroid administration is not beneficial. The pulmonary function of recumbent animals must be monitored closely. If hypoventilation is suspected, an arterial blood gas analysis should be performed to determine whether mechanical ventilation is necessary. Animals should be turned and passive range of motion exercises and massage of limbs should be performed at least four times a day. If pulmonary function is unaffected, with adequate supportive care most animals will recover over a period of 3–6 weeks. However, the need for mechanical ventilation, the presence of aspiration pneumonia, and severe muscle atrophy with development of contractures all worsen the outcome.

PROTOZOAL NEURITIS

Definition/overview

Infection with the protozoal organisms *Toxoplasma gondii* and *Neospora caninum* can cause an intense polyradiculoneuritis in dogs, accompanied by a myositis.

Etiology

Protozoal infection.

Pathophysiology

Clinically significant protozoal infections affect young or immunocompromised dogs. Dogs are both definitive and intermediate hosts for *Neospora* spp., with cattle, sheep, goats, and other mammals also acting as intermediate hosts. Cats are the definitive host for *Toxoplasma* spp., with most mammals serving as intermediate hosts. Infection can occur transplacentally (common for *N. caninum*), by ingestion of protozoal cysts from infected secondary hosts, and by ingestion of oocysts shed in feces (common for toxoplasmosis).

Clinical presentation

Clinical signs can be extremely variable as a result of infection of muscle, peripheral nerve, and the CNS. Typically, the hindlimbs are affected first and the combination of myositis and neuritis causes rigid extension of the limbs, with severe muscle atrophy and contractures developing quickly. However, multifocal CNS signs can be present and a cerebellar syndrome has also been reported.

Diagnosis

Definitive diagnosis can be made by identification of the organisms in muscle or nerve biopsies, combined with serology. Serology alone can be confusing with a high rate of false-positive titers, particularly in the case of toxoplasmosis. PCR analysis of CSF may provide a more specific diagnosis but the sensitivity of this test is unknown.

Management

Treatment of protozoal infections can be attempted using clindamycin. However, a combination of trimethoprim/sulfadiazine and pyremethamine is more effective at actually killing the organisms, and penetrates the CNS well. Animals on this protocol can be supplemented with folic acid; azithromycin can be added as it is effective at killing intracellular organisms. Prognosis depends on the severity of clinical signs and muscle contractures. Recovery of normal function is unlikely, although institution of treatment can prevent progression of signs. If treatment is initiated while signs are still mild, the prognosis is better, but relapses can occur.

TOXIC DISEASES

BOTULISM

Definition/overview

Botulism intoxication can result in an acute onset of rapidly progressive diffuse neuromuscular signs. Multiple dogs can be involved at the same time depending on the source and accessibilty of the toxin.

Etiology

There are several forms of the botulinum toxin produced by *Clostridium botulinum*, but botulinum C is the only form associated with canine disease.

Pathophysiology

Botulism is caused by absorption of the botulinum toxin following ingestion of spoiled carrion or raw meat. The botulinum toxin produced by *C. botulinum* is taken up at the neuromuscular junction and prevents synaptic release of acetylcholine at the neuromuscular junction of cholinergic nerves. Botulinum toxins, like tetanospasmin, are zinc endopeptidases, and botulinum C binds to the presynaptic protein SNAP 25.

Clinical presentation

Botulism causes LMN tetraparesis that starts in the hindlimbs as mild weakness, but progresses to tetraplegia in severe cases. CNs are often involved, producing facial paresis, dysphonia, megaesophagus, and regurgitation. Autonomic signs such as mydriasis and dry eye are variably present. Onset of signs usually occurs over 2–4 days and is often preceded by a history of dietary indiscretion (usually consuming spoiled meat) and vomiting or diarrhea. Botulism is extremely rare in cats.

Diagnosis

History and clinical signs are indicative of the disease. Electrophysiologic studies may be supportive of the diagnosis. Reduced motor nerve conduction velocity has been reported suggesting that there is a concurrent neuropathy. Definitive diagnosis is difficult to establish. The presence of botulinum toxin in the serum, feces, or vomitus may be detected using a specific antitoxin to perform a neutralization test in mice, and use of an ELISA has been reported, demonstrating an increase in serum titers to botulinum neurotoxin type C, 3 weeks after onset of signs. Typically, the toxin is no longer detectable by the time neurologic signs are evident.

Management

Treatment is supportive and recovery occurs over a period of approximately 3 weeks. Recumbent dogs should be turned regularly, kept clean and dry, and their bladder expressed if necessary. Megaesophagus and regurgitation should be managed by intermittent suction of the esophagus by means of a nasoesophageal tube, antacids (e.g. famotidine) to decrease acidity of stomach contents (decreases esophagitis and effects of aspiration), and antibiotics for aspiration pneumonia if necessary. Ampicillin, aminoglycosides, erythromycin, ciprofloxacin, and imipenum interfere with neuromuscular conduction and should be avoided. If megaesophagus is present, the dog should be fed while held or propped with the head up, and that position maintained for approximately 30 minutes after feeding. Arterial blood gas analysis should be performed to check for hypoventilation in tetraplegic animals and in animals that may have aspirated. Passive range of motion exercises and massage should be performed every 6 hours while the animal is recumbent. If pulmonary function is not adversely affected, dogs have a good prognosis with adequate nursing. If aspiration pneumonia or hypoventilation develops, the prognosis is grave, but recovery can occur if appropriate ventilatory support can be provided.

TICK PARALYSIS

Definition/overview

Attachment of a tick is associated with an acute onset of progressive diffuse neuromuscular disease. It is encountered commonly in the USA and more severe forms occur in Australia and Africa.

Etiology

In the USA, *Dermacentor andersoni* and *D. variabilis* are the primary ticks involved. In Australia, the disease is produced by *Ixodes holocyclus*.

Pathophysiology

Certain species of female ticks contain a toxin within their saliva that causes presynaptic blockade of acetylcholine release and a flaccid tetraplegia.

Clinical presentation

Signs appear after the tick has been attached for 3–5 days and progress over 1–3 days. They usually resolve within an equal period following removal of the tick, except in the case of the Australian tick, where signs can progress following tick removal.

Diagnosis

Diagnosis is based on identifying the tick on physical examination, particularly in large long-haired animals.

Management

Tick removal manually or using an insecticide can lead to recovery within 24 hours.

MYASTHENIA GRAVIS

Definition/overview

Immune-mediated myasthenia gravis (MG) is a relatively common neuromuscular disease affecting dogs and, occasionally, cats. Acquired MG has been observed in dogs older than 3 months of all breeds, but particularly in German Shepherd Dogs, Golden Retrievers, and Labrador Retrievers. In one report, the relative risk of acquired MG in different breeds of dog was highest in Akitas. Newfoundlands and Great Danes may be predisposed to a familial form of acquired MG. A bimodal age of onset (<5 years and >7 years) has also been reported in affected dogs, and spayed females may have heightened risk. In cats, Abyssinians and the closely related Somalis seem to be overrepresented and gender is not a risk factor in cats.

Etiology

MG is an immune-mediated disease.

Pathophysiology

MG is characterized by failure of neuromuscular transmission due to a reduction in the number of functional nicotinic AChRs on the postsynaptic membrane of the neuromuscular junction. This deficiency of functional receptors reduces the sensitivity of the postsynaptic membrane to the neurotransmitter acetylcholine. Acquired canine MG is an immune-mediated disease caused by production of autoantibodies (predominantly IgG) directed against muscle AChRs at the neuromuscular junction. Based on experimental and human clinical studies, MG involves both B and T cells. Complement-mediated destruction of the postsynaptic membrane of the neuromuscular junction and antibody-induced blockade of AChR function occur.

Clinical presentation

Several forms of MG have been described in dogs including:

- Focal MG, with regurgitation, megaesophagus, and/or dysphagia being the only clinical signs. The incidence ranges from 26% to 43% of all cases of MG.
- Generalized MG, with severe exercise intolerance and megaesophagus, is reported in up to 57% of dogs with MG (**Figure 14.79**).
- An acute fulminating form of generalized MG with a rapid onset of paralysis and megaesophagus.

Up to 43% of dogs with MG may not have clinically detectable limb muscle weakness. Approximately 7% of dogs with MG have generalized weakness without esophageal or pharyngeal dysfunction. Generalized weakness without megaesophagus or dysphagia occurs in approximately 30% and 20% of feline cases, respectively. Generalized weakness associated with thymoma occurs in approximately 26% of cats with MG, while focal forms of MG, including megaesophagus and dysphagia, without signs of generalized weakness, occur in approximately 15% of affected cats. While affected dogs may develop a stiff choppy gait, in which the stride shortens until they crouch in sternal recumbency and rest their head on their forepaws, cats with MG are usually hypotonic, 'floppy', and reluctant to walk. After rest, dogs walk normally for a short period before repeating the cycle. Many animals have facial weakness (repeated stimulation of the palpebral reflex causes it to diminish) and are unable to close their eyelids (accompanied by lack of menace and absent palpebral reflex). Third eyelids may be protruded. Neurologic examination may reveal normal sensation and intact tendon reflexes but diminished withdrawal

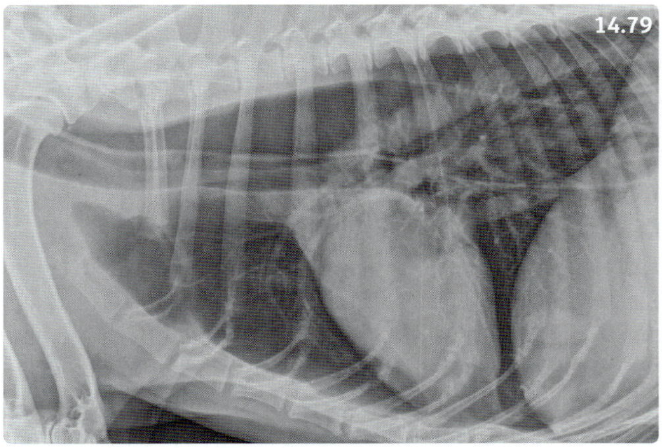

Figure 14.79 Lateral thoracic radiograph of a dog with megaesophagus.

reflexes, poor postural reactions, and proprioceptive deficits. There is a greater incidence of mediastinal thymoma in cats with MG (25.7%) than in dogs (3.4%).

Diagnosis

A presumptive diagnosis of MG may be made by the resolution of muscle weakness following IV injection of edrophonium chloride (0.1 mg/kg in dogs, with a maximum 5 mg dose; 0.2–1.0 mg total dose in cats). This test may be useful in diagnosing focal myasthenia if a decreased or absent palpebral reflex responds to edrophonium. A negative test does not rule out MG – either focal or generalized. Occasionally, this test causes a cholinergic crisis of bradycardia, profuse salivation, miosis, dyspnea, cyanosis, and limb tremors, which can be reversed with atropine (0.05 mg/kg IV). Electrodiagnostics in the form of repetitive stimulation and single fiber EMG can assist in the diagnosis, although the tests lack sensitivity and specificity. However, lengthy anesthesia is necessary and this may be contraindicated in a critical patient.

Diagnosis of MG is confirmed in both dogs and cats by the demonstration of circulating AChR antibodies in a serum sample. Reactive antibodies can usually be demonstrated in the sera of approximately 98% of dogs with acquired MG and in most affected cats. Antibody elevations in dogs and cats are specific for MG, whether it is acquired, paraneoplastic, or concurrent with another autoimmune disease. In the absence of immunosuppressive therapy, there is a good correlation in dogs between the clinical course of MG and the AChR antibody titer. Immunosuppressive therapy for longer than 7–10 days will lower antibody titers, so a thorough history is important to establish prior medication administration. Antibody titers may be negative early in the course of disease and so retesting is suggested if clinical signs were recent in onset. Seronegative MG may occur if low-titer and high-affinity antibodies are bound to muscle AChRs in a range undetectable by the standard serum assay.

Management

Treatment should begin with oral anticholinesterase drugs (pyridostigmine bromide 0.5–3 mg/kg q12–8h). The drug dosage should be started at the low end to avoid cholinergic crisis, and can then be modified based on response. As noted above, cholinergic crisis manifests itself as a combination of bradycardia, profuse salivation, urination, diarrhea, dyspnea (bronchospasm, bronchosecretion), miosis, cyanosis, and limb tremors. If oral treatment is not possible due to severe regurgitation, injectable neostigmine can be given (0.04 mg/kg IM q6h).

If limb muscle strength has not returned to normal following anticholinesterase treatment or if intolerable side-effects of cholinergic excess are noted, and if there is no evidence of aspiration pneumonia, alternate day low-dose corticosteroid therapy should be initiated (0.5 mg/kg PO q48h). Immunosuppressive dosages of corticosteroids should be avoided early in the disease, as this can exacerbate weakness, but the steroid dose can be increased every 2 weeks up to an immunosuppressive daily dose (2 mg/kg) if necessary. Once a state of clinical remission is achieved, the dose is reduced by 50% every 2–4 weeks while monitoring carefully for relapse. If there is no response to immunosuppressive doses of corticosteroids, azathioprine can be added to the regimen (2 mg/kg PO q24h).

MYOPATHIES

NONINFLAMMATORY MYOPATHIES: ACQUIRED

ENDOCRINE MYOPATHIES

STEROID MYOPATHY

Definition/overview

Chronic corticosteroid therapy may result in dramatic muscle atrophy and weakness, particularly in dogs. Steroid myopathy may be overlooked in patients receiving steroid treatment for disorders that produce weakness, such as inflammatory myopathies or CNS diseases.

Etiology

Chronic corticosteroid therapy.

Pathophysiology

The major actions of glucocorticoids are to increase muscle protein catabolism and inhibit synthesis of myofibrillar proteins. Protein synthesis is inhibited primarily in type II muscle fibers and so net protein loss is greatest in these fibers. Inhibition of protein synthesis is dependent on the dose of steroids administered. Steroid myopathy is also associated with alterations in muscle carbohydrate metabolism, due in part to steroid-induced insulin resistance.

Clinical presentation

Animals with steroid myopathy commonly have other clinical signs of glucocorticoid excess; skin and hair coat changes are typical. Patients rarely develop severe clinical weakness with <4 weeks of steroid administration. Muscle atrophy, particularly of the masticatory muscles, may occur within 2 weeks of steroid therapy (**Figure 14.80**). It has been reported that steroid myopathy

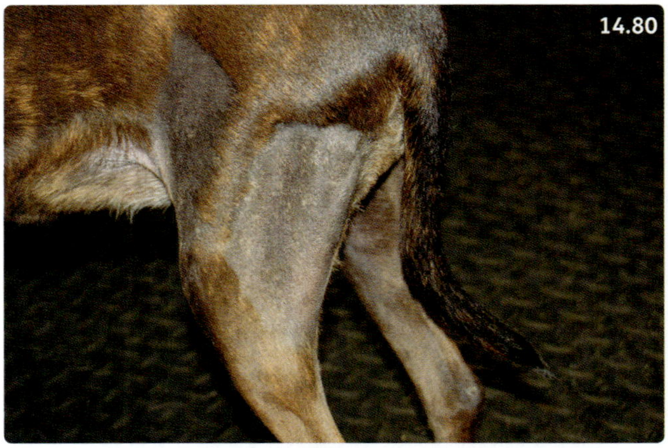

Figure 14.80 Marked hindlimb muscle atrophy is seen in this dog confirmed to have an underlying steroid myopathy.

is more common after administration of the fluorinated corticosteroids such as triamcinolone, betamethasone, and dexamethasone.

Diagnosis

Diagnosis of steroid myopathy necessitates exclusion of other causes of generalized muscle disease, in addition to evidence of long-term steroid administration and muscle biopsy confirmation of disease. The typical pattern of type II fiber atrophy may be identified early in the course of steroid myopathy with muscle biopsy.

Management

The treatment of choice for iatrogenic steroid myopathy is steroid dose reduction. Obviously, this can only be achieved if the condition that warranted treatment with corticosteroids is safely controlled. Conversion to a non-fluorinated steroid preparation and alternate day treatment are recommended. Improvement may be seen but can take many weeks or longer. Because of the catabolic effect of corticosteroids, optimizing nutritional status is important. Protein supplementation in patients with a loss of muscle mass is recommended. Physical therapy or mild exercise may be useful in prevention and treatment of muscle weakness and wasting in patients receiving glucocorticoids. Androgens can partially antagonize the catabolic actions of glucocorticoids.

CUSHING'S MYOPATHY

Definition/overview

A myopathy has been described in dogs with spontaneous hyperadrenocorticism. A pseudomyotonia is most often seen.

Etiology

Hyperadrenocorticism.

Pathophysiology

The myopathy found in Cushing's disease has been attributed to glucocorticoid excess, as described above for steroid myopathy. It has been suggested that elevated levels of ACTH may also be myopathic.

Clinical presentation

Most affected dogs are middle aged; females are predisposed. Poodles and the smaller breeds are also overrepresented. Affected dogs often, but not always, have characteristic signs of hyperadrenocorticism, in addition to generalized muscle atrophy, but with a stiff gait and hypertrophy of the proximal appendicular muscles. Of the cats that have been reported with Cushing's syndrome, the majority are middle aged or older (average 10–11 years) and are usually of mixed breed. Approximately 70% of the cats are female. No distinct myopathy has been reported in these cats but muscle wasting is a prominent finding. Some dogs will have generalized muscle weakness and atrophy on presentation rather than generalized stiffness.

Diagnosis

Diagnosis necessitates exclusion of other causes of generalized muscle disease, in addition to biochemical confirmation of Cushing's disease and muscle biopsy evidence of type II myofiber atrophy. There may be mild serum CK elevation in some dogs. The pathologic changes have been described as dystrophic.

Management

Signs can resolve in some dogs over a period of months when they are treated for their primary disease, but deficits can persist. Improvement in motor function appears unlikely but may be inversely related to the duration of disease prior to therapy. Dietary and rehabilitation treatments should also be instituted, as for steroid myopathy.

HYPOTHYROID MYOPATHY

Definition/overview

A myopathy occurs in dogs associated with spontaneous or experimentally induced hypothyroidism.

Etiology

Hypothyroidism.

Pathophysiology
In general, hypothyroidism affects carbohydrate, protein, and lipid metabolism within muscle. Muscle glycogenolysis is impaired, protein synthesis and degradation are decreased, causing net protein catabolism, and muscle uptake of triglycerides is reduced. Thyroid hormone imbalance has been determined to contribute to abnormalities of cellular energy generation in striated muscle through multiple carnitine-dependent mitochondrial biochemical pathways, supported in part by the fact that chronic hypothyroidism in dogs is associated with a marked reduction of skeletal muscle-free carnitine.

Clinical presentation
Neuromuscular signs, including stiffness, weakness, reluctance to move, and muscle wasting, may be the first indication of an underlying endocrine disorder. Typical clinical signs of hypothyroidism, including lethargy, weight gain, seborrhea, and alopecia, may or may not be clinically evident.

Diagnosis
Serum CK concentrations may be normal, especially in the first 6 months of the disease, or significantly elevated. Aspartate aminotransferase and lactate dehydrogenase activities can also be elevated. Prominent histopathologic alterations include variation in muscle fiber size with type II fiber atrophy and an increased population of type I fibers, and multifocal nemaline rod inclusions.

Management
The only effective treatment is to restore the patient to a euthyroid state. Once this is achieved, the prognosis for recovery can be good and be achieved in a few weeks. It is reasonable to institute physical therapy to limit disuse atrophy and joint contractures. There is no evidence that dietary manipulation improves muscle function in this disease.

NONINFLAMMATORY MYOPATHIES: DYSTROPHIC

MUSCULAR DYSTROPHY

Definition/overview
Muscular dystrophies are a heterogeneous group of inherited, degenerative, mostly noninflammatory disorders characterized by progressive muscle weakness, muscle atrophy or hypertrophy, gait abnormalities, and muscle contractures beginning in the first few months of life. While over 30 muscular dystrophies have been identified to date in humans, only a small number have been characterized in dogs and cats. The muscular dystrophies were originally characterized based on phenotypic features such as pattern of inheritance and the distribution of muscle involvement. With the advent of the molecular age, most have been shown to occur due to mutations of genes that code for proteins in the dystrophin–glycoprotein complex that spans the muscle cell membrane. Dystrophin and its associated glycoproteins connect the contractile apparatus in the muscle to the sarcolemma, providing mechanical stability.

Etiology
Muscular dystrophy in dogs and cats is most commonly associated with dystrophin deficiency. In some cases, dystrophin is present but is abnormal.

Pathophysiology
Dystrophin links the myofiber cytoskeleton to the extracellular matrix and is crucial in stabilization of muscle fiber membranes during contraction. The dystrophin gene is located on the X-chromosome; thus, dystrophin deficiency is an X-linked recessive trait transmitted by a female carrier. Females may be asymptomatic or expressing carriers, or be homozygous for the disease, produced from mating carriers and affected males. Homozygous females have elevated CK levels and comparable histologic lesions to those seen in affected male dogs.

Clinical presentation
Dystrophin deficiency has been documented in several breeds of dogs including Golden Retriever, Rottweiler, German Short-haired Pointer, Irish Terrier, Groenendaeler Shepherd Dog, Japanese Spitz, Samoyed, Miniature Schnauzer, Brittany, Rat Terrier, Old English Sheepdog, Pembroke Welsh Corgi, Cavalier King Charles Spaniel, Weimaraner, and Labrador Retriever, and in Domestic Shorthair cats. Clinical signs usually develop in the first 6 months of life and are rapidly progressive, although a slower disease course has been documented in some dogs. Affected dogs may demonstrate remarkable phenotypic variation, with some dogs dying within the first few days of life and others living well into adulthood.

A deficiency of dystrophin in dogs manifests primarily in males, causing generally diffuse muscle atrophy and hypertrophy of certain muscle groups (cranial sartorius, semimembranosus, semitendinosus, and tongue muscles), and with generalized muscle hypertrophy or atrophy in cats (**Figure 14.81**). Affected animals can be weak

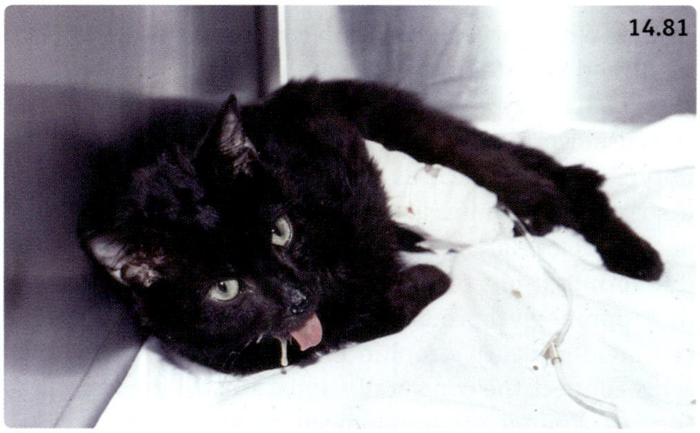

Figure 14.81 Muscular dystrophy in a young cat showing excessive salivation associated with hypertrophy of its tongue. (Courtesy M. Schaer and F. Gaschen)

at birth and ineffectual sucklers, necessitating nutritional supplementation; as affected animals age they become more evidently exercise intolerant. Dogs have a characteristic plantigrade posture with the paws laterally rotated and tarsi held close together. While walking they may advance the hindlimbs simultaneously ('bunny hop') and abduct the forelimbs. Dysphagia, regurgitation, and dyspnea may occur as a result of hypertrophy of the lingual, pharyngeal, and esophageal musculature and the diaphragm. Cardiomyopathy may result in heart failure.

Diagnosis

The serum CK concentration is usually markedly elevated (10,000–100,000 IU/l). EMG reveals complex repetitive discharges. A dystrophic phenotype, characterized early in the course of disease by small group muscle fiber necrosis and regeneration, and more chronically by fibrosis and fatty deposition, is typically present on histopathology of muscle biopsy specimens. An absence of or decreased amount of dystrophin on immunohistochemistry and immunoblotting of muscle specimens confirms the diagnosis. Recently, MRI has been used to characterize the dystrophic muscle. Gene sequencing is routinely done in humans to identify specific mutations for the sake of genetic counseling and targeted therapies. However, mutations have been identified in only a few of the canine conditions.

Management

There is no specific treatment. Prednisone (0.5 mg/kg q24h) could have benefit in affected dogs. However, this has not been substantiated by clinical studies. If steroids are used, they should be combined with physical therapy. The prognosis is poor.

NONINFLAMMATORY MYOPATHIES: NONDYSTROPHIC CONGENITAL MYOPATHIES

The nondystrophic congenital myopathies are defined by distinctive morphologic abnormalities in skeletal muscle biopsies including centronuclear and myotubular myopathies, the core myopathies, and protein accumulation myopathies including nemaline rod and myofibrillar myopathies. The genetic basis for some of these myopathies is known in dogs.

CENTRONUCLEAR MYOPATHY (PREVIOUSLY KNOWN AS LABRADOR RETRIEVER MYOPATHY, TYPE 2 FIBER DEFICIENCY, AUTOSOMAL RECESSIVE MUSCULAR DYSTROPHY)

Definition/overview

Centronuclear myopathies in humans are heterogeneous forms of inherited muscle disorders that share common clinical and histologic features. Hallmarks of the disease include generalized muscle weakness, ptosis, ophthalmoplegia externa, absence of the patellar reflex in Labrador Retrievers, muscular atrophy predominantly affecting type 1 myofibers, nuclei centralization, and pale central zones with variably staining granules.

Etiology

This is an autosomal recessively inherited myopathy. A short interspersed repeat element (SINE) exonic insertion in the *PTPLA* gene leads to multiple splicing defects.

Pathophysiology

Historically, this disorder has been referred to as a polyneuropathy, muscular dystrophy, myotonia, and a hereditary myopathy. The precise etiology was unknown and there was much debate about whether it represented a myopathy or a neuropathy, as characteristics of both were observed. Investigation of chronic pathologic changes in a group of Labrador Retrievers with a similar phenotype demonstrated that the muscle pathology became more obviously myopathic with time and central nuclei were evident. The term centronuclear myopathy was proposed for this disease, as the majority of muscle fibers display centrally placed nuclei, with disorganized sarcoplasmic architecture over the long term.

Clinical presentation

Yellow, chocolate, and black Labrador Retrievers from 8 weeks to 11 months of age exhibit a stiff 'bunny-hopping' gait with an abnormal 'low' head and neck posture and exercise intolerance. Tendon reflexes are absent or reduced. The signs are exacerbated by cold ambient temperature, exercise, or excitement but tend to stabilize at 1 year of age. Affected dogs often have reduced muscle mass and a poor conformation, and working strains of Labrador Retriever are overrepresented.

Diagnosis

Serum CK activity is normal or only mildly elevated. EMG reveals fibrillation potentials, positive sharp waves, and complex repetitive discharges. Nerve conduction studies are normal. Pathologic changes within muscle biopsy specimens are variable and can include both neuropathic and myopathic abnormalities. There is usually dramatic variation in myofiber size, with small and large group atrophy. A few fibers display centrally placed nuclei and this percentage increases over the long term. A type II fiber deficiency has been described. Genetic testing provides the definitive diagnosis and a DNA based test is now available for identification of affected dogs and carriers (http://www.labradorcnm.com).

Management

Supportive therapy and avoidance of cold are advised until the condition stabilizes. The disease itself is not lethal and so the prognosis is fair, but dogs always have reduced exercise tolerance and will not be able to perform as working dogs. The condition tends to stabilize at approximately 1 year of age.

INHERITED MYOPATHY IN GREAT DANES (PREVIOUSLY NAMED CENTRAL CORE MYOPATHY, CORE-LIKE MYOPATHY)

Definition/overview

A hereditary, noninflammatory myopathy with distinct histologic myopathic features has been described in young Great Dane dogs, affecting both sexes. While it was originally described as a 'central core myopathy', the histochemical characteristics differ from this disease in humans. Now the disease is termed 'inherited myopathy of Great Danes', potentially until an underlying cause has been identified.

Etiology

An autosomal recessive mode of inheritance is most likely. New unpublished studies have recently confirmed that this myopathy now belongs in the centronuclear/myotubular group of myopathies.

Clinical presentation

Clinical dysfunction can be seen to affect both males and females from 6–19 months of age (median age of onset is 7 months), and consists of progressive muscle wasting, exercise intolerance, general body tremors, and collapse exacerbated by excitement or exercise. All affected dogs have fawn or brindle coat coloration. Affected dogs are usually stunted when compared to their littermates. The generalized muscle atrophy is usually mild to moderate and particularly affects the biceps femoris, quadriceps, temporalis, gluteal, supraspinatus, and infraspinatus muscles. The dogs 'tuck' their legs under their abdomen and have an extended tail carriage; when they walk or run they are short strided with a stiff hindlimb gait, beginning to 'bunny hop' as they get faster. The tremors are present at rest and get worse with any movement or excitement. The neurologic examination is unremarkable but some dogs have been described with reduced reflexes. Myalgia has not been described in any dogs.

Diagnosis

Serum CK activity has been noted to be normal to increased (up to 26-fold). EMG reveals fibrillations and positive sharp waves in all muscles. Diagnosis is easily made by examination of muscle biopsy specimens that show well-defined central cytoarchitectural changes that are highlighted by localization of oxidative enzyme activity.

Management

There is no known treatment at present and the disease is usually progressive and fatal, although survival for up to 55 months has been described.

HYPOKALEMIC MYOPATHY

Definition/overview

Hypokalemic myopathy is seen in cats and, very rarely in dogs, resulting from one of the following: reduced potassium intake; increased potassium entry into the cells; increased potassium loss from the body; familial disorder of electrolyte regulation (seen in Burmese kittens)

Etiology

Acute or chronic hypokalemia.

Pathophysiology

Hypokalemia significantly affects muscle membrane activity and therefore muscle function. The myocyte becomes increasingly refractory to depolarization in a hypokalemic environment. Eventually, the muscle cell membrane suddenly becomes permeable to sodium ions and membrane hypopolarization occurs, inducing an acute onset of severe weakness.

Clinical presentation

Clinical signs of muscle weakness in the cat become evident with any cause of potassium depletion, and include generalized weakness and ventroflexion of the neck (**Figures 14.82, 14.83**). The most severely affected patients exhibit profound exercise intolerance accompanied by collapse. The weakness can ultimately result in paralysis and is progressive until the potassium deficit is corrected. The neurologic examination is within normal limits.

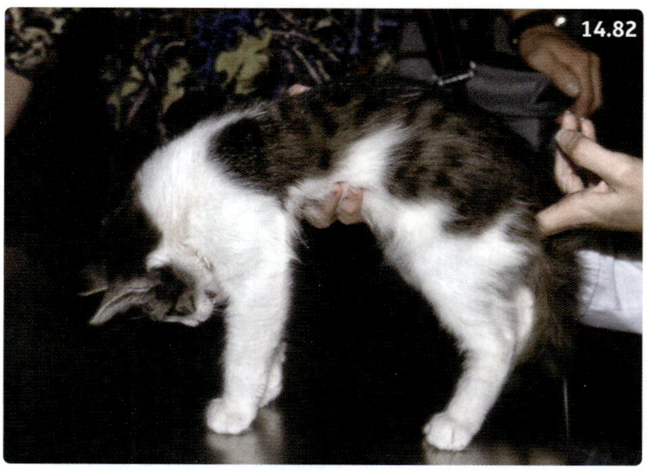

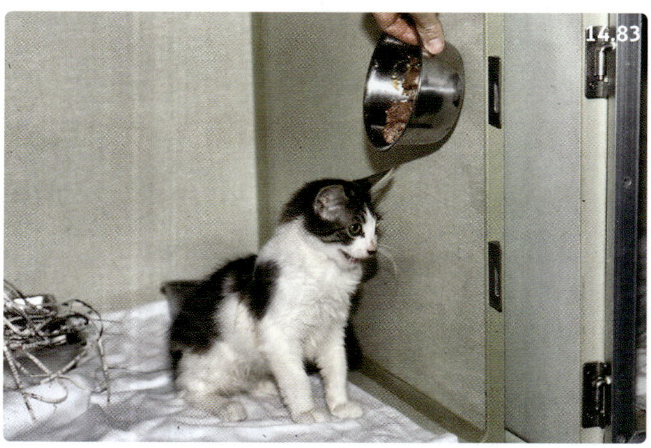

Figures 14.82, 14.83 (14.82) Young kitten with hypokalemic myopathy showing its muscular weakness. (14.83) The same kitten 24 hours later after potassium supplementation. (Courtesy M. Schaer)

Diagnosis

The serum potassium level is often 1.5–3.5 mEq/l. Serum CK is often 500–10,000 IU/l. Chronic kidney disease and adrenocortical aldosteronomas in cats with urine loss of potassium should be ruled out with serum biochemistry and urine evaluations, as well as imaging assessments of the structure and function of the kidney and adrenal glands. The dietary potassium content should be investigated; diets should be at least 0.6% rich in potassium. Hyperthyroidism should also be ruled out. Electrophysiology may be normal or have areas of fibrillations and positive sharp waves. Histologic examination of muscle biopsies may be normal or show muscle fiber necrosis with little or no evidence of inflammation.

Management

Potassium gluconate (2–4 mEq PO q12h) may be used in all animals. The dosage is adjusted until the serum potassium levels are normal. Adequate diet may be enough if insufficient potassium was the initiating cause, but potassium supplementation may be needed for life in cats with renal disease. Spironolactone is helpful for treating aldosterone-secreting tumors and adrenocortical hyperplasia involving the zona glomerulosa. Adrenalectomy is a definitive treatment for the adrenal tumor unless metastasis has occurred. Severely affected cats may be treated with IV potassium chloride (0.2–0.4 mEq/kg/hour diluted in IV fluids) with constant cardiac monitoring. Higher doses might even be required. Prognosis can be good if the potassium levels can be regulated or supplemented.

MYOTONIA CONGENITA

Definition/overview

Myotonia is a clinical sign defined as prolonged contraction or delayed relaxation of a muscle after voluntary movement or after mechanical or electrical stimulation.

Etiology

Myotonia congenita is commonly due to diminished chloride conductance across the muscle membrane.

Pathophysiology

As the chloride channel contributes approximately two-thirds of the resting membrane conductance, a fall in chloride channel conductance significantly compromises the resting membrane potential. During normal muscle activation–depolarization, potassium ions accumulate in the sarcoplasmic reticulum and increase the probability of further depolarizations, which is 'buffered' in the presence of normal high-chloride conductance. Loss of this conductance tips the balance towards potassium-induced after-depolarization bursts that manifest as myotonia. In some cases this is due to genetic defects in skeletal muscle ion channels. Sodium, calcium, and potassium channel abnormalities have all been documented in people with similar muscle dysfunctions and likely exist in veterinary medicine.

Clinical presentation

Myotonia is characterized by muscle stiffness without cramping and muscle dimpling after palpation. Congenital myotonia has been described in the Chow Chow (suspected autosomal recessive), Miniature Schnauzer (autosomal recessive), Australian Cattle Dog, Jack Russell Terrier, and in a series of related domestic kittens. Dental and craniofacial abnormalities were exhibited in affected Miniature Schnauzers. Single cases of congenital myotonia have been reported in a Great Dane, a Staffordshire Terrier, and a Cocker Spaniel. In dogs, clinical signs of muscle stiffness are evident at the time of first ambulation and are progressive; however, the signs can improve with exercise. Myotonia is accompanied by difficulty in rising, splaying of the limbs, a 'bunny-hopping' gait, muscle hypertrophy, regurgitation, and stridor. Hypertrophied skeletal muscles are painless on palpation. Similar clinical signs have been documented in cats.

Diagnosis

Routine laboratory evaluations, including serum CK concentration, are usually normal. Electrophysiologic findings are characterized by waxing and waning myotonic discharges sounding like a 'revving' motorcycle. Muscle biopsy evaluation may reveal muscle hypertrophy or a type I fiber predominance without inflammation. For detection of the mutant allele in affected and carrier Miniature Schnauzers, a DNA-based test on whole blood has been developed and is available at the University of Pennsylvania. A novel mutation of the CLCN1 gene associated with hereditary myotonia has also been identified in the Australian Cattle Dog and a DNA test is now available.

Management

Treatment is directed at decreasing the repetitive activity in the muscle by using antagonists to voltage-gated sodium channels. These drugs include extended-release procainamide (40–50 mg/kg PO q8–12h), quinidine, phenytoin, and mexilitine (8.3 mg/kg PO q8h). The treatment has been documented to improve but not normalize the condition, therefore the prognosis depends on the severity of the clinical signs in the individual animal.

MISCELLANEOUS MYOPATHIES AND CAUSES OF COLLAPSE

EXERCISE-INDUCED COLLAPSE IN LABRADOR RETRIEVERS

Definition/overview

A syndrome of exercise intolerance and collapse has been observed in young adult (often 7 months to 2 years old) Labrador Retrievers of either sex and any color, especially those used in field trials.

Etiology

A genetic mutation identified in the dynamin 1 gene (*DNM1*) is responsible for this disorder in Labrador Retrievers.

Pathophysiology

Dynamin 1 is expressed almost exclusively in the brain and spinal cord, where it plays a key role in synaptic vesicle endocytosis at the presynaptic terminal membrane. The mutant protein results in a temperature dependent reversible loss of motor function. It appears that this is an autosomal recessive disease.

Clinical signs

Affected dogs are normal at rest and with normal activity. They are usually very well muscled, athletic, and excitable. The earliest gait abnormalities seen in exercising dogs with exercise-induced collapse (EIC) usually include a 'rocking' or forced gait, with a wide-based hindlimb stance. Dogs that can still walk after exercise exhibit a characteristic crouched hindlimb gait with long strides and a base-wide posture when turning. Ataxia is usually noted after 5–15 minutes of strenuous activity, often followed by an episode of collapse, panting, and distress Patellar reflexes are lost during this time and this finding may persist beyond recovery to a normal gait. The dogs usually return to normal after 10–20 minutes of rest, especially if passive cooling actions such as fans are used. A small percentage of dogs have died during the exercise period. Although dramatic elevations in body temperature after exercise (>41.5°C) have been reported, normal Labrador Retrievers demonstrate similar such elevations without collapse.

Affected dogs are significantly more tachycardic and have more severe respiratory alkalosis after exercise compared with normal dogs. Although a few dogs with EIC have been documented with mild elevations in serum CK levels after exercise, they are not compatible with dystrophic or myonecrotic muscle. Muscle biopsy characteristics and sequential lactate and pyruvate concentrations are normal when evaluated. A similar syndrome has been seen in working Border Collies, Golden Retrievers, and Australian Shepherd Dogs, although it is likely that a different genetic mutation is responsible.

Diagnosis

Apart from severe alkalosis on arterial blood gas analysis, all clinicopathologic (including lactate:pyruvate ratios), electrophysiologic, and histopathologic tests are normal. A genetic test is now available for identification of affected and carrier dogs of the Labrador Retriever, Chesapeake Bay Retriever, and Curly Coated Retriever breeds http://www.vdl.umn.edu/services-and-fees/canine-neuromuscular/index.htm.

Management

The condition is not progressive and so a normal life span should be expected if the dogs are not heavily exercised. Exercise restriction is the only advice given at this time regarding treatment, especially when ambient temperatures are high. Hunting dogs may be less affected in cold weather. Genetic testing can be used to guide breeding programs.

FIBROTIC MYOPATHY

Definition/overview

This acquired, usually nonpainful disorder associated with a fibrous band within a muscle has been reported sporadically in dogs affecting specific muscle groups including the muscles of the medial thigh (gracilis, semimembranosus, or semitendinosus), sartorius, infraspinatus, and iliopsoas. It is most commonly seen in German Shepherd Dogs, usually male, with an age range from 8 months to 9 years. Similar disorders have been reported in the Dobermann, Rottweiler, St. Bernard, Boxer, and Old English Sheepdog. Fibrotic myopathy of the semitendinosus has been reported in a cat.

Etiology

Active dogs seem to be susceptible to this disorder and recent studies in dogs suggest that fibrotic myopathy may be related to muscle injury from excessive activity, including jumping and sprinting.

Pathophysiology

Fibrotic myopathy has been called gracilis or semitendinosus myopathy, although any of the hamstring muscles can be affected, and a similar disease has been described affecting the infraspinatus, sartorius, and iliopsoas muscles. A fibrous band can be palpated within the affected muscle belly and can extend the length of the muscle. It is proposed that muscle strain causes inflammation, edema, and localized hemorrhage, which leads to fibrosis. Increased angulation (flexion) at the stifle in normal German Shepherd Dogs may predispose these dogs to increased hamstring stress during physical activity, explaining their overrepresentation.

Clinical presentation

This may be a unilateral or bilateral disease and signs depend on the muscle group involved. While onset in some dogs is acute, the gait deficit appears to be insidious in most dogs and is best seen when dogs are 'trotting'.

- **Gracilis myopathy**. In dogs with gracilis and/or semimembranosus or semitendinosus muscle involvement, the hindlimb gait is characterized by a shortened stride with a rapid medial rotation of the paw, external rotation of the hock, and internal rotation of the stifle during the mid-to-late swing phase of the stride, resulting in the paw being slapped to the ground prematurely. The gait anomaly results from restricted abduction of the coxofemoral joint and reduced extension of the stifle and hock.
- **Iliopsoas fibrotic myopathy**. This has been associated with chronic progressive lameness, flexion contracture of the coxofemoral joints, severe pain, and decreased femoral reflexes.
- **Infraspinatus myopathy**. Fibrotic contracture of the infraspinatus muscle, a rare musculotendineous disorder mainly affecting hunting dogs, begins as an acute onset of a painful nonweight-bearing lameness. Following this onset, the initial pain and lameness improve over a period of 1–4 weeks, after which a characteristic circumducted gait abnormality develops in the forelimb accompanied by elbow adduction with external rotation of the distal part of both forelimbs.

Diagnosis

The gait is characteristic of the disease and neurologic examination is usually normal. Tight fibrous cords are palpable in affected muscles. Atrophy or swelling may be associated with this disease when affecting the infraspinatus muscles. Serum CK levels may be normal or moderately elevated in some animals. Absence of myoelectrical activity in the band during EMG evaluation is consistent with total replacement of muscle fibers by dense connective tissue. Ultrasonography, CT, and MRI can all be useful for diagnosing muscle fibrosis in the specific muscles affected by this disease.

Management

Prognosis is guarded to poor, since the condition in dogs tends to recur within several months following surgical resection of the fibrous band, or transection, partial excision, or complete resection of the affected muscle. However, tenectomy has been described to improve gait and provide pain relief associated with iliopsoas muscle contracture, as it has with bilateral infraspinatus contractures. Nonsurgical treatment (e.g. corticosteroids, NSAIDs, acupuncture) is usually ineffective. Nonsurgical rehabilitation, including therapeutic ultrasound and cross-fiber friction massage, resulted in mild improvement in several dogs (slight increase in range of motion of the stifle and less crossing-over of hindlimbs). However, gracilis and semitendinosus fibrosis does not appear to be painful and simply causes a gait deficit: dogs can live with these diseases without a problem.

EXERTIONAL RHABDOMYOLYSIS, MALIGNANT HYPERTHERMIA, AND RHABDOMYOLYSIS

Definition/overview

Rhabdomyolysis is a clinical syndrome consisting of acute muscle necrosis with swollen painful muscles causing weakness and collapse. With the exception of racing Greyhounds and sled dogs, exertional rhabdomyolysis (ER) is rare. Malignant hyperthermia (MH) has been reported in various breeds of immature and mature dogs: St. Bernards, Border Collies, Labrador Retrievers, Pointers, Spaniels, Greyhounds, and animals crossbred with Dobermanns.

Etiology

MH is a hereditary disorder of skeletal muscle, with collapsing episodes triggered by exposure to halothane, depolarizing muscle relaxants, and occasionally stress or exercise. Rhabdomyolysis may also occur sporadically in dogs as a complication of prolonged convulsive seizures (and extreme muscle exertion), infections including babesiosis and neosporosis, heat stroke, and MH. Rhabdomyolysis has also been reported following various intoxications and envenomations, and as an idiopathic disorder in dogs.

Pathophysiology

In racing Greyhounds exhibiting ER, severe lactic acidosis leading to muscle cell swelling, local ischemia, muscle cell necrosis, and myoglobinuria (**Figure 14.84**) with nephropathy has been proposed as a likely sequence of events in the pathogenesis. The final common pathophysiologic mechanism resulting from direct injury to the sarcolemma or failure of energy supply to the muscle is an uncontrolled rise in free intracellular calcium concentration and activation of calcium-dependent proteases. These abnormalities result in destruction of myofibrils and lysosomal digestion of muscle fiber contents (myonecrosis). In MH, the underlying defect in calcium (Ca) homeostasis occurs at the level of the skeletal muscle sarcoplasmic reticulum, where there is hypersensitive and heightened ligand-gating of the Ca-release channel. Most variants of MH are known to be caused by a mutation in the gene on chromosome 1 encoding the skeletal muscle calcium release channel (ryanodine receptor 1: RYR1).

Clinical presentation

Clinical signs of ER may occur during or within 24–48 hours of a race or trial and are characterized by extreme distress, hyperpnea, and generalized muscle pain, especially over the back and hindquarters, which may appear swollen and firm. Limbs may be rigidly tonic and affected dogs may have a 'hunchback' appearance and refuse to walk. Myoglobinuria and death within 48 hours are common in severe, acute cases. Typical manifestations of collapse associated with MH include a rapidly progressive elevation in body temperature, tachycardia, hypercarbia, and rhabdomyolysis.

Diagnosis

Clinical signs associated with an acute episode of exertion should prompt suspicion. Serum CK may be markedly elevated. Urinalysis should be performed to rule out subsequent myoglobinuria (**Figure 14.84**). EMG investigation will be normal in acute muscle disease. Muscle biopsy will confirm rhabdomyolysis but, as time is of the essence for the treatment of this disease, it is rarely advised.

Management

Treatment for rhabdomyolysis is mainly supportive, with intensive fluid therapy being necessary to maintain normal renal function. The systemic complications of rhabdomyolysis should be identified and individually addressed. Multimodal drug therapy including dantrolene, analgesics, antibiotics, and mannitol has been described with a beneficial effect. Frequent blood gas analyses, biochemistry, and urine analyses are advised,

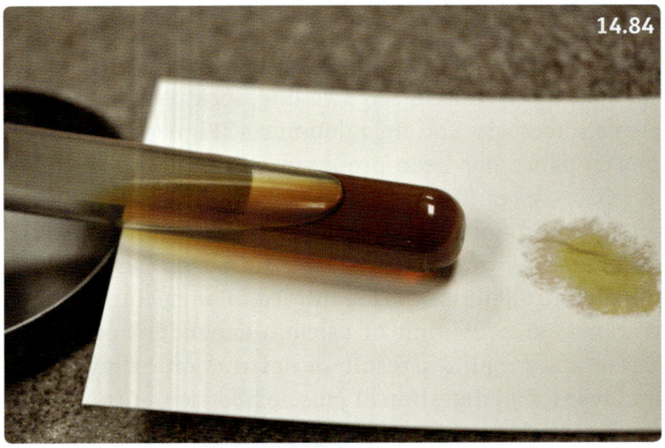

Figure 14.84 A urine sample showing myoglobinuria. (Courtesy M. Schaer)

to monitor systemic acid–base status as well as kidney function. The prognosis is guarded.

It is essential to remove triggering agents in the treatment of MH. This needs to be combined with symptomatic treatment. Stomach lavage with iced water, body surface cooling, and IV administration of cold isotonic saline solution may be beneficial. Dantrolene can prevent a MH crisis or reverse anesthetic-induced MH if given early enough (3–5 mg/kg IV). As for rhabdomyolysis, the prognosis is guarded.

INFLAMMATORY MYOPATHIES: INFECTIOUS

Definition/overview

Infection can occasionally cause diffuse muscle and/or nerve disease and may be part of a systemic disease.

Etiology

Inflammatory myopathies have been associated with protozoal, viral, rickettsial, and, rarely, bacterial infections.

Pathophysiology

Infections causing myopathies in dogs and cats are usually multisystemic. Protozoal and viral infections often become clinical in young animals in situations of immune compromise. Older animals may have concurrent infections or neoplastic diseases affecting local immunocompetence.

Clinical presentation

Signs seen in these patients are not specific but represent diffuse muscle disease; they include marked weight loss, weakness, exercise intolerance, generalized muscle atrophy, muscle pain (myalgia) and, in the late stages of disease, contractures and recumbency.

Diagnosis

Diagnosis of an inflammatory myopathy necessitates muscle biopsy. Elevations of serum CK and abnormal needle EMG can be nonspecific findings. Definitive etiologic diagnosis may be difficult as it relies on the identification of organisms within the tissues, specifically with molecular or immunohistochemical methods; however, *Toxoplasma* and *Neospora* spp. are often seen within the muscle. The interpretation of serologic titers is particularly difficult in the acute stages of disease, because a single positive result only implies exposure to the disease, rather than clinical infection.

Management

The prognosis for most infectious inflammatory myopathies is guarded, but partial function may remain if treatment is initiated early in the course of the disease. Clindamycin treatment is recommended for protozoal myositis and this has been reported to be successful but may require months of administration. If CNS infection is suspected, additional antimicrobials should be considered such as the trimethoprim–sulfa drugs. If treatment is not initiated until the disease has reached a state of recumbency, it is unlikely that the patient will walk again. Intense physiotherapy may be needed in addition to specific antibiotics, especially in young patients that are continuing to grow in the face of severe muscle contractures caused by the infections.

INFLAMMATORY MYOPATHIES: IMMUNE-MEDIATED

IDIOPATHIC POLYMYOSITIS

Definition/overview

Idiopathic polymyositis is a generalized inflammatory myopathy affecting dogs and, less commonly, cats, not associated with any other systemic connective tissue disease or infectious cause.

Etiology

Immune-mediated dysfunction.

Pathophysiology

Tissue inflammation arises due to immune-mediated damage by CD8+ T lymphocytes. Several genes involved with innate and adaptive immunity are upregulated in this disease, as are those involved in proinflammatory and anti-inflammatory pathways. Circulating autoantibodies against an unidentified sarcolemmal antigen supporting a humoral immune component have been reported in

Newfoundlands and Boxers. Autoantibodies to a 42-kDa molecule in striated muscle have been documented in Pembroke Welsh Corgis.

Clinical presentation

Progressive exercise intolerance with acute exacerbation of weakness may occur, but the disease may initially be episodic; marked weight loss is often reported by the owner. A stiff, uncomfortable gait in all limbs is often accompanied by an arched thoracolumbar spine (kyphosis) and a ventroflexed neck. Commonly, multiple skeletal muscles are affected, but it can manifest as a focal disease affecting pharyngeal, laryngeal, esophageal, or, infrequently, tongue muscle groups, causing dysphagia, dysphonia, and stridor, or regurgitation. Myalgia may be present but this is not a consistent finding. Pyrexia may be a feature of the disease or a consequence of aspiration pneumonia. Any age and breed of dog and cat may be affected. However, breed-specific variants of polymyositis affect Newfoundlands, Boxers, Pembroke Welsh Corgis, and, recently, Hungarian Vizslas. The disease affecting Vizslas is marked by pharyngeal dysphagia, megaesophagus, and masticatory muscle atrophy, although exercise intolerance has also been described. Dysphagia and megaesophagus are more commonly seen in Newfoundlands with inflammatory myopathy when compared with other dogs. Corgis present with severe tongue atrophy, facial muscular atrophy, and occasional gait abnormalities.

Diagnosis

Diagnosis is based on identification of at least three of the following, including a confirmatory muscle biopsy:

- Appropriate clinical signs.
- Elevation of serum CK concentration (at least 5–10 times the upper reference range) (CK can be low in end-stage disease). CK is not always elevated during active muscle disease; this seems to depend on distribution of cellular infiltrates and degree of muscle damage.
- Compatible electrophysiologic findings.
- Negative infectious disease titers.
- Inflammatory muscle biopsy (critical for the diagnosis); demonstration of mononuclear cell infiltration into muscle and invasion of cells into apparently non-necrotic fibers.

Management

Early and aggressive institution of immunosuppressive therapy is essential for a good clinical outcome. The prognosis can be good unless there is concurrent megaesophagus or pharyngeal dysfunction, or if therapy is not initiated until after there has been severe myofiber loss or fibrosis. Robust muscle regeneration has been documented in the face of significant inflammation and fibrosis, suggesting that muscle can survive if treatment can be initiated prior to regenerative capacity of the muscle being exhausted. Long-term treatment is usually required. The serum CK concentration should be monitored and immunosuppressive therapy continued until the CK returns to the reference range and clinical signs have resolved.

RECOMMENDED FURTHER READING

De Lahunta A, Glass E, Kent M (2015) *Veterinary Neuroanatomy and Clinical Neurology*, 4th edn. Elsevier, St. Louis.

De Risio L, Platt SR (2014) *Canine and Feline Epilepsy: Diagnosis and Management*. CABI Publishing, Wallingford.

Lorenz MD, Coates J, Kent M (2010) *Handbook of Neurology* 5th edn. Elsevier, St. Louis.

Platt SR, Garosi L (2012) *Small Animal Neurological Emergencies*. Manson Publishing, London.

Platt SR, Olby N (2012) *BSAVA Manual of Canine and Feline Neurology*, 4th edn. British Small Animal Veterinary Association, Gloucester.

Chapter 15

Bone and joint disorders

Steven M. Fox

INTRODUCTION

These are exciting times in veterinary medicine, particularly for those with an interest in musculoskeletal disorders. As a result of an ever expanding knowledge base, pets are living longer and the human–animal bond has never been stronger. Senior dogs are becoming recognized as a group with special needs and pain management is gaining recognition as a foundation of our practice ethics. The discovery of cyclo-oxygenase-1 and cyclo-oxygenase-2 has revived interest in identifying and designing nonsteroidal anti-inflammatory drugs (NSAIDs), which have found increasing use in the treatment of pain and inflammation. Nutritional management, exercise, and physical therapy, long ignored in veterinary medicine, are now being recognized as rational treatment adjuncts. Disease processes are being recognized as more complex than previously appreciated, and it follows that treatment must embrace similar complexity. The quest for greater understanding must always be a driving force for the practitioner.

History

Making a clinical diagnosis is often assisted by noting the correlation of clinical signs to a time course (**Figure 15.1**). This can only be done by recording an accurate history. Whereas traumatic injuries present with an acute severity that rapidly diminishes, autoimmune diseases are often episodic in clinical presentation and neoplasia generally presents with vague signs that become progressively worse with time.

Examination

Dogs and cats with skeletal diseases most often present with lameness, swelling, or a combination of the two. After recording a thorough history and conducting a comprehensive physical examination, radiography is often the most informative diagnostic aid. To determine the most probable cause of the problem, the clinician must identify the pathophysiologic disease mechanisms involved that are associated with the clinical presentation and, thereafter, derive a diagnosis. Trying to determine a cause of the problem without identifying the pathophysiologic disease mechanisms involved leads to an overdependence on diagnosis by previous experience, thereby restricting the capacity to diagnose disease processes never personally encountered.

The Problem Oriented Medical Record is designed for a logical approach to problem solving. Additionally, to avoid overlooking possible differential diagnoses, many find it helpful to screen for disease processes using the DAMNIT acronym of pathophysiology:

- **D**egenerative disorders.
- **A**nomalies, autoimmunity.
- **M**etabolic disorders.
- **N**eoplasia, nutritional disorders.
- **I**nflammation (infectious or noninfectious), immune disorders, iatrogenic disorders, idiopathic.
- **T**oxicity (endogenous or exogenous), trauma (internal or external).

The following conditions should be considered under the heading of musculoskeletal disorders:

- Degenerative disorders. Degenerative joint disease (DJD), canine hip dysplasia, intervertebral disk disease, cauda equina syndrome.

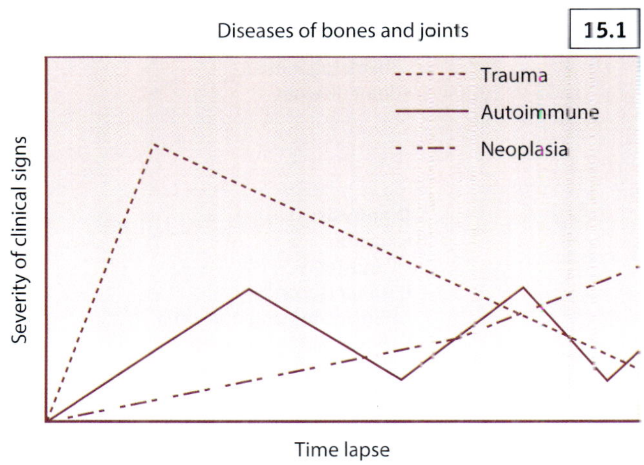

Figure 15.1 The correlation between clinical signs and a time course.

- Anomalies. Agenesis, luxation, ectrodactyly, osteochondrodysplasia, elbow dysplasia (ununited anconeal process, fragmented coronoid process), growth arrests, growth plate disorders, retained cartilage core.
- Autoimmunity.
- Metabolic disorders. Hyperparathyroidism, hyperadrenocorticism.
- Neoplasia. Osteosarcoma, chondrosarcoma, hemangiosarcoma, fibrosarcoma, synovial cell sarcoma.
- Nutritional disorders. Nutritional hyperthyroidism, hypervitaminosis A, hypovitaminosis D.
- Inflammation. Osteomyelitis, diskospondylitis, arthritis.
- Immune disorders. Systemic lupus erythematosus (SLE).
- Iatrogenic disorders. Synostosis.
- Idiopathic. Avascular necrosis of the femoral head (Legg–Calvé–Perthes disease), hypertrophic osteopathy, bone cyst, multiple cartilaginous exostoses, osteochondrosis, panosteitis, craniomandibular osteopathy, hypertrophic osteodystrophy.
- Toxicity. Lead poisoning.
- Trauma. Fracture, luxation, cruciate ligament rupture.

Many skeletal diseases are predisposed to specific areas of long bones, which makes disease rule outs logical by region of bone affected (**Figure 15.2**). Bone diseases that affect the epiphysis include infectious arthritis (with extension to subchondral bone), joint tumors (fibrosarcoma, synovial sarcoma [with extension to adjacent bone]), osteochondrosis (proximal humerus, medial humeral condyle, and lateral femoral condyle), osteoarthrosis (with subchondral bone sclerosis and/or epiphyseal 'cysts'), primary bone tumors (with extension to the epiphysis), and erosive polyarthritis (rheumatoid [with periarticular and subchondral bone lysis]). Alterations of the physis may be seen with traumatic injury or fracture, hematogenous dissemination of infection, and nutritional or endocrine disorders. Diseases that may affect the metaphysis include primary bone tumors (osteogenic sarcoma, chondrosarcoma, and fibrosarcoma), primary hemangiosarcoma of bone, disseminated osteomyelitis, metastatic tumors, and hypertrophic osteodystrophy. Lesions of the diaphysis can result from canine panosteitis, metastatic tumors, bone infarction, disseminated osteomyelitis, primary hemangiosarcoma of bone, and hypertrophic osteopathy (hypertrophic pulmonary osteoarthropathy). It must be appreciated that some skeletal diseases are characterized by unpredictable anatomic location and variable distribution.

DEGENERATIVE DISORDERS

DEGENERATIVE JOINT DISEASE

Definition/overview

DJD is a total joint disease, with joint cartilage degeneration. Surface fibrillation and fissures ultimately result from an initial increase in cartilage swelling followed by dehydration and reduction in concentration of matrix proteoglycan. This leads to deformation under loading, with less elastic return and, consequently, more contact pressure on subchondral bone (**Figure 15.3**).

Pathophysiology

Autoimmunity and the phagocytosis of immune complexes, leading to the release of substances deleterious

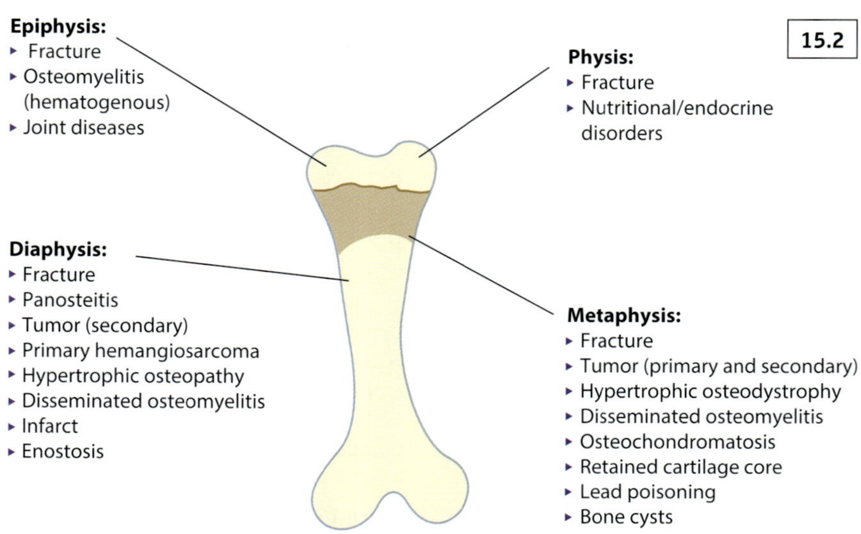

nutritional or endocrine disoders. Diseases tumors, bone infraction, disseminated osteomyelitis, primary

Figure 15.2 Bone diseases affecting long bones.

to the affected joint, play an important role in the pathogenesis of DJD, although the exact role of specific immune responses is not known.

Clinical presentation

Affected animals usually present with lameness or gait change. Once the affected joints are identified and examined, radiographs are taken to support the diagnosis.

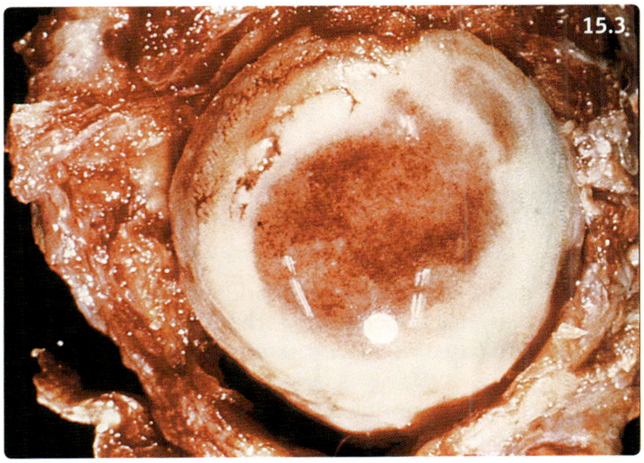

Figure 15.3 Eburnation of the femoral head resulting from DJD. Chondromalacia attributed to a decrease in sulfated mucopolysaccharide content is the earliest sign of degeneration, followed by fibrillation–exposure of the collagen framework through the loss of ground substance. Fibrillation progresses to eburnation as subchondral bone becomes sclerotic from mechanical pressure and/or the effect of the synovial fluid.

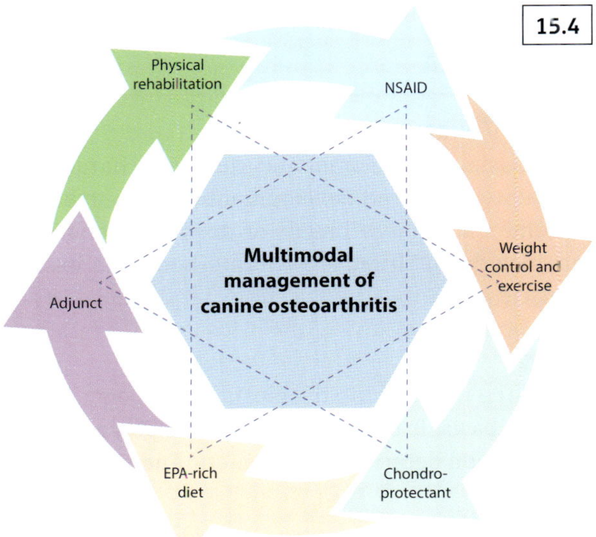

Figure 15.4 The multimodal management of canine osteoarthritis integrates six different elements: NSAIDs; weight control and exercise; a chondroprotectant; an eicosapentaenoic acid-rich diet; an adjunct; and physical rehabilitation. (From Fox SM (2013) *Pain Management in Small Animal Medicine*. CRC Press, Boca Raton).

Diagnosis

Characteristic radiographic features of DJD include subchondral bony sclerosis, subchondral cyst formation, joint space narrowing, and intra-articular or periarticular osteophyte formation. Arthroscopy can be both diagnostic and a treatment option. Arthroscopically observed morphologic changes gives the clinician an appreciation for early treatment of these disorders.

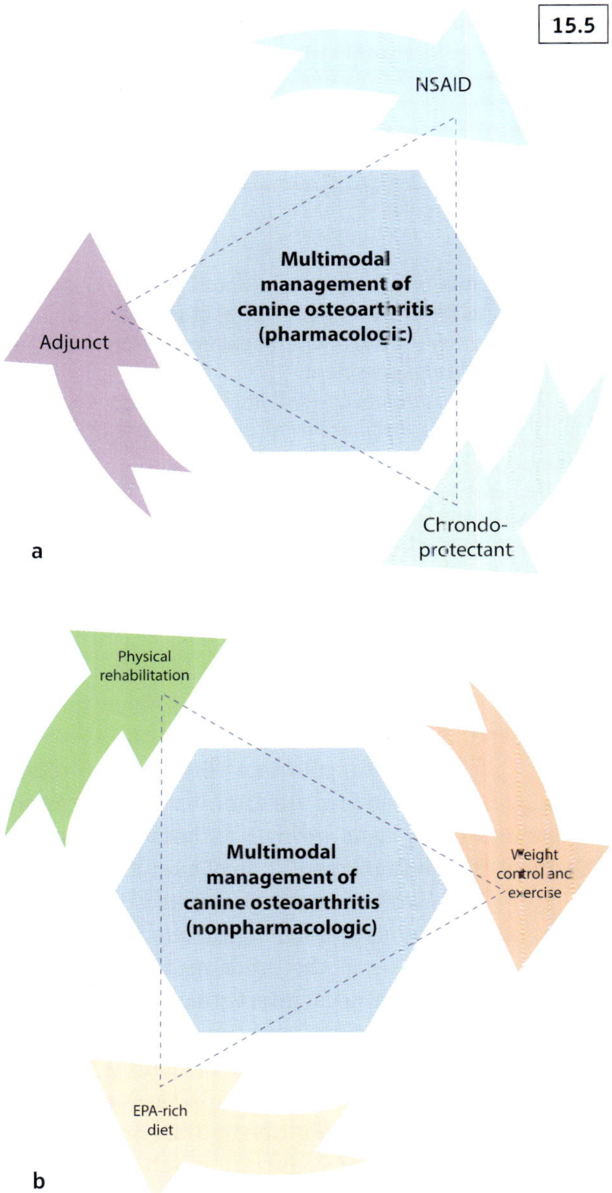

Figures 15.5a, b (15.5a) The pharmacologic (medical) management of osteoarthritis is achieved with a NSAID, a chondroprotectant, and analgesic adjuncts. (15.5b) The nonpharmaceutical management of osteoarthritis comprises weight control/exercise, an eicosapentaenoic acid-rich diet, and physical rehabilitation. (From Fox SM (2013) *Pain Management in Small Animal Medicine*. CRC Press, Boca Raton)

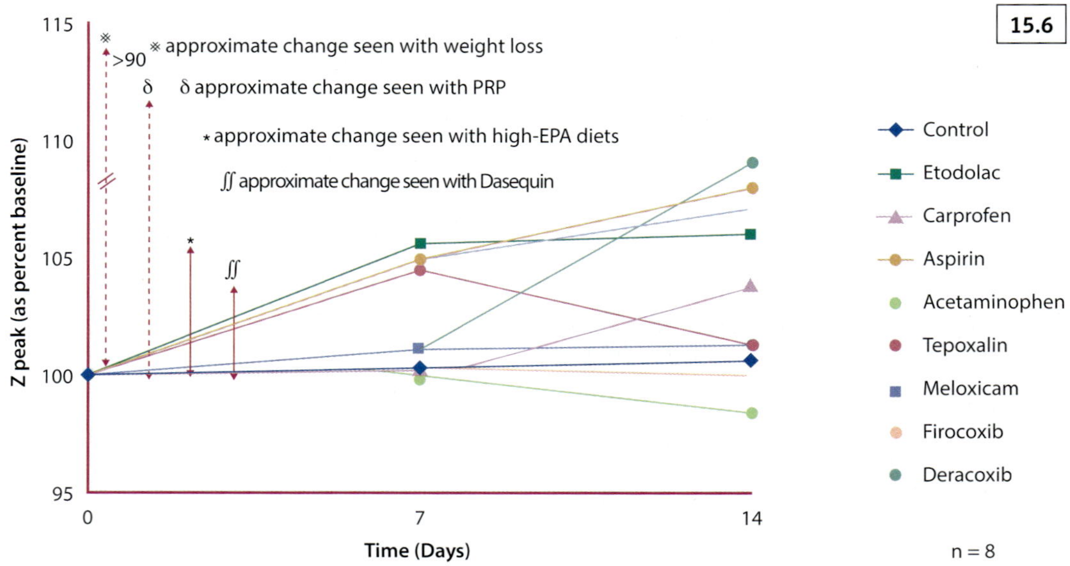

Figure 15.6 Relative efficacy of several contemporary NSAIDs used in veterinary medicine to treat osteoarthritis as assessed by force plate gait analysis (FPGA). Every dog in this study responded to a NSAID, but not every dog responded to each NSAID. Comparative responses from different treatment modalities (different studies) are further superimposed on this NSAID response graphic. All the studies used FPGA for assessment.
Millis DL (2006) Nonsteroidal anti-inflammatory drugs, disease-modifying drugs, and osteoarthritis. A multimodal approach to treating osteoarthritis. *Symposium Proceedings, Western Veterinary Conference*. (Comparing relative efficacy of various NSAIDs by force plate gait analysis in cruciate deficient dogs.)
※ Clinician's Update™ (2005) Canine osteoarthritis: overview, therapies, & nutrition. *Supplement to NAVC Clinician's Brief®*. April 2005.
δ Fahle MA, Ortolano GA, Guercia V *et al.* (2013) A randomized controlled trial of the efficacy of autologous platelet therapy for the treatment of osteoarthritis in dogs. *J Am Vet Med Assoc* **243(9)**:1291–1297.
* Millis DL (2005) Effects of feeding omega-3 fatty acids on force plate gait analysis in dogs with osteoarthritis: 3-month feeding study, 2003. Hill's Clinical Evidence Report. Technical Information Services.
∬ Millis DL (2010) Dasuquin's efficacy may be similar to that of NSAIDs in dogs. Joint Health: a roundtable discussion. Supplement. *Vet Med* **105(11)**:10.

Management

Treatment goals are to alleviate discomfort, retard the development of further deterioration, and restore affected joints to as near normal as possible. Optimal management is with implementation of a multimodal regimen (**Figure 15.4**), which is best approached through the six points of two overlapping triangles, one representing nonmedical treatment and the other medical treatment (**Figures 15.5a, b, 15.6**). Surgical intervention may be appropriate, especially in correcting conditions of instability.

Two recent additions to the adjunct modality in consideration for management of canine DJD are implementation of a piprant class drug and radiosynoviorthesis. In 2013 the World Health Organization defined a newly recognized class of drug that acts as a prostaglandin receptor antagonist. The prototypic drug grapriprant is an analgesic, anti-inflammatory agent that acts as an EP4 prostaglandin receptor antagonist. Radiosynoviorthesis is an intra-articular radionuclide therapy, for which Sn-117m is showing promise for its therapeutic effects in animal models of inflammatory arthritis.

HIP DYSPLASIA

Definition/overview

Hip dysplasia, a developmental disorder characterized by hip laxity, pain, and development of osteoarthritis, is more common in large breeds of dogs. Nongenetic risk factors include nutrition, growth rate, body size, exercise, and muscle mass.

Etiology

Although the cause of hip dysplasia is unknown, it has a hereditary basis. It is considered to be a polygenic trait, with expression determined by genetic and environmental factors.

Pathophysiology

At birth the hip is normal. With development, congruity of the femoral head and the acetabulum is lost, resulting in increased amounts of synovial fluid and hypertrophy of the round ligament of the head of the femur. Articular cartilage deteriorates, synovitis ensues, and the

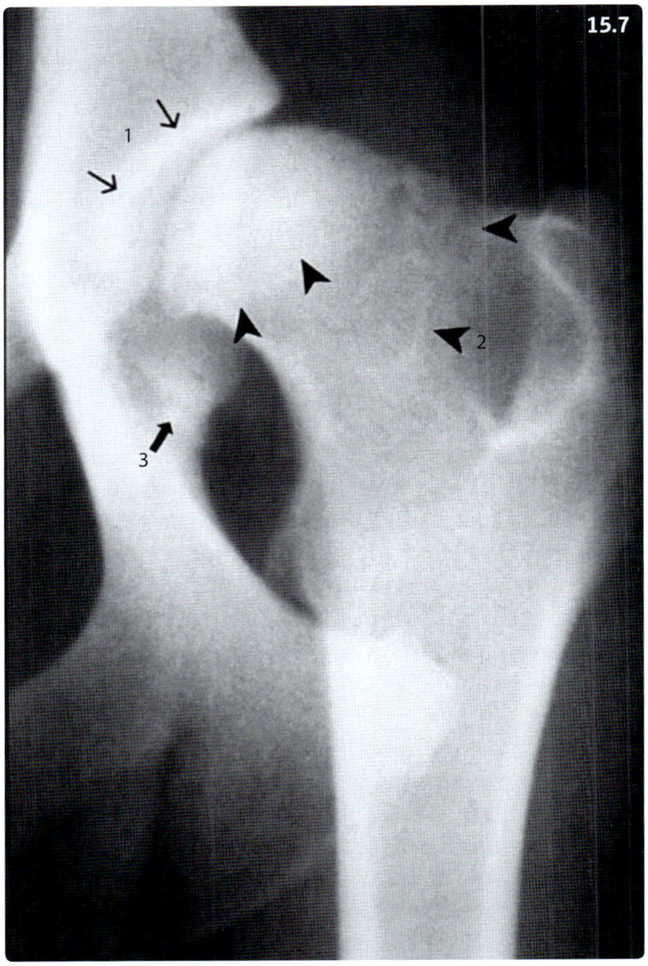

Figure 15.7 Moderate hip dysplasia. Less than 40% dorsal rim acetabular cover of the femoral head and secondary changes: 1, sclerosis of the cranial acetabular margin; 2, osteophyte build up at femoral neck capsule attachment (Morgan's line or caudolateral curvilinear osteophyte); and 3, caudal acetabular rim osteophyte deposition.

joint capsule thickens. With further progression of joint incongruity, bone changes occur and osteophytes form surrounding the joint (**Figure 15.7**). Discomfort in the early stages of the disease is associated with stretching or tearing of fibers in the joint capsule and the round ligament, while that in advanced disease is from osteoarthritis (**Figures 15.8, 15.9**).

Clinical presentation

Signs of decreased activity and various degrees of joint discomfort are seen at two stages of the afflicted dog's life; between 4 and 12 months of age, and over 5 years. Affected dogs will often bunny hop (run with both hindlimbs moving together), prefer to sit rather than stand, demonstrate decreased motility and range of motion, posture abnormally to toilet, and may show changes in eating trends and behavior.

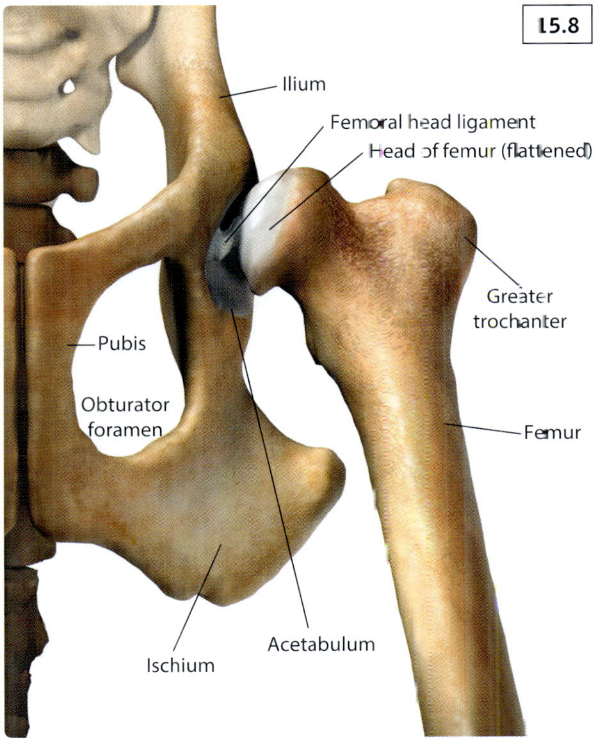

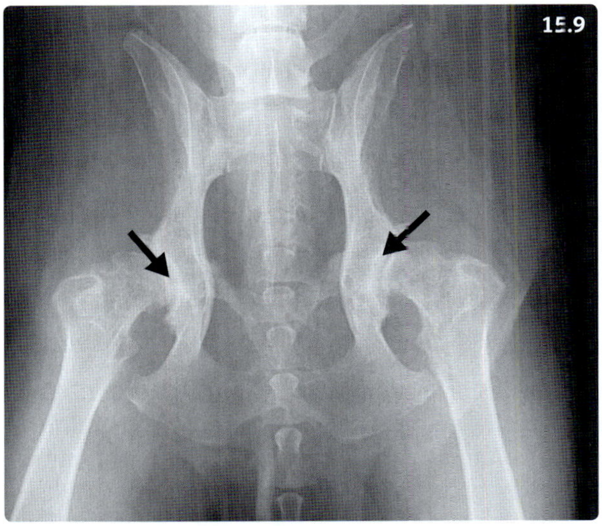

Figures 15.8, 15.9 (15.8) Illustration of hip dysplasia showing femoral head luxation, shallow acetabulum, and femoral head conformation change. (15.9) Poor acetabular cover to the femoral head (arrows).

Differential diagnosis

Degenerative myelopathy, lumbosacral disease, stifle instability, fracture, luxation.

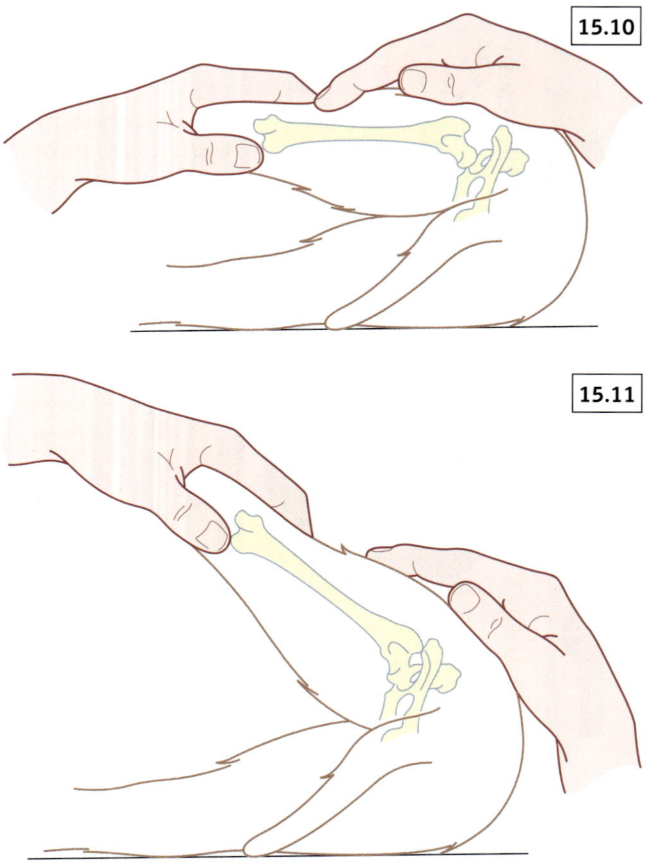

Figures 15.10, 15.11 Physical examination for the Ortolani sign. In 15.10, the coxofemoral joint is subluxated by driving the femoral shaft dorsal to the long axis of the spine. In 15.11, with the coxofemoral joint subluxated, the femur is abducted until the femoral head 'clunks' back into the acetabulum. The palpable (and often audible) clunk is considered a positive Ortalani sign. (Adapted from Fox SM (1987) A symposium on hip dysplasia. *Veterinary Medicine* **82(7):**683–716.)

Diagnosis

Diagnosis is made by physical (**Figures 15.10, 15.11**) and radiographic examination. Comparing a lame limb with the contralateral limb and observing the dog ambulate at different gaits and on different surfaces, as well as on steps, can be helpful during the physical examination.

Management

Available treatments (conservative or surgical) vary widely depending on the age of the animal, the pathologic condition of the joint, the expectation of function, the surgical skill of the clinician, and the financial resources of the owner. Conservative management consists of formulated exercise, weight loss, EPA-rich diets, and judicious use of analgesics and NSAIDs. Nutraceuticals have gained popularity as adjunct therapy for DJD; however, their evidence base remains indecisive.

For the immature animal, pectineal myectomy, pubic symphysiodesis, pelvic osteotomy, and femoral osteotomy are procedures frequently performed, while femoral head and neck excision and total hip replacement are most often performed in the mature animal. With the exception of pectineal myectomy and femoral head and neck excision, these surgeries require both special equipment and training.

INTERVERTEBRAL DISK DISEASE

(See also Chapter 14: Disorders of the nervous system and muscle.)

Definition/overview

Intervertebral disk degeneration and protrusion or extrusion of disk material into the vertebral canal cause the most common neurologic syndrome in dogs. The disease is particularly common in chondrodystrophoid breeds, which present with spinal-associated pain, ataxia, paresis, and even paralysis or myelomalacia.

Etiology

The cause of intervertebral disk degeneration is unknown. With aging, the center of the intervertebral disks, the nucleus pulposus, loses the stainability by safranin-O stain, suggesting a reduced amount of proteoglycans. The outer layer of the intervertebral disk, the annulus fibrosus, shows cracks or fissures, and the nucleus protrudes peripherally through these fissures. Changes progress with aging and result in a mass of protruded nucleus in the spinal canal causing spinal cord compression. With advanced aging, all intervertebral disk tissues are forced out of the intervertebral disk space and bone-to-bone contact of the vertebral endplates causes irregular margins. At the same time, spondylosis deformans (new bone formation around the intervertebral disks) progresses. The protruded mass in the spinal canal may eventually become calcified or even ossified. Although articular cartilage is made of hyaline cartilage and intervertebral disks are composed of fibrocartilage, both are cartilaginous tissues and similar cellular and structural changes are seen with aging.

Pathophysiology

Hansen type I disk lesions with early chondroid degeneration of the disk, disk mineralization, and acute onset are typical for ages 3–6 years (**Figure 15.12**). Dachshunds are most commonly affected, although Shih Tzus, Pekingese, Lhaso Apsos, Welsh Corgis, and Beagles are at significant risk. Hansen type II disk lesions are more typical in non-chondrodystrophoid dogs, often between 8 and 10 years old (**Figure 15.13**). Type II lesions are more slow and insidious, with fibroid degeneration and little mineralization.

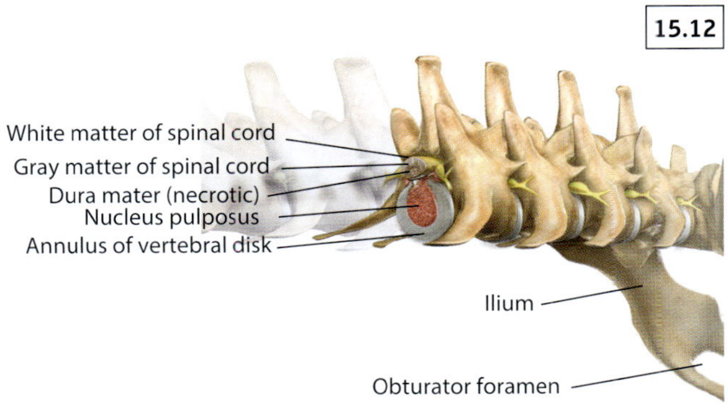

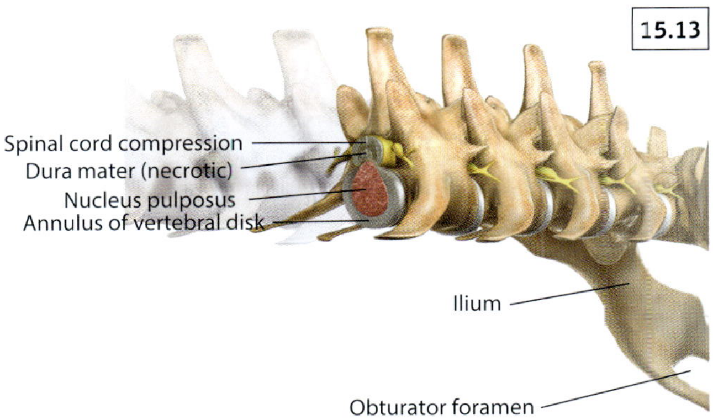

Figures 15.12, 15.13 Intervertebral disk herniation: type I (15.12) and type II (15.13).

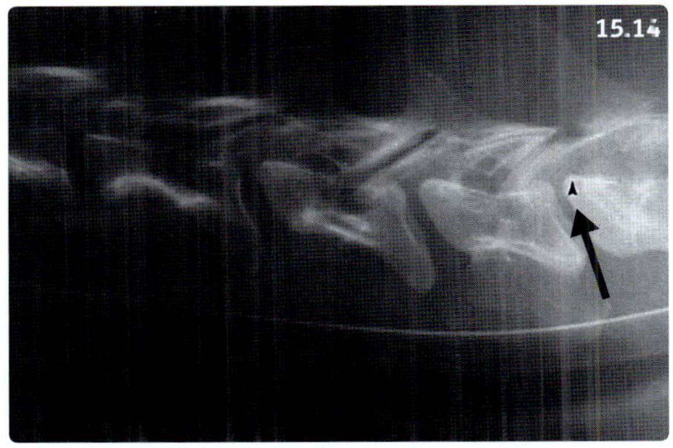

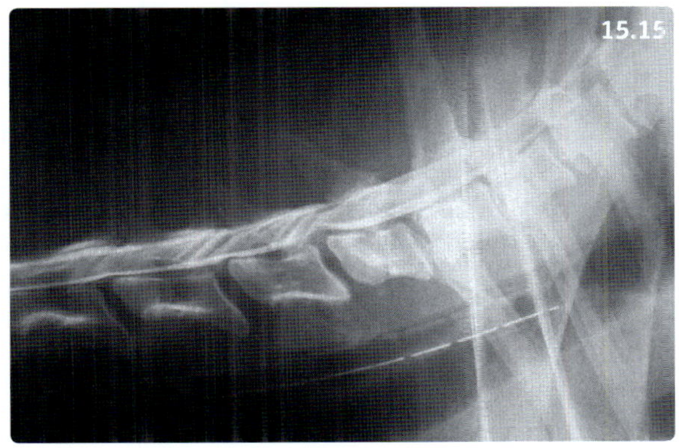

Figures 15.14, 15.15 Intervertebral disk disease (C6/7) (arrow) in a female Dobermann (15.14, plain film; 15.15, myelogram). Protrusion or extrusion of disk material is suggested radiographically by (1) narrowing of the intervertebral disk space; (2) narrowing of the space between the paired cranial and caudal articular facets; (3) decreased size or a change in shape of the neural foramen; (4) increased density in the area of the neural foramen; and (5) presence of calcified disk material within the spinal canal. Note the dorsal 'tipping' of the C7 leading edge in the plain film.

Clinical presentation

Protrusions or extrusions can occur laterally, dorsally, or ventrally. Lateral protrusions and extrusions may occasionally cause clinical signs, but in most cases dorsal disk protrusions are clinically significant, manifesting as meningeal irritation and compression of the nerve root or spinal cord. Back pain (68%), nonambulatory paraparesis (77%), and upper motor neuron signs (90%) prevail. The effects of lower motor neuron disease are a flaccid urinary bladder, which is easily expressed, and overflow incontinence.

Differential diagnosis

Diskospondylitis, fracture, vertebral spondylosis, neoplasia, fibrocartilaginous embolism.

Diagnosis

Diagnosis is made from patient data, history, and physical examination. Localization of the lesion(s) is made by neurologic examination and radiographic studies. Survey radiographic findings include narrowing, wedging, or collapse of the intervertebral disk space and articular facets, narrowing of the intervertebral foramen, and calcified material within the vertebral canal (**Figures 15.14–15.16**). Myelography studies are almost always

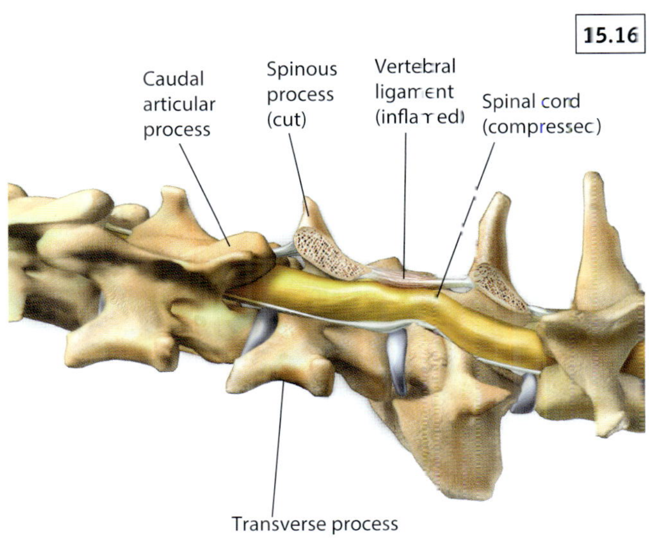

Figure 15.16 Illustration of the cervical vertebrae as associated with wobbler disease.

required, particularly in assessing for multiple lesion sites. MRI has been reported to be the best method for early recognition of disk degeneration in dogs, and CT is becoming more widely used with increased accessibility.

Management

Considerable controversy surrounds treatment. Conservative therapy relies on forced rest to resolve the inflammation and stabilize the ruptured disk by fibrosis. Conservative management consists of restricted exercise, weight loss, and judicious use of analgesics and NSAIDs. The judicious use of anti-inflammatory drugs and muscle relaxants is secondary to cage rest in this treatment choice. Worsening of clinical signs due to overactivity is common in dogs treated with medication alone.

Surgical management is subdivided into prophylactic and therapeutic procedures. While prophylaxis involves surgical removal of the nuclear material from the intact disk, treatment relies on removal of the herniated nuclear material from the vertebral canal or intervertebral foramen.

CAUDA EQUINA SYNDROME

Definition/overview

A number of pathologic disorders (acute disk extrusions at the L6/L7 and L7/S1 level, spondylosis and acquired stenosis of L7/S1, and the congenital stenotic canal syndrome of L6/L7 and L7/S1) are collectively referred to as the cauda equina syndrome. This syndrome encompasses all possible causes of compression, destruction, displacement, inflammation, or vascular compromise of the nerve roots, often captured in various names such as lumbosacral spondylopathy, lumbosacral stenosis, lumbosacral malformation/malarticulation, degenerative lumbosacral stenosis, lumbosacral disease, and lumbosacral spondylolisthesis.

Etiology

Suggested causes include conformation, physical activity, vertebral malformation, and genetic predisposition. The most common cause is degenerative lumbosacral stenosis (**Figure 15.17**), where soft tissue and bony changes impinge on the nerve roots or vasculature of the cauda equina.

Pathophysiology

The lumbosacral joint is a site of considerable force transfer, with flexion being the main movement. Abnormal lumbosacral motion due to degenerative changes leads to compensatory skeletal changes such as lumbosacral endplate sclerosis, osteophytes of articular facets, hypertrophy of the interarcuate ligament and articular facet joint capsule, and bulging of the dorsal annulus. The aftermath is compression of the terminal spinal cord and adjacent nerve roots within the vertebral canal.

15.17

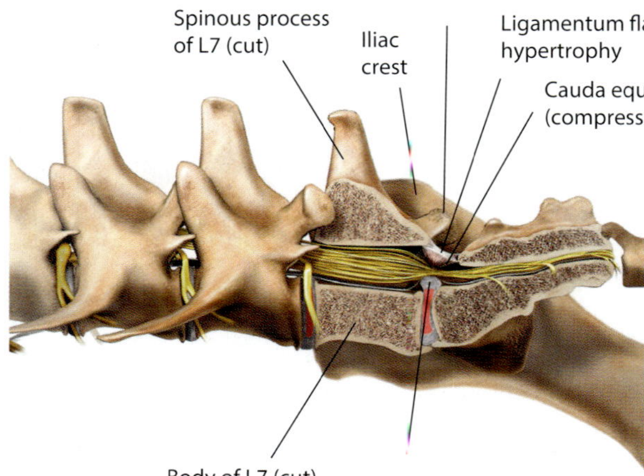

Figure 15.17 Illustration of degenerative lumbosacral stenosis.

Clinical presentation

Neurologic signs may include back pain, lameness, proprioception deficits, atrophy of muscles with sciatic nerve innervation, progressive paraparesis, tail weakness, urinary then anal sphincter disturbances, and paresthesia. Lower back pain, accentuated by clinician manipulation, is a cardinal feature of this disease. The German Shepherd Dog is the most commonly affected breed. Affected dogs often maintain a characteristic posture, flexing their lumbosacral joint to increase the diameter of the vertebral canal and intervertebral foramina, thereby decreasing nerve root compression.

Differential diagnosis

Degenerative myelopathy, thoracolumbar disk disease, peripheral neuropathies and myopathies, coxofemoral arthrosis, stifle instability, semitendinosus/gracilis muscle contracture, prostatic/urogenital disease.

Diagnosis

Due to the multifaceted etiology of this syndrome, a thorough physical and neurologic examination followed by survey radiographs (**Figures 5.18, 15.19**) and myelography and/or epidurography studies may be required for a diagnosis. Lumbosacral pain can usually be elicited by applying digital pressure on the spinous processes of L7 and S1 with the dog standing. Extension of the hips (lordosis test) can be done simultaneously to elicit a response. Digital palpation of the lumbosacral joint per rectum may

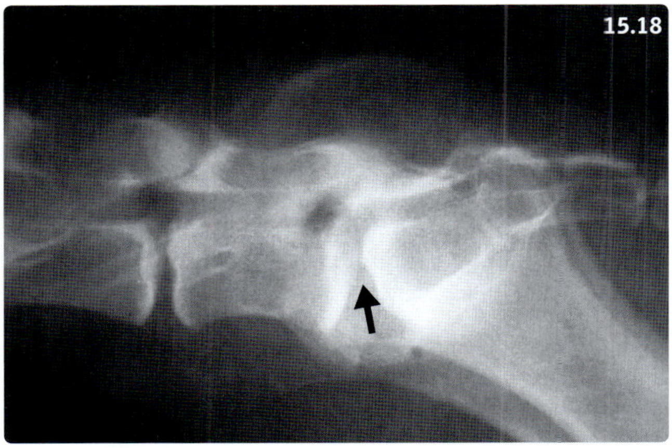

Figure 15.18 Cauda equina in a 10-year-old female German Shepherd Dog presented for pain when defecating. Cauda equina syndrome may result in entrapment of one or more of the terminal lumbar nerve roots. Survey radiographic findings such as sclerosis, vertebral malalignment, and/or spondylosis of the lumbosacral joint may be suggestive of this diagnosis (arrow).

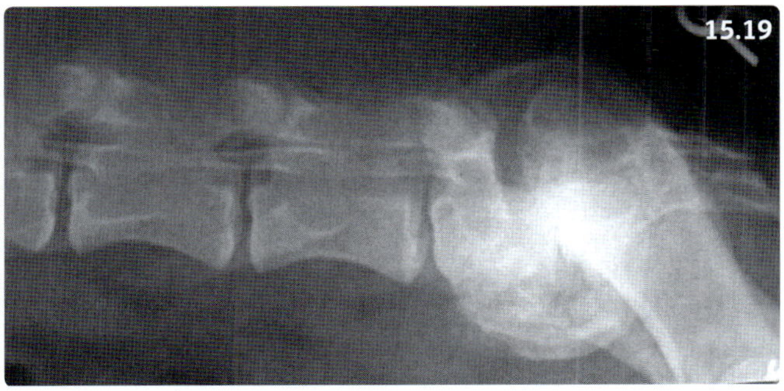

Figure 15.19 Cauda equina syndrome may lead to entrapment of terminal lumbar nerve roots. Radiographs often show sclerosis, vertebral malalignment, and spondylosis of the lumbosacral joint.

further pinpoint the source of pain. Neurogenic intermittent claudication refers to the presentation of clinical signs associated with exercise. In this situation the dilated radicular blood vessels crowd the adjacent nerve root in the stenotic intervertebral foramen or lateral recess, causing intermittent ischemia of the nerve.

MRI appears to be superior to CT for detecting spinal stenosis caused by soft tissue proliferation and for recognizing early disk degeneration; however, MRI (like CT) is expensive and relatively inaccessible.

Management

Surgical treatment is the best option when the pain is continuous or there are neurologic deficits, and progression of clinical signs with conservative treatment may negatively affect the prognosis. Surgical treatment is via decompression by dorsal laminectomy or fixation–fusion of the lumbosacral joint.

ANOMALIES

ECTRODACTYLY

Definition/overview

Skeletal growth disorders that are apparent at birth or manifest later in young animals are of two main types: generalized dysplasias and localized malformations of individual bones. Ectrodactyly (Gr. ectro = congenital absence) (split hand or lobster claw deformity) is an abnormal limb development with metacarpal bone separation (**Figure 15.20**), digit contracture, digit aplasia, metacarpal hypoplasia, and metacarpal fusions. The condition is usually unilateral.

Etiology

In the cat, ectrodactyly is caused by a dominant gene with variable expression.

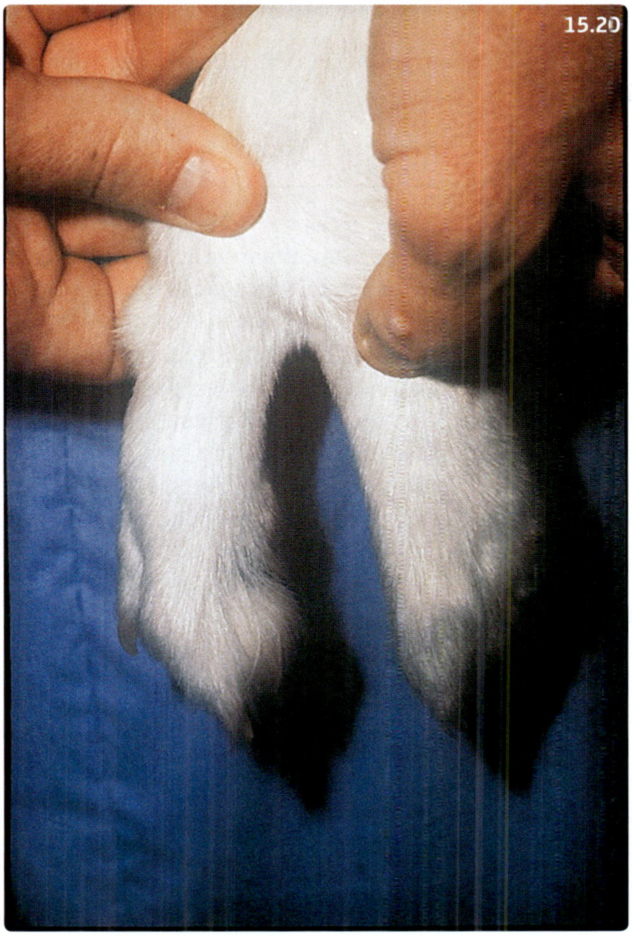

Figure 15.20 A number of congenital anomalies may affect the digits. Here a syndactyly of digits 2/3 and 4/5 is seen as metacarpals 3 and 4 are separated at the level of the metacarpal heads. (Courtesy the late M.S. Bloomberg)

Pathophysiology

The cleft between metacarpal bones may terminate just below the carpus or extend proximally through the carpus, separating the radius and ulna entirely.

Clinical presentation

Ectrodactyly presents as absence of the central digit or incomplete fusion of three digits. There are many variations of this condition, but typically the third digit and metacarpal bone are absent, which produces a deep cleft dividing the paw into ulnar and radial parts. Concomitant congenital elbow luxation is common.

Differential diagnosis

Congenital amputation.

Diagnosis

Diagnosis is made by physical examination and supporting radiographs.

Management

Reconstructive surgery or arthrodesis can improve function.

OSTEOCHONDRODYSPLASIA

Definition/overview

Osteochondrodysplasia is an abnormality of cartilage or bone growth and development. In achondroplasia, endochondral ossification of all long bones is retarded, resulting in shortened and deformed limbs. Hypochondroplasia is similar to achondroplasia; however, the condition is less severe. The Bulldog, Boston Terrier, Pug, Pekingese, Japanese Spaniel, and Shih Tzu are achondroplastic, while the Dachshund, Basset Hound, Beagle, Welsh Corgi, Dandi Dinmont Terrier, Scottish Terrier, and Skye Terrier are hypochondroplastic.

Etiology

In most osteochondrodyplasias there is a known or suspected genetic basis, and autosomal recessive inheritance is common.

Pathophysiology

There are a number of syndromes of chondrodystrophia fetalis in animals, some of them inherited, and all of them result in disproportionate dwarfism. Dwarfism of chondrodystrophia fetalis is differentiated from primordial dwarfism by disproportionate body form. As a result of an endochondral ossification defect, one or more long bones grows in retardation.

Clinical presentation

Animals may exhibit dwarfism and there may be reduced limb length relative to the trunk because of the discrepant development of the axial and appendicular skeleton.

Differential diagnosis

When the condition affects one or more limbs, particularly the forelimbs, bilateral premature closure of the physes (radial/ulnar) can be a differential diagnosis of concern. Genetic anomalies tend to be symmetrical. Premature physeal closure can be bilateral, and closure of the distal ulnar physis is more sensitive to insult than the radial physis.

Diagnosis

Serial radiography of the long bone physes during the rapid growth phase is often diagnostic for premature physeal closure as a differential.

Management

Correction of severe deformities is unrewarding.

ELBOW DYSPLASIA: UNUNITED ANCONEAL PROCESS/FRAGMENTED CORONOID PROCESS

Definition/overview

The term elbow dysplasia describes generalized osteoarthrosis of the elbow joint, specifically including the conditions of ununited anconeal process (UAP) and fragmented coronoid process (FCP) (**Figure 15.21**).

Etiology

Because these two diseases, together with osteochondritis dissecans (OCD) of the medial humeral condyle, overlap, the common etiology of osteochondrosis has been proposed. Skeletally immature large and giant breed dogs are affected and the condition is often bilateral. The etiology of UAP and FCP is most often accepted to be incongruous growth of the radius and ulna. The anconeus develops from a separate ossification center only in large dogs and will normally come to union with the parent ulna by 20 weeks of age. If this union has not occurred by this time, it is considered ununited.

Pathophysiology

It is proposed that if the radius grows faster than the ulna in large breed dogs, it places abnormal distractive forces

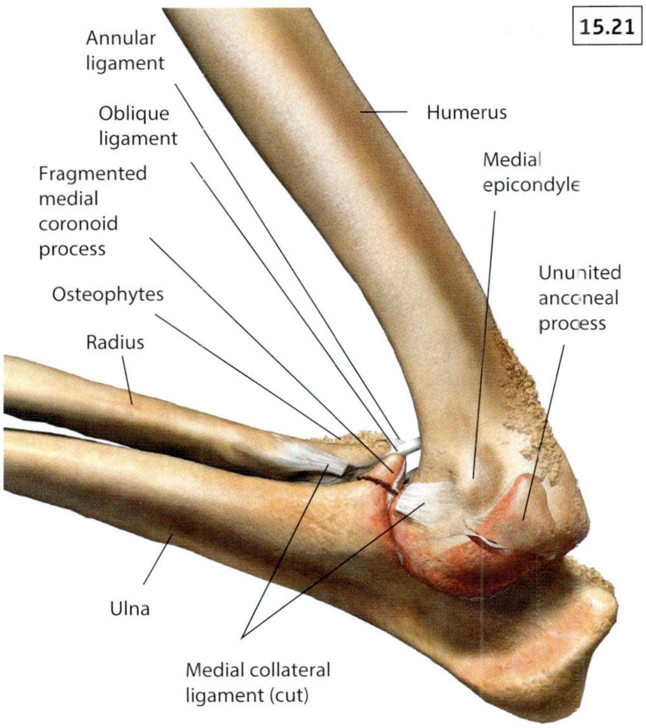

Figure 15.21 Elbow dysplasia is often a manifestation of FCP and/or UAP.

on the anconeus through the distal end of the humerus, destabilizing the cartilaginous attachment of the anconeus to the ulna and therefore preventing its normal ossification.

In contrast, if the ulna grows faster than the radius, more weight than normal is placed on the medial ulnar coronoid. Normally the coronoid processes, together with the radial head, bear the compressive forces from the distal humerus. With asynchronous growth, the lateral aspect of the medial ulnar coronoid suffers damage and can become fragmented.

Clinical presentation

Both UAP and FCP lead to forelimb lameness with an abnormal gait. Affected dogs often hold the elbow close to their body and outwardly rotate their foot. Joint effusion may be present and the dog resents elbow manipulation, especially hyperextension and pronation of the antebrachium.

Differential diagnosis

Luxation/subluxation, OCD (distal humeral condyle/humeral head), biceps brachii muscle/tendon disease.

Diagnosis

UAP is diagnosed radiographically by a hyperflexed lateral radiograph of the elbow revealing failure of the anconeal process to fuse with the proximal ulna in a dog older than 5 months of age (**Figure 15.22**). CT is a helpful diagnostic aid; however, a definitive diagnosis of the type and severity of the different conditions comprising elbow dysplasia is obtained through arthroscopy.

Primary lesions associated with a fragmented medial coronoid process are extremely difficult to see radiographically (**Figures 15.23, 15.24**). Therefore, a diagnosis of fragmented medial coronoid process is often made based on breed, age, history, clinical signs, and physical examination. Secondary changes such as osteophyte deposition proximal to the anconeal process, caudal to the distal humeral condyle, and anterior to the radial head are radiographic findings consistent with a fragmented medial coronoid process of long standing (**Figure 15.25**). The diagnosis of FCP is often one of exclusion.

Management

Treatment for UAP is surgical; either removal or attachment of the process. Surgery to include fragment removal and lesion curettage is the treatment of choice for FCP. Prognosis for both conditions is dependent on the severity of secondary changes at the time of treatment. The surgical technique of total elbow replacement was introduced in 2004, with a success rate of approximately 80% in a limited number of cases.

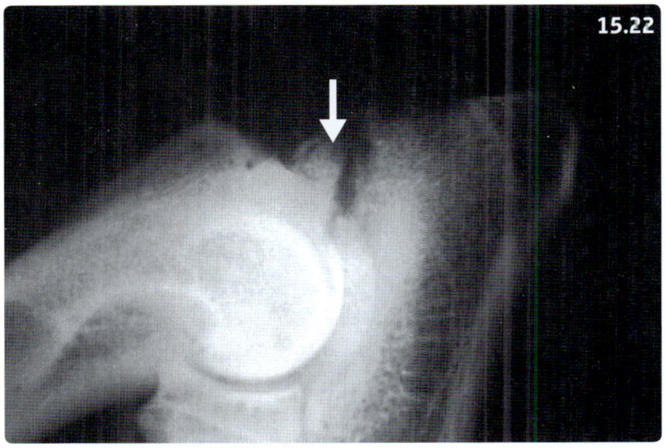

Figure 15.22 Ununited anconeal process (arrow) is best demonstrated in a hyperflexed lateral radiograph, which avoids the overlapping density of the medial humeral epicondyle. A diagnosis is made when the anconeus has not fused by 5 months of age.

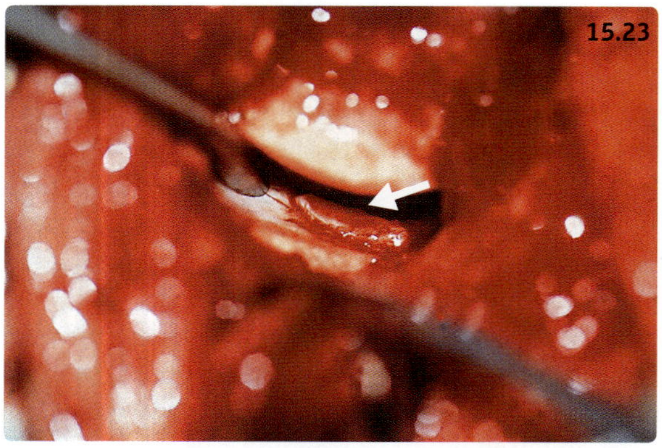

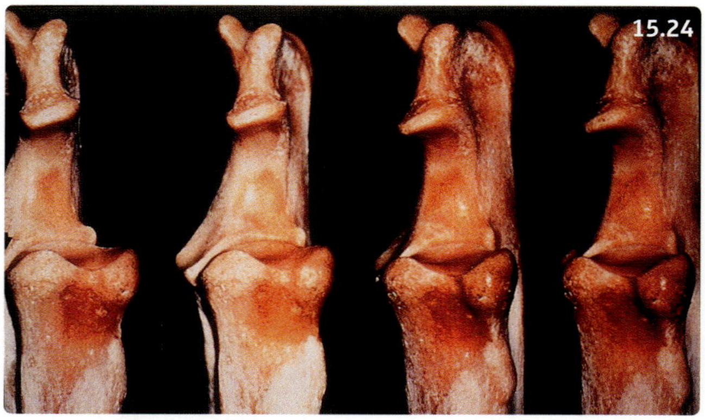

Figures 15.23, 15.24 The separate coronoid fragment is rarely identified because it usually occurs on the lateral aspect of the medial coronoid process. (15.23) An intraoperative view (arrow). (15.24) Sequential views made along an arc around the elbow joint demonstrate the difficulty with radiographic identification of the coronoid lesion, as other bony structures always silhouette this area. The presence of secondary joint disease may be the only radiographic evidence of the fragmented coronoid. Periarticular osteophytes may be observed on the proximal margin of the anconeal process, coronoid process, medial humeral epicondyle, or cranial proximal radius. Sclerosis of the subchondral bone of the ulnar trochlear notch, a widened humeral–ulnar trochlear notch, and a widened humeral–ulnar joint space may be observed. Comparison radiographs of both elbows are extremely helpful because the lesions are often subtle.

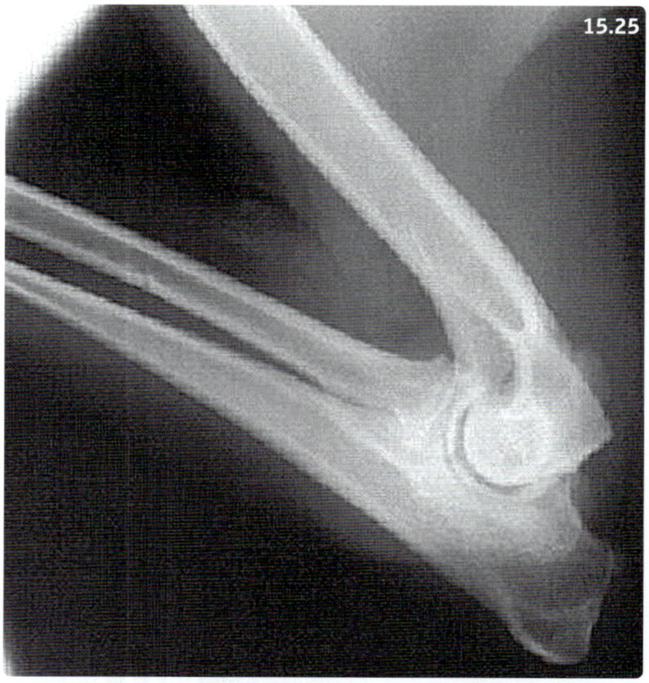

Figure 15.25 Radiographic signs of elbow dysplasia include osteophyte deposition within the anconeal process, at the leading edge of the radial head, and on the medial humeral condyle, as well as sclerosis of the trochlear notch of the ulna.

Conservative management consists of NSAIDs. Chondroprotectants are also used, often in combination with NSAIDs.

GROWTH DEFORMITIES

Definition/overview

Trauma is the most common origin of growth deformities, due to the exuberant nature of puppies.

Etiology

Long bones grow in length through the process of endochondral ossification, which occurs at the growth plate or physis. Alterations in this normal process lead to growth deformities, which are most frequently seen in the antebrachium. The most common cause of premature growth cessation is trauma to the distal ulnar physeal plate; large and giant breeds are most commonly affected.

Pathophysiology

Following trauma, asymmetric growth of the physis leads to valgus (**Figure 15.26**) or varus (**Figure 15.27**) deformation of the limb. The severity of disfigurement is dependent on the growth potential remaining after the physeal trauma. The antebrachium is predisposed to growth deformity because of the two-bone system and the architecture of the distal ulnar physis.

Clinical presentation

Three deformities of the radius result from premature closure of the distal ulnar physis: lateral deviation (valgus), cranial bowing (curvus) (**Figure 15.28**), and external rotation (supination). Caudolateral subluxation of the radial carpal joint results, with stretching of the medial

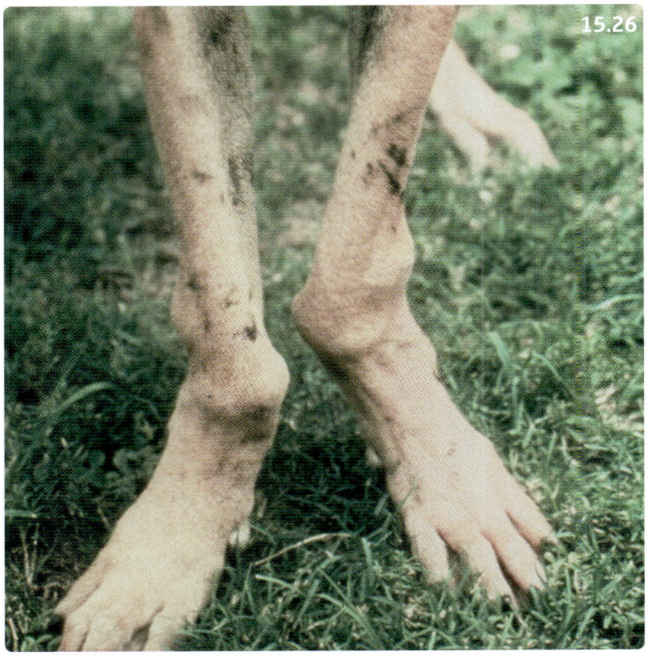

Figure 15.26 Valgus deformation of the carpus resulting from premature closure of the distal ulnar physes.

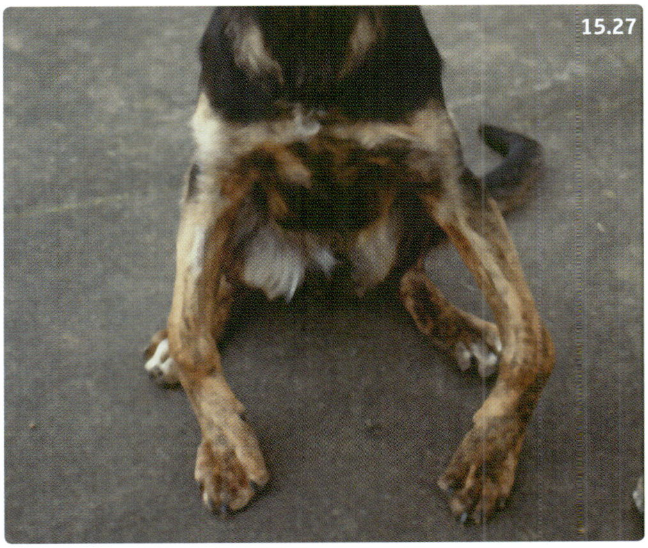

Figure 15.27 Young dog with varus deformation of the carpal joints resulting from premature closure of the distal radial physes.

soft tissue supporting structures. The radial head may also luxate the humeral condyles from the trochlear notch of the ulna. Abnormal articulations, resulting in

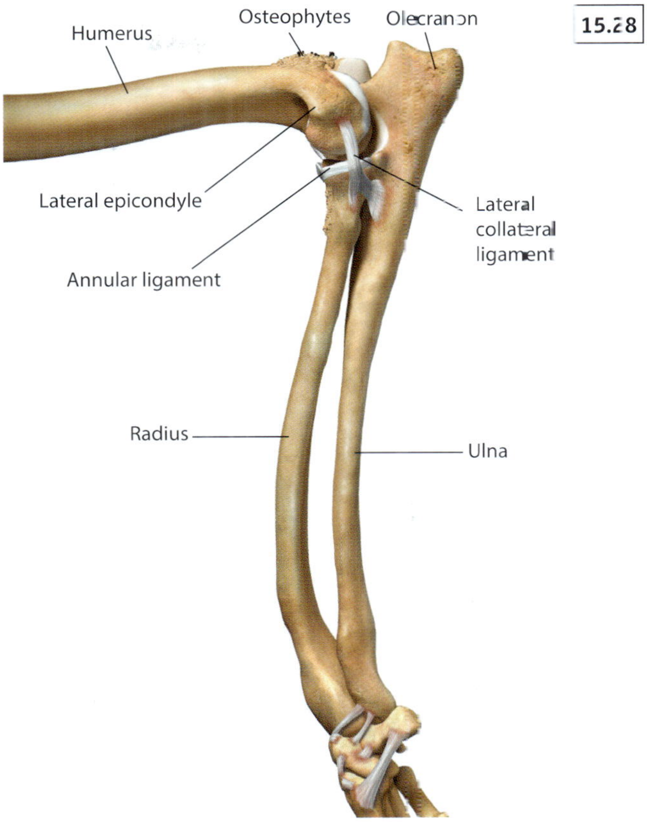

Figure 15.28 Radius curvus can lead to disfigurement of the entire antebrachium, including the elbow and carpus.

irreversible degenerative osteoarthritis in the carpal and elbow joints, may be sequelae. In the severe condition, the patient appears to be walking on its mediopalmar metacarpals. Elbow luxation can be very painful for the patients.

Differential diagnosis

Congenital deformity, ligamentous trauma, luxation, fracture.

Diagnosis

Diagnosis is by radiography of the carpal and elbow joints (**Figures 15.29, 15.30**), comparing them with the contralateral limb if that limb is normal. The condition is predictable when closure of the distal ulnar physis precedes that of the distal radial physis and significant growth remains before skeletal maturation.

Management

Surgical reconstruction.

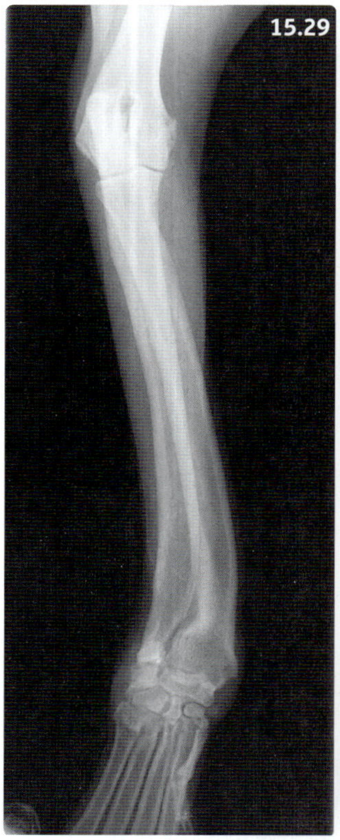

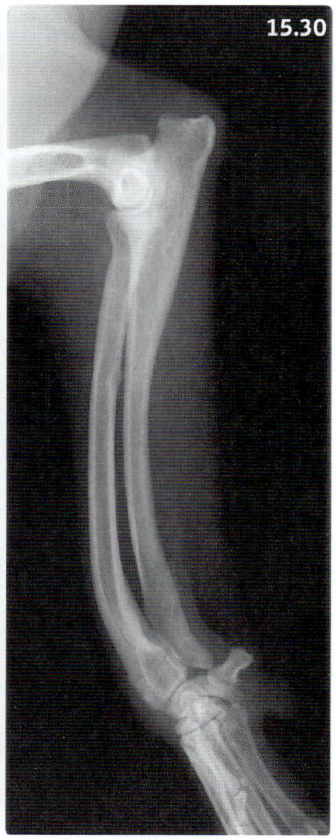

Figures 15.29, 15.30 Anterior (15.29) and lateral (15.30) views showing the radiographic changes commonly seen with premature closure of the distal ulnar growth plate (remodeling of the anconeal process with sclerosis; elbow luxation with shallowing of the trochlear notch; anterior radial bowing; anterior and medial subluxation of the distal radius with increased angulation of the radiocarpal joint; and secondary arthritic changes).

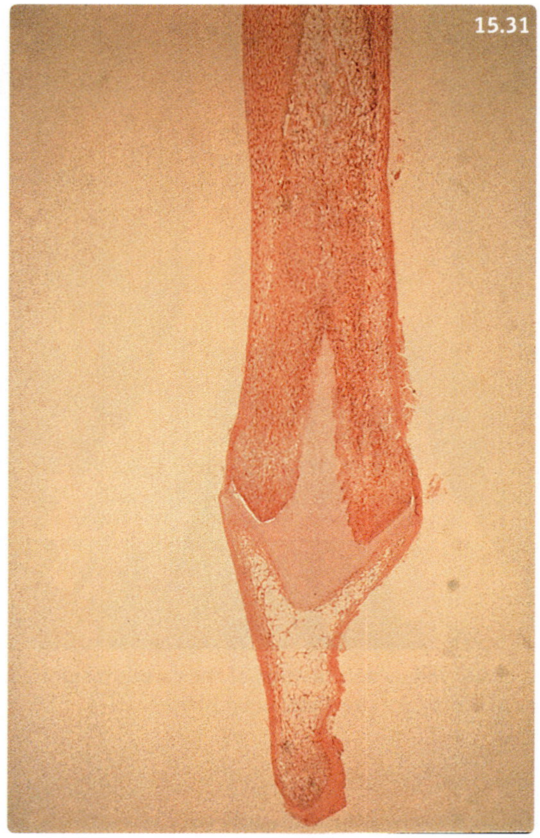

Figure 15.31 Histologically, retained cartilage core, as seen here, is a failure of normal endochondral ossification within the distal ulna. Radiographically, an inverted radiolucent cone may be observed extending proximally from the distal ulnar physis into the metaphysis. This condition may lead to deformation of the carpus as is seen in the condition radius curvus.

RETAINED ENDOCHONDRAL CARTILAGE CORE

Definition/overview

Retained endochondral cartilage core occurs in the distal ulnar metaphysis of immature large and giant breed dogs, appearing as a radiolucent inverted cone.

Etiology

The etiology of the disorder is not understood. The core is a result of improper mineralization (**Figure 15.31**); fortunately, most cases of retained endochondral cartilage core do not persist long enough to produce a deformity. This same condition may be seen in the lateral femoral condyle, leading to genu valgum, a predisposition to 'knock-knees' and lateral patellar luxation.

Pathophysiology

In Great Dane pups, formation of cartilage core in the distal ulnar and tibial metaphyses has been associated with feeding excess calcium.

Clinical presentation

The condition is often self-resolving and an incidental radiographic finding; however, it may be associated with varying degrees of growth retardation after 5 months of age.

Diagnosis

Radiography of the distal ulna. A radiolucent core of cartilage 5–10 mm wide and 2–6 cm long extending from the distal ulnar physis into metaphyseal bone is pathognomonic.

Management

Reconstructive surgery is the treatment of choice for deformities resulting from retained endochondral cartilage core.

METABOLIC DISORDERS

PANOSTEITIS

Definition/overview

Panosteitis is a disease of the fatty bone marrow with secondary involvement of bone.

Etiology

The cause is poorly understood; some authors have implicated a viral role.

Pathophysiology

Medullary enostosis and occasional subperiosteal new bone formation are characteristic of this self-limiting disease in young, large, or giant breeds of dogs, which may last up to 18 months. Pain may be due to disturbance of endosteal and periosteal elements, vascular congestion, or high intramedullary pressure. German Shepherd Dogs are most commonly affected.

Clinical presentation

Clinical signs of lameness usually appear in immature dogs, with a prevalence in males, but onset has been documented as late as 5 years of age. Episodic lameness lasts 2–3 weeks, with bouts persisting for 2–9 months. Lameness may range from mild to severe, involve one or more bones, and be persistent or intermittent. Other signs include anorexia, lethargy, pyrexia, and weight loss. The ulna is most commonly affected, although the radius, humerus, femur, and tibia may also show involvement.

Clinical signs are usually associated with pain, which can be elicited with deep palpation of the affected bone and which often self-resolves by the time the dog reaches 18–20 months of age. Mild depression, inappetence, and weight loss may occur in severely affected patients.

Differential diagnosis

Osteochondrosis, elbow dysplasia, fractures, ligamentous injury, immune-mediated arthritides, Lyme disease, bacterial endocarditis.

Diagnosis

The earliest radiographic abnormality seen is an increase in intramedullary density (**Figures 15.32–15.35**). Initially unifocal with indistinct margins, lesions coalesce as the disease progresses. There is no correlation between radiographic signs, degree of lameness, and amount of pain elicited on deep palpation of the limb.

Management

Treatment with analgesics (NSAIDs) and supportive care yields excellent results, although the course of treatment may be prolonged.

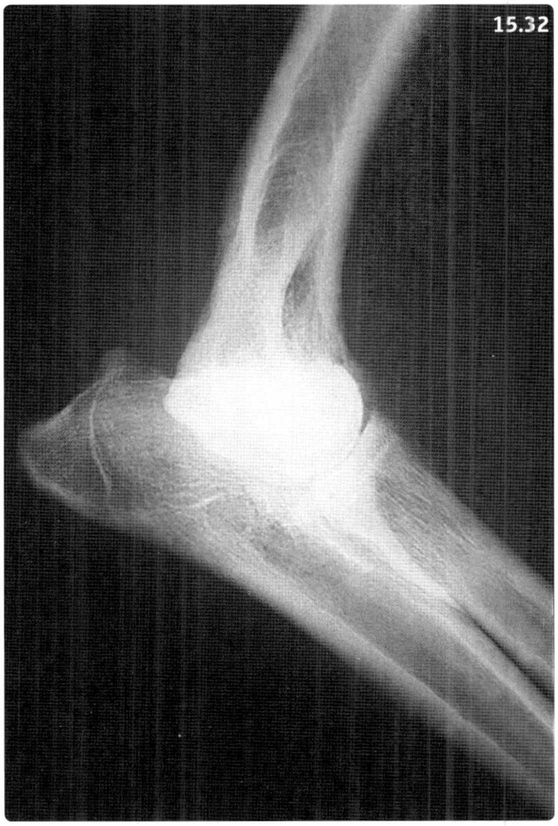

Figure 15.32 Radiographic findings of panosteitis center around the nutrient foramina. The early phase begins with an increase in endosteal and medullary density, with blurring of the normal trabecular pattern. In the second phase the densities tend to coalesce, become patchy and mottled, and fill the medullary canal. After 4–6 weeks the medullary canal regains a normal or decreased density and cortical thickening may persist. A differential diagnosis list should include bone neoplasm and hematogenous osteomyelitis.

15.33

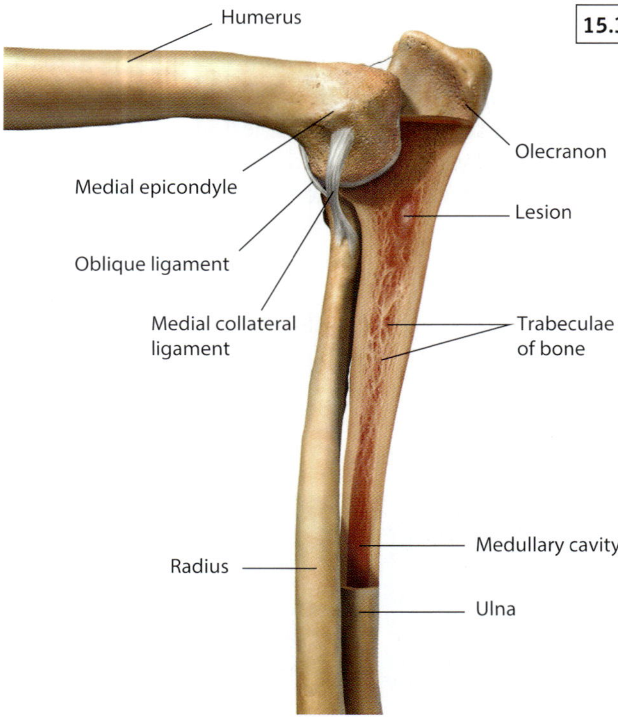

15.35

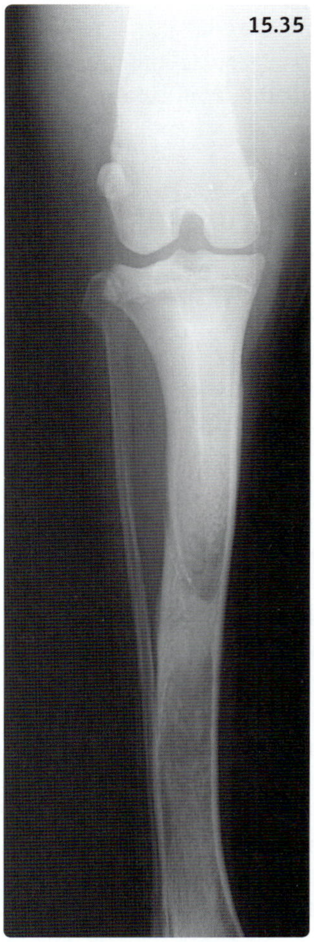

15.34

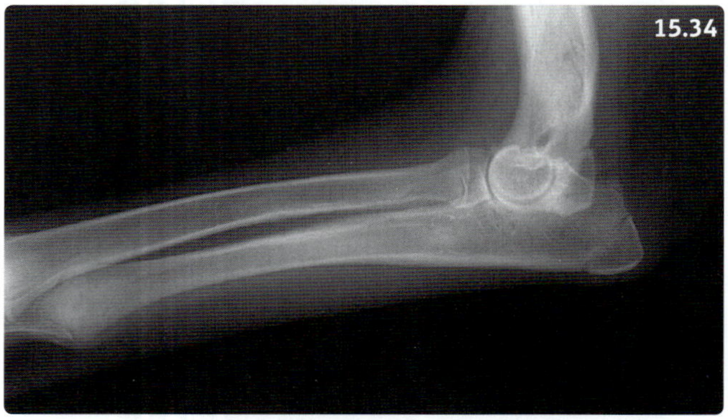

Figures 15.33–15.35 Radiography of panosteitis reveals areas of increased density within the medullary canal. The disease is most commonly seen in long bones such as the tibia and ulna.

OSTEOCHONDROSIS

Definition/overview

Osteochondrosis is an endochondral ossification defect, the term denoting a dissecting lesion between articular cartilage and underlying bone. Once articular cartilage dissects free from the underlying calcified tissue, the lesion of OCD has formed.

Etiology

The etiology of the disease is multifactorial, with genetic, nutritional, and environmental contributions.

Pathophysiology

Local matrix degeneration secondary to defects in the nutritional supply to the cartilage is likely to be responsible for the lesions. The degeneration produces areas of epiphyseal cartilage that are prone to stress-induced necrosis. Once the chrondrocytes have died, the surrounding cartilage matrix is unable to mineralize and therefore blood vessels with their accompanying osteogenic mesenchyme fail to penetrate the cartilage and normal ossification is prevented.

Clinical presentation

Clinical signs of lameness appear between 4 and 12 months of age, mostly in large and giant breeds of dogs. Bones affected include the humeral head, medial humeral condyle, femoral condyles, and talus.

Differential diagnosis

Intra-articular (osteochondral) fractures, elbow dysplasia, panosteitis, periarticular ligamentous injury.

Diagnosis

The typical lesion appears radiographically as a flattened radiolucent defect in the subchondral bone immediately beneath the articular cartilage. Free-floating, mineralized cartilage fragments ('joint mice') may also be present within the affected joint (**Figures 15.36, 15.37**).

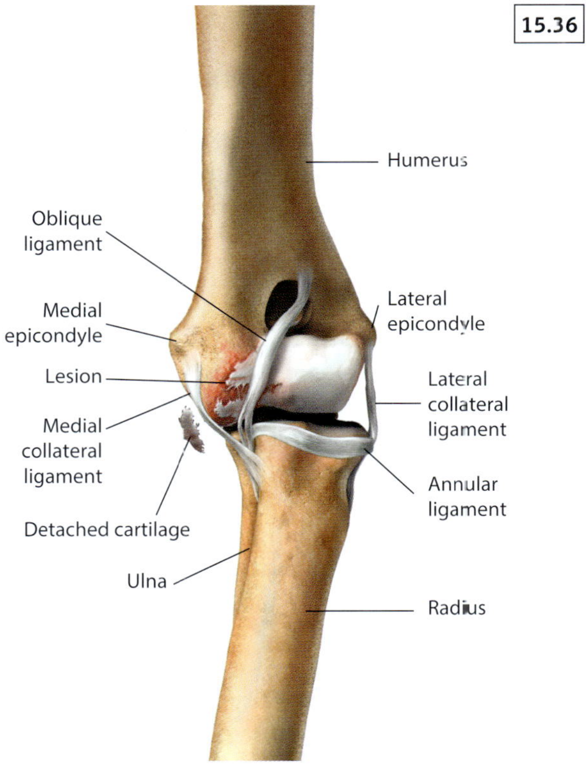

Figure 15.36 Humeral head osteochondrosis appears grossly with fibrillation and eburnation, and may include joint mice, as seen in this case. Also note the thickened joint capsule, which may manifest clinically as restricted range of motion.

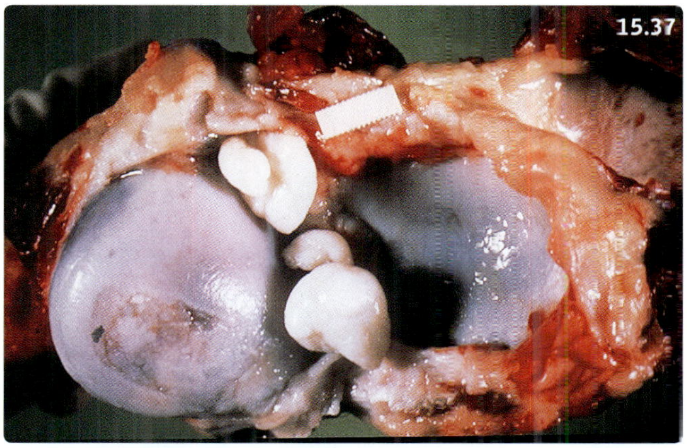

Figure 15.37 Humeral head osteochondrosis appears grossly with fibrillation and eburnation and may include joint mice, as seen in this case. Also note the thickened joint capsule, which might manifest clinically as restricted range of motion.

Management

Treatment is surgical. Pain and lameness in a dog with radiographic evidence of osteochondrosis are an indication for surgical exploration. All loose cartilage fragments, including joint mice, are removed from the joint and the lesion is curettaged to stimulate the articular surface defect to heal by fibrocartilage formation. Although clinical severity is not correlated with radiographic findings, the prognosis is based on secondary changes. Shoulder and stifle lesions typically yield a better prognosis than elbow and tarsus lesions. Although not curative, NSAIDs are useful to treat symptomatically the pain associated with DJD.

CRANIOMANDIBULAR OSTEOPATHY

Definition/overview

Craniomandibular osteopathy is a proliferative nonneoplastic disease of the flat bones in the skull, where mandibular lamellar bone is resorbed and juvenile bone is produced. Scottish Terriers and West Highland White Terriers between 3 and 6 months of age are most commonly affected (**Figure 15.38**).

Etiology

The condition is inherited in West Highland White Terriers and there may be a genetic predisposition in Scottish Terriers. However, as the condition occurs sporadically in other breeds, there may be several causes.

Pathophysiology

The disease is characterized by resorption of existing lamellae, vascular fibrous stroma in place of marrow spaces, proliferation of coarse trabecular bone beyond

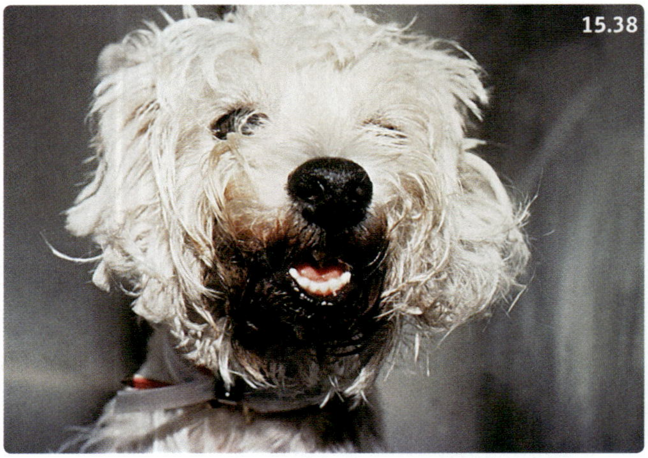

Figure 15.38 This young West Highland White Terrier has severe osteoproliferative pathology involving the mandible and temporomandibular joint. (Courtesy M. Schaer)

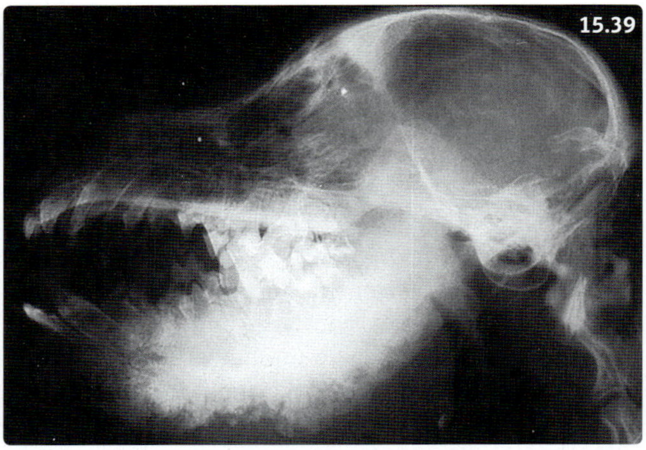

Figure 15.39 Lateral radiograph showing pronounced mandibular periosteal proliferation. (Courtesy M. Schaer)

normal periosteal boundaries, and infiltration by inflammatory cells at the periphery of new bone. New primitive bone shows a mosaic pattern of cement lines.

Clinical presentation

Animals are usually presented because of pain on opening the mouth, although lethargy, anorexia, pyrexia, excess salivation, prehension difficulties, lymphadenopathy, temporal muscle atrophy, weight loss, and dehydration may also be seen. The clinical course may fluctuate, with periods of remission and exacerbation.

Differential diagnosis

Osteomyelitis, traumatic periostitis, neoplasia.

Diagnosis

Skull radiographs demonstrate bilaterally symmetrical periosteal lesions involving the mandible and temporal bones. Osseous proliferation of the mandible or tympanic bulla and periosteal new bone formation may be seen around the temporomandibular junction (**Figure 15.39**).

Management

Craniomandibular osteopathy is a self-limiting disease for which treatment is directed at supporting the animal (with inclusion of analgesic therapy) until the condition regresses. In severely affected nonresolving cases, resection of the condyloid process of the mandible or a partial hemimandibulectomy may be considered. NSAID treatment can reduce pain and discomfort. The poorest prognosis is associated with deposition of bone surrounding the temporomandibular joint. Prolonged glucocorticoid therapy can slow disease progression if started early.

HYPERPARATHYROIDISM

(See also Chapter 11: Endocrine disorders.)

Definition/overview

Hyperparathyroidism results from increased production and release of parathyroid hormone (PTH) and its subsequent metabolic role in bone resorption. Bone is replaced by fibrous tissue. Primary hyperparathyroidism associated with hyperplasia or neoplasia of the parathyroid glands is the less common form, while secondary hyperparathyroidism is more common in dogs and is associated with renal disease or a nutritional deficiency.

Etiology

Excessive synthesis and secretion of PTH may be due to hyperplasia of the parathyroids either directly (adenomas, carcinomas) or by nonendocrine changes in calcium and phosphate hemostasis (e.g. diets deficient in calcium or rich in phosphate).

Pathophysiology

PTH promotes mineral resorption from bone to correct imbalances in blood calcium and phosphate concentrations. Generalized osteopenia may occur in adults.

Clinical presentation

Clinical signs reflect the severity of the primary problem and skeletal involvement is often first manifest in bones of the skull and jaw. Loss of lamina dura dentes may lead to loosening of teeth and mastication problems, while resorption of alveolar bone, seen radiographically

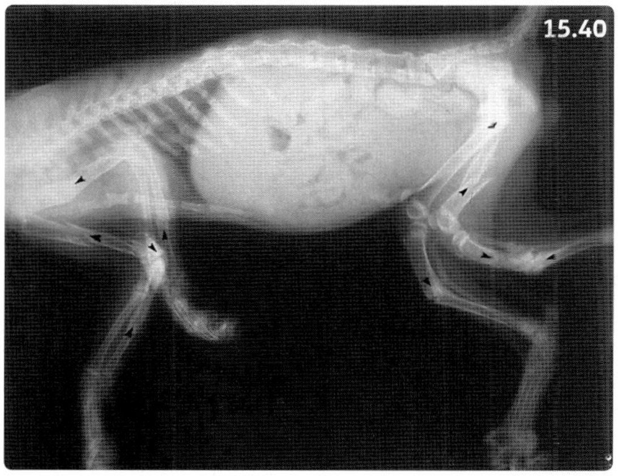

Figure 15.40 Hyperparathyroidism may cause extensive bony demineralization that involves the skull, vertebral column, and long bones. Pathologic fractures may result from extensive loss of mineral in the long bones and vertebral bodies. In dogs there is a tendency for renal secondary hyperparathyroidism to cause more severe bone loss in the skull, while nutritional secondary hyperparathyroidism causes more severe changes in the long bones, as shown in this radiograph. (Courtesy B.R. Jones)

as demineralization, can lead to pathologic fractures (**Figure 15.40**). Signs of associated hypercalcemia may include muscle weakness, nephrocalcinosis, urolithiasis, constipation, anorexia, vomiting, polyuria, or polydipsia.

Differential diagnosis
Dietary insufficiencies, renal disease.

Diagnosis
With nutritional secondary hyperparathyroidism in young animals, radiographs may show thin long bone cortices and an apparently abnormally wide medullary cavity.

Management
Prognosis is based on successful treatment of the underlying cause. While bisphosphonates have been used to decrease the hypercalcemia, surgical excision of parathyroid adenoma or adenocarcinoma is the treatment of choice for primary hyperparathyroidism. Two to 4 months may be required for cortical thickness to return to normal and complications are generally related to delayed fracture union or malunions.

HYPERTROPHIC OSTEODYSTROPHY

Definition/overview
Hypertrophic osteodystrophy (HOD) (metaphyseal osteopathy) is a metaphyseal bone disease of immature large and giant breeds of dogs. Although all bones are susceptible, the distal radius and ulna are most commonly affected. Metaphyses are widened due to perimetaphyseal swelling and bone deposition.

Etiology
The cause of the disease is unknown. Hypotheses including the influence of hypovitaminosis C, dietary oversupplementation, and infectious organisms have not been validated. HOD has been diagnosed in a number of different dog breeds. Weimaraners appear to have a strong heritable predisposition, and an immune mechanism is likely involved.

Pathophysiology
The pathogenesis is obscure; however, a disturbance of the metaphyseal blood supply leads to a failure or delay in ossification of the hypertrophic zone of the metaphyseal growth plate. The disease is usually bilaterally symmetrical and episodic. Some cases recover within a few days, but others have one or more relapses over several weeks before recovery.

Clinical presentation
Presenting signs involve some degree of lameness where the metaphyseal region of the long bones may be swollen, warm, and painful on palpation (**Figure 15.41**). The disease may be accompanied by depression, inappetence, and variable pyrexia.

Differential diagnosis
Panosteitis, elbow dysplasia, OCD, polyarthritis, septic metaphysitis, retained cartilage core, canine osteochondrodysplasia.

Diagnosis
Necrosis and resorption of the metaphyseal trabeculae may be seen radiographically as an irregular radiolucent line in the metaphyses adjacent to the growth plates (**Figure 15.42**). Subperiosteal new bone formation (likely hematoma mineralization) may be mild or extensive in the area of the metaphyseal growth plate.

Management
Treatment is largely supportive, with rest, analgesics, anti-inflammatory drugs, and attention to a proper diet. Vitamin C supplementation has no efficacy. Antibiotics may be indicated for treatment of secondary infection, if identified. Animals with mild lesions have a good to excellent prognosis, while the severely affected carry a guarded

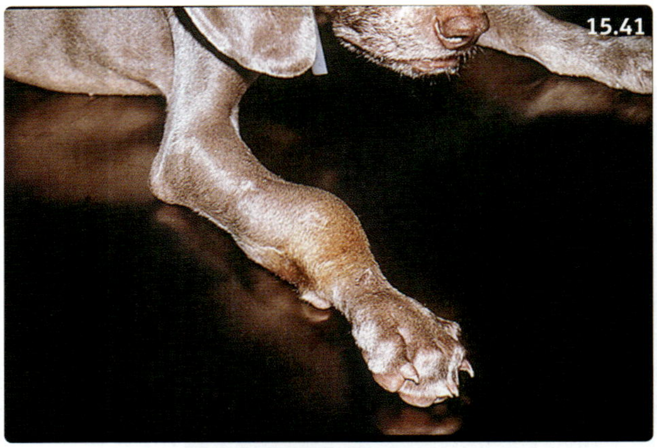

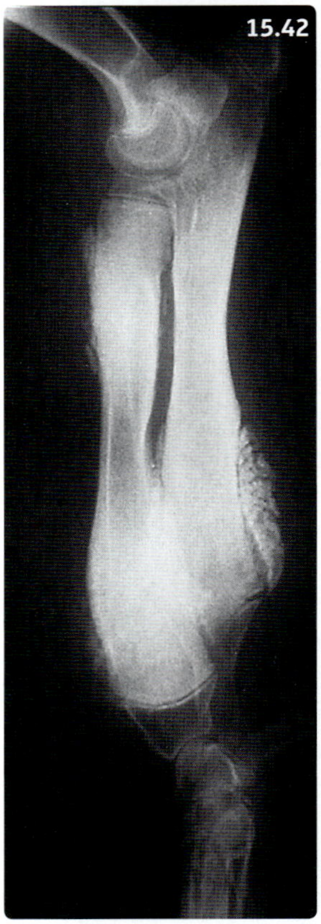

Figures 15.41, 15.42 This approximately 2–3-month-old Weimaraner puppy (15.41) suffered from severe debilitating effects of hypertrophic osteodystrophy. Note the marked swelling of the carpal metaphyseal region (15.42). Bacterial physitis with sepsis was also present. (Courtesy M. Schaer)

prognosis (death and euthanasia are not uncommon). There is no specific treatment for the disease, although anti-inflammatory analgesia (NSAIDs) can be palliative and physical rehabilitation activities may be beneficial. In one study of Weimaraners, treatment with corticosteroids was superior to treatment with NSAIDs, suggesting that the immune suppressive action of corticosteroids may be preferential for achieving remission.

HYPERADRENOCORTICISM

(See also Chapter 11: Endocrine disorders.)

Definition/overview

Hyperadrenocorticism is found in the presence of Cushing's disease or with chronic excessive administration of glucocorticoids.

Etiology

There are several recognized causes of hyperadrenocorticism: a pituitary tumor, which synthesizes and secretes excess adrenocorticotrophic hormone (pituitary-dependent hyperadrenocorticism [PDH]); adrenocortical tumors, which randomly secrete excessive cortisol independently of the pituitary (adrenocortical-dependent); and administration of excessive glucocorticoids (e.g. drugs for skin, ear, and eye conditions [iatrogenic]).

Pathophysiology

Osteoporosis of the spine and long bones can be associated with this disease in dogs, as calcium absorption from the gut, urinary excretion of calcium, normal production of bone matrix, and fibroblast as well as osteoblast proliferation and differentiation are affected.

Clinical presentation

Poodles, Dachshunds, Boston Terriers, Boxers, and Beagles have been reported to be at higher risk than other breeds. In general, endogenous hyperadrenocorticism affects middle aged to old animals; however, the iatrogenic form can be seen in young dogs. Severity of signs varies depending on the duration and degree of cortisol excess. The most apparent signs are polyuria and polydipsia, polyphagia, and a pendulous abdomen. Lethargy, muscle weakness, muscle atrophy, panting, obesity, hyperpigmentation, calcinosis cutis, and facial nerve palsy can also occur. Cats show similar signs and are commonly poorly controlled diabetics as well.

Differential diagnosis

Hypothyroidism, acromegaly, renal disease, hepatopathy, diabetes mellitus, ligament rupture.

Diagnosis

Radiography will reveal the extent of bone involvement (**Figure 15.43**). A urine cortisol:creatinine ratio is a very

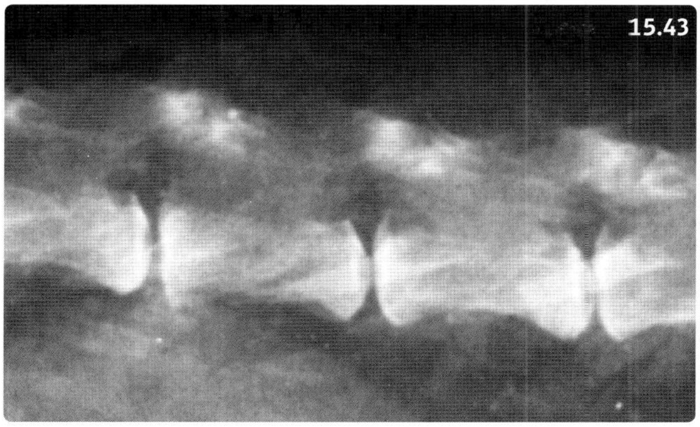

Figure 15.43 Lumbar vertebrae showing osteopenia. (Courtesy M. Schaer)

practical screening test. A diagnosis of hyperadrenocorticism is made by dexamethasone suppression testing or ACTH response testing. Abdominal radiography, ultrasonography, CT, and MRI are all useful in differentiating PDH from adrenal tumors.

Management

Surgery is not an option. Medical management for treating both PDH and adrenal tumors in dogs is with o,p'-DDD. Trilostane is now used commonly for treating PDH in dogs and cats.

NEOPLASIA

Bone neoplasms may arise from bone tissue elements or they may invade bone by local extension or distant metastasis. The majority of primary bone tumors are malignant. While the most frequent clinical signs in dogs and cats with appendicular bone tumors are pain or lameness referable to the primary tumor, signs of axial skeletal neoplasms reflect the tumor location. Radiographic findings such as periosteal new bone formation and bone destruction may support a diagnosis of neoplasia, but a definitive diagnosis is made histologically from a bone biopsy. Primary bone tumors and bone metastases are infrequent in cats.

SQUAMOUS CELL CARCINOMA

Definition/overview

Squamous cell carcinoma (SCC) is a common tumor involving the skin in both the dog and cat, and it is a common feline neoplasm involving bone. SCCs are usually found in nonpigmented or lightly pigmented skin.

Etiology

Primary lesions occur on the skin and may arise *de novo* or from overexposure to sunlight. Cats are predisposed to this type of cancer because of a lack of skin pigmentation and a desire to seek sunlight. The lesions are highly erosive and deeply infiltrative and, although late to metastasize, may spread to bone. SCC in cats occurs frequently in the oral cavity and less frequently involves the digits.

Pathophysiology

Unknown; however, SCC can metastasize almost anywhere.

Clinical presentation

The most common cutaneous locations for SCC in the dog are the toes, scrotum, nose, limbs, and anus, while the nose, eyelids, lips, and pinnae are common locations in the cat. Lesions vary from a red firm plaque to a cauliflower-like ulceration and they may appear as sequelae to crusts, ulcers, or masses that may have been present for months and been unresponsive to conservative treatment. SCC located deep to teeth can be a reason for premature tooth loosening.

Differential diagnosis

Draining abscessation, nail bed infection/osteomyelitis, eosinophilic granuloma, mast cell tumor, cutaneous lymphosarcoma.

Diagnosis

Biopsy or cytology.

Management

Superficial tumors are treated by surgery, cryosurgery, or irradiation. Digits with tumor involvement should be amputated. Cisplatin and mitoxantrone have provided remission (generally only for a short duration) where surgical excision is incomplete, the mass is nonresectable, or the patient has metastasis. When lesions are advanced and bone involvement is present, the prognosis is guarded.

PAROSTEAL OSTEOSARCOMA IN THE CAT

Definition/overview

Parosteal osteosarcoma is the second most common bone tumor in the cat.

Etiology

The cause is unknown.

Pathophysiology

Typically, the lesions appear as a mixed proliferative or lytic pattern in the metaphyseal region of the affected bone. The formation of periosteal bone in adjacent tissue leads to the development of Codman's triangle, comprising proliferation of the periosteum and mild destruction of cortical tissue.

Clinical presentation

Lesions are slow growing, but affected sites can elicit pain.

Differential diagnosis

Metastatic lesion, other primary bone tumor, osteomyelitis.

Diagnosis

Radiographically, parosteal tumors appear less aggressive than periosteal tumors. The lesions are moderately well-circumscribed and lysis of the cortex is usually mild. Biopsy specimens must be evaluated carefully for areas of tumor cells, as lesions may be misdiagnosed as reactive bone, chondroma, or osteoma.

Management

Frequently, amputation of the affected limb or area of tumor will be curative.

OSTEOSARCOMA

Definition/overview

Osteosarcoma is the most frequently reported (70–80%) primary bone tumor in cats. Solitary osteolytic metaphyseal long bone lesions in older cats are considered osteosarcoma until proven otherwise; these lesions tend to be less aggressive than canine osteosarcoma.

Osteosarcoma is the most common (85%) bone tumor in the dog. At greatest risk are the Saint Bernard, Great Dane, Golden Retriever, Irish Setter, Dobermann, and German Shepherd Dog.

Etiology

The cause is unknown. The association of osteosarcoma with metaphyseal bone, however, suggests that neoplastic transformation may result from aberrant bone growth or differentiation. Some dogs may be genetically predisposed, as mutation and inactivation of the p53 tumor suppressor gene have been found.

Pathophysiology

No pathophysiologic pathway has been identified. Osteosarcomas have been reported at locations where metallic implants have been used for fracture fixation, as well as at previous fracture sites or where there is chronic inflammation.

Clinical presentation

The majority of osteosarcomas originate in the metaphyses of long bones, with a higher frequency in the forelimbs. Tumors are most prevalent away from the elbow and around the stifle. Animals usually present with swelling and lameness of the affected limb. Swelling may or may not involve soft tissue. The tumor is seen arising on the outer surface of the cortex of the humerus, femur, frontal bones, and ramus of the mandible. Although osteosarcomas generally do not cross articular cartilage, adjacent bones can be affected, but generally through periarticular soft tissue or if the tumor is a telangiectatic osteosarcoma. Owing to the sudden onset of swelling and pain, a non-neoplastic orthopedic problem can be mistakenly assumed.

Differential diagnosis

Metastatic lesion, other primary bone tumor, osteomyelitis. Osteosarcoma should be ruled out in any large breed dog presenting with sudden lameness.

Diagnosis

A presumptive diagnosis can be made by radiography, which may reveal Codman's triangle and the proliferative or lytic pattern of the metaphyseal bone region (**Figure 15.44**). Pain is often elicited with deep palpation over the site. If treatment is considered, the extent of disease metastasis should be determined by a radiographic survey of the thorax or skeleton. A small percentage (5–10%) of affected animals have detectable lung lesions. Diagnosis is made by bone biopsy.

Management

Wide surgical excision or amputation is the treatment of choice. The tumor grows rapidly and treatment is unrewarding. Cisplatin is the chemotherapy of choice for treatment of osteosarcoma in dogs (toxic to cats). However, microscopic metastasis is common by the time of diagnosis. Survival is <6 months with limb amputation and <18 months if there is additional chemotherapy. Osteosarcoma in cats is less aggressive and amputation alone yields a median survival of >4 years. Since osteosarcoma is often associated with considerable

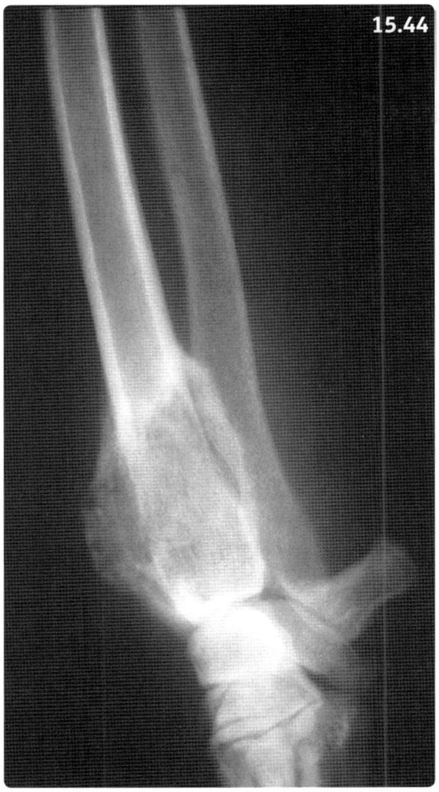

Figure 15.44 Osteosarcomas may produce a localized soft tissue swelling containing mineralized foci. In this case the carpus was swollen. There is extensive bony destruction, with the cortex eroded at several sites.

pain, management with NSAIDs may be appropriate for dogs. Furthermore, there is some speculation that COX-2-specific NSAIDs manifest antitumor mechanisms. Adjunctive analgesics such as opioids, N-methyl-d-aspartate antagonists, and ion channel regulators may be necessary to control the pain.

CHONDROSARCOMA

Definition/overview

Chondrosarcoma is the second most common bone tumor in dogs (**Figure 15.45**). Lesions can originate in the ribs (most common primary rib tumor), long bones, extra-skeletal sites, nasal cavity, vertebrae, facial bones, pelvis, digits, and os penis. The nasal cavity is commonly affected. This tumor is uncommon in cats.

Etiology

The cause is unknown, although lesions can occur in cases of multiple cartilaginous exostosis.

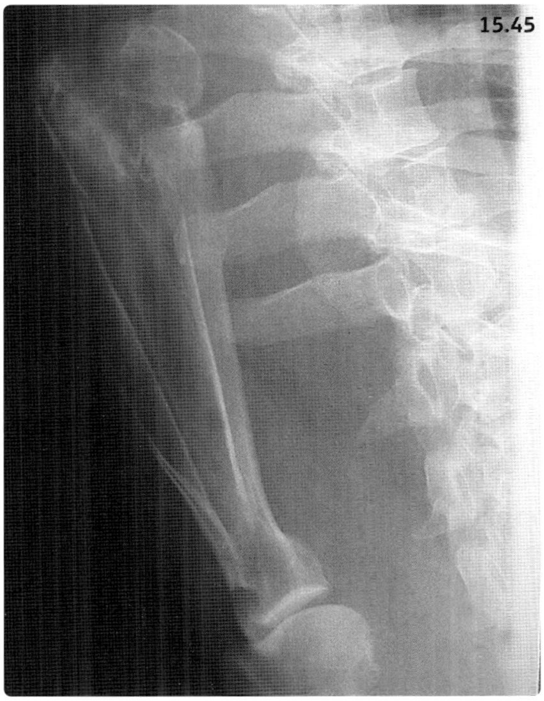

Figure 15.45 Chondrosarcoma of the proximal scapula characterized by both destruction and proliferation. (Courtesy I.A. Robertson)

Pathophysiology

Anaplastic cartilage cells between and within the tumors show various stages of differentiation and maturation. Metastasis may occur in any tissue, but most commonly in lung tissue.

Clinical presentation

Chondrosarcoma occurs commonly in ribs, nasal bones, and the pelvis. Pain on palpation of the lesion is common and swelling may occur at the tumor site. Intrathoracic extension of tumors may give rise to pleural effusion.

Differential diagnosis

Other primary bone tumors, osteomyelitis.

Diagnosis

Diagnosis is based on biopsy and histopathologic examination.

Management

The prognosis is good to guarded if complete excision of the tumor is accomplished. Chemotherapy with cisplatin is appropriate for nonresectable tumors; however, response of chondrosarcomas to radiation and chemotherapy is poor.

VASCULAR TUMORS OF BONE

Definition/overview

Primary vascular tumors of bone are infrequently encountered, but they are virtually all malignant. Any bone may be affected, but the axial skeleton is more frequently affected than the appendicular skeleton. Hemangiosarcoma of the bone is more common in the dog than in the cat, and the German Shepherd Dog is most frequently at risk.

Etiology

Hemangiosarcoma is a malignancy of vascular endothelial cells or their precursors.

Pathophysiology

These tumors rapidly metastasize via hematogenous routes to the liver and lungs. They can rupture, leading to acute hemorrhage and sudden death.

Clinical presentation

History and presenting signs are similar to those for osteosarcoma. Osteolysis is the dominant radiographic feature.

Differential diagnosis

Telangiectatic osteosarcoma (**Figures 15.46–15.48**).

Diagnosis

Radiographically, hemangiosarcomas show massive destruction, often involving one-half or more of the entire bone shaft. Destruction tends to remain confined within the medullary cavity with both proximal and distal expansion. Marked periosteal new bone formation is not characteristic but may be seen (**Figure 15.49**), and pathologic fractures may occur. Hemangiosarcomas often have vascular spaces and biopsy for diagnosis may be nondiagnostic. Therefore, it is prudent to biopsy at the periphery of the tumor to obtain distinct cores of tissue.

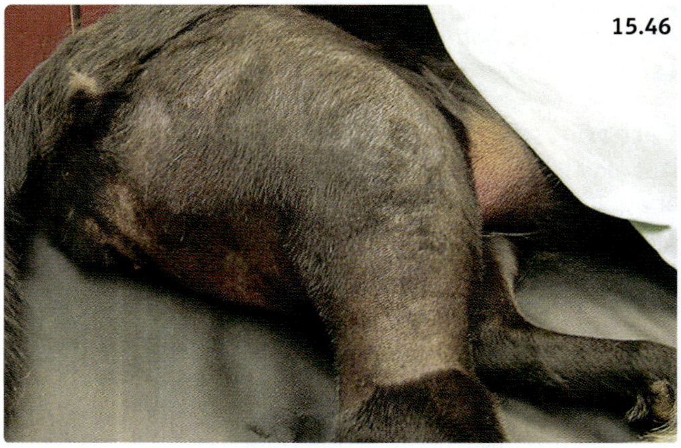

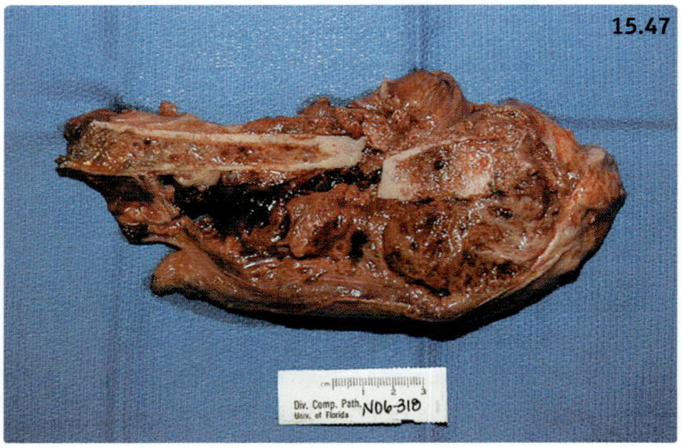

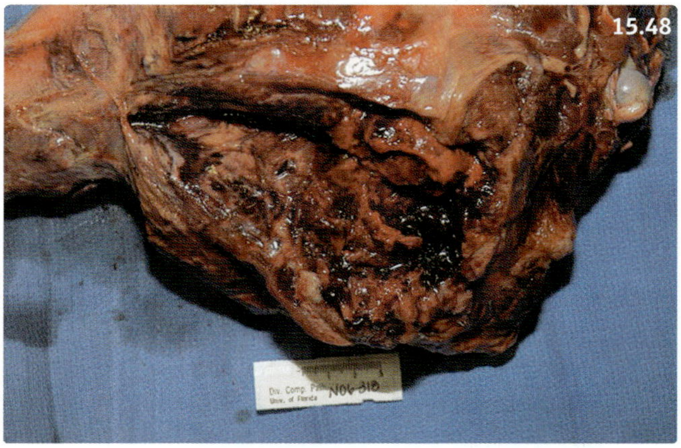

Figures 15.46–15.48 This dog was lame on her right hindlimb for several weeks before she had a sudden onset of hemorrhagic swelling in the thigh muscle region (15.46). Radiographs showed considerable osteolysis of the femur. The primary differential diagnosis included a hemangiosarcoma, but histopathology showed the lesion to be a telangiectatic osteosarcoma that had hemorrhaged into the thigh muscles (15.47, 15.48). (Courtesy M. Schaer)

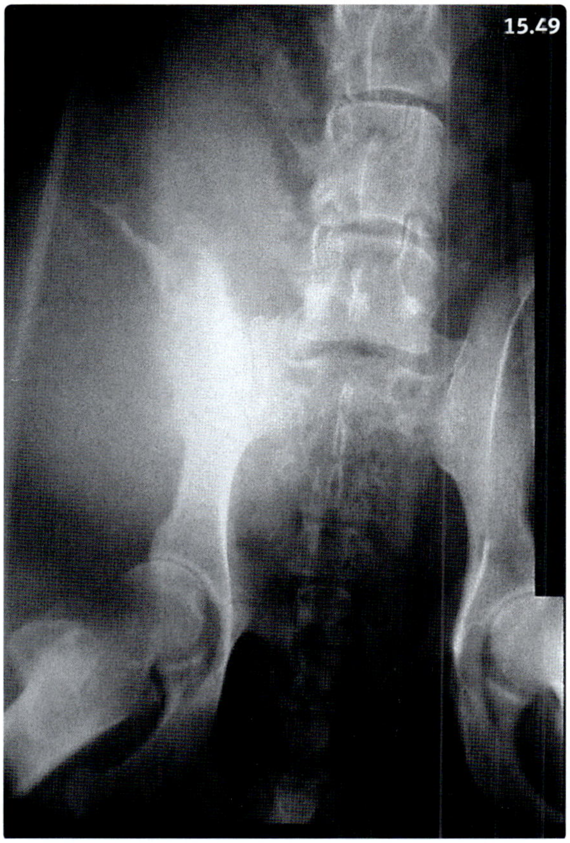

Figure 15.49 Pelvic hemangiosarcoma. This lesion is characterized by soft tissue swelling and periosteal proliferation.

Management

Affected dogs must be thoroughly staged with thoracic and abdominal radiography, bone scintigraphy, or bone survey radiography. Prognosis is poor irrespective of surgical excision and adjunct chemotherapy.

FIBROSARCOMA

Definition/overview

Primary fibrosarcoma of bone originates from the fibrous components of the medulla and is the third most common primary bone neoplasm in dogs. Primary fibrosarcoma of bone is rare in cats; parosteal or soft tissue origin is more common and axial skeleton sites are more common than appendicular sites. This neoplasm tends to be locally invasive but late to metastasize.

Etiology

Unknown.

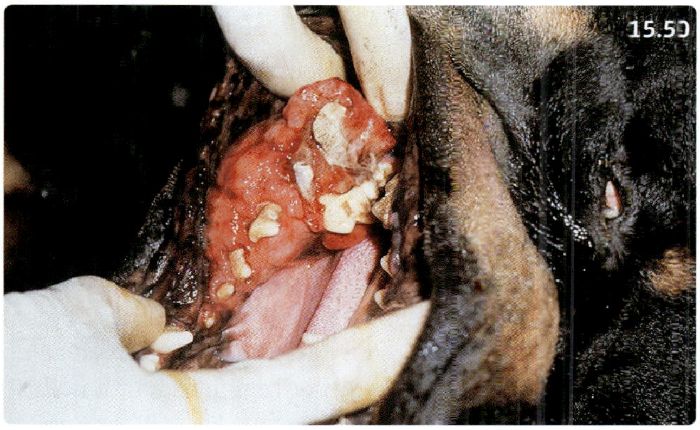

Figure 15.50 Mandibular fibrosarcoma in an 8-year-old Rottweiler.

Pathophysiology

This fibroblastic tumor produces bundles of collagenous fibers but no neoplastic bone, osteoid, or cartilage either in the primary tumor or its metastases. It is often difficult to determine if the tumor is primarily a bone neoplasm or a soft tissue neoplasm invading bone. Fibrosarcomas produce bone lysis with minimal reactive bone response.

Clinical presentation

Animals with oral lesions (**Figure 15.50**) usually present with fleshy, pink, firm, sessile masses in the palate or gingiva, which deeply infiltrate soft tissue and bone. Long bones may have swelling, typically at a metaphyseal site, and the site is often painful to palpation.

Differential diagnosis

Osteomyelitis, other primary bone tumors (osteosarcoma, chondrosarcoma, hemangiosarcoma).

Diagnosis

Biopsy specimens should be carefully examined as it is difficult to distinguish fibroblastic osteosarcoma from fibrosarcoma.

Management

Treatment is with surgical excision and the prognosis is guarded. There is no suggestion that chemotherapy may be advantageous.

SYNOVIAL CELL SARCOMA

Definition/overview

Synovial cell sarcoma is the most frequent tumor of soft tissue that involves adjacent bones.

Etiology

This tumor may arise from precursor mesenchymal cells outside the synovial membrane of articular structures.

Pathophysiology

The biological behavior of this tumor is variable. Synovial cell sarcoma is a disease of middle aged to older dogs, and is rarely reported in cats. Joints most commonly involved are the stifle, elbow, carpus, tibiotarsal, and phalangeal joints. Nearly half of affected patients ultimately develop metastasis involving the lungs or regional lymph nodes.

Clinical presentation

Examination of the affected joint may reveal swelling, pain, and a decreased range of motion. Joint swelling typically involves both sides of the joint.

Differential diagnosis

Primary bone tumor, osteoarthritis, osteomyelitis, villonodular synovitis.

Diagnosis

Radiographic evidence of a destructive lesion involving bones on both sides of a joint suggests synovial sarcoma, and both the stifle and the elbow are sites of predilection (**Figures 15.51–15.54**). A biopsy of both the soft tissue lesion and associated bone is diagnostic. Regional lymph node cytology may also be diagnostic.

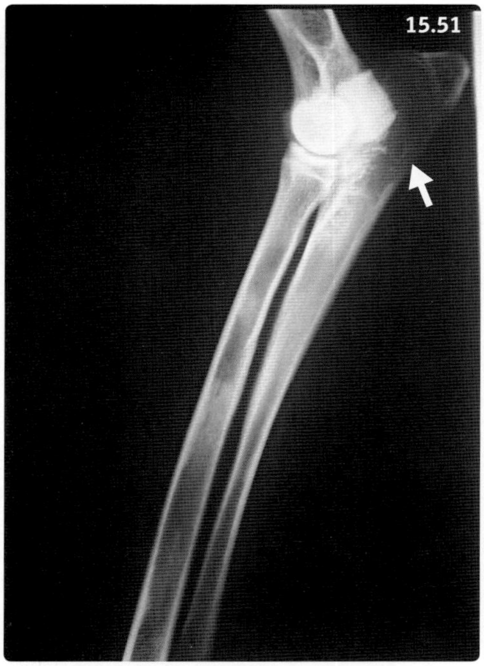

Figure 15.51 Synovial cell sarcoma with soft tissue swelling of the elbow and erosion of the olecranon (proximal ulna) (arrow). Synovial cell sarcoma is most often seen in the elbow and stifle. The tumor usually crosses the joint space. The lesion is predominantly osteolytic, periosteal proliferation is minimal, and soft tissue mineralization is rare. (Courtesy A.M. Walker)

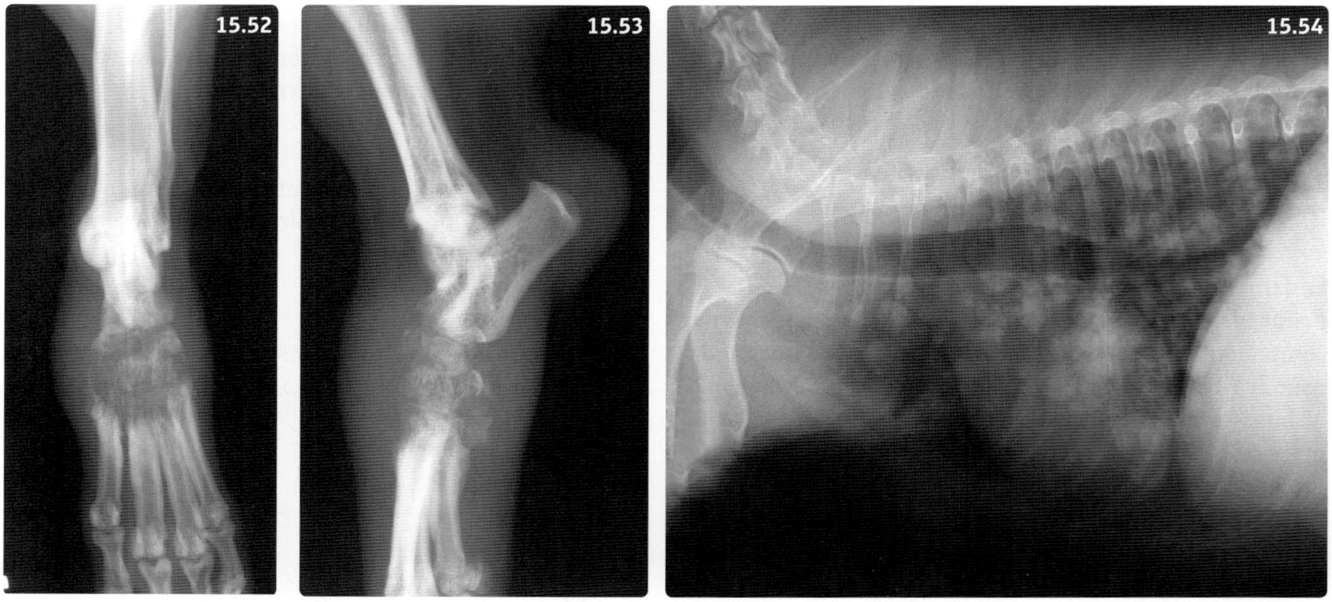

Figures 15.52–15.54 Radiographic lesions diagnosed as synovial cell sarcoma of the tarsometatarsal joint, with metastatic lesions in the thorax. (Courtesy B. Poteet)

Management

The prognosis after surgery is variable, with recurrence being not uncommon. Survival after excisional biopsy and combination chemotherapy has been reported; however, metastasis occurs in up to 50% of cases.

NUTRITIONAL DISORDERS

RICKETS/OSTEOMALACIA

Definition/overview

Inadequate supplies of cholecalciferol or vitamin D result in rickets or osteomalacia (adult equivalent), diseases affecting the hypertrophic zone of metaphyseal growth plates.

Etiology

Likely causes include dietary deficiency (hypovitaminosis D), impaired absorption or an inadequate concentration of minerals from the diet, and an inborn error in the metabolism of vitamin D. Dogs and cats are mainly dependent on vitamin D from their diet due to an inability to synthesize cholecalciferol in skin exposed to ultraviolet light.

Pathophysiology

There is a failure of mineralization of cartilage and osteoid. The costochondral junctions and metaphyses may be enlarged so that the joints appear swollen.

Clinical presentation

Immature animals with rickets or mature animals with osteomalacia may be presented with lameness, difficulty rising, a stiff gait, limb bowing, pathologic fractures, or sudden paralysis.

Differential diagnosis

Hyperparathyroidism.

Diagnosis

Radiographic signs may be similar to hyperparathyroidism and commonly include radiolucent cortical bone due to poor mineralization, thin cortices, bowed diaphyses, and a loss of lamina dura dentes.

Management

Treatment consists of proper dietary supplementation with adequate but not excessive amounts of calcium, phosphorus, and vitamin D, and repair of any pathologic fractures.

HYPERVITAMINOSIS A

Definition/overview

Hypervitaminosis A is a disease of cats that consume large amounts of raw liver.

Etiology

Excessive and prolonged intake of vitamin A either from supplements or liver-rich diets.

Pathophysiology

The condition is characterized by cervical and thoracic bridging exostoses and limb joint periarticular ankylosis, especially in the elbow.

Clinical presentation

Animals may present with irritability, poor grooming, lethargy, depression, gingivitis, and lameness. In the early stages the lesions are painful and they may ankylose, leading to abnormal posture and neck stiffness.

Differential diagnosis

Nutritional secondary hyperparathyroidism, hypovitaminosis D.

Diagnosis

Radiographically there is evidence of exostoses and enthesophytes in the cranial and thoracic vertebrae, particularly in older affected animals (**Figures 15.55–15.57**). There may also be enthesophytes around limb joints (e.g. the elbow or shoulder).

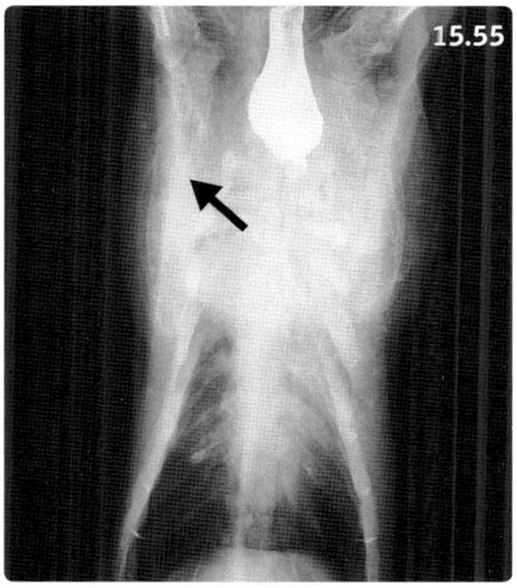

Figure 15.55 Thoracic rhabdomyosarcoma and long-standing hypervitaminosis A. The tumor caused esophageal obstruction, as shown on this barium esophagram. The hypervitaminosis A causes the bony proliferation, as shown by the arrow. (Courtesy M. Schaer)

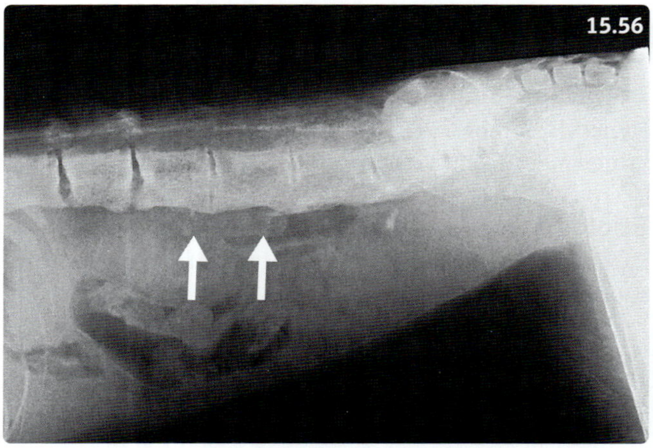

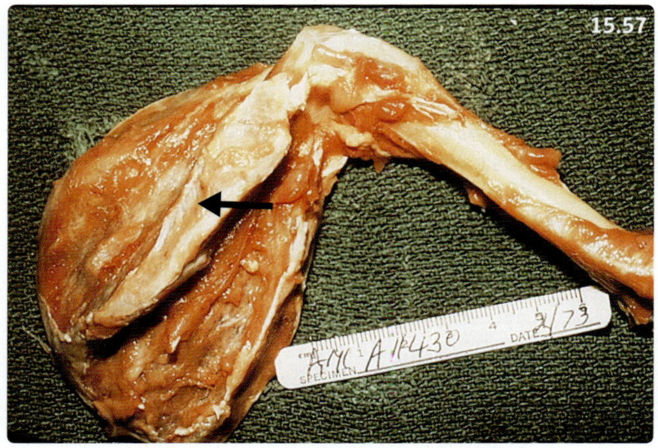

Figures 15.56, 15.57 Radiograph (15.56) and postmortem specimen (15.57) from an aged cat with thoracic rhabdomyosarcoma and long-standing hypervitaminosis A. Note the characteristic bone thickening involving the lumbar vertebrae, pelvis, and scapulae (arrows). (Courtesy M. Schaer)

Management

Treatment is aimed at avoidance of excess vitamin A. In elderly cats, despite bone remodeling, there may be rigidity from anklyosis. In young animals, bone growth may be permanently affected.

INFLAMMATION

SUPPURATIVE OSTEOMYELITIS

Definition/overview

Suppurative osteomyelitis is a bacterial (rarely fungal) contamination of bone leading to the formation of pus.

Etiology

About half of infections are caused by *Staphylococcus aureus*, whereas polymicrobial infections can be caused by *Streptococcus* spp. and gram-negative bacteria such as *Pseudomonas* spp., *Klebsiella* spp., *Escherichia coli*, and *Proteus* spp. Sometimes, anaerobic bacteria are involved. Bone is relatively resistant to infection unless there is a concurrent soft tissue injury, bone necrosis, sequestration, fracture instability, implanted foreign material, altered host defenses, or some combination.

Pathophysiology

Associated soft tissue changes are visible within 24 hours. These include swelling and loss of fascial planes; sometimes, a fistulous tract may develop. Bone changes, bony lysis, areas of periosteal new bone formation, or presence of a sequestrum do not become apparent until 10–14 days after introduction of the infection. Bacteriologically, the most frequent organism isolated in the dog and cat with osteomyelitis is *S. aureus*.

Clinical presentation

In acute conditions, animals may present with signs of systemic illness including inappetence, dullness, weight loss, and pyrexia. Affected periosteum and surrounding muscle may appear swollen and painful and feel hot. In chronic conditions, animals may present with fibrosis, muscle atrophy, lymphadenopathy, and contracture.

Differential diagnosis

Neoplasia, bone cysts, HOD, medullary bone infarction.

Diagnosis

Diagnosis is usually determined from the history, physical examination, microbiology, and radiology. Radiography reveals swelling of soft tissue (**Figures 15.58, 15.59**) in acute cases but no osseous changes, whereas in chronic cases there is evidence of formation of periosteal new bone, which appears as radially oriented, spiculated, and extensive growth. Bone resorption leads to lysis of the medulla, rounding of the ends of fractured bones, and thinning of the cortex. Osteomyelitis can virtually be diagnosed by the presence of sequestra. Bacterial culture should confirm the diagnosis and determine antibacterial selection.

Management

Drugs that readily cross the capillary membrane of bone and are widely distributed in interstitial fluid include beta-lactams (cephalosporins, penicillins),

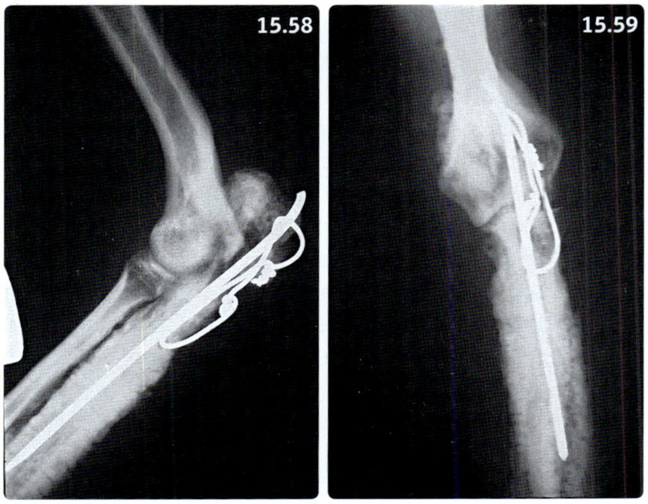

Figures 15.58, 15.59 Postoperative radiographs showing typical features of osteomyelitis.

aminoglycosides, and quinolones. Acute osteomyelitis is usually cured after 4–6 weeks of antibacterial treatment, whereas such treatment is pointless in chronic cases without débridement and surgical removal of sequestra. Antibiotic-impregnated beads have been used in chronic cases. Recurrence of infection may require repeated sequestrectomy, débridement, microbiologic culturing, drainage, fracture stabilization, bone grafting, or implant removal.

DISKOSPONDYLITIS

(See also Chapter 14: Disorders of the nervous system and muscle.)

Definition/overview

Diskospondylitis (vertebral osteomyelitis) usually involves a hematogenous spread of coagulase-positive staphylococcal bacteria (may also be fungal) that localizes in the vertebral metaphysis and extends to the adjacent disk. Common primary sites of infection are skin, heart, and urinary tract. The disease is common in dogs but rare in cats. Large dogs are most commonly affected and predisposed sites are L7/S1, the caudal cervical area, and the mid-thoracic spine.

Etiology

Organisms associated with diskospondylitis are *Staphylococcus aureus*, *Staphylococcus intermedius*, *Brucella canis*, *Streptococcus* spp., *Escherichia coli*, *Pasteurella multocida*, *Actinomyces viscosus*, *Norcardia* spp., *Mycobacterium avium*, *Aspergillus* spp., *Paecilomyces variotii*, *Mucor* spp.,

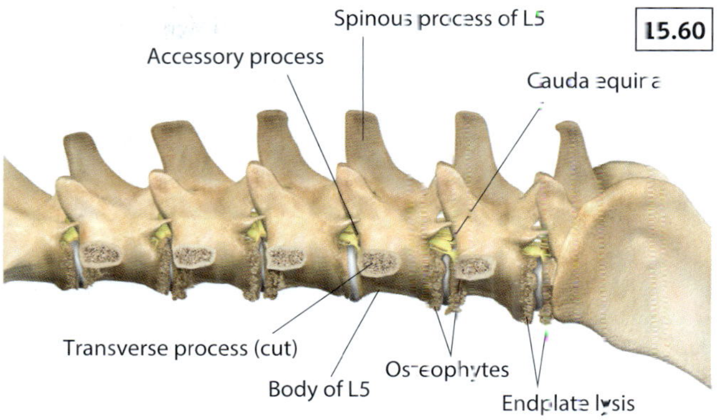

Figure 15.60 Illustration of diskospondylitis, where new bone production is appearing in adjacent vertebrae.

and *Fusarium* spp. Occasionally the cause is foreign body migration or extension of local soft tissue infection caused by bite wounds (cats).

Pathophysiology

Early lesions may comprise only lytic areas in affected vertebral endplates, whereas advanced lesions show both bone lysis and extensive new bone production (**Figure 15.60**). Neurologic dysfunction is usually associated with spinal cord compression caused by proliferation of bone and fibrous tissue or meninges infection.

Clinical presentation

Progressive clinical signs include both systemic illness such as anorexia, depression, and pyrexia, and neurologic signs such as hyperesthesia or paralysis. Focal or multifocal areas of spinal pain are a common presenting sign.

Differential diagnosis

Intervertebral disk disease, vertebral fracture/luxation, spondylosis deformans, neoplasia, brucellosis.

Diagnosis

Diagnosis is usually made by radiography; collapse of the disk followed by lysis at the vertebral endplate (**Figures 15.61–15.63**). Lysis is a distinguishing feature from spondylosis deformans, but it is also seen in neoplasia of the spine. However, vertebral neoplasia is uncommon at endplates and seldom involves adjacent vertebrae. Hemograms are often normal. Urine cultures are positive in about 25% of patients and serologic testing for *B. canis* should be performed.

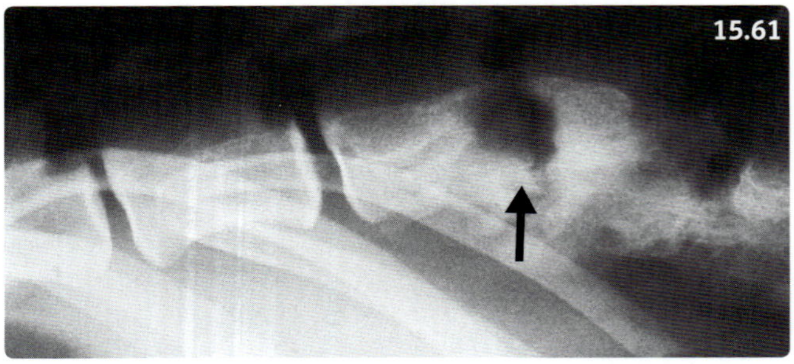

Figure 15.61 Diskospondylitis in a 4-year-old male Rottweiler. Intradiskal osteomyelitis (diskospondylitis) originates in or near the intervertebral disk and extends to the adjacent vertebra (arrow). This disease is first seen with a loss of the densely calcified cortical border of the vertebral body, progressing to lysis of the vertebral endplates and, subsequently, the vertebral bodies.

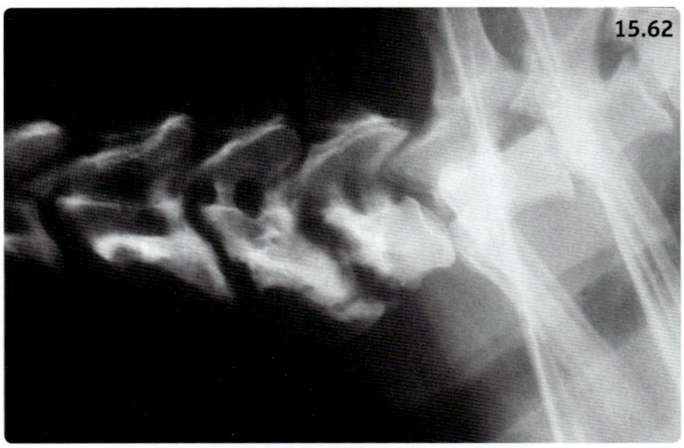

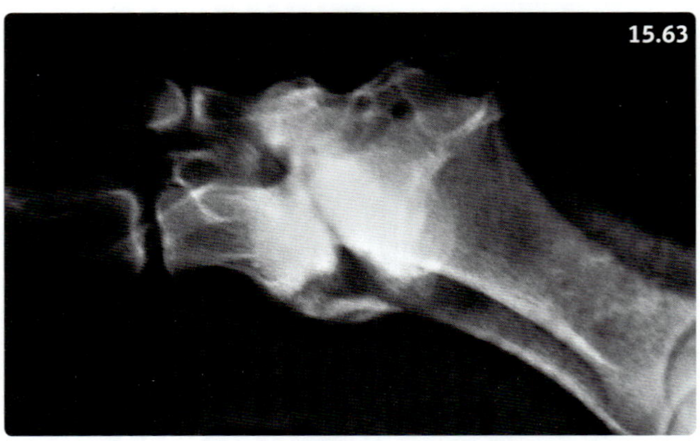

Figures 15.62, 15.63 Lateral cervical and lumbosacral radiographs depicting *Aspergillus* spp. diskospondylitis at the C6/C7 and lumbosacral interspaces in a 7-year-old male Airedale. (Courtesy M. Schaer)

Management

Treatment is based on antibiotic selection from both blood and urine culture and analgesics for pain-induced distress. *Streptococcus* spp. or *Staphylococcus* spp. are assumed if these cultures are negative. Lactamase-resistant antibiotics such as cefadroxil or cloxacillin are generally effective, and most dogs respond immediately. Brucellosis is treated with tetracycline and streptomycin or a fluoroquinolone. Animals failing to improve within 5 days should be reassessed by lesion curettage and culture. Extended treatment may be necessary for up to 6 months.

ARTHRITIS

Definition/overview

Arthritis is an inflammatory disease of the joints characterized by cellular infiltrates and inflammatory changes in the synovial membrane and synovial fluid. Clinical manifestations are due to both persistent inflammatory reactions resulting from deposition and phagocytosis of immune complexes and release of damaging lysosomal enzymes within the joint. The cause and source of immune complexes are unknown. Noninfective inflammatory arthropathies, including the immune-mediated arthritides, are subdivided as erosive and nonerosive. Nonerosive arthritides can be further subdivided as follows:

- Systemic lupus erythematosus.
- Plasmacytic–lymphocytic synovitis.
- Polyarthritis/polymyositis syndrome.
- Idiopathic polyarthritis.
- Drug-induced arthritis.
- Hepatopathic arthritis.
- Enteropathic arthritis.
- Arthritis associated with malignant neoplasia.

Canine rheumatoid arthritis (RA) is a progressive inflammatory polyarthropathy characterized by erosion and destructive changes in the joint that involves both cellular and immune interactions. Characteristic signs are generalized stiffness and shifting limb lameness accompanying systemic signs such as fever, lethargy, and inappetence. The most severely affected joints are the carpal, tarsal, and interphalangeal joints, although the stifle, elbow, and hip are commonly affected.

Polyarthritis is a specific disease entity in the young Greyhound (**Figures 15.64, 15.65**) and mature cat. Chronic progressive polyarthritis of cats is etiologically linked to feline syncytium-forming virus, a common retrovirus

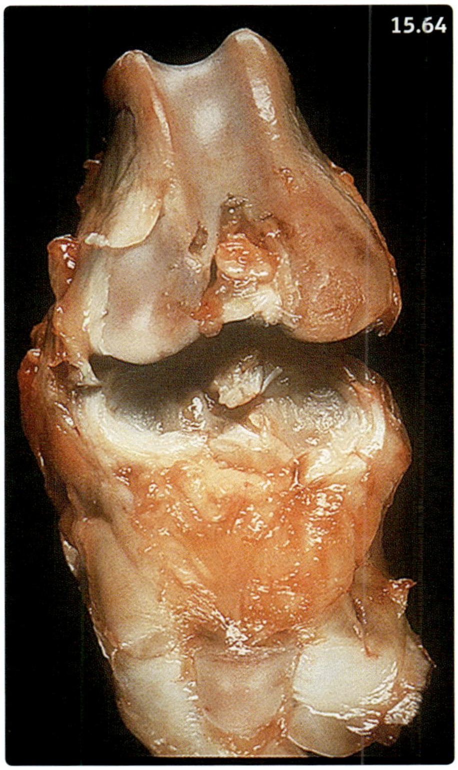

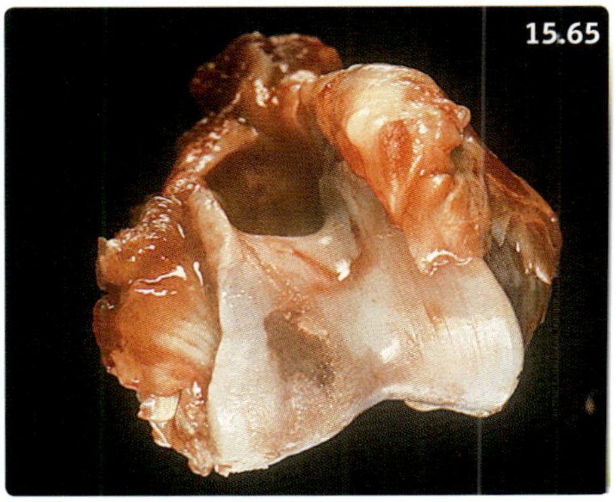

Figures 15.64, 15.65 Gross specimen from a Greyhound with polyarthritis. (15.64) The cartilage of the trochlear groove has a rough surface, and the red and blue caste to the cartilage identifies the subchondral bone beneath thin, translucent cartilage. The synovium is hypertrophic. (15.65) The distal humerus has a granular, rough cartilagenous surface with linear score marks, cartilage cracks, and a deep erosion. (Courtesy the late M.S. Bloomberg)

infection, and all cats with this disease are serologically and virologically positive for this infection (high incidence of false-positive tests). Cats can also acquire a calicivirus-associated arthritis from natural infection and by vaccination.

SLE is a multisystem autoimmune disease characterized by the formation of autoantibodies against a wide array of self-antigens and circulating immune complexes. Although polyarthritis is a frequent feature of SLE in both dogs and cats, it is more likely to be a predominant clinical disease in dogs, whereas cats tend to manifest other systemic signs.

Etiology

Joints are common destinations for blood-borne microbial pathogens because the synovium and subchondral bone are highly perfused. Additionally, the synovium is a highly phagocytic organ, therefore a common site for trapping blood-borne microbes and immune complexes. Urinary tract and skin infections are less common in cats than in dogs, and acquired heart valve disease is quite rare; therefore, infectious arthritis is less common in the cat. Organisms commonly involved in joint infections in dogs include *Staphylococcus* spp., *Streptococcus* spp., *Erysipelothrix* spp., *Corynebacterium* spp., coliforms, *Pasteurella* spp., *Salmonella* spp., and, occasionally, *B. canis*. In cats the usual offending organisms are *Pasteurella multocida* and hemolytic strains of *E. coli*.

Erosive arthritis

In RA, immune complexes in the synovium and synovial fluid probably initiate the inflammatory reaction.

Nonerosive arthritis

Etiologically diverse, nonerosive, noninfectious arthritis occurs in both dogs and cats. Immune complexes in the synovial membrane (resulting in a type III immune reaction) are believed to result in joint disease. In idiopathic nondeforming arthritis the origin and nature of the antigens in the complexes are unknown. The antigens in SLE are of nuclear origin; the antigens in enteropathic arthritis probably originate from the inflamed bowel; and antigens in arthritis secondary to chronic infectious disease or neoplasia originate from the offending microorganisms or from the tumor cells. The cause of SLE is unknown.

Polyarthritis may be a manifestation of drug-induced vasculitis. Fever and stiffness may be seen from the time of first administration or as late as 3 weeks after drug initiation. Skin rash may or may not occur concurrently. Intolerance to trimethoprim–sulfa, penicillins, erythromycin, lincomycin, and cephalosporins is most common. Drug withdrawal yields rapid resolution of signs.

Pathophysiology

Damaged joints are more likely to accommodate blood-borne pathogens. Larger dogs, older dogs, and proximal rather than distal joints are more commonly affected.

Prostatitis, cystitis, pyelonephritis, pyodermas, and oral infections can all be accompanied by septicemia, leading to arthritis. Complications include osteomyelitis, fibrous or bony ankylosis, and secondary joint disease.

Erosive arthritis

Canine RA is more severe in the carpal and tarsal joints. In the early stages the disease is often accompanied by fever, malaise, anorexia, and lymphadenopathy, while renal amyloidosis can be a complication of long-standing disease. In the central region of the joint, pannus arising from granulation tissue in the underlying marrow cavity causes cartilage destruction. Ankylosis in advanced lesions is common in the intercarpal and intertarsal joints.

Nonerosive arthritis

This joint disease tends to be cyclic, affecting one or more joints. Biopsy of the synovial membranes shows a nonvillous hyperplasia, sparse mononuclear cell infiltrates, moderate neutrophil infiltrate, and fibrin exudation.

In SLE the production of autoantibodies to nonorgan-specific nuclear and cytoplasmic antigens and to cell- and organ-specific antigens results from an immunoregulatory defect. Resultant immune complexes are deposited in the glomerular basement membrane, synovial membrane, skin, blood vessels, and other sites. Complement is activated by the immune complexes, leading to tissue injury and inflammation. Furthermore, a direct cytotoxic effect of autoantibodies against membrane-bound antigens contributes to tissue damage.

Clinical presentation

Animals with septic arthritis are usually painful on palpation, and redness as well as swelling may be observed in the overlying skin and soft tissue. Fever is common. Pointing abscessation and draining tracts may also be present (**Figure 15.66**).

Erosive arthritis

Canine RA is a disease of mainly small dogs, manifesting initially as a shifting lameness with soft tissue swelling around involved joints. The disease is often accompanied by fever, malaise, anorexia, and lymphadenopathy in the early stages, while renal amyloidosis can complicate long-standing disease. Excessive amounts of synovial fluid may be present, which is generally discolored and turbid and yields a typically poor and friable mucin clot.

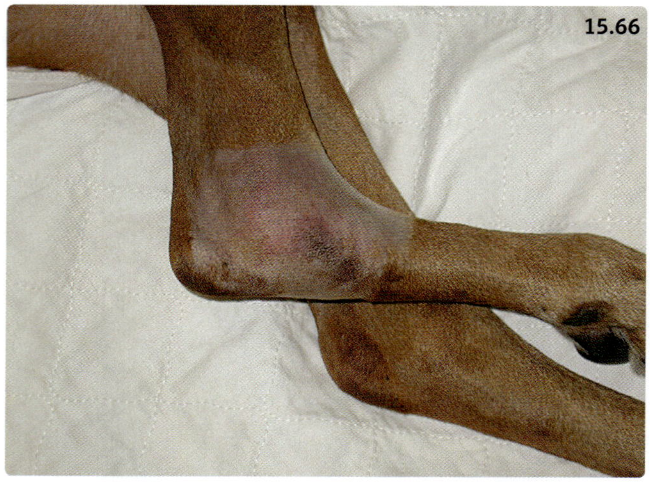

Figure 15.66 This patient had been treated with high doses of prednisone for an earlier diagnosis of pemphigus vulgaris. The immunosuppresive doses of this drug very likely predisposed her to a monoarticular *Salmonella* spp. joint infection that responded well to aspiration and intensive antimicrobial treatment. (Courtesy M. Schaer)

Nonerosive arthritis

The clinical and radiographic findings of polyarthritis demonstrate the inflammatory nature of the disease and simulate those of RA (narrowed joint space, periarticular osteophytes, subchondral sclerosis, and capsular swelling). The history is one of cyclic fever, including anorexia, lameness, stiffness, and malaise. Muscle atrophy may also be noted.

Differential diagnosis

Lyme disease (*Borrelia burgdorferi*), mycoplasmosis (often associated with immunocompromise), rickettsiosis (polyarthritis is a prominent feature), ehrlichiosis (nonerosive polyarthritis, always thrombocytopenia, triad of thrombocytopenia, fever, and lymphadenopathy).

Erosive arthritis

Neoplasia, immunologic cause.

Nonerosive arthritis

Neoplasia, infectious disease, trauma.

Diagnosis

Synovial fluid from septic joints is often bloody and the presence of toxic, ruptured, and degranulated neutrophils should suggest a bacterial infection. Although slight periosteal proliferation of bone adjacent to the joint space may be seen in late-stage arthritis, early stages are characterized by thickened synovial membrane, distended joint capsule with displacement of adjacent fascial planes, and widening of the joint space from joint effusion. Aspiration of the joint is necessary for a diagnosis by cytology and culture.

Erosive arthritis

No single test can diagnose canine RA, including the presence of rheumatoid factors in the blood. A prominent radiographic lesion is the progressive destruction of subchondral bone in the more central areas and at the area of synovium attachment (**Figures 15.67, 15.68**). A characteristic finding in canine RA is the presence in synovial fluid of mononuclear cells containing IgG.

Nonerosive arthritis

Diagnosis is complicated by the cyclic nature of the disease; therefore, consideration must be made of a clinical history with antibiotic-nonresponsive cyclic fever, malaise, anorexia, and lameness. Joint fluid with a neutrophilia of 5,000–100,000 cells/µl, yet sterile for bacteria, viruses, *Mycoplasma*, and *Chlamydia* is diagnostic. Diagnosis of SLE is based on a positive ANA or lupus erythematosus test, or both, and two major signs of polyarthritis, proteinuria, dermatitis, hemolytic anemia, leukopenia, thrombocytopenia, or polymyositis.

Management

Treatment of bacterial arthritis is dictated by identification of the causative organism and determination of antibiotic sensitivities. Concurrent cultures of joint fluid, serum, and urine may optimize isolation of the pathogen(s). Generally, continued administration of appropriate antibiotics for 2 weeks or more after the resolution of clinical signs is curative. Drainage of the suppurative exudate helps prevent lysosomal-caused joint damage. The majority of cases of bacterial arthritis are monoarticular.

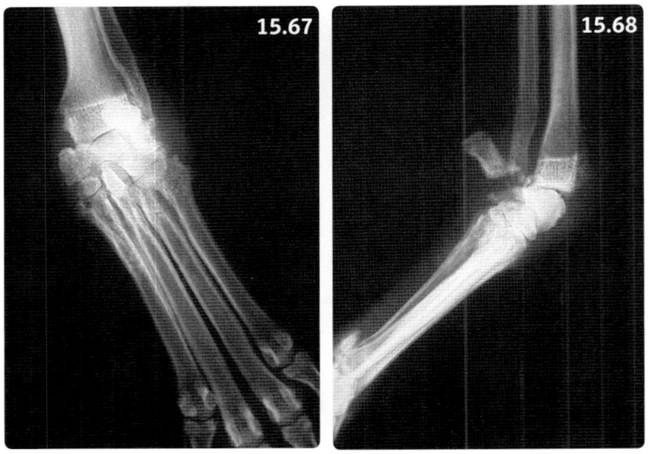

Figures 15.67, 15.68 Erosive polyarthritis in the carpus of a 7-year-old male Whippet. Radiographic investigations of patients with polyarthritis often reveal slightly large joints with soft tissue swelling, periarticular osteophytes, osteclysis of the distal portion of the radius and radial carpal bone, and loss of joint space. (Courtesy A.M. Walker)

Erosive arthritis

Treatment of RA with corticosteroids, anti-inflammatories, and gold salts has been used, but the effect is merely palliative. If the condition is identified in the early stages, it can be arrested with combination immunosuppressive drug therapy, whereas in advanced conditions adjunctive joint arthrodesis may be necessary.

Nonerosive arthritis

Glucocorticoids alone or in combination with immunosuppressive drugs provide remission; however, recurrence of illness is common when therapy is discontinued. Treatment of SLE is directed at controlling the abnormal immune response and reducing the inflammation. Corticosteroids are the foundation of treatment with adjunctive cytotoxic immunosuppressive drugs for additional improvement or when the patient is steroid intolerant.

The most commonly encountered immune disorders affecting the skeletal system are SLE and immune-mediated polyarthropathy. When there is doubt as to whether an arthritis is due to a tick-borne or immune etiology, it is rational to first treat with tetracycline or doxycycline for at least 5 days before initiating treatment with immunosuppressive therapy. A favorable response is expected in 2–4 days if the arthritis is due to spirochetes or rickettsiae.

IATROGENIC DISORDERS

SYNOSTOSIS

Definition/overview

Synostosis of the radius and ulna is not a developmental disease, but rather an iatrogenic restriction in the relative growth of the proximal ulna.

Etiology

A restriction in the relative growth of the proximal ulna is usually associated with a callus spanning the radius and ulna after inadequate fracture reduction.

Pathophysiology

Synostosis is usually associated with a bridging callus following inadequate reduction of radial or ulnar fractures. The condition may also be caused by transfixation of both bones with pins or screws during internal fixation before skeletal maturity. Where considerable growth follows transfixation, a relative overgrowth of the proximal radius occurs, with proximal displacement of the humeral condyles and trochlear notch deformation.

Clinical presentation

Synostosis presents as an antebrachial deformity that may also include luxation or subluxation of the elbow joint.

Differential diagnosis

Traumatic premature physeal closure.

Diagnosis

Radiographic finding is of bone bridging two synchronously growing bones, such as the radius and ulna in a growing animal (**Figure 15.69**).

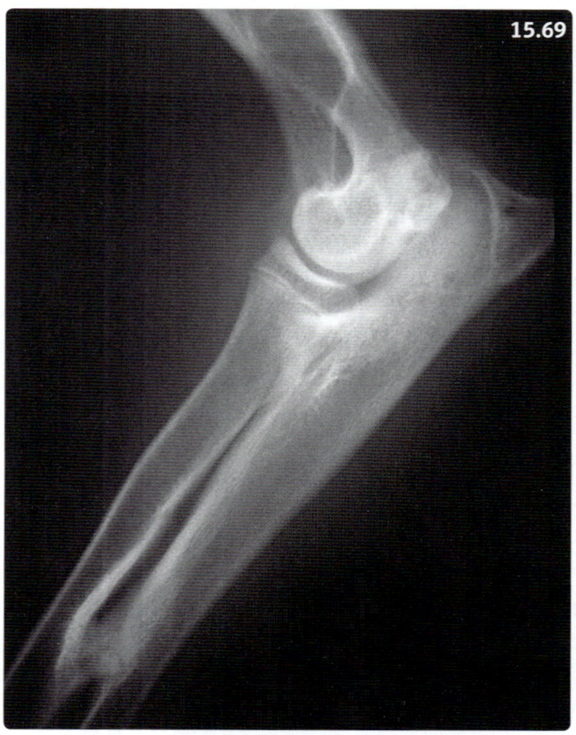

Figure 15.69 Synostosis of the radius and ulna in a young German Shepherd Dog. The synostosis (within the diaphysis) resulted in a relative overgrowth of the proximal radius compared with the ulna, producing elbow incongruity and an ununited anconeal process. (Courtesy the late M.S. Bloomberg)

Management

Treatment of synostosis is based on the degree of malformation and the potential for further bone growth. Surgery consists of removal of the growth constraint and realignment of the elbow joint if appropriate. Bridging callus can be resected and the defect filled with autogenous fat graft to prevent re-formation.

IDIOPATHIC

LEGG–CALVÉ–PERTHES DISEASE

Definition/overview

Legg–Calvé–Perthes disease (aseptic necrosis of the femoral head) is a disease of small, immature dogs seen most commonly in Cairn Terriers, West Highland White Terriers, Manchester Terriers, Miniature Pinschers, and Poodles. Spontaneous degeneration of the femoral head and neck (**Figure 15.70**) is followed by collapse of the coxofemoral joint and osteoarthritis.

Etiology

The cause of Perthes disease is unknown, although in the Manchester Terrier a multifactorial inheritance pattern with a high degree of heritability has been identified.

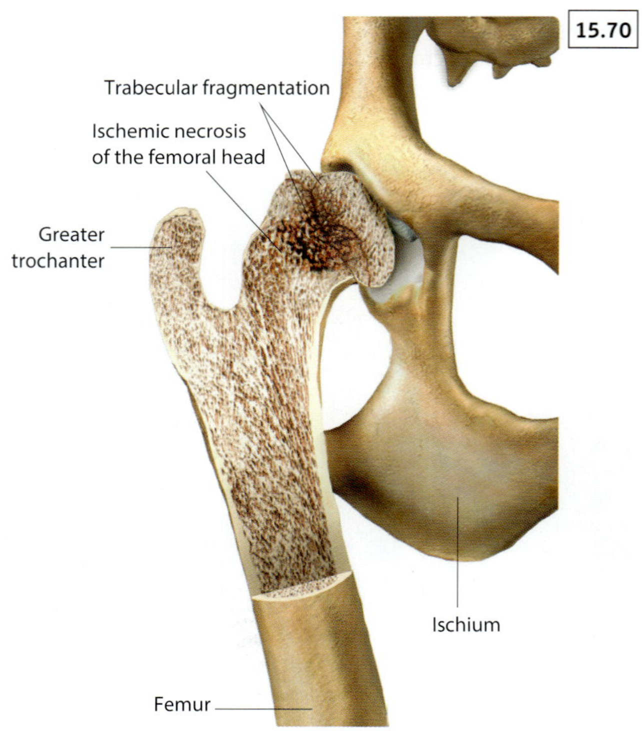

Figure 15.70 Illustration of Legg–Calvé–Perthes disease depicting collapse of the femoral head and neck areas.

Pathophysiology
A major part of the blood supply to the capital epiphysis of the femur becomes compromised and the ischemic portion becomes necrotic. Necrosis of subchondral bone leads to collapse and deformation of the femoral head under normal weight bearing.

Clinical presentation
Perthes disease is usually unilateral and associated with thigh muscle atrophy and pain in the hip.

Differential diagnosis
Luxating patella, coxofemoral luxation.

Diagnosis
Diagnosis is confirmed by radiographic findings that include radiolucent areas of the proximal femoral epiphysis (**Figure 15.71**), epiphyseal deformity, thickening of the femoral neck, and increased width of the hip joint space.

Management
Pathology is usually advanced by the time dogs are presented with clinical signs. The surgical procedure of femoral head and neck ostectomy is recommended as a salvage procedure.

BONE CYSTS

Definition/overview
Simple bone cysts are benign bone lesions occurring only in large breed dogs. The distal radius and/or ulna is affected most often.

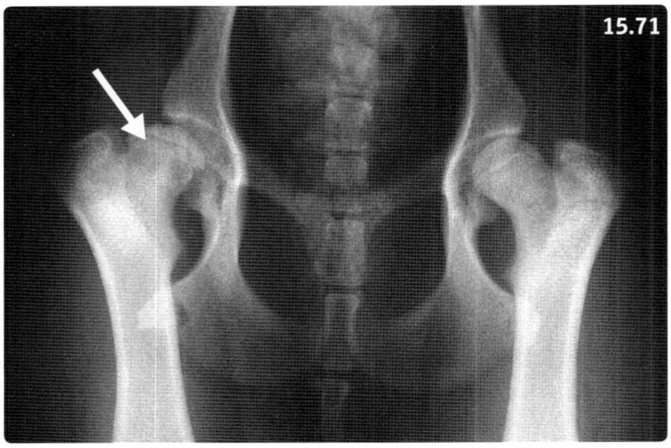

Figure 15.71 Unilateral Perthes disease in a 6-month-old female Fox Terrier presented for right hindlimb lameness. This radiograph shows lysis of the femoral head (arrow).

Etiology
The etiology is unknown but may involve intramedullary metaphyseal hemorrhage or local disturbance of bone growth.

Pathophysiology
Lesions occur in metaphyses and adjacent diaphyses of long bones. They are lined by thin membranes and contain serosanguineous fluid.

Clinical presentation
Affected dogs either have no clinical signs referable to the lesion or have an associated lameness. Pain, swelling, and joint stiffness may be evident in the area of the bone cyst and the cyst may predispose to a pathologic fracture.

Differential diagnosis
Atypical bone neoplasia, fibrous dysplasia of bone, aneurysmal bone cyst.

Diagnosis
Radiographically, bone cysts appear as radiolucent defects with cortical thinning (**Figures 15.72, 15.73**). Periosteal reaction is absent and the lesion may consist of several chambers. Fine needle aspiration biopsy and cytologic examination may prove diagnostic.

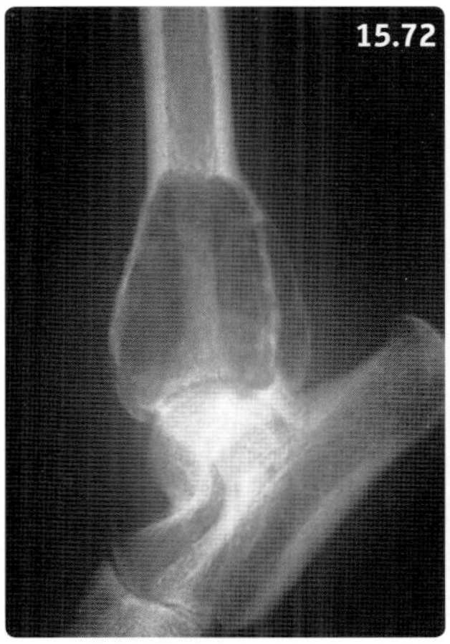

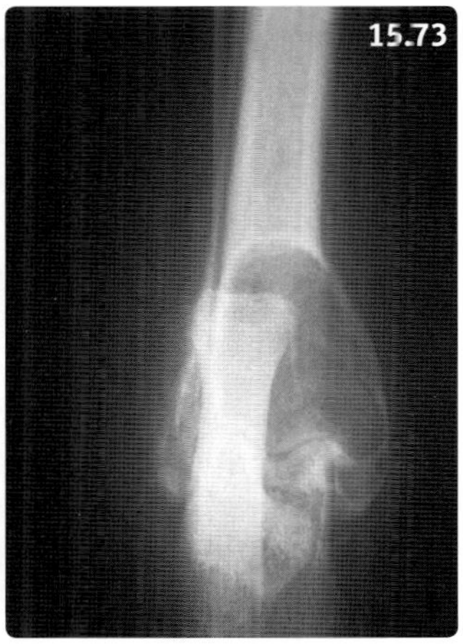

Figures 15.72, 15.73 An aneurysmal bone cyst is seen in the distal tibia of a mature male Sheltie. This is a rare neoplasm and has produced bony lysis with minimal cortical or periosteal reaction. The bone has expanded with a thin cortex, and a pathologic fracture may ensue. (Courtesy S. Newell)

Management
Drainage, curettage, autogenous grafting, and drilling with multiple holes have all been used to treat bone cysts. Left untreated, bone cysts have the potential for inciting a pathologic fracture.

SECONDARY HYPERTROPHIC OSTEOPATHY

Definition/overview
Hypertrophic osteopathy (pulmonary osteoarthropathy, hypertrophic pulmonary osteoarthropathy, hypertrophic pulmonary osteopathy) is a secondary pathologic disease frequently associated with some form of pulmonary disease and characterized by bilateral symmetrical swellings in the distal extremities of all four limbs. It is a disease of older dogs and the majority of bones in the limb may show a diffuse periosteal reaction. Bone changes usually begin distally and spread proximally.

Etiology
The cause is unknown and the disease is not restricted to primary thoracic neoplasia.

Pathophysiology
This disease involves increased blood flow to the distal extremities, then overgrowth of connective tissue and subsequent osteoneogenesis. It is proposed that a neural reflex originating in the thorax affects connective tissue and periosteum of the limbs.

Clinical presentation
Diseased patients are stiff and reluctant to move. Limbs are often painful, warm, and swollen (**Figure 15.74**). Primary thoracic disease may manifest with cough, abnormal lung sounds, dyspnea, or cardiac displacement.

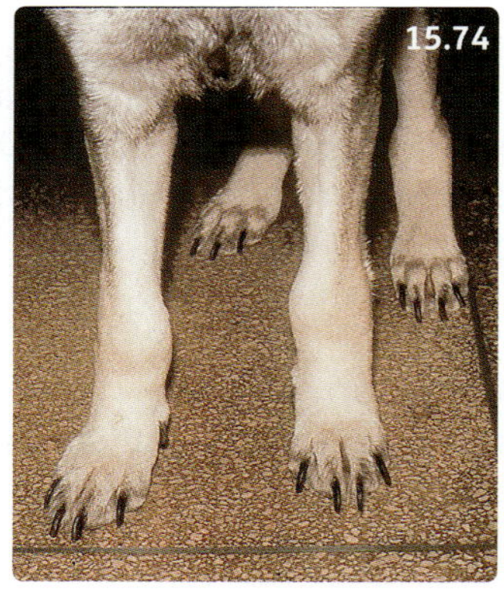

Figure 15.74 This 11-year-old female spayed German Shepherd Dog has hypertrophic osteopathy as a result of renal carcinoma metastasizing to its chest. Note the distal appendigeal swellings. (Courtesy M. Schaer)

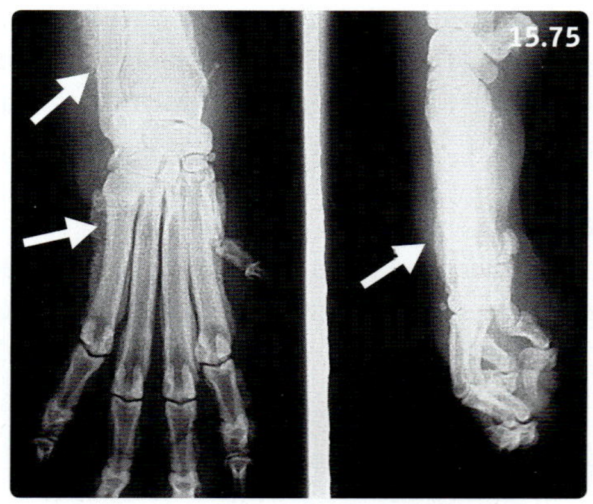

Figure 15.75 Hypertrophic osteopathy was diagnosed in this 11-year-old female spayed German Shepherd Dog. All four distal extremities were involved. The radiograph shows the periosteal proliferation involving the distal foreleg (arrows). (Courtesy M. Schaer)

Differential diagnosis
Osteomyelitis, metastatic neoplasia.

Diagnosis
Radiographic examination reveals early involvement of the metacarpal and metatarsal bones (**Figure 15.75**), with subsequent progression of periosteal reaction recognized in more proximal long bones and joints. Radiographic studies should include films of the thoracic and abdominal cavities to rule out pulmonary or abdominal (e.g. bladder rhabdomyosarcoma or liver adenocarcinoma) disease. Skeletal recognition of hypertrophic osteopathy signals other disease processes; therefore, interrogative diagnostics should follow if hypertrophic osteopathy is suspected.

Management
Clinical signs typically resolve within 1–2 weeks of successful treatment for the primary cause, although resolution of the bony lesions may take months. Relief of lameness may be gained with intrathoracic vagotomy on the ipsilateral side to the bony lesion(s).

MULTIPLE CARTILAGINOUS EXOSTOSES

Definition/overview
Multiple cartilaginous exostoses (osteochondromatosis, diaphyseal aclasis, hereditary multiple exostoses), reported in both dogs and cats, is a disease manifestation of endochondral ossification where partially ossified

protrusions arise from the cortical surfaces of bones. The vertebrae, ribs, and long bones are most frequently affected in dogs.

Etiology
The condition may be inherited as an autosomal dominant trait in dogs. Differentiation to cartilage and bone of chondrocytes displaced from the metaphyseal growth plate is believed to be the cause, and growth of the exostoses usually ceases with skeletal maturation. In the cat, feline leukemia virus has been associated with osteochondromas. Transformation of cartilaginous exostoses into osteosarcoma and chondrosarcoma has been reported.

Pathophysiology
Protuberances consist of cancellous bone covered by a surface of hyaline cartilage; they arise in the metaphyseal region of bones by endochondral ossification. As growth continues, exostoses may finally become located in the diaphysis.

Clinical presentation
Clinical signs may include paresis due to spinal cord compression or pain from exostoses touching adjacent tissue. Superficial exostoses may be palpated.

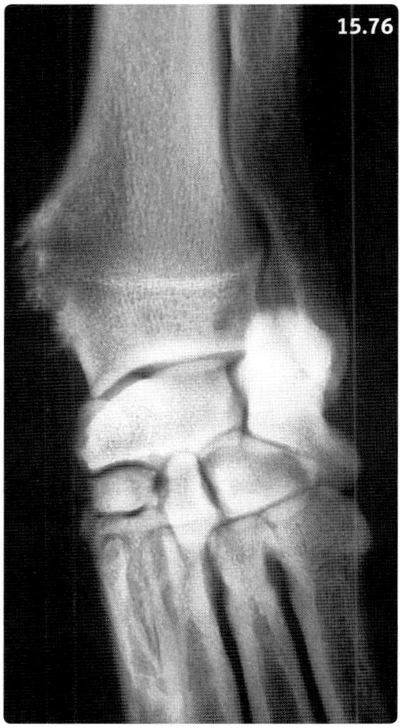

Figure 15.76 Cartilaginous exostoses observed on the medial aspect of the distal radial metaphysis.

Differential diagnosis
Neoplasia, fracture callus.

Diagnosis
Radiographs reveal bony masses with a smooth thin shell arising from the cortical surfaces of the appendicular or axial skeleton (**Figures 15.76, 15.77**). The expanding exostoses may lead to skeletal deformation. Periodic radiographic evaluation is advised, with the consideration that chronic lesions may transform to bone neoplasia.

Management
The extent of the lesion dictates treatment, and surgical excision may be indicated if the lesion interferes with function.

TOXICITY AND TRAUMA

LEAD POISONING

Definition/overview
Skeletal signs are usually absent with lead poisoning, but in some affected young dogs radiography reveals 'lead lines' in the bones.

Etiology
Plumbism is a disease caused by the ingestion of lead-containing materials, mainly paint.

Pathophysiology
Lead toxicity may result in gastrointestinal, neurologic, and hematologic abnormalities. Radiographic 'lead lines' result from accumulation of thick mineralized trabeculae at the metaphyseal sites because of impaired osteoclastic activity.

Clinical presentation
Gastrointestinal signs of vomiting, diarrhea, anorexia, and abdominal pain tend to predominate over central nervous system (CNS) signs of lethargy, hysteria, seizures, and blindness.

Differential diagnosis
Hypervitaminosis D, hyperphosphatemia, bismuth toxicity.

Diagnosis
Radiographically, dense sclerotic 'lead lines' may be seen in the metaphysis of long bones of immature dogs (**Figure 15.78**). They are most apparent in the distal radius and ulna. Chronic toxicity of vitamin D, phosphorus, or bismuth can cause a similar radiographic lesion.

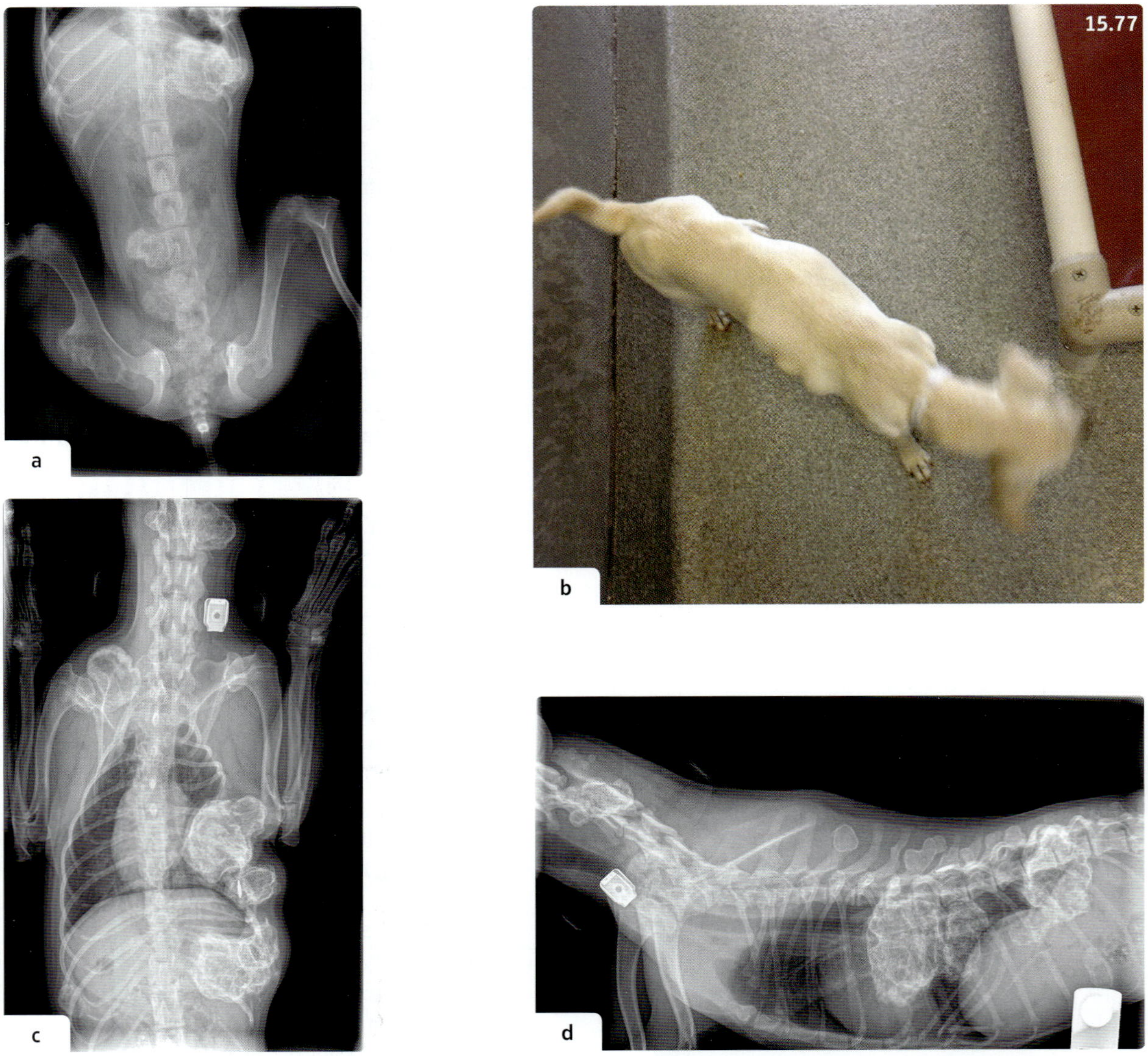

Figures 15.77a–d These images depict a young mixed-breed dog with diffuse cartilaginous exostoses showing the external masses and their radiographic appearance at various costochondral sites. (Courtesy H. Campbell and A. Alvarez)

Management

Skeletal signs may persist following treatment for toxicity.

LUXATIONS

Definition/overview

The majority of joint luxations are traumatic, although congenital luxations (**Figure 15.79**) do occur in both dogs and cats. Femoropatellar luxation is frequently diagnosed in small dogs and occasionally in large dogs and cats (**Figures 15.80, 15.81**). The condition varies from complete, irreducible luxation of the patella and severe lameness to mild instability without associated clinical signs. Grading is made from 1–4 based on the severity of the condition and clinical signs.

Etiology

In dogs the smaller breeds are more commonly affected with congenital luxations owing to disruption of supporting joint structures or anatomic developmental failures. With congenital absence of the patella within the femoral trochlear groove, the trochlear groove fails to develop, resulting in a convex surface rather than a concave surface.

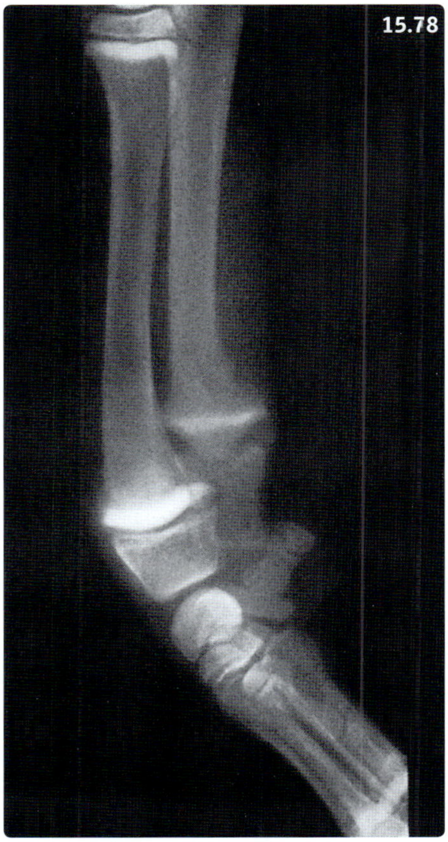

Figure 15.78 'Lead lines' seen in the metaphysis of an immature dog. (Courtesy B.R. Jones)

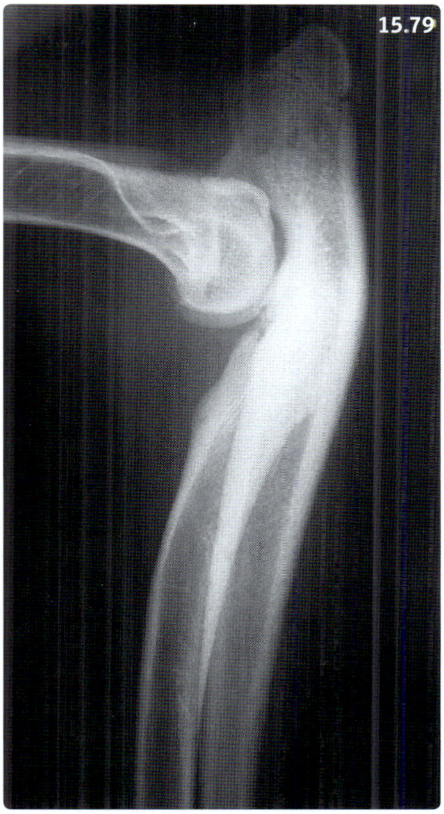

Figure 15.79 Congenital joint luxations, such as this elbow, often accompany other anomalies and are best treated by 'salvage' procedures.

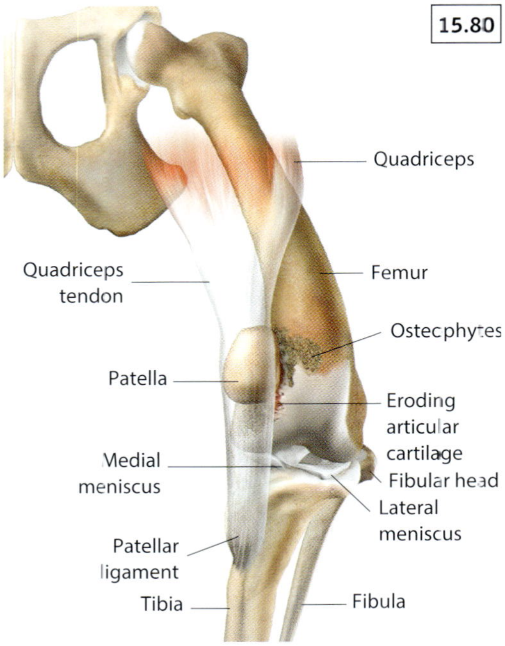

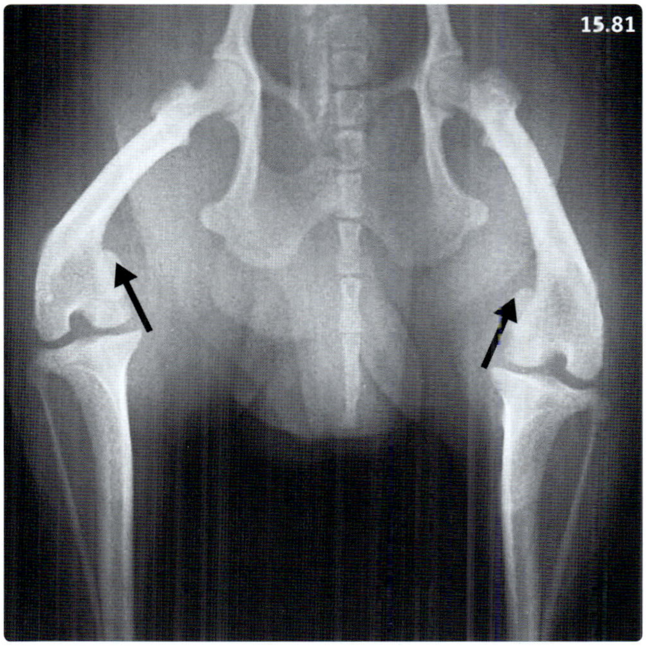

Figures 15.80, 15.81 Illustration (15.80) and radiograph (15.81) of medial patella luxation, a common developmental anomaly in small breed dogs.

Pathophysiology

Agenesis of or an underdeveloped trochlear groove and lack of supporting joint structures (such as the fabellopatellar ligament) allows easy luxation with joint extension. In doing so, the patella rides over the trochlear ridge (medial more common than lateral). Articular cartilage of both this ridge as well as the articular surface of the patella may become eburnated to subchondral bone. Ultimately, DJD leads to chronic osteoarthritis. In Grades 3 and 4, severe bony deformities may be present, including marked internal tibial rotation and an S-shaped curve of the distal femur and proximal tibia.

Clinical presentation

Grade 1 luxations are often incidental findings during physical examination, where the patella can be manually luxated. Grade 2 luxations present with a history of intermittent lameness, resolving spontaneously with patella reduction. Owners often report that the dog suddenly skips and carries the limb without apparent pain, flexes and extends the joint several times, and is then able to bear weight normally thereafter. In this case the animal is allowing the patella to pop back into place by forcing the limb into extension. With a Grade 3 luxation the owner frequently reports that the dog shows a 'crouched' gait, since the dog often uses the limb in a semiflexed, internally rotated position. Grade 4 is a nonreducible luxation of the patella. The tibia is often rotated from 60 to 90 degrees relative to the sagittal plane, and limb disfiguration often accompanies abnormal gait. Patella luxation often occurs bilaterally.

Differential diagnosis

Premature physeal closure, cranial cruciate ligament rupture, collateral ligament disruption, tibial tubercle avulsion fracture, patellar tendon rupture.

Diagnosis

Diagnosis is most often apparent on physical examination, and it can be confirmed radiographically. Acute lameness in a dog with chronic luxation is usually caused by rupture of the cranial cruciate ligament, as cranial stifle support from the straight patella ligament is lacking. Every small breed dog should be examined for patella luxation.

Management

Surgical correction for congenital luxations is often disappointing due to the rapid anatomic changes in the growing dog and inevitable DJD. An exception is the condition of luxating patella in the dog, where surgical correction is rewarding. Surgical methods include wedge section sulcoplasty, trochleoplasties, tibial tuberosity transposition, and antirotational techniques. Additionally, uncomplicated traumatic luxations most often carry a favorable prognosis if treated promptly.

CRANIAL CRUCIATE LIGAMENT RUPTURE

Definition/overview

Rupture of the cranial cruciate ligament (**Figure 15.82**) is frequently associated with hindlimb lameness in dogs (especially large breeds of older, overweight females), contributing to its recognition as the major cause of stifle joint DJD. Injury leaves the animal with partial to complete instability of the joint (**Figure 15.83**).

Etiology

The majority of dogs with cranial cruciate ligament rupture have a chronic course rather than a history of distinct trauma. Degeneration of the ligament may be caused by aging, conformational abnormalities, immune-mediated processes, and limb immobilization or loss of tone due to

15.82

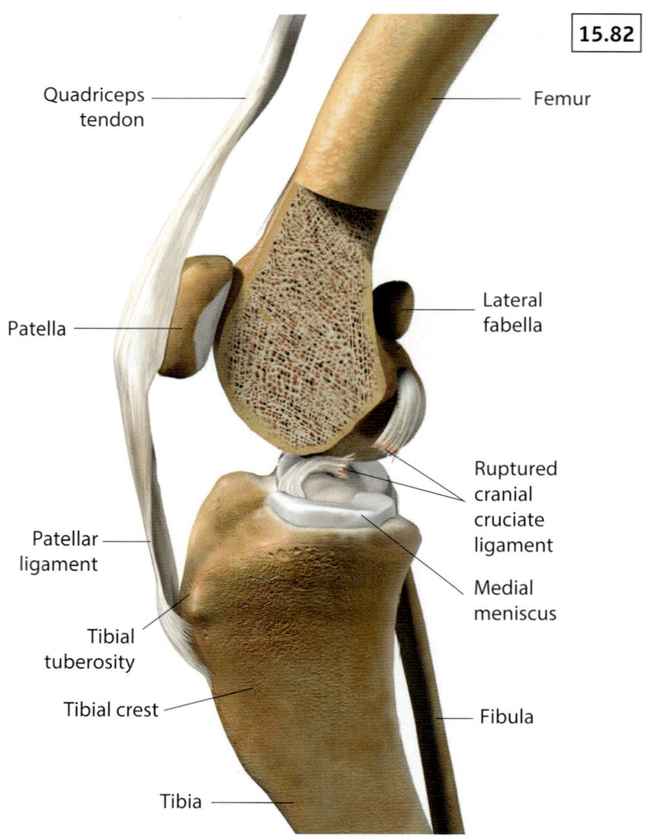

Figure 15.82 Illustration depicting a torn cranial cruciate ligament.

irregular use. Speculation suggests tibial plateau angle as an etiologic factor.

Pathophysiology

Immune-mediated arthritis, lymphocytic–plasmacytic synovitis, and septic arthritis may predispose the ligament to rupture. Cranial cruciate ligament strength deteriorates with aging, correlating with loss of fiber bundle organization and metaplastic changes of cellular elements. Tears may occur in total or in part (approximately 30% of patients with stifle lameness) and osteoarthritis soon follows. Cranial cruciate ligament compromise results in additional stress on the menisci, which frequently tear (>50% of patients), thus contributing to joint osteoarthritis.

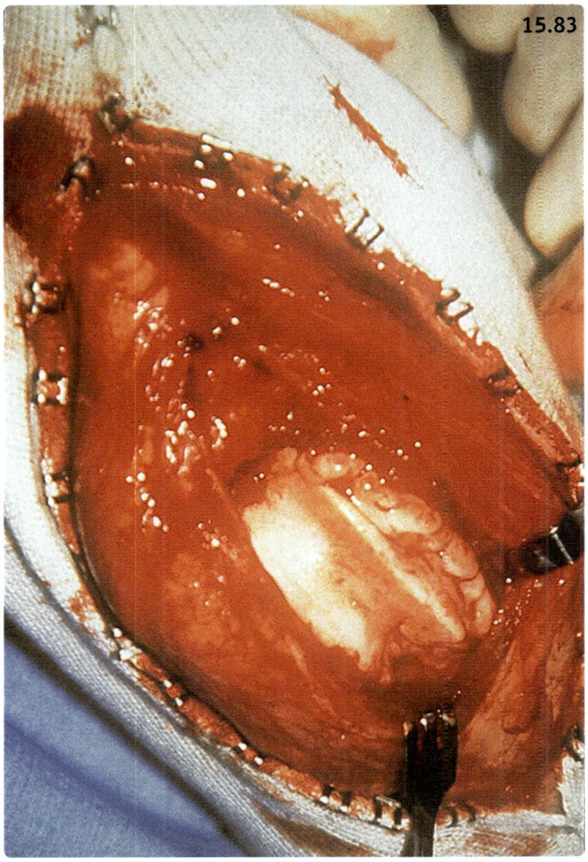

Figure 15.83 Cranial cruciate ligament rupture is a common presentation in clinical practice. In larger breeds of dog, surgical stabilization is important in order to minimize the progression of degenerative joint disease, demonstrated by osteophyte deposition on the lateral aspect of this femoral condyle. (Courtesy late M.S. Bloomberg)

Clinical presentation

A common presenting sign is lameness of the hindlimb. Acute traumatic ligament rupture is accompanied by severe lameness and occasional nonweight-bearing. Lameness subsides in 3–5 weeks as muscle atrophy progresses. In contrast, dogs with chronic disease have a more insidious history of lameness, often intermittent and exacerbated by exercise. Joint effusion is characteristic. Subtle weight shifts during standing and difficulty rising can also suggest cruciate disease.

Differential diagnosis

Patellar luxation, meniscal injury, collateral ligament compromise, hip dysplasia, skeletally immature dog (have some degree of drawer sign), osteochondrosis of the femoral condyle (**Figure 15.84**), neoplasia (synovial cell sarcoma).

Diagnosis

High-quality radiographs often demonstrate joint effusion and early signs of DJD (**Figures 15.85–15.88**). Joint effusion may cause cranial displacement of the

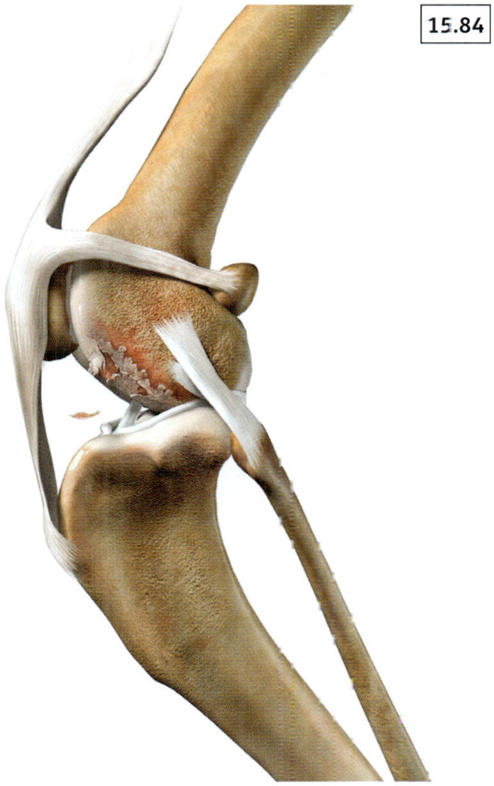

Figure 15.84 Osteochondrosis dissecans of the femoral condyle is a differential diagnosis for stifle lameness; however, the condition does not present with cranial drawer motion.

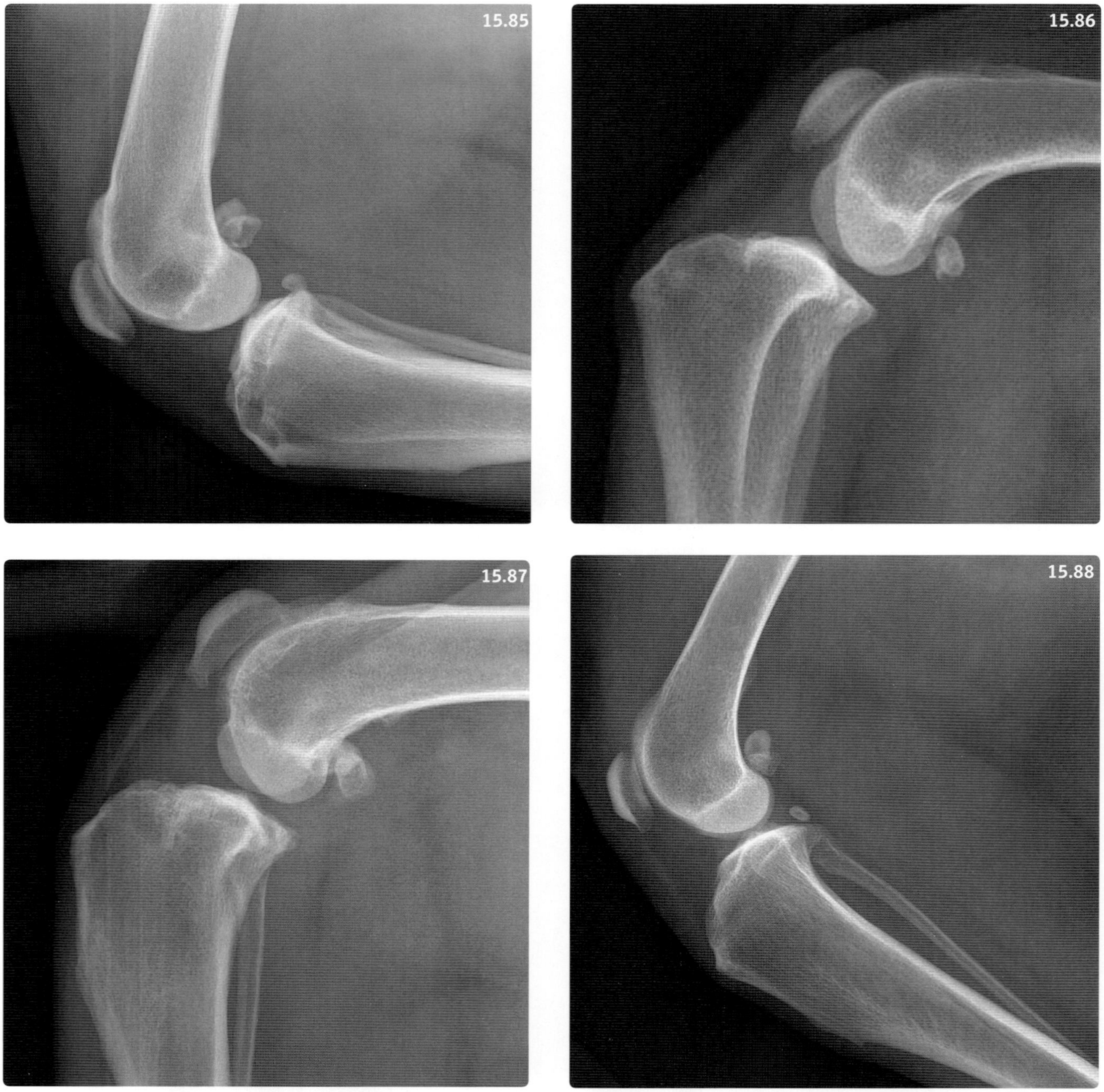

Figures 15.85–15.88 Radiographs showing the relative displacement of the fat pad in mild (15.85), moderate (15.86), and severe (15.87) cranial cruciate ligament rupture, contrasted with the normal joint (15.88). (Courtesy B. Poteet)

infrapatellar fat pad, and osteophyte deposition is commonly observed on the distal pole of the patella in more chronic cases. A bow-legged conformation, internal rotation of the tibia, or straight stifle increases suspicion of cruciate disease. Thickening of the medial joint capsule is characteristic of long-standing disease. Cranial drawer motion is the hallmark of cruciate compromise and may be detected by the cranial drawer test in either flexion or extension. The tibial compression test is also diagnostic. Partial tears of the craniomedial band of the ligament are identified by palpation when cranial tibial displacement is prevented by extension, but abnormal cranial drawer motion is evident in flexion. Due to periarticular fibrosis, cranial drawer motion may be difficult to elicit in dogs with chronic cruciate disease.

Management

Treatment options are influenced by the animal's weight, age, intended use, concurrent medical problems, economic considerations, and veterinary surgical training. Dogs >15 kg body weight clearly benefit from surgical therapy, while smaller dogs and cats are often treated conservatively.

Conservative therapy is basically restriction of activity and use of NSAID analgesics. Leash walking and swimming are appropriate exercise activities. The objectives of surgery are joint stabilization and minimizing secondary DJD.

Hundreds of surgical methods of joint stabilization have been described, suggesting that no one method is ideal. At present, extracapsular stabilization, tibial plateau leveling osteotomy techniques, and tibial tuberosity advancement are in favor. Irrespective of the technique for stabilization, the joint must be inspected for meniscal damage. The frequency of meniscal damage increases with chronicity and is as great as 80% in dogs with complete tears.

ADVANCED DIAGNOSTIC TECHNIQUES

Increasingly sophisticated tests for the diagnosis of musculoskeletal disorders have become available over recent years. Patient history and physical examination continue to be the mainstay; however, arthroscopy, CT, and MRI are becoming more integrated into our diagnostic offerings. In addition, nuclear scintigraphy, ultrasonography, and gait analysis are techniques for special interests.

Magnetic resonance imaging

MRI offers excellent contrast and resolution, providing the ability to differentiate between adjacent joint structures.

Indications

Any soft tissue structure that can be placed within the magnetic field. Common uses include:

- CNS diseases of the brain and spinal cord; peripheral nerve root diseases.
- Orthopedic conditions of tendons, ligaments, joint capsule, connective tissue, and bone marrow.
- Nasal, oral, and auditory diseases.

Contraindication

Cases precluding general anesthesia.

Advantages

- Helpful in early disease detection.
- Assists in chemotherapy and radiation therapy planning.
- Noninvasive.
- Higher contrast makes MR image quality superior to that of reconstructed CT images.
- Chemically maps body tissues.
- Excellent detection of tissue hemorrhage and edema.
- Allows image acquisition in any anatomic plane.
- Paramagnetic contrast medium is very safe.
- Allows detection of diskospondylitis before radiographic detection.
- More accurate detection of tumor invasion to adjacent structures.
- Absence of ionizing radiation.
- High sensitivity in detecting abnormal bone marrow.

Disadvantages

- Highly motion sensitive.
- Resolution inferior to that of CT images.
- Cannot image body areas containing metal.
- Limited availability.
- Very expensive purchase and maintenance.

Computed tomography

The newest CT technology is spiral or helical scanning. In CT the patient continuously moves through a gantry on a motorized couch, while the x-ray tube rotates continually during the patient transit. This gives a volumetric representation of the resulting pixels that allows for 3-D reconstruction. Multiple slices (1–64) are taken per rotation. The technique is very fast, requiring approximately 10 seconds to do an entire canine thorax.

Indications

- Any body part can be assessed, provided it can fit within the gantry.
- Skull and CNS lesions most often assessed in veterinary patients.

Contraindication

Cases precluding general anesthesia.

Advantages

- Excellent resolution (down to 0.1 mm diameter) and detail.

- Excellent image contrast, with 2,000 shades of gray.
- Any areas of mineral and gas are detectable, where they are unseen in conventional radiographs.
- Noninvasive.

Disadvantages

- General anesthesia required.
- Limited availability.
- Large doses of ionizing radiation.
- Limited gantry size.
- Expense.

Arthroscopy

Arthroscopy has revolutionized orthopedic surgery since its veterinary acceptance in the 1970s. In the equine species, arthroscopy has replaced many arthrotomies. A characteristic value of arthroscopy is that this procedure can serve as both a diagnostic and treatment technique at the same time. The technique is implemented as an adjunct to a thorough orthopedic and radiographic examination.

Advantages

- Is routinely available at surgical referral centers.
- Offers a minimally invasive technique, with few complications.
- Provides a detailed view and magnification of intra-articular structures and lesions.

Disadvantages

- Requires a substantial financial investment and long learning curve.
- Has limited application in the smaller breeds.
- Is associated with a low frequency of complications, the most common of which is perhaps iatrogenic cartilage damage associated with instrument insertion and manipulation.

FURTHER READING

Barr FJ, Kirberger RM (2006) *BSAVA Manual of Canine and Feline Musculoskeletal Imaging*. British Small Animal Veterinary Association, Gloucester.

Houlton JEF, Cook JL, Innes JF *et al.* (2006) (eds.) *BSAVA Manual of Canine and Feline Musculoskeletal Disorders*. British Small Animal Veterinary Association, Gloucester.

Johnston SA (1997) Osteoarthritis. Joint anatomy, physiology, and pathobiology. *Vet Clin North Am Small Anim Pract* **27(4)**:699–723.

Levine D, Millis DL, Marcellin-Little DJ *et al.* (2005) Introduction to veterinary physical rehabilitation. *Vet Clin North Am Small Anim Practice* **35(6)**:1247–1254.

Renberg WC, Roush JD (2001) Lameness. *Vet Clin North Am Small Anim Pract* **33(1)**.

Safra N, Johnson EG, Lit L *et al.* (2013) Clinical mainifestations, response to treatment, and clinical outcome for Weimaraners with hypertrophic osteodystrophy. *J Am Vet Med Assoc* **242**:1260–1266

Scott HW, McLaughlin R (2007) *Feline Orthopedics*. Manson Publishing, London.

Chapter 16

Hematologic disorders

Katie M. Boes & Rose E. Raskin

INTRODUCTION

Blood disorders occur commonly in dogs and cats, often secondary to systemic disease or injury. History, physical examination, and laboratory diagnostic tests are crucial for recognition and complete characterization of these disorders. Complete blood count (CBC) and bone marrow evaluation are the laboratory diagnostic tests most often used.

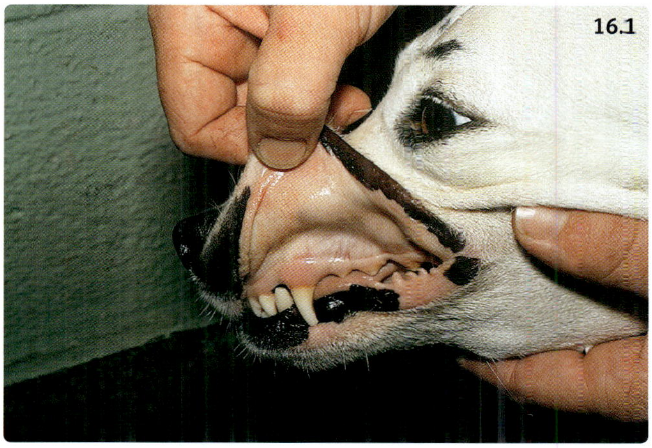

Figure 16.1 Marked pallor. (Courtesy M. Schaer)

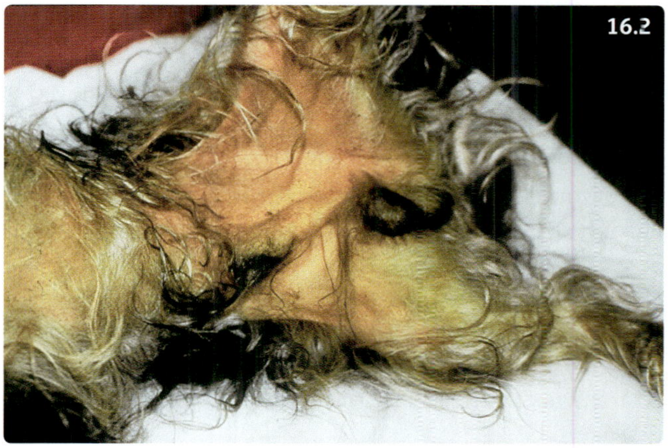

Figure 16.2 Icterus demonstrated by yellow skin discoloration. (Courtesy J. Thompson)

ERYTHROCYTE DISORDERS (NON-NEOPLASTIC)

ANEMIA

Definition/overview

Anemia is one of the most frequent hematologic abnormalities encountered in practice. It is not a disease, but rather the reflection of a disease state.

Etiology

The three general causes of anemia are erythrocyte loss (hemorrhage), lysis (hemolysis), and decreased production (hypoplasia or aplasia).

Pathophysiology

A decreased red blood cell (RBC) mass leads to insufficient oxygen delivery to vital organs, and subsequent decreased aerobic metabolism, energy production, and tissue function. Cellular and tissue injury can occur with more severe or prolonged anemia.

Clinical presentation

Common historical signs of anemia include lethargy, depression, weakness, exercise intolerance, and hyporexia. Recumbency, seizures, syncope, and coma may occur with severe anemia. Pale mucous membranes are a common physical examination finding (**Figure 16.1**). With moderate to severe anemia, heart murmur, tachycardia, tachypnea, and dyspnea may be appreciated. Icterus (**Figure 16.2**) may occur with hemolytic anemia or internal hemorrhage, whereas intravascular hemolytic anemia can cause red plasma (hemolysis, **Figure 16.3**) and urine (hemoglobinuria) in addition to icterus. Hemorrhage into the thoracic and abdominal cavities may cause dyspnea and abdominal enlargment, respectively. Occasionally, anemia may be discovered during routine blood evaluation, even when the animal appears clinically normal. Sedentary animals, especially cats, often have a moderate anemia that goes unnoticed for

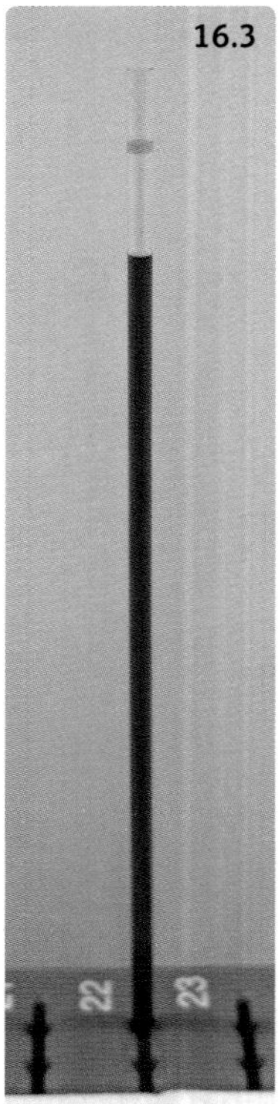

Figure 16.3 Red plasma and PCV of 0.14 l/l (14%) in an animal with intravascular hemolysis.

long periods of time. Splenomegaly and hepatomegaly frequently occur due to increased extravascular hemolysis or extramedullary hematopoiesis.

Differential diagnosis

Trauma with blood loss, platelet or clotting factor deficiency, hemoparasitism, infectious diseases, neoplasia, immune-mediated disease, drug or plant toxicosis, chronic organ disease, inflammation.

Diagnosis

A complete history and physical examination should evaluate for trauma or surgery, sites of blood loss, drug or toxin exposure, concurrent disease, and duration of disease.

Complete blood count

Anemia is identified by a decreased packed cell volume (PCV), hematocrit (Hct), RBC count, or hemoglobin (Hgb) concentration. The PCV is the most accurate and least expensive method of documenting anemia. It is performed by centrifuging a microhematocrit tube filled with anticoagulated whole blood for 5 minutes at 12,000–15,000 g, and then measuring the RBC volume as a percentage of the total blood volume. Erroneous PCV results may occur with inadequate mixing of blood before filling the microhematocrit tubes, excessive EDTA, and inadequate centrifugation.

The plasma of the spun microhematocrit tube should be evaluated for lipemia, hemolysis, or icterus, since this may help identify the cause of the anemia, disease states, or potential biochemical interferences. The plasma protein or total solids concentration should be determined by refractometer.

The Hct may be calculated from the mean cell volume (MCV) and RBC by a hematology analyzer (Equation 1), or it may be measured by conductivity by some blood gas instruments. The Hct is similar to the PCV, except the PCV is typically greater than the Hct by 1–3 percentage units due to trapped plasma between RBCs in the microhematocrit tube. The calculated Hct is inaccurate when the MCV or RBC results are erroneous, whereas the conductivity Hct may be affected by factors that alter the electrical conductivity of blood, such as excessive EDTA, excessive or deficient blood particles (e.g. leukocytosis, thrombocytosis, hyperproteinemia, or hypoproteinemia), or electrolyte disturbances.

$$\text{Equation 1: Hct} = \text{MCV} \times \text{RBC count}/10$$
$$\text{Example: MCV} = 50\ \text{fl; RBC count} = 8.00 \times 10^6/\mu l$$
$$\text{Hct}\ (\%) = 50 \times 8.00/10 = 40$$

Hgb concentration is typically determined using a spectrophotometer by the cyanmethemoglobin method or a cyanide-free method. Artifactual increases may occur with gross lipemia, excessive Heinz bodies, or some monoclonal gammopathies.

The RBC count is usually performed by an automated cell counter or, less commonly, by a hemocytometer. The RBC count may be inaccurate with inadequate mixing of the sample, clots in the sample, *in-vitro* hemolysis, RBC agglutination, and marked thrombocytosis.

The mean cell hemoglobin (MCH) and mean cell hemoglobin concentration (MCHC) are calculated RBC indices (Equations 2 and 3) that help classify the type of anemia as normochromic (normal MCH and MCHC) or hypochromic (decreased MCH and MCHC). When these values are discrepant, MCHC is the preferred index for interpretation. Decreased values reflect the presence of young RBCs (reticulocytes) or abnormal hemoglobinization (e.g. iron deficiency). Increased levels occur artifactually from hemolysis, lipemia, Heinz bodies, or paraproteins.

MCV may be determined directly by automated cell counters or calculated (Equation 4). MCV reflects RBC size and may be categorized as macrocytic (increased MCV), microcytic (decreased MCV), or normocytic (normal MCV). An increased MCV may occur with underfilled EDTA tubes, RBC regeneration, feline leukemia virus (FeLV) infection, breed variation (Toy and Miniature Poodle dogs),

RBC agglutination, and hyperosmolarity. Decreased MCVs are observed with iron deficiency, liver disease, portosystemic shunts, breed variation (Akita and Shiba dogs), young animals, and hypo-osmolarity.

Equation 2: MCH = Hgb × 10/RBC count
Equation 3: MCHC = Hgb × 100/Hct
Equation 4: MCV = Hct x 10/RBC count
Example: Hgb = 12.0 g/dl; RBC count = 7.00 × 10^6/µl; Hct = 30%
MCH (pg) = 12.0 × 10/7.00 = 17.1
MCHC (g/dl) = 12.0 × 100/30 = 40
MCV (fl) = 30 × 10/7.00 = 43

Blood smear evaluation of RBCs involves qualification of changes in size (anisocytosis), shape (poikilocytosis), and color (chromasia). The presence of abnormal red cells (e.g. nucleated precursors, basophilic stippling, infectious parasites, and Heinz bodies) or red cell arrangement (e.g. agglutination and rouleaux) should be noted.

Reticulocyte counts

Reticulocytes are young RBCs that contain more RNA and less Hgb than mature RBCs. Most reticulocytes develop into mature RBCs in the bone marrow, and are subsequently released into peripheral circulation. However, low numbers of reticulocytes are present in blood under normal hematologic conditions. Increased numbers of reticulocytes in blood (reticulocytosis) are seen with tissue hypoxia, and the presence or absence of reticulocytosis classifies the anemia as regenerative or nonregenerative, respectively.

Reticulocyte counts may be determined by automated hematology analyzers or by manual methods. For manual reticulocyte count quantification, equal volumes of blood and 0.5% new methylene blue stain are incubated together for 15–20 minutes at room temperature. Then, a routine blood smear is made and allowed to dry. The numbers of aggregated (dogs and cats) and punctate (cats) forms per 1,000 erythrocytes are counted to determine the reticulocyte percentage (Retic%) (**Figures 16.4, 16.5**). The absolute reticulocyte count (Retic#) is the more accurate reflection of RBC regeneration, and is calculated from the Retic% and RBC count (Equation 5).

Equation 5: Retic# = RBC count × Retic% × 10,000
Example: RBC count = 3.00 × 10^6/µl; Retic% = 3.5%
Retic# (/µl) = 3.00 × 3.5 × 10,000 = 105,000

Dogs normally have 0–1% reticulocytes (0–80,000/µl) in blood. In normal cats, aggregated reticulocytes range from 0% to 0.4% (0–30,000/µl) and punctate reticulocytes are <5% (<500,000/µl). Aggregated reticulocytes represent the most active or recent form of regeneration in the dog and cat, and are identified as polychromatophils in Romanowsky-stained smears. Punctate reticulocytes in cats do not stain as polychromatophilic cells and they represent past regeneration that occurred in the prior 2–4 weeks.

Note: The absolute reticulocyte count is the best method to identify regeneration. In the absence of a reticulocyte count, increased polychromasia on a Romanowsky-stained blood smear is the only RBC morphology that is specific for regeneration. Within the monolayer, dogs normally have 0–1 polychromatophils/100× objective field, and cats have no to rare polychromatophils/100× objective field. Greater numbers reflect regeneration.

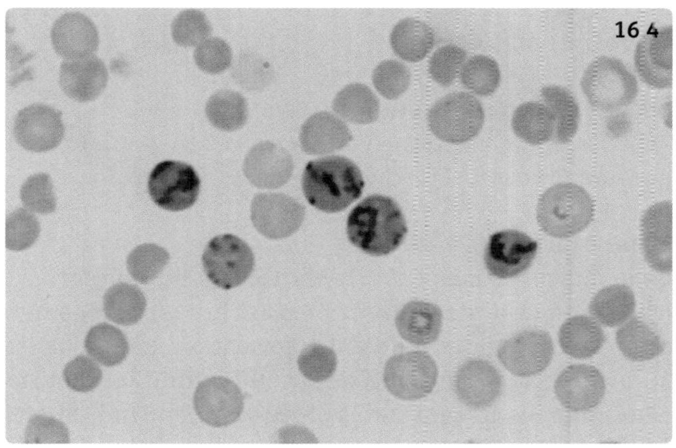

Figure 16.4 New methylene blue-stained blood smear from a dog, showing five aggregated reticulocytes.

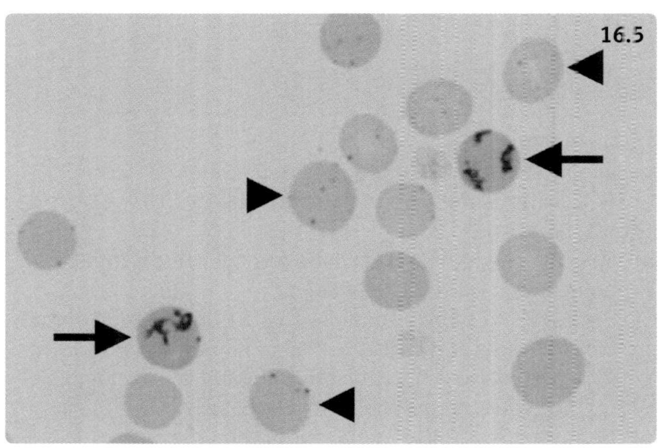

Figure 16.5 Feline aggregated (arrows) and punctate (arrowheads) reticulocytes demonstrated by new methylene blue stain.

When the RBC count is not available, the PCV may be used to calculate the corrected reticulocyte percentage (CRP, Equation 6). A CRP value >1% indicates increased RBC regeneration. Once initiated in the bone marrow, regeneration may take at least 3 days before reticulocytes appear in circulation.

Equation 6: CRP = Retic% × (patient's Hct)/(average Hct for species)

Example (dog): Retic% = 3.5%; patient's Hct = 20; average Hct for dogs = 45%

CRP (%) = 3.5 x 20/45 = 1.6

Example (cat): Retic% = 2.5%; patient's Hct = 20; average Hct for cats = 35%

CRP (%) = 2.5 x 20/35 = 1.4

Biochemical profiles

Biochemical profiles may reveal disease that can affect the ability to regenerate erythrocytes, especially diseases of the liver and kidney.

Fecal examination and urinalysis

These tests are performed to determine sources of blood loss and function of the kidney.

Bone marrow evaluation

Bone marrow evaluation (**Table 16.1**) is best performed when both aspirate and core biopsies are taken together, since each provides different information. Results must always be compared with a recent CBC (within 24 hours) to determine the current status of regeneration. Indications for bone marrow evaluation include persistent cytopenia(s) of unknown etiology, diagnosing leukemia or infectious myelitis, and cancer staging. This is a sterile procedure often performed with only local anesthesia; however, sedation with reversible or general anesthesia may be used.

Sites frequently used in dogs include the dorsal ilium, humerus (best for obese animals), and femur (small dogs or puppies). Sites frequently used in cats include the humerus, femur, and dorsal ilium by transilial or perpendicular approach (**Figures 16.6–16.8**). Specialized needles are preferred for the collection process and the procedures are well established.

Classifying the general cause of anemia

The above tests help classify the cause of anemia as hemorrhage, hemolysis, or decreased RBC production (**Table 16.2**).

16.6

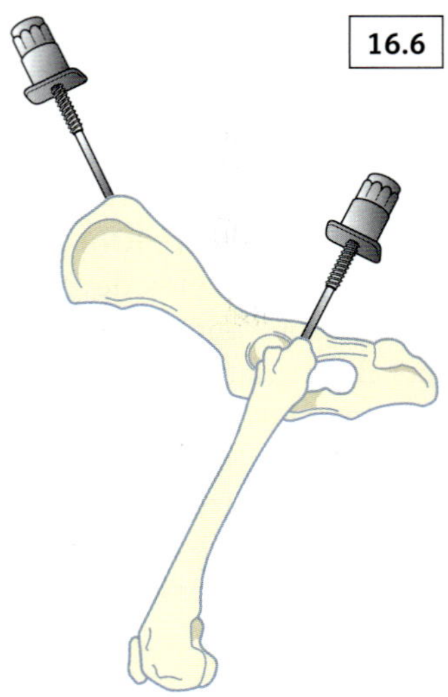

Figure 16.6 Bone marrow sites for aspiration and core biopsy using the dorsal crest of the ilium and the proximal femur. The parallel approach to the ilium is best for aspiration biopsy in medium or large sized breeds having an easily palpable crest protuberance.

Table 16.1 Bone marrow aspiration and core biopsy procedures for the dog and cat.

Aspiration biopsy	Core biopsy
Equipment: • Illinois sternal disposable needle, 15–18 G, 2.5–5 cm (1–2 inches) long (Cardinal Health, Dublin, OH) Procedure: • Pass the needle with its stylet a few millimeters into the bone until it is firmly embedded • Place a 12 ml syringe coated with 5% EDTA solution onto the biopsy needle and collect 1–2 ml of bloody material • Place the marrow material into a plastic Petri dish and pick up the glistening particles with a pipette • Gently express this material out of the tube onto a glass slide • Make a squash preparation by laying a second slide on the first and pulling them horizontally apart	Equipment: • Jamshidi aspiration/biopsy disposable needle, 11–13 G, 5–10 cm (2–4 inches) long (Cardinal Health, Dublin, OH) Procedure: • Pass the needle with stylet through the skin and subcutaneous tissues • Remove the stylet while advancing the needle 0.5–1.5 cm into the bone, depending on the size of the animal • Twist the instrument sharply to cut the sample and withdraw the needle slowly • Remove the core sample and roll it onto a glass slide for cytologic examination; following this, place sample in 10% buffered formalin for histologic fixation

16.7

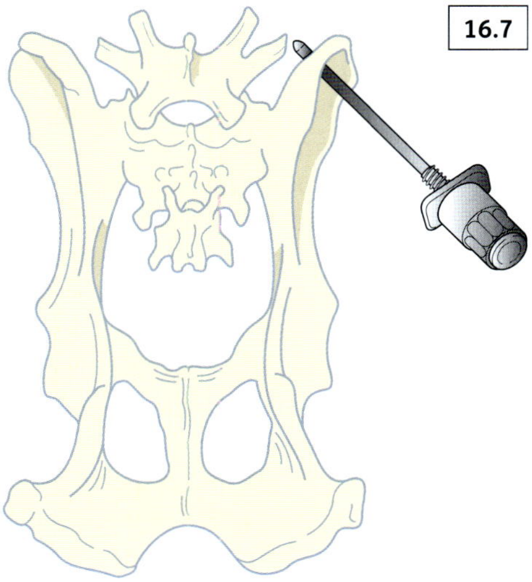

Figure 16.7 Bone marrow site for the transilial approach for core biopsy in a cat or small dog.

16.8

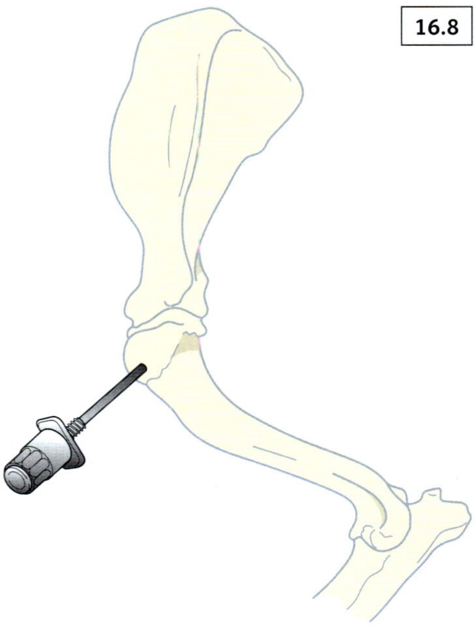

Figure 16.8 Bone marrow site for aspiration and core biopsy using the anterior or lateral side of the proximal humerus. This site is especially helpful in obese animals.

Historical and physical support for hemorrhage includes a history of trauma or surgery or the observation of bleeding wounds, petechiae, ecchymoses, heavy external or intestinal parasitism, epistaxis, hemoptysis, melena, hematochezia, hemorrhagic effusions, or hematuria. Hemorrhage typically causes regenerative anemia, but nonregenerative anemia may occur with peracute hemorrhage prior to the release of reticulocytes from the bone marrow (preregenerative anemia), or with chronic external blood loss leading to iron deficiency. Proportionate decreases in albumin and globulin concentrations, termed panhypoproteinemia, support hemorrhage as the cause of anemia since proteins are also lost with extravasation of whole blood. An increased urea nitrogen concentration relative to creatinine concentration can occur with excessive intestinal absorption of protein due to gastric or small intestinal hemorrhage.

Excessive destruction of mature RBCs results in regenerative anemia unless the hemolysis is peracute, and therefore preregenerative. Support for hemolysis as the cause of anemia includes yellow plasma or mucous membranes (icterus), red plasma (hemolysis), and hemoglobin in the urine (hemoglobinuria). Since icterus may occur with other disease processes (e.g. liver disease or obstructional cholestasis), it is not pathognomonic for hemolysis. Panhypoproteinemia is not an expected finding of hemolysis.

Decreased RBC production causes nonregenerative anemia. Therefore, reticulocyte counts are typically within normal limits or decreased. Icterus or hemolysis does not typically occur, but icterus may occur with nonregenerative immune-mediated hemolytic anemia (IMHA) or if there is concurrent liver or cholestatic disease. Nonregenerative anemia is not directly linked with panhypoproteinemia.

Table 16.2 Indicators of general categories of anemia.

	Blood loss	Hemolysis	Decreased production
Clinical	Hemorrhage; trauma	Icteric plasma and mucous membranes; red plasma	
CBC	Reticulocytosis; increased polychromasia; decreased plasma proteins	Reticulocytosis, increased polychromasia; increased MCHC	No reticulocytosis, no polychromasia; other cytopenias
Chemistry	Increased BUN vs. creatinine; panhypoproteinemia; hyperbilirubinemia (internal hemorrhage)	Hyperbilirubinemia	
Urinalysis	Red urine with RBCs in sediment; bilirubinuria (internal hemorrhage)	Golden-orange urine; red urine without RBCs in sediment; bilirubinuria	

Management

Principles of transfusion therapy

Blood transfusion depends on the etiology, severity, and chronicity of the anemia. Whole blood or packed RBCs (RBCs without plasma) may be administered when the anemia is not caused by a coagulopathy. If a coagulopathy is causing the anemia, then whole blood or plasma should be given, if warranted (see Chapter 17: Disorders of hemostasis). Rapid decreases in RBC mass can cause more severe clinical signs and patient outcomes since physiologic compensation mechanisms are more easily overwhelmed. However, slow daily decreases in PCV of 0.01–0.03 l/l (1–3%) may not cause clinical signs of dyspnea or weakness. Generally, replacement therapy may not be warranted until the PCV drops below 0.20–0.25 l/l (20–25%), since compensatory mechanisms begin to fail at lower RBC masses. When the PCV reaches 0.10 l/l (10%), transfusion therapy becomes imperative.

Pretransfusion testing should be performed to ensure efficacy of treatment and patient safety. Pretransfusion compatibility testing includes blood typing and cross-matching. Blood typing detects antigen on the cell surface, while cross-matching detects the presence of antibody on the cell surface.

Dogs do not have naturally occurring RBC alloantibodies. Therefore, dogs develop alloimmune RBC antibodies when they are exposed to foreign RBCs during pregnancy, parturition, or blood transfusion. At least 12 dog erythrocyte antigens (DEAs) have been identified, but DEAs 1.1, 1.2, 4, 7, and Dal are most likely to induce alloantibody formation. Blood typing and cross-matching are not essential prior to a nonparous patient's first blood transfusion, but administering DEA 1.1-positive blood to a DEA 1.1-negative dog will reduce the blood donor pool if subsequent blood transfusions are needed. Alloantibodies develop 4 days after the first transfusion; therefore, a cross-match should be performed if additional transfusions are given after this timeframe.

Cats have three major RBC types: type A, type B, and type AB. Type A is the most prevalent blood type in the US, with type B cats more commonly identified in Europe and Australia; type AB cats are rare. Exotic breeds of cats, including Abyssinians, Birmans, Persians, Himalayans, and Rexes, have an increased prevalence of type B blood. RBC alloantibodies occur naturally in cats, except in type AB cats, which do not produce A or B alloantibodies. At a minimum, all cats should be blood typed prior to their first blood transfusion to ensure they receive appropriate type A or type B blood. However, only typing for A and B antigens carries a slight risk of not identifying other natural occurring alloantibodies, such as the recently identified Mik antigen. If blood typing is not available, a cross-match should be performed. Similar to dogs, cross-matching should be performed if blood is administered 4 or more days after the first transfusion.

During cross-match testing, incompatibility between patient and donor manifests itself as hemolysis and/or agglutination in either the major or minor cross-matches (**Table 16.3**). If the donor autocontrol displays either hemolysis or agglutination, it is best not to use it. If the donor autocontrol displays these changes, the major and minor cross-match results will be difficult, if not impossible, to interpret. A major cross-match incompatibility indicates that the donor's blood may not be used. However, incompatibility in the minor cross-match may not prevent use of the donor's blood if a better match cannot be found. The decision is up to the clinician, and the blood transfusion should be carefully monitored.

Table 16.3 Standard cross-matching procedures used to detect transfusion incompatibility.

- Collect from each patient and donor, 1 tube for serum (red top) and 1 tube for cells (purple top)
- Wash cells 3 times in 0.9% saline
- Add 4.8 ml saline to 0.2 ml RBCs to make a 4% cell suspension
- Red cells and serum mixtures are:
  - Major cross-match: donor RBCs (0.1 ml or 2 drops) + patient serum (0.1 ml or 2 drops)
  - Minor cross-match: patient RBCs (0.1 ml or 2 drops) + donor serum (0.1 ml or 2 drops)
  - Donor control: donor cells (0.1 ml or 2 drops) + donor serum (0.1 ml or 2 drops)
  - Patient control: patient cells (0.1 ml or 2 drops) + patient serum (0.1 ml or 2 drops)
- Incubate each mixture in a glass tube for 15 minutes at 37°C (98.6°F) to evaluate compatibility. Additional incubations at room temperature and 4°C (39.2°F) may be performed to identify cold agglutinins and hemolysins
- Centrifuge tubes at 280 g for 1 minute
- Examine the supernatant for hemolysis in all cross-matches, including autocontrols. Report the presence of hemolysis relative to autocontrols
- Examine cell suspension for gross and microscopic agglutination in all cross-matches, including autocontrols. Agglutination is defined as the collection of three or more RBCs. Report the presence of agglutination relative to autocontrols

Efficacy of the blood transfusion is assessed by measuring the Hct, PCV, or Hgb prior to and after the administration of whole blood or packed RBCs. Intermittently measuring the patient's vital signs (e.g. body temperature, heart rate, respiratory rate, and blood pressure) during and several hours after a transfusion promotes early identification of transfusion-related adverse events. The transfusion should be discontinued if severe signs are noted (e.g. urticaria, vomiting, diarrhea, or collapse).

Blood transfusion

The goal of transfusion therapy is to provide the anemic patient with sufficient oxygen-carrying particles (erythrocytes or oxyglobin solution) to alleviate clinical signs of hypoxia, but with as little product as necessary so as to reduce the likelihood of transfusion reactions and volume overload. Smaller dosages may be needed in chronic anemias due to the presence of physiologic compensation and internal blood loss anemia, since hemorrhaged RBCs will re-enter the circulation (approximately 50% over 24 hours). Massive transfusions (e.g. 90 ml/kg in 24 hours or 45 ml/kg in 3 hours in the dog) may be required for acute, marked decreases in RBCs, such as acute external hemorrhage. In these cases, the patient should be monitored for hypocalcemia and hypomagnesemia secondary to citrate anticoagulant administration.

In general, the optimal component for normovolemic patients (e.g. normovolemic blood loss anemia, anemia of chronic kidney disease, anemia of bone marrow failure, and hemolytic anemia) is packed RBCs. Hypovolemic blood loss anemia is best treated with packed RBCs and hypertonic fluids (e.g. crystalloid or colloid solutions) in separate lines and into different veins. However, whole blood or oxyglobin solution are alternate components that can be given to any patient, and product availability often dictates which component will be administered. Initial dosages are 6–10 ml packed RBCs/kg, 10–15 ml packed RBCs in additive solution/kg, or 10–20 ml whole blood/kg.

Appropriate filters and administration sets must be used to retain clotted blood or debris. The blood does not need to be warmed prior to administration. For the first 30 minutes, the initial rate of administration should be kept slow (e.g. 0.25 ml/kg) in order to observe any incompatibility reactions. After initial transfusion, normovolemic patients can receive rates of 10–20 ml/kg/hour, but hypovolemic patients with acute anemia can receive rates up to 60 ml/kg/hour. Slow transfusion rates are recommended for patients with cardiac disease, but any transfusion should be given within 4 hours of initiating treatment. If not initially hemolyzed, transfused RBCs have a half-life of approximately 21–35 days.

REGENERATIVE ANEMIA

Regenerative anemia is anemia with increased numbers of reticulocytes in the blood. It identifies the cause of the anemia as RBC loss from blood vessels or RBC destruction. Depending on the severity of hemorrhage or hemolysis, the regenerative response may be mild to strong. In some cases, the anemia may occur so rapidly that the animal may have too little time to mount a regenerative response by the time the condition is recognized. A period of 2–3 days is necessary for RBC maturation, once the stimulation from hypoxia has occurred. Therefore, anemia due to hemorrhage or hemolysis may appear nonregenerative during this preregenerative phase. Sequential CBCs can help differentiate preregenerative anemia from nonregenerative anemia.

ACUTE BLOOD LOSS

Definition/overview

Whole blood is lost from the blood vessels. Hemorrhage may be internal (e.g. abdominal, thoracic, or pericardial cavities) or external (e.g. gastrointestinal [GI] tract or environment).

Etiology

Common causes of blood loss include trauma, surgery, external and internal parasitism, gastric ulcers, tumors of the GI and urinary systems, splenic rupture, coagulation abnormalities, marked thrombocytopenia, and phlebotomy (**Table 16.4**).

Pathophysiology

Large volumes of blood must be lost before appreciable changes occur in the number of erythrocytes or the PCV. The immediate loss of blood results in little or no change to the PCV, owing to the concurrent and proportional loss of RBCs and plasma. In an attempt to increase blood volume and pressure, the body redistributes fluid from the extravascular space to the intravascular space over the course of several hours to days. This results in a lowered

Table 16.4 Common causes of blood loss.

Trauma
Surgery
External and internal parasitism
Gastric ulcers
Tumors of the gastrointestinal and urinary systems
Splenic rupture
Coagulation abnormalities

PCV and plasma protein concentration. Physiologic alterations to acute blood loss include preservation of perfusion of the brain, heart, and viscera by restricting blood flow to less essential tissues such as the skin.

Clinical presentation

Animals with acute blood loss of >20% of normal blood volume have pale, dry mucous membranes and decreased capillary refill time (CRT). This is the result of several hemodynamic mechanisms directing blood away from less essential tissue to preserve perfusion of important organs such as the brain and heart. Animals usually present with cardiovascular signs such as tachycardia, as the heart compensates in an attempt to maintain cardiac output. Blood losses of 30–40% of normal blood volume cause decreased cardiac output and hypotension, and cardiovascular collapse occurs. Such animals are usually immobile and have a rapid pulse and cold extremities and skin. Blood losses of >50% normal blood volume cause shock and death within hours.

Differential diagnosis

Disorders of hemostasis, hemolytic conditions, and intracavitary hemorrhage.

Diagnosis

A CBC, with assessment of erythrocyte morphology, reticulocyte count, and calculation of red cell indices, are the most important laboratory data to obtain from anemic animals. Other diagnostic tests include physical examination for external wounds or parasites, fecal floatation, fecal occult blood, buccal mucosal bleeding time and coagulation testing, total protein, urinalysis, abdominal and thoracic imaging, body cavity fluid analysis, and endoscopy.

Management

Blood or oxyglobin solution transfusions should be considered when acute hemorrhage causes the PCV to drop to 0.2–0.25 l/l (20–25%) in the dog or cat. The cause of the hemorrhage should be appropriately treated.

HEMOLYTIC ANEMIA

Hemolytic anemia is most commonly a result of immune-mediated destruction, RBC parasites, oxidant-induced injury, or mechanical fragmentation (microangiopathy). Blood smear evaluation has a critical role in differentiating the causes of hemolysis (**Table 16.5**), and therefore the appropriate disease treatment.

PRIMARY (IDIOPATHIC) IMMUNE-MEDIATED HEMOLYTIC ANEMIA

Definition/overview

IMHA is antibody-mediated RBC destruction. It is subclassified into primary (idiopathic) IMHA and secondary IMHA. The primary form is characterized by a dysregulated immune system that produces antibodies against unaltered RBC surface antigens in the absence of an identifiable cause. Secondary IMHA may occur as a sequela to infection, drugs, or neoplasms that typically alter RBC

Table 16.5 Potential erythrocyte abnormalities with main causes of hemolysis.

	Immune-mediated	Infectious	Oxidant-induced	Microangiopathy
Ghost cells	✔	✔	✔	✔
Agglutination	✔	✔		
Spherocytes*	✔	✔		
RBC parasites		✔		
Heinz bodies			✔	
Eccentrocytes			✔	
Methemoglobinemia			✔	
Schistocytes				✔
Acanthocytes				✔
Keratocytes				✔

*Spherocytes are difficult to identify in cats since their red cells normally lack central pallor.

surface antigens. Primary IMHA is the most common form of IMHA in dogs, but the majority of feline IMHAs are secondary.

Etiology

The etiology of primary IMHA is unknown, but regulatory T-lymphocyte dysfunction, defects in central or peripheral tolerance, cross-reactivity with self- and foreign antigens, and exposure of hidden antigens have been implicated. It may be associated with systemic lupus erythematosus (SLE) or other autoimmune disease.

Pathophysiology

Antibodies of the IgG subclass are most commonly implicated in canine IMHA, but IgM antibodies and complement may also contribute to disease. The variable fragment of the antibody binds the RBC surface antigen, marking it for removal by the monocyte–macrophage system, or activating the classical complement pathway. Splenic macrophages, and to a lesser degree hepatic macrophages (Kupffer cells), bind the constant fragment of the RBC-bound antibody. The macrophages either completely phagocytize the RBC and remove it from circulation, or only phagocytize a part of the RBC membrane. Completely phagocytized RBCs are digested, and the hemoglobin is converted to bilirubin, which results in clinical icterus and hyperbilirubinemia. The partially phagocytized RBC remains in circulation, but with an abnormal RBC morphology (spherocyte). Therefore, spherocytes on a blood smear indicate RBC lysis by macrophages (extravascular hemolysis). Activation of the classical complement pathway can lead to membrane attack complex formation and subsequent RBC lysis within the blood vessel (intravascular hemolysis). The lysed RBC releases its intracellular contents into the plasma, which results in hemoglobinemia and subsequent hemoglobinuria if the haptoglobin savage system is overwhelmed. The lysed RBC membranes can be visualized on a blood smear as ghost cells. *In-vivo* agglutination of RBCs occurs when IgM or high titers of IgG molecules cause bridging of RBCs.

Common causes of death in canine IMHA are tissue hypoxia due to anemia, and thromboembolic disease, including disseminated intravascular coagulation (DIC) and pulmonary thromboembolism.

Clinical presentation

Primary IMHA may occur in dogs of any signalment, but young adult to middle-aged dogs, females, and several breeds (American Cocker Spaniel, Bichon Frise, Collie, English Springer Spaniel, Finnish Spitz, Miniature Pinscher, Miniature Schnauzer, Old English Sheepdog, and Poodle) have an increased risk of disease. In dogs, the mean age is 5–6 years, with a reported range of 1–13 years. In feline IMHA, young, male, mixed breed and Domestic Shorthair cats are overrepresented.

Clinical signs vary with the severity and duration of onset of the anemia, but often include lethargy, depression, weakness, and anorexia. Collapse, vomiting, diarrhea, tachypnea, and polydipsia are less common. Multisystemic hemorrhages may occur secondary to DIC, whereas red urine may occur with intravascular hemolysis.

Pale mucous membranes are the most common physical examination finding, but patients may also exhibit tachycardia, tachypnea, icterus, and fever. A systolic heart murmur may occur from increased turbulences due to low red blood cell content. Due to extravascular phagocytosis, splenomegaly and/or hepatomegaly may be detected. If the patient's autoantibodies are primarily active below normal core body temperatures (cold agglutinins) then clinical signs may be most prominent at the cooler extremities, particularly necrosis of the tail, ear tips, nose, and nail bed (**Figure 16.9**).

Differential diagnosis

Hemorrhage or other causes of hemolysis, including infectious hemolytic anemia, oxidant-induced hemolytic anemia, congenital erythrocyte defects, hypophosphatemia, envenomation, mechanical fragmentation, and hemophagocytic histiocytic sarcoma.

Diagnosis

CBC often reveals severe to moderate (0.05–0.3 l/l [5–30%]) anemia with evidence of regeneration (reticulocytosis and polychromasia) and support for regeneration (increased MCV, decreased MCHC, anisocytosis, nucleated RBCs in circulation [metarubricytosis, rubricytosis, or normoblastemia], Howell–Jolly bodies, basophilic stippling, and siderocytes). Identification of agglutination

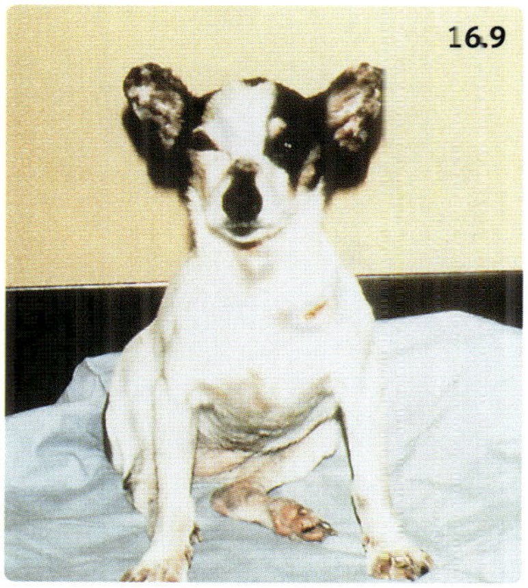

Figure 16.9 Cold agglutinin disease demonstrating necrotic ear tips. (Courtesy J. Thompson)

or spherocytes confirms an immune-mediated etiology for the anemia (**Figures 16.10–16.12**); however, spherocytes are difficult to appreciate in cats since their RBCs normally lack central pallor. The saline test is helpful in distinguishing agglutination from rouleaux. A drop of physiologic saline is mixed with a drop of blood, and then examined as a wet mount. The dilution will reduce rouleau formation, but agglutinated RBCs remain in tight clusters (**Figures 16.13, 16.14**). Ghost cells may be seen with intravascular hemolysis (**Figure 16.15**). The leukogram is often inflammatory, and is characterized by moderate to marked neutrophilia, regenerative left shift, variable lymphocyte counts, and monocytosis. Neutrophil toxicity is usually absent or mild. Neutrophils may contain hemosiderin, and monocytes may exhibit erythrophagocytosis. Thrombocytopenia is present in 25–70% of dogs with IMHA, and may be due to concurrent immune-mediated platelet destruction (Evan's syndrome) or DIC.

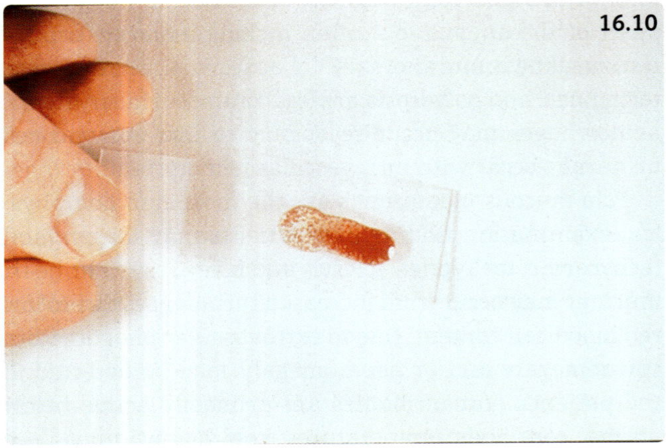

Figure 16.10 Gross appearance of macroscopic agglutination. (Courtesy J. Thompson)

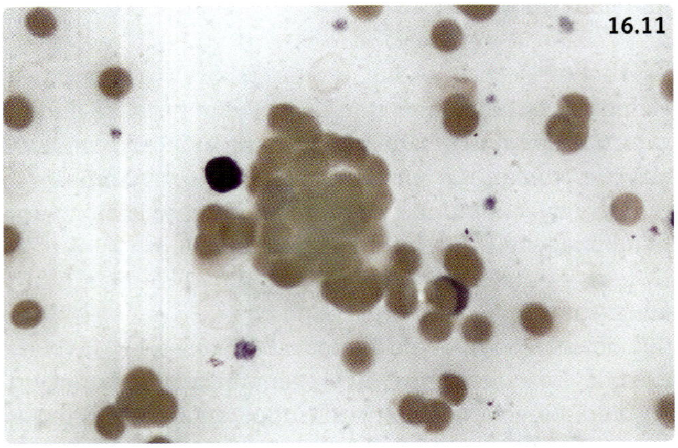

Figure 16.11 Microscopic RBC agglutination on a Romanowsky-stained blood smear.

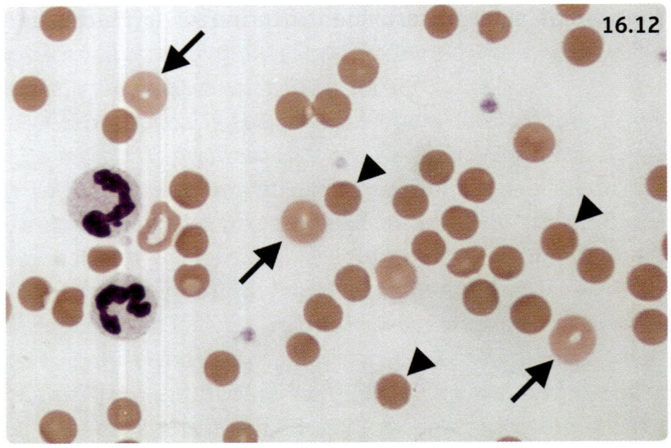

Figure 16.12 Compared with normal RBCs (arrows), spherocytes (arrowheads) are more eosinophilic, appear smaller, and lack central pallor.

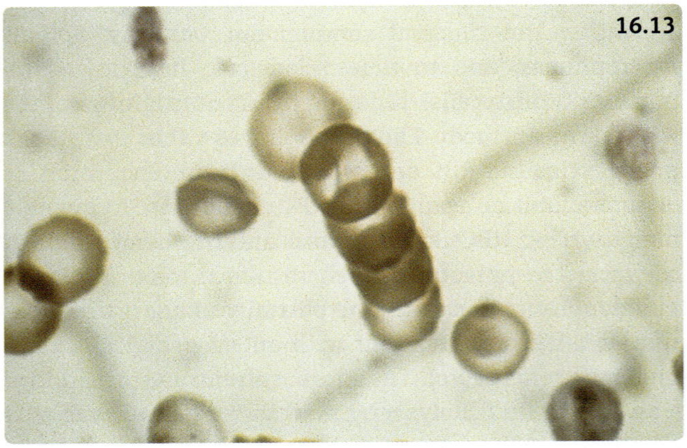

Figure 16.13 Rouleaux formation in a wet mount of blood before the addition of saline to dilute or reduce cell adherence. (Courtesy J. Thompson)

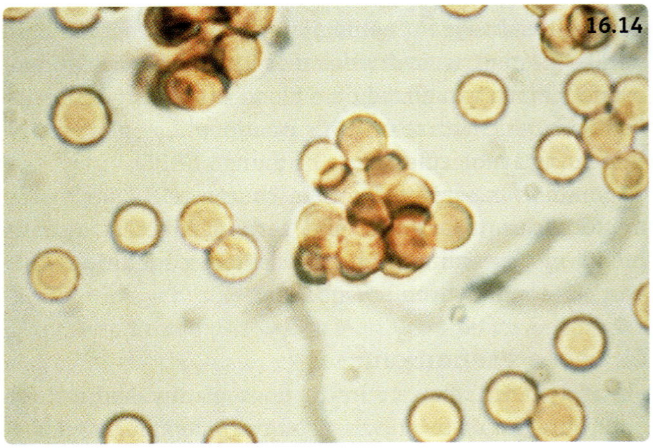

Figure 16.14 Wet mount of blood demonstrating tight red cell clusters following addition of saline, indicating true agglutination. (Courtesy J. Thompson)

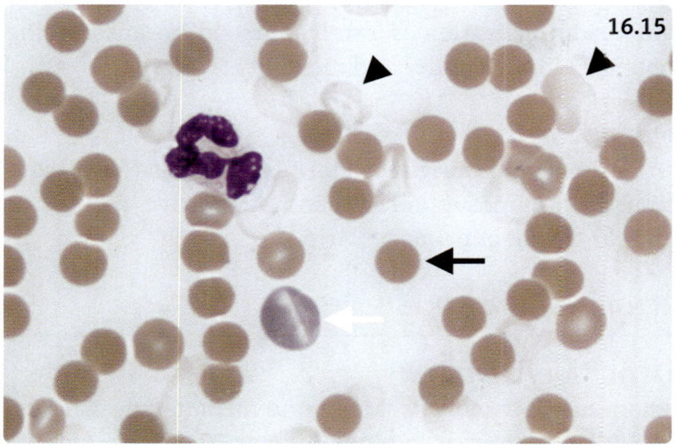

Figure 16.15 Blood smear from a dog with immune-mediated hemolytic anemia shows spherocytes (black arrow), ghost cells (arrowheads), and one polychromatophil (white arrow).

Serum biochemistry findings may include hyperbilirubinemia due to enhanced RBC destruction, and elevations in ALT and AST activities with hypoxic liver injury. ALP activity may be increased with cholestasis and, in the dog, stress.

Urine may be golden yellow or orange due to bilirubinuria or red due to hemoglobinuria. Proteinuria may be attributed to hemoglobinuria or renal injury secondary to immune complex deposition, hypoxia, or hemoglobin nephropathy. Cylindruria may present as Hgb or granular casts.

A direct antiglobulin test or Coombs test identifies antibody and complement on the surface of RBCs, and is used to diagnose IMHA in the absence of agglutination. The Coombs test may be positive in up to 75% of animals with IMHA. For this test, the patient's washed RBCs are combined with antiglobulin reagent. This reagent contains species-specific antibodies that bind complement and the Fc portion of the patient's antibodies. When the patient's complement and antibodies are bound to the patient's RBCs, the antiglobulin reagent creates antibody bridges, and induces RBC agglutination. Agglutination, when observed, is diagnostic for the presence of antibody-coated erythrocytes. A positive Coombs test may also occur with secondary hemolytic anemias, lymphoproliferative disorders, and immune-mediated thrombocytopenia. False-negative results occur with the recent use of corticosteroids or low levels of antibody present on the red cell surface.

Additional tests, such as diagnostic imaging and serologic testing for blood-borne infectious agents, should be pursued to rule out causes of secondary IMHA.

Management

Specific treatment of IMHA is directed at immune suppression, and may involve one or more of the following drugs.

Parenterally administered dexamethasone (0.1–0.2 mg/kg IV q12h) is preferred by many clinicians in the initial management scheme if the patient is unable to receive oral medications. Oral prednisone or prednisolone can be given at a dose of 2 mg/kg for 2–4 weeks. If the PCV is stable, the dose is decreased to 1 mg/kg/day for 2–4 weeks; then, if the PCV is still stable, the dose is decreased to 1 mg/kg every other day for 2–4 weeks, gradually tapered to the lowest effective dose, and maintained on this low alternate day dose for 9–12 months. Treatment for IMHA should probably always include glucocorticoids given in the proper dosage for the appropriate duration. Relapse most often arises when too little is given for too short a time. Side-effects of glucocorticoid therapy include panting, polyuria, polydipsia, polyphagia, alopecia, cutaneous atrophy, vacuolar hepatopathy, and iatrogenic hyperadrenocorticism.

Azathioprine is typically reserved for severe cases of IMHA (intravascular hemolysis, persistent RBC agglutination, or nonregenerative anemia), when the animal is not neutropenic (<2,000/µl) or thrombocytopenic (<80,000/µl). The dosage for dogs is 2 mg/kg/day PO for 1–2 weeks, then 1–2 mg/kg PO every other day; for cats it is 0.3 mg/kg PO every 1–2 days. Although side-effects of azathioprine therapy are infrequent, they may include acute pancreatitis, hepatotoxicosis, bone marrow toxicosis, and GI disease.

Cyclosporine is traditionally reserved for refractory IMHA that fails to respond to corticosteroid and azathioprine therapy. The current recommended starting dose for dogs is 5–10 mg/kg PO q12–24h. Trough plasma levels around 100–300 ng/ml are suggested, and may be monitored every 2–4 weeks. Treatment with cyclosporine may be discontinued after remission occurs for at least 2 weeks. Cyclosporine side-effects include vomiting, gingival hyperplasia, hair loss, and papilloma-like skin lesions.

Cyclophosphamide was used for more severe cases, but its adverse side-effects have decreased its popularity. It may take 1–2 weeks before a significant benefit is seen. The dosage for dogs is 50 mg/m^2 every other day, and for cats it is 200 mg/m^2 every 2 weeks.

Other treatment options may include blood transfusions or splenectomy. Administration of aspirin (0.5 mg/kg PO q24h) has been suggested to prevent thromboemboli in dogs.

Danazol reduces the immune response when used at a dosage in dogs of 7.5 mg/kg PO q12h. The drug is not recommended in cats, as it may be hepatotoxic. In refractory cases, mycophenolate mofetil (10 mg/kg PO q12h, side-effects include diarrhea) or leflunomide (4 mg/kg PO q24h) may be useful.

Prognosis

In general, there is guarded to poor prognosis for long-term survival in dogs. While 50–88% of dogs with IMHA are discharged from the hospital, most die or are euthanized within the subsequent 2 months. Negative prognostic indicators are the presence of severe disease (liver, kidney), thrombocytopenia, SLE, intravascular hemolysis, RBC agglutination, prolonged coagulation times (PT and aPTT), left shift, marked leukocytosis, and icterus. Primary feline IMHA has a 24–32% mortality rate, and relapse occurs in 16–19% of cases.

DRUG-INDUCED IMMUNE HEMOLYTIC ANEMIA

Definition/overview

Red cell destruction is secondary to an adverse or idiosyncratic drug reaction.

Etiology

Substances known to induce immune hemolytic anemia include levamisole, carprofen, cephalosporin antibiotics, griseofulvin, propylthiouracil, and methimazole.

Pathopyhysiology

Drug-induced immune hemolytic anemia (DIIHA) may be drug-dependent or drug-independent. Drug-dependent IHA occurs only in the presence of the inciting drug. In these cases, the immune reaction is directed at the drug, which is bound to RBC surface antigens. Drug-independent IHA may occur in the absence of the inciting drug and is likely secondary to immune system stimulation.

Clinical presentation

Signs are similar to animals with primary IMHA.

Differential diagnosis

Similar to primary IMHA.

Diagnosis

Diagnosis is based on a history of administering a drug known to induce IMHA, the presence of laboratory findings consistent with IMHA, and the absence of other causes of secondary IMHA (e.g. erythrocytic parasites). The diagnosis is confirmed when clinical signs resolve when the drug is withheld, but then reappear with subsequent administration of the drug. However, confirmation via readministration is rarely pursued because of the potential for morbidity and mortality.

Management

Drugs known to cause secondary IMHA should be discontinued. Immunosuppressive and supportive therapy is similar to that of primary IMHA.

ALLOIMMUNE HEMOLYSIS

Definition/overview

Alloimmune hemolysis is immune-mediated destruction of RBCs that express foreign antigens. The most common forms of alloimmune hemolysis in small animal medicine are hemolytic transfusion reactions and neonatal isoerythrolysis (NI).

Etiology

See Principles of transfusion medicine.

Pathophysiology

In dogs, sensitization occurs at least 4 days after initial antigen exposure. A major hemolytic transfusion reaction occurs when a blood recipient receives a blood product containing a DEA to which the recipient has been sensitized, causing hemolysis of the donated RBCs. NI rarely occurs in dogs, but most commonly involves a DEA 1.1-positive puppy ingesting colostrum that contains DEA 1.1-antibodies from a previously sensitized DEA 1.1-negative bitch.

Since RBC alloantibodies occur naturally in cats, transfusion reactions may occur on the initial exposure to blood. The naturally occurring anti-B antibodies in type A cats are weak hemolysins and agglutinins, reducing the donated RBC half-life to 2.1 days. However, type B cats produce anti-A antibodies that are strong hemolysins and agglutinins, which can induce severe and life-threatening hemolytic transfusion reactions. NI is most commonly seen in kittens, wherein type A or type AB kittens ingest colostrum that contains type A antibodies from a type B queen.

Clinical presentation

Clinical signs in affected animals are similar to those with primary IMHA, except for the additional historical findings of receiving a blood transfusion or nursing from the dam. Clinical signs can occur within minutes to days of receiving a blood product or hours to days after ingesting colostrum. In NI, puppies and kittens are born healthy and nurse normally, then become pale and weak within 1–2 days after birth; reluctance to nurse, failure to thrive, dyspnea, hemoglobinuria, icterus, tail tip necrosis, and death may also occur.

Differential diagnosis

Similar differential diagnoses to primary IMHA.

Diagnosis

The blood product recipient's temperature, heart rate, respiratory rate, blood pressure, and PCV should be monitored during the transfusion for signs of an adverse reaction. Evidence of hemolytic transfusion reaction includes hemolyzed plasma and red urine. Blood typing and cross-matching, if not already performed, can help confirm a hemolytic transfusion reaction. Clinical signs of nonhemolytic transfusion reactions, such as vomiting, diarrhea, abdominal pain or facial swelling, should also be monitored.

NI should be suspected in pale, icteric 1–2-day-old kittens and puppies. For a definitive diagnosis of NI, the dam's serum or colostrum can be cross-matched against the sire's or neonate's washed RBCs, or by blood typing the queen and tom or kitten.

Management

Blood transfusion reactions can be avoided or reduced by blood typing and cross-matching prior to blood product administration. Starting the transfusion at a slower rate can help lessen the severity of the reaction if a reaction were to occur. The blood transfusion may be stopped once clinical signs of a reaction have been identified, or the transfusion may be slowed if the reaction is mild.

If NI is identified, puppies and kittens should not be allowed to nurse from their dam, and should be fed a milk replacement formula. Blood typing queens and toms prior to breeding can prevent disease.

HEMOPLASMOSIS

(See also Chapter 21: Infectious diseases.)

Definition/overview

Hemotropic mycoplasmosis (hemoplasmosis, formerly hemobartonellosis) is an infectious hemolytic disease of mammals caused by small, pleomorphic bacteria that parasitize the surface of RBCs. Acute hemolytic anemia is most common in cats, whereas dogs typically require immunosuppression, splenectomy, or splenic pathology to manifest clinical signs of disease.

Etiology

Carrier animals are the source of infection. The hemoplasmas of feline erythrocytes are *Mycoplasma haemofelis*, '*Candidatus* Mycoplasma haemominutum', and '*Candidatus* Mycoplasma turicensis' Dogs may be infected by *Mycoplasma haemocanis* or '*Candidatus* Mycoplasma haematoparvum'. Potential routes of transmission include cat fighting, biting arthropods (ticks in dogs and fleas in cats), periparturient transmission, or blood transfusions. Splenectomy, immunosuppression, or stress can cause recrudescence of latent infections

Pathophysiology

Hemoplasmas cause hemolysis by inducing secondary IMHA, the 'innocent bystander effect', and causing direct RBC lysis. An acute bacteremic phase usually occurs 1 week to 2 months after infection. This phase involves cyclical bacteremia persisting for weeks to months. An immune response elicited by the infected erythrocytes causes them to be rapidly sequestered in the spleen and other tissues, where they become phagocytized. Bacteria may be shed from the sequestered erythrocytes and thus re-enter the blood circulation.

Clinical presentation

Clinical signs include those generally observed with hemolytic anemia (see primary IMHA). Fever is cyclical and corresponds to high levels of bacteremia. Canine hemoplasmosis and the small form of feline hemoplasmosis are often not associated with clinical disease unless other conditions exist.

Differential diagnosis

Similar differential diagnoses to primary IMHA.

Diagnosis

CBC, biochemical, and urinalysis abnormalities are almost identical to primary IMHA, except that *Mycoplasma* organisms may be observed on the surface of RBCs or in the background of the smear if there is a delay between sample collection and blood smear preparation. However, bacteremia is cyclical during the acute phase, so absence of visible organisms does not rule out infection. Organisms are rare or inapparent during preparasitemic, recovery, and carrier phases. Blood films should be well stained without precipitate to minimize any confusion in identifying the parasite. Cats often have coccoid or ring shapes, whereas dogs mostly have linear chain forms (**Figures 16.16, 16.17**). Polymerase chain reaction (PCR)-based tests can identify infections when organisms are not microscopically apparent. A positive Coombs test may be observed. Bacterial consumption of glucose in a blood sample may cause *in-vitro* hypoglycemia with heavy bacterial loads.

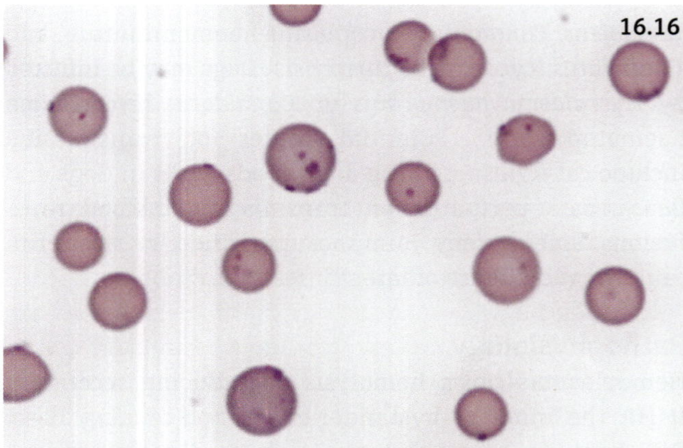

Figure 16.16 Blood smear from cat with coccoid and ring forms of *Mycoplasma haemofelis*.

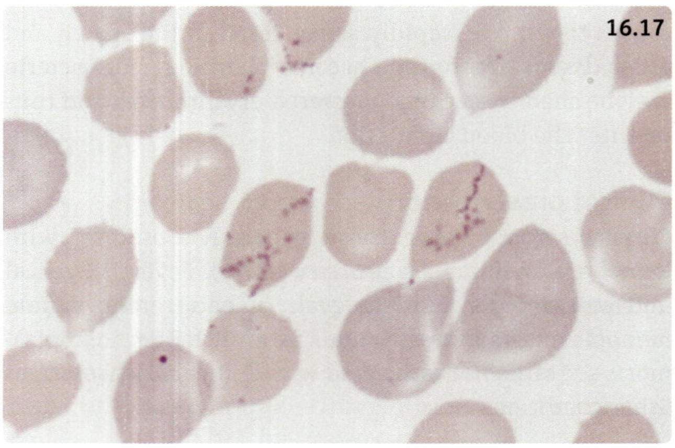

Figure 16.17 *Mycoplasma haemocanis* forms chains on the surface of dog erythrocytes.

Management

Treatment involves blood transfusion if the anemia is severe. Prednisolone (2 mg/kg PO q12h) may be necessary initially to suppress the severe immune-mediated destruction of red cells. Doxycycline is the preferred antibiotic: dogs (5 mg/kg PO q12h for 3 weeks); cats (1–3 mg/kg PO q12h for 3 weeks). Doxycycline administration in cats should be followed by 5 ml of water in order to avoid esophageal irritation. Tetracycline (22 mg/kg PO q8h for 3 weeks) can be given, but this may cause fever and GI disease in cats, so the drug dosage or form of tetracycline may need to be modified. Enrofloxacin (5–10 mg/kg PO q24h) has shown efficacy in cats, but large doses can cause blindness. Blood donor animals should be screened for hemoplasma infection by PCR.

Prognosis

If the animal survives the initial hemolytic crisis, there is a good long-term prognosis. Even with antibiotic therapy, animals that recover may become latent carriers, and there is potential for disease recrudescence during times of immune compromise or stress.

BABESIOSI

(See also Chapter 21: Infectious diseases.)

Definition/overview

Babesiosis is a tick-borne protozoal disease affecting erythrocytes of dogs (*Babesia canis*, *Babesia gibsoni*). *Babesia felis* has not been reported in North American cats, but is reported in Africa and southern Asia.

Etiology

Ixodid ticks are the major vectors of *Babesia* spp., although there have been cases of infection through blood transfusion and transplacental transmission. Sporozoites are transmitted through the tick's saliva during a blood meal, but the parasite needs to feed for at least 2 days before transmission occurs. Infection is also thought to occur through dog fighting.

Pathophysiology

Babesia organisms become engulfed by erythrocytes, in which the parasites multiply to merozoites capable of infecting other erythrocytes. The incubation period is 10–12 days. Hosts are usually able to mount an effective immune response at this stage. If not, infected animals may develop a severe hemolytic anemia, hypotensive shock, and multiple organ dysfunction syndrome. Direct RBC lysis and secondary IMHA contribute to the anemia. Animals may relapse following therapy and affected dogs often remain carriers.

Clinical presentation

Babesiosis is common in kennel conditions and is especially associated with Greyhounds and American Pit Bull Terriers. The animal may have a history of immune compromise (e.g. cancer chemotherapy) or splenectomy. Clinical signs in affected animals are similar to those with primary IMHA.

Differential diagnosis

Similar differential diagnoses to primary IMHA.

Diagnosis

CBC, biochemical, and urinalysis abnormalities are almost identical to primary IMHA, except that *Babesia* organisms may be observed within RBCs as clear, tear-drop-shaped organisms, sometimes in pairs. *B. canis* is often large (**Figure 16.18**), while *B. gibsoni* is much smaller

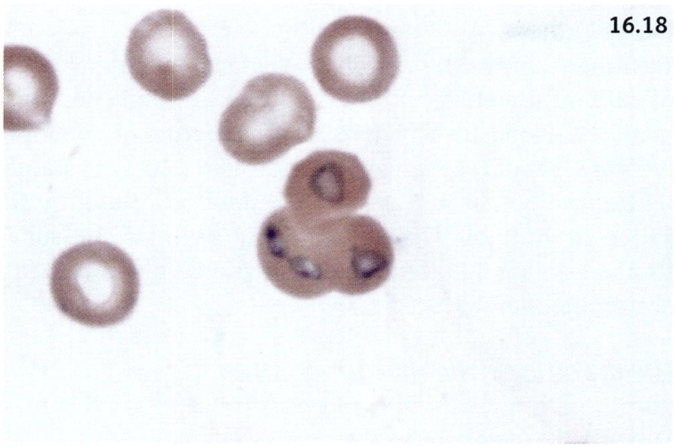

Figure 16.18 Singular or paired tear-drop-shaped organisms of *Babesia canis* in three agglutinated erythrocytes.

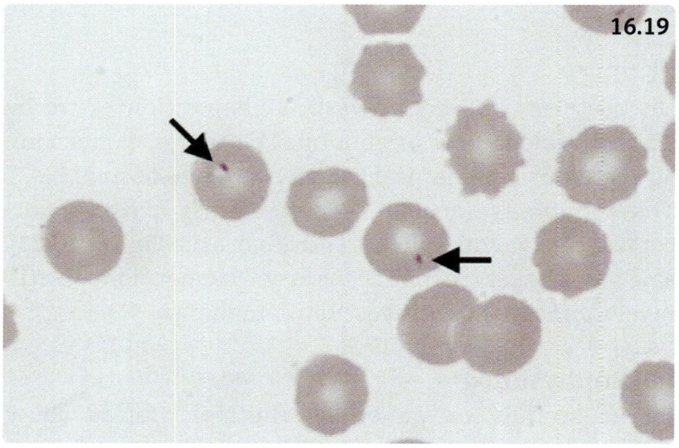

Figure 16.19 Two small *Babesia gibsoni* (arrows) organisms in canine erythrocytes.

(**Figure 16.19**). An indirect fluorescent antibody (IFA) serum test is available, which, when titers are high, indicates current infection. The most sensitive and specific test for genus, species, and subspecies is the PCR-based assay. Concurrent infections with *Ehrlichia canis* may occur. A Coombs test may be positive, as in IMHA. In severe cases, DIC may be present.

Management

Treatment primarily involves imidocarb dipropionate 12% (Imizol®) at a dose of 6.6 mg/kg IM given once with a repeat dose in 2 weeks. This clears the large form infection but may only reduce the severity of the small form infection. Additionally, diminazene aceturate (Berenil®) (3–7 mg/kg IM given once), phenamidine isethionate (15 mg/kg SC q24h for 2 days), or an atovaquone (13.5 mg/kg PO q8h administered with a fatty meal for 10 consecutive days) and azithromycin (10 mg/kg PO q24h for 10 consecutive days) combination can be given. Supportive therapy (e.g. blood transfusion) should be given when indicated.

Prognosis

Despite treatment, animals should be considered infected for life. A high incidence of relapse is reported.

OXIDANT-INDUCED HEMOLYTIC ANEMIA

Definition/overview

Irreversible damage occurs to erythrocytes when the normal protective antioxidant mechanisms are exceeded, resulting in the formation of Heinz bodies or eccentrocytes.

Etiology

Oxidative agents that cause precipitation of Hgb and fusion of RBC membranes produce Heinz bodies and eccentrocytes, respectively. Causes of oxidant-induced hemolytic anemia include onions, garlic, Chinese chives, zinc (e.g. pennies, toys, zippers, galvanized wire, and zinc phosphide rodenticides), acetaminophen (paracetamol), methylene blue (in old urinary antiseptics), vitamin K3, methionine, topical benzocaine, propofol, mothball ingestion, propylene glycol, and skunk spray. Heinz body formation in cats has also been associated with diabetic ketoacidosis, hyperthyroidism, and lymphoma.

Pathophysiology

Accelerated red cell destruction involves intravascular fragmentation and extravascular phagocytosis by the spleen. Feline RBCs are predisposed to oxidant damage because of their Hgb structure.

Clinical presentation

Clinical signs of affected animals are similar to those with acute primary IMHA.

Differential diagnosis

Similar differential diagnoses to primary IMHA.

Diagnosis

Diagnosis is made by the observation of hemolytic anemia (regenerative anemia, icterus, hemolysis, hemoglobinuria, and/or ghost cells) with many Heinz bodies and/or eccentrocytes on a blood smear. On Romanowsky-stained blood smears, Heinz bodies are large, pale-staining areas in erythrocytes, or blunt projections from the membrane surface (**Figure 16.20**); there is only one Heinz body per RBC. On new methylene blue-stained wet mounts or dried blood smears, Heinz bodies are dark blue spots within RBCs (**Figure 16.21**). Eccentrocytes are RBCs with densely packed Hgb on one side of the cell and a thin colorless portion, or hemighost, on the opposite side (**Figure 16.22**). When the hemighost fragments off from the RBC, the remaining RBC is termed a pyknocyte. With zinc toxicosis, abdominal radiographs may reveal ingestion of a metal object.

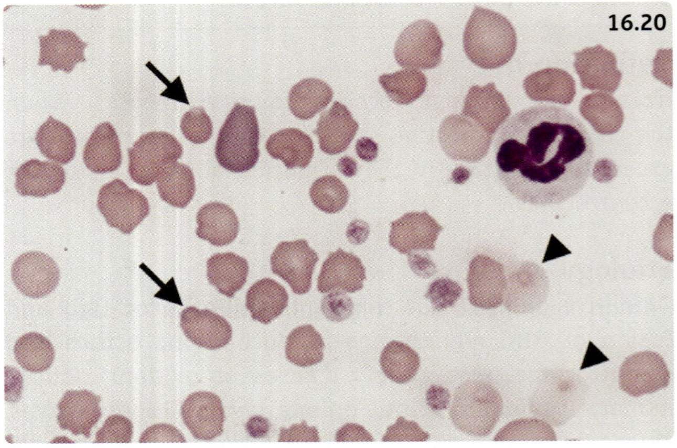

Figure 16.20 Heinz bodies in intact erythrocytes (arrows) and ghost cells (arrowheads) in a cat with oxidant-induced hemolytic anemia.

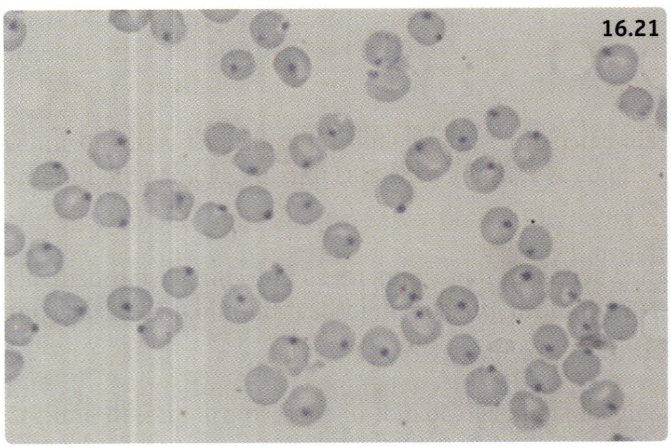

Figure 16.21 Heinz bodies are basophilic round structures with new methylene blue stain.

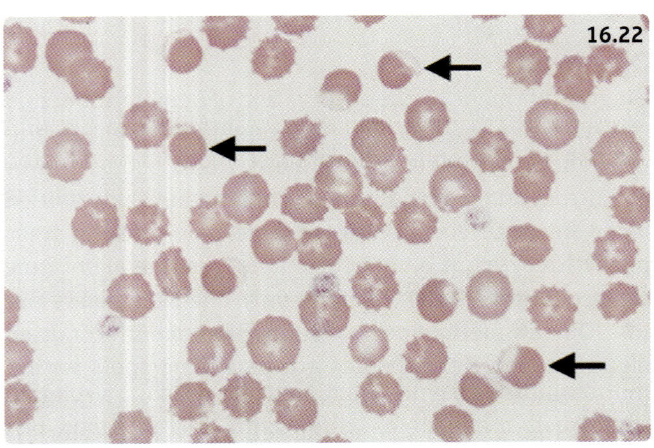

Figure 16.22 Eccentrocytes (arrows) in a dog receiving a continuous rate infusion of propofol.

Management

Treatment primarily involves removal of the source of oxidant. Emetics can be used if recent ingestion has occurred. Blood transfusions or other forms of supportive care should be given as indicated. Acetylcysteine (Mucomyst®) (140 mg/kg of a 5% solution diluted with saline IV initially, then give 70 mg/kg [of a 5% solution] q4–6h for 3–5 treatments) should be given to treat acetaminophen-induced toxicity.

MICROANGIOPATHIC HEMOLYTIC ANEMIA

Definition/overview

Microangiopathic hemolytic anemia is due to mechanical fragmentation of normal RBCs in an abnormal vasculature system.

Etiology

Diseases that cause intravascular deposition of fibrin, turbulent blood flow, or abnormal blood vessel morphology can cause mechanical fragmentation of normal RBCs. These diseases include DIC, vasculitis, hemangiosarcoma, heart valvular defects, dirofilariasis (**Figure 16.23**), splenic disease, hepatic disease, glomerulonephritis, myelofibrosis, and intravascular lymphoma.

Pathophysiology

Fibrin strands or abnormal rheologic forces cause shearing or lysis or RBCs. The RBC fragments, including schistocytes, acanthocytes, and keratocytes, are removed from circulation by the monocyte–macrophage system.

Differential diagnosis

Blood loss, IMHA, oxidant-induced hemolysis, infectious hemolytic anemia, liver disease, disorders of lipid metabolism.

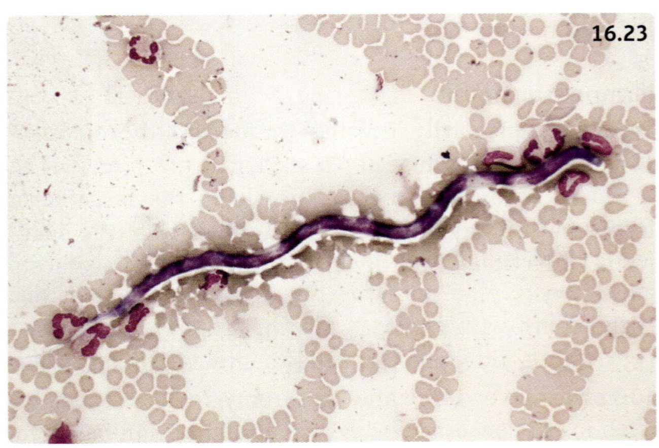

Figure 16.23 Microfilaria in a dog with *Dirofilaria immitus* infection.

Clinical presentation

The clinical presentation varies depending on the cause of the RBC fragmentation.

Diagnosis

Microangiopathic hemolytic anemia is typically a regenerative anemia with evidence of RBC fragmentation on blood smear evaluation (e.g. schistocytes, acanthocytes, keratocytes) (**Figure 16.24**). The degree of anemia is typically mild, but may be moderate to rarely severe. Marrow erythropoiesis may be able to compensate for the degree of hemolysis, so RBC regeneration and/or anemia may not be present. Diagnosis of the underlying disease may include CBC with blood smear evaluation, heartworm antigen test, serum biochemical and urine analysis, coagulation panel, abdominal and thoracic imaging, and bone marrow biopsy.

Management

Management is directed at resolving the underlying cause of the microangiopathy.

PYRUVATE KINASE DEFICIENCY

Definition/overview

Pyruvate kinase (PK) deficiency is a congenital deficiency in glycolytic enzymes. The condition has been documented in dogs (Basenji, Beagle, West Highland White Terrier, Cairn Terrier, American Eskimo Dog, Miniature Poodle, Chihuahua, and Pug) and cats (Abyssinian, Somali, and Domestic Shorthair cats).

Etiology

PK deficiency is an autosomal recessive trait due to a variety of mutations in the erythrocyte PK gene.

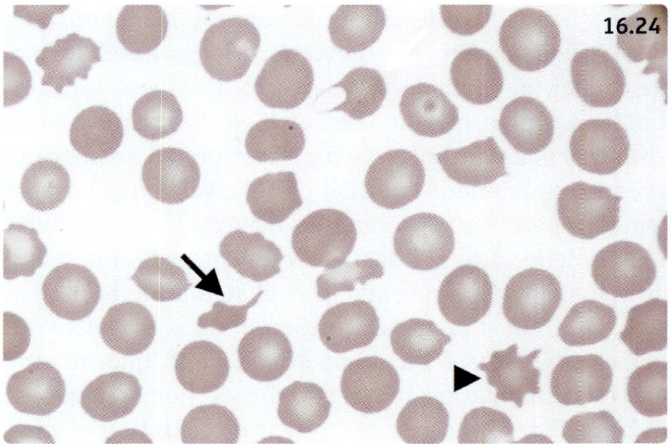

Figure 16.24 This dog with disseminated intravascular coagulation has circulating schistocytes (black arrow), acanthocytes (arrowhead), and keratocytes (white arrow).

Pathophysiology

PK is an enzyme in the glycolytic pathway that is necessary for the anaerobic production of adenosine triphosphate (ATP). Therefore, energy metabolism is markedly impaired in PK-deficient RBCs, leading to shortened RBC life spans and hemolytic anemia. Persistent anemia causes increased intestinal absorption of iron and subsequent hepatic (hemosiderosis, hemochromatosis, cirrhosis, and failure) and bone marrow (myelofibrosis and osteosclerosis) injury.

Clinical presentation

Heterozygotes show no clinical signs. Homozygotes often present in their youth with pale mucous membranes, exercise intolerance, tachycardia, and splenomegaly. Cats may not present until they are at an advanced age, or with intermittent hemolytic anemia.

Differential diagnosis

Phosphofructokinase deficiency, IMHA, oxidant-induced hemolysis, mycoplasmosis, babesiosis.

Diagnosis

Diagnosis is suggested by the presence of hemolytic anemia with an intense reticulocytosis (15–50%) and frequent nucleated red cells in a young dog (**Figure 16.25**). Splenectomy results in marked poikilocytosis with schistocytes and acanthocytes. Dogs may also show biochemical signs of liver injury or failure, as well as hematologic evidence of marrow failure (e.g. neutropenia and thrombocytopenia). PCR-based tests are available for the Basenji, West Highland White Terrier, Beagle, Dachshund, Toy Eskimo, and Cairn Terrier dog breeds, as well as Abyssinian and Somali cats. Definitive diagnosis for other breeds requires PK isoenzyme characterization.

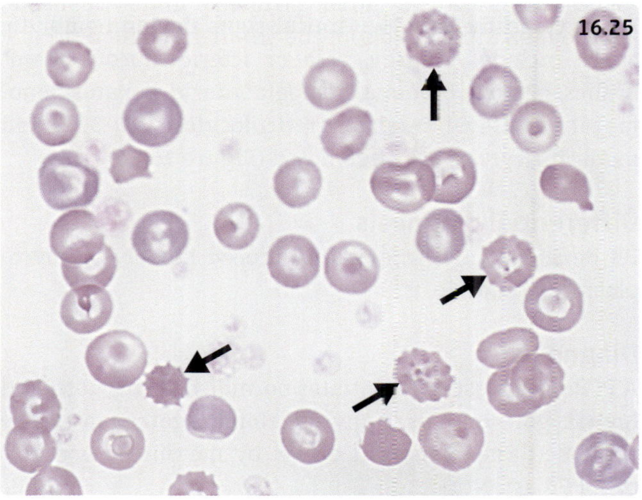

Figure 16.25 Pyruvate kinase deficiency in a dog showing polychromasia and several echinocytes (arrows).

Management

There is no specific treatment.

Prognosis

Dogs usually die between 1 and 5 years of age.

PHOSPHOFRUCTOKINASE DEFICIENCY

Definition/overview

Phosphofructokinase (PFK) deficiency is a congenital deficiency in glycolytic enzymes. It has been identified in English Springer Spaniels, American Cocker Spaniels, and mixed-breed dogs.

Etiology

A nonsense mutation of the muscle-type PFK gene leads to truncation of M-type PFK enzyme, which is structurally unstable and rapidly degrades.

Pathophysiology

Decreased PFK in RBCs leads to decreased glycolysis and anaerobic ATP generation, as well as decreased concentrations of 2,3-diphosphoglycerate (2,3-DPG). Energy metabolism is impaired in PFK-deficient RBCs, leading to a shortened RBC life span and hemolytic anemia. The 2,3-DPG deficiency causes an increase in intracellular pH, and RBCs are especially fragile under alkaline conditions, such as hyperventilation-induced alkalemia.

Clinical presentation

Heterozygote dogs show no clinical signs. Homozygote dogs have persistent compensated hemolytic anemia with sporadic episodes of intravascular hemolysis. Animals between episodes of hemolytic crises appear clinically normal or may have a decreased muscle mass; Hct is typically 30–45%. Clinical signs during hemolytic crises include lethargy, pale or icteric mucous membranes, hemoglobinemia, hemoglobinuria, hepatosplenomegaly, and fever. Persistent reticulocytosis (10–30%) and metarubricytosis are often noted (**Figure 16.26**).

Differential diagnosis

PK deficiency, IMHA, oxidant-induced hemolysis, mycoplasmosis, babesiosis.

Diagnosis

A PCR-based test differentiates normal, heterozygote, and homozygote animals of any age. Homozygotes can also be identified after 3 months of age by measuring erythrocyte PFK activity.

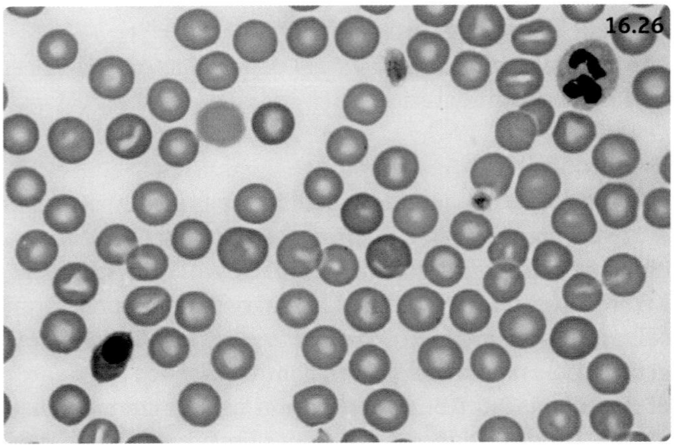

Figure 16.26 Polychromasia and metarubricytosis in a dog with phosphofructokinase deficiency. (Courtesy H. Tvedten.)

Management

Management is directed at avoiding situations that could lead to hyperventilation, such as excessive exercise, excitement, or high temperatures.

Prognosis

Dogs may have a normal life span if properly managed.

OTHER CAUSES OF HEMOLYTIC ANEMIA

Other rare congenital hemolytic anemias have been documented. Feline erythropoietic porphyria has been reported in a family of Siamese cats that had hemolytic anemia, photosensitivity, and renal disease. A hereditary nonspherocytic hemolytic anemia has been identified in three related Beagles that exhibited persistent regenerative mild anemia (Hct, 30–39%). Idiopathic hemolytic anemia has been documented in 13 Abyssinian and five Somali cats with regenerative moderate to marked anemias (Hct, 5–25%).

Uncommon to rare causes of acquired hemolytic anemia include snake envenomation, hypophosphatemia, hemophagocytic histiocytic sarcoma, L-sorbose intoxication, and hypo-osmolality. Hematologic changes also noted with snakebites include spherocyte formation, echinocytosis, and coagulation abnormalities. Marked hypophosphatemia, typically ≤1.0–1.5 mg/dl, may cause intracellular ATP depletion, loss of RBC membrane integrity, and subsequent hemolysis. Severe hypophosphatemia has been associated with insulin administration in dogs and cats with diabetes mellitus, feline idiopathic hepatic lipidosis, and enteral alimentation in dogs and cats. Hemophagocytic histiocytic sarcoma is a malignant proliferation of macrophages that exhibit marked erythrophagocytic activity.

The neoplasm occurs with high incidence in Bernese Mountain Dogs, Golden Retrievers, Rottweilers, and Labrador Retrievers; it is rare in cats. Affected animals often present with Coombs-negative regenerative anemia, thrombocytopenia, hypoalbuminemia, hypocholesterolemia, and diffuse splenomegaly. Oral ingestion of L-sorbose, a sugar substitute, by dogs may cause intravascular hemolytic anemia secondary to glycolysis inhibition and decreased production of ATP within erythrocytes. Dogs with inherited high Na-K-ATPase activity in their RBCs (e.g. Japanese Akitas and Japanese Shibas) are resistant to hemolysis. Hypo-osmolar hemolysis may occur with rapid IV infusion of hypotonic fluids.

NONREGENERATIVE ANEMIA

A poorly regenerative or nonregenerative anemia is generally due to decreased RBC production in the bone marrow. Causes of regenerative anemia (hemorrhage and hemolysis) appear initially nonregenerative since the bone marrow requires at least 3–4 days to undergo erythroid hyperplasia and release greater numbers of reticulocytes.

PREREGENERATIVE ANEMIA

CYTAUXZOONOSIS

Definition/overview

Cytauxzoonosis, caused by *Cytauxzoon felis*, is a highly fatal protozoal disease of wild and domestic cats in the southern USA. It is a tick-borne disease whose natural reservoir host is the bobcat, and possibly Florida panthers.

Etiology

Cytauxzoon felis is transmitted by *Dermacentor variabilis* and *Amblyomma americanum* ticks. The organism is a piroplasm hemoparasite of the family Theileriidae.

Pathophysiology

Macrophages infected with schizonts, a large membrane-bound structure containing numerous merozoites, line and occlude blood vessels throughout the body. This leads to tissue ischemia and hypoxia, organ dysfunction, and DIC. Schizonts release merozoites, which infect erythrocytes, and cause hemolysis.

Clinical presentation

Initial clinical signs include anorexia, dehydration, and lethargy, with gradual development of fever. This progresses rapidly to icterus, moderate nonregenerative anemia, leukopenia, thrombocytopenia, and splenomegaly. The nonregenerative nature of the anemia is thought to represent a preregenerative state wherein the bone marrow has not had adequate time to respond to the acute onset of hemolysis. Regeneration is poorly documented since cats usually die within 1 week after clinical signs are recognized.

Differential diagnosis

Other infectious agents, neoplasia, organ failure, DIC.

Diagnosis

Diagnosis is generally made postmortem by histologic identification of large schizonts in macrophages lining the sinusoids and veins of many tissues. Terminally, blood films may contain small (1–2 mm in diameter) ring or 'safety pin' structures within erythrocytes (**Figure 16.27**).

Management

Traditionally, diminazene aceturate (2 mg/kg IM, repeated in 7 days) or imidocarb dipropionate (2 mg/kg IM, repeated in 2 weeks) has been used to treat cytauxzoonosis. However, a recent clinical trial achieved a 60% survival rate with atovaquone (15 mg/kg PO q8h for 10 days) and azithromycin (10 mg/kg PO q24h for 10 days) compared with a 26% survival rate with imidocarb dipropionate (3.5 mg/kg IM). Supportive therapy may include fluid therapy and heparin (100–200 U/kg SC q8h). Atropine (0.04 mg/kg, repeated in 7 days) is recommended prior to treatment with imidocarb to reduce the immediate toxic effects of this drug. Blood transfusions are necessary for those cats with severe anemia.

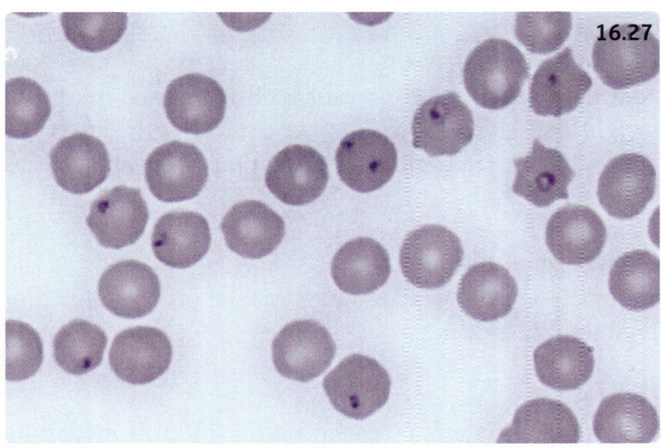

Figure 16.27 Blood smear with multiple organisms from a cat infected with *Cytauxzoon felis*. (Courtesy N. Weinstein)

Prognosis
Traditionally, cats have a guarded to grave prognosis despite the use of antibiotics and supportive care. However, a high survival rate may be achieved with contemporary therapy.

SELECTIVE ERYTHROID HYPOPLASIA OR APLASIA

Selective erythroid hypoplasia or aplasia is decreased or absent RBC production in the bone marrow without decreased production of other hematopoietic cells. Therefore, neutropenia and thrombocytopenia due to decreased production are not present.

ANEMIA OF INFLAMMATORY OR CHRONIC DISEASE

Definition/overview
Inflammatory or chronic disease is the most frequent cause of nonregenerative anemia. The anemia is usually mild to moderate in severity. Once recognized, it is of little clinical significance.

Etiology
Almost any chronic disorder can initiate this anemia, including infectious diseases, immune-mediated diseases, toxicities, and neoplasms.

Pathophysiology
The mechanism may involve decreased erythropoiesis, reduced iron availability through sequestration in macrophages, and decreased RBC survival. Studies have shown that cytokines, such as tumor necrosis factor (TNF), interferon-gamma, and interleukin (IL)-1, inhibit erythropoietin synthesis and decrease the responsiveness of progenitor cells to growth factors.

Clinical presentation
Affected animals may present with prolonged anorexia, weight loss, and weakness. Other clinical signs reflect the actual source of chronic inflammation or organ systems affected.

Differential diagnosis
Iron deficiency anemia, neoplasia, organ failure, preregenerative anemia.

Diagnosis
Laboratory findings often indicate a mild to moderate, normocytic, normochromic anemia, inflammatory leukogram, low serum iron, low total iron-binding capacity, and increased serum ferritin and bone marrow stores of iron. The bone marrow is usually hypocellular, with a normal to increased myeloid:erythroid ratio. The MCV may be normal to slightly decreased.

Management
Treatment is directed at the underlying disease, and not the anemia. Iron supplementation does not effectively reverse this form of anemia.

ANEMIA OF CHRONIC KIDNEY DISEASE

(See also Chapter 12: Nephrology/urology.)

Definition/overview
The peritubular interstitial cells in the renal cortex produce erythropoietin (EPO) at a rate inversely proportional to the oxygen content (and therefore RBC mass) of blood.

Etiology
The anemia is primarily due to EPO deficiency, with minor contributions from decreased marrow responsiveness to EPO and decreased RBC survival. Concurrent hemorrhage caused by uremic ulcers may contribute to the anemia.

Pathophysiology
Inadequate EPO and reduced response to EPO lead to decreased erythropoiesis. Uremic toxins may damage RBCs, and decrease RBC life span.

Clinical presentation
Patients may present with weakness, weight loss, inappetence, and pale mucous membranes. In addition, they may display vomiting, diarrhea, polyuria, and polydipsia.

Differential diagnosis
Gastric ulcers, chronic liver disease, chronic inflammation, neoplasia, iron deficiency.

Diagnosis
Diagnosis of renal failure involves the presence of azotemia and an abnormal urinalysis. The major hematologic abnormality is normocytic, normochromic nonregenerative anemia. Abnormal RBCs called burr cells (**Figure 16.28**) are associated with chronic kidney disease.

Management
A recombinant form of human erythropoietin (Epogen®) has been used in dogs and cats to promote proliferation and differentiation of red cell precursors. Dogs: initial dose of 150 U/kg SC or IV, three times a week; cats: initial dose of 100 U/kg SC or IV, 2–3 times a week. These initial doses are given until a low normal hematocrit is reached (37% [0.37 l/l] in dogs and 30% [0.30 l/l] in cats).

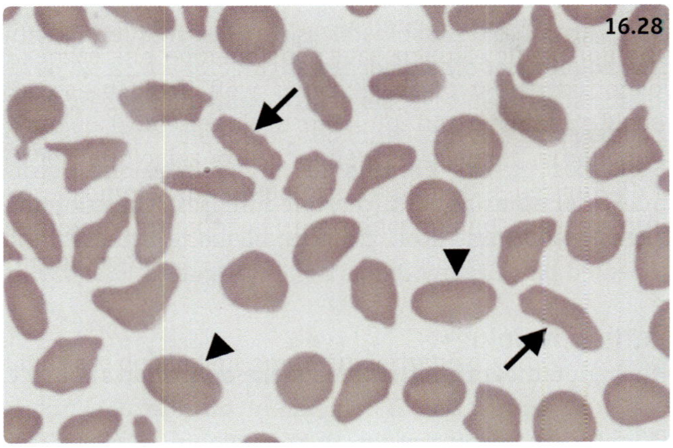

Figure 16.28 Burr cells (arrows) and ovalocytes (arrowheads) are elongate erythrocytes with and without ruffled borders, respectively.

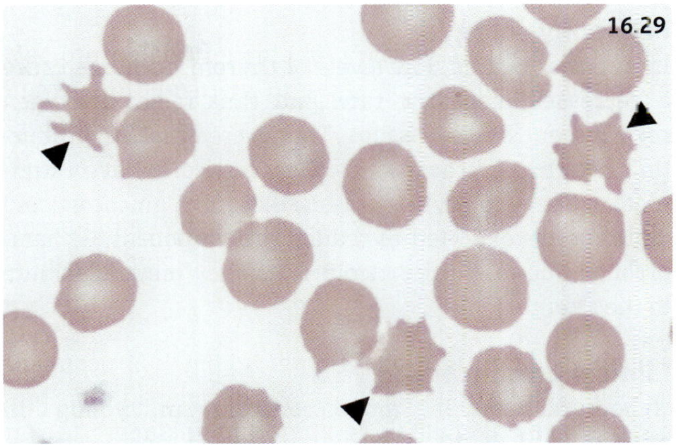

Figure 16.29 Three acanthocytes (arrowheads) with multiple irregularly shaped cytoplasmic projections.

The dose is then reduced to 1–2 times weekly for 3 weeks. After this, the maintenance dosage is adjusted to the animal and is usually given once per week. Maintenance involves periodic monitoring of the hematocrit and detection of any side-effects. Most side-effects occur from an immune reaction to the human erythropoietin and nonregenerative IMHA.

ANEMIA OF CHRONIC LIVER DISEASE

(See also Chapter 9: Liver disorders.)

Definition/overview

Decreased liver functional mass may influence red cell production, survival, or loss.

Etiology

Chronic liver failure or portosystemic shunts may cause a significantly decreased liver functional mass. The liver produces a small percentage of EPO.

Pathophysiology

Mechanisms for nonregenerative anemia may include anemia of chronic/inflammatory disease, decreased RBC life span due to defective protein and lipid metabolism, iron sequestration due to decreased production of iron transport proteins, and EPO deficiency. Iron sequestration may cause microcytosis. Concurrent blood loss secondary to decreased liver production of clotting factors may contribute to the anemia.

Clinical presentation

Patients may present with weakness, weight loss, inappetence, and pale mucous membranes. In addition, they may display vomiting, diarrhea, polyuria, and polydipsia.

Differential diagnosis

Chronic kidney disease, chronic inflammation in other sites, neoplasia.

Diagnosis

The anemia is typically mild to moderate, normocytic, and normochromic; microcytosis is occasionally noted. Blood smears often reveal acanthocytes (**Figure 16.29**) or budding fragmentation. Laboratory findings suggestive of hepatic disease include elevated serum liver enzymes (ALT, ALP, GGT), increased serum bile acid levels, and hyperbilirubinemia. Indicators of liver failure include decreases in serum glucose, BUN albumin, and cholesterol concentrations, as well as prolonged clotting times and increased serum bile acid and ammonium levels. Abdominal imaging and liver biopsy may help identify the cause of the liver disease.

Management

Treatment is directed at the underlying liver disease, and not the anemia.

ANEMIA OF ENDOCRINE DISORDERS

(See also Chapter 11: Endocrine disorders.)

Definition/overview

Hypothyroidism and hypoadrenocorticism may cause mild to moderate nonregenerative anemia in dogs. Anemia due to hyperestrogenism is discussed elsewhere (see Generalized marrow hypoplasia or aplasia).

Etiology

Anemia is secondary to hypothyroidism and hypoadrenocorticism.

Pathophysiology

In hypothyroidism, low levels of thyroid hormone cause a decreased metabolic rate, and thus reduced oxygen requirement by the tissues. This decreases EPO production, and then erythropoiesis. Glucocorticoids have a stimulatory effect on erythropoiesis; therefore, glucocorticoid deficiency is expected to reduce erythropoiesis. GI hemorrhage due to glucocorticoid deficiency may contribute to the anemia.

Clinical presentation

Hypothyroidism is most common in young to middle aged (4–10 years), large breed dogs, particularly Golden Retrievers, Dobermanns, Irish Setters, and Miniature Schnauzers. Clinical signs include lethargy, exercise intolerance, mental dullness, obesity, dermatologic changes, and reproductive disturbances. Dogs with hypoadrenocorticism are frequently young to middle aged with an increased incidence in Standard Poodles, West Highland White Terriers, Great Danes, Bearded Collies, and Portuguese Water Dogs. Clinical signs include anorexia, vomiting, diarrhea, weight loss, polydipsia, polyuria, melena, dehydration, acute weakness, and collapse.

Differential diagnosis

Organ failure, chronic inflammation, neoplasia, drug toxicosis.

Diagnosis

Hypothyroidism and hypoadrenocorticism produce mild to moderate normocytic, normochromic nonregenerative anemia. Dogs with hypoadrenocorticism and GI hemorrhage may have regenerative anemia. Other clinicopathologic abnormalities associated with hypoadrenocorticism include: lack of a stress leukogram; lymphocytosis; eosinophilia; decreased sodium, chloride, glucose, and cholesterol values; increased potassium, calcium, BUN, creatinine, and phosphorus results; and poorly concentrated urine (urine specific gravity <1.030). Definitive diagnoses of hypothyroidism and hypoadrenocorticism are based on history, clinical signs, and endocrine testing (total T4 and TSH concentrations and adrenocorticotropic hormone [ACTH] stimulation test, respectively).

Management

Treatment is aimed at correcting the endocrine abnormality, since the degree of anemia is generally mild.

IRON DEFICIENCY ANEMIA

Definition/overview

This condition produces a poorly regenerative anemia due to deficient Hgb synthesis. It occurs most commonly with chronic external blood loss, and less frequently with inadequate dietary intake.

Etiology

Etiologies include chronic GI hemorrhage (neoplasia, intestinal parasites, or ulcerative diseases), chronic cutaneous blood loss (fleas, ticks, or bleeding tumors), and repeated phlebotomy (blood donor animals).

Pathophysiology

Hemoglobin synthesis is dependent on iron availability, and RBC maturation is dependent on adequate intracytoplasmic concentrations of hemoglobin. During times of iron deficiency, RBCs undergo additional mitoses to form smaller cells (microcytes) in an attempt to reach optimal intracytoplasmic concentrations of hemoglobin. With continued iron unavailability, the microcytes are no longer able to obtain optimal intracytoplasmic hemoglobin concentrations, thereby forming hypochromic cells. RBCs formed during times of iron deficiency are more fragile and less deformable, and therefore lyse easily in circulation. This leads to decreased RBC life spans, and the formation of keratocytes, acanthocytes, and schistocytes.

Clinical presentation

Clinical signs of iron deficiency are nonspecific and include insidious fatigue and exercise intolerance that develops over weeks to months. Owners may report pica as the animal licks or chews at unusual substances to try to compensate for the iron loss. Physical examination may reveal a systolic murmur, gallop rhythm, pale mucous membranes, and bounding pulses. Melena or hematochezia is usually present, whereas heavy parasitism is less common.

Differential diagnosis

Parasitism, neoplasia, organ failure, chronic disease or inflammation.

Diagnosis

Diagnosis is based on history and the presence of a microcytic hypochromic anemia that is nonregenerative or poorly regenerative for the degree of anemia. The MCV usually decreases prior to the MCHC, and so the MCHC may be within normal limits at the time of presentation. Erythrocytes in blood smears may appear small (microcytes) with increased central pallor (hypochromasia) (**Figure 16.30**). Microcytes and hypochromasia are observed in blood prior to changes in the MCV and MCHC, since the latter represent average cell values. Poikilocytosis may be prominent in the form of schistocytes, acanthocytes, keratocytes, codocytes, and elliptocytes (**Figure 16.31**). Thrombocytosis occurs in 50% of

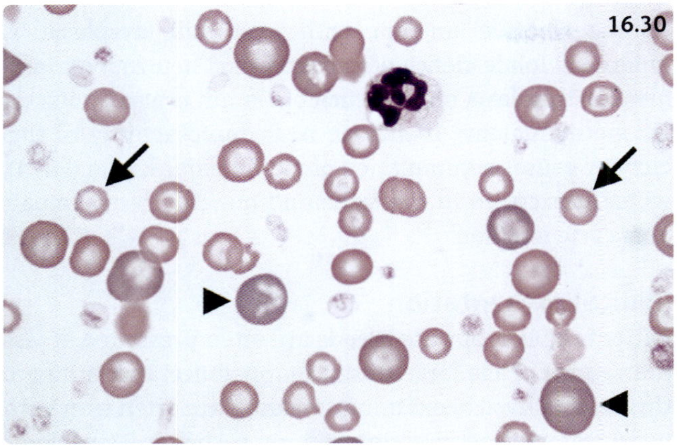

Figure 16.30 Iron deficient erythrocytes are small with increased central pallor (arrows). Regeneration is present in early stages of iron deficiency anemia (arrowheads).

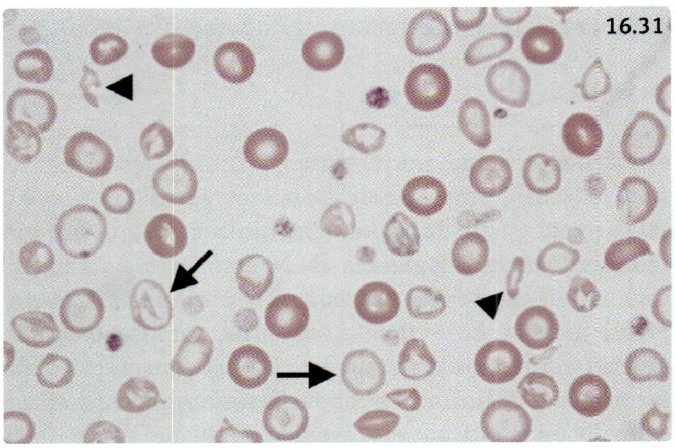

Figure 16.31 Late stage iron deficiency anemia with marked hypochromasia (arrows) and no polychromatophils. Iron deficient erythrocytes are fragile and prone to fragmentation (arrowheads).

canine cases. Iron profiles have a decreased serum iron level (in cats <10.7 µmol/l [60 µg/dl]; in dogs <14.3 µmol/l [80 µg/dl]), normal to increased level of transferrin (measured as total iron-binding capacity), and decreased serum ferritin concentration. Percent saturation of transferrin in iron deficient animals is often <19% (normal is about 33%). Bone marrow examination shows decreased iron stores in the dog, and marked erythroid proliferation. Absence of bone marrow iron stores is a normal finding in the cat.

Management

Treatment involves correction of the inciting cause for the blood loss, and iron supplementation. Ferrous sulfate is given at a rate of 4–6 mg of iron/kg/day orally in divided doses. Therapy is continued for several weeks to months until the PCV and MCV return to normal.

NONREGENERATIVE IMMUNE-MEDIATED HEMOLYTIC ANEMIA

Definition/overview

Immune-mediated destruction of erythroid precursors occurs within the bone marrow, resulting in moderate to marked anemia without reticulocytosis. The bone marrow may reveal a near complete absence of erythroid precursors (pure red cell aplasia [PRCA]) or erythroid hyperplasia with maturation arrest (ineffective erythropoiesis).

Etiology

Similar to the more common regenerative IMHA, immune-mediated destruction of erythroid precursors may be primary/idiopathic or secondary. Primary nonregenerative IMHA is more common in dogs. Potential causes of secondary PRCA include vaccination of dogs with a modified live parvovirus vaccine and administration of recombinant human EPO.

Pathophysiology

Immune-mediated destruction of erythroid cells may occur at any level of maturation. If hemolysis is directed at erythroid stem cells, there is PRCA. If hemolysis is directed at later erythroid precursors, there is marked proliferation of stages prior to the targeted developmental stage, and near absence of those after. This is termed 'maturation arrest', and is indicative of either ineffective erythropoiesis or an early marrow response to anemia (preregenerative anemia). Therefore, preregenerative anemia should be ruled out prior to diagnosing ineffective erythropoiesis.

Clinical presentation

History and physical examination findings are similar to those seen in animals with regenerative primary IMHA, except that red plasma and urine are not expected and icterus is less frequent.

Differential diagnosis

Iron deficiency anemia, anemia of renal failure, drug toxicosis, anemia of chronic disease.

Diagnosis

Hematologic findings include moderate to severe normocytic, normochromic nonregenerative anemia (Hct, 5–26%). Spherocytes and agglutination are present in 15–54% and 0–5% of cases, respectively. Mature and band neutrophils are often increased, but neutrophils may be within the reference interval or decreased. Platelets may be increased, decreased, or within the reference interval. A direct

Coombs test is often positive. Bone marrow findings are dependent on the RBC stage that is being destroyed, and may reveal erythroid hypoplasia (including pure red cell aplasia) or erythroid hyperplasia with maturation arrest. Increased numbers of lymphocytes and plasma cells are common, and may compose up to 60% and 33% of the total marrow cells, respectively. Serum ALT activity is commonly increased due to hypoxia-induced liver injury, but the total serum bilirubin concentration is only increased in less than one-quarter of cases. Concurrent immune-mediated disorders, such as polyarthritis, positive antinuclear antibody titers, and the presence of antimegakaryocyte antibodies, support an immune-mediated etiology.

Management

Treatment is similar to regenerative primary IMHA.

Prognosis

More than 70% of dogs and cats are expected to recover. However, response to treatment may take weeks to months.

FOLATE OR COBALAMIN (VITAMIN B12) DEFICIENCY

Definition/overview

Folate and cobalamin are acquired through the diet and intestinally absorbed. Both are needed for DNA synthesis. Unlike most other tissues, the bone marrow is particularly susceptible to inhibition of DNA synthesis, as the hematopoietic cells are constantly produced.

Etiology

Folate deficiency has been experimentally produced in cats fed a folate-deficient diet. However, dogs are highly resistant to folate deficiency. Congenital cobalamin deficiency is an autosomal recessive trait in Giant Schnauzer dogs due to a cobalamin receptor complex defect. It has also been documented in a Beagle, a Border Collie, and in Australian Shepherd Dogs. Drug-induced folate deficiency is associated with anticonvulsants (phenobarbital, primidone), sulfonamides (sulfasalazine, trimethoprim–sulfadiazine), and antineoplastic agents by impairing its absorption or production. Serum folate and/or cobalamin levels may be decreased in dogs and cats with various GI, hepatic and/or pancreatic disorders, but this very rarely results in anemia.

Pathophysiology

Folate and cobalamin are required for DNA synthesis. Deficiencies in folate and/or cobalamin impair hematopoiesis, especially erythrocyte and neutrophil production. Nonregenerative anemia with erythroid dysplasia is typical of folate deficiency; concurrent neutropenia and myeloid dysplasia often occur. Cobalamin is also a cofactor for methylmalonyl coenzyme A. Reduced activity of this enzyme causes accumulation of methymalonic acid (MMA), which is excreted in the urine and may indirectly impair urea cycle function.

Clinical presentation

Patients of appropriate breeds are often presented at less than a year of age for lethargy, inappetence, and failure to thrive. On physical examination, dogs are often thin with poorly developed muscle mass or cachexia. Neurologic signs may be apparent if urea cycle impairment has caused hyperammonemia.

Differential diagnosis

Myelodysplastic syndrome, drug-induced dysplasias.

Diagnosis

Erythrocyte changes with congenital cobalamin deficiency include normocytic, normochromic anemia (Hct, 21–36%), anisocytosis, poikilocytes, and nucleated erythrocytes with fully hemoglobinized cytoplasm and immature nuclei (megaloblasts). Neutropenia with hypersegmented neutrophils is frequently present, but neutrophilia may occur. Platelet concentrations are typically normal, and giant platelets may be present. In the bone marrow, both erythroid hypoplasia and hyperplasia have been documented, but erythroid and myeloid dysplasia is a consistent finding. Specific tests include measurement of serum folate and cobalamin concentrations, as well as urine MMA concentrations.

Management

Dogs with congenital cobalamin deficiency have been successfully treated with parenteral cobalamin supplementation (1 mg SC q1–2months, or 20 µg/kg SC q2weeks).

Prognosis

Dogs with congenital cobalamin deficiency have a good prognosis for recovery.

OTHER CAUSES OF SELECTIVE ERYTHROID HYPOPLASIA OR APLASIA

Dyserythropoiesis in English Springer Spaniels is characterized by microcytic normochromic nonregenerative anemia with polymyopathy, megaesophagus, and cardiomegaly.

GENERALIZED MARROW HYPOPLASIA OR APLASIA

APLASTIC ANEMIA

Definition/overview

The marrow consists of fat, and is nearly void of all hematopoietic cells along with peripheral pancytopenia

Etiology

A variety of etiologies have been implicated, including infectious agents (e.g. canine parvovirus, feline panleukopenia virus, canine distemper virus [CDV], *Ehrlichia canis*, FeLV, and feline immunodeficiency virus [FIV]), drugs (e.g. trimethoprim–sulfadiazine, antineoplastic drugs, estradiol, phenylbutazone, fenbendazole, quinidine, cephalosporins, and griseofulvin), hyperestrogenism (e.g. Sertoli cell and granulosa cell tumors), whole body irradiation, and idiopathic immune-mediated stem cell destruction.

Pathophysiology

Stem cells or progenitor cells are targeted and destroyed, leading to decreased production of all hematopoietic precursors (granulocytic, erythroid, and megakaryocytic) with subsequent pancytopenia.

Clinical presentation

The clinical presentation is partially dependent on the cause of the aplastic anemia. Specifically, animals with hyperestrinism may exhibit alopecia, feminization, or cryptorchidism. Clinical signs attributable to cytopenias include those associated with anemia (e.g. lethargy, weakness, pale mucous membranes), neutropenia (e.g. fever, infection, sepsis), and thrombocytopenia (e.g. petechial hemorrhages, epistaxis).

Differential diagnosis

Idiopathic myelofibrosis, myelophthisic neoplasia, infectious myelitis, FeLV infection.

Diagnosis

Minimal diagnostics include a CBC and bone marrow aspirate and core biopsies. The diagnosis of aplastic anemia is based on the presence of nonregenerative anemia, neutropenia, and thrombocytopenia with concurrent marked erythroid and megakaryocytic hypoplasia/aplasia in the bone marrow, which is nearly replaced with adipose tissue. The cytopenias are often moderate to severe. In CDV infections, erythrocytes or leukocytes may contain one or more pale blue spots in the cytoplasm when stained with methanolic Romanowsky-type stains. However, these inclusions stain a deep purple color with an aqueous Romanowsky stain such as Diff-Quik® (**Figures 16.32a–d**). Additional diagnostics should be directed at identifying the underlying cause for the aplastic anemia and include historical inquires of drug, radiation, or toxin exposure, testing for specific infectious agents, and evaluation for estrogen-secreting neoplasms.

Management

Specific treatment is directed at the underlying cause of the aplastic anemia, and includes cessation of myelotoxic drug administration, toxin removal, antiviral therapy, doxycycline administration for chronic *E. canis* infection, and surgical removal of estrogen-secreting neoplasms. Immune suppression may be attempted for idiopathic aplastic anemia. Supportive therapy may include blood transfusions for anemia or DIC, broad-spectrum antibiotics for neutropenia-induced bacterial infections, and bone marrow stimulants.

Prognosis

The prognosis is guarded to poor, but complete clinical recovery is possible.

INFILTRATIVE BONE MARROW DISEASE (MYELOPHTHISIS)

Definition/overview

Replacement of normal hematopoietic tissue in the bone marrow is termed myelophthisis.

Etiology

The marrow may be replaced by collagen (myelofibrosis), inflammatory cells (e.g. infectious myelitis due to histoplasmosis, other fungal infections, or toxoplasmosis), or neoplastic cells (e.g. hematopoietic or metastatic neoplasms).

Pathophysiology

Mild infiltrates or focal lesions within the bone marrow produce minimal peripheral blood changes. Cytopenia occurs if the involvement is diffuse and severe. Myelofibrosis usually occurs as a result of marrow damage produced by inflammation, necrosis, neoplasia, and toxic agents and may be seen in the terminal stages of PK deficiency. Myelofibrosis is also associated with myelodysplastic syndrome and acute myelogenous leukemia in cats or with chronic myeloid neoplasia in dogs and cats.

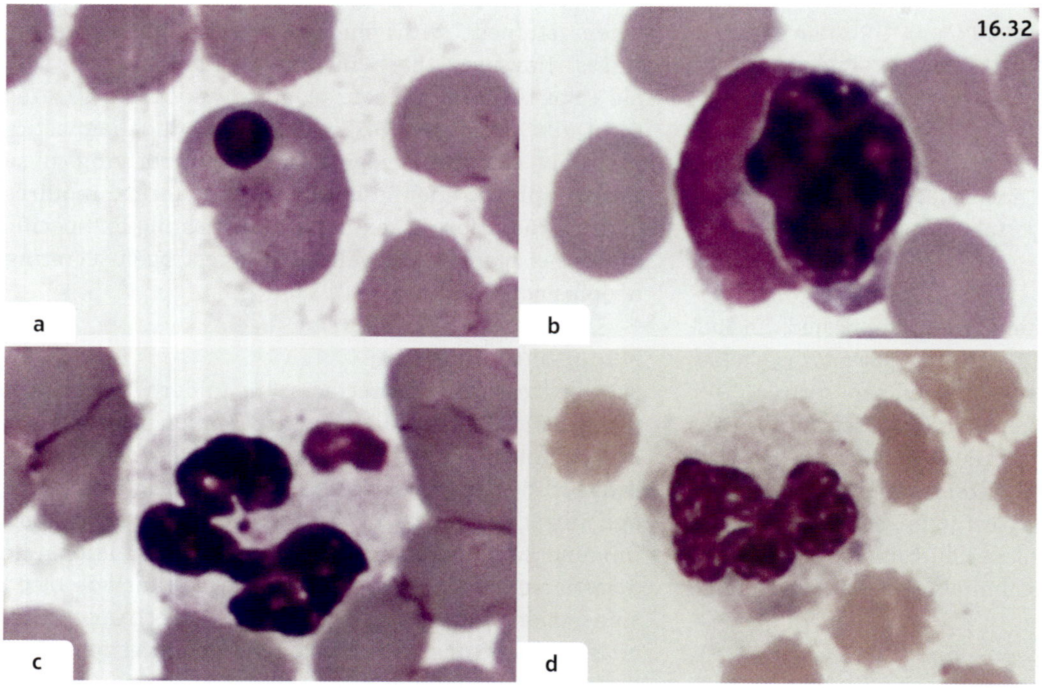

Figures 16.32a–d. Canine distemper viral inclusions in an erythrocyte (a), lymphocyte (b), and neutrophils (c and d). Vibrant magenta staining occurs with aqueous Romanowsky staining (a–c), but methanolic Romanowsky stains impart a light pink–blue appearance (d).

Clinical presentation

Animals are often presented with pale mucous membranes, fever, and bleeding, occasionally accompanied by hepatomegaly, splenomegaly, and lymphadenopathy.

Differential diagnosis

Drug toxicosis, myelodysplastic syndrome, hematolymphatic neoplasia, endogenous hyperestrogenism.

Diagnosis

Myelophthisis is likely if there is bicytopenia or pancytopenia (anemia, neutropenia, and thrombocytopenia) with circulating neoplastic cells, or evidence of systemic infection (e.g. fungal or protozoal organisms seen in blood smears or in tissue biopsies). Dacryocytes may be observed on blood smears (**Figure 16.33**). However, definitive diagnosis of an infiltrative process requires bone marrow examination by both aspirate and core biopsies. Bone marrow aspiration attempts on fibrotic marrow usually produce 'dry taps' (e.g. blood alone without marrow particles). In such cases, bone marrow core biopsy is diagnostic (**Figure 16.34**).

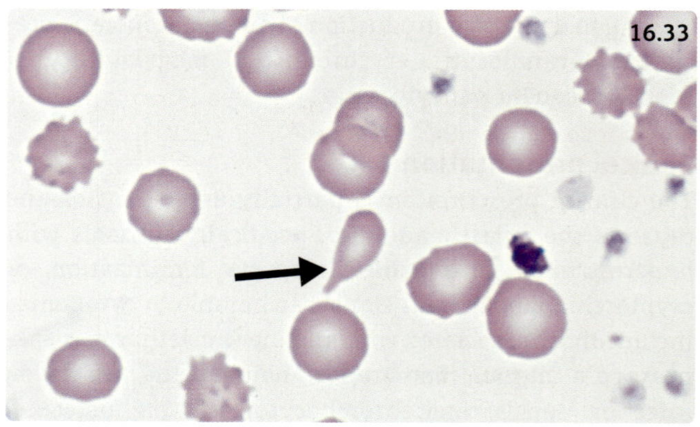

Figure 16.33 Dacryocyte (arrow) from the blood of a dog with myelofibrosis.

Management

Treatment is directed at the underlying cause of the cytopenia and may include immunosuppressive, antibiotic, or antineoplastic therapy for idiopathic myelofibrosis, infectious myelitis, or neoplasia, respectively. Supportive care, including antibiotics, blood transfusions, anabolic steroids, and glucocorticoids, is often required in severe cases. The condition may be reversible.

FELINE LEUKEMIA VIRUS-ASSOCIATED ANEMIA

Definition/overview

Anemia is a major non-neoplastic complication of FeLV infection in cats. The anemia is variable in severity and regenerative status, and is dependent on the underlying mechanism.

Etiology

FeLV infects hematopoietic stem cells and the supporting marrow stromal cells.

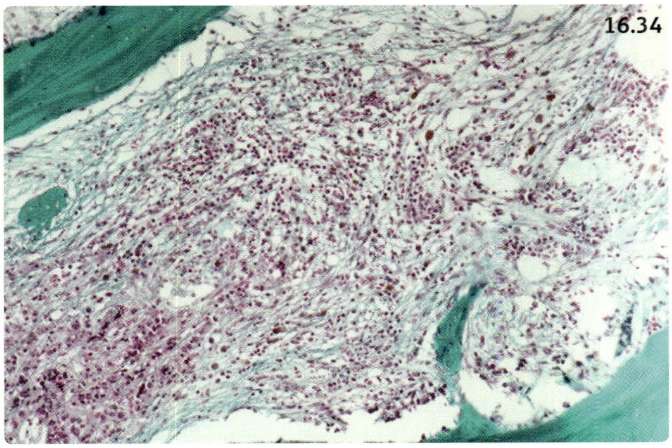

Figure 16.34 Bone marrow core section with trichrome stain for collagen (in green). Note the tight fibrillar arrangement of connective tissue, demonstrating myelofibrosis.

Pathophysiology

Most FeLV-associated anemias are nonregenerative. Mild to moderate nonregenerative anemia may occur secondary to anemia of chronic disease. More severe nonregenerative anemia is expected with selective erythrocyte hypoplasia, PRCA, erythroid leukemia, or neoplastic myelophthisis. PRCA is associated with FeLV-C infection. When the virus infects erythroid precursors, it may cause either selective erythroid precursor damage (erythroid hypoplasia or PRCA) or neoplastic transformation of erythroid precursors. Erythroid neoplastic transformation leads to proliferation of abnormal erythroid cells with defective metabolism, function, and proliferation. These dysfunctional neoplastic cells fail to mature or prematurely die within the marrow, resulting in ineffective erythropoiesis in the marrow and anemia in the peripheral blood. Defective mitosis may cause macrocytic RBCs. Approximately 10% of FeLV-associated anemias are regenerative. Virus-induced immune suppression may allow secondary hemoplasmosis and infectious hemolytic anemia. FeLV may induce expression of foreign antigens on erythrocyte surfaces, thereby inciting IMHA. Hemorrhage may occur secondary to thrombocytopathia or suppressed platelet production causing marked thrombocytopenia (<50,000 platelets/µl).

Clinical presentation

Clinical presentation is dependent on the severity and cause of the anemia. Affected cats with moderate to marked nonregenerative anemia often exhibit a chronic wasting disease characterized by pale mucous membranes, lethargy, and anorexia.

Differential diagnosis

Lymphoma, systemic mycoses or other chronic inflammatory conditions, other viral infections, chronic kidney disease.

Diagnosis

Most FeLV-associated anemias are mild to severe, normocytic to macrocytic, normochromic, and nonregenerative or poorly regenerative. Nucleated erythrocytes in circulation with inadequate RBC regeneration (inappropriate metarubricytosis) or nucleated erythrocytes with asynchronous maturation (megaloblasts) may be noted. Concurrent neutropenia and thrombocytopenia occur with aplastic anemia, leukemia, or myelophthisis. Bone marrow findings vary from PRCA to erythroid hypoplasia to erythroid neoplasia (myelodysplastic syndrome or acute myeloid leukemia-M6). Concurrent findings with regenerative anemia may include hemotropic mycoplasma infection or marked thrombocytopenia. A definitive FeLV association is diagnosed with positive ELISA or IFA tests.

Management

Treatment will vary depending on the presence of concurrent conditions such as neoplasia, hemoplasmosis, FIV infection, or FIP. Hematologic abnormalities due to defective production are mostly irreversible. However, marrow hypoplasia may be cyclical, so temporary life support may be considered during times of cytopenias. Supportive care might include blood transfusions, antibiotics, appetite stimulants, and anabolic steroids. FeLV-associated PRCA may respond to immunosuppressive drugs.

Prognosis

Cats with PRCA often relapse with cessation of treatment, whereas those with aplastic anemia typically do not respond to treatment. Regardless of the cause, regenerative FeLV-associated anemias tend to respond favorably to treatment.

ERYTHROID DYSPLASIA

BONE MARROW DYSCRASIA OF POODLES

Definition/overview

Bone marrow dyscrasia is a hereditary disorder of Toy and Miniature Poodles characterized by erythrocyte macrocytosis without anemia or reticulocytosis.

Etiology

The underlying etiology is unknown.

Pathophysiology
Measurements of folate or vitamin B12 are normal, and there is no response to therapeutic doses of vitamin B12. The abnormality appears to originate from the bone marrow, as precursors are dysplastic.

Clinical presentation
There are no associated clinical signs, and the dysplastic findings are usually incidental.

Differential diagnosis
Myelodysplastic syndrome, drug-induced dysplasia, vitamin deficiency dysplasia, causes of regenerative anemia.

Diagnosis
Diagnosis is based on the breed and hematologic findings of normal PCV and reticulocyte results, macrocytosis (MCV >80 fl), inappropriate metarubricytosis with megaloblasts, Howell–Jolly bodies, and neutrophil hypersegmentation and gigantism (**Figure 16.35**).

Management
Treatment is not required.

Prognosis
The dyscrasia does not have any negative clinical effects.

LEAD POISONING

(See also Chapter 20: Clinical toxicology.)

Definition/overview
Young animals are particularly susceptible to lead poisoning because it is absorbed quickly and may cross the blood–brain barrier in larger amounts than in older animals. Dietary calcium may increase lead absorption.

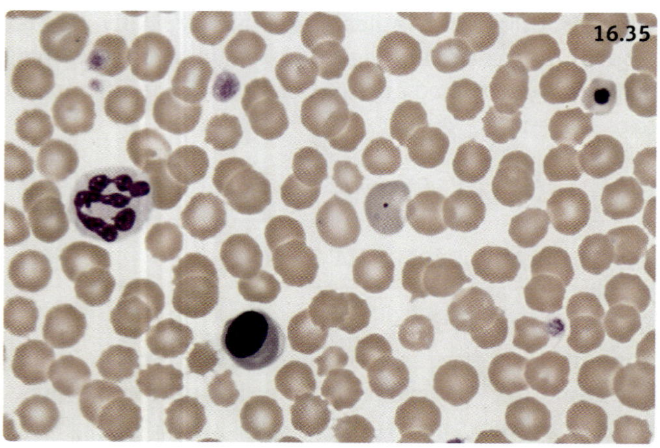

Figure 16.35 Blood from a Poodle with marrow dyscrasia demonstrating a hypersegmented neutrophil, inappropriate metarubricytosis, and nuclear fragments within erythrocytes. The MCV was 99.1 fl (reference range, 66.4–77.4) without reticulocytosis.

Etiology
Causes of lead poisoning include lead shot, especially if it is embedded in tissue in or near joints, and ingestion of lead-containing paint, linoleum, plumbing solder, and window caulking.

Pathophysiology
This condition causes a mild anemia in some cases, possibly due to increased RBC fragility and abnormal erythropoiesis. Lead primarily affects heme synthesis, causing defective maturation.

Clinical presentation
Most clinical signs involve lethargy, anorexia, and GI (vomiting and diarrhea) and neurologic (hysteria and seizures) disturbances. Other signs include blindness, polyuria, polydipsia, abdominal pain, aggression, dementia, pica, megaesophagus, and coma.

Differential diagnosis
Iron deficiency, FeLV infection, drug toxicosis, neurologic disorders, GI disorders, splenic neoplasia (e.g. hemangiosarcoma).

Diagnosis
Diagnosis is often based on a history of exposure to lead and increased lead concentrations in heparinized blood. The most consistent hematologic findings are nucleated RBCs with normal or slightly decreased PCV and no RBC regeneration (54% of cases have inappropriate metarubricytosis). When present, the anemia is often normocytic and normochromic, but may be microcytic and hypochromic. Basophilic stippling is present in 25% of dogs with lead poisoning (**Figure 16.36**). Bone marrow aspirates or core biopsies are characterized by maturation arrest at the metarubricyte stage.

Management
Treatment involves removal of the source of lead, including surgical removal of GI foreign bodies, and administration of calcium EDTA diluted to 10 mg/ml using 5% dextrose (25 mg/kg SC q6h for 5 days). If initial blood lead levels are high (>100 µg/dl), then a second chelation treatment should be considered to reduce concentrations below 40 µg/dl.

Prognosis
Despite dramatic clinical signs, reported mortality rates are low (5.6–15%) in treated dogs.

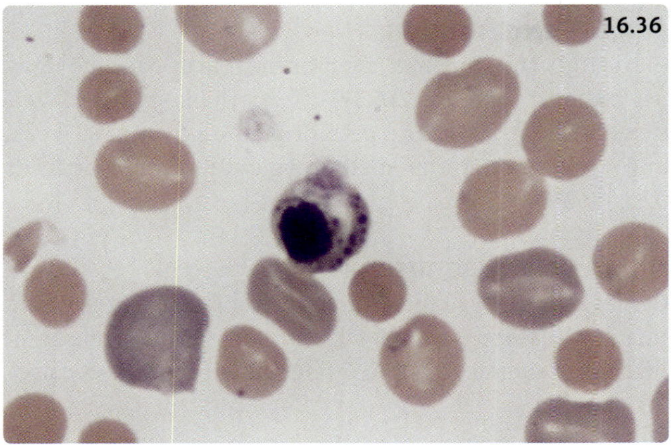

Figure 16.36 Basophilic stippling in a nucleated erythrocyte from a dog with lead poisoning.

ERYTHROCYTOSIS

Erythrocytosis is an increased RBC concentration in peripheral blood that is detected by an increased PCV, Hct, RBC count, or Hgb concentration. Erythrocytosis may be relative (i.e. there is hemoconcentration or redistribution of RBCs in circulation) or absolute, indicating that there is an increased RBC mass due to increased RBC production. Absolute erythrocytosis is further classified as primary or secondary. If the erythroid proliferation is independent of EPO levels, then the absolute erythrocytosis is primary, or an erythroid neoplasm. Secondary absolute erythrocytosis is characterized by EPO-induced erythroid hyperplasia. Polycythemia is sometimes used interchangeably with erythrocytosis, but is also used to indicate an absolute erythrocytosis. Polycythemia vera (PV) is a neoplastic proliferation of hematopoietic cells that produces mature erythrocytes.

RELATIVE ERYTHROCYTOSIS

Definition/overview

The increased RBC concentration is due to redistribution of fluid or RBCs.

Etiology

Etiologies include dehydration, excitement, and endotoxic shock.

Pathophysiology

Fluid loss from the blood vessels causes a relative increase in the proportion of RBCs. Fluid may be lost from the body with dehydration or shifted into the interstitial tissues with endotoxic shock. The spleen contracts during an excitement/physiologic response to epinephrine, releasing erythrocytes from the splenic sinusoids into peripheral circulation.

Clinical presentation

Dehydrated patients may present with tacky mucous membranes and prolonged CRTs and skin tents. Animals with epinephrine-induced physiologic response are often young, healthy animals that are easily excited.

Differential diagnosis

Causes of absolute erythrocytosis (heart disease, chronic pulmonary disease, hyperthyroidism, renal neoplasms, nonrenal neoplasms, PV, acute erythroid leukemia).

Diagnosis

Diagnosis is based on the CBC, history, and physical examination. The hemogram indicates a red cell mass (PCV, Hct, Hgb, and/or RBC) that exceeds the normal reference range for that species or breed. Greyhounds normally have a high PCV of 0.6 l/l (60%). Highly concentrated urine, azotemia, and concurrent increases in serum total protein, sodium, and chloride concentrations may be present with dehydration. Epinephrine release may also cause an excitement leukogram (mild mature neutrophilia and lymphocytosis), thrombocytosis, and hyperglycemia.

Management

Dehydrated patients may require fluid therapy. Treatment is not necessary for excitement-induced erythrocytosis, as the response often declines within 30 minutes.

SECONDARY ABSOLUTE ERYTHROCYTOSIS

Definition/overview

Secondary erythrocytosis involves overproduction of EPO or an EPO-like substance. The erythrocytosis is appropriate if it is in response to hypoxia and inappropriate if oxygen transport and tissue utilization are normal.

Etiology

Causes of secondary appropriate erythrocytosis include hypoxia (e.g. caused by high altitude, chronic pulmonary disease, cardiac disease with right-to-left shunting, hyperthyroidism, or chronic methemoglobinemia). Secondary inappropriate erythrocytosis is caused by tumors that produce erythropoietin (e.g. renal lymphoma, renal carcinoma, and renal fibrosarcoma) and renal disease (e.g. pyelonephritis).

Pathophysiology

As a physiologically appropriate response to hypoxia, EPO production is stimulated in cardiopulmonary disorders. When the hypoxic stimulation is absent, an inappropriate production of EPO or EPO-like substance occurs related to tumor development or renal disease.

Marked erythrocytosis can cause blood hyperviscosity and, subsequently, poor tissue perfusion.

Clinical presentation

Signs may be acute despite the chronic nature of the disorder. Initial findings are dependent on the initiating disease and the presence of hyperviscosity. Findings directly resulting from the erythrocytosis may include erythema, splenomegaly, and bright red mucous membranes. Clinical signs associated with hyperviscosity include functional abnormalities of the CNS and hemorrhage (epistaxis, hyphema, or GI bleeding).

Differential diagnosis

PV, relative erythrocytosis.

Diagnosis

Diagnosis of hypoxia is based on history and evidence of lung disease, right-to-left shunting heart disease, hyperthyroidism, or renal disease. Urinalysis, radiography, ultrasonography, or biopsy can exclude renal disease. Serum total thyroxine can identify hyperthyroidism. Serum EPO levels are currently measured by radioimmunoassay and ELISA methods.

Management

Treatment of secondary erythrocytosis often involves removal of the inciting cause (e.g. nephrectomy). Phlebotomy is indicated if there are signs of hyperviscosity.

METHEMOGLOBINEMIA

Definition/overview

Methemoglobin may be produced in amounts that exceed normal protective antioxidant mechanisms. This form of Hgb is unable to bind and carry oxygen. Normal amounts are generally <1% of Hgb.

Etiology

Methemoglobinemia occurs most commonly from exposure to oxidative agents mentioned under Heinz body formation (p. 695). Rarely, a hereditary deficiency of methemoglobin reductase (cytochrome-b5 reductase) may cause methemoglobinemia. The latter has been documented in several dog breeds and a DSH cat.

Pathophysiology

The erythrocyte antioxidant pathways are overwhelmed, which results in heme oxidation from the ferrous (Fe^{2+}) to the ferric (Fe^{3+}) state. Hemoglobin within the ferric state is termed methemoglobin and is unable to bind oxygen, producing a state of hypoxia.

Clinical presentation

Clinically, the mucous membranes appear blue–gray or cyanotic (**Figure 16.37**) if methemoglobin levels exceed 0.2 l/l (20%). The patient is often dyspneic, weak, and ataxic when the methemoglobin content exceeds 0.5 l/l (50%).

Differential diagnosis

Causes of multisystemic hypoxia without anemia (e.g. pulmonary disease, right-to-left cardiac shunts), causes of hemolytic anemia (e.g. IMHA, hemoplasmosis, babesiosis).

Diagnosis

The appearance of dark red or chocolate-colored blood, even after exposure to air, is diagnostic for the condition and is readily visible by a spot test on filter paper. When normal blood is exposed to air it becomes bright red, while the blood of affected animals remains dark red if the methemoglobin content exceeds 10% (**Figure 16.38**). Methemoglobin content is measured by spectrophotometry by a CO-oximeter or at specialized laboratories; the pulse oximeter cannot cannot detect methemoglobinemia. Other erythrocyte changes may include mild secondary polycythemia in animals with methemoglobin reductase deficiency, or regenerative anemia, Heinz bodies, and eccentrocytes in animals with oxidant-induced hemolytic anemia.

Management

Treatment is similar to that for Heinz body anemia. The source of oxidant should be removed with emetics if recent ingestion has occurred. For acetaminophen (paracetamol)-induced toxicity, acetylcysteine (Mucomyst®) is given initially IV at 140 mg/kg of a 5% solution diluted with saline, and then 70 mg/kg (of a 5%

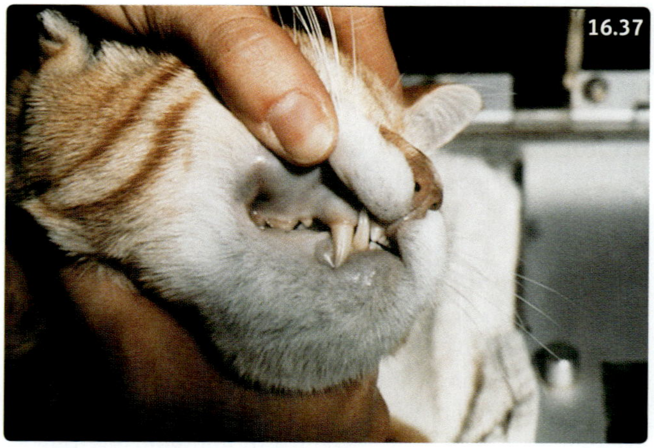

Figure 16.37 This cat with methemoglobinemia as a result of acetaminophen toxicity has blue–gray gums. (Courtesy S. Ford)

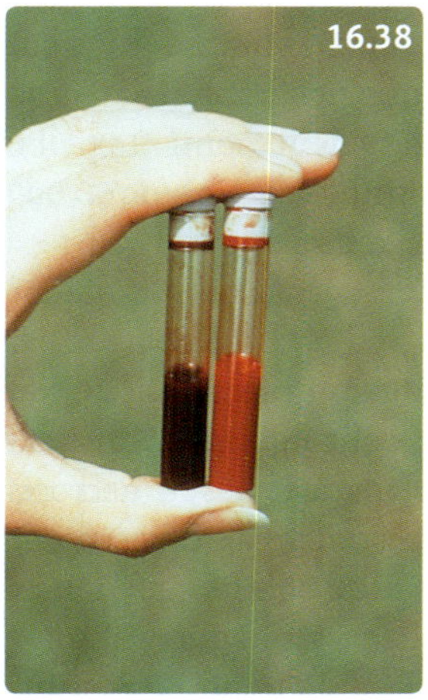

Figure 16.38 Two tubes of blood recently exposed to air. The tube on the left remains a dark color compared with normal blood in the right tube, indicating methemoglobinemia. (Courtesy J. Harvey)

solution) q4h for 3–5 treatments. In addition, sodium ascorbate (vitamin C) may further reduce methemoglobin levels. A dose of 100–500 mg/day IV is recommended for dogs, and a dose of 100 mg/day IV is recommended for cats (see Chapter 20). Therapy is usually not required for animals with the reductase enzyme deficiency.

LEUKOCYTE DISORDERS (NON-NEOPLASTIC)

LEUKOCYTOSIS

Leukocytosis is an increased concentration of the collective white blood cell (WBC) concentration above its reference interval. It does not distinguish which leukocyte type is increased.

Note: Some hematology analyzers (e.g. impedance analyzers) cannot distinguish nucleated RBCs (nRBCs) from WBCs. Therefore, the WBC count represents the sum of WBCs and nRBCs, and should be considered the total nucleated cell count (TNCC) in these cases. If a metarubricytosis is present, the corrected WBC (cWBC) count can be calculated using the TNCC and a blood smear quantification of nRBCs (nRBCs/100 WBCs): cWBC = TNCC × 100/(100 + nRBCs/100 WBCs).

NEUTROPHILIA

Neutrophilia is defined as a neutrophil concentration above the upper reference interval, which is generally >11,500/μl in the dog and >12,500/μl in the cat. Common causes of neutrophilia are excitement, stress, and inflammation, whereas uncommon to rare causes include paraneoplastic syndromes, myeloid leukemia, and canine leukocyte adhesion deficiency (CLAD).

Note: When attempting to distinguish the cause of the neutrophilia as inflammation or noninflammatory (excitement or stress), the presence of one or more of the following observations supports an inflammatory etiology: neutrophilia >2–3 times the upper reference limit, presence of left shift, or neutrophil toxicity.

PHYSIOLOGIC NEUTROPHILIA

Definition/overview

Physiologic (excitement or shift) neutrophilia is a transiently increased neutrophil concentration associated with epinephrine release during a fight or flight response.

Etiology

Epinephrine is released during times of morbid fear, strenuous exercise, or excitement.

Pathophysiology

There are two leukocyte pools within blood, one that is adhered to endothelial cells (marginal pool) and one that is free flowing and not adhered to endothelial cells (circulating pool). The circulating pool is sampled during a blood draw, but the marginal pool is not. In dogs, there are equal numbers of marginal and circulating neutrophils, whereas cats have three times more neutrophils in the marginal pool relative to the circulating pool. Epinephrine release causes decreased adherence of leukocytes to endothelial cells, causing neutrophils and lymphocytes to shift into the circulating pool. The effect is more common and greater in cats in which a three-fold increase may occur compared with a two-fold increase in dogs. There is no left shift associated with this response. Cell counts return to normal within 30 minutes.

Clinical presentation

Physiologic neutrophilia is most common in young, healthy cats. Physical signs of excitement may be observed in the waiting or examination room.

Differential diagnosis

Inflammation, corticosteroid-induced conditions.

Diagnosis

Concurrent abnormalities attributed to epinephrine release include relative erythrocytosis, lymphocytosis, thrombocytosis, and hyperglycemia. If a physiologic response is suspected, blood counts should be repeated after the animal has adjusted to the surroundings. The presence of a left shift or toxicity in neutrophils supports an inflammatory etiology.

Management

Removing the animal from the environmental stimulus should suppress the excitement response within 30 minutes.

CORTICOSTEROID-INDUCED NEUTROPHILIA

Definition/overview

The neutrophilia may be related to exogenous administration or endogenous release of glucocorticoids or ACTH.

Etiology

The neutrophilia may be secondary to stress, hyperadrenocorticism (Cushing's syndrome), or exogenous administration of glucocorticoids or ACTH.

Pathophysiology

Neutrophils shift from the marginal to the circulating pool and are released from the bone marrow storage pool. The magnitude and duration of the effect depend on the type of corticosteroid given. After a single dose of prednisone, neutrophil counts will rise within 4–8 hours and return to baseline within 24 hours.

Clinical presentation

Signs will reflect the underlying condition. Hair loss, polydipsia, polyuria, polyphagia, swollen abdomen, and recurrent bacterial infections are often present with hyperadrenocorticism.

Differential diagnosis

Physiologic neutrophilia, inflammation.

Diagnosis

History and physical examination findings are consistent with an underlying, stress-inducing disease or hyperadrenocorticism. The neutrophilia is typically mild without a left shift, although minimal left shifts rarely occur in dogs. Lymphopenia is the most consistent laboratory finding, but eosinopenia, monocytosis, and hyperglycemia may also occur. Hypersegmented neutrophils may be seen with hyperadrenocorticism or exogenous glucocorticoid administration. Dogs may have increased serum ALP activity.

Management

Treatment should be aimed at the underlying cause.

INFLAMMATORY NEUTROPHILIA

Definition/overview

Inflammation causes increased mobilization of neutrophils from the bone marrow to the site of tissue inflammation. The main indicators of inflammation are increased numbers of immature neutrophils in the blood, termed a left shift, and neutrophil toxicity. A marked inflammatory neutrophilia that exceeds 50,000 neutrophils/μl is called a leukemoid response.

Etiology

The etiology can involve infectious or noninfectious sources. Infectious agents include bacteria, fungi, protozoa, or rickettsiae. Noninfectious conditions involve tissue necrosis such as necrotizing pancreatitis, neoplasia, thrombosis, and burns. A leukemoid response may be associated with IMHA, pancreatitis, pyelonephritis, pyometra, peritonitis, pneumonia, hepatozoonosis, and malignant neoplasms with necrotic centers, especially carcinomas. Canine granulocytopathy syndrome is a rare condition of Irish Setter dogs characterized by recurrent life-threatening bacterial infections, pyrexia, and leukemoid response with impaired neutrophil bactericidal activity.

Pathophysiology

Inflammatory conditions produce cytokines, such as granulocyte colony-stimulating factor (G-CSF) and granulocyte/macrophage colony-stimulating factor (GM-CSF), which promote release of neutrophils from the bone marrow and stimulate granulopoiesis.

Clinical presentation

Sites of inflammation may be apparent from physical examination or diagnostic procedures. Signs will reflect the underlying condition. Pyrexia is often present.

Differential diagnosis

Physiologic neutrophilia, corticosteroid-induced neutrophilia, hematopoietic leukemia.

Diagnosis

Diagnosis of inflammatory neutrophilia is based on a careful history and CBC evaluation. The most specific hematologic indicators of inflammation are the presence of a left shift or neutrophil toxicity.

Management

Treatment will depend on the inciting cause.

OTHER CAUSES OF NEUTROPHILIA

Paraneoplastic neutrophilia is caused by production of G-CSF by neoplasms, such as rectal adenomatous polyp, renal tubular carcinoma, and fibrosarcoma. CLAD is a genetic disorder characterized by marked neutrophilia and recurrent, life-threatening infections due to the inability of neutrophils to exit blood vessels and enter tissues. Both paraneoplastic neutrophilia and CLAD tend to produce neutrophilias that exceed 50,000/µl.

EOSINOPHILIA

Eosinophils are identified by pink–orange cytoplasmic granules that are round and variably sized in dogs and small and rod-shaped in cats. In some Greyhounds, Golden Retrievers, and Shetland Sheepdogs, and, rarely, cats, eosinophils may have granules that do not stain with Romanowsky stains and are termed gray eosinophils (**Figure 16.39**). Eosinophilia is defined as an eosinophil concentration above the upper reference interval, which is generally >1,250/µl in the dog and >1,500/µl in the cat. Non-neoplastic eosinophilia is due to inflammation, hypoadrenocorticism, or paraneoplastic response.

INFLAMMATORY EOSINOPHILIA

Definition/overview

Eosinophilia may be seen with tissue parasitism or allergic (hypersensitivity) disorders.

Etiology

Peripheral eosinophilia may result from infiltration of the skin, respiratory tract, and alimentary tract by such parasites as *Ancylostoma* spp., *Trichuris vulpis*, *Toxocara canis*, *Dirofilaria immitis* (see **Figure 16.23**), *Acanthocheilonema* (formerly *Dipetalonema*) *reconditum*, *Aelurostrongylus abstrusus*, *Eucoleus* (formerly *Capillaria*) spp., *Filaroides* spp., and *Paragonimus kellicotti*. Hypersensitivity reactions can occur from the effects of fleas, food, grasses, and nonspecific allergens. Many idiopathic eosinophilic conditions are thought to be hypersensitivity reactions, including feline eosinophilic granuloma complex and canine eosinophilic bronchopneumopathy.

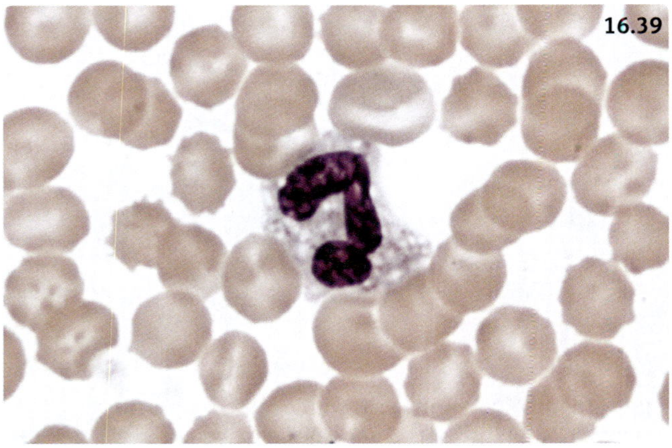

Figure 16.39 Canine eosinophil with poorly staining granules (gray eosinophil).

Pathophysiology

T cell-dependent eosinophils are associated with parasitic infections and hypersensitivities. This type of eosinophilia is mediated by soluble factors, especially IL-5 and GM-CSF. The production of IgE causes mast cell degranulation and release of chemical mediators that attract eosinophils.

Clinical presentation

Signs reflect the organ systems affected, such as skin rashes, diarrhea, coughing, and scratching.

Differential diagnosis

Hypoadrenocorticism, paraneoplastic eosinophilia, hypereosinophilic syndrome, leukemia.

Diagnosis

Diagnosis of parasitism or hypersensitivities includes history, physical examination, food trials, skin tests, serology (e.g. heartworm antigen test), and evaluations of blood smears for microfilaria (see **Figure 16.23**), fecal floats and sediment, tracheobronchial washes, and cytologic or histologic biopsies.

Management

Treatment is aimed at the underlying cause. Treatment for allergic conditions usually involves elimination of the allergen, along with antihistamine and glucocorticoid administration.

HYPOADRENOCORTICISM (ADDISON'S DISEASE)

(See also Chapter 11: Endocrine disorders.)

Definition/overview

Glucocorticoids (e.g. cortisol) and mineralocorticoids (e.g. aldosterone) are hormones produced by the adrenal cortex. Deficient production of these hormones leads to hypoadrenocorticism. Eosinophilia is present in 20% of dogs with hypoadrenocorticism.

Etiology

Hypoadrenocorticism in dogs is typically a result of immune-mediated destruction of the adrenal cortex. Pituitary disease causing ACTH deficiency is uncommon.

Pathophysiology

The pathophysiology of eosinophilia is not completely known, but probably involves cortisol deficiency.

Clinical presentation

Young to middle aged dogs (mean, 4 years; range, 4 months to 14 years) are predisposed, especially Standard Poodles, Portuguese Water Dogs, and Nova Scotia Duck Tolling Retrievers. Animals are often presented for anorexia, vomiting, lethargy, depression, weakness, weight loss, diarrhea, shivering or shaking, polyuria, polydipsia, and/or abdominal pain. There may be weight loss, fasting hypoglycemia, GI hemorrhage, dehydration, bradycardia, and weak femoral pulses. More severe signs of aldosterone deficiency include hypovolemic shock, collapse, and severe dehydration.

Differential diagnosis

Inflammation, paraneoplastic eosinophilia, hypereosinophilic syndrome, leukemia

Diagnosis

Diagnosis is often based on history, physical examination findings, and blood tests for electrolytes and basal and post-ACTH cortisol levels. The most consistent hematologic abnormality is lack of a stress leukogram in a clinically ill animal. Less frequently, lymphocytosis and eosinophilia are observed.

Management

Acute cases of hypoadrenocorticism are treated with appropriate IV fluids, along with administration of glucocorticoids and mineralocorticoids.

PARANEOPLASTIC EOSINOPHILIA

Definition/overview

Paraneoplastic syndromes are disorders caused by neoplasms, but are not a direct result of the physical presence of the tumor in the organ or tissue.

Etiology

Tumor-associated eosinophilia has been reported in dogs with fibrosarcoma, anaplastic mammary carcinoma, T-cell lymphoma, or mast cell tumors, as well as in cats with mast cell tumors or lymphoma.

Pathophysiology

Tumor production and release of GM-CSF, IL-5, histamine, or chemotactic mediators enhance eosinophilopoiesis.

Clinical presentation

Signs reflect the organ systems affected by the neoplasm and often involve one or more tissue masses in the skin, lymphatic system, or urogenital system.

Differential diagnosis

Inflammation, hypoadrenocorticism, hypereosinophilic syndrome, leukemia.

Diagnosis

Diagnosis of a paraneoplastic eosinophilia requires normalization or reduction of the eosinophil concentration in response to tumor removal.

Management

Treatment will reflect the underlying disease and may include surgery, radiation therapy, or chemotherapy.

HYPEREOSINOPHILIC SYNDROME IN CATS

Definition/overview

Hypereosinophilic syndrome is an uncommon form of peripheral eosinophilia in cats accompanied by severe infiltration of eosinophils into many organs, often including the GI tract, liver, spleen, lymph nodes, and lung. It is difficult to differentiate from chronic eosinophilic leukemia, and at least in human medicine, it is now considered a form of chronic leukemia.

Etiology

The etiology is unknown.

Pathophysiology

There is often evidence of intestinal thickening and involvement of the bone marrow that resembles leukemia of well-differentiated eosinophils. Counts have been reported to exceed 50,000/µl (**Figure 16.40**).

16.40

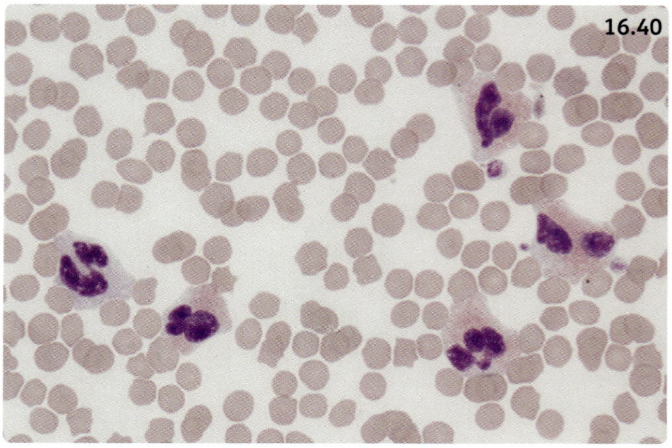

Figure 16.40 Blood from a cat with hypereosinophilic syndrome. Note the four eosinophils and one neutrophil (far left).

Clinical presentation

Clinical signs may include anorexia, weight loss, fever, vomiting, diarrhea, and lymphadenopathy. Death results from organ dysfunction caused by tissue infiltration.

Differential diagnosis

Inflammation, paraneoplastic eosinophilia, eosinophilic leukemia.

Diagnosis

Diagnosis is based on history, physical examination, presence of multisystemic involvement, and ruling out other causes of eosinophilia with fecal examination, diagnostic imaging, and heartworm testing. Bone marrow evaluation establishes the number of eosinophil precursor cells and the degree of marrow involvement. Tissue biopsies show eosinophilic infiltrates.

Management

Prednisolone (1–3 mg/kg PO q12h), with or without hydroxyurea (7.5 mg/kg PO q12h), has been used to reduce eosinophil numbers and clinical signs.

Prognosis

Cats often respond poorly to chemotherapy for long-term control.

BASOPHILIA

Basophilia is defined as an increased blood basophil concentration above the upper reference interval, generally >200/µl in the dog and cat. With the exception of hypoadrenocorticism and hypereosinophilic syndrome, non-neoplastic causes of basophilia are similar to those for eosinophilia: inflammation due to parasitic infections or hypersensitivities, and paraneoplastic basophilia due to mast cell neoplasia or other malignancies. Marked basophilia with atypical leukocytes in the circulation or bone marrow should suggest basophilic leukemia.

It is important to note that basophil granules in dogs and cats stain poorly. In these cases the cells may be mistaken for toxic neutrophils in dogs or faded eosinophils in cats. In addition, basophilia must be distinguished from circulating mast cells in the dog.

LYMPHOCYTOSIS

Lymphocytosis is an increased concentration of lymphocytes in blood, usually >4,800/µl in the dog and >7,000/µl in the cat. Young animals within the first year of life typically have higher lymphocyte concentrations relative to adults, so appropriate reference intervals should be used.

Note: The general classifications of lymphocytosis are reactive (physiologic, chronic inflammation, hypoadrenocorticism) and neoplastic. Reactive lymphocytosis tends to be mild to moderate in severity (e.g. <15,000/µl in dogs and <20,000/µl in cats), consists of lymphocytes of varying morphology, and normalizes when the underlying disorder is appropriately treated. Neoplastic lymphocytosis has varying presentations, but may be mild to marked in severity, consist of a single lymphocyte morphology, and persists without immunosuppressive or cancer chemotherapy.

PHYSIOLOGIC LYMPHOCYTOSIS

Definition/overview

Physiologic (excitement or shift) lymphocytosis is a transient lymphocytosis associated with epinephrine release during a fight or flight response.

Etiology

Epinephrine is released during times of morbid fear, strenuous exercise, or excitement.

Pathophysiology

Epinephrine release causes lymphocytes to shift from the marginal pool to the circulating pool.

Clinical presentation

Physiologic lymphocytosis is most common in healthy, young animals, especially cats. Affected animals appear excited or have a history of strenuous muscular exertion.

Differential diagnosis

Chronic inflammation, hypoadrenocorticism, lymphoid neoplasia.

Diagnosis

The lymphocytosis is typically less than two-fold above the upper reference limit. Concurrent laboratory abnormalities may include relative erythrocytosis, mature neutrophilia, thrombocytosis, and hyperglycemia. If a physiologic response is suspected, blood counts should be repeated after the animal has adjusted to the surroundings.

Management

Removing the animal from the environmental stimulus should suppress the excitement response.

CHRONIC INFLAMMATORY LYMPHOCYTOSIS

Definition/overview

Chronic antigenic or cytokine stimulation results in lymphoid hyperplasia.

Etiology

Chronic inflammation of an infectious or noninfectious etiology can cause lymphoid hyperplasia and subsequent lymphocytosis. In particular, lymphocytosis involving intermediate-sized granular lymphocytes (**Figure 16.41**) has been associated with *Ehrlichia canis* infection in dogs. Modified live vaccines may also produce lymphocytosis about 1 week post immunization.

Pathophysiology

Antigen presenting cells, such as macrophages and dendritic cells, process and present inciting antigens to T lymphocytes. B cell development often requires co-stimulatory signals from T-helper cells, along with cytokines, for activation and differentiation into plasma cells that produce antibodies against the inciting antigen.

Clinical presentation

Signs reflect the underlying inflammatory condition.

Differential diagnosis

Excitement, hypoadrenocorticism, lymphoid neoplasia.

Diagnosis

There is typically a mixed lymphoid population of small and large lymphocytes of varying morphology. Slightly enlarged lymphocytes with deeply basophilic cytoplasm (reactive lymphocytes) may be noted (**Figure 16.42**). Hyperglobulinemia due to a polyclonal gammopathy and plasma cell infiltration of tissues may also occur (**Figure 16.43**). The presence of intermediate-sized lymphocytes characterized by abundant pale blue cytoplasm with or without granules suggests T cell stimulation (see **Figure 16.41**). Maximum lymphocytosis in extreme immune reactions is usually <15,000/µl in dogs and <20,000/µl in cats.

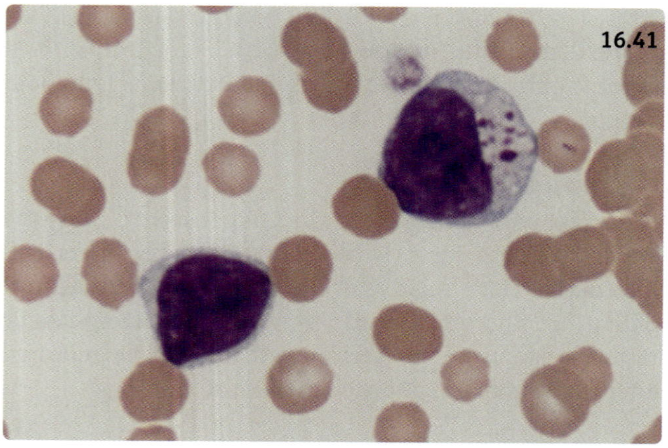

Figure 16.41 Compared with a small lymphocyte (left), a large granular lymphocyte (right) has a moderate amount of basophilic cytoplasm containing several coarse pink–purple granules.

Management

Treatment should be aimed at the underlying cause.

HYPOADRENOCORTICISM

(See also Chapter 11: Endocrine disorders.)

Definition/overview

Glucocorticoids (e.g. cortisol) and mineralocorticoids (e.g. aldosterone) are hormones produced by the adrenal cortex. Deficient production of these hormones leads

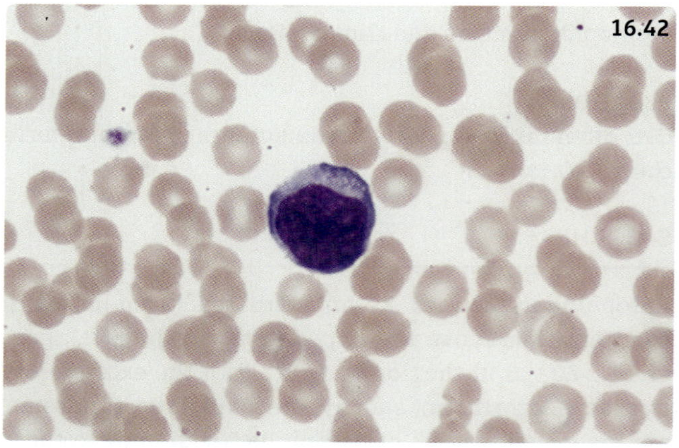

Figure 16.42 A reactive lymphocyte with a moderate amount of deeply basophilic cytoplasm and a perinuclear pale zone (Golgi apparatus).

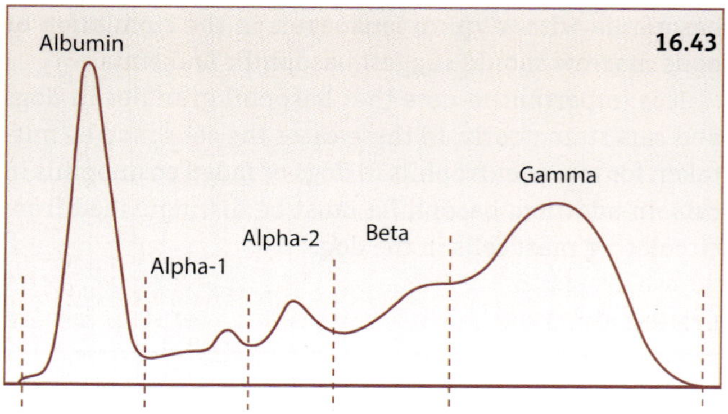

Figure 16.43 Serum protein electrophoretic tracing with a broad peak in the gamma region indicating the presence of a polyclonal gammopathy in a case of canine ehrlichiosis.

to hypoadrenocorticism. Lymphocytosis is present in 10–20% of dogs with hypoadrenocorticism.

Etiology

Hypoadrenocorticism in dogs is typically a result of immune-mediated destruction of the adrenal cortex. Pituitary disease causing ACTH deficiency is uncommon.

Pathophysiology

Corticosteroids cause lymphocytes to leave the circulation and enter lymphoid tissues. A lack of glucocorticoids inhibits this redistribution and allows lymphocyte numbers to increase in the circulation.

Clinical presentation

Animals present with lethargy, decreased tolerance to stress, weakness, and GI symptoms such as anorexia, vomiting, diarrhea, and abdominal pain. There may be weight loss, fasting hypoglycemia, dehydration, bradycardia, and weak femoral pulses. Vascular collapse is possible because of impaired vascular compensation for hypovolemia.

Differential diagnosis

Physiologic lymphocytosis, chronic inflammation, lymphoid leukemia.

Diagnosis

Diagnosis is often based on history, physical examination findings, and blood tests for electrolytes and basal and post-ACTH cortisol levels. Lack of a stress leukogram in a visibly ill dog is the most consistent hematologic abnormality.

Management

Acute cases of hypoadrenocorticism are treated with appropriate IV fluids, along with administration of glucocorticoids and mineralocorticoids.

MONOCYTOSIS

Monocytosis is defined as a blood monocyte concentration above the upper reference interval, generally >1,350/µl in the dog and >850/µl in the cat. It most frequently results from an increased demand for monocytes and tissue macrophages, which function in the defense against infectious agents, phagocytosis of damaged cells and debris, and secretion of many important biologically active molecules. Monocytes are not stored in the bone marrow during production, but are immediately released. However, they may marginate in blood vessels for short periods of time or enter tissues from the circulating pool. Monocytes entering the tissues are transformed into macrophages, which can persist for days to months. Myeloid leukemia should be considered when monocyte counts exceed 15,000/µl or immature monocytoid forms are predominant.

CORTICOSTEROID-INDUCED MONOCYTOSIS

Definition/overview

Monocytosis can be induced by glucocorticoids, especially in dogs.

Etiology

Monocytosis may be secondary to stress, hyperadrenocorticism (Cushing's syndrome), or exogenous administration of glucocorticoids or ACTH.

Pathophysiology

Monocytes shift from the marginal pool to the circulating pool within the vasculature. The leukogram alterations occur within 4–8 hours of a single dose of glucocorticoids and counts return to baseline within 24 hours.

Clinical presentation

Signs will reflect the underlying condition. Hair loss, polydipsia, polyuria, polyphagia, distended abdomen, and recurrent bacterial infections are often present with hyperadrenocorticism.

Differential diagnosis

Chronic inflammation, myeloid leukemia.

Diagnosis

Diagnosis is based on history, physical examination, and diagnostic imaging; however, the presence of concurrent mature neutrophilia, lymphopenia, and eosinopenia suggests corticosteroid effects.

Management

Treatment is directed at the underlying disease. If exogenous glucocorticoids are the cause, readjustment of the dose or cessation of administration should be considered.

CHRONIC INFLAMMATORY MONOCYTOSIS

Definition/overview

Monocytosis may occur with acute or chronic inflammation. However, the monocytosis associated with acute conditions is secondary to stress, whereas chronic inflammatory monocytosis results from monocytic hyperplasia.

Etiology
Inflammatory diseases that cause a high demand for tissue macrophages may produce monocytosis. These include immune-mediated disorders, tissue necrosis, foreign body reactions, and mycobacterial or fungal infections.

Pathophysiology
Inflammatory conditions produce cytokines, such as GM-CSF, macrophage colony-stimulating factor, and IL-3, which stimulates marrow production of monocytes.

Clinical presentation
Signs will reflect the underlying inflammatory condition.

Differential diagnosis
Corticosteroid-induced monocytosis, myeloid leukemia.

Diagnosis
Other hematologic abnormalities with chronic inflammation may include neutrophilia, neutrophil left shifting, toxic neutrophils, and lymphocytosis.

Management
Treatment is aimed at the inciting cause.

MASTOCYTEMIA

Mast cell precursors are produced in the bone marrow as nongranular mononuclear cells. They travel through peripheral blood to complete their maturation in tissues. As such, mast cell precursors cannot be distinguished from other mononuclear cells in blood. Mastocytemia is therefore defined as the presence of mast cells in peripheral blood, since the observance of any mast cells in blood is abnormal. Hematology analyzers cannot identify mast cells, so blood smear evaluation is imperative to identify mastocytemia. Mast cells are identified by the presence of purple cytoplasmic granules and a round nucleus (**Figure 16.44**), and should be distinguished from basophils, which have segmented nuclei. Methanolic Romanowsky stains are preferable to aqueous Romanowsky stains for identification of mast cells, since their granules are soluble in the latter stains and may not be visible. Mastocytemia typically indicates disseminated mast cell neoplasia (systemic mastocytosis) in cats, but most dogs with mastocytemia have disease other than mast cell neoplasia. Feline mast cell neoplasms often exhibit erythrophagocytosis.

Note: When present, mast cells tend to localize within the feathered edge of the blood smear.

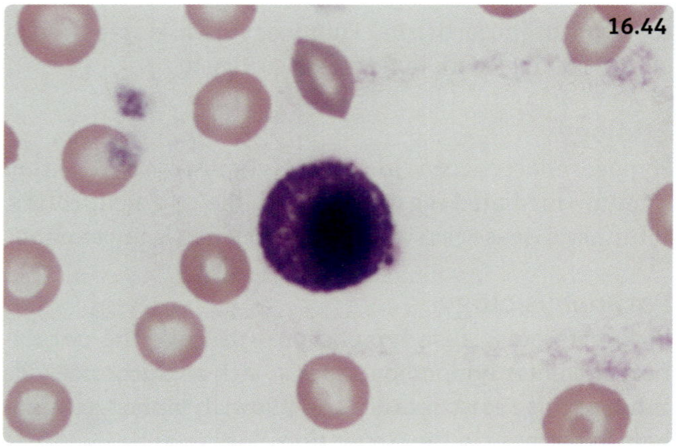

Figure 16.44 Mast cells are identified by dark purple cytoplasmic granules and a round nucleus.

REACTIVE MASTOCYTEMIA

Definition/overview
Non-neoplastic conditions that present with mast cells in blood are termed mastocytemia.

Etiology
Mastocytemia in dogs is associated with inflammatory disease (parvovirus enteritis, hypersensitivities, acute pancreatitis), regenerative anemia, neoplasms other than mast cell tumors, and trauma.

Pathophysiology
It is suggested that inflamed tissues, such as the GI tract or skin, may release these mast cells more readily than normal.

Clinical presentation
Signs are dependent on the underlying disorder.

Differential diagnosis
Mast cell neoplasia.

Diagnosis
History, physical examination, diagnostic imaging, and tissue biopsies are necessary to rule out mast cell neoplasia.

Management
Treatment will reflect the underlying condition.

LEUKOPENIA

Leukopenia is a decreased concentration of all WBCs combined. Leukopenia may be due to decreases in neutrophils or lymphocytes. Because of their normally low concentrations in blood, decreases in monocytes, eosinophils, or basophils tend not to cause leukopenia. Monocytopenia and basopenia are not clinically significant in dogs and cats.

NEUTROPENIA

Neutropenia is decreased blood neutrophils, often <3,000/µl in the dog and <2,500/µl in the cat. It may result from excessive tissue demands, redistribution within the vasculature, peripheral destruction, or decreased production.

Note: Patients with neutrophil concentrations <500–1,000/µl are at risk for secondary, life-threatening infection, termed neutropenic sepsis; prophylactic administration of broad-spectrum antibiotics should be considered in these cases.

INFLAMMATORY NEUTROPENIA

Definition/overview

Tissue utilization of neutrophils exceeds bone marrow production of neutrophils during times of severe inflammation.

Etiology

Causes of severe inflammation are typically infectious, and include gram-negative septicemia, severe enteritis, systemic mycoses, and systemic protozoal infections.

Pathophysiology

Neutrophil migration into inflamed tissues exceeds the release of neutrophils from the bone marrow.

Clinical presentation

Signs are often indicative of infectious disease, including anorexia, pyrexia, and lethargy. Additional signs are dependent on the affected tissues or organs.

Differential diagnosis

Myelosuppression, endotoxemia, immune-mediated neutropenia, hemophagocytic syndrome, cyclic hematopoiesis.

Diagnosis

Diagnosis is based on history, complete physical examination, tests for infectious diseases, and cytology or histopathology of bone marrow. The presence of a left shift or neutrophil toxicity supports inflammation, but a mild left shift or slight toxicity may be seen with other causes of neutropenia. Sequential evaluation of the leukogram should exclude cyclic or transient neutropenia.

Management

Treatment is directed at the inciting cause.

REDISTRIBUTION NEUTROPENIA

Definition/overview

Increased margination of circulating neutrophils can result in neutropenia.

Etiology

Endotoxins from gram-negative sepsis produce a transient neutropenia.

Pathophysiology

After a single exposure to endotoxin, neutrophils rapidly shift from the circulating pool to the marginal pool for 1–3 hours. The neutropenia is short lived since endotoxins also stimulate release of neutrophils from the bone marrow, and neutropoiesis within the bone marrow.

Clinical presentation

Signs of gram-negative infection include pyrexia, anorexia, lethargy. However, given the peracute time frame for the neutropenia, redistribution neutropenia is often no longer present on presentation of the animal.

Differential diagnosis

Myelosuppression, severe inflammation, immune-mediated neutropenia, hemophagocytic syndrome, cyclic hematopoiesis.

Diagnosis

Diagnosis is based on history, complete physical examination, tests for infectious diseases, and cytology or histopathology of bone marrow. Sequential evaluation of the leukogram may reveal a normal or increased neutrophil concentration with or without signs of inflammation (e.g. left shift, neutrophil toxicity).

Management

Treatment for sepsis involves appropriate antibiotics.

PERIPHERAL DESTRUCTION NEUTROPENIA

Definition/overview

Neutropenia may be due to immune targeting of neutrophil antigens (immune-mediated neutropenia) or nonspecific destruction of hematopoietic cells by dysregulated phagocytes (hemophagocytic syndrome).

Etiology

Drugs responsible for suspected immune-mediated neutropenia include antithyroid drugs (e.g. thiouracil, methimazole) and cephalosporins. Hemophagocytic syndrome is caused by inappropriate activation of normal macrophages secondary to infectious (canine parvovirus, bacterial sepsis, ehrlichiosis, blastomycosis, and Lyme disease), neoplastic (lymphoid neoplasia and myelodysplastic syndrome), or immune-mediated (SLE) disease. Idiopathic hemophagocytic syndrome has also been described.

Pathophysiology

The disorder may involve antibody directed against surface antigens on the cell itself, or antibody directed toward drug antigens attached to the neutrophil as an 'innocent bystander'. Autoantibodies may also produce defects in neutrophil function.

Clinical presentation

Signs may reflect those of immune-mediated, infectious, or neoplastic diseases.

Differential diagnosis

Other immune-mediated hematologic disorders, SLE, immune-mediated arthritis, neoplasia, drug-induced myelosuppression, severe systemic inflammation, endotoxemia, hypersplenism, cyclic hematopoiesis, myelophthisis.

Diagnosis

Diagnosis of immune-mediated neutropenia requires detection of antineutrophil antibodies on the cells or in serum. However, such assays are not widely available and are not specific for immune-mediated neutropenia. Immune-mediated neutropenia is more commonly diagnosed by excluding other causes of neutropenia, and demonstrating improvement with appropriate therapy. Hemophagocytic syndrome may cause bicytopenia or pancytopenia. Cytologic or histologic tissue biopsies reveal many phagocytic macrophages. An underlying disease may be identified with a complete diagnostic work up, including physical examination, thoracic and abdominal imaging, and fluid and tissue biopsies.

Management

Immune-mediated neutropenia may be resolved by stopping administration of the inciting drug and commencing immunosuppressive therapy. Treatment for hemophagocytic syndrome is directed at the inciting disease.

DECREASED PRODUCTION NEUTROPENIA

Definition/overview

Decreased neutrophil production may occur with certain drugs, infectious agents, myelophthisis, and irradiation that affect the bone marrow. It is diagnosed by demonstrating bone marrow hypoplasia (**Figure 16.45**).

Etiology

Drugs that cause neutropenia due to myelotoxicity include estrogens, chloramphenicol, trimethoprim–sulfadiazine, griseofulvin, and cancer chemotherapeutic agents. Antineoplastic agents that can cause neutropenia include cyclophosphamide, chlorambucil, busulfan, mephalan, cisplatin, cytosine arabinoside, methotrexate, mitoxantrone, doxorubicin, and hydroxyurea. Cephalosporins and certain NSAIDs have been associated with myelotoxicity. Reduced granulopoiesis may be associated with such viruses as FeLV, FIP virus, feline panleukopenia virus, and canine parvovirus. *Ehrlichia canis* infection, when severe, may also cause bone marrow hypoplasia. Leukemia, myelitis (systemic histoplasmosis), or idiopathic myelofibrosis may cause myelophthisis.

Pathophysiology

Normal hematopoietic precursors may be crowded out with myelophthisis. Irradiation, drugs, and infectious agents destroy rapidly dividing precursor cells. Aplastic anemia and myelofibrosis may be idiopathic.

Note: If there is generalized marrow injury, cells with short circulating life spans decrease prior to those with

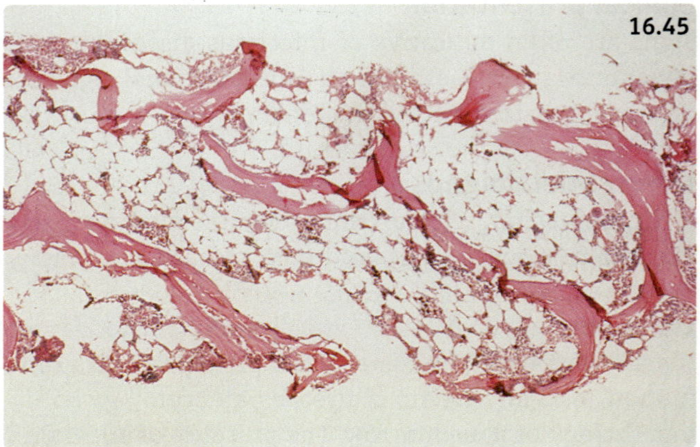

Figure 16.45 Bone marrow histologic section showing the hypocellularity and increased fat infiltration seen in conditions such as myelosuppression.

longer life spans. Neutrophils circulate for hours, platelets circulate for days to weeks, and erythrocytes circulate for months. Therefore, neutropenia often precedes other cytopenias, but moderate to marked anemia is appreciated for months after the initial insult.

Clinical presentation

Signs may include those due to severe neutropenia (severe bacterial infections or sepsis) with or without signs of marked thrombocytopenia (multisystemic hemorrhage) and anemia (lethargy, pale mucous membranes). Other signs reflect the animal's underlying condition.

Differential diagnosis

Cyclic hematopoiesis, severe systemic inflammation, endotoxemia, hemophagocytic syndrome, immune-mediated neutropenia.

Diagnosis

Diagnosis of the underlying disorder may require a thorough history and physical examination, blood tests for viral disease and organ health (CBC, serum chemistry, and urinalysis), diagnostic imaging, tissue biopsy, bone marrow evaluation, and bacterial culture.

Management

Treatment requires cessation of myelotoxic drugs and supportive care, particularly antibiotics. The use of recombinant canine G-CSF (5 µg/kg SC q24h) has shown promise in reducing the severity of drug-induced myelosuppression in the dog and cat. Specific treatment is dependent upon the underlying disorder.

CYCLIC HEMATOPOIESIS

Definition/overview

Congenital cyclic hematopoiesis is an inherited autosomal recessive disorder of gray Collies characterized by periodic fluctuations in neutrophils and, to a lesser extent, in monocytes, platelets, and reticulocytes. Nonhereditary cyclic hematopoiesis may involve other breeds of dogs. Cyclic neutropenia in cats has been associated with FeLV infection.

Etiology

The molecular basis of the genetic defect in dogs is unknown, but seems to be associated with a defect in the intracellular trafficking of neutrophil elastase. FeLV infection is associated with cyclic neutropenia in cats.

Pathophysiology

In gray Collies, cyclic differentiation of stem cells toward committed lineages results in 11–14 day cycles of erythrocyte, neutrophil, monocyte, and platelet production. Decreases in blood neutrophil concentrations are most prevalent given their shorter circulating life spans. Dogs with nonhereditary cyclic hematopoiesis have variable cycle lengths from 10–29 days. Cats infected with FeLV have neutrophil cycle lengths reported to range from 8–16 days.

Clinical presentation

Clinical signs during neutropenic episodes include lethargy, pyrexia, anorexia, arthritis, keratitis, diarrhea, and respiratory infections. Affected Collies present with other distinctive features such as abnormal hair pigmentation, bilateral scleral ectasia, enteropathy, and gonadal hypoplasia.

Differential diagnosis

Severe systemic inflammation, noncyclic myelosuppression from drugs, infections, or irradiation, immune-mediated neutropenia, hemophagocytic syndrome, endotoxemia.

Diagnosis

Diagnosis is based on history, signalment, clinical signs, and cyclic decreases in cell counts. Carrier animals can be determined only by test mating. All affected dogs have a diluted coat color. Amyloidosis is commonly found in many tissues.

Management

Antibiotics and supportive care are necessary during neutropenic cycles. Experimental treatment for dogs with the 'gray Collie syndrome' involves bone marrow transplantation and administration of lithium carbonate (21–26 mg/kg/day) or recombinant canine G-CSF (5 µg/kg/day). Cyclic neutropenia in FeLV-infected cats can respond to prednisone.

Prognosis

Most affected dogs die within 6 months following chronic recurrent infections.

EOSINOPENIA

Eosinopenia is defined as an eosinophil concentration less than the lower reference interval, generally <100/µl in the dog. Since the cat may normally lack eosinophils, it is difficult to recognize reduced numbers. Eosinopenia often results from decreased production or redistribution.

CORTICOSTEROID-INDUCED EOSINOPENIA

Definition/overview

Eosinopenia can be induced by exogenous administration or endogenous release of glucocorticoids or ACTH.

Etiology

Eosinopenia may be secondary to stress, hyperadrenocorticism (Cushing's syndrome), or exogenous administration of glucocorticoids or ACTH.

Pathophysiology

Implicated mechanisms are intravascular lysis, decreased bone marrow release, enhanced margination, and reduced bone marrow production. Eosinopenia occurs within 1–6 hours of a single dose of glucocorticoids and counts return to baseline within 24 hours.

Clinical presentation

Signs reflect the underlying condition. Hair loss, polydipsia, polyuria, polyphagia, swollen abdomen, and recurrent bacterial infections are often present with hyperadrenocorticism.

Differential diagnosis

Generalized marrow hypoplasia or aplasia.

Diagnosis

History and physical examination findings are consistent with an underlying disease. Other leukogram changes attributed to stress include neutrophilia without a left shift, lymphopenia, and monocytosis. However, hematologic evidence of inflammation (left shift, neutrophil toxicity) may occur if the underlying disease is inflammatory. Hypersegmented neutrophils may be seen with hyperadrenocorticism or exogenous glucocorticoid administration. Dogs may have increased serum ALP activity.

Management

Treatment is directed at the underlying disease. Levels will normalize in one day after a single dose of corticosteroids is given.

LYMPHOPENIA

Lymphopenia is defined as a blood lymphocyte concentration less than the lower reference interval, generally <1,000/μl in the dog and <1,500/μl in the cat. Mechanisms include redistribution into lymphoid tissues, decreased production, infection-induced destruction, obstruction of lymph flow, and increased loss through lymphatic vessel damage.

CORTICOSTEROID-INDUCED LYMPHOPENIA

Definition/overview

Lymphopenia often accompanies stress, hyperadrenocorticism, or exogenous glucocorticoid or ACTH administration. This is the most common cause of lymphopenia.

Etiology

Endogenous or exogenous corticosteroids produce an absolute lymphopenia or a normal value reduced from a previous lymphocytosis.

Pathophysiology

The immediate effect of glucocorticoids is lymphocyte redistribution to lymphoid tissues. Prolonged or high doses of glucocorticoids cause lympholysis and lymphoid hypoplasia. Lymphopenia is transient as cell counts return to normal within 1–3 days following drug withdrawal.

Clinical presentation

Signs reflect the underlying condition. Hair loss, polydipsia, polyuria, polyphagia, swollen abdomen, and recurrent bacterial infections are often present with hyperadrenocorticism.

Differential diagnosis

Systemic infections, generalized lymphadenopathy, chylothorax, lymphangiectasia, severe combined immunodeficiency (SCID).

Diagnosis

Other leukogram changes attributed to glucocorticoids include neutrophilia without a left shift, eosinopenia, and monocytosis. However, concurrent inflammation (left shift, neutrophil toxicity) may be present. Hypersegmented neutrophils may be seen with hyperadrenocorticism or exogenous glucocorticoid administration. Dogs may have increased serum ALP activity.

Management

The underlying cause should be treated. If drug induced, the dosage may be adjusted or stopped.

LYMPHOID HYPOPLASIA

Definition/overview

Decreased lymphocyte production occurs with certain viral infections, immunosuppressive drugs, generalized lymphadenopathy, or whole body irradiation.

Etiology

Etiologies include viruses (CDV, FeLV, FIV, parvoviruses), drugs (chemotherapeutics), generalized lymphadenitis (systemic fungal infections), multicentric lymphoma, and whole body irradiation.

Pathophysiology

There is direct lympholysis or lymphoid tissue destruction.

Clinical presentation

Signs reflect the affected organ systems.

Differential diagnosis

Corticosteroids, chylothorax, lymphangiectasia, SCID.

Diagnosis

Diagnosis of the underlying disease is based on history, physical examination, serology for the specific viral infections, and tissue biopsy.

Management

Treatment is directed toward the underlying cause.

ALTERED LYMPH FLOW

Definition/overview

Obstruction of lymph flow or loss of lymphatic fluid from the body interferes with the recirculation of lymphocytes.

Etiology

Lymph flow may be obstructed by generalized lymphadenitis (systemic fungal infections) or multicentric lymphoma. Lymphocytes can be lost from the body with repeated drainage of chylous effusions or through loss of lymph into the GI tract with lymphangiectasia and protein-losing enteropathy (PLE).

Pathophysiology

Blocked lymph flow or lymph loss prevents lymphocyte recirculation.

Clinical presentation

Signs are dependent on the underlying disease. Chylous effusions typically cause dyspnea, and there will be a history of repeated effusion drainage. Signs associated with PLE include weight loss and diarrhea.

Generalized lymphadenomegaly is expected with lymphadenitis and multicentric lymphoma.

Differential diagnosis

Corticosteroids, viral infections, SCID.

Diagnosis

Diagnosis is based on history, physical examination, and laboratory and imaging tests. Chylous effusions are identified by body cavity fluid analysis. They tend to be white with high triglyceride and lymphocyte concentrations. Hypoproteinemia, hypocholesterolemia, and GI hemorrhage can occur with PLE; intestinal biopsy or empirical therapy may reveal the underlying disease. Lymphoma and systemic fungal infections are typically diagnosed by cytologic or histologic biopsy of lymph nodes or other diseased tissue.

Management

Treatment is directed at the underlying disease.

SEVERE COMBINED IMMUNODEFICIENCY

Definition/overview

Congenital defects in lymphocyte development result in lymphoid aplasia and subsequent marked lymphopenia and hypoglobulinemia. The disease is rare, but has been documented in Basset Hounds, Cardigan Welsh Corgis, Jack Russell Terriers, and Frisian Water Dogs.

Etiology

The deficiency in Basset Hounds and Cardigan Welsh Corgis is X-linked due to separate mutations in an IL receptor. An autosomal recessive mode of inheritance occurs in Jack Russell Terriers due to mutated DNA-dependent protein kinase. Frisian Water Dogs have a mutation of RAG1.

Pathophysiology
Defective lymphocyte development results in immune incompetence, which becomes fatal when maternal antibodies wane. There is depressed T cell function, low IgG and IgA concentrations, and variable IgM concentrations. Affected animals usually die from infectious disease.

Clinical presentation
Puppies may be small, thin, and inactive. Signs of recurrent infections occur as bacterial pyoderma and otitis externa within the first 6 weeks of life. Mucopurulent ocular and nasal discharges are common. Lymphadenopathy is not present. Death may occur within 50 hours of administering a modified live vaccine.

Differential diagnosis
Viral infections, PLE, exogenous corticosteroids.

Diagnosis
Diagnosis is based on the history of high morbidity and mortality in puppies from the same breeding pair of dogs. Affected puppies have lymphopenia, hypoglobulinemia, and depressed T lymphocyte function. Necropsy reveals profound lymphoid hypoplasia.

Management
Antibiotics may be administered, but death due to infectious disease is expected. Bone marrow transplantation is the only means to regain immune competence. Carrier animals should not be bred.

Prognosis
Mortality occurs when maternal antibodies wane at 8–14 weeks of age.

ABNORMAL NUCLEAR MORPHOLOGY

INFLAMMATORY LEFT SHIFT

Definition/overview
A left shift is defined as an increase in immature neutrophils over the reference interval. Immature neutrophils include band neutrophils (bands), metamyelocytes, myelocytes, and promyelocytes. The shift is considered 'degenerative' when immature neutrophils outnumber segmented neutrophils or when a left shift occurs in the presence of neutropenia. A degenerative left shift indicates severe tissue inflammation that has overwhelmed the bone marrow's ability to produce neutrophils. Any left shift that is not degenerative is termed 'regenerative', meaning that neutropoiesis is able to meet or exceed peripheral demand.

Etiology
A left shift is usually caused by a systemic inflammatory lesion, such as in pyometra, pneumonia, large neoplasm, or immune-mediated disorders (e.g. IMHA). A degenerative left shift is typically a result of severe infectious disease.

Pathophysiology
Inflammatory cytokines (e.g. IL-1, IL-6, IL-8, GM-CSF, and G-CSF) enhance neutrophil release from the bone marrow into blood. Release is sequential in that bands enter the blood before metamyelocytes and earlier stages. With continued inflammation, cytokines stimulate neutrophil production, taking 5–7 days for a myeloblast to mature into a segmented form. A left shift may accompany acute or chronic inflammation.

Clinical presentation
Signs reflect the affected organ system.

Differential diagnosis
Pelger–Huët anomaly, myelodysplastic syndrome, granulocytic leukemia.

Diagnosis
Blood smear evaluation shows increased numbers of immature neutrophils, particularly band neutrophils (**Figure 16.46**). Sites of inflammation can be determined by history, physical examination, biochemical profile, urinalysis, diagnostic imaging, and biopsies.

Management
Treatment is directed toward the underlying cause.

Prognosis
Animals with degenerative left shifts tend to have poorer outcomes relative to those with regenerative left shifts. Worsening of the left shift is a negative prognostic indicator, whereas dampening or resolution of a left shift indicates clinical improvement.

PELGER–HUËT ANOMALY

Definition/overview
This non-neoplastic developmental abnormality is an inherited disorder in dogs and cats involving all granulocytes.

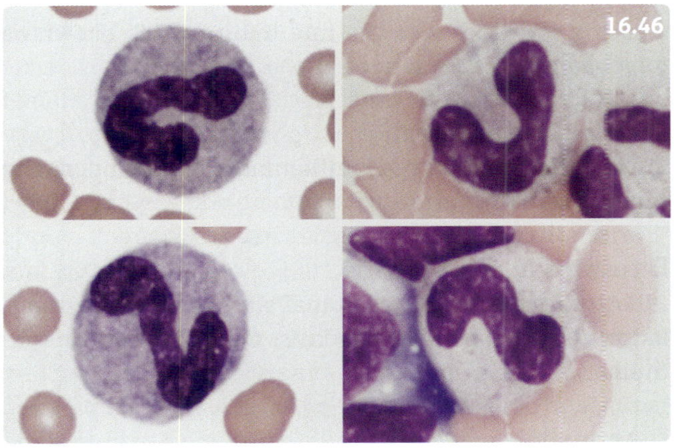

Figure 16.46 Band neutrophils from a cat (left) and dog (right) lack nuclear segments, and have slightly open chromatin. The two feline neutrophils display cytoplasmic basophilia (toxicity).

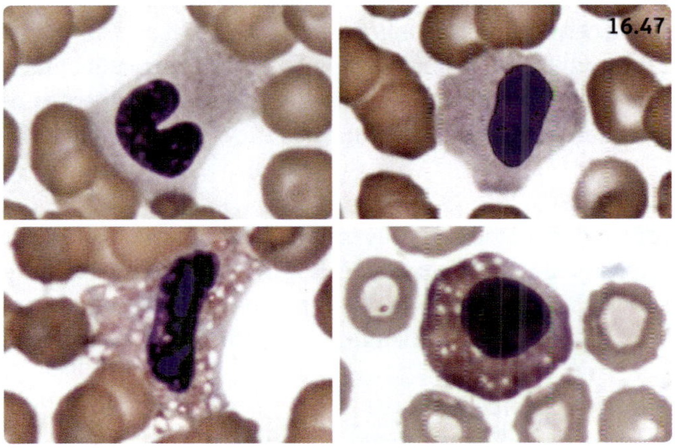

Figure 16.47 Nuclei of neutrophils (top) and eosinophils (bottom) fail to segment with Pelger–Huët anomaly. However, the chromatin pattern is dense, indicating nuclear maturity.

Etiology
Pelger–Huët anomaly is inherited in an autosomal dominant manner due to a mutated lamin B receptor. Affected dog breeds include, but are not exclusive to, Australian Heelers, Australian Shepherd Dogs, Basenjis, Border Collies, Cocker Spaniels, Coonhounds, German Shepherd Dogs, and Samoyeds. It has been reported in one family of Domestic Shorthair cats.

Pathophysiology
This condition is suggested to be a stem cell defect, since megakaryocytes may also appear hyposegmented.

Clinical presentation
Chondrodysplasia has been recognized in a stillborn homozygous kitten. Heterozygote kittens may be stillborn or viable. Heterozygote dogs do not present with signs of infection.

Differential diagnosis
Inflammatory left shift, myelodysplastic syndrome, granulocytic leukemia.

Diagnosis
Diagnosis is based on the appearance of blood leukocytes that have mature chromatin (condensed, coarse, and patchy) and nuclear shapes that reflect immaturity (band, indented, or round) (**Figure 16.47**). The cytoplasm undergoes normal maturation. Pelger–Huët anomaly is frequently found during routine preoperative screening.

Note: The significance in diagnosing Pelger–Huët anomaly is that it is not interpreted as a degenerative left shift due to severe inflammation.

Management
No treatment is necessary.

Prognosis
Leukocyte function in dogs is not impaired and there is no predisposition to infection or immunodeficiency. The homozygous condition found in the cat is lethal and may be associated with skeletal deformities and increased susceptibility to infection.

HYPERSEGMENTATION

Definition/overview
Hypersegmentation is defined as a neutrophil with more than five nuclear segments, and it indicates aging or dysplasia.

Etiology
Hypersegmentation is seen with delayed sample analysis, glucocorticoid administration, hyperadrenocorticism, hyperthermia (e.g. heat stroke, malignant hyperthermia), CLAD, dysplastic processes (Poodle macrocytosis, vitamin B12 deficiency), and myeloid leukemias.

Pathophysiology
Hypersegmentation occurs as part of the normal aging process, and reflects a prolonged transit time in blood. Dysplastic and neoplastic processes are due to abnormal neutrophil maturation.

Clinical presentation
Signs reflect the underlying condition.

Differential diagnosis

Hyperadrenocorticism, exogenous glucocorticoids, heat stroke, malignant hyperthermia, CLAD, Poodle macrocytosis, vitamin B12 (cobalamin) deficiency, myeloid leukemia.

Diagnosis

Affected neutrophils present with five or more distinct nuclear lobes on blood smears (**Figure 16.48**). Blood smears should be made at the time of sample acquisition to prevent *in-vitro* neutrophil aging and hypersegmentation.

Management

Treatment is directed toward the underlying cause.

ABNORMAL CYTOPLASMIC MORPHOLOGY

NEUTROPHIL TOXICITY

Definition/overview

In addition to a left shift, neutrophils may exhibit toxic change during times of inflammation.

Etiology

Antibiotic responsiveness suggests a bacterial cause, but toxic change may also be found in cases of sterile inflammation or drug toxicity.

Pathophysiology

Toxic change is a result of a shortened maturation time or direct toxic injury to developing neutrophils. Döhle bodies represent lamellar aggregates of rough endoplasmic reticulum. Persistent ribosomes cause diffuse cytoplasmic basophilia. Foamy cytoplasmic vacuolation occurs with dispersed organelles. Enhanced primary granule staining contributes to the fine red granules known as toxic granulation.

16.48

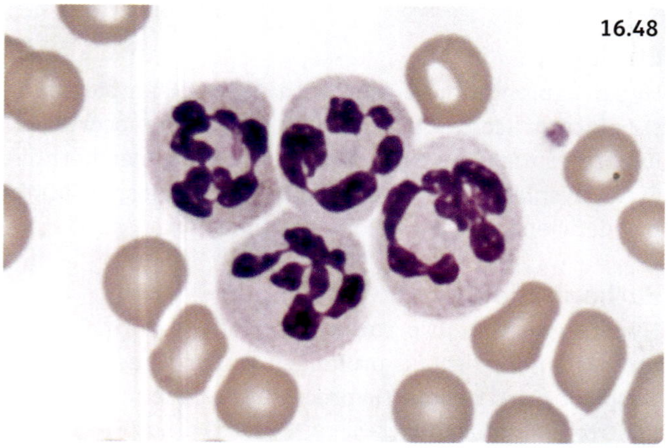

Figure 16.48 Hypersegmented neutrophils in a dog with canine leukocyte adhesion deficiency.

Clinical presentation

Signs reflect the site of inflammation or underlying condition.

Differential diagnosis

EDTA storage artifact, lysosomal storage disease, granulation syndrome in Birman cats, Chédiak–Higashi syndrome in cats.

Diagnosis

Neutrophil toxicity is diagnosed via blood smear evaluation (**Figures 16.49a–d**). Tests for specific infectious agents and immune-mediated disorders may be indicated.

Management

Treatment is directed toward the underlying illness.

Prognosis

Reduction of toxic changes implies a favorable prognostic indicator.

LYSOSOMAL STORAGE DISEASES

Definition/overview

Lyosomal storage diseases are a group of inheritable disorders caused by enzyme deficiencies that result in intralysosomal accumulations of undigested molecules. All these diseases are rare in dogs and cats.

Etiology

Lysosomal storage diseases produce granules or vacuoles in leukocytes include fucosidosis, GM1 gangliosidosis, GM2 gangliosidosis, alpha-mannosidosis, mucopolysaccharidosis (MPS) I, MPS IIIB, MPS VI, and MPS VII.

Pathophysiology

As lysosomes become engorged with degradation material they compress surrounding organelles and impair cellular respiration and function. Waste products build up and damage the cell.

Clinical presentation

Signs will vary with the type of enzyme deficiency, but may include failure to thrive, growth retardation, seizures, ataxia, corneal clouding, hepatosplenomegaly, cardiac murmurs, renal dysfunction, and skeletal abnormalities.

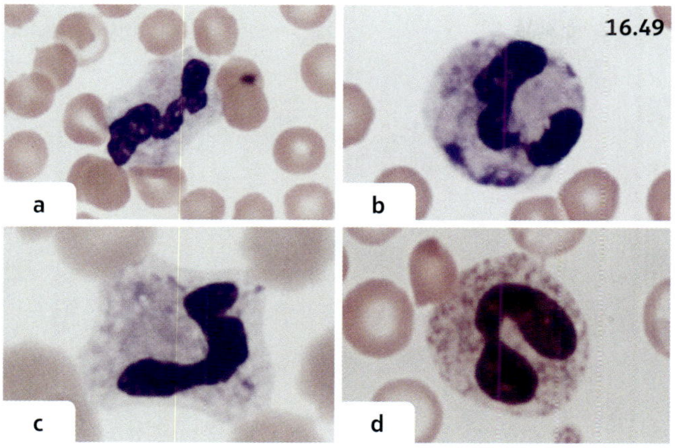

Figures 16.49a–d Signs of neutrophil toxic change include diffuse cytoplasmic basophilia (a–c), cytoplasmic aggregates of basophilia termed Döhle bodies (b, c), foamy cytoplasm (a, c), and prominent pink primary granules or toxic granulation (d).

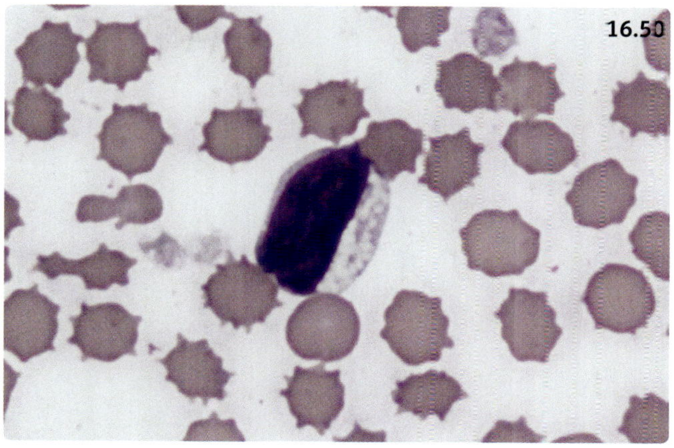

Figure 16.50 Vacuolated lymphocyte from a cat with lysosomal storage disease, consistent with mannosidosis

Differential diagnosis

EDTA storage artifact, toxic granulation, granulation syndrome in Birman cats, Chédiak–Higashi syndrome in cats.

Diagnosis

Cytoplasmic granules or vacuoles are present in leukocytes depending on the type of enzyme deficiency (**Figures 16.50, 16.51**). Storage diseases associated with leukocyte inclusions include fucosidosis, GM1 gangliosidosis, GM2 gangliosidosis, alpha-mannosidosis, MPS I, MPS IIIB, MPS VI, and MPS VII. A urine spot test is used to screen for glycosaminoglycans, while a cell enzyme activity test is diagnostic. DNA-based tests are available for some diseases with known mutations.

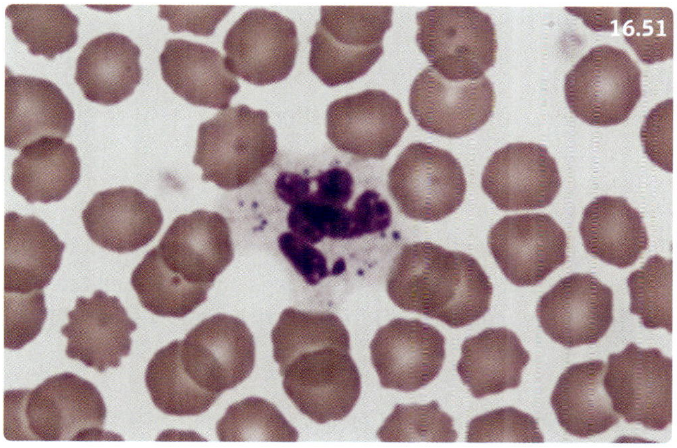

Figure 16.51 Granulated neutrophils in a dog with mucopolysaccharidosis I.

Management

Experimentally, bone marrow transplantation has been used to treat some of these disorders. Affected animals should not be bred.

Prognosis

Without bone marrow transplantation, these diseases are progressive and fatal.

ABNORMAL NEUTROPHIL GRANULATION IN BIRMAN CATS

Definition/overview

Abnormal neutrophil granulation is a genetic anomaly recognized in some Birman cats without associated clinical disease.

Etiology

The disorder is inherited in an autosomal recessive manner.

Pathophysiology

The pathophysiology is poorly understood, as neutrophil ultrastructure and function are normal.

Clinical presentation

There are no signs associated with this disorder.

Differential diagnosis

Toxic granulation, lysosomal storage disease.

Diagnosis

Diagnosis is based on the presence of fine, pink granules within the cytoplasm of neutrophils (**Figure 16.52**).

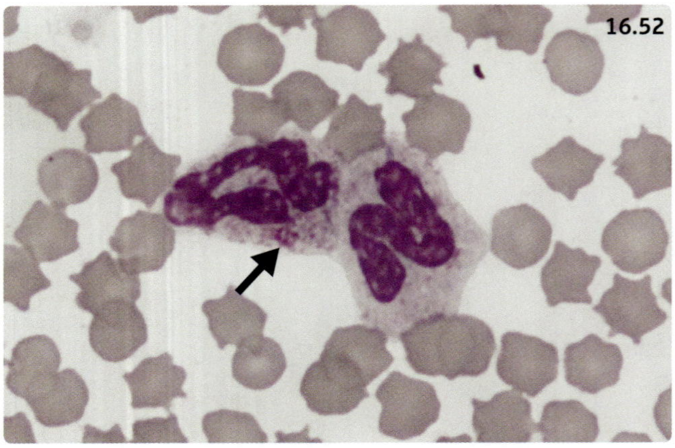

16.52

Figure 16.52 Fine pink granules (arrow) in a neutrophil from a Birman cat.

Management
No treatment is required.

Prognosis
There are no known negative effects.

FELINE CHÉDIAK–HIGASHI SYNDROME

Definition/overview
Feline Chédiak–Higashi syndrome is a rare, inherited disorder of blue-smoke Persian cats with yellow eye color.

Etiology
The disorder is inherited as an autosomal recessive trait and caused by a mutant lysosomal docking protein, LYST.

Pathophysiology
Granule defects are present in leukocytes, melanocytes, and platelets, leading to abnormal and enlarged lysosomal granules in leukocytes, decreased neutrophil chemotaxis, bleeding diathesis, and oculocutaneous color dilution.

Clinical presentation
Affected cats may be photophobic with cataract formation. There is increased bleeding time due to platelet granule defects.

Differential diagnosis
Cytoplasmic toxicity, lysosomal storage disease.

Diagnosis
Diagnosis is based on signalment, physical examination, and characteristic large, pink to magenta neutrophil granules (**Figure 16.53**) that are positive with peroxidase and Sudan black B stains. Neutropenia may also be present.

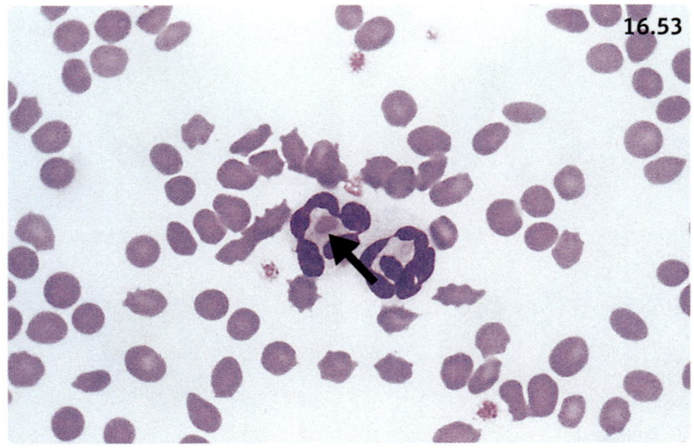

16.53

Figure 16.53 Feline Chédiak–Higashi syndrome presenting as large lavender cytoplasmic structures (arrow) within granulocytes. (Courtesy J. Harvey)

Management
Supportive therapy (e.g. blood transfusions, antibiotics) should be given as needed. Neutrophil chemotaxis has been reported to improve following administration of canine G-CSF in cats. Neutrophil and platelet function can be restored with bone marrow transplantation.

Prognosis
Life expectancy can exceed 10 years.

INFECTIOUS AGENTS

(See also Chapter 21: Infectious diseases.)

A variety of infectious agents may be found within leukocytes during examination of the blood or bone marrow. These include bacterial (**Figures 16.54, 16.55**), rickettsial, protozoal (**Figure 16.56**), and fungal organisms, or CDV inclusions (see **Figure 16.32**).

EHRLICHIOSIS

Definition/overview
Disease is caused by a variety of rickettsial bacteria, which are primarily transmitted by ticks.

Etiology
Causative agents in the dog include *Ehrlichia canis*, *Ehrlichia ewingii*, *Anaplasma phagocytophilum*, and, rarely, *Ehrlichia chaffeensis*. *A. phagocytophilum* and *E. canis* appear to infect cats. Disease is commonly termed ehrlichiosis no matter which genus is causing infection.

Pathophysiology
In the acute phase of the disease, replication of the organism occurs within the leukocytes, with hematogenous spread, vasculitis, and thrombocytopenia. In the chronic

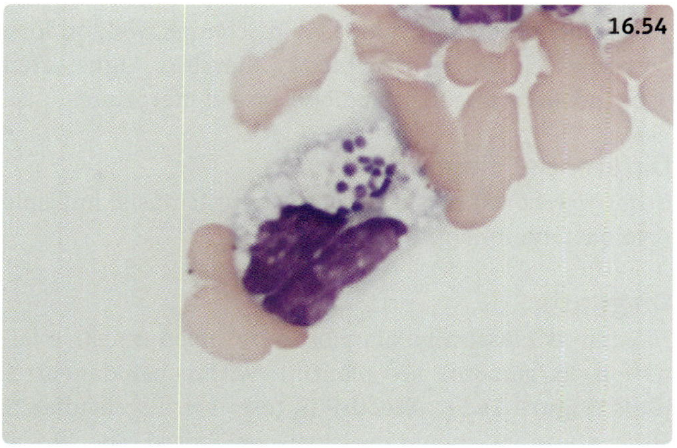

Figure 16.54 Blood smear from a dog with sepsis showing bacteria within a toxic neutrophil. Culture of the blood, liver, and lungs grew *Salmonella cholerasuis* subspecies *arizonae*.

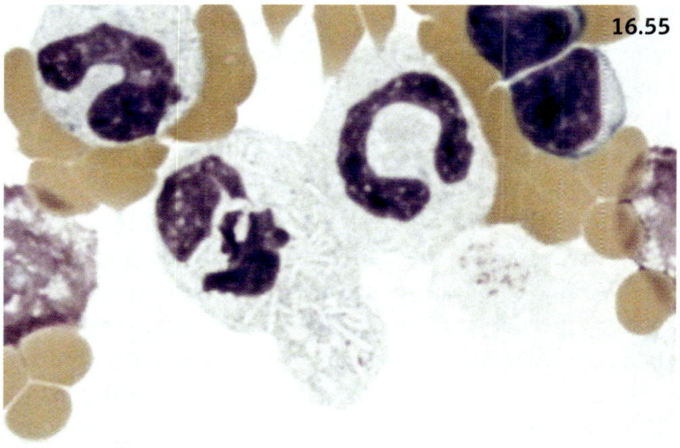

Figure 16.55 Circulating feline neutrophils with multiple intracytoplasmic nonstaining linear shapes identified as *Mycobacterium* spp.

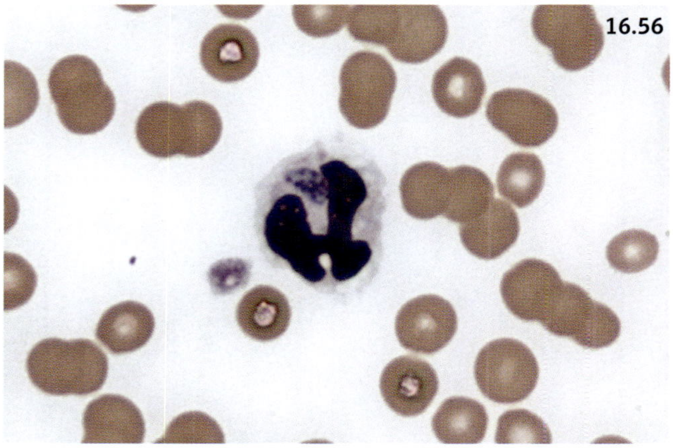

Figure 16.56 Blood neutrophil containing a tachyzoite in a cat with toxoplasmosis.

phase of *E. canis* infection, there is an ineffective immune response by the host leading to pancytopenia related to hypoplasia of the bone marrow. Because of the long life span of erythrocytes, thrombocytopenia and neutropenia often occur before anemia.

Clinical presentation

Acute signs include fever, anorexia, lethargy, lymphadenomegaly, hepatosplenomegaly, lameness, stiffness, and joint swelling. More severe signs include hemorrhage (e.g. epistaxis, melena, and petechiation), neurologic signs, vomiting, diarrhea, coughing, and cardiac arrhythmias. Emaciation may occur with chronic *E. canis* infection. Feline disease presents as vague illness with fever, weight loss, lymphadenopathy, and tick infestation. However, most clinical signs seen with canine ehrlichiosis have also been identified in cats.

Differential diagnosis

Chronic inflammation, organ failure, other infectious agents, drug-induced injury.

Diagnosis

Acute disease in dogs and cats most consistently causes thrombocytopenia and mild nonregenerative anemia. With chronic canine infection, hyperglobulinemia, pancytopenia, or large granular lymphocytosis (see **Figure 16.41**) is possible. The gammopathy is typically polyclonal, but is rarely monoclonal. Blood smear evaluation may show intracytoplasmic bacterial colonies (morulae) in mononuclear cells (*E. canis* and *E. chaffeensis*) or granulocytes (*E. ewingii* or *A. phagocytophilum*) during acute infection (**Figure 16.57**). Aspiration of enlarged lymph nodes reveals reactive lymphoid hyperplasia, and neutrophilic polyarthropathy is observed on synovial fluid analysis. In the absence of visualizing morulae,

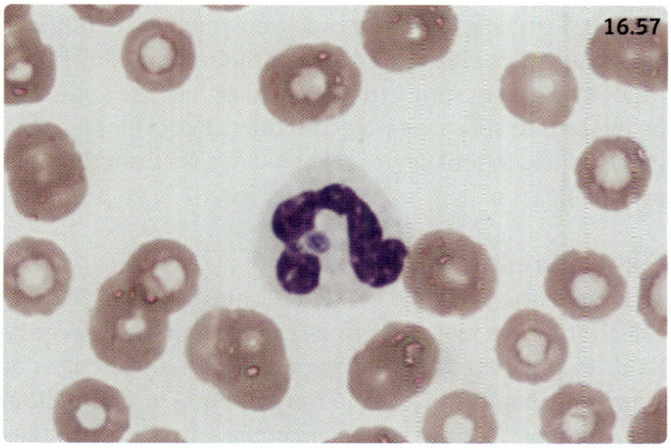

Figure 16.57 *Ehrlichia ewingii* morula in a canine neutrophil.

diagnosis is best determined by positive or rising serum titers. For canine infections, serologic screening tests include an in-house ELISA test and IFA testing performed at reference laboratories. Serologic titers by immunoblot and DNA detection by PCR are confirmatory tests. In cats, seropositivity by IFA is most commonly used, but some cats may have low or negative titers.

Management

The recommended treatment for canine or feline ehrlichiosis is doxycycline (10 mg/kg PO q24h for 28 days). Clinical improvement is expected within 24–48 hours after initiating therapy, but dogs with pancytopenia due to chronic *E. canis* infection do not respond to treatment.

HEPATOZOONOSIS

Definition/overview

This tick-borne disease of dogs, domestic cats, and wild canids is found in Africa, Southern Europe, Italy, the Middle East, Asia, and in the US Gulf Coast states from Texas to Georgia. Infections in cats are found in India, Africa, the Middle East, and California in the USA.

Etiology

The disease is caused by ingestion of *Rhipicephalus sanguineus* ticks that are infested with the protozoan organism *Hepatozoon canis*. Another species, *Hepatozoon americanum*, is also prevalent in the USA and is transmitted by *Amblyomma maculatum*.

Pathophysiology

Ingested ticks release sporozoites, which penetrate the intestinal wall and are carried by blood and lymph to the lungs, spleen, liver, or muscle, where cysts are formed. The schizonts within the cyst develop into merozoites or meronts, which eventually become gametocytes or gamonts that infect leukocytes or endothelial cells. Following a blood meal containing infected leukocytes, the organism develops into sporozoites within the tick. Development of gametocytes in leukocytes takes 4–5 weeks from the time of tick exposure.

Clinical presentation

Tick infestation may be evident. Clinical signs of *H. canis* infection range from subclinical to chronic, and severity tends to correlate with the dog's immune status. Signs of overt disease include fever, lethargy, anorexia, depression, and anemia. *Hepatozoon americanum* infection includes additional signs of muscle atrophy, hyperesthesia, stiff gait, mucopurulent oculonasal discharge, weight loss, polydipsia, polyuria, and bloody diarrhea. Signs often wax and wane due to periodic release of merozoites.

Differential diagnosis

Other tick-borne diseases such as ehrlichiosis, multiple myeloma, lymphoma.

Diagnosis

H. canis is classically diagnosed by blood smear evaluation, as gamonts are plentiful within blood neutrophils (**Figure 16.58**). Blood PCR tests are also available. *H. americanum* should be suspected based on clinical signs, marked neutrophilia (leukemoid response), and the observance of chronic periosteal hypertrophic proliferation on radiographs. In contrast to *H. canis*, only rare gamonts are present in the blood (<0.1% of WBCs). Muscle biopsy is the diagnostic standard, but schizonts may also be observed within pyogranulomatous lesions of the lung, liver, spleen, and lymph nodes. Serology using IFA and blood PCR tests are also available.

Management

Treatment is aimed at improving clinical signs, as therapy is not curative, and relapses are expected. *H. canis* infections are typically treated with imidocarb diproprionate (5–6 mg/kg SC q2weeks) until gamonts are no longer visible on blood smears for 2–3 consecutive months. It is suggested that dogs with *H. americanum* infection receive a triple combination of trimethoprim–sulfadiazine (15 mg/kg PO q12h), clindamycin (10 mg/kg PO q8h), and pyrimethamine (0.25 mg/kg PO q24h) for 14 days, or toltrazuril sulfone (10 mg/kg PO q12h) for 14 days. The triple combination or toltrazuril sulfone is followed by 2 years

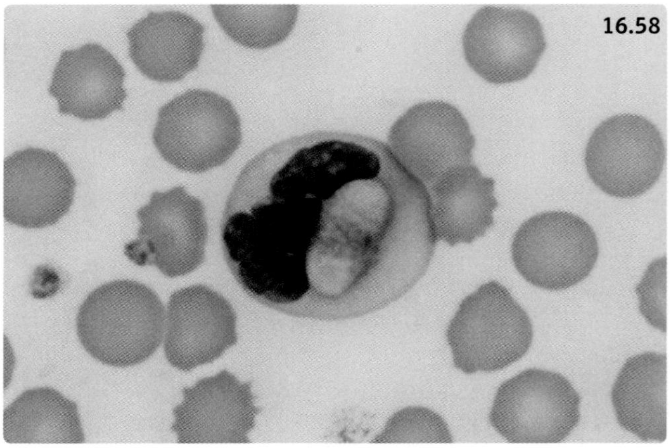

Figure 16.58 A large, ovoid, nonstaining *Hepatozoon canis* gamont within a neutrophil.

of decoquinate (10–20 mg/kg PO q12h). NSAIDs are indicated to reduce pain.

LEISHMANIASIS

Definition/overview

Leishmaniasis is an infrequent protozoal disease in dogs, and is rarely found in cats. It is caused by *Leishmania* spp. History usually indicates travel outside the US to Mediterranean and Middle East countries (e.g. Greece, Spain, or Italy). The disease is also present in Central and South America and Asia. Endemic foci in Oklahoma and Texas have been reported, as well as a research colony in Ohio.

Etiology

Sandflies are the vectors of *Leishmania* spp. Rodents and dogs are the primary reservoirs for human infection, and cats are probably incidental hosts.

Pathophysiology

The parasite produces visceral or cutaneous manifestations. Promastigotes are disseminated throughout the body, likely within macrophages. Nonflagellate forms called amastigotes develop and multiply within macrophages, infecting new cells. Signs can develop from 3 months to 7 years after infection.

Clinical presentation

Clinical signs in dogs develop over months and include exercise intolerance, weight loss, lethargy, polydipsia, anorexia, diarrhea, vomiting, polyphagia, epistaxis, melena, sneezing, coughing, and fainting. Physical examination findings involve lymphadenopathy, alopecia, ulcerative dermatitis, fever, cachexia, lameness, and conjunctivitis. Cutaneous nodules are mostly seen in cats.

Differential diagnosis

Multiple myeloma, lymphoma, immune-mediated arthritis.

Diagnosis

The most consistent laboratory findings are mild to moderate nonregenerative anemia, hyperglobulinemia due to polyclonal gammopathy, hypoalbuminemia, decreased albumin:globulin ratio, and proteinuria. Rarely, monoclonal gammopathy is reported. Half or fewer cases will present with thrombocytopenia, azotemia, and increased serum ALP and ALT activities; leukocytosis or leukopenia may occur. High serum antibodies with appropriate clinicopathologic signs are confirmatory, but low or negative serum antibodies warrant further testing, namely cytology or histopathology. Characteristic organisms are present in macrophages of the bone marrow, lymph nodes, spleen, liver, kidney, and skin (**Figure 16.59**). Amastigotes are recognized by the presence of a small purple nucleus and a perpendicular rod-shaped kinetoplast in Romanowsky-stained smears. Other tests include tissue culture and detection of leishmanial DNA by PCR, which has high diagnostic sensitivity and specificity.

Management

Therapy and prognosis depend on the patient's clinical stage and antibody titers. Antimicrobial options include meglumine antimoniate (75–100 mg/kg SC q24h) for 4–8 weeks, allopurinol (10 mg/kg PO q12h) for at least 6–12 months, or miltefosine (2 mg/kg PO q24h) for 4 weeks. Meglumine antimoniate and allopurinol may also be given in combination. Complete staging, therapy, and prognostic guidelines have been described (see Recommended further reading). The disease in zoonotic and infected dogs can serve as a reservoir in the presence of the appropriate sandfly vectors. In endemic areas, euthanasia of infected dogs is part of the eradication program, although this is controversial.

HISTOPLASMOSIS

Definition/overview

Histoplasmosis is the second most commonly reported systemic fungal infection in cats. In dogs, the disease is common in geographic areas of high prevalence such as the mid-Atlantic, south central, and Mississippi regions of the USA.

Etiology

The causative fungal agent, *Histoplasma capsulatum*, is commonly found as a mycelial form in soil rich with bird or bat manure. It occurs predominantly within the Mississippi region of the USA. Cats housed

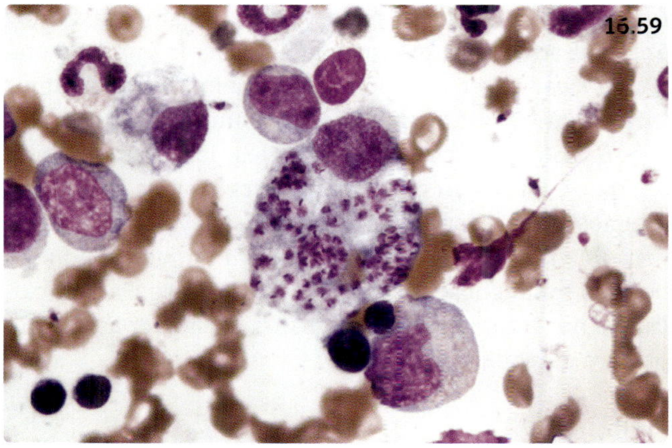

Figure 16.59 *Leishmania* amastigotes within a bone marrow macrophage from a dog.

exclusively indoors are thought to acquire infection through household dust or potting soil.

Pathophysiology

Infection is by inhalation or ingestion of infective conidia. After transmission, infective conidia transform to the yeast phase and are engulfed by mononuclear phagocytes and disseminated throughout the body in lymph and blood. Multisystemic disease is common in infected cats. In persistently infected organs there is granulomatous inflammation.

Clinical presentation

The mean age of feline patients is 3.9 years, and most dogs are under 5 years of age. Clinical findings in cats frequently include depression, weight loss, emaciation, fever, pale mucous membranes, organomegaly, respiratory signs (dyspnea, tachypnea, abnormal lung sounds, chronic cough), and ocular signs. Less frequent signs are soft tissue swelling, joint effusion, lameness, vomiting, diarrhea, or CNS involvement. Canine patients show similar signs to cats, but GI involvement is more frequent.

Differential diagnosis

Mycobacterial infection, protozoal infection, other systemic fungal agents, neoplasia.

Diagnosis

Routine laboratory tests are not specific for histoplasmosis but may reflect the extent of systemic involvement. Some cats may develop pancytopenia due to marrow infection. Hypercalcemia associated with granulomatous disease is infrequent. Yeast forms are found within monocytes/macrophages of the blood, bone marrow, lung, lymph node, liver, rectal scrapings, spleen, effusions, tracheal or bronchoalveolar washes, and, rarely, within cerebrospinal fluid (**Figure 16.60**). The organism may also be found within neutrophils and, rarely, in eosinophils. They are oval structures measuring 2–4 microns and having a thin clear space or halo around them. Granulomatous inflammation and organisms are found on histopathology. A *Histoplasma* urine antigen test is currently being validated for use in cats; preliminary studies show high diagnostic sensitivity (17/18). A *Blastomyces* urine antigen test cross-reacts with *Histoplasma* antigens and may be used to diagnose systemic fungal disease. Fungal culture is not recommended because it is hazardous for laboratory personnel.

Management

Treatment should be continued for 4–6 months to be most effective. The current drug of choice is itraconazole (10 mg/kg PO q24h) in dogs or cats with disseminated histoplasmosis. In cats, the oral solution is more consistently absorbed than the capsules, so administration of itraconazole capsules may require more frequent dosing (10 mg/kg PO q12h).

A combination of itraconazole and amphotericin B is used in severe disseminated forms. Amphotericin B is given at 0.25–0.5 mg/kg IV three times weekly for 2–3 months. Ketoconazole (10 mg/kg PO q12h) has lower potency against *Histoplasma*, but may be considered if there are financial constraints.

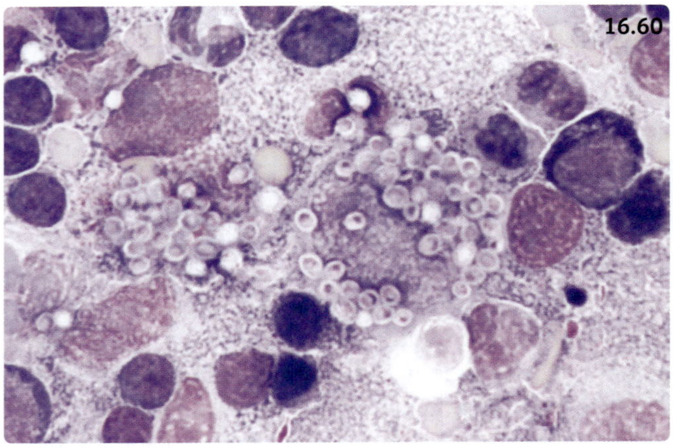

Figure 16.60 Bone marrow smear from a cat with systemic histoplasmosis. There are numerous small, round to ovoid yeasts within two macrophages.

PLATELET DISORDERS (NON-NEOPLASTIC)

Platelets are anucleate cells produced in the bone marrow from the cytoplasmic shearing of megakaryocytes. Platelets are a critical component of hemostasis, and will therefore primarily be presented in the next chapter (Chapter 17: Disorders of hemostasis). However, causes of non-neoplastic thrombocytosis and dysplasia are offered here.

REACTIVE THROMBOCYTOSIS

Definition/overview

A non-neoplastic thrombocytosis is termed reactive thrombocytosis.

Etiology

Etiologies include exercise and epinephrine, inflammation, iron deficiency, recovery from thrombocytopenia, blood loss, nonhemic neoplasia, vincristine and vinblastine, and splenectomy.

Pathophysiology

Exercise and epinephrine cause splenic contraction and increased blood flow, which leads to redistribution of platelets from the spleen and lungs into circulating blood. Other etiologies cause enhanced platelet production. For example, inflammatory cytokines, especially IL-6, stimulate thrombopoietin production and, subsequently, thrombopoiesis.

Clinical presentation

Signs are dependent on the underlying disorder.

Differential diagnosis

Essential thrombocythemia, primary myelofibrosis, PV.

Diagnosis

Diagnosis is based on an increased platelet concentration in the presence of an underlying cause for reactive thrombocytosis. Epinephrine release also causes erythrocytosis, neutrophilia, lymphocytosis, and hyperglycemia. Moderate to marked neutrophilia, a left shift, or the observation of toxic neutrophils supports inflammation. Blood loss is identified by anemia and decreases in albumin and globulin concentrations. Microcytic hypochromic nonregenerative or poorly regenerative anemia suggests iron deficiency. History and physical examination findings are also helpful. Persistent, marked thrombocytosis without an underlying etiology should raise concern for leukemia.

Management

Treatment is directed at the underlying cause.

MACROTHROMBOCYTOPENIA

Definition/overview

Macrothrombocytopenia (thrombocytopenia with giant platelets) is an inherited disorder of Cavalier King Charles Spaniels, as well as Norfolk and Cairn Terriers, without hemorrhage or clinical signs. The giant platelets have diameters greater than those of RBCs.

Etiology

The disorder is caused by a mutant beta1-tubulin gene.

Pathophysiology

The mutant beta1-tubulin forms unstable dimers, which results in altered platelet formation and the release of large platelets. Small numbers of giant platelets result in a normal or near normal total platelet mass in the blood.

Clinical presentation

Macrothrombocytopenia is typically an incidental finding when the patient presents for routine evaluation or for other disease.

Differential diagnosis

Immune-mediated thrombocytopenia, DIC, megakaryocytic leukemia.

Diagnosis

Diagnosis is based on the presence of thrombocytopenia and giant platelets in affected dogs (**Figure 16.61**). Median measurements in one study of platelets in Cavalier King Charles Spaniels compared with other breeds were 2.5–3.75 µm and 1.25–2.5 µm, respectively. The reduced platelet count is partially related to giant platelets being missed by automated hematology analyzers with small thresholds. Platelet counts measured by platelet mass (e.g. QBC hematology analyzer) better reflect the true platelet concentration. Studies indicate that male dogs have significantly lower platelet counts than females of the breed.

Management

Treatment is not warranted for affected dogs.

Prognosis

The disorder is not known to affect hemostasis.

DYSPLASTIC DISORDERS

Dysplastic disorders are characterized by developmental changes within the erythrocytes, granulocytes, and platelets. The etiology may be related to inheritable,

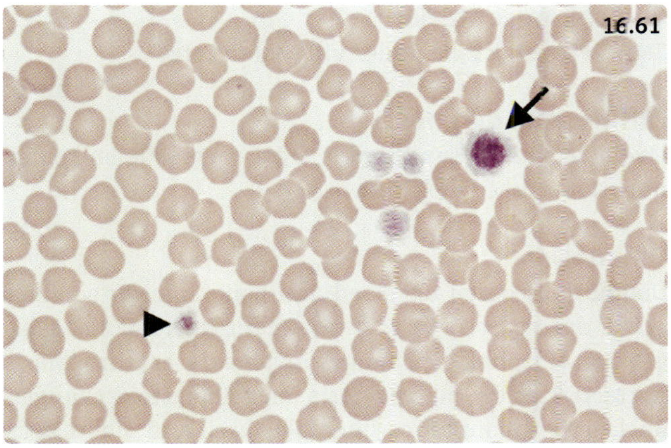

Figure 16.61 The platelets of Cavalier King Charles Spaniel dogs with macrothrombocytopenia range from normal (arrowhead) to giant (arrow) in size.

infectious, drug-induced, and nutritional conditions. While dysplastic disorders often affect multiple hematopoietic lineages, abnormal growth of one cell line typically results in the patient's clinical manifestations. For this reason, select dysplastic disorders are included with the cell lineage that is chiefly deregulated. Disorders that primarily present as erythroid dysplasia include iron deficiency anemia, FeLV infection, Poodle marrow dyscrasia, folate or cobalamin (vitamin B12) deficiency, and lead poisoning. Manifestations of leukocyte dysplasias are Pelger–Huët anomaly, cyclic hematopoiesis of gray Collies, and leukocyte granule abnormalities. The most common platelet dysplastic disorders are macrothrombocytopenia of Cavalier King Charles Spaniels and vincristine-associated macrothrombocytes. Previously considered a preleukemic dysplasia, myelodysplastic syndrome is now considered a form of myeloid neoplasia, and will be addressed in the corresponding section.

DRUG-INDUCED DYSPLASIA

Definition/overview

Antibiotics and antineoplastic agents can produce reversible morphologic changes in blood cells.

Etiology

Drugs implicated are azathioprine, cyclophosphamide, cytosine arabinoside, vincristine, and chloramphenicol.

Pathophysiology

The drugs disrupt the normal production of erythroid cells within hours to days following administration. The mechanism is not related to folate deficiency.

Clinical presentation

Signs will reflect the underlying conditions.

Differential diagnosis

Myelodysplastic syndrome, acute myeloid leukemia, nutrition-related dysplasia.

Diagnosis

Diagnosis is based on blood and bone marrow samples taken during routine post-treatment hematologic evaluations. Morphologic changes involve dyserythropoiesis characterized by macrocytosis, megaloblastoid changes, nuclear fragmentation, sideroblastosis, and siderocytosis. Folate concentrations are within normal limits.

Management

Normal morphology of hematopoietic cells occurs several days after cessation of drug therapy.

HEMATOPOIETIC MALIGNANCIES

Hematopoietic malignancies include neoplasms of lymphoid cells (lymphocytes and plasma cells), myeloid cells (erythrocytes, nonlymphoid leukocytes, and megakaryocytes), and uncommitted stem cells (acute undifferentiated leukemia). Lymphoid neoplasms are more common than those of myeloid origin.

LYMPHOID NEOPLASIA

Malignant lymphoid conditions may originate from tissues such as lymph nodes, alimentary tract, thymus, spleen, liver, skin, and eye, or from the bone marrow. The term leukemia is used when neoplastic cells appear in blood or bone marrow, while lymphoma designates lymphoid neoplasia arising from the other sites. Primary leukemia originates from the bone marrow progenitor cells, while secondary or metastatic lymphoid leukemia occurs as a late and advanced stage of the disease. Lymphoid leukemia is further classified based on the maturity of the neoplastic cells. Acute lymphoid leukemia denotes a predominance of immature cells, namely blast cells, whereas small mature lymphocytes present in chronic lymphocytic leukemia. A neoplasm of plasma cells arising from the bone marrow is called myeloma, whereas nonmarrow sites are referred to as plasmacytomas. Lymphoid neoplasms, arranged in descending frequency of occurrence, are lymphoma, plasmacytoma, plasma cell myeloma, chronic lymphocytic leukemia, and acute lymphoblastic leukemia.

LYMPHOMA

Definition/overview

Lymphoma (the preferred term over lymphosarcoma) is the most common hematopoietic tumor of dogs and cats. Multicentric disease is more common in dogs and usually involves the peripheral lymph nodes, spleen, and liver. Other sites of canine lymphoma include alimentary, thymic, cutaneous disease, and miscellaneous extranodal locations in decreasing frequency. Thymic lymphoma is most common in young, FeLV-positive cats, while alimentary lymphoma is more common in older cats. Cats may also develop multicentric, renal, and cutaneous lymphoma.

Etiology

Prior to widespread FeLV testing and vaccination programs, about 60–80% of feline cases were associated with FeLV infection. However, positive FeLV antigenemia is only identified in 10–20% of contemporary cases. Strong evidence for a retroviral etiology in dogs does not exist. Environmental exposure is also considered a possible etiology. The Boxer, Bulldog, Bull Mastiff, Golden Retriever, and Labrador Retriever dog breeds are overrepresented.

Pathophysiology

Lymphoma originates in peripheral lymphoid tissues, which causes local tissue injury and dysfunction. Over time, neoplastic cells will infiltrate widely into a variety of sites, which often include multiple lymph nodes, spleen, liver, and bone marrow.

Clinical presentation

Clinical signs often involve nonpainful swellings of superficial lymph nodes. Splenomegaly or hepatomegaly may be present, along with internal lymphadenomegaly. Mediastinal or thymic masses can produce dyspnea, pleural effusion, or effects associated with hypercalcemia such as polydipsia and polyuria. Cutaneous lesions can arise as a mild eczematous pruritic plaque and progress to a nodular lesion. Weight loss, vomiting, and inappetence often suggest an advanced stage with worse prognosis.

Differential diagnosis

For generalized lymphadenopathy: disseminated infections, immune-mediated disorders, and other hematopoietic tumors. For alimentary disease: lymphocytic–plasmacytic enteritis, other neoplasms, granulomatous bowel disease, and hypereosinophilic syndrome should be considered. For cutaneous disease: pyoderma, other infectious or immune-mediated disease, parasitic infestation, and other neoplasms should be considered.

Diagnosis

Hematology often reveals anemia of chronic disease, but a full CBC with blood smear evaluation is recommended to assess for concurrent blood loss or hemolysis, FeLV-associated macrocytosis, myelophthisis-associated cytopenias, and circulating atypical lymphocytes suggestive of stage V disease (**Figure 16.62**). Bone marrow aspiration is performed for staging, prognosis, and cases in which lymphoma is suspected, but otherwise not proven.

Serum biochemical abnormalities include hypercalcemia in 15% of dogs with lymphoma due to parathyroid hormone-related peptide production by neoplastic cells, azotemia with renal infiltration, elevated liver enzyme activity due to hepatic involvement, or hyperglobulinemia and monoclonal gammopathy with some B cell lymphomas. Cats should be screened for retrovirus (FeLV and FIV) infection for diagnostic, prognostic, and husbandry purposes.

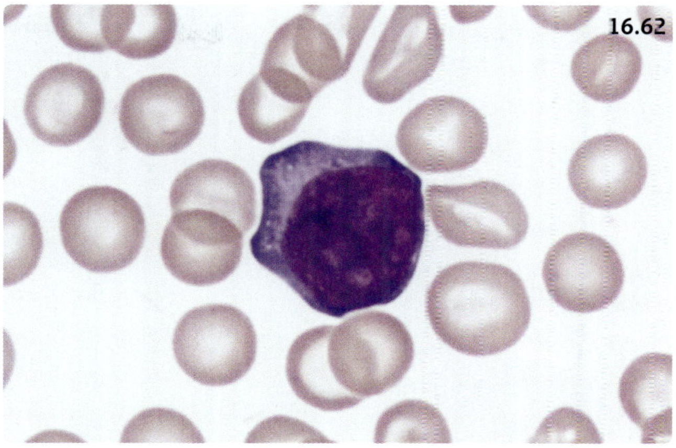

Figure 16.62 A lymphoblast in a dog with stage V lymphoma. Note the cell's large size, immature chromatin, and nucleoli.

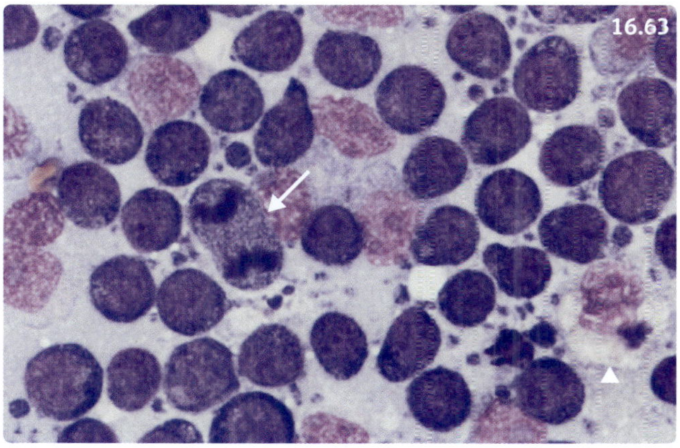

Figure 16.63 Cytologic preparation of large cell lymphoma in a dog. The neoplastic lymphocytes are large with open chromatin and prominent nucleoli. Mitotic figures (arrow) and macrophages (arrowhead) are frequent.

Imaging, including radiographs, ultrasound, and CT, may be important for diagnosis, clinical staging, and monitoring response to treatment. In particular, cranial mediastinal lymphadenopathy in dogs negatively correlates with remission and survival duration.

Lymphoma is frequently diagnosed from fine needle aspirates of lymph nodes or other affected tissues or fluids; these usually disclose a homogeneous population of lymphoblasts (**Figure 16.63**). Lymphoma of large granular lymphocytes has characteristic pink granules (**Figure 16.64**) and is most associated with splenic origin. If cytology is equivocal in distinguishing extreme lymphoid hyperplasia from early lymphoma, a surgical biopsy may provide a definitive diagnosis based on changes in normal follicular architecture.

Advanced diagnostic techniques may be pursued in cases where a diagnosis cannot be obtained by cytology or histopathology, and for determining immunophenotype

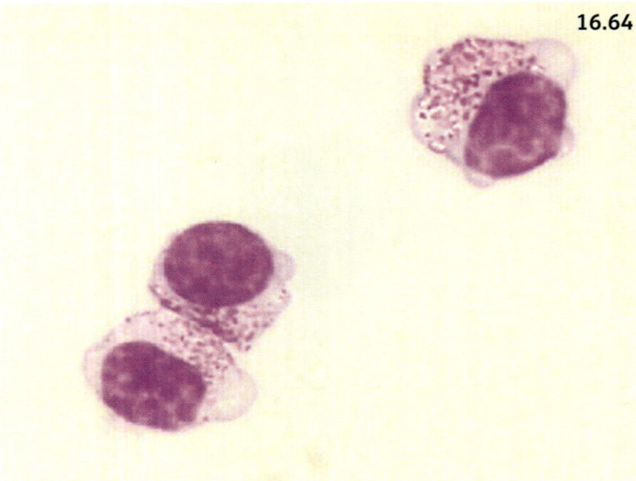

Figure 16.64 Cells from a cat with large granular lymphoma containing abundant magenta coarse cytoplasmic granules. Methanolic Romanowsky stain.

(B, T, or null cell). In these cases, immunocytochemistry, immunohistochemistry, flow cytometry, or PCR for antigen receptor rearrangement may be rewarding.

Management

In general, lymphoma requires systemic therapy. 'CHOP'-based protocols involve combination chemotherapies of cyclophosphamide (C), doxorubicin (hydroxydaunorubicin [H]), vincristine (Oncovin [O]), and prednisone (P). The University of Wisconsin-Madison CHOP protocols are commonly recommended (see Recommended further reading). Prior to administering any potentially myelotoxic drug, a CBC should be performed to assess neutrophil and platelet concentrations. Rare cases of solitary lymphoma may be treated with surgery or radiation therapy.

In dogs, doxorubicin (30 mg/m^2 IV q3weeks for 5 treatments) is the most effective single agent chemotherapeutic drug for lymphoma. For owners that opt for oral medication, lomustine (CCNU; 70 mg/m^2 PO q3weeks) and prednisone (initially at 2.0 mg/kg PO q24h) can be given. However, response rates and remission durations are typically less than for CHOP-based protocols or doxorubicin. Breeds at risk for P-glycoprotein drug transport abnormalities, including Collies and Shetland Sheepdogs, should undergo MDR1 gene mutation analysis prior to chemotherapy.

Unlike dogs, single agent doxorubicin is not effective in cats. Cats with small cell GI or hepatic lymphoma can be administered oral chlorambucil (2 mg q48h or 20 mg/m^2 q2weeks) and immunosuppressive and tapering doses of oral prednisone. This protocol offers remission and median survival times of approximately 2 years.

After remission is achieved, relapse with a more drug-resistant form eventually occurs. At this time, rescue therapy may be pursued. While the response rate is high, the length of response is generally half that of the induction therapy. Many protocols have been reported, and the complexity and toxicity of the chemotherapies often requires consultation with a veterinary oncologist.

Prognosis

Untreated dogs and cats survive an average of 4–6 weeks after lymphoma diagnosis, but individual survival is dependent on tumor location and grade. Remission rates for combination CHOP chemotherapy are 75–90% for dogs and 60–70% for cats, with median survival times of 12 months in dogs and 7 months in cats. In 25% of patients, this may extend to 2 years survival. Response rates and lengths vary, and are dependent on prognostic factors. In general, poor prognostic indicators for canine lymphoma include T-cell phenotype, presenting with clinical signs of disease (WHO substage b), heavy bone marrow infiltration (WHO stage V), and presence of cranial mediastinal lymphadenopathy. A high histopathology grade tends to give high initial response rates, but reduced overall survival. Prior steroid treatment is associated with shortened response durations. General positive prognostic factors in cats include negative FeLV status, low histopathology grade, lack of clinical disease at presentation, addition of doxorubicin to treatment protocols, and complete response to therapy.

CHRONIC LYMPHOCYTIC LEUKEMIA

Definition/overview

Chronic lymphocytic leukemia (CLL) has a slow and protracted course of months to years. It occurs mostly in middle aged to older dogs (mean 10 years), with a higher frequency in females. This form of leukemia occurs infrequently in cats.

Etiology

An etiology has not been definitively proven.

Pathophysiology

Phenotypically mature lymphocytes proliferate, and there is an increase in the stem cell compartment. In dogs, about 70% are of T cell origin (CD8+, CD4+), with the remainder B cells or null cells. CLL arises from mature cells, but one form with granular morphology has been shown to develop initially from the spleen. Generally, the malignancy spreads into liver, spleen, and lymph nodes late in the disease. Cases of B cell origin may present with increased gamma globulins, with resulting hyperviscosity owing to paraprotein overproduction.

Clinical presentation

Clinical signs include lethargy, inappetence, vomiting, mild to absent lymphadenomegaly, organomegaly, and fever. Polyuria, polydipsia, hemorrhage, lameness, and collapse may also occur. Routine screening may detect asymptomatic disease.

Differential diagnosis

Canine ehrlichiosis, other infectious diseases, post-vaccinal responses in young dogs.

Diagnosis

There is marked lymphocytosis of mature, small lymphocytes with condensed chromatin (**Figure 16.65**). Cell counts range from 10,000 cells/µl to 300,000 cells/µl or more. A subset of CLL has granular lymphocyte morphology with an increased amount of pale blue cytoplasm and fine to coarse cytoplasmic pink granules. In dogs, lymphocyte counts exceeding 25,000/µl in blood or greater than 15% in bone marrow strongly suggest a malignant process. Mild normocytic, normochromic nonregenerative anemia is common. Neutropenia and thrombocytosis occur late in disease with myelophthisis. Biopsy with histopathology may better document the infiltration into nodal tissues by neoplastic lymphocytes, with loss of tissue architecture. Causes of chronic systemic disease (e.g. ehrlichiosis, leishmaniasis) should be ruled out. Flow cytometry or PCR for antigen receptor rearrangement can demonstrate malignancy in equivocal cases.

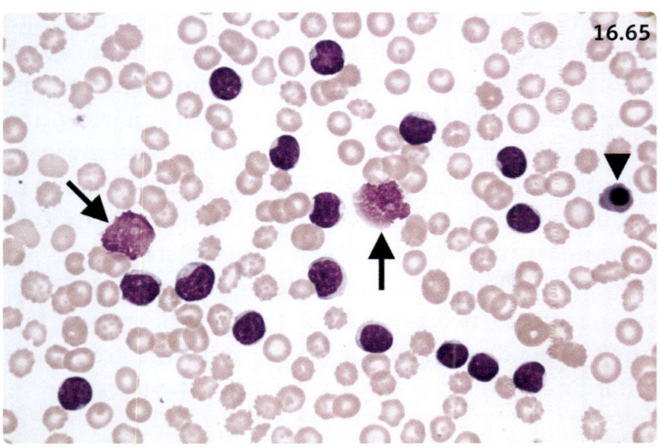

Figure 16.65 Chronic lymphocytic leukemia in a dog with a lymphocytosis of 183,000 cells/µl. The lymphocytes are small (i.e. ≤1.5 times the diameter of a RBC) with mature, dense chromatin. There are also two lysed cells (arrows) and one metarubricyte (arrowhead).

Management

Chemotherapy to reduce the neoplastic cell population is warranted when clinical or hematologic signs are present. Drugs include chlorambucil (dogs: 0.2 mg/kg PO q24h for 10 days, then 0.1 mg/kg PO q24h; cats: 2 mg/cat PO q48h) and prednisone (2 mg/kg PO q24h), with adjustment of dosing based on response.

Prognosis

Prognosis is generally good with survival in the range of 2 or more years, but progression to acute lymphoblastic leukemia is likely.

ACUTE LYMPHOBLASTIC LEUKEMIA

Definition/overview

Acute lymphoblastic leukemia is a rapidly progressive disorder that occurs mostly in middle aged dogs (mean 6 years) and in cats with FeLV infection.

Etiology

Viral agents (FeLV) or environmental exposure are possible causes.

Pathophysiology

The bone marrow or peripheral blood contains morphologically immature precursor cells or lymphoblasts. Acute lymphoblastic leukemia is thought to arise from the bone marrow and later spreads to the liver, spleen, and other tissues.

Clinical presentation

Clinical signs include lethargy, anorexia, vomiting, and diarrhea over several weeks. Neurologic signs may occur with marked thrombocytopenia. Hepatosplenomegaly occurs, but lymph node involvement is minimal to none.

Differential diagnosis

Stage V lymphoma, acute myeloid leukemia without maturation, acute undifferentiated leukemia.

Diagnosis

Hematologic abnormalities include increased numbers of immature lymphoid cells in the blood or bone marrow (**Figure 16.66**), nonregenerative anemia, neutropenia, thrombocytopenia, and an occasional monoclonal gammopathy. Flow cytometry may be useful to confirm an acute leukemia phenotype (CD34+), as well as lymphoid origin, since acute myeloid leukemia appears morphologically similar. Approximately 10% of cases are confined to the bone marrow without detectable blood involvement

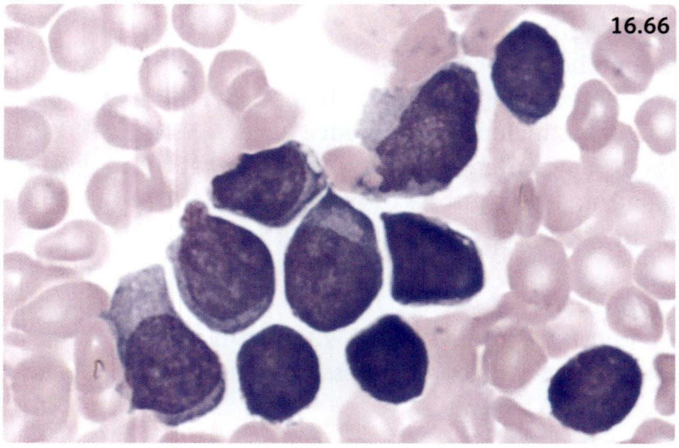

Figure 16.66 Acute lymphoblastic leukemia from a dog bone marrow. Note the large (i.e. ≥2.5–3 times the diameter of a RBC) immature cells with high nuclear to cytoplasmic ratio, finely stippled chromatin, and round to ovoid nuclei that contain multiple prominent nucleoli.

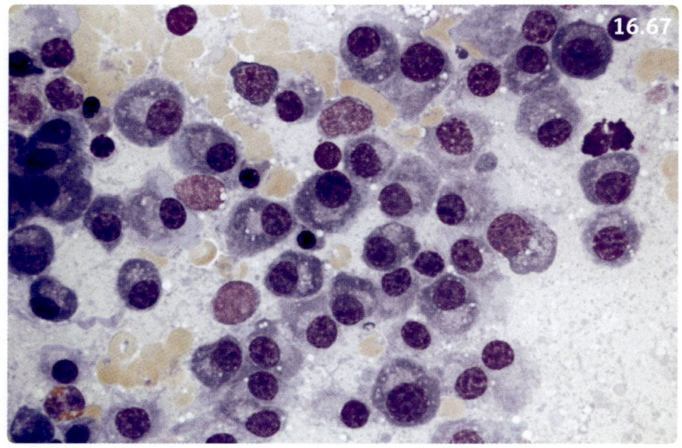

Figure 16.67 Aspirate preparation from a lytic bone lesion in a dog with multiple myeloma showing many plasma cells with abundant basophilic cytoplasm, prominent perinuclear pale zones, and peripherally placed nuclei with clumped chromatin.

(aleukemic leukemia). Bone marrow evaluation is warranted in these cases and in cases with low numbers of circulating blasts (subleukemic leukemia). PCR tests for B- or T-cell antigen receptor rearrangement are available for difficult to diagnose cases.

Management

Treatment most often involves the same combination chemotherapy used for lymphoma. The prognosis is poor, with median survival (untreated or treated) being less than 3 months.

MULTIPLE MYELOMA

Definition/overview

Multiple myeloma (MM, plasma cell myeloma) is a malignant disease of bone marrow plasma cells.

Etiology

The etiology is unknown.

Pathophysiology

Malignant plasma cells produce a clonal or, rarely, biclonal population of immunoglobulins (M proteins or paraproteins), light chains (Bence-Jones proteins), or heavy chains (heavy chain disease). These proteins may inhibit platelet function, causing bleeding diathesis, or result in hyperviscosity syndrome, renal failure, amyloidosis, or cryoglobulinemia. Infiltration into the bone marrow by neoplastic plasma cells produces hematologic cytopenias. The destruction of bone by osteoclast-activating factors released by tumor cells results in lytic lesions and hypercalcemia. Bone pain and pathologic fractures are common sequelae. Plasma cell dysfunction can lead to immunodeficiency and increased susceptibility to infection.

Clinical presentation

Clinical signs may be vague and variable, with lethargy, anorexia, and lameness. Paresis, bone pain, blindness, bleeding from mucous membranes, or polydipsia and polyuria can occur.

Differential diagnosis

Ehrlichiosis, lymphoma, primary bone tumors, osteomyelitis.

Diagnosis

The four diagnostic features of MM are (1) hyperproteinemia (hyperglobulinemia) with a monoclonal gammopathy, (2) osteolytic lesions, particularly in the spine, (3) >20% plasma cells in aspirates (**Figure 16.67**) or histology sections of lytic bone lesions or bone marrow, and (4) Bence-Jones proteinuria. Bence-Jones proteinuria is infrequent in dogs and cats, and these light chains of antibodies are best identified by electrophoresis of concentrated urine. Urine protein reagent strips will not detect light chain proteinuria. Confirmation of the diagnosis requires two to three of the four diagnostic features, depending on the level of confidence from each criterion.

Management

Combination therapy in dogs and cats with melphalan (0.1 mg/kg PO q24h for 10 days, then 0.5 mg/kg q24h) and prednisone (0.5 mg/kg PO q24h for 10 days, then 0.5 mg/kg q48h). Patients should be monitored for myelosuppression with biweekly CBCs for the first 2 months, and then monthly thereafter. Depending on which complications of MM are present, additional therapy may include plasmapheresis for hyperviscosity, fluid therapy for renal failure, orthopedic stabilization of pathologic fractures, and antibiotics for immunodeficiency. Hypercalcemia, if present, typically resolves within 2–3 days of initiating chemotherapy.

Prognosis

While complete elimination of disease is rarely achieved, chemotherapy is effective at reducing tumor burden, improving clinical signs, and reducing serum globulin concentrations. In dogs, there is 43% complete remission, 49% partial remission, and median survival of 540 days with melphalan and prednisone therapy. Extensive bone lesions, light chain proteinuria, hypercalcemia, and anemia are considered poor prognostic indicators. Cats transiently respond to chemotherapy, but relapse relatively early (median survival of 83–183 days).

PLASMACYTOMA

Definition/overview

Extramedullary plasmacytoma is a neoplastic proliferation of plasma cells that arises from tissues other than the bone marrow. The cells may be benign or malignant.

Etiology

The etiology is unknown.

Pathophysiology

Neoplastic plasma cells proliferate in the tissues. Malignant neoplasms may cause local and systemic tissue injury. Monoclonal gammopathies are less common than with MM.

Clinical presentation

Canine cutaneous plasmacytomas are frequently dome-shaped, erythremic, hairless masses of the digits, lips, and ears. Oral plasmacytomas may cause difficulty drinking, eating, or breathing. Dogs with GI plasmacytoma may present with vague signs of alimentary involvement.

Differential diagnosis

Other cutaneous neoplasms, lymphoplasmacytic hyperplasia or inflammation, abscesses.

Diagnosis

Diagnosis requires cytologic or histopathologic biopsy. For noncutaneous plasmacytomas, additional diagnostics (survey radiographs, bone marrow aspirate, serum electrophoresis) are important to ensure the lesion is solitary.

Management

Solitary plasma cell tumors are treated with surgical excision and/or external beam radiotherapy.

Prognosis

Canine cutaneous and oral plasmacytomas tend to be benign. Other plasmacytomas are potentially malignant, with metastases occurring months to years after initial diagnosis.

MYELOID (NONLYMPHOID) NEOPLASMS

Myeloid leukemias are clonal proliferations of erythroid, granulocytic, monocytic, and megakaryocytic cells. The 2008 WHO Classification of Tumors of Hematopoietic and Lymphoid Tissues divides myeloid neoplasms into three broad categories: myelodysplastic syndrome (MDS), myeloproliferative neoplasia (MPN), and acute myeloid leukemia (AML). The main differences between the new and previous classification schema are that MDS was previously considered a premalignancy, and that lower percentages of blasts are currently required for an acute leukemia designation. A consensus classification system for canine and feline myeloid neoplasms has not been established. Erythremic myelosis is a historical term that refers to erythroid leukemia of cats. Under the conventional classification, it encompasses MDS and erythroid subcategories of AML.

MYELODYSPLASTIC SYNDROME

Definition/overview

MDS is characterized by persistent peripheral cytopenia(s), normocellular to hypercellular marrow, dysplasia in one or more cell lines, and <20% blast cells in the marrow.

Etiology

Affected cats may be seropositive for FeLV. Other causes are idiopathic and may involve environmental effects or genetic predisposition.

Pathophysiology

MDS often precedes acute leukemia by several weeks to months. Increased apoptosis is considered the mechanism for cytopenias in the face of marrow proliferation.

Clinical presentation

Clinical signs involve chronic infections, lethargy due to anemia, and hemorrhage.

Differential diagnosis

Chronic myeloid leukemia, immune-mediated nonregenerative anemia, drug-induced dysplasia, nutrition-related dysplasia.

Diagnosis

Other causes of dysplasia (e.g. drugs, breed-associated) should be excluded. Diagnosis requires one or more cytopenias, normocellular to hypercellular marrow, <20% marrow myeloblasts, and myelodyplasia. Dysplastic changes in the blood or bone marrow include macrocytosis, megaloblastosis (**Figure 16.68**), nuclear fragmentation, abnormal cytoplasmic granulation, neutrophil hypersegmentation (**Figure 16.69**) or hyposegmentation, micromegakaryocytes or macrothrombocyte formation, and cell gigantism.

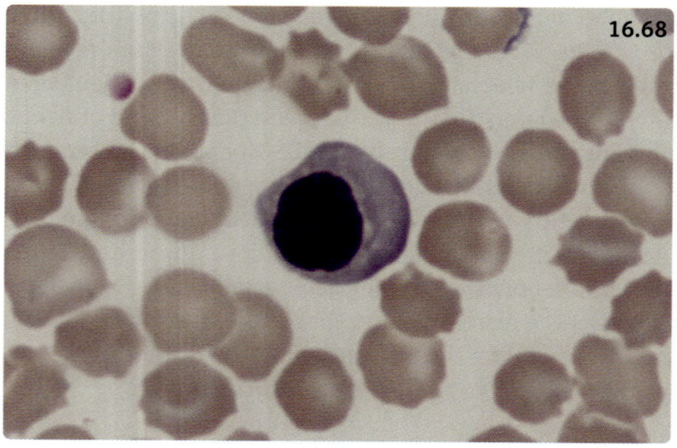

Figure 16.68 Inappropriate metarubricytosis and a dysplastic erythroid cell (megaloblast) in blood from a dog with myelodysplastic syndrome.

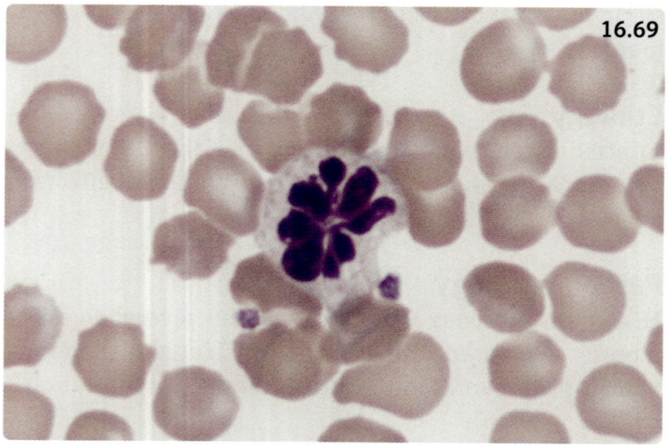

Figure 16.69 Dysplastic hypersegmented neutrophil from a dog with myelodysplastic syndrome.

Management

As the condition may persist for long periods of time without major clinical disease, treatment is usually supportive and includes antibiotics and blood transfusions as needed. Dyserythropoiesis in the dog may respond to recombinant human EPO (100 U/kg SC q48h for 10 days). Immune suppression may be attempted, but cancer chemotherapy is typically unrewarding.

Prognosis

Progression to AML is expected.

MYELOPROLIFERATIVE NEOPLASMS

Definition/overview

MPNs (chronic myeloproliferative disease/disorders) consist of persistent, unexplained increases in one or more myeloid lineages with a predominance of morphologically mature neoplastic cells. MPNs in small animals include primary myelofibrosis, chronic granulocytic leukemia, essential thrombocythemia, PV, and chronic myelomonocytic leukemia, and all are uncommon conditions.

Etiology

Feline MPN may be associated with FeLV infection.

Pathophysiology

Genetic mutations lead to cell proliferation and prolonged cell survival. BCR–ABL translocations have been documented in dogs with chronic monocytic leukemia and chronic myelomonocytic leukemia. The leukemia slowly effaces the marrow, leading to a chronic disease course, and cytopenias of other cell lines later in disease. Hyperviscosity syndrome is a potential complication of PV.

Clinical presentation

Animals with leukocyte proliferations often have no clinical signs until late-stage disease. Therefore, animals may appear healthy and diagnosis may be made with routine health screens. Late-stage disease consists of organ and marrow effacement, resulting in organomegaly, pallor if anemia is present, sepsis due to neutropenia or nonfunctional neutrophils, and hemorrhage from thrombocytopenia. Clinical signs in patients with PV relate to increased RBC mass and blood hyperviscosity. Mucous membranes are dark red (**Figure 16.70**) because of PCVs of 0.65–0.82 l/l (65–82%). Splenomegaly is usually not present. Polyuria, polydipsia, hemorrhage, and neurologic disorders occur in 50% of canine cases. Clinical signs of essential thrombocythemia include splenomegaly

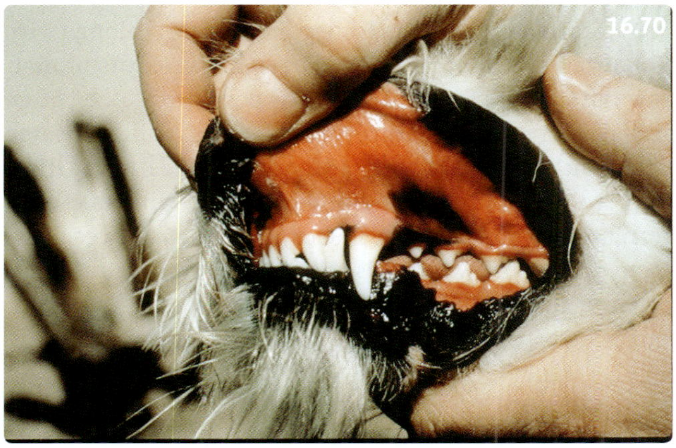

Figure 16.70 Brick red gums in a dog with polycythemia vera. (Courtesy J. Harvey)

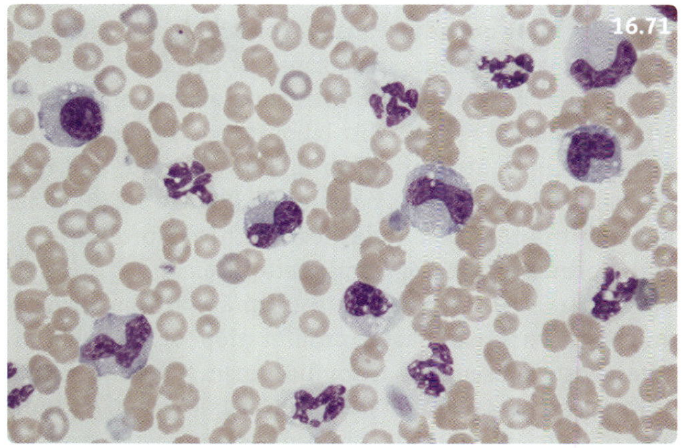

Figure 16.71 Chronic myelomonocytic leukemia in a dog with 116,491 neutrophils/µl and 26,277 monocytes/µl.

and platelet function abnormalities such as spontaneous bleeding and thromboembolism.

Differential diagnosis

For PV: causes of relative, appropriate absolute, and inappropriate absolute erythrocytosis. For proliferations of neutrophils and monocytes: causes of leukemoid response. For proliferations of eosinophils and basophils: hypersensitivity reactions, parasitic infections, and hypereosinophilic syndrome. For essential thrombocythemia and primary myelofibrosis: causes of reactive thrombocytosis.

Diagnosis

Since routine genetic testing is not available in veterinary medicine, these leukemias are diagnoses of exclusion. General features for all MPNs are persistent (>3 months) unexplained increases in one or more cell lines and relatively few blast cells in the bone marrow (<20% of all nucleated cells).

The subclassification is dependent on which cell lines are increased. Proliferations of neutrophils and/or monocytes include chronic myelogenous leukemia, chronic myelomonocytic leukemia, and chronic monocytic leukemia (**Figure 16.71**). Leukocyte counts are often markedly elevated (40,000–200,000/µl), and monocyte counts often exceed 4,000/µl (**Figure 16.72**). Neutrophilic leukemia must be differentiated from causes of a leukemoid inflammation, such as pyometra and pyelonephritis. Chronic eosinophilic leukemia is characterized by a high eosinophil count (often >50,000/µl) with a shift towards immaturity. It may be difficult to differentiate this malignancy from reactive hypereosinophilic conditions (e.g. allergies, parasitism, eosinophilic inflammatory diseases, mast cell tumors, and certain lymphomas). Chronic basophilic leukemia is mostly reported in the dog. It has been associated with thrombocytosis and anemia. Cytochemical staining with omega-exonuclease is helpful in identifying basophil precursors when cytoplasmic granulation is not apparent. Mature and immature basophils are increased in the blood or bone marrow, and tissue infiltration may occur. Basophilic leukemia must be differentiated from mast cell leukemia.

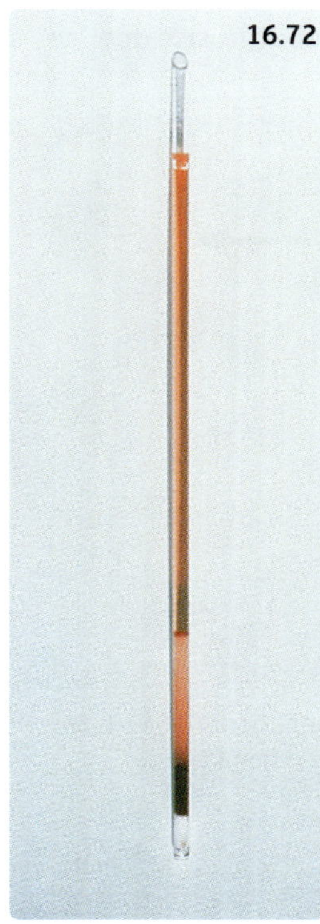

Figure 16.72 Large buffy coat present in a cat with acute myeloblastic leukemia displaying marked leukocytosis. (Courtesy J. Harvey)

PV, a proliferation of erythrocytes (primary erythrocytosis), occurs infrequently in dogs and cats. Diagnosis requires ruling out other causes of erythrocytosis. Arterial blood gas evaluations are normal, with no evidence of hypoxemia. Erythropoietin levels are absent or reduced when measured at specialist laboratories. Leukocyte and platelet counts are normal to mildly elevated, and in a few cases basophilia has been noted (**Figure 16.73**). Bone marrow examination indicates erythroid proliferation with normal morphology and maturation.

Essential thrombocythemia (primary thrombocythemia) is a rare neoplastic proliferation of megakaryocytes with subsequent thrombocytosis. Platelet counts are persistently above 600,000/µl (usually >1,000,000/µl) and platelet morphologic abnormalities may be present (**Figure 16.74**). Neutrophilia or basophilia may also be observed.

Primary myelofibrosis (chronic idiopathic myelofibrosis) causes persistent thrombocytosis due to a proliferation of atypical megakaryocytes along with enhanced granulopoiesis with variable amounts of marrow fibrosis (see **Figure 16.34**). The peripheral blood often has concurrent immature granulocytes and nucleated erythroid cells, termed a leukoerythroblastic reaction. Erythrocytes may display poikilocytosis with tear-drop formation or dacryocytosis (see **Figure 16.33**) resulting from the marrow fibrosis. Bone marrow aspiration is often difficult and is related to the presence of myelofibrosis, so core biopsy is required to confirm the diagnosis.

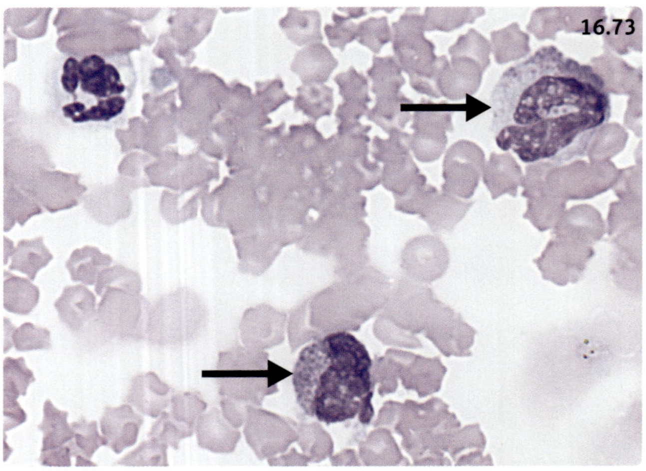

Figure 16.73 Feline blood with high hematocrit (0.64 l/l [64%]) and basophils (arrows) in a case of polycythemia vera.

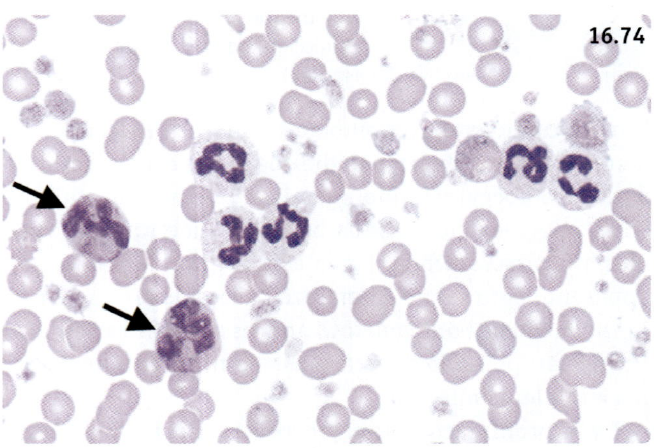

Figure 16.74 Essential thrombocythemia in a dog having numerous, occasionally atypical, platelets along with frequent basophils (arrows).

Management

Treatment is not required until clinical signs or cytopenias of non-neoplastic cells develop. Hydroxyurea is most commonly used, and has produced successful reductions in leukemic cell counts. In dogs, hydroxyurea is initially given at a dosage of 20–25 mg/kg PO q12h until there is a significant reduction in the neoplastic cell counts. For white cell neoplasms, the dosage is dropped to 10–15 mg/kg PO q24h or 50 mg/kg PO q2–3weeks when the leukocyte concentration is <20,000 cells/µl. For PV, once the PCV is below 0.6 l/l (60%), hydroxyurea can be tapered to the lowest effective frequency based on monitoring of the PCV. Lower initial doses of hydroxyurea (10–15 mg/kg PO q12h) should be used in cats due to their greater risk for myelotoxicity. Phlebotomy (15–20 ml/kg/day) provides immediate relief for PV. Supportive care (e.g. antibiotics, blood transfusions, and fluids) should be given when indicated.

Prognosis

Survival of months to years is expected, but eventual drug refractoriness or blast transformation is possible.

ACUTE MYELOID LEUKEMIA

Definition/overview

AML is a proliferation of immature nonlymphoid hematopoietic cells that often results in myelophthisis and poor prognosis.

Etiology

FeLV is associated with feline AML, especially the erythroid subtypes.

Pathophysiology

Immature myeloid cells proliferate rapidly and efface the bone marrow, resulting in life-threatening cytopenia. Neoplastic cells often disseminate hematologically to the tissues, causing widespread organ infiltration. BCR–ABL translocation has been documented in one dog with acute myeloblastic leukemia.

Clinical presentation

Clinical signs include organomegaly, pale mucous membranes, sepsis, and hemorrhage from thrombocytopenia.

Differential diagnosis

Lymphoid leukemia, recovery following viral, toxin, or drug-induced leukopenia.

Diagnosis

Diagnosis is often made on a CBC and blood smear review. Peripheral blood findings often include immature myeloid cells and blast cells, as well as decreases in one or more cell lines due to myelophthisis. Thrombocytopenia-induced hemorrhage may also contribute to the low red cell mass. Bone marrow evaluation may be performed in cases with low or no circulating blasts or when AML subtype classification is desired. Flow cytometry or other special diagnostic techniques (e.g. cytochemistry on the blood or bone marrow) may be required to identify the myeloid lineage of poorly differentiated leukemia.

Within the marrow, there is hypercellular marrow, ≥20% blast cells, and variable proportions of myeloid cells. AML subtypes with a predominance of myeloblasts include acute myeloblastic leukemia minimally differentiated (AML-M0), acute myeloblastic leukemia without maturation (AML-M1), acute myeloblastic leukemia with maturation (AML-M2), and acute promyelocytic leukemia (AML-M3). Monocyte differentiation is observed in acute myelomonocytic leukemia (AML-M4, **Figure 16.75**), acute monoblastic leukemia (AML-M5a), and acute monocytic leukemia (AML-M5b). Leukemias with erythroid differentiation (**Figure 16.76**) are acute erythroleukemia (AML-M6a) and acute erythroleukemia with erythroid predominance (AML-M6b). Acute megakaryoblastic leukemia (AML-M7) has a prominent megakaryoblast component. Cytochemical staining of blast cells is variably positive for peroxidase, Sudan black B, chloroacetate esterase, leukocyte ALP, and acid phosphatase. When rebounding from neutropenia, such as that following feline panleukopenia infection, the blood may appear neoplastic owing to the presence of large numbers of myeloblasts in the bone marrow. Persistent hematologic abnormalities must occur to confirm leukemia. Regenerative attempts following leukopenia are generally evident after 7–10 days for nonleukemic conditions.

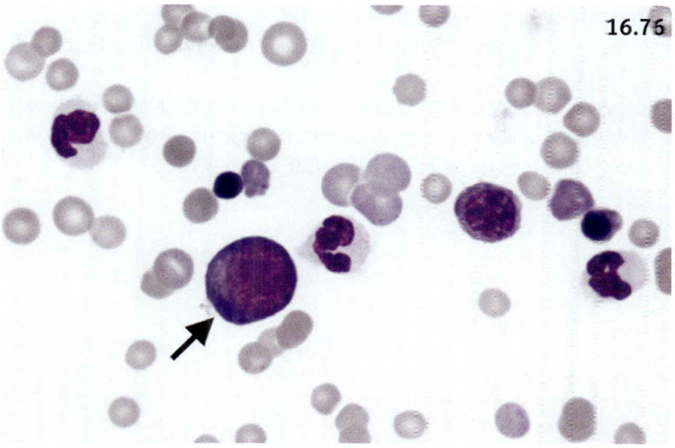

Figure 16.76 Acute erythroleukemia in a FeLV-positive cat. There are three segmented neutrophils and four nucleated erythroid precursors, the largest of which is an erythroblast or rubriblast (arrow).

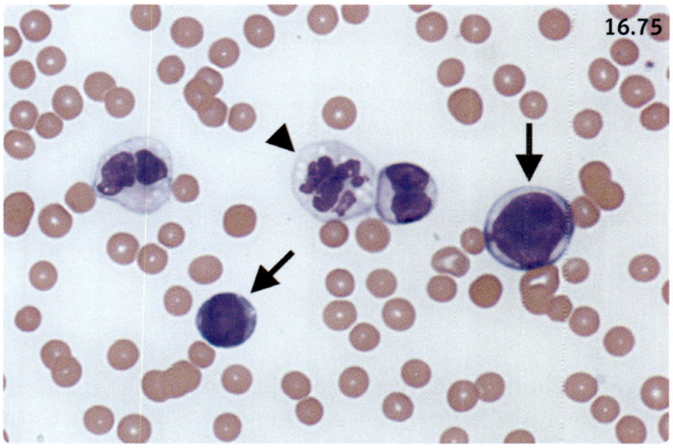

Figure 16.75 Blood from a dog with acute myelomonocytic leukemia with arrows indicating immature myeloid cells (myeloblasts) and an atypical segmented cell (arrowhead).

Management

In general, AML is poorly responsive to any chemotherapy protocol. If therapy is pursued, lymphoma protocols may be attempted, along with aggressive supportive care for cytopenias.

Prognosis

The prognosis is poor, as AML therapeutic response rates are low and overall survival times are short.

RECOMMENDED FURTHER READING

Harvey JW (2012) *Atlas of Veterinary Hematology: A Diagnostic Guide and Color Atlas*. Elsevier, St. Louis.

Messick JB (2012) (ed.) Hematology. *Vet Clin North Am Small Anim Pract* **42:**1–218.

Solano-Gallego L, Koutinas A, Miró G *et al.* (2009) Directions for the diagnosis, clinical staging, treatment and prevention of canine leishmaniosis. *Vet Parasitol* **165:**1–18.

Thrall MA, Weiser G, Allison R *et al.* (2012) (eds.) *Veterinary Hematology and Clinical Chemistry*, 2nd edn. Wiley-Blackwell, Ames

University of Wisconsin-Madison (2012) *UW-Madison Lymphoma Protocol for Dogs*. https://uwveterinarycare.wisc.edu/wp-content/uploads/2012/10/k9_chop.pdf.

University of Wisconsin-Madison (2012) *UW-Madison Lymphoma Protocol for Cats*. http://uwveterinarycare.wisc.edu/wp-content/uploads/2012/10/feline_chop.pdf.

Weiss DJ, Wardrop KJ (2010) (eds.) *Schalm's Veterinary Hematology*, 6th edn. Wiley-Blackwell, Ames.

Chapter 17

Disorders of hemostasis

Bobbi Conner

INTRODUCTION

Hemostasis refers to the process that minimizes blood loss following injury. It encompasses aspects of primary hemostasis, secondary hemostasis (usually thought of as clotting or coagulation), as well as the induction of local vasoconstriction that serves to limit loss of blood. Although not technically part of the hemostatic process, fibrinolysis is the important final step of the process that functions to return blood flow to its pre-injury state by removing the clot once it has served its purpose. All phases of hemostasis and fibrinolysis commence as part of a delicately balanced system that, when dysregulated this can lead to excessive hemorrhage or inappropriate thrombosis. An understanding of the normal physiology is, therefore, crucial to an understanding of the pathology when imbalances occur.

PRIMARY HEMOSTASIS

Primary hemostasis refers to the formation of the initial, relatively unstable, platelet plug. Although platelets are the major element of primary hemostasis, the vessel wall, von Willebrand factor (vWF), and several other proteases also play important roles in successful plug formation. The process is commonly divided into three major phases: platelet adhesion, activation, and aggregation.

In health, platelet adhesion occurs following compromise of the vascular endothelium, which exposes subendothelial collagen. Under high shear conditions, such as the ones present in small and medium arteries, platelets adhere to collagen via vWF, which binds to the platelet membrane glycoprotein (GP) Ib-IX-V. In contrast, under comparatively low shear stress conditions in large arteries and veins, platelets bind to collagen via fibronectin and laminin. Once adhered, platelets become activated by one of any number of pathways. Many platelet activators have been identified and their relative importance varies between species (**Table 17.1**). The final step in platelet activation involves release of granule contents, platelet shape change, and expression of GP IIb/IIIa, which mediates binding of fibrinogen and platelet aggregation (**Figure 17.1**).

The release of granule contents during activation is an important step in the recruitment of additional platelets to the developing plug, as well as factors important for additional adhesion and aggregation. Some of the alpha granule contents include fibronectin, clotting factors

Table 17.1 Relative activities of platelet activators in various species. NI, no information available.

	Man	Dog	Rat	Calf	Horse	Pig	Sheep
Thrombin	++++	++++	+++	++	++++	NI	NI
ADP	+++	+++	+++−	++	++++	+++	++
TXA2	+++	+++	NI	+	++++	++	++
PAF	NI	NI	NI	NI	++++	++	+++
Serotonin	++	++	+	NI	NI	NI	NI
Epinephrine	+	++	NI	+	NI	NI	NI
Ristocetin	+++	+++	NI	NI	+++	NI	++++
Collagen	+++	+++	NI	++	++++	NI	NI

ADP, adenosine diphosphate; TXA2, thromboxane A2; PAF, platelet activating factor.

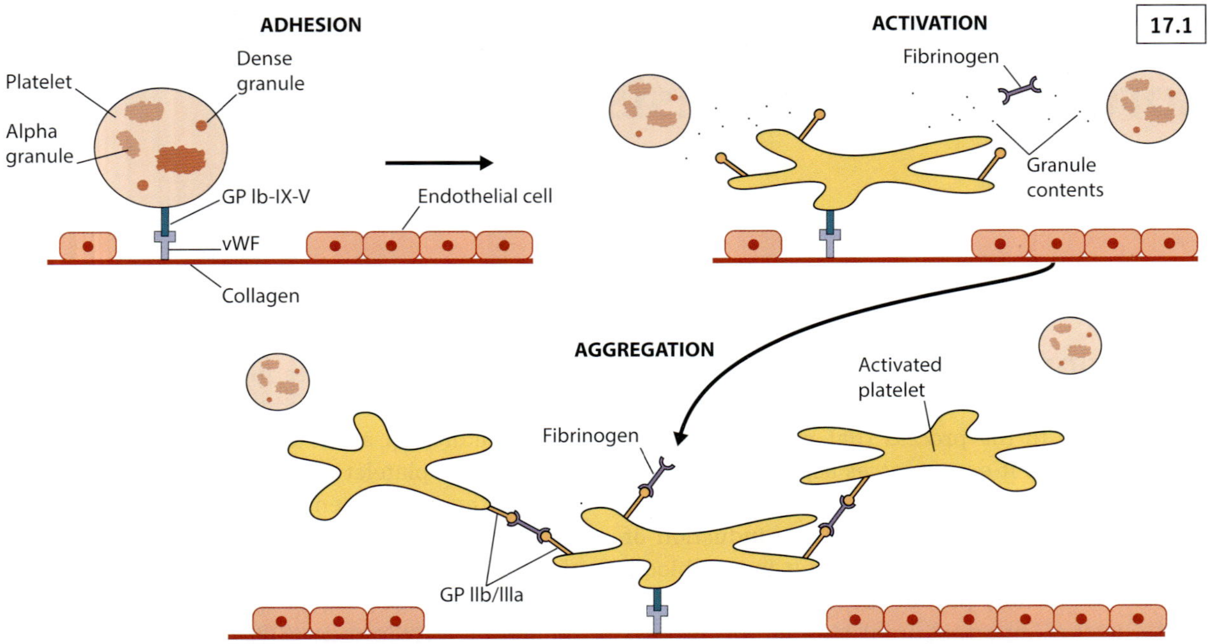

Figure 17.1 Platelet adhesion, activation, and aggregation. During adhesion, platelets bind to exposed subendothelial collagen. Platelet activation leads to shape change and increased exposure of glycoprotein (GP) IIb/IIIa as well as release of granule contents to recruit additional platelets. Platelet aggregation is mediated by GP IIb/IIIa and fibrinogen under low-shear stress conditions.

(F) V and VIII, as well as vWF. Dense granules contain adenosine triphosphate (ADP), histamine, epinephrine, serotonin, and calcium, among others. Most of the granule contents play some role in hemostasis, although many are also pro-inflammatory substances, such as interleukin-1 and other cytokines.

Activated platelets begin to aggregate via GP IIb/IIIa (also called integrin αIIb/β3) and fibrinogen (**Figure 17.1**) under low-shear stress conditions; vWF and GP Ib-IX-V or GP IIb/IIIa mediate aggregation under high-shear stress.

Inhibitors of platelet activation and aggregation, such as prostacyclin, nitric oxide, and ecto-ADPase, are released by or expressed on the surface of intact endothelial cells and are important for preventing platelet plug formation in the absence of vascular damage as well as limiting the spread of the platelet plug beyond the damaged endothelium.

SECONDARY HEMOSTASIS (COAGULATION)

Traditionally, coagulation has been understood – and taught – as a series of protease reactions, describing two separate, redundant pathways leading to a final common pathway with thrombin as the end-product. In the past few decades, our knowledge about how coagulation happens *in vivo* has increased and vastly improved our understanding of the complex process of clot formation and regulation. The previous 'cascade' model of coagulation has largely been replaced by the cell-based model. This has shed new light on both normal coagulation pathways as well as (and in particular) on why the process sometimes becomes deranged. Parallel to our growing understanding of coagulation there has been greater awareness of imbalances that often lead to increased morbidity and mortality. An understanding of the normal balance of clot formation and breakdown is crucial to the identification and safe treatment when these systems go awry.

The cascade model of coagulation (**Figure 17.2**) is not an accurate reflection of the *in-vivo* process, yet it has value in helping to interpret some of the diagnostic tests commonly employed in veterinary medicine when trying to sort out a bleeding disorder. Separating some of the serine proteases into the intrinsic, extrinsic, and common pathways can be useful when evaluating the prothrombin time (PT) and partial thromboplastin time (PTT) tests that are run as part of a standard coagulation profile. The intrinsic factors – FXII, FXI, FIX, FVIII – are necessary for a normal PTT test; the extrinsic factors – tissue factor (TF) and FVII – are needed for a normal PT test; and the common pathway factors – FX, FV, FII, and FI – are required for both tests to be normal.

The cell-based model of coagulation underscores the important role that cells (platelets and endothelial cells in particular) play in successful and balanced coagulation. It also illustrates that the cascade model is overly simplistic and a poor reflection of the *in-vivo* process.

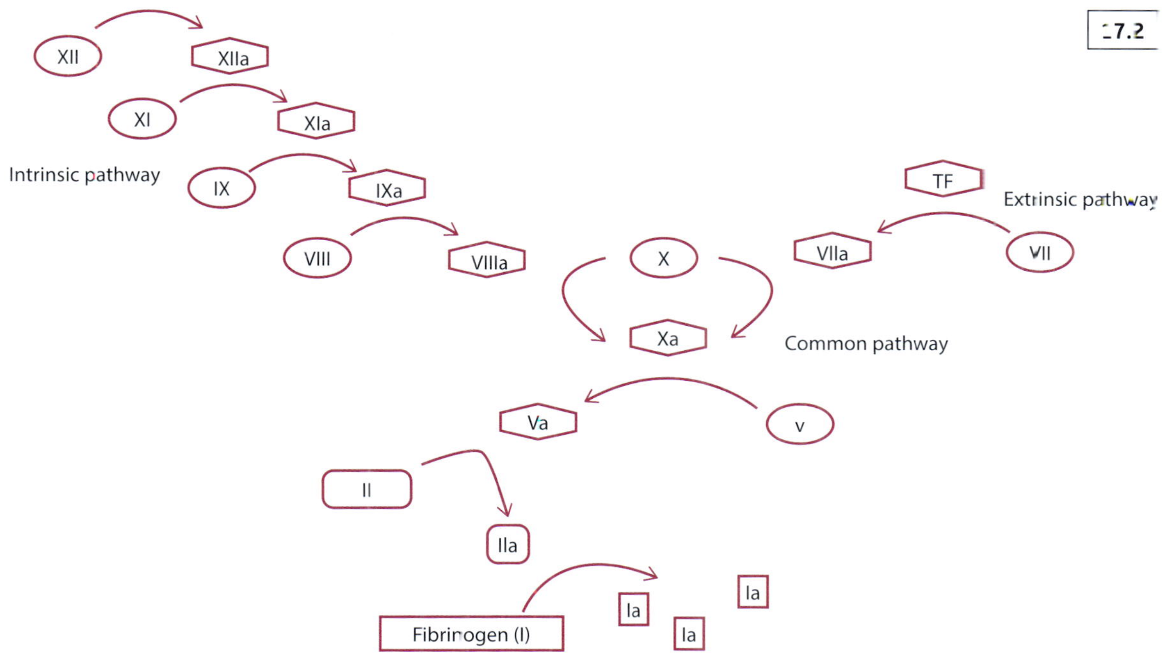

Figure 17.2 Depiction of the traditional coagulation cascade. Activated clotting factors are denoted with an 'a'. II, prothrombin; IIa, thrombin; Ia, fibrin.

Based on our current understanding, rather than two overlapping, redundant pathways to thrombin and fibrin formation, coagulation is now described in terms of initiation, amplification, and propagation.

Initiation of coagulation occurs when TF becomes exposed to circulating activated FVII (FVIIa) – this is essentially the 'extrinsic pathway' from the cascade model. TF and FVIIa combine to activate FX, which in turn activates and binds FV to form the prothrombinase enzyme. Prothrombinase will cleave prothrombin, yielding thrombin. Thrombin has a number of physiologic functions, but its most important coagulation function is the conversion of fibrinogen into fibrin. Fibrin monomers will spontaneously polymerize into a fibrin meshwork. With this process, it may seem that the intrinsic pathway is not necessary for clot formation; however, we know that patients with hemophilia A or B (FVIII or FIX deficiency, respectively) have a bleeding tendency. This is because the amount of thrombin and fibrin produced at the end of this initiation process is relatively small; the process must be amplified. Thrombin has a positive feedback effect by activating FV, FVIII, and FXI, as well as activating platelets, which will provide the scaffolding on which the developing clot will form, and FXIII, which will help to stabilize the final clot by cross-linking with fibrin. The activation of FVIII and FXI will enhance the 'intrinsic pathway' to yield more FX and therefore prothrombinase, setting the stage for more thrombin formation during the propagation phase (**Figure 17.3**).

Factor XII deficiency (also called Hageman factor deficiency) has been reported rarely in dogs, cats, and people. It is associated with a prolonged PTT without a bleeding disorder. Among other inconsistencies, this finding led researchers to question the validity of the traditional coagulation cascade and, ultimately, the development of the cell-based model of coagulation.

A number of factors are in place to keep coagulation in check. Circulating antithrombin (AT) will inactivate FVIIa, FIXa, FXa, FXIa, FXIIa, and, to a greater extent, thrombin. The activity of AT is enhanced >2,000-fold by the addition of unfractionated heparin (UH). Thrombomodulin also participates in the prevention of excessive clot formation. Thrombomodulin is expressed on endothelial cell surfaces and binds to thrombin. The thrombin–thrombomodulin complex will then activate protein C. Once activated, protein C, along with one of its cofactors, protein S, will inactivate FVa and FVIIIa.

FIBRINOLYSIS

Fibrinolysis, or the degradation of fibrin, is crucial for restoration of normal blood flow following vessel wall repair, when the hemostatic clot is no longer needed. The fibrinolytic system relies on precise control, as imbalances can

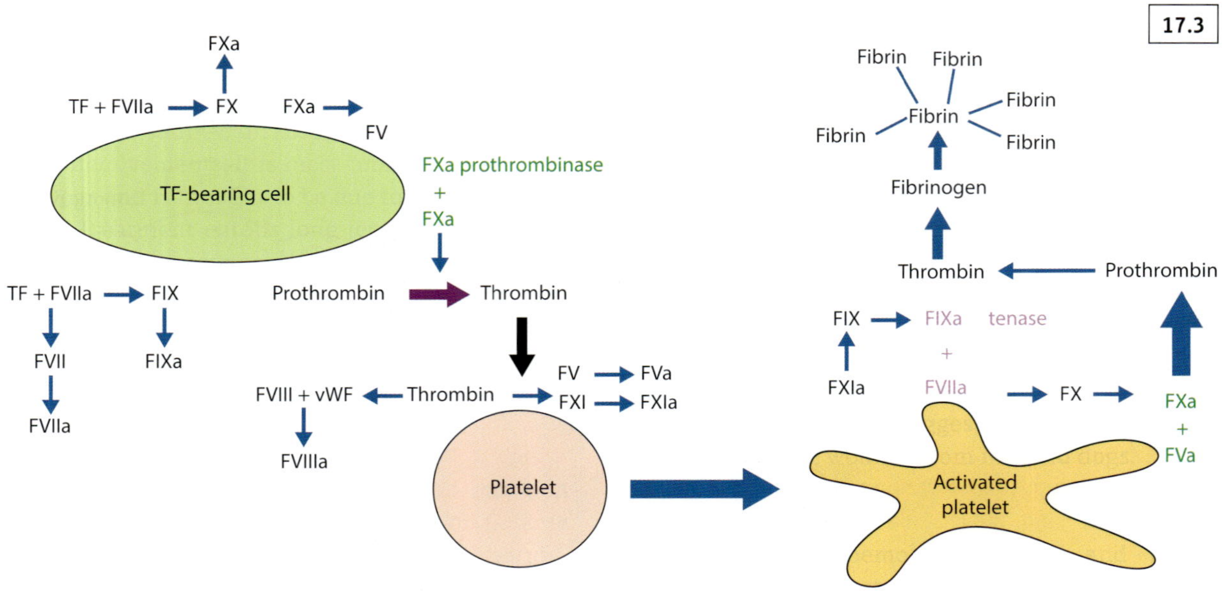

Figure 17.3 Depiction of the cell-based model of coagulation. F + Roman numeral denotes the corresponding clotting factor. F + Roman numeral + a denotes the activated clotting factor. TF, tissue factor.

lead to hemorrhage (hyperfibrinolysis) or propagation of thrombosis (hypofibrinolysis). Fibrinolysis is part of a larger balancing act between pro- and anticoagulation, but as a subsystem it is also regulated by activators and inhibitors.

Cross-linked, polymerized fibrin is the primary and most clinically relevant substrate when considering fibrinolysis; the protease of interest – plasmin – is the enzyme responsible for thrombus degradation. Plasmin is generated by the activation of the zymogen plasminogen by a plasminogen activator, either tissue-type plasminogen activator (tPA) or urokinase/urine-type plasminogen activator (uPA). Plasminogen is inserted into the developing clot and may be bound to fibrin for days before it becomes activated by tPA and converted to plasmin.

When formed appropriately, clots serve the important function of preventing excessive blood loss following injury; therefore, early or excessive fibrinolysis must be prevented. A number of inhibitors of the fibrinolytic system act to either prevent activation of plasminogen, or inhibit plasmin, once formed. The activity of tPA and uPA will be blunted by plasminogen activator inhibitor 1 (PAI-1), preventing the activation of plasminogen into plasmin. Alpha$_2$-antiplasmin (α_2AP) and thrombin activatable fibrinolysis inhibitor (TAFI) both interfere with binding of plasminogen and plasmin to fibrin, thereby preventing the breakdown of fibrin.

The breakdown of fibrinogen, fibrin monomers, and cross-linked fibrin will all yield fibrin degradation products (FDPs) that are indistinguishable from one another. D-dimers, on the other hand, only result from the breakdown of cross-linked fibrin. D-dimers are therefore more specific for clot formation and breakdown.

DISORDERS ASSOCIATED WITH BLEEDING (HYPOCOAGULATION)

PRIMARY HEMOSTATIC DISORDERS

THROMBOCYTOPENIA

Thrombocytopenia is an abnormally reduced number of circulating platelets, generally <100,000 platelets/µl (reference ranges may vary). Causes of thrombocytopenia generally fall into one of five broad categories: (1) reduced production; (2) consumption; (3) destruction; (4) sequestration; or (5) loss. Splenic sequestration or blood loss alone rarely cause clinically significant thrombocytopenia.

REDUCED PRODUCTION

Definition/overview

Reduced platelet production by the bone marrow is a common cause of thrombocytopenia in dogs and cats.

Etiology

Causes for reduced bone marrow thrombopoiesis may include infectious agents (e.g. *Ehrlichia canis*, canine distemper virus, feline leukemia virus), drugs or toxins (e.g. chemotherapeutic drugs, linezolid, sulfonamides, estrogen), and disorders that crowd the bone marrow (myelophthisis).

Pathophysiology

Thrombopoietin (THO) is produced primarily in the liver and stimulates megakaryocyte (platelet precursor) production and differentiation in the bone marrow. Once released into the bloodstream, THO binds to a platelet surface receptor, where it is subsequently degraded. This results in blood THO concentrations that are inversely related to platelet concentration. Fewer platelets in circulation lead to less THO breakdown and more is available to reach the bone marrow. When platelet numbers are high in circulation, THO concentration (and therefore platelet production) falls. If the bone marrow is unable to respond to THO, platelets will not be replenished.

Clinical presentation

Patients may be presented with signs consistent with a primary hemostatic disorder, including petechial or ecchymotic hemorrhages (**Figures 17.4–17.7**). These occur commonly on the gums, the pinnae, and the ventral abdomen, but may occur anywhere on the skin or other mucous membranes. Other mucosal hemorrhages may be seen clinically as melena, hematemesis, epistaxis, or hematuria (**Figures 17.8–17.10**), or other less common locations (**Figure 17.11**). Clients and veterinary staff may appreciate excessive bruising or prolonged bleeding from venepuncture or catheter sites. Additionally, patients may have clinical signs referable to the underlying disease process.

Diagnosis

A reduced number of circulating platelets will be diagnosed and confirmed with a complete blood count (CBC) and blood smear (**Figure 17.12**). Identification of a primary disorder (e.g. *E. canis*) may lead to suspicion of a cause for the reduced platelet production or consumption; however, bone marrow disorders are diagnosed on a bone marrow aspirate or biopsy. (See Destruction for more detail on platelet evaluation on a blood smear and Chapter 16, Hematologic disorders, for bone marrow aspiration procedure.)

Management

Successful management of the underlying disease often leads to a return of normal platelet production. Withdrawal of the causative toxin or drug is also warranted in cases of exposure. If bleeding occurs secondary to severe thrombocytopenia, transfusion of platelet products may be valuable. There is no evidence to support the transfusion of platelet products in the absence

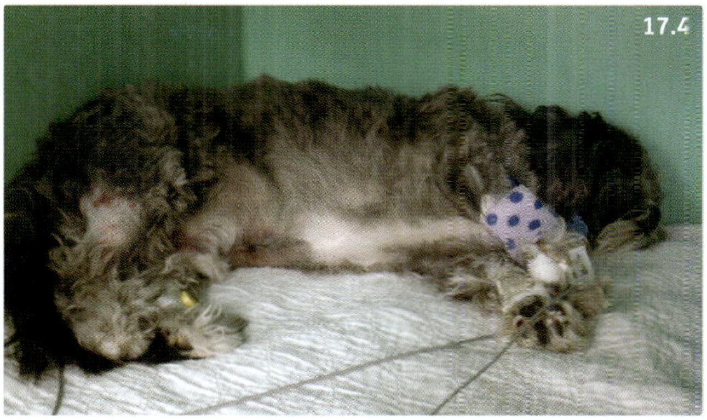

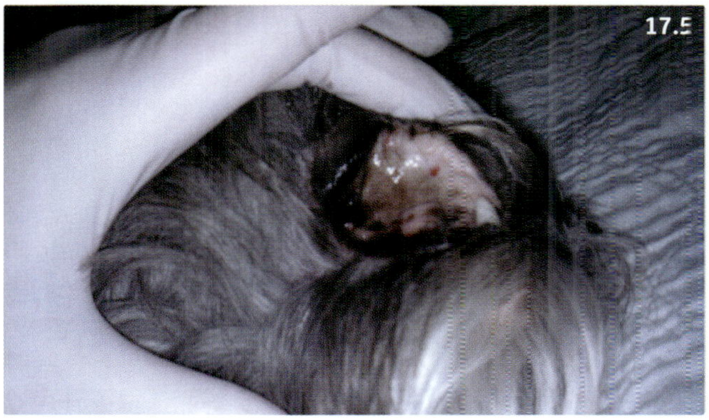

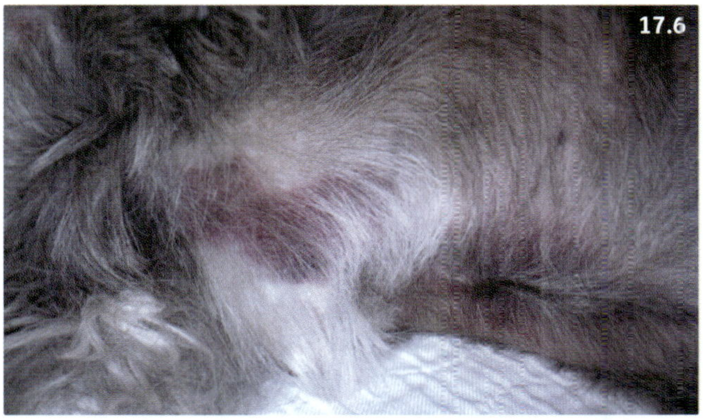

Figures 17.4–17.6 A 4-year-old male castrated Shih Tzu with immune-mediated thrombocytopenia. Note the petechiae and ecchymoses on the ventral abdomen, hindlimb, and gums.

of clinically significant bleeding or before emergency invasive procedures.

To date, neither commercially available fresh or stored platelet products nor in-house prepared fresh platelet products have proven efficacy for reducing or preventing hemorrhage in thrombocytopenic veterinary patients. The cost–benefit of these products must be carefully considered and prophylactic platelet transfusions should be avoided except when invasive procedures must be performed (e.g. emergency surgery). Additional studies on

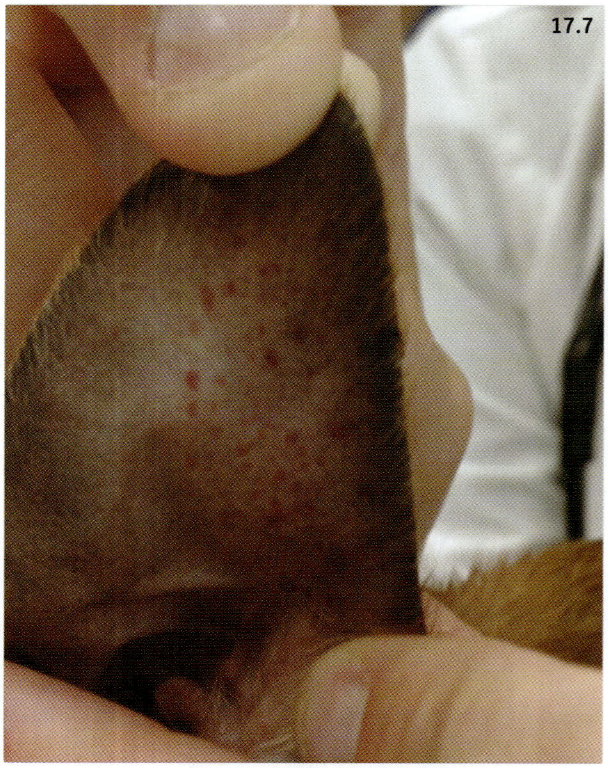

Figure 17.7 Petechiae on the pinna of a dog with severe thrombocytopenia.

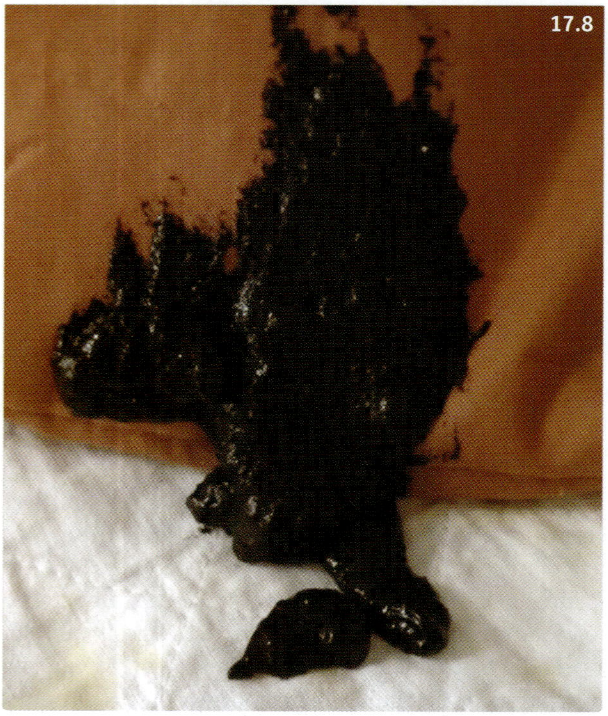

Figure 17.8 Melena. Note the very dark brown to black color and tarry texture.

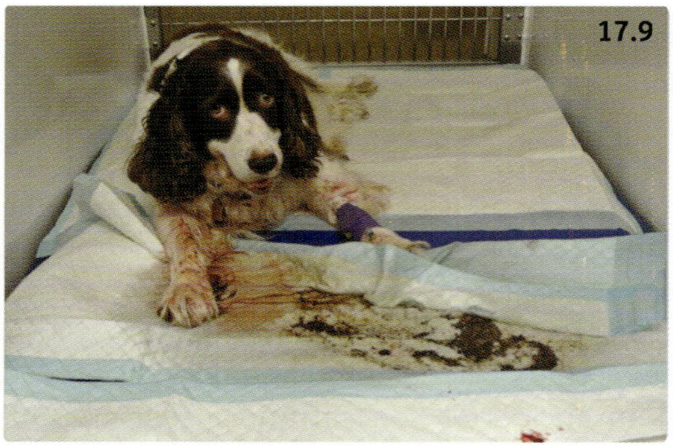

Figure 17.9 Springer Spaniel with hematemesis. Note the coffee ground appearance of the vomitus and the blood staining on the forelimb.

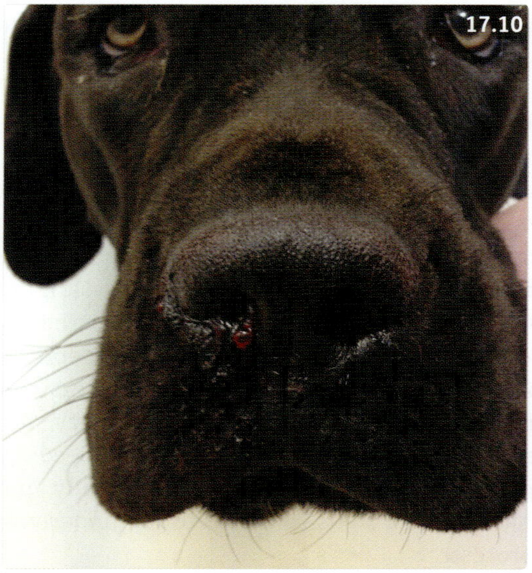

Figure 17.10 Mastiff with epistaxis.

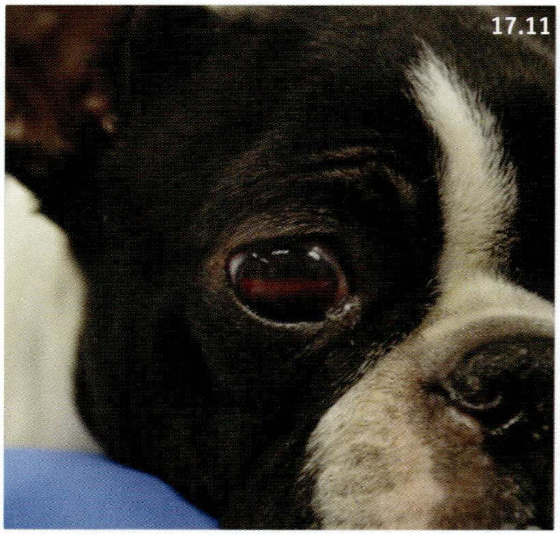

Figure 17.11 Hyphema in a dog with severe thrombocytopenia. (Courtesy M. Schaer)

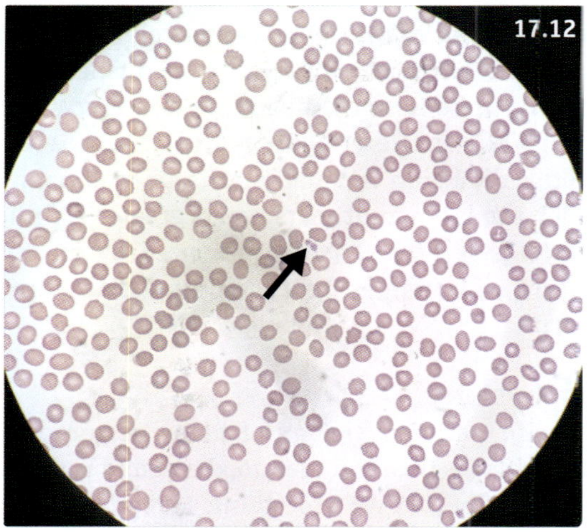

Figure 17.12 Blood smear from a dog with severe thrombocytopenia. Two platelets are seen in the center of the field (arrow). The average number of platelets seen per 5–10 fields is then multiplied by 15 × 10^3/µl to yield a platelet estimate.

the effectiveness of these products in veterinary medicine are needed.

Prognosis

Outcomes for dogs and cats with reduced platelet production will vary depending on the severity and response to treatment of the underlying disease process.

CONSUMPTION

Consumptive processes are typified by disseminated intravascular coagulation (DIC), a complex syndrome of coagulation activation triggered by a number of inflammatory conditions. This will be discussed in detail later in the chapter. Endothelial damage or dysfunction can also lead to consumption of platelets in the absence of DIC.

LOSS

Hemorrhage may also lead to loss of platelets, although this is generally seen as only a relatively mild reduction in platelet count, and the platelet count typically rebounds when the hemorrhage is controlled.

Massive hemorrhage requires massive transfusion (generally defined as either replacement of the patient's total blood volume in less than 24 hours or 50% of the total blood volume within 3 hours). Most protocols for massive transfusion in people recommend blood is replaced with various ratios of component therapy; for example, 3 units of packed red blood cells: 2 units of fresh frozen plasma: 1 unit of fresh platelet concentrate. Similar protocols have not been evaluated in veterinary patients.

DESTRUCTION

Definition/overview

Immune-mediated platelet destruction is a common cause of thrombocytopenia in dogs, but is less common in cats.

Etiology

Immune-mediated platelet destruction is often categorized as primary (autoimmune, mediated by direct antiplatelet antibodies) or secondary (mediated by antibodies directed against cell-surface antigens from infectious agents, tumors, or some drugs).

Pathophysiology

Both humoral and cell-mediated immunologic mechanisms are described in immune-mediated thrombocytopenia. It may be associated with a variety of inflammatory diseases that may serve as a 'trigger' for the immunologic response, including various infectious and neoplastic diseases.

Platelets are necessary for maintenance of endothelial intercellular junctions. When platelet numbers are extremely low, these junctions are compromised, leading to petechiae and ecchymoses. When platelets are normal in number, but function is impaired – as with antiplatelet drugs and thrombocytopathias – petechiae are rarely seen, but excessive bruising and mucosal bleeding may occur.

Clinical presentation

All causes of thrombocytopenia may present with clinical signs referable to a disorder of primary hemostasis, including petechiae, ecchymoses, or mucosal bleeding. Clinical signs of the associated or causative disease process may also be present. Primary or secondary immune-mediated thrombocytopenia may be associated with fever.

Differential diagnosis

Thrombocytopathy, endothelial dysfunction.

Diagnosis

Thrombocytopenia is identified with a CBC and confirmed via evaluation of a direct blood smear (see **Figure 17.12**). At 100× magnification, platelets should be counted; the average number of platelets seen per 5–10 fields is then multiplied by 15 × 10^3/µl to yield a platelet estimate. Review of the feathered edge for platelet clumps is important; if significant clumping is seen, the platelet estimate should be considered the minimum platelet count. Screening for infectious and neoplastic diseases is recommended in most cases. Antiplatelet antibody testing is neither sensitive nor specific and is not necessary. Bone marrow aspiration is not routinely recommended, unless a hematologic malignancy is suspected.

Management

The mainstay of treatment for immune-mediated platelet destruction remains immunosuppressive corticosteroids. Prednisone should be initiated at 2 mg/kg/day, although dosages up to 4 mg/kg/day may be needed in small dogs that do not initially respond to treatment. Dexamethasone (or dexamethasone sodium phosphate) may be used initially in patients that cannot tolerate oral medications. It should be dosed at 0.2–0.3 mg/kg/day of dexamethasone IV. Adjunctive therapy with human immunoglobulin is commonly employed in people and may reduce platelet recovery time in dogs. Vincristine has also been recommended to shorten platelet recovery time in dogs. Other adjunctive immunosuppressive drugs may be initiated at the clinician's discretion; however, investigations in veterinary medicine are lacking.

Prognosis

Survival rates of dogs with immune-mediated thrombocytopenia are around 80–85%, with similar rates reported in cats (far fewer reports overall). A relapse rate of ~10% in dogs can also be expected. Response times in dogs range from 1 to 15 days after initiation of immunosuppressive therapy. Relapse is not uncommon, therefore close monitoring of these patients' platelet counts should be done whenever there is a reduction in the prednisone treatment dose and every 2–3 months while on maintenance doses.

THROMBOCYTOPATHIA

Definition/overview

Thrombocytopathia (also referred to as thrombopathia) refers to an abnormality of platelet function. This could be from altered platelet adhesion or activation or, more commonly, from altered or reduced platelet aggregation.

Etiology

Thrombocytopathias may be acquired or inherited. Acquired disorders have been described with various infectious diseases, metabolic disorders (liver disease and uremia), various neoplasms, or they may be iatrogenic secondary to platelet-inhibiting drugs (e.g. aspirin, clopidogrel). More than 10 inherited platelet disorders have been described in veterinary medicine. The most common of these is von Willebrand disease (vWD). Three forms of vWD are described: type I is characterized by an overall reduction in small and large vWF multimers (of which the large multimers are of greater significance in hemostasis); type II is characterized by an absence of the large multimers; and type III is the absence of all multimers.

Pathophysiology

The specific pathophysiology of many acquired thrombocytopathias is poorly understood. Uremia is associated with disruptions of vWF processing. Liver disease is associated with reduced platelet aggregation, although the precise mechanism is unclear. Reduced or absent vWF leads to impaired adhesion and aggregation.

Clinical presentation

Patients with a thrombocytopathia may be clinically indistinguishable from a thrombocytopenic patient; however, if the platelet count is normal, there is a tendency for mucosal bleeding rather than petechiae or ecchymoses.

Differential diagnosis

Thrombocytopenia, endothelial dysfunction.

Diagnosis

Clinical suspicion is raised when mucosal bleeding or petechiae occur in the absence of severe thrombocytopenia. A buccal mucosal bleeding time will be prolonged despite normal or near-normal platelet numbers. Advanced platelet analysis is necessary to further differentiate thrombocytopathy from endothelial disorders. Platelet function analysis and platelet aggregometry are the most commonly used tests for identifying platelet function disorders, and are commercially available at outside laboratories. Viscoelastic testing (i.e. sonoclot, thromboelastography, and thromboelastometry) may be available to some clinicians and can provide some insight into platelet function. Suspicion of vWD can be confirmed with direct measurement of vWF using an ELISA.

Management

Acquired thrombocytopathias are generally reversed when the underlying condition is effectively treated. If life-threatening bleeding occurs, transfusion of blood products may be of use. Choice of product may depend on the known or suspected pathophysiology. For vWD, fresh frozen plasma or cryoprecipitate will provide vWF to treat bleeding or prevent hemorrhage when surgery is needed. A single dose of desmopressin acetate at 1 μg/kg IV will stimulate release of vWF from endothelial stores in type I vWD, and it may have a role in other thrombocytopathias as well. Repeated doses are not effective as stores become depleted. Transfusion of platelet-containing blood products may be needed in some cases of thrombocytopathia until the underlying disease can be identified and treated.

Prognosis

Dogs and cats with type I vWD can have varying degrees of bleeding, but with client education directed at minimizing the chance of injury and preoperative planning, dogs can be well-managed for years, whereas the prognosis for dogs with type III disease is grave because of a severe bleeding tendency. Type II disease has a guarded prognosis because of its intermediate tendency for bleeding. Prognosis for animals with acquired thrombocytopathy will depend on the severity of the underlying disease and response to therapy. In general, platelet dysfunction returns to normal when the causative disease is controlled or reversed.

VASCULAR/ENDOTHELIAL DYSFUNCTION

Definition/overview

In health, the endothelium participates in the homeostatic mechanisms maintaining vascular integrity, including normal anticoagulation, as well as the regulation of vascular tone. In inflammatory conditions, particularly sepsis, dysfunction of the endothelium leads to imbalances of coagulation and impaired maintenance of vascular tone.

Vasculitis is commonly confused with endothelial dysfunction. Vasculitis refers to direct inflammation (infiltration by white blood cells) of the blood vessels. This is not a feature of endothelial dysfunction. The term vasculopathy is sometimes used to describe the latter condition and is more appropriate that the commonly misused term vasculitis.

Etiology

Endothelial dysfunction has been implicated in human diseases as varied as Alzheimer's disease and sleep apnea to hypertension and diabetes mellitus. In veterinary medicine, it is most commonly suspected in systemic inflammatory diseases, such as sepsis, severe trauma, and pancreatitis.

Pathophysiology

Probably in response to exposure to various inflammatory cytokines, nitric oxide and prostacyclin production and release by the endothelium are impaired, leading to vasodilation and reduced platelet inhibition. This may contribute to the development of DIC. Reduced or increased platelet adhesion and activation may occur. Reduced platelet aggregation may also be seen.

Clinical presentation

Clinical signs may vary to include dysfunction of platelet function, causing petechiae or excessive bleeding; however, increased risk of thrombosis is generally more likely with endothelial dysfunction. A coagulation disorder is frequently accompanied by loss of regulation of vascular tone leading to hypotension.

Differential diagnosis

Thrombocytopenia, thrombocytopathy, DIC.

Diagnosis

Reliable diagnostic tests for endothelial dysfunction are lacking. Clinical suspicion and resolution of signs with successful treatment of the underlying disease are suggestive of vascular endothelial dysfunction.

Management

Treatment of the causative disease is paramount. Supportive treatment for bleeding or thrombosis may be needed in some cases.

Prognosis

Diseases causing endothelial dysfunction are generally severe systemic inflammatory conditions with variable prognoses. If rapid identification and treatment of the primary disease process does not occur, prognosis will be guarded.

SECONDARY HEMOSTATIC DISORDERS

INHERITED SECONDARY HEMOSTATIC DISORDERS (HEMOPHILIAS)

Definition/overview

Hemophilia A is a deficiency of FVIII and is the most common inherited deficiency of coagulation in veterinary medicine. Hemophilia B is a deficiency of FIX and occurs much less frequently than hemophilia A. Hageman factor (FXII) deficiency has been described in both cats and dogs. Deficiencies in other clotting factors and fibrinogen are rarely reported.

Etiology

Both hemophilia A and hemophilia B are X-linked recessive traits, making them a disease of males almost exclusively. Factor XII deficiency has an autosomal recessive inheritance pattern.

Pathophysiology

Factors VIII and IX are crucial in the amplification of thrombin formation, and their absence or severe reduction may lead to clinically significant bleeding. Mild reductions in factor concentrations correspond to a milder bleeding diathesis. Factor XII does not play a crucial role in coagulation *in vivo*, and its absence is not associated with clinical bleeding.

Clinical presentation

Depending on the severity of the factor deficiency, patients with hemophilia A or B may present with spontaneous bleeding or bleeding of varying degrees following surgery or trauma. Patients with FXII deficiency do not exhibit abnormal bleeding.

Differential diagnosis

Acquired coagulopathy, DIC, vWD.

Diagnosis

Prolongation of a PTT test with a normal PT test in the presence of unexpected bleeding is suggestive of hemophilia A or B (**Figure 17.13**). Prolongation of PTT in the absence of bleeding may be suggestive of FXII deficiency. Confirmation and differentiation requires quantification of individual factors and is available at selected veterinary reference laboratories.

Management

Hemophilia A or B may not require regular therapy other than careful avoidance of trauma. Prior to surgery and other invasive procedures, or after accidental trauma, a transfusion of fresh frozen plasma (10–20 ml/kg) is appropriate for hemophilia A or B. If available, cryoprecipitate (1 unit/10 kg) may be used for hemophilia A, but not hemophilia B. Packed red blood cells (RBCs) (in addition to fresh frozen plasma) or fresh whole blood may be needed if significant bleeding occurs. Therapy is not needed for FXII deficiency.

17.13

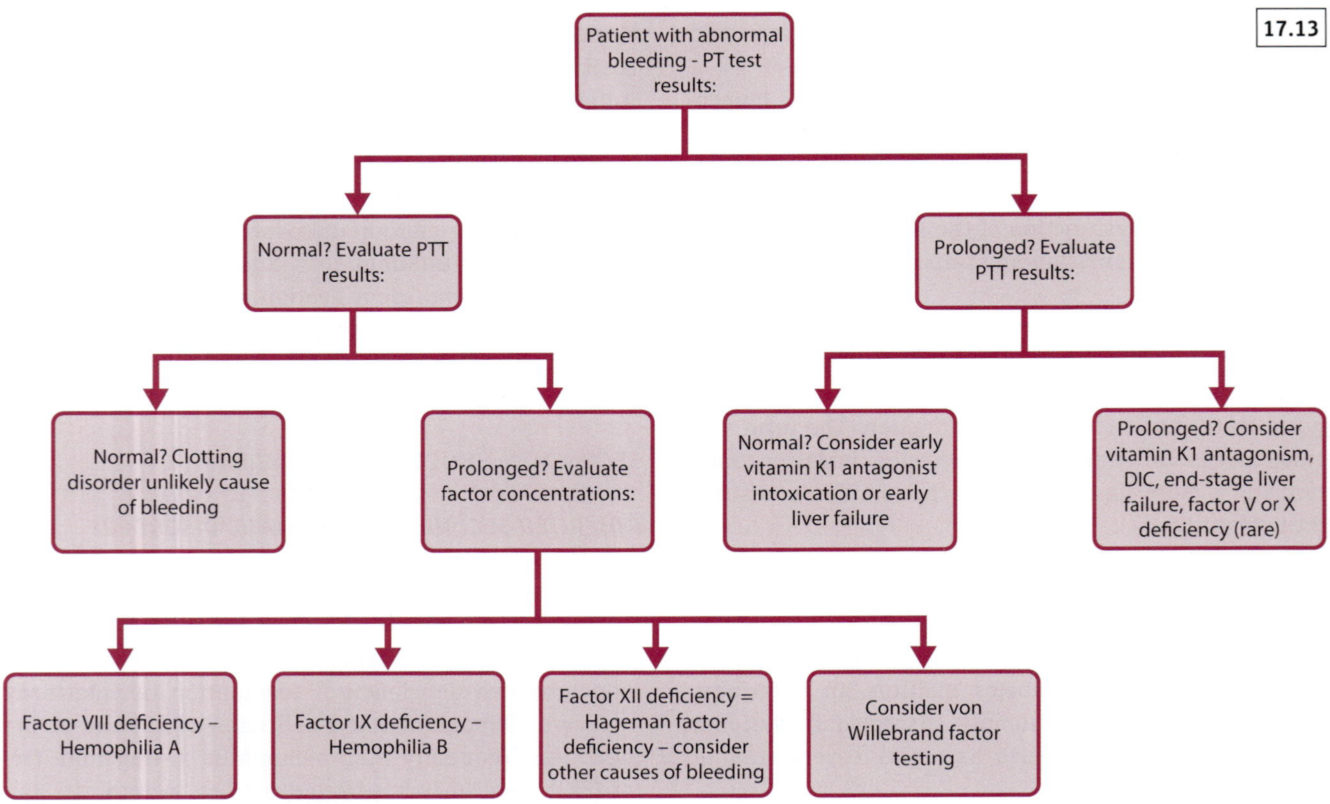

Figure 17.13 Differential diagnoses chart for results of prothrombin time (PT) and partial thromboplastin time (PTT) tests.

Prognosis

Prognosis is good for many patients with hemophilia A or B once the diagnosis has been confirmed and appropriate precautions are taken. If the factor deficiency is severe and causes frequent spontaneous bleeding, long-term management may be more difficult. Breeders should be alerted to the diagnosis and education provided to discontinue further breeding with the carrier bitch. Prognosis for FXII deficiency is excellent.

ACQUIRED SECONDARY HEMOSTATIC DISORDERS

Definition/overview

Acquired disorders of coagulation are caused by an insufficient quantity or impaired function of one or more essential clotting factors, which can occur secondary to disease, injury, or intoxication.

Etiology

The most common simple acquired coagulopathy in veterinary medicine is intoxication by one of the many types of anticoagulant rodenticides, mostly coumarins. Other diseases or syndromes associated with complex acquired coagulopathies (DIC, liver disease, sepsis, trauma) will be discussed later in this chapter. As the use of therapeutic anticoagulants becomes more common in veterinary medicine, the risk of iatrogenic coagulopathy or accidental overdose may increase.

Pathophysiology

The toxic mechanism of anticoagulant rodenticides involves disruption of the vitamin K cycle in mammals (**Figure 17.14**). Reduced vitamin K is a cofactor for the enzyme γ-glutamyl carboxylase, which is necessary to convert FVII, FIX, FX, prothrombin, protein C, and protein S to their functional zymogen forms. During this process, reduced vitamin K is converted to vitamin K epoxide. Coumarins, including warfarin, and the noncoumarin anticoagulant rodenticides antagonize the enzyme vitamin K epoxide reductase, which is necessary for vitamin K recycling. When reduced vitamin K stores become depleted, nonfunctional zymogens are released into the circulation, preventing normal clot formation.

17.14

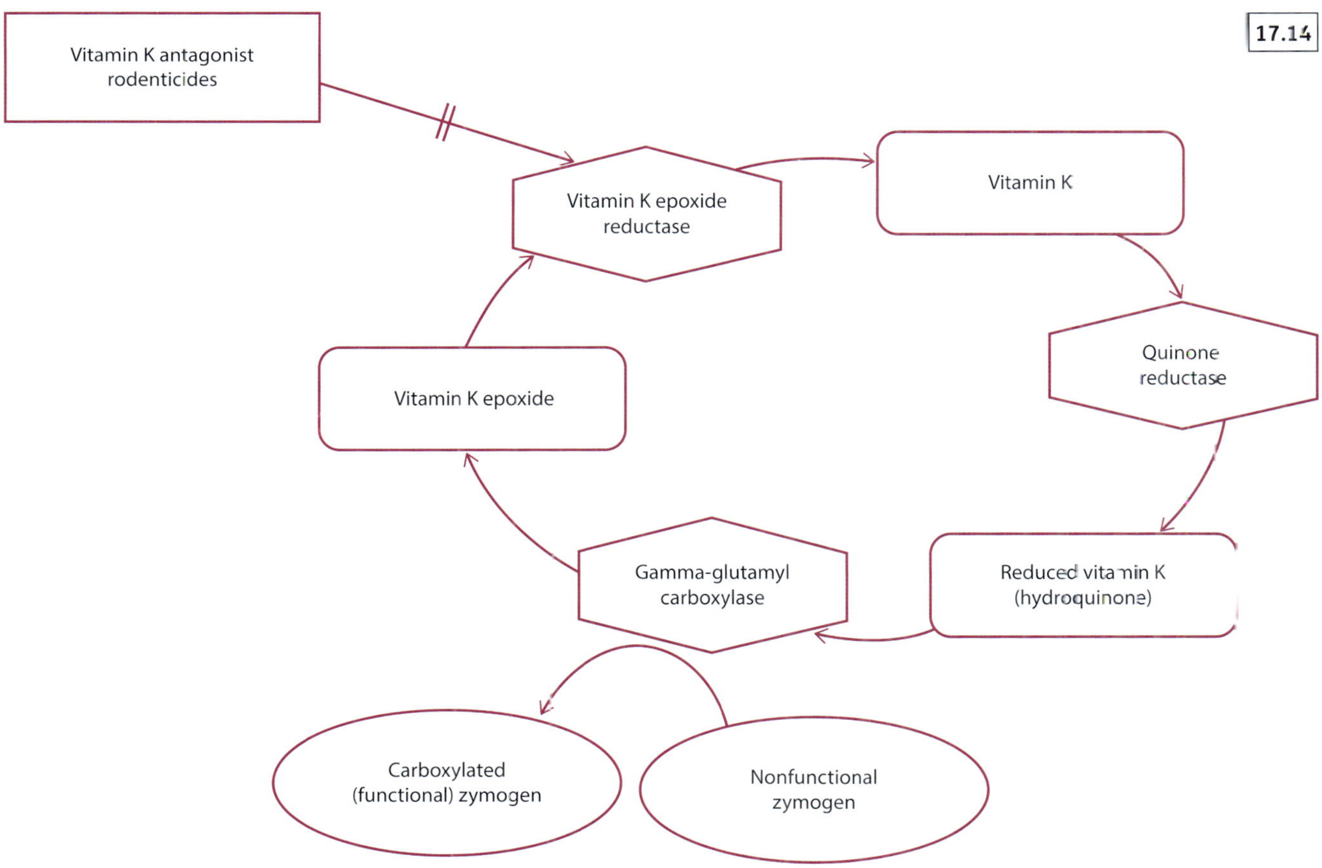

Figure 17.14 The vitamin K cycle. Arrow with two crossed lines indicates inhibition.

Clinical presentation

In the case of witnessed or suspected ingestion of anticoagulant rodenticide, patients are presented without clinical signs if evaluated within 2–3 days of ingestion. If ingestion is not suspected or treatment is not sought, patients are often presented with signs referable to the location and severity of bleeding. General signs of anemia (pallor, weakness, collapse) may be accompanied by signs such as respiratory distress, hemoptysis, abdominal distension, hematuria, vaginal bleeding, and epistaxis. Uncommon presentations such as lameness may mislead clinicians, delaying a timely diagnosis.

Differential diagnosis

Severe liver disease, DIC, iatrogenic anticoagulant overdose, congenital coagulopathy.

Diagnosis

Clinical suspicion is confirmed with prolongation of PT and PTT tests (see **Figure 17.13**). Occasionally, the clinician may note a prolonged PT prior to prolongation of PTT, reflecting the more rapid depletion of functional FVII prior to the other factors, because it has the shortest half-life of the procoagulant factors. Thrombocytopenia is commonly recognized at the time of diagnosis, and may be severe in some cases. A proteins induced by vitamin K antagonism (PIVKA) test is commercially available and will identify the nonfunctional zymogens in circulation, in many cases confirming the suspicion of exposure. False-positive results may occur with severe liver dysfunction. A positive response to therapy is also supportive of a diagnosis.

Not all rodenticides cause coagulopathy. Other rodenticides have a toxic mechanism of hypercalcemia (calciferols causing hypervitaminosis D), phosphine gas production (metal phosphides), or disruption of oxidative phosphorylation, causing irreversible neurologic damage (bromethalin). Clinicians should not assume that 'rat poison' necessarily refers to the anticoagulants and, whenever possible, the package or other information on the toxin ingested should be requested and investigated.

Management

Shortly after ingestion, gastrointestinal (GI) decontamination may be curative. Induction of emesis is recommended if ingestion is believed to have occurred within 1–2 hours of hospital presentation. Activated charcoal may be indicated to reduce absorption. Once signs of bleeding occur, GI decontamination is of no value. Actively bleeding patients should be treated with fresh frozen plasma or cryo-poor plasma (the supernatant remaining after separation of cryoprecipitate – it contains all of the factors impaired by coumarins). An initial dose of plasma of 10–20 ml/kg will halt bleeding in many patients and should be given if the patient's status is deemed critical, which is often the case if hemorrhage is present. Additional doses may be considered on the basis of persistent bleeding or persistently prolonged PT and PTT times. Definitive therapy with vitamin K1 (phytonadione) supplementation should begin as soon as possible in all cases of known or suspected exposure, but after samples have been collected for coagulation testing. The PIVKA test will not be affected by the administration of vitamin K1. Because anaphylaxis due to the cremophor excipient (polyethoxylated castor oil) found in some preparations (especially in the USA) can accompany a bolus IV injection of vitamin K1, the recommended dose of 5 mg/kg of phytonadione (vitamin K1) given by this route should not exceed a rate of 1 mg per minute. This is not a concern in countries where cremophor is not used for vitamin K injectable preparations. In less urgent situations, parenteral vitamin K1 can be given at 5 mg/kg SC using a 25-gauge needle or an oral preparation formulation can be given by mouth. The IM route of administration is contraindicated because of the excessive bleeding that can occur with this route of administration, causing hematoma and pain. Once the patient is stabilized, 3–5 mg/kg/day (given once or divided into twice daily dosing) of oral vitamin K1 supplementation should be administered, usually with a fatty treat (e.g. peanut butter, cheese), which increases vitamin K1 absorption. Normalization of clotting time tests may take up to 12–24 hours with vitamin K1 supplementation alone, so close monitoring of the bleeding patient should occur for the first day, and fresh frozen plasma should be administered as needed to control clinical signs. If the IV form is used, clotting times are normalized in 20–30 minutes. Duration of therapy needed varies with the generation of rodenticide ingested. The half-lives of coumarins range from hours to weeks. If the specific product ingested is not known, treatment should be provided for 2–4 weeks and the clotting times (PT alone is sufficient) rechecked 48–72 hours following cessation of vitamin K1 supplementation. Other specific therapies may be needed on a case-by-case basis, depending on the location of the bleeding (e.g. careful thoracocentesis in the patient with hemothorax, although this procedure is only necessary if severe dyspnea is present, since most patients will tolerate hemothorax and eventually resorb all of the blood into their circulation).

Vitamin K1 (phytonadione) is active in the production of functional clotting factors, and is the form that must be supplemented in anticoagulant rodenticide intoxication. Vitamin K2 (also sometimes called menaquinone) is the most common form found in animal products and some over-the-counter supplements. Vitamin K2 will not effectively treat anticoagulant rodenticide intoxication.

Prognosis

Prognosis following anticoagulant rodenticide ingestion is good to excellent. If the patient can be treated prior to development of bleeding, vitamin K1 supplementation is a successful antidote. Bleeding is generally controlled with a combination of transfusion with fresh frozen plasma and vitamin K1 supplementation. Bleeding into some locations may lead to life-threatening complications (e.g. intracranial hemorrhage), but this is rare.

DISORDERS OF FIBRINOLYSIS

INHERITED DISORDERS

Definition/overview

Very little has been published regarding fibrinolytic disorders in veterinary species.

Etiology

Disorders of increased fibrinolysis in people are generally caused by a deficiency or dysfunction of α_2AP, PAI-1, or FXIII, or elevated production/release of tPA or uPA. These disorders may lead to a delayed bleeding phenotype. Alternatively, a thrombotic tendency from impaired fibrinolysis may be seen in people with a deficiency or dysfunction of plasminogen, fibrinogen, or tPA, or with elevated concentrations of PAI-1 or TAFI. Reduced circulating α_2AP has been demonstrated in Greyhounds with a propensity for delayed bleeding after trauma or surgery. A heritable component is presumed, but has not yet been elucidated.

Pathophysiology

α_2AP is an important inhibitor of fibrinolysis. It interferes with the binding of plasminogen and plasmin to fibrin, preventing premature fibrin breakdown.

Clinical presentation

Patients with an inherited disorder causing hyperfibrinolysis develop a delayed bleeding phenotype. Primary and secondary hemostatic mechanisms are intact. Lack of α_2AP is associated with normal initial clot formation, with hemorrhage usually occurring 1–3 days following injury or surgery.

Differential diagnosis

Acquired disorders of primary or secondary hemostasis, DIC, liver disease, trauma, sepsis.

Diagnosis

Direct measurement of the enzymes and regulators can confirm suspicion of an inherited disorder of fibrinolysis, although testing of all components of fibrinolysis is not readily available or validated in veterinary species. Commercial assays are available to measure α_2AP, plasminogen, FXIII, and fibrinogen and these should be evaluated in a patient suspected of a disorder of fibrinolysis. Additional testing may be available at select laboratories.

Management

Antifibrinolytics such as tranexamic acid (TXA) and epsilon aminocaproic acid (EACA) have been used successfully in people with hyperfibrinolysis as well as in limited reports in animals. If a hyperfibrinolytic disorder is confirmed or strongly suspected, administration of EACA or TXA may be considered. A starting dose of 15 mg/kg IV or PO q8h of EACA for 5 days postoperatively has been shown to be beneficial in Greyhounds with fibrinolytic disorders. Dosages up to 40 mg/kg PO q8h have been reported without obvious complications. There is evidence in people that TXA may be more effective than EACA; however, in the USA, there are few FDA-approved indications for it and it can be difficult and expensive to procure for veterinarians. In people, a dose of approximately 25 mg/kg PO q6–8h is recommended during the perioperative period. Dose reduction is recommended in cases of renal insufficiency because of reduced clearance. The primary adverse side-effect of either EACA or TXA is thrombosis; therefore, these drugs should be used with extreme caution in patients with increased thrombotic risk. Antifibrinolytics are contraindicated in DIC. Fresh frozen plasma (10–20 ml/kg) will also provide a source of α_2AP and other fibrinolysis inhibitors in patients with a deficiency.

Prognosis

If identified, an inherited disorder of fibrinolysis can be managed with careful planning of surgery. Early evidence in Greyhounds suggests EACA as a promising treatment for dogs with a disorder of fibrinolysis. Although unproven, breeders should be educated on the likelihood of a genetic cause for hyperfibrinolysis in Greyhounds and appropriate preventive measures should be recommended whenever possible.

ACQUIRED FIBRINOLYTIC DISORDERS

Disorders leading to altered fibrinolysis can and do occur in veterinary species, generally as part of a complex coagulopathy seen with systemic injury and inflammation.

These will be discussed in more detail in the complex hemostatic disorders section later in the chapter.

DISORDERS ASSOCIATED WITH THROMBOSIS (HYPERCOAGULATION)

Overview

Arterial and venous thromboses are increasingly recognized as complications of various diseases in veterinary medicine. Far more has been published on thromboembolic disease in people, but it is unclear how much of this can be extrapolated to animals. The general principles of risk factors leading to thrombosis likely hold true. **Virchow's triad** refers to the three primary risk factors for the development of thrombosis: (1) abnormal blood flow; (2) endothelial injury or dysfunction; and (3) hypercoagulability. It is generally believed that the presence of two or three of these factors increases the risk of thrombosis. However, there is no evidence that the presence of only one risk factor is insufficient for inappropriate thrombus formation. Further, diagnosis of altered blood flow and endothelial injury is elusive at best, nearly impossible at worst. Much attention has, therefore, been focused on identification of hypercoagulability in an attempt to provide insight into the development of thromboembolic complications. There is strong evidence in people that the development of venous and arterial thrombi is somewhat different and each is associated with different diseases.

VENOUS THROMBOTIC DISORDERS

Definition/overview

The occurrence of a blood clot (thrombus) that develops within a vein in the absence of injury is referred to as venous thrombosis. Thromboembolism refers to a vessel obstructed by all or part of a thrombus that developed at another site in the circulation and became dislodged.

Etiology

Pathologic processes can overwhelm the normal balance of hemostasis and excessive thrombin formation may occur.

Pathophysiology

Development *in situ* of a thrombus frequently occurs at sites associated with vascular damage or increased blood turbulence or stasis. Factors promoting hypercoagulability include circulating TF expressed on microparticles or monocytes associated with many neoplasms, depletion of normal anticoagulant mechanisms (AT loss in protein-losing nephropathy or enteropathy), and probably many pathways that have not yet been elucidated. Inflammatory conditions are frequently associated with hypercoagulability; the reciprocal activation of the hemostatic and inflammatory systems is now well recognized. Many diseases have been associated with thrombosis in veterinary species (**Table 17.2**). Insertion of IV catheters can also increase the risk of thromboembolic disease; careful consideration of catheter location and size should include these risks. Removal of catheters that are no longer needed, dysfunctional, or associated with thrombophlebitis (**Figure 17.15**) should be prompt.

In people, pulmonary embolism has a clear association with deep vein thrombosis (DVT), making it a primarily venous disorder. Given the rarity of DVT in dogs and cats, it is as yet unclear in veterinary species if the same is true or if pulmonary thrombi develop *in situ* (**Figures 17.16, 17.17**). Many of the diseases associated with pulmonary embolism in dogs are also associated with venous thrombosis in other sites, suggesting a similar pathogenesis to that seen in people.

Table 17.2 Selected diseases associated with thrombosis in people and animals.

People	Dogs and/or Cats
Surgery	Atrial fibrillation
Trauma	(Hypertrophic) cardiomyopathy
Immobility	Hypothyroidism
Cancer	Protein-losing nephropathy
Chemotherapy and/or radiation therapy	Trauma
Venous compression	Hyperadrenocorticism
Increasing age	Cancer
Inflammatory bowel disease	Diabetes mellitus
Nephrotic syndrome	Infective endocarditis
Obesity	Immune-mediated hemolytic anemia
Central venous catheterization	Sepsis
Cardiac disease	

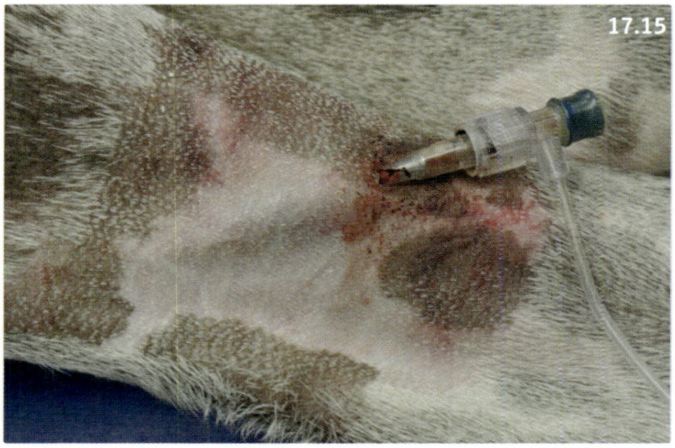

Figure 17.15 Thrombosis associated with an intravenous catheter. Note the swelling associated with the vein just proximal to the catheter insertion site.

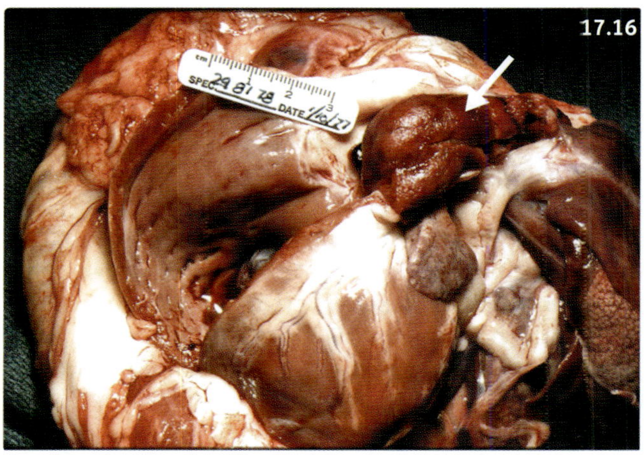

Figure 17.16 Large pulmonary artery thrombus (arrow) in a dog with glomerular nephropathy secondary to amyloidosis. (Courtesy M. Schaer)

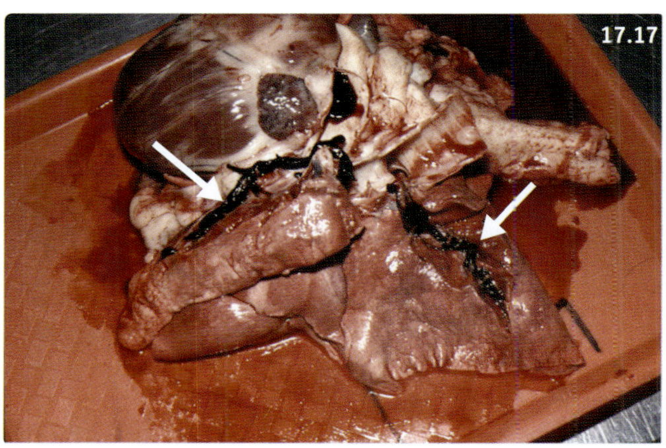

Figure 17.17 Multiple pulmonary thromboses (arrows) in a dog with immune-mediated hemolytic anemia. (Courtesy M. Schaer)

Clinical presentation

Many thrombi are clinically silent and only recognized on postmortem examination. If clinical signs develop, they are generally referable to the location of the thrombus. Severe signs may include respiratory distress, cardiovascular collapse, regional edema, abdominal pain, ascites, and lameness (**Figures 17.18–17.20**).

Differential diagnosis

Differential diagnoses will be variable depending on the location of the thrombus. When pulmonary thromboembolism (PTE) is suspected, other pulmonary diseases must be ruled out, including pneumonia, heartworm disease, pulmonary hypertension, and cardiogenic pulmonary edema.

Diagnosis

Antemortem diagnosis may be difficult in some cases, but various imaging modalities are often needed to confirm the presence of a thrombus. Abdominal ultrasound can be helpful for detecting portal and splenic vein thrombosis as well as caval thrombosis. Pulmonary thromboemboli can be challenging to identify, but CT is often helpful. Thoracic radiographs are frequently inconclusive for confirming PTE, although a large thrombus can cause a grossly enlarged pulmonary artery. Echocardiography is often helpful for identifying evidence of pulmonary hypertension or primary cardiac disease. Coagulation testing may add supportive evidence for the presence of thromboembolic disease, but is not definitive. Elevated D-dimer concentration or hypercoagulability seen on viscoelastic coagulation tests can increase suspicion.

Management

Control of the underlying disease process is crucial for managing thromboembolic complications. When a disease with known thromboembolic risk is identified, thromboprophylaxis warrants consideration. Protocols have not been established in veterinary medicine; however, when venous thrombosis predominates, therapies directed at coagulation may be preferable. UH or low-molecular-weight heparin (LMWH) may be considered for in-hospital or at-home use (**Table 17.3**). Ideally, therapy should be adjusted based on the results of anti-FXa activity, which is a commercially available assay that measures the amount of inhibition caused by either UH or LMWH. For treatment of thromboembolic disease, a more aggressive strategy may be needed. A combination of either UH or LMWH and antiplatelet therapy may be considered. Newer drugs are continuously being developed, and several oral anticoagulants have recently become available for use in people. Safety and efficacy are not

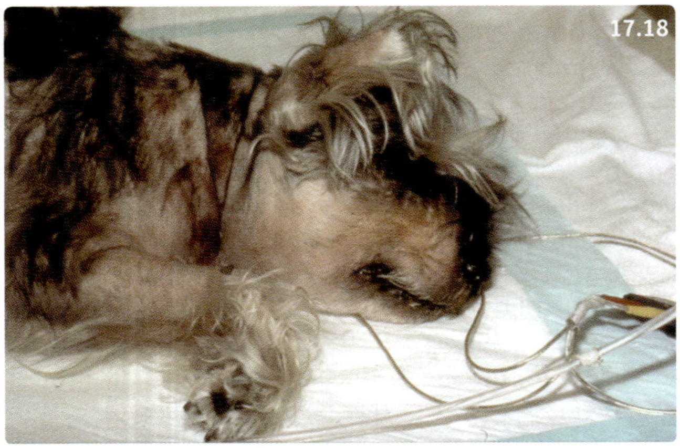

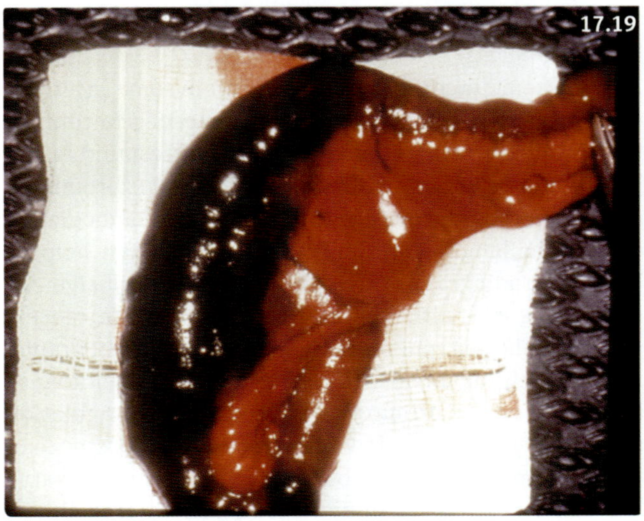

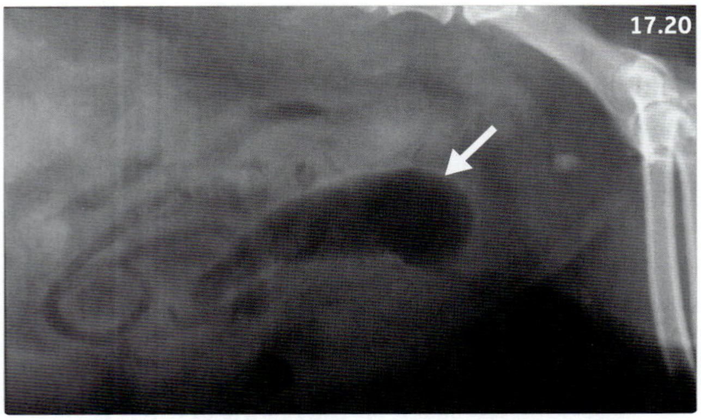

Figures 17.18–17.20 Dog with anterior vena caval thrombosis secondary to disseminated intravascular coagulation. (17.18) Head and neck swelling. Note the concurrent ecchymotic hemorrhages over the neck. (17.19) Area of ischemic bowel found at postmortem examination. (17.20) Lateral abdominal radiograph showing severe dilation of the jejunal segment in the ventral abdomen (arrow), which was attributed to intestinal infarction secondary to disseminated intravascular coagulation. (Courtesy M. Schaer)

yet known in veterinary species, but these new drugs may offer a promising alternative to frequent daily injections. In some cases, surgical thrombectomy may be an option, but requires specialized surgical training and facilities. Additionally, depending on the location (main pulmonary artery), surgery might be a severe risk to the patient. Antifibrinolytics are occasionally considered, but carry significant risk of bleeding when used systemically and have not yielded positive results in the few published reports in the veterinary literature. Antifibrinolytics remain the standard of care in people with acute thromboembolic disease. Lack of efficacy in dogs and cats may be related to inappropriate dosing or administration or significant delays between occurrence and treatment.

Because blood coagulation represents only one-third of the components contributing to thrombosis, other strategies can and should be employed to prevent thrombosis beyond drug therapy. Whenever possible, controlled exercise should be encouraged in hospitalized veterinary patients. Even several short walks a day for patients that are able to could make a big difference in preventing thrombosis. Additionally, passive range of motion exercises and massage can stimulate blood flow in patients that cannot walk frequently or at all. In general, the importance of encouraging even small amounts of activity in patients that can tolerate it should not be underestimated. This may be used alone or as an adjunct to the pharmacologic interventions discussed above.

Prognosis

Outcome following development of thromboembolic complications can vary widely, but may be devastating in some cases, making thromboprophylaxis an attractive strategy to employ while the predisposing disease is being treated or managed. Studies in people suggest a significant benefit when thromboprophylaxis is employed in patients with known risk factors. It is not yet clear if this is also true in veterinary patients. Early evidence evaluating clot prevention strategies in dogs with immune-mediated hemolytic anemia shows potential, but further studies are needed to determine true efficacy and the best treatment practices.

ARTERIAL THROMBOTIC DISORDERS

Definition/overview

Most arterial thromboses of dogs and cats occur in the distal aorta (**Figures 17.21**, **17.22**), although there have been a few reports of thrombi identified at other locations.

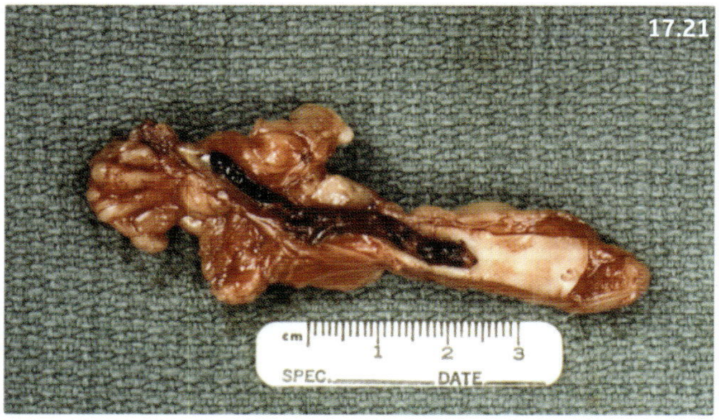

Figure 17.21 Distal aortic ('saddle') thrombus in a cat with hypertrophic cardiomyopathy. (Courtesy M. Schaer)

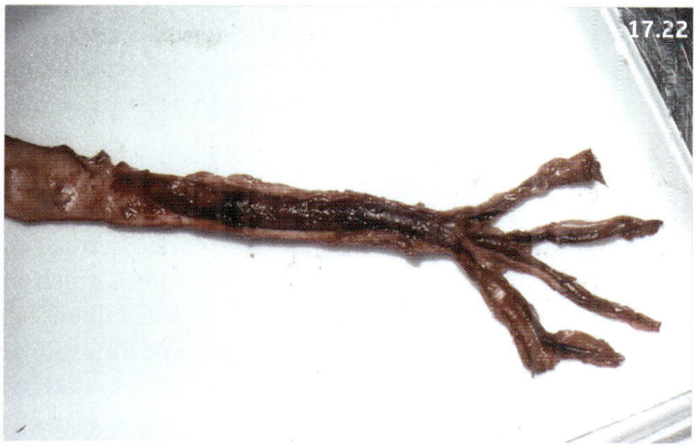

Figure 17.22 Distal aortic ('saddle') thrombus in a dog. The underlying cause was not identified. (Courtesy M. Schaer)

Etiology

In cats, there is a clear association with hypertrophic cardiomyopathy (HCM), but arterial thrombosis has also been associated with other forms of cardiomyopathy, hyperthyroidism, and cancer. In dogs, the comorbidities identified with aortic thromboembolism are more varied, and include hypothyroidism, protein-losing nephropathy, hyperadrenocorticism, neoplasia, and diabetes mellitus. Hypothyroidism and protein-losing nephropathy are the most frequently reported comorbidities.

Pathophysiology

It is generally accepted in cats that HCM predisposes to development of thrombus formation in the left atrium, which then embolizes to the distal aorta or, less frequently, a brachial artery, causing hindlimb or forelimb dysfunction, respectively. In dogs, the development is less clear, and it is unknown whether *in-situ* thrombus formation versus embolus from a distant site occurs.

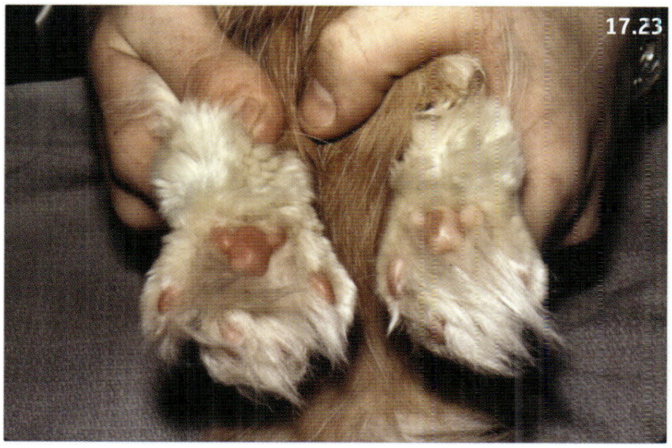

Figure 17.23 Paw pads from a cat with aortic thromboembolism. Note the difference in color between the pads, the pad on the right showing acrocyanosis compared with the pad on the left. (Courtesy M. Schaer)

Clinical presentation

In cats, once the embolus becomes occlusive, clinical signs rapidly become evident and often include severe paresis or paralysis of the affected limb(s), often with accompanying pain. Hypothermia and tachycardia or bradycardia are also frequently present. Around two-thirds of cats have concurrent tachypnea or respiratory distress. As many as one-third of cats will have no abnormalities detected on cardiac auscultation. Absent femoral and pedal pulse with cool foot pads of the affected limb(s) is commonly observed (**Figure 17.23**). Dogs frequently have a more insidious onset, sometimes with a long history (months) of lameness in the affected limb. Absent or weak pulses in the affected limb are common. The term 'intermittent claudication' is used if the signs are associated with temporary vascular occlusion or vasospasm associated with a small thrombus that causes partial obstruction.

Differential diagnosis

Spinal cord disease, neuromuscular disease, orthopedic disease.

Diagnosis

In cats, a diagnosis of arterial thromboembolism is frequently made based on results of physical examination and a few clinical tests confirming absence of blood flow to the affected limb(s). Echocardiography frequently confirms the presence of cardiomyopathy. Results of blood work may be variable, but aspartate aminotransferase and creatine kinase are typically elevated, although not specific for thromboembolism. In dogs, presence of an aortic thrombus is generally confirmed with ultrasound or CT.

Management

Treatment of the underlying disease concurrent with therapy directed at reducing embolus/thrombus size or preventing further thrombus formation is recommended. The available evidence suggests that systemic fibrinolytic therapy in cats is generally unsuccessful, but study designs have not been maximized for success. Surgical or transarterial thrombectomy methods may be more successful, but further evaluation of these more invasive techniques is needed. Most commonly, clinicians aim to prevent further clot development while the natural process of fibrinolysis dissolves the clot. A combination of anticoagulation with heparin and antiplatelet therapy may be warranted in these cats (**Table 17.3**). Bleeding is an uncommon complication of anticoagulant and antiplatelet therapy. Some evidence in cats suggests clopidogrel to be superior to aspirin in cats with thromboembolic disease. Clopidogrel and aspirin are synergistic in people, and combination therapy may be beneficial in veterinary species as well. Concurrent management of heart failure is frequently needed. Pain relief is also important in cats with thromboembolism. Similar treatment protocols are appropriate for dogs with arterial thromboembolism. A combination of UH or LMWH with one or more antiplatelet drugs is recommended for most cases.

Prognosis

Prognosis for cats with aortic thromboembolism is guarded to poor. Around two-thirds of cats do not survive the initial insult, and there is a high rate of re-embolization. Reperfusion tissue injury can be a potentially devastating complication. Long-term survival reportedly ranges from a few weeks to a little over a year. For dogs, the prognosis may depend on the underlying disease and success of treatment. For diseases that can be reversed or controlled, signs associated with thromboembolic disease can be successfully reversed as well.

COMPLEX HEMOSTATIC DISORDERS

DISSEMINATED INTRAVASCULAR COAGULATION

Definition/overview

DIC is a syndrome characterized by systemic intravascular activation of coagulation within the circulation.

Etiology

DIC is always secondary to an underlying disease process. It has been difficult to describe, but in recent years its pathogenesis has become better understood. Virtually

Table 17.3 Commonly used antithrombotic drugs.

Drug	Mechanism of action	Dose recommendation	Comments
Unfractionated heparin	Thrombin, FXa inhibition	600–900 units/kg/day, starting dose	Can be given as a CRI or divided into daily subcutaneous doses q8h; dose should be adjusted as needed
Dalteparin	FXa inhibition	Dog: 150 units/kg SC q8h Cat: 100 units/kg SC q4h *For feline ATE: 100 units/kg SC q12–24h	The half-life of dalteparin is much shorter in cats, limiting its usefulness in this species; a reduced frequency may be of benefit in cats with ATE
Enoxaparin	FXa inhibition	Dog: 0.8 mg/kg SC q6h Cat: 1.5 mg/kg SC q6h	Further studies are needed to ensure adequate dosing in dogs and cats
Warfarin	Vitamin K1 antagonism	Dog: 0.22 mg/kg PO q12h Cat: 0.1–0.2 mg/kg PO q24h	Starting dose recommendations for both dogs and cats; treatment must be carefully monitored and dosing adjusted accordingly
Aspirin	Cyclo-oxygenase inhibition	Dog: 1 mg/kg PO q24h Cat: 1 mg/kg PO q72h	Studies in dogs have shown that very low-dose aspirin may be safely combined with prednisone usage
Clopidogrel	ADP-receptor antagonist	Dog: 2–4 mg/kg PO q24h Cat: 18.75 mg per cat q24h	Dosage in dogs is extrapolated and efficacy studies are still needed

FXa, activated factor X; CRI, constant rate infusion; ATE, arterial thromboembolism; ADP, adenosine diphosphate.

any systemic inflammatory disease could lead to the development of DIC. Some examples include sepsis, severe trauma, pancreatitis, neoplasia, hepatic failure, as well as some toxins and envenomations.

Snake venom composition can vary significantly between species (and even within species), but many snake venoms do contain molecules that can alter hemostasis, and they are referred to as hemostatins. Whether a venom component inhibits or activates coagulation depends on the molecule in question. Because of the variety of hemostatins found in different snake venoms, the coagulopathy that occurs from snakebites can also vary widely. Veterinarians are encouraged to become familiar with the species of venomous snakes in their region and learn what, if any, hemostatic alterations should be expected and how they should be managed.

Pathophysiology

DIC is characterized by simultaneous thrombin generation and depression of inhibitory mechanisms, such as AT and the protein C system. This leads to widespread fibrin deposition, potentially obstructing the microvasculature and causing ischemia and, ultimately, organ failure. Later in the syndrome, the massive consumption of platelets and clotting factors can lead to hemorrhage (**Figure 17.24**). Impaired fibrinolysis also contributes to an enhanced intravascular fibrin deposition in most cases. Some patients with DIC have simultaneous bleeding and thrombosis, making it a complex clinical challenge (see **Figures 17.18–17.20**, **Figure 17.25**).

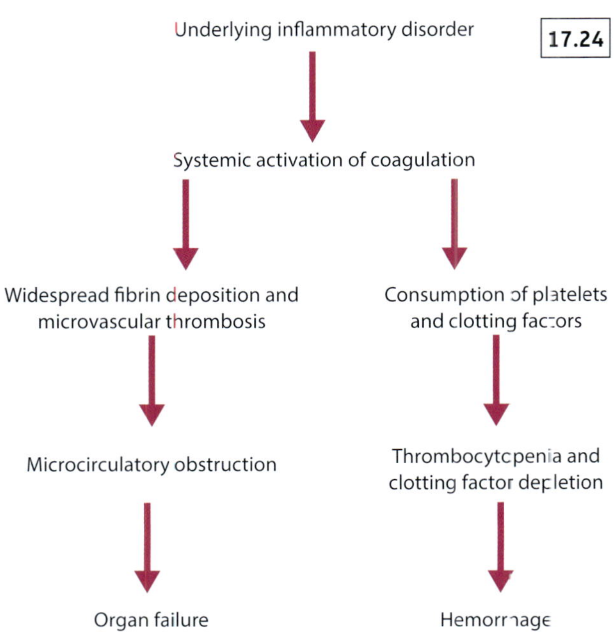

Figure 17.24 The pathways and clinical picture associated with disseminated intravascular coagulation.

Clinical presentation

Most patients with DIC will not have obvious signs of bleeding until late in the syndrome. In the early prothrombotic phase, organ failure unrelated to the causative disease process may develop, such as acute kidney injury, acute onset of respiratory distress, hepatic dysfunction, or neurologic deficits. Concomitant with organ dysfunction is often evidence of consumption of platelets and clotting factors that late in the syndrome may be seen as petechiae, excessive bleeding from venepuncture or catheter sites, or overt spontaneous hemorrhage, particularly from mucosal sites.

Differential diagnosis

Coagulopathy of liver disease, coagulopathy of trauma, multiple organ dysfunction syndrome.

Diagnosis

A number of algorithms have been published for a diagnosis of DIC in people, but no universally accepted schema yet exists for veterinary patients. The first criterion that must be met for a diagnosis of DIC is the presence of a disease capable of inducing the condition. This circular definition is a large part of why DIC has been so confusing and elusive. Broadly, any disease causing a widespread inflammatory response might be capable of inducing DIC. Several diagnostic tests are recommended to aid in the identification of DIC, most commonly the presence of two or more of thrombocytopenia, prolonged clotting times

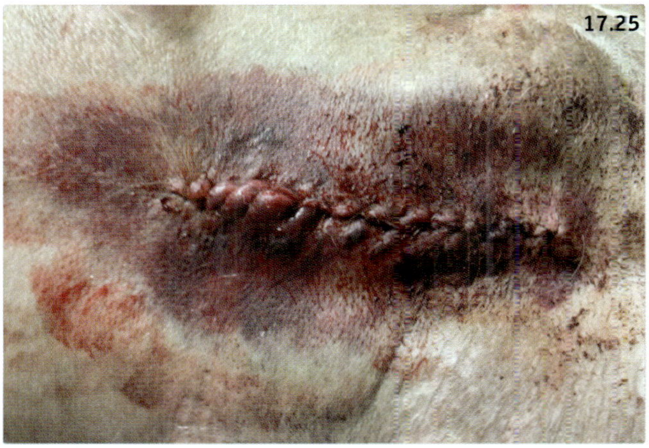

Figure 17.25 Postoperative bleeding and excessive bruising in a dog with disseminated intravascular coagulation.

(PT, PTT, activated clotting time), elevated D-dimer or FDP concentration, or hypofibrinogenemia. Other markers may include schistocytosis or a reduction of the natural anticoagulants (AT or protein C). A significant decline in platelet count and/or fibrinogen concentration, even in the absence of overt thrombocytopenia or hypofibrinogenemia, may be an early marker of DIC in patients with a predisposing condition.

Patients with complex hemostatic disorders should generally not be treated on the basis of laboratory results alone. Traditional tests of coagulation are poor predictors for risk of bleeding and thrombosis.

Management

The only true successful strategy for treating DIC is control and reversal of the causative disease. Management of the complications may be needed in some cases. Once signs of active hemorrhage have occurred, transfusion of blood products is appropriate. Fresh frozen plasma (10–20 ml/kg) should be given to correct bleeding caused by consumption of clotting factors. RBCs should be provided as needed in anemic patients to support perfusion and oxygenation. Transfusion of platelet-containing products is rarely needed, but may help reduce bleeding in patients with severe thrombocytopenia (<20,000 platelets/µl). In patients that are not actively bleeding, but in which an invasive procedure is unavoidable, correction of prolonged clotting times is warranted. If surgery or other invasive procedure is not necessary, however, transfusion of blood products to correct laboratory coagulation abnormalities is neither warranted nor recommended. Antifibrinolytic drugs are typically contraindicated in patients with DIC, even those with active bleeding, although this may be somewhat controversial. In the early, nonhemorrhagic stage of DIC when thrombosis predominates, antithrombotic therapy may be considered. If thromboembolism is documented, aggressive anticoagulation strategies are warranted (**Table 17.3**).

Prognosis

Although DIC has traditionally been associated with a hopeless prognosis, improved understanding of the pathogenesis can allow early detection and aggressive supportive care. The prognosis when overt DIC develops should be considered guarded to poor, but when treatment for DIC is provided in parallel with definitive treatment of the underlying disease, favorable outcomes are often achieved.

SEPSIS

Definition/overview

It is well established that sepsis in people is associated with a prothrombotic state. Degree of coagulopathy is an independent predictor of mortality in people with severe sepsis and septic shock.

Etiology

Sepsis is defined as bacterial infection with systemic signs of inflammation. Severe sepsis reflects septic patients with evidence of organ dysfunction, and septic shock refers to septic patients with refractory hypotension. All septic patients have some degree of coagulation derangements, ranging from subclinical to overt DIC (see above).

Pathophysiology

Many mechanisms emerge in the inflammatory process to lead to a prothrombotic state in sepsis. Cytokine-mediated cross talk between the inflammatory and hemostatic systems is well documented. The most important of these effects in sepsis include early and inappropriate activation of the TF–FVIIa pathway leading to initiation of thrombin formation, as well as extensive platelet activation. At the same time, endogenous anticoagulant pathways are impaired, specifically AT and protein C activities. These processes combine to generate an environment that fosters development of the micro- and macrothrombosis that contributes to multiple organ dysfunction and failure.

Clinical presentation

Most of the signs of thrombosis in sepsis will be clinically inapparent, especially to the clinician who is not looking for them. All patients diagnosed with sepsis should be presumed to have some degree of coagulation derangement. Patients that have progressed to a severe consumptive coagulopathy may present with signs of hemorrhage.

Differential diagnosis

DIC, coagulopathy of liver failure.

Diagnosis

Regular (every 1–2 days) evaluation of coagulation is recommended for patients with severe sepsis or septic shock to determine the degree of derangement present. At a minimum, this should include a platelet count and some evaluation of the coagulation system (PT, PTT, activated clotting time, thrombin time). Ideally, it would also include evaluation of fibrinogen concentration, AT and/or protein C concentration, D-dimer or FDP measurement, and viscoelastic testing (thromboelastography, thromboelastometry, or sonoclot). Early recognition of alterations may help guide supportive therapy or provide an indication of disease progression.

Management

Approaches to avoid morbidity associated with coagulopathy in human septic patients have been disappointing. Provision of recombinant activated protein C was a promising therapy that ultimately has been unsuccessful in improving outcomes for people with severe sepsis or septic shock. Some experimental data suggest a benefit of heparin therapy; however, this has not yet been substantiated by clinical trials. Septic patients with overt thrombosis should be treated as described for other causes of thrombosis (**Table 17.3**); however, the risk of bleeding complications may be higher in this population. Nonpharmacologic measures to reduce the risk of thrombosis should be considered and employed whenever possible. Early ambulation in the postoperative period may reduce the risk of venous stasis; when this is not possible, tissue massage and passive range of motion should be contemplated. Patients with hemorrhagic tendencies may need fresh frozen plasma or platelet transfusions, especially if invasive procedures are necessary.

Prognosis

Severe sepsis and septic shock are associated with a high mortality rate in people and companion animals. Coagulopathies can significantly contribute to poor outcomes. Aggressive treatment of the source of the sepsis combined with supportive care is still the best approach to achieving satisfactory results.

LIVER DISEASE

Definition/overview

Coagulation abnormalities are common in dogs and cats with acute and chronic liver disease and can lead to both hemorrhagic and prothrombotic tendencies.

Etiology

Any disease that reduces the functional capacity of the liver may have an effect on primary hemostasis, secondary hemostasis, and fibrinolysis. Toxic, infectious, congenital, and neoplastic diseases have all been associated with hemostatic derangements in veterinary patients.

Pathophysiology

The liver is directly and indirectly involved in the regulation of all phases of hemostasis. Thrombocytopenia and thrombocytopathia are both recognized in dogs and cats with liver disease, although the exact mechanisms are unknown. Reduced hepatic thrombopoietin production occurs in people, and may occur in animals with liver disease as well. The liver produces all of the pro- and anticoagulant proteins needed for secondary hemostasis, and the diseased liver often has reduced capacity for this. Similarly, most of the pro- and antifibrinolytic proteins are produced in the liver. The final balance of hemostasis in a patient with liver disease may rest anywhere on the coagulation spectrum, resulting either in clinical bleeding, thrombosis, both, or neither. In addition, alterations in portal blood flow may promote venous stasis and thrombosis.

Clinical presentation

Despite frequent abnormalities in coagulation testing results for patients with liver disease, spontaneous bleeding is rarely reported in dogs and cats (or people) with even severe liver disease. Some exceptions include severe, acute hepatotoxicity, as may be seen with aflatoxicosis or amanita toxicity. In people with advanced liver failure (as with cirrhosis), prothrombotic tendencies predominate. An individual patient may develop a variety of clinical signs ranging from petechiae and GI bleeding to respiratory distress or abdominal pain and ascites from PTE or portal vein thrombosis, respectively.

Differential diagnosis

DIC.

Diagnosis

Traditional tests of coagulation are inadequate for thoroughly evaluating hemostatic abnormalities in patients with hepatic dysfunction. PT and PTT results do not reliably predict bleeding episodes, probably because they do not account for likely reductions in the natural anticoagulants AT and protein C, among others. Thromboelastography (**Figure 17.26**) and other viscoelastic testing modalities have shown promise for providing a more global assessment of coagulation and have been used successfully for this purpose in people. In particular, thromboelastography may have a role in identifying patients with hyperfibrinolysis, as sensitive and specific tests for fibrinolysis are not readily available.

Management

It is important for clinicians to remember that correction of laboratory abnormalities is not the goal of treatment for patients with coagulopathy associated with liver disease. As with DIC, treatment should be aimed at correcting clinical abnormalities. Transfusion of blood products

17.26

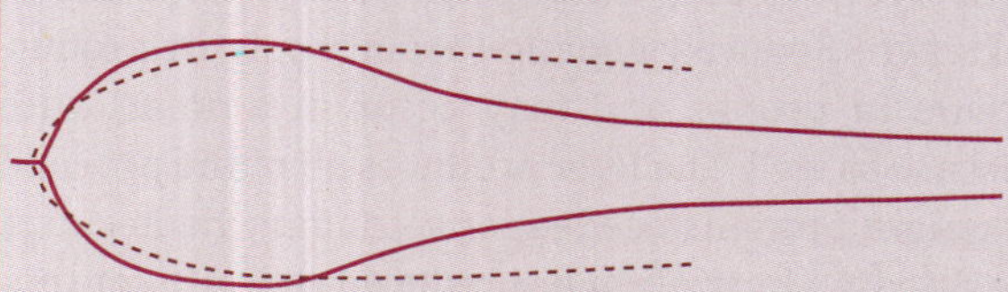

R	K	Angle	MA	G	LY30	LY60	A	PMA	CI
min	min	deg	mm	d/sc	%	%	mm	0.0	
4.2	2.4	59.0	49.6	4.9K	12.5	35.2	11.8		
3–9	2–8	27–59	39–59	3.2K–7.2K	0–2	0–8			

Figure 17.26 Thromboelastography tracing of a dog with hyperfibrinolysis secondary to acute liver failure (solid line). Note how the tracing regresses back to baseline after initial divergence. Compare this with a normal tracing (dashed line) in which the tracing does not return to baseline.

is warranted in patients that are actively bleeding, while antithrombotics are appropriate for patients with evidence of thrombosis. Fresh frozen plasma (10–20 ml/kg) may be used to halt significant bleeding. Component therapy should be considered where available (e.g. cryoprecipitate rather than fresh whole blood or fresh frozen plasma for patients with severe hypofibrinogenemia). Heparin and/or antiplatelet drugs should be initiated in patients with thrombosis (**Table 17.3**). The effect of UH might be compromised in the absence of AT production by the diseased liver, but this is not a concern when using LMWH products. The value of antifibrinolytic drugs in people with liver disease is still uncertain and has not been evaluated in veterinary patients. It might be considered if a hyperfibrinolytic state was the suspected cause of bleeding or invasive procedures are needed. EACA (15 mg/kg IV or PO q8h) may be given in the perioperative period.

Prognosis

Patients with a reversible acute or chronic liver disease often do very well, even if hemostatic derangements have developed. Patients with irreversible liver disease that progress to developing clinically significant hemostatic abnormalities, including chronic DIC, carry a guarded to poor prognosis.

TRAUMA

Definition/overview

Coagulopathy of trauma (CoT; also called acute coagulopathy of trauma, traumatic coagulopathy, and trauma-induced coagulopathy) is a recently recognized phenomenon in which hemostatic derangements contribute to the secondary injury in patients with severe blunt and penetrating trauma.

Etiology

Hypocoagulability and hyperfibrinolysis are the hallmark features of CoT; however, the exact mechanisms by which these occur have not yet been clearly elucidated. Several theories have been proposed, ranging from CoT being a variation of DIC to a physiologic 'overreaction' to endothelial damage promoting anticoagulant and profibrinolytic activity to counteract the prothrombotic state induced by traumatic inflammation.

Pathophysiology

It is generally agreed that at least two key factors combine to initiate CoT. Tissue injury and tissue hypoperfusion lead to hypocoagulation and hyperfibrinolysis, probably via endothelial damage and increased exposure to thrombomodulin, which combines with thrombin to activate protein C, a potent endogenous anticoagulant and indirect promoter of fibrinolysis. Additional features of CoT have been proposed and debated, and include systemic inflammation, hypothermia, and metabolic acidosis. After initiation of classic resuscitative strategies, hemodilution and dilution of clotting factors may also contribute to CoT, although some pretreatment hemodilution occurs from extracellular fluid shifting.

Clinical presentation

It can be difficult for the clinician to distinguish ongoing hemorrhage from direct trauma/laceration of blood vessels and the possible development of CoT. Of course, persistent oozing or bleeding despite adequate mechanical hemostasis (i.e. ligation) or bleeding at sites distant from the trauma, including IV catheter sites, might increase the suspicion of CoT and motivate clinicians to perform diagnostic tests.

Differential diagnoses

DIC, pre-existing coagulopathies.

Diagnosis

Evidence of hypocoagulability and hyperfibrinolysis is supportive of a diagnosis of CoT, although accepted testing protocols are lacking in human and veterinary medicine. Prolongations of PT and/or PTT >1.5 times the mean of the reference interval are consistent with a diagnosis of CoT. This does not account for the dynamic nature of CoT, nor does it allow for assessment of fibrinolysis. Thromboelastography or other viscoelastic tests are likely better suited for CoT evaluation. Hypocoagulable thromboelastography tracings offer support of a diagnosis of CoT, and evidence of hyperfibrinolysis will add valuable information to the overall picture.

Thromboelastography evaluates blood clot parameters in whole blood. The classic tracing consists of an initial divergence that reflects initiation of clot formation, followed by the speed of clot development. The width of the tracing reflects overall strength of the final clot. During fibrinolysis, the tracing returns to baseline (**Figure 17.26**).

Management

Treatment recommendations continue to change as new studies emerge. Current therapy involves treating the clinical signs of hemorrhage with blood products as dictated by results of coagulation testing (e.g. transfusion of fresh frozen plasma for ongoing hemorrhage and prolonged clotting times). Tranexamic acid therapy has shown great promise for reducing mortality in human patients suffering from severe trauma, but benefit is lost if it is not given within 3 hours of the trauma. Whether this can be extrapolated to veterinary patients is unclear, and safety and efficacy studies are needed.

Prognosis

Overall survival rates for dogs and cats (~70–90% survival) that are presented to veterinary hospitals following trauma are quite good, although evidence suggests the presence of CoT is associated with worse outcomes. Aggressive treatment to stop ongoing hemorrhage and vigilant monitoring of hemostasis may allow for better provision of timely supportive care.

RECOMMENDED FURTHER READING

Brooks MB, Catalfamo JL (2013) Current diagnostic trends in coagulation disorders among dogs and cats. *Vet Clin North Am Small Anim Pract* **43**:1349–1372.

Glas-Greenwalt P (1996) *Fibrinolysis in Disease: Molecular and Hemovascular Aspects of Fibrinolysis*. CRC Press, Boca Raton.

Kavanagh C, Shaw S, Webster C (2011) Coagulation in hepatobiliary disease. *J Vet Emerg Crit Care* **21**:589–604.

Marder VJ, Aird WC, Bennett JS *et al.* (2013) (eds) *Hemostasis and Thrombosis*, 6th edn. Lippincott Williams & Wilkins, Philadelphia.

McMichael M (2005) Primary hemostasis. *J Vet Emerg Crit Care* **15**:1–8.

Mousa SA (2010) *Anticoagulants, Antiplatelets, and Thrombolytics*, 2nd edn. Humana Press, New York.

Michelson AD (2013) *Platelets*, 3rd edn. Elsevier, London.

Palmer L, Martin L (2014) Traumatic coagulopathy. Part 1: Pathophysiology and diagnosis. *J Vet Emerg Crit Care* **24**:63–74.

Palmer L, Martin L (2014) Traumatic coagulopathy. Part 2: Resuscitative strategies. *J Vet Emerg Crit Care* **24**:75–92.

Smith SA (2009) The cell-based model of coagulation. *J Vet Emerg Crit Care* **19**:3–10.

Chapter 18

Dermatologic disorders

Diane T. Lewis

INTRODUCTION

History

A careful history and complete physical examination of the patient are essential. It is important to establish the age at onset, region of the body first affected, earliest symptoms, and progression of the disease, how the disease has changed, initial seasonality, and how pruritus correlates with the presence or resolution of lesions. Flea bite hypersensitivity often begins in the caudal trunk and hindlimb regions and may progress to involve the entire body. Pruritus associated with allergies may decrease when the patient is treated with appropriate antibiotics for a staphylococcal folliculitis or appropriate antifungals for *Malassezia* dermatitis. Autoimmune diseases usually involve the face, with variable involvement of the trunk or extremities, while staphylococcal folliculitis may be limited to the trunk. Miliary dermatitis in cats may begin as a localized or generalized disease.

Because certain diseases have a heritable basis, note should be made of the breed. Some diseases are more common in young animals (e.g. food or flea allergy, demodicosis, dermatophytosis) while others are more common in middle aged to older animals (e.g. endocrinopathies, neoplasia). The habitat of the animal should be noted. Is it likely that fleas or other ectoparasites will survive in the environment? What is the status of coexistent pets in the household? Are people in the household affected?

Response to previous treatment is useful in attempting to define the list of differential diagnoses only when therapy has been used at appropriate dosages, for proper time periods, and not used simultaneously with other drugs or treatments.

Examination

The skin should be examined in a systematic fashion. The degree and distribution of pruritus and the nature and distribution of primary lesions and those secondary lesions that are diagnostically significant (**Figures 18.1–18.18**) should be assessed.

All mucous membranes, oral cavity, eyelids, eyes, mouth, lip margins, nasal planum, lymph nodes, the inguinal and axillary areas, the interdigital spaces, the claws and clawbeds, the footpads (**Figure 18.19**), the perineum, and the ear canals should be inspected.

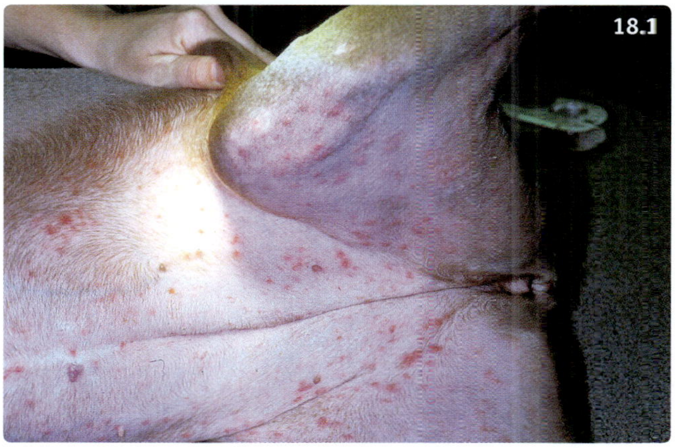

Figure 18.1 Classification of dermatologic lesions. Papule.

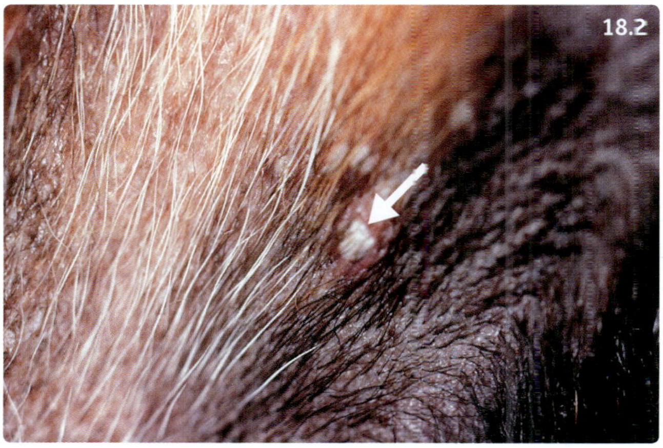

Figure 18.2 Classification of dermatologic lesions. Pustule (arrow).

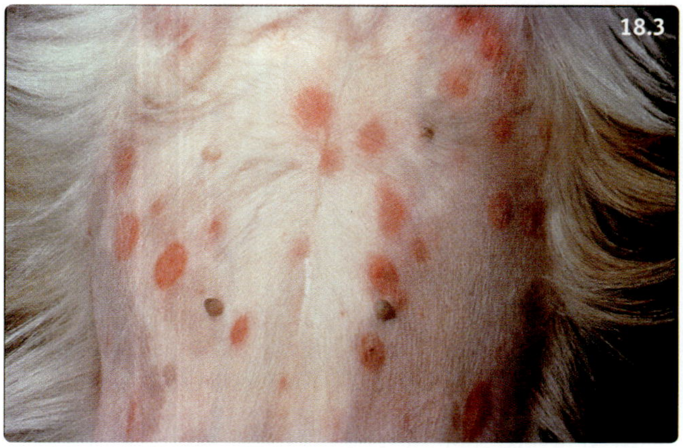

Figure 18.3 Classification of dermatologic lesions. Macule.

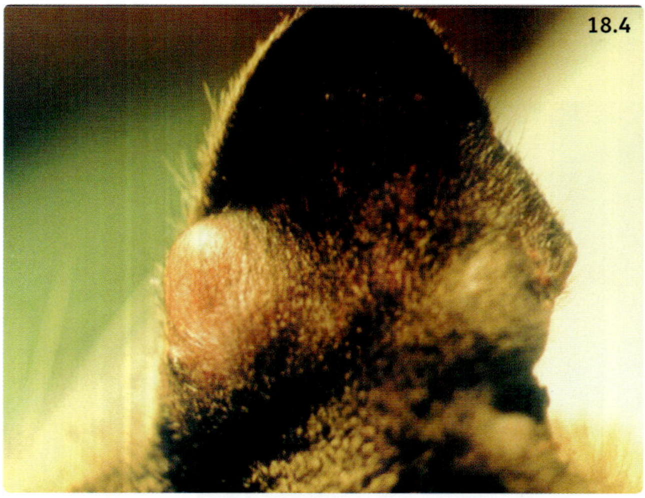

Figure 18.4 Classification of dermatologic lesions. Nodule.

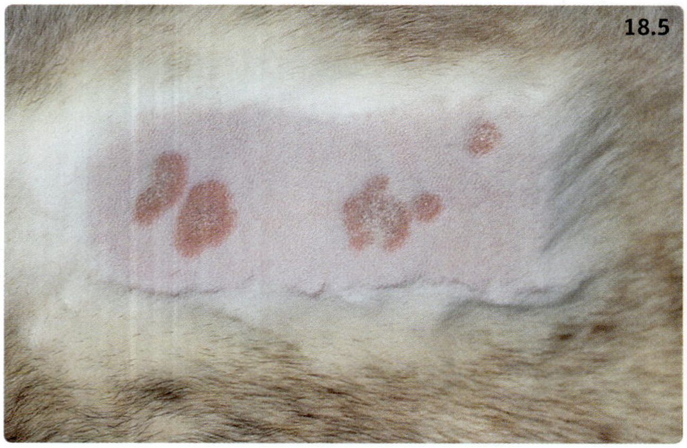

Figure 18.5 Classification of dermatologic lesions. Plaque.

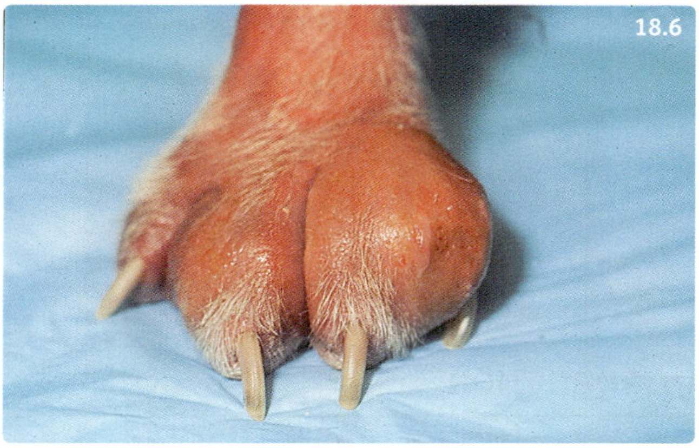

Figure 18.6 Classification of dermatologic lesions. Tumor.

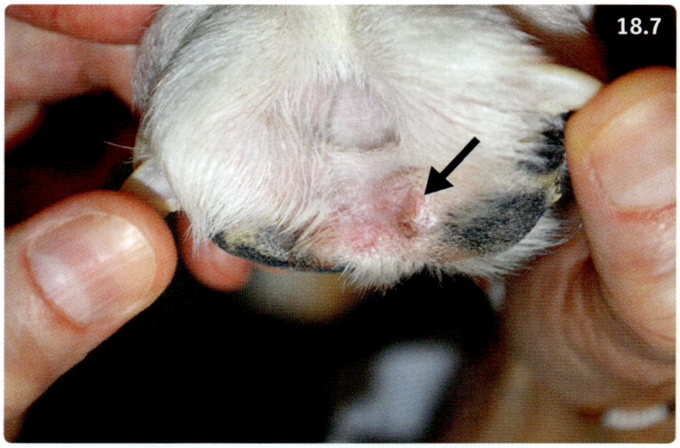

Figure 18.7 Classification of dermatologic lesions. Bulla (arrow).

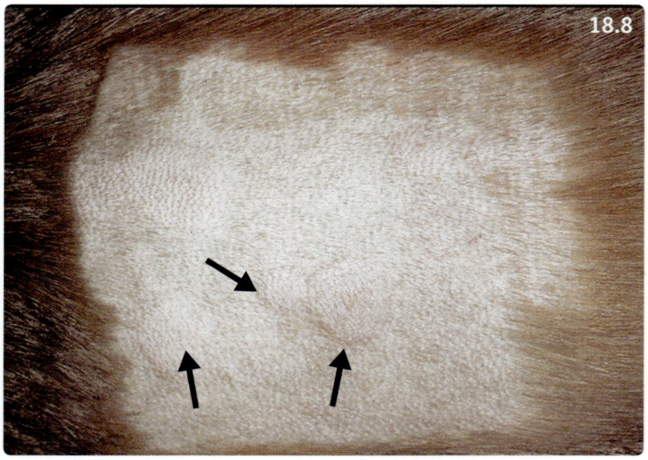

Figure 18.8 Classification of dermatologic lesions. Wheal (arrows).

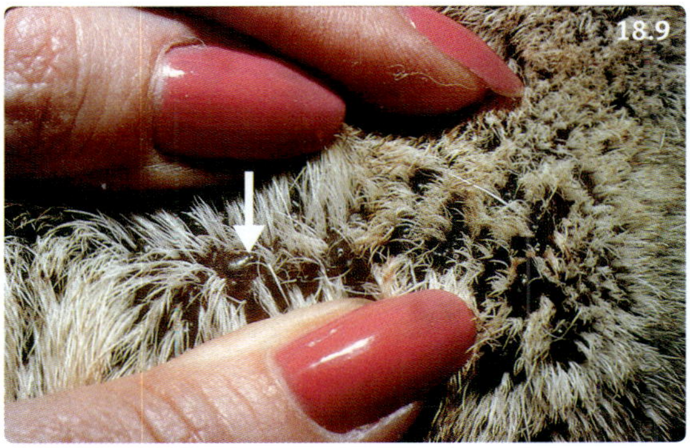

Figure 18.9 Classification of dermatologic lesions. Vesicle (arrow).

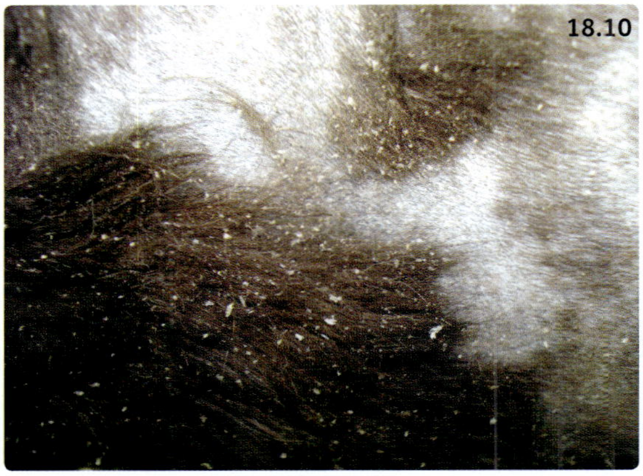

Figure 18.10 Classification of dermatologic lesions. Scale.

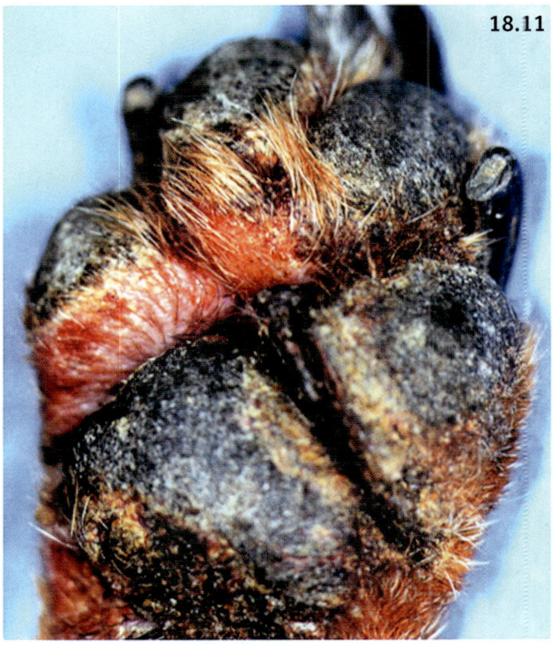

Figure 18.11 Classification of dermatologic lesions. Crust.

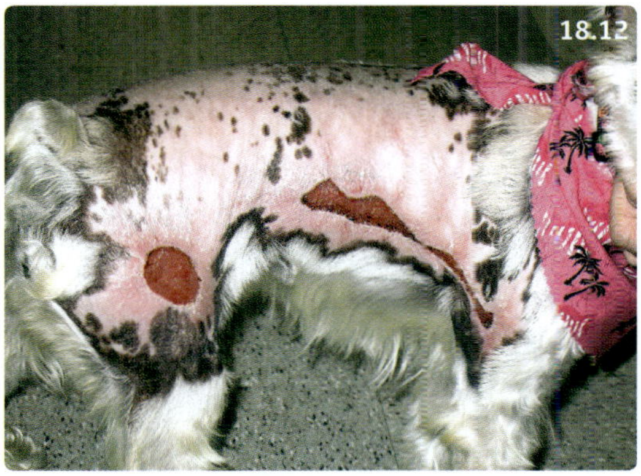

Figure 18.12 Classification of dermatologic lesions. Scar.

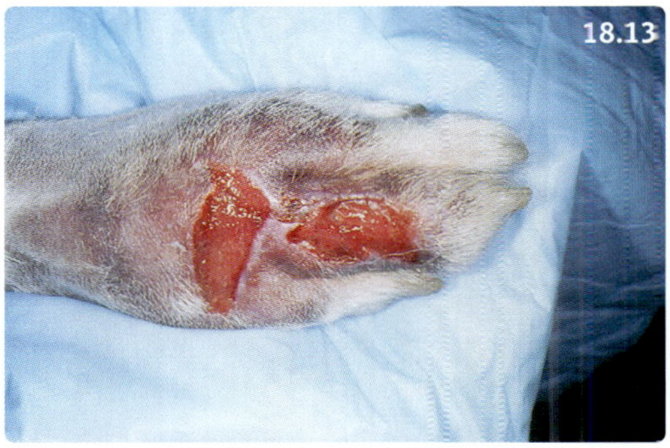

Figure 18.13 Classification of dermatologic lesions. Ulcer.

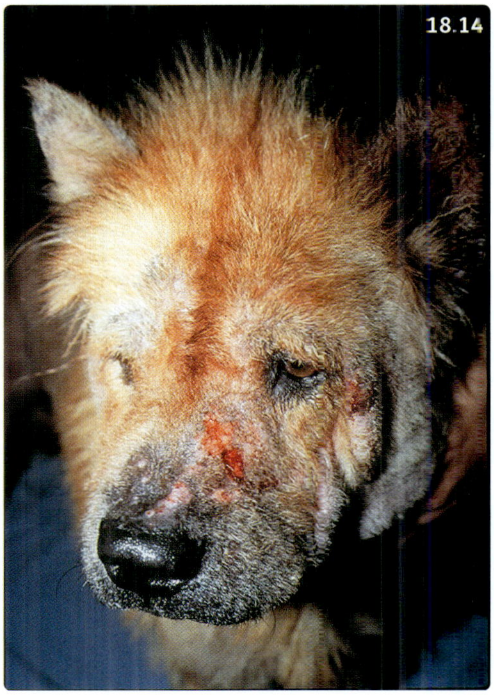

Figure 18.14 Classification of dermatologic lesions. Excoriation.

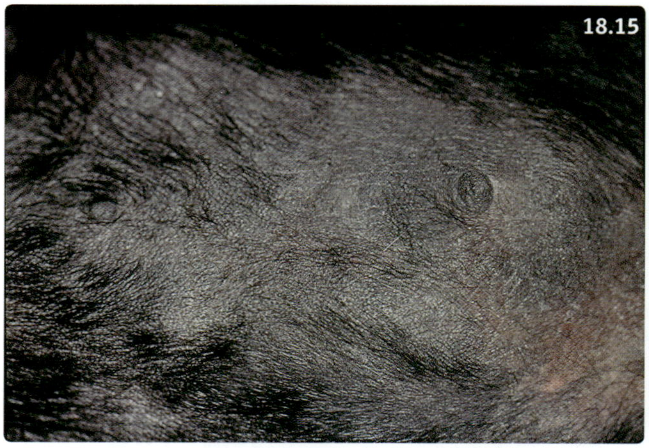

Figure 18.15 Classification of dermatologic lesions. Lichenification.

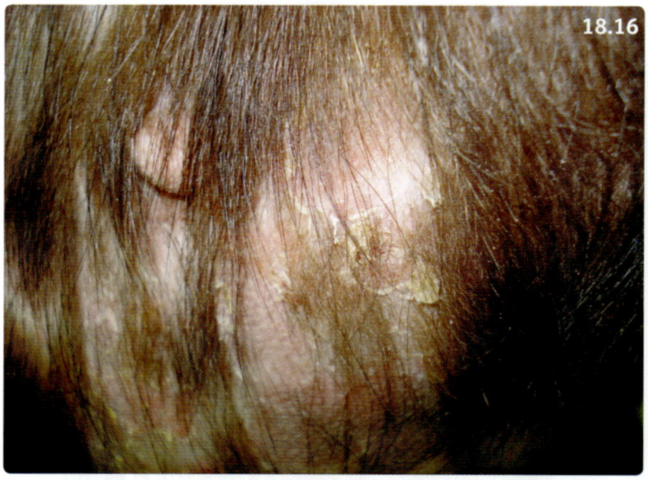

Figure 18.16 Classification of dermatologic lesions. Epidermal collarette.

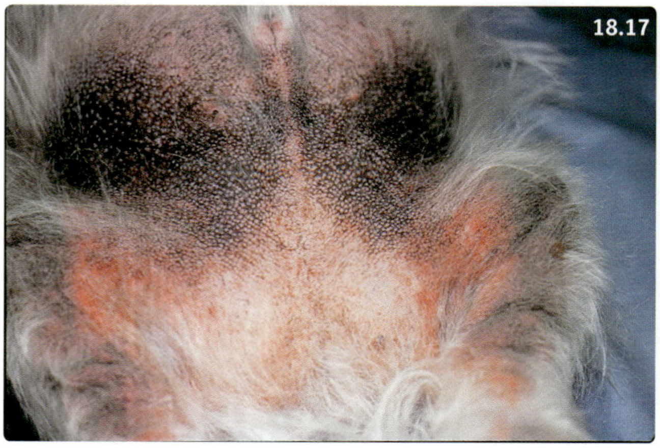

Figure 18.17 Classification of dermatologic lesions. Hyperpigmentation.

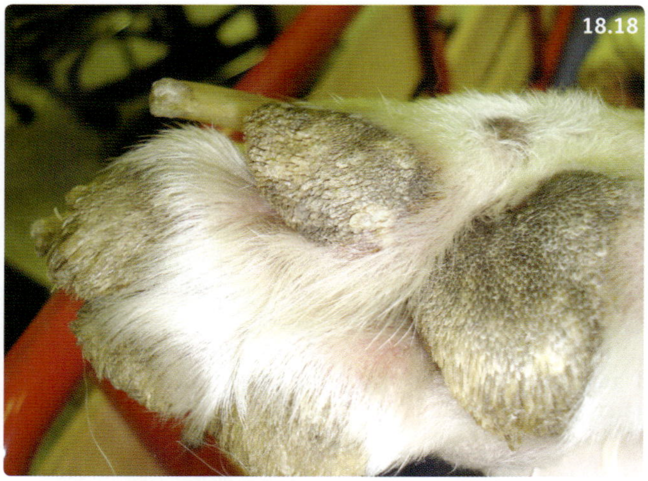

Figure 18.18 Classification of dermatologic lesions. Hyperkeratosis.

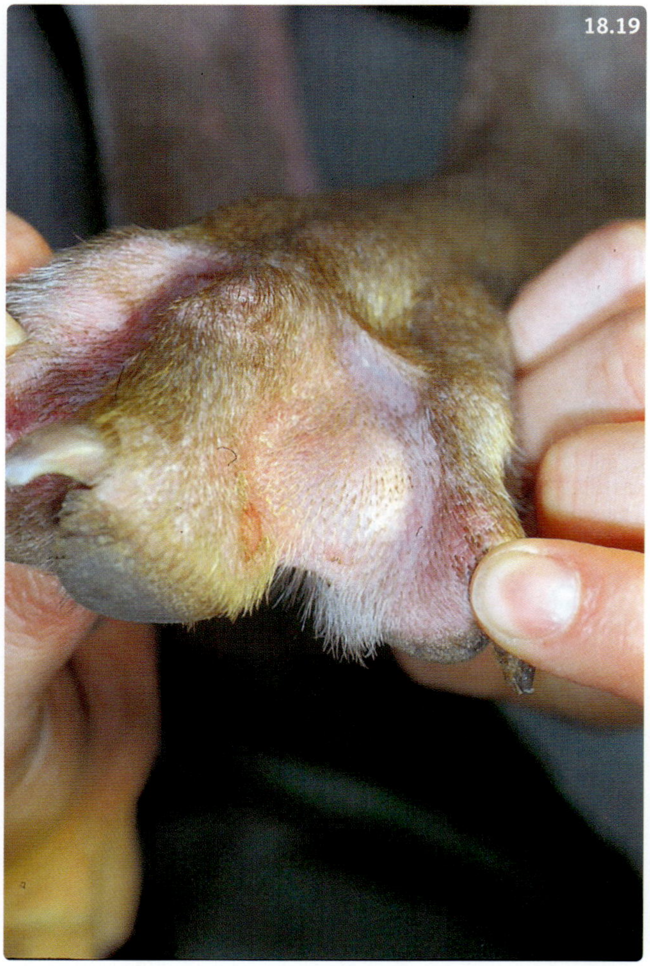

Figure 18.19 Examination of the feet. This must be included in any dermatologic examination.

Honey-colored crusts, epidermal collarettes, and circular areas of alopecia are seen more commonly in dogs and cats than is their predecessor, the pustule. When confined to the trunk, these secondary lesions more often indicate a staphylococcal folliculitis rather than dermatophytosis. Should these lesions involve the face, ears, or footpads, an autoimmune disease might be considered. A positive scratch reflex, elicited by rubbing the pinna or scratching the lateral thorax, may indicate scabies (**Figure 18.20**). Pruritus of the dorsolumbar, antebrachial, or umbilical areas would indicate flea bite hypersensitivity.

After considering the patient's history and physical and dermatologic examination findings, diagnostic investigations may be ordered (**Table 18.1**).

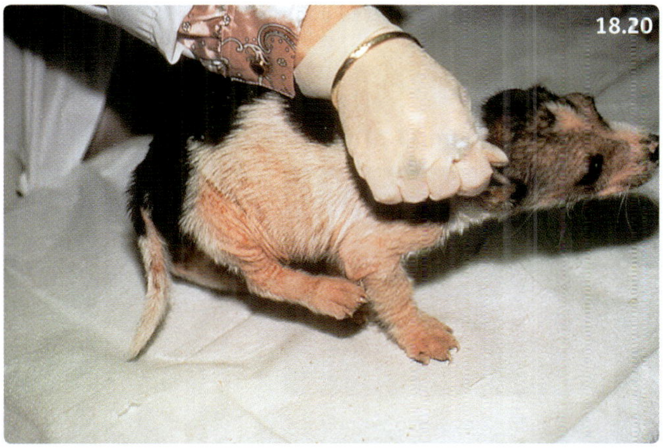

Figure 18.20 Pinnal–pedal scratch reflex elicited in a puppy with canine scabies. (Courtesy S.R. Merchant)

Table 18.1 Investigations used in dermatologic diseases of the dog and cat.

Test	Equipment	Method	Comments
Skin scraping (**Figures 18.21, 18.22**) 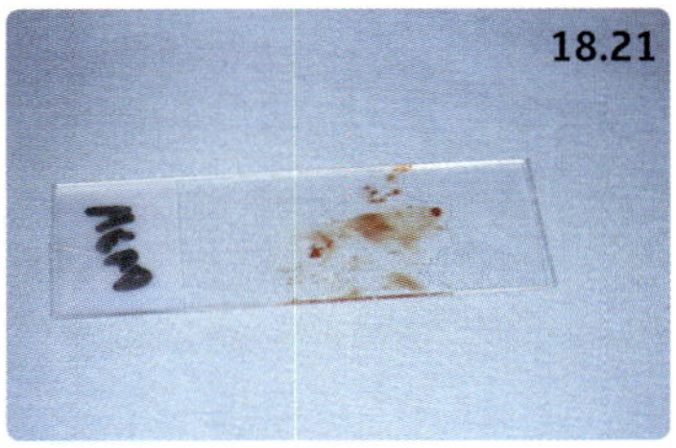 **Figure 18.21** Glass slide with material collected from a deep skin scraping of a lesion from a dog. Adequate deep skin scrapings contain a large amount of blood. Skin scrapings of a lesion should be done on every dermatologic patient. 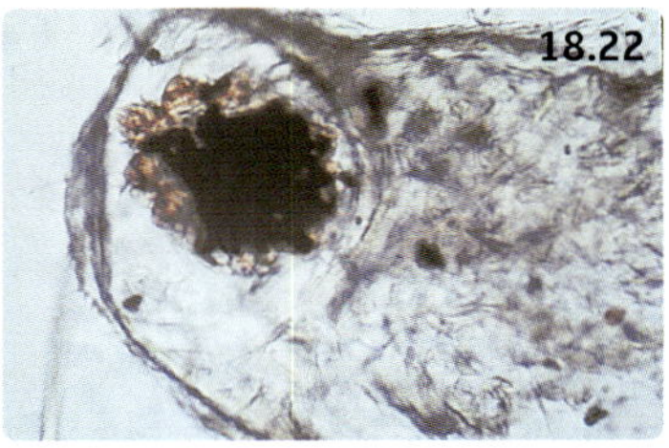 **Figure 18.22** *Notoedres cati* adult mite in stratum corneum. (Case material UFVMC)	Glass slide, #10 scalpel blade, microscope, mineral oil, clippers, coverslips	Superficial: scrape broad area. Deep: capillary oozing, squeeze site, scrape and pluck hairs	Adult parasites, eggs, and feces may be noted

(*Continued*)

Table 18.1 Investigations used in dermatologic diseases of the dog and cat. (*Continued*)

Test	Equipment	Method	Comments
Wood's lamp (**Figure 18.23**) 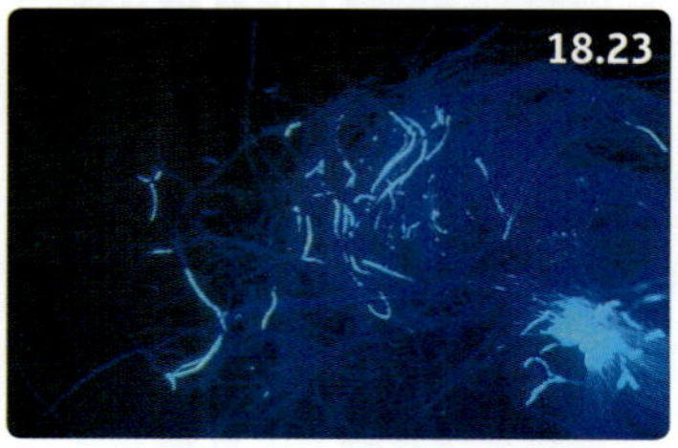 **Figure 18.23** A positive Wood's lamp examination displays fluorescence of individual hairs. Scale, crust, and certain medications will fluoresce in the absence of true dermatophytosis. A negative Wood's lamp examination is inconclusive for dermatophytosis. (Courtesy A. Mundell)	Ultraviolet light with cobalt or nickel filter may assist in collecting hairs for culture	Apple-green fluorescence of individual hairs	Negative examination inconclusive; crust and medications will fluoresce
Fungal culture (**Figure 18.24**) 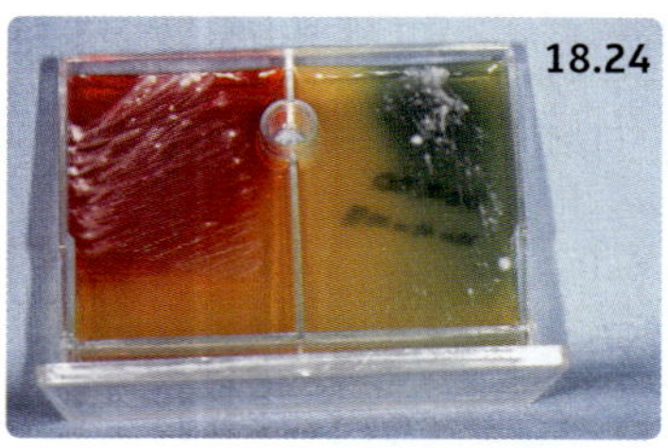 **Figure 18.24** False-positive DTM culture from a cat with a surface yeast infection. Any suspicion of dermatophyte growth on the culture plate MUST be confirmed by microscopic identification of macroconidia. Nondermatophytic fungi and yeast may turn the culture media red, concomitant with colony growth.	DTM, toothbrush, hemostats, alcohol, glass slide, acetate tape, lactophenol cotton blue	Plucked hairs; toothbrush collection of hairs; claw shavings	Must identify any suspicious colonies
Acetate tape preparations (**Figures 18.25, 18.26**) 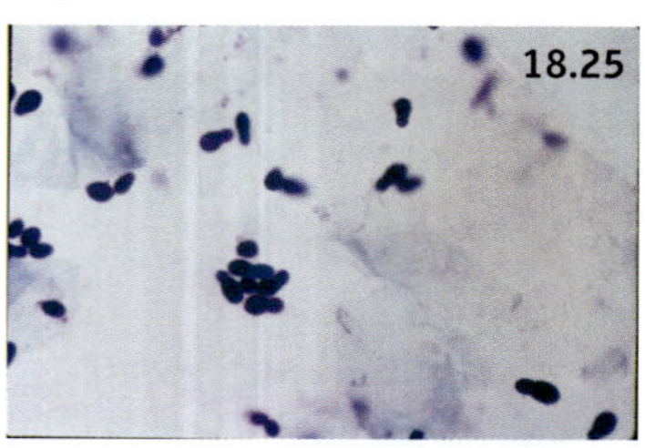 **Figure 18.25** Cytology of budding yeast of *Malassezia pachydermatis* from a dog with *Malassezia* dermatitis.	Acetate tape, glass slides, Diff-Quik® stain, immersion oil	Apply tape to lesion; stain tape for yeast and bacteria; apply to glass slide	Yeast and bacteria: use ×100; ectoparasites: do not stain, use ×10

Test	Equipment	Method	Comments
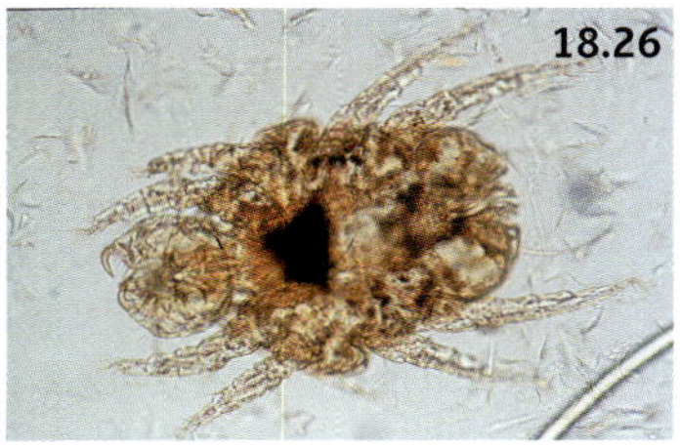 **Figure 18.26** *Cheyletiella* spp. adult mite. Note the diagnostic hook-like mouth parts.			
Pustule cytology (**Figures 18.27, 18.28**) 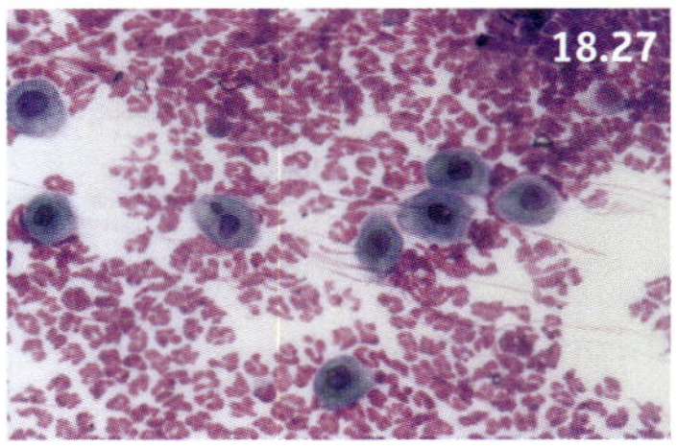 **Figure 18.27** Cytology from a pustule containing numerous acantholytic cells without polymorphonuclear intracellular cocci is suspicious of, but not diagnostic for, pemphigus foliaceus. (Courtesy S.R. Merchant) 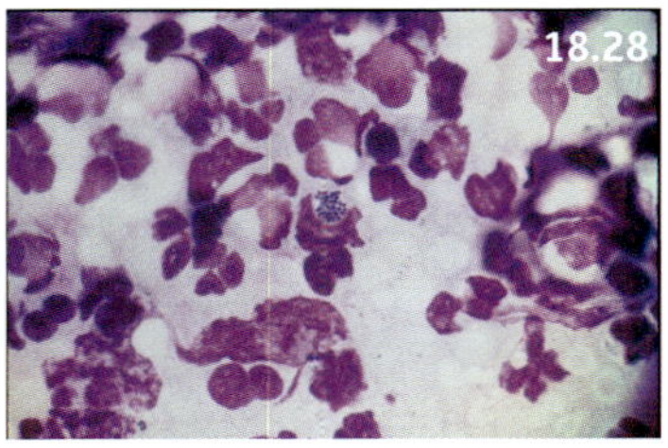 **Figure 18.28** Cytology from a pustule containing neutrophils with intracellular cocci. (Courtesy S.R. Merchant)	Glass slides, Diff-Quik® stain, 25-gauge needle, immersion oil	Smear pustule contents onto glass slide and stain	Look for intracellular cocci and acantholytic cells
Skin biopsy	10% formalin in containers, suture, 6 mm biopsy punch, needle drivers, scissors, #10 scalpel blade and handle, forceps, pieces of tongue depressor, local anesthetic	Punch biopsy for small (4 mm) lesions; elliptical biopsy for larger lesions or for tissue culture	When the cutaneous lesions are unusual or do not respond to routine therapy, use nonulcerative lesions or primary lesions supply extensive history to veterinary dermatopathologist

(*Continued*)

Table 18.1 Investigations used in dermatologic diseases of the dog and cat. (*Continued*)

Test	Equipment	Method	Comments
Intradermal allergy test	Allergens, syringes and needles, diluent, histamine	Intradermal injections	For ASIT, not for food allergy; withdraw antihistamines and cortisone
Serum allergy test	Syringe, needles, tubes	Venepuncture and serum separation	For ASIT, not for food allergy; may need to withdraw antihistamines and cortisone preparations; low reliability
Hematologic, biochemical, serologic, fecal flotation, endocrine therapy, ANA tests	Syringe, needles, tubes, special reagents	Venepuncture; serum; urine via cystocentesis; plasma required	Screens for systemic disease; monitors immunosuppressive drug therapy; detects surface mite ingestion
Microbiologic bacterial culture	Culturettes	Material in pustule, bulla, under crust or collarette	Prior antibiotic withdrawal unnecessary
Mycobacterial, anaerobic, subcuta-neous culture	Sterile biopsy supplies	Aseptic dermal/subcutaneous tissue acquisition	Culture not recommended for blastomycosis, histoplasmosis, coccidioidomycosis

DTM, dermatophyte test medium; ASIT, allergen-specific immunotherapy; ANA, antinuclear antibody.
Underlying medical or surgical problems should be investigated appropriately.

BACTERIAL INFECTIONS

SKIN FOLD PYODERMA (INTERTRIGO)

Definition/overview

Intertrigo is an inflammatory condition that occurs at sites of skin folds.

Etiology

Anatomic defects at certain body sites predispose to intertrigo. Areas prone to skin fold pyoderma include the face, vulva, lip folds, body, flank, and tail fold.

Pathophysiology

Friction, abrasion, poor ventilation, and excess surface secretions lead to maceration of the skin and secondary inflammation, with colonization by bacterial and yeast microorganisms.

Clinical presentation

Skin fold pyoderma is characterized by exudative, odiferous, erythematous lesions within skin folds (**Figure 18.29**). Lesions may be present at the lip, facial, vulvar, hock, flank, or tail fold areas.

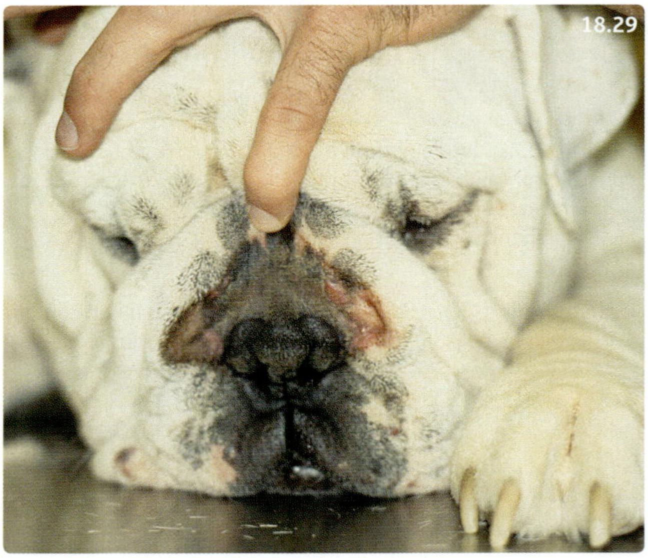

Figure 18.29 Nasal fold pyoderma in an English Bulldog. (Case material UFVMC)

Differential diagnosis

Atopic dermatitis (AD), food hypersensitivity, demodicosis, *Malassezia pachydermatis* infection, epitheliotropic lymphoma.

Diagnosis

The presence of bacteria or yeast should be determined. Skin scrapings and tape strips or impression smears of affected areas should rule out infection with *Demodex canis* and *M. pachydermatis*, respectively (**Table 18.2**).

Management

This will be a lifelong problem. Palliative therapy includes clipping long hair, cleansing with antibacterial and/or antifungal wipes, shampoos appropriate antibiotic (**Table 18.3**) or antifungal creams. Phytosphingosine solutions may be helpful. Surgical ablation of the

Table 18.2 Predisposing causes of pyoderma.

	Cause	Investigation
Pruritic	Flea bite hypersensitivity	Flea eradication, IDAT flea antigen
	Food hypersensitivity	Novel single protein prescription or home-cooked diet for 12 weeks
	Atopic dermatitis	History, rule out other causes of pruritus, IDAT
	Canine scabies	Response to therapy, SSS
	Cheyletiellosis	SSS, tape preparations
	Demodicosis	DSS, hair plucks
Nonpruritic	Hypothyroidism	FT4ed, TSH, TT4
	Hyperadrenocorticism (endogenous, atypical, or iatrogenic)	ACTH stimulation test, LDDST
	Food hypersensitivity	Novel single protein prescription or home-cooked diet for 12 weeks
	Reproductive hormone imbalance	Rule out early Cushing's and other endocrine causes, ACTH stimulation test and hormone levels, neuter
	Keratinization disorder (primary or secondary)	Rule out allergic causes, response to topical/other therapy
	Demodicosis	DSS, hair plucks
	Occult neoplasia	Thorough search
	Nutritional imbalance	Response to optimal diet
	Severe metabolic disease	Thorough search
	Immune system abnormality (deficiency or immaturity)	Thorough search
	Environmental factors	History, rule out other causes
	Concurrent autoimmune disease	Skin biopsy, rule out infectious cause
	Concurrent dermatophytosis	Dermatophyte culture
	Idiopathic	Rule out all other causes

SSS, superficial skin scrape; DSS, deep skin scrape; IDAT, intradermal allergy test; LDDST, low-dose dexamethasone suppression test; FT4ed, free T4 by equilibrium dialysis; TSH, thyroid-stimulating hormone; TT4, total T4; ACTH, adrenocorticotropic hormone.

Table 18.3 Antibiotic therapy for dermatologic disorders.

Generic	Species	Dose (mg/kg)	Route	Interval (hours)
Amoxicillin–clavulanate	C	10–20	PO	12
	D	13.75–25	PO	12
Azithromycin	C	7–15	PO	12–24
	D	5–10	PO	12–24
Cefadroxil	C	22–35	PO	24
	D	22–35	PO	12
Cefovecin	B	8	SC	q14d
Cefpodoxime	C	5–10	PO	12–24
	D	10	PO	24
Cephalexin	B	22–30	PO	12
Chloramphenicol	C	15–20	PO	12
	D	40–60	PO	8
Ciprofloxacin	C	20	PO	24
	D	10–30	PO	24
	D	5–15	PO	12
Clarithromycin	C	7.5	PO	12
	D	5–10	PO	12
Clindamycin	C	5–11	PO	12
	C	11–33	PO	24
	D	11–33	PO	24
	D	11	PO	12
Doxycycline	B	5–10	PO	12–24
Enrofloxacin	C	5	PO	24
	D	5–15	PO	24
Erythromycin	B	15–25	PO	12
Lincomycin	C	15–22	PO	12
	D	15	PO	8
	D	22	PO	12
Marbofloxacin	B	2.75–5.5	PO	24
Minocycline	B	5–25	PO	12–24
Moxifloxacin	B	10	PO	24
Ormetoprim/sulfadimethoxine	D	55 day 1 27.5 day 2	PO	24
Pradofloxacin	C	7.5	PO	24
	D	3–5	PO	24
Rifampin	B	5–10	PO	12
Tetracycline	B	15–20	PO	8
Trimethoprim/sulfadiazine	B	10	PO	12
		15–30	PO	12–24

D, dog; C, cat; B, dog and cat; PO, per os; SC, subcutaneous.

anatomic defect and weight reduction, if obese, offer a potential cure.

PYOTRAUMATIC DERMATITIS (ACUTE MOIST DERMATITIS, HOT SPOT)

Definition/overview

Pyotraumatic dermatitis involves acute inflammation and exudation of skin that has been damaged by chewing, scratching, or licking.

Etiology

Pyotraumatic dermatitis is very common in hot weather and especially in dogs with thick, long hair coats. Underlying diseases associated with pyotraumatic dermatitis include flea bite hypersensitivity, otitis externa, ectoparasites, ocular disease, food hypersensitivity, contact dermatitis, AD, and anal sac disease.

Pathophysiology

Licking, chewing, or scratching in response to pruritus or pain initiates erythematous, swollen, exudative lesions that spread peripherally and are worsened by further self-trauma (**Figure 18.30**).

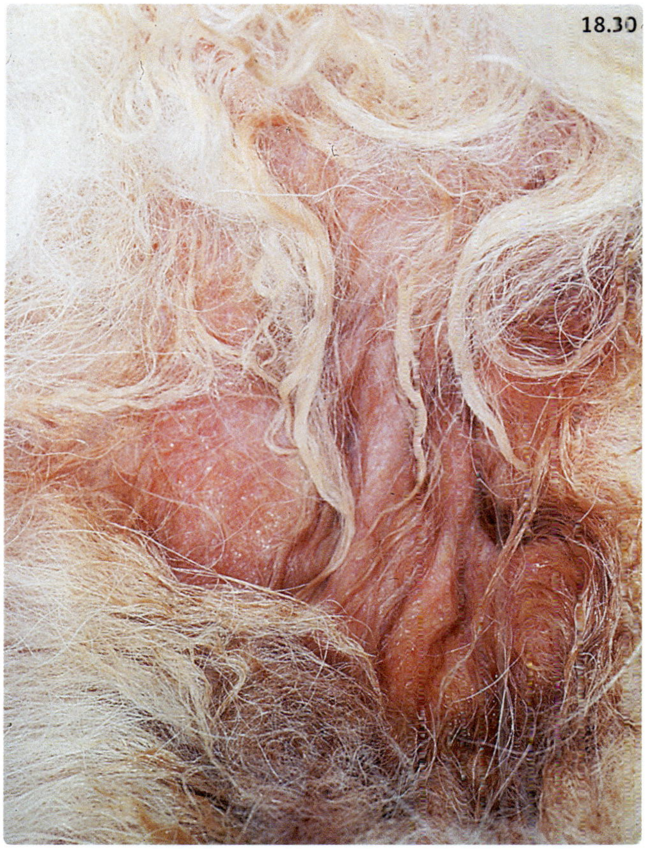

Figure 18.30 Acute moist dermatitis of the ventral neck in a Pyrenean Mountain Dog. (Case material UFVMC)

Clinical presentation

Affected animals typically lick or scratch persistently at an area of skin. The periaural and the dorsal and dorsolateral lumbosacral regions are commonly affected. The skin is erythematous and moist and may be exudative. Alopecia or thinning of the hair may be evident later in the condition.

Differential diagnosis

Superficial burn, clipping or grooming, flea bite hypersensitivity, AD, calcinosis cutis, irritant contact dermatitis, folliculitis and furunculosis, food hypersensitivity, demodicosis, dermatophytosis, anal sac disease.

Diagnosis

Clipping the hair coat allows visualization of the extent of the lesion and identification of satellite lesions associated with pyotraumatic folliculitis (**Figure 18.31**). Underlying causes should be investigated and corrected.

Management

The goals of therapy of pyotraumatic dermatitis are to clip the hair and clean the lesions, break the itch cycle, and remove underlying causes. Papules or pustules surrounding the lesion indicate that folliculitis and furunculosis may be present and warrant appropriate systemic antibiotic therapy (**Table 18.3**).

IMPETIGO (PUPPY PYODERMA)

Definition/overview

Impetigo is a subcorneal pustular disease of prepubertal dogs.

Etiology

Impetigo is often associated with poor husbandry conditions. *Staphylococcus* spp. are usually isolated from subcorneal pustules.

Pathophysiology

Impetigo is not contagious and may occur for no apparent reason. In some young dogs it may be associated with parasitism, poor nutrition, or infectious diseases.

Clinical presentation

Nonfollicular pustules are localized to the sparsely haired skin of the ventral abdomen and occasionally the axilla in puppies aged 2–9 months (**Figure 18.32**). Ruptured pustules appear as small yellowish crusts or epidermal collarettes. Pruritus may be present.

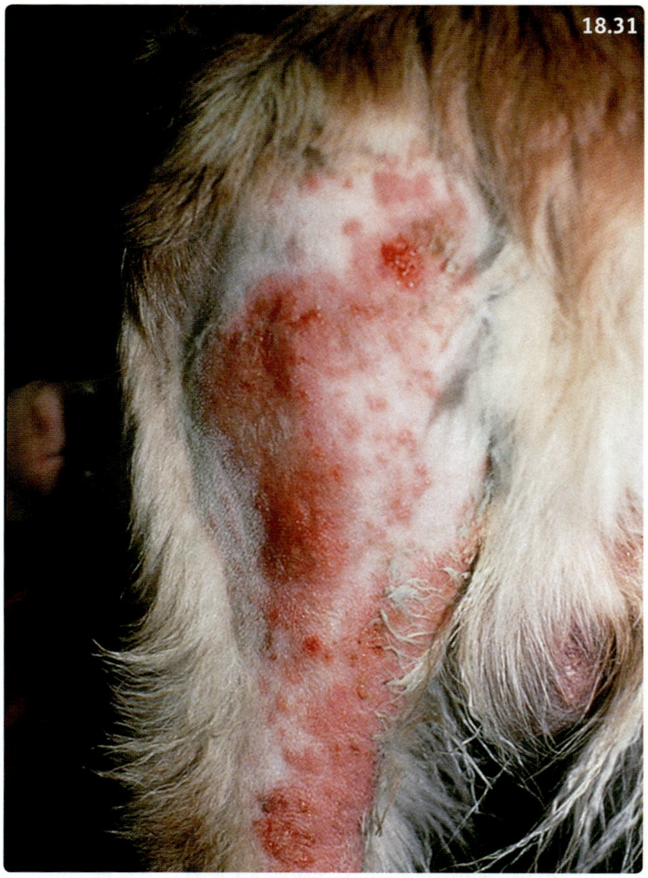

Figure 18.31 Pyotraumatic folliculitis in a Golden Retriever. Clipping of the hair coat allows identification of large, papular satellite lesions at the periphery of the lesion.

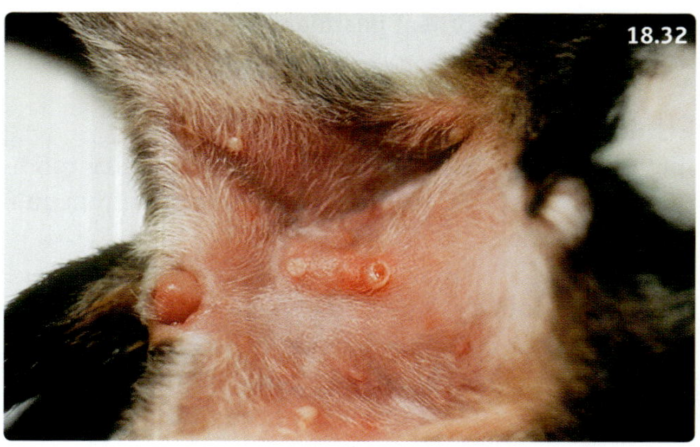

Figure 18.32 Large, nonfollicular pustules in a puppy with impetigo. (Courtesy C.S. Foil)

Differential diagnosis

Contact irritant dermatitis, demodicosis, dermatophytosis, food hypersensitivity.

Diagnosis

Diagnosis is based on the identification of cocci from impression smears of the pustule contents.

Management

Impetigo is considered a self-limiting disease and usually requires only topical antibacterial baths combined with general health care. Severe or persistent cases may benefit from systemic antibiotics for 10–14 days. Cultures should be performed if antibacterial treatment fails.

MUCOCUTANEOUS PYODERMA

Definition/overview

Mucocutaneous pyoderma (MCP) affects the lips, perioral skin, and occasionally other mucocutaneous areas of dogs.

Etiology

The etiology of MCP is unknown, although bacterial infections play a role. Underlying diseases such as hypersensitivities and endocrinopathies may predispose dogs to MCP.

Pathophysiology

The mechanisms that lead to MCP are not understood. Antibiotics improve the condition, while relapse is common.

Clinical presentation

Erythema, swelling, and crusting of the lips and perioral skin are evident and can lead to fissures, erosions, ulceration, and depigmentation (**Figure 18.33**). Salivary staining, exudate, and odor may occur. The planum nasale, nares, prepuce, and perianal areas can be affected. German Shepherd Dogs may be overrepresented.

Differential diagnosis

Lip fold intertrigo, cutaneous (discoid) lupus erythematosus (CLE), demodicosis, zinc-responsive dermatosis or generic dog food dermatosis, pemphigus foliaceus or pemphigus erythematosus, cutaneous T-cell (epitheliotropic) lymphoma.

Diagnosis

Location of lesions and response to appropriate, extended antibiotic therapy (bacterial culture and sensitivity if indicated), followed by histopathology of a skin biopsy confirm the diagnosis. Histopathologic changes

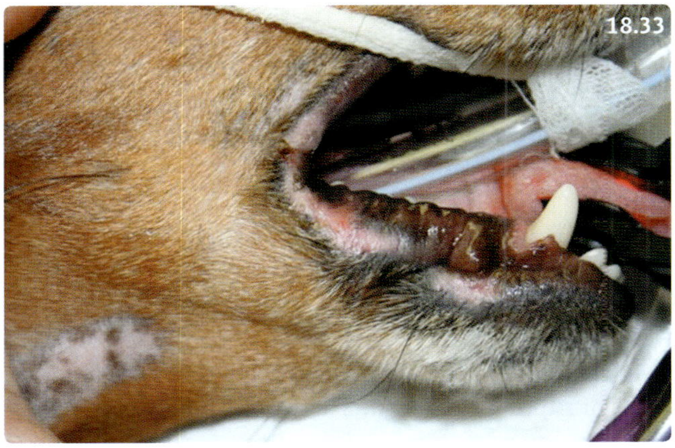

Figure 18.33 Depigmentation and erosion on the lips and perioral area of a mixed-breed dog with mucocutaneous pyoderma. (Case material UFVMC)

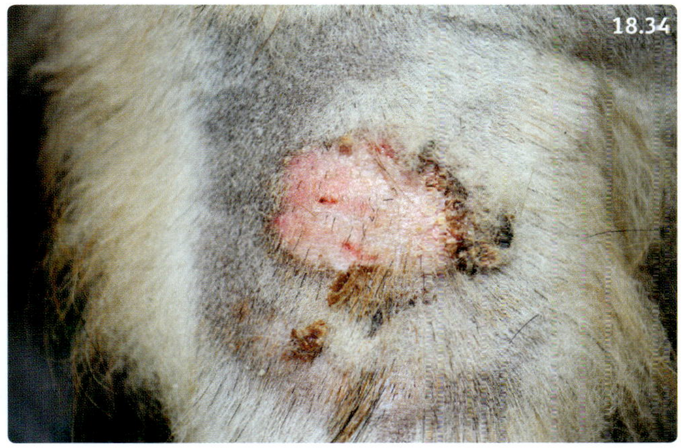

Figure 18.34 Patch of circular alopecia and erythema rimmed by a subtle crust in a dog with staphylococcal folliculitis due to food hypersensitivity.

can be confused with CLE, so antibiotic treatment is recommended prior to biopsy.

Management

Extended use of systemic antibiotics for *Staphylococcus* species and topical mupirocin may temporarily clear the disease, but relapses are common (**Table 18.3**). A search for underlying causes (e.g. food hypersensitivity or hypothyroidism) is indicated. Maintenance therapy with antibacterial wipes, topical mupirocin, and ophthalmic antibacterial preparations for affected eyelids aid in managing recurrences.

STAPHYLOCOCCAL FOLLICULITIS

Definition/overview

Staphylococcal folliculitis is a bacterial infection of the hair follicles. Methicillin resistance is prevalent.

Etiology

The most common causes of staphylococcal folliculitis are endocrinopathies, hypersensitivities, and ectoparasites. *Staphylococcus pseudintermedius*, *S. schleiferi schleiferi* and *S. schleiferi coagulans* predominate; *S. aureus* may also be found.

Pathophysiology

Changes to the cutaneous microenvironment lead to the development of conditions favoring the growth of pathogenic staphylococci.

Clinical presentation

Staphylococcal folliculitis is extremely common in canine patients presented for skin disease. Because the clinical signs are often similar to the circular lesions of ringworm in people, dogs with staphylococcal folliculitis (**Figure 18.34**) are often mistakenly treated for ringworm (dermatophytosis). Lesions of circular alopecia, a moth-eaten appearance to the hair coat, epidermal collarettes, honey-colored crusts, papules, pustules, macules, and crusted plaques are typical for staphylococcal folliculitis in the dog (**Figure 18.35**). Superficial spreading pyoderma refers to the presence of large (1–3 cm) erythematous macules with peripheral collarettes of keratin.

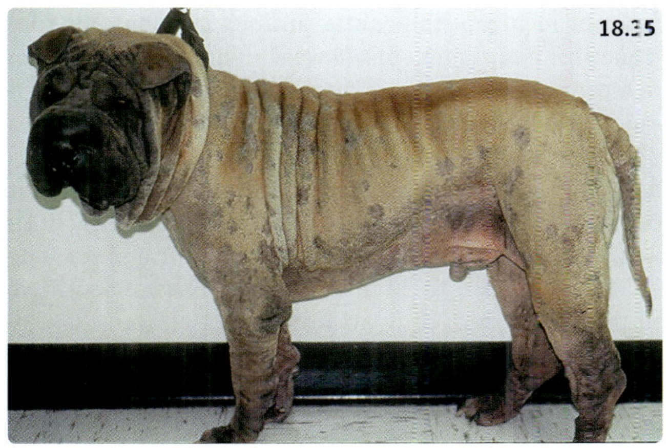

Figure 18.35 Circular areas of alopecia in a Shar Pei with staphylococcal folliculitis due to atopic dermatitis.

Differential diagnosis

Demodicosis, dermatophytosis, pemphigus foliaceus, dermatophilosis, *Malassezia pachydermatis* infection.

Diagnosis

Diagnosis is initially based on the identification of lesions. Neutrophils and intracellular cocci may be identified from cytologic (see **Figure 18.28**) examination of pustule contents or impression smears from crusts or collarettes. Bacterial culture and sensitivity of an intact pustule, papule, under a crust or collarette, or sterile tissue sample should correctly identify the pathogen to the species level, provided the laboratory is experienced with *S. schleiferi*, *S. pseudintermedius*, and *S. aureus* identifications. Deep skin scrapings should always be performed to rule out demodicosis.

Management

After initial suspicion of staphylococcal folliculitis and appropriate antibiotic therapy for a minimum of 3–4 weeks (**Table 18.3**), the patient is re-examined while still receiving antibiotics, with antibiotics continued 1 week past lesion resolution and full hair regrowth. In cases of recurrent folliculitis, antibiotics should be continued for a minimum of 4–8 weeks, with re-examination determining when treatment can be stopped. It is important to discern a true recurrence of folliculitis from a nonresponse based on re-examining patients while they are still receiving antibiotics. If the folliculitis responds but quickly relapses once antibiotics are discontinued, antibiotic therapy has not been continued for long enough. Oxacillin resistance indicates resistance *in vivo* to the entire class of β-lactam antibiotics regardless of *in-vitro* results. Penicillin binding protein 2a testing can confirm this result. Daily topical antibacterial therapy is an important aspect of managing methicillin resistant infections (1:10 dilute bleach made fresh daily) as an effective antibiotic may not be available for use or side-effects may preclude the use of an otherwise culture sensitive antibiotic. The use of vancomycin or linezolid is not recommended in veterinary patients. Corticosteroids and oclacitinib are not recommended in the initial management of folliculitis for three reasons:

- It is important to assess the degree of residual pruritus once the folliculitis has cleared.
- Corticosteroids may contribute to folliculitis for several months after discontinuation. Relapses are more common and more severe with corticosteroid usage.
- Corticosteroids will mask the clinical signs of folliculitis, not allowing adequate assessment of its resolution, and may cause secondary problems.

To minimize the recurrence of folliculitis, the predisposing cause(s) must, if possible, be identified and treated. Pet owners should be informed of the importance of hand washing and environmental surface cleaning to reduce transmission of staphylococcal organisms to susceptible individuals. The mouth is the recommended site to sample for MRSA investigation.

DEEP PYODERMA AND FURUNCULOSIS

Definition/overview

Deep pyoderma is a bacterial infection of the dermis that may result from the extension of infection through the walls of ruptured hair follicles (furunculosis).

Etiology

Deep pyoderma and furunculosis are the result of a hair follicle rupturing into the dermis, with subsequent liberation of keratin. This liberated keratin acts as a foreign body within the dermis to perpetuate the cycle of inflammation. Underlying causes of deep pyoderma include flea bite or food hypersensitivity, AD, demodicosis, hypothyroidism, hyperadrenocorticism, obesity, breed, over-aggressive grooming, callus trauma, abnormal weight bearing and ambulation, and idiopathy.

Pathophysiology

Hemorrhagic bullae, ulcers, fibrosis, scarring, and cellulitis with draining fistulous tracts may result (**Figure 18.36**).

Clinical presentation

Malaise, inappetence, fever, and lymphadenopathy may be present. Regionalized furunculosis can be noted on

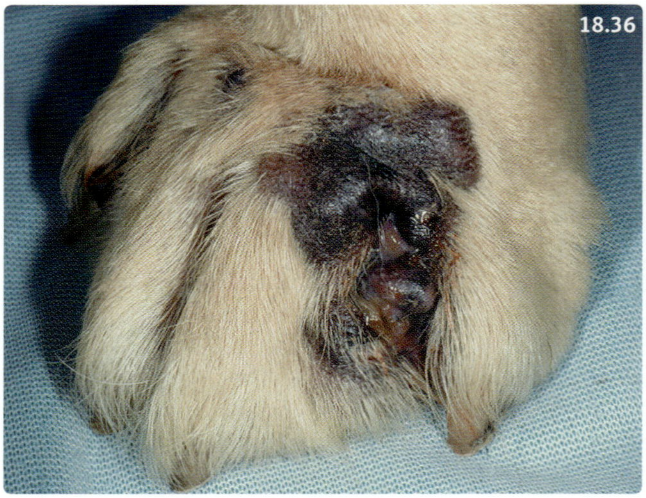

Figure 18.36 Interdigital bulla with draining tracts in a 2-year-old Labrador Retriever with staphylococcal furunculosis due to food hypersensitivity.

the chin (canine chin acne) and at callus, pressure point, or interdigital areas. Due to their stubby and bristly hair shafts, shortcoated breeds of dogs may be more prone to a generalized furunculosis. An acute onset *Pseudomonas* furunculosis may occur following bathing or water immersion.

Differential diagnosis

Demodicosis, nocardiosis, panniculitis (infectious or sterile), deep fungal infection, mast cell tumor, foreign body, histiocytosis, sterile granuloma/pyogranuloma syndrome.

Diagnosis

Sterile preparation of skin for culture and sensitivity of tissue or an unopened bulla is required to determine a causative agent. Furunculosis is more often associated with *Staphylococcus* spp., but occasionally gram-negative bacteria may be isolated alone. Finding organisms within neutrophils or macrophages on cytology of exudate may aid determination of a causative organism yielded from culture.

Management

In mixed staphylococcal and gram-negative infections, treating the staphylococci and ignoring the gram-negative bacteria is usually adequate. Systemic antibiotics are often required for 3–6 months and longer, as lesions may relapse if antibiotics are stopped prematurely (**Table 18.3**). Occasionally, lesions may be sterile. Underlying diseases must be investigated. German Shepherd Dogs can develop a severe, deep pyoderma of the hindlimbs and dorsal lumbosacral area. Topical tacrolimus or oral cyclosporine may be helpful for sterile lesions. Lifetime therapy with antibacterial shampoos, sprays, wipes, and ointments and oral antibiotics is often required. Focal areas of interdigital lesions may be amenable to laser or surgical ablation.

ABSCESSES AND CELLULITIS

Definition/overview

An abscess is a localized collection of purulent material in the dermis or subcutaneous tissues. Cellulitis is more extensive and often dissects through tissue layers.

Etiology

Oral or epidermal flora are introduced by inoculation during penetration of the skin by teeth, claws, or foreign bodies. In dog bites, typical pathogens are *Staphylococcus pseudintermedius* and *Escherichia coli*, whereas in cat bites these are *Pasteurella multocida*, β-hemolytic streptococci, *Porphyromonas* spp. and *Fusobacterium* spp. Cellulitis may develop secondary to demodicosis or abscessed tooth roots in dogs.

Pathophysiology

Abscess formation results from tissue damage and local infection 2–4 days after a traumatic wound when the wound site becomes promptly sealed.

Clinical presentation

Subcutaneous abscesses and cellulitis are common in cats, especially intact males. Abscesses are most often present on the face, limbs, base of the tail, or back, and are the result of cat bite wounds. Symptoms of fever, lameness, depression, or pain may be noted.

Differential diagnosis

Penetrating foreign body, panniculitis nocardiosis or actinomycosis, subcutaneous and deep mycoses, feline leprosy, rapidly growing (atypical/opportunistic) mycobacterial infection, canine demodicosis, *Rhodococcus* or L-form bacteria, neoplasia, cuterebriasis or dracunculiasis, dermatophytic pseudomycetoma.

Diagnosis

A complete history and examination of the site of the abscess usually lead to the diagnosis. Recurrent formation of abscesses necessitates a more thorough investigation to determine the cause. If an underlying immunosuppression or endocrinopathy is suspected, appropriate tests should be conducted. Other tests include cytologic examination of exudate and fungal, mycobacterial, aerobic, and anaerobic bacterial culture and sensitivity of tissue.

Management

Adequate drainage and amoxicillin–clavulanate should resolve cat bite abscesses in 10–14 days. Any abscess that does not heal or recurs should be investigated for feline immunodeficiency virus (FIV), feline leukemia virus (FeLV), and opportunistic mycobacteria, the latter especially if present in the inguinal or lumbar areas (**Figure 18.37**). Deep tissue wedges (which should include subcutaneous fat) should be submitted promptly for mycobacterial culture. Additionally, aerobic, anaerobic, and fungal culture of tissue may be indicated in recurrent cases. Adding clindamycin or metronidazole to the therapy can help most anaerobic infections.

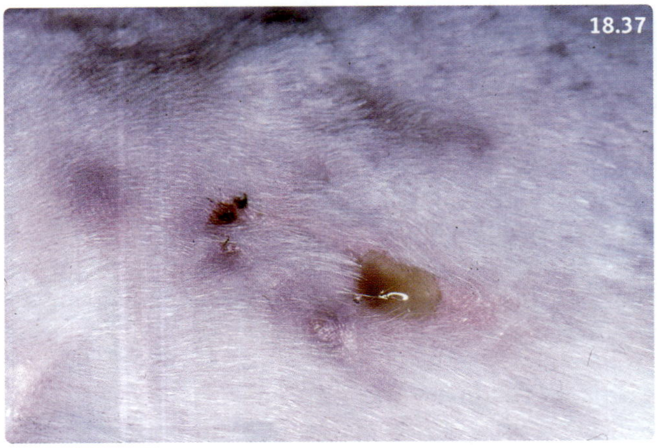

Figure 18.37 Punctate ulcers and draining tracts on the ventral abdomen of a 6-year-old Domestic Shorthair cat with panniculitis due to *Mycobacterium smegmatis.*

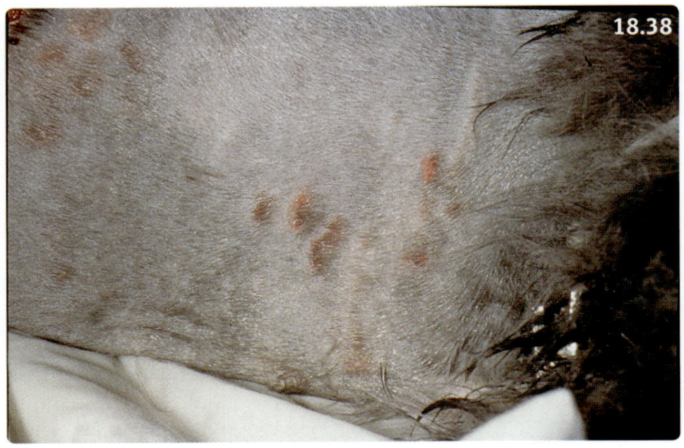

Figure 18.38 Erythematous plaques and nodules in a 1-year-old Persian cat with generalized dermatophytosis and pseudomycetoma due to *Microsporum canis*.

FUNGAL AND YEAST INFECTIONS

DERMATOPHYTOSIS

Definition/overview

Dermatophytosis is a fungal infection of the skin, hair, or claw with zoonotic (or reverse zoonotic) potential.

Etiology

Dermatophytosis is caused by infection with species of keratinophilic fungi. In dogs and cats the fungi most commonly implicated are *Microsporum canis, M. gypseum*, and *Trichophyton* spp. *M. persicolor* has been reported.

Pathophysiology

A cell-mediated and humoral response is elicited after infection. Any type of microtrauma (fleas, mites, aggressive grooming or clipping of hair coat) is a risk factor for infection when infective spores are present. The inflammatory reaction leads to increased epidermal proliferation. Persian cats may develop a nodular phase of furunculosis.

Clinical presentation

In cats, lesions may range from alopecia, scale, miliary dermatitis, or nodules (dermatophytic pseudomycetoma) (**Figure 18.38**) to none at all (asymptomatic carriers). In dogs, lesions may include papules, pustules, alopecic nodules (kerion), and draining tracts. Dermatophytosis is more common in very young or old animals, immunosuppressed animals, and in cattery situations. Yorkshire Terriers and longhaired cats may be predisposed to *M. canis* dermatophytosis.

Differential diagnosis

- **Regional/generalized lesions.** In cats: flea bite hypersensitivity, telogen/anagen defluxion, demodicosis, psychogenic alopecia. In dogs: demodicosis, staphylococcal folliculitis, autoimmune diseases, deep mycotic lesions.
- **Focal lesions.** In cats: cat bite abscess, cheyletiellosis, demodicosis. In dogs: staphylococcal folliculitis, demodicosis, defects in keratinization, alopecia after injection.

Diagnosis

Although not a common disease, dermatophytosis is an overdiagnosed disease when clinical signs or color change on dermatophyte test medium (DTM) alone are used. Once hair or scale applied to fungal culture medium exhibits nonpigmented colony growth concomitant with red color change, the colony MUST be identified microscopically to confirm the presence of a dermatophyte. PCR identification of isolates identified as *T. mentagrophytes* is recommended, as they may be otherwise incorrectly identified. Nondermatophytes may cause the red color change similar to a dermatophyte (see **Figure 18.24**). Identification of the dermatophyte assists the veterinarian, the client, and the patient in the following ways:

- It avoids a false-positive diagnosis of dermatophytosis and unnecessary treatment.
- The source of the dermatophyte may be identified and removed or treated, and the potential need for environmental decontamination can be evaluated.
- Along with signalment and clinical presentation of the patient, dermatophyte identification guides

the selection of appropriate therapy – systemic and topical or topical alone.

- Culture of hair on DTM is recommended for all cats presented for skin disease and for all dogs with evidence of primary lesions. Culture of tissue is recommended when fungal or hyphal structures present in tissue cannot be readily identified on histopathologic examination and culture of hair or scale is negative.

Management

In all cases of generalized dermatophytosis and dermatophytosis in longhaired cats, twice weekly topical treatments (lime sulfur, ketoconazole, miconazole, climbazole, accelerated hydrogen peroxide, 1:10 bleach, or enilconazole rinses) should be used together with systemic antifungal agents (itraconazole, ketoconazole, fluconazole, or terbinafine). Clipping away affected hair and burning the clippings is recommended to decrease environmental and human exposure, but this may not be needed if thorough application of topical solutions can be done. Colloidal silver, silver sulfadiazine, hypochlorous acid, and lufenuron have not been found to be effective in the treatment and prevention of dermatophytosis. Treatment should be continued for at least 6 weeks and until two fungal cultures 1 week apart are negative. In cases of *M. canis* infection, to prevent fomite carriage, false-positive fungal cultures, and decrease transmission risk, owners should mechanically remove debris from the environment and wash all surfaces once or twice weekly with 1:10 bleach or accelerated hydrogen peroxide (products with label efficacy for *T. mentagrophytes*), allowing a 10 minute contact time. Patient confinement to easily cleaned areas is helpful.

MALASSEZIA DERMATITIS

Definition/overview

Malassezia dermatitis is a pruritic condition associated with the presence of the yeast *Malassezia pachydermatis.*

Etiology

Increased numbers of yeast organisms or a hypersensitivity to surface yeast may be associated with diseases that may induce seborrheic conditions on the skin. Predisposing factors for *Malassezia* dermatitis include hypothyroidism, hyperadrenocorticism, flea bite hypersensitivity, food hypersensitivity, AD, staphylococcal folliculitis, primary keratinization disorders, long-term glucocorticoid therapy, and breed (Terriers, Basset Hound, Poodle, American Cocker Spaniel, Shih Tzu, Dachshund, English Setter).

Pathophysiology

The precise pathogenesis is unclear, although *M. pachydermatis* thrives in areas of skin with increased lipid content and may be more prevalent in geographic regions where ambient humidity is high.

Clinical presentation

Moist, erythematous, hyperpigmented, lichenified (acanthosis nigricans) lesions typify those of *Malassezia* dermatitis and are often located in the ventral neck fold, axilla, lip fold, ears, claw folds, and interdigital spaces (**Figure 18.39**). Pruritus is present and often constant. *Malassezia* dermatitis in cats may be associated with hypersensitivities, otitis externa, feline acne, generalized keratinization defects, FIV, thymoma, and exfoliative erythroderma.

Differential diagnosis

Demodicosis, AD, flea bite hypersensitivity, food hypersensitivity, sarcoptic mange, staphylococcal folliculitis, idiopathic defects in keratinization, cutaneous adverse drug reaction, allergic contact dermatitis, cutaneous T-cell (epitheliotropic) lymphoma.

Diagnosis

Peanut-shaped budding yeasts are visible on acetate tape preparations from affected skin (see **Figure 18.25**). While numbers per high-power (×100) field should be noted, the presence of any yeast in a clinically affected dog merits treatment.

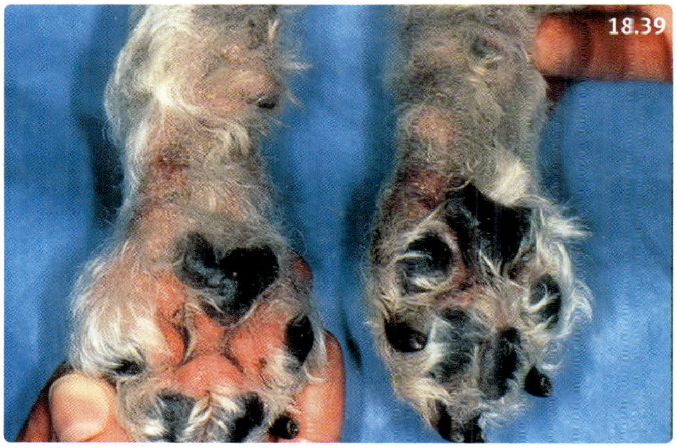

Figure 18.39 Erythematous pododermatitis due to *Malassezia pachydermatis* in a 10-year-old Poodle with hypothyroidism.

Management

Topical degreasing shampoos and antifungal treatment with oral ketoconazole, fluconazole, itraconazole, or terbinafine is necessary. It is important to investigate and correct underlying diseases, as mentioned above, to minimize recurrence.

PARASITIC DERMATOSES

CANINE DEMODICOSIS

Definition/overview

Demodicosis, an intrafollicular parasitic disease caused by demodicid mites, is probably the most serious non-neoplastic dermatologic condition in animals.

Etiology

Demodicosis is caused by *Demodex canis, D. folliculorum,* and *D. injai*. A hereditary factor predisposes an animal to develop juvenile-onset demodicosis.

Pathophysiology

Typically, the mites reside in the hair follicles, although some have been found in apocrine and sebaceous glands adjacent to follicles. Mites feed mostly on follicular debris and cells and occasionally on sebum. It seems that lymphocyte suppression, possibly influenced by secondary bacterial infection, allows the mites to proliferate.

Clinical presentation

Lesions comprise one or several areas of either scaling, thinning of hair, hyperpigmentation, alopecia, or erythema with alopecia (**Figure 18.40**). Lesions may appear on any part of the body, but typically affect the face and forelimbs. About 10% of localized cases progress to generalized disease. Juvenile-onset demodicosis is limited to onset at <18–24 months of age and is considered hereditary. Adult-onset demodicosis occurs after 2 years of age and is often associated with an underlying disease (iatrogenic or endogenous hyperadrenocorticism, hypothyroidism, infectious diseases).

Differential diagnosis

Color dilution alopecia, alopecia areata, sebaceous adenitis, staphylococcal folliculitis or furunculosis, injection site reaction, deep fungal infection, cutaneous T-cell lymphoma, pemphigus foliaceus, cutaneous adverse drug reaction, sterile granuloma/pyogranuloma syndrome, zinc-responsive dermatosis, dermatophytosis, *Malassezia* dermatitis, endocrine or keratinization disorders.

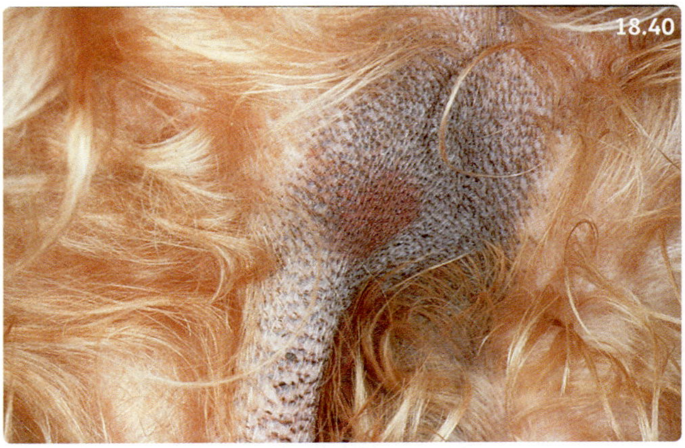

Figure 18.40 Patch of perifollicular hyperpigmentation and comedones in a 5-year-old Afghan Hound with adult-onset generalized demodicosis.

Diagnosis

Determining the extent of disease in demodicosis is one of the most important steps in diagnosis. Acquiring deep skin scrapings and hair plucks from five body sites is helpful in determining the extent of disease (lip fold, fore- and hindfeet, two additional areas – preferably lesions) (**Table 18.4**). Noting which life cycle stages are present and their relative numbers can give the veterinarian an idea as to the activity of the disease (**Figure 18.41**) (numerous eggs, few adults – active disease; numerous dead adults, no eggs – less active disease, potentially a better prognosis).

Generalized disease involves positive skin scrapings from more than one body region. Localized disease is limited to a few lesions in one body region. Skin scrape sites can be re-scraped biweekly to assess response to therapy. A skin biopsy may be necessary in the Shar Pei and in cases of pododermatitis if skin scrapings are negative.

Management

The most effective therapies to date include topical amitraz weekly (250 ppm), oral milbemycin daily (2 mg/kg), and oral or parenteral ivermectin daily (300–600 µg/kg). Ivermectin sensitive animals can be identified by testing (www.vetmed.wsu.edu/depts-VCPL/test.aspx). Topical imidacloprid–moxidectin weekly has also been effective. Appropriate miticidal therapy should be continued until three consecutive negative deep skin scrapings are achieved 2 weeks apart, rather than until the dog is clinically normal. Affected animals should be neutered as soon as practical and prior to complete resolution of disease.

Table 18.4 Common external parasites affecting the skin of dogs and cats.

Parasite	Depth of skin scraping	Location	Treatment
Cheyletiella	S	Trunk	I, P, L, A, I-M, F
Notoedres	S	Head	I, L, A, I-M
Sarcoptes	S	Ear margin, elbows, hocks	I, L, M, A, Se, I-M
Otodectes	S	Head, rump	I, P, I-M
Demodex (dog)	D*	Face, feet, trunk	I, M, A, I-M
Demodex (cat)	D, S	Head, trunk	A, L, I-M

S, superficial; D, deep; I, ivermectin; P, pyrethrin; L, lime sulfur; A, amitraz; I-M, imidacloprid–moxidectin; M, milbemycin; F, fipronil; Se, selamectin.
*, hair plucks are also useful.

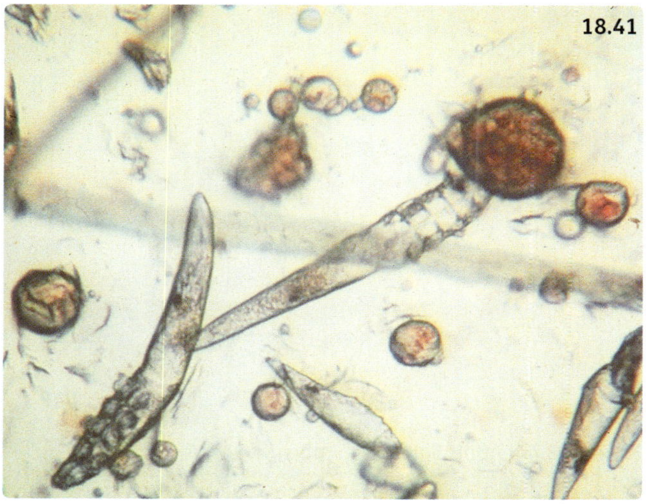

Figure 18.41 Adult and larval stages of *Demodex canis*.

Identifying and treating secondary bacterial infections helps minimize them as a contributing factor of demodicosis. When furunculosis is present, intact bulla or tissue culture with antibiotic sensitivity is financially prudent due to the long duration of antibiotic therapy required.

Generalized juvenile-onset demodicosis is hereditary and can be a serious and expensive disease to treat. Fifteen percent of dogs will never be cured. All dogs with juvenile-onset generalized demodicosis must be neutered as soon as practical. Dogs treated for localized demodicosis with systemic agents intended for generalized disease should also be neutered. This may be especially important with the use of afoxolaner and fluralaner medications in young dogs. Dogs from litters affected by demodicosis should not be bred. Mature dogs that develop generalized demodicosis may have an associated endocrine abnormality. Corticosteroids, cyclosporine A, and oclacitinib are contraindicated in dogs with any form of demodicosis.

FELINE DEMODICOSIS

Definition/overview

Feline demodicosis is an uncommon parasitic disease caused by increased numbers of demodicid mites in the skin.

Etiology

Feline demodicosis is caused by a follicular mite *Demodex cati* (which looks similar to *D. canis*), a surface mite *D. gatoi* (shorter with a blunt, rounded abdomen), and an as yet unnamed species larger than *D. gatoi* (**Figure 18.42**). An inapparent carrier state and contagiousness between cats has been reported with *D. gatoi*.

Pathophysiology

Some cases of feline demodicosis caused by *D. cati* have been associated with food hypersensitivity, feline acne, FIV, diabetes mellitus, and actinic dermatitis.

Clinical presentation

Cats may present with pruritus and hair pulling, localized or symmetrical alopecia, erythema, and excoriations.

Differential diagnosis

Staphylococcal folliculitis/furunculosis, psychogenic alopecia, dermatophytosis, AD, food hypersensitivity, flea bite hypersensitivity, infestation with *Cheyletiella* spp. or *Notoedres cati*, contact dermatitis.

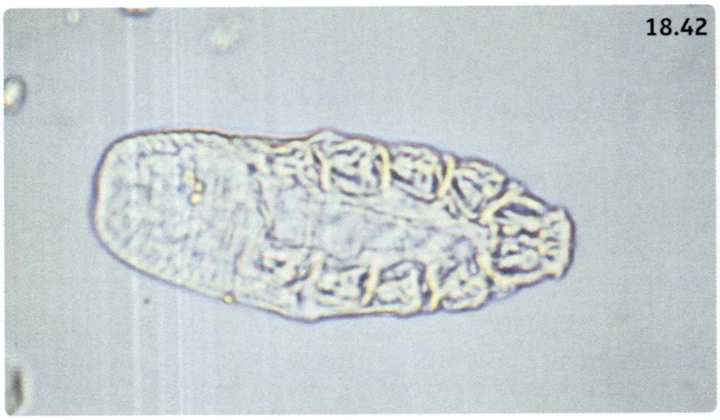

Figure 18.42 Adult mite of *Demodex gatoi*. (Courtesy S.R. Merchant)

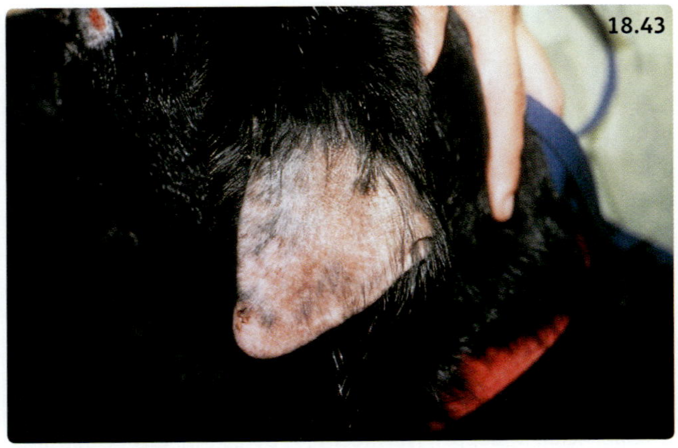

Figure 18.43 Pinnal alopecia due to canine scabies in a Labrador Retriever.

Diagnosis

If superficial skin scrapings are negative for *D. gatoi*, consider fecal floatation and scraping other household cats, as they may be asymptomatic carriers. Deep skin scrapings are necessary for *D. cati* identification.

Management

Topical treatment with weekly imidacloprid–moxidexctin or 2% lime sulfur, or daily oral ivermectin should be considered in any cat that presents with the above symptoms and continued for 6 weeks. Failing this, 125 ppm amitraz may be used weekly as a dip and continued for 3 weeks after a skin scraping has given negative results. All cats in the household should be treated simultaneously when *D. gatoi* is found or suspected. Occasionally, pruritus may persist after mites are no longer present, possibly due to a persistent hypersensitivity response or to what has become a compulsive behavior. A short course of oral glucocorticoids after miticidal therapy may stop the excessive grooming behavior.

CANINE SCABIES

Definition/overview

Canine scabies (sarcoptic mange) is a contagious dermatosis of dogs, and rarely cats, caused by the mite *Sarcoptes scabiei* var. *canis*.

Etiology

Caused by the highly contagious mite *S. scabiei* var. *canis*, sarcoptic mange is one of the most pruritic skin diseases of dogs. The mite has also been reported to cause disease in cats, foxes, and humans.

Pathophysiology

Most of the pruritus may be caused by a hypersensitivity reaction to the mite and its secretions.

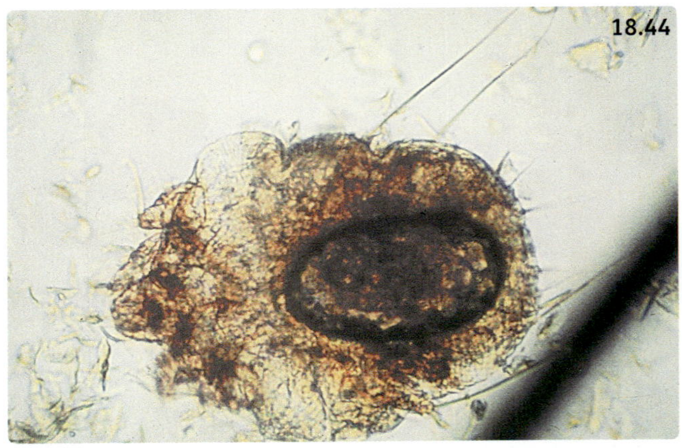

Figure 18.44 Adult *Sarcoptes scabiei* var. *canis* mite.

Clinical presentation

Canine scabies is a ventrally distributed disease, with the ear margins, elbows, hocks, and abdomen typically involved (**Figure 18.43**). The pinnal–pedal reflex may be positive in 25–90% of dogs with scabies (see **Figure 18.20**).

Differential diagnosis

Flea bite hypersensitivity, AD, food hypersensitivity, *Malassezia* dermatitis, otodectic dermatitis, cheyletiellosis, *Pelodera strongyloides* dermatitis.

Diagnosis

Apart from puppies, fewer than 25–50% of dogs with symptoms of sarcoptic mange are positive for mites on superficial skin scrapings (**Figure 18.44**). The diagnosis is often ultimately made by response to appropriate therapy. Although ELISA serology is not perfect and may result in treatment delay, a negative result has high predictive value.

Management

The most effective therapies are topical lime sulfur rinses (weekly × 6), ivermectin (PO, pour-on, or SC weekly × 4), milbemycin (every other day for 14 days or weekly × 4), selamectin or imidacloprid–moxidectin (three times, 2 weeks apart), and topical amitraz rinses (weekly × 6). All in-contact animals must be treated, as well as the environment, fomites, and bedding.

OTODECTIC ACARIASIS

Definition/overview

Otodectic acariasis is a contagious, parasitic, zoonotic, otic, or cutaneous disease caused by the psoroptid mite *Otodectes cynotis*.

Etiology

O. cynotis is the most common cause of otitis externa in young cats. Its incidence in dogs is lower. The mites can also transiently affect humans.

Pathophysiology

Otodectes mites feed on epidermal debris and tissue fluid, exposing the host to mite antigen. The ear canal epidermis becomes irritated, producing excessive cerumen and blood.

Clinical presentation

Ear pruritus with black, granular debris in the external ear canal is a common symptom. *O. cynotis* may also exist outside of the ear canal and be a cause of head and tail pruritus, especially in cats (**Figure 18.45**). Papules, crusts, and excoriations may be evident.

Differential diagnosis

Foreign bodies, bacterial infection, *Malassezia* infection, *Pseudomonas* spp. infection, defects in keratinization, autoimmune diseases, hypersensitivities, dermatophytosis.

Diagnosis

Diagnosis may be made by visualization of the mites in the ear canal, mineral oil ear swabs or on skin scrapings or acetate tape preparations (**Figure 18.46**). However, mites may be difficult to demonstrate in the ear canal, as immunity to the salivary antigens of the mite may develop and the ensuing inflammation may destroy the mites or cause them to leave the ear canal.

Management

Aural and topical parasiticides applied to the ears and entire body, respectively, at varying intervals, for a total of 30 days are required. Ivermectin (oral weekly, pour-on or SC biweekly), selamectin, and imidacloprid–moxidectin biweekly are also effective. All in-contact animals must be treated as well.

CHEYLETIELLOSIS

Definition/overview

Cheyletiellosis is a variably pruritic, contagious, and zoonotic dermatosis of dogs and cats caused by *Cheyletiella* spp. mites living on the skin surface.

Etiology

Cheyletiella yasguri (dogs), *C. blakei* (cats), and *C. parasitovorax* (rabbits) are obligate parasites that may travel freely among various host species.

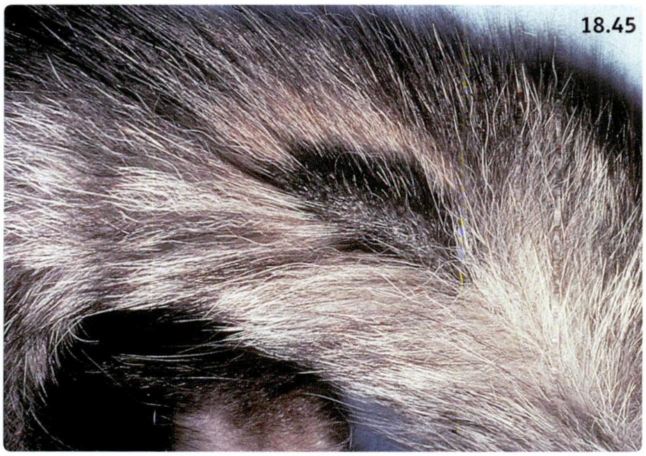

Figure 18.45 Tail alopecia and scale due to *Otodectes cynotis* dermatitis in a cat. (Courtesy C.S. Foil)

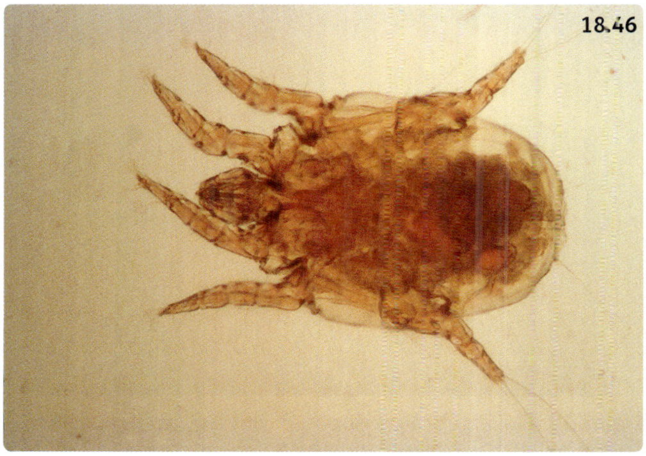

Figure 18.46 Adult *Otodectes cynotis* mite from the ear of a cat. (Courtesy E. Greiner)

Pathophysiology

The mites live in the keratin layer, moving rapidly in pseudotunnels of epidermal debris and periodically attaching themselves to pierce the skin and engorge with tissue fluid and lymph. Eggs are bound to hairs. When eggs are shed, they can act as an environmental reservoir of infection.

Clinical presentation

Symptoms can range from none to intense pruritus with or without dorsal scaling, papules, or crusts (**Figure 18.47**). Through grooming, cats may efficiently remove scale, mites, and eggs, initially leaving only alopecia.

Differential diagnosis

Flea bite hypersensitivity, pediculosis, demodicosis, otodectic acariasis, keratinization disorder, intestinal parasitism, malnutrition, scabies, food hypersensitivity.

Diagnosis

Direct observation of mobile mites in scale collected from the affected animal and placed on a dark surface ('walking dandruff') is diagnostic. Mites and eggs can be difficult to detect, but they may be found on microscopic examination of superficial skin scrapings, on acetate tape impression placed on a mineral oil slide, or on fecal floatation. A negative result does not rule out the possibility of *Cheyletiella* infestation. The adult mites have characteristic crescent-shaped hooks on the accessory mouthparts (see **Figure 18.26**). Lack of response to appropriate therapy may lessen the likelihood of cheyletiellosis.

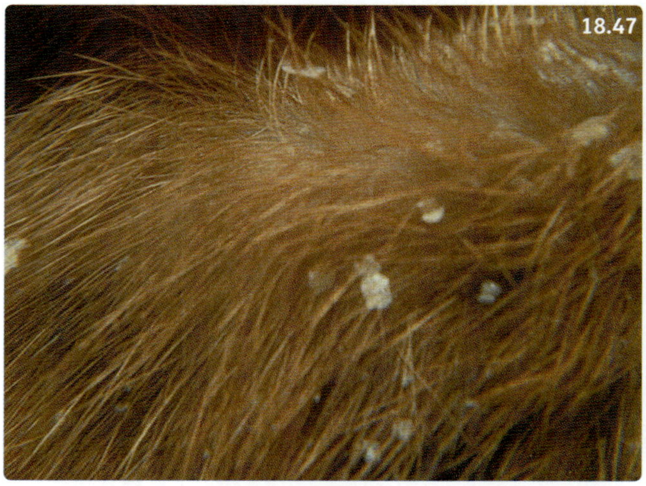

Figure 18.47 Large scale associated with *Cheyletiella* in the hair coat of a dog. (Case material UFVMC)

Management

The infested animal's bedding and all fomites should be treated with a pyrethroid-containing product. All in-contact animals should also be treated. Weekly pyrethroid (caution in cats) or lime sulfur rinses, biweekly ivermectin (oral or injectable), selamectin, imidacloprid–moxidectin, fipronil (not for use in rabbits), or milbemycin weekly have been effective when used for 6–8 weeks. If nasal sequestration of mites occurs, ivermectin should be considered.

TROMBICULOSIS

Definition/overview

Trombiculosis is a pruritic, papular, crusting dermatitis caused by species of mites (chiggers) of the family Trombiculidae.

Etiology

The six-legged larval stage (**Figure 18.48**) infests dogs and cats from summer through autumn/fall. Species involved include *Neotrombicula autumnalis* (harvest mite), *Eutrombicula alfreddugesi* (North American chigger), *Walchia americana*, *Leptotrombidium subquadratum* (S. Africa), and *Straelensia cynotis*.

Pathophysiology

Adult chigger mites live in decaying plant material. The six-legged red larvae are parasitic and feed on animals, causing severe irritation.

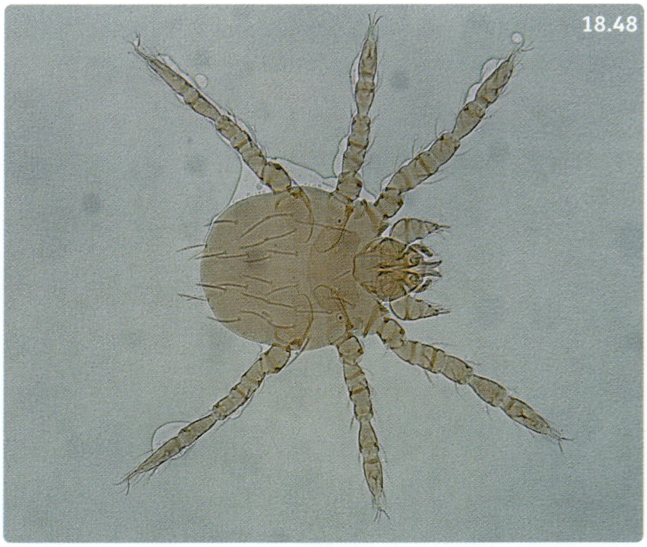

Figure 18.48 Larval stage of the chigger mite *Eutrombicula cinabaris*. (Courtesy E. Greiner and C. Welbourn)

Clinical presentation
Papules and crusts with intense or little pruritus are present in body areas in contact with the ground (feet, head, ears, ventrum). The red larvae may be noted as well.

Differential diagnosis
Insects and other causes of pruritus, AD, food hypersensitivity, allergic contact dermatitis, demodicosis, staphylococcal folliculitis, dermatophytosis.

Diagnosis
Finding the red larvae at affected areas is diagnostic. Affected animals will have a history of environmental contact, but careful examination may be necessary to find the mite larvae in thick coated pets. Microscopic examination in mineral oil will allow identification of the mites.

Management
Treatment with ectoparasiticidal sprays is effective. A short course of oral glucocorticoid can be used if pruritus is severe. Weekly or biweekly application of 0.25% fipronil spray or oral ivermectin can help prevent reinfestation in animals with continued exposure to the mites.

HYPERSENSITIVITIES

CANINE ATOPIC DERMATITIS

Definition/overview
AD results from a genetic predisposition to become sensitized to environmental allergens.

Etiology
Canine AD is a multifaceted disease due to a combination of genetic and environmental factors affecting the immune response and skin barrier function.

Pathophysiology
The pathophysiology is still unclear in animals. Defective epidermal barrier function allows environmental allergens to penetrate the skin. A decrease in transforming growth factor beta (TGFβ) could lead to a lack of tolerance to the allergens, allergen processing by Langerhans cells and activation of T helper (Th)-2 lymphocytes. Subsequent overproduction of interleukin-4 and B-cell class switching increases allergen-specific IgE. Mast cell degranulation leads to cutaneous inflammation which causes self-trauma, secondary infections, and further inflammation via Th-1 lymphocytes.

Clinical presentation
AD usually affects young adult dogs (onset at 1–3 years old), with initially a seasonal pruritus. It is important to discern the presence, intensity, and frequency of itch in the absence of infection; the aspect, distribution, and progression of cutaneous lesions; flea eradication programs; and previous treatment and effect. Pruritus (usually corticosteroid responsive) should be evident and affect one or more of the following areas: face, extensor and flexor skin surfaces, axilla, pinna, anal, or inguinal area (**Figure 18.49**).

Differential diagnosis
Sarcoptic mange, cheyletiellosis, pediculosis, contact allergic dermatitis, food hypersensitivity, flea bite hypersensitivity, *Pelodera strongyloides* dermatitis, *Malassezia* dermatitis, staphylococcal folliculitis, xerosis.

Diagnosis
Diagnosis of AD is based on compatible historical and clinical information, as well as ruling out infections, infestations, and food hypersensitivity. Secondary diseases (e.g. otitis externa/media, staphylococcal folliculitis, acute moist dermatitis, keratinization disorder, *Malassezia* dermatitis, flea bite hypersensitivity [common in dogs with AD], acral lick dermatitis [ALD], and fibropruritic nodules [noted in some dogs with flea bite hypersensitivity]) may also contribute to the pruritic threshold in the atopic patient, and these can be recurrent problems that must be continually addressed. Intradermal allergy testing (IDAT) is used to prepare allergen-specific immunotherapy (ASIT), not to diagnose AD. Serum allergy

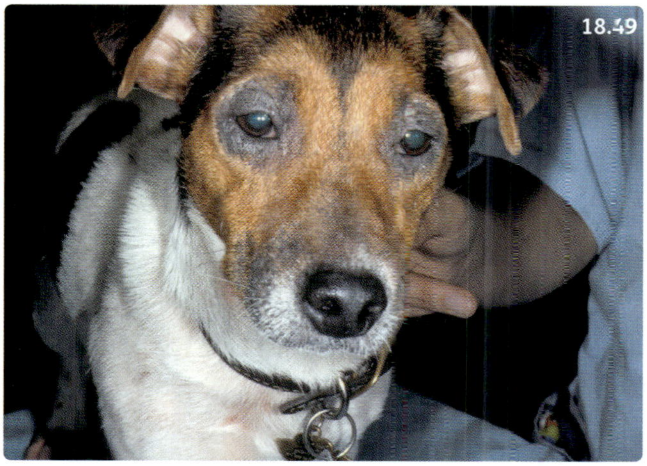

Figure 18.49 Periocular alopecia, hyperpigmentation and lichenification in a 3-year-old Jack Russell Terrier with atopic dermatitis.

testing by competent laboratories may be used if IDAT is unavailable.

Management

Allergen avoidance is difficult at best. ASIT is preferred over long-term symptomatic therapy as it is a more specific therapy, side-effects are less likely to occur, and it is the only therapy with the potential for a 'cure' in 15% of patients. Allergy symptoms tend to become year-round in many climates. Sublingual or subcutaneous ASIT based on IDAT is effective in decreasing pruritus or reducing the need for other medications in 60–80% of dogs, although results can take up to 12 months. ASIT promotes production of Treg cells and tolerance to allergens. It is ideal to begin ASIT early in the course of the disease. Serum IgE allergy testing results vary widely between and within laboratories. Ceramide application is an important aspect of skin barrier repair in people, although studies on clinical efficacy are lacking in dogs.

Symptomatic therapy includes the use of antihistamines (**Table 18.5**) and essential fatty acids (EFAs); a novel single-protein prescription or home-cooked diet; topical antipruritic therapy (colloidal oatmeal, glucocorticoid, capsaicin, pramoxine, tacrolimus); oral alternate day corticosteroids; oral pentoxifylline, cyclosporine, or oclacitinib; frequent cool water baths to remove

Table 18.5 Antihistamine therapy for dermatologic disorders.

Generic	Species	Dose (mg/kg)	Route	Interval (hours)
Amitriptyline	C	0.5–1	PO	12–24
	D	1–2	PO	12
Cetirizine	C	1 (or 5 mg/cat)	PO	12–24
	D	1 (or 10–20 mg/dog)	PO	12–24
Chlorpheniramine	C	2–4 mg/cat	PO	8–12
	D	4–8 mg/dog	PO	8–12
Clemastine	C	0.34–0.68 mg/cat	PO	12
	D	0.05–1.5	PO	12
Clomipramine	C	0.25–1	PO	12–24
	D	2–4	PO	24 or ÷ 12
Cyproheptadine	C	1–4 mg/cat	PO	12–24
	D	0.5–2	PO	8–12
Diphenhydramine	B	2–4	PO	8–12
Doxepin	C	0.5–1	PO	12–24
	D	0.5–5 (max 50 mg/dog)	PO	12
Fexofenadine	C	10–15 mg/cat	PO	12–24
	D	2–5 (up to 18)	PO	12–24
Hydroxyzine	B	2	PO	12
Loratadine	C	5 mg/cat	PO	24
	D	0.5	PO	24
Trimeprazole+prednisolone	D	1 tablet/5 kg	PO	12–24–48

D, dog; C, cat; B, dog and cat; PO, per os.

environmental allergens; as well as managing secondary staphylococcal and *Malassezia* skin or ear infections. Short-term oral oclacitinib antipruritic therapy may be especially useful to allow appropriate corticosteroid and antihistamine withdrawal prior to IDAT. Affected dogs should not be used for breeding.

FELINE ATOPIC DERMATITIS

Definition/overview

AD is an inherited predisposition to develop hypersensitivity to inhaled or percutaneously absorbed allergens.

Etiology

Feline AD results from a genetic tendency to become sensitized to environmental allergens.

Pathophysiology

Although the pathogenesis of AD is unclear in cats it has immune dysfunction similarities to canine and human AD.

Clinical presentation

Feline AD causes a variety of clinical signs. Symmetrical alopecia, miliary dermatitis, eosinophilic plaques, indolent ulcer, pruritus of the head, neck, ventral abdomen, limbs, feet, and generalized pruritus are most commonly noted (**Figure 18.50**). Onset of clinical signs usually occurs between 1 and 3 years of age and rarely before 1 year. Domestic mixed, Abyssinian, and Devon Rex breeds may be overrepresented.

Differential diagnosis

Flea bite hypersensitivity, food hypersensitivity, *Notoedres cati*, cheyletiellosis, pediculosis, *Otodectes cynotis*, biotin deficiency, EFA deficiency, intestinal parasite hypersensitivity, staphylococcal folliculitis, dermatophytosis, *Malassezia* dermatitis, demodicosis.

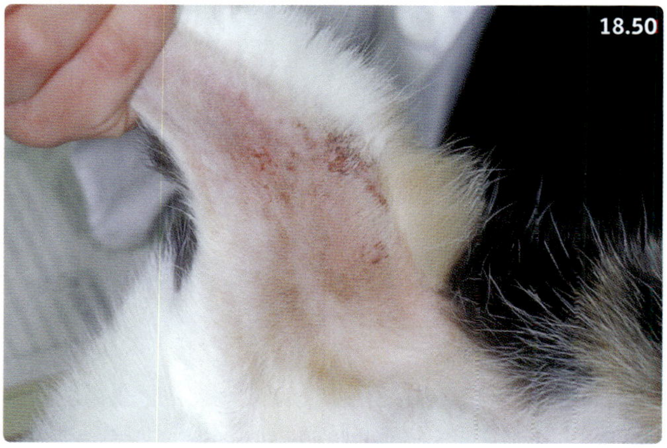

Figure 18.50 Erythema, excoriations, and alopecia in the axilla of a 4-year-old Domestic Shorthair cat with atopic dermatitis. (Case material UFVMC)

Diagnosis

As in the dog, a careful clinical history, physical examination, and ruling out of infectious and other allergic causes of pruritus assist in the diagnosis of AD in the cat. IDAT can identify allergens for oral or sublingual ASIT and the best opportunity for treatment success.

Management

EFA supplementation, antihistamines, intermittent oral or topical glucocorticoids, oral cyclosporine A, ASIT, antibiotics and antifungals to control secondary cutaneous infections, as well as enhanced flea eradication, afford an animal every opportunity to improve. Topical tacrolimus or oral pentoxifylline may be useful as well. ASIT may be beneficial in patients with asthma.

FLEA BITE HYPERSENSITIVITY

Definition/overview

Flea bite hypersensitivity is a pruritic dermatosis due to an immediate and/or delayed cell-mediated response to several proteins present in flea saliva.

Etiology

Hypersensitivity to *Ctenocephalides felis felis* is probably the most common and the most underdiagnosed cause of skin disease in dogs and cats worldwide.

Pathophysiology

An immediate type I hypersensitivity, a late phase IgE-mediated reaction, a cutaneous basophil hypersensitivity, and a delayed cell-mediated hypersensitivity may all be responsible for flea bite hypersensitivity.

Clinical presentation

Clinical signs in the dog include a papular, pruritic dermatitis of the tailhead, lumbar, perineum, hindlimb, dorsal antebrachium, or umbilical areas. Fibropruritic nodules and pyotraumatic dermatitis may be present on the dorsal and lateral trunk. In the cat, symptoms may be similar or include miliary dermatitis, symmetric alopecia, indolent ulcer, and eosinophilic plaque.

Common secondary problems include otitis externa and staphylococcal folliculitis. A vigilance for these problems, as well as enhanced flea eradication, must be maintained in order to keep pruritus below its threshold in the flea hypersensitive pet.

Differential diagnosis
Cheyletiellosis, pediculosis, sarcoptic mange, trombiculosis, staphylococcal folliculitis, ectopic *Otodectes cynotis* infestation, *Lynxacarus radovsky* infestation, dermatophytosis, food hypersensitivity.

Diagnosis
Diagnosis is achieved ultimately by resolution of symptoms with enhanced flea eradication. Improvement may be expected after 3 months. Many of the newer flea adulticides, combined with insect development inhibitors or insect growth regulators, make flea eradication quite feasible in a closed environment, although monthly administration is not sufficient. A diagnosis supportive of flea bite hypersensitivity can be made with compatible clinical signs, the presence of fleas or flea feces, recent evidence of *Dipylidium caninum*, or a positive intradermal skin or serum allergy test. Absence of fleas does not eliminate flea bite hypersensitivity as a diagnosis. Other household pets should be inspected for fleas, and inquiries made about feral cats and local wildlife that carry fleas into the environment.

Evidence of fleas will be difficult to find in the flea hypersensitive patient. An animal that displays a negative immediate intradermal allergy test (IDAT) with flea antigen may still be hypersensitive. The patient can be observed for delayed IDAT reactions in 24–48 hours. Because of the unavailability of an effective flea repellent, it is very difficult to rule out flea bite hypersensitivity as the cause of an animal's skin disease.

Management
By virtue of their constant obsessive grooming, pruritic animals remove most fleas from themselves. An adult flea survives less than 24–48 hours on an allergic animal. Even very minimal exposure to flea saliva may be sufficient to perpetuate pruritus in the hypersensitive patient. Other animals (especially cats and wildlife) as well as humans may carry adult fleas into the environment and seed the environment with pre-adult fleas, which then emerge continuously to affect the allergic pet. All animals in the environment must be included in the flea eradication plan. Topical flea products with repellent activity are required in many hypersensitive dogs. Environmental flea eradication is often necessary as well. Secondary bacterial and yeast infections must be continually identified and controlled. The judicious use of short-term topical and oral glucocorticoids can relieve intense and excessive pruritus, but larger dosages are often required with each successive flea season. Oral oclacitinib or microemulsified cyclosporine A may be beneficial in some patients with low flea numbers.

ALLERGIC CONTACT DERMATITIS

Definition/overview
Allergic contact dermatitis is a papular, macular dermatosis of sparsely haired body regions.

Etiology
The condition results from an individual predisposition to develop sensitivity to contactants.

Pathophysiology
Allergic contact dermatitis is a cell-mediated, type IV hypersensitivity reaction to percutaneous absorption of environmental or medicinal haptens (fibers, topical medications [e.g. neomycin], nickel, cement, plants [e.g. Commelinaceae], dog foods [rice flour]).

Clinical presentation
Erythematous macules and papules (**Figure 18.51**) may be present at the muzzle, ventral interdigital, perineal, pinnal, axillary, or inguinal areas depending on the nature of the offending agent. Pruritus is often marked.

Differential diagnosis
Irritant contact dermatitis, AD, food hypersensitivity, *Malassezia* dermatitis, staphylococcal folliculitis, dermatophytosis, demodicosis, scabies, insect hypersensitivity, pemphigus, hookworm dermatitis, *Pelodera* dermatitis.

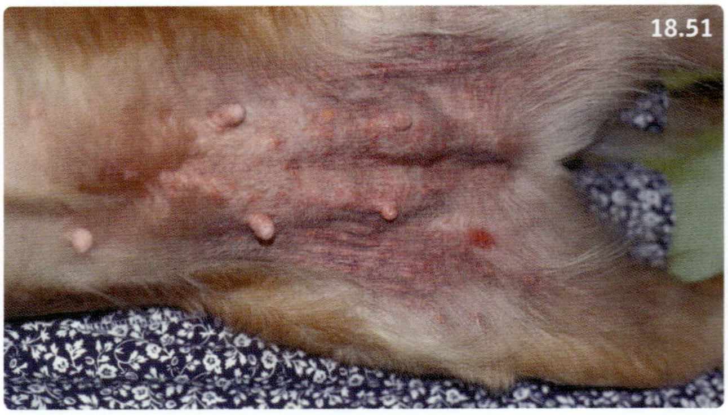

Figure 18.51 Multifocal papules and erythema on the ventral abdomen of a 5-year-old Golden Retriever with allergic contact dermatitis. (Case material UFVMC)

Diagnosis

Diagnosis is based on history, clinical signs, excluding other diseases, provocative testing, patch testing, and histopathology of lesions.

Management

The animal must be prevented from contacting the offending agent. Pentoxifylline (15–30 mg/kg PO q8h) has been useful in preventing the allergic reaction when given 48 hours prior to exposure. A favorable response can be seen with oral cyclosporine (5 mg/kg PO q24h). Corticosteroids may give symptomatic relief but usually require higher doses over time. Systemic antibiotics and antifungals may be necessary for secondary bacterial and yeast infections.

FOOD HYPERSENSITIVITY

Definition/overview

Food hypersensitivity is a nonseasonal hypersensitivity caused by a dietary substance.

Etiology

Food hypersensitivity is an abnormal immunologic response to an ingested food ingredient, flavoring, or additive.

Pathophysiology

While the pathomechanism of food hypersensitivity is not clear, complex immediate and delayed hypersensitivity reactions are incriminated. Food hypersensitivity is not usually associated with a change in diet. Most patients have been eating the offending diet for over 2 years.

Foodstuffs most commonly incriminated include: beef, dairy products, lamb, poultry products, wheat, soy, corn, rice, and eggs in dogs; and fish, dairy products, beef, and eggs in cats.

Clinical presentation

Self-trauma and secondary staphylococcal folliculitis and *Malassezia* dermatitis may be evident; however, food hypersensitivity is not always dramatically pruritic (**Figures 18.52**, **18.53**). Symptoms may mimic flea bite hypersensitivity. Otitis externa or a recurrent staphylococcal folliculitis or *Malassezia* dermatitis may be the only symptom. Cats commonly display pruritus of the head and neck (**Figure 18.54**). Pruritus may or may not be responsive to glucocorticoids. Between 19% and 35% of dogs and 21–30% of cats may have concurrent hypersensitivities including atopic, flea bite, contact, and endoparasitic dermatitis.

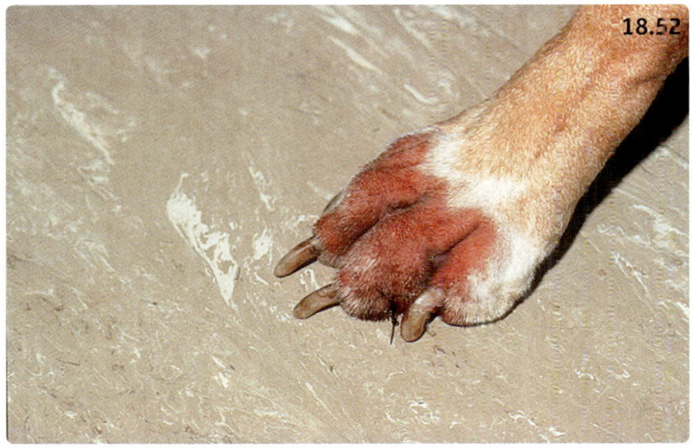

Figure 18.52 Erythematous pododermatitis in a dog with food hypersensitivity.

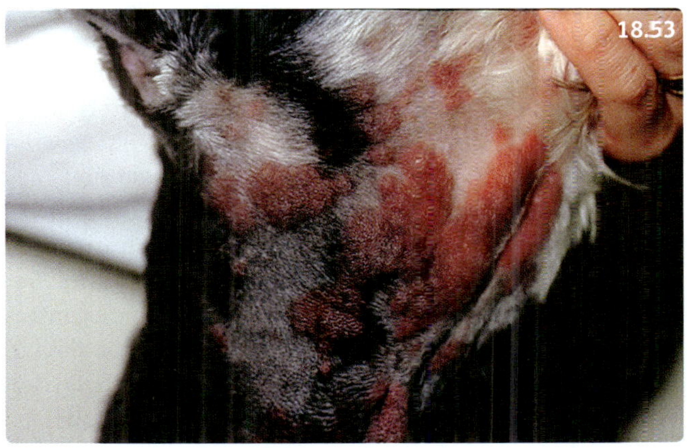

Figure 18.53 Erythematous wheals on the neck of a dog with food hypersensitivity.

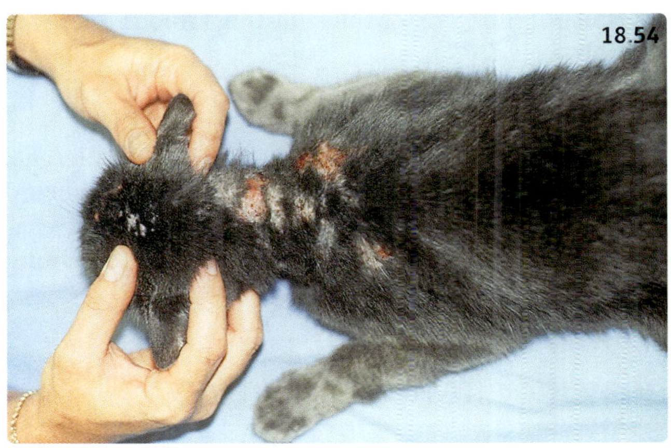

Figure 18.54 Erosions and ulceration on the dorsum of the head and neck in a Domestic Shorthair cat with food hypersensitivity. (Case material UFVMC)

Common secondary problems in food hypersensitive patients include otitis externa, keratinization disorders, anal pruritus, staphylococcal folliculitis, and *Malassezia* dermatitis.

Differential diagnosis

Dogs: flea bite hypersensitivity, cutaneous adverse drug reaction, AD, ectoparasitism, staphylococcal folliculitis, allergic contact dermatitis, defects in keratinization. Cats: flea bite hypersensitivity, cutaneous adverse drug reaction, ectoparasitism, AD, dermatophytosis, idiopathic miliary dermatitis, psychogenic alopecia, staphylococcal folliculitis, feline acne.

Diagnosis

Diagnosis can only be achieved by resolution of symptoms while the patient receives a reliable, novel protein diet (a protein and carbohydrate source that has not been fed previously) over a period of 6–12 weeks. Over-the-counter diets are not recommended due to the potential for ingredient cross-contamination. Secondary skin infections and otitis media must be appropriately identified and resolved prior to, or in the early phase of, a food trial. Nutritionally balanced home-cooked diets are ideal, as they do not contain preservatives or other additives. Treats, human food, chew toys, flavored nutritional supplements, flavored antibiotics, toothpastes, and flavored heartworm or flea preventives must be discontinued or replaced during the trial diet. Cats with access to the outdoors are unable to reliably complete a food trial. Provocation confirms the diagnosis. Animals should be challenged with their old diet and observed for 1–14 days (or longer depending on original symptom recurrence rate) for an exacerbation of symptoms (otitis, folliculitis, pruritus). Serum, hair, or saliva testing for food allergy is invalid.

Management

Management depends on identification of the allergen, as determined by provocation studies. The diet should be complete and balanced and highly digestible, containing limited antigens and none of the offending ingredient(s).

MOSQUITO BITE HYPERSENSITIVITY

Definition/overview

Mosquito bite hypersensitivity is a local hypersensitivity response of cats to mosquito bites.

Etiology

Lesions are the direct result of mosquito bites.

Pathophysiology

An underlying immediate and delayed hypersensitivity reaction to mosquito antigen results in a diffuse eosinophilic dermatitis with collagen degeneration.

Clinical presentation

Cats present with alopecic, erosive, ulcerative patches on the bridge of their nose, which may extend to the nasal planum (**Figure 18.55**). Additional lesions may be present at the lateral elbows, periorbital areas, footpads, and ear pinnae. Indoor or outdoor cats may be affected.

Differential diagnosis

Pemphigus foliaceus, pemphigus erythematosus, AD, food hypersensitivity, flea bite hypersensitivity, dermatophytosis, demodicosis, herpesvirus, squamous cell carcinoma (SCC), mast cell tumor, CLE, cryptococcosis, idiopathic eosinophilic granuloma.

Diagnosis

The history of a seasonal dermatitis, exposure to mosquitoes, and histopathology of the lesion is diagnostic.

Management

Prevention of exposure to mosquitoes is ideal. Mosquito repellents may be helpful and include pyrethrin-based

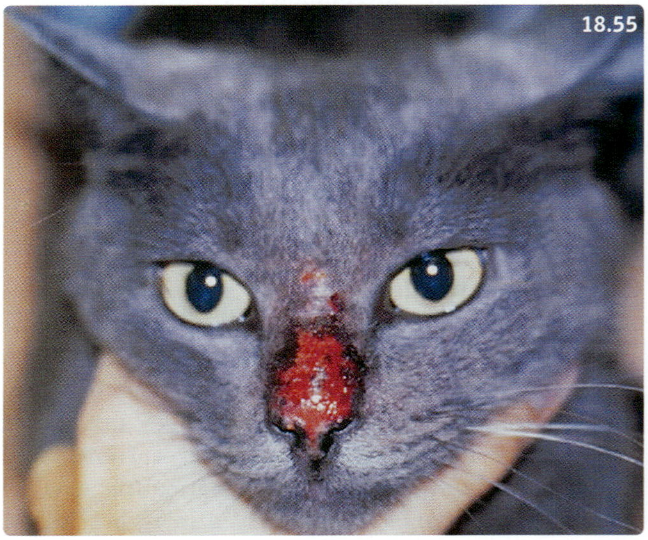

Figure 18.55 Erosions and ulceration of the nasal planum and bridge of the nose in a Domestic Shorthair cat with mosquito bite hypersensitivity.

gel or picaridin solution. Other non-DEET products must be applied several times daily (10% citronella, cedar, and lemongrass oils or 2% soybean oil). Oral or repositol corticosteroids will temporarily resolve the lesions.

CORNIFICATION DISORDERS

CANINE SEBORRHEA

Definition/overview

Canine seborrhea is a symptom of chronic disease characterized by scaliness, greasiness, and, often, inflammation of the skin. Disorder of cornification (DOC) is the preferred terminology.

Etiology

The proliferation, differentiation, or desquamation of the surface and follicular epidermis can be altered by any disease affecting the skin (secondary DOC) or it may be an inherited primary DOC.

Pathophysiology

Although incompletely understood, the inflammation is due to numerous causes: endocrinopathies (iatrogenic or endogenous); deficiency, excess, or imbalance of essential nutrients; variation in transepidermal water loss. An alteration of lipid content of skin may affect the production and maintenance of the epidermis and sebaceous glands (secondary seborrhea). Primary seborrhea is an inherited DOC (e.g. vitamin A-responsive dermatosis).

Clinical presentation

Primary DOC begins at a young age and is seen in certain breeds (American Cocker and English Springer Spaniels, Labrador Retrievers, West Highland White Terriers, German Shepherd Dogs, Basset Hounds, Dachshunds, Shar Peis, and Schnauzers). Secondary DOC begins at the age that the underlying disease begins (**Figure 18.56**).

Seborrheic dermatitis presents with greasiness and/or flakiness complicated by inflammation. Generalized or localized erythema, lichenification, hyperkeratosis, scale, and crust often affect body fold areas (lip, neck, antecubital, axillary, inguinal, interdigital, flank, anterior hock). Pruritus is usually only present with hypersensitivities and/or staphylococcal folliculitis or *Malassezia* dermatitis. Ceruminous otitis externa is common.

Differential diagnosis

Primary (inherited defect in cornification [e.g. vitamin A-responsive, ichthyosis]) vs. secondary to underlying diseases: hypersensitivities (flea, food, atopic dermatitis); external parasites (*Demodex*, *Cheyletiella*, *Sarcoptes*), leishmaniasis; endocrine (hypothyroidism, iatrogenic or endogenous hyperadrenocorticism, hyperestrogenism, hyper-/hypoandrogenism); malnutrition secondary to internal parasites; lipid abnormalities (diet, pancreatic insufficiency, liver disease, malabsorption, or other systemic disease), staphylococcal folliculitis, dermatophytosis, *Malassezia* dermatitis, excessive bathing (low or high humidity); cutaneous T-cell lymphoma, paraneoplastic syndromes.

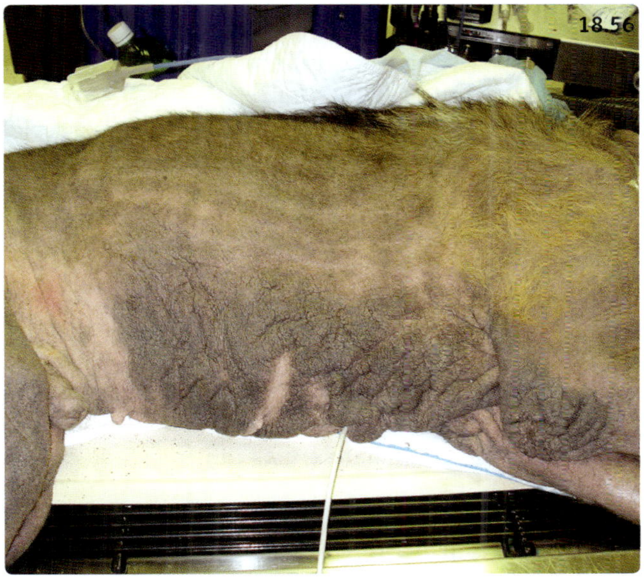

Figure 18.56 Secondary seborrhea (alopecia, hyperpigmentation, lichenification, *Malassezia* dermatitis) due to atopic dermatitis in a German Shepherd Dog. (Case material UFVMC)

Diagnosis

Diagnosis is based on breed, age of onset, and identification of, or ruling out, secondary causes of seborrhea. A skin biopsy, when infections are cleared, may reveal characteristic features of an underlying or primary disease but often may not.

Management

Identifying and correcting underlying diseases and infections are paramount. The use of degreasing, but not overly drying, shampoos or moisturizing agents, as well as necessary antimicrobial systemic and aural agents, are the mainstay of therapy and may be required for an extended period of time. Clipping the hair coat often allows more effective visualization and topical treatment of the skin.

CANINE EAR MARGIN DERMATOSIS

Definition/overview
Canine ear margin dermatosis is a common disorder of keratinization seen in Dachshunds and other breeds with pendulous ears.

Etiology
A hereditary basis is suspected.

Pathophysiology
Follicular casts adhere to the skin and hairs of the medial and lateral pinnal margins. With progression, head shaking, or scratching, the hard crusts can crack and fissure the ear tissue.

Clinical presentation
Variable alopecia, scale, crust, and keratinous debris are present at the pinnal margins (**Figure 18.57**). Pruritus is not often a symptom.

Differential diagnosis
Hypothyroidism, scabies, vasculitis.

Diagnosis
A superficial skin scraping can rule in scabies while histopathology can confirm the diagnosis and rule out vasculitis.

Management
Control may be achieved with regular lifelong use of antiseborrheic shampoos (benzoyl peroxide, sulfur, salicylic acid, and others) and moisturizers. Inflamed lesions may benefit from hydrocortisone and/or antibiotic creams or ointments.

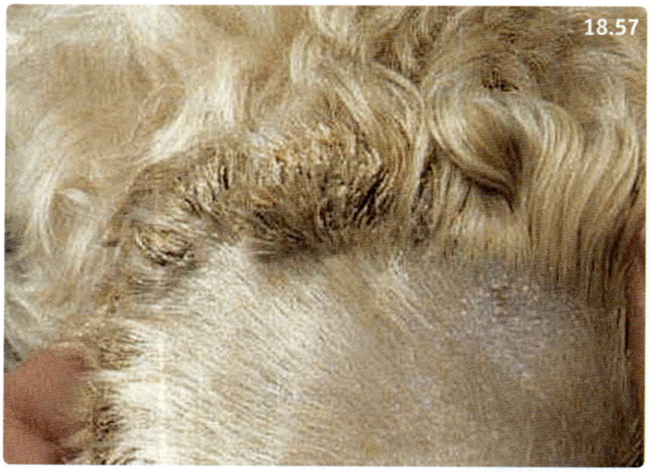

Figure 18.57 Thickened, hyperkeratotic crusts and follicular casts along the pinnal margins of a 2-year-old Cockapoo dog with ear margin dermatosis. (Courtesy R. Calvert)

NASODIGITAL HYPERKERATOSIS

Definition/overview
This condition is associated with excessive amounts of stratum corneum, confined to the planum nasale and footpads.

Etiology
Nasodigital hyperkeratosis results from an increased production, or retention, of keratinized tissue. Nasodigital hyperkeratosis in the idiopathic form occurs most commonly in old dogs.

Pathophysiology
There is increased production, or retention, of keratinized tissue as an idiopathic change or due to a variety of skin disorders.

Clinical presentation
Nasal hyperkeratosis presents as a thickened, fissured accumulation of dry, horny tissue confined to the planum nasale (**Figure 18.58**). Pedal hyperkeratosis is more variable in its presentation, often extensively affecting the cranial edges of the footpads.

Differential diagnosis
Pemphigus foliaceus, canine distemper virus or *Leishmania* infection, zinc-responsive dermatosis, generic dog food dermatosis, superficial necrolytic dermatitis (necrolytic migratory erythema), cutaneous adverse drug

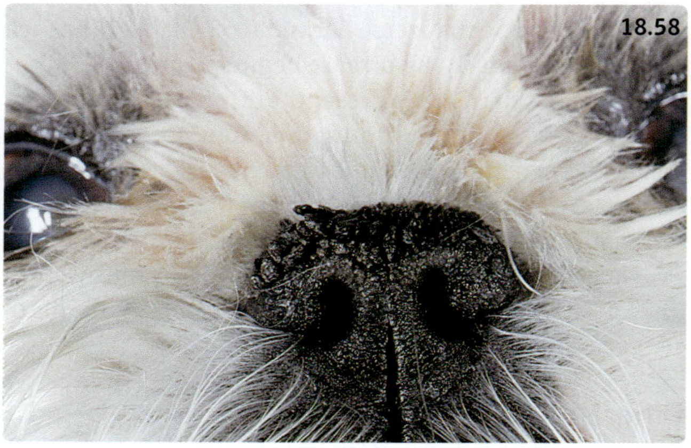

Figure 18.58 Hyperkeratosis of the nasal planum in a dog with idiopathic nasodigital hyperkeratosis. (Case material UFVMC)

reaction, systemic lupus erythematosus (SLE), cutaneous T-cell lymphoma, contact dermatitis, CLE, familial pad hyperkeratosis, papillomavirus, hereditary nasal parakeratosis of Labrador Retrievers.

Diagnosis

If the lesions occur in an old dog with no other skin or systemic problems, diagnosis can be made on clinical findings. If any other skin lesions are present or if the dog is young to middle aged, other disorders must be considered and excluded. A skin biopsy can confirm idiopathic nasodigital hyperkeratosis.

Management

Hydration and application of topical keratolytic agents (propylene glycol, salicylic acid, sodium lactate, urea, tretinoin) may improve the condition, but treatment must be lifelong. Oral synthetic retinoids and zinc supplementation may be of some benefit.

FELINE ACNE

Definition/overview

Feline acne is characterized by the formation of comedones and other lesions on the chin and perioral area.

Etiology

Multiple factors that lead to a localized keratinization defect of hair follicles and hyperplasia of the sebaceous glands may result in feline acne, or the condition may be idiopathic. Aggravating factors include poor grooming habits, a seborrheic predisposition, stress, viral influences, and immunosuppression.

Pathophysiology

Feline acne occurs relatively frequently in the cat. It is considered a disorder of keratinization that is commonly complicated by secondary bacterial or yeast infection.

Clinical presentation

Comedones on the chin, lower lip, or upper lip are early lesions of feline acne (**Figure 18.59**). Folliculitis, furunculosis, or cellulitis may develop, as evidenced by papules, pustules, bullae, and draining tracts.

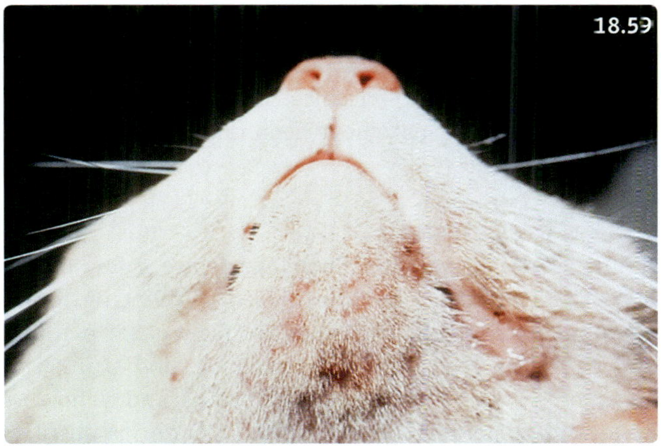

Figure 18.59 Papules, pustules, and comedones on the chin of a cat with feline acne. (Courtesy S.R. Merchant)

Differential diagnosis

Contact dermatitis, folliculitis (*Pasteurella*, β-hemolytic *Streptococcus*, *Staphylococcus*), *Malassezia* dermatitis, eosinophilic granuloma, dermatophytosis, demodicosis, trauma, AD, food hypersensitivity.

Diagnosis

Diagnosis is based on the presence of classic lesions on the chin and lips. *Demodex*, *Malassezia*, secondary bacteria, dermatophytosis, other fungi, and the chin form of eosinophilic granuloma may need to be ruled out.

Management

Treatment is lifelong and can include gentle topical application of antiseborrheic shampoos, metronidazole, clindamycin, mupirocin, vitamin A acid (isotretinoin), and systemic antibiotics. Although mupirocin can be helpful, nephrotoxicity can occur if topical mupirocin in a polyethylene glycol base is applied over large areas of the cat.

AUTOIMMUNE DISORDERS

PEMPHIGUS FOLIACEUS

Definition/overview

Pemphigus foliaceus is the most common autoimmune skin disease in the dog and cat. It is characterized by loss of keratinocyte cohesion.

Etiology

Antikeratinocyte membrane autoantibodies cause loss of adhesion between keratinocytes (acantholysis), with subsequent intraepidermal pustule formation.

Pathophysiology

Pemphigus antibody binds to antigen on the keratinocyte adhesion molecule, which hydrolyzes the adhesion molecule. Loss of intercellular cohesion results. Acantholysis and vesicle formation, followed quickly by neutrophil or eosinophil influx, yields a pustule. Genetics, topical or systemic medications, vaccines, neoplasia, and chronic hypersensitivity disease have been implicated in the disease onset.

Clinical presentation

Akitas, Chow Chows, and Dachshunds are a few of the breeds considered to be predisposed to this transiently pustular disease that starts on the face, nasal planum, and ears. The feet, clawbeds, footpads, and trunk can be involved singly or together. Erosions and yellow or honey-colored crusts are more often evident as pustules rupture easily (**Figure 18.60**). Scale, alopecia, erythema, and epidermal collarettes can be seen as well.

Differential diagnosis

Staphylococcal folliculitis, dermatophytosis, demodicosis, zinc-responsive dermatosis, SLE, dermatomyositis, cutaneous T-cell lymphoma, superficial necrolytic dermatitis (necrolytic migratory erythema), dermatophilosis, pemphigus erythematosus, CLE, cutaneous adverse drug reaction, and leishmaniasis should be considered, depending on which clinical signs predominate.

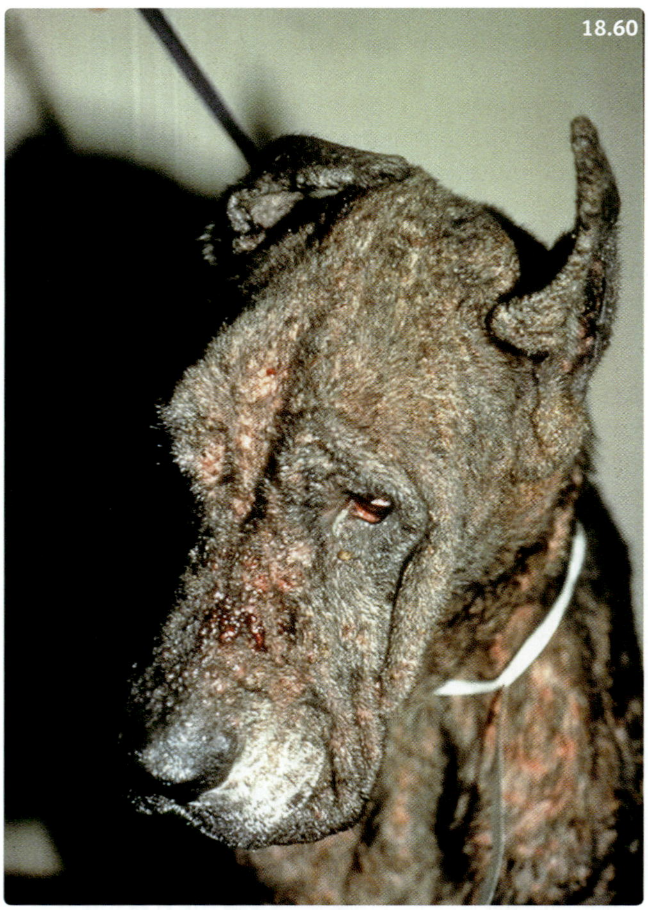

Figure 18.60 Generalized crusted papules, pustules, and draining tracts in a 2-year-old Great Dane with pemphigus foliaceus and furunculosis due to *Staphylococcus pseudointermedius*.

Diagnosis

History, physical examination, pustule cytology (see **Figure 18.27**), skin biopsy, dermatophyte culture. Staphylococcal folliculitis and dermatophytosis can mask or mimic, respectively, the histopathologic changes of pemphigus foliaceus. Many dermatologists recommend appropriate treatment for staphylococcal infection prior to biopsy to remove this potentially confusing component for the pathologist. Immunopathologic testing is not necessary for a diagnosis.

Management

The extent of treatment depends on the severity of the disease. Some patients may only require topical glucocorticoids, or tetracycline and niacinamide, but the majority require immunosuppressive doses of prednisolone, dexamethasone, or triamcinolone and either alternate day azathioprine (or mycophenolate mofetil) (dogs) or chlorambucil (cats) (**Table 18.6**). Leflunomide has been successful in otherwise difficult cases. Close monitoring of the patient for side-effects of therapy is imperative. Ten percent of patients do not respond to treatment. Animals that survive 1 year often have a good prognosis. A response to treatment should be evident after 2 weeks of immunosuppressive therapy and maintenance therapy is hopefully achieved in 4 months. Treatment is lifelong.

CUTANEOUS (DISCOID) LUPUS ERYTHEMATOSUS

Definition/overview

CLE is a benign variant of SLE, usually confined to the face.

Etiology

CLE is the second most common autoimmune skin disease of dogs. It is exacerbated by ultraviolet (UV) light.

Pathophysiology

UV light induces expression of nuclear and cytoplasmic antigens on keratinocytes. Antibodies are produced to these antigens and deposited at the basement membrane. Epidermal basal cells become damaged, leading to subepidermal vesicle formation and immune

Table 18.6 Anti-inflammatory/immunosuppressive therapy for dermatologic disorders.

Generic	Species	Dose (mg/kg)	Route	Interval (hours)
Corticosteroids				
Dexamethasone	C	0.125–1	PO	12–24
	D	0.07–0.9	PO	24 or ÷ 12
Methylprednisolone	C	2–6	PO	24
	D	0.8–1.5	PO	12–24
Prednisolone	C	1.2–6	PO	24
	D	0.5–2	PO	24
Triamcinolone	B	0.05–0.6	PO	24–72
Others				
Azathioprine	D	1.5–2.5	PO	48
Chlorambucil	B	0.1–0.2	PO	24–48
Cyclosporine A (microemulsified)	C	7	PO	24–48
	D	5	PO	24–48
Dapsone	D	1	PO	8
Interferon alpha	C	30–300	PO/SC	24
	D	20,000–1.5 MU/kg	PO/SC	24–72
Interferon gamma	D	5,000–10,000 U/kg	SC	3 times a week for 4 weeks; every 7 days for 4 weeks
Interferon omega	C	1–1.5 MU/kg	SC	24–96
	D	500 IU/15 kg	PO	24
Leflunomide	B	2–4	PO	24
Lomustine	B	50–90 mg/m2	PO	21–42 days
	C	10 mg total	PO	21–42 days
Mycophenolate mofetil	D	7–14	PO	8
Niacinamide	D	250–500 total	PO	8
Oclacitinib	D	0.4–0.6	PO	12 × 14 days, 24 subsequent
Pentoxifylline	C	100 mg total	PO	12
	D	10–30	PO	8–12
Piroxicam	D	0.3	PO	24–48
Tetracycline	D	250–500 total	PO	8

D, dog; C, cat; B, dog and cat, PO, per os; SC, subcutaneous.

complex deposition at the basement membrane zone of the epidermis. CLE may be related to exfoliative CLE (formerly German Shorthaired Pointer lupoid dermatosis), vesicular CLE (formerly ulcerative dermatosis of Shetland Sheepdogs), and symmetric lupoid onychitis.

Clinical presentation

Gray–white depigmented macules and loss of cobblestone appearance of nasal planum may be the earliest signs. Generalized nasal planum depigmentation, secondary erosion, ulceration, and crusting may ensue (**Figure 18.61**). The eyelids, lips, and ear pinnae may also be affected and, rarely, footpads and genitalia. Collies, German Shepherd Dogs, Shetland Sheepdogs, and their crosses are predisposed.

Differential diagnosis

MCP, nasal pyoderma, pemphigus foliaceus, pemphigus erythematosus, dermatomyositis, uveodermatologic syndrome, SLE, cutaneous T-cell lymphoma, cutaneous adverse drug reaction, vitiligo, contact irritant dermatitis, fungal infections.

Diagnosis

Histopathology of nonulcerated lesions after appropriate extended antibiotic treatment for MCP can aid in the diagnosis, as these two disorders are similar histopathologically. An antinuclear antibody test should be negative, although false-positive results are not uncommon from nasal planum or footpad samples. Immunopathologic testing is not necessary for a diagnosis.

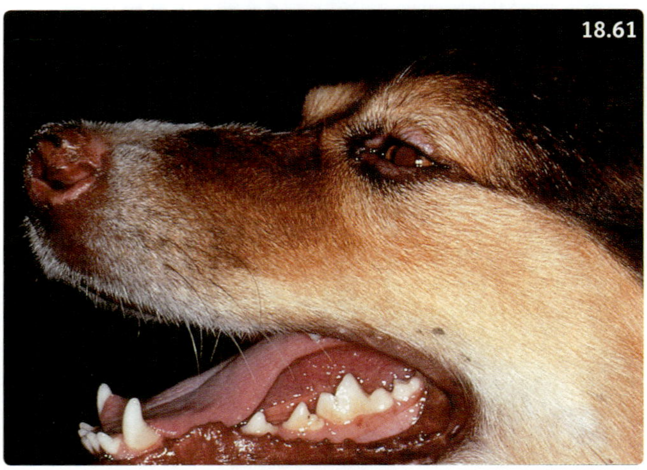

Figure 18.61 Depigmentation and erosions of the nasal planum and eyelid in an Australian Shepherd Dog with cutaneous lupus erythematosus.

Management

Extended oral antibiotic therapy for *Staphylococcus* spp. infections is usually indicated initially (**Table 18.3**). Depending on the severity of the CLE lesions, treatment can be successful with topical glucocorticoids or topical tacrolimus, applying sunscreen, and avoiding UV exposure, trial of oral tetracycline/niacinamide, and supplementing with vitamin E and EFAs. In severely ulcerated patients, systemic immunosuppression (prednisone, azathioprine) is indicated to reduce alar cartilage destruction (**Table 18.6**).

METABOLIC DISORDERS

NECROLYTIC MIGRATORY ERYTHEMA/ SUPERFICIAL NECROLYTIC DERMATITIS/ METABOLIC EPIDERMAL NECROSIS/ HEPATOCUTANEOUS SYNDROME

Definition/overview

Necrolytic migratory erythema (NME) is a rare condition in older dogs and cats associated with hepatocutaneous syndrome (HCS) or glucagonoma syndrome (GS).

Etiology

Cirrhosis, infectious or drug-induced (e.g. phenobarbital) hepatitis, hepatic or pancreatic neoplasia, or gastrointestinal disorders result in the clinical signs of NME.

Pathophysiology

While not completely understood in both HCS and GS, lesions of NME are believed to be caused by the catabolic and gluconeogenic effects of excessive glucagon and its resulting hypoaminoacidemia. Many dogs have diabetes mellitus subsequently. Hypoalbuminemia due to chronic hepatic or other disease may result in zinc and EFA deficiencies as well and contribute to symptoms of NME.

Clinical presentation

The age of onset is variable from 4–16 years old. Hyperkeratotic footpads with or without fissuring or ulceration are the most common cutaneous lesions. Erythematous, ulcerative plaques on the distal limbs, elbows, perioral, periocular, scrotal, prepuce, or perivulvar areas may also occur frequently (**Figure 18.62**). Secondary staphylococcal folliculitis and/or *Malassezia* dermatitis can be present. Lameness, lethargy, anorexia, and weight loss may be noted by owners. Polyuria and polydipsia due to diabetes mellitus can be evident.

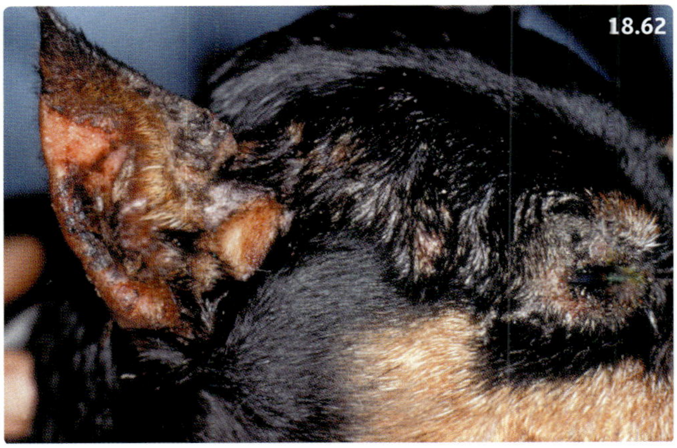

Figure 18.62 Periocular, perioral, and pinnal crusting and erosions in a 9-year-old Miniature Pinscher dog with necrolytic migratory erythema due to infectious cholangiohepatitis.

Differential diagnosis

Pemphigus foliaceus, cutaneous T-cell lymphoma, zinc responsive dermatosis, toxic epidermal necrolysis, dermatophytosis, demodicosis, contact irritant dermatitis, and SLE should be considered. Additionally, in cats, exfoliative dermatosis due to thymoma or FeLV- or FIV-associated disease must be suspected.

Diagnosis

A skin biopsy from a nonulcerated lesion will give the diagnosis of NME. The underlying cause must be uncovered by a thorough diagnostic work up, which will include a complete blood count, serum chemistry panel, urinalysis, fasting and postprandial bile acids, abdominal ultrasound, and liver biopsy or exploratory celiotomy for pancreatic neoplasia. Amino acid and glucagon profiles do not always correlate with disease severity and may be abnormal in other diseases. Immunohistochemistry of neoplastic tissue for glucagon, and other markers, can be performed.

Management

The prognosis is poor unless a correctable underlying disease is identified (**Figure 18.63**). Staphylococcal folliculitis and *Malassezia* dermatitis should be treated if present (caution with hepatic drug metabolism). Otherwise, IV administration of amino acids is the most effective treatment, although it usually only yields temporary improvement. Symptoms may improve for 3 months between treatments. A high-quality protein diet is recommended for nonencephalopathic dogs. Egg yolks (3–6 per day), zinc, EFA, and oral amino acid supplementation can be helpful. While prednisone can encourage zinc and EFA absorption, it must be considered only against the risks of its use (diabetes, infections). Topical antimicrobial shampoo therapy is indicated and can provide some temporary comfort. Appropriate medication for pain and lameness due to footpad involvement can be helpful.

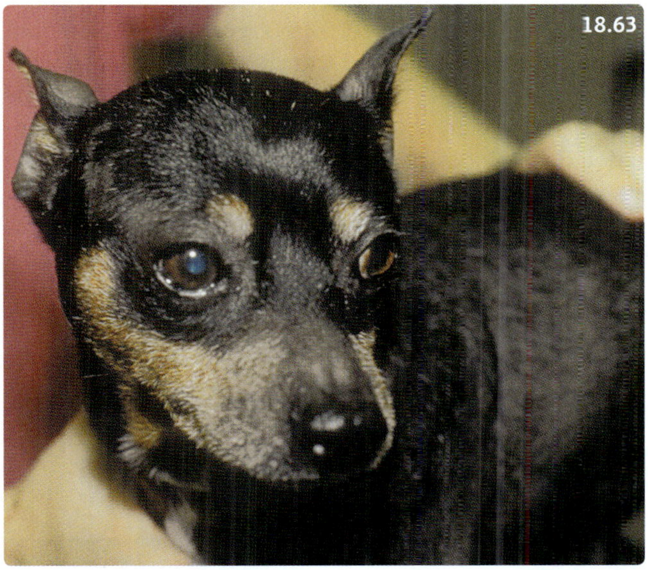

Figure 18.63 Marked improvement in cutaneous lesions of the dog in Figure 18.62 after treatment with amoxicillin/clavulanate for *E. coli* cholangiohepatitis.

PSYCHOGENIC DERMATOSES

CANINE ACRAL LICK DERMATITIS

Definition/overview

Canine ALD manifests as continued or chronic licking of a focal area on a distal extremity.

Etiology

The cause of most psychogenic dermatoses is unknown. Underlying causes of ALD include hypersensitivities (food, flea, AD), neurogenic, bacterial, *Demodex*, dermatophytosis, orthopedic conditions, and previous trauma. In many cases there is no obvious underlying physical cause and lesions may result from boredom, separation anxiety, lack of environmental stimulation, and psychic stressors (e.g. a change in the usual routine of a household member).

Pathophysiology

Canine ALD is an animal model of obsessive-compulsive disorder of humans. Constant licking over the anterior carpus or metatarsus produces a thickened, firm, oval plaque with an erosive surface (**Figure 18.64**). Boredom is often the major cause of this disease, but it is important to rule out other causes for the lesion and determine whether infection preceded the licking or was superimposed on an underlying condition.

Clinical presentation

The most common manifestation is a well-circumscribed, alopecic, erosive or ulcerative plaque that is peripherally hyperpigmented and localized to the distal limb. It is more common in large breed dogs. Several lesions may be present. Local lymphadenopathy is not evident. Purulent or serosanguineous fluid is not usually expressed by digital pressure.

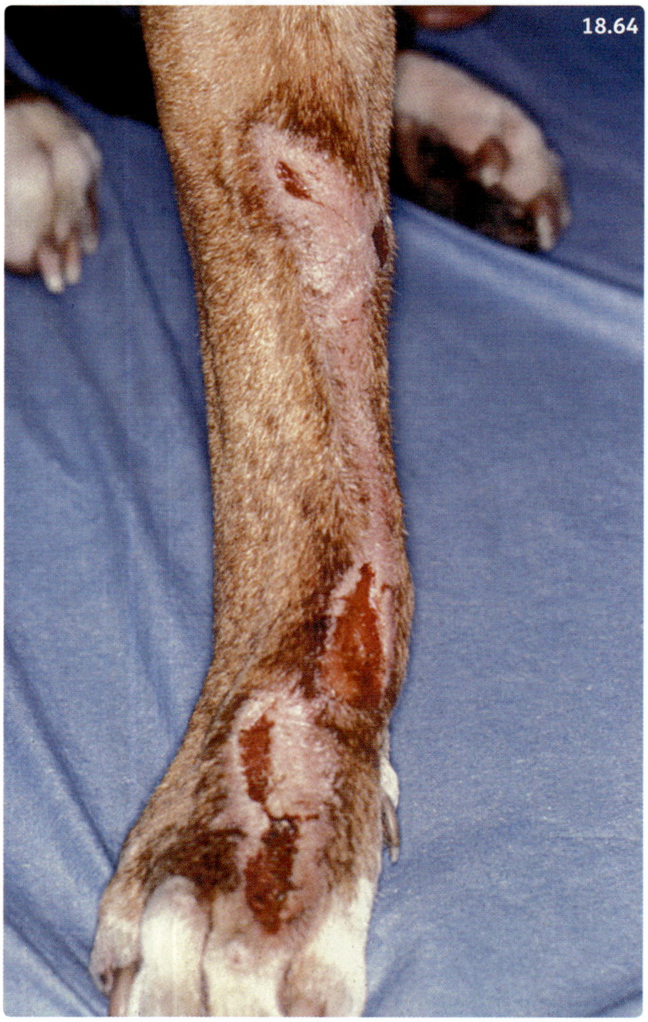

Figure 18.64 Well-demarcated alopecic and ulcerative plaques on the forelimb of a Pit Bull Terrier with anesthesia of the cutaneous branch of the radial nerve and acral lick dermatitis 9 months after being struck by a motor car. (Courtesy C.S. Foil)

Differential diagnosis

Localized folliculitis/furunculosis, demodicosis, fungal, mycobacterial, or oomycete granuloma, reaction to referred pain from underlying osteoarthroses, cutaneous neoplasia.

Diagnosis

Diagnosis is based on history and signalment, clinical signs, skin scrapings, and dermatophyte culture. Treatment should commence for staphylococcal folliculitis/furunculosis and hypersensitivities. Biopsy can be performed for histopathology, aerobic culture and sensitivity considered (**Table 18.7**), and the involved limb radiographed to rule out osteoarthritis.

Management

After skin scraping and fungal culture of the lesion, most dogs can be treated empirically for staphylococcal folliculitis/furunculosis. Because of chronic fibrotic changes in the dermis, the infection should be treated for a minimum of 8–12 weeks. If a response does not occur within 2–4 weeks, however, aerobic culture and sensitivity must be considered. The underlying cause must also be treated. Behavior modification can be used as necessary and/or an Elizabethan or similar collar or barrier. Additional options include: topical antipruritics (flucinolone/dimethyl sulfoxide, lidocaine gel followed by capsaicin); intralesional corticosteroids; systemic narcotics or narcotic antagonists; anxiolytic agents; tricyclic antidepressants; progestogens; or acupuncture.

If treatment is unsuccessful, further diagnostics are in order. However, in many of these cases a guarded prognosis is warranted.

FELINE PSYCHOGENIC ALOPECIA

Definition/overview

Feline psychogenic alopecia is an uncommon disorder that manifests as loss of hair on the limbs or trunk. Psychodermatoses may affect both crossbred and pedigree cats.

Etiology

Any change in a cat's environment may cause it to overgroom. Siamese cats may be overrepresented.

Pathophysiology

Feline psychogenic alopecia, by itself, is an uncommon cause of alopecia. More often, cats may transfer repetitive licking and self-induced hair loss caused by a pruritic stimulus such as a hypersensitivity into a psychogenic

Table 18.7 Canine acral lick dermatitis: biopsy or culture?

When to biopsy	When to culture
Unusual lesion appearance	No response to initial therapy
Unusual location	Rapid onset and progression of lesion
No response to therapy	
Rapid onset and progression of lesion	

component. In the cat, stressful stimuli are thought to release a melanocyte-stimulating hormone, which leads to increased grooming and endorphin production. Endorphins may play an addictive role in this stereotypic behavior of overgrooming.

Clinical presentation

Bilaterally symmetric alopecia or localized areas of alopecia (**Figure 18.65**) (especially on the medial forelimbs) may be evident in cats with psychogenic alopecia.

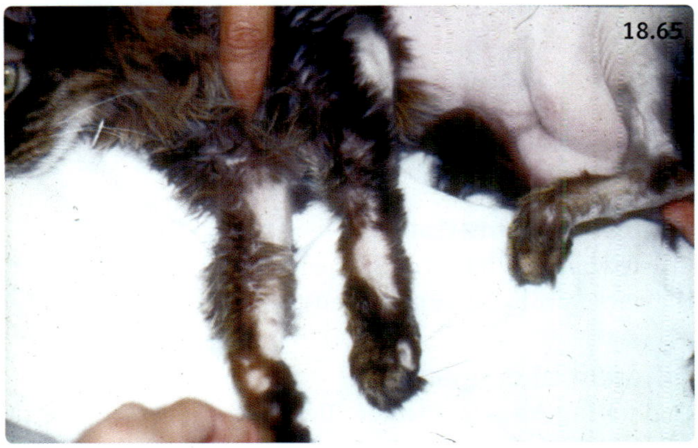

Figure 18.65 Psychogenic alopecia on the limbs and trunk of a Domestic Longhair cat. (Case material UFVMC)

Differential diagnosis

Flea bite or food hypersensitivity, demodicosis, AD, telogen defluxion secondary to internal disease, urinary tract infection, ectoparasites.

Diagnosis

Psychogenic alopecia is overdiagnosed in cats. Diagnostic investigation should include a comprehensive history (environment [indoor cats more common], presence of aggressive household companions, additions or deletions to the household), temperament of the patient (shy or nervous cats predisposed), and exclusion of underlying pruritic disorders. A minimum database should include superficial and deep skin scrapings, fecal floatation, fungal culture of hairs, acetate tape preparation cytology, complete and thorough flea eradication, food elimination diet(s), and identification of stress factors. Further ectoparasite trial therapy (*Cheyletiella*, *Otodectes*, *D. gatoi*) and a 30-day trial with an Elizabethan, or similar, collar to assess hair regrowth capability can be considered.

Management

Treatment is aimed at modifying/removing stress factors, decreasing the patient's response to stress, referral to a feline behaviorist, exercise, and owner education (mild cases). Medical therapy may reduce the cat's response to stress. Tricyclic antidepressants, tranquilizers, and narcotic antagonists have been used with varying success. A pruritic disease must always be considered and appropriately excluded.

MISCELLANEOUS DISORDERS

FELINE MILIARY DERMATITIS

Definition/overview

Feline miliary dermatitis is a cutaneous reaction pattern of small crusted, millet-sized papules caused by numerous diseases.

Etiology

Feline miliary dermatitis is not a single disease but rather a manifestation of various underlying diseases, usually allergic, the most common of which is flea bite hypersensitivity.

Pathophysiology

The lesion is a result of a focal influx of eosinophils, with subsequent serum exudation. It is a cutaneous reaction to many underlying diseases.

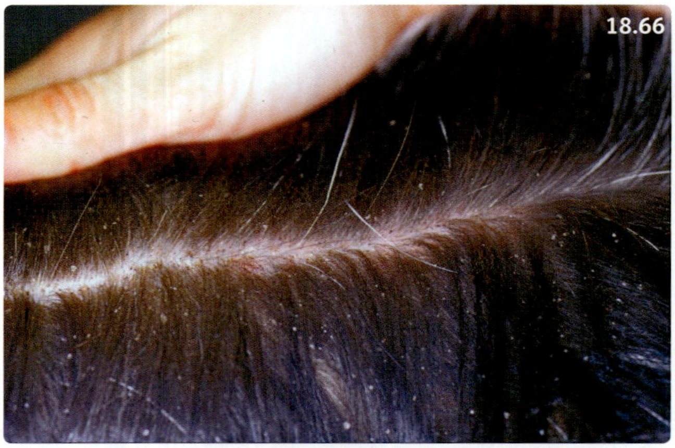

Figure 18.66 Erythematous papules and scale on the trunk of a cat with miliary dermatitis due to flea bite hypersensitivity. (Case material UFVMC)

Clinical presentation

Crusted papules (**Figure 18.66**) may be distributed around the neck, focally, or generalized on the trunk.

Differential diagnosis

Underlying causes include flea bite hypersensitivity, AD, food hypersensitivity, cutaneous adverse drug reaction, intestinal parasite hypersensitivity, *Cheyletiella*, *Otodectes*, *Notoedres*, *Demodex*, lice, chiggers, *Lynxacarus*, pemphigus foliaceus, staphylococcal folliculitis, dermatophytosis, and biotin or EFA deficiency.

Diagnosis

Diagnosis is based on a comprehensive history, physical examination, ear cytology, superficial and deep skin scrapings, fecal floatation, acetate tape preparation, complete and prolonged flea eradication, DTM culture, aerobic culture and response to antibiotics, histopathology of lesions, novel protein elimination diet, and ruling out infectious causes and hypersensitivities.

Management

Treatment is aimed at removing the primary cause. Repositol methylprednisolone (20 mg/cat q3–6 months) in patients without cardiac disease, prednisolone (2.2 mg/kg PO on alternate days), amoxicillin–clavulanate, or oral microemulsified cyclosporine A may give short-term relief while the primary cause is resolving (**Table 18.6**).

FELINE EOSINOPHILIC GRANULOMA COMPLEX

Definition/overview

The eosinophilic granuloma complex (EGC) comprises a group of cutaneous lesions in cats that are the result of underlying hypersensitivities. All forms should be diagnosed and treated similarly.

Etiology

EGC is secondary to an underlying hypersensitivity condition (flea, mosquito, food, atopic dermatitis), which may be complicated by staphylococcal or *Malassezia* colonization.

Pathophysiology

Uncontrolled recruitment of eosinophils is thought to lead to the release of potent inflammatory agents. If allowed to accumulate, these agents may initiate a local inflammatory response and collagen necrosis.

FELINE EOSINOPHILIC PLAQUE

Clinical presentation

Feline eosinophilic plaque is an intensely pruritic, well-circumscribed, ulcerated or eroded plaque often present in the inguinal, medial thigh, mucocutaneous junctions, or ventral abdominal regions (**Figure 18.67**). These lesions may be single or multiple and are associated with hypersensitivity conditions (especially flea bite hypersensitivity).

Differential diagnosis

Cutaneous neoplasia (mast cell tumor, SCC, cutaneous T-cell lymphoma), trauma, AD, food hypersensitivity, bacterial, mycobacterial, or fungal granulomas, cutaneous viral disease.

Diagnosis

Diagnosis is made on clinical signs, histopathology of the lesion to rule out neoplasia or viral disease, and an exhaustive search for underlying hypersensitivity. Ectoparasites, dermatophytosis, staphylococcal folliculitis, and *Malassezia* dermatitis should be excluded.

Management

Treatment of the underlying hypersensitivity is imperative. Intense flea eradication for a minimum period of 3 months is necessary (even in geographic regions where fleas are not considered to be prevalent). Repositol methylprednisolone acetate on two or three occasions 2 weeks apart, high doses of oral prednisolone, microemulsified cyclosporine A, or topical hydrocortisone aceponate will usually allow resolution of the lesion once the hypersensitivity is controlled. Leflunomide has been effective in otherwise poorly responsive patients (**Table 18.6**).

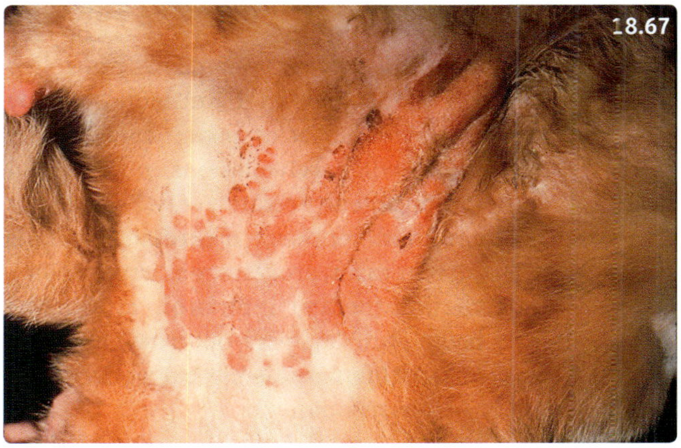

Figure 18.67 Multiple coalescing eosinophilic plaques in a Domestic Shorthair cat. (Courtesy S.R. Merchant)

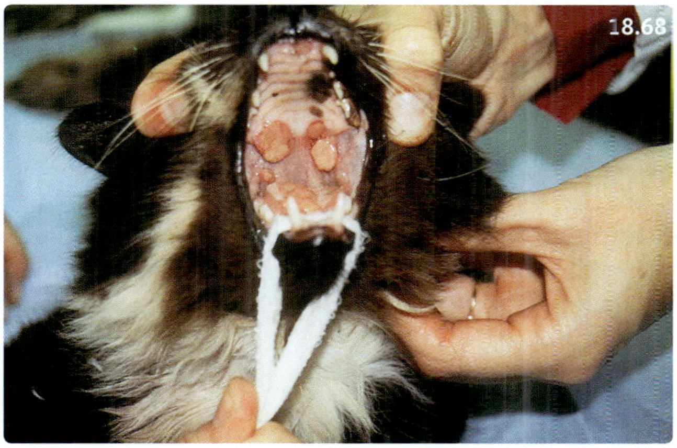

Figure 18.68 Multiple nodules on the tongue and hard and soft palates of a Domestic Longhair cat with pharyngeal granuloma and flea bite hypersensitivity.

FELINE EOSINOPHILIC GRANULOMA

Definition/overview

A clinical and histopathologic syndrome of EGC of the cat.

Etiology

A hypersensitivity reaction is suspected to be responsible.

Pathophysiology

While the exact cause is unknown, collagen degeneration with variable granulomatous inflammation occurs. Tissue collagen is considered to be an innocent bystander and not the specific target. Tissue eosinophilia is present in early lesions.

Clinical presentation

Feline eosinophilic granuloma has three clinical manifestations:

- The linear form is a firm, raised, linear lesion present on the distal hindlimb or abdomen of young cats or as ulceration with white foci of the footpads. Pruritus may or may not be evident.
- The pharyngeal form is a verrucous or smooth nodule present in the mouth or pharynx of older cats (**Figure 18.68**). It is often associated with indolent ulcer. Dysphagia or respiratory obstruction may be evident.
- The chin form is manifest as chin edema, which may wax and wane and be asymptomatic (**Figure 18.69**).

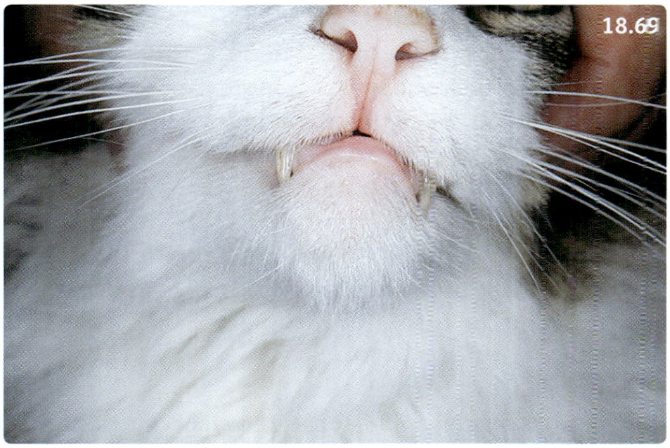

Figure 18.69 Edema of the chin in a cat with the chin form of eosinophilic granuloma. (Case material UFVMC)

Differential diagnosis

Cutaneous neoplasia (mast cell tumor, SCC, cutaneous T-cell lymphoma), staphylococcal folliculitis, bacterial or fungal granuloma, demodicosis, trauma, feline cowpox infection, AD, food hypersensitivity, plasma cell pododermatitis, sterile granuloma/pyogranuloma syndrome.

Diagnosis

Diagnosis of any of these forms is based on clinical signs and histopathology of the lesions. Ectoparasites, staphylococcal folliculitis, and dermatophytosis should be excluded.

Management

Repositol methylprednisolone acetate or oral prednisolone, triamcinolone, or dexamethasone may aid resolution of the pharyngeal and chin forms (**Table 18.6**). Intensive, lifelong flea eradication is necessary. Underlying hypersensitivity conditions must be diagnosed and controlled. Amoxicillin–clavulanate for 30 days is useful (**Table 18.3**).

FELINE INDOLENT ULCER

Definition/overview
Indolent lip ulcers are the most common of the dermatoses included in the EGC.

Etiology
A combined genetic and hypersensitivity predisposition is suspected. A heritable form of feline indolent ulcer has been described.

Pathophysiology
While the exact underlying cause is unknown, flea bite hypersensitivity and a genetic predisposition are implicated. Spontaneous improvement has been reported, as well as resolution, with complete flea eradication.

Clinical presentation
Feline indolent ulcer is a unilateral or bilateral, well-circumscribed, dish-shaped ulcer located on the upper lip, lower lip, and rarely on the skin (**Figure 18.70**). It may be associated with pharyngeal eosinophilic granuloma.

Differential diagnosis
Cutaneous neoplasia (SCC), trauma, feline cowpox, herpesvirus, calicivirus, FeLV infections, AD, food hypersensitivity, cryptococcosis.

Diagnosis
Diagnosis is made on histopathology of the lesion to rule out SCC and a search for underlying hypersensitivities. Ectoparasites and dermatophytosis should also be excluded. Acetate tape preparations for bacteria and yeast can be helpful.

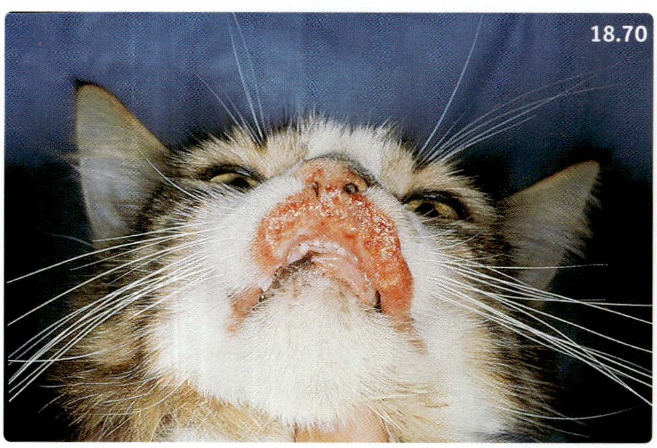

Figure 18.70 Extensive ulceration of the upper lip in a Domestic Longhair cat with an indolent ulcer due to flea bite hypersensitivity. (Case material UFVMC)

Management
The underlying hypersensitivities should be controlled with an intense flea eradication trial. Antibiotic therapy (amoxicillin with clavulanic acid, potentiated sulfonamides) for 3–6 weeks will resolve lesions in some cats. Repositol methylprednisolone acetate every 2 weeks for three treatments is often necessary if cardiac disease is not present. In resistant cases, progestagens, cryosurgery, laser surgery, radiation therapy, interferon, or immune stimulants may be helpful. Cats may 'outgrow' the disorder at 2–3 years of age. Leflunomide has been effective in otherwise poorly responsive patients.

ACTINIC DERMATITIS

Definition/overview
Actinic dermatitis is induced by solar damage to lightly or nonpigmented and sparsely haired skin.

Etiology
Actinic dermatitis is caused by chronic keratinocyte exposure to UV light.

Pathophysiology
Chronic exposure to UVA and UVB light leads to a progressive decrease in the number of Langerhans cells in the epidermis and monoclonal malignant transformation of keratinocytes. Solar irradiation may result in epidermal dysplasia, carcinoma in situ, invasive SCC, or cutaneous hemangioma and hemangiosarcoma.

Clinical presentation
The earliest clinical sign is erythema of the exposed area. Subsequently, hyperkeratosis, crust, induration, and plaques may develop on the pinnae (**Figure 18.71**),

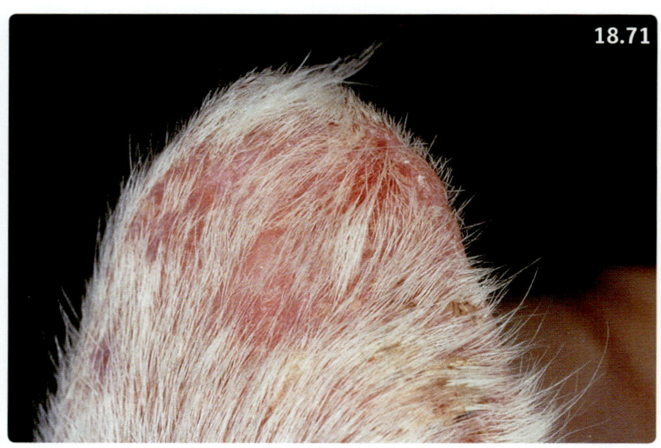

Figure 18.71 Erythema, alopecia, and crusts in a white Domestic Shorthair cat with feline solar dermatitis and actinic keratoses.

eyelids, or nose of white or lightly pigmented cats, and on the nose and abdomen (**Figure 18.72**) of lightly pigmented dogs. Dogs may develop actinic comedones and erythematous nodules, which may become secondarily infected and rupture. Invasive SCCs may develop from these premalignant actinic keratoses. With chronic solar damage, cutaneous hemangioma or hemangiosarcoma may occur.

Differential diagnosis

Dermatomyositis, uveodermatologic syndrome, cutaneous adverse drug reaction, cutaneous neoplasia, demodicosis, dermatophytosis, CLE, staphylococcal folliculitis/furunculosis, pemphigus foliaceus or erythematosus, sterile granuloma/pyogranuloma syndrome.

Diagnosis

Diagnosis is made on a history of sun exposure, the color of the affected skin of the cat or dog, and histopathology of infection-free, nonulcerated skin lesions.

Management

Affected animals must be protected (avoidance, sunscreens, UV protective body suits) from the UV radiation of the sun (including window exposure) between 9 am and 4 pm daily to slow the progression of premalignant actinic dermatitis and actinic keratoses. Surgical amputation of the pinnae prevents development of SCC in that area. CO_2 laser ablation and radiation therapy have been successful. Topical imiquimod is helpful in small superficial lesions. Other treatments that have varying success include cryosurgery, topical 5-fluorouracil (toxic to cats), oral acitretin, oral firocoxib (dogs), and hyperthermia of lesions. Waterproof, high-SPF, non-zinc sunscreen that protects against UVA and UVB should be applied 10–15 minutes before sun exposure. Because tattoo ink is deposited in the dermis, it is not photoprotective for keratinocytes. Staphylococcal folliculitis/furunculosis must be completely treated.

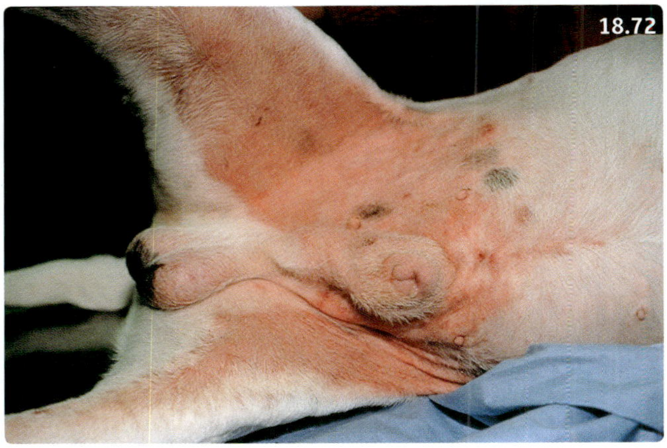

Figure 18.72 Erythematous plaques on the ventral abdomen of an 8-year-old Bull Terrier with solar dermatitis.

CANINE JUVENILE CELLULITIS/JUVENILE STERILE GRANULOMATOUS DERMATITIS AND LYMPHADENITIS (PUPPY STRANGLES)

Definition/overview

Canine juvenile cellulitis is a granulomatous condition that primarily affects the submandibular lymph nodes and the skin of the pinnae and face.

Etiology

The cause is unknown. There is, however, the possibility of both an immunologic abnormality and a hereditary component.

Pathophysiology

An underlying immune dysfunction is suspected as the cause of the condition. There is an increased occurrence in certain breeds of dogs (Dachshunds and Golden Retrievers).

Clinical presentation

Young dogs usually 3–16 weeks of age are affected. Edema and/or pustules can be present on the face, lips, pinnae (**Figure 18.73**), eyelids, prepuce, or anus. Crusts and draining tracts also occur. Lymphadenopathy, fever, depression, and joint pain are often noted. Entire litters or an adult dog may be affected.

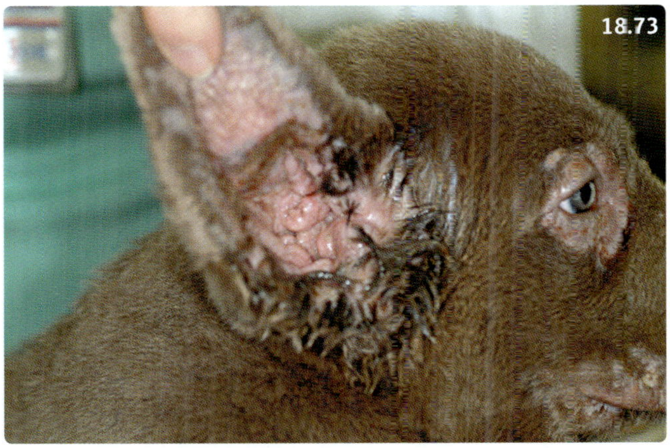

Figure 18.73 Hyperplasia, edema, and pustules of the aural canal and pinna, periocular and perioral alopecia, erosions, and crusts in a 3-month-old silver Labrador Retriever with juvenile cellulitis. (Case material UFVMC)

Differential diagnosis
Demodicosis, staphylococcal folliculitis/furunculosis, sterile granuloma/pyogranuloma syndrome, angioedema due to a reaction to an insect bite or vaccine, pemphigus foliaceus, cutaneous adverse drug reaction, dermatophytosis, causes of otitis externa.

Diagnosis
A deep skin scraping must be performed to rule out demodicosis as the etiology. Once demodicosis has been excluded, most cases can be diagnosed on clinical signs and age of onset. Cytology (pyogranulomatous inflammation with no microorganisms) and histopathology of lesions will also assist in the diagnosis.

Management
Immunosuppressive doses of oral corticosteroids, followed by a slow taper, will often resolve lesions, but in some patients lesions can recur when corticosteroids are discontinued or the dosage is reduced. Evidence of secondary bacterial infection justifies the use of appropriate antibiotics.

OTITIS EXTERNA

Definition/overview
Otitis externa is an inflammation of the epithelial lining of the external ear canal.

Etiology
Otitis externa can result from numerous causes. Predisposing factors increase the risk of otitis externa and assist primary or perpetuating factors to cause disease. Primary factors directly cause otitis externa. The most common primary factors are hypersensitivities, keratinization disorders, and *Otodectes* infestation. Primary factors must be controlled to aid in resolution of otitis externa.

Perpetuating factors prevent resolution of otitis externa and may be the major reason for poor response to treatment or recurrence regardless of the predisposing or primary causes.

Pathophysiology
Initially, the ear canal becomes swollen and erythematous. Sebaceous gland hyperplasia and apocrine gland dilatation develop, causing excessive cerumen production with altered composition. Continued inflammation can lead to permanent changes such as ear canal cartilage calcification (**Figure 18.74**), fibrosis, and occlusion of the ear canal.

Clinical presentation
Otitis media has been found to be present in 80–85% of dogs with chronic otitis externa. Erythema, hyperpigmentation, and lichenification may be present on the pinna and external ear canal to varying degrees. Pain, pruritus, odor, and exudate are often evident (**Figure 18.75**). Ear canal cartilage may not be pliable on palpation.

Differential diagnosis
Foreign bodies, *Otodectes cynotis*, bacterial and/or yeast infections, defects in keratinization, autoimmune diseases, food hypersensitivity, AD, hypothyroidism, hyperadrenocorticism, juvenile cellulitis.

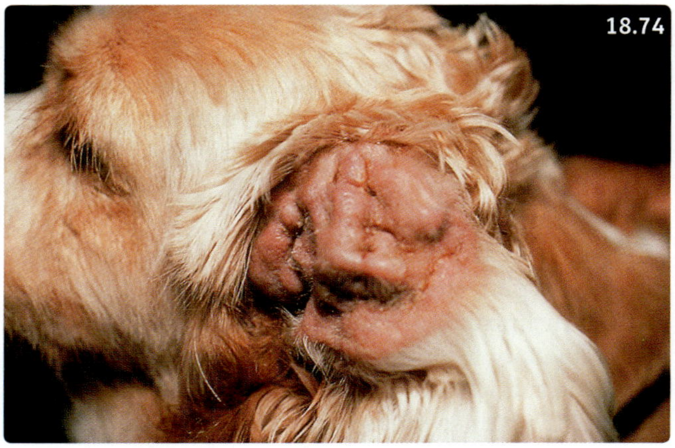

Figure 18.74 Severe aural canal hyperproliferation with aural cartilage calcification in an 8-year-old Cocker Spaniel with end-stage otitis externa and otitis media due to food hypersensitivity.

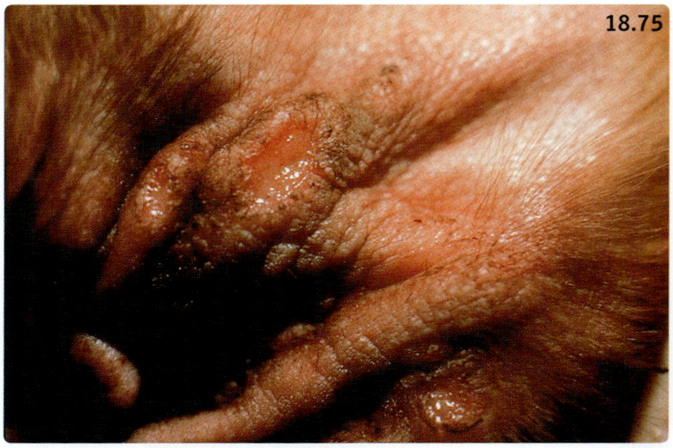

Figure 18.75 Aural ulcers of the vertical canal and pinna due to *Malassezia pachydermatis* in a 4-year-old Golden Retriever with atopic dermatitis.

Diagnosis
A thorough search for underlying causes is warranted. Ear cytology is useful for selecting topical medications in early cases. Normal radiographs of the tympanic bullae do not rule out otitis media. CT (fine bony detail) or MRI (soft tissue detail) yield better results for imaging the ear. Otoscopic examination may enhance the suspicion of otitis media if an abnormal tympanic membrane, or no tympanic membrane, is visualized. Pain on palpation of the bullae, recurrent otitis externa, or evidence of neurologic abnormalities may further one's suspicions of otitis media.

Management
Treatment of otitis externa and otitis media is aimed at removing exudate, using topical antimicrobials and systemic antimicrobials (if otitis externa is severe and in all cases of otitis media) based on cytology and/or culture and sensitivity from the appropriate areas of the ear canal for an appropriate length of time (6–8 weeks for otitis media). Surgery (usually total ear canal ablation with lateral bulla osteotomy) is indicated to alleviate stenosis of the ear canal, remove tumors or polyps, and to manage medically resistant otitis media such as that associated with mineralized ear canals. Surgery does not replace a thorough search for predisposing and primary factors. If these factors are not identified and controlled, treatment will be a failure and recurrence must be expected.

SEBACEOUS ADENITIS

Definition/overview
Sebaceous adenitis is an uncommon idiopathic scaling and alopecic dermatosis of dogs and cats caused by sebaceous gland destruction.

Etiology
An autosomal recessive mode of inheritance is suspected for the Standard Poodle and Akita, although the exact etiology is uncertain.

Pathophysiology
A heritable inflammatory destruction of sebaceous glands results in the absence of sebum and subsequent scaling and follicular plugging. Young adult to middle aged dogs are affected.

Clinical presentation
Two syndromes exist:

- In longhaired breeds (Standard Poodles, Samoyeds, and Akitas), bilaterally symmetrical follicular casts, hyperkeratosis, and silvery scale on the dorsal muzzle, head, ears, neck, and thorax predominate. Secondary staphylococcal folliculitis and furunculosis may be evident. Otitis externa is common.
- In shortcoated breeds such as Vizslas, nodules and alopecic, annular, scaling plaques develop (**Figure 18.76**).

In both syndromes pruritus is not usually a complaint unless staphylococcal folliculitis is present. Any breed of dog can be affected with sebaceous adenitis.

Differential diagnosis
Primary seborrhea, ichthyosis, vitamin A responsive dermatosis, demodicosis, dermatophytosis, staphylococcal folliculitis/furunculosis, hypothyroidism, follicular dysplasia.

Diagnosis
Multiple skin specimens from scaly areas without alopecia are best to document active sebaceous gland inflammation on histopathology.

Management
Response to treatment varies with the breed of animal and severity of disease. Control may be achieved in mild cases with keratolytic shampoos and emollient rinses. Daily application of 75% propylene glycol in water until improvement is seen may be effective, although labor intensive. Poodles have improved with daily then weekly mineral bath oil soaks followed by shampooing. Oral cyclosporine A, vitamin A, isotretinoin, or acitretin are more often used. A response may be seen after 4–8 weeks of therapy. Affected animals should not be used for breeding.

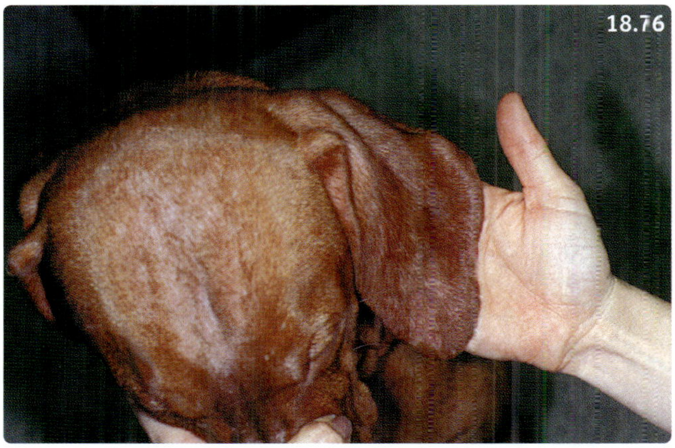

Figure 18.76 Irregular, patchy alopecia with variable erythema on the head and pinna of a 3-year-old Vizsla with sebaceous adenitis. (Case material UFVMC)

OVERVIEW OF SELECTED SKIN TUMORS

CUTANEOUS T-CELL (EPITHELIOTROPIC) LYMPHOMA

Definition/overview

Cutaneous T-cell lymphoma is a cutaneous neoplasia characterized by the presence of epitheliotropic T lymphocytes.

Etiology

Clones of CD8+ T lymphocytes infiltrate the epithelium of the epidermis, hair follicles, apocrine glands, and oral mucosa.

Pathophysiology

Malignant transformation of one or several clones of epitheliotropic T lymphocytes occurs, with subsequent infiltration into the epidermis, dermis, and oral mucosa.

Clinical presentation

Cutaneous T-cell lymphoma generally occurs in older dogs and, occasionally, in cats. Depigmentation of the nasal planum, muzzle, lips, and eyelids may be noted (**Figure 18.77**). Gingivitis may be the earliest sign. Excessive scale, erythema, ulcerations, and nodules occur later in the disease.

Differential diagnosis

Dermatophytosis, keratinization disorders, dental disease, staphylococcal folliculitis, cheyletiellosis, regressing histiocytoma.

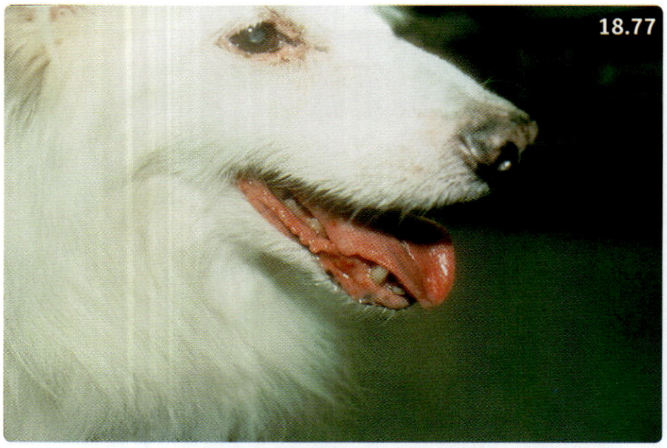

Figure 18.77 Depigmentation of the eyelids, nasal planum, and lips, as well as loss of cobblestone architecture of nasal planum and oral erosions, in a 9-year-old Spitz with cutaneous T-cell lymphoma.

Diagnosis

Histopathology of nonulcerated lesions containing epidermis is usually diagnostic (**Table 18.8**).

Management

Excision of solitary lesions may be curative. Chemotherapeutic protocols with lomustine or leflunomide may prolong survival. Responses have been observed in a few patients who have failed lomustine therapy using oral cyclophosphamide, vincristine, doxorubicin, and prednisone. In general, the prognosis is extremely poor as most patients are diagnosed late in the disease process. Early diagnosis and treatment may yield better results.

HISTIOCYTOMA

Definition/overview

Histiocytoma is a tumor originating from a CD34+ progenitor cell of the Langerhans or dendritic cell system.

Etiology

It is a common, benign neoplasm of young dogs and, rarely, of cats, with an unknown cause. Histiocytoma may be a reactive hyperplasia rather than a true neoplasm.

Clinical presentation

Usually solitary nodules on the head, pinnae, or extremities. May be multiple in some patients and may involve draining lymph nodes or spread internally in rare cases. Histiocytomas are usually small, firm, button- or dome-shaped (**Figure 18.78**), well-circumscribed, and occasionally ulcerated.

Differential diagnosis

Cutaneous reactive histiocytosis, any cutaneous neoplasm, dermatophytic kerion.

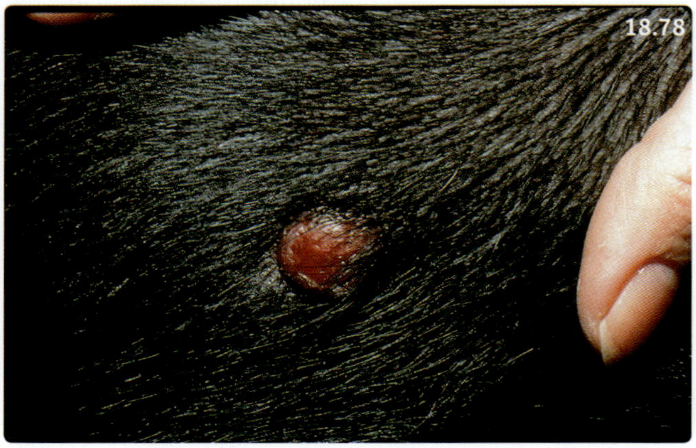

Figure 18.78 Alopecic, slightly erosive, raised, flat (button-shaped) nodule of histiocytoma in a Labrador Retriever.

Table 18.8 Common neoplastic and non-neoplastic skin tumors of the dog and cat.

Tumor	Characteristic lesion	Location	Diagnosis	Treatment
Squamous cell carcinoma	Erosion, ulceration, plaque	Ear, nose, trunk, clawbed	Histopathology	Sx, C, R, I
Mast cell tumor	Nodule	Any	Histopathology, cytology	Sx, R, C, CCS, H1, H2, H, D
Sebaceous adenoma	Nodule (wart-like)	Trunk, head	Histopathology	Sx, vitamin A
Cutaneous T-cell lymphoma	Depigmentation, erosion, ulceration, plaque, nodule, gingivitis	Oral cavity, trunk	Histopathology	CCS, Le, Lo, CHOP, Sx, R
Histiocytoma	Nodule	Foot, face, trunk	Histopathology, cytology	None
Fibropruritic nodule	Nodule	Rump	Histopathology	Flea eradication
Perianal gland adenoma	Nodule	Perianal region	Histopathology, cytology	Sx, neuter

Sx, surgical excision; C, cryosurgery; R, radiation; CCS, corticosteroids; H1, H1 blocker; H2, H2 blocker; H, hyperthermia; D, deionized water; I, imiquimod; Le, leflunomide; Lo, lomustine; CHOP, cyclophosphamide, doxorubicin, vincristine, prednisone.

Diagnosis

The age of the patient (young) and the location (head or distal extremities) and appearance of the nodule (button-like) usually give a high index of suspicion. Subsequent regression or histologic examination confirms the diagnosis (**Table 18.8**). Intraepithelial tumor cells may be noted on histology and confused with cutaneous T-cell lymphoma. The presence of lymphocytes within the nodule signals regression.

Management

Most of these tumors regress on their own in 2–8 weeks. Surgical excision is usually curative. Immunosuppression is contraindicated.

MAST CELL TUMOR

Definition/overview

Mast cell tumors (MCTs) are common cutaneous neoplasms in dogs and cats that originate from dermal mast cells.

Etiology/pathophysiology

The etiology of mast cell neoplasia is unknown, although experimental transmission has been successful in dogs. Mast cells may release numerous vasoactive amines, most notably histamine and heparin, which elicit paraneoplastic effects of gastric ulceration and coagulopathies. Palpation of lesions may result in release of amines and local edema, inflammation, and flushing.

Clinical presentation

While MCTs are more common in older dogs, they can occur at any age. Predisposed breeds include Boxers, Boston Terriers, English Bulldogs, Labrador Retrievers, and Shar Peis. MCTs are usually solitary, but they may be multicentric. The trunk, extremities (**Figure 18.79**), then the head are predilection sites for dogs. Multiple histiocytic MCTs have been described in Siamese kittens and cutaneous mastocytosis has occurred in puppies. In cats (**Figure 18.80**), lesions more often occur on the head and neck in older cats, with males and Siamese cats predisposed. Tumors may be soft or firm, large or small, plaque or nodule, generally alopecic or occasionally pin-feathered (see **Figure 18.6**).

Differential diagnosis

Histiocytoma, lipoma, SCC, fungal or bacterial granuloma, other cutaneous neoplasm.

Diagnosis

Impression smears or aspirates may give a tentative diagnosis. Anaplastic and histiocytic mast cells may not contain distinctive granules and histologic examination would be necessary (**Table 18.8**). MCTs may be confused with other round cell tumors or eosinophilic plaques.

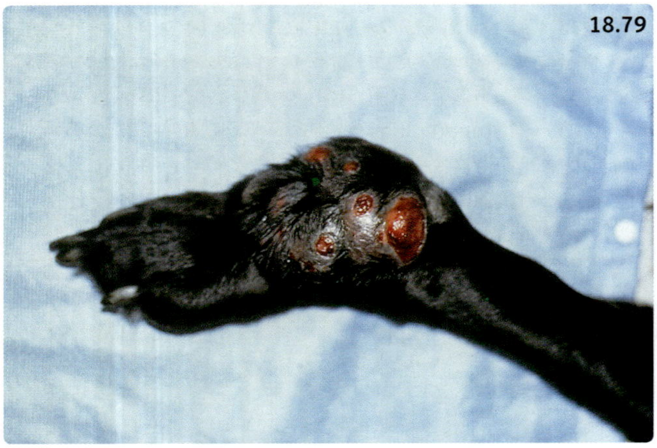

Figure 18.79 Ulcerative, alopecic nodule on the carpus of a 9-year-old Labrador Retriever with a mast cell tumor. (Case material UFVMC)

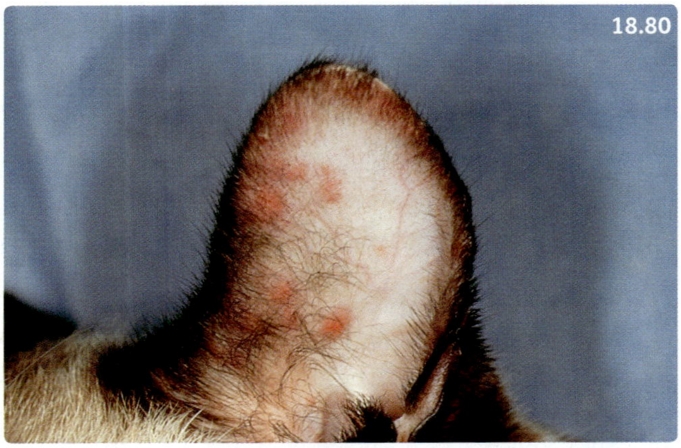

Figure 18.80 Erythematous papules and nodules on the pinna of a 1-year-old Siamese cat due to a mast cell tumor.

Special stains may be employed to stain the metachromatic granules, although less well-differentiated tumors require histochemical markers for diagnosis. Determination of local and systemic involvement should then be done (regional lymph nodes, spleen, liver, mesenteric lymph nodes, other cutaneous sites, bone marrow).

Management

A combination of wide surgical excision, cryosurgery, chemotherapy, external beam megavoltage radiotherapy, or immunotherapy is employed, as well as oral histamine blocking agents. Metastasis to regional lymph nodes, spleen, liver, and bone marrow occurs in 50% of dogs. Tumors arising from the perineum or genitalia, digits, and mucocutaneous sites are more commonly aggressive.

Well-differentiated MCTs often have a better prognosis, but all tumors should be considered potentially malignant. Mast cells may be found in lymph node and bone marrow aspirates and buffy coat smears from normal dogs and dogs with hypersensitivities or ectoparasites. Histopathology of draining lymph nodes is recommended.

H1 and H2 blockers and prednisone are recommended to counteract the effects of histamine and other vasoactive amines. Glucocorticoid drugs may reduce swelling preoperatively, so wide (at least 2 cm margins and one fascial plane) surgical excision might be more readily achieved. Further therapy using lomustine, prednisone, and vinblastine is predicated on presence of metastasis.

PAPILLOMATOSIS

(see also Chapter 21: Infectious diseases, Dogs)

Definition/overview

Papillomas are common cutaneous epidermal neoplasms (warts) caused by papillomaviruses.

Etiology

At least 15 types of papillomaviruses have been identified in dogs; these are site and tissue specific. The viruses are environmentally stable for up to 2 months. Viral proteins interfere with control of cell proliferation, thus inducing cell growth.

Pathophysiology

Papillomaviruses are transmitted by direct contact and fomites to damaged skin. Papillomaviruses may also be responsible for certain types of SCC in dogs and cats. Glucocorticoids and immunosuppression cause recrudescence of latent infections. Solitary papillomas of cats may not be caused by papillomaviruses, although two types of papillomaviruses do occur in cats.

Clinical presentation

Five syndromes exist in dogs:

- Canine oral papillomatosis affects the oral cavity, face, and eyes of young dogs, with papules that progress to fronding hyperkeratotic nodules (**Figure 18.81**).
- Cutaneous papillomas affect the head, eyelids, and feet of older Cocker Spaniels and Kerry Blue Terriers. They are pedunculated, fronded, alopecic masses (<0.5 cm).
- Cutaneous inverted papillomas occur on the ventral abdomen and groin of young adult dogs (**Figure 18.82**). These firm, raised nodules have a central pore opening to the skin.

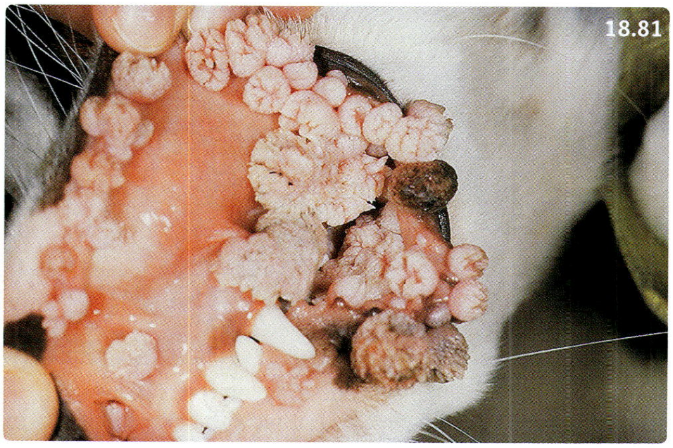

Figure 18.81 Multiple, exophytic, verrucous nodules in a 4-month-old Llewelyn Setter with oral and cutaneous papillomatosis. (Case material UFVMC)

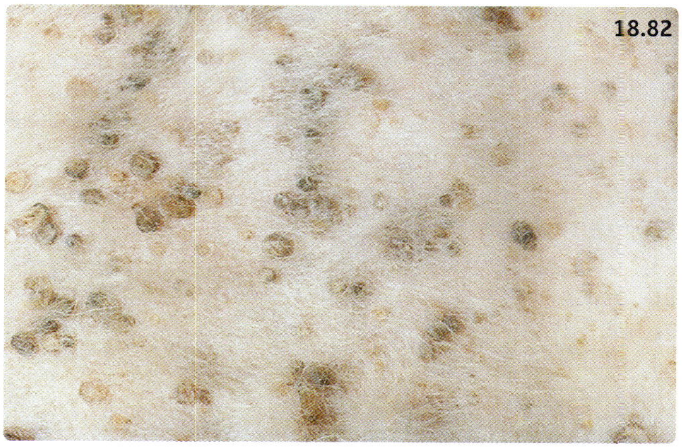

Figure 18.82 Multiple, variably hyperpigmented, hyperkeratotic nodules on the trunk of a Poodle with endophytic squamous papillomas. (Case material UFVMC)

- Multiple pigmented, papular, cutaneous papillomas were reported from the ventrum of an adult Boxer receiving glucocorticoids long term. Regression occurred after the glucocorticoids were discontinued.
- Multiple pigmented plaques have occurred in Miniature Schnauzers and Pugs as an autosomal dominant pattern (pigmented epidermal nevi). Lesions consisted of melanotic macules and plaques. These are precursors to Bowen's disease (multicentric SCC in situ).

Multiple viral papillomas occur in cats on the head, neck, dorsal thorax, ventral abdomen, and proximal limbs. They begin as melanotic macules, then plaques, which become scaly and seborrheic. Oral lesions on the dorsal tongue may occur in 6–9-month-old kittens. These are pink, soft plaques.

Differential diagnosis

Dogs: infundibular keratinizing acanthoma, cutaneous horn, lentigo, melanoma, sebaceous gland adenoma. Cats: cutaneous horn, melanoma, dilated pore (of Winer), mast cell tumor.

Diagnosis

Diagnosis may be made on history and clinical appearance and confirmed on histology of the lesion. Cutaneous horns may overlie papillomas. Sebaceous adenoma and sebaceous hyperplasia are commonly clinically misdiagnosed as papillomas.

Management

Cellular immunity is responsible for papilloma regression. Vaccines may be effective in prevention, but they have no therapeutic benefit. SCCs can arise at injection sites. Regression often occurs in 3–5 months and correlates with a strong antibody response. Cryo- or electrosurgery, or CO_2 laser ablation may give relief from large, foul-smelling lesions that interfere with mastication.

SQUAMOUS CELL CARCINOMA

Definition/overview

SCCs are common malignant neoplasms of keratinocytes in dogs and cats.

Etiology/pathophysiology

Although not clear, the etiology of SCC may be solar induction or, rarely, associated with previous severe damage to the epidermis in the form of thermal injury, frostbite, or chronic infections. Multicentric SCCs in situ (Bowen's disease) of cats may contain papillomavirus antigen.

Clinical presentation

In dogs, proliferative or ulcerative lesions occur on the trunk, digits, and face. Cutaneous horns may develop on ulcerative lesions. Dogs that sunbathe may have multiple lesions on the ventral trunk. Dogs with white, short hair coats on the ventrum have the highest incidence of solar-induced SCC. Subungual SCC (clawbed) usually affects a single digit and causes pain, swelling, exudate and loss of, or misshapen, claw. Subungual SCC more often affects black-coated breeds of dogs.

In cats, actinic damage accounts for the majority of tumors, as white cats are at increased risk of SCC. Common sites for the ulcerative or erosive lesions include the external nares, pinnae, eyelids, and lips (**Figure 18.83**).

Multicentric SCCs in situ are not actinic and are seen in older cats and dogs. Lesions occur in darkly

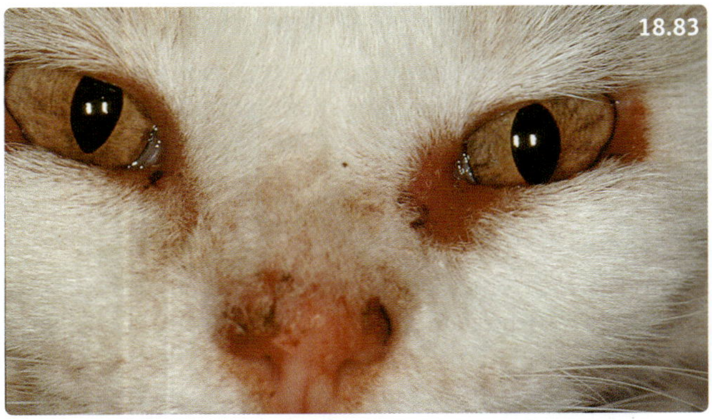

Figure 18.83 Erosions and ulcerations of the eyelids and nares with patchy alopecia of the nasal bridge of a white Domestic Shorthair cat with squamous cell carcinoma.

pigmented skin. Melanotic, hyperkeratotic macules and plaques may be verrucous.

Differential diagnosis

Various neoplastic, infectious, granulomatous disorders.

Diagnosis

While cytology may yield a presumptive diagnosis, definitive diagnosis can be made on histopathology (**Table 18.8**). Clawbed or lip lesions may be mistaken for paronychia or indolent ulcer, respectively.

Management

SCCs are generally locally invasive and slow to metastasize. However, subungual SCCs are more aggressive and 22% metastasize to regional lymph nodes. Early diagnosis and aggressive surgical amputation are imperative. Pinnectomy and nosectomy, cryosurgery, noninvasive brachytherapy, hyperthermia, photodynamic therapy, and laser therapy are viable options for SCC.

Multicentric SCCs in situ in cats usually respond to CO_2 laser therapy or topical 5% imiquimod cream. Synthetic oral retinoids have yielded variable responses. Piroxicam and firocoxib have also been used.

SELECTED DERMATOSES OF DOGS AND CATS

RAPIDLY GROWING (OPPORTUNISTIC OR ATYPICAL) MYCOBACTERIA

Characteristic lesion

Nodule(s), purpuric macules, draining tract (**Figure 18.84**).

Location

Inguinal, lumbar.

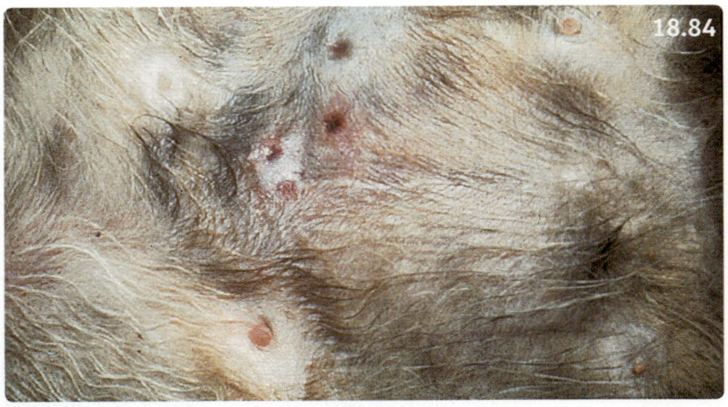

Figure 18.84 Punctate ulcers and draining tracts in the abdominal and inguinal regions of a cat with panniculitis due to opportunistic mycobacteriosis (*M. fortuitum*).

Diagnosis

Biopsy and mycobacterial tissue culture (including panniculus), mycobacterial speciation, and sensitivity.

STERILE NODULAR PANNICULITIS

Characteristic lesion

Nodule, draining tract, or ulcer in area of panniculus (**Figure 18.85**).

Location

Trunk.

Diagnosis

Biopsy, aerobic, anaerobic, mycobacterial, fungal tissue cultures (include panniculus).

CALCINOSIS CUTIS

Characteristic lesion

Erythematous plaque (**Figure 18.86**) or coalescing (white) papules with pruritus.

Location

Inguinal, dorsal neck, axillae.

Diagnosis

Biopsy, history of cortisone use.

FELINE IDIOPATHIC ULCERATIVE DERMATOSIS

Characteristic lesion

Ulcer (**Figure 18.87**).

Location

Dorsal neck and shoulders.

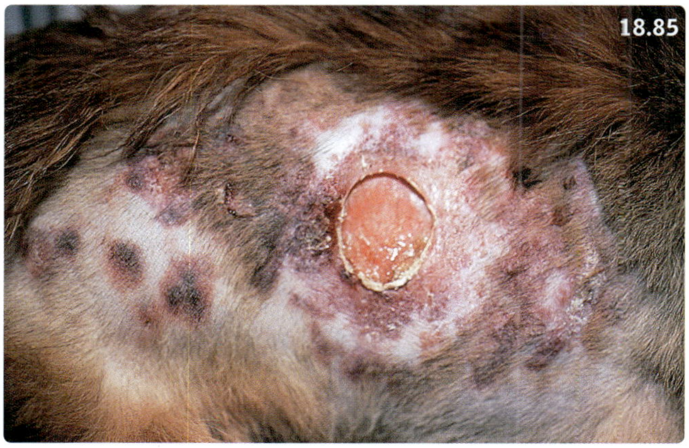

Figure 18.85 Purpuric nodules and ulceration in a 1-year-old Pomeranian with sterile nodular panniculitis. (Courtesy S.R. Merchant)

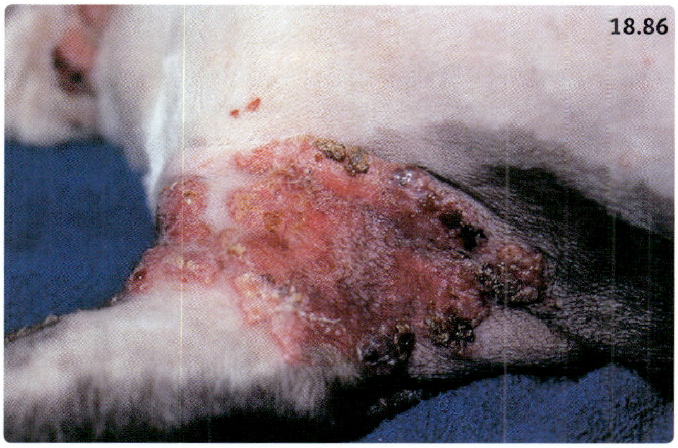

Figure 18.86 Erythematous, firm plaque of calcinosis cutis in a 10-year-old female spayed Boston Terrier with iatrogenic hyperadrenocorticism. (Case material UFVMC)

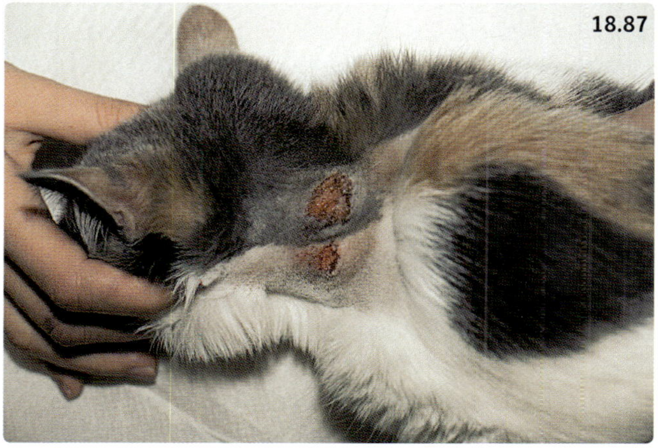

Figure 18.87 Ulcers on the dorsal neck of a cat with feline idiopathic ulcerative dermatosis.

Diagnosis
Biopsy; rule out food hypersensitivity, injection reaction SCC, panniculitis, contact irritant, burn.

PLASMA CELL PODODERMATITIS

Characteristic lesion
Swelling, deflation, erosion, or ulceration (**Figure 18.88**).

Location
Footpads.

Diagnosis
Biopsy.

DERMATOMYOSITIS/ISCHEMIC DERMATOPATHY

Characteristic lesion
Scarring alopecia (**Figure 18.89**).

Location
Pressure points, ear tips, tail tip, bridge of nose.

Diagnosis
Biopsy (skin and muscle), electromyography.

POST-RABIES VACCINE PANNICULITIS

Characteristic lesion
Alopecia, hyperpigmentation (**Figure 18.90**).

Location
Site of prior subcutaneous rabies vaccine.

Diagnosis
Biopsy; include panniculus.

CUTANEOUS ADVERSE DRUG REACTION

Characteristic lesion
Any lesion type, erythematous plaque, macule, papule, pustule, erosion, ulceration, urticaria, angioedema, vasculitis, lichenoid. (**Figure 18.91**).

Location
Inguinal, dorsal neck, face, any location.

Diagnosis
Biopsy, history of any type of medication use (including nutraceuticals and/or herbal products)

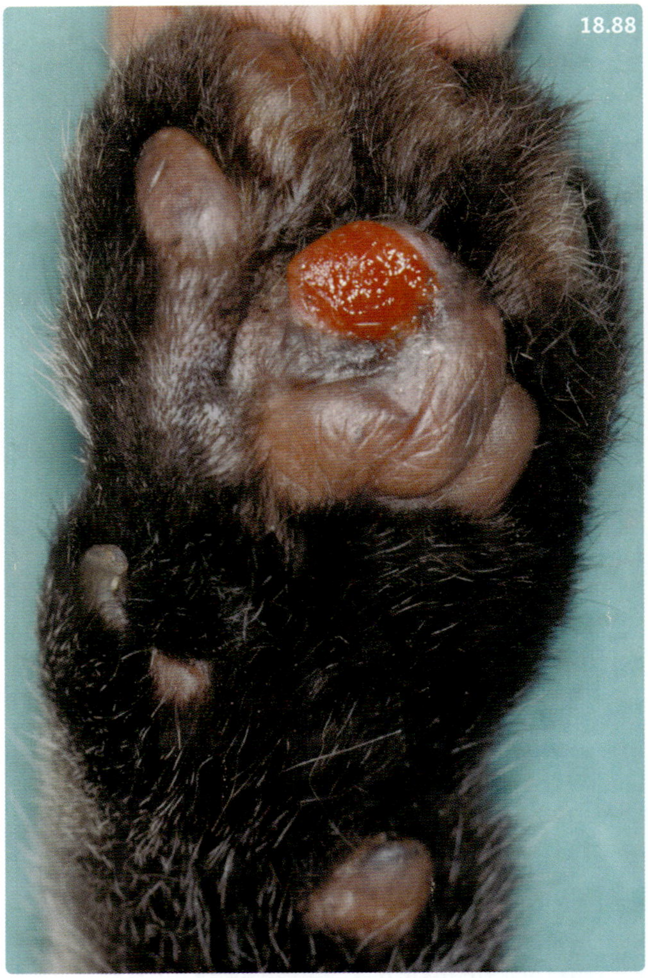

Figure 18.88 Ulcer and deflation of the metacarpal footpad in a cat with plasma cell pododermatitis.

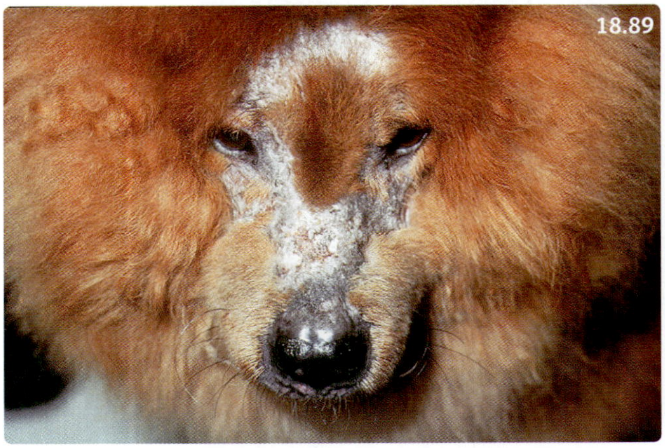

Figure 18.89 Symmetrical scarring alopecia, scale, and hyperpigmentation in a Chow Chow with dermatomyositis.

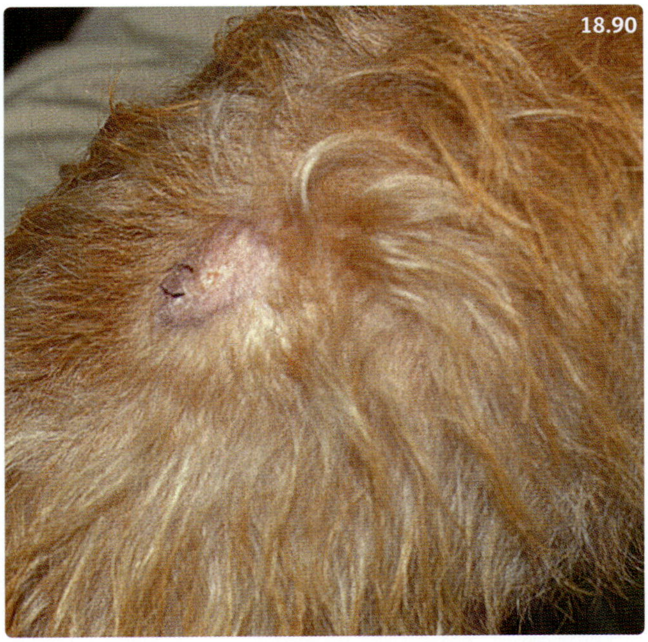

Figure 18.90 Patch of alopecia and hyperpigmentation in an 8-month-old Terrier mix with post-rabies vaccine panniculitis.

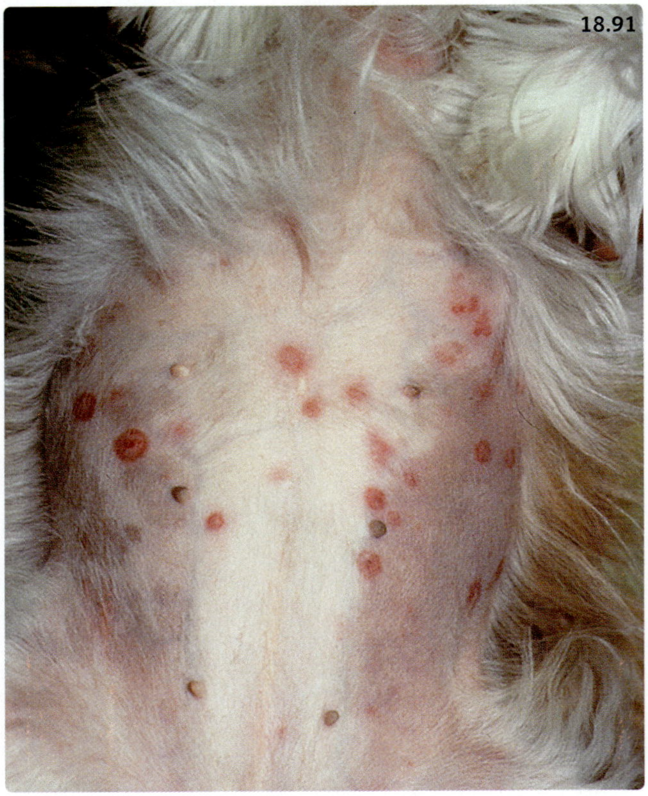

Figure 18.91 Erythematous macules in a 4-year-old female Shih Tzu with a cutaneous drug reaction to cephalexin.

VASCULITIS

Characteristic lesion

Ulceration (**Figure 18.92**).

Location

Pinnae, footpads, philtrum, tail, claws, elbow, lips

Diagnosis

Biopsy, history, breed, diascopy, body region, dermatologic examination, search for underlying causes (drugs, vaccines, food, insect, vector-borne, lupus, idiopathic).

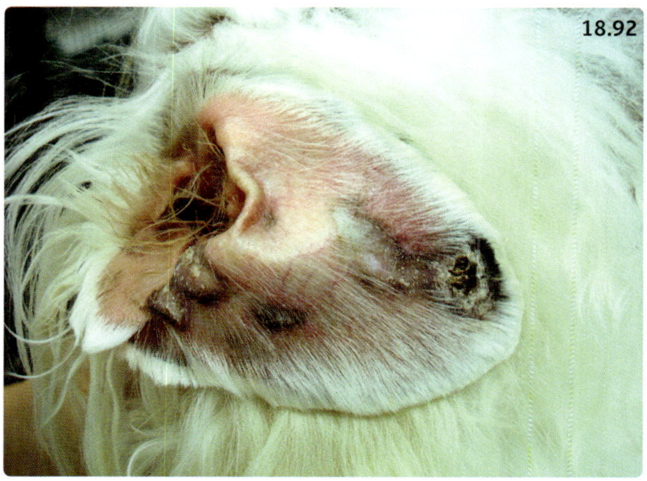

Figure 18.92 Chronic lesions in a dog with pinnal vasculitis: ear tip necrosis, circular to linear scarring, alopecia, and hyperpigmentation. (Case material UFVMC)

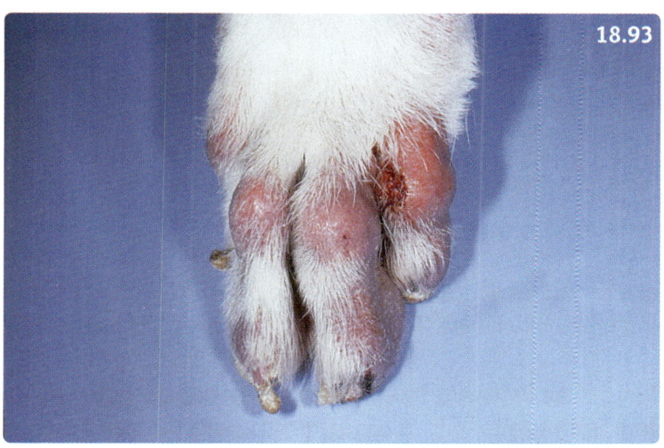

Figure 18.93 Onychodystrophy and onychomadesis of multiple claws with erythematous, alopecic, ulcerative pododermatitis in a mixed-breed dog with symmetric lupoid onychitis.

LUPOID ONYCHITIS

Characteristic lesion

Onychomadesis, onychorrhexis, erythematous, alopecic ulcerative dermatitis (**Figure 18.93**).

Location

Claws and surrounding skin.

Diagnosis

Cytology of clawbeds, aerobic culture and sensitivity, fungal culture of claw or tissue, biopsy of claw, food elimination diets.

RECOMMENDED FURTHER READING

Gold RM, Patterson AP, Lawhon SD (2013) Understanding methicillin resistance in staphylococci isolated from dogs with pyoderma. *J Am Vet Med Assoc* **243:**817–824.

Greene CE (2012) *Infectious Diseases of the Dog and Cat*, 4th edn. Elsevier Saunders, St. Louis.

Gross TL, Ihrke PH, Walder EJ *et al.* (2005) (eds.) *Skin Diseases of the Dog and Cat: Clinical and Histopathological Diagnosis*, 2nd edn. Blackwell Science, Oxford.

Jackson H, Marsella R (2012) *BSAVA Manual of Canine and Feline Dermatology*, 3rd edn. British Small Animal Veterinary Association, Gloucester.

Koch SN, Torres SMF, Plumb DC (2012) *Canine and Feline Dermatology Drug Handbook*. Wiley-Blackwell, Ames.

Marsella R, Sousa CA, Gonzales AJ *et al.* (2012) Current understanding of the pathophysiologic mechanisms of canine atopic dermatitis. *J Am Vet Med Assoc* **241:**194–207

Miller WH, Griffin CE, Campbell KL (2013) *Muller & Kirk's Small Animal Dermatology*, 7th edn. Elsevier Saunders, St. Louis.

Mueller RS, Bensignor E, Ferrer L *et al.* (2012) Treatment of demodicosis in dogs: 2011 Clinical Practice Guidelines. *Vet Dermatol* **23:**86–96.

Chapter 19

Ocular manifestations of systemic diseases

Dennis E. Brooks & Megan L. Sullivan

INTRODUCTION

Ophthalmic examination of animals with systemic disease is an important diagnostic method of categorizing and differentiating systemic disease processes. Infectious, neoplastic, autoimmune, nutritional, toxic, and metabolic diseases may all have early and prominent ocular manifestations. Visual status may also be important to owners attempting to decide how aggressively they wish to pursue diagnostic and therapeutic options in the treatment of systemic diseases.

BACTERIAL INFECTIONS

(See also Chapter 21: Infectious diseases.)

BACTEREMIA

Definition/overview

Bacteremia due to *Staphylococcus* spp., *Streptococcus* spp., *Escherichia coli*, and other bacteria can cause anterior or posterior uveitis, endophthalmitis, chorioretinitis, and optic neuritis. The ocular disease occurs from inflammation of the tissue from seeding of the iris, ciliary body, or choroid with bacteria. Bacterial embolization occurs in pyometra, prostatitis, pancreatitis, bacterial endocarditis, periodontal disease, and salmonellosis, or as an immune-mediated phenomenon associated with circulating antigen–antibody complexes (chronic inflammatory disease processes). Bacterial meningitis can be associated with ocular signs.

LEPTOSPIROSIS

Definition/overview

Dogs with leptospirosis may have conjunctival hemorrhages, icterus, and hyphema and signs of anterior uveitis due to an immunologic reaction and/or direct infection of the uvea. Leptospirosis causes mild or inapparent ophthalmic signs in cats. It is considered a zoonotic disease. The penicillin class of drugs and doxycycline effectively treat this condition.

BRUCELLOSIS

Definition/overview

Brucella canis in dogs causes ophthalmic signs of recurrent corneal edema, anterior uveitis, chorioretinitis, optic neuritis, endophthalmitis, and secondary glaucoma. The organism can be cultured from aqueous and vitreous, and titers detected in serum and aqueous humor. It is a zoonotic disease diagnosed by bacteriologic culturing. Systemic therapy with oral tetracycline and intramuscular streptomycin is recommended, although relapses can occur.

LYME DISEASE

Definition/overview

Borreliosis (Lyme disease), caused by the spirochete *Borrelia burgdorferi*, is transmitted by the tick *Ixodes dammini*. It is associated with orbital disease, conjunctivitis, corneal edema, anterior uveitis, retinal petechiae, chorioretinitis, and retinal detachment (RD) in dogs. Systemic doxycycline is the antibiotic of choice for borreliosis.

CLOSTRIDIAL DISEASE

Definition/overview

Clostridium botulinum type C in dogs, due to ingestion of the bacterium in contaminated food, causes systemic muscular weakness and mydriasis. *Clostridium tetani* infects skin wounds and releases a potent neurotoxin, which is associated with nictitans protrusion in dogs and cats, and a unique smiling/sneering appearance in cats due to spasm of the facial musculature. Dogs and cats are not as easily infected as other species such as horses, humans, and sheep, but they certainly can become infected with tetanus.

BARTONELLOSIS

Definition/overview

Bartonella henselae is the causative agent for human 'cat scratch disease'. *Bartonella vinsonii (berkhoffii)* and *B. clarridgeiae* and *B. elixbethae* cause naturally occurring disease in dogs and cats, with *B. henselae*, *B. koehlerae*, and *B. weissii* also infecting cats, and are considered emerging zoonotic agents. These gram-negative, intracellular rods cause blepharitis, conjunctivitis, anterior uveitis (**Figures 19.1, 19.2**), hyphema, and RD due to vascular hypertension. Chorioretinitis in cats and dogs also occurs. Lymphadenopathy and conjunctival ulceration may be present. The infection is flea related in cats and tick related in dogs, and has a high incidence in hot and humid climates. The bacteria adhere to and penetrate red cells, thus making every organ system vulnerable to hematogenous spread. Treatment of systemic bartonellosis in dogs and cats involves the use of systemic antibiotics such as azithromycin, enrofloxacin, or doxycycline for several weeks.

MYCOPLASMA

Definition/overview

Mycoplasma spp. are considered a rare cause of conjunctivitis in cats. They are also isolated from normal cats.

Etiology

Mycoplasma felis, *M. gatae*, and *M. arginini* are a cause of conjunctivitis in catteries and research colonies where stress may contribute to disease. *Mycoplasma canadense*, *M. cynos*, *M. lipophilum*, and *M. hyopharyngis* are also reported. The disease is not self-limiting in all cases.

Pathophysiology

Conjunctival cytology reveals a predominantly neutrophilic response. *Mycoplasma* organisms are coccoid or coccobacillary basophilic clusters found in focus at the level of the cell membrane. Herpesvirus infection may predispose to mycoplasmal conjunctivitis.

Clinical presentation

Initially, conjunctivitis may be unilateral, with the opposite eye usually becoming affected in 7–14 days. Early in the disease the ocular discharge is serous, with chemosis, hyperemia, and blepharospasm also present. With time, the exudate increases, becoming mucopurulent and the chemosis more severe. The thick exudate may adhere to the conjunctiva and appear as a pseudomembrane. The nictitans may become hyperemic and swollen, and protrude. Papillary hypertrophy of the conjunctiva may occur.

Differential diagnosis

Conjunctivitis is found in many types of eye diseases. It may be infectious (herpes, calicivirus, *Mycoplasma*, and *Chlamydia* in cats) or noninfectious. It may be primary or be secondary to ulcerative keratitis, episcleritis, glaucoma, anterior uveitis, eyelid disease (entropion,

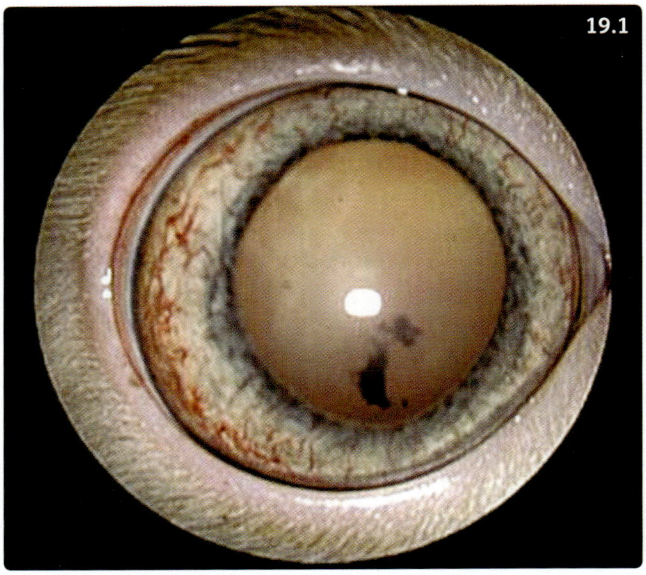

Figure 19.1 Rubeosis iridis, corneal haze, lens opacity, and pigment on the lens capsule in the eye of a cat with bartonellosis. The pupil is dilated from topically administered atropine.

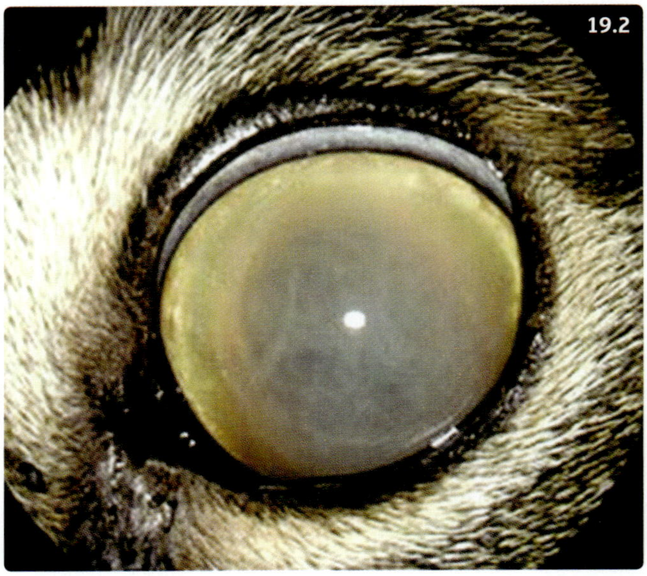

Figure 19.2 Fibrin in the anterior chamber obscures the pupil in this cat with bartonellosis.

ectropion, blepharitis), orbital cellulitis, nasolacrimal duct obstruction, keratoconjunctivitis sicca (KCS), atopy, environmental irritation, and neoplasia (lymphoma).

Diagnosis

A red eye with no other findings tends to be the basis on which conjunctivitis is diagnosed. The *Mycoplasma* organisms can be cultured or the diagnosis made based on finding the characteristic cytologic inclusions.

Management

Treatment of conjunctivitis due to *M. felis* consists of application of topical antibiotic ophthalmic ointment for several weeks. Effective antibiotics include tetracycline and chloramphenicol.

VIRAL INFECTIONS

(See also Chapter 21: Infectious diseases.)

FELINE CALICIVIRUS

Definition/overview

Calicivirus conjunctivitis is suspected when conjunctivitis accompanies oral ulcers in cats. The calicivirus is not as pathogenic to the conjunctiva as feline herpesvirus (FHV). Specific topical antiviral preparations are not available for viruses other than herpesvirus.

RABIES

Definition/overview

Rabies in dogs and cats may show as pupillary dilation, uveitis, slowed palpebral and corneal reflexes, and photophobia due to neurologic dysfunction.

CANINE HERPESVIRUS

Definition/overview

Dogs infected with canine herpesvirus may have a transient bilateral conjunctivitis, panuveitis, dendritic ulcerative keratitis, cataracts, and optic neuritis progressing to optic nerve atrophy. Retinal dysplasia may be found in infected pups. Therapy for dogs with corneal ulcers utilizes antiviral medications.

CANINE DISTEMPER VIRUS

Definition/overview

Ocular signs have been observed in animals with acute and chronic infection with canine distemper virus (CDV).

Etiology

Canine distemper is caused by a large RNA morbillivirus. The virus is spread mainly by inhalation of aerosolized respiratory viral particles or other infected secretions such as urine. Widespread vaccination of dogs has markedly decreased the incidence of canine distemper. It can also generate an immune response in cats.

Clinical presentation

Clinical signs of CDV infection can vary with the age and immune status of the dog and the strain of the virus. CDV infection has systemic features ranging from mild to severe coughing, dyspnea, lethargy, anorexia, vomiting, diarrhea, and central nervous system (CNS) signs. Ocular signs include serous to mucopurulent bilateral ocular discharge, chorioretinitis, RD, KCS (**Figures 19.3–19.8**) (which may last 4–8 weeks or be permanent), corneal ulcers, optic neuritis (sudden blindness), and cortical blindness. Chronic retinochoroidopathies are seen as areas of increased tapetal reflectivity (gold-medallion lesions) and altered pigmentation in tapetal and non-tapetal fundic areas. Perivascular cuffing of retinal vessels and axonal demyelination are present histologically.

Differential diagnosis

Tables 19.1–19.3.

Diagnosis

Conjunctival scrapings reveal mononuclear leukocytes and giant cells initially, then neutrophils. Intracellular inclusion bodies in conjunctival epithelial cells may be noted. Immunofluorescence of conjunctival smears may be positive 5–10 days post infection, although the virus disappears 21–28 days post infection.

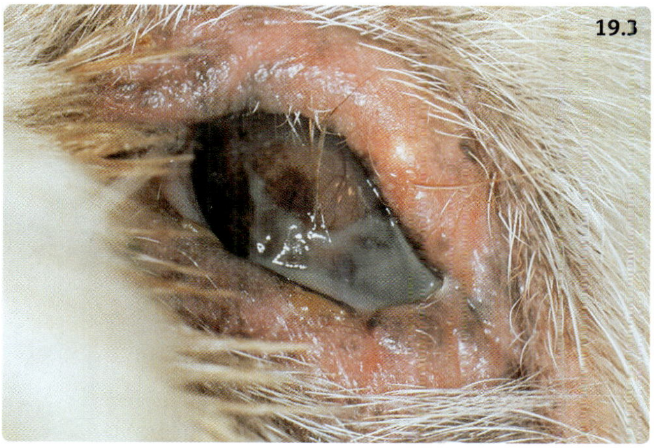

Figure 19.3 Pigmentary keratitis, mucoid discharge, and lid margin blepharitis are associated with KCS in this dog.

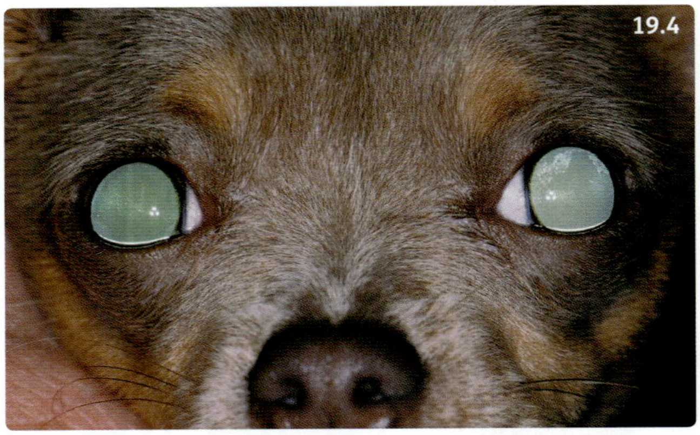

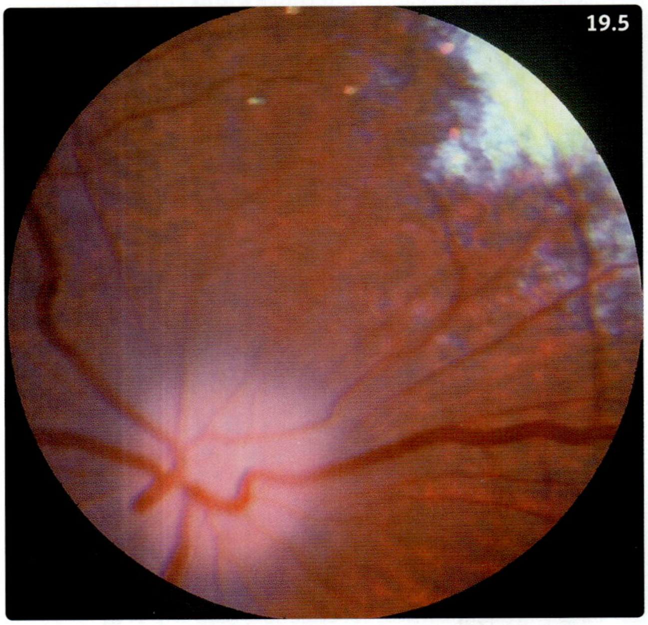

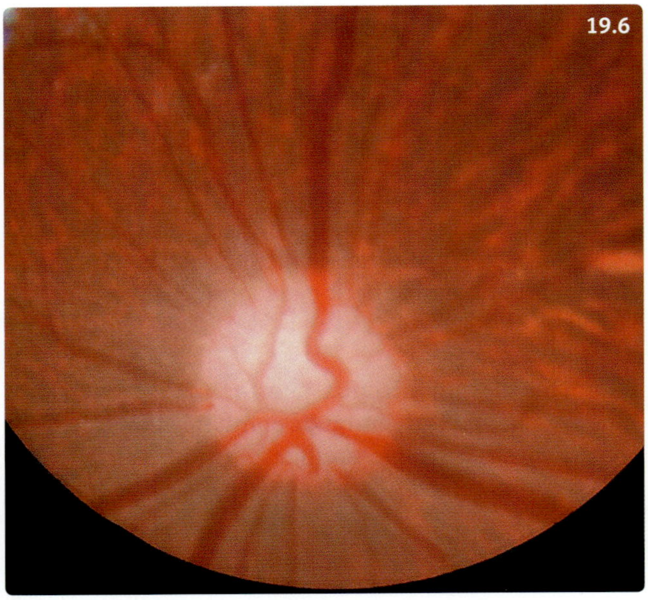

Figures 19.4–19.6 Dog with optic neuritis from canine distemper. (19.4) Note the dilated pupils. (19.5) The blurred edges of the optic disk indicate active optic neuritis. (19.6) Optic nerve atrophy is present 2 months later.

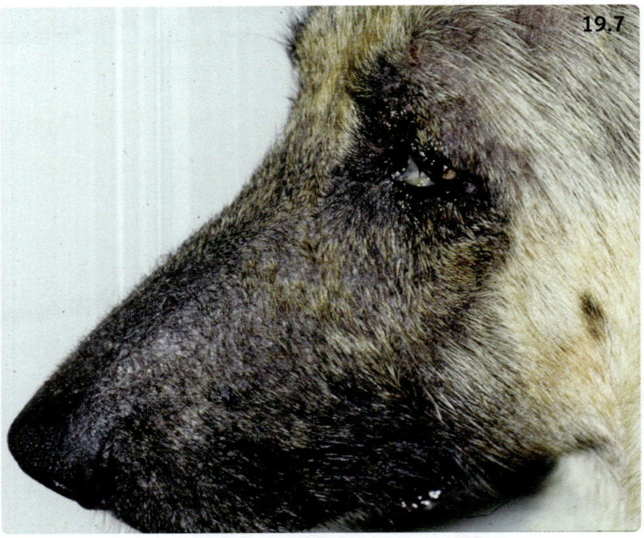

Figure 19.7 KCS and demodicosis are present in this dog with canine distemper.

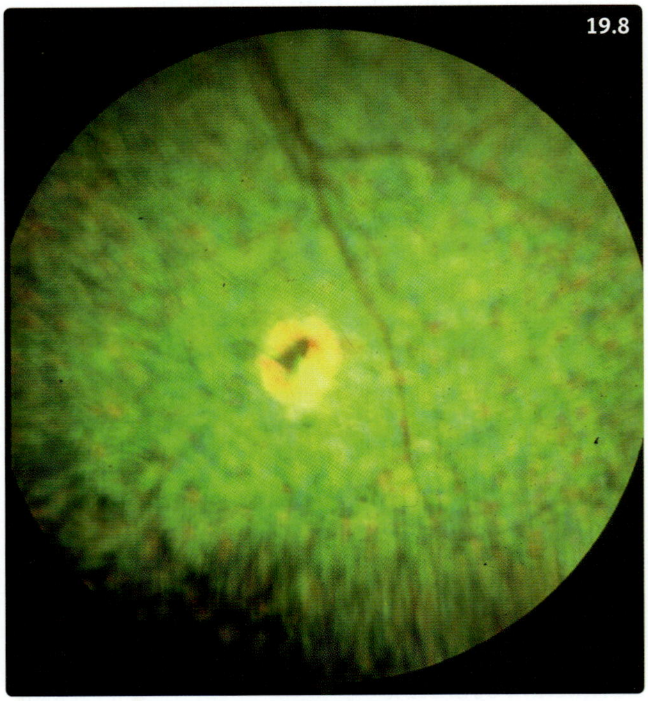

Figure 19.8 A focal area of chorioretinitis from distemper is found in this dog.

Table 19.1 Etiologies of optic neuritis.

Etiologies
Vascular embarrassment/ischemia
Idiopathic
Canine distemper
Reticulosis
Fungal (cryptococcosis, blastomycosis)
Toxoplasmosis
Neoplasia (especially squamous cell carcinoma, lymphosarcoma, nasal tumors, meningiomas)
Toxins (lead, arsenic, thallium, ethyl/methyl alcohol, chlorinated hydrocarbon)
Septicemia
Vitamin A deficiency
Feline infectious peritonitis
Orbital inflammation
Trauma (e.g. after proptosis of globe)

Table 19.2 Etiologies of keratoconjunctivitis sicca.

Etiologies
Loss of lacrimal tissues: • Congenital/breed-related • Idiopathic atrophy • Iatrogenic removal of nictitans gland
Secondary reaction to chronic conjunctivitis or blepharitis
Secondary reaction to systemic disease (canine distemper, feline herpes, leishmaniasis)
Drugs (atropine, several sulfonamides, general anesthesia)
Loss of innervation (e.g. traumatic, infectious, iatrogenic, neoplastic)
Idiopathic
Immune-mediated
Radiation

Table 19.3 Etiologies of chorioretinitis.

Etiologies
Dogs
Viral: distemper
Bacterial: any septicemia or bacteremia (e.g. leptospirosis, brucellosis)
Rickettsial: ehrlichiosis, Rocky Mountain spotted fever, borrelia
Fungal: aspergillosis, blastomycosis, histoplasmosis, cryptococcosis
Algal: geotrichosis, protothecosis
Parasites: ocular larval migrans, toxoplasmosis, leishmaniasis, neosporosis
Cats
Viral: FeLV, FIV, FIP
Bacterial: any septicemia
Fungal: cryptococcosis, histoplasmosis
Parasites: toxoplasmosis, ophthalmomyiasis, ocular larval migrans

Reverse-transcriptase polymerase chain reaction (PCR) assays have been shown to be both sensitive and specific for detection of CDV.

Management

Treatment is aimed at controlling secondary infections, although ribavirin inhibits CDV replication *in vitro*. Supportive treatment improves the chance for recovery and quality of life. Vaccination is the key to preventing CDV infection.

INFECTIOUS CANINE HEPATITIS

Definition/overview

Canine adenovirus 1 (CAV-1) may cause ocular signs including anterior uveitis and corneal edema in naturally infected dogs, and in dogs vaccinated with the modified live canine adenovirus type I vaccine. Due to the potential reaction to CAV-1, newer vaccines now contain CAV type 2 to minimize the incidence of this condition.

Etiology

CAV-1 is a DNA adenovirus.

Pathophysiology

The corneal edema is a result of an Arthus-type hypersensitivity reaction in the corneal endothelium rather than direct viral replication. Classically 14–21 days post vaccination or 10–21 days following natural infection, a severe, generally unilateral anterior uveitis with aqueous flare, hypotony, and corneal edema ('blue eye') appears in affected eyes (**Figure 19.9**). The anterior uveitis generally resolves over a 2–3-week period, although persistent corneal edema can occur.

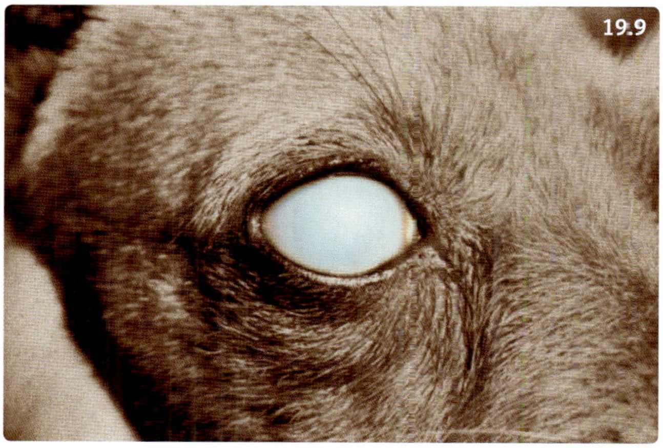

Figure 19.9 Infectious canine hepatitis causes immune-mediated damage to the corneal endothelium and corneal edema ('blue eye').

Clinical presentation

Ocular complications include bullous keratopathy, keratoconus/keratoglobus, phthisis bulbi, and secondary glaucoma. Complications are most likely to occur in the Afghan Hound.

Differential diagnosis

Table 19.4.

Diagnosis

Diagnosis is based on the clinical history and signs, and immunohistochemistry for CAV-1 and detection of viral DNA using PCR in infected ocular tissue.

Management

Therapy is symptomatic and includes topically administered corticosteroids, hyperosmotics, atropine, and nonsteroidal anti-inflammatory drugs.

Table 19.4 Etiologies of anterior uveitis.

Exogenous: • Trauma • Perforating wounds or exogenous introduction of infection • Intraocular surgery
Endogenous: • Extension of disease from cornea or sclera • Ulcerative keratitis • Interstitial keratitis
Infectious: • Canine hepatitis • Systemic mycoses – blastomycosis • *FeLV • *FIP, FIV, FeSV, herpesvirus, toxoplasmosis, cryptococcosis • Brucellosis, leishmaniasis • Septicemia in general • Leptospirosis
Parasitic: • Dirofilariasis, eosinophilia in dogs • Toxoplasmosis • *Toxocara canis*
Hypersensitivity: • Lens-induced uveitis • Unknown antigenic response • Hepatitis vaccine reaction
Intraocular neoplasia (lymphoma particularly)
Idiopathic
Immune-mediated

*Common causes in cats.

FELINE HERPESVIRUS (RHINOTRACHEITIS)

Definition/overview

FHV-1 is a double-stranded DNA virus that is highly species specific. FHV-1 has marked tropism for the conjunctival epithelium and less so for the corneal epithelum. The virus is spread from cat to cat through fomites, aerosolization, or direct contact.

Etiology

Herpesvirus is the major cause of respiratory disease and associated conjunctivitis in cats. It is estimated that >90% of cats are seropositive to the virus with as many as 80% of infected cats remaining latently infected on a life-long basis. Approximately 45% of these latently infected cats shed virus throughout their life. Cats with chronic herpetic conjunctivitis may also be feline immunodeficiency virus (FIV) positive.

Pathophysiology

FHV-1 infects the epithelial surfaces of the respiratory tract and conjunctiva and, to a lesser degree, the corneal epithelium, and then ascends by axons of sensory neurons to the trigeminal ganglion to establish life-long latency with a potential for recrudescence. Cytolytic pathology and immune-mediated disease are associated with FHV-1 infection. FHV-1 was isolated from the conjunctiva, cornea, uveal tract, retina, optic nerve, ciliary ganglion, pterygopalatine ganglion, trigeminal ganglion, brainstem, visual cortex, cerebellum, and olfactory bulb of infected cats during the acute phase. Trigeminal and cranial cervical ganglia harbor latent virus in the latent phase.

Clinical presentation

Early signs of herpesvirus conjunctivitis include a bilateral serous ocular discharge that becomes mucopurulent with time (**Figures 19.10–19.15**). Secondary bacterial infections enhance the mucopurulent exudate.

Dendritic corneal and conjunctival ulcers from viral induced cytolysis and larger geographic immune-mediated stromal ulcers can be associated with FHV (**Figures 19.16–19.19**). Symblepharon and iridocyclitis are also noted in some infected cats. KCS may develop with time. Corneal sequestration and eosinophilic keratitis are also associated with herpes in cats.

Differential diagnosis

Conjunctivitis is found in many types of eye diseases. It may be infectious (herpesvirus, calicivirus, *Mycoplasma* and *Chlamydia* in cats) or noninfectious. Conjunctivitis may be primary or be secondary to ulcerative keratitis, anterior uveitis, eyelid disease, orbital cellulitis, nasolacrimal duct obstruction, KCS, atopy, environmental irritation, and neoplasia (lymphoma).

Diagnosis

Immunofluorescent antibody (IFA) testing of conjunctival or corneal scrapings for herpesvirus and *Chlamydia* is available at many laboratories. Because it is an IFA test, prior fluorescein staining may yield false positives, so scrapings should be taken before staining. Positive IFA tests are more common early in the course of the disease.

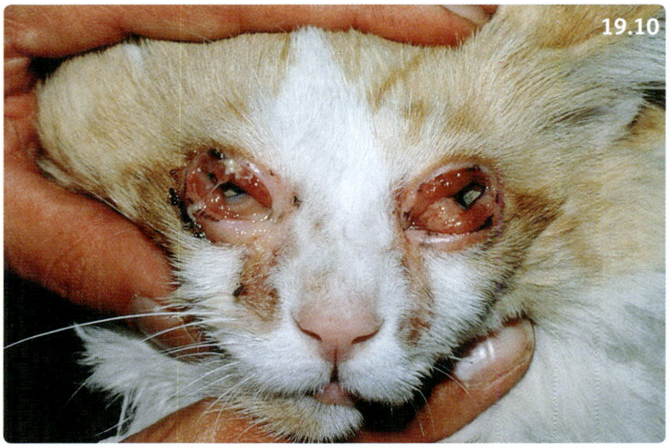

Figure 19.10 Bilateral conjunctival chemosis, hyperemia, and a slight mucoid discharge are found in this cat with herpesvirus.

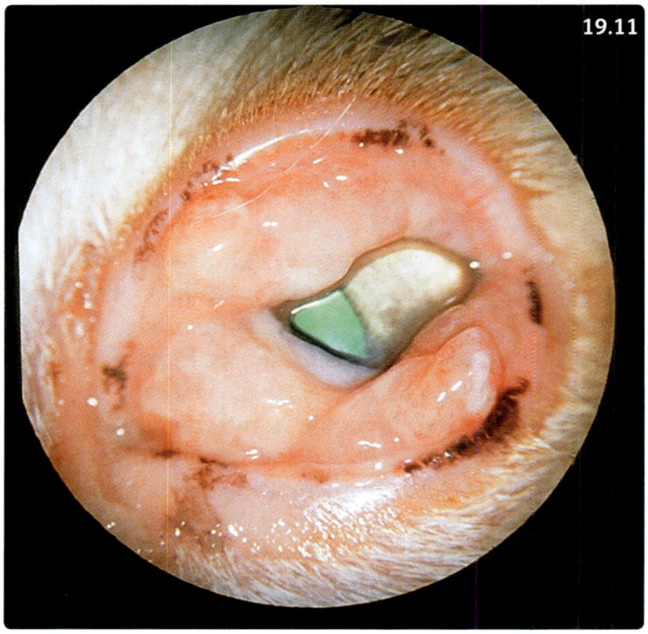

Figure 19.11 Chemosis is so severe in this cat with herpesvirus that the cornea can be barely seen.

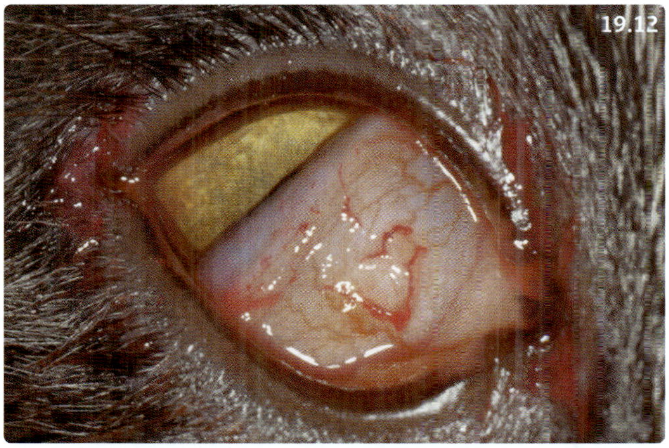

Figure 19.12 Dendritic rose bengal-positive lesions of the third eyelid conjunctiva are present in this cat with herpesvirus.

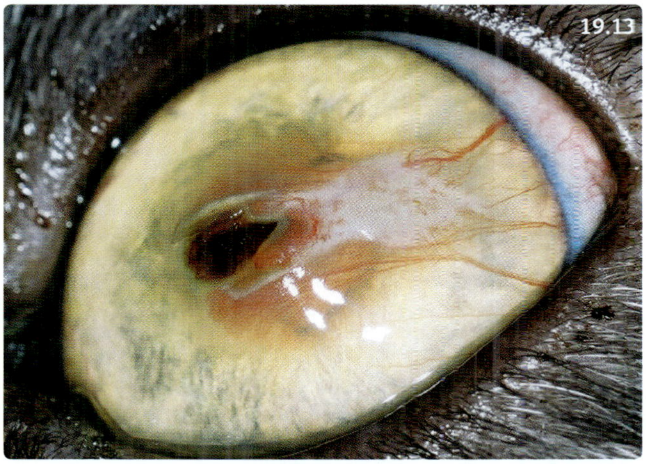

Figure 19.13 The dark corneal lesion with corneal fibrosis and vascularization is a corneal sequestrum and is associated with feline herpesvirus.

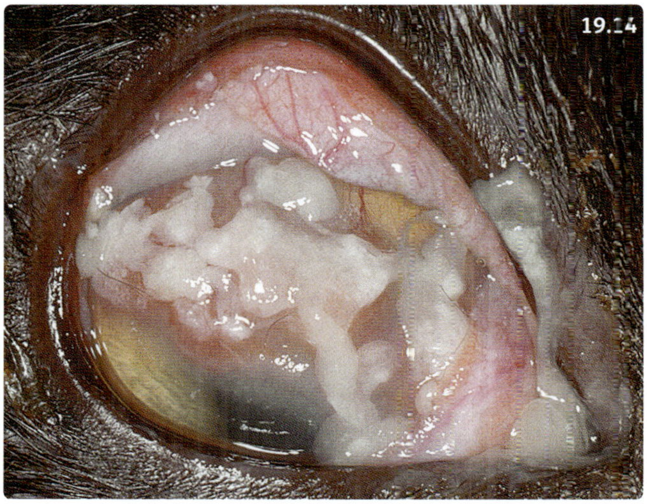

Figure 19.14 Eosinophilic keratitis is associated with feline herpesvirus in this cat.

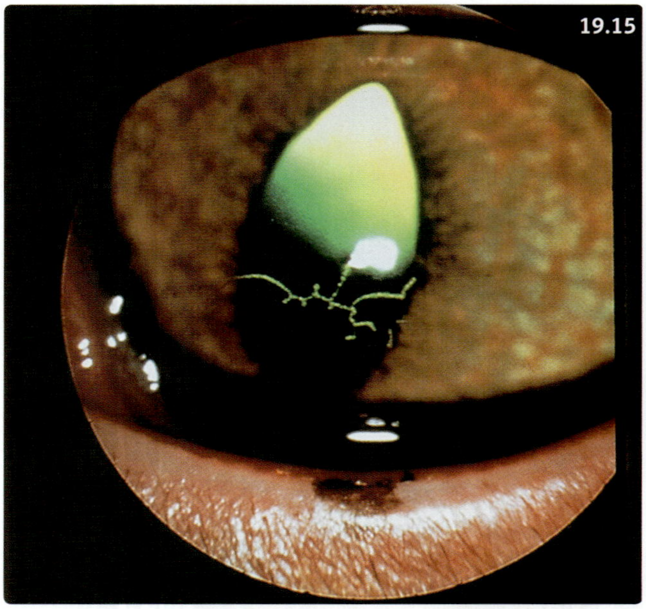

Figure 19.15 Linear, dendritic corneal ulcers are unique to feline herpesvirus.

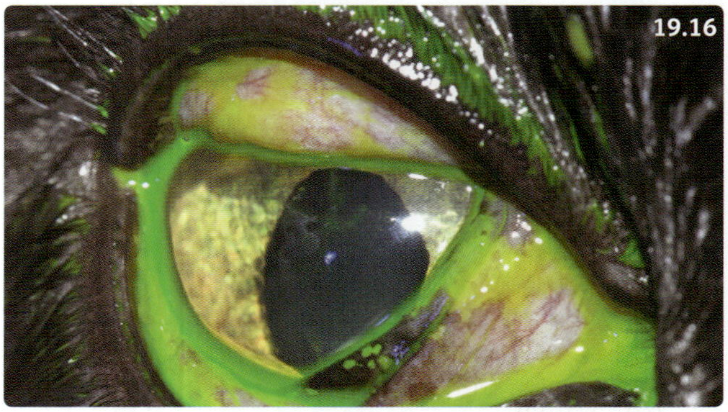

Figure 19.16 Herpetic dendritic ulcers staining positive for fluorescein and conjunctival chemosis are present in the eye of this cat.

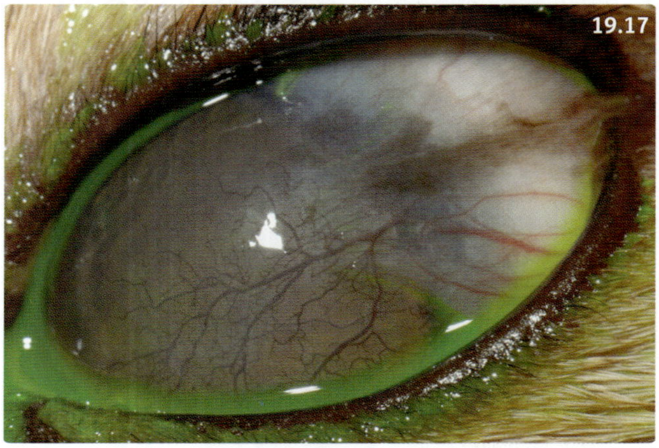

Figure 19.17 Symblepharon from herpesvirus is present in this cat.

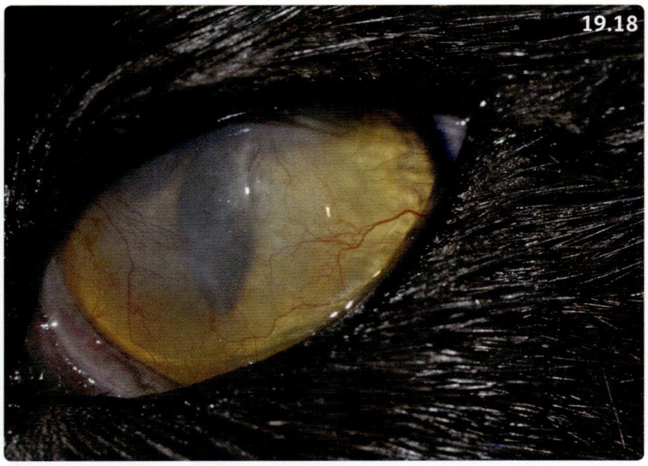

Figure 19.18 Generalized stromal keratitis is caused by FHV-1 in this cat.

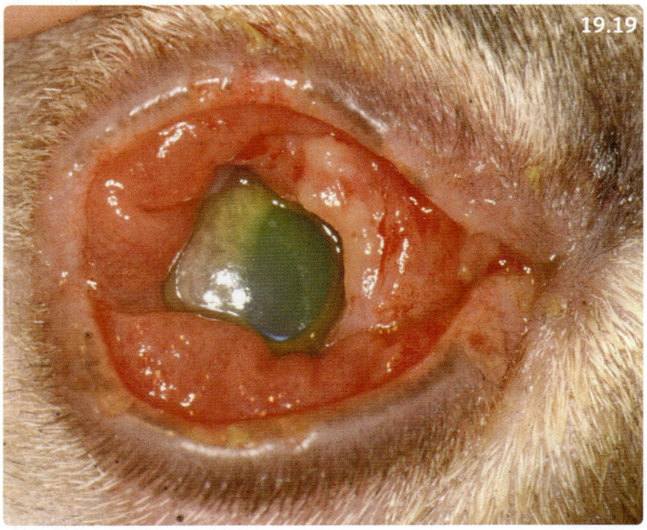

Figure 19.19 Severe conjunctival hyperemia and chemosis caused by FHV-1 in a cat.

PCR and reverse-transcriptase PCR testing are more accurate than the IFA tests. Although the extreme sensitivity (and specificity) of PCR has improved detection of virus, it has also confirmed that virus can be demonstrated in up to 31% of apparently normal cats.

Clinically, keratoconjunctivitis with dendritic branching corneal ulcers is diagnostic of herpesvirus infection (**Figures 19.15, 19.16**). Herpetic keratitis in the cat may or may not be associated with upper respiratory disease. Lymphocytes generally predominate early and large mononuclear cells are not uncommon. Neutrophils and giant epithelial cells are seen with chronic or secondary infection. Intranuclear inclusion bodies are seen very rarely, if ever, in clinical cases.

Management

Therapy for herpesvirus conjunctivitis consists of topical antiviral preparations and broad-spectrum antibiotics to control the secondary bacterial infection. The efficacy of the antiviral medication in controlling the herpesvirus conjunctivitis (without corneal involvement) is variable. Herpesvirus vaccines are available for cats; however, herpesvirus conjunctivitis can occur in vaccinated cats. Recurrent herpesvirus may be associated with the immunosuppression by FIV/FeLV.

Antiviral agents should be prescribed when ocular signs are severe, persistent, or recurrent, or when there is corneal ulceration, although topical antivirals and other ophthalmic medications are often irritating to affected cats.

Initial treatment includes topical cidofovir q12h or topical idoxuridine (0.5%) or trifluorothymidine (1%) 5 times a day. Oral L-lysine (500 mg q12h) can reduce virus shedding in latently infected cats. Oral famciclovir (90 mg/kg PO q8h) for 3 weeks can improve ocular and systemic FHV disease.

Acyclovir (200 mg PO q8h) is useful in combination with interferon. Systemic interferon may be beneficial in cats that are refractory to other therapies. Alpha-2 interferon may be administered (3 U/ml/cat PO q24h for the life of the cat, or 30 U/ml/cat PO q24h for 7 days, off 7 days, on 7 days, etc.).

Client education is important. Herpesvirus infection may be chronic and recurrent, especially during times of stress. Recurrent and chronic herpes infections may suggest systemic immunosuppression so cats should be evaluated for FeLV and FIV.

FELINE INFECTIOUS PERITONITIS

Definition/overview

Effusive (wet) and non-effusive (dry) forms of feline infectious peritonitis (FIP) are known. The dry (noneffusive or parenchymatous) form of FIP is associated with the most ocular changes (32% of dry cases have ocular lesions).

Etiology

FIP is caused by a coronavirus.

Pathophysiology

The virus replicates in oropharyngeal tissues and at the tips of intestinal villi. Dissemination of the virus in macrophages leads to pyogranulomatous lesions in a variety of tissues. Granulomatous lesions in the dry form are often found outside the abdomen and thorax, especially in the CNS and eye. A fatal Arthus-type immune reaction of cats is associated with infection with the FIP virus.

Clinical presentation

There is increased risk of development of disease in young cats and in Abyssinians, Bengals, Birmans, Himalayans, Ragdolls, and Rexes. Ocular signs may occur without concurrent systemic signs or may be prodromal to systemic signs. The ocular signs are often bilateral. There have been several cases of remission in cats with ocular signs only and high FIP antibody titers. Clinical signs include pyogranulomatous anterior and posterior uveitis, aqueous flare, 'mutton fat' keratic precipitates, hypopyon, synechiae, secondary glaucoma, RDs, choroiditis, retinal hemorrhages (**Figures 19.20–19.23**), vasculitis with pyogranulomatous sheathing or cuffing of retinal vessels, and optic neuritis.

Differential diagnosis

Tables 19.2 and **19.3**.

Diagnosis

Diagnosis can be aided by clinical pathologic alterations, with the total plasma protein frequently >7.8 g/dl and a polyclonal gammopathy and elevated serum fibrinogen present. Anterior chamber paracentesis reveals protein, fibrin, neutrophils, erythrocytes, and mononuclear cells. Serology and PCR are not reliable. Reverse-transcriptase PCR and a direct IFA test may aid diagnosis of FIP.

19.20

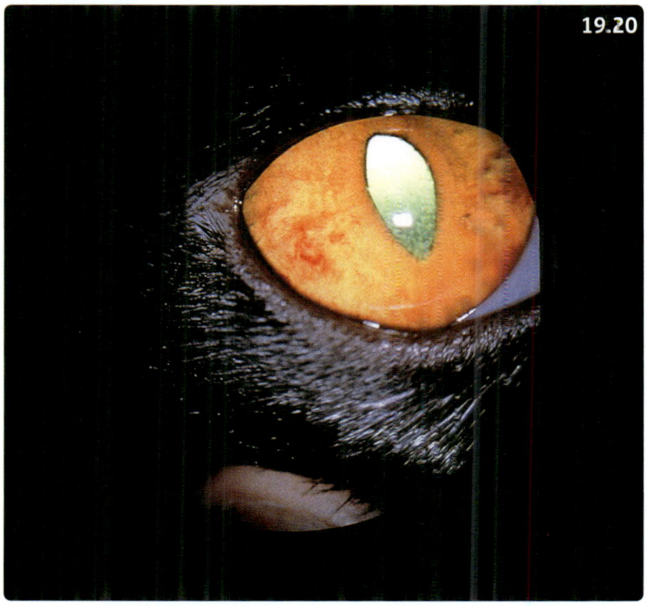

Figure 19.20 Rubeosis iridis or iris neovascularization is found in this cat with FIP.

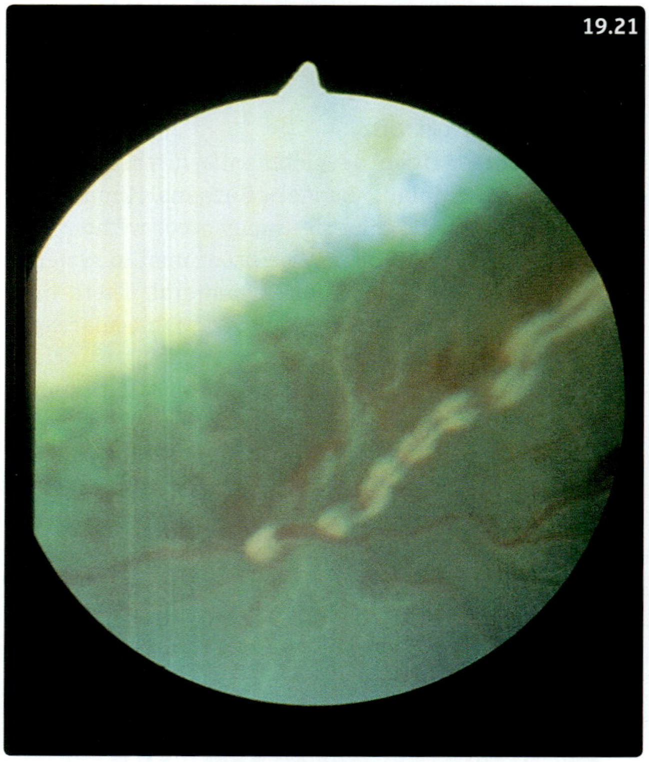

Figure 19.21 Perivascular cuffing, retinal edema, and retinal hemorrhage are noticed in the retina of a cat with FIP. (Courtesy B. Spiess)

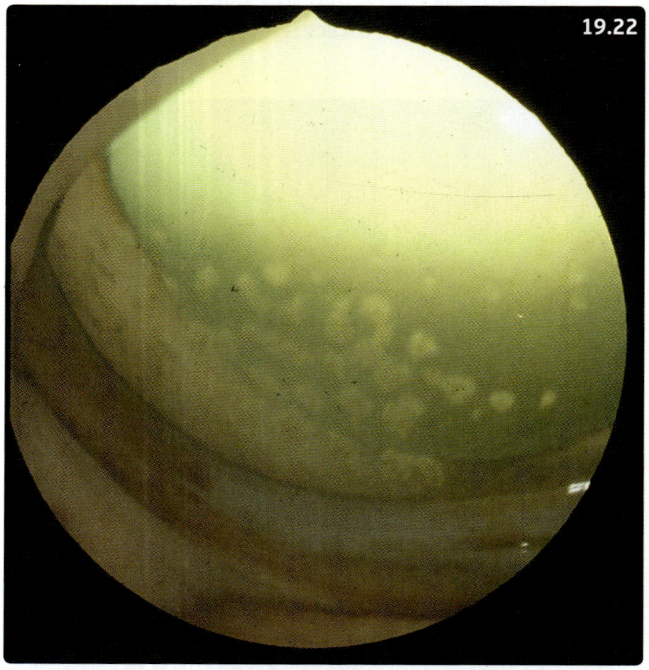

Figure 19.22 This cat with FIP has 'mutton fat' keratic precipitates.

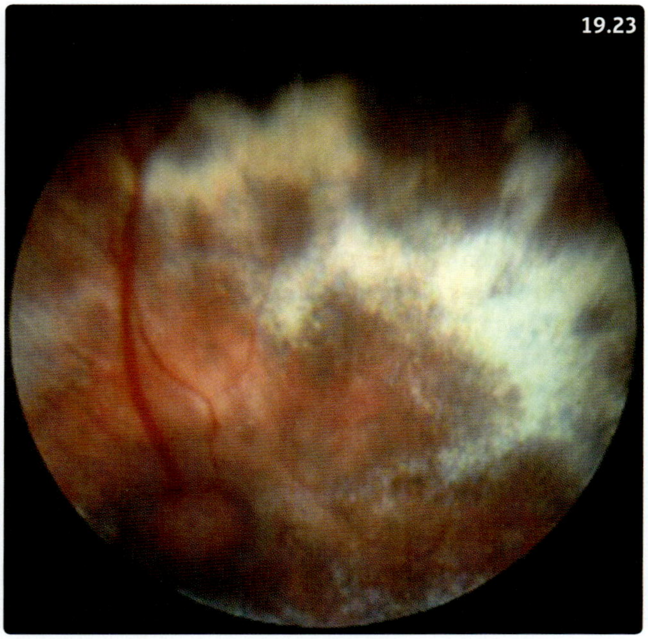

Figure 19.23 Focal regions of granulomatous and pigmented chorioretinitis are noticed in this cat with FIP.

Management

Therapy for FIP is symptomatic for the anterior uveitis and systemic problems. Tumor necrosis factor-alpha neutralizing antibody may have some benefit for therapy.

FELINE LEUKEMIA VIRUS

Definition/overview

FeLV causes anterior uveitis (one or both eyes), retinitis, cataracts, irregular or asymmetrical pupils, and secondary glaucoma.

Etiology

FeLV is a retrovirus whose genetic material is transmitted from host to host as RNA. Anterior chamber or vitreal paracentesis may reveal neoplastic cells in cases of lymphosarcoma, but is usually nonspecific as to the etiology.

Pathophysiology

Retinal changes include hemorrhages (**Figure 19.24**), pale retinal vessels (anemia), leukemic infiltrates appearing as multifocal gray opacities, and RDs. Infection with FeLV appears to cause little in the way of ocular disease with the exception of its role in lymphosarcoma. The uveal tract is a common site for metastasis of leukemic lymphocytes. Cats with ocular lymphosarcoma may present initially with signs of mild uveitis, including miosis, aqueous flare and keratic precipitates, or subtle iridal masses. As the disease progresses, the iris becomes greatly thickened and distorted with the infiltration of tumor cells. Glaucoma is a common sequela as lymphoma cells infiltrate the iridocorneal angle.

Clinical presentation

Corneal changes are uncommon, but include keratitis, edema, and a keratopathy appearing as a wide opaque band of neoplastic stromal lymphoid cells. Conjunctivitis with proliferation of lymph follicles may be noted. Horner's syndrome associated with mediastinal lymphosarcoma in FeLV-positive cats has been noticed. Isolated iridal tumor formation may occur. Abnormal pupillary light reflexes ('spastic pupil') have also been associated with FeLV infection of the ciliary ganglia and short ciliary nerves.

Differential diagnosis

Tables 19.2 and **19.3**.

Diagnosis

The ELISA is an excellent in-hospital screening test with good sensitivity. Confirmatory indirect IFA testing should be performed on a peripheral blood smear of ELISA-positive cats. Recently, a PCR test has been used for the detection of FeLV antigen. FeLV antigens are present in corneal tissue and all potential donors should be tested prior to transplantation.

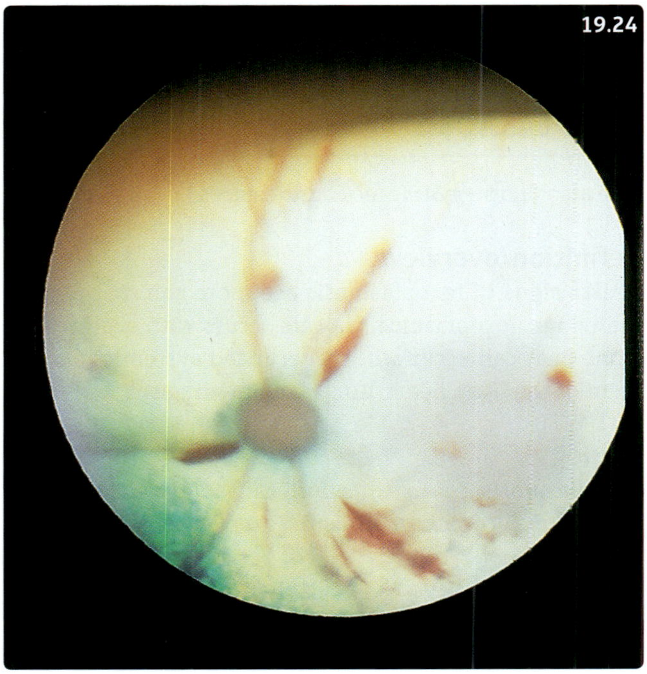

Figure 19.24 Linear flame hemorrhages of the nerve fiber layer and a focal exudative retinal detachment are noticed in this FeLV-positive cat.

Management

Therapy for FeLV includes management of opportunistic infections and supportive therapy. Cats with an increased risk of exposure to FeLV should be vaccinated regularly.

FELINE PANLEUKOPENIA VIRUS

Definition/overview

Feline panleukopenia virus is a parvovirus known to cause cerebellar hypoplasia and retinal dysplasia, with retinal rosette formation, loss of normal retinal layered architecture, and reduced thickness of the neural retina in kittens. Focal retinal dysplasia appears as sharply defined hyperreflective areas in the tapetal fundus and depigmented areas in the nontapetal fundus. Optic nerve hypoplasia may also occur with the feline panleukopenia virus.

FELINE IMMUNODEFICIENCY VIRUS

Definition/overview

FIV is a lentivirus. FIV infection results in progressive loss of $CD4^+$ T-helper cells early in the infection, followed by depletion of $CD8^+$ T cells in the advanced stages of the disease. Anterior uveitis (**Figure 19.25**), lens luxation, pars planitis, and conjunctivitis are reported with FIV. Anterior uveitis and chorioretinitis are the most common ocular findings in cats co-infected with both FIV and *Toxoplasma gondii*. Currently marketed PCR assays for the detection of FIV lack sensitivity and vary significantly in accuracy. Positive serum antibody titers for toxoplasmosis are more common in FIV-positive cats.

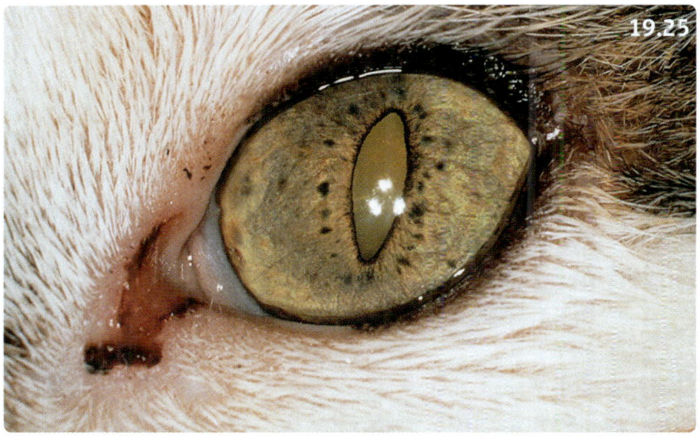

Figure 19.25 Iridal hyperpigmentation is associated with chronic uveitis due to FIV in this cat.

FELINE SARCOMA VIRUS

Definition/overview

Feline sarcoma virus is associated with uveal melanoma and anterior uveitis in cats.

PROTOZOAL INFECTION

LEISHMANIASIS

Definition/overview

Leishmaniasis is of major public health significance in Central and South America, the Mediterranean region, Africa, and Asia. The visceral and cutaneous forms are associated with blepharitis, keratitis, conjunctivitis, KCS, anterior uveitis, rubeosis iridis, and severe panuveitis. Dogs are more commonly affected than cats.

Etiology

Leishmania spp. are diphasic protozoan parasites. Dogs are considered important primary reservoirs of *Leishmania* spp., and sandflies (*Phlebotomus* or *Lutzomyia* spp.) are the vectors. Naturally occurring leishmaniasis has been increasingly reported in cats in the last few years. Feline leishmaniasis is generally caused by *L. mexicana* in Texas, *L. major* in Egypt, and *L. (Viannia) panamensis* in Brazil. *L. infantum*, a causative agent of feline leishmaniasis in southern France and Italy, also causes leishmaniasis in dogs.

Pathophysiology

Transmission to vertebrates is via bites from infected sandflies. The incubation period may be a few months to between 3 and 4 years. Over 80% of infected dogs have ocular lesions with both eyes affected. The inflammation is mononuclear with the organism found in histiocytes.

Clinical presentation

Melting ulcerative keratitis, KCS, blepharitis, exudative panuveitis, optic neuritis, and secondary glaucoma are reported with *Leishmania* infections (**Figure 19.26**).

Differential diagnosis

Tables 19.3 and **19.4**.

Diagnosis

The *Leishmania* organism can be diagnosed with histopathologic or immunoperoxidase evaluation of cutaneous or ocular biopsy specimens, PCR of anticoagulated blood, or isolation of the organism from the subcutaneous tissue, bone marrow, or lymph node aspirates. Serologic tests are available that use ELISA and indirect IFA testing.

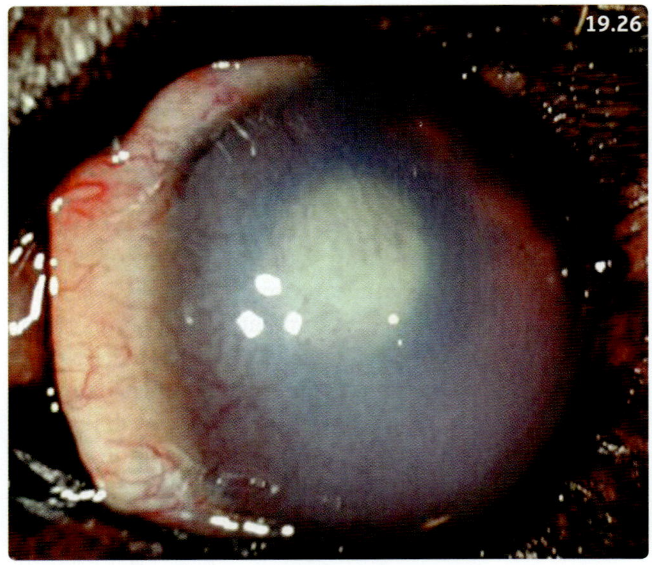

Figure 19.26 Leishmaniasis is causing keratouveitis in this dog from Italy. (Courtesy A. Guandalini)

Management

Allopurinol combined with sodium stibogluconate has been successful for the treatment of canine leishmaniasis, but prognosis is always guarded. Symptomatic therapy is used for the ocular lesions.

TOXOPLASMOSIS

(See also Chapter 21: Infectious diseases.)

Definition/overview

Ocular signs of toxoplasmosis are more common in cats than dogs. Toxoplasmosis in cats occurs with ocular signs alone or it can occur with generalized systemic involvement of the liver, heart, lungs, and meninges.

Etiology

Toxoplasmosis is an infection caused by the obligate intracellular coccidian parasite *Toxoplasma gondii*.

Pathophysiology

Oral ingestion of tissue cysts or oocysts results in spread of *Toxoplasma* organisms to extraintestinal organs via the blood or lymph. Focal necrosis of the heart, eye, and brain results due to proliferation of *T. gondii*. Uveitis secondary to toxoplasmosis may result from rapid replication of tachyzoites within ocular tissue or from deposition of immune complexes within uveal tissue. Intraocular production of antibodies specific for *T. gondii* has been reported, and the organism has been identified within the uveal tract by histopathology and in the aqueous humor by PCR.

Clinical presentation

The uveitis is frequently documented as multiple foci of retinitis or retinochoroiditis (**Figure 19.27**) with varying degrees of anterior uveitis in cats. In dogs, chorioretinitis, optic neuritis, and, less frequently, anterior uveitis and inflammation of extraocular muscles are present.

Differential diagnosis

Tables 19.3 and **19.4**.

Diagnosis

The presumptive diagnosis of toxoplasmosis can be made in cats with signs of uveitis and a positive serum titer, although ocular toxoplasmosis in cats is not associated with markedly elevated titers. Histologic demonstration of the parasite is the sole definitive means of confirmation. ELISA tests for detection of IgM antibodies and toxoplasma antigen have been developed for diagnosis of toxoplasmosis. Levels of the IgM class of antibody rise and fall over approximately 3–4 months after infection whereas those of the IgG class of antibody may rise more slowly and remain elevated in cats for years after exposure to *T. gondii*. Fecal examination for *Toxoplasma* oocysts can be useful to determine if the cat is shedding and potentially infectious for other animals or humans.

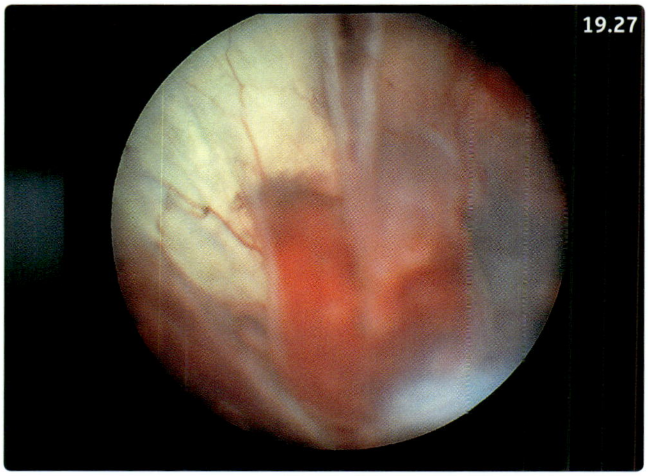

Figure 19.27 Extensive retinal hemorrhage and detachment are associated with intraocular toxoplasmosis in this cat.

Management

Owners should be instructed in basic hygienic rules to prevent toxoplasmosis. It is a zoonotic disease. Treatment for toxoplasmosis includes antimicrobial agents (sulfadiazine, pyrimethamine, clindamycin) and supportive therapy. In case of localized ocular involvement, the standard treatment for uveitis is also definitively indicated.

FUNGAL DISEASES

(See also Chapter 21: Infectious diseases.)

Systemic mycotic infections that commonly involve the eyes include cryptococcosis, histoplasmosis, blastomycosis, and coccidioidomycosis. Inhalation is believed to be the primary route of infection, with hematogenous spread to the eye. Diagnosis is based on clinical and ocular signs, radiographs, stained smears from tissue samples, ocular paracentesis, peripheral lymph node aspirates and serology. Miscellaneous fungi/yeasts causing conjunctivitis, endophthalmitis, keratitis, and/or chorioretinitis include *Nocardia* spp., *Candida* spp., *Geotrichum* spp., *Aspergillus* spp., *Sporotrichum* spp., and *Paecilomyces* spp. *Candida* has caused corneal ulcers in cats. The systemic aspergillosis (*Aspergillus terreus*) of German Shepherd Dogs often has ocular manifestations.

CRYPTOCOCCOSIS

Definition/overview

Cryptococcosis is an opportunistic systemic fungal infection. It is not a contagious disease. Cats are more frequently affected than dogs with cryptococcosis, which is considered to be the most common feline systemic fungal infection. Dog breeds typically affected include American Cocker Spaniels, Dobermanns, Great Danes, and Labrador Retrievers.

Etiology

Cryptococcosis is caused by the saprophytic yeast-like organism *Cryptococcus neoformans*. *C. neoformans* is associated with soil enriched with avian feces containing high levels of nitrogen. Birds such as pigeons are considered to be significant vectors of *Cryptococcus* spp. The organism is most commonly inhaled from the environment.

Pathophysiology

Cryptococcosis may infect the eye by hematogenous means or by extension from the nose or CNS. The organisms may be found in the ocular tissues, including the vitreous.

Clinical presentation

Cats have respiratory, CNS, ocular, and skin lesions, while dogs have mainly CNS and ocular lesions. Dogs may also show gastrointestinal (GI) and neurologic signs. The ocular signs of cryptococcosis in cats include dilated, nonresponsive pupils, exudative RDs, granulomatous chorioretinitis (**Figure 19.28–19.31**), optic neuritis, and anterior uveitis. Dogs may show exudative granulomatous chorioretinitis, optic neuritis, and dilated pupils.

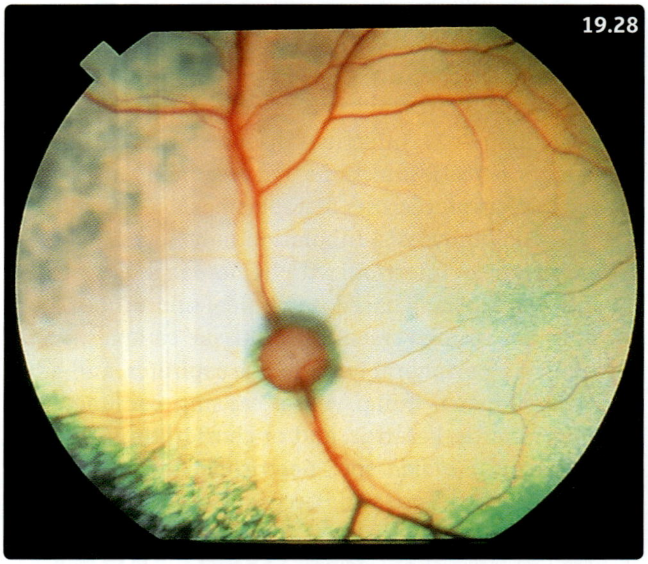

Figure 19.28 A large, focal, granulomatous lesion with hyperpigmented regions caused by cryptococcosis in a cat.

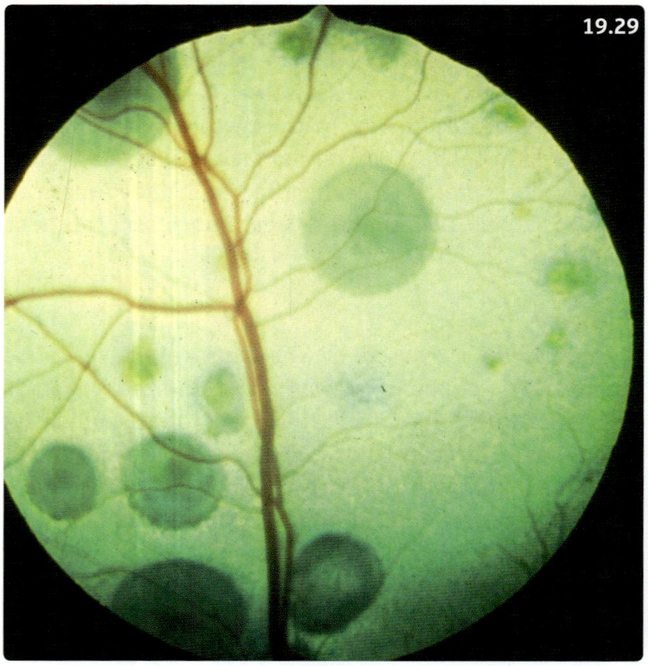

Figure 19.29 Inactive focal regions of chorioretinitis in a cat with cryptococcosis.

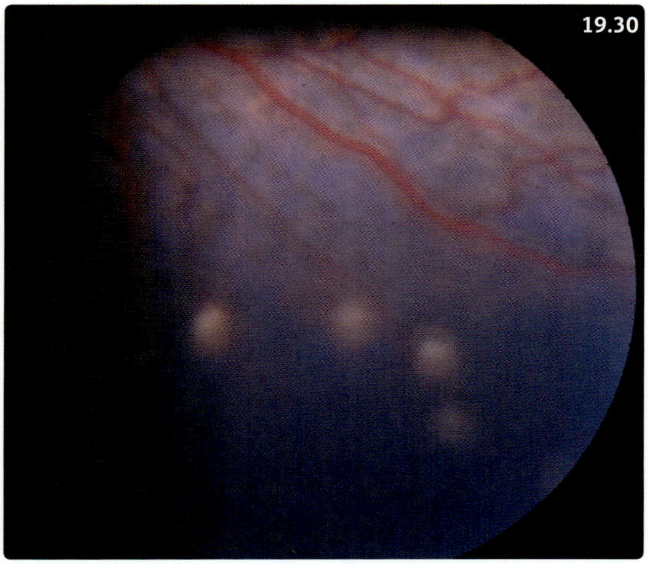

Figure 19.30 Fuzzy white areas in the nontapetal region of this cat with cryptococcosis indicate active chorioretinitis.

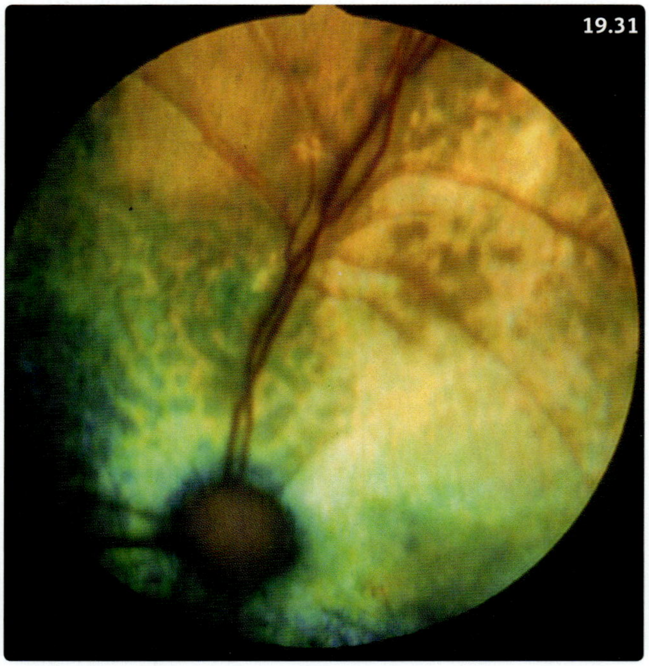

Figure 19.31 Tapetal discoloration is present with chorioretinitis in this cat with cryptococcosis.

Differential diagnosis
Tables 19.3 and **19.4**.

Diagnosis
Diagnosis is based on identification of the organism by cytology or histology. Organisms may be identified in subretinal or vitreal aspirates, or cerebrospinal fluid (CSF) tap. A latex agglutination test against capsular antigens is available.

Management
Cryptococcosis has been treated in cats with ketoconazole, combination amphotericin B and 5-flucytosine therapy, and 5-flucytosine alone. Combination amphotericin B/5-flucytosine therapy or fluconazole is recommended for dogs. Itraconazole can also be used to treat cryptococcosis in dogs and cats.

COCCIDIOIDOMYCOSIS

Definition/overview
Coccidioidomycosis is a systemic fungal infection found in dogs, and rarely in cats. It is not a contagious disease. It appears to be a posterior segment disease, which can extend to the anterior segment.

Etiology
Coccidioidomycosis is caused by a dimorphic fungus *Coccidioides immitis*, found in the alkaline soil of the dry climate of the southwestern USA, western Mexico, and central America. Infection is through inhalation of arthrospores from the environment.

Pathophysiology
Hematogenous and lymphatic dissemination of endospores causes disseminated disease. The eye is one of several organs that are most commonly affected. A granulomatous uveitis, either unilateral or bilateral, is most common. The cornea, iridocorneal angle, ciliary body, retina, and choroid are affected. Hyphema and vitreal hemorrhage may be present.

Clinical presentation
Systems affected include the respiratory tract, skin, bone, joints, heart, testicles, eyes, and CNS. Ocular signs may appear first, and consist of granulomatous panuveitis, secondary glaucoma, orbital cellulitis, keratitis, retinitis, and RDs (**Figure 19.32**).

Differential diagnosis
Tables 19.3 and **19.4**.

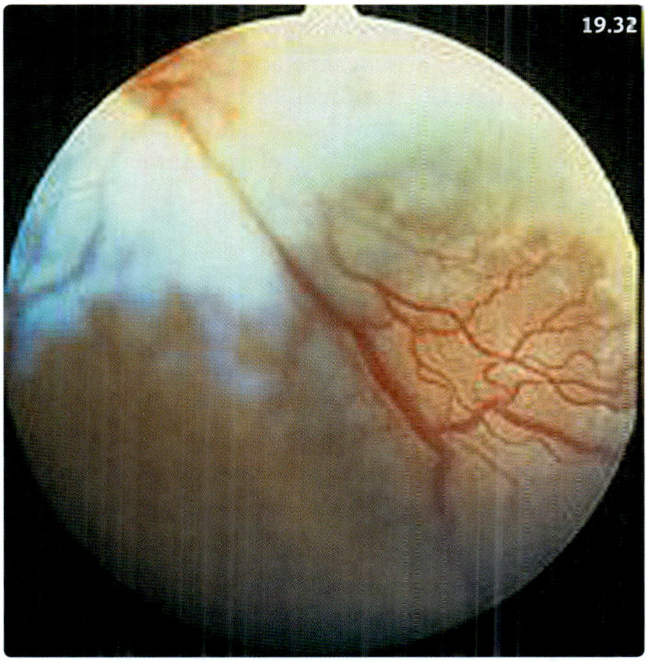

Figure 19.32 A large chorioretinal granuloma caused by *C. immitis* is present in the nontapetum of this dog.

Diagnosis
Vitreous aspiration may reveal endospores. Serologic tests are available in endemic areas.

Management
Oral ketoconazole and itraconazole are the current treatments of choice for coccidioidomycosis. Long-term use of ketoconazole in dogs has been found to be associated with the development of cataracts. Cats have been successfully treated with fluconazole.

HISTOPLASMOSIS

Definition/overview
Histoplasmosis is a systemic fungal infection of dogs and cats. It is a primary respiratory disease with dissemination to liver, spleen, intestine, lymph nodes, CNS, and bone. Histoplasmosis is widespread in alkaline soils of North and South America, but particularly in the Ohio, Mississippi, and Missouri River valleys.

Etiology
Histoplasmosis is caused by the dimorphic fungus *Histoplasma capsulatum*. Infective conidia are either inhaled or ingested. Young hunting breeds of dogs may have an increased risk.

Pathophysiology

Dissemination is hematogenous or via the lymphatics to the lungs, GI tract, liver, bone marrow, and eyes, resulting in a granulomatous inflammatory response. The choroid appears to be a preferred target region in the eye.

Clinical presentation

Ocular signs in dogs and cats include granulomatous chorioretinitis (**Figures 19.33–19.37**), optic neuritis, and RD with some signs of anterior uveitis.

Differential diagnosis

Tables 19.3 and **19.4**.

Diagnosis

Normocytic, normochromic, nonregenerative anemia is the most common hematologic abnormality. The organism may occasionally be seen in circulating mononuclear cells and eosinophils. Definitive diagnosis is based on identification of the organism, usually by cytology, biopsy, and culture.

Management

Early or mild cases may respond to ketoconazole or itraconazole alone. Combined treatment with amphotericin B and ketoconazole or itraconazole is preferred in patients with severe or fulminating disease.

BLASTOMYCOSIS

Definition/overview

Blastomycosis is a systemic fungal infection that usually originates in the lungs and then disseminates to other organ systems. All systems of the body may be infected. The disease affects dogs more than cats. Bluetick Coonhounds, Treeing-walker Coonhounds, Pointers, and Weimaraners have been reported to have the highest risk of *Blastomyces dermatitidis* infection.

Etiology

Blastomycosis is caused by the dimorphic fungus *B. dermatitidis*. Infection usually occurs by inhalation of infective conidiophores from the environment. Water and soil contamination play an important role in the spread of blastomycosis.

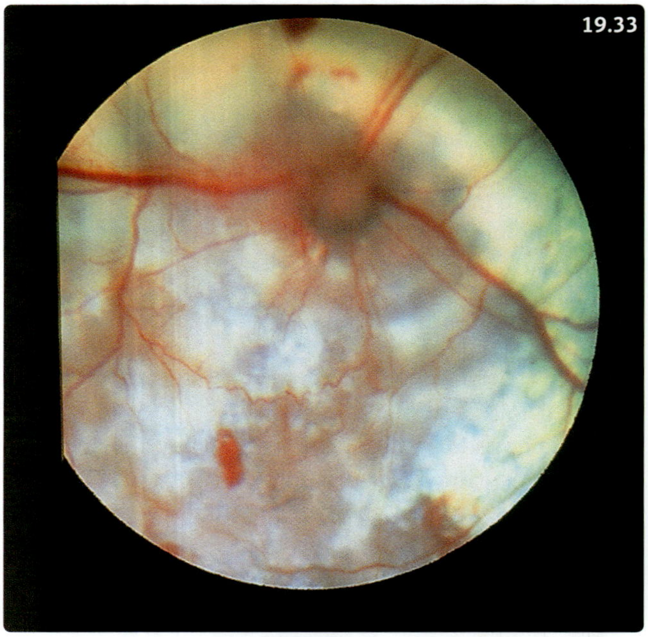

Figure 19.33 Retinal hemorrhage, elevation of retinal vessels, and peripapillary retinal edema due to histoplasmosis-induced chorioretinitis in a cat.

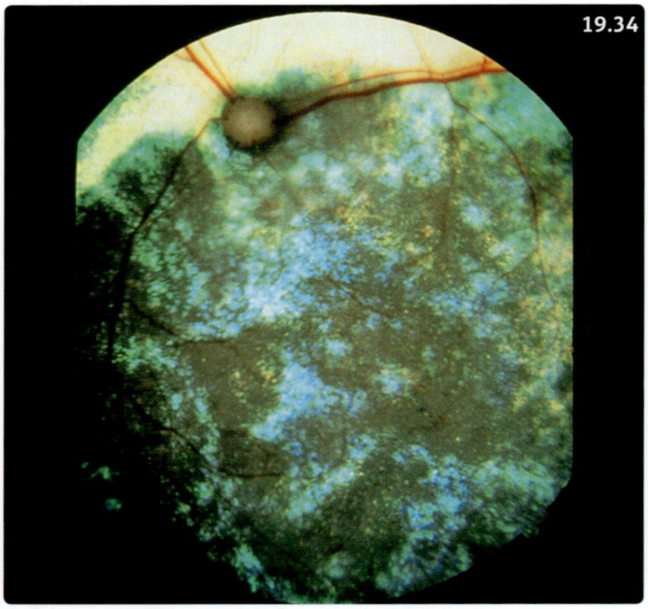

Figure 19.34 Resolution of the retinal edema and chorioretinitis, with subsequent retinal hyperpigmentation, following itraconazole therapy for histoplasmosis in the cat in Figure 19.33.

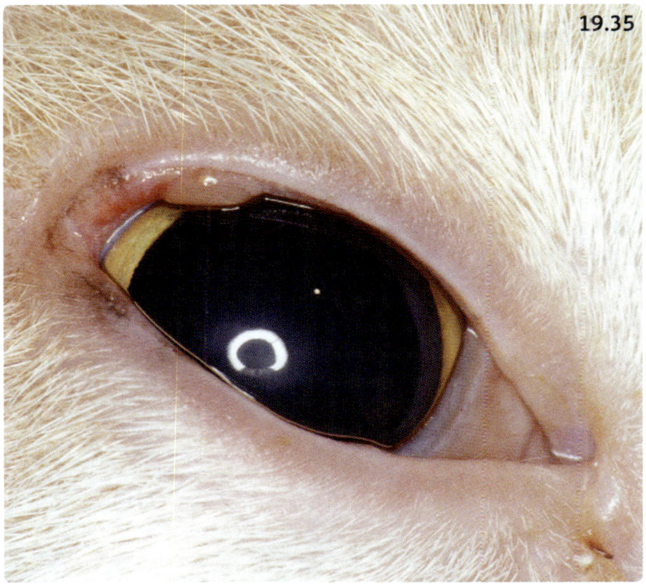

19.35

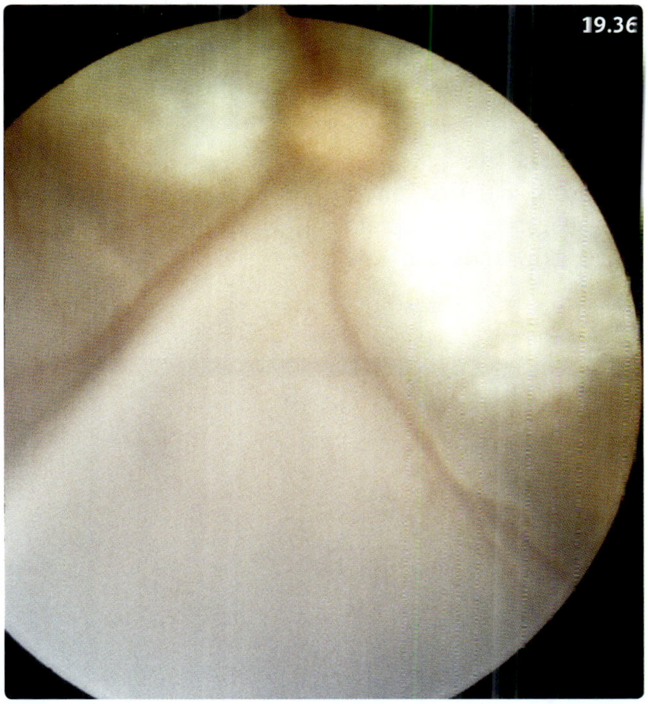

19.36

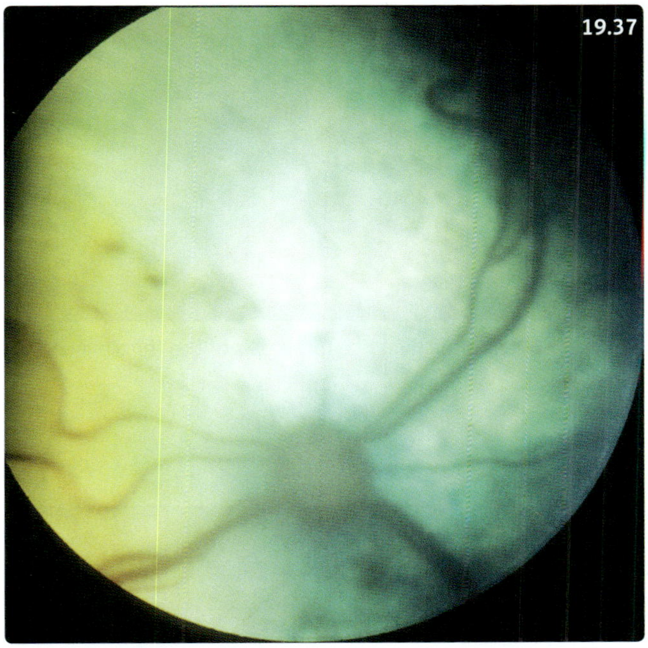

19.37

Figure 19.35–19.37 Cat with histoplasmosis. (19.35) Histoplasmosis is present as a lump in the upper lid of this cat. (19.36) A large fold of retina ventral to the optic disk indicates retinal detachment due to the histoplasmosis. (19.37) The contralateral eye has diffuse retinal edema and early detachment caused by histoplasmosis.

Pathophysiology

Alveolar macrophages phagocytize the conidia. These cells may be transported into the pulmonary interstitium from where they gain access to the vascular system and lymphatics. Hematogenous and lymphatic dissemination leads to pyogranulomatous disease. The eyes are commonly affected in both dogs and cats.

Clinical presentation

Ocular signs include conjunctivitis (**Figure 19.38**), corneal edema, corneal vascularization, anisocoria, anterior uveitis (**Figure 19.39**), secondary glaucoma, exophthalmos (retrobulbar inflammation), granulomatous chorioretinitis (**Figures 19.40–19.42**), RD, and optic neuritis (**Figure 19.43**).

Differential diagnosis

Tables 19.1, 19.3 and **19.4**.

Diagnosis

Diagnosis is based on the cytologic identification of the characteristic organisms within infected lymph nodes, skin, and eyes.

Management

Itraconazole, ketoconazole, and amphotericin B are effective in treating some cases of canine blastomycosis. Systemic corticosteroids combined with an antifungal may also be necessary to successfully treat blastomycosis. Itraconazole, ketoconazole, and etoconazole/amphotericin B can be used to treat blastomycosis in the cat.

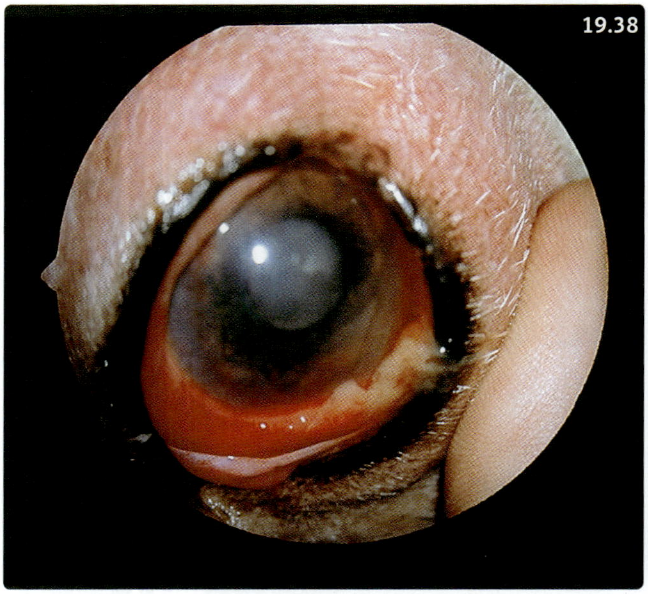

Figure 19.38 Severe iridocyclitis and conjunctivitis in a dog with blastomycosis.

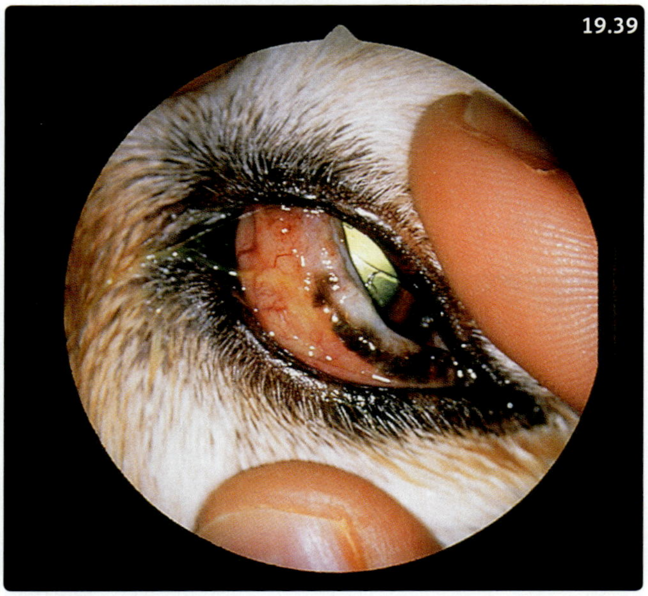

Figure 19.39 Conjunctival blastomycosis of the third eyelid in a dog.

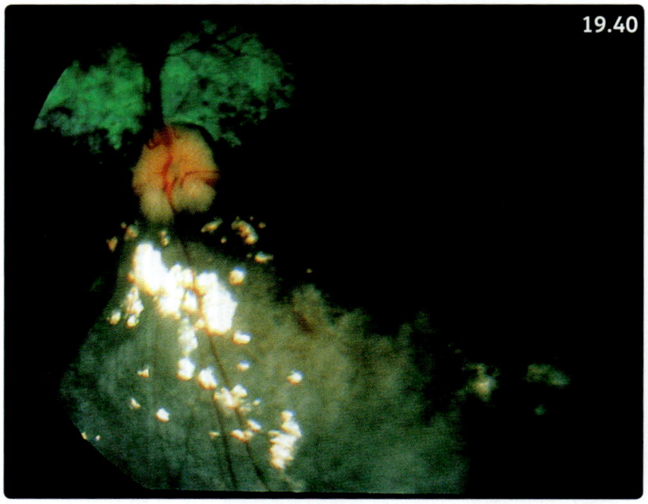

Figure 19.40 A large subretinal granuloma with multiple hyperreflective foci indicates active chorioretinitis in the nontapetum and optic neuritis in this dog with blastomycosis.

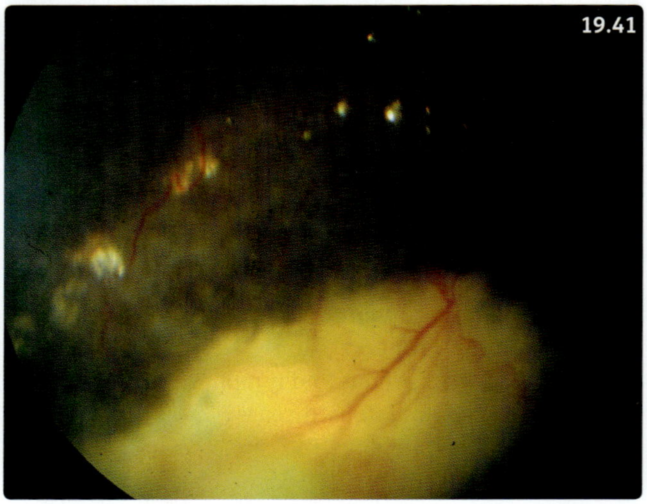

Figure 19.41 A large yellow retinal abscess from blastomycosis is present in this dog.

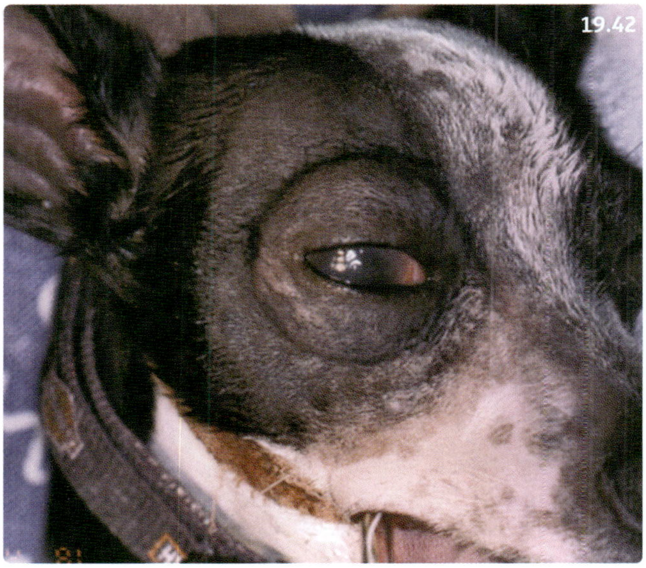

Figure 19.42 Periorbital swelling from blastomycosis-induced endophthalmitis.

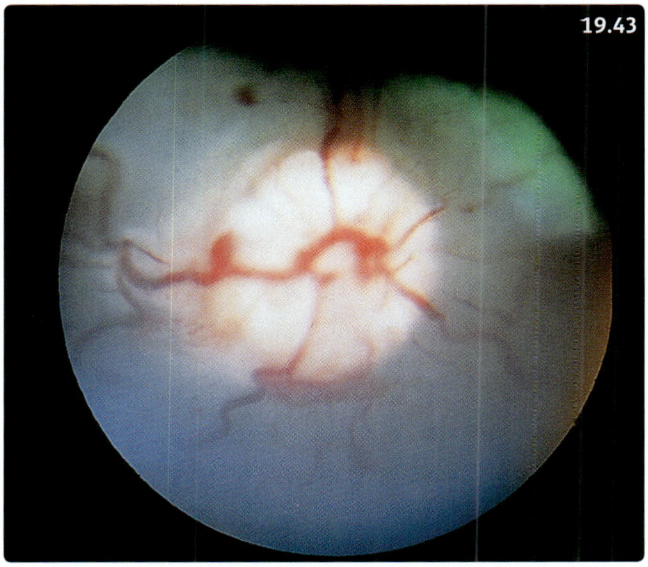

Figure 19.43 Optic neuritis, peripapillary retinal edema, and retinal hemorrhages in a dog with blastomycosis.

ASPERGILLOSIS

Definition/overview

Aspergillosis is caused by the filamentous fungus *Aspergillus* spp. Animals are infected opportunistically after inhaling *Aspergillus* spores. Disseminated aspergillosis has been reported to cause panuveitis, chorioretinitis, exudative RDs, and endophthalmitis (**Figures 19.44, 19.45**). German Shepherd Dogs are at increased risk. Diagnosis is made based on identification and culture of urine sediment, serum, synovial fluid,

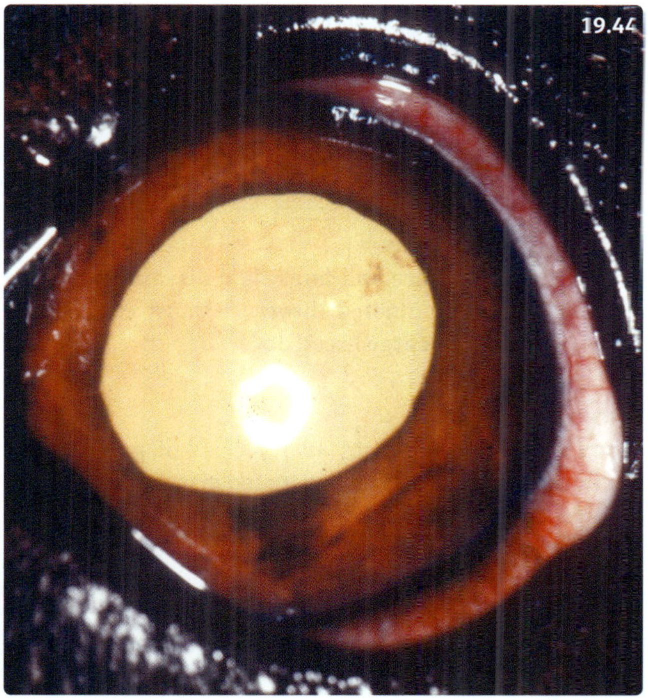

Figure 19.44 Bilateral vitreal haze in a dog with aspergillosis.

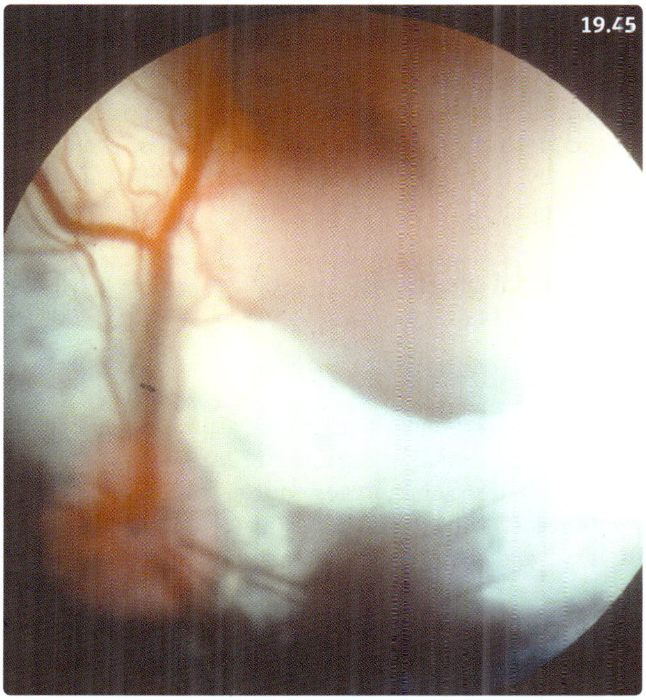

Figure 19.45 Severe active granulomatous chorioretinis caused by aspergillosis in the dog in Figure 19.44.

vitreous, lymph node, or intervertebral disk fine-needle aspirate biopsy specimens. Treatment is directed at eliminating the organism by administering amphotericin B, itraconazole, or fluconazole IV. Regardless, the prognosis for recovery from disseminated aspergillosis is poor.

ALGAE

PROTOTHECOSIS

Definition/overview

Protothecosis is a rare and fatal algal disease in the dog and cat. The disseminated disease is most common in Collies, Boxers, and large breed dogs.

Etiology

Protothecosis is caused by two species of green algae, *Prototheca zopfii* (causes disseminated disease) and *P. wickherhamii* (associated with skin disease). These organisms are found in animal wastes and sewage. They are transmitted by ingestion of contaminated food, soil, or water.

Clinical presentation

Systemic features in dogs include intermittent or protracted bloody diarrhea, CNS signs, skin lesions, lymphadenopathy, and respiratory and renal signs. Cats are reported to have skin lesions only. Ophthalmic signs are severe in >50% of the reported cases in dogs, and include focal, diffuse, granulomatous chorioretinitis (**Figures 19.46–19.48**), vitreal exudate, RDs and degeneration, retinal hemorrhage, and panuveitis. The ocular signs may be the initial clinical abnormality, and are usually bilateral.

Differential diagnosis

Tables 19.3–19.6.

Diagnosis

Diagnosis is by clinical signs, tissue aspiration, histologic and cytologic examination, and culture. Because colitis is one of the more common systemic signs associated with protothecosis, any dog with a history of hemorrhagic diarrhea and ocular lesions should be considered to be a candidate for this diagnosis.

Management

Amphotericin B and itraconazole were effective in two cases, but most systemic infections are fatal.

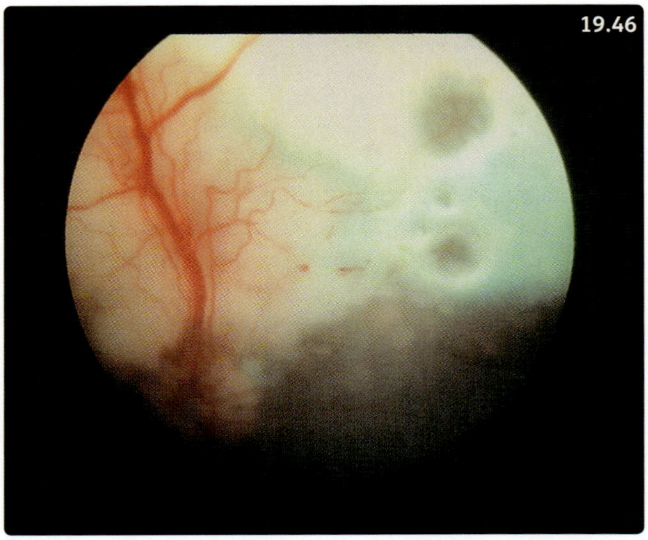

Figure 19.46 A subretinal granuloma elevates the retinal vessels dorsal to the optic disk. Focal hyperpigmented areas of chorioretinitis are also found in this dog with protothecosis.

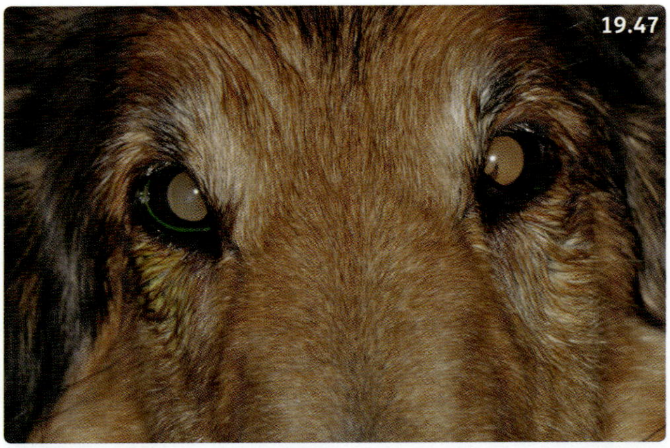

Figure 19.47 Bilateral vitreal haze in a dog with protothecosis.

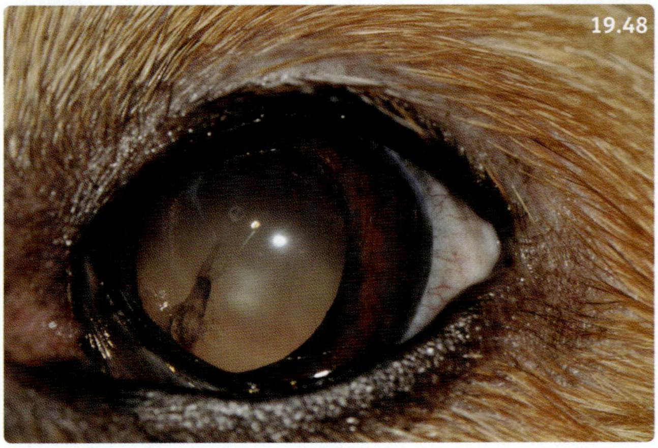

Figure 19.48 Note the anterior uveitis and vitreal opacification from protothecosis in the dog in Figure 19.47.

Table 19.5 Etiologies of sudden blindness.

Bilateral dilated and nonresponsive pupils: • Optic neuritis/GME • Retinal detachments • Acute glaucoma • Postictal (transient blindness) • Sudden acquired retinal degeneration • Ivermectin toxicosis Normal pupils and light reflexes (cortical blindness): • Congenital (hydrocephalus, lissencephaly, storage disease) • Metabolic (hypoglycemia, hepatic encephalopathy) • Toxic (lead poisoning) • Nutritional (thiamine deficiency) • Traumatic/vascular (embolus) • Hypoxic: postictal, respiratory or cardiac arrest • Infectious (canine distemper, toxoplasmosis, FIP) • Neoplastic (e.g. reticulosis, meningioma) • Idiopathic Normal pupils and light reflexes: • Cataracts

Table 19.6 Etiologies of retinal detachments.

Associated with Collie eye anomaly, retinal dysplasias Systemic infectious diseases: mycoses, FIP, toxoplasmosis, lymphosarcoma/FeLV, and other intraocular inflammatory diseases Neoplastic disease causing solid detachment Traction detachments associated with vitreoretinal adhesions Trauma Vitreal degeneration Sudden decreases in intraocular pressure Serous or fluid detachments (vasculitis, uremia, vascular hypertension) Extraocular pressure Retinal holes

RICKETTSIA

EHRLICHIA CANIS

(See also Chapter 21: Infectious diseases.)

Definition/overview

Ehrlichiosis is a tick-borne systemic disease known to be caused by a variety of rickettsial species. Several species of *Ehrlichia* are known to infect the dog, although *E. canis* is the most common. *E. canis* infection is associated with acute, subclinical, and chronic phases.

Etiology

E. canis is a small pleomorphic rickettsial organism that infects circulating mononuclear cells. The brown dog tick, *Rhipicephalus sanguineus*, is the arthropod vector of *E. canis*.

Pathophysiology

The prevalence of ocular lesions in canine ehrlichiosis has been reported as 10–37% and they are typically bilateral. Ocular lesions result from platelet deficiency, vasculitis, or both. Chronic disease occurs in those dogs unable to mount an effective immune response to the organism. Neurologic signs consistent with meningoencephalitis are typical of dogs with disease manifestations that develop during chronic infection.

Clinical presentation

Systemic features include lymphadenopathy, fever, nasal discharge, thrombocytopenia, and pancytopenia, with an underlying vasculitis. The ophthalmic signs include tortuous retinal vessels with gray perivascular circular retinal foci in the early stages. Chorioretinitis and retinal vasculitis appearing as dark gray spots with surrounding hyperreflectivity in the tapetal fundus, subretinal hemorrhages, RD, optic neuritis, and papilledema are found in the later stages. Anterior uveitis, iridal petechiae, hyphema, and keratic precipitates may also be prominent (**Figures 19.49, 19.50**).

Differential diagnosis

Tables 19.4 and **19.6–19.8**.

Diagnosis

In the clinical setting, a diagnosis of ehrlichiosis is usually made on the basis of clinical signs, hematologic abnormalities, and serology. Nonregenerative anemia and thrombocytopenia are the predominant hematologic findings. Diagnosis of ehrlichiosis also involves direct visualization of morulae in peripheral blood smears, detection of *E. canis* antibodies, or PCR amplification of *Ehrlichia* spp. DNA.

Management

Tetracycline and doxycycline are used for systemic therapy. Anterior uveitis is treated with topical corticosteroids and atropine.

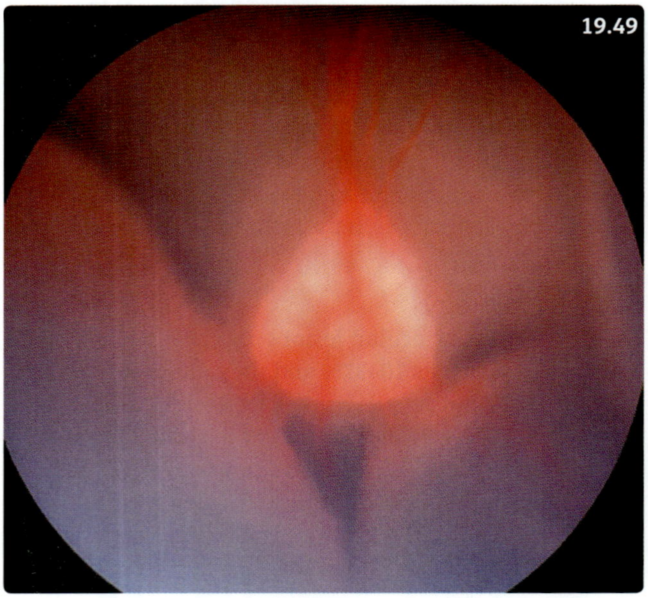

Figure 19.49 Retinal detachment involves nearly the entire retina in this dog with ehrlichiosis.

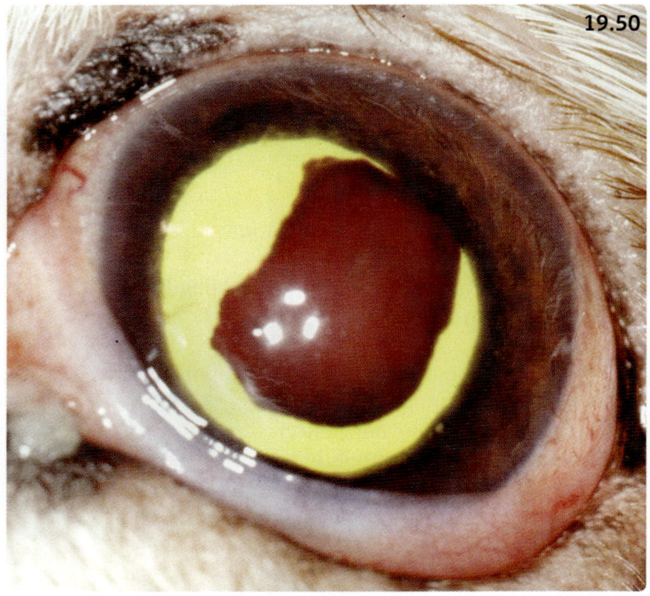

Figure 19.50 A blood clot is attached to the anterior lens capsule in this dog with ehrlichiosis.

Table 19.7 Etiologies of hyphema.

Uveitis associated with viral/bacterial/parasitic/fungal/ immune-mediated diseases
Congenital anomalies
Trauma (blunt trauma to head or globe, penetrating wounds of globe)
Intraocular tumors
Coagulopathies
Hyperviscosity syndromes
Hypertension
Retinal detachment
Glaucoma

Table 19.8 Etiologies of retinal hemorrhage.

Trauma
Bleeding disorders
Blood parasites
Hyperviscosity syndromes
Retinal inflammation
Neoplasia and lymphoreticular diseases
Congenital retinal/vascular anomalies
Hypertension
Severe anemia

ROCKY MOUNTAIN SPOTTED FEVER

Definition/overview

Rocky Mountain spotted fever (RMSF) is a rickettsial disease of several vertebrate species that is transmitted by ticks of the genus *Dermacentor.*

Etiology

RMSF is caused by *Rickettsia rickettsii*, the type species of the spotted fever group rickettsiae.

Pathophysiology

After entering the circulatory system, the rickettsiae replicate in the endothelial cells of capillaries and small blood vessels. Direct damage to the endothelial cells leads to vascular inflammation, necrosis, and increased vascular permeability. This process results in extravasation of fluid and blood cells into the extravascular fluid space. Varying degrees of damage are shown by the extent of ocular abnormalities.

Clinical presentation

RMSF has ocular signs of scleral injection/edema, anterior uveitis, hyphema, retinal edema, and focal retinal petechiae associated with a mucopurulent oculonasal discharge, cough, lymphadenopathy, muscle and joint pain, vasculitis, splenomegaly, and thrombocytopenia (**Figure 19.51**).

Differential diagnosis

Tables 19.4 and **19.6–19.8**.

Diagnosis

Diagnosis is based on direct immunofluorescent testing for the organism, serologic testing, PCR, or rickettsial culture.

Management

Tetracyclines are used for systemic therapy. Anterior uveitis is treated with topically administered corticosteroids and atropine.

CHLAMYDIA

Definition/overview

Chlamydia felis, the cause of feline 'pneumonitis', produces a mild conjunctivitis in cats. Along with FHV-1 it is the most common infectious cause of conjunctivitis in cats, and is considered a zoonotic disease. Dogs may be a reservoir for infection in cats. *C. psittaci* genotype C infection in dogs can cause keratoconjunctivitis. Clinically induced infections with *C. abortus* have also led to conjunctivitis. *C. psittaci* and *C. abortus* are both zoonotic.

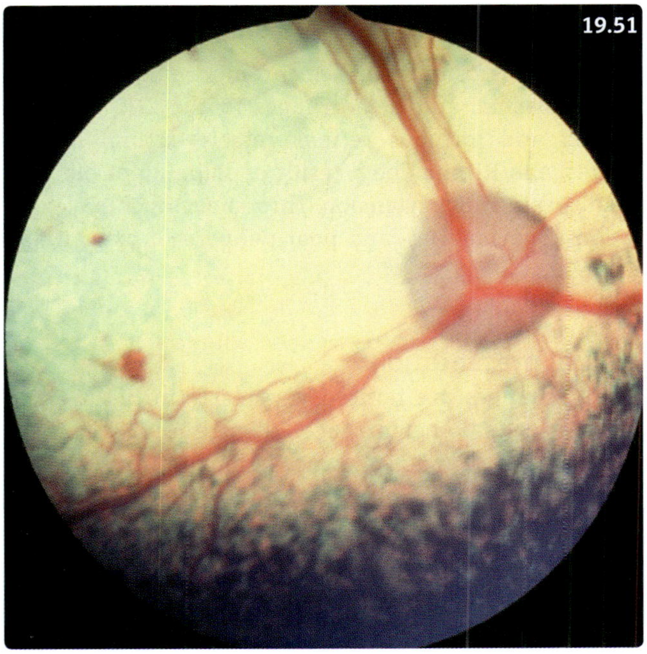

Figure 19.51 Multiple deep retinal focal hemorrhages are present in this dog with Rocky Mountain spotted fever.

Etiology

C. felis is an obligate intracellular bacterium that contains both DNA and RNA.

Pathophysiology

Ocular disease results from host cell lysis that occurs during the release of *Chlamydia* elementary bodies. Intracytoplasmic inclusions known as elementary bodies within conjunctival epithelial cells and neutrophils may be noticed in conjunctival cytologic scrapings early in the disease.

As the disease progresses, the discharge becomes mucoid and then mucopurulent, the chemosis decreases, and the conjunctiva becomes hyperemic and thickened. Follicular conjunctivitis occurs in chronic untreated cases. If untreated, infection with *C. felis* can produce chronic conjunctivitis. Asymptomatic carrier states can exist, and are likely significant in spreading the organism within a population.

Chlamydophilosis may be complicated by co-infection with other microorganisms including *Mycoplasma* spp., *Bordetella bronchiseptica*, feline calicivirus, FHV-1, and FIV.

Clinical presentation

Initially, the disease is unilateral, becoming bilateral in 7–14 days. Early in the disease, the conjunctiva is chemotic, glistening, and grayish-pink, and the ocular discharge is serous. Sneezing is also present early in the disease. Severe blepharospasm occurs and may cause a secondary spastic entropion.

Differential diagnosis

Conjunctivitis is found in many types of eye diseases. It may be infectious (herpesvirus, calicivirus, *Mycoplasma* and *Chlamydia* in cats) or noninfectious.

Diagnosis

Diagnosis of chlamydophilosis has been established by using a variety of ELISAs or using cell culture. *Chlamydia* spp. can be cultured in many types of mammalian and avian cells. Finding the characteristic inclusion body within the conjunctival epithelial cell cytoplasm on cytologic examination of Giemsa-stained conjunctival smears may be helpful in lending support for a diagnosis of chlamydophilosis. However, inclusions are typically only detectable during early infection, and in some cases not at all. PCR assays have become available for the diagnosis of *C. felis*.

Management

Treatment of chlamydial conjunctivitis consists of topical tetracycline, erythromycin, rifampin, fluoroquinolones, or azithromycin for several weeks. Systemic therapy may also be necessary. Vigorous therapy should be continued for several weeks after clinical signs subside. Follicular conjunctivitis is treated by anesthetizing the cat and rupturing the follicles by vigorously rubbing with a gauze sponge or scraping with a surgical blade. Topical tetracycline and corticosteroids are then applied, unless the corneal epithelium is damaged. Recurrence of disease is common in catteries and research colonies due to the short immunity to *C. felis*. *C. felis* may cause disease in humans; therefore, owners and technicians are advised to exercise care and observe strict hygiene when handling or treating infected cats. Vaccination may be necessary to prevent reoccurrence.

NEMATODIASIS

Ocular filariasis is associated with immature canine heartworms (*Dirofilaria immitis*) in the anterior chamber or vitreous. Signs of anterior uveitis are evident, and the photophobic filarid fourth-stage larva may move from the anterior to posterior chamber. The immature heartworm must be surgically removed to be curative. Ocular larval migrans (*Toxocara canis* and *Balisascaris procyonis*) causes anterior uveitis and focal chorioretinitis. Visual impairment is generally mild. Diagnosis is by serologic testing and larval identification. Treatment involves surgical removal of the larvae and anthelmintics and anti-inflammatories.

MISCELLANEOUS SYSTEMIC DISEASES

Ocular manifestations of hypercalcemia from hyperparathyroidism, neoplasia, renal failure, and hypoadrenocorticism may be associated with white, perilimbal calcium crystals on the conjunctiva, corneal calcification, corneal degeneration, and cataracts. Sustained hypocalcemia due to primary hypoparathyroidism, postparturient hypocalcemia, acute kidney injury or chronic kidney disease, acute pancreatitis, and intestinal malabsorption can cause focal punctate to linear cataracts to form in the anterior and posterior cortices of the lens of dogs and cats.

HYPERVISCOSITY SYNDROME

Definition/overview

Hyperviscosity syndrome results from abnormal microcirculatory changes due to increased serum viscosity. The severity of hyperviscosity syndrome is linked to the size, shape, type, and concentration of large molecules (e.g. imunoglobulins [IgG and IgM]) in the bloodstream. (See Appendix: Clinical cases.)

Etiology

Hyperviscosity may be caused by monoclonal gammopathy (multiple myeloma, macroglobulinemia, lymphocytic leukemia), polycythemia, renal disease, hepatic tumors, and extreme leukocytosis (>100,000/µl).

Pathophysiology

The hyperviscosity results in thromboembolism, sludging of plasma, and hemorrhages in the CNS and eye. Dilated and tortuous retinal vessels, retinal hemorrhages, and RD may be a result of sludging of blood in small vessels, hypertension, thrombocytopenia, coagulation abnormalities, and poor delivery of oxygen and nutrients.

Clinical presentation

Ocular changes are noticed very early in disease and include retinal hemorrhage (**Figure 19.52**), retinal venous dilatation and segmentation, retinal vascular tortuosity, 'box-carring' of retinal vessels, microaneurysms of the retina, subretinal hemorrhage, RD (**Figures 19.53–19.55**), perivascular retinal folding, and papilledema. Anterior uveitis and secondary glaucoma may also be present.

Differential diagnosis

Tables 19.3, **19.4** and **19.8**.

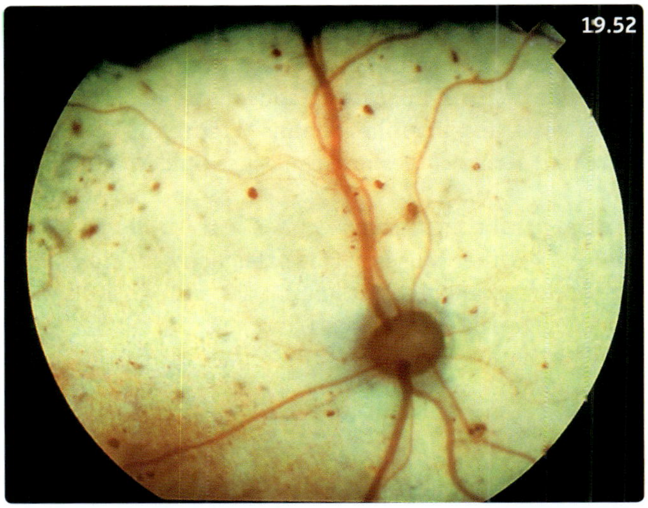

Figure 19.52 Multiple focal retinal hemorrhages and a small, peripheral, serous retinal detachment in an 18-year-old Siamese cat with hyperviscosity syndrome.

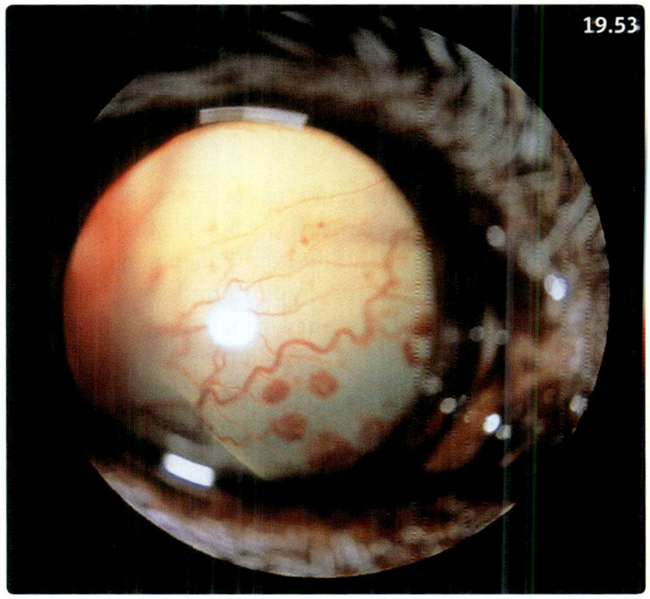

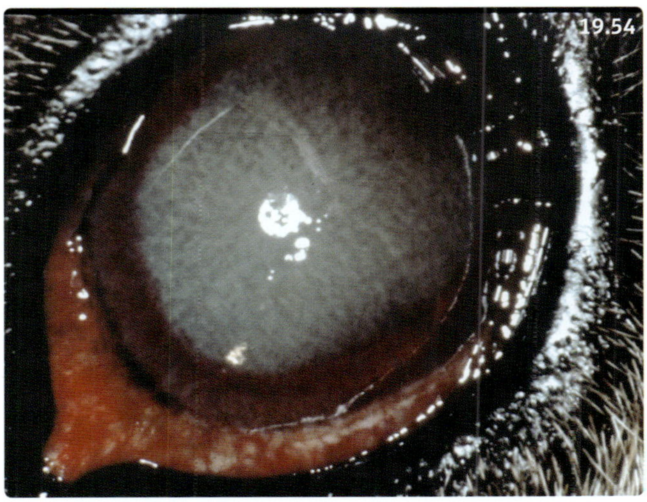

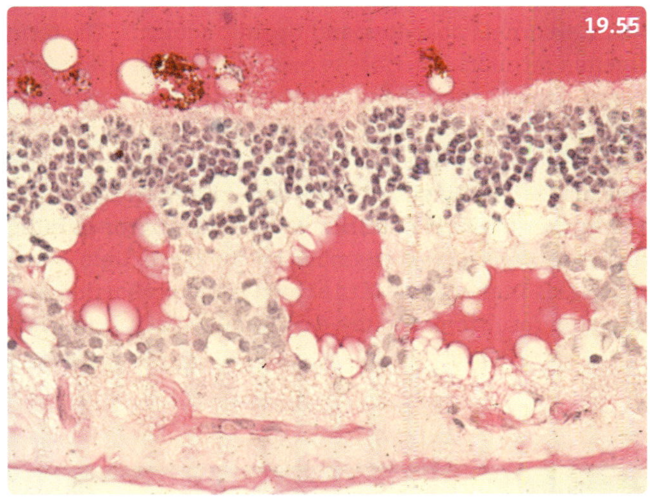

Figures 19.53–19.55 Dog with macroglobinemia and hyperviscosity syndrome. (19.53) Note the undulating retinal detachment with retinal hemorrhages in the dilated pupil. (19.54) Note the corneal edema from secondary glaucoma. (19.55) Histology. The right retina is detached with a large amount of PAS-positive subretinal fluid present. Intraretinal PAS-positive deposits, retinal vessel dilatation, and retinal pigment epithelium hyperplasia are noted. (×250)

Diagnosis

A coagulation assessment (platelet count, partial thromboplastin time, prothrombin time), serum protein electrophoresis, and serum viscosity measurements should be undertaken. Animals should undergo a thorough anterior segment and funduscopic examinations.

Management

Plasmapheresis may be used to treat the hyperviscosity. Specific antineoplastic therapy directed at the underlying disease is indicated.

HYPERLIPIDEMIA

Definition/overview

Hyperlipidemia is an increase in plasma concentration of triglycerides and/or cholesterol. Hyperlipidemia represents an abnormal finding in fasted dogs and cats, and, when present, is indicative of either increased production or reduced degradation of lipoproteins. Hypothyroidism, diabetes mellitus, hyperadrenocorticism, pancreatitis, and renal (e.g. nephrotic syndrome) as well as hepatic (e.g. cholestasis) diseases can be associated with hyperlipidemia. Both primary and secondary hyperlipidemias may show ocular signs. Dogs and cats are commonly affected.

Etiology

Hyperlipidemia in dogs may be primary as an idiopathic hyperlipoproteinemia in the Beagle, Briard, Collie, Miniature Schnauzer, and Shetland Sheepdog, or be secondary to diabetes mellitus, hypothyroidism, pancreatitis, lipoprotein lipase deficiency, renal and liver disease, or Cushing's disease. Hyperlipidemia can occur in cats for several reasons, including postprandial hyperlipidemia, diabetes mellitus, exogenous corticosteroid administration, megestrol acetate administration, nephrotic syndrome, lipoprotein lipase deficiency, idiopathic hyperchylomicronemia, and familial hyperchylomicronemia.

Pathophysiology

Altered lipid metabolism leads to lipemia of ocular blood vessels, corneal opacities, and lipemic aqueous. The term lipemia retinalis describes excess lipid within the retinal vessels, thus giving them a pale appearance. In both cats and dogs, it is the large, triglyceride-rich lipoproteins (e.g. low-density lipoproteins) that produce a visible lipemia. Hyperlipidemia may also manifest with lipids in the anterior chamber. A prerequisite for gaining access to the anterior chamber by the large, lipid-laden molecules is alteration of the blood–aqueous barrier, presumably resulting from pre-existing uveitis. It is unclear, however, whether the lipids incite or are the result of uveitis.

Clinical presentation

Increased triglycerides may result in brain dysfunction, acute pancreatitis, lipid-laden aqueous humor with anterior uveitis, and lipemia retinalis (**Figures 19.56–19.59**). Increased serum cholesterol can cause lipid keratopathy.

Differential diagnosis

Table 19.4. Other causes of corneal opacity, including corneal ulcers, scars, and inflammatory cellular infiltrates, must also be ruled out.

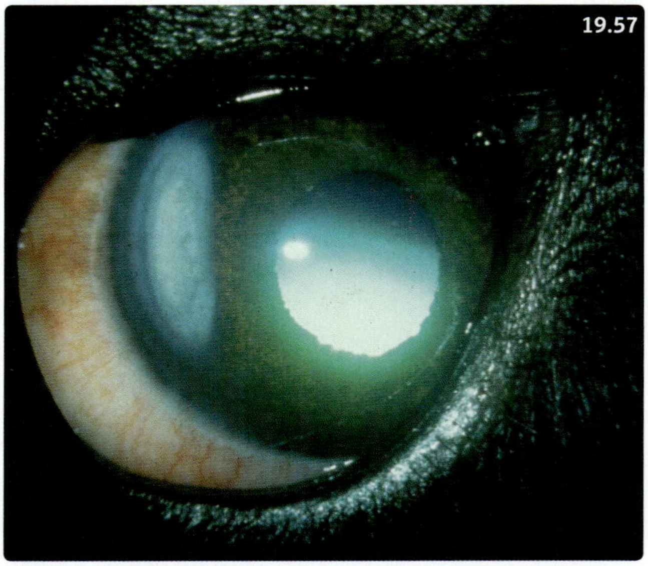

Figure 19.57 Lipidosis of the cornea in a hypercholesterolemic Dobermann.

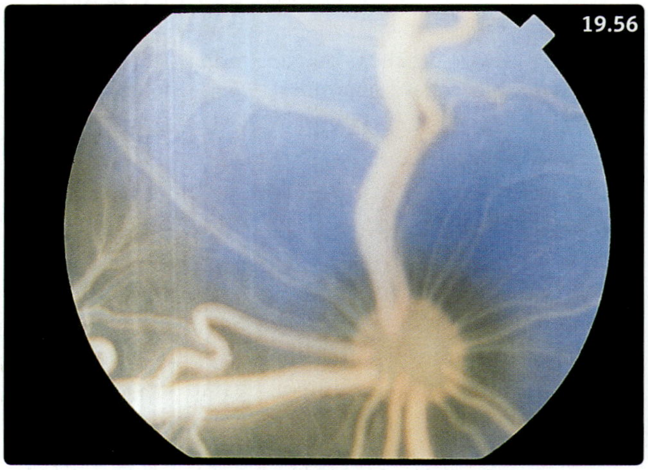

Figure 19.56 Lipemia retinalis in a kitten with a lipoprotein lipase deficiency.

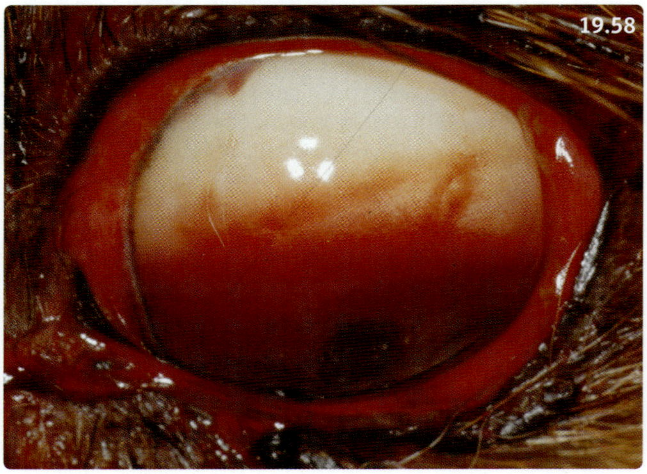

Figure 19.58 Hyphema and lipid aqueous in a lipemic dog with anterior uveitis.

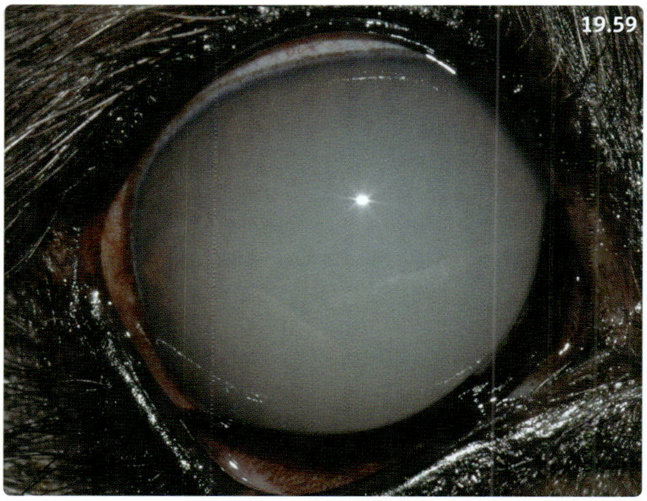

Figure 19.59 Lipemic aqueous in a dog.

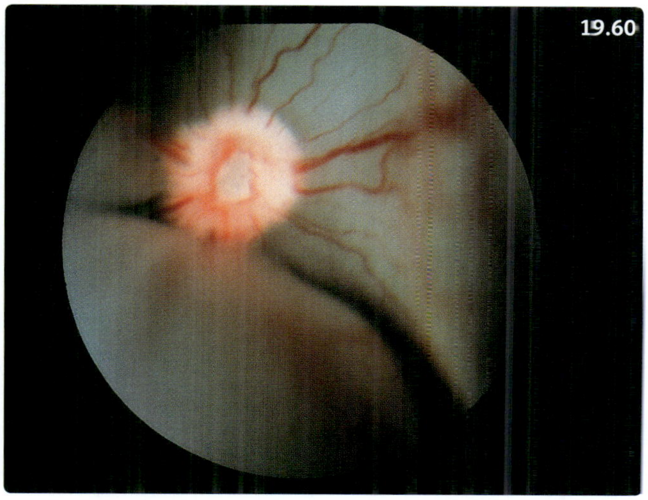

Figure 19.60 Exudative retinal detachment in a dog with nephrotic syndrome.

Diagnosis

Diagnosis is based on measurement of specific serum lipoproteins by electrophoresis or ultracentrifugation.

Management

Lipid-laden aqueous and lipemia retinalis resolve with resolution of the primary disorder and dietary modifications (low-fat diet), if necessary. Iridocyclitis should be treated if present. Corneal lipid accumulation may not resolve. Only a limited number of lipid lowering drugs have been used in dogs, with varying degrees of success for persistent hyperlipidemia. These include gemfibrozil, fish oils, cholestyramine, and lovastatin.

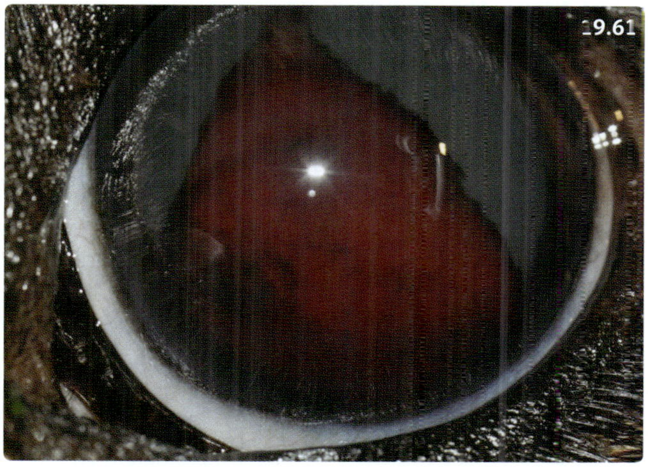

Figure 19.61 Hyphema shown in one of both eyes from a dog with immune-mediated hemolytic anemia and thrombocytopenia.

SYSTEMIC VASCULAR DISEASE

RDs associated with systemic hypertension due to chronic kidney disease are common in older cats and noticed in dogs (**Figure 19.60**). RDs result in blindness, but vision may return if the hypertension responds to medical treatment and dietary adjustment.

ANEMIA

Definition/overview

Ocular manifestations of severe anemia in cats and dogs include conjunctival pallor, pale attenuated retinal vasculature, varying degrees of retinal hemorrhage, and subtle changes in tapetal reflectivity. Retinal hemorrhages are more likely to be observed, however, and are more dramatic if accompanied by thrombocytopenia. The lack of red blood cells renders vascular endothelial cells hypoxic, thereby increasing vascular fragility and allowing retinal hemorrhages to occur in cats and dogs. The tapetal reflection is generally normal, which differentiates the retinal vessel attenuation from anemia from the attenuation found with retinal degeneration. Thrombocytopenia is more likely to cause ocular lesions such as hyphema and anterior uveitis in dogs (**Figures 19.61, 19.62**).

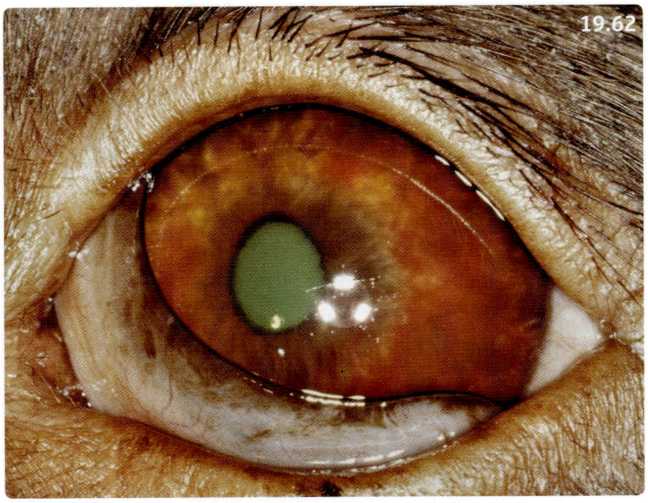

Figure 19.62 Iritis from thrombocytopenia in a dog.

ARTERIAL HYPERTENSION

(See also Chapter 12: Nephrology/urology.)

Definition/overview

Repeatable measurements of systolic pressure exceeding 160 mmHg and/or diastolic blood pressure measurements >100 mmHg are considered arterial hypertension. Blindness is one of the most common presenting complaints with this disorder, as the eye is particularly sensitive to the effects of high blood pressure. Hypertensive retinopathy in many cats is a slow, insidious process. Vision may be spared if the process is identified and controlled before severe ocular disease develops. Consequently, old cats with diseases such as chronic kidney disease and hyperthyroidism should be screened for systemic hypertension.

Etiology

Arterial hypertension in dogs and cats has been associated with old age, chronic anemia, hypercholesterolemia, athero-/arteriosclerosis, high salt diets, obesity, and idiopathic essential hypertension. Secondary hypertension in dogs is now recognized as being a common complication of renal disease (60–80% of cases), hyperadrenocorticism (59–86% of cases), pheochromocytoma (>50% of cases), diabetes mellitus, primary hyperaldosteronism, hypothyroidism, and hyperthyroidism.

Hypertensive cats have been shown to have a greater prevalence of retinal lesions (48%) compared with normotensive cats (3%). In addition, cats with retinopathies had higher blood pressure (262 ± 34 mmHg) than hypertensive cats without retinal lesions (221 ± 34 mmHg). Cats over 8 years of age should have their fundi examined for lesions related to hypertension.

Pathophysiology

Renal pathology causes an increase in renin–angiotensin–aldosterone activity, which, in combination with increased plasma levels of norepinephrine, causes peripheral vasoconstriction. Incoming arterial and capillary blood at high pressure causes vasospasm, tissue hypoxia of the capillary beds allowing changes in vessel permeability, and exudation of fluid, plasma, or blood, resulting in development of infarcts and end organ damage.

The consequence of ocular vascular hypertensive changes is an initial vascular constriction in the retinal arterioles in response to increased blood pressure, which when sustained, results in occlusion and ischemic necrosis of the vessel walls with resultant increased vascular permeability. The ocular circulation is not tolerant of such changes in its microcirculation.

Clinical presentation

Ocular features in cats and dogs with hypertension include retinal arteriolar tortuosity, preretinal hemorrhage, retinal edema, perivasculitis, anterior uveitis, vitreal and anterior chamber hemorrhage, RDs, and retinal atrophy (**Figures 19.63–19.73**). In severe cases, irreversible blindness occurs.

Differential diagnosis

Tables 19.3–19.5 and **19.8**.

Diagnosis

Diagnosis is based on serial measurements of blood pressure. A complete blood count (CBC), urinalysis, and serum biochemical profiles should be undertaken in all patients.

Management

Treatment includes salt restricted diets, diuretics, and calcium channel blockers such as amlodipine. Eyes with RD and little hemorrhage may reattach and recover vision if the RD has been present for less than 2–3 weeks.

HEMORRHAGIC RETINOPATHY

Definition/overview

Hemorrhage with retinal disease may be manifested as preretinal bleeding in the vitreous, superficial linear retinal hemorrhages, small circular focal deep retinal areas of hemorrhage, and large, dark subretinal hemorrhages.

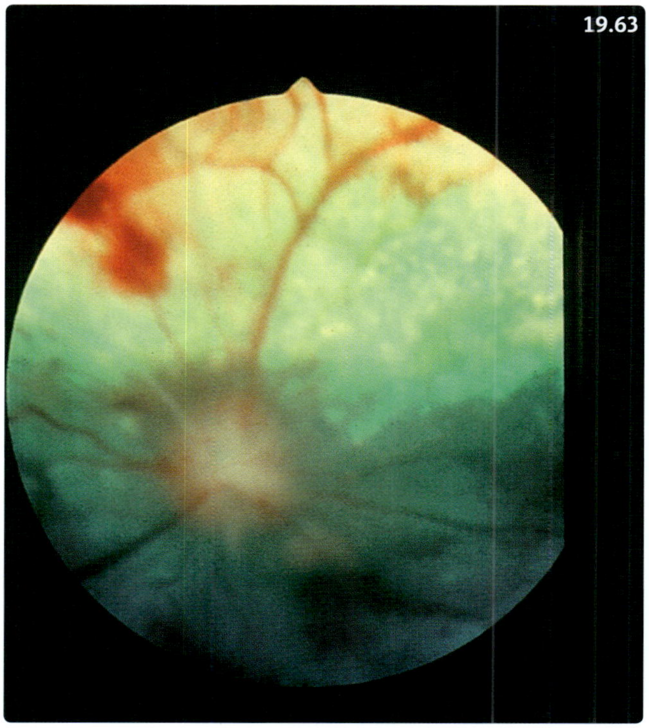

Figure 19.63 Retinal hemorrhages, vitreal haze, retinal edema, and optic neuritis in a dog with renal failure and hypertension.

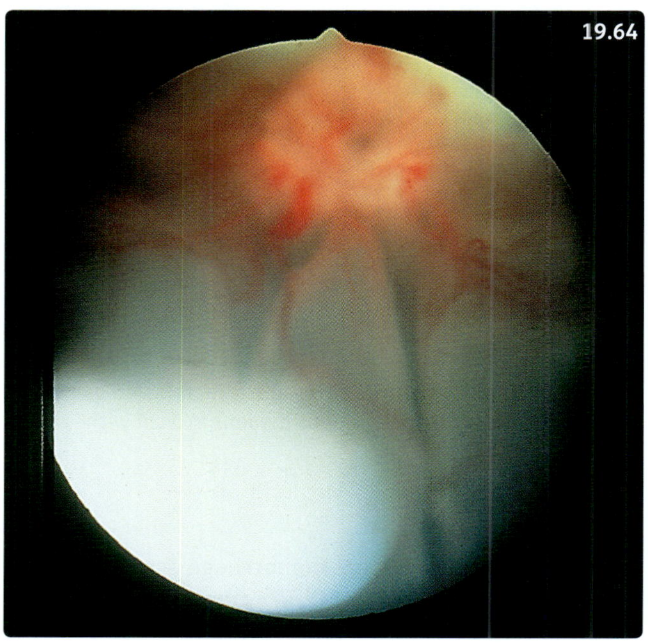

Figure 19.64 Extensive retinal folding and detachment and preretinal hemorrhages in a dog with systemic hypertension.

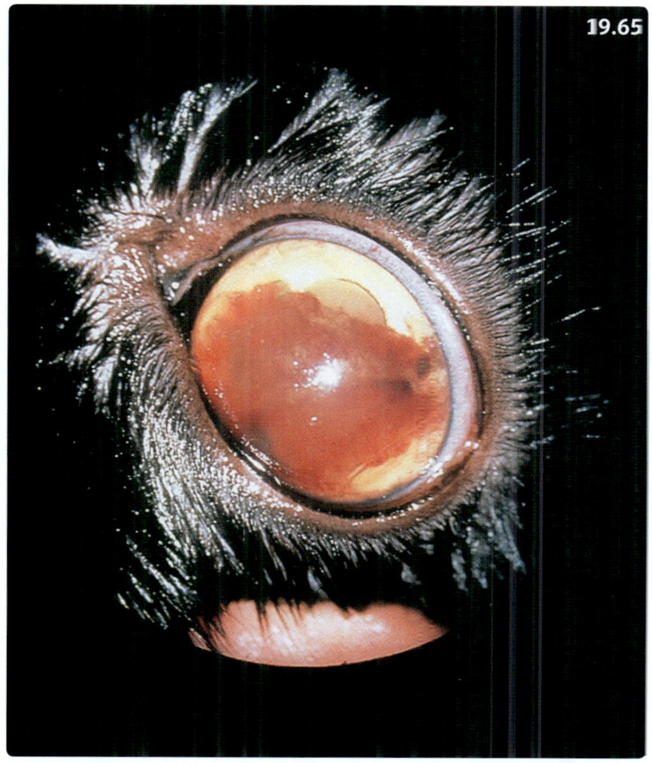

Figure 19.65 Hyphema is present in this cat with systemic hypertension.

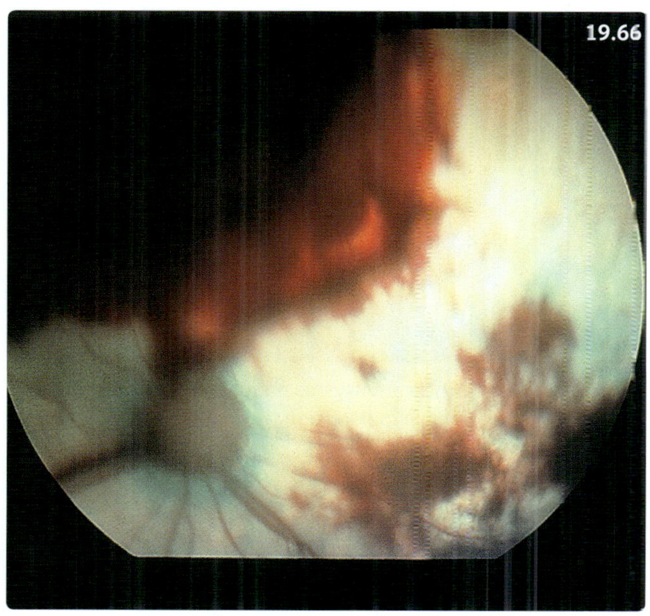

Figure 19.66 Hypertensive retinopathy manifested by dorsal vitreal hemorrhage and intraretinal hemorrhage in a cat.

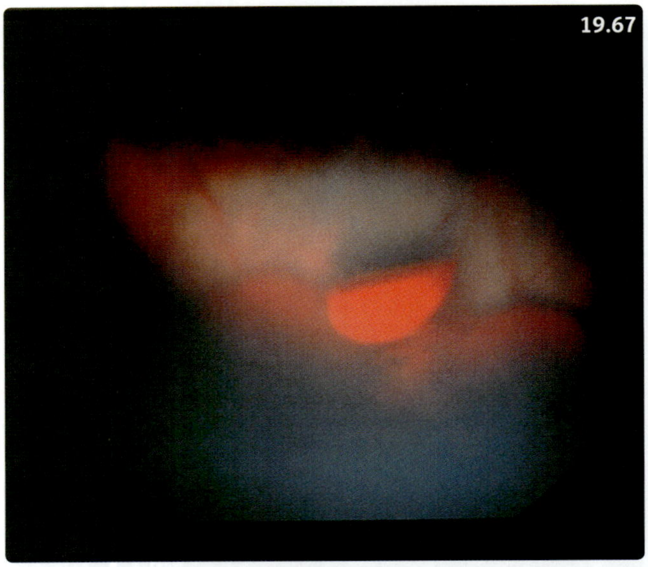

Figure 19.67 Preretinal 'keel boat' hemorrhage in a cat with hypertensive retinopathy.

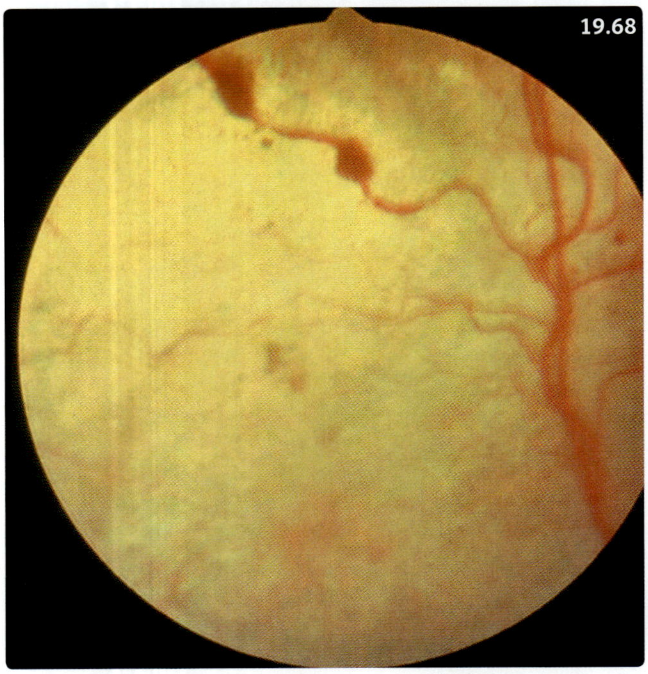

Figure 19.68 Arteriolar aneurysms are present in the retina of this dog with systemic hypertension.

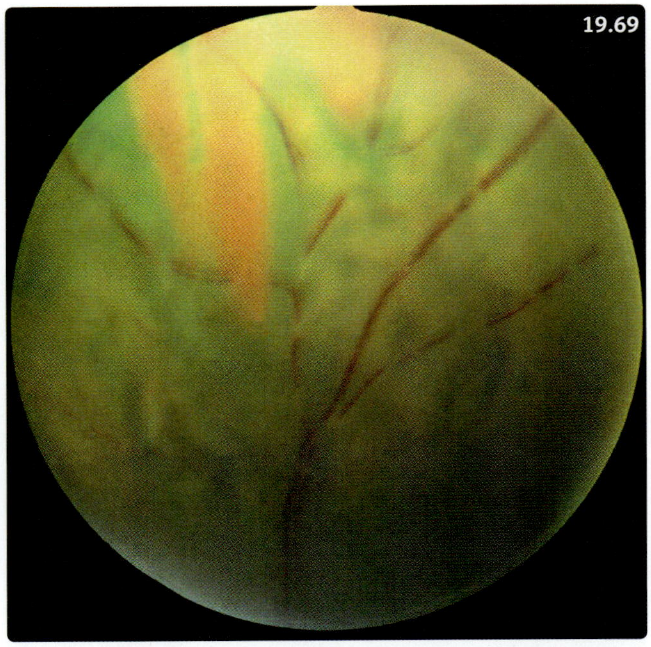

Figure 19.69 'Box carring' of retinal vessels indicates that the retinal tissue pressure is elevated and retinal perfusion reduced in this cat with systemic hypertension.

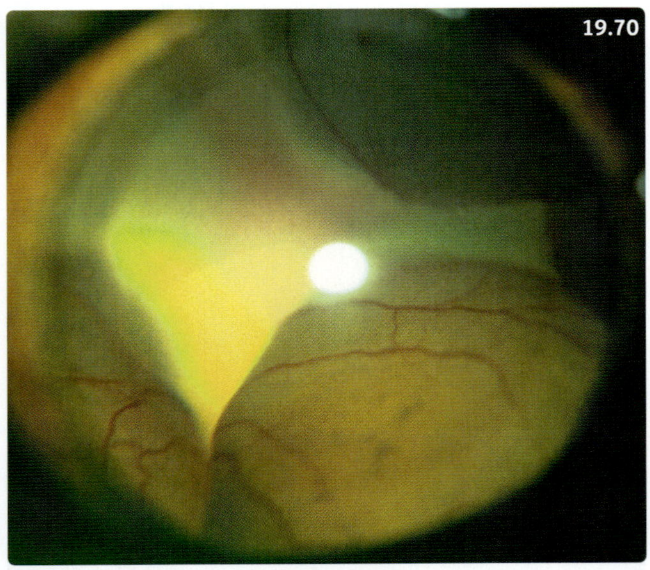

Figure 19.70 Bullous retinal detachment manifested as folds of opaque tissue posterior to the lens in a cat with hypertension.

Etiology

Hemorrhagic retinopathy is seen associated with anemia, systemic hypertension, coagulopathies, and systemic infections. The cat has an apparently unique predisposition to the development of small multifocal areas of intraretinal and preretinal hemorrhage associated with severe anemia (**Figure 19.74**). Lymphosarcoma, reticuloendotheliosis with thrombocytopenia, chronic bleeding from a duodenal ulcer, FIP, and hemobartonellosis are other causes for hemorrhagic retinopathy in cats.

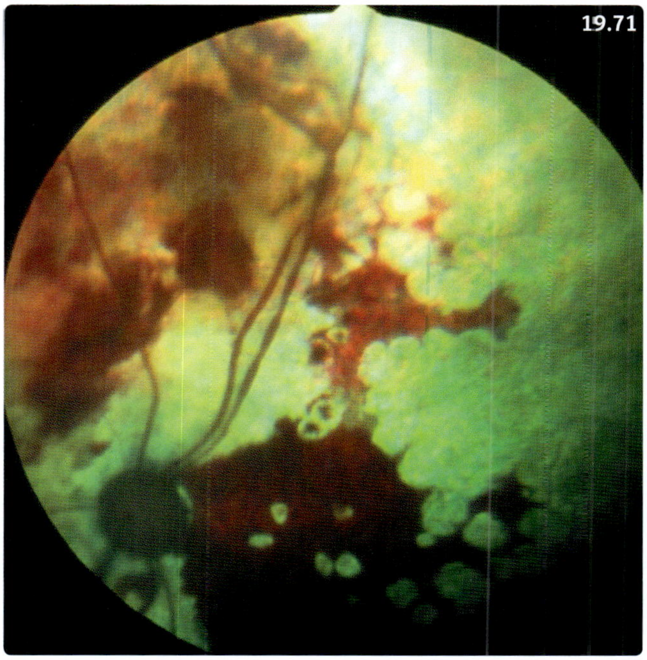

Figure 19.71 Vitreal and retinal hemorrhages obscure the optic disk in a dog with immune-mediated thrombocytopenia.

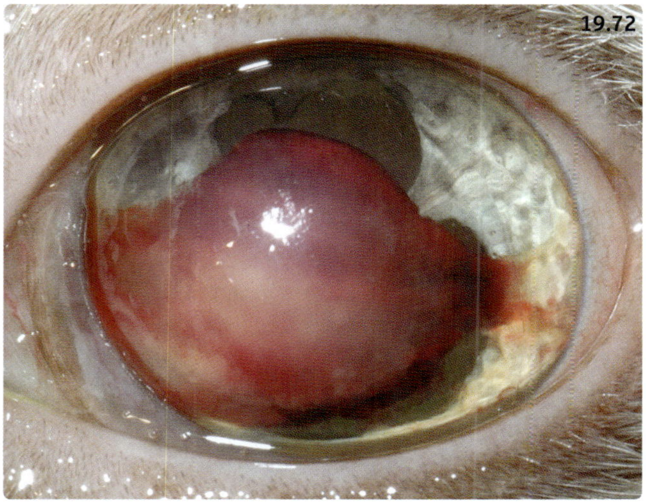

Figure 19.72 Hyphema is present in a dog with vascular hypertension.

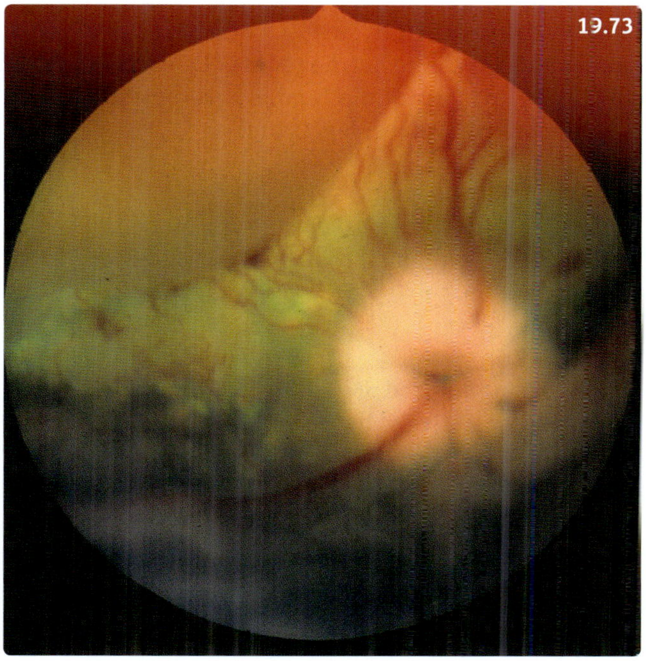

Figure 19.73 Retinal detachment and retinal hemorrhages in a dog with vascular hypertension.

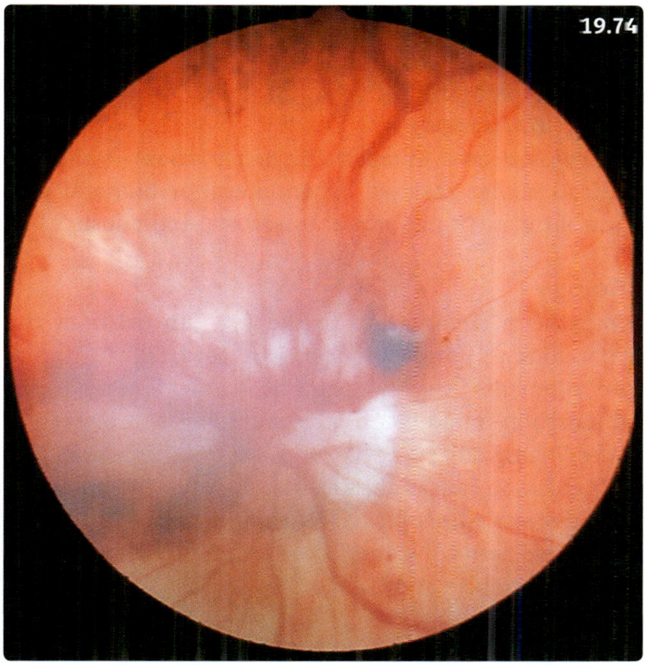

Figure 19.74 Vitreal and retinal hemorrhage obscure the fundus in a cat with systemic hypertension.

Pathophysiology

Vascular constriction in retinal arterioles in response to increased blood pressure results in occlusion and ischemic necrosis of the vessel walls, with a resultant increase in retinal vascular permeability and possible hemorrhage. Choroidal vascular changes result in subretinal fluid accumulation and RD.

Clinical presentation

Retinal and vitreal hemorrhages may be observed bilaterally in all regions of the fundus in a majority of cats with hemoglobin values <5 g/100 ml.

Differential diagnosis

Tables 19.5, 19.6 and **19.8**. Systemic hypertension should be ruled out with any ocular hemorrhage or RD of unknown origin.

Diagnosis

Repeated systolic blood pressure measurements >160–180 mmHg are indicative of hypertension.

Management

Functional vision is not usually affected in mildly hypertensive cats, and treatment is normally directed against the primary cause of anemia or hypertension. Massive vitreal hemorrhage generally results in irreversible blindness. Antihypertensive agents including beta-adrenergic blockers, diuretics, angiotensin converting enzyme inhibitors, vasodilators, and calcium channel blockers may be beneficial.

HORNER'S SYNDROME

Definition/overview

Horner's sydrome (sympathetic denervation) in the dog and cat is characterized by unilateral or bilateral prolapse of the nictitans, ptosis, anisocoria, and miosis.

Etiology

Sympathetic denervation to the eye can occur at the hypothalamus, brainstem/cervical cord, T1–T3 spinal cord segments, vagosympathetic trunk, cranial cervical ganglion, middle ear, ophthalmic branch of cranial nerve V, long ciliary nerve, and iris dilator muscle. The most common causes of Horner's syndrome include anterior mediastinal neoplasia, brachial plexus injury, otitis media, and cervical trauma. It is commonly idiopathic in Golden Retrievers and Collies.

Pathophysiology

Loss of sympathetic innervation causes a lack of tone in the orbital smooth muscle so that the eye retracts slightly, producing enophthalmos. Loss of innervation to the muscle of the upper eyelid (Muller's muscle) and sympathetically innervated tissue in the lower eyelid results in narrowing of the palpebral fissure and incomplete elevation of the upper eyelid, or ptosis. Lack of sympathetic tone and enophthalmos results in protrusion of the nictitans, which is most prounounced in cats. Reduction of normal sympathetic tone to the iris dilator muscle results in the anisocoria and miosis in the affected eye **(Figure 19.75)**.

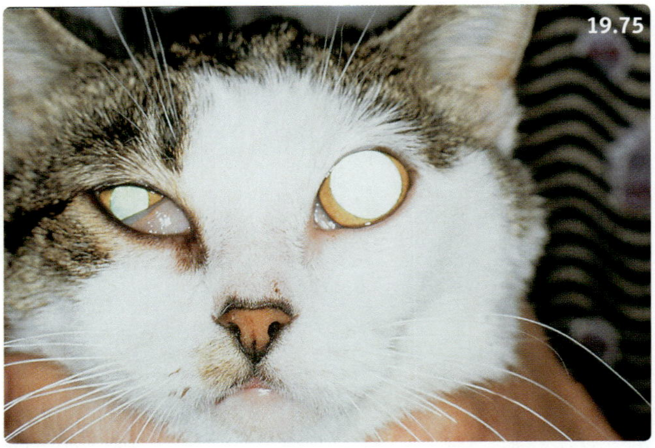

Figure 19.75 Miosis, nictitans protrusion, and ptosis are found on the right side of a cat with Horner's syndrome caused by neoplastic involvement of the right middle ear.

Clinical presentation

The Horner's miotic pupil is not pinpoint in room light. Constriction still occurs and dilation in dark light occurs, but not as much dilation as a normal pupil (no dilation beyond the size of the pupil with a resting iris sphincter muscle). The causative lesion can occur anywhere along the sympathetic chain. Intraocular pressure is normal and vision is present unless the pupil is obstructed by the protrusion of the nictitans.

Differential diagnosis

Uveitis can cause nictitans prominence when dogs and cats do not feel well, when the eye is painful, and a miotic pupil is found with aqueous flare in uveitis. Conjunctivitis and blepharospasm may be present with many eye diseases.

Diagnosis

Diagnosis is based on a complete physical examination and neurologic, otoscopic, and ophthalmologic examinations. Topically administered adrenergics such as 2.5% phenylephrine will restore the pupil to normal size, reposition the nictitans, and minimize the ptosis if the sympathetic lesion is postganglionic.

Management

The disorder spontaneously resolves in some patients.

FELINE DYSAUTONOMIA OR FELINE DILATED PUPIL SYNDROME

Definition/overview

Feline dysautonomia or feline dilated pupil syndrome (Key–Gaskell syndrome or feline autonomic neuropathy) is much more common in Europe than the USA. A similar syndrome is found in young, large breed dogs living in rural areas of the midwestern USA.

Etiology

The cause is unknown, although lesions in the autonomic ganglia are consistent with a toxic cause. The bacterium *Clostridium botulinum* may be important in the pathogenesis of feline dysautonomia

Pathophysiology

Parasympathetic and sympathetic ganglia are equally affected. There is depletion of neuronal cell bodies, with many remaining neurons showing an atypical homogeneous cytoplasm, eccentric pyknotic nuclei, and dissolution of Nissl substance. Autonomic nerves show axonal degeneration but peripheral nerves are comparatively spared. Ultrastructural changes include derangement of the rough endoplasmic reticulum, with cisternae lacking ribosomes and distended with flocculent material. Stacks of smooth membranous profiles are evident but no normal Golgi bodies.

Clinical presentation

Clinical signs include dilated, nonresponsive pupils with some cats showing dysphagia, prolapsed nictitans, constipation, bradycardia, decreased tear production (Schirmer tear tests may be as low as 0–2 mm/min), regurgitation due to megaesophagus, vomiting, and dysuria. Ataxia and poor proprioception may also occur.

Differential diagnosis

Table 19.2. Dilated pupils are associated with glaucoma and retinal and optic nerve diseases.

Diagnosis

Diagnosis should be suspected from the characteristic clinical signs and a definitive diagnosis confirmed by the presence of lesions in the autonomic ganglia. Urinary catecholamines are reduced. Pharmacologic testing can support the diagnosis. Pilocarpine (1%) topically constricts the pupil in affected cats, while topical echothiophate iodide (0.06%) and physostigmine (0.25%) will cause miosis in normal cats but not dysautonomic cats. Epinephrine at a concentration of 1:10,000 will induce retraction of the prolapsed third eyelid.

Management

Treatment includes supportive therapy with fluids laxatives, and dietary management. Topical parasympathomimetics may be beneficial. Recovery rates are poor

CANINE UVEODERMATOLOGIC SYNDROME

Definition/overview

Ocular manifestations of canine uveodermatologic syndrome (Vogt–Koyanagi–Harada [VKH])-like) are reported most often in the Akita, Australian Shepherd Dog, Beagle, Fila, Chow, Dachshund, Golden Retriever, Irish Setter, Old English Sheepdog, Saint Bernard, Samoyed, Shetland Sheepdog, and Siberian Husky dogs.

Etiology

This is an autoimmune condition directed against melanin of neural crest (skin, hair, anterior uvea) and neuroectodermal (retina) origin.

Pathophysiology

This syndrome is considered to be an immune-mediated reaction to melanin that affects various organs containing melanocytes. It is similar to VKH syndrome in people, although neurologic signs are rare in dogs. Skin lesions are the result of a Th1-mediated inflammatory response while ocular lesions are the result of a Th2-mediated inflammatory response. The role of certain dog leukocyte antigen class II gene alleles may be important regarding the pathogenesis of VKH-like syndrome in Akitas.

Clinical presentation

Severe, bilateral panuveitis (**Figures 19.76–19.82**) and hypotony, with secondary cataracts, glaucoma, RDs, and blindness are common. Iris and retinal depigmentation and poliosis/vitiligo of the face and muzzle are noticed. Ocular lesions appear before the skin lesions. Dermal and hair depigmentation (vitiligo and poliosis, respectively) develop either gradually or rapidly, and they may be ulcerative in nature. The lesions are usually restricted to the face, involving the eyelids, nasal planum, and lips, but the scrotum and footpads are other areas of possible dermal involvement.

Differential diagnosis

Table 19.2.

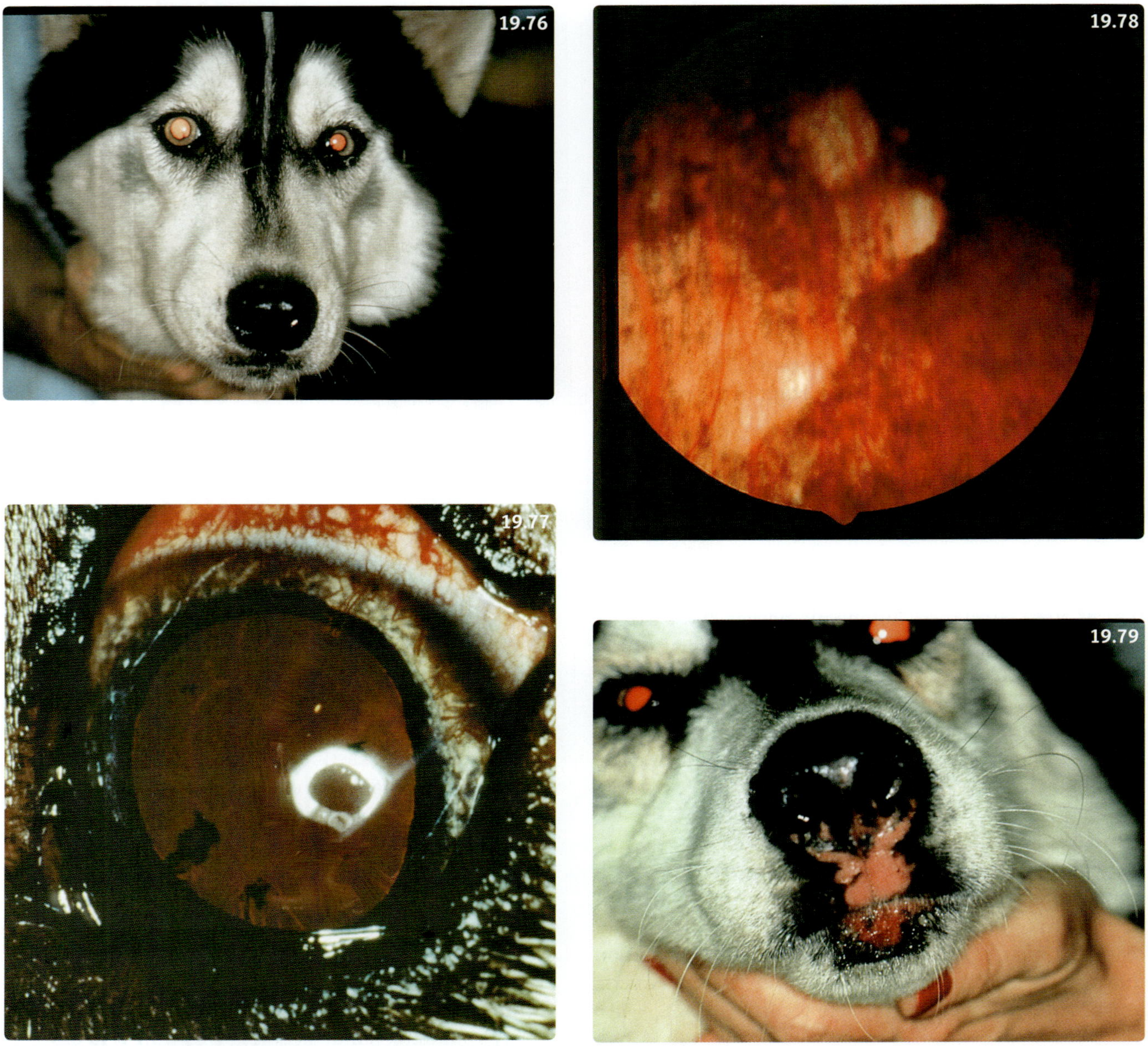

Figure 19.76–19.79 Husky dog with uveodermatologic (UVD) syndrome. (19.76) Iris color change due to iridocyclitis of the right eye. (19.77) Iridocyclitis and secondary glaucoma in the eye. (19.78) Focal depigmentation of the retinal pigment epithelium due to chorioretinitis. (19.79) Depigmentation of the nose accompanies a relapse of UVD syndrome in this dog.

Diagnosis

There is no specific diagnostic test for uveodermatologic syndrome. The diagnosis is made on the basis of clinical signs and histopathologic examination of skin biopsies. Skin biopsy specimens have lichenoid dermatitis, histiocytes, and small mononuclear cells as well as giant cell infiltrations. The level of melanin in the epidermis and hair follicles is decreased. Special stains should be requested in the presence of granulomatous infiltrates in an attempt to identify microorganisms. Other tests include a CBC, antinuclear antibody (ANA) test, Coombs test, and serologic testing for leishmaniasis.

Management

Short-term success with systemically administered corticosteroids or azathioprine is good, but recurrence is common. Topical treatment of the uveitis is required.

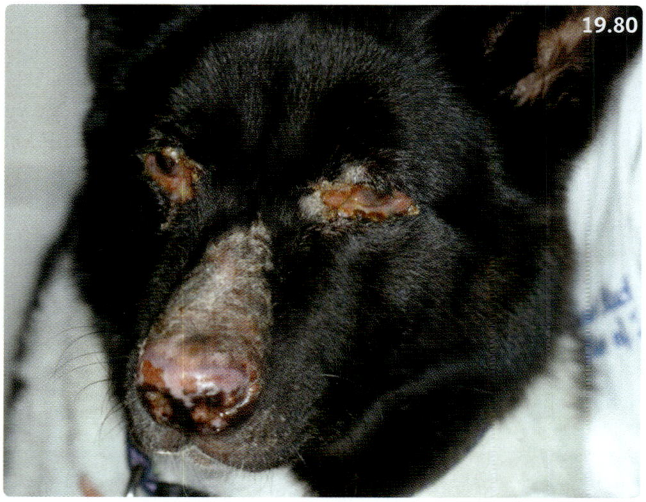

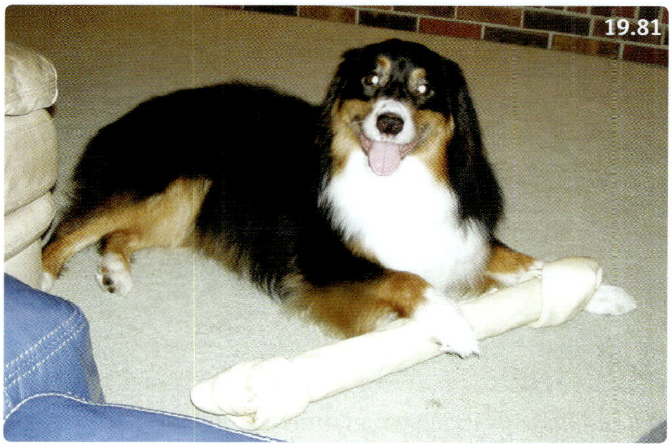

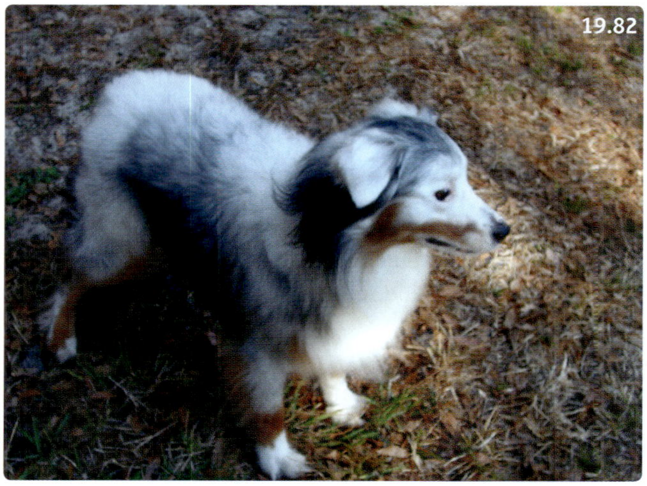

Figure 19.80–19.82 Uveodermatologic (UVD) syndrome. (19.80) The nose, periocular skin, and eyes are involved in this Akita. (19.81) Photograph of a 'normal' dog that eventually developed coat depigmentation of ocular lesions from UVD, as shown in 19.82.

GRANULOMATOUS MENINGOENCEPHALITIS

(See also Chapter 14: Disorders of the nervous system and muscle.)

Definition/overview

Granulomatous meningoencephalitis (GME) can be seen alone as a primary ocular disease or, more commonly, in conjunction with CNS disease. It is probably the most common inflammatory disease of the canine nervous system. The ocular signs may occur before CNS signs. The disease is typically seen in young small breeds, although any breed or age of dog may be affected.

Etiology

GME is an idiopathic, nonsuppurative inflammatory disease.

Pathophysiology

GME is characterized by the proliferation of reticuloendothelial elements and lymphoplastic infiltration of blood vessels of the CNS, the ciliary body, and the choroid. Perivascular infiltrates are composed of a heterogeneous population of major histocompatibility complex class-II antigen-positive macrophages and mainly CD3 antigen-positive lymphocytes, supporting a hypothesis of T-cell-mediated, delayed type hypersensitivity or an autoimmune disease.

Clinical presentation

Ocular features include acute, bilateral blindness with widely dilated, nonresponsive pupils. Uveitis, optic neuritis (hyperemic, swollen, elevated optic disk, disk hemorrhage, peripapillary engorged vessels), retinal inflammation (white perivascular cuffs and yellow–white patches), RD, and secondary glaucoma are common. The eye may appear normal if the optic nerve involvement is posterior to the globe (**Figures 19.83, 19.84**).

Differential diagnosis

Tables 19.1 and **19.4–19.6**.

Diagnosis

Diagnosis can only be confirmed at necropsy or by brain biopsy. MRI and analysis of CSF (increased CSF protein and pleocytosis) may enable a tentative diagnosis to be made.

Management

Treatment involves aggressive use of immunosuppressive corticosteroids often with added immunosuppression using cytosine arabinoside or cyclosporine A. Gradual

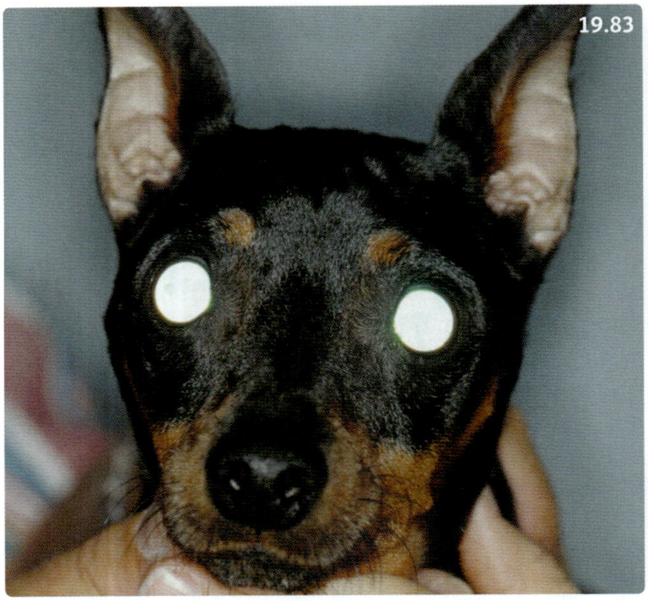

Figure 19.83 Dilated, nonresponsive pupils are present in a Miniature Pinscher with optic neuritis from granulomatous meningoencephalitis.

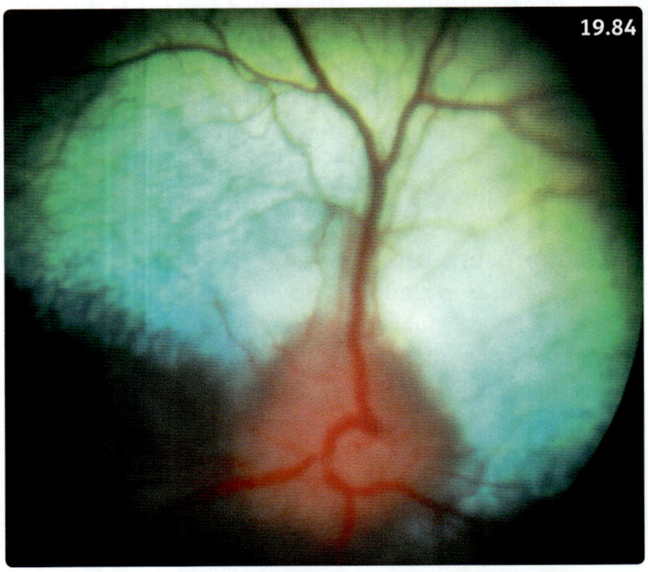

Figure 19.84 A swollen optic disk indicating optic neuritis that was associated with granulomatous meningoencephalitis.

improvement and temporary remission are possible with the judicious use of immunosuppressants.

LYMPHOSARCOMA

Definition/overview

Lymphosarcoma is the most common intraocular tumor of dogs and cats. It is a secondary ocular tumor, and is usually bilateral.

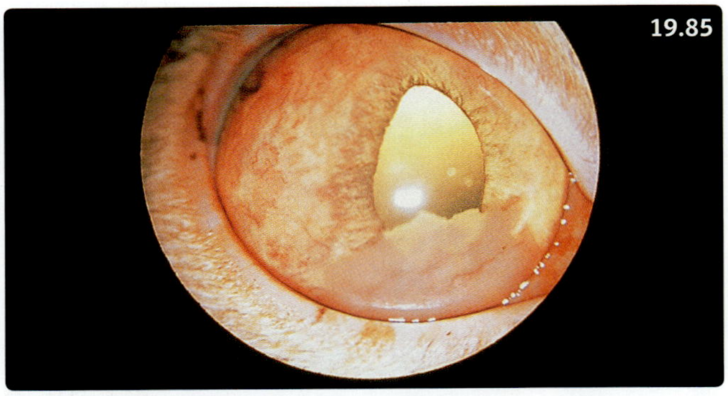

Figure 19.85 Intraocular lymphosarcoma manifests as hypopyon in this cat.

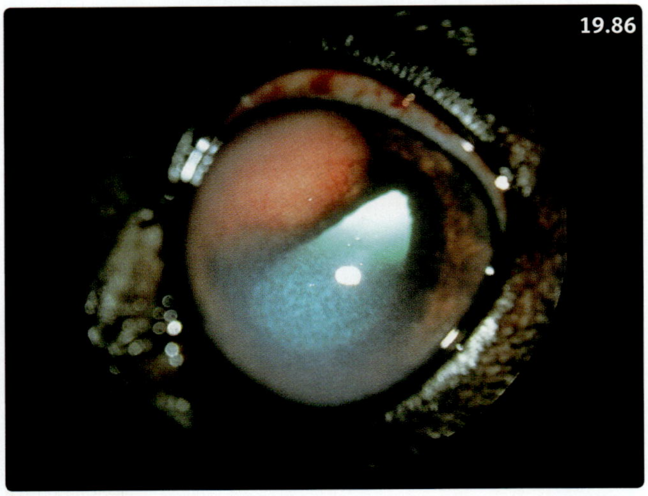

Figure 19.86 Iridal lymphosarcoma and corneal edema in a dog.

Etiology

This is a metastatic neoplastic disease to the eye and its adnexa. Cats may be positive for FeLV.

Pathophysiology

Systemic involvement precedes or accompanies ocular lymphosarcoma. Lymphosarcoma with ocular involvement equates to advanced disease and translates to a shorter survival period for the dog.

Clinical presentation

Lymphosarcoma in dogs and cats **(Figures 19.85–19.88)** may manifest as corneal edema, centrally migrating white bands of neoplastic cells, stromal hemorrhage, corneal vascularization, anterior uveitis with hyphema, hypopyon, keratic precipitates and secondary glaucoma, and tortuous retinal vessels, retinal hemorrhages, perivascular sheathing, RD, or retinal tissue infiltration by tumor cells **(Figures 19.89–19.94)**. Cats may have cranial nerve dysfunction.

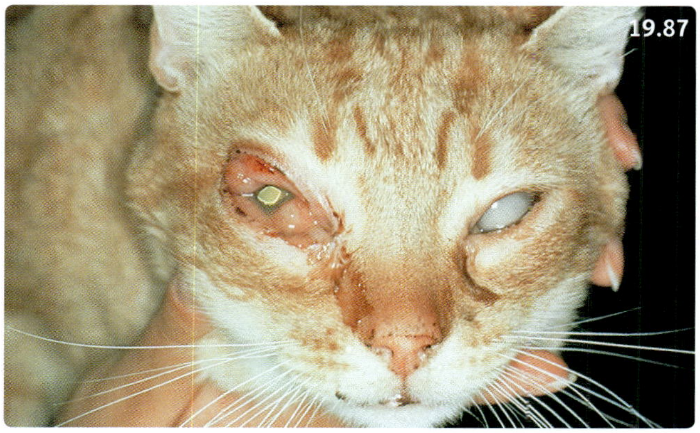

Figure 19.87 Conjunctival lymphosarcoma masquerades as conjunctivitis in the right eye of this cat. A cataract is present in the left eye.

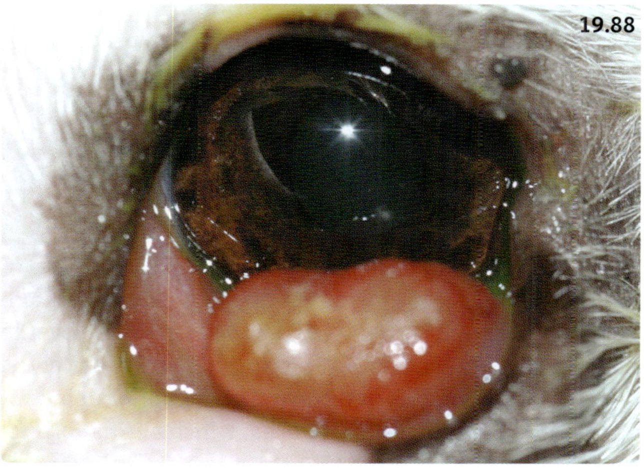

Figure 19.88 This mass on the third eyelid in a dog is lymphoma.

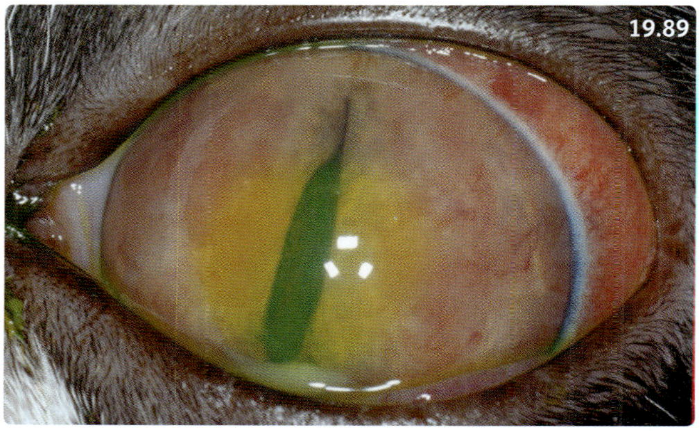

Figure 19.89 Iris thickening is severe in this cat.

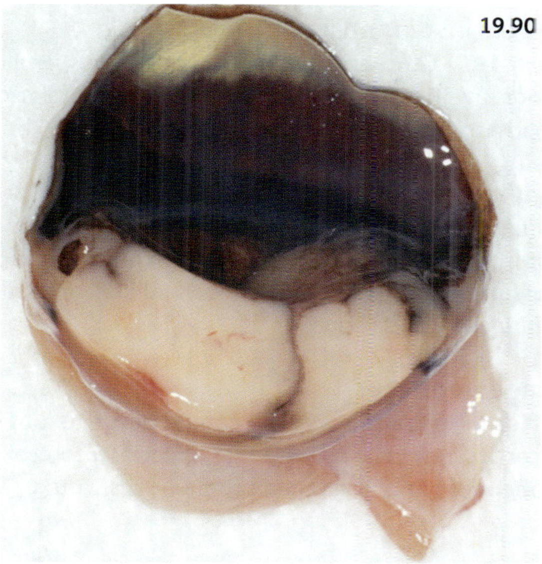

Figure 19.90 Iris lymphoma caused the iris swelling in the cat in Figure 19.89.

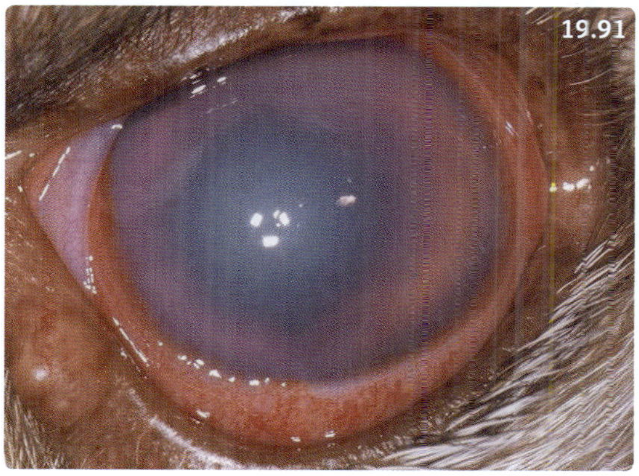

Figure 19.91 Iridocyclitis from lymphoma is present in this mixed-breed dog.

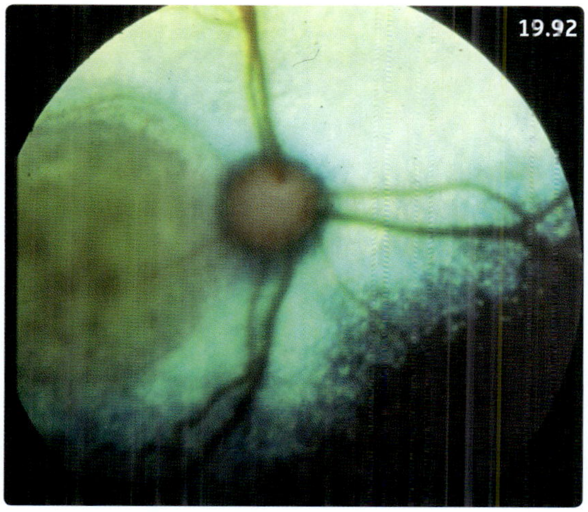

Figure 19.92 Lymphosarcoma invasion of the choroid causes a focal retinal detachment in this cat.

Differential diagnosis

Tables 19.3–19.6 and **19.8**. Conjunctivitis, hyphema, anterior uveitis, RD, and glaucoma may be caused by lymphosarcoma.

Diagnosis

Lymphadenopathy combined with bilateral anterior uveitis or intraocular hemorrhages should cause suspicion of lymphoma. Enlarged lymph nodes should be investigated by fine-needle aspiration.

Management

Anterior uveitis and hyphema should be treated by topical corticosteroids and atropine. Medical protocols for treatment of lymphosarcoma should be instituted.

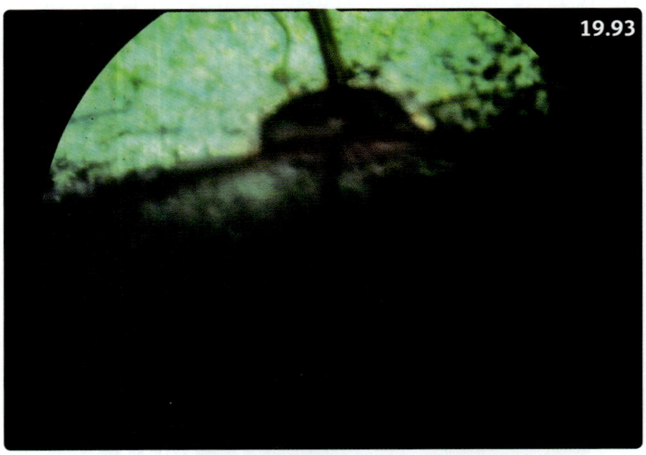

Figure 19.93 Orbital lymphoma pressing on the globe indents the eye and distorts the optic nerve head.

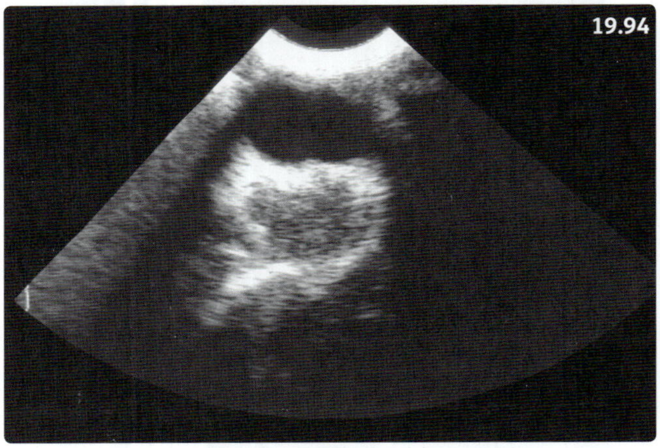

Figure 19.94 Ultrasound demonstrates the tumor presence behind the globe in the dog in Figure 19.93.

DIABETES MELLITUS

(See also Chapter 11: Endocrine disorders.)

Definition/overview

There is a high incidence of cataracts in diabetic dogs, with many cataracts apparently developing rapidly over days to weeks. Most diabetic dogs form cataracts within 12–16 months after diagnosis.

Etiology

In dogs, inciting factors include obesity, immune-mediated insulitis, pancreatitis, infection, genetic predisposition, and insulin-antagonistic diseases. In cats, obesity-induced carbohydrate intolerance and amyloid deposition in islet cells are potential factors.

Clinical presentation

The most common ocular manifestation of diabetes mellitus in small animals is acute formation of cataracts, often associated with sudden blindness. Diabetic cataracts in dogs begin at the lens equator. Diabetic cataracts in cats involve the posterior cortex initially. Diabetic dogs may have KCS, reduced corneal sensitivity, and reduced tear film breakup times (**Figures 19.95–19.97**).

Pathophysiology

The cataracts form during periods of hyperglycemia when glucose enters the lens and is converted by the enzyme aldose reductase (AR) to sorbitol as the glycolytic enzyme hexokinase is saturated. Lens sorbitol dehydrogenase (SD) activity is also reduced, which allows sorbitol

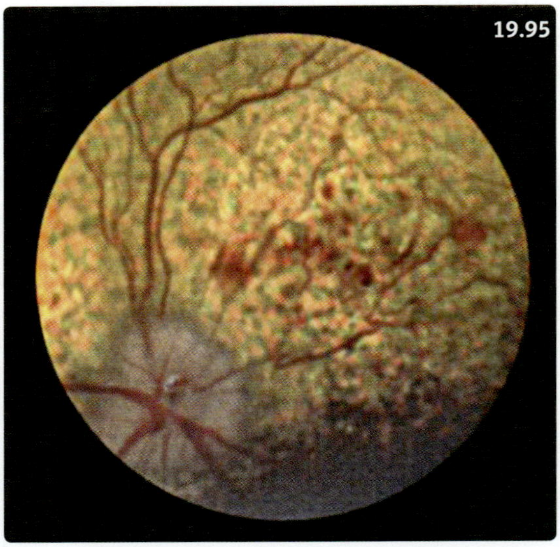

Figure 19.95 Retinal hemorrhages are present in this dog with diabetic retinopathy.

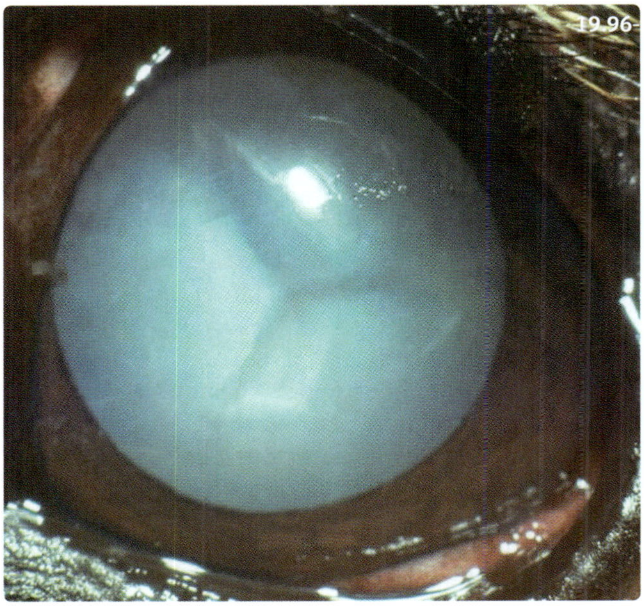

Figure 19.96 A mature cataract with prominent lens Y suture involvement is caused by diabetes in this dog.

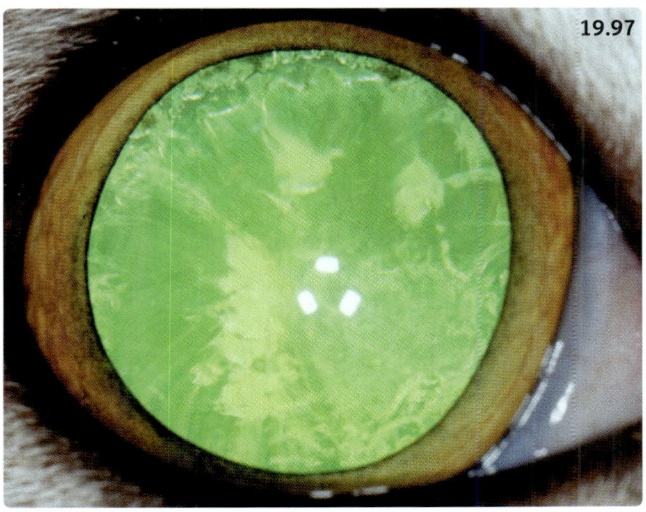

Figure 19.97 Posterior cortical changes are present in the lens of this diabetic cat.

to accumulate in the lens. The sorbitol osmotically draws water into the lens, and the lens fibers swell and rupture to result in cataracts.

The cat lens generally has less age-matched activity of both AR and SD than that present in the lens of dogs, but the ratio of AR to SD is higher in the cat lens than the dog. Sorbitol should thus accumulate more quickly in diabetic cat lenses than in dogs, but the incidence of diabetic cataracts is actually lower clinically in diabetic cats than diabetic dogs. This may be a result of diabetes being primarily a disease of cats >7 years of age who have little AR

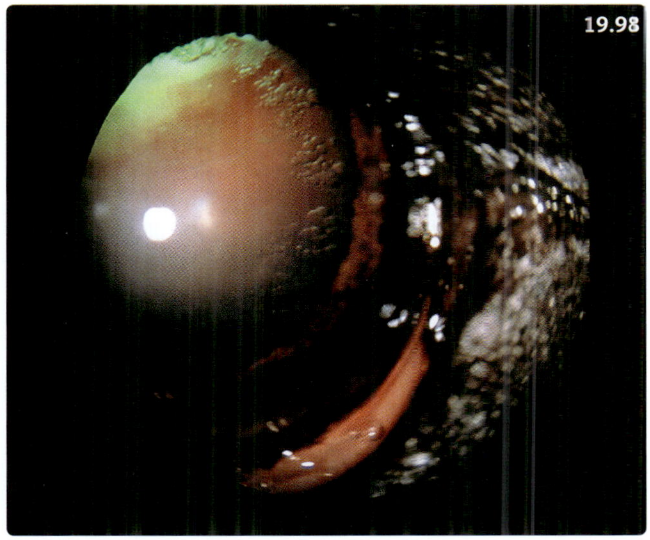

Figure 19.98 Lens fibers in the equatorial lens cortex swell and appear as 'water clefts' in this dog with diabetes.

activity in their aging lens. AR lens activity is highest in young cats (<4 years).

Ischemic changes in the retina of chronically diabetic dogs and cats can result in retinal vessel aneurysms and retinal hemorrhages. These changes may be masked by the rapid cataract formation.

Differential diagnosis

Cataracts may be a hereditary condition in specific breeds. They may also be caused by, aging, advanced retinal degeneration, anterior uveitis, diseases causing hypocalcemia, radiation therapy, and milk replacers in puppies and kittens. Atopy is also associated with cataract development in humans, and may also play an important role in cataract formation in dogs living in subtropical environments.

Diagnosis

Early cataractous changes appear as vacuoles **(Figure 19.98)** in the subepithelial equatorial cortex, which progress to mature, intumescent cataractous lenses with prominent Y-suture clefting. Anterior uveitis is also found in some canine diabetics. Diabetic retinopathy is slow to develop in diabetic dogs and cats.

Management

Surgery is necessary to treat the cataracts of controlled diabetic patients, and is very successful at restoring sight.

LACRIMAL SYSTEM MANIFESTATIONS OF SYSTEMIC DISEASE

ACUTE AND CHRONIC KERATOCONJUNCTIVITIS SICCA

Definition/overview

KCS is a disease associated with reduced secretions from the lacrimal and third eyelid glands. Most cases of chronic conjunctivitis in dogs are caused by KCS.

Etiology

KCS in dogs is associated with canine distemper, trauma, irradiation, and drug toxicity (**Figure 19.99**). It most commonly results from immune-mediated dacryoadenitis. Canine immune-mediated KCS has also been associated with atopy, hypothyroidism, hyperadrenocorticoidism, systemic lupus erythematosus (SLE), rheumatoid arthritis, diabetes mellitus, chronic active hepatitis, and pemphigoid disorders. FHV infection is associated with KCS in cats.

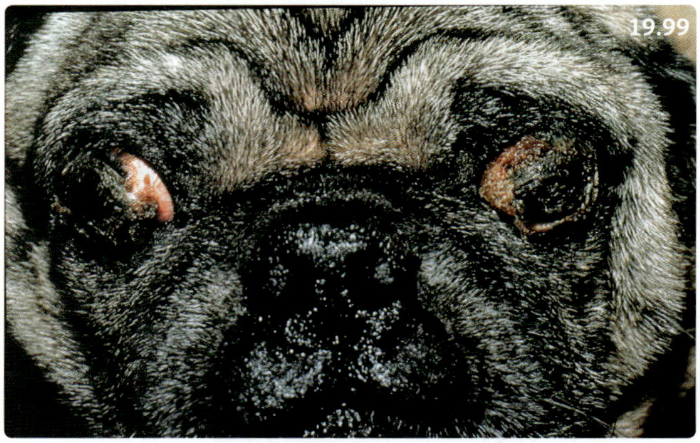

Figure 19.99 Severe keratitis from keratoconjunctivitis sicca in a Pug.

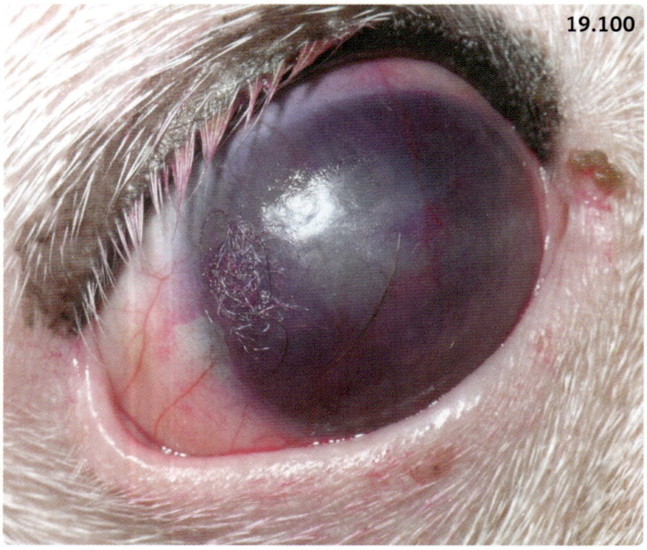

Figure 19.100 Rose Bengal is retained in a dog with KCS. The corneal reflection is dull rather than shiny.

Pathophysiology

The tri-layered precorneal tear film is critical for maintaining optical clarity and providing nutrition to the cornea. Lack of tears results in painful corneal and conjunctival degeneration, and often blindness.

Clinical presentation

Blepharospasm, conjunctivitis, chemosis, mucoid to mucopurulent ocular discharge, corneal pigmentation and vascularization, and corneal ulcers can be present (**Figures 19.100, 19.101**). Cats seem less affected by low tear levels than dogs.

Differential diagnosis

Table 19.2. KCS is often confused with bacterial conjunctivitis.

Diagnosis

Decreased Schirmer tear test levels are diagnostic (<10 mm/minute). Concurrent corneal ulcers must be identified.

Management

Topically administered cyclosporine A, tacrolimus, or pimecrolimus, artificial tears, and antibiotics are effective at controlling KCS in up to 80% of dogs with KCS.

SJÖGREN'S-LIKE SYNDROME

Definition/overview

Sjögren's syndrome is a systemic autoimmune disease directed against glandular tissues. It is characterized by

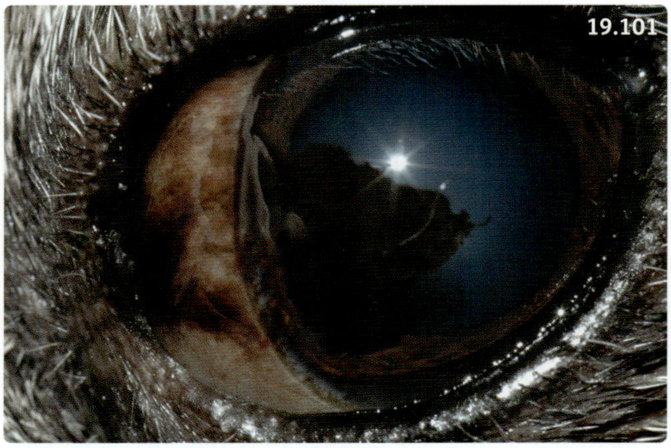

Figure 19.101 The cornea is pigmenting in response to a lack of tears in KCS.

KCS, xerostomia, lymphoplasmacytic dacryoadenitis, and lymphocytic sialoadenitis.

Etiology

Sjögren's syndrome is frequently associated with human autoimmune disease (rheumatoid arthritis, SLE, thyroiditis). A similar syndrome to Sjögren's syndrome has recently been recognized in dogs (KCS associated with SLE, hypothyroidism, diabetes mellitus, other immune disorders, and xerostomia) and cats.

Pathophysiology

There is immune-mediated destruction of the lacrimal and salivary glands.

Clinical presentation

Sjögren's syndrome is characterized by KCS (xerophthalmia) and xerostomia (dry mouth) (**Figures 19.102, 19.103**).

Differential diagnosis

Table 19.2.

Diagnosis

Clinical signs (KCS, keratitis, conjunctivitis), presence of other immune-mediated systemic diseases (e.g. pemphigus) associated with salivary signs, positive ANA test.

Management

Treatment is the same as for KCS, with additional identification and management of concurrent autoimmune diseases.

SYSTEMIC DISEASE ASSOCIATED WITH INFLAMMATORY MYOPATHY

MASTICATORY MUSCLE MYOSITIS

(See also Chapter 8: Digestive diseases [Pharynx to anorectum].)

Definition/overview

Eosinophilic masticatory muscle myositis is an inflammatory disorder involving the muscles of mastication. Masticatory myositis typically affects young to middle aged adult dogs and predominantly medium to large breeds dogs such as German Shepherd Dogs and Weimaraners.

Etiology

The cause is unknown but an immune-mediated reaction is possible. Neutrophils and eosinophils infiltrate the temporalis and pterygoid muscles to cause pronounced masticatory muscle fiber swelling and subsequent fibrosis.

Pathophysiology

The 2M muscle fibers in the masticatory muscles contain a unique type of myosin, which is specifically involved in immune-mediated reactions. The pathogenesis is not understood, although autoantibodies against type 2M muscle fibers are present in the circulation and tissue. Bacteria containing antigens similar to type 2M muscle fibers may initiate the myositis. Exophthalmos results from inflammatory swelling

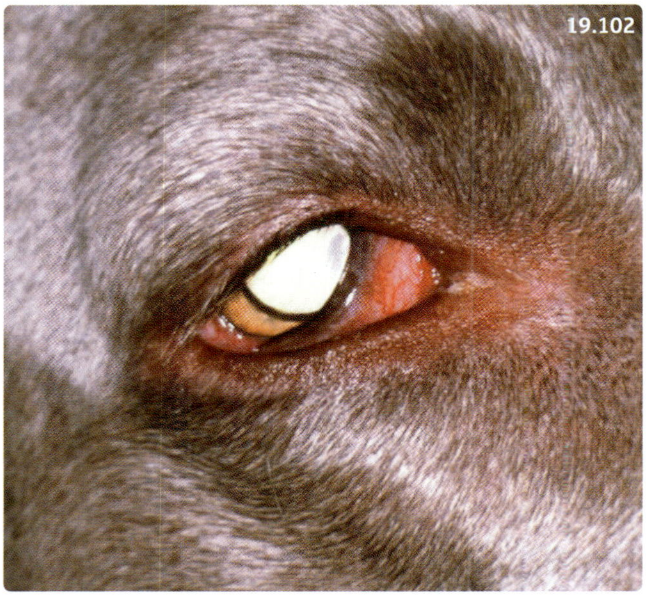
19.102

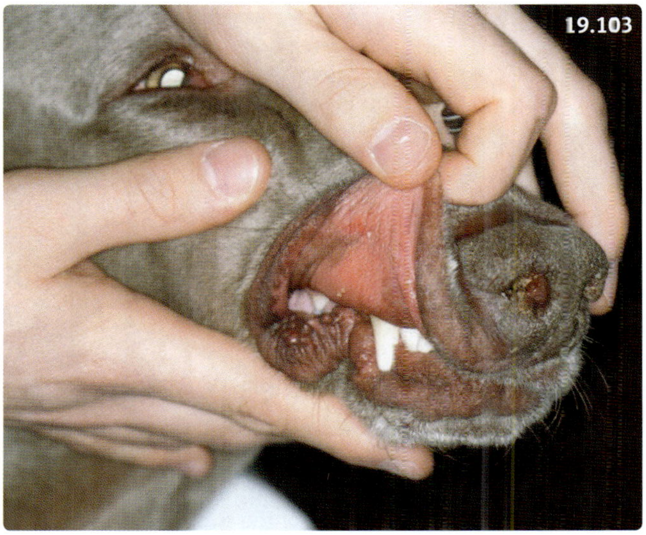
19.103

Figures 19.102, 19.103 Sjögren's syndrome. (19.102) KCS in a Weimaraner with Sjögren's syndrome. (19.103) Xerostomia is also present.

of the muscles of mastication forcing orbital fat and the globe anteriorly to cause the exophthalmos (**Figures 19.104, 19.105**).

Clinical presentation

Masticatory muscle myositis of the masseter, pterygoid, and temporalis muscles may cause acute, painful exophthalmos that is followed by chronic muscle atrophy with enophthalmos and nictitans protrusion. Pain is elicited when opening the mouth. Most dogs present with anorexia and depression, although tonsillitis, submandibular and prescapular lymphadenopathy, and pyrexia may occur.

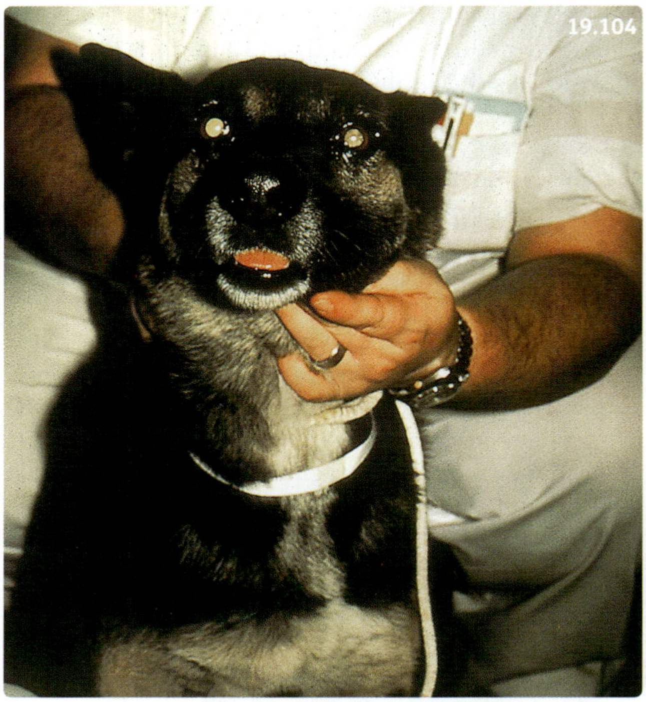

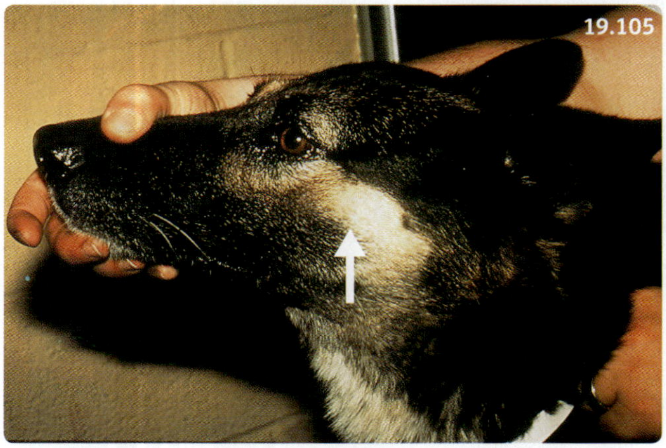

Figures 19.104, 19.105 A 3-year-old female German Shepherd Dog with eosinophilic myositis. (19.104) The frontal view shows exposure conjunctivitis as a result of the swollen extraocular muscles causing exophthalmos. (19.105) The side view shows the swollen muscles (arrow). (Courtesy M. Schaer)

Differential diagnosis

Orbital cellulitis and orbital neoplasia.

Diagnosis

Diagnosis is based on electromyelography, which reveals abnormal spontaneous pathologic activity in the temporal and masseter muscles, peripheral eosinophilia, elevated serum creatine kinase, temporalis muscle biopsy, and the demonstration of serum 2M autoantibodies. MRI detects widespread, symmetrical, and inhomogeneously hyperintense areas in the masticatory muscle.

Management

Systemically administered corticosteroids are indicated in acute disorders. Uncontrolled myositis leads to painful masticatory muscle atrophy. Therapy may be life-long.

EXTRAOCULAR MUSCLE MYOSITIS

Definition/overview

Extrocular muscle myositis is common in 8–10-month-old Golden Retrievers.

Etiology

The specific cause of this focal inflammatory myositis is unknown at present.

Pathophysiology

Extraocular muscle myositis is an immune-mediated disease directed against the type I myofibers of the extraocular muscles. The pressure on the optic nerve from the swollen extraocular muscles can severely reduce optic nerve axoplasmic flow.

Clinical presentation

The clinical signs are bilateral in most dogs. A generally nonpainful chemosis precedes exophthalmos in 81% of cases, and optic nerve impingement with optic neuritis may occur to cause blindness (**Figures 19.106–19.109**).

Differential diagnosis

Table 19.1. Orbital cellulitis and orbital neoplasia.

Diagnosis

Diagnosis is by serum and muscle biopsy for detection of type I myofiber antibodies.

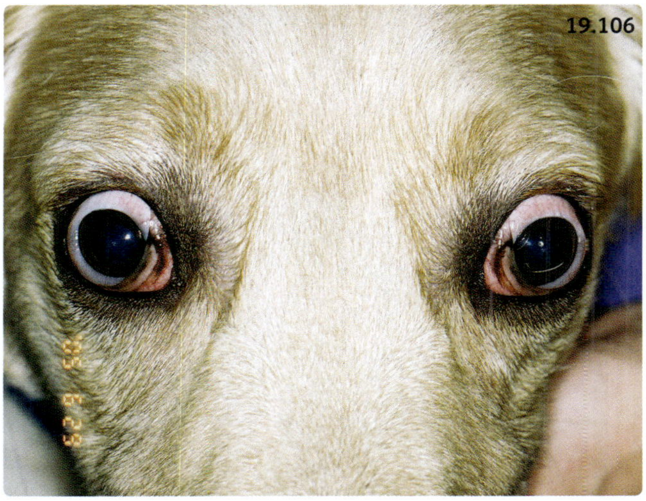

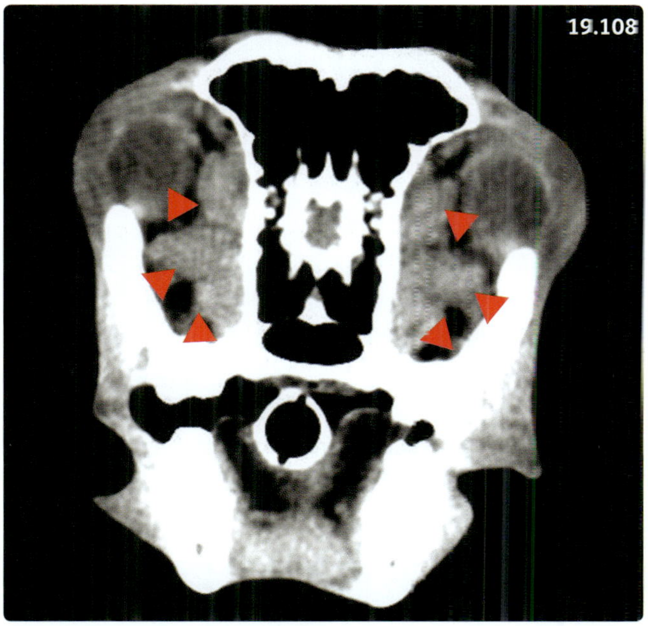

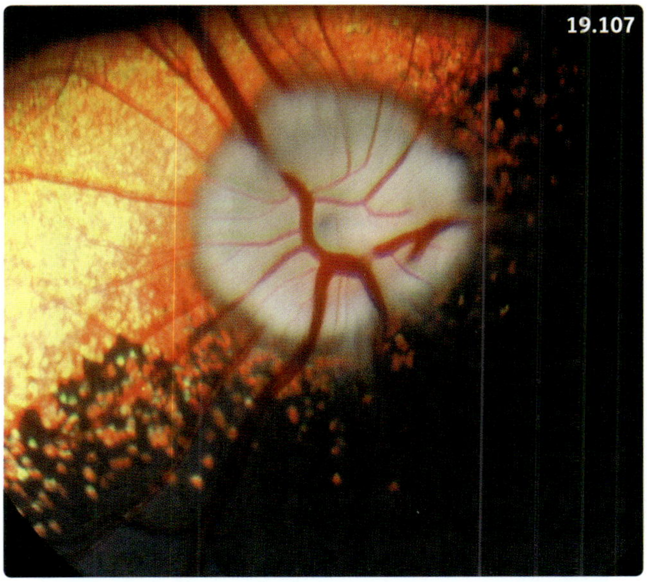

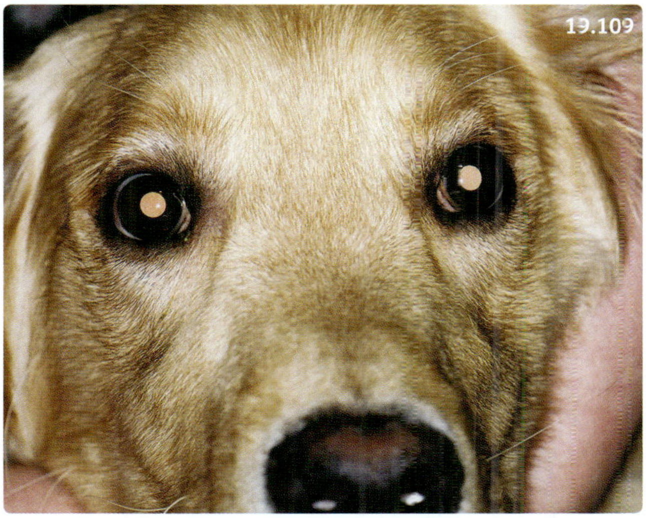

Figures 19.106–19.109 Young Golden Retriever with extraocular muscle myositis. (19.106) Bilateral exophthalmos due to the extraocular muscle myositis. (19.107) The optic disk is slightly swollen. (19.108) MRI shows bilateral extraocular muscle swelling (arrowheads). (19.109) Four months later, therapy for the extraocular myositis has reduced the exophthalmos.

Management

Treatment is the same as for masticatory muscle myositis.

METASTATIC AND MULTICENTRIC NEOPLASIA OF THE ORBIT

Definition/overview

Metastatic and multicentric neoplasia of the orbit is common in dogs and cats.

Etiology

Most orbital tumors are primary and highly malignant.

Pathophysiology

Malignant cell types predominate, with any widely metastatic tumor potentially involving the orbit.

Clinical presentation

Progressive, often painless slow exophthalmos with varying amounts of strabismus and exposure keratitis are the most common clinical signs (**Figures 19.110–19.116**).

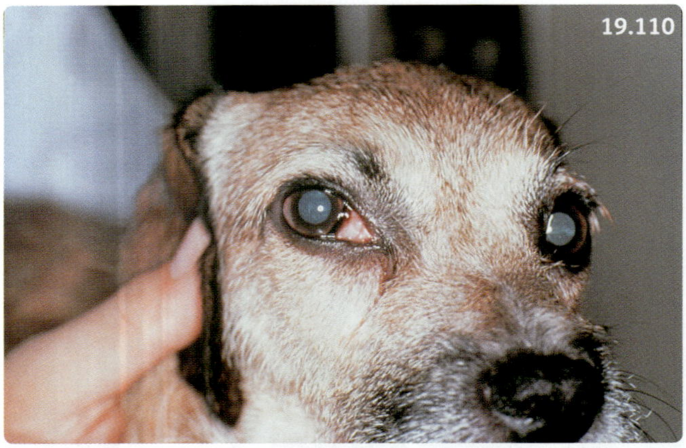

Figure 19.110 A retrobulbar fibrosarcoma causing exophthalmos, nictitans protrusion, and strabismus in this dog.

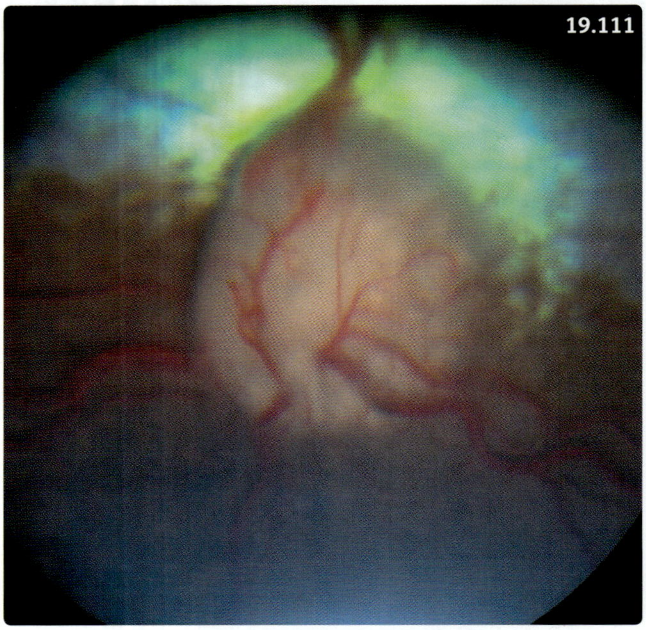

Figure 19.111 An optic nerve meningioma in the orbit has caused distortion of the optic disk in this old Labrador Retriever.

Acute-onset exophthalmos is associated with orbital inflammatory diseases such as retrobulbar abscesses/cellulitis. Exophthalmos with pain on attempting to open the mouth usually indicates a retrobulbar abscess or cellulitis, with swelling behind the last upper molar on the affected side also often observed. Dogs with orbital tumors undergoing necrosis can have the same clinical signs as dogs with orbital abscesses/cellulitis. Orbital infections due to systemic coccidioidomycosis, blastomycosis, and cryptococcosis are reported, but orbital cellulitis/abscessation is generally a localized infection.

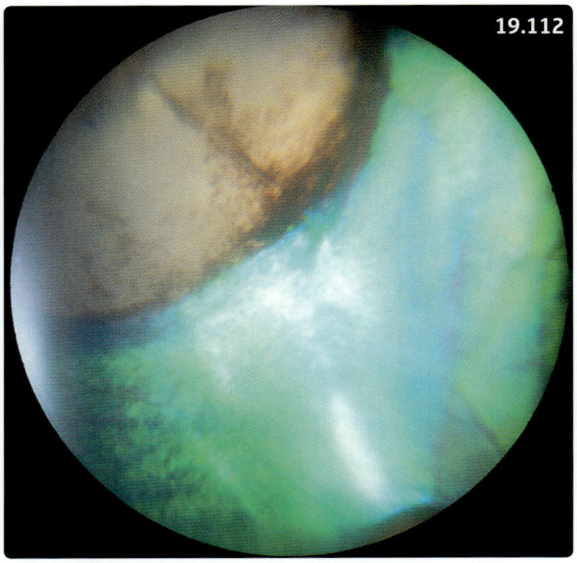

Figure 19.112 This pale focal retinal lesion in a cat is a ciliary body tumor that has metastasized to the retina.

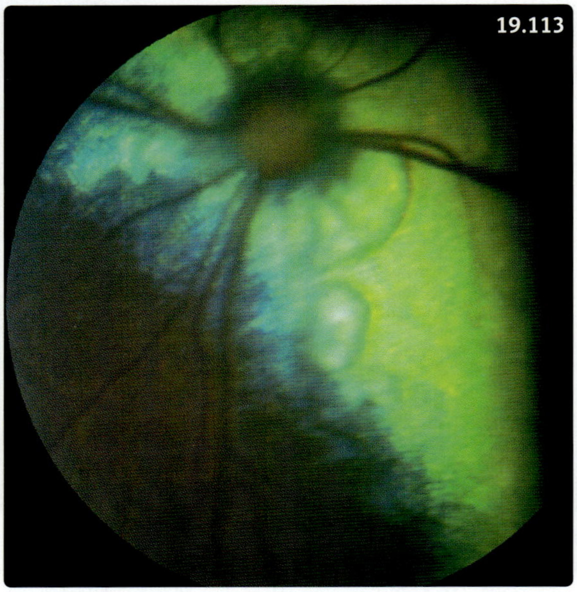

Figure 19.113 Orbital osteosarcoma has caused focal peripapillary retinal detachments in this aged cat.

Differential diagnosis

Orbital abscesses/cellulitis, salivary gland mucoceles, orbital varices.

Diagnosis

Cytologic examination and culture of discharge or aspirates from the orbit, biopsy of masses, exploration of fistulous tracts, ultrasonography, and MRI and CT are very valuable in evaluating orbital diseases.

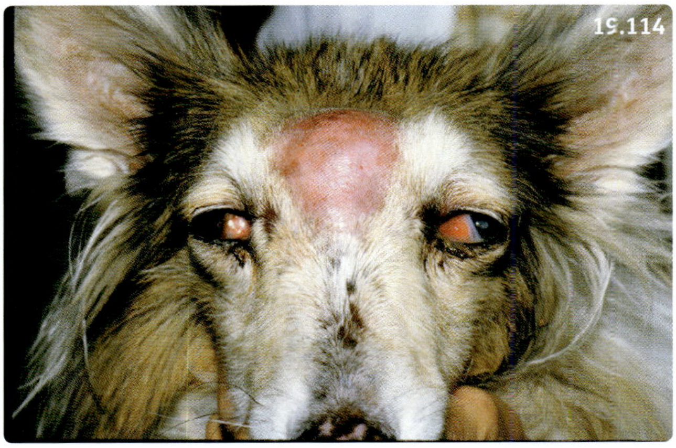

Figure 19.114 Third eyelid protrusion occurring bilaterally from a brain tumor.

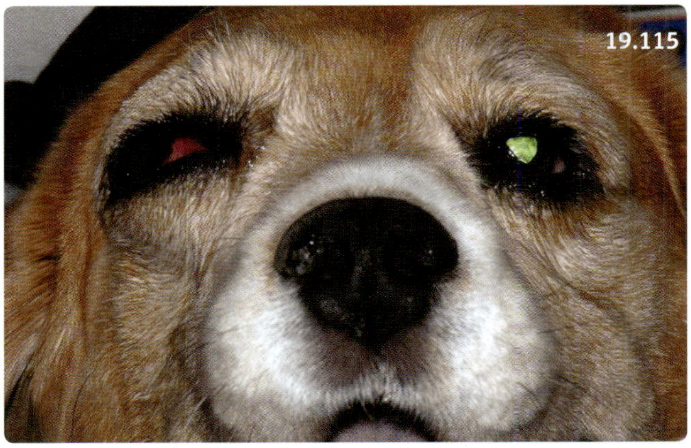

Figure 19.115 Slowly progressive exophthalmos in this dog was due to a right-sided retrobulbar mass of the orbit and nasal cavity.

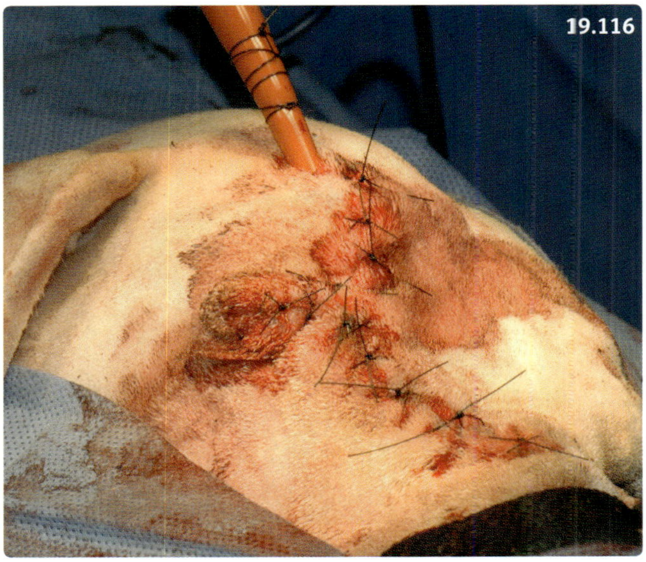

Figure 19.116 The globe and mass were removed in the dog in Figure 19.115. The mass was a squamous cell carcinoma.

Management

Early exenteration is generally the therapy of choice unless the orbital tumor is well circumscribed. The prognosis is poor for dogs with orbital neoplasia.

CONJUNCTIVAL MANIFESTATIONS OF SYSTEMIC DISEASE

Definition/overview

Many systemic diseases of dogs and cats have nonspecific conjunctival manifestations. Mild hypoxia in cardiovascular disorders is manifested as conjunctivitis with dilation and darkening of conjunctival vessels. Conjunctival petechiation may be seen in cases of infectious endocarditis. Conjunctival venous engorgement may be noticed with congestive heart failure. Anemia may be seen as pallor or hemorrhage of the conjunctiva. Hyperviscosity syndromes are associated with conjunctival congestion. Conjunctival petechiae and ecchymoses are found with immune-mediated thrombocytopenia and coumarin (warfarin) toxicity. Icterus of the conjunctiva is found with liver diseases. Systemic tumors such as lymphoma may masquerade as simple conjunctivitis.

Calcification deposition of the subepithelial cornea, termed calcific band keratopathy, is reported in dogs with hyperadrenocorticoidism. Lymphoma cells can directly invade the corneal stroma of dogs to cause keratitis, a migrating white band, vascularization, and stromal hemorrhage. The anterior uvea is commonly infiltrated with tumor cells, resulting in moderate to severe uveitis. Aqueous flare, hypopyon, miosis, and keratic precipitates may be found.

LIPID KERATOPATHY

Definition/overview

Lipid keratopathy may be induced in hypercholesterolemic states by corneal trauma, ulcers, and surgery. Corneal lipidosis is reported in Shelties, Collies, German Shepherd Dogs, and Dobermanns.

Etiology

Lipid keratopathy in the dog is associated with hyperlipidemia, hypothyroidism, pancreatitis, diabetes mellitus, and spontaneous hyperlipidemia.

Pathophysiology

Lipid keratopathy is characterized by peripheral and central crystalline corneal stromal opacities (**Figure 19.117**). Corneal lipidosis generally does not completely regress.

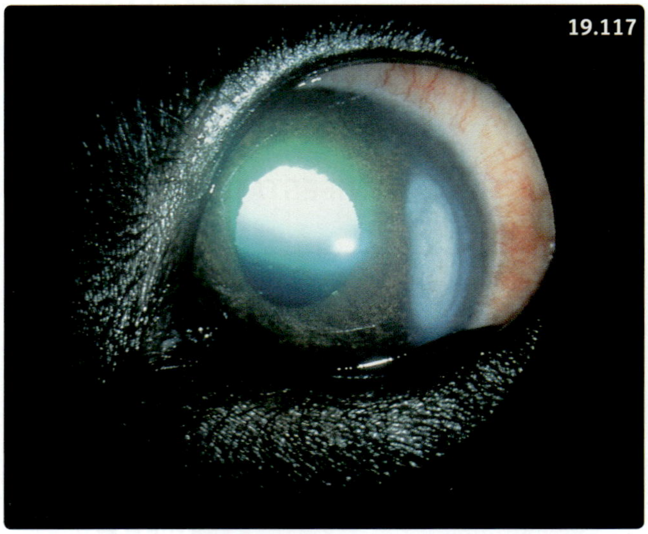

Figure 19.117 A limbal infiltrate of lipids accompanies elevated serum triglycerides in this dog with hypothyroidism.

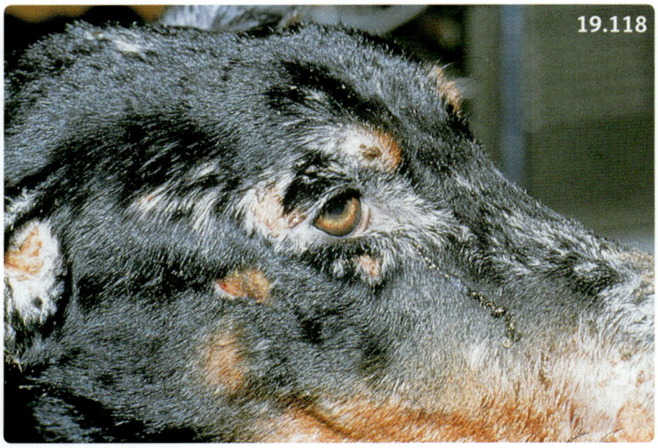

Figure 19.118 Alopecia and crustiness of the face and eyelids in a dog with systemic lupus erythematosus.

Clinical presentation

Lipid keratopathy appears as a bilateral, silver or blue-gray, complete ring at the limbus. The central cornea may be affected in advanced cases. Vascularization of the cornea may speed lipid deposition.

Differential diagnosis

Rule out causes of corneal opacity including corneal ulcers, edema, scars, and inflammatory cellular infiltrates.

Diagnosis

Dogs with lipid keratopathy should have a serum lipid profile performed and be screened for thyroid function, pancreatitis, and diabetes mellitus.

Management

Low fat diets may be beneficial in reducing the corneal opacity. Keratectomy is necessary if vision is significantly affected by the opacification.

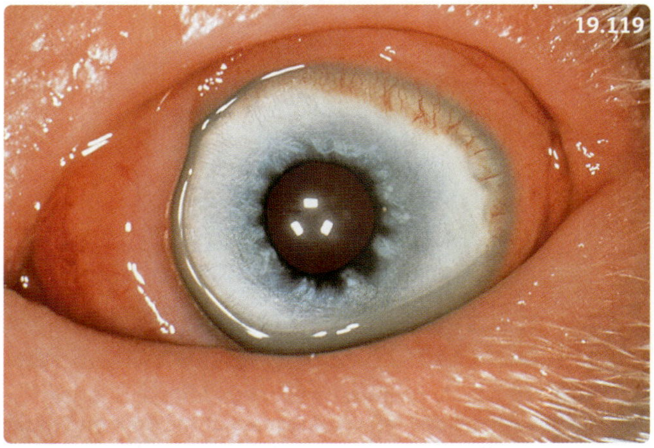

Figure 19.119 Blepharoconjunctivitis in a dog with demodicosis.

EYELID MANIFESTATIONS OF SYSTEMIC DISEASE

Definition/overview

Chronic blepharitis may be associated with systemic endocrine imbalances such as hypothyroidism. Bacterial, fungal, parasitic, allergic, and neoplastic (lymphoma and mast cell tumors) diseases may affect the eyelids (**Figures 19.118–19.122**). Atopy, exposure to contact allergens, and autoimmune conditions are reported. Juvenile pyoderma

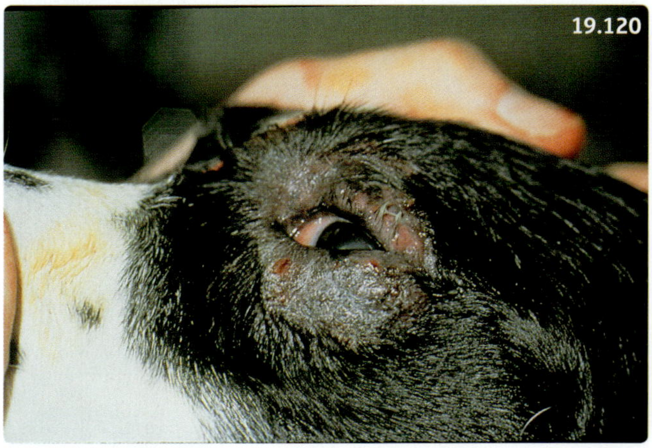

Figure 19.120 Redness, alopecia, and swelling of the eyelids in a dog with blepharitis, KCS, and hypothyroidism.

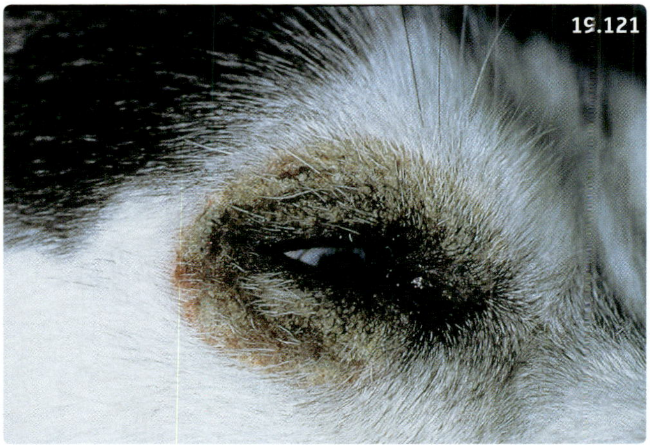

Figure 19.121 Zinc-responsive dermatosis in a Husky dog with bilateral blepharitis.

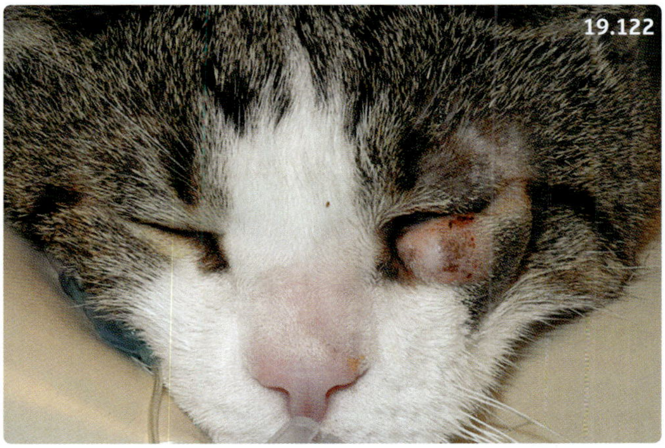

Figure 19.122 This mast cell tumor of the left lower lid of a cat was responsive to strontium radiation.

can affect the lids of puppies. Predisposed breeds include the Dachshund, Golden Retriever, Labrador Retriever, Gordon Setter, and Lhasa Apso. Papillomatous eyelid growths in young dogs may be associated with oral papillomatosis. Demodicosis causing deep lid pyoderma is reported in dogs and cats (**Figure 19.123**).

Bilateral and symmetrical hyperkeratotic 'crustiness' of the lids is found in Huskies and Malamutes with zinc-responsive keratosis. An inherited inability to absorb zinc from the intestines causes the problem. Oral and parenteral elemental zinc supplementation is beneficial and will be required for the life of the patient.

Ocular manifestations of Ehlers–Danlos syndrome reported in the cat have been linked to excessive laxity of the eyelid skin and include entropion with secondary blepharospasm and keratoconjunctivitis (**Figure 19.124**).

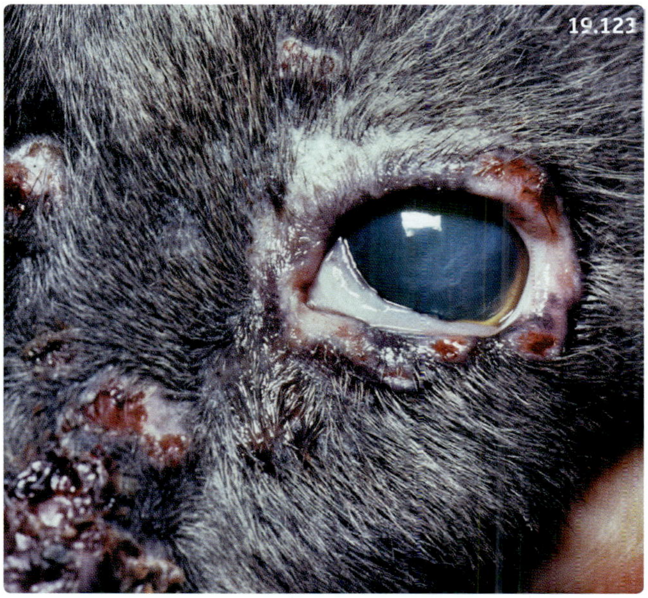

Figure 19.123 Blepharitis in a cat due to *Demodex* spp. infestation.

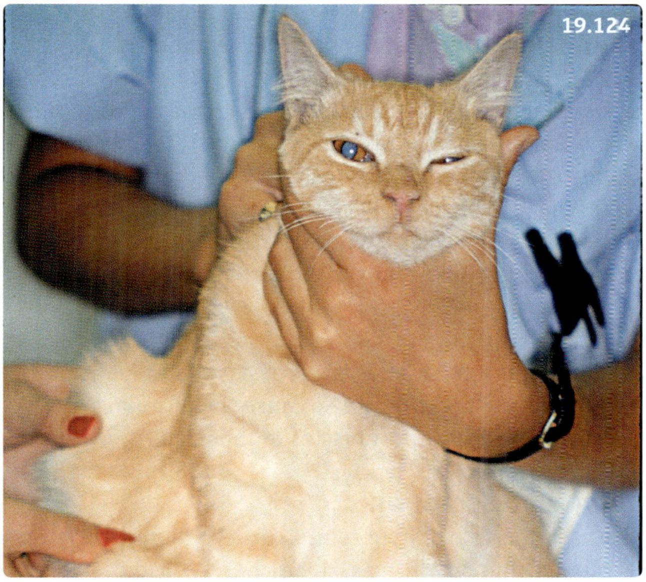

Figure 19.124 This cat has left-sided blepharospasm and Ehlers–Danlos-associated cataracts.

Pemphigus foliaceus is the most common immune-mediated dermatologic condition affecting the feline eyelid, and is also found in dogs. Pemphigus foliaceus, pemphigus erythematosus, pemphigus vulgaris, food hypersensitivity, and atopy may also affect the lids of cats and dogs.

UVEAL MANIFESTATIONS OF SYSTEMIC DISEASES

INFLAMMATION OF THE ANTERIOR UVEA

Definition/overview

Inflammation of the anterior uvea (iris and ciliary body) is termed anterior uveitis or iridocyclitis. Inflammation of the posterior uvea or choroid is termed choroiditis. It is often useful to discuss inflammation of the anterior uvea as a distinct entity from the choroid, but inflammation of one region is generally associated with some degree of inflammation of the other region. Panuveitis is inflammation of the entire uveal tract, with endophthalmitis also involving the anterior chamber and vitreous. Anterior and posterior uveitis disrupt the protective blood–ocular barrier and allow blood and blood-derived compounds access to transparent nonvascular regions of the eye such that vision can be compromised.

Etiology

Infectious and noninfectious neoplastic, immune-mediated, and metabolic systemic diseases can cause uveitis. Uveitis in cats is caused by systemic diseases such as FIP, FHV, FeLV-associated disorders, FIV, feline sarcoma virus (FeSV), toxoplasmosis, and systemic mycotic infections. Other causes for feline uveitis include bacteria (tuberculosis) and hypersensitivity reactions. Uveitis in dogs is caused by algae, bacteria, fungi, immune-mediated diseases, metabolic diseases, parasites (**Figure 19.125**), neoplasms, viruses, and rickettsiae.

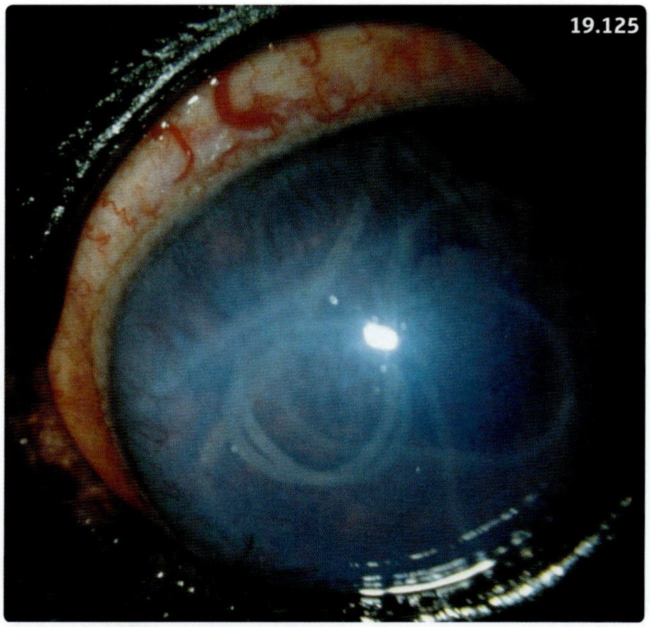

Figure 19.125 Heartworm larvae are motile and causing uveitis in this dog.

Pathophysiology

Inflammatory mediators are released that disrupt the blood–ocular barrier and also cause the pupillary sphincter muscles and ciliary muscles to constrict.

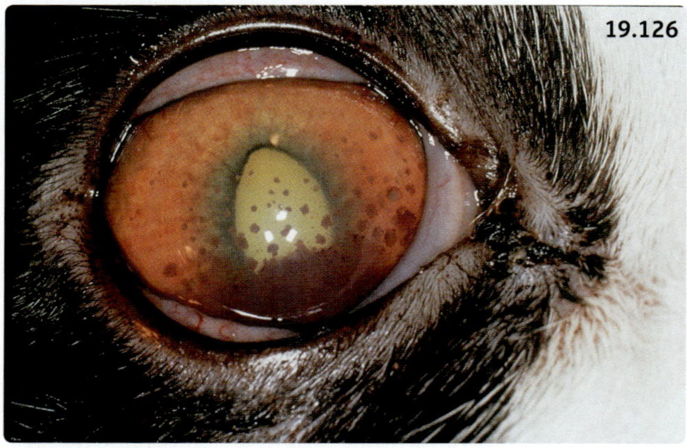

Figure 19.126 Keratic precipitates and hyphema in a cat with anterior uveitis from FIP.

Clinical presentation

Miosis, conjunctival hyperemia, corneal edema, hypotony, hyphema, hypopyon, iris color change, iridal swelling, keratic precipitates (adherence of clusters of mononuclear inflammatory cells to the corneal endothelium), and pain may be found with anterior uveitis. Cataracts, deep corneal stromal vascularization, endophthalmitis, lens luxation, rubeosis iridis, iris bombé, and secondary glaucoma are adverse sequelae. Choroiditis is associated with decreased vision, choroidal effusion, choroidal granulomas, optic neuritis, RD, retinal hemorrhage, and vitreal opacification (**Figures 19.126–19.131**).

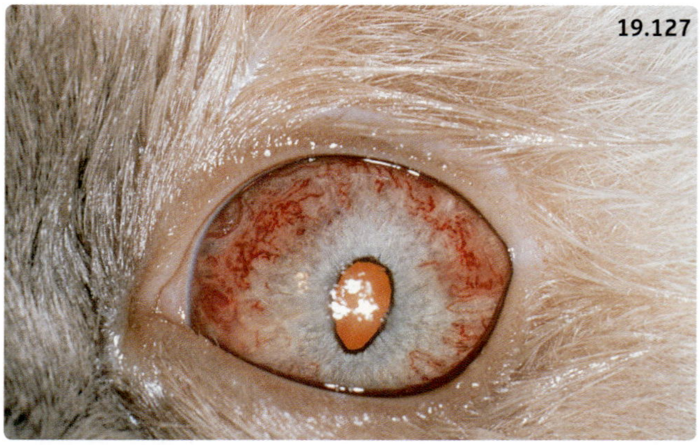

Figure 19.127 Iridal neovascularization (rubeosis iridis) in a cat with extreme anemia due to thrombocytopenia.

Differential diagnosis

Tables 19.4 and **19.7**.

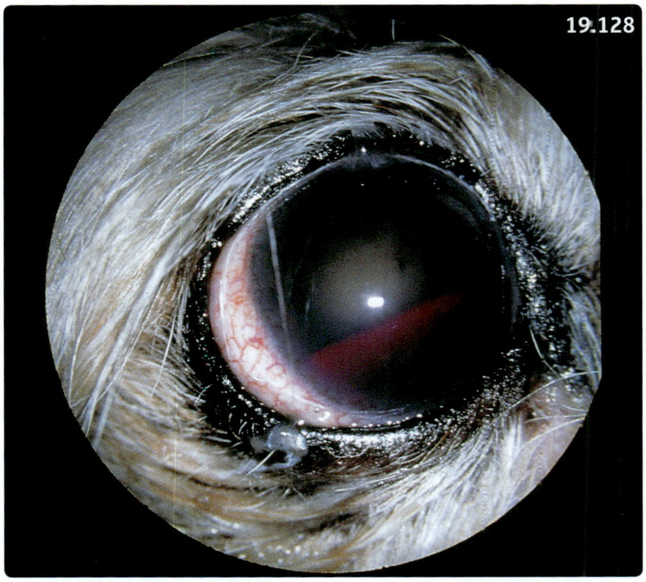

Figure 19.128 Hyphema due to renal hypertension indicates anterior uveitis in this dog.

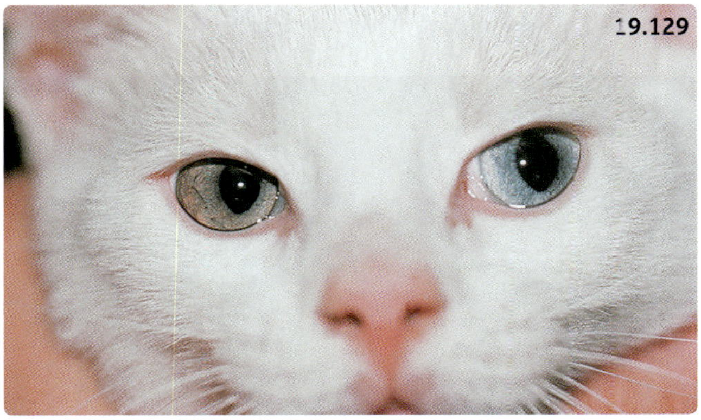

Figure 19.129 An iris color change from blue to brown in the right eye of this cat may be caused by anterior uveitis or iridal neoplasia.

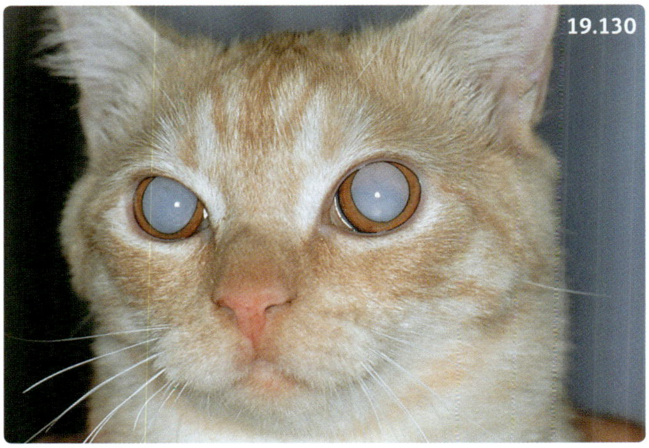

Figure 19.130 Cataracts may occur secondary to uveitis or they may induce uveitis.

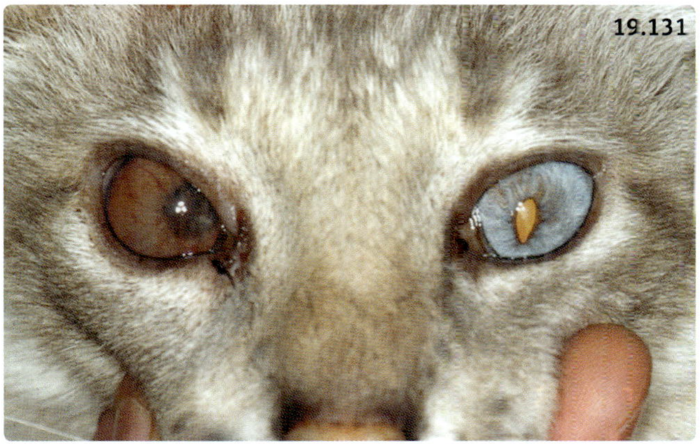

Figure 19.131 Iris color change and rubeosis in the right eye of a cat with chronic uveitis.

Diagnosis

Complete physical and ocular examinations are important in animals with uveitis since they may provide diagnostic clues to the etiology. Other diagnostic considerations are a CBC, blood chemistries, serologic tests, and aqueous humor analysis. Cytologic evaluation and bacterial culture of aqueous and vitreous aspirates may help characterize the etiology of the uveitis. The uveitis may be unilateral or bilateral in multiple system diseases.

Managment

Acute unilateral uveitis can be treated empirically. Bilateral or chronic uveitis is usually due to infection and should be treated accordingly.

RETINAL AND OPTIC NERVE MANIFESTATIONS OF SYSTEMIC DISEASES

Definition/overview

Neuronal ceroid lipofuscinosis (Batten's disease) is reported in the English Setter, Tibetan Terrier, the American Bulldog, American Cocker Spaniel, Australian Blue Heeler, Border Collie, Chihuahua, Dachshund, Dalmatian, Miniature Schnauzer, Polish Owczarek Nizinny, and Saluki. Ceroid is deposited in neurons of the CNS and in the retina and retinal pigment epithelium. Blindness and neurologic signs occur concurrently. Ophthalmoscopic lesions have not been noted in the English Setter and Tibetan Terrier, but mild tapetal hyperreflectivity, mild retinal vascular attenuation, and optic disk pallor have been noted as early as 2.5 years of age in affected Miniature Schnauzers.

Fucosidosis is an autosomal recessive glycoproteinosis occurring in the English Springer Spaniel.

The disease is produced by a deficiency of the lysosomal enzyme α-L-fucosidase. While retinal ganglion cells are vacuolated from the accumulation of substrate, ophthalmoscopic lesions have not been reported with the visual impairment in the affected English Springer Spaniels.

The retinal dystrophy of the Briard dog is caused by a defect in polyunsaturated fatty acid metabolism. Plasma arachidonic acid levels are elevated to twice normal levels in American Briards with this congenital night blindness.

CHORIORETINITIS

Definition/overview

Posterior uveitis involves the choroid and cannot be clinically distinguished from retinitis. It is therefore usually described as chorioretinitis.

Etiology

Chorioretinitis in the cat is frequently caused by toxoplasmosis, FIP, cryptococcosis, histoplasmosis, and blastomycosis. Toxoplasmosis and cryptococcosis commonly involve only the posterior segment, although anterior and posterior uveitis may occur. Granulomatous choroiditis in cats can also be associated with several *Mycobacterium* species. Chorioretinitis in dogs is caused by distemper, leptospirosis, brucellosis, Rocky Mountain spotted fever, aspergillosis, blastomycosis, coccidioidomycosis, histoplasmosis, protothecosis, toxoplasmosis, leishmaniasis, and primary and secondary neoplasia. Potentially toxic drugs such as ivermectin can also cause chorioretinitis.

Clinical presentation

The signs of retinal or chorioretinal inflammation include edema, infiltration with inflammatory cells and granuloma formation, hemorrhage, and possible exudative detachment (**Figure 19.132**). In dogs, retinal exudates, hemorrhage, and RD are a sequelae to chorioretinitis (**Figures 19.133, 19.134**).

Differential diagnosis

Table 19.3.

Diagnosis

Chorioretinal scars, characterized by hyperreflective areas in the tapetal region, are observed in normal healthy cats and dogs and are an indication of a previous subclinical inflammatory process (**Figure 19.135**).

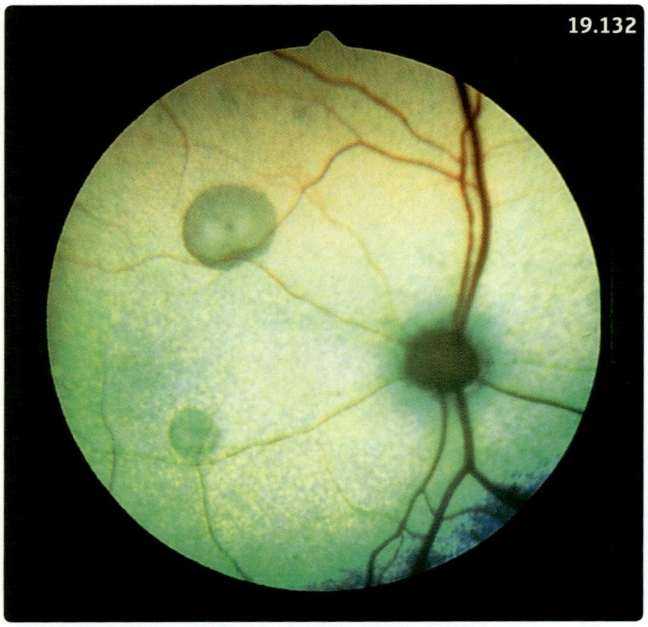

Figure 19.132 Focal, sharply delineated areas of inactive chorioretinitis in a cat.

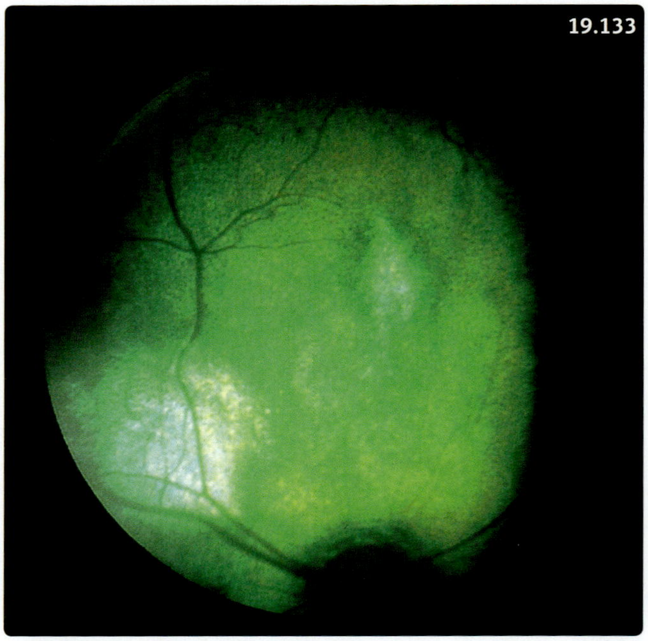

Figure 19.133 Inactive chorioretinitis is manifested as a focal yellow area with a hyperpigmented center in the green tapetum of this dog.

Management

Treatment is determined by the inciting cause. Systemic therapy is necessary for treatment of retinal diseases.

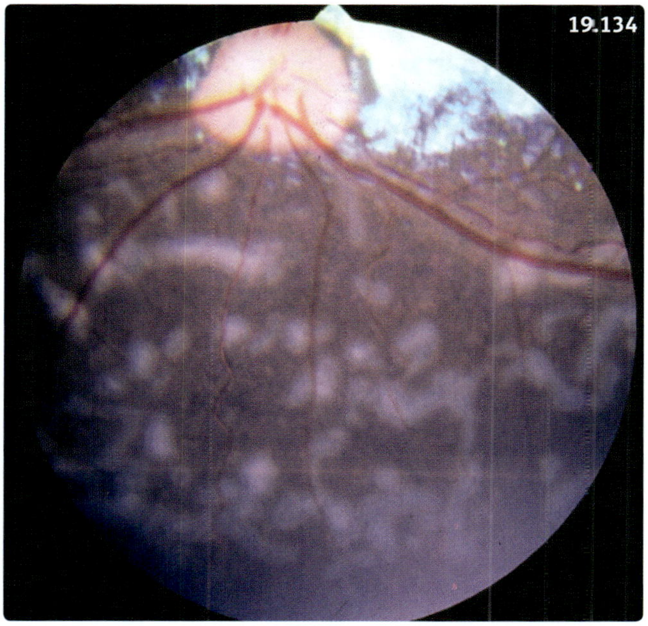

Figure 19.134 Chorioretinitis post ivermectin ingestion is present in this Border Collie.

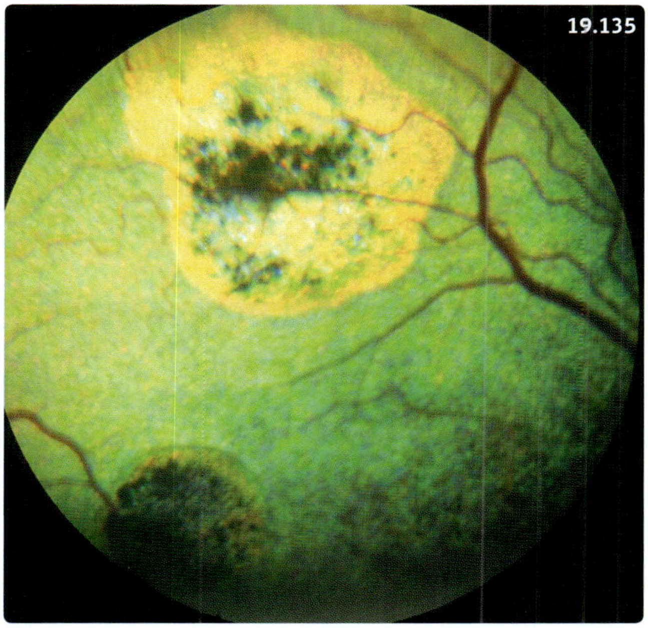

Figure 19.135 Hyperreflective areas of retinal atrophy with pigmentation from inactive chorioretinitis in a cat.

RETINAL DETACHMENT

Definition/overview

RD occurs with separation of the inner nine layers of the neurosensory retina from the single outer retinal pigment epithelium (RPE).

Etiology

Bilateral RD suggests a systemic problem. Optic nerve colobomas, severe retinal dysplasia, systemic hypertension due to renal or cardiac failure, intraocular neoplasia and chorioretinitis may cause RD. The condition can be breed associated in Lhasa Apsos and large breed dogs.

Pathophysiology

The neurosensory retina may be pushed away from the RPE by accumulation of chorioretinal inflammatory or neoplastic exudate in the subretinal space (exudative RD), or the retinal tissue may be torn, with retinal holes forming, and the retina can be pulled away from the RPE by vitreal traction from vitreal inflammation or hemorrhage (rhegmatogenous RD). Retinal tears can occur spontaneously in Lhasa Apsos.

Clinical presentation

The pupils are fixed and dilated if the RD is complete. Small detachments are not associated with blindness, but total RD is a serious problem with a poor visual outcome in most cases.

Differential diagnosis

Tables 19.3, **19.5**, and **19.6**.

Diagnosis

Ophthalmic examination reveals dilated pupils (if bilateral), blood vessels located behind the lens, leukocoria, vitreous degeneration and/or hemorrhage, and an opaque, folded retina. Ocular ultrasound is diagnostic of RD in eyes with cataracts.

Management

Systemic medical therapy may be curative in exudative RD of short duration (e.g. cats with systemic hypertension-induced RD). Rhegmatogenous RD requires advanced microsurgery. The inciting systemic cause of the RD must be identified and treated.

OPHTHALMOMYIASIS

Definition/overview

Ophthalmomyiasis interna refers to the presence of dipteran fly larva in the eye.

Etiology

Ophthalmomyiasis is caused by the sheep nasal botfly (*Oestrus ovis*), warble fly (*Cuterebra* spp.), or the cattle warble fly (*Hypoderma bovis*). Larvae gain access to the eye via the blood or via direct migration through the tissues of the eye.

Pathophysiology
Larval migration and/or death incite mild to severe inflammation of the ocular tissues.

Clinical presentation
Anterior uveitis and RDs may also occur with ophthalmomyiasis. Cats are more commonly affected than dogs. The presence of arcuate or linear areas of depigmention in the tapetal and nontapetal fundus may be due to traumatic, degenerative, or inflammatory disease of the retina, RPE, and choroid **(Figure 19.136)**. Clinical findings of ophthalmomyiasis are usually incidental.

Differential diagnosis
Tables 19.3–19.6.

Diagnosis
Ophthalmomyiasis is evident as curvilinear tracks of retinal degeneration and retinal hemorrhage in dogs and cats. Larvae may be noticed floating in the vitreous or actively migrating in the retina.

Managment
Most cases are incidental findings and require no therapy. Surgical removal of vitreal larvae can be done to remove a source of inflammation.

FELINE NUTRITIONAL RETINAL DEGENERATION OR TAURINE RETINOPATHY

Definition/overview
Diets deficient in the amino acid taurine cause retinal degeneration and dilated cardiomyopathy in cats.

Etiology
Feline nutritional retinal degeneration occurs in cats that are fed commercial dog food and special diets formulated for dogs. Improperly formulated vegetarian cat diets can result in blindness in cats. This problem is unusual in outdoor cats that hunt.

Pathophysiology
Taurine is an essential amino acid for cats with long-term deficiency causing severe retinal lesions. A taurine intake of 110 mg/kg body weight per day is needed to maintain normal retinal structure and function.

Clinical presentation
Early lesions appear as bilateral, focal, hyperreflective regions in the area centralis. If taurine continues to be deficient in the diet, the retinal lesions progress to symmetrical, horizontal, band-shaped hyperreflective areas dorsal to the optic disk **(Figures 19.137–19.141)**, with advanced stages appearing as diffuse generalized retinal atrophy and having complete blindness.

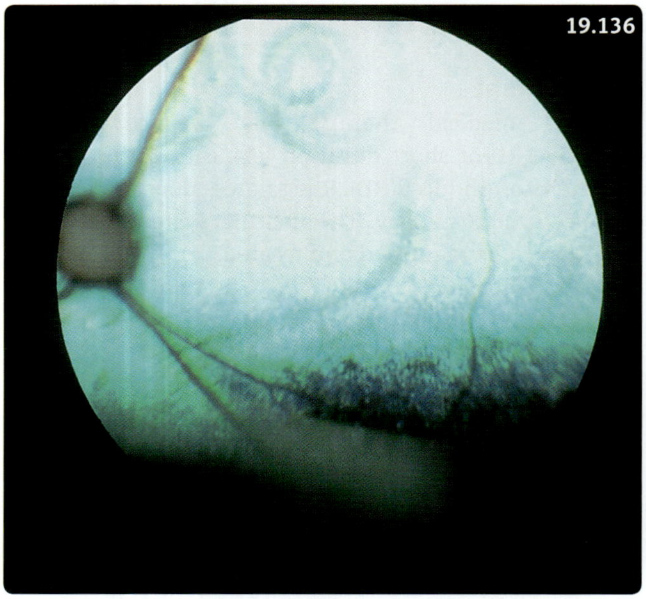

Figure 19.136 Curvilinear tracks due to ophthalmomyiasis in a cat.

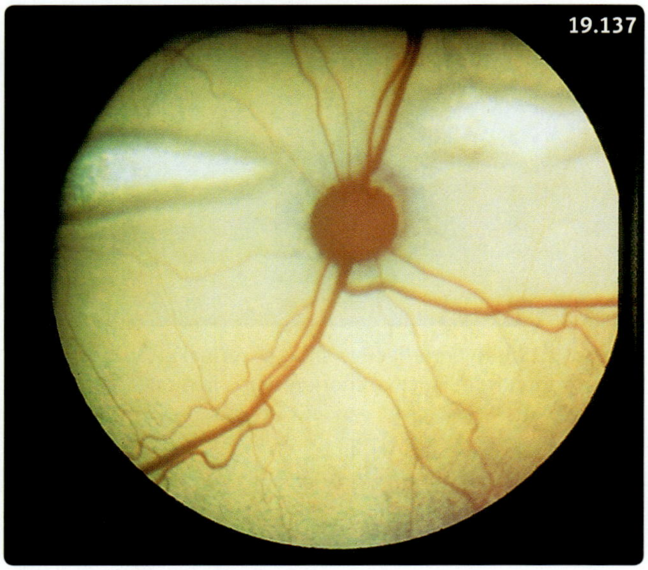

Figure 19.137 A nearly complete horizontal band of hyperreflectivity dorsal to the optic disk is found in a cat with early taurine retinopathy.

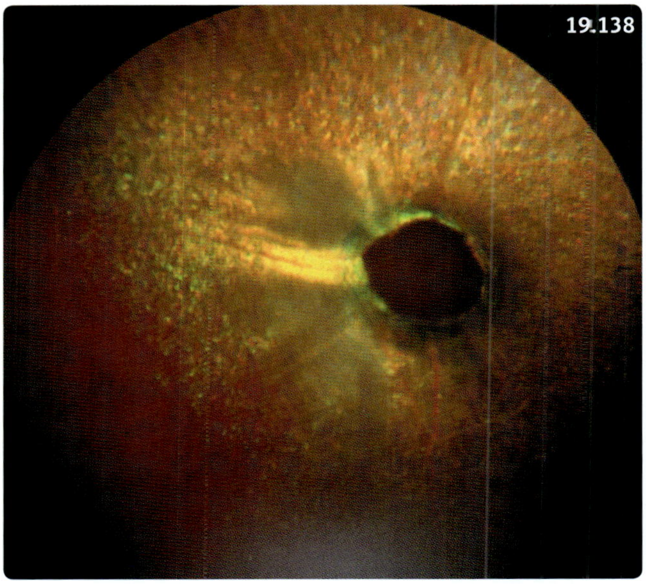

Figure 19.138 Retinal and optic nerve atrophy, caused by home-formulated 'vegan' cat diet, is present bilaterally in this cat

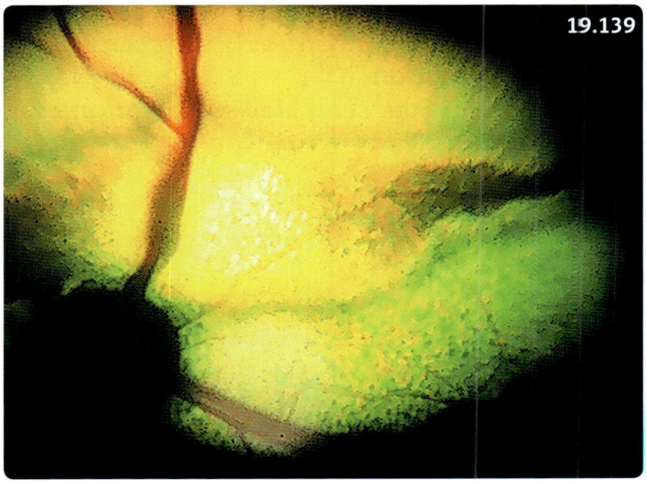

Figure 19.139 Feline central retinal degeneration (FCRD) is manifested as a hyperreflective band dorsal to the optic disk in this cat. FCRD may be related to dietary taurine deficiency.

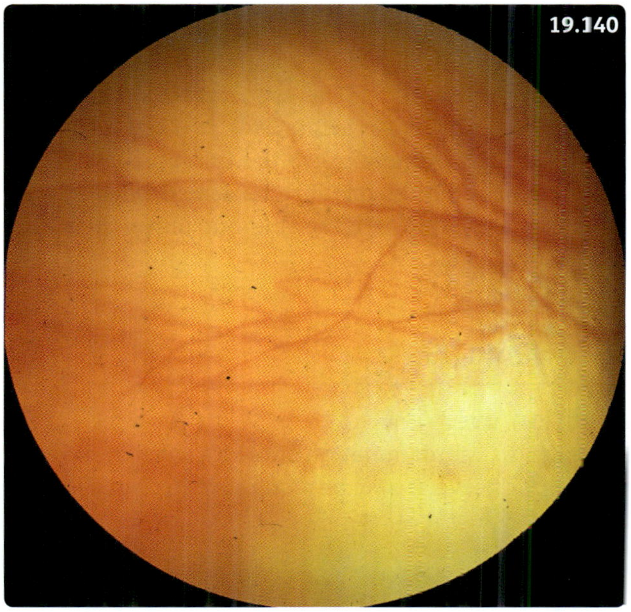

Figure 19.140 Choroidal vessel attenuation is present in this cat with advanced feline taurine retinopathy.

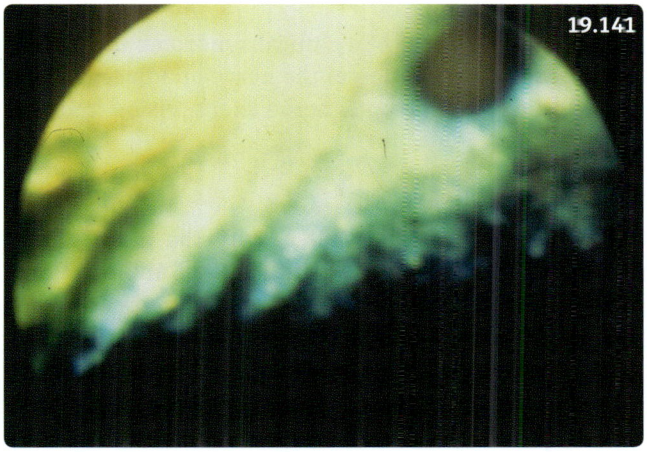

Figure 19.141 Generalized tapetal hyperreflectivity with tapetal striping due to conformation of the atrophic retina to the choroidal vessels is present in this cat with advanced feline taurine retinopathy.

Differential diagnosis

Tables 19.3, **19.5** and **19.8**.

Diagnosis

Measurement of plasma taurine levels is necessary to determine if taurine deficiency is present (a level <20 nmol/ml is critically low).

Management

Restoration of vision with taurine supplement is dependent on the degree of damage. The degeneration in early cases can be arrested if adequate amounts of taurine are included in the diet. However, taurine supplementation is of no value restoring vision in eyes with advanced retinal degeneration and blindness.

ENROFLOXACIN RETINOPATHY

Definition/overview

Enrofloxacin, a fluoroquinolone antibiotic, has recently been associated with a rare adverse ophthalmic reaction causing an acute, irreversible, retinal degeneration in cats. Pupils are fixed and dilated and the tapetum is hyperreflective. Vision loss is acute and follows enrofloxacin administration. The reported estimated incidence of this adverse reaction is 1 in 122,414 treated cats, or 0.0008%. Adherence to the manufacturer's current recommendation for enrofloxacin dosage in cats (2.5 mg/kg PO q12h) is advisable but may still be too high for aged cats.

OPTIC NEURITIS

Definition/overview

Optic neuritis is inflammation of the intraocular or intraorbital optic nerve. It may be a manifestation of systemic illness.

Etiology

Causes include idiopathic, immune, infectious, inflammatory, and neoplastic disorders.

Pathophysiology

Optic neuritis is more of a clinical syndrome than a single disease. Inflammation of the nerve or adjacent tissue causes damage to the optic nerve axons, vision loss, and optic nerve atrophy.

Clinical presentation

The optic disk appears swollen, with the peripapillary retina displaying evidence of RD. Retinal and optic disk hemorrhages and a vitreal haze may be present. The pupil is fixed and dilated, and vision absent.

Differential diagnosis

Tables 19.1, 19.5, and **19.6.** Intraorbital optic neuritis must be differentiated from glaucoma, RD, cataracts, and sudden acquired retinal degeneration, a retinal disease associated with sudden blindness and elevated intraocular glutamate.

Diagnosis

Diagnosis is based on elimination of possible causes, a CBC, serum chemistry profile, urinalysis, screening for infectious diseases, heartworm antigen test, thoracic radiography, and analysis of CSF.

Management

Oral corticosteroids are the drugs of choice in idiopathic cases. Many cases, however, relapse.

PAPILLEDEMA

Definition/overview

Papilledema is noninflammatory swelling of the optic nerve head. Papilledema results in optic nerve atrophy and blindness if the inciting condition cannot be eliminated.

Etiology

Papilledema is caused by partial obstruction of axoplasmic flow associated with increased intracranial pressure, and is rarely reported in dogs. Vision is present. Papilledema is also seen in dogs with elevated intraocular pressure in early glaucoma, and dogs with compression of the optic nerve by retrobulbar tumors.

Pathophysiology

Sustained mechanical trauma to the optic nerve axons or ischemia to any part of the optic nerve can reduce axoplasmic flow. Axoplasmic flow of both fast and slow components becomes reduced at the lamina cribrosa in papilledema.

Clinical presentation

Dilated pupils and optic nerve head swelling are present, but vision is maintained.

Differential diagnosis

Tables 19.1 and **19.5**.

Diagnosis

Elevation and hyperemia of the optic disk, blurring of the disk margin, filling in of the optic cup, and protrusion of the disk into the vitreous are found ophthalmoscopically with papilledema.

Management

Resolution of the elevated intracranial or intraocular pressure can aid animals with papilledema.

LYSOSOMAL STORAGE DISEASES

Definition/overview

Several lysosomal storage diseases have been identified in cats and dogs. Storage diseases are characterized by an accumulation of metabolic by-products within lysosomes, the cellular organelles that degrade complex macromolecules. Specific lysosomal storage diseases are normally named according to the specific accumulated product.

Because this excess material is a normal cellular component, the histopathologic changes result from physical distortion of affected cells rather than from a toxic effect. Most lysosomal storage diseases with known modes of inheritance are inherited as an autosomal recessive trait.

ALPHA-MANNOSIDOSIS

Definition/overview

Alpha-mannosidosis is a member of the inherited oligosaccharidoses described in Persian, Domestic Shorthair, and Domestic Longhair cats that results from a deficiency in acidic alpha-mannosidase. Ocular abnormalities described in affected cats include progressive corneal and lenticular opacification and resting nystagmus.

GLOBOID CELL LEUKODYSTROPHY

Definition/overview

Globoid cell leukodystrophy, or Krabbe's disease, is a member of the inherited sphingolipidoses described in the cat that result from a deficiency in galactocerebrosidase activity. The substrate galactocerebroside (i.e. galactosylceramide), a constituent of myelin, and another metabolite of myelin turnover, psychosine (galactosyl sphingosine), accumulate. Ocular manifestations of this disease in cats include lack of vestibular ocular reflexes and signs associated with visual deficits including diminished pupillary light reflexes and reduced menace responses. Galactocerebrosidosis is an autosomal recessive trait in West Highland White and Cairn Terriers. Clinical signs of globoid cell leukodystrophy in dogs are generally rapidly progressive and develop at a young age (2–6 months). Visual deficits and blindness may result late in the course of disease, but ophthalmoscopic lesions have not been observed.

GM1-GANGLIOSIDOSIS

Definition/overview

GM1-gangliosidosis is caused by a deficiency of a lysosomal hydrolase, beta-galactosidase, which produces an accumulation of GM1-ganglioside in the cerebral cortex and visceral organs. Ganglion cell swelling is the main ocular sign in cats. With respect to dogs, GM1-gangliosidosis is an autosomal recessive condition seen in Alaskan Huskies, English Springer Spaniels, mixed breed-Beagles, Portugese Water Dogs, and Shiba Inus. Abnormal ocular findings in dogs with this disease are limited to: (1) central corneal clouding, as has been observed in Shiba Inus and Portugese Water Dogs; (2) vision disturbances, as seen in Shiba Inus and Portugese Water Dogs; (3) strabismus, as has been observed in mixed breed-Beagles and Huskies; and (4) nystagmus, as has been observed in English Springer Spaniels, Portugese Water Dogs, and Huskies.

GM2-GANGLIOSIDOSIS

Definition/overview

GM2-gangliosidosis is caused by a deficiency of hexosaminidase. Clinical signs include ataxia, immobility, blindness, and dysphagia and finally seizures or generalized myoclonus (5 months of age), quadriplegia (6 months of age), and death prior to 8 months of age in cats. Variant forms of GM-2 gangliosidosis have been reported in the Japanese Spaniel, the German Shorthair Pointer, and the Golden Retriever.

MUCOLIPIDOSIS II

Definition/overview

Mucolipidosis II, or inclusion cell disease, is caused by deficient activity of the enzyme N-acetylglucosamine-1-phosphotransferase. Ocular abnormalities detected in cats affected with mucolipidosis II include, from early to late lesions, absent menace response, diminished pupillary light reflexes, and dilated pupils by 4 months of age. Initially, retinal development appears normal until 2.5 months of age, at which time dorsal retinal degeneration develops followed by progressive end-stage generalized retinal degeneration and blindness by 3.5 months of age.

MUCOPOLYSACCHARIDOSES

Definition/overview

The mucopolysaccharidoses (MPS) are a group of diseases characterized by defective metabolism of mucopolysaccharides (glycosaminoglycans). Three types of MPS have been identified in cats (MPS I, VI, and VII). Corneal clouding is the most debilitating ocular manifestation.

Five types of MPS have been identified in dogs (MPS I, II, III, VI, and VII). Corneal opacities are also seen with these conditions in dogs.

RECOMMENDED FURTHER READING

Aroch, I, Ofri R, Sutton GA (2013) Ocular manifestations of systemic diseases. In: *Slatter's Fundamentals of Veterinary Ophthalmology*, 5th edn. (eds. DJ Maggs, PE Miller, R Ofri R) Elsevier, St. Louis, pp. 394–436.

Cullen CL, Webb AA (2013) Ocular manifestations of systemic disease. Part 1: the dog. In: *Veterinary Ophthalmology*, 5th edn. (ed. KN Gelatt) John Wiley and Sons, Ames, pp. 1897–1977.

Cullen CL, Webb AA (2013) Ocular manifestations of systemic disease. Part 2: the cat. In: *Veterinary Ophthalmology*, 5th edn. (ed. KN Gelatt) John Wiley and Sons, Ames, pp. 1978–2036.

Martin CL (2010) *Ophthalmic Disease in Veterinary Medicine*. Manson Publishing, London.

Part 3

Multisystemic disorders

Chapter 20 **Clinical toxicology**
Lisa A. Murphy & Kenneth J. Drobatz

Chapter 21 **Infectious diseases**
Richard B. Ford & Annette Litster

Chapter 22 **Immunologic disorders**
Michael J. Day

Chapter 20

Clinical toxicology

Lisa A. Murphy & Kenneth J. Drobatz

INTRODUCTION

Animals can come into contact with an endless variety and type of toxins. This chapter contains some of the more common toxins reported in veterinary medicine and also some of the not-so-common toxins. Relatively speaking, toxins are less common than spontaneous diseases, but a toxin should always be considered in any sick or abnormally behaving animal. The chapter is broken down into seven major categories of toxins: insecticides, rodenticides, plants, over-the-counter medications, household products, metals, and human foods. Each toxin is consistently broken down into common names (if applicable), source, type of toxin, a brief synopsis of the pathophysiology of the toxin, clinical signs, differential diagnosis, basis of a diagnosis of the toxin, and finally clinical management of the toxicity. The authors have purposely kept the discussion concise, clinically relevant, and easy to use.

INSECTICIDES

ANTICHOLINESTERASE INSECTICIDES

Common names

Common organophosphates (OPs) include disulfoton, terbufos, chlorpyrifos, fenthion, diazinon, and malathion. Common carbamates include aldicarb, carbofuran, methomyl, propoxur, and carbaryl.

Source

OP and carbamate insecticides are commonly used on plants, animals, and soil, and in and around the home for insect control. Products are typically formulated as sprays, powders, and granules.

Type of toxin

OP and carbamate insecticides interfere with the normal breakdown of acetylcholine at cholinergic receptor sites.

Pathophysiology

The stimulatory neurotransmitter acetylcholine acts at cholinergic nerve synapses and neuromuscular junctions. Normally, acetylcholine is catabolized by acetylcholinesterase or other cholinesterases (ChE). OP and carbamate insecticides directly bind and inhibit ChE (**Figure 20.1**). Toxicity is the result of postsynaptic overstimulation due to the accumulation of acetylcholine.

Clinical signs

There are two clinical syndromes of OP intoxication: an acute syndrome and an intermediate syndrome. The acute syndrome is much more common.

Acute syndrome

Clinical signs of acute syndrome can be grouped into three categories: muscarinic, nicotinic, and central nervous system (CNS) signs:

- The traditional mnemonic that has been used to identify the acute muscarinic signs is SLUD (Salivation, Lacrimation, Urination, Defecation), which reflects stimulation of the parasympathetic nervous system. A more complete mnemonic is DUMBELS (Diarrhea, Urination, Miosis, Bronchospasm/Bradycardia, Emesis, Lacrimation, and Salivation). Other muscarinic signs include anorexia, coughing, difficulty breathing, and abdominal pain. Stimulation of the parasympathetic nervous system can be modified by concurrent stimulation of the sympathetic nervous system, resulting in sympathetic signs such as mydriasis or tachycardia, but this is less common.
- Nicotinic signs include generalized muscle stiffness, tremors, or weakness/paralysis (**Figures 20.2, 20.3**).
- CNS signs include restlessness, hyperactivity, depression, coma, and/or seizures (**Figure 20.4**).

Not all signs will be present in every case. The onset of signs from exposure varies depending on the dose, route

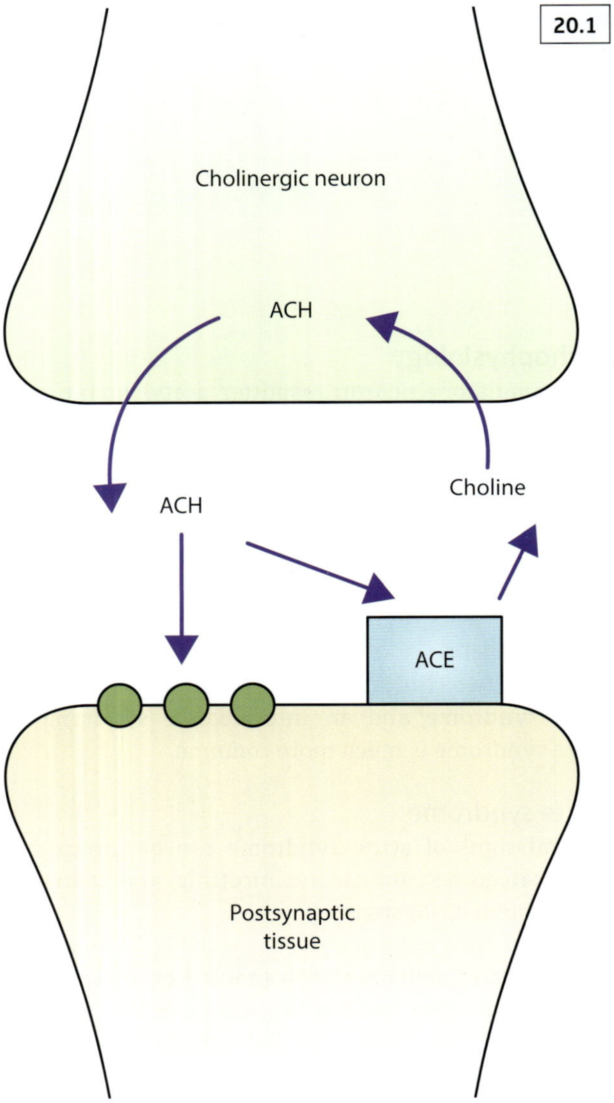

Figure 20.1 Normally, acetylcholine (ACH) is catabolized by acetylcholinesterase (ACE) at the myoneural junction. When the enzyme is inhibited, the parasympathomimetic signs from acetylcholine excess cause the characteristic muscarinic and nicotinic signs of organophosphate intoxication. (Courtesy M. Schaer)

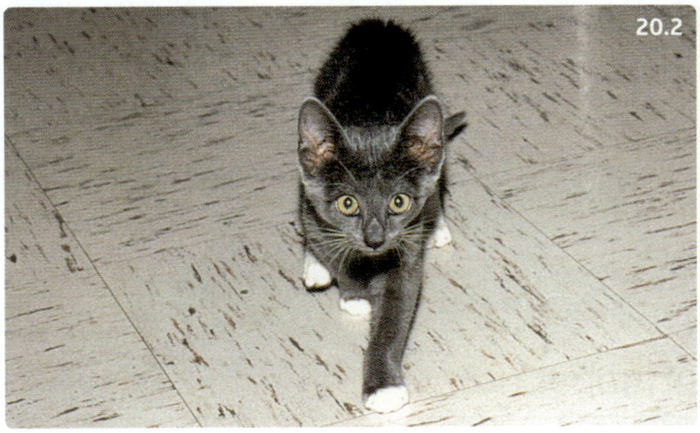

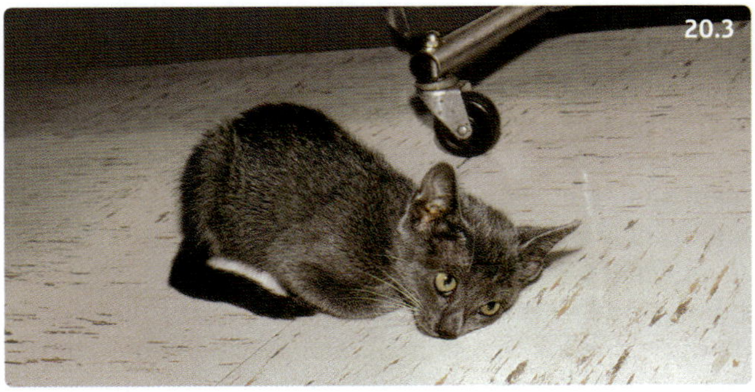

Figures 20.2, 20.3 One minute this kitten (20.2) was walking around normally with minimal muscular exertion, the next it was showing signs of muscular fatigue (20.3). This was due to chronic organophosphate intoxication. (Courtesy M. Schaer)

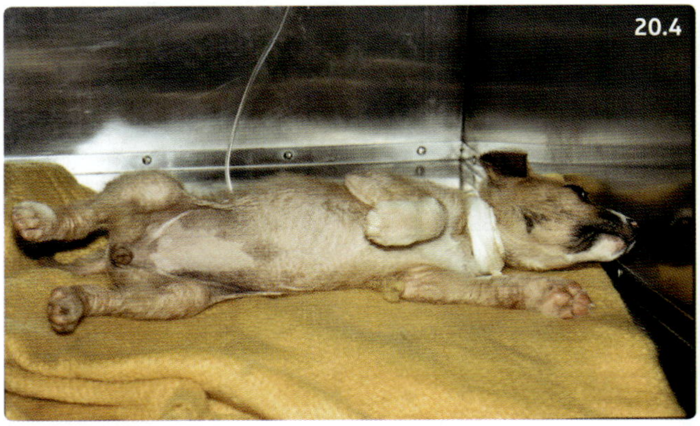

Figure 20.4 This puppy is seizuring from the nicotinic effects of acute organophosphate intoxication. (Courtesy M. Schaer)

of exposure, and the formulation of the toxin. It can range from minutes to hours.

Intermediate syndrome

Intermediate syndrome may occur with or without the acute syndrome and is thought to occur as a result of downregulation of the cholinergic receptors. It has been recognized in dogs and cats and clinical signs include loss of appetite, diarrhea, weakness (**Figure 20.5**), muscle tremors, altered behavior, abnormal posture, mental depression, and even death. These signs may occur days after the exposure.

Differential diagnosis

Any condition that can result in tremors, tonic/clonic seizures, or vomiting, or gastrointestinal (GI) signs of vomiting and diarrhea, should be considered. The combination of GI signs with the neurologic signs makes acetylcholinesterase inhibition highly likely.

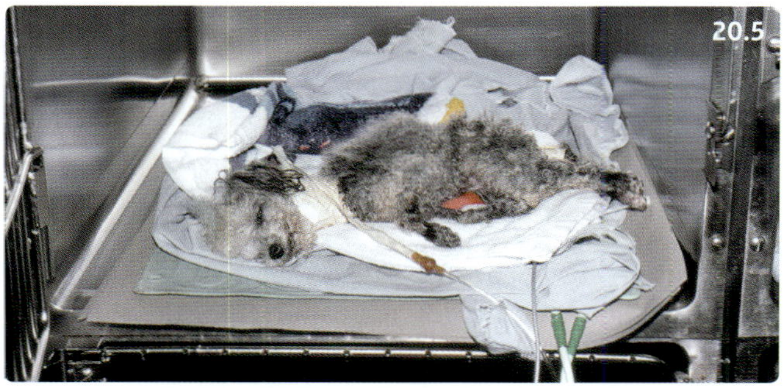

Figure 20.5 This Poodle is very weak and moribund from chronic organophosphate intoxication. A history of exposure to the poison would be vital for an expedient diagnosis for this dog. (Courtesy M. Schaer)

Diagnosis

History of exposure with compatible clinical signs is adequate for a working diagnosis and warrants therapy for acetylcholinesterase inhibition. Response to treatment can be supportive of a diagnosis. Measuring acetylcholinesterase activity in heparinized whole blood allows for a premortem diagnosis. Fresh whole blood is best or refrigerated heparinized whole blood if analysis is delayed. Depressed activity may occur with anemia. Activity <50% of normal is suspicious of intoxication, while activity <25% is diagnostic.

Stomach contents, vomited material, or samples of the suspected material that was ingested may also be assessed for the actual toxin.

Carbamate binding of acetylcholinesterase is reversible and this may occur in stored blood, resulting in a false-negative result. Keeping the blood sample refrigerated will help minimize this problem.

Management

If ingestion is recent, decontamination procedures (e.g. emesis induction, activated charcoal/cathartic, bath) should be done.

Specific therapy

Atropine sulfate (0.1–0.5 mg/kg: give 1/4 of the dose IV and the rest SC). Most clinicians start with 0.2 mg/kg slow IV and give the higher dose to animals with more severe muscarinic signs. Repeat doses are usually lower and can be titrated based on heart rate, pupil size, and amount of salivation. Over-atropinization should be avoided.

Protopam chloride or pralidoxime chloride (2-PAM) (10–20 mg/kg very slowly IV, or may be given IM or SC q8–12h) can reverse the binding of the OP to the acetylcholinesterase (carbamates have reversible binding and this therapy is not necessary). 2-PAM may not be effective if 'aging' has occurred. The longer OPs are bound to acetylcholinesterase, the more irreversible is the binding. There is no way to predict if irreversible binding has occurred, so 2-PAM should be given to see if clinical signs improve. If they do not, then it is unlikely that 2-PAM will be helpful.

Nonspecific therapy

Nicotinic signs (muscle tremors) and CNS signs (seizures) can be treated with diazepam (0.05–1.0 mg/kg IV).

FIPRONIL

Common names

Trade names for fipronil-containing products include Combat, Frontline, Maxforce, and Termidor.

Source

Fipronil is approved for use on dogs and cats for flea and tick control. Other common uses include insect control in the home and on crops and golf courses. Available fipronil formulations include spot-ons, sprays gels, and granular products.

Type of toxin

Fipronil is a phenylpyrazole insecticide.

Pathophysiology

Fipronil appears to act as a noncompetitive blocker of gamma-aminobutyric acid (GABA). This blockade causes neural excitement and death in insects. Because the shape of mammalian and insect GABA receptors is different, fipronil is much less toxic in mammals.

Clinical signs

Relatively rare and most are mild. Topical hypersensitivity skin reactions are the most commonly reported adverse effects. Hypersalivation or vomiting may occur.

Differential diagnosis

Local skin hypersensitivity reaction.

Diagnosis

Analysis of hair and skin where drug is applied can confirm exposure. Skin reaction at the site of application is suggestive of hypersensitivity to fipronil.

Management

No specific antidote exists. Treatment is symptomatic and supportive. Bathe the dermal exposure area with mild dishwashing detergent. Symptomatic treatment for skin hypersensitivity reactions includes bathing with a pet shampoo +/– corticosteroids or antihistamines.

IMIDACLOPRID

Common names
Trade names include Advantage, Marathon, and Premise.

Source
In addition to its agricultural uses, imidacloprid is used around the home for termites and on dogs and cats for flea control. Available formulations include powders, granules, sprays, and spot-on products.

Type of toxin
Imidacloprid is a chloronicotinyl nitroguanide insecticide.

Pathophysiology
Imidacloprid causes insect death by competitively blocking nicotinic acetylcholine receptors, resulting in a blockade of normal impulse transmission. Imidacloprid is not degraded by acetylcholinesterase. Imidacloprid is useful for the control of fleas and other insects, but is not active against ticks.

Clinical signs
Relatively rare and if present tend to be mild. Hypersalivation or vomiting may occur. Nicotinic signs such as muscle tremors, twitching, weakness, or cramps would be expected if toxicity occurs. A local skin hypersensitivity reaction also occurs.

Differential diagnosis
Clinical signs of toxicity are quite rare. If nicotinic signs are present, electrolyte changes (hypocalcemia) or toxins that cause muscle tremors should be considered.

Diagnosis
History of exposure and compatible clinical signs.

Management
Dermal exposure can be treated by bathing the toxin exposed area with a mild dishwashing detergent. The clinical signs of ingestion of the topically applied product (hypersalivation, vomiting) can be treated by administering a diluent such as milk or water.

SELAMECTIN

Source
Selamectin is marketed as Revolution® for use against fleas, ticks, heartworms, and mites in dogs, and fleas, heartworms, mites, hookworms, and roundworms in cats.

Type of toxin
Selamectin is a semisynthetic avermectin derived from a precursor avermectin produced by a bioengineered strain of *Streptomyces avermitilis.*

Pathophysiology
Selamectin causes paralysis in target organisms due to increased permeability of neuronal chloride channels. Rapid influx of chloride ions into neurons results in flaccid paralysis. Mammalian chloride channels are less sensitive and less accessible to selamectin.

Clinical signs
Clinical signs are relatively rare. A reversible, localized alopecia has been reported in cats. Other signs include disorientation, lethargy, anorexia, hypersalivation, vomiting, diarrhea, muscle tremors, pruritus/urticaria, erythema, and tachypnea. Rarely, seizures and ataxia occur in dogs. Severely affected dogs may become progressively weaker and comatose.

Differential diagnosis
If there are CNS/neurologic signs, other toxins, metabolic abnormalities (e.g. hypocalcemia, hypoglycemia, hypernatremia, hyponatremia, hepatic encephalopathy), or primary brain disease (encephalitis, neoplasia) should be considered.

Diagnosis
Detection of selamectin in the blood or tissues such as liver or adipose tissue will indicate exposure. Ideally, brain concentration of selamectin is what should be measured, but this is not possible antemortem. Compatible clinical signs with recent exposure can support a diagnosis. Dogs that lack P-glycoprotein in the blood–brain barrier have greater susceptibility to toxicity (e.g. Collies, other herding breeds). Dogs receiving drugs that inhibit P-glycoprotein may be more susceptible to toxicity: ketoconazole, cyclosporine A, verapamil.

Management
No specific antidote exists. Decontamination for oral ingestion within 2–3 hours (emesis induction, activated charcoal, cathartic). Treatment is primarily supportive: IV fluids, nutrition, and good nursing care for animals that are recumbent and not responsive. Close monitoring of ventilation should be provided in comatose patients. Full recovery can occur despite the severity of the signs.

IVERMECTIN

Source

A semi-synthetic macrocytic lactone derived from *Streptomyces avermitilis*. It is an antiparasitic drug that is effective against a broad spectrum of external and internal parasites of both large and small animals.

Type of toxin

Avermectins function by potentiating glutamate-gated chloride channels and gamma-aminobutyric acid (GABA)-gated chloride channels in the nervous system.

Pathophysiology

The actions on the gated chloride channels lead to nerve dysfunction and the clinical signs in intoxicated animals. The enhanced release of GABA at presynaptic nerve terminals blocks postsynaptic stimulation of adjacent neurons by acting as an inhibitory neurotransmitter, which causes paralysis and eventual death of the parasite. Unfortunately, these same effects can occur in animals that become intoxicated with this agent. Major adverse signs are seen in Collie dogs and other dogs in the sheepdog group because they have a deletion mutation in the multidrug resistance (mdr1) gene, thus allowing for sustained neurologic impairment that can culminate in death.

Clinical signs

The clinical signs are mainly neurologic, which can cause the patient to have a multitude of neurologic abnormalities. These signs include blindness, dementia, seizures, and ventilatory impairment. The clinical signs can last for several days, but in the sheepdog breeds they can last for weeks, with some dogs requiring ventilator support for 2 or more weeks.

Differential diagnosis

Any disease, injury, drug, or toxin that can adversely affect the CNS.

Diagnosis

The history is of utmost importance because it will reveal the animal's access to the parasitide. Dog owners might provide information of giving their horse's ivermectin formulation to their pet or the dogs might have been in the same area where horses were recently dewormed with the agent, thus providing a means of ingesting the ivermectin from amounts that are spilt onto the ground or remnants of the drug that come out in the feces, which are subsequently ingested by the dog.

Treatment

Treatment is generally supportive, using IV crystalloid for systemic support and anticonvulsants as indicated. If the animal was observed to ingest the ivermectin, rapid induction of vomiting using apomorphine might be very helpful followed by several doses of orally administered activated charcoal.

The use of IV lipid emulsions is theoretically effective because of the high lipid solubility of avermectins. The high lipid solubility is the main reason for the drug's long action in cases of intoxication because it is stored in the fat tissue and then slowly released into the circulation. By giving the lipid emulsion IV (Intralipid® 20% [A 20% IV fat emulsion], Baxter Healthcare Corp.) a 'lipid sink' is theoretically created and the drug will become partitioned into a lipid compartment in the blood stream. The recommended dose is 4.0 ml/kg as a bolus IV, followed by a maintenance rate of 3.0 ml/kg/hour for 4 hours.

The IV lipid emulsion has also been used to treat permethrin intoxication.

LUFENURON

Source

Lufenuron is commonly used to control fleas on pets and on field crops. It has also been used to treat cutaneous fungal infections in dogs and cats.

Type of toxin

Lufenuron is a benzophenyl urea insect development inhibitor.

Pathophysiology

The drug does not affect adult fleas, but is ovicidal and larvicidal. Lufenuron blocks chitin synthetase, disrupting the synthesis and deposition of chitin.

Clinical signs

Extremely rare. Vomiting, lethargy/depression, pruritus/urticaria, diarrhea, dyspnea, anorexia, and reddened skin are reported clinical signs.

Differential diagnosis

Skin hypersensitivity reaction. Any potential causes for vomiting/diarrhea.

Diagnosis

Exposure with compatible clinical signs is supportive.

Management
Decontamination for oral ingestion within 2–3 hours (emesis induction, activated charcoal, cathartic). Supportive care.

NITENPYRAM

Source
Nitenpyram was developed for use against fleas as an oral adulticide.

Type of toxin
Nitenpyram is a neonicotinoid, systemically active drug.

Pathophysiology
Nitenpyram is a nicotinic acetylcholine receptor agonist that is insect specific. It does not inhibit acetylcholinesterase.

Clinical signs
Nitenpyram is extremely safe and toxicity is very rare. As fleas die the animal may become pruritic, but this is not considered to be toxicity.

Differential diagnosis
Not applicable as toxicity is very rare.

Diagnosis
Recent exposure with compatible clinical signs.

Management
Decontamination of the GI tract if exposure is recent (within 3 hours) followed by activated charcoal and a cathartic. Supportive care.

N,N-DIETHYL-M-TOLUAMIDE

Common names
N,N-Diethyl-M-toluamide (DEET) is the active ingredient in products such as Cutters and Deep Woods Off.

Source
DEET is an insect repellent marketed for mosquito, fly, and tick control on pets, clothing, and humans. Available formulations include sprays, creams, lotions, sticks, and gels, ranging in DEET concentration from 5% to 100%.

Pathophysiology
The toxicologic mechanisms of action of DEET have not been well described.

Clinical signs
Hypersalivation, vomiting, hyperexcitability, muscle tremors, ataxia, and seizures.

Differential diagnosis
For CNS signs consider neoplasia, trauma, infection, metabolic disturbances (e.g. hypoglycemia, sodium concentration disorders, hepatic encephalopathy) or congenital neurologic disorders. Other possible toxins include lead, metaldehyde, acetylcholinesterase inhibitors, mycotoxins, or macrolide antiparasitic products.

Diagnosis
Blood, urine, tissue, or stomach content concentrations of DEET indicate exposure. Exposure with compatible clinical signs is suggestive of toxicity.

Management
Treatment is supportive as there is no antidote for DEET intoxication. Rinse the animal with soap and water vigorously if a topical preparation was used. If the DEET has been ingested, vomiting should be induced followed by oral activated charcoal once the vomiting has ceased. IV crystalloid fluid support is highly recommended. Anticonvulsants (diazepam, midazolam) should be given if seizures ensue. Ventilation and oxygen support should be provided if indicated.

PYRETHRINS/PYRETHROIDS

Source
Products containing pyrethrins and pyrethroids are widely available, marketed under a vast number of trade names, for flea and tick control in cats and dogs. Formulations include dips, sprays, spot-ons, shampoos, and mousses.

Type of toxin
Natural pyrethrum extract is derived from *Chrysanthemum cinerariaefolium* and related plants. Pyrethroids are synthetic products, formulated to provide enhanced stability and potency.

Pathophysiology
Pyrethrins and pyrethroids affect neuronal sodium ion channels. By increasing the length of depolarizing action potentials, these compounds cause repetitive nerve firing. Sensory nerve fibers are especially susceptible to stimulation.

Clinical signs

Much more common in cats compared with dogs. Often results from inappropriate use of a cat product or applying canine formulation to a cat. Hypersalivation, tremors, ear and facial twitching, ataxia, pruritus, vomiting, and agitation are the most common clinical signs. Muscle tremors can be severe and appear as if the animal is seizuring, but the majority are alert and aware of their surroundings during these seizure-like episodes (**Figure 20.6**). Allergic reactions manifested by pruritus and hyperemia have been reported.

Differential diagnosis

Other neurotoxins such as metaldehyde, caffeine, theobromine, illicit drugs (amphetamines, cocaine), mycotoxins, acetylcholinesterase inhibitors, and carbamates. Also trauma, metabolic disturbances (e.g. hypoglycemia, sodium disorders, hypocalcemia, hepatic encephalopathy), neoplasia, infections, inflammatory brain lesions.

Diagnosis

Compatible clinical signs after recent exposure are adequate for a working clinical diagnosis. Analysis of hair can confirm exposure, but is generally not necessary.

Management

Decontamination of skin by bathing animal. If topical formulation is ingested by a cat, then GI decontamination and administration of activated charcoal is warranted. Muscle tremor control is best achieved by administration of methocarbamol (55–220 mg/kg slow IV bolus). Doses may be repeated as needed to control tremors, but the total dose should not exceed 330 mg/kg/day. (**Note:** Anecdotally, total doses greater than this have been administered in severe or protracted cases without obvious adverse clinical signs.) Diazepam (0.5–5.0 mg/kg IV, titrating to effect) may also be used to control tremors. Supportive care.

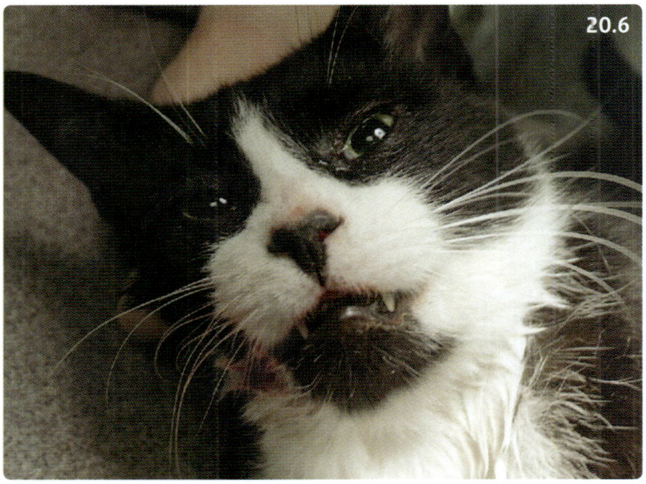

Figure 20.6 This cat has neurologic signs from pyrethroid intoxication. It showed signs of neuromuscular twitching and a variable degree of altered consciousness. (Courtesy M. Schaer)

METALDEHYDE

Source

Snail and slug baits available under various trade names as pellets, granules, liquids, or powders contain metaldehyde. In some countries, metaldehyde is also sold as solid or pelletized fuel for camping stoves and lamps.

Type of toxin

Metaldehyde is a tetramer of acetaldehyde.

Pathophysiology

Acid hydrolysis of metaldehyde in the stomach results in the formation of acetaldehyde, but acetaldehyde residues were not detected in the serum of orally exposed rats. Metaldehyde is absorbed intact from the GI tract but once absorbed, its metabolic fate is largely unknown. Studies in mice have shown a significant decrease in GABA concentrations in the brain. Monoamine oxidases, norepinephrine, and 5-hydroxytryptamine may also contribute to the effects of metaldehyde.

Clinical signs

Seizures, muscle tremors, tachycardia, hyperthermia, mydriasis, hypersalivation, ataxia, panting, severe depression, coma, and death due to respiratory failure.

Differential diagnosis

Other toxins that affect the nervous system including strychnine, bromethalin, acetylcholinesterase inhibitors, pyrethrins/pyrethroids, and mycotoxins. Metabolic conditions such as hypoglycemia, hypocalcemia, or hepatic encephalopathy. CNS trauma, neoplasia, infection, encephalitis, or congenital disorders.

Diagnosis

Chemical analysis of serum, stomach contents, vomitus, urine, or liver tissue. Analysis of material that was ingested. Exposure with compatible clinical signs is the basis of most working clinical diagnoses.

Management

GI decontamination procedures (emesis, gastric lavage, cleansing enemas followed by activated charcoal and a cathartic) should be applied appropriately. Fluid therapy will help control increased body temperature and maintain hydration in severely affected cases. Methocarbamol (55–220 mg/kg slow IV bolus) can be given to control tremors. (**Note:** According to the manufacturer the daily dose should not exceed 330 mg/kg, but anecdotally this dose has been exceeded in severe cases without obvious adverse clinical effects.) Most animals respond well to methocarbamol. Diazepam (0.5–5 mg/kg IV, titrated to effect) can be given to control tremors/seizures. If the seizures are not controlled with methocarbamol or diazepam, pentobarbital (2–4 mg/kg slow boluses to effect [to control tremors, not to anesthetize if possible]) should be considered. Propofol administered by CRI can be given instead of pentobarbital. When administering a combination of sedatives, make sure the airway is protected and ventilation is adequate.

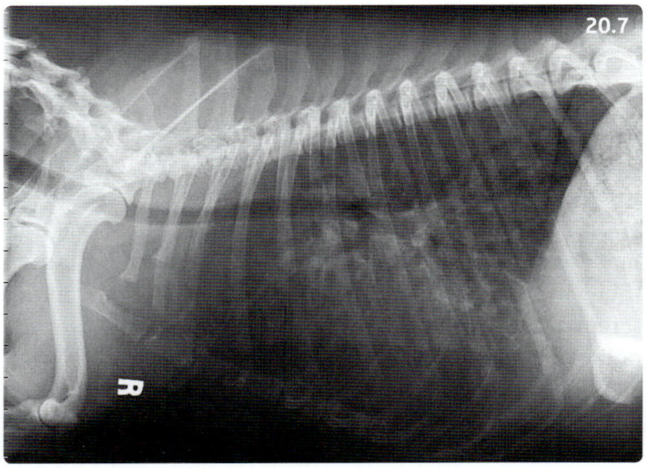

Figure 20.7 This radiograph shows intrapulmonary hemorrhage along with bleeding into the wall of the trachea, which caused luminal attenuation. (Courtesy M. Schaer)

RODENTICIDES

ANTICOAGULANT RODENTICIDES

(See also Chapter 17: Disorders of hemostasis.)

Common examples

Warfarin, chlorphacinone, bromadiolone, brodifacoum.

Source

Anticoagulant rodenticides are the most common type of rodenticides designed to kill rats, mice, gophers, and other rodents. These products are readily available as pellets, wax blocks, and tracking powders. These baits may then be mixed with foodstuffs, inadvertently attracting pets instead.

Type of toxin

Anticoagulant rodenticides cause coagulopathies by depleting vitamin K1 hydroquinone.

Pathophysiology

Vitamin K1 hydroquinone is converted to vitamin K1 epoxide during the synthesis of clotting factors II, VII, IX, and X. Vitamin K1 epoxide is then converted back to vitamin K1 quinone. Anticoagulant rodenticides stop the 'recycling' of vitamin K1 by inhibiting vitamin K1 (2,3)-epoxide reductase.

Clinical signs

Vomiting, diarrhea, lethargy, generalized weakness, respiratory distress, bleeding (can be from anywhere) (**Figures 20.7–20.12**), pale mucous membranes, altered mentation/seizures (if bleeding into brain occurs, but this is extremely rare; **Figure 20.13**).

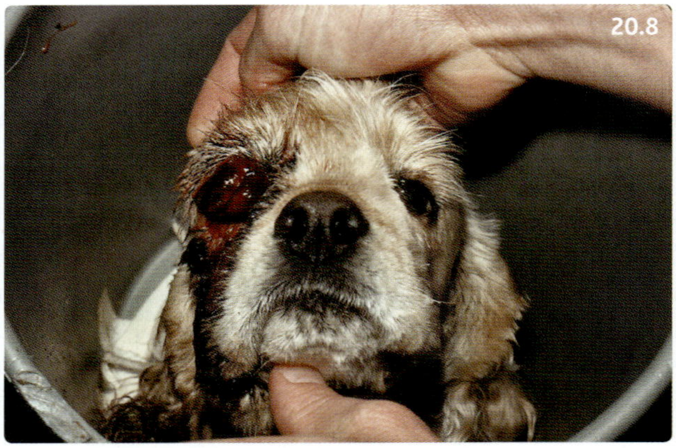

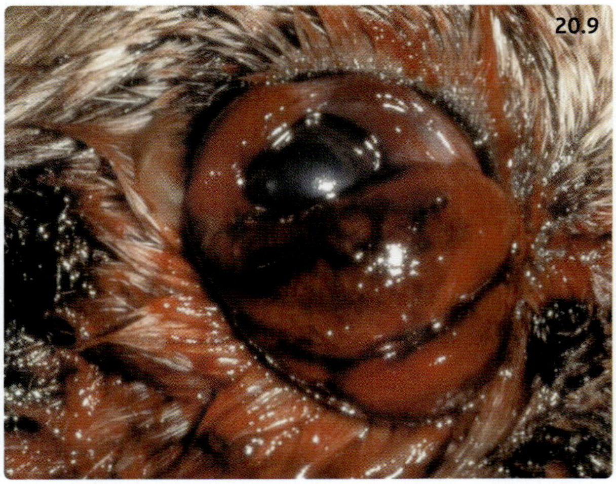

Figures 20.8, 20.9 This Cocker Spaniel shows marked conjunctival hemorrhage as its only bleeding site from warfarin intoxication. (Courtesy M. Schaer)

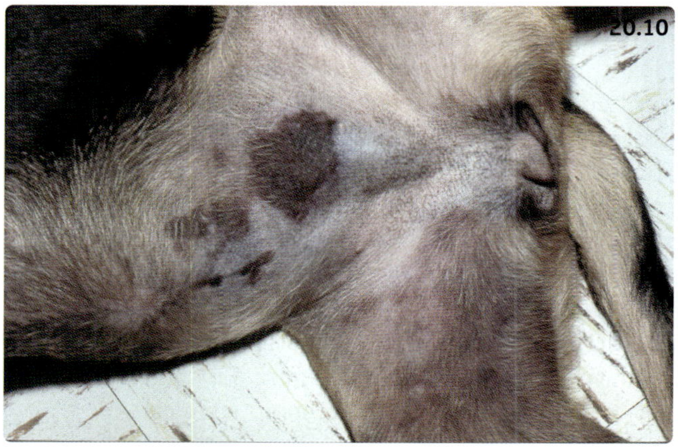

Figure 20.10 Ecchymotic hemorrhages caused by anticoagulant rodenticide ingestion are shown in this dog. (Courtesy M. Schaer)

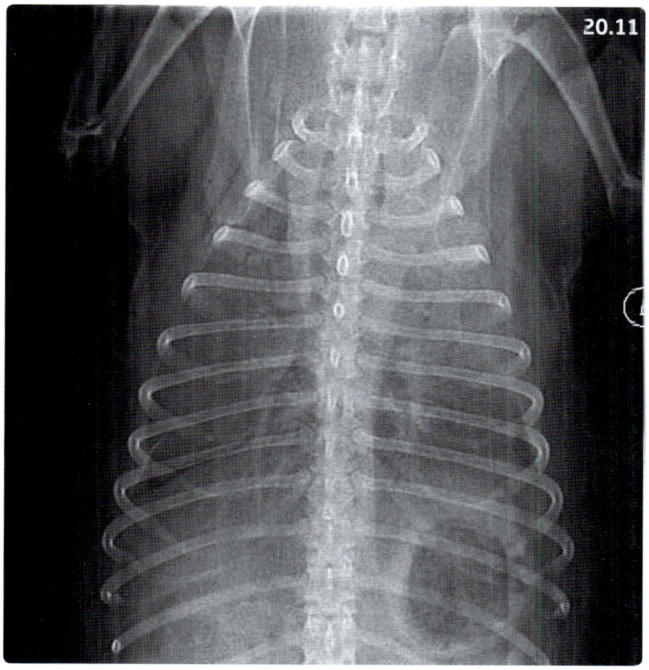

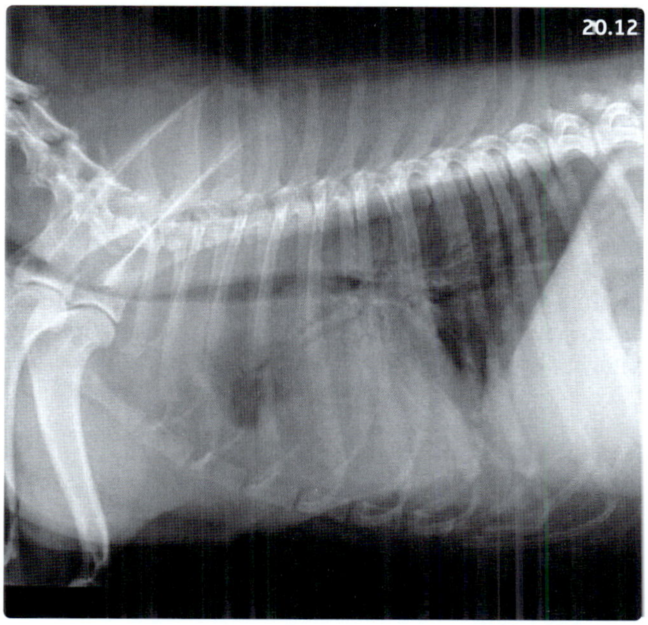

Figures 20.11, 20.12 These radiographs show marked pulmonary and pleural hemorrhage caused by 2nd generation anticoagulant rodenticide ingestion. The effusion will require approximately 5–7 days to resolve (Courtesy M. Schaer)

Differential diagnosis

Disseminated intravascular coagulation (typically these animals are systemically ill as well), congenital bleeding disorders, thrombocytopenia, or severe liver disease (usually other signs of liver disease are present once the coagulation factors are not being produced).

Diagnosis

History of exposure with compatible clinical signs is adequate for a working diagnosis. Analysis of blood for anticoagulant rodenticides is definitive.

Management

Recent exposure (within hours of ingestion)

Induce emesis. Administer activated charcoal with a cathartic. There are two further options to choose from:

- Administer vitamin K1 (2.5 mg/kg PO q12h) empirically for 4 weeks (if given with higher-fat food, will enhance absorption, but this is not necessary). Recheck prothrombin time (PT) 48–72 hours after final dose of vitamin K1. If PT is prolonged, administer vitamin K1 for 2 further weeks and follow same PT recheck procedure. For very large dogs, vitamin K1 can be expensive.
- Do not administer vitamin K1. Check PT 48 hours after exposure. If PT is within reference range, then it is unlikely that the animal ingested a toxic amount of the rodenticide and no further therapy is necessary. If PT is prolonged, begin vitamin K1 therapy as indicated above in the empirical vitamin K1 therapy protocol.

If animal is actively bleeding

Bleeding can occur anywhere in the body, but it is most commonly noted in the pleural space and lung parenchyma. Perform PT and partial thromboplastin time to

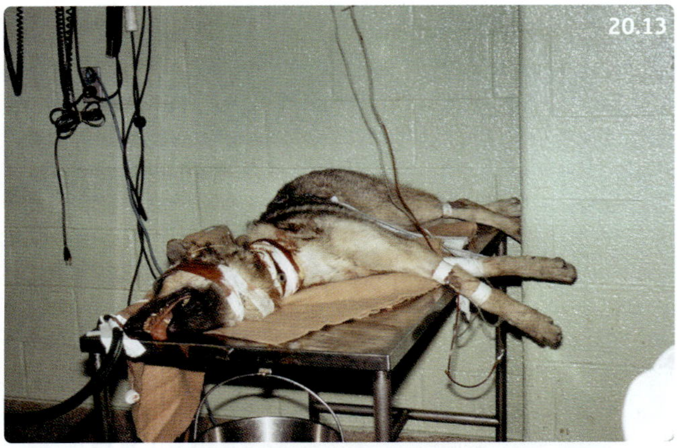

Figure 20.13 This German Shepherd Dog suffered severe brainstem hemorrhage from anticoagulant rodenticide poisoning and died. (Courtesy M. Schaer)

confirm coagulopathy. Administer 10–20 ml/kg of fresh frozen plasma IV. (**Note:** All venepuncture sites can form large hematomas; therefore, avoid the jugular veins.) If fresh frozen plasma is not available, consider fresh whole blood. If anemic, also administer packed red blood cells (RBCs) or fresh whole blood. Administer 5 mg/kg vitamin K1 SC using a small needle or administer 5 mg/kg vitamin K1 PO if tissue perfusion is good. If tissue perfusion is poor, GI absorption may be inadequate. Do not administer vitamin K1 IM as a severe hematoma may develop. Avoid administration IV as an anaphylactoid type reaction may occur.

It takes about 12–24 hours for vitamin K1 to have its effect on coagulation. Once the animal is stable and coagulation parameters are corrected, discharge the animal with vitamin K1 therapy as indicated in the empirical vitamin K1 administration protocol above.

BROMETHALIN

Source
Bromethalin has been in use as a rodenticide since the 1980s.

Type of toxin
Bromethalin and its primary metabolite, desmethylbromethalin, are uncouplers of oxidative phosphorylation.

Pathophysiology
Uncoupling of oxidative phosphorylation decreases ion channel pump activity; bromethalin has also been shown to induce lipid peroxidation in the brains of rats. Cerebral edema and increased cerebrospinal fluid pressures are seen in lethally poisoned animals.

Clinical signs
Most clinical signs are associated with the CNS. Signs will vary depending on time of exposure to presentation and dose. Onset and progression of clinical signs will vary from hours to days, with higher dose exposures requiring a shorter time period for onset of signs. Clinical signs include hindlimb ataxia/paresis that can progress to hindlimb paralysis. Other CNS signs can include anisocoria, behavioral changes, positional nystagmus, loss of bark, muscle tremors, focal motor to generalized seizures, and even stupor or coma. Abdominal distension secondary to generalized ileus has been noted in cats.

Differential diagnosis
Any condition that causes CNS signs including head trauma, neoplasia, intracranial hemorrhage or embolism, infections, inflammatory conditions, and other CNS toxins.

Diagnosis
Primarily based on history of exposure and compatible clinical signs. Chemical confirmation from adipose tissue, brain, liver, kidney, and other tissues is definitive for exposure and diagnostic in the face of compatible clinical signs.

Management
This is a deadly toxin and aggressive decontamination should be applied in cases of recent exposure. Emesis should be induced (exposure within 2–3 hours) as soon as possible in animals that do not have contraindications for this procedure (e.g. altered mentation, seizures, respiratory difficulty, upper airway disease).

If emesis is contraindicated, gastric lavage should be performed. Oral activated charcoal combined with a cathartic should be given following emesis induction. Sorbitol or sodium sulfate are appropriate cathartics. Magnesium sulfate should be avoided in animals with renal disease or animals with CNS depression, which often occurs with bromethalin intoxication (increased brain magnesium levels may contribute to the CNS depression). Bromethalin is excreted into the GI tract and goes through enterohepatic recirculation; therefore, repeated doses of activated charcoal with a cathartic should be given every 4–6 hours. Hydration should be monitored as repeated doses of a cathartic can result in dehydration.

If CNS signs are evident, mannitol (0.5–1.0 g/kg slow IV) should be administered. Furosemide (1–2 mg/kg IV q6h) and high doses of dexamethasone (2 mg/kg IV) have been recommended. These treatments have met with limited success in treating animals that develop CNS signs after bromethalin ingestion.

CHOLECALCIFEROL

Common names
Rodenticides containing cholecalciferol include Quintox®.

Source
Cholecalciferol (vitamin D3) can be found in rodenticides and multivitamins.

Type of toxin
With normal dietary intakes, cholecalciferol is converted to various metabolites that are eventually eliminated, primarily through the bile and feces. After massive intakes, excessive concentrations of cholecalciferol metabolites exert metabolic effects.

Pathophysiology
The active cholecalciferol metabolites calcifediol and calcitriol produce hypercalcemia and hyperphosphatemia through two mechanisms: (1) increasing calcium and phosphorus absorption from the intestines and (2) stimulating calcium and phosphorus release from bone. Once the plasma calcium × phosphorus product is greater than 60, soft tissue mineralization may occur.

Clinical signs
Anecdotally, the frequency of toxicity associated with this poison is decreasing. Clinical signs are related to hypercalcemia and include lethargy/depression, anorexia, weakness, vomiting (occasionally hematemesis), polydipsia/polyuria, constipation, melena, and dehydration.

Differential diagnosis
Any disease that causes hypercalcemia should be considered.

Diagnosis
Hypercalcemia with recent exposure is adequate for a working diagnosis. More supportive but not exclusively diagnostic evidence includes measuring the variables associated with calcium metabolism (i.e. serum intact parathyroid hormone [PTH], ionized calcium, 25-hydroxyvitamin D3, and 1,25-dihydroxyvitamin D3). With cholecalciferol intoxication PTH is decreased, 25-hydroxyvitamin D3 is increased, and 1,25-dihydroxyvitamin D3 is normal.

Management
GI decontamination followed by activated charcoal and a saline cathartic should be carried out if ingestion was within the last 6–8 hours. Blood calcium concentration should be monitored every 24 hours for several days after exposure (between 2 and 6 days). If hypercalcemia is already present, GI decontamination is not necessary unless the animal was recently exposed to more toxin based on the owner's history.

Treatment for hypercalcemia should be administered at presentation. This can include:

- Saline diuresis.
- Furosemide (2–6 mg/kg IV in the dog or 1–4 mg/kg in the cat q8–12h).
- Prednisolone (2 mg/kg PO q12h). (**Note:** Make sure neoplastic causes of hypercalcemia have been ruled out.)
- Salmon calcitonin (4–6 IU/kg SC q6h) until calcium stabilizes.
- Pamidronate disodium (1.3–2 mg/kg slow IV over 2–4 hours, given two times 4 days apart) has been shown to be effective in controlling experimentally induced cholecalciferol intoxication in dogs. (**Note:** Pamidronate disodium and salmon calcitonin should not be administered concurrently.)
- Dietary calcium restriction.

Treatment is continued at home once the serum calcium concentration is stabilized. Oral furosemide and prednisolone in conjunction with a low-calcium diet may be necessary for weeks with some cholecalciferol ingestions. Calcium concentrations are monitored to determine when therapy can be discontinued.

STRYCHNINE

Source
Often considered restricted-use pesticides, strychnine baits are used to control many nuisance animal species. Pet animals may be exposed accidentally or maliciously.

Type of toxin
Strychnine is an alkaloid isolated from the seeds of *Strychnos nux-vomica* and *Strychnos ignatii*.

Pathophysiology
Strychnine blocks the inhibitory actions of glycine, leading to excessive neuronal stimulation with highly exaggerated reflex arcs.

Clinical signs

Clinical signs are primarily referable to lack of inhibition of muscle reflexes resulting in extensor muscle spasms and tetany. The speed of onset and severity of clinical signs are proportional to the amount of toxin ingested. Larger amounts result in faster onset of signs (usually within minutes to an hour). Earliest signs include nervousness, anxiety, tachypnea, and hypersalivation. Ataxia, muscle spasms, and stiffness followed by generalized convulsions are characterized primarily by tonic extensor muscle spasms (opisthotonus). The severity of the muscle contractions may be increased with noise stimulation. Death can result from respiratory paralysis.

Differential diagnosis

Any toxin or disorder that can result in CNS signs primarily characterized by tonic muscle spasms (e.g. metaldehyde, penitrem A [moldy food], theobromine, nicotine, caffeine, amphetamines, cocaine, chlorinated hydrocarbons), tetanus, hypocalcemia.

Diagnosis

Exposure with compatible clinical signs is adequate for a working diagnosis. Analysis for the toxin in vomitus or gastric lavage contents is necessary to confirm ingestion/exposure. Analysis of the substance that was ingested confirms exposure. Strychnine can sometimes be detected in urine and blood.

Management

The GI tract must be decontaminated (induce emesis or gastric lavage) if exposure was recent and the animal does not have clinical signs associated with strychnine ingestion. Decontamination is followed with activated charcoal and a cathartic. The convulsions should be controlled:

- Pentobarbital (3–15 mg/kg to effect, but give very slowly IV as full effect of each dose is delayed by a few minutes).
- Diazepam (0.5–5 mg/kg IV to effect). If this is effective, it can be followed by a CRI (usually start with the dose that controlled the convulsions at that rate/hour). The dose is adjusted as needed to control muscle spasms.
- Methocarbamol (55–220 mg/kg slow IV bolus). Generally, do not exceed 330 mg/kg/day. Anecdotally, this dose has been exceeded without obvious clinical problems.

Ventilation should be monitored. If ventilation is inadequate, positive pressure mechanical ventilation should be administered. Minimize any sensory stimulation. Provide supportive care (IV fluids, control temperature, monitor acid–base status, good nursing care).

ZINC PHOSPHIDE

Common names

Brand names for zinc phosphide include Sweeney's Poison Peanuts, Mole Guard, and ZP Tracking Powder.

Source

Zinc phosphide is a dark gray powder that has been formulated into various rodenticide pellets, baits, and tracking powders.

Type of toxin

Under acidic conditions or in the presence of water, zinc phosphide is rapidly converted to highly toxic phosphine gas. The odor of phosphine gas has been described as rotten fish or rotten eggs.

Pathophysiology

Phosphine gas inhibits oxidative phosphorylation and also causes lipid peroxidation and other cellular damage.

Clinical signs

Onset of vomiting occurs within 15 minutes to 1 hour after ingestion. Other signs include depression, anorexia, and hematemesis. The vomitus can smell like rotten fish or be garlicky, which indicates phosphine gas (use caution). Due to the rapid corrosive effect of the toxin, the animal may have acute abdominal pain. Respiratory signs include respiratory distress with harsh sounds. Neurologic signs include vocalization, convulsions, generalized muscle fasciculations, tremors, exaggerated response to stimuli, and disorientation. Tachycardia or bradycardia may be noted. Abdominal pain can result in irritability and agitation.

Differential diagnosis

- GI signs. Gastric ulcer, GI foreign body, pancreatitis, intussusception, gastritis, peritonitis, or any systemic disease that can result in vomiting.
- Respiratory signs. Congestive heart failure, pneumonia, pulmonary thromboembolism, pulmonary hemorrhage, neurogenic pulmonary edema or acute respiratory distress syndrome.
- Neurologic signs. Epilepsy, distemper, postictal neurologic changes, other neurotoxins, intracranial neoplasia, encephalitis, hepatic encephalopathy, hypoglycemia, hyperosmolar nonketotic diabetes, electrolyte changes (hypernatremia, hyponatremia, hypocalcemia), severe acidemia, or severe uremia.

Diagnosis

History of exposure with compatible clinical signs. Definitive identification of phosphine gas is difficult, as it rapidly dissipates in air. Tissue samples or samples of material ingested, vomitus, or stomach contents should be rapidly collected, placed in airtight containers, and frozen. The samples are then submitted to the toxicology laboratory.

Management

There are no specific antidotes for zinc phosphide toxicity. Animals with this toxicity are critically ill. Supportive critical care should be applied and should specifically address the respiratory, cardiovascular, neurologic, and renal systems. Additionally, attention to the GI effects should be applied.

PLANTS

EASTER LILIES

Common names

Acute kidney injury (AKI) in cats has been associated with members of the Liliaceae family, including Easter lilies (*Lilium longiflorum*), tiger lilies (*Lilium tigrinum*), rubrum or Japanese showy lilies (*Lilium speciosum* and *Lilium lancifolium*), and various daylilies (*Hemerocallis* species). Plants such as peace lilies (*Spathiphyllum* species) and calla lilies (*Zantedeschia* species) should not be confused with members of the Liliaceae family.

Source

Lilium species are usually found inside the home as potted plants or cut flowers. *Hemerocallis* species are common garden plants in many regions.

Type of toxin

The toxic principle has not been identified.

Pathophysiology

Affected cats develop AKI with renal tubular necrosis. The basement membrane remains intact, meaning that tubular epithelial cells can regenerate with prompt and aggressive treatment.

Clinical signs

The most common clinical signs are vomiting, depression, anorexia, dehydration, and hypothermia. Less commonly reported are disorientation, ataxia, facial and paw edema, dyspnea, and seizures.

Differential diagnosis

The clinical signs of depression, anorexia, dehydration, and hypothermia are seen with a variety of diseases that cause systemic illness in cats. Therefore, the clinician must be open to numerous possibilities.

Diagnosis

Diagnosis is based on compatible clinical signs and clinical pathology evidence of renal dysfunction after witnessed ingestion of the toxic plant. There is currently no specific test to identify the presence of the toxin in the body.

Management

These plants are extremely toxic, therefore with known recent exposure, GI decontamination procedures should be rapidly administered (induced emesis followed by activated charcoal and a cathartic). Immediate IV fluid administration is necessary to correct dehydration and maintain diuresis at 2–3 times fluid maintenance requirements. This is continued for 24–72 hours.

Renal parameters, acid–base and electrolyte concentrations, and urine output should be monitored. Dialysis (hemodialysis or peritoneal dialysis) should be provided if anuric AKI develops. Most cats tend to do well if treated before dehydration and anuria develop.

GRAPES AND RAISINS

Common names

Various *Vitus* species are cultivated worldwide for use as fresh fruit, raisins, juice, and wine.

Source

Toxic ingestions in dogs have involved raisins and grapes from various sources, including vines on the owners' property and grocery stores.

Type of toxin

The toxic principle involved has not been identified.

Pathophysiology

In 10 dogs that developed AKI after ingesting grapes or raisins, all had renal proximal tubular degeneration and/or necrosis with intact basement membranes. Mineralized tubular debris or casts were also present. Five of the 10 cases showed evidence of epithelial regeneration.

Clinical signs

Clinical signs are relatively nonspecific and include vomiting, anorexia, diarrhea, lethargy/depression, and abdominal pain.

Differential diagnosis
The clinical signs are nonspecific and can be associated with nearly any systemic disease; therefore, the clinician must be open to numerous possibilities. Clinical pathology findings of AKI encompass a variety of conditions associated with this problem including ethylene glycol, heavy metals, nephrotoxic antibiotics (e.g. aminoglycosides), nonsteroidal anti-inflammatory drugs, and leptospirosis.

Diagnosis
The actual toxin responsible for renal injury has not been identified, therefore specific analytic tests are not available. Evidence of AKI after ingestion is the strongest evidence currently available for a diagnosis.

Management
Recent ingestion should be treated with GI decontamination procedures (emesis/gastric lavage) followed by activated charcoal with a cathartic. IV fluid therapy should be administered immediately to correct dehydration and maintain diuresis for at least 48–72 hours. Urine output, renal clinical pathology parameters, acid–base, and electrolytes should be monitored.

MUSHROOMS

Source
Dogs and cats may encounter various mushroom species growing in their environment, and may occasionally be exposed to hallucinogenic mushrooms used illicitly by humans.

Type of toxin
- *Amanita*, *Conocybe*, *Galerina*, and *Pholiotina* species: amatoxins.
- *Cortinarius* species: orellanine.
- *Tricholoma* species.
- Muscimol and ibotenic acid.
- Monomethylhydrazine.
- Muscarine.
- Psilocybin and psilocin.

Pathophysiology
- Amatoxins inhibit mammalian nuclear RNA polymerases involved in transcription of DNA to messenger RNA. Primary target organs are the GI tract, kidney, and liver, with clinical signs beginning after a latent period of several hours.
- Orellanine is a nephrotoxin producing renal tubular dilatation and necrosis, arterial muscle hyperplasia, epithelial flattening, and interstitial edema and fibrosis.
- Muscimol and ibotenic acid act as false neurotransmitters, appearing to cross the blood–brain barrier using an active transport system.
- Monomethylhydrazine-containing mushrooms are most commonly associated with acute or delayed GI signs.
- Muscarine efficiently binds acetylcholine receptors throughout the body, initiating muscarinic-type signs.
- Psilocybin and psilocin are structurally similar to serotonin, with both exerting serotonergic properties in the peripheral and central nervous systems.
- Certain mushroom species associated primarily with gastroenteritis due to hypersensitivities, irritant reactions, and some other unknown mechanisms include *Chlorophyllum molybdites*, *Gomphus floccosus*, *Rhodophyllus rhodopolius*, and *Rhodophyllus sinatus*.

Clinical signs
The clinical signs can be quite varied depending on the type of mushroom ingested. A variety of organ systems can be affected including the GI tract (vomiting, diarrhea, abdominal pain), nervous system (muscarinic-type effects, excitation, hallucinations), kidney (AKI signs), liver (signs associated with hepatic failure such as encephalopathic signs, bleeding, and icterus), and RBCs (methemoglobinemia, hemolysis).

Differential diagnosis
Because so many organ systems can be involved, the differential diagnosis list is quite long depending on the mushroom ingested and the organ system affected. Therefore, the clinician must always have an index of suspicion when an animal presents acutely ill in an area where mushroom exposure is possible. The clinician should be familiar with the types of mushrooms present in the geographic area where he/she practices.

Diagnosis
Diagnosis is based on known ingestion of a specific mushroom and compatible clinical signs. Owners should bring in the potential offending mushroom for identification if ingestion was witnessed or if there is an acute onset in an ill pet where mushroom toxicity is possible based on the clinical findings.

Management
Try to identify the ingested mushroom so that specific therapy can be anticipated. If ingestion was recent, GI decontamination should be performed (induce emesis,

perform gastric lavage) followed by activated charcoal with a cathartic. Repeated doses of activated charcoal with a cathartic may be necessary in some mushroom toxicities where enterohepatic recirculation is possible.

Most management is supportive and should be tailored to the individual animal depending on the organ systems affected and the clinical signs that are present.

OVER-THE-COUNTER MEDICATIONS

ACETAMINOPHEN

Common names

Tylenol, Paracetamol, Anacin-3.

Source

As an analgesic and antipyretic human drug, acetaminophen is available in many prescription and over-the-counter products, both alone and in combination with other ingredients.

Type of toxin

The toxicity of acetaminophen is the result of the formation of the reactive metabolite N-acetyl p-benzoquinoneimine (NAPQI).

Pathophysiology

In most species, acetaminophen is metabolized and excreted primarily by glucuronidation and, to a lesser extent, by sulfation. As these pathways become saturated, increasing amounts of NAPQI are formed (**Figure 20.14**). Cats are especially sensitive to acetaminophen because they lack glucuronyl transferase. In addition, the cat's sulfation pathway is very inefficient. Due to rapid binding by NAPQI, glutathione stores in the liver and RBCs are rapidly depleted, leaving them vulnerable to NAPQI-induced oxidative damage.

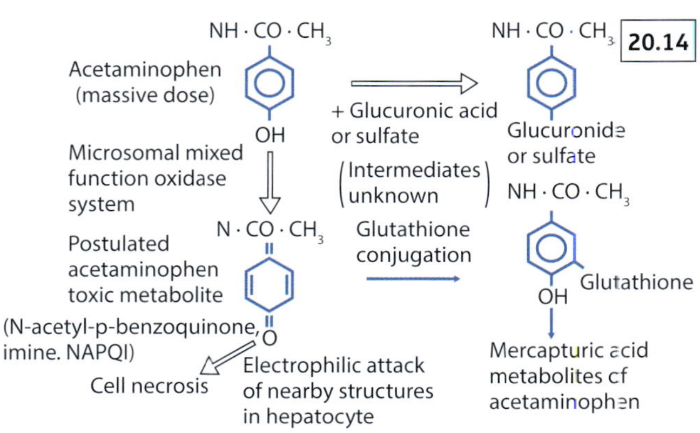

Figure 20.14 Acetaminophen is highly toxic to cats because of their inability to metabolize it to harmless waste products. (Adapted from Black M (1987) Hepatotoxic and hepatoprotective potential of histamine (H2)-receptor antagonists. *Am J Med* **83(Suppl 6A):**68–75.)

Clinical signs

Clinical signs in the cat are most commonly due to the hematological effects and include increased respiratory rate, respiratory distress, pale/muddy/cyanotic mucous membranes (**Figures 20.15, 20.16**), hypothermia, icterus,

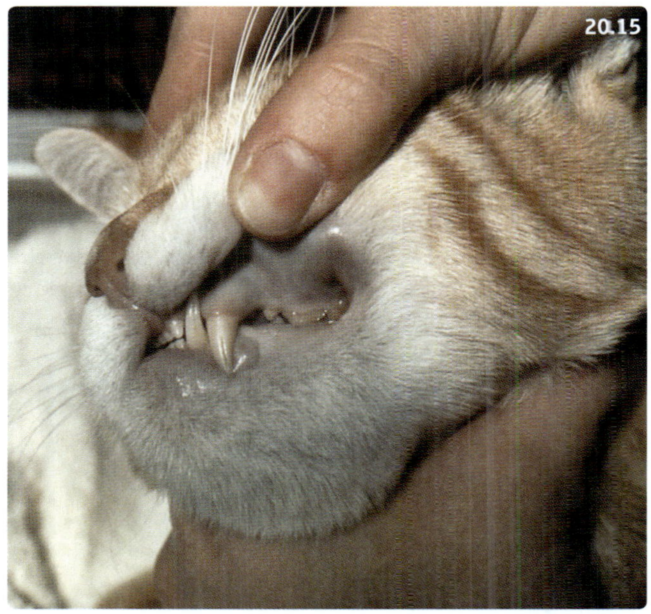

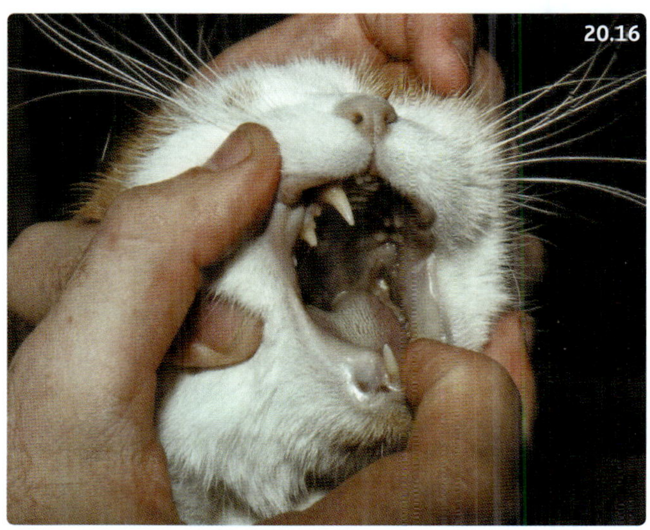

Figures 20.15, 20.16 Methemoglobinemia formation causes cyanotic mucous membranes. (Courtesy M. Schaer)

facial (**Figure 20.17**) and paw edema, depression, and vomiting.

Clinical signs in the dog are most often referable to the hepatotoxic effects and include vomiting, anorexia, tachycardia, tachypnea, abdominal pain, and icterus. Rarely, dogs can exhibit the hematologic effects without evidence of liver injury.

Differential diagnosis

Other causes of methemoglobinemia include other toxins such as nitrites, nitrobenzene, phenacetin, naphthalene, phenol and cresol, sulfites, and topically applied benzocaine. Methemoglobin reductase deficiency has been reported in cats. This can result in higher concentrations of methemoglobin and can demonstrate similar clinical signs except for the facial and paw edema. Acute hepatic injury can be due to a variety of toxins as well as pancreatitis and leptospirosis.

Diagnosis

History of exposure and compatible clinical signs are the basis for the majority of diagnoses made in veterinary medicine. The presence of acetaminophen in plasma, serum (**Figures 20.18, 20.19**), or urine (**Figure 20.20**) can be detected and measured (more commonly available in human diagnostic laboratories).

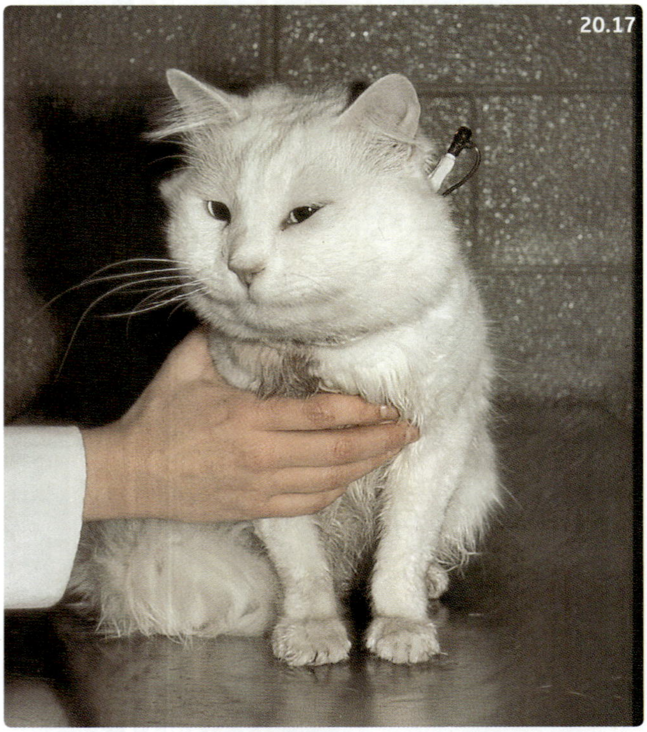

20.17

Figure 20.17 Facial edema is a characteristic sign of acetaminophen intoxication in the cat. It might be caused by endothelial pathology allowing for plasma leakage into the interstitial space. There is no known reason for the swelling to occur in the head region. (Courtesy M. Schaer)

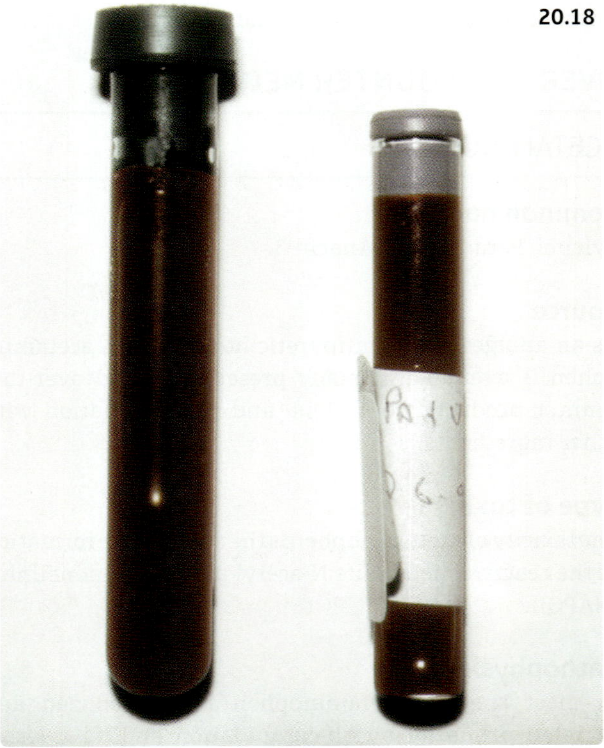

20.18

Figure 20.18 Blood tubes showing marked methemoglobinemia causing the blood to have a characteristic chocolate brown color. (Courtesy M. Schaer)

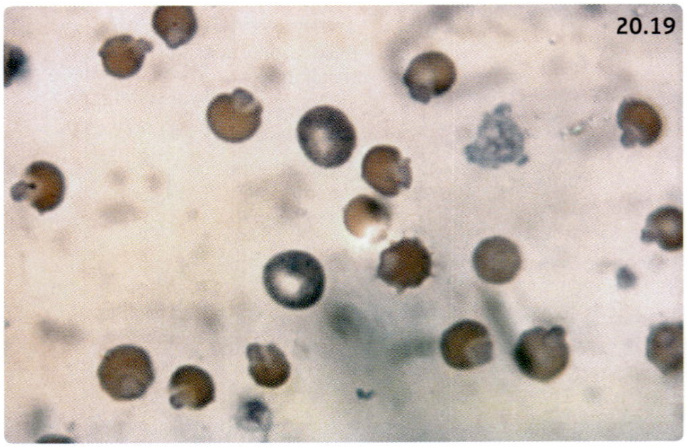

20.19

Figure 20.19 Heinz body hemolytic anemia is caused by acetaminophen intoxication. Glucocorticoid treatment is not indicated for this type of hemolysis. (Courtesy M. Schaer)

Management

If ingestion is very recent, decontamination of the GI tract (emesis induction, gastric lavage) is indicated, but most cats are presented after clinical signs develop and absorption of a toxic amount has taken place. Administration of activated charcoal may help prevent absorption of any toxin remaining in the GI tract if ingestion occurred within 4–6 hours of presentation.

Supportive care with supplemental oxygen and IV fluids is needed to maintain hydration. A transfusion of packed RBCs should be administered if anemia develops and clinical signs attributable to anemia are evident. Alternatively, a hemoglobin-based oxygen carrier can be administered (Oxyglobin®, if available).

N-acetylcysteine (140 mg/kg IV or PO initially, followed by 70 mg/kg IV or PO q6h for an additional 5–7 treatments) serves as a glutathione precursor and is considered an antidote for acetaminophen toxicity.

S-Adenosylmethionine (SAMe) has also been suggested as a potential adjunctive treatment for dogs and cats with acetaminophen toxicity.

Ascorbic acid (30 mg/kg PO q6h for 6 treatments) has been advocated to promote reduction of methemoglobin. Cimetidine (a cytochrome P-450 inhibitor) has also been advocated, although this has not been evaluated or described rigorously in clinical veterinary medicine. New methylene blue has also been suggested as a therapy to reduce methemoglobin, but it is not routinely used and has a very narrow margin of safety in cats (**Figures 20.21, 20.22**).

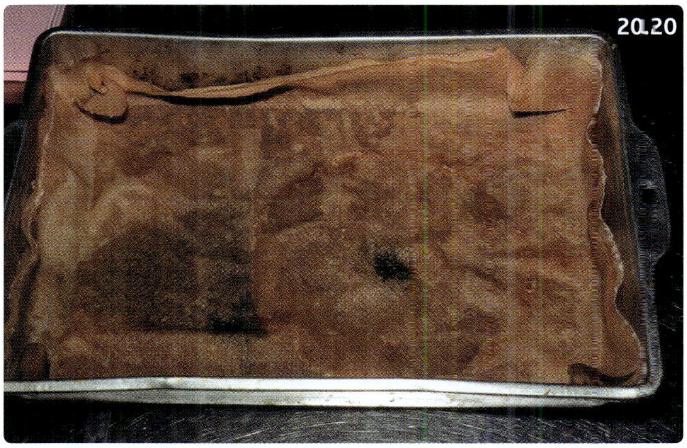

Figure 20.20 Acetaminophen-induced hemolysis causes this hemoglobinuria. The green pigment is an acetaminophen urine metabolite. (Courtesy M. Schaer).

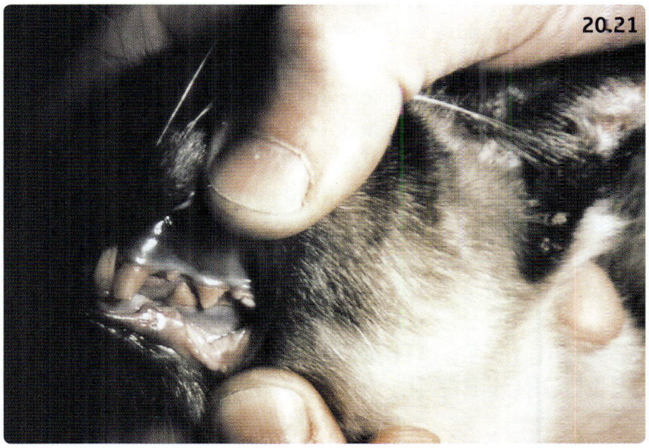

Figure 20.21 Methylene blue caused blue pigment deposition in the tissues of this Siamese cat. It is no longer used as a urinary antiseptic in cats. (Courtesy M. Schaer)

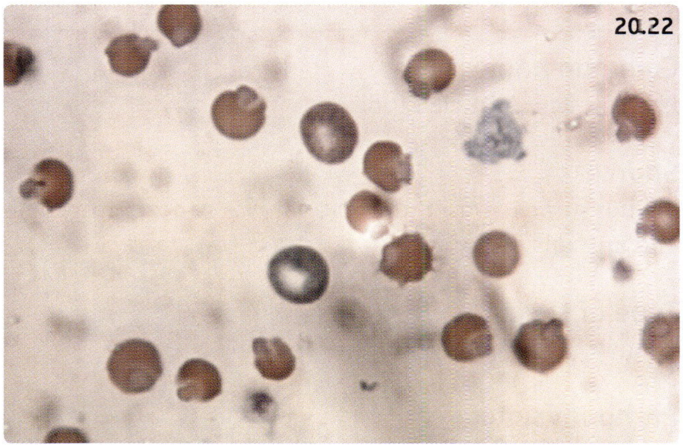

Figure 20.22 Methylene blue ingestion can accentuate the blood reticulocytes and cause Heinz body hemolytic anemia in the cat. (Courtesy M. Schaer)

COUGH AND COLD MEDICATIONS (ANTIHISTAMINES, PSEUDOEPHEDRINE)

Source

Pseudoephedrine is a common ingredient in over-the-counter decongestants and cold medications. Pseudoephedrine has also been used as a substitute for phenylpropanolamine in the treatment of urinary incontinence in dogs.

Type of toxin

Pseudoephedrine is a sympathomimetic drug that is structurally similar to amphetamines.

Pathophysiology

The exact mechanism of action is unknown, but it is believed that pseudoephedrine causes the release of norepinephrine, leading to adrenergic stimulation.

Clinical signs
Most common are signs associated with CNS stimulation such as agitation, tachycardia, tremors, disorientation, and seizures. Hyperthermia, mydriasis, and vomiting are other signs associated with toxicity.

Differential diagnosis
Any drugs that act as CNS stimulants, tremorgenic toxins, organophosphates, pyrethrins/pyrethroids, strychnine, caffeine, cocaine, methylxanthines, hypocalcemia, pheochromocytoma, hyperthyroidism, or CNS disease.

Diagnosis
History of exposure and compatible clinical signs.

Management
Some clinicians feel that emesis induction should be avoided with this toxicity due to the potential for stimulation of seizures. If agitation is present, phenothiazines such as chlorpromazine or acepromazine are recommended. Start at low doses and gradually increase to effect. Tachycardia can be treated with beta-blockers (e.g. esmolol, propranolol).

Supportive care with IV fluids and monitoring is necessary. Temperature should be monitored if elevated due to muscle tremors/agitation/hyperactivity. The animal should be cooled with cool water baths/fans.

TOPICAL MEDICATIONS (CALCIPOTRIENE, 5-FLUOROURACIL, VITAMIN D, ZINC OXIDE)

CALCIPOTRIENE

See Cholecalciferol intoxication.

5-FLUOROURACIL

Common names
Fluorouracil, Adrucil, Efudex.

Source
5-Fluorouracil is used to treat various cancers in people and animals.

Type of toxin
5-Fluorouracil is a pyrimidine analog.

Pathophysiology
Cytotoxic 5-fluorouracil metabolites, produced primarily in the liver, disrupt RNA and inhibit thymidylate synthase. In addition to neoplasms, tissues with high rates of cellular metabolism such as GI mucosa and bone marrow are most sensitive to the effects of 5-fluorouracil. A fatal outcome is not uncommon.

Clinical signs
Severe and sustained seizures, GI signs (vomiting, diarrhea), mucositis, and signs associated with leukopenia and thrombocytopenia.

Differential diagnosis
Bone marrow suppression due to any cause, intracranial and extracranial causes of seizures, any toxins that cause seizures.

Diagnosis
Exposure and compatible clinical pathology findings (leukopenia, thrombocytopenia). One report describes echinocytosis.

Management
If ingestion is recent, the GI tract should be decontaminated (emesis/gastric lavage) and further absorption prevented (activated charcoal).

Once animals have compatible clinical signs, supportive care similar to any animal that has chemotherapy-induced clinical abnormalities should be provided (i.e. IV fluid to maintain hydration/electrolyte balance, antiemetics). Broad-spectrum antibiotics should be provided if leukopenia is diagnosed. Blood transfusion is necessary if anemia develops from thrombocytopenia-associated hemorrhage.

VITAMIN D

See Cholecalciferol intoxication.

ZINC OXIDE

See Zinc intoxication.

HOUSEHOLD PRODUCTS

SOAPS AND DETERGENTS

Common names
Soaps and detergents are classified according to their chemical structure. True soaps are salts of fatty acids obtained from animal or vegetable sources; detergents are surfactants that contain ingredients such as phosphates, silicates, or carbonates. Detergents are further classified as nonionic, anionic, or cationic depending on their charge in solution.

Source
This group includes hand and bar soaps, shampoos, dishwashing liquids and powders, and laundry detergents.

Type of toxin
Soaps and detergents work as surfactants, helping to remove dirt and emulsify grease.

Pathophysiology
The majority of bar and liquid hand soaps and nonionic detergents cause mild GI irritation only. The high alkalinity of anionic dishwashing detergents can cause severe corrosive lesions. Intravascular hemolysis seen in patients with impaired liver function is thought to be related to effects of detergent in the bloodstream. Quaternary ammonium compounds are cationic detergents that can cause both local and systemic effects (**Figure 20.23**). Local effects include corrosive damage to the GI tract. The exact mechanism of action for the systemic effects is unknown, but these detergents appear to be able to paralyze neuromuscular junctions of striated muscle.

Clinical signs
Most soaps are low in toxicity but can be irritating to the GI tract, resulting in vomiting and diarrhea. Some soaps contain alkali and result in corrosive injury. Ocular irritation occurs if the eyes are exposed.

Differential diagnosis
Gastroenteritis due to any cause, pancreatitis, GI foreign body.

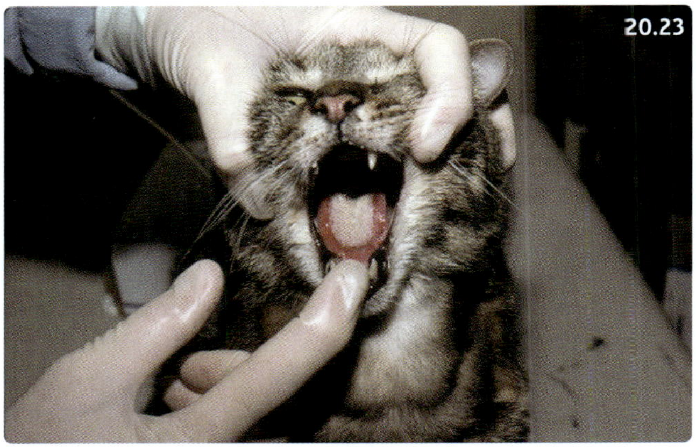

Figure 20.23 The lingual ulceration in this cat was caused by accidental contact with a quarternary ammonium cleaning agent that was used on the cage floor and inadequately wiped clean. (Courtesy M. Schaer)

Diagnosis
History of exposure with compatible clinical signs is suggestive.

Management
If ingestion is recent and in a large quantity (>20 g/kg and not a corrosive-containing soap), then emesis can be induced. Otherwise a diluent such as milk or water should be administered. Supportive care with IV fluids should be given if vomiting and diarrhea are profuse. Copious flushing of the eyes with water or eye irrigating solution is necessary if there is ocular irritation. Staining for corneal ulcers can be performed, but this is not a common problem.

NONANIONIC DETERGENTS (e.g. SHAMPOOS, HAND/DISHWASHING AGENTS)

Clinical signs
Similar to noncorrosive soap ingestion, as described above.

ANIONIC DETERGENTS (DISHWASHING DETERGENTS, LAUNDRY DETERGENTS, RARELY SOME HAIR SHAMPOOS)

Clinical signs
- Ingestion. Primarily GI signs manifested by vomiting, diarrhea, and abdominal discomfort. Intravascular hemolysis may occur in animals with liver dysfunction.
- Dermal exposure. Relatively rare, but prolonged or repeated exposure can result in skin irritation.
- Ocular exposure. Ocular irritation, corneal ulcer or opacity. Conjunctivitis.

Differential diagnosis
- Ingestion. Soap ingestion, other detergent ingestion, early corrosive ingestion, gastroenteritis due to any cause, pancreatitis, GI foreign body, nearly anything that can cause GI signs.
- Dermal exposure. Other topical irritants, dermatitis, contact hypersensitivity.
- Ocular exposure. Conjunctivitis due to any cause, trauma.

Diagnosis
History of exposure and compatible clinical signs.

Management

- Ingestion. Dilute with milk or water. Activated charcoal to prevent absorption if large quantities have been ingested. IV fluids to maintain hydration and electrolyte balance if vomiting and diarrhea are profuse. Monitor for hemolysis if large quantity was ingested.
- Dermal exposure. Bathe and rinse exposed areas.
- Ocular exposure. Copious flushing of exposed eyes with water or eye irrigating solutions. Stain for corneal ulcer. If present, treat appropriately.

CATIONIC DETERGENTS (GERMICIDES, FABRIC SOFTENERS, SANITIZERS)

Clinical signs

- Ingestion. Hypersalivation, vomiting (+/– hematemesis), muscle fasciculations, depression, increased body temperature, collapse, seizures, or coma. Irritation/ulceration of the oral, pharyngeal, and gastric mucosal membranes.
- Dermal exposure. Skin irritation and ulceration; the full effects of the dermal exposure may not be immediately evident. It can sometimes take 2–3 days to see the full effects on the skin.
- Ocular exposure. Ocular irritation, which may range from mild to severe with deep corneal ulceration.

Differential diagnosis

- Ingestion. Gastroenteritis, gastric/esophageal ulceration, pancreatitis, GI foreign body, corrosive ingestion.
- Dermal exposure. Other topical irritants, dermatitis, contact hypersensitivity.
- Ocular exposure. Conjunctivitis due to any cause, corneal trauma.

Diagnosis

Exposure with compatible clinical signs.

Management

- Ingestion. Do not induce vomiting to avoid re-exposing esophagus to the detergent. Administer oral diluents such as water, milk, or egg whites. Activated charcoal and a saline cathartic can be given. Severity of injury may range from mild GI irritation to severe ulceration and perforation that could result in hypovolemic and/or septic shock. If esophageal or gastric perforation has occurred, surgery will be required after cardiovascular stabilization. If perforation has not occurred, supportive care with IV fluids, gastroprotectants, pain management, and nutritional supplementation should be provided. Esophageal stricture may be a long-term sequela.
- Dermal exposure. Rinse affected area thoroughly with soap and water.
- Ocular exposure. Lavage exposed eye(s) with isotonic saline for 20–30 minutes. Eyes should be assessed for corneal ulcers and if present, treated appropriately.

COMMON HOUSEHOLD CHLORINE BLEACHES

Common names

Most household bleaches contain 3–6% sodium hypochlorite. Swimming pool chlorines may contain 50% hypochlorite.

Source

Hypochlorite bleaches are commonly used as disinfectants and water purifiers.

Type of toxin

Household bleaches are mild to moderate GI irritants.

Pathophysiology

The corrosive nature of a hypochlorite bleach is due to its strong oxidizing potential. In the acidic environment of the stomach, hypochlorous acid is formed, which is able to penetrate mucous membranes.

Clinical signs

- Ingestion can cause mild to moderate mucosal irritation manifested by hypersalivation, oropharyngeal irritation, vomiting, and abdominal pain.
- Inhalation of fumes can cause respiratory signs such as coughing, retching, and difficulty breathing.
- Ocular exposure. Similar to cationic detergents, but problems may not be as severe depending on concentration of sodium hypochlorite.

Differential diagnosis

- Ingestion. Gastroenteritis, gastric/esophageal ulceration, pancreatitis, GI foreign body, corrosive ingestion.
- Dermal exposure. Other topical irritants, dermatitis, contact hypersensitivity.
- Inhalation. Upper respiratory tract infection, pneumonia, collapsing trachea.
- Ocular exposure. Conjunctivitis due to any cause, corneal trauma.

Diagnosis

History of exposure and compatible clinical signs.

Management

Management is similar to that for cationic detergents, although the injuries associated with common household chlorine bleaches tend to be not as severe at the more common lower sodium hypochlorite concentrations.

ETHYLENE GLYCOL

Source

Ethylene glycol is the main ingredient in most antifreeze products. Small concentrations of ethylene glycol are also present in some paints.

Pathophysiology

Metabolism of ethylene glycol to glycolaldehyde, glycolic acid, glyoxalic acid, and oxalic acid leads to metabolic acidosis, AKI, and cardiopulmonary failure.

Clinical signs

Initial signs (30 minutes to 12 hours after ingestion) include primarily neurologic changes such as ataxia, altered mentation, seizures, and coma (**Figures 20.24, 20.25**). Other signs include vomiting, polydipsia, and polyuria. Later signs (36–72 hours after ingestion: 12–24 hours in cats) are due to uremia secondary to AKI. Renal pain on abdominal palpation may also be noted.

Differential diagnosis

- Neurologic changes. Hepatic encephalopathy, neurotoxins, hypoglycemia, severe electrolyte changes (hyponatremia, hypernatremia, hypocalcemia), encephalitis, intracranial neoplasia, hyperosmolar nonketotic diabetes, intracranial infection (e.g. viral, protozoan, rickettsial, bacterial), head trauma, or stroke.
- Any potential cause of AKI (**Figures 20.26, 20.27**).

Diagnosis

History of exposure with compatible clinical signs is adequate to begin therapy, since this toxin acts rapidly and irreversible devastating effects can occur prior to obtaining a definitive confirmation (see below). Calcium oxalate crystals may be detected in the urine within 6 hours after ingestion and lend strong support to the diagnosis (**Figures 20.28, 20.29**). The absence of these crystals does not rule out ethylene glycol intoxication. Oxalate crystals can also be found in the kidneys (**Figure 20.29**), where they can cause a hyperechoic pattern with ultrasonography (**Figure 20.31**).

The presence of ethylene glycol in blood or urine can be detected using a specific ethylene glycol test kit, although the reliability of the kit has been questioned (**Figure 20.32**). Ethylene glycol is usually not detectable in blood or urine 2–3 days after ingestion. Suspicion of ethylene glycol in blood can be made from detecting a high osmolar gap or high anion gap acidosis, but these are not specific for ethylene glycol.

Using a Wood's lamp and detecting fluorescence on some noningested material or urine may suggest ethylene glycol intoxication because many antifreeze solutions contain a fluorescent dye. This test may be positive in the urine up to 6 hours after ingestion. A negative test does not rule out ethylene glycol ingestion.

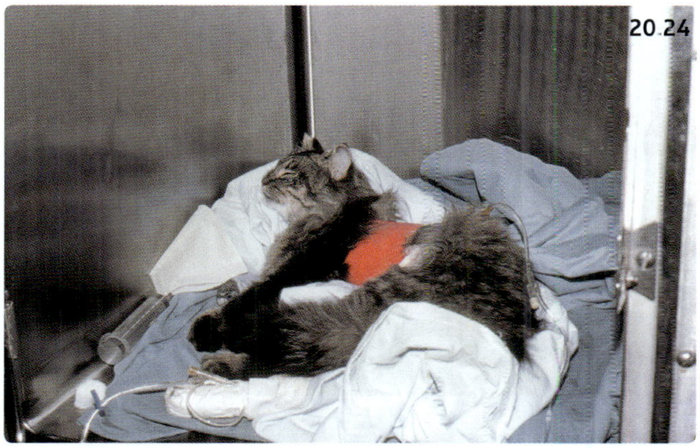

Figure 20.24 This cat is in a stupor caused by the central nervous system toxic effects of the glycoaldehyde metabolite of ethylene glycol. The prognosis is usually grave at this stage of disease. (Courtesy M. Schaer)

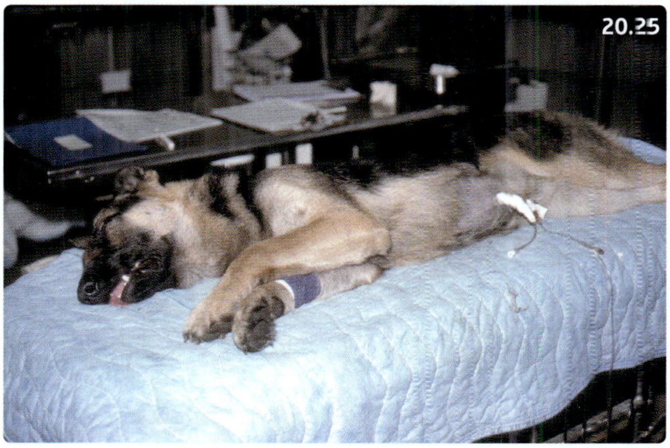

Figure 20.25 This German Shepherd Dog puppy is comatose and anuric from the combined effects of glycoaldehyde and oxalate crystalluria, respectively, caused by antifreeze ingestion. (Courtesy M. Schaer)

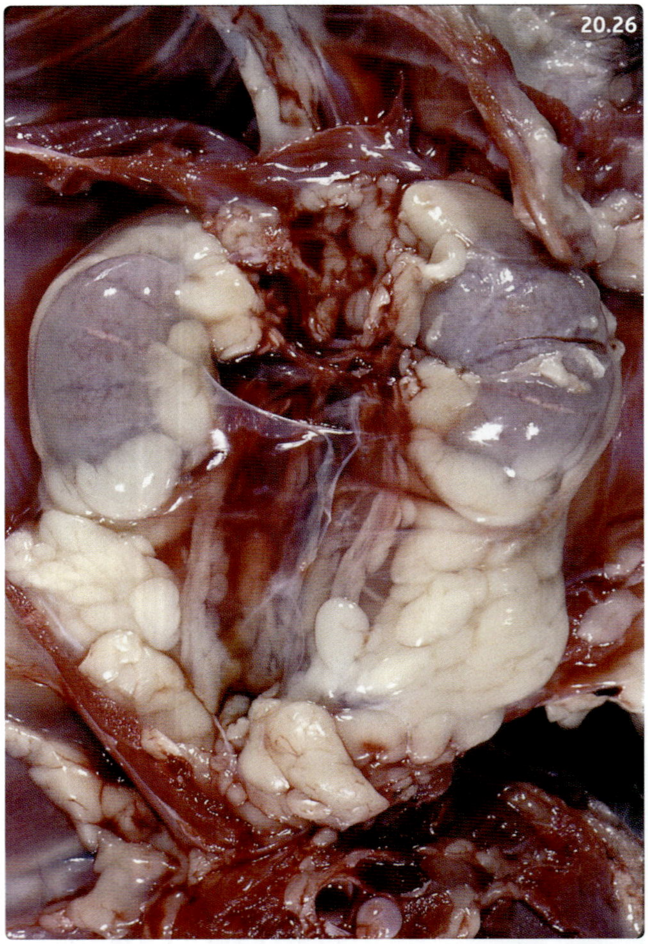

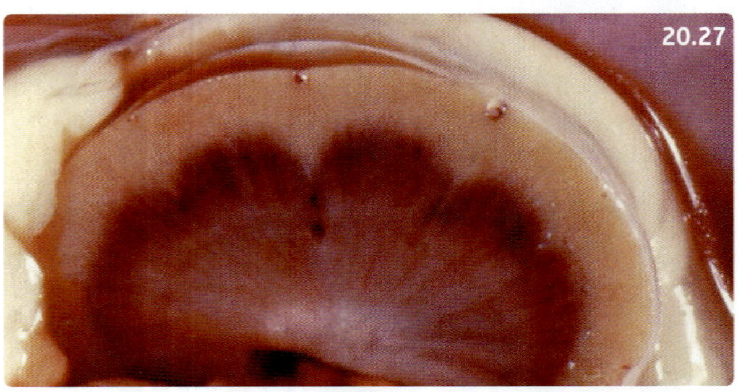

Figures 20.26, 20.27 (20.26) Post-mortem view of swollen kidneys in a cat that had ethylene glycol-caused irreversible renal tubular damage. (20.27) Close up view of one of the kidneys showing the subcapsular edema, which is rarely seen by the clinician. (Courtesy M. Schaer)

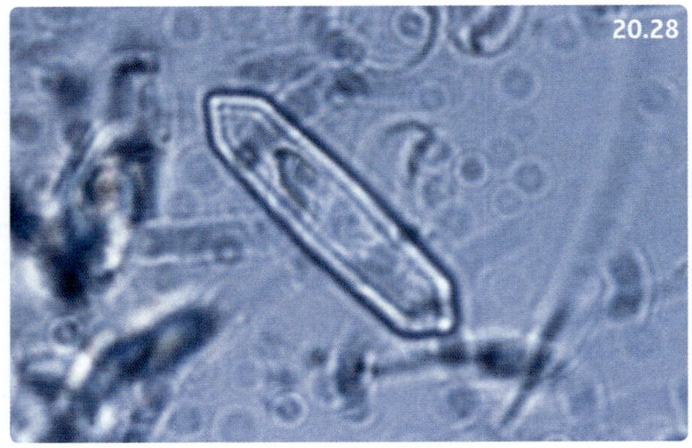

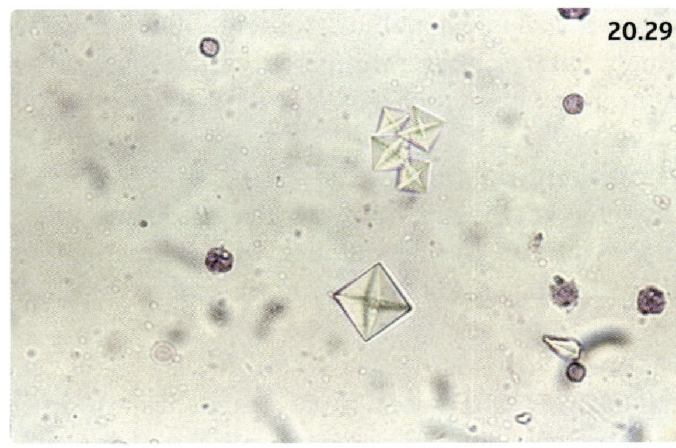

Figures 20.28, 20.29 A microscopic view of a urine sediment showing monohydrate (20.28) and dihydrate (20.29) oxalate crystals. (Courtesy M. Schaer)

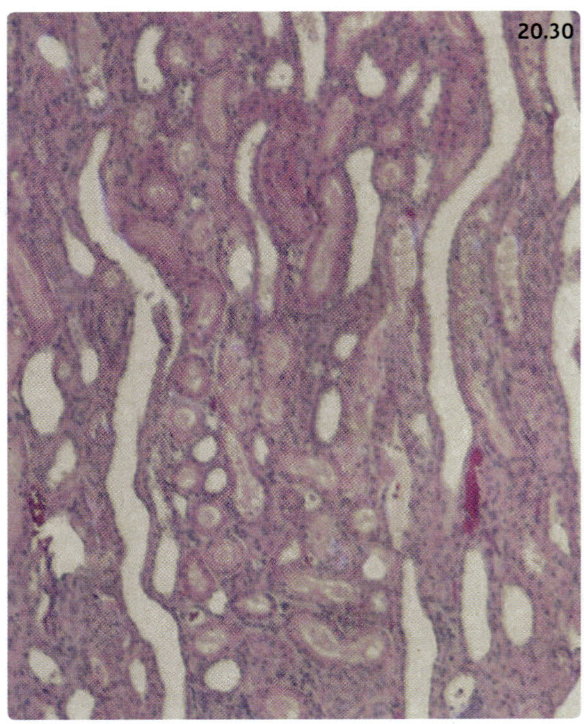

Figure 20.30 Histopathologic view of a cat kidney showing oxalate deposits in the renal tubules. (Courtesy M. Schaer)

Management

Ethylene glycol is absorbed and metabolized rapidly; therefore, management should begin immediately if ingestion is suspected. Because absorption is so rapid, gastric elimination (emesis) is usually not effective, but it can be tried if there are no contraindications to doing

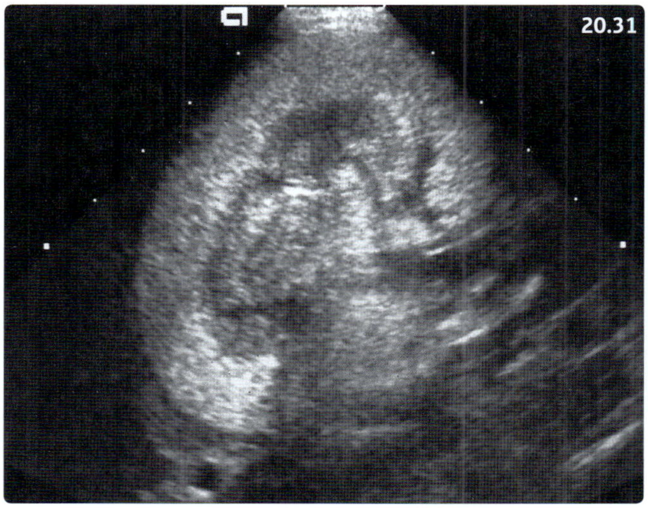

Figure 20.31 The deposit of large amounts of oxalate crystals in the kidney causes a characteristic ultrasonographic image with hyperechogenicity of the renal cortex. (Courtesy M. Schaer)

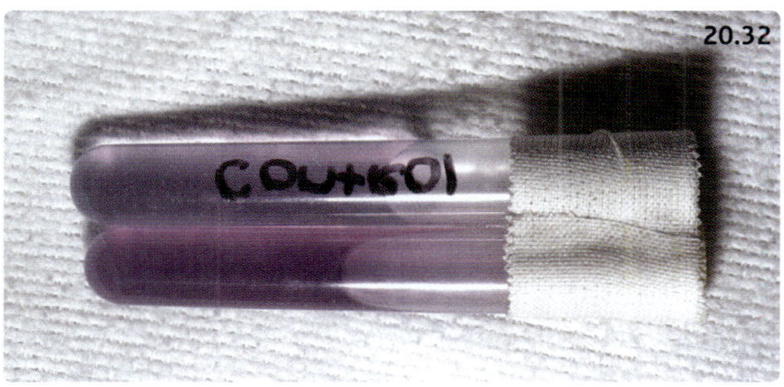

Figures 20.32 An ethylene glycol kit is commercially available for detecting ethylene glycol in the blood. The dark tube is a positive test. (Courtesy M. Schaer)

this. If ingestion is recent (within hours), the ideal therapy is hemodialysis to remove the toxin, but this is available only in a small number of referral veterinary hospitals.

Inhibition of conversion of ethylene glycol to its toxic metabolites is the mainstay of therapy. The drug of choice was 4-methylypyrazole (fomepizole) (no longer available as a veterinary drug in the USA):

- Dogs: 20 mg/kg IV followed by 15 mg/kg IV at 12 and 24 hours and 5 mg/kg IV at 36 hours. This therapy is not effective if given after the ethylene glycol has been metabolized and AKI is present.
- Cats: 125 mg/kg IV then 31.25 mg/kg IV at 12, 24, and 36 hours after the initial bolus. Note the comparatively much higher dose for the cat than the dog.

Ethanol may be used if 4-methylpyrazole is not available, but it is not considered as efficacious and has more side-effects (**Figure 20.33**):

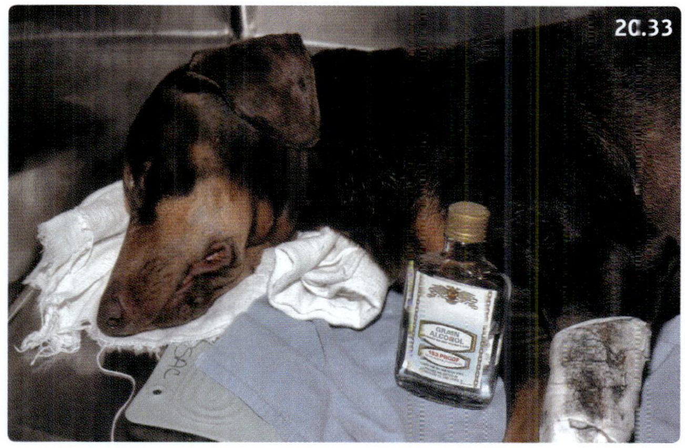

Figure 20.33 Administering ethyl alcohol as an antidote can cause marked inebriation and possible alcohol intoxication. (Courtesy M. Schaer)

- Dogs and cats: 1.3 ml/kg of 30% ethanol IV bolus followed by 0.42 ml/kg/hour for 48 hours.

Supportive care with IV fluids and monitoring urine output, blood urea nitrogen, creatinine, electrolytes, and acid–base balance is also recommended.

BATTERIES

Source

Batteries ranging from small button or disk batteries up to the large D size are used in remote controls, smoke alarms, clocks, watches, and toys.

Type of toxin

Alkaline batteries contain potassium hydroxide or sodium hydroxide. Disk, nickel–cadmium, mercuric oxide, and silver batteries are generally alkaline. Ingested lithium batteries can generate current and produce alkali. Acidic dry cell batteries contain ammonium chloride and manganese dioxide.

Pathophysiology

Ingestion of batteries may cause several types of injury: acid or alkali burns; current-induced tissue necrosis; metal toxicity from the battery casings; GI obstruction.

Clinical signs

Clinical signs are primarily related to GI tract irritation/ulceration/perforation and can range from no signs to anorexia, vomiting/regurgitation, abdominal pain, hypersalivation, retching, fever, difficulty breathing, hypovolemia, and septic shock.

Differential diagnosis
Ingestion of caustic substances, esophageal or GI foreign body, esophageal stricture or rupture, gastroenteritis, pancreatitis, septic peritonitis, and intussusception.

Diagnosis
History of ingestion and radiographic confirmation.

Management
The principles of critical care should be applied if the animal is severely compromised secondary to esophageal or GI perforation. Surgical or endoscopic removal of the battery may be necessary. If esophageal or gastric ulceration is present, GI protectants (e.g. sucralfate, H2 blockers, proton pump inhibitors) should be provided. Feeding tubes and nutritional support will be necessary if the animal is unable to eat.

MOTHBALLS

Source
Mothballs contain either naphthalene or paradichlorobenzene. Naphthalene is found in 'old-fashioned' mothballs. In addition to mothballs, paradichlorobenzene is also found in deodorizer cakes.

Type of toxin
Naphthalene is a bicyclic aromatic hydrocarbon, naturally found as a component of petroleum and coal. Paradichlorobenzene is an organochlorine insecticide.

Pathophysiology
Metabolism of naphthalene by the liver can produce epoxides or quinines that cause cellular damage. Paradichlorobenzene is oxidized then rapidly conjugated for excretion. Paradichlorobenzene is considered less toxic than naphthalene.

Clinical signs
- Naphthalene-containing mothballs. Similar to acetaminophen ingestion in cats: vomiting, methemoglobinemia, hemolytic anemia, hemoglobinuria, and possible liver damage.
- Paradichlorobenzene-containing mothballs. Acute abdomen (vomiting and abdominal pain), tremors, seizures, and possible liver or kidney injury.

Differential diagnosis
- Naphthalene-containing mothballs. Any oxidant type toxin: zinc, acetaminophen, and onions; immune-mediated hemolytic anemia.
- Paradichlorobenzene-containing mothballs. Acute abdomen signs: pancreatitis, GI foreign body, gastric ulceration, or intussusception; neurologic signs: other neurotoxins, general causes of seizures.

Diagnosis
Both naphthalene and paradichlorobenzene types: history of exposure and compatible clinical signs.

Management
- Naphthalene-containing mothballs. Gastric decontamination if ingestion is recent (emesis followed by activated charcoal with a cathartic). Give 4 mg/kg (dogs) or 1.5 mg/kg (cats) of 1% methylene blue IV (discontinue if hemolysis occurs). Supportive care with IV fluids and blood transfusions as indicated.
- Paradichlorobenzene-containing mothballs. Gastric decontamination if ingestion is recent (emesis followed by activated charcoal with a cathartic). IV fluids to induce diuresis. Symptomatic supportive care. Diazepam to control seizures or tremors.

METALS

LEAD

Source
Even though lead-based household paints are no longer commonly in use, pets may be exposed to lead paint chips and dusts in older homes, especially during remodeling projects. Other lead sources include lead solder, leaded gasoline, some soils, lead-containing toys, lead bullets and shot, and weights from fishing tackle and curtains.

Pathophysiology
The duodenum is the primary site of lead absorption (**Figure 20.34**); absorbed lead is then transported to soft tissues (liver, kidney, brain) and bone. Chronic lead exposure inhibits heme synthesis, resulting in mild to moderate anemia. Acute lead exposure increases intracytoplasmic calcium levels, causing cell death and neuronal impairment.

Clinical signs
Primarily GI and neurologic signs. GI signs in order of decreasing frequency include vomiting, anorexia, diarrhea, and abdominal pain (**Figures 20.35, 20.36**). Neurologic signs include seizures, hysteria, lethargy, ataxia, blindness, and jaw champing.

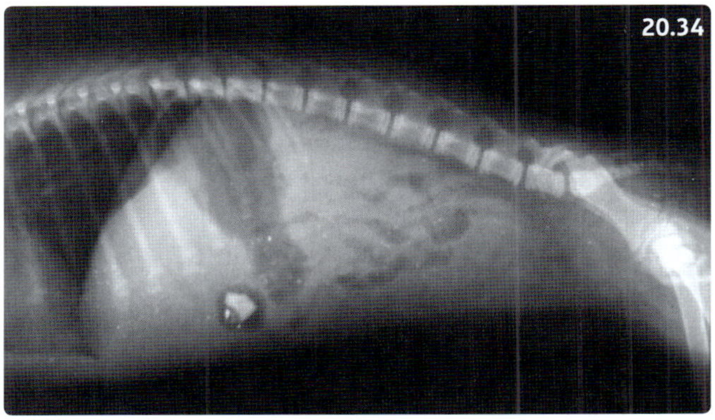

Figure 20.34 This lateral abdominal radiograph shows a metallic density in the duodenum. This was ingested paint that contained lead. Lead lines are visible at the endplates of the vertebral bodies, which prompted the radiograph shown in Figure 20.36. A diagnosis of lead poisoning is often made indirectly until the blood level results return from the laboratory. (Courtesy M. Schaer)

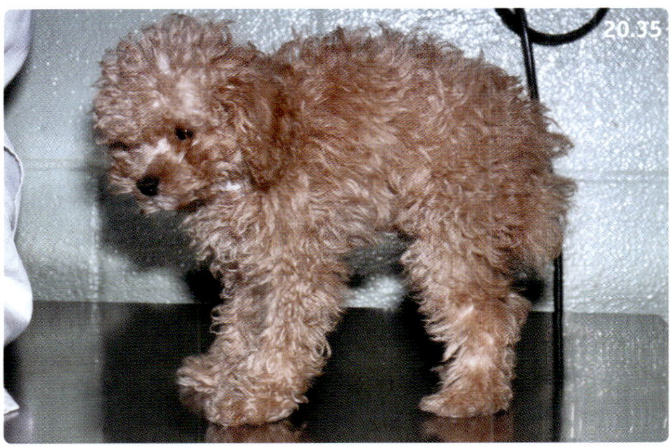

Figure 20.35 This Poodle puppy had lead colic from contaminated paint chip ingestion. Note the tucked abdominal posture. (Courtesy M. Schaer)

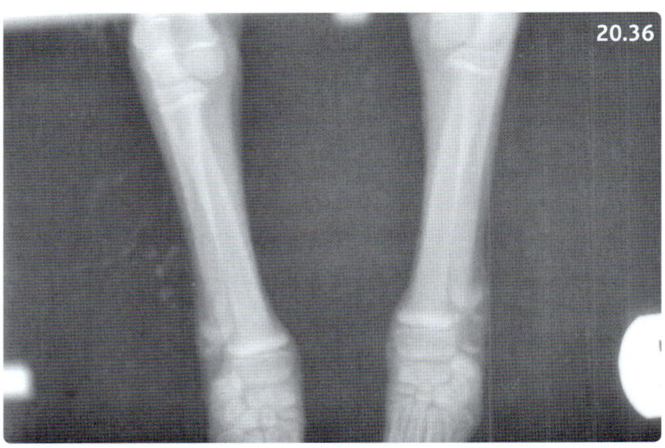

Figure 20.36 Radiograph of the Poodle puppy in Figure 20.35 showing increased radiographic density of it growth plates as a result of lead deposition.

Differential diagnosis

- GI signs. Pancreatitis, GI foreign body, intussusception, parvovirus enteritis, intestinal parasitism, gastroenteritis or GI ulceration.
- Neurologic signs. Other neurotoxins distemper, epilepsy, hypoglycemia, hepatic encephalopathy, or electrolyte changes (severe hyponatremia, hypernatremia, or hypocalcemia).

Diagnosis

History of exposure and compatible clinical signs is supportive for the diagnosis but not definitive. Finding increased nucleated RBCs without signs of red cell regeneration is supportive, along with exposure history and compatible clinical signs (**Figure 20.37**).

Definitive diagnosis

Whole blood lead concentration above 2.88 μmol/l (60 μg/dl [0.6 ppm]) is definitive. Whole blood lead concentration between 1.44 and 2.5 μmol/l (30 and 50 μg/dl [0.3 and 0.5 ppm]) with compatible clinical signs is also definitive.

Management

IV diazepam should be given if seizures are present and IV mannitol if seizures are severe or persistent. IV fluids should be given to maintain fluid, electrolyte, and acid–base balance.

The GI tract should be decontaminated if a lead source is present. Surgical removal of large metallic GI foreign bodies may be required. If flecks of lead paint are present in the GI tract, enemas can be used to remove the flecks from the colon. A sulfate-containing cathartic that might chelate the lead in the GI tract can be administered (e.g. magnesium sulfate, sodium sulfate).

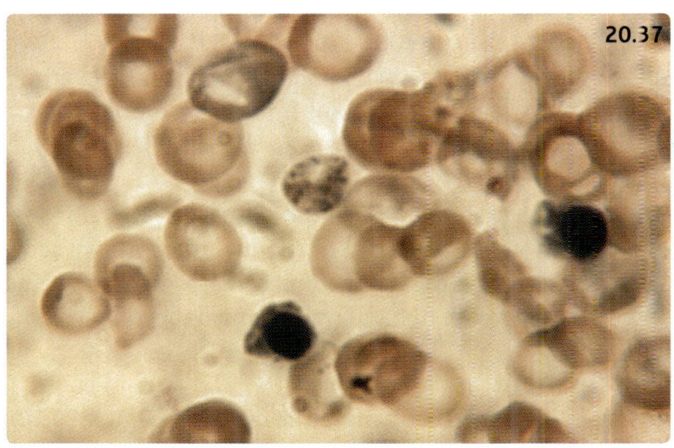

Figure 20.37 Nucleated RBCs and basophilic stippling are characteristic hematologic changes caused by plumbism (lead poisoning). (Courtesy M. Schaer)

The lead in the blood can be chelated using dimercaptosuccinic acid (succimer) at 10 mg/kg PO q8h for 10 days or, if Succimer is not available, calcium EDTA (100 mg/kg/day SC divided q6h for 2–5 days). However, calcium EDTA has potential nephrotoxic effects, so the total dose should not exceed 2 g/day. The calcium EDTA should be diluted with 5% dextrose to a concentration of 10 mg/ml to reduce the pain of the injection. Hydration with fluid diuresis should be maintained during calcium EDTA therapy.

Clinical signs should improve within 24–48 hours after starting therapy. Blood lead concentrations should be repeated 2–3 weeks after cessation of chelation therapy.

Owners should be warned about the potential for human exposure and referred to their family doctor.

ZINC

Source
Common sources of zinc include USA pennies minted after 1982, galvanized metal objects, and zinc oxide ointments.

Type of toxin
The exact mechanism of zinc toxicity is unknown.

Pathophysiology
Organs that accumulate the highest concentrations of zinc following ingestion include the liver, kidney, pancreas, and RBCs. Intravascular hemolysis is the most common manifestation of zinc toxicity.

Clinical signs
Vomiting is an extremely common clinical sign (nearly 90% of dogs with zinc toxicity). Other signs primarily relate to hemolysis and include weakness, lethargy, tachypnea, pale mucous membranes, rapid heart rate, and pigmenturia.

Differential diagnosis
All potential causes of hemolytic anemia including immune-mediated and oxidant injury (e.g. onions).

Diagnosis
Hemolytic anemia and identification of a GI metallic foreign body warrant retrieval of the metallic foreign body. Most foreign bodies are in the stomach. Increased blood zinc levels with evidence of hemolysis confirm the diagnosis.

Management
The metallic foreign body should be removed (**Figure 20.38**). Supportive care with IV fluids and blood transfusions is given as indicated. Most cases resolve within 2–3 days after the zinc source is removed.

IRON

Source
Iron is found in relatively small amounts in most multivitamin products, although prenatal vitamins and supplements used to treat iron-deficient conditions may contain much higher amounts. Most ingestions of multivitamins do not represent significant iron exposures in pet animals, although massive ingestions or those involving products containing higher quantities of iron could potentially result in severe clinical signs.

Type of toxin
The highly reactive nature of iron, which allows it to play a major role in biologic redox reactions, also makes unbound iron potentially toxic.

Pathophysiology
Iron toxicosis is due to both direct effects on the GI mucosa and excessive unbound iron in the circulation.

Clinical signs
The three major organ systems affected are the GI, cardiovascular, and central nervous systems. GI signs include vomiting, hematemesis, diarrhea (bloody, melena), and abdominal pain. Cardiovascular signs include cardiovascular collapse/shock. Neurologic signs include depression, and muscle tremors. Severe hepatic injury can occur with severe intoxication (**Figure 20.39**).

GI signs generally occur within the first 6 hours of ingestion. This can be followed by apparent recovery for the next 24 hours, but then GI signs return and the more severe signs associated with the nervous system and cardiovascular collapse can occur.

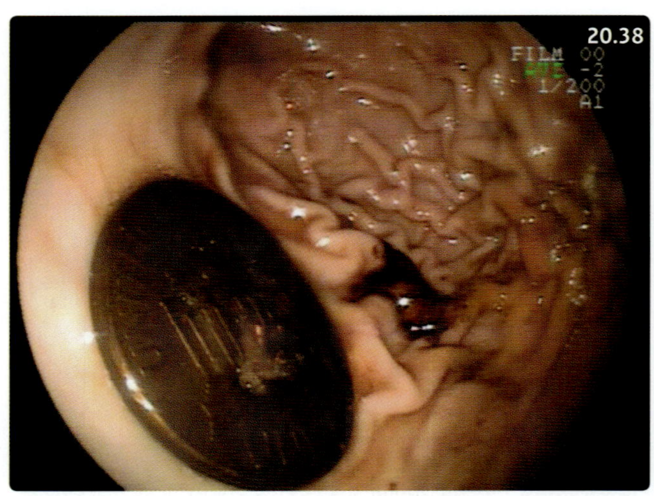

Figure 20.38 Gastroscopic removal of a zinc-containing USA penny. (Courtesy M. Schaer)

Differential diagnosis

Gastroenteritis, intestinal ulcers, pancreatitis, bacterial enteritis, corrosive ingestion, intestinal foreign body, intussusception, viral enteritis, and distemper.

Diagnosis

Total iron binding capacity and serum iron concentration should be measured 4–6 hours after ingestion to get an accurate representation of a consistent serum concentration. Poisoning does not occur unless serum iron concentration exceeds serum iron binding capacity.

Management

GI decontamination (emesis induction/gastric lavage) is necessary if ingestion was recent. Activated charcoal and saline cathartics have not been shown to be helpful. In animals with clinical signs:

- Aggressive IV fluid resuscitation if in shock.
- IV fluids to maintain hydration and electrolyte balance.
- GI protectants (sucralfate).
- Chelation therapy if severe intoxication. Deferoxamine (if ingestion was within the last 12 hours): CRI at 15 mg/kg/hour (monitor for cardiac arrhythmias/hypotension). If CRI is not possible, IM injections (40 mg/kg q4–8h), although this is not considered as effective as CRI. Continue chelation therapy until serum iron concentration is below 300 µg/dl (53.7 µmol/l) or measured serum iron concentration is below the serum iron binding capacity.

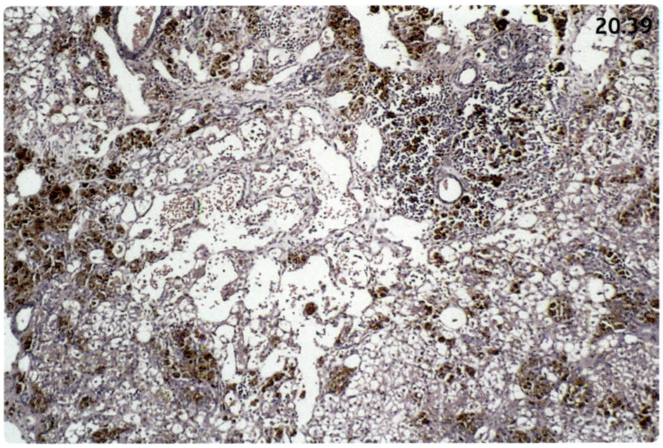

Figure 20.39 Histopathologic signs caused by adverse effects of iron in the liver. The parenchymal pathology is extensive. (Courtesy M. Schaer)

HUMAN FOODS

ALLIUM SPECIES

Source

Various types of onions, garlic, scallions, leeks, chives, and products containing powdered or granulated onions and garlic.

Type of toxin

Allium spp. contain organosulfur compounds that cause oxidant injury to RBCs.

Pathophysiology

Oxidation of the sulfhydryl groups of hemoglobin results in Heinz body formation, oxidation of membrane lipid and sulfhydryl groups, and methemoglobin formation. As a result, RBC membranes become less deformable and more fragile, resulting in hemolysis.

Clinical signs

Common clinical signs include lethargy, weakness, anorexia, pigmenturia, and pale mucous membranes (**Figure 20.40**).

Differential diagnosis

Zinc toxicity, immune-mediated hemolytic anemia, RBC parasites.

Diagnosis

Clinical history of ingestion of an *Allium* spp., compatible clinical signs, and the presence of Heinz body anemia and methemoglobinemia all support a diagnosis of *Allium* toxicity.

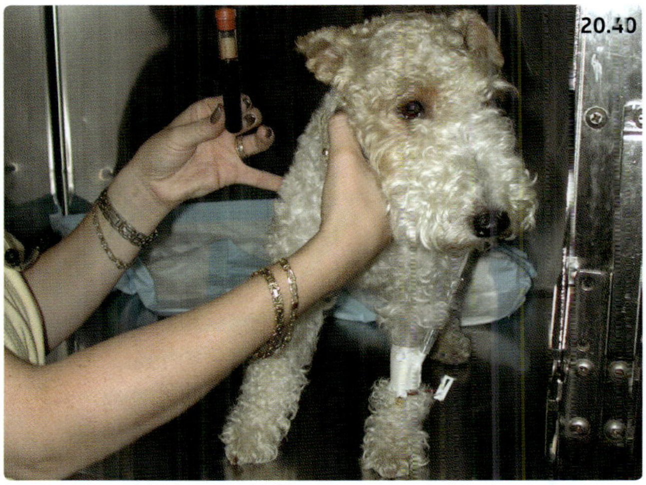

Figure 20.40 A urine sample from an onion-intoxicated dog showing methemoglobinuria.

Management
Vomiting can be induced in asymptomatic animals within 1–6 hours of ingestion, followed by activated charcoal once vomiting has been controlled. Treatment is supportive with the administration of IV fluids and packed RBC transfusions as needed.

XYLITOL

Source
Xylitol is an artificial sweetener most commonly found in sugarless gum and other 'sugar-free' items such as, peanut butter, candies, mints, nicotine gums, chewable vitamins, baked goods, and some oral care products.

Type of toxin
Induces insulin synthesis and release in dogs.

Pathophysiology
The exact mechanism by which xylitol stimulates the synthesis and release of insulin in dogs is unknown. The resulting hyperinsulinemia primarily results in hypoglycemia and potentially hypokalemia and hypophosphatemia. Increased ALT and AST may also occur secondary to liver damage. The exact cause of the hepatotoxicity has not been determined, but possible mechanisms include cellular ATP depletion, excessive reactive oxygen species, and binding of anti-xylitol antibodies to hepatic vessels. A dosage of >0.1g/kg can induce hypoglycemia; >0.5 g/kg may also potentially cause hepatotoxicity.

Clinical signs
The most common clinical signs are depression, vomiting, ataxia, and seizures. When hepatotoxicity has occurred, ecchymoses, icterus, and GI hemorrhages have also been noted.

Differential diagnosis
Insulin overdose, oral hypoglycemia medication ingestion, insulin-like secreting tumors, insulinoma, liver failure, hypoadrenocorticism, acute hepatic necrosis, portocaval shunt.

Diagnosis
Clinical history of ingestion of a xylitol-containing product combined with hypoglycemia and/or increased ALT and AST support a diagnosis of xylitol toxicosis. Routine toxicology screening tests for the detection of xylitol are not available, so it is important to rule out other possible differential diagnoses.

Management
If ingestion was within 1–6 hours of presentation and there are no contraindications, induction of vomiting is recommended. Activated charcoal is not administered as it binds poorly to xylitol.

Hypoglycemic animals should receive 0.25–0.5 g/kg of 50% dextrose diluted with saline, then continued IV fluids containing 2.5–5% dextrose. Small frequent meals should also be provided if the patient is able to eat without vomiting. Antiemetics and GI protectants should be added if vomiting is present or persistent.

In cases of severe acute hepatic necrosis, provide supportive care (see Chapter 9: Liver disorders). Although their efficacy has not been definitively proven for this use, medications that support liver function (SAMe, vitamin C, vitamin E, silymarin, *N*-acetylcysteine) may be beneficial. Vitamin K1 and/or fresh or fresh-frozen plasma transfusions may be indicated if severe coagulopathies are present.

METHYLXANTHINES

Source
These naturally occurring alkaloids are found in beverages, foods, and some dietary supplements. Chocolate contains caffeine and theobromine. Unsweetened and dark chocolate contains higher levels of methylxanthines than milk or white chocolate. Caffeine is also present in coffee, tea, other beverages, and herbal supplements containing guarana (*Paullinia cupana*). Another potential source of caffeine is cocoa bean hulls, which are sometimes used as mulch.

Type of toxin
Methylxanthines produce positive inotropic and chronotropic effects on the heart, cerebral vasoconstriction, renal vasorelaxation, and GI smooth muscle relaxation.

Pathophysiology
The clinical signs appear to be related to competitive inhibition of cellular adenosine receptors. Cellular calcium reuptake inhibition and competition for benzodiazepine receptors may also be involved. The significant amount of fat in many chocolate products may also cause GI upset and/or pancreatitis. The half-life of caffeine and theobromine in dogs is 4.5 and 17.5 hours, respectively.

Clinical signs
The most common signs in dogs include vomiting, restlessness, tachycardia with or with cardiac arrhythmias, tachypnea, polyuria, hyperthermia, tremors, and

seizures. Death may occur due to arrhythmias or respiratory failure (**Figures 20.41, 20.42**).

Differential diagnosis

Pseudoephedrine, amphetamines, antihistamines, cocaine, other causes of seizures.

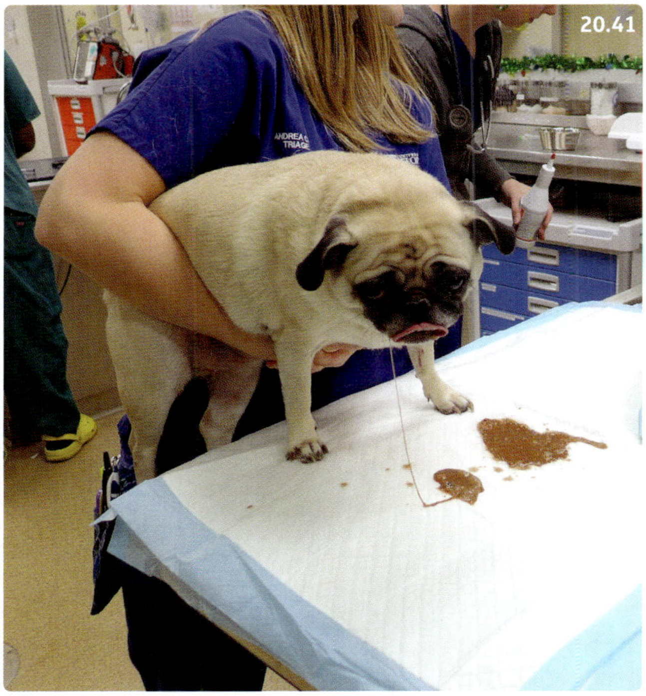

20.41

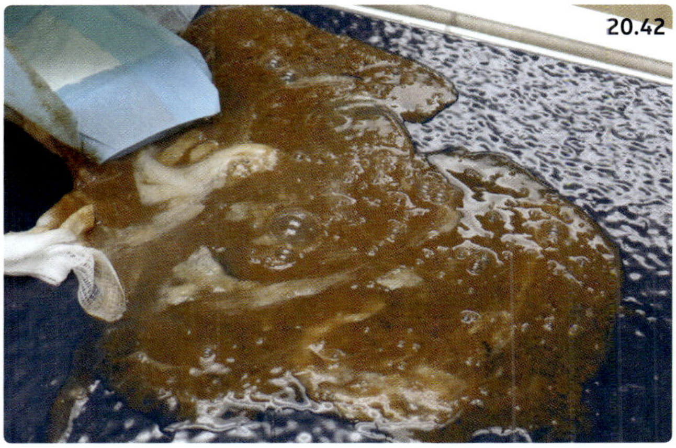

20.42

Figures 20.41, 20.42 This Pug shows nausea and vomiting after ingesting a large amount of dark chocolate. (Courtesy M. Schaer)

Diagnosis

Clinical history of ingestion of a caffeine and/or theobromine-containing product and compatible clinical signs support a diagnosis of methylxanthine intoxication. Some laboratories may be able to screen stomach contents, serum, plasma, or urine for methylxanthines.

Management

Emesis may be induced in asymptomatic dogs and cats if the ingestion has been recent; however, gastric lavage may be more effective for breaking down and removing large masses of chocolate from the stomach. Activated charcoal can be given after either procedure, and multiple doses may be beneficial due to the long half-life of theobromine. Electrolytes should be monitored in animals with diarrhea and those receiving multiple doses of activated charcoal.

IV fluids should be administered following significant exposure to enhance excretion of caffeine, and other treatments should be tailored to any signs that develop. Tremors may be controlled with diazepam or methocarbamol, and seizures may additionally require phenobarbital or gas anesthesia.

Tachyarrhythmias may be treated with beta-blockers or lidocaine, and atropine can be used for bradycardia. Prognosis is generally good for patients that receive timely care.

RECOMMENDED FURTHER READING

Gupta RC (2007) Ivermectin and selamectin. In: *Veterinary Toxicology: Basic and Clinical Principles*. (ed. RC Gupta) Academic Press, New York.

Khan SA, Hooser SB (2012) (eds.) Common toxicologic issues in small animals. *Vet Clin North Am Small Anim Pract* **42(2):**xi–xii.

Kidwell JH, Buckley GJ, Allen AE *et al.* (2014) Use of lipid emulsion for treatment of ivermectin toxicosis in a cat. *J Am Anim Hosp Assoc* **50(1):**59–61.

Macintire DK, Drobatz KJ, Haskins SC *et al.* (2005) *Manual of Small Animal Emergency and Critical Care Medicine*. Lippincott Williams and Wilkins, Philadelphia.

Peterson ME, Talcott PA (2006) (eds.) *Small Animal Toxicology*, 2nd edn. Elsevier Saunders, St. Louis.

Plumb DC (2011) (ed.) *Plumb's Veterinary Drug Handbook*, 7th edn. Blackwell Publishing, Ames.

Poppenga RH, Gwaltney-Brant SM (2011) (eds.) *Small Animal Toxicology Essentials*. Wiley-Blackwell, Chichester.

Chapter 21

Infectious diseases

Richard B. Ford & Annette Litster

INTRODUCTION

Today, access to an impressive array of diagnostic testing platforms, whether performed at the point of care or through commercial laboratories, has proven to be among the most significant factors influencing how veterinarians manage infectious disease risk and the level of care that can be provided to the individual patient. Advanced diagnostic technology has not only increased our awareness of the spectrum of infectious agents capable of causing clinical illness in companion animals, it has made it quite clear that co-infection (i.e. simultaneous infection with two or more pathogens in the same patient at the same time) is prevalent in veterinary medicine and can be a major turning point in the outcome.

The significance of co-infection in veterinary patients is most apparent to the clinician who is attempting to establish a diagnosis of infectious disease. Traditional textbooks, including this one, provide descriptions of characteristic clinical manifestations associated with single pathogens. Yet when faced with the sick patient, clinical signs alone frequently may not fit a conventional clinical description that leads to a diagnosis. The astute clinician must be able to assimilate historical and clinical information, along with knowledge of diagnostic test availability, interpretation, and testing limitations, to arrive at a diagnostic conclusion and prescribe a rational treatment regimen in the infected patient.

The discussion on infectious diseases that follows is not intended to be comprehensive. Instead, the diseases presented in this chapter represent the most common infections encountered in dogs and cats seen in clinical practice. Updates on practical, accessible, diagnostic testing protocols, treatment recommendations, and prevention/vaccination are included.

Part 1: The dog

Richard B. Ford

BACTERIAL AND SPIROCHETAL INFECTIONS

CANINE INFECTIOUS RESPIRATORY DISEASE

Definition/overview

Canine infectious respiratory disease (CIRD) is the descriptive term that replaces 'kennel cough' in the veterinary literature. Previous descriptive terms include canine cough, canine croup, and infectious tracheobronchitis. Nonetheless, each of these terms refers to a contagious, acute-onset, upper respiratory tract infection characteristically manifesting as cough. Occasionally, lower respiratory disease (bronchopneumonia) will result and may become life-threatening, particularly in young dogs. CIRD can occur in dogs of any age; risk is particularly high among co-housed dogs (e.g. boarding kennels, day care facilities, dog parks).

Etiology

Because clinical manifestations vary according to the primary infecting agent, or combination of agents, CIRD is also described as a respiratory syndrome. *Bordetella bronchiseptica* is commonly implicated as the principal cause of kennel cough; however, it is by no means the exclusive, nor is it the most virulent, pathogen involved. The pathogenic agents implicated in CIRD are summarized in **Table 21.1**.

Pathophysiology

Bacterial pathogens

Among the pathogens implicated in CIRD, *B. bronchiseptica* has received the most attention. *B. bronchiseptica* is a gram-negative coccobacillus that has the unique ability to

Table 21.1 The most common respiratory pathogens implicated in canine infectious respiratory disease.

Bacterial agents
Bordetella bronchiseptica
Streptococcus equi subspecies *zooepidemicus*
Mycoplasma spp. (*Mycoplasma cynos* is frequently implicated)
Viral agents
Canine parainfluenza virus
Canine adenovirus-2
Canine influenza virus
Canine distemper virus
Canine respiratory coronavirus
Canine pneumovirus

live on the respiratory epithelium as a commensal (normal flora) organism. For reasons not fully understood, these 'innocent' bacteria are able to transition into highly pathogenic organisms. *Bordetella* virulence is linked to a gene complex (Bvg) capable of expressing multiple, well-defined virulence factors (toxins) that cause serious, rapid injury to respiratory epithelium. Because *B. bronchiseptica* can be recovered from the respiratory tract of healthy dogs, it poses significant risk in dogs exposed to a viral respiratory pathogen, as co-infected dogs appear to have significantly more severe disease than dogs infected by a single respiratory pathogen.

More recently, *Streptococcus equi* subspecies *zooepidemicus*, a gram-positive bacterium, has been recognized as an important cofactor in the pathophysiology of CIRD. Although not a commensal organism in dogs/cats, *S. zooepidemicus* is capable of colonizing upper respiratory epithelial cells of dogs and cats. It appears to be a significant cofactor in upper respiratory infections of dogs and cats and has been attributed to fatal necrohemorrhagic pneumonia in outbreaks of CIRD in shelters

Viral pathogens

Canine parainfluenza virus (CPiV) is perhaps best recognized for its ability to cause inflammation of the tracheal and laryngeal epithelium. Vocal fold swelling increases the resistance to airflow during exhalation, resulting in the so-called 'goose honk' cough. In contrast to *B. bronchiseptica*, CPiV is a short-lived, although highly contagious, respiratory pathogen in dogs.

Canine influenza virus (CIV) is an H3N8 virus that is known to have been derived from the equine influenza virus. Virus shedding is generally limited to less than 14 days post infection. Experimentally infected dogs demonstrate fever and mild inflammation involving tracheal epithelium. Viral pneumonitis is uncommon. Clinical infection is generally considered to be mild unless the dog is co-infected. Bacterial pathogens (discussed above) in combination with CIV can result severe respiratory disease and death.

Other viral respiratory pathogens (**Table 21.1**) are associated with CIRD. Canine distemper virus (CDV) is not commonly implicated as a primary agent of CIRD because respiratory disease is just one of the severe systemic manifestations that occur in unvaccinated dogs. Canine adenovirus-2 (CAV-2), canine respiratory coronavirus (CRCoV), and canine pneumovirus (CPnV) infections appear to occur less commonly and may actually be most important as cofactors in CIRD.

Clinical presentation

Clinical signs vary based on the individual agent responsible for infection in clinically affected dogs. The clinical history typically reveals recent exposure to other dogs.

Viral pathogens tend to be associated with clinical signs ranging from an acute-onset, highly contagious cough with expectoration of mucus that typically lasts 1–2 weeks to mild or no clinical signs (seroconversion only). Although coughing may persist for several weeks, dogs tend to effectively clear infectious viruses within 2 weeks following onset of signs.

Bacterial pathogens tend to be associated with not only cough, but systemic illness characterized by mucoid to mucopurulent nasal and ocular discharge, fever, and loss of appetite. Other clinical findings include orthopnea, dyspnea, and even life-threatening pneumonia, particularly in young animals. Clinical signs can persist for several days or longer depending on treatment administered.

Clinical illness associated with individual pathogens, however, does not necessarily represent the spectrum of clinical manifestations encountered in practice. For example, reports of dogs with confirmed CIV infection indicate that some simply seroconvert without developing significant respiratory signs, while others die.

However, it is unlikely that agents implicated in CIRD, acting alone, cause such severe or life-threatening respiratory disease; CIRD likely results from the complex interaction between:

- Host.
- Multiple respiratory pathogens acting together (viral and bacterial).
- Environmental factors.

The occurrence of co-infection explains, at least in part, why predicting clinical outcomes of CIRD in individual dogs can be difficult, and it explains why well vaccinated dogs still develop kennel cough.

Differential diagnosis

Importantly, *B. bronchiseptica* infection, in the absence of culture, is difficult to distinguish from any acute bacterial pneumonia, whether primary or secondary to an underlying viral infection (e.g. CIV, CDV, CpiV infection).

Diagnosis

Clinical diagnosis of CIRD is commonly established on the basis of history and clinical signs. Establishing a definitive diagnosis of CIRD is complicated by at least three factors: (1) isolation of the individual agent(s) involved entails laboratory-based isolation capabilities not available in practice; (2) the duration of clinical illness tends to be relatively short-lived; and (3) most of the agents implicated have been recovered from healthy (noncoughing) dogs.

However, some laboratories do provide individual test capability (e.g. culture, PCR) for individual agents implicated in CIRD. Tests must be requested on an individual basis. Currently, a comprehensive 'CIRD panel' is not available.

Management

Treatment/prognosis

In most cases, clinical signs progress rapidly, justifying the need for antimicrobial intervention before bacterial isolates can be identified. Empiric treatment of affected puppies is indicated. Doxycycline (liquid) (2.5–5.0 mg/kg PO q12h for 5–7 days) is recommended. Alternative antimicrobials include amoxicillin–clavulanate (12.5–25 mg/kg PO q12h for 10 days [(minimum]), and trimethoprim–sulfonamide (15 mg/kg PO q12h for 10 days [minimum]).

Healthy, but coughing, dogs may receive short-term treatment with a corticosteroid to reduce inflammation of the respiratory epithelium and manage coughing paroxysms. Treatment should be limited to 5 days without risk of complications and should be supplemented with an antimicrobial. Predisolone (0.5 mg/kg PO once or twice daily) is usually sufficient to reduce the intensity of cough.

Doxycycline, like tetracycline, can yellow the enamel of developing permanent teeth (**Figure 21.1**). This complication can be minimized in puppies by limiting the duration of treatment to less than 10 days. In puppies, a clinical response to treatment should be detectable within 24–72 hours.

The prognosis for affected dogs is good to excellent. Many infections resolve spontaneously within 10–14 days. Clinical signs may persist beyond the time of viral shedding. Infected puppies appear to be at greater risk for developing complications associated with CIRD (e.g. bronchopneumonia). Outcomes are directly related to the severity of disease at the time antimicrobial therapy is started and any co-infecting pathogens.

Aggressive intervention with antimicrobial therapy is critical in the effective management of outbreaks. Other factors influencing outbreaks include the ability to depopulate the facility, cleanliness of the facilities, ventilation (12–16 complete air exchanges per hour are recommended), and the ability to provide supportive care in the form of rehydration, nutrition, and cleaning of nasal discharges.

Prevention

In the USA, routine vaccination of dogs at risk for exposure is indicated and generally effective in reducing severity of cough in challenged dogs, despite the inability to immunize dogs against each of the known CIRD pathogens. **Table 21.2** lists the vaccines available in the USA for pathogenic viruses and bacteria associated with CIRD. This vaccination recommendation might be altered in different parts of the world because of factors such as incidence or economics.

Several types of vaccine (**Tables 21.3** and **21.4**) are available for administration to dogs by the intranasal,

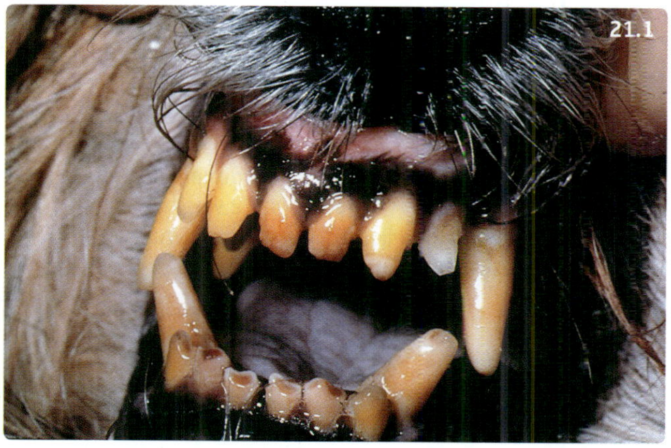

Figure 21.1 Tetracycline labeling of the enamel in an adult dog subsequent to extended administration of the antibiotic during puppyhood.

Table 21.2 Vaccines (available in the USA) for prevention against known CIRD pathogens.

B. bronchiseptica
Canine parainfluenza virus
Canine adenovirus-2
Canine distemper virus
Canine influenza virus

Table 21.3 Initial vaccination recommendations for dogs based on the 2011 American Animal Hospital Association (AAHA) Vaccination Guidelines.

Core vaccines	Administration	First booster
MLV or recombinant distemper + MLV parvovirus + MLV adenovirus-2 (administered as a combination product)	3 doses are recommended between 6 and 16 weeks of age **Example:** 8 weeks, 12 weeks, and 16 weeks of age	Administer a single dose (of a combination product) not later than 1 year following the last dose in the initial series. **Note:** A minimum interval of 2 weeks between any 2 doses of vaccine is recommended
Canine parainfluenza virus option: In the USA and Canada, canine parainfluenza virus vaccine is commonly administered in combination with the above vaccines as DA2PPi (see below)		
Rabies (killed) (1-year and 3-year products are available)	Administer a single dose of rabies vaccine not earlier than 12 weeks of age (State/Local/Provincial law applies)	Schedule a second dose of rabies vaccine to be administered not later than 1 year following administration of the first dose, regardless of the dog's age at the time the initial dose is administered. (State/Local/Provincial law applies)
Noncore vaccines	**Administration**	**Booster recommendations**
B. bronchiseptica + canine parainfluenza virus (IN only) (some IN products may also contain CAV-2 antigen)	Single dose (intranasal) at 12 or 16 weeks of age. (Optional: some authors recommended 2 doses at 12 and 16 weeks of age.) IN vaccines may be administered as early as 3 to 4 weeks of age	When risk of exposure is sustained, administer a single dose 1 year following the last dose administered
B. bronchiseptica only (monovalent) Three options are available: • Parenteral (killed-bacterin) • IN (avirulent live) • Intraoral (avirulent live)	Parenteral (SC): 2 doses are required, 2–4 weeks apart. Intraoral: The manufacturer recommends a single initial dose	When risk of exposure is sustained, administer a single dose 1 year following the last dose administered
Leptospirosis (killed) 4-serovar (2-way leptospirosis vaccines are not recommended by either AAHA or the American College of Veterinary Internal Medicine)	2 initial doses, 2–4 weeks apart **Note:** It is not recommended to administer the first dose prior to 12 weeks of age. **Note**: Small breed dogs: consider delaying initial doses until the core vaccine series has been completed	Where risk of exposure is sustained, administer a single dose 1 year following completion of the initial 2-dose series
Lyme disease (recombinant or killed)	2 initial doses, 2 to 4 weeks apart **Note**: Small breed dogs: consider delaying initial doses until the core vaccine series has been completed	Where risk of exposure is sustained, administer a single dose 1 year following completion of the initial 2-dose series. Option: For dogs residing in endemic regions, administration of the first booster 6 months following completion of the initial 2-dose series is a reasonable alternative schedule. An additional booster is recommended at 1 year following completion of the initial series, with annual vaccination recommended thereafter
Canine influenza virus (killed)	2 initial doses, 2–4 weeks apart are required	Manufacturer recommends annual re-vaccination where risk of exposure is sustained Duration of immunity has not been established

MLV, modifield live virus; IN, intranasal.
Note: Canine coronavirus vaccination is not recommended.
Note: *Crotalus atrox* (Western Diamondback rattlesnake) vaccine should only be used in dogs with a defined risk for exposure. Follow the manufacturer's recommendations for dosing.

Table 21.4 Booster recommendations for adult dogs.

- After completing the initial series of core vaccines (distemper + parvovirus + adenovirus-2) it is recommended to administer a single dose (combination vaccine) at intervals of every 3 years (or longer).
  Note: Substantial data exist to demonstrate that dogs derive protective immunity for at least 5 years following administration of modified live virus core vaccines (in the absence of maternally derived antibody).
- Rabies boosters. In the USA, all States currently recognize and accept the use of '3-year' rabies vaccine in dogs.
  Note: Some local municipalities may mandate stricter requirements (annual booster) for rabies vaccination.
- Noncore vaccines: administer annually where risk of exposure is sustained.

oral, and parenteral (subcutaneous) route. The constituents and the routes of administration of commercially available vaccines vary. The route of vaccine administration indicated by the manufacturer must be strictly adhered to.

Although not indicated for the prevention of signs of CIRD in individual pets, doxycycline (5 mg/kg PO q24h for 5 days) has been empirically administered to all dogs entering a large animal shelter experiencing high rates (>50%) of acute-onset cough. Follow-up over a 30-day period indicated:

- Rapid and substantial reduction in incidence of CIRD within the population.
- Higher placement rates.
- Reduced euthanasia rates.
- Lower operating costs.

Anecdotal observations suggest that empirical, daily administration of a broad-spectrum antibiotic may be of benefit in managing endemic respiratory disease associated with bacteria among shelter-housed dogs. While the cost of doxycycline may prohibit implementing programmatic treatment of all dogs entering a shelter, other less expensive, broad-spectrum antibiotics are available and may augment attempts to reduce the frequency or severity of CIRD in populations of co-housed dogs.

Nosodes are liquid homeopathic preparations, sometimes called homeopathic vaccines, containing minute amounts of infectious material (tissue/discharge) collected from actively infected, unvaccinated animals. Intended for oral administration, proponents of nosodes claim efficacy in not only preventing but also treating infectious diseases in dogs and cats. Nosodes are not recommended for the treatment or prevention of CIRD because:

- Values for composition, concentration, and purity of ingredients are not standardized.
- Nosodes are not subject to regulatory oversight.
- No studies have been published documenting either safety or efficacy.

Public health implications

Human bordetellosis (*Bordetella pertussis*) is among the most common respiratory infections of children and immunocompromised adults and has recently reappeared in children in unusually high numbers. *B. bronchiseptica* can, in fact, infect the respiratory tract of humans. Several cases of human *B. bronchiseptica* pneumonia have been documented in children and immunocompromised adults. The risk of transmission from dogs to humans is considered to be low.

Although human influenza viruses have been documented to infect the respiratory tract of dogs, there is no evidence that CIV is transmitted from dogs to humans.

LYME BORRELIOSIS (BORRELIOSIS; CANINE LYME DISEASE)

Definition/overview

In the USA, Lyme borreliosis, caused by the spirochete *Borrelia burgdorferi*, is the most common vector-borne disease reported to occur in humans, 300,000 humans are estimated to be infected annually. Canine Lyme disease is likely to be among the most common vector-borne diseases of dogs living in the USA and Canada, although prevalence data are not available.

Similar to the incidence of Lyme borreliosis in humans, the highest rates of infection in dogs are reported from the northeastern USA, especially from Virginia to Southern Maine, the upper Midwest, particularly Wisconsin and eastern Minnesota, and northwestern California. However, there are increasing reports of dogs with a positive test for Lyme borreliosis living in fringe areas of traditional Lyme-endemic regions. Movement of infected ticks by migratory ground-feeding birds, and possible climatic changes, are believed responsible for the spread of canine Lyme disease in the USA and Canada (and in other countries). In addition, positive cases have been reported in geographic regions of the USA (e.g. Denver, Colorado) where ticks are not present. Such infections are likely to be associated with pet travel into endemic regions.

Vector ticks are found throughout Japan, Europe, and Eurasia, with most documented cases found in Scandinavian countries and central Europe. Various species of *Borrelia*, in addition to *B. burgdorferi*, are implicated. These differences may account for the variation in clinical signs seen in different parts of the world.

Etiology

Lyme borreliosis is a tick-borne infection capable of affecting a wide spectrum of mammalian and avian hosts. The principal vectors of *B. burgdorferi* are generally associated with the *Ixodes ricinus* complex of ticks (**Figure 21.2**). The *Ixodes* species ticks that transmit the infection have a 2-year life cycle. Infected nymph ticks are considered the most likely source of infection for humans. In dogs, the slow-feeding adult tick has been implicated as the primary source for infection. Although other tick species, fleas, flies, and mosquitoes have been found to be infected in nature, their role in transmitting the infection is considered to be insignificant.

Pathophysiology

Clinical disease depends on the host's inflammatory response to *B. burgdorferi*, manifested primarily in the limb joints of affected dogs. Unique biochemical or hematologic changes have not been associated with canine Lyme disease. Rarely, dogs will develop an acute-onset glomerulonephritis, associated with proteinuria, which frequently culminates in death. Cytologic assessment of synovial fluid may show leukocyte counts from 2,000 to 100,000 nucleated cells/ml, typical of suppurative polyarthritis.

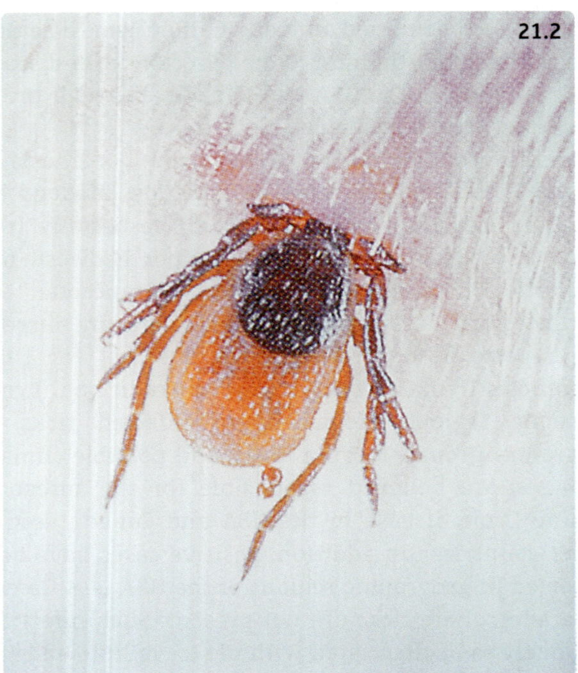

Figure 21.2 The *Ixodes* species of ticks is the vector of Lyme disease. (From Kassira JP (1997) (ed.) *Images in Clinical Medicine*. Selections from the *New England Journal of Medicine*, with permission.)

Clinical presentation

Sustained tick attachment and feeding (at least 50 hours) is required for effective transmission. Infection, however, is uncommonly associated with development of clinical signs. Characteristic clinical signs of naturally infected dogs include: fever, shifting-leg lameness and joint swelling (associated with nonerosive polyarthritis), joint pain, malaise, and decreased appetite. Generalized illness might be associated with Lyme nephritis (see below). In experimentally infected dogs, clinical signs develop between 2 and 5 months following tick exposure. Clinical signs may not develop for several months following exposure to ticks. Lameness may manifest in different limbs at different times throughout infection. It is estimated that at the time of testing approximately 15–20% of Lyme-positive dogs manifest clinical signs of lameness. In practice, it is feasible that nonclinical, but positive, dogs may eventually develop signs over time. Also, healthy Lyme-positive dogs, if untreated, may become reinfected and more susceptible to manifesting clinical signs.

Lyme nephropathy

A small number of large breed dogs have been reported to develop acute-onset protein-losing glomerulonephritis attributed to *B. burgdorferi* infection. Clinical signs are consistent with acute kidney injury. Treatment is generally not successful.

Lyme nephropathy is a rare, but often fatal, syndrome associated with *B. burgdorferi* infection in dogs. This rapidly progressive renal disease is characterized by glomerulonephritis, tubular necrosis, and lymphocytic–plasmacytic interstitial nephritis.

Believed to be an immune-mediated disease, the pathogenesis of Lyme nephropathy remains unknown. The most commonly affected breeds include Labrador Retrievers, Golden Retrievers, and Shetland Sheepdogs; however, any breed or mixed-breed dog may be affected.

A critical factor in the diagnosis of Lyme nephropathy is proteinuria, and assessing every seropositive patient for proteinuria (including a urine protein:creatinine [UP:UC] ratio) is an important component of laboratory evaluation.

In one study, only 30% of affected dogs had been vaccinated for Lyme borreliosis, which suggests that vaccination is not an inciting factor. This highlights the fact that Lyme nephropathy is the consequence of natural infection, not vaccination.

Differential diagnosis

Dogs presented for Lyme borreliosis manifest a variety of clinical signs ranging from, most commonly, acute lameness and polyarthritis, to an acute-onset febrile illness with nonspecific signs. Rarely, primary renal, neurologic, dermatologic, or cardiac signs are observed. Therefore, the differential diagnosis can include other causes of polyarthropathy, various types of bone infections, and immune-mediated polyarthropathy. An array of other disorders can be listed in the list of differentials depending on the particular organ system adversely affected.

Diagnosis

There are no discrete hematologic or biochemical abnormalities that are diagnostic of canine Lyme disease. Serologic (antibody) testing is predominantly used in veterinary medicine to diagnose infection. Since the introduction of the first point-of-care ELISA C6 antibody test (Snap 3Dx® and Snap 4Dx®) several other commercially available tests have become available.

In veterinary medicine, it must be emphasized that there is no single pathognomonic diagnostic test for canine Lyme borreliosis. For over 10 years, point-of-care tests (Snap4×® and Snap4D× Plus®) have been available to detect antibodies to the highly conserved C6 peptide of *B. burgdorferi*. With high sensitivity and specificity, this rapid assay is an excellent surveillance tool for identifying dogs that are infected with, not simply 'exposed' to, *B. burgdorferi*, and is particularly valuable to screen dogs within areas where Lyme disease is emerging. None of the commercial Lyme disease vaccines causes false-positive C6 test results. A positive test, however, cannot be used to predict the clinical outcome of an infected dog.

Because the majority of dogs infected with *B. burgdorferi* have no clinical signs at the time of testing, use of the laboratory-based, quantitative C6 assay (Lyme Quant C6® Test) has been proposed as a way to monitor response to treatment of nonclinical seropositive dogs (see Management).

Another laboratory-based diagnostic test (AccuPlex4®), introduced in 2012, has the ability to detect five different antibody responses to *B. burgdorferi* infection (OspA, OspC, Ospf, p39, and OspF). The test also reportedly differentiates between natural exposure and vaccination as well as distinguishing early from chronic infection.

Limitations to this testing platform include an inability to:

- Distinguish acutely infected dogs from those vaccinated with a whole-cell (inactivated) vaccine.
- Reliably distinguish between dogs with a positive test result for chronic infection (OspF) and those that have been treated and reinfected.
- Consistently and reliably detect vaccine-induced antibody (OspA); therefore, at this time, these results should not be considered when interpreting a report.

Diagnosis of Lyme borreliosis is based on the presence of all three of the following factors: (1) positive serology results (C6, OspC, or OspF); (2) clinical and/or laboratory findings consistent with Lyme borreliosis; and (3) a reasonable history of exposure to *Ixodes* species ticks.

The laboratory assessment of any patient found to have serum antibodies against *B. burgdorferi* should include: hematology; serum biochemistry profile; urinalysis; UP:UC ratio to assess proteinuria.

With uncomplicated Lyme borreliosis, hematologic and biochemical abnormalities are unlikely. However, seropositive dogs are at risk for co-infection with other vector-borne pathogens and may have underlying laboratory abnormalities (e.g. thrombocytopenia, anemia, hypoalbuminemia).

Positive C6 antibody test results are highly indicative of infection but are not predictive for development of clinical signs in healthy dogs. Unlike immunofluorescent antibody (IFA) testing, prior vaccination does not cause false-positive test results for C6 antibody. The quantitative C6 antibody test has been introduced and this may be useful in assessing the likelihood of clinical signs developing in a healthy dog with a positive ELISA Snap test and assessing the antibody response to therapy. Treatment of dogs with a high concentration of C6 antibody (>30 units) may be indicated. Seropositive dogs and cats can only be assessed as having seroreactivity to *B. burgdorferi*. Diagnostic confirmation is based, instead, on detection of the organism in culture specimens of tissues or body fluids. These tests are uncommonly performed in clinical practice.

Management

Treatment/prognosis

Treatment with an oral antimicrobial is indicated in any patient meeting the above criteria, and oral doxycycline is the preferred therapeutic approach to canine Lyme borreliosis. Optional treatment regimens are listed in **Table 21.5**. Most authors agree that dogs exhibiting lameness and/or myalgia resulting from *B. burgdorferi* infection will rapidly improve within 3–5 days.

It is important not to discontinue treatment earlier than recommended, even if clinical signs rapidly resolve. Also, although clinical signs may rapidly resolve with treatment, none of the antimicrobials outlined in **Table 21.5** are known to eliminate *B. burgdorferi* from tissue.

Indications for treating the seropositive patient with no clinical signs or laboratory abnormalities are less clear than those for treating patients clearly affected by Lyme disease (see above). While treatment guidelines for healthy but antibody-positive dogs have not been published, the following options for this particular patient population can be considered:

- **Response to therapy.** One option for monitoring these dogs is to perform the laboratory-based quantitative C6 test. Dogs with pretreatment quantitative titers ≥30 U/ml can be monitored for response to treatment by measuring reduction in C6 antibody concentration 6 months after treatment. Dogs that experience reductions in antibody ≥50% have responded to treatment.
- **Observe nontreated dogs.** Because laboratory-based antibody tests cannot predict clinical disease, conducting routine or quantitative serology is generally not useful in seropositive patients with no clinical signs or laboratory abnormalities.
- **Vaccination of seropositive dogs.** Because natural infection does not induce protective immunity, it is reasonable to recommend vaccination of seropositive dogs, particularly those living in endemic regions, to prevent reinfection. If a seropositive dog manifests clinical signs, vaccination may be given following completion of the recommended treatment period. If clinical signs are not present, vaccination may be administered at the time of testing. There is no known therapeutic value associated with vaccinating a seropositive dog.

Prevention

Despite the fact that infection with *B. burgdorferi* does not consistently cause clinical illness, canine Lyme borreliosis is a disease to prevent, not to treat. Prevention consists of three components.

Limit exposure to ticks

Reducing or eliminating exposure to infected ticks is the core strategy to preventing canine Lyme borreliosis. Even in regions where tick exposure is considered minimal, administration of an oral or topical tick preventive is critical. The recommendation for widespread practice of adequate tick control extends beyond the control of Lyme disease because the same measures will prove beneficial in preventing an array of other tick-borne diseases.

Vaccinate at-risk dogs

In regions of the USA and Canada known to be endemic for ticks infected with *B. burgdorferi*, dogs should be vaccinated annually. Vaccination is not routinely recommended for dogs living in nonendemic regions (e.g. Colorado, Utah, New Mexico, western Canada). Instead, appropriate use of tick preventives reasonably manages exposure risk.

All vaccines immunize by stimulating antibody to the OspA antigen, which is ingested by ticks while they feed (on the dog), binding to spirochetes in the mid-gut of the ticks and preventing transmission of *B. burgdorferi* (**Tables 21.3** and **21.4**).

Based on results of *in-vitro* studies, some products (whole-cell bacterins) claim provision of expanded protection due to the addition of OspC antigen. However, OspC antibody has not yet demonstrated *in-vivo* protection against infection when independent from the OspA antibody.

Table 21.5 Treatment recommendations for dogs with Lyme disease.

Antimicrobial	Dosage	Recommended treatment period
Preferred treatment		
Doxycycline	10 mg/kg PO q24h (or 5 mg/kg PO q12h)	4–6 weeks (1 month minimum)
Optional treatment		
Minocycline	25 mg/kg PO q24h	4–6 weeks (1 month minimum)
Cefovecin	8 mg/kg SC	2 doses at 14-day interval
Amoxicillin	20 mg/kg PO q8h	1 month (minimum)
Azithromycin	25 mg/kg PO q24h	1 month (minimum)

Avoid at-risk regions

Encourage owners to avoid traveling with their dogs to regions inhabited by the *Ixodes* tick. However, if dogs must travel to, or reside within or in the periphery of, Lyme endemic regions, especially during periods of increased tick activity (spring/summer/fall), highly recommend application of a tick preventive as well as vaccination.

Public health implications

Lyme borreliosis in dogs is not considered to be a source of infection for humans. Since humans and pets are incidental hosts for the vector tick, dogs and cats appear to be sentinel hosts, rather than reservoir hosts, for human infection.

CANINE BOTULISM

Definition/overview

Botulism is a neurologic disorder of dogs and humans caused by intoxication of botulinum neurotoxin produced by *Clostridium botulinum*.

Etiology

Botulism is a neuroparalytic disease; it is not the result of a bacterial infection. The highly potent neurotoxin is produced by the gram-positive bacterium *C. botulinum*.

Pathophysiology

Following ingestion of the preformed toxin, botulinum toxin binds rapidly and irreversibly to membrane receptors at the neuromuscular junction. Clinical signs are associated with interruption of acetylcholine release, resulting in lower motor neuron and parasympathetic dysfunction.

Clinical presentation

Initially, affected dogs develop progressive, symmetric weakness, beginning with the hindlimbs and progressing to the forelimbs (**Figure 21.3**). Quadriplegia may result, although a tail wag is maintained. Neurologic examination characteristically reveals hyporeflexia and hypotonia. Pain sensation is maintained. Cranial nerve abnormalities include mydriasis, decreased pupillary light response, decreased jaw tone, salivation, diminished palpebral reflexes, and weak vocalization. Mentation is generally normal. Severely affected dogs may experience difficulty breathing, associated with decreased muscular tone. Affected patients appear to have decreased swallowing reflexes and should be considered predisposed to aspiration pneumonia. Respiratory paralysis or secondary respiratory/urinary tract infections may culminate in death in a small number of patients.

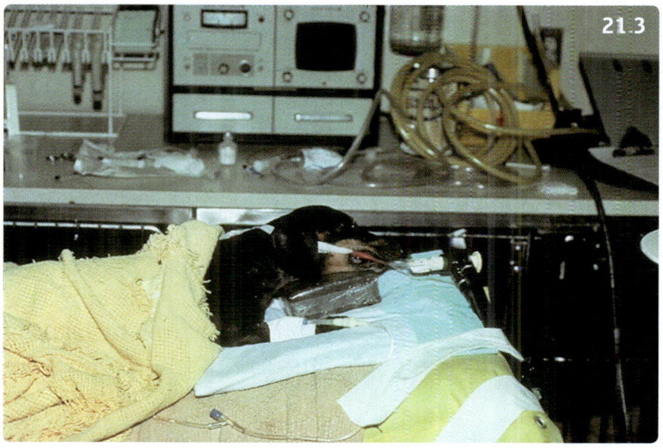

Figure 21.3 The toxin of *Clostridium botulinum* can cause a severe bulbar and lower motor neuron paralysis, causing impaired respiration and requiring life-preserving ventilatory support. (Courtesy M. Schaer)

Differential diagnosis

Rabies is an important differential among dogs with overt signs of botulism toxicity. In addition, CNS neoplasia, tetanus, and other forms of poisoning should be considered.

Diagnosis

Diagnosis is based on clinical signs. Results of laboratory profiles, including analysis of cerebrospinal fluid (CSF), are normal. Diagnostic confirmation is based on identification of botulinum toxin in serum, feces, vomitus, or samples of the suspect food. However, identification of the *C. botulinum* organism from feces is not necessarily diagnostic. In clinical practice, attempts to confirm the presence of toxins must be coordinated with the laboratory to verify specimen type, volume, and preparation.

Management

Treatment/prognosis

The principal treatment of botulism entails a commitment to extended supportive care. Affected dogs require assistance in eating, drinking, and moving. Significant effort is required to prevent the occurrence of decubital sores and to prevent urine and fecal contamination of skin. Antibiotics should not be routinely utilized in affected patients unless a secondary bacterial infection is diagnosed (e.g. aspiration pneumonia).

Antitoxin does not constitute effective therapy when clinical signs are present, since botulinum toxin is already bound to membrane receptors. Antitoxin type C can be administered to asymptomatic dogs suspected of recent (within 1 hour) ingestion of contaminated food and ongoing intestinal absorption of botulinal toxin.

Clinical signs may persist for as long as 3 weeks. If appropriate supportive care can be provided, the prognosis is good and recovery, if it occurs, is complete. Recovery of head, neck, and forelimb muscle function occurs first, followed by the hindlimbs.

Prevention

The most important means of preventing botulism is to prevent access to contaminated food, especially raw meat. The botulinum toxin is easily destroyed by heating food to 80°C (176°F) for 30 minutes or to 100°C (212°F) for 10 minutes.

Public health implications

Botulism is not transmitted from dogs to humans.

CANINE BRUCELLOSIS

Definition/overview

Canine brucellosis is the clinical manifestation of infection with *Brucella canis*, a gram-negative aerobic coccobacillus. Although dogs are susceptible to natural infection with *B. abortus* and *B. suis* following ingestion of contaminated placentas and aborted fetuses of livestock, the dog does not play a significant role in the transmission of these infections. However, *B. canis* is excreted in high concentrations from vaginal discharges and semen, and these are the most likely source of infection among dogs.

Etiology

Oronasal contact with aborted material and breathing are the most likely means of transmitting the infection among dogs. Seminal fluid and urine of male dogs has also been incriminated as a source of infection.

Pathophysiology

The ability of *B. canis* to localize in nonreproductive tissues such as the intervertebral disk is responsible for the clinical manifestations of *B. canis* infection (e.g. diskospondylitis). The eyes, kidneys, and meninges may also be affected subsequent to immune-complex deposition. Antibody is not protective. Cell-mediated immunity plays the most important role in protecting against the consequences of infection.

Clinical presentation

Among adult females, abortion of dead puppies is the primary clinical finding in dogs with brucellosis. In most cases, bitches usually abort between 45 and 60 days of gestation without other signs of clinical illness. Subcutaneous edema, congestion, and hemorrhage are reported in the dead puppies. A brown or greenish-gray vaginal discharge may persist for up to 6 weeks following abortion. Failure of conception is commonly reported in dogs with *B. canis* infection; however, this is an unreliable diagnostic sign since numerous causes of failure to conceive exist. Puppies that are born live may demonstrate generalized peripheral lymphadenomegaly for as long as 4–6 months. Hyperglobulinemia may also be observed.

In adult males, *B. canis* infection is not frequently associated with overt clinical signs. Careful examination may indicate the presence of nonpainful epididymitis. Testicular enlargement and orchitis are uncommon. In chronically affected males, testicular atrophy may be apparent.

Nonreproductive abnormalities associated with *B. canis* infection are less common yet are more likely to be associated with clinical signs. Spinal pain, paresis, and even ataxia may occur in dogs with diskospondylitis (**Figure 21.4**). Osteomyelitis has been reported in the appendicular skeleton and is associated with lameness. Rarely, anterior uveitis and corneal edema may be observed alone or in combination with other clinical signs.

Differential diagnosis

Among male dogs, clinical signs of brucellosis are not likely to be apparent. Among females, vaginitis and/or open pyometra should be considered. Occasionally, dogs will present with acute neurologic signs consistent with intervertebral disk disease or diskospondylitis.

Diagnosis

In adult males and females, laboratory diagnosis of *B. canis* infection is usually based on serologic testing. Although hyperglobulinemia is a common finding among chronically infected dogs, it is not diagnostic. Examination of semen may reveal abnormalities as early as 5 weeks post infection. A variety of morphologic abnormalities (e.g. immature sperm, swollen midpieces, deformed acrosomes) are apparent in the sperm along with aggregates

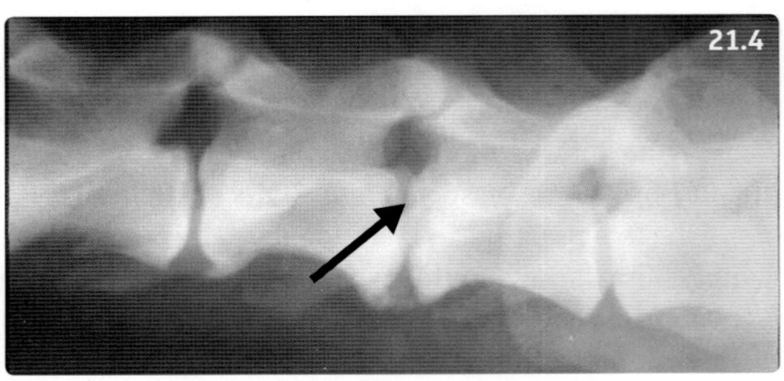

Figure 21.4 Radiograph depicting diskospondylitis in a dog, which can be caused by *Brucella canis*.

of inflammatory cells (neutrophils) and macrophages. By 20 weeks post infection, more that 90% of sperm are abnormal. Aspermia may ultimately result.

A variety of serologic tests can be performed to rule a diagnosis in or out:

- 2-Mercaptoethanol rapid slide agglutination test (ME-RSAT) is the recommended initial, in-office screening test for detection of antibodies. False-positive test results are common; however, there is a good correlation between a negative test and lack of infection. Therefore, the ME-RSAT is most useful in identifying patients that do not have brucellosis.
- The tube agglutination test (TAT) is commonly used to confirm infection in dogs with a positive ME-RSAT. However, lack of availability and diagnostic specificity diminish the value of the TAT as a diagnostic test.
- The agar gel immunodiffusion test is the recommended confirmatory test in dogs found to be positive by the ME-RSAT or TAT. This test is limited by the number of laboratories capable of performing the procedure.
- Although indirect IFA testing and ELISA assays are being evaluated as diagnostic tests for *B. canis*, these tests are not in widespread use today and may not be available to most clinicians.
- *B. canis* may be isolated from whole blood cultures in affected dogs as early as 4 weeks following oronasal infection. Concurrent or prior antibiotic therapy will diminish bacterial numbers in blood. Occasionally, cultures of urine collected by cystocentesis may yield *B. canis*.
- Polymerase chain reaction (PCR) testing of whole blood samples (not serum) has proven to be more sensitive than blood culture or serologic testing. Additionally, PCR testing of vaginal swab samples may be used to confirm positive test results.

Management

Treatment/prognosis

Treatment is difficult owing to the organism's persistence within cells. Relapses are therefore common once antimicrobials are discontinued, necessitating repetitive courses. Combination antimicrobial therapy, especially dihydrostreptomycin combined with either tetracycline or minocycline, has consistently been recommended in the treatment of brucellosis. However, the restricted availability of dihydrostreptomycin in some countries, combined with the fact that *B. canis* is an intracellular bacterium, makes the successful treatment of canine brucellosis particularly difficult.

Administration of doxycycline (12.5 mg/kg PO q12h for 4 weeks) or minocycline (same dose as doxycycline) plus streptomycin (20 mg/kg IM q24h on treatment weeks 1 and 4) has provided the best results in experimentally infected dogs. Recurrence of bacteremia may develop weeks or months following discontinuation of antibiotic therapy. Gentamicin (2.5 mg/kg IM or SC q12h on treatment weeks 1 and 4) has been used in lieu of streptomycin when administering combination therapy.

Ocular infection with *B. canis* is difficult to treat. If vision has been lost in one eye, enucleation is indicated. Multiple drug therapy using both topical products (prednisolone, gentamicin, cyclosporine) and oral or parenteral antimicrobials (rifampin, doxycycline, gentamicin, or a fluoroquinolone) is indicated. Attempts to treat dogs with CNS infections have not been successful.

In addition to antibiotics, infected pets should be neutered to diminish the chances of infecting other dogs or humans. Among dogs used in breeding programs, isolation and elimination from the breeding program are recommended at the time diagnosis is confirmed. Among those dogs that cannot be maintained as pets, euthanasia is justified.

Prevention

There is currently no effective vaccine available for preventing *B. canis* infection in dogs. The risk of infection is greatest among dogs utilized in breeding programs or maintained in breeding kennels. Quarantine procedures should be in place in breeding facilities prior to the admission of new dogs. At least two negative serotests (ME-RSAT or TAT) should be documented at 1-month intervals prior to entry into a breeding program.

Public health implications

Although the total number of human infections caused by *B. canis* is small, canine brucellosis must be regarded as a zoonotic infection. Both natural and laboratory acquired infections are reported. Caution should be taken when handling aborted tissues and discharges from dogs suspected of having brucellosis.

INFECTIOUS TRACHEOBRONCHITIS

See Viral infections.

LEPTOSPIROSIS

(See also Chapter 12: Nephrology/urology.)

Definition/overview

Leptospirosis is an important clinical and zoonotic disease of worldwide significance known to occur in dogs, humans, and many other animal species. Numerous serovars of *Leptospira interrogans* have been recognized, at least 10 of which are considered potentially important for dogs. Serogroups most often implicated in dogs worldwide include canicola, icterohaemorrhagiae, grippotyphosa, pomona, and bratislava. In the USA, killed vaccines are available for *L. canicola*, *L. icterohaemorrhagiae*, *L. grippotyphosa*, and *L. pomona*. Other vaccine serovars might be available in different parts of the world.

Etiology

Leptospires are long, flexible, filamentous bacteria. Over 250 serovars and serogroups of leptospirosis have been classified; approximately 10 are known to infect and cause disease in dogs. Leptospirosis is transmitted to dogs through direct contact with infected urine, bite wounds, ingestion of infected tissues/fluids, and by venereal and placental transfer. Organisms may be excreted in the urine of recovered dogs intermittently for several months following initial infection. The organism is not known to persist for extended periods in voided urine. Although cats may develop leptospirosis, the incidence of infection is much lower than that of the dog and infection is typically mild or subclinical.

Pathophysiology

Clinical illness is associated with the penetration of leptospires through mucous membranes, with subsequent spread and replication in other tissues, especially the kidney, liver, spleen, eyes, and genital tract. Although clinical signs may be mild, death, associated with disseminated intravascular coagulation (DIC), can occur rapidly. Colonization of leptospires in the kidney occurs in most infected animals. Even following treatment and apparent clinical recovery, infectious leptospires may be excreted for several weeks or months in the urine.

Clinical presentation

Leptospirosis occurs most commonly in outdoor adult dogs, although dogs of any age are susceptible. The severity of infection varies according to age, environment, and serovar. Acute infections are characterized by fever and muscle tenderness. Vomiting, weakness, and coagulopathies, with hematemesis, hematochezia, melena, epistaxis, and petechiation, characterize the clinical picture of DIC. The most common clinical signs associated with leptospirosis include lethargy, depression, anorexia, and vomiting. A variety of additional clinical signs include weight loss, nonlocalizing pain, arthralgia, posterior paresis, and labored breathing. Icterus is more commonly encountered in dogs with acute leptospirosis (**Figure 21.5**).

Differential diagnosis

Acute-onset signs associated with leptospirosis may manifest as any one of several serious systemic illnesses including acute kidney injury/chronic kidney disease, acute hepatitis, neoplasia, adverse drug reaction, polyarthritis, myositis (e.g. canine toxoplasmosis), pneumonia, and spinal cord injury.

Diagnosis

Fever (39.4°–40.0°C [103°–104°F]) associated with shivering and muscle tenderness is among the earliest clinical signs seen during the acute infection. Leukocytosis and thrombocytopenia characterize the hematologic abnormalities in canine leptospirosis. Increased serum urea nitrogen and creatinine associated with varying degrees of renal failure are commonly encountered. Young dogs with acute-onset icterus or renal failure should be

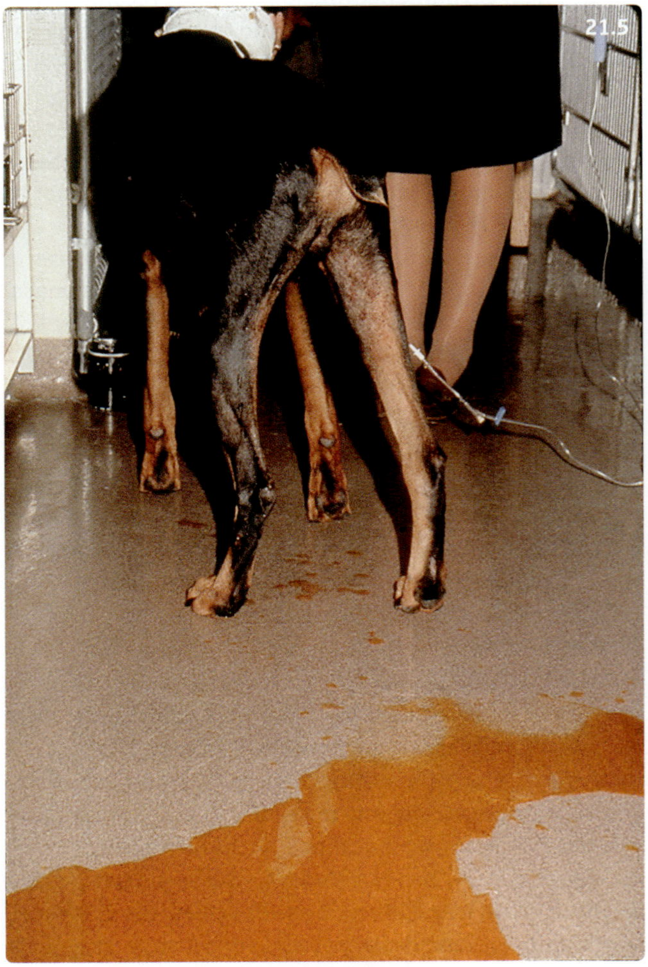

Figure 21.5 Bilirubinuria in an icteric dog with leptospirosis-induced hepatitis. The urine of dogs infected with leptospirosis can remain infectious for several weeks or months following clinical recovery.

considered suspect for leptospirosis. Considering the public health implications of this disease, an effort should be made to confirm the diagnosis.

In practice, the diagnosis of leptospirosis is typically based on presenting signs and clinician intuition. Conventional diagnostic tests for leptospirosis require submission of at least one sample of blood/urine to an appropriately equipped laboratory. Because results may require several days to obtain, testing is seldom done. At the time of writing, efforts to license a rapid, point-of-care diagnostic test are in progress (see below).

The so-called 'gold standard' method of diagnosing leptospirosis is the microscopic agglutination test (MAT). This test entails adding serial dilutions of serum to a known concentration of live organisms. The dilution at which 50% of spirochetes agglutinate *in vitro* defines the titer. Documentation of a rising titer in two samples 3–4 weeks apart is recommended for establishing a diagnosis of leptospirosis. However, due to the rapid onset of signs in clinically affected dogs, two samples are seldom submitted from the same patient. Less sensitive, but used most often, is a single titer where the highest titer considered to be above that caused by vaccine is regarded as the infecting organism. However, there are shortcomings to the MAT. Reference ranges for seropositivity, based on a single sample, can vary among laboratories; interpretation requires subjective assessment of the degree of agglutination, and cross-reactivity among the various serovars tested is common. Observation of live spirochetes in fresh urine, evaluated by dark field microscopy, can confirm infection. However, this test is uncommonly performed in dogs today.

A growing number of laboratories are able to perform PCR testing on blood (for acute disease) and fresh urine (carrier state) on dogs suspected as having leptospirosis. Most laboratories request that both blood and urine be submitted on individual patients and that samples are express mailed to the laboratory.

An ELISA-based assay to detect *Leptospira* antibody in blood is currently available (Idexx Laboratories). At the time of writing, samples must be submitted to a designated laboratory for testing. Results are reported to be available within 48 hours. In the near future, a rapid, point-of-care assay is expected to become available for in-hospital testing of dogs suspected of having leptospirosis. Antibody tests do not distinguish among various serogroups.

Postmortem examination of tissues does not guarantee ready confirmation of diagnosis. Although it is possible to culture leptospires from fresh, macerated kidney, the number of organisms present in the tissue is low and identification can be difficult.

Management

Treatment/prognosis

Dogs with clinical signs associated with leptospirosis require hospitalization and intensive supportive therapy. Fluid replacement with polyionic IV-administered fluids should be used to correct deficits associated with vomiting and diarrhea. In animals with spontaneous bleeding, plasma or fresh whole blood transfusions are indicated. Low-dose heparin administration is indicated for dogs considered to have DIC. Osmotic diuretics (e.g. mannitol) may be required after euhydration is restored and any co-existing hypotension is corrected in oliguric patients (<2 ml of urine produced/kg/hour). Failure to induce diuresis with osmotic diuretics justifies administration of dopamine (5 μg/kg/minute IV) or furosemide (2–6 mg/kg IV).

Antibiotic therapy should begin immediately. Today, doxycycline (5 mg/kg PO or IV q12h for up to 3 weeks) is the preferred antimicrobial treatment for dogs with leptospirosis. Doxycycline has been recommended for the treatment of both the initial phase of infection and the carrier state. Doxycycline is primarily excreted in the feces and can be administered to dogs in renal failure.

Alternative antimicrobials include: amoxicillin (22 mg/kg PO q8–12h for 2 weeks) or penicillin G (25,000–40,000 U/kg SC or IV q12h for 2 weeks). Penicillin does not eliminate the carrier state. Aminoglycosides are strictly contraindicated in dogs with renal disease associated with leptospirosis. Ampicillin, first-generation cephalosporins, and chloramphenicol have not been effective.

The prognosis for dogs with clinical leptospirosis is highly variable. Dogs with acute onset of clinical signs associated with icterus and DIC have a poor prognosis. Dogs with subacute leptospirosis, with evidence of mild renal disease, have a fair prognosis for recovery if treatment is instituted early and maintained for a minimum of 2 weeks.

Prevention

Killed leptospiral bacterins are available for *L. canicola*, *L. icterohaemorrhagiae*, *L. grippotyphosa*, and *L. pomona* (**Table 21.3**). With little exception, the current vaccines do not provide cross-protection against other disease-producing serovars recognized in dogs. Vaccination against leptospirosis is indicated in dogs considered to be at risk of exposure. Veterinarians recommending leptospirosis vaccine should only administer a four-serogroup vaccine. Annual administration of booster vaccines to adult dogs deemed to be at risk of exposure is indicated. When vaccination of puppies is indicated, two doses are recommended 3–4 weeks apart, beginning at not less than 12 weeks of age. It should be noted that leptospirosis bacterins are often associated with acute adverse events, especially in small breed dogs (<10 kg [22 lb] body weight) and in dogs <12 weeks of age.

Public health implications

Contaminated urine of dogs with leptospirosis is infectious for humans and other susceptible animal species. Individuals who must handle dogs considered to be suspect for leptospirosis should wear latex gloves at all times, particularly when handling urine or urine-contaminated items. Floors and cages contaminated with urine of dogs with leptospirosis should be washed with a detergent and treated with an iodine-based disinfectant. Most cases of human leptospirosis, however, occur subsequent to occupational, recreational, or avocational activities. Seasonal flooding, rather than contact with dogs, is recognized as a major risk factor for human leptospirosis.

TETANUS

Definition/overview

Clostridium tetani is a gram-positive, anaerobic, spore-forming bacillus capable of producing a potent neurotoxin subsequent to the introduction of spores into wounds. In contrast to horses and humans, dogs are considered to be several hundred times more resistant to the effects of tetanus toxin; cats are considered to be approximately 12 times more resistant to tetanus toxin than dogs. As a result of this natural resistance, the prevalence of tetanus in dogs and cats is low.

Etiology

Resistant spores of *C. tetani* can be found in the environment, particularly in rich soil. Spores enter the body through contaminated wounds.

Pathophysiology

The neurotoxin produced by the *C. tetani* spores binds irreversibly to inhibitory interneurons of the brain and spinal cord, where it prevents the release of glycine and gamma-aminobutyric acid. Recovery from tetanus depends on the development of new axon terminals.

Clinical presentation

Evidence of localized or general muscle stiffness characteristically develops within 5–10 days from the onset of wounding. In cats, however, the onset of signs may be delayed for up to 3 weeks because of their inherent resistance to the neurotoxin.

Tetanus in dogs can be characterized as localized or generalized. Localized tetanus occurs more commonly in dogs (and less often in cats). Stiffness usually begins in the limb closest to the wound site. Gradually, the opposite extremity becomes involved. With time, localized tetanus can become generalized.

Extreme muscle rigidity, a stiff gait, or an inability to walk characterizes generalized tetanus (**Figure 21.6**). Extreme body temperature can result from excessive muscular activity. The patellar reflex may be accentuated but, because of muscle stiffness, may be difficult to assess. In advanced stages of the disease, enophthalmos and protrusion of the third eyelid will develop. The ears are typically held erect, the lips are drawn, and the forehead appears wrinkled. Hypertonus of masticatory muscles is responsible for trismus (also called 'lockjaw').

Affected dogs and cats are particularly reactive to tactile or auditory stimulation. Opisthotonus or generalized convulsions may develop subsequent to even mild provocation. Pain and hyperthermia associated with muscle spasms justify the use of muscle relaxants in managing affected patients.

Differential diagnosis

Muscle rigor and conformational changes associated with localized and generalized tetanus are characteristic of the disease. Differential diagnoses that should be considered include rabies and trauma, particularly trauma involving the CNS.

Diagnosis

Diagnosis of tetanus is based on the history of a recent wound and clinical signs. Physical evidence of a wound or skin penetration may not be apparent on physical

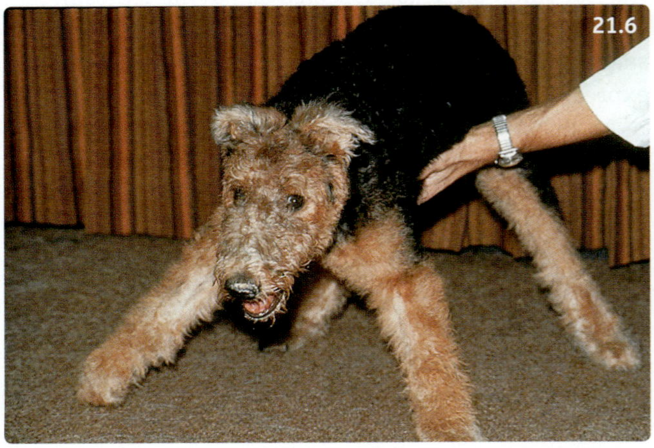

Figure 21.6 Generalized tetanus in this 5-month-old Airedale is characterized by profound limb and neck rigidity, erect ears, and trismus.

examination. Neutrophilic leukocytosis with a left shift may be the only hematologic abnormality present. Creatine kinase may be particularly elevated in animals with generalized muscle spasms. Although serum antibody titers to tetanus toxin have been used to document a diagnosis, this test has limited value in clinical practice. In addition, attempting to isolate *C. tetani* from a wound infection is not recommended as a diagnostic procedure. The organism is present in low numbers and must be grown under strict anaerobic conditions for as long as 12 days.

Management

Treatment/prognosis

Once clinical signs of tetanus have developed, treatment centers around providing intensive supportive care until clinical signs resolve. In patients that develop generalized tetanus, treatment may entail 3–4 weeks of hospitalization in a facility capable of providing 24-hour a day care.

The following elements of intervention and supportive care are recommended in patients with tetanus:

- Antitoxin. Antitetanus equine serum, administered IV, is recommended in patients identified during the earliest stages of clinical signs associated with tetanus. Antitoxin is able to neutralize only unbound toxin or toxin that has yet to be formed. Because antitoxin is associated with anaphylaxis, 0.1 ml of antitoxin should be administered SC or intradermally 15–30 minutes prior to IV administration. Antitoxin hypersensitivity is indicated by the development of a wheal at the site of injection; false test results are known to occur. Affected patients should be pretreated with a glucocorticoid or an antihistamine prior to administration of the IV dose.
- Antimicrobial therapy. Penicillin G and metronidazole are indicated for the treatment of *C. tetani* infection. Penicillin G may be given at doses ranging from 20,000 to 100,000 U/kg IV, IM, or SC q6–12h for at least 10 days. Although preferred over penicillin G, metronidazole must be administered IV or PO at 10 mg/kg q8h for at least 10 days.
- Muscle relaxation. Pentobarbital (or an adequate alternative anesthetic drug) may be administered (3–15 mg/kg IV q2–6h depending on response). It is not unusual to continue this level of sedation throughout the period that clinical signs are manifest. Alternatively, phenothiazines are especially helpful in controlling the hyperexcitable state. Chlorpromazine (0.5–2.0 mg/kg IV or PO q8–12h) may be used alone or with barbiturates. Narcotics are not indicated in the treatment of dogs with tetanus.
- Surgery. Careful evaluation and débridement of any obvious wound is indicated in patients with tetanus. The author has encountered cases in which dogs had become impaled on sticks, resulting in rapid-onset localized tetanus. Prompt removal of foreign material from infected wounds is clearly indicated and may result in rapid resolution of clinical signs.
- Supportive care. The most critical issue in managing any patient with tetanus is the time and ability to administer long-term supportive care. Affected patients must be maintained in an area where noise suppression is possible and soft bedding can be provided to prevent decubital sores. Oral hyperalimentation is necessary since most animals cannot prehend or swallow. Animals being tube fed are at risk of developing aspiration pneumonia. In addition, constant management of urine and feces to prevent contamination and irritation of skin is required. Patients with generalized tetanus are particularly susceptible to hyperthermia associated with muscle spasm. The ability to provide sedation and muscle relaxation over a 24-hour period, for as long as 2–4 weeks, is imperative. Hiatal hernia and megaesophagus have been reported in animals with tetanus. Further complications such as rhabdomyolysis-induced acute kidney injury, sepsis, and respiratory distress associated with laryngeal spasm are possible.

The prognosis for patients with tetanus is directly related to the degree of systemic involvement. Dogs with tetanus that is localized to a peripheral limb have a commensurately better prognosis than those with generalized tetanus. The extended duration of treatment and associated costs of that treatment may be significant limiting factors.

Prevention

Although tetanus toxoid is available, it is generally administered as treatment to those animals with acute-onset signs. The natural resistance of dogs and cats to tetanus does not justify routine vaccination.

Public health implications

Tetanus in dogs and cats is not a zoonotic disease.

VIRAL INFECTIONS

ADENOVIRUS-1 INFECTIONS (INFECTIOUS CANINE HEPATITIS)

Definition/overview

CAV-1, the cause of infectious canine hepatitis (ICH), is one of two adenoviruses capable of causing clinical illness in dogs; it has a worldwide distribution. CAV-1 is genetically distinct from CAV-2, one of the causative agents in the infectious tracheobronchitis complex. CAV-1 is a resilient virus capable of existing outside of the host, at room temperature, for periods of days to months.

Etiology

CAV-1 is transmitted among dogs, particularly among those under 1 year of age, by oronasal contamination. After replicating in the tonsils, regional lymph nodes, and lymphatics, viremia quickly develops. The virus principally targets liver and vascular endothelial cells, although the kidney and eye are typically affected as well. Although virus may persist in the kidney for several months post infection, urine contamination does not appear to be an important source of infection for susceptible dogs.

Pathophysiology

Subsequent to exposure, transient viremia is associated with rapid dissemination of the virus. The cytotoxic effects of the virus are most pronounced in the liver, kidney, and eye. There appears to be a good correlation between antibody titer and protection from infection. However, dogs determined to be immune to CAV-1 challenge are still considered susceptible to respiratory infection caused by CAV-2. On the other hand, dogs that are immune to CAV-2 are protected against CAV-1 infection. Pyelonephritis, chronic hepatitis, DIC, anterior uveitis, and corneal edema may be observed independently from other clinical signs.

Clinical presentation

Although CAV-1 has a worldwide distribution, confirmed CAV-1 infection is regarded as an uncommon to rare infection among dogs in the USA today. Although infections are most likely to occur in dogs younger than 1 year of age, the most severe infections occur in dogs from birth to 3 weeks of age. The disease rapidly progresses to death within hours following the onset of signs.

Initial clinical findings include fever, tachycardia, enlarged tonsils, coughing associated with bronchopneumonia, and cervical lymphadenopathy commonly associated with edema of the head and neck. Despite its name, ICH is not characteristically associated with icterus. Clouding of the cornea and evidence of anterior uveitis generally develop during clinical recovery.

Differential diagnosis

Poisoning, especially among fatal cases, pneumonia, lymphoma, sepsis, leptospirosis, and acute hepatitis associated with icterus.

Diagnosis

Leukopenia, with lymphopenia and neutropenia, and thrombocytopenia are characteristic hematologic findings in acutely infected dogs. Liver enzymes (ALT, AST, and serum AP) are variably increased during the acute viremic stage of the disease. Coagulation defects consistent with DIC are possible.

On postmortem examination, dogs that have died of acute ICH will typically manifest edema and hemorrhage of superficial lymph nodes and subcutaneous tissue, particularly in the area of the neck. Examination of the abdominal contents reveals petechiae, and ecchymotic hemorrhages are commonly seen on all serosal surfaces. The gallbladder is characteristically thickened and edematous. Icterus is uncommon. Ocular lesions characteristic of anterior uveitis and corneal opacification (edema) may also be present.

Diagnostic confirmation of the acutely infected dog is based on virus isolation. Since the kidney is the most persistent site of virus localization, CAV-1 is likely to be isolated from urine for at least 6 months following initial infection in dogs that survive the acute infection. Alternatively, cytologic examination of hepatic aspirates or impressions of hepatic biopsies are most likely to reveal the presence of inclusion bodies.

Management

Treatment/prognosis

Specific antiviral therapy is not available for ICH, therefore supportive treatment in the form of IV fluid therapy, management of DIC, and administration of IV glucose to counter the effects of hypoglycemia is indicated. Animals that recover from the acute phase of the disease are at some degree of risk for developing chronic hepatic fibrosis.

The prognosis for ICH in puppies is poor, since the virus can be spread through contact with infectious secretions, contaminated feeding utensils, or hands. The infection is readily transmitted to susceptible puppies following exposure.

Prevention

Commercially available CAV-2 vaccines, for parenteral administration only, are recommended for routine use in vaccination protocols (**Tables 21.3** and **21.4**). It should be noted that a CAV-2 vaccine is currently offered in combination with *B. bronchiseptica* and canine parainfluenza for intranasal (mucosal) administration. However, when administered by the intranasal route, CAV-2 vaccine provides protection against respiratory infections only and is not intended to protect against CAV-1.

Public health implications

Canine adenoviruses do not pose a risk to human health.

CANINE INFLUENZA

(See also Canine infectious respiratory disease.)

Definition/overview

Canine influenza is a highly contagious viral respiratory infection of dogs first described as a clinical disease in a racing Greyhound kennel in Florida in 2005. Mortality among infected dogs is low. While clinical infections have only recently been described, serologic studies suggest that canine infections may have been present for several years.

Etiology

It has been confirmed that canine influenza resulted from interspecies transmission of an entire equine influenza A (H3N8) virus (documented as a cause of equine respiratory disease for over 40 years) to the dog (i.e. the virus sequence corresponds with the H3 hemaglutinin and the N8 neuraminidase subtype). Sequence analyses of virus isolated from lung tissue of Greyhounds that died from hemorrhagic bronchopneumonia in 2003 indicated that viruses had infected Greyhounds prior to 2004. Further studies comparing the equine and canine influenza viruses have shown that only four amino acid changes differentiate the equine and canine viruses.

Pathophysiology

Following infection, canine influenza virus concentrates in epithelium of the lower respiratory tract, including the trachea and bronchi. Pulmonary edema and congestion develop, with subsequent suppurative (secondary bacterial) bronchopneumonia. Necrosis of epithelial cells lining the trachea and bronchial glands is reported. The virus may also cause lymphocytic or neutrophilic rhinitis. Viral shedding is limited to 7–10 days post infection.

Clinical presentation

In January 2005, an outbreak of respiratory disease occurred in 22 racing Greyhounds at a Florida racetrack. Two clinical syndromes were reported: a mild cough, with fever, lasting 10–14 days with subsequent recovery (14 dogs); and peracute death associated with extensive lower respiratory tract hemorrhage (eight dogs [36%]) involving the lungs, mediastinum, and pleural space. The incubation period in dogs is 2–5 days after exposure before clinical signs appear. Infected dogs may shed virus for 7–10 days from the initial day of clinical signs. Nearly 20% of infected dogs will not display clinical signs and these will become the silent shedders and spreaders of the infection. Histology of the lungs revealed suppurative bronchopneumonia as well as bronchiolitis and tracheitis. Since then sporadic reports of infection, predominantly from dogs housed in animal shelters, have occurred. At the time of writing, enzootic infections are not being reported.

Differential diagnosis

Apparently, many dogs with H3N8 infection are subclinical. Those that do develop clinical disease are most likely to present with signs consistent with infectious tracheobronchitis ('kennel cough'). More severely affected dogs could present with signs of pneumonia similar to those associated with CDV infection, deep mycoses, or bacterial pneumonia.

Diagnosis

No point-of-care rapid assay is available for the diagnosis of canine influenza. Because clinical signs are vague and easily confused with other causes of lower respiratory disease, clinical diagnosis of recent infection is predicated on documenting a ≥four-fold rise in antibody titer over a 2–4 week period. A single, positive titer only denotes prior exposure. PCR and antigen-capture ELISA tests are available, but samples must be collected during the 7–10 days following infection. Beyond that period, viral shedding likely to have ended.

Management

Treatment/prognosis

Treatment for dogs with a cough, with or without nasal discharge, entails isolation from other dogs for at least 7–10 days, exercise restriction until the cough subsides, and supportive antimicrobial therapy to prevent secondary bacterial respiratory infection. Intensive therapy is indicated for dogs with clinical pneumonia. Supplemental oxygen therapy is indicated, as is IV fluid and antimicrobial therapy. Combination antibiotic therapy (e.g. ampicillin + clindamycin) is indicated to provide maximum coverage against a wide range of opportunistic bacteria. The addition of a bronchodilator in patients with bacterial pneumonia is controversial. If available, methylxanthine bronchodilators such as extended release theophylline preparations (5–10 mg/kg PO q18–24h) have been advocated as needed. Nebulization and coupage are also recommended. However, effective nebulization requires use of equipment that will deliver water particles between 0.5 and 3.0 micrometers. Vaporizers and humidifiers are not adequate.

Prevention

Inactivated (killed) CIV vaccines are currently available. Vaccination does not prevent infection nor shedding of virus following exposure. However, vaccination will mitigate the severity of disease and decreases the period of virus shedding among exposed/infected dogs. Considering the relatively low prevalence of clinical disease, the need for administering vaccine will likely depend on defined risk of exposure. Dogs considered to be at greatest risk for exposure to CIV are those housed in animal shelters, boarding facilities, dog day-care centers, pet stores, and dog shows.

Public health implications

Although human influenza viruses have been recovered from dogs and cats, CIV is not considered to represent a threat to human health.

CANINE CORONAVIRUS

Definition/overview

Canine coronavirus (CCV) is a single-stranded RNA virus that has been associated with outbreaks of diarrhea in young dogs. Dogs of all ages are susceptible, but the clinical disease is more likely to become apparent in puppies under 6 weeks of age. Although CCV is highly contagious and capable of spreading rapidly among susceptible dogs, the overall incidence of disease is considered to be low. Furthermore, the severity of clinical signs is limited to mild, transient enteritis.

Etiology

CCV is transmitted among young dogs by the fecal–oral route; contamination of the environment is the primary source of exposure.

Pathophysiology

The virus penetrates enterocytes located on villus tips. The incubation period is 1–4 days.

Clinical presentation

A clinical diagnosis of CCV enteritis is based on a history of acute-onset diarrhea in young dogs, especially puppies (**Figure 21.7**). Feces are described as orange in color and malodorous, and may contain blood. Only in the most severe cases will dehydration and electrolyte imbalances follow. Infected dogs will occasionally develop vomiting. However, the clinical signs associated with CCV infection are especially difficult to distinguish from other causes of infectious enteritis (e.g. canine parvovirus [CPV]).

Differential diagnosis

CCV infection can mimic several causes of mild enteritis of puppies associated with soft stool (e.g. intestinal parasites, dietary indiscretion, and food intolerance). Canine rotavirus is a reasonable differential diagnosis, although confirmation of infection is difficult to establish. Any puppy with acute-onset diarrhea, with or without vomiting, should be evaluated for CPV infection. Affected puppies should be examined for the presence of intussusception.

Diagnosis

Confirmation of CCV infection is based on isolation of the virus in fresh feces or visual evidence of virus using electron microscopy. Such testing is limited to experienced laboratories capable of performing these tests. On histopathology, small intestinal lesions of CCV infection

21.7

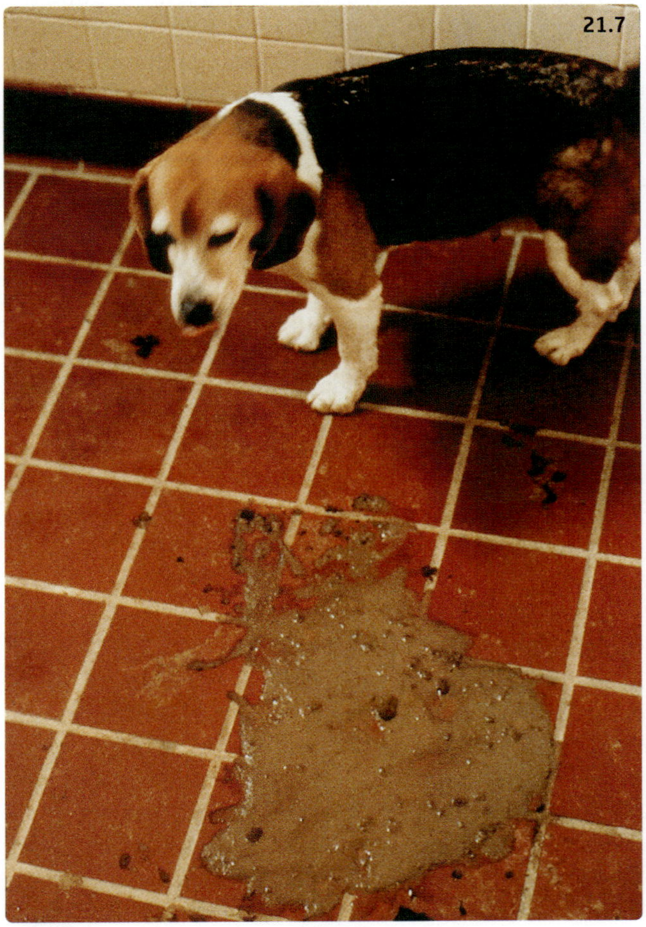

Figure 21.7 Diarrhea is a common sign of canine coronavirus infection. (Courtesy Pfizer Ltd.)

are classically described as atrophy and fusion of intestinal villi, with deepening of the intestinal crypt. Recently, PCR testing has become commercially available to private practices. However, considering that CCV is such a minor pathogen in the spectrum of agents causing infectious diarrhea in dogs, the value of diagnostic test results may not be relevant.

Management

Treatment/prognosis

Supportive therapy is the mainstay of treatment. CCV infection inconsistently causes clinical disease. When present, disease is typically mild and self-limiting. In the worst cases, electrolyte and fluid replacement is indicated to counter the effects of fluid loss and dehydration, acidosis, and rarely shock. In most cases, therapeutic intervention is not required. The prognosis for recovery without treatment is excellent.

Prevention

Although both killed and modified live CCV vaccines are currently available, their effectiveness in preventing disease in dogs has been questioned. Parenterally administered vaccines do not eliminate replication of CCV in the intestine subsequent to challenge. Furthermore, the value of vaccinating adult animals is limited by the fact that natural resistance to the disease occurs with age. Since 2003, canine vaccination guidelines have recommended against the routine use of coronavirus vaccine in pet dogs as well as dogs housed in shelters.

Public health implications

CCV is not zoonotic.

CANINE ORAL PAPILLOMA INFECTION (PAPILLOMATOSIS)

(See also Chapter 18: Dermatologic disorders.)

Definition/overview

The canine oral papillomavirus (COPV) is a large DNA virus unique to the dog. Although humans, cattle, and even cats have been reported with viral papillomas, viruses belonging to this family are considered to be species specific. COPV is associated with the development of benign, transmissible tumors involving the head, oral cavity, and eyelids. Dogs 2 years of age and younger appear to be most susceptible. There is no sex or breed predilection. Malignant transformation of papillomavirus-induced tumors is extremely rare.

Etiology

Canine papillomatosis is a benign mucocutaneous tumor caused by infectious papillomavirus. The highly species-specific virus is responsible for the development of large papillomas (also called warts or verruca vulgaris) in and around the mouth. The virus is transmissible to other dogs.

Pathophysiology

The tumors induced by COPV are the result of infection of the basal cells of the stratum germinativum, which leads to acanthosis and hyperkeratosis. The incubation period ranges from 4–8 weeks following infection. Tumors typically persist for 1–5 months, after which they undergo spontaneous regresssion.

Clinical presentation

Diagnosis of infectious papillomatosis is based on physical examination findings and the clinical history. The disease is most likely to occur in young dogs, while the tissues most likely to be affected are the oral mucosa, labial margins, and tongue (**Figure 21.8**). Less commonly affected are the palate, pharynx, epiglottis, and esophagus. Alternatively, individual eyelid papillomas may develop on the margin of the eyelids of one or both eyes. Associated signs include halitosis, hypersalivation, minor bleeding of affected tissue, and discomfort. Trauma to proliferating tumors caused by toenails and teeth may actually serve to spread the tumors within and around the oral cavity. Secondary oral ulceration and infection may develop. Dogs experiencing high tumor concentration or a particularly large tumor may find it difficult or painful to eat and, consequently, become malnourished.

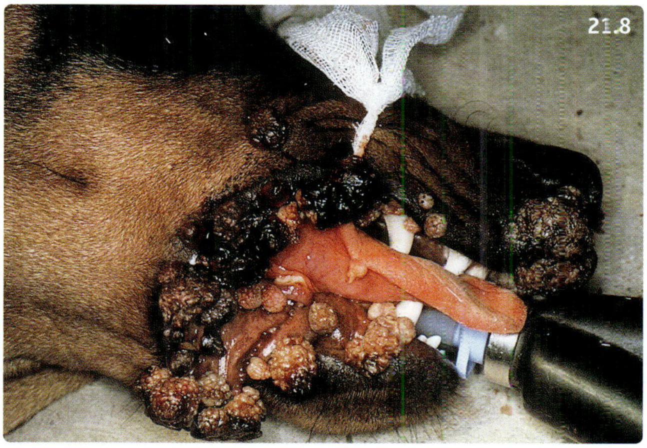

Figure 21.8 Advanced viral oral papillomatosis in a young Dobermann.

Differential diagnosis

Benign and malignant oral neoplasms (e.g. epulides, fibroma, hemangioma, hemangiopericytoma, and histiocytoma).

Diagnosis

Diagnostic confirmation of papillomatosis is based on biopsy and gross appearance of these benign tumors.

Management

Treatment/prognosis

In most cases the virus-induced tumor burden is not sufficiently large to warrant treatment. Spontaneous regression of tumors is common by 1–5 months following their initial appearance. It is not known why these tumors spontaneously regress or how they spread. Occasionally, surgical excision, cryosurgery, or electrosurgery is indicated to remove large oral tumors. It has been reported that simply crushing 5–15 of the tumors may provoke spontaneous regression and, thereby, shorten the course of disease. The use of systemic and lesional or intralesional treatment with chemotherapeutic agents has not been uniformly effective in dogs. The prognosis for recovery is excellent without specific therapeutic intervention.

Prevention

There is currently no licensed biological agent for use in dogs to prevent canine viral papillomatosis. Experimentally, a recombinant vaccine has demonstrated protection against viral challenge, but prospects for a commercial vaccine are unknown. Most dogs develop natural resistance to infection by 2 years of age.

Public health implications

COPV is unique to the dog and, as such, presents no risk to human health.

CANINE DISTEMPER VIRUS (DISTEMPER, 'HARD-PAD DISEASE')

Definition/overview

CDV, recognized worldwide, is a single-stranded RNA virus that belongs to the genus *Morbillivirus*. The virus is relatively unstable at room temperature. It is especially susceptible to ultraviolet light, drying, and temperatures >50–60°C (122–140°F). At freezing temperatures the virus is reported to survive for several weeks. Most routine disinfection procedures effectively destroy CDV.

Etiology

Animals infected with CDV readily transmit the disease through infectious microdroplets or, less often, by aerosol. Among vaccinated populations, CDV is particularly rare. In unvaccinated populations, however, CDV poses a significant health threat, particularly to dogs between 3 and 6 months of age as maternal antibody concentration wanes. Unvaccinated dogs of all ages are susceptible.

Pathophysiology

The initial infection of CDV begins as the virus invades the epithelium of the upper respiratory tract. The virus spreads quickly to local lymphatics, tonsils, and bronchial lymph nodes. Subsequently, CDV spreads to epithelial and CNS tissues within the first week of infection. The humoral immune response following infection correlates with clearance of the virus. Dogs that recover from acute CDV infection are likely to derive several years of immunity as a result. Dogs that fail to mount a significant immune response experience rapid spread of the virus to the skin, the exocrine and endocrine glands, and the GI, respiratory, and genitourinary tracts.

Clinical presentation

Clinical signs of CDV infection range from mild to severe, depending on virus strain, environmental factors, and the individual patient's response to the infection. Clinical signs may be limited to the upper respiratory tract, therefore coughing and nasal discharge may be present. Unvaccinated puppies are most susceptible to severe systemic signs such as pneumonia, diarrhea, dehydration, and anorexia. Vomiting is a common finding in the early stages of infection. If complicated by the presence of intestinal parasites, puppies may develop intussusception.

Neurologic signs typically begin 1–3 weeks following recovery from the acute illness. Neurologic signs associated with CDV infection are characteristically progressive, resulting in rapid deterioration (**Figure 21.9**). Patients that survive the neurologic disease may experience permanent complications (seizures, vestibular disease, tetraparesis, and myoclonus). Enamel hypoplasia (**Figure 21.10**) may develop if CDV infection occurs prior to the eruption of permanent teeth.

Additional clinical signs include anterior uveitis and optic neuritis (associated with sudden-onset blindness), as well as retinal degeneration and necrosis involving both the tapetal and nontapetal fundus. On funduscopic examination, chronic inactive retinal lesions are seen as hyperreflective areas in the tapetum, often called 'gold medallion lesions' (**Figure 21.11**). CDV infection in young

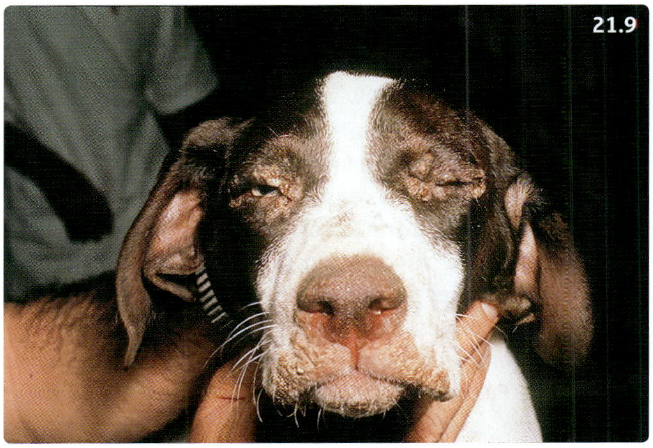

Figure 21.9 A 3-year-old unvaccinated Pointer presented with acute-onset seizures followed by progressive neurologic signs and eventual coma.

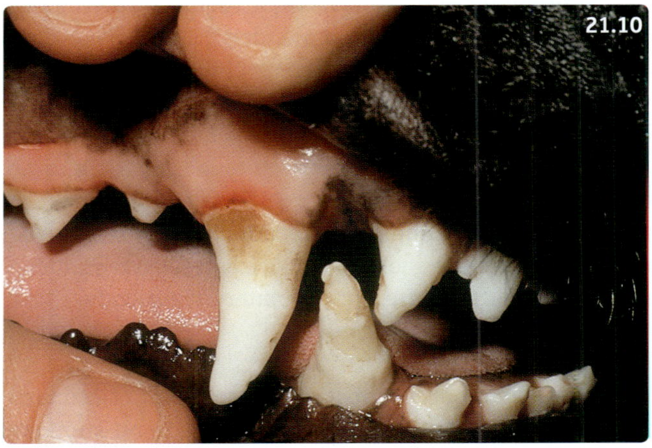

Figure 21.10 Enamel hypoplasia in a 1-year-old dog that recovered from CDV infection at 3–4 months of age.

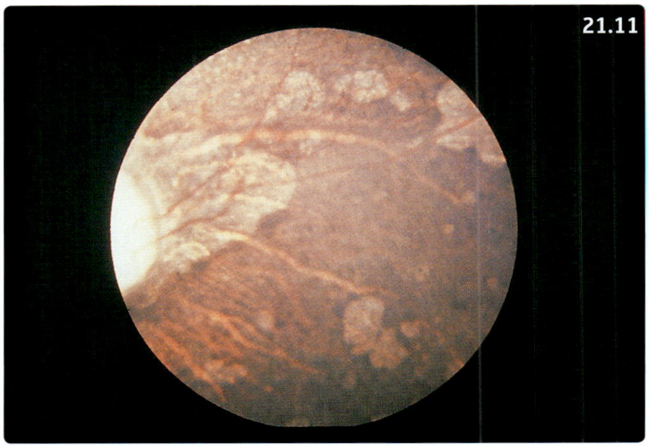

Figure 21.11 Hyperreflective tapetum in a dog that recovered from CDV infection.

dogs has been associated with metaphyseal osteosclerosis of the long bones. CDV RNA transcripts have been identified in bone lesions of dogs with hypertrophic osteodystrophy (HOD). These finding have raised concern over the association between HOD and the use of modified live virus (MLV) distemper vaccines.

The absence of a reliable antemortem test for CDV dictates that a clinical diagnosis be predicated on the basis of clinical signs and history. Dogs with severe illness have the most characteristic clinical features of CDV infection. However, mild clinical illness caused by CDV may be limited to respiratory or ocular disease, making a clinical diagnosis of distemper difficult.

Differential diagnosis

While a rare disease among vaccinated dogs, canine distemper is associated with a complex array of clinical signs, depending on the individual animal. Alternative diseases to consider include, most importantly, rabies, pneumonia (a common secondary event), *B. bronchiseptica* infection, idiopathic epilepsy, hypoglycemia, CNS trauma, and renal failure.

Diagnosis

Hematologic changes described in experimental CDV infection, including lymphopenia, thrombocytopenia, and regenerative anemia, are not consistently seen in clinical cases. Occasionally during acute infections it is possible to demonstrate distemper inclusions in stained peripheral blood smears (especially lymphocytes and, occasionally, granulocytes) (**Figure 21.12**). Examination of buffy coat smears and bone marrow aspirates may increase the chances of detecting inclusions. In

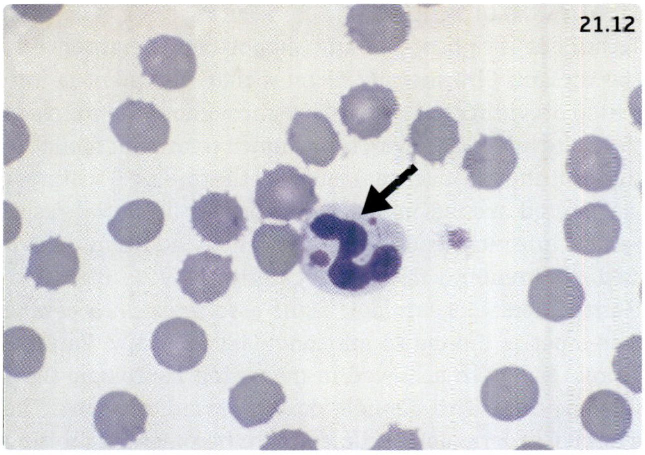

Figure 21.12 Distemper inclusion body (arrow) in a peripheral blood neutrophil collected from a dog with acute CDV infection.

addition, inclusion bodies may be identified in cytologic preparations of conjunctival epithelium. (**Note:** CDV inclusions are best elucidated in blood films stained with a quick Romanowski-type stain [e.g. Diff-Quik®]. Inclusion bodies in blood films stained with conventional Wright's stain may not be visible.)

Examination of CSF may reveal an increased intracranial pressure causing a rapid flow rate of CSF, increased protein concentration (>0.25 g/l [25 mg/dl]), and lymphocytes. These changes are characteristic of, but not unique to, CDV encephalomyelitis. Distemper-specific IgG in the CSF may be used to diagnose CDV infection. Vaccine-induced CDV antibody is not normally detected in CSF.

Although other diagnostic tests for CDV infection have been described (immunocytology, the use of ELISA to detect serum IgG and IgM antibodies, and virus isolation), special facilities and sample preparation are required. Within households where CDV infection is suspected and other dogs are at risk, postmortem examination is the most effective means of confirming CDV infection. Emphasis should be placed on evaluation of the white matter in both the cerebrum and cerebellum.

Real-time PCR technology is commercially available for the detection of CDV RNA. Samples can be submitted as whole blood, serum, pharyngeal swabs, or CSF. Results may be available within 1–3 days. However, it is important to understand that the exceptional sensitivity of PCR technology may limit the diagnostic value of the assay. Dogs recently vaccinated (MLV vaccine) may have false-positive test results. Also, there is concern that, at least in some dogs able to overcome infection, the RNA detected may not define live, replicating (or infectious) virulent virus.

Management

Treatment/prognosis

Treatment is nonspecific and supportive. The absence of specific anti-CDV therapy dictates that treatment is limited to providing supportive care throughout the course of the acute infection. There is no known treatment modality that will alter the eventual course of the disease. Treatment is centered around managing secondary bacterial respiratory infection and conjunctivitis. In addition, provision of parenteral fluids and calories may be indicated. Management of neurologic signs associated with canine distemper is limited to anticonvulsant therapy. Variable success has been achieved in managing neurologic signs in some dogs with a single dose of dexamethasone. The extent of progression of clinical signs becomes the limiting factor in the prognosis of dogs with CDV infection. Once neurologic signs become evident, the prognosis is commensurately poor and euthanasia is frequently justified.

Prevention

Highly effective modified live and recombinant (canarypox vectored) CDV vaccines are available. These products have an excellent safety record and are considered to be highly efficacious. While most manufacturers recommend three doses of vaccine between 6 and 16 weeks of age, the duration of immunity (DOI) following the initial booster vaccination (1 year following the last of the initial series inoculations) has been documented to persist for at least 5 years. Current guidelines recommend triennial administration of booster vaccine in adult dogs. Furthermore, dogs recovering from natural infection are expected to be immune for several years. Rarely, dogs vaccinated with the Rockborn strain of CDV have been reported to develop post-vaccinal encephalitis. Furthermore, postvaccinal encephalitis has been reported in neonatal puppies subsequent to the vaccination of pregnant dogs at or near parturition. Vaccination of pregnant dogs is not recommended.

Earlier concerns that concurrent CPV vaccine and CDV would predispose vaccinated dogs to encephalitis have not been substantiated. Currently, there is no established risk to administering both antigens simultaneously to the same dog. In high-risk environments such as animal shelters, administration of a single dose of recombinant CDV vaccine to puppies has been shown to induce a protective immune response despite the presence of maternal antibody.

Public health implications

Despite older reports that multiple sclerosis of humans might be linked to CDV exposure, there is no supporting documentation for either measles or distemper virus involvement in human multiple sclerosis. CDV infection is not considered to be zoonotic.

CANINE PARVOVIRUS INFECTION

(See also Chapter 8: Digestive diseases [pharynx to anorectum].)

Definition/overview

CPV was first recognized in the late 1970s as a truly new virus infection of dogs capable of causing rapid-onset, severe viral enteritis and, in young dogs, myocarditis. CPV is a small DNA virus that reproduces best in rapidly dividing cells such as the myocardium of puppies and intestinal epithelium. The virus is resilient and may remain on clothing, floors, and utensils for periods of 5 months or longer. The virus is particularly resistant to detergents and most disinfectants. Sodium hypochlorite (one part household bleach to 30 parts water) is an effective disinfectant providing prolonged contact with contaminated surfaces can be achieved.

CPV enteritis is among the most common, highly contagious diseases of dogs. Since clinical infections first became apparent, genetic alterations in the dog have resulted in new viral strains. Today, in the USA and Japan, the CPV-2b strain of CPV predominates. In Europe and the Far East, both CPV-2a and CPV-2b are known to infect dogs.

Etiology

The transmission of CPV to susceptible dogs occurs by way of oronasal exposure, usually with contaminated feces. Subsequent to the initial viremia, CPV localizes in the epithelium of the small intestine, the tongue, and the oral and esophageal mucosae, as well as in lymphoid tissues including the bone marrow. Virus has been isolated from lungs, spleen, liver, kidney, and myocardium. Clinical signs of infection are related to the actual tissues affected. In the clinical setting, enteritis and myocarditis (in young dogs) predominate.

Pathophysiology

The virus replicates in the lymphoid tissue of the oropharynx, thymus, and mesenteric lymph nodes, from where it disseminates to the intestinal crypts of the small intestine. Viremia, lasting 1–5 days after infection, is followed by localization of the virus, mainly in the epithelium lining the oral cavity, tongue, esophagus, small intestine, and lymphoid tissue.

Clinical presentation

Clinical signs associated with CPV infection in dogs are highly variable and may range from inapparent infection to acute fatal disease. Most dogs, subsequent to exposure, develop subclinical infection and recover without showing significant clinical disease. The most severely affected dogs are younger than 12 weeks of age.

Vomiting, diarrhea (frequently associated with blood), anorexia, and dehydration characterize acute CPV enteritis. Alternatively, CPV myocarditis can develop in puppies younger than 8 weeks of age (**Figure 21.13**). Today, puppies with myocardial disease associated with CPV infection are rare. Affected dogs are either found dead or die following a brief episode of discomfort and dyspnea. Examination of the heart and lungs reveals cardiomegaly and pulmonary edema. CPV myocarditis can occur in the absence of enteritis. Hypercoagulability and thrombosis formation are reported in dogs with naturally occurring CPV infection.

Differential diagnosis

The clinical signs associated with enteric CPV infection are not unique. Affected dogs should also be evaluated for intussusception, intestinal obstruction (foreign body), acute-onset manifestation of chronic kidney disease, poisoning or toxicity, intestinal parasitism, and hypoadrenocorticism (Addison's disease).

Diagnosis

In the clinical setting, a diagnosis of CPV infection is based on clinical signs, hematology, and point-of-care test platforms capable of detecting CPV antigen in feces. In the acute disease, profound leukopenia and lymphopenia will develop within 7–10 days following exposure. Severe diarrhea may be associated with gram-negative sepsis.

All young dogs presented with acute-onset diarrhea should be evaluated using an ELISA fecal antigen test. Although these tests are highly specific (few false-positive results), the period during which parvovirus can be detected in feces appears limited. A negative test result does not necessarily rule out CPV infection.

Pathologic confirmation of CPV infection is based on histologic evaluation of the distal duodenum and jejunum. Necrosis of crypt epithelium characterizes the lesion. The myocardium, especially the ventricles, should be evaluated for nonsuppurative myocarditis, with infiltrates of lymphocytes and plasma cells evaluated in puppies that die of acute respiratory distress.

Management

Treatment/prognosis

IV replacement of fluid and electrolytes is the principal goal of treatment in dogs with CPV enteritis. Antimicrobial agents (e.g. ampicillin, 10–20 mg/kg IV q6–8h daily for 5 days) are indicated. Alternatively, enrofloxacin (5 mg/kg PO q24h) can be given to dogs older than 6 months of age. The use of motility modifiers in the treatment of

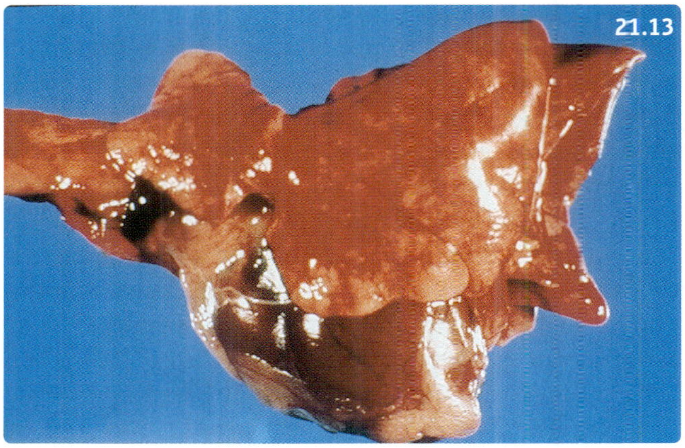

Figure 21.13 Viral myocarditis in conjunction with CPV in dogs is associated with ventricular arrhythmias, congestive heart failure, pulmonary edema, and death.

dogs with CPV enteritis is controversial. Metoclopramide (0.2–0.4 mg/kg SC q8h) can be given as needed to control vomiting. Narcotic antispasmodics (e.g. diphenoxylate HCl) can be administered but are generally not recommended. The administration of human recombinant granulocyte-colony stimulating factor (G-CSF) has been recommended in treating panleukopenic patients. The dosage of G-CSF ranges from 5 to 100 mg/kg SC q24h for not longer than 3 weeks. As a general recommendation, food should be withheld for 1–2 days following the cessation of vomiting. Small amounts of water are introduced, followed by the introduction of a highly digestible, low-fat diet.

The prognosis for recovery from CPV infection following the first 7 days of enteritis is good to excellent in the absence of secondary complications (e.g. sepsis). The prognosis of puppies with CPV-induced myocarditis is poor to grave.

Prevention

The immunity derived subsequent to recovery from natural infection is reported to be a minimum of 20 months and possibly for life. There is a strong correlation between serum antibody titer and protection.

Today, all CVP vaccines are attenuated (modified live) virus and provide excellent immunity in most dogs (**Table 21.4**). Current vaccination recommendations are the same as those for CDV. Three doses of vaccine are recommended between 6 and 16 weeks of age. A booster dose is administered 1 year later, then every 3 years thereafter.

There are several potential reasons for vaccinated dogs to remain susceptible to infection; maternally derived antibody interference with vaccination in young dogs and genetically predisposed non- and low-responders (to vaccination) are among the most important. Subsequent to vaccination, transient lymphopenia (4–6 days) and shedding of vaccine virus are possible. Dogs tested with the ELISA fecal antigen test may actually have a transiently positive test result during the time of vaccine virus shedding. Although annual vaccination is recommended for adult dogs, there is evidence to support the fact that the DOI subsequent to the first booster vaccination persists for 3 years or longer.

During the initial enzootic of CPV infection in the USA (late 1970s and early 1980s), the incidence of infection in Dobermanns and Rottweilers appeared to be significantly greater than in other breeds. The reason behind this increased susceptibility is based on the fact these breeds (or lines within these breeds) were genetic non-responders. It is generally agreed today that Dobermanns and Rottweilers do not have significantly greater risk than other breeds.

Public health implications

CPV is not zoonotic and poses no threat to human health.

CANINE RABIES

(See also Chapter 14: Disorders of the nervous system and muscle.)

Definition/overview

With descriptions of 'mad dogs' dating back to the 23rd century BC, rabies is regarded as one of the oldest infectious diseases known to infect humans and animals. The disease is caused by a fragile, enveloped RNA virus of the family Rhabdoviridae. While clinical rabies virus infection is considered to be uniformly fatal, conventional disinfectants, ultraviolet light, and heat easily destroy rabies virus.

Etiology

Several routes of transmission have been documented. Inoculation of infectious saliva into a susceptible animal through a bite wound is the most common means of rabies transmission. Airborne transmission and transplacental rabies infection have been documented in some species; however, these are not uniformly important in the transmission of rabies to companion animals. The incidence of dog and cat rabies correlates with the incidence of wildlife rabies. Furthermore, the frequency of human rabies exposures associated with rabid cats is increasing at a greater rate than that of dogs.

The vectors for rabies vary throughout the world and include dogs, skunks, red and Arctic foxes, raccoons, bats, cats, wolves, mongooses, jackals, and cows. In North America, rabies infection has been sustained within a variety of wildlife reservoirs. Skunks, coyotes, raccoons, and foxes comprise the majority of wildlife carnivores known to harbor the rabies virus. Although a small percentage of bats throughout the USA are known to carry rabies virus, bat rabies has been primarily implicated in human infections for the past several decades. Bats have only rarely been implicated in transmitting infection or infectious virus to cats and dogs.

Rodents, rabbits, and hares are uncommonly affected with rabies, and no human cases of rabies have ever been associated with these species. Bite wounds to humans by any of these species are not routinely regarded as rabies exposure.

Pathophysiology

Clinical rabies has been conventionally classified into two major types: furious ('mad' or hyperexcitable, or psychotic) and paralytic ('dumb' rabies). However, the clinical signs of rabies are highly variable and do not necessarily fit into one classification. The usual incubation period following exposure in dogs is 3–8 weeks; incubation periods as long as 6 months have been reported.

Clinical presentation

Initially, dogs will manifest signs of nervousness, anxiety, and seeking solitude. If a bite wound is present, most animals will demonstrate irritation and pruritus at the site of viral entry. Dogs typically manifest clinical illness for 1–10 days following the onset of signs. Dogs with furious rabies become progressively restless and demonstrate hyperexcitability in response to auditory and visual stimuli. They may bite at imaginary objects or develop pica. In the terminal phase, progressive disorientation and grand mal seizures develop.

Progressive lower motor neuron paralysis or cranial nerve deficits are the first recognizable signs in dogs with paralytic ('dumb') rabies (**Figure 21.14**). The dog may be observed to have a change in the tone of the bark associated with laryngeal paralysis. Excess salivation and dysphagia are seen in conjunction with a so-called 'drop jaw'. The appearance of choking prompts owners/veterinarians to attempt to remove a foreign body from the oral cavity, resulting in significant exposure to infectious saliva. Once paralysis develops, death follows from respiratory failure within 2–4 days.

Differential diagnosis

Rabies is a principal differential diagnosis in any dog with an acute-onset neurologic disorder associated with behavior change, particularly among dogs that do not have a vaccination history. Other diseases that present with signs similar to rabies include CDV infection and other causes of encephalitis, sepsis, tetanus, botulism, and intracranial neoplasia.

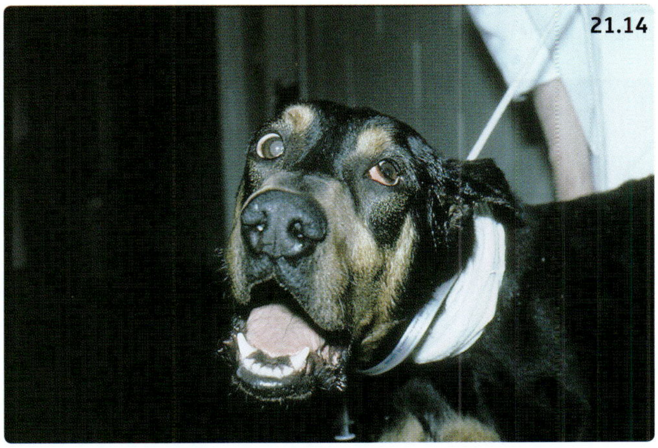

Figure 21.14 Progressive lower motor neuron paralysis with cranial nerve deficits similar to those shown here can be early signs of 'dumb' rabies in the dog. (Courtesy M. Schaer)

Diagnosis

A diagnosis of rabies may be presumed on the basis of clinical signs. The fact that other infectious diseases (e.g. CDV infection or idiopathic epilepsy) may manifest indistinguishable clinical signs justifies including rabies as a differential diagnosis in any animal with unexplainable neurologic or behavioral signs. There is no antemortem diagnostic test considered sufficiently accurate to confirm rabies infection.

Direct IFA testing of nervous tissue is the most common method utilized today to confirm rabies infection. Because this method requires thin touch impressions of the brain and cerebellum, severely traumatized or decomposed tissues may invalidate this test. Prompt, proper handling of specimens is critical for ensuring an accurate diagnosis.

A number of other diagnostic methods have been described. PCR testing of nervous system tissue, histologic identification of Negri bodies (intracytoplasmic inclusions), and mouse inoculation are still available, but are less sensitive than direct IFA testing of nervous tissue.

The head (or body) of an animal suspected of having rabies should be chilled on wet ice or refrigerated as soon after death or euthanasia as possible. The tissue must not be frozen. If it is necessary to ship the head (or body), it is recommended that approved shipping containers available from public health or animal control officials are utilized. If it does become necessary to remove the head of a suspect animal, extreme care should be taken to avoid direct contact with any body fluids or tissues (especially brain tissue).

Management

Treatment/prognosis

No attempt should be made to provide primary care for a dog or cat suspected of having rabies. In dogs, cats, and humans, rabies is regarded as a uniformly fatal disease.

Prevention

Only killed (inactivated) virus vaccines are currently available for use in dogs. Administering rabies vaccine in accordance with state and local statutes is recommended for all dogs. The first dose of vaccine may be given as early as 12 weeks of age. Regardless of age at the time of initial inoculation, all dogs should be boosted with a single dose of rabies vaccine at 1 year following the initial dose. Booster vaccinations should be given every year or every 3 years thereafter depending on local statutes and manufacturer recommendations. General recommendations for vaccinating dogs against rabies are outlined in **Table 21.4**. Where required, veterinarians are expected to follow state, provincial, or local law. Serologic testing can be done to establish an individual dog's response to vaccination. Such testing may be required prior to shipment of dogs to rabies-free countries or regions of the world. **Important:** A rabies antibody titer is not a legal index of immunity in lieu of vaccination.

Public health implications

Virtually all strains of rabies virus can infect humans. Humans exposed to infectious saliva of any rabid animal are considered to be at risk of developing rabies. However, determining whether or not 'exposure' has actually occurred can be difficult and is typically determined by criteria established by state or local health departments. In many locations, human and animal exposure is defined in law.

The ability to specifically identify and capture the animal involved, knowledge of any contact with saliva, knowledge of whether the attack was provoked or unprovoked, and knowledge of rabies prevalence in the geographic area are criteria that are commonly taken into consideration prior to recommending post-exposure immunoprophylaxis of humans. In any event, a bite wound from any domestic or wild animal should be treated aggressively by washing thoroughly as soon after the exposure as possible. Irrigation of the wound with large quantities of a 20% aqueous soap solution or quaternary ammonium solution (e.g. benzalkonium chloride) is recommended. Ethanol in concentrations of 43% or higher can be applied to open wounds. Post-exposure immunoprophylaxis in humans consists of the administration of human rabies immunoglobulin and human diploid cell vaccine.

FUNGAL, RICKETTSIAL, AND PROTOZOAL INFECTIONS

EHRLICHIOSIS AND ANAPLASMOSIS

(See also Chapter 16: Hematologic disorders, and Chapter 19: Ocular manifestations of systemic diseases.)

Definition/overview

Ehrlichiosis is a tick-borne systemic disease that occurs worldwide and is known to be caused by a variety of rickettsial species in the genus *Ehrlichia* (reclassified in 2001). Several species of *Ehrlichia* are known to infect the dog, although *Ehrlichia canis*, the cause of canine monocytotropic ehrlichiosis, is the most common cause of the disease in dogs. Variations of the clinical disease (e.g. granulocytotropic ehrlichiosis [*Ehrlichia ewingi*] and infectious canine cyclic thrombocytopenia) have been recognized and are associated with different species of *Ehrlichia*.

Anaplasmosis, another tick-borne systemic disease, is known to cause a spectrum of clinical signs similar to that of ehrlichiosis. *Anaplasma phagocytophilum* (formerly *Ehrlichia equi*), the cause of canine granulocytotropic anaplasmosis, is likely to produce the most common form of clinical anaplasmosis in dogs.

Etiology

The brown dog tick *Rhipicephalus sanguineus* is the arthropod vector of *E. canis* (**Figure 21.15**). Although vector ticks do not serve as reservoirs of infection, they are able to harbor infectious organisms for over 1 year and can transmit the infection to susceptible dogs for at least 155 days following infection.

A. phagocytophilum is a gram-negative obligate intracellular parasite. Subsequent to the reclassification of ehrlichiae, the term 'granulocytic ehrlichiosis' has been replaced with granulocytotropic anaplasmosis. Occurrence of infection follows the distribution of *Ixodes* spp. tick vectors, and is similar to that of canine Lyme borreliosis.

Pathophysiology

Canine monocytotropic ehrlichiosis is characterized by a reduction in cellular blood elements. *E. canis* is characterized by three distinct phases of infection: acute (weeks), subclinical (months to years), and chronic (months). During the acute phase the organism multiplies within circulating mononuclear cells and the mononuclear phagocytic tissues of the liver, spleen, and lymph nodes. Infected cells are transported in the blood to other tissues, particularly meninges, lung, and kidney, where

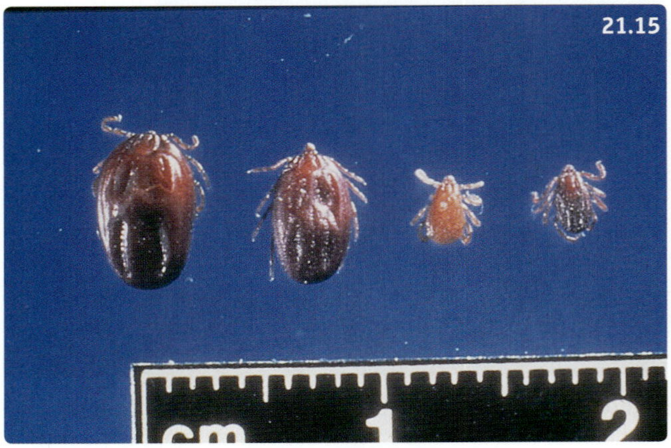

Figure 21.15 The nymphal and adult life stages of the brown dog tick *Rhipicephalus sanguineus*. (Courtesy D.J. Meyer)

they attach to the vascular endothelium, causing vasculitis and infection of the subendothelial tissue. During this phase thrombocytopenia develops subsequent to platelet consumption, sequestration, and destruction. Anemia develops progressively owing to suppression of erythropoiesis and accelerated destruction of erythrocytes. During the subclinical phase there is variable persistence of the thrombocytopenia, leukopenia, and anemia. Chronic disease occurs in those dogs unable to mount an effective immune response to the organism.

The actual mechanism whereby *A. phagocytophilum* causes clinical disease is unknown. The bacteria enter neutrophils by endocytosis, where they become incorporated into phagosomes. Morulae are formed within the phagosome subsequent to replication. Infection occurs only after an extended feeding time by the *Ixodes* tick lasting at least 24–48 hours. Clinical signs develop 1–2 weeks following infection. Acute and chronic phases of infection are described.

Clinical presentation

Classically, canine monocytotropic ehrlichiosis is categorized into three phases. The acute phase begins following a 1–3-week incubation period and lasts for 2–4 weeks. Clinical signs of illness are varied and include fever, nasal discharge, decreased appetite, weight loss, and lymphadenomegaly. Clinical signs typically resolve spontaneously. During the subclinical phase, at 40–120 days post infection, clinical signs are absent, although the infection is still established. The subclinical phase can persist for several years. In some dogs a chronic phase of infection will develop and is characterized by either vague signs of illness or more severe hematologic impairment associated with bone marrow suppression. Profound pancytopenia may develop. Spontaneous bleeding, characterized as dermal petechiae or ecchymoses, is common. Epistaxis is most frequently reported by owners. In other cases, profound neurologic signs such as seizures, ataxia, vestibular dysfunction, and anisocoria, as well as hyperesthesia, have been observed.

The spectrum of clinical signs associated with ehrlichiosis is further complicated by the fact that they can vary dramatically depending on the species involved. Clinical findings range from polyarthritis associated with immune complex arthritis or hemarthrosis, to atrophy of skeletal muscles, enlarged peripheral lymph nodes, edema, and lethargy.

Clinical signs associated with granulocytotropic anaplasmosis are vague and indistinct. It is currently not known whether all infections lead to the development of clinical signs. Most dogs are reported to develop fever and lethargy, with associated anorexia. Generalized, nonlocalizing pain is described in most dogs. Dogs may appear weak, stiff, or lame. Discrete joint pain is uncommon. Thrombocytopenia and granulocytopenia are spontaneous and are not part of the clinical presentation. Immunity from natural infection appears short-lived and reinfection is possible.

Differential diagnosis

Immune-mediated thrombocytopenia is an important differential diagnosis to consider when evaluating a patient suspected of having ehrlichiosis, but not granulocytotropic anaplasmosis. Affected dogs may also have concurrent immune-mediated hemolytic anemia. The presence of other clinical signs (neurologic signs, peripheral limb edema) and laboratory findings (leukopenia) significantly expands the list of differential diagnoses. Dogs with granulocytotropic anaplasmosis may appear to have Lyme borreliosis, toxoplasmosis (myositis), systemic lupus erythematosus, bacteremia/sepsis, or any of a multitude of system disorders.

Diagnosis

In the clinical setting, a diagnosis of ehrlichiosis is usually made on the basis of clinical signs, hematologic abnormalities, and serology. It has been suggested that infections are more common among German Shepherd Dogs. Nonregenerative anemia and thrombocytopenia are the predominant hematologic findings. Approximately one-third of affected dogs will manifest leukopenia. Pancytopenia is a less common finding and is more likely to occur in the chronic phase of disease. Pancytopenia is reported to occur more often in German Shepherd Dogs. Although thrombocytopenia is consistently reported in all stages of ehrlichiosis, the absence of thrombocytopenia cannot be used to rule out the infection. Serologic confirmation of ehrlichiosis is based on the results of an indirect IFA test. Antibody may be detected in serum as early as 7 days following the initial infection. However, some dogs may not seroconvert until 28 days post infection. Depending on the laboratory and methodology used, a single titer may be used to establish infection/exposure. It should be noted that infection cannot be confirmed by the presence of a single 'positive' antibody titer alone. Clinical signs and laboratory findings must be considered in the light of serology results. Following treatment, antibody titers may decline in 6–9 months. In other dogs, titers are sustained for several years despite the absence of clinical signs. A canine rapid assay (ELISA) test is available as a point-of-care test for *E. canis* antibody (Snap 3Dx® and Snap 4Dx®). While the test has high sensitivity and specificity for detecting antibody, a positive test result confirms exposure, not infection. Test results must be considered in the light of the patient's clinical presentation.

Among dogs that have died of ehrlichiosis, histopathologic findings include perivascular plasma cell infiltrates in several organs (e.g. lung, brain, kidney, lymph node, bone marrow, and spleen). Morulae (intracytoplasmic inclusions) are rare but have been observed in mononuclear phagocytic cells and bone marrow (**Figure 21.16**).

Diagnosis of canine granulocytotropic anaplasmosis has generally been limited to those cases in which morulae can be visualized. Recently, a canine rapid assay (ELISA) test has become available in the USA for the detection of antibody to *Anaplasma* (Snap 4Dx®). A positive test result for *Anaplasma* antibody does not confirm the infection. Clinicians must consider the clinical signs along with test results before initiating treatment.

Management

Treatment/prognosis

Although several inexpensive drugs are available, the success of treatment of ehrlichiosis is generally dependent on the severity of disease and the ability to treat early in the course of infection. Dogs with chronic ehrlichiosis are particularly difficult to treat and have a commensurately poor prognosis. Doxycycline (5–10 mg/kg PO q12h for 10–21 days) is the preferred treatment for acute infection. Significant clinical improvement may be noted within 1–2 days. However, the treatment duration is justifiably extended to 6 weeks depending on clinical response. The cost of treatment combined with the dramatic resolution of clinical signs justifies the empiric administration of antibiotic to treat ehrlichiosis in the absence of a confirmed diagnosis. In fact, a presumptive diagnosis of ehrlichiosis can be based on response to therapy.

Alternatively, minocycline (10 mg/kg PO q12h) can be given for 10 days with similar results expected. Tetracycline and oxytetracycline are still considered effective, but they should be given three times daily and may be associated with mild side-effects. Since the tetracyclines, including doxycycline, will produce yellow discoloration of erupting teeth, it is feasible to recommend chloramphenicol (15–25 mg/kg PO, IV, or SC q8h) for at least 2 weeks in dogs less than 6 months of age.

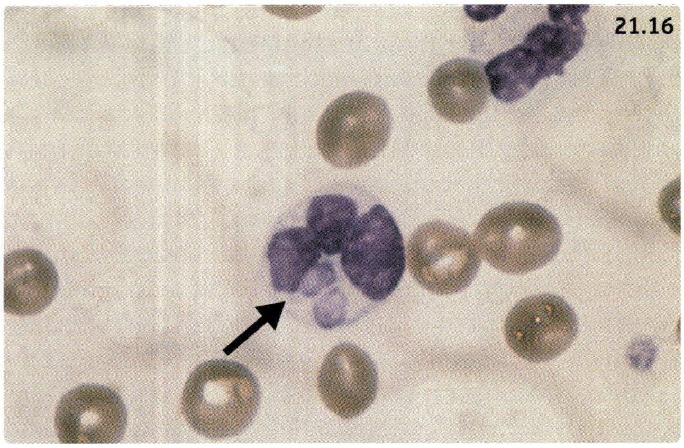

Figure 21.16 This blood smear, taken from a dog with ehrlichiosis, shows an *Ehrlichia* sp. morula (arrow) within the cytoplasm of a neutrophil. (Courtesy D.J. Meyer)

Failure to respond to conventional oral antimicrobial therapy may denote the presence of a resistant infection. Imidocarb dipropionate (5 mg/kg IM once, repeated in 2–3 weeks) is recommended.

The role of short-term corticosteroid therapy in the early treatment of ehrlichiosis is controversial. In the clinical setting it may be difficult quickly to distinguish between immune-mediated thrombocytopenia and ehrlichiosis. As a result, initial empiric therapy of thrombocytopenic dogs is justified and includes both immunosuppressive levels of prednisolone (1–2 mg/kg PO q12h for 7–10 days) plus administration of an appropriate antimicrobial (e.g. doxycycline).

The recommended treatment for canine granulocytotropic anaplasmosis is doxycycline (5–10 mg/kg PO q12h for 10 days).

Prevention

There is currently no vaccine available for the prevention of ehrlichiosis or anaplasmosis. Short-term preventive measures include oral administration of tetracycline (6.6 mg/kg/day) or doxycycline (10 mg/kg/day) for dogs living in endemic areas. In addition, efforts to manage tick infections using oral or topical acaricidal products are recommended.

Public health implications

Canine ehrlichiosis is not a zoonotic disease. However, it should be noted that humans are also susceptible to ehrlichiosis subsequent to contact with vector ticks. It is not known whether dogs play a significant role in carrying the ticks capable of infecting humans. Although dogs, cats, and humans can be naturally infected with *E. equi*, the role of domestic pets in the transmission of disease to humans has not been established.

CANINE NASAL ASPERGILLOSIS

(See also Chapter 4: Respiratory disorders.)

Definition/overview

Aspergillus fumigatus is a ubiquitous, saprophytic fungus capable of colonizing tissue within the nasal cavity and frontal sinuses. Rarely, disseminated aspergillosis can develop in dogs, with German Shepherd Dogs (between the ages of 2 and 8 years) being the most common breed affected.

Nasal aspergillosis is hypothesized to occur in immunocompromised dogs. However, other factors, particularly nasal foreign bodies and trauma, are likely to play an important role. Nasal aspergillosis is most likely to occur in dogs without concomitant disease. *A. fumigatus* infection is associated with the production of a dermonecrotic endotoxin that is presumed to cause turbinate necrosis and erosion of the planum nasale (**Figure 21.17**). *Penicillium* infection is frequently described in conjunction with *Aspergillus* infection; however, nasal penicilliosis has not been characterized.

Etiology

Aspergillosis is caused by several species of fungus of the genus *Aspergillus. A. fumigatus*, the most commonly implicated species in aspergillosis, grows abundantly in rotting vegetation and wood chips, compost, sewage, and moldy hay. Some species live mainly in soil. The fungus produces many small spores, which can become airborne and inhaled.

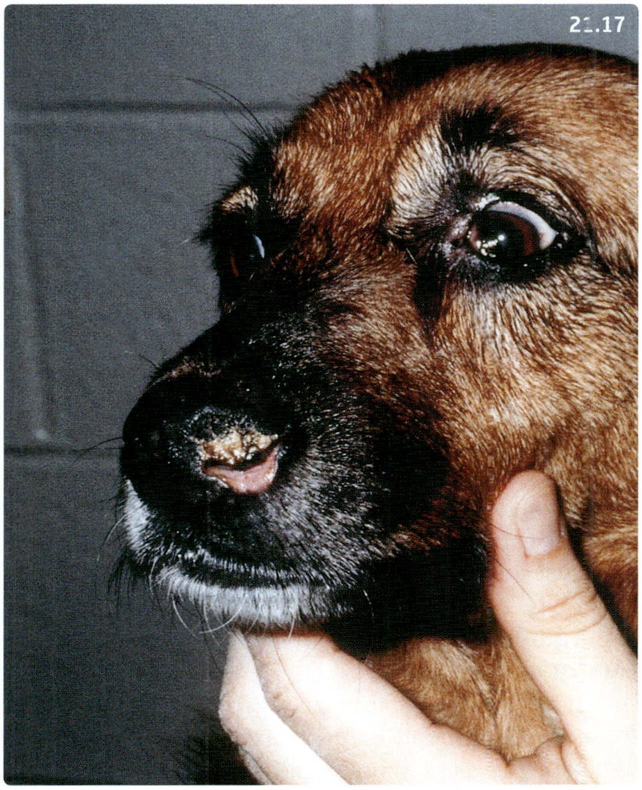

Figure 21.17 Erosion of the planum nasale in a 4-year-old mixed-breed dog with nasal aspergillosis of at least 6 months' duration.

Pathophysiology

Colonization is usually prevented by a local immune response to inhaled spores involving IgA and tissue macrophages. Due to their size (2–3 µm), airborne conidia penetrate no further than the nasal epithelium. Adhesion systems have been recognized that allow the conidia to adhere to and penetrate epithelial cells. A toxic metabolite, gliotoxin, inhibits phagocytosis, thereby facilitating recognition by innate immune mechanisms.

Clinical presentation

Nasal mycosis is most likely to occur in dogs that are 3 years of age or younger, although dogs of any age may be affected. Profuse mucopurulent nasal discharge that is not responsive to antimicrobials, intermittent epistaxis, ulceration of the external nares (planum nasale), and facial pain are the most common clinical signs seen in dogs with an established infection. Radiographic or CT evaluation of the nasal cavity (occlusal view) typically reveals an intact vomer, with evidence of turbinate destruction and fluid density in one or both nasal cavities (**Figure 21.18**).

Differential diagnosis

Nasal aspergillosis is a complex diagnosis to confirm in clinical practice. Several intranasal disorders such as foreign body, oronasal fistula, cryptococcosis (rare in dogs), and neoplasia should be ruled out. Bacterial rhinitis is a common secondary manifestation of intranasal disease, regardless of the cause, and should not be considered a primary diagnosis.

Diagnosis

Diagnostic confirmation of nasal mycosis is based on identification of the fungus in conjunction with clinical signs. The fact that either *Aspergillus* spp. or *Penicillium* spp. may occur as contaminants in the nasal cavity of the dog precludes making a diagnosis strictly on the basis of cytologic examination or a positive fungal culture. Radiographic or CT features, combined with visualization of lesions in the nasal cavity (rhinoscopy) and serology, are the principal criteria used to make a diagnosis of nasal mycosis.

The quality of a rhinoscopic examination is dependent on the quality of equipment available and the experience of the endoscopist. A 3–5 mm diameter flexible pediatric bronchoscope with a suitable biopsy channel is the preferred instrument for examining the nasal cavity (**Figures 21.19–21.21**). Biopsies of appropriate lesions should be evaluated cytologically, by fungal culture, as well as with histopathology and appropriate special

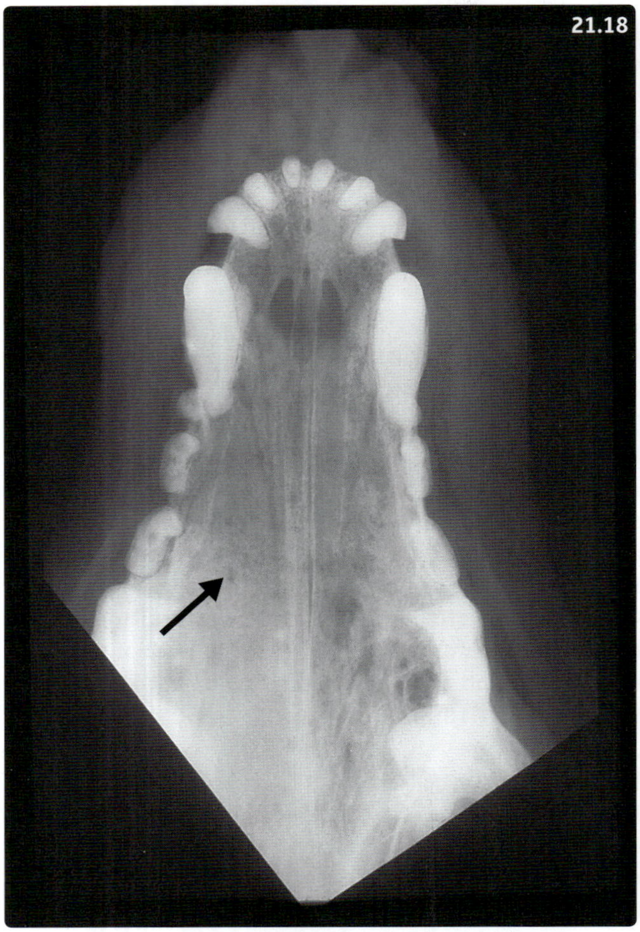

Figure 21.18 Occlusal radiographic projection of the nasal cavity of a dog with a 7-month history of nasal discharge not responsive to antibiotics. Note the loss of turbinate detail (arrow).

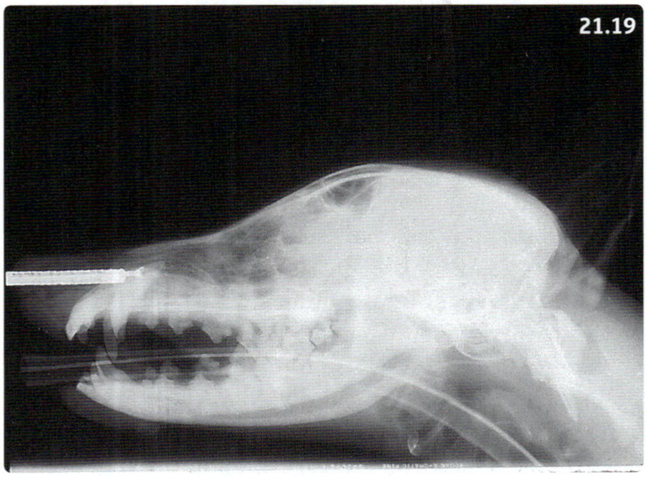

Figure 21.19 Lateral radiographic projection of the nasal cavity of a dog during rhinoscopy with a 5 mm bronchoscope.

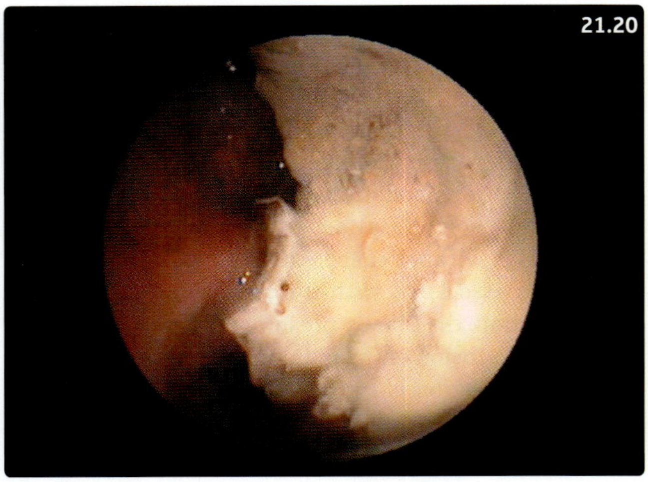

Figure 21.20 Rhinoscopic view of nasal aspergillosis showing a characteristic fungal granuloma. (Courtesy M. Schaer and K. Cooke)

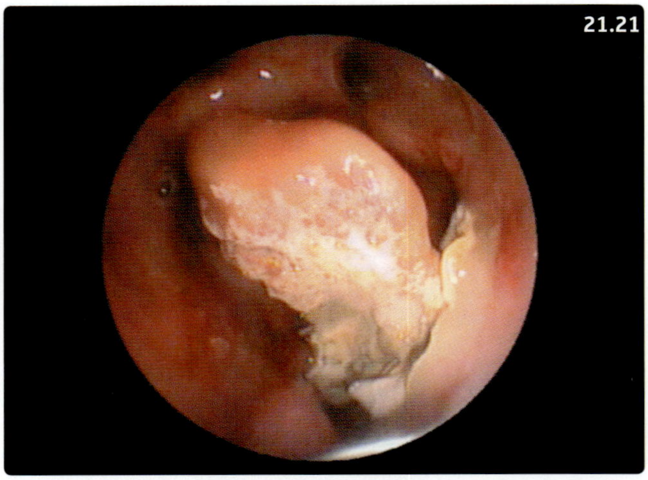

Figure 21.21 Rhinoscopic view of nasal aspergillosis showing fungal rhinitis (white plaque). (Courtesy M. Schaer and K. Cooke)

staining. A limited number of laboratories offer serologic testing as a means of diagnosing both *Aspergillus* and *Penicillium* infection. In the author's experience, serologic evidence of nasal mycosis is less reliable than direct visualization, culture, and cytology.

Management

Treatment/prognosis

Systemic therapy (itraconazole, 5 mg/kg PO q12h for 10 weeks [minimum] or fluconazole, 2.5–5.0 mg/kg PO q12h for 10 weeks [minimum]) for nasal aspergillosis has generally been associated with poor success rates and high costs. Enilconazole emulsion has been recommended for introduction into the nasal cavities and

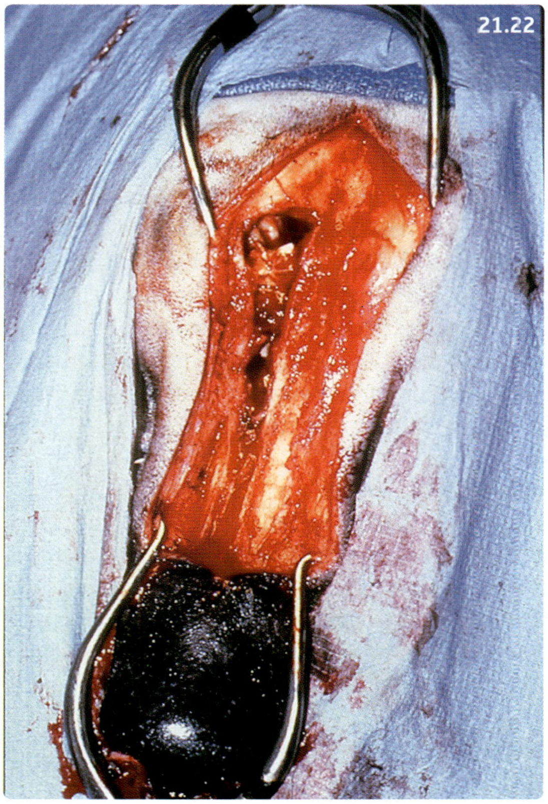

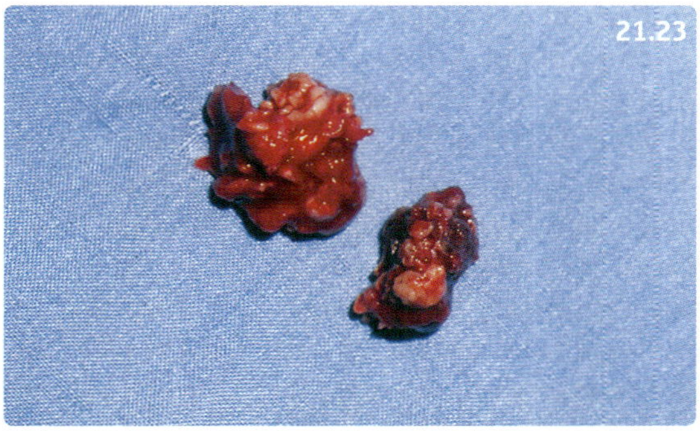

Figures 21.22, 21.23 *Aspergillus* fungal granulomas surgically removed from the nasal cavity of a dog. (Courtesy M. Schaer)

frontal sinuses by way of surgically implanted tubes. Although the treatment success rate approaches 90% in affected dogs, the need to irrigate the nasal cavity twice daily for 7 days, combined with the discomfort experienced by the patient, makes this a difficult procedure to perform routinely.

Topical treatment with the antifungal agent clotrimazole is recommended. Treatment can be performed in clinical practice, it is not expensive, and it has a high rate of success following a single treatment. The clotrimazole treatment protocol entails filling the left and right nasal cavities with commercially available 1% clotrimazole liquid (flush); gel and cream preparations are also available and may be indicated in the management of advanced frontal sinus infections.

The patient is prepared so that the clotrimazole liquid can be administered over a 1-hour period directly into the nasal cavity. The posterior nares (choanae) are occluded, thereby preventing seepage of the compound into the nasopharynx. The clinician is encouraged to become completely familiar with this technique prior to attempting treatment.

Rhinotomy and turbinectomy have also been advocated in surgical texts for the treatment of nasal aspergillosis. Today, most authors agree that medical management of aspergillosis with clotrimazole infusion into the nasal cavity is the preferred method of treatment. Surgical treatment is indicated only if all other methods have failed (**Figures 21.22, 21.23**); it is generally reserved for removal of large granulomas and mycetoma.

The prognosis for recovery from nasal aspergillosis approaches 90% in patients treated with clotrimazole infusion. Approximately 15–20% of patients will require a second treatment. Left untreated, the infection will progress and can, in advanced cases, penetrate the cribriform plate and infect the meninges and/or brain. Resolution of clinical signs following treatment, rather than a decrease in antibody titer, is the best means of evaluating the response to treatment. Antibody titers are known to persist for as long as 5 years following the successful treatment of nasal aspergillosis. The prognosis following resolution of clinical signs appears to be quite good, as recurrence is uncommon.

Treatment is most likely to fail when fungal granulomas are located within the frontal sinus. An optional treatment for these cases includes performing sinusotomy and curettage followed by infusing clotrimazole directly into the frontal sinuses.

Prevention

There is no vaccine currently available for use in companion animals to prevent aspergillosis or penicilliosis. Since the organism is a ubiquitous fungus, it is clinically impractical to advise owners to avoid pet contact with the organism.

Public health implications

Although humans as well as dogs can acquire aspergillosis, the infections in dogs are not considered to be zoonotic.

Editors' note: There is a systemic form of aspergillosis in dogs caused by *Aspergillus terreus* that causes polysystemic disease including the formation of fungal granulomas in the kidney, diskospondylitis, uveitis, and other tissue involvements. It is most common in German Shepherd Dogs and is thought to be due to an immunoincompetency. Treatment entails long-term systemic antifungal drugs, but the prognosis is usually poor.

BABESIOSIS

(See also Chapter 16: Hematologic disorders.)

Definition/overview

Canine babesiosis refers to disease caused by infection with *Babesia canis* (larger piroplasms) and/or *Babesia gibsoni* (smaller piroplasms). Infection follows inoculation with sporozoites transmitted in the saliva of infected ticks. Infections are recognized throughout much of the world, particularly southern Europe, Africa, Asia, North America, Central America, and South America. Infections are most likely to occur in dogs <1 year of age.

Etiology

The disease is transmitted by a variety of tick vectors, including *Rhipicephalus sanguineus*. Recently, *Dermacentor variablilis*, the American dog tick, has been recognized as a competent vector. Once infected, the *Babesia* organisms multiply within erythrocytes. Transplacental transmission is suspected to occur and has been associated with the 'fading puppy' syndrome. Infection may also result from transfusion of contaminated blood. Interestingly, infection with *B. gibsoni* may result from fighting between dogs. A higher than expected incidence is reported in the American Staffordshire Terrier and American Pit Bull Terrier.

Pathophysiology

Erythrocytes parasitized by *Babesia* are destroyed by replication of the organism within the cells or by immune-mediated reactions against the parasite or self-antigens. The resulting destruction of erythrocytes leads to anemia. The incubation period is usually from 10 days to 3 weeks. Subclinical carrier dogs used as blood donors are excellent sources of infection for blood recipients.

Clinical presentation

Acute-onset (severe) hemolytic anemia, associated with fever, decreased appetite, splenomegaly, and lethargy, are the most common clinical findings reported. Although chronic infections can occur, they are uncommon and poorly characterized. Sudden death is a possible consequence of acute-onset *Babesia* infection associated with hypotensive shock and hypoxia. In addition to hemolytic anemia and splenomegaly, thrombocytopenia and lymphadenomegaly have been observed. The variation in clinical signs that may be manifested depends on the tissues affected. Mild to severe pulmonary disease, vomiting, diarrhea, ulcerative stomatitis, significant hemorrhage, myositis and rhabdomyolysis, and CNS signs are also reported. Subclinical infections are also reported.

American Staffordshire Terriers and American Pit Bull Terriers are two breeds having a relatively high prevalence of infection and this has been reported in many countries. Recent studies suggest transmission may occur subsequent to bite wounds from infected dogs.

Differential diagnosis

Immune-mediated hemolytic anemia and thrombocytopenia are important differential diagnoses for acute-onset signs associated with babesiosis in dogs. However, affected dogs should also be evaluated for other tick-borne diseases (e.g. ehrlichiosis, Rocky Mountain spotted fever [RMSF]).

Diagnosis

Diagnostic confirmation is frequently based on visual identification of the organisms within infected erythrocytes using routine staining methods (**Figure 21.24**). Merozoites can be detected within erythrocytes (peripheral blood smear) by 1–3 weeks following infection. Serology may prove useful in identifying *B. canis* antibody, which cross-reacts with *B. gibsoni* antibody. Detection of antibody titers to *Babesia* spp., using the indirect IFA test, can be performed. Since intraerythrocytic organisms can be difficult to enumerate, the use of antibody titers to document infection is relevant in the clinical setting. Depending on the laboratory used and the methodology,

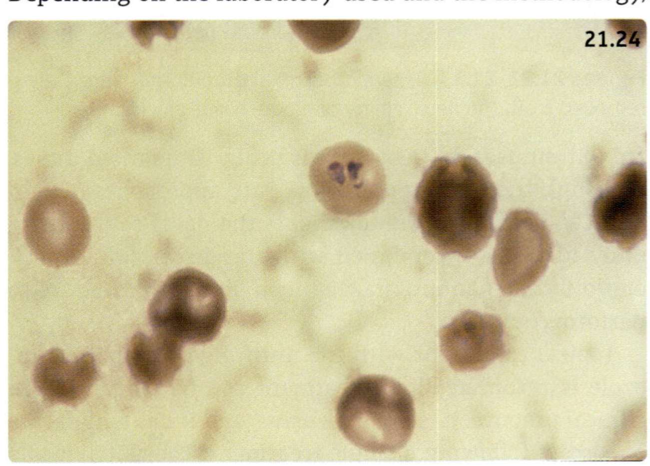

Figure 21.24 Canine *Babesia* organisms shown as intraerythrocytic protozoal organisms.

a single serum titer of 1:80 or higher is generally regarded as sufficient to diagnose *B. canis* infection. A titer of 1:320 or higher is required to diagnose *B. gibsoni* infection. While some university and commercial laboratories are offering PCR assays for the detection of babesiosis in dogs, test results may vary among laboratories, as test standards have not been defined. Also, low specificity (false-positive test results) remain problematic. To avoid false-negative test results, dogs should be tested as early in the course of infection as possible and prior to the initiation of treatment.

Management

Treatment/prognosis

Although a wide variety of drugs has been advocated for treating babesiosis throughout the world, the two most effective drugs, diminazene aceturate and phenamidine isethionate, are not approved for use in the USA. Relapses may occur as the organism can persist even after treatment. A single dose of imidocarb dipropionate (7.5 mg/kg IM) has been effective against *B. canis* only. Alternatively, administration of two doses of imidocarb dipropionate (6 mg/kg IM), 2 weeks apart, has also been recommended.

Quinuronium sulfate (0.25 mg/kg SC given twice over a 2-day interval) has resulted in resolution of clinical signs. Concurrent administration of corticosteroids (1–2 mg/kg q12h) may be necessary for periods of 2–3 weeks. However, sustained corticosteroid treatment may result in exacerbation of the disease. Given the acute systemic impact of *B. canis* infection, the prognosis of dogs with confirmed infection is poor. Treatment is not expected to clear the infection completely.

Clinical reports support a breed predilection among Greyhounds for *B. canis (vogeli)* infection. Although clinical illness is uncommon, the significance of the infection is as yet undetermined.

Natural infection with *B. gibsoni* has been effectively treated in dogs using a combination of atovaquone (13.3 mg/kg PO q8h) with azithromycin (10 mg/kg PO q24h) for 10 days.

Clindamycin is the recommended treatment for *B. microti* infection in humans. In dogs, anecdotal reports suggest resolution of clinical signs associated with babesiosis using doses ranging from 25 to 50 mg/kg/day. Supplemental babesiacidal therapy is still recommended.

Prevention

Efforts to prevent infection are based on the ability adequately to control tick infestations. Routine topical administration of an acaricide (e.g. fipronil) or oral administration (e.g. afoxolaner) combined with environmental control constitutes the most effective means of preventing infection. An attenuated *B. canis* vaccine is available in Europe. Reports on efficacy vary. The vaccine does not prevent infection, but appears to mitigate severity of clinical signs once infection occurs. There is currently no licensed vaccine available in the USA.

Public health implications

Although canine babesiosis is not regarded as a risk to humans, infected dogs do represent a reservoir of infectious organisms that, in the presence of the vector ticks, could result in human exposure. However, *B. microti* is the most common organism affecting humans in the USA. Infections are generally considered to be mild and self-limiting or can be treated with clindamycin.

ROCKY MOUNTAIN SPOTTED FEVER

Definition/overview

Rickettsiae belonging to the spotted fever group (SFG) are responsible for the tick-borne infection of dogs and people known as Rocky Mountain spotted fever (RMSF). Despite its name, RMSF occurs throughout the USA, in parts of western Canada, and in Mexico and Central and South America. Today, the majority of cases reported in humans and dogs are from the eastern USA. Although four SFG species of *Rickettsia* have been isolated from ticks, *R. rickettsii* is the SFG species known to infect humans and animals in the western hemisphere.

Etiology

This obligate intracellular parasite is transmitted through the bite of either of two ticks: *Dermacentor andersoni* or *D. variabilis*.

Pathophysiology

Subsequent to inoculation through the bite of an infected tick, the rickettsiae replicate in vascular endothelium, producing a significant vasculitis within small arteries and venules. Subsequent loss of plasma may culminate in the formation of edema in the brain, lungs, and skin. In addition, microvascular hemorrhage, thrombocytopenia, and DIC may result. In a small number of animals, infection culminates in shock and death.

Clinical presentation

Clinical disease associated with SFG rickettsial infection is most likely to occur in young dogs (<2 years of age) presented between the months of March and October (in the northern hemisphere). A breed predilection has been recognized, with the German Shepherd Dog having a particularly high incidence of infection.

Fever associated with myalgia/arthralgia, decreased appetite, and a history of known tick exposure are among the most common findings in dogs with RMSF. Other signs resulting from widespread vasculitis include edema and hyperemia of the lips and ears. In males, scrotal edema and epididymal swelling may be present. In addition, petechial and ecchymotic hemorrhages may be seen on mucous membranes and during funduscopic examination. Overt, spontaneous bleeding may be noted in severely affected animals. In advanced cases, evidence of cardiovascular, neurologic, and renal damage may be present and this represents some of the most common causes of death or permanent organ dysfunction. Severe cases can terminate from shock, DIC, or meningoencephalitis.

Differential diagnosis

Dogs with RMSF may present with a wide spectrum of clinical signs consistent with those associated with other tick-borne diseases (e.g. ehrlichiosis and babesiosis). If presented for spontaneous bleeding and/or epistaxis, patients should be evaluated for immune-mediated thrombocytopenia, von Willebrand disease, or rodenticide toxicity. Canine distemper, polyarthritis, and brucellosis (among male dogs with orchitis/epididymitis) should also be considered.

Diagnosis

Hematologic findings are relatively unremarkable in dogs with RMSF. However, thrombocytopenia is among the most consistent laboratory abnormalities reported in infected dogs. (RMSF is not usually associated with platelet counts <75,000/ml. In the clinical setting this information may be helpful in distinguishing RMSF from dogs with immune-mediated thrombocytopenia, which usually have platelet counts <50,000/ml.) Hypercholesterolemia is reported to be a consistent finding among infected dogs, but it does not represent a reliable diagnostic criterion. Although a number of slight biochemical abnormalities are reported, the incidence is highly variable, depending on the severity and location of infection. Severely infected animals may have cardiac involvement, during which ECG abnormalities may be detected: ST-segment and T-wave depressions, as well as premature ventricular contractions.

Although considerable effort has been made to develop serologic tests that will reliably diagnose RMSF, acute and convalescent titers are still recommended as the most reliable means of confirming a diagnosis. However, IgG titers for RMSF antibody are not expected to rise significantly until 2–3 weeks post infection. For this reason, the clinician is advised to prescribe empiric antimicrobial therapy on the basis of clinical signs and history rather than wait for laboratory results on paired serum samples. Using a single IgM RMSF antibody titer may have some advantage in obtaining early diagnostic confirmation on the basis of a single titer. However, the availability of this assay does limit its practical application in clinical practice. If available, laboratories that provide direct IFA staining of infected tissues offer the advantage of an early, single sample diagnosis.

Although death from RMSF is uncommon, the most common findings include petechial and ecchymotic hemorrhages throughout most tissues in addition to hemorrhagic lymphadenomegaly. Rickettsiae are not detected by routine histologic staining methods.

Management

Treatment/prognosis

The decision to treat RMSF should be based on history, physical findings, and evidence of moderate thrombocytopenia. Several drugs are available. Doxycycline (10–20 mg/kg PO q12h for 7–10 days) is the primary recommendation for treating RMSF in dogs and humans. Alternatively, tetracycline (22–30 mg/kg PO q8h for 7–10 days) can be used. Other antibiotics have not proven to be efficacious and may actually lead to increased morbidity (and death). Tetracycline is more likely than doxycycline to label (or stain) dental enamel when administered for 10 days or longer to puppies less than 6 months of age.

Response to therapy can be dramatic, with improvement noted within 24–72 hours following the onset of antibiotic therapy. In severely affected cases, supportive care of dogs is centered around the management of shock, spontaneous bleeding, or evidence of cardiac or renal disease. However, administration of IV fluid therapy may actually contribute to rapid onset pulmonary or cerebral edema due to increased vascular permeability associated with the infection.

Prevention

Currently there is no vaccine available for the prevention of RMSF in dogs. However, natural immunity subsequent to infection with *R. rickettsii* has been reported to persist for as long as 3 years post infection. Management of tick infestation in dogs is still the best method of preventing RMSF. The routine use of the excellent topical acaricidal drugs available today is the best means of preventing RMSF.

Public health implications

Although RMSF is frequently cited as a zoonotic disease, infection is not transmitted directly from infected dogs to humans. Although dogs may serve as a reservoir of infectious ticks, dogs with RMSF do not pose a direct threat to humans. It should be noted that human infection can potentially occur subsequent to removal of infectious ticks from dogs. Direct contact with infectious hemolymph is a potential source of infection for people.

SYSTEMIC MYCOSES

Definition/overview

The systemic (or deep) mycoses are those infections in dogs and cats caused by *Blastomyces dermatitidis* (blastomycosis), *Coccidioides immitis* (coccidioidomycosis), *Cryptococcus neoformans* (cryptococcosis), and *Histoplasma capsulatum* (histoplasmosis). Each of the organisms listed can be isolated from soil within specific geographic regions throughout the world. Despite the mapping of endemic areas within the USA, the frequency with which pets travel throughout the country suggests that both dogs and, less commonly, cats can be presented with clinical disease outside of defined endemic areas. Since humans and animals share the environment in which soil contamination exists, it is not unusual to see the prevalence of animal infections correspond to the prevalence of human infections.

Etiology

The respiratory tract is the primary route of exposure among susceptible dogs and cats. Given the ubiquitous nature of the organisms in soil, it is obvious that many more animals will be exposed than will become clinically ill.

Pathophysiology

In susceptible animals, primary infection generally begins in the lung once the organism reaches the terminal airways. From there, dissemination to multiple organs is possible. In the clinical setting it is the particular organ or organ systems infected that are responsible for the clinical signs. It is still unclear why some animals, subsequent to exposure, develop severe disseminated disease, while others remain healthy. It has been suggested that disseminated disease is a consequence of exposure in immunocompromised animals. Although antibody does develop in response to infection, it is not protective. Recovery from mycotic disease is attributed to cell-mediated immunity.

Clinical presentation

In the few reported cases of systemic mycosis in cats there appears to be no age, breed, or sex predilection to infection. In dogs, however, infection is most likely to occur between 1 and 5 years of age. In most cases, clinical signs include weight loss, decreased appetite, and lethargy. Since the respiratory tract is the portal of entry, clinical signs of pneumonia, including cough and dyspnea, are reported (**Figures 21.25–21.30**). Systemic signs include diarrhea, lameness, abdominal effusion, skin lesions,

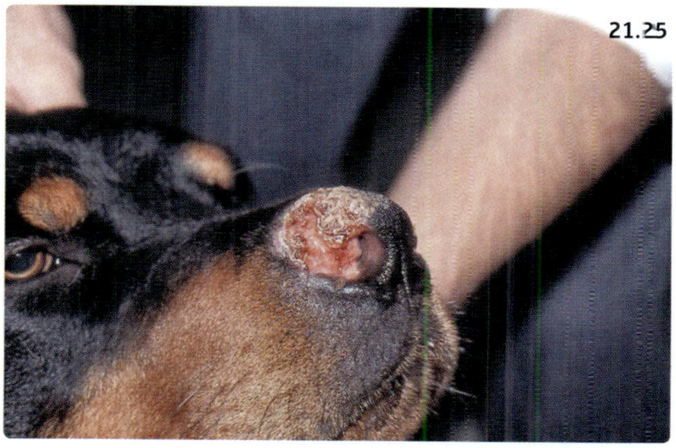

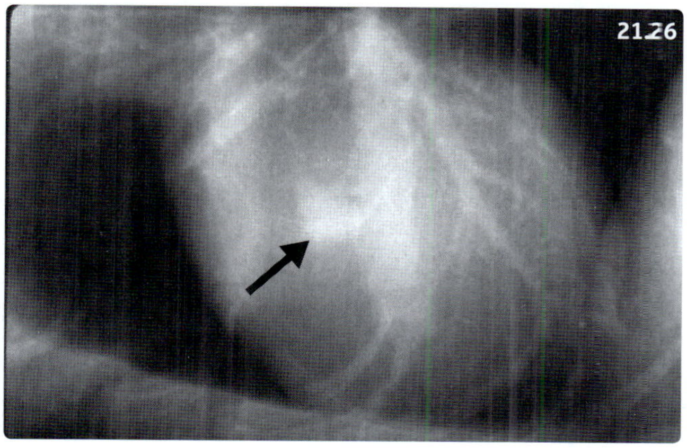

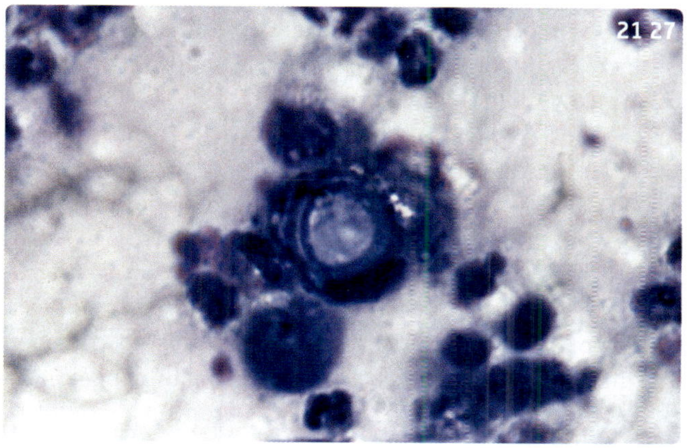

Figure 21.25–21.27 (21.25) *Blastomyces dermatitidis* nasal granuloma on the nares of a young Rottweiler dog. (21.26) Chest radiograph of the same dog showing a solitary fungal granuloma in the dog's lung (arrow). (21.27) Microscopic appearance of a *Blastomyces* spore taken on a 'touch prep' sample from the dog's nasal lesion. (Courtesy M. Schaer)

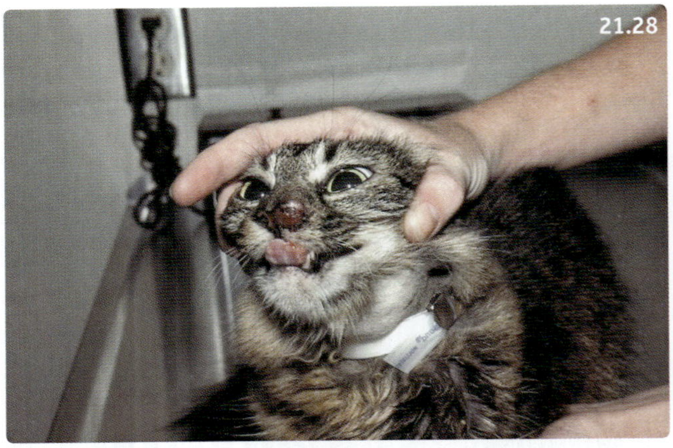

Figure 21.28 Cryptococcal granulomas involving the tongue and nares of this Domestic Shorthair cat. (Courtesy M. Schaer)

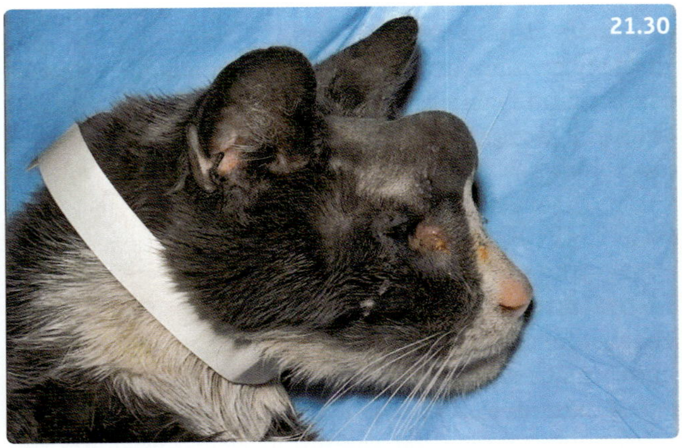

Figure 21.30 A solitary cryptococcal granuloma involving the nasal cavity and growing outward through the nasal bone of this 17-year-old diabetic cat. (Courtesy M. Schaer)

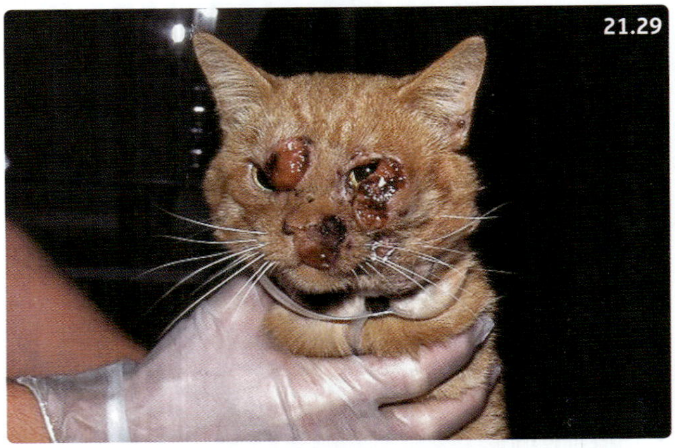

Figure 21.29 Several cryptococccal granulomas on the face of a cat. (Courtesy M. Schaer)

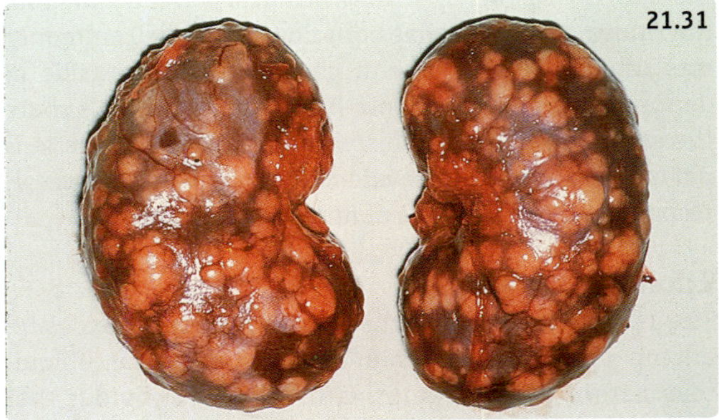

Figure 21.31 Granulomas associated with disseminated histoplasmosis in the kidneys of a dog.

renal (**Figure 21.31**) or hepatic failure, and ocular disease (**Figure 21.32**), but the signs vary depending on the particular organism involved.

Differential diagnosis

The list of differential diagnoses appropriate for dogs with clinical signs associated with any of the systemic mycoses is extensive, depending on the primary organ system(s) involved. However, cachexia associated with neoplasia is one of the most important differentials to consider. Pneumonia, sepsis, enteritis, hepatic insufficiency, and polyarthritis are among the other differentials that apply.

Diagnosis

Bone marrow and other tissues are important sources for obtaining samples for a cytologic diagnosis (**Figures 21.33, 21.34**). In dogs and cats with overt clinical signs and external manifestations of disease, it is practical, in the clinical

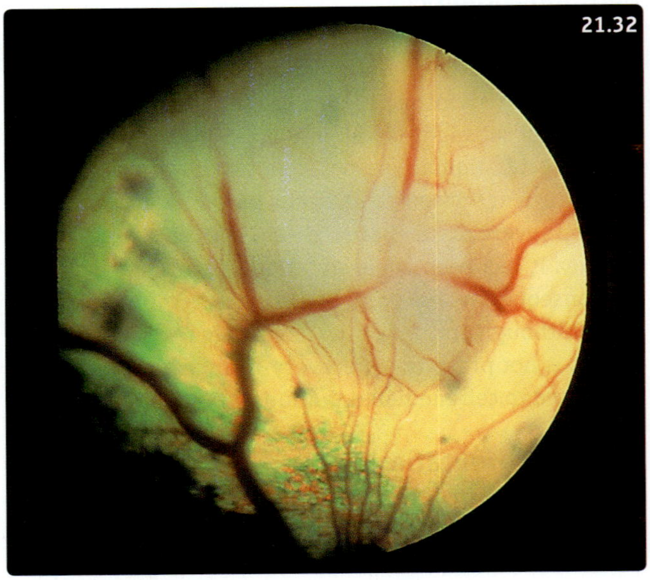

Figure 21.32 Subretinal exudates associated with blastomycosis in a dog.

setting, to identify the specific organism involved. The predominant clinical findings and the preferred tissue for identification of organisms are summarized in **Table 21.6**. If it is not possible to identify the specific organism, serologic testing is indicated. However, only a limited number of laboratories are able to perform serologic testing for systemic mycoses. Results of serologic testing, regardless of the causative organisms, must be interpreted carefully, since the serologic response to infection is variable. The serum latex agglutination test can be used for detecting cryptococcal antigen.

Thoracic radiographs are indicated in any dog or cat suspected of having a systemic mycotic infection. A diffuse, miliary to nodular interstitial pulmonary infiltrate is a common clinical finding, particularly in animals with signs of respiratory disease (**Figure 21.35**). The most common sites of biopsy for cytologic evaluation and diagnosis for each of the major systemic mycoses are summarized in **Table 21.6**.

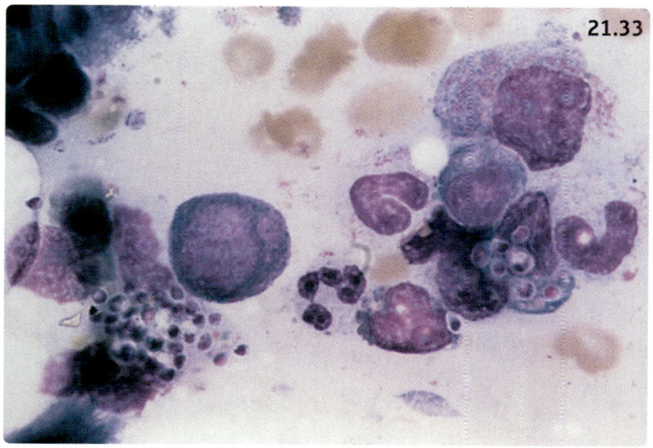

Figure 21.33 Clusters of *H. capsulatum* in the macrophages in the bone marrow of dog with diffuse histoplasmosis.

Management

Treatment/prognosis

Over the last 10 years, the introduction of more effective antifungal agents has greatly improved the prognosis for those animals fortunate enough to receive treatment. However, the cost associated with treatment and the severity of clinical signs associated with the infection may ultimately determine the prognosis. The treatment protocols for both dogs and cats infected with each of the four systemic mycoses described in this section are summarized in **Table 21.7**.

Prevention

There is currently no vaccine available for any of the systemic fungal infections known to occur in the dog and cat. Given the ubiquitous nature of the organisms in soil, preventing exposure is extremely difficult in endemic areas. Chemical decontamination of the soil with formaldehyde solution is possible, but this is impractical for treating large areas.

Public health implications

Despite the fact that both humans and animals can be infected with each of the organisms discussed in this section, there is no known transmission from dogs or cats to humans or other animals. None of the systemic mycoses discussed in this section are considered zoonotic diseases.

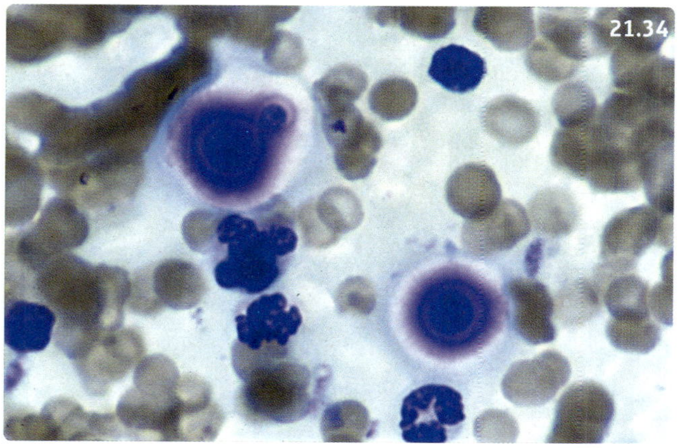

Figure 21.34 A cytology specimen stained with new methylene blue showing *Cryptococcus neoformans* spores. Note the thick capsule and the daughter spore. (Courtesy M. Schaer)

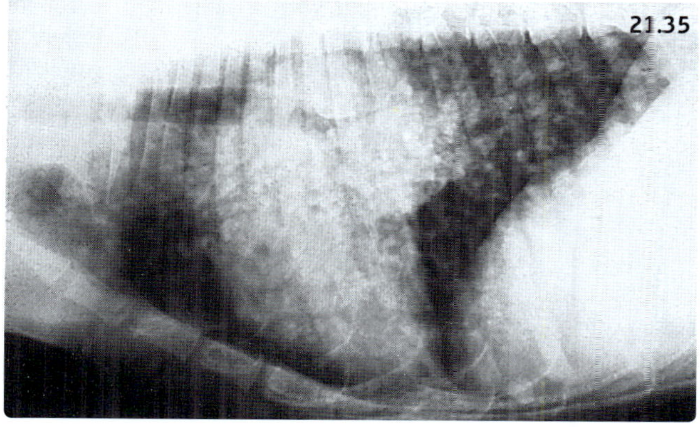

Figure 21.35 Lateral radiograph of a 2-year-old dog with a diffuse interstitial lung pattern characteristic of mycotic pneumonia.

Table 21.6 Summary of the major clinical signs and recommended biopsy sites for systemic mycotic infections in dogs and cats.

	Canine		Feline	
Mycotic infection	**Presenting signs**	**Recommended biopsy site**	**Presenting signs**	**Recommended biopsy site**
Histoplasmosis	Inappetence, weight loss, and fever (unresponsive to antimicrobials). Large bowel diarrhea (chronic), hematochezia, tenesmus. Hepatomegaly and splenomegaly. Diffuse interstitial lung pattern with increased hilar density on thoracic radiographs	Rectal biopsy (mucosal) or rectal mucosal scraping. Bone marrow aspiration/biopsy. Fine-needle aspiration of lung, liver, spleen. Bronchoalveolar lavage may be helpful when other procedures are not diagnostic	Dyspnea, tachypnea, possible abnormal lung sounds. Enlarged lymph nodes. Splenomegaly, hepatomegaly	Bone marrow aspiration/biopsy. Fine-needle aspiration of lung and/or lymph node
Cryptococcosis	The American Cocker breed is overrepresented in North America. Weight loss and lethargy (common). Multifocal CNS signs predominate: head tilt, nystagmus, facial paralysis, paresis, ataxia, circling, seizures. Ocular signs include granulomatous chorioretinitis, retinal hemorrhage, and optic neuritis	Cytologic examination of CSF and/or fluid obtained by paracentesis from the inside of the eye. New methylene blue or Gram stain is preferred over Wright's and India ink	Cryptococcosis is the most common systemic mycotic infection in cats in North America. Upper respiratory signs predominate: sneezing with mucoid nasal discharge not responsive to antimicrobials. A polypoid mass may be visible at the external nares. Mandibular lymphadeno-megaly Subcutaneous papules or nodules	Cytologic examination of exudate from the nose and skin stained with new methylene blue or Gram stain is preferred over Wright's and India ink
Blastomycosis	Lymphadenomegaly, lethargy, anorexia and weight loss. Dry, adventitial lung sounds, with variable cough. Interstitial lung pattern Uveitis and retinal detachment are seen in up to 40% of dogs. Multifocal subcutaneous abscesses. Lameness associated with fungal osteomyelitis may be the only presenting sign in up to 30% of dogs	Fine-needle aspiration of enlarged lymph nodes and other affected body sites. Cytopathology of skin lesions or exudate (conventional stains may be used)	Uncommon in cats. When present, signs are similar to those seen in dogs. Dyspnea, weight loss, draining skin lesions, and visual impairment are most commonly reported	Fine-needle aspiration of enlarged lymph nodes and other afected body sites. Cytopathology of skin lesions or exudate (conventional stains may be used)

(continued)

	Canine		Feline	
Mycotic infection	**Presenting signs**	**Recommended biopsy site**	**Presenting signs**	**Recommended biopsy site**
Coccidioidomycosis	Fever, decreased appetite, and weight loss are common. Cough with mild to inapparent respiratory tract infection. Draining skin lesions. Keratitis, uveitis, acute blindness. Lameness associated with long bone pain and bone swelling (may be associated with a draining tract in skin	Skin biopsy involving tissue affected with microabscesses. Multiple biopsies may be required. **Note:** Attempting to culture *C. immitis* in practice is not recommended	Similar to the dog. Skin lesions without evidence of a bone lesion are most common. Respiratory signs are rare	Skin biopsy involving tissue affected with microabscesses. Multiple biopsies may be required. **Note:** Attempting to culture *C. immitis* in practice is not recommended

Table 21.7 Recommended and alternative treatment protocols for systemic mycotic infections in dogs and cats.

Mycotic infection	Canine	Feline
Histoplasmosis	Itraconazole (10 mg/kg PO q12–24h for 4–6 months; oral solution is recommended). **Alternatives:** Fluconazole (2.5–5.0 mg/kg PO q12–24 for 4–6 months) or amphotericin B (deoxycholate) (0.25–0.5 mg/kg IV only administered on alternate days until a cumulative dose of 5–10 mg/kg is achieved)	Itraconazole (10 mg/kg PO q12h for 4–6 months (oral solution is recommended). **Alternatives:** Fluconazole (2.5–5.0 mg/kg PO q12–24 for 4–6 months) or amphotericin B (deoxycholate) (0.25–0.5 mg/kg IV only administered on alternate days until a cumulative dose of 4–8 mg/kg is achieved)
Cryptococcosis	Fluconazole (5–15 mg/kg PO q12–24h for at least 6 and up to 18 months). **Alternatives:** Flucytosine (50–75 mg/kg PO q8h for 1–12 months plus amphotericin B (deoxycholate) (0.25–0.5 mg/kg IV only administered on alternate days until a cumulative dose of 5–10 mg/kg is achieved). (Recommended for patients with CNS involvement.) **Note:** Amphotericin B is the only drug that is fungicidal	Itraconazole (10–20 mg/kg PO q24h for at least 6 and up to 18 months). **Alternatives:** Fluconazole (2.5–5.0 mg/kg PO q12–24h for 6–10 months) or flucytosine (75 mg/kg PO q12h for 1–9 months) plus amphotericin B (deoxycholate) (0.1–0.5 mg/kg IV only administered on alternate days until a cumulative dose of 4–8 mg/kg is achieved). (Recommended for patients with CNS involvement.) **Note:** Amphotericin B is the only drug that is fungicidal
Blastomycosis	Itraconazole (5 mg/kg PO q12h for 5 days, then 5 mg/kg q24h for 2 months or at least until 1 month following resolution of signs. **Alternatives:** Fluconazole (5 mg/kg PO q12h for 2 months or at least until 1 month following resolution of signs)	Itraconazole (5 mg/kg PO q12h for 2 months or at least until 1 month following resolution of signs)

(continued)

Table 21.7 Recommended and alternative treatment protocols for systemic mycotic infections in dogs and cats. *(Continued)*

Mycotic infection	Canine	Feline
	or amphotericin B (deoxycholate) (0.25–0.5 mg/kg IV only administered on alternate days until a cumulative dose of 5–10 mg/kg is achieved)	**Alternative:** Amphotericin B (deoxycholate) (0.1–0.5 mg/kg IV only administered on alternate days until a cumulative dose of 4–8 mg/kg is achieved)
Coccidioidomycosis	Ketoconazole (5–15 mg/kg PO q12h for 8–12 months). **Alternatives:** Amphotericin B (deoxycholate) (0.25–0.5 mg/kg IV only administered on alternate days until a cumulative dose of 5–10 mg/kg is achieved) or Itraconazole (5 mg/kg PO q12h for 8–12 months)	Ketoconazole (50 mg [total] PO q12h; expect to treat for up to 12 months). **Alternative:** Itraconazole (25–50 mg [total] PO q12–24h for 8–12 months)

RECOMMENDED FURTHER READING

Ettinger SJ, Feldman EC (2010) (eds.) *Textbook of Veterinary Internal Medicine*, 7th edn. Elsevier Saunders, St. Louis.

Greene CE (2011) (ed.) *Infectious Diseases of the Dog and Cat*, 4th edn. Elsevier Saunders, St. Louis.

King LG (2004) (ed.) *Textbook of Respiratory Disease in Dogs and Cats*. Elsevier Saunders, St. Louis.

Plumb DC (2015) (ed.) *Plumb's Veterinary Drug Handbook*, 8th edn. Blackwell Publishing, Ames.

Part 2: The cat

Annette Litster

BACTERIAL INFECTIONS

FELINE ACTINOMYCOSIS AND NOCARDIOSIS

Definition/overview

Actinomycosis and nocardiosis are rare chronic infections, reported in both dogs and cats, caused by a variety of anaerobic (actinomycosis) and aerobic (nocardiosis) actinomycetes.

Etiology

Actinomyces spp. and *Nocardia* spp. are branching, filamentous, gram-positive bacteria. The organisms are ubiquitous and can be found in the oral cavity of cats as well as in soil. Infections are opportunistic and usually occur subsequent to mechanical disruption of mucosal barriers, such as inoculation of skin with contaminated plant material or, less often, bite wounds. Actinomycosis is more prevalent, especially in cats, than nocardiosis.

Pathophysiology

Entry and spread of infection depend on the host's immunocompetence. In both infections, hematologic and biochemical findings are nonspecific and typical of any pyogenic inflammatory process. There is usually a leukocytosis with a left shift.

Clinical presentation

Feline actinomycosis

Feline actinomycosis is most often associated with subcutaneous cat bite abscess formation or pyothorax. A viscous, opaque exudate is characteristic.

Feline nocardiosis

Feline nocardiosis infections are characterized by suppurative or pyogranulomatous inflammation that can be localized (cutaneous–subcutaneous, pulmonary) or disseminated (systemic). The cutaneous form is the most common and often presents as fistulous tracts with serosanguineous discharge.

Differential diagnosis

Penetrating (subcutaneous) injury and neoplasia are among the most important differential diagnoses for actinomycosis. Pneumonia (bacterial, parasitic, viral, or protozoal [toxoplasmosis]) is an important differential diagnosis for nocardiosis. As *Actinomyces* spp. and *Nocardia* spp. are opportunistic pathogens, all infected cats should be tested for feline leukemia virus (FeLV) and feline immunodeficiency virus (FIV).

Diagnosis

Feline actinomycosis

Recovery of multiple bacterial pathogens from the exudate is common. Cytology of the exudate may reveal so-called sulfur granules, which can occasionally be visualized without microscopy (**Figures 21.36, 21.37**). Cytologic assessment of exudates is complicated by the presence of mixed bacterial populations. *Actinomyces* in the exudate may be difficult to visualize, but they should appear as gram-positive filamentous organisms. Attempts to culture *Actinomyces* spp. from exudates are complicated by bacterial overgrowth. In addition, specimens need to be processed anaerobically. However, the high degree of susceptibility of *Actinomyces* to antimicrobial therapy could preclude the need to confirm the antimicrobial susceptibility profile.

Feline nocardiosis

Although local infections can cause abscess formation containing the gram-positive filamentous organisms, the presence of mixed bacterial populations from subcutaneous abscesses is, unlike actinomycosis, rare. Microscopically, filaments are finer than fungal filaments (<1 µm) and can be identified using Bourke's modification of Gram stain. Filaments do not stain with Romanowsky stains.

Management

Treatment/prognosis

Both diseases are best treated with surgical drainage and débridement of affected areas, except in cases where infection is disseminated. Treatment with antimicrobials is essential for weeks to months because of the limited drug penetration of granulomas.

Feline actinomycosis

Penicillin G (100,000 U/kg IV or SC q6–8h) or penicillin V (phenoxymethyl penicillin, 40 mg/kg PO q8h) is the recommended treatment for feline actinomycosis. Antimicrobial penetration of the granulomas is difficult and, therefore, dictates extended therapy. Once effective drainage has been established, treatment should continue for a minimum of 2 weeks or as long as necessary for clinical and microbiological cure. Once treatment has been initiated, the volume of discharge is frequently reduced. The clinician should attempt to identify the extent of draining tracts and the possibility of a foreign body within the wound site or tract. Treatment is significantly complicated by infections associated with migrating foreign bodies. Animals that fail to respond to initial drainage and antimicrobial therapy should undergo exploratory surgery in an attempt to identify the underlying cause. Assuming that effective drainage can be established, the inciting foreign material removed, and antibiotic therapy administered appropriately, the prognosis for cure is excellent.

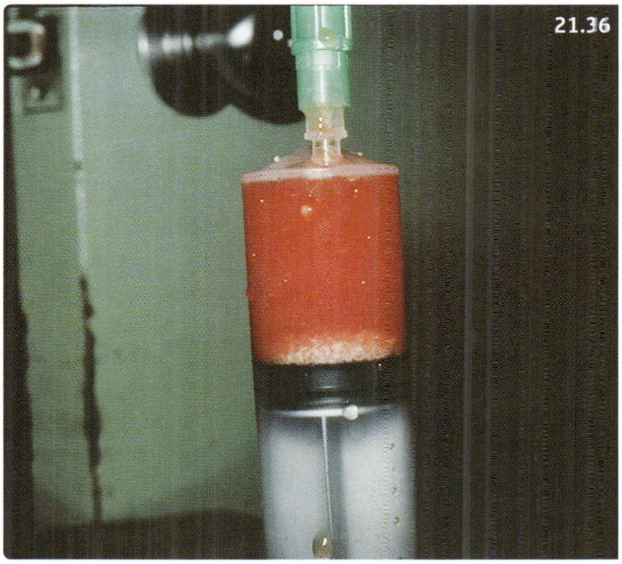

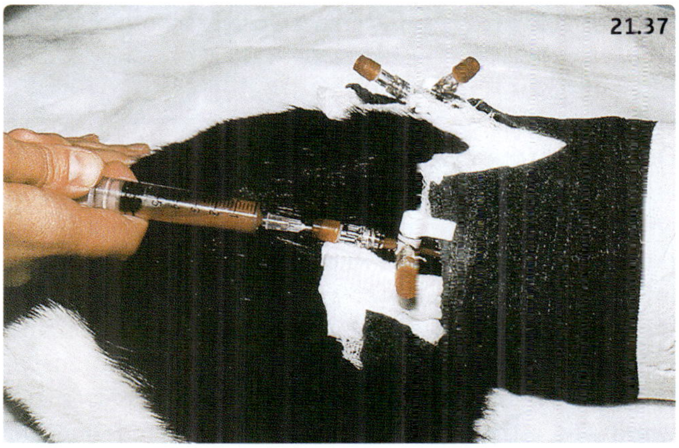

Figures 21.36, 21.37 (21.36) Suppurative exudate containing 'sulfur' granules, taken from a feline patient with suppurative pleuritis caused by *Actinomyces* infection, is shown in the syringe. (21.37) The cat in 21.36 is having thoracic exudate aspirated through chest tubes.

Feline nocardiosis

Feline nocardiosis has a considerably poorer prognosis than actinomycosis. Sulfonamides are the recommended drugs in the management of nocardiosis (sulfadiazine 80 mg/kg PO q8h and sulfisoxazole 50 mg/kg PO q8h). Doxycycline (5–10 mg/kg PO q12–24h, with water to follow), in combination with amoxicillin (20 mg/kg PO q12h) and/or clarithromycin (62.5–125 mg/cat PO q12h) and amikacin (15–20 mg/kg IV q24h) have also been used to treat feline nocardiosis. Amoxicillin–clavulanate and fluoroquinolones are not effective. Although response to therapy may be noted within 7–10 days following the onset of treatment, extended treatment periods of 2 months or longer are usually required. In addition to potential adverse reactions to long-term sulfonamide administration, not all nocardial isolates are sensitive to sulfonamides. Cats that do not have easily resectable nocardial lesions have an extremely poor prognosis.

Prevention
There is currently no vaccine on the market for the prevention of either actinomycosis or nocardiosis in cats.

Public health implications
Although human cases of actinomycosis and nocardiosis are reported, human infections are not directly transmitted from infected dogs or cats. Individuals handling material from draining wounds should use normal routine precautions to avoid inadvertent contact with infectious material.

FELINE BARTONELLOSIS

Definition/overview
Feline bartonellosis is generally attributed to infection with the bacteria *Bartonella* (previously *Rochalimaea*), and the most common isolate in cats is *B. henselae*. Although infected cats rarely show obvious clinical signs of illness, the relationship between feline *B. henselae* infection and human cat scratch disease (CSD) has prompted intensive research. Over 20 species of *Bartonella* are now recognized worldwide, although their role as pathogens in feline and human disease is still poorly understood.

Etiology
Bartonellae are small, gram-negative bacteria that are arthropod (flea) transmitted. Studies of cats infected with *B. henselae* and *B. clarridgeiae* have demonstrated transmission of infection between cats by fleas; transmission of *B. henselae* by the tick *Ixodes ricinus* has also been reported.

Pathophysiology
A prolonged (>1 year), fluctuating bacteremia occurs in infected cats, which are usually young (<2 years old). When the infection is first acquired, animals may have a transient lymphadenopathy and low-grade fever. Despite the duration of bacteremia, there seem to be no long-lasting effects.

Clinical presentation
In the small number of feline cases documented, bartonellosis was described as a self-limiting, febrile illness lasting for 2–3 days, with clinical signs of lethargy, unresponsiveness to environmental stimuli, and mild postural reaction deficits in all limbs. In all cases the clinical signs resolved without the administration of antimicrobial therapy. Chronically bacteremic cats are typically healthy, as cats act as reservoirs of infection for the host-adapted *B. henselae*. A number of studies have attempted to link clinical signs or laboratory abnormalities with *Bartonella* seropositivity, including hyperglobulinemia, urinary tract disease, hematuria, CNS disease, and osteoarthritis, but the strength of evidence in these reports has been variable. Additionally, response to treatment for *Bartonella* has been documented in case reports of feline uveitis, endocarditis, and myocarditis.

Differential diagnosis
Since experimental infections have demonstrated transient pyrexia, mild anemia, localized or generalized lymphadenopathy, and/or mild CNS signs, bartonellosis could reasonably be included in the differential diagnosis list for cats with any of those presenting signs. FeLV and FIV testing is indicated.

Diagnosis
Seropositivity (IFA or ELISA) is common among healthy cats and generally only denotes prior exposure to any of several genetic varieties of *Bartonellae*. Therefore, serology is more useful to exclude *Bartonella* from the differential diagnosis list. Currently, blood or tissue culture remains the preferred means of confirming the diagnosis, but these tests might need to be performed repeatedly to avoid false-negative results. Positive serologic results do not appear to be related to bacteremia. PCR testing can be performed on blood, aqueous humor, oropharyngeal swabs, and CSF or tissue aspirates, and submission of multiple specimen types from a single case increases test sensitivity.

Management
Treatment/prognosis
Although marbofloxacin (5 mg/kg PO q12–24h for 6 weeks) or doxycycline (10 mg/kg PO q12–24h for 2–4 weeks; give 5 ml water or food immediately following administration) is the recommended treatment, failure to clear infection is still common. Azithromycin (10 mg/kg PO q24h for 7 days, followed by 10 mg/kg PO q48h for 6–12 weeks) and amoxicillin–clavulanate (62.5 mg/kg PO q12h for 2 months) have also been reported to resolve infection. However, because clinical disease is seldom associated with infection, the value of treating infected cats may be limited to households in which cats reside with immunocompromised humans.

Prevention

There is currently no vaccine available for bartonellosis in cats. However, effective flea and tick management is deemed to be a prudent means of minimizing the risk of infection. Blood donors should be screened for *Bartonella* antibodies.

Public health implications

A variety of clinical disorders in humans (e.g. bacillary angiomatosis, bacillary peliosis, relapsing fever, neuroretinitis, uveitis, endocarditis, and neurologic disorders), as well as CSD, have been associated with *Bartonella* spp. infection. Infections are most profound in people with human immunodeficiency virus (HIV) infection and other causes of immunosuppression. Although infections do develop in immunocompetent individuals, these infections tend to be subclinical or localized to regional lymph nodes.

There is a strong relationship between *B. henselae* infection and human CSD. Despite the fact that CSD in humans has for years been associated with cat scratches, there is considerable speculation as to the actual means of transmission between cats and humans. Currently it appears that feline saliva is not an effective means of transmitting *B. henselae* to humans. However, there is increased awareness of the important role played by fleas in human infections, so the risk of exposure to arthropod vectors, not only to cats, should be considered in suspected human infections.

FELINE BORDETELLOSIS

Definition/overview

Documentation that *Bordetella bronchiseptica* is a significant and primary respiratory disease of cats is distinctly lacking in the clinical literature, although its status as a primary pathogen has been documented in experimental infections of specific pathogen free cats. The most compelling evidence supporting *B. bronchiseptica* as a respiratory pathogen in naturally infected cats is limited predominantly to clusters of kittens with concurrent viral upper respiratory infection, especially calicivirus. In these cases *B. bronchiseptica* infection was associated with severe, frequently fatal, bronchopneumonia in kittens. Bordetellosis could also be considered in the differential diagnosis list for cats presented with acute or chronic coughing.

Etiology

B. bronchiseptica is an aerobic, gram-negative coccobacillus associated with respiratory infections in a variety of species, including humans, dogs, and pigs. The organism is frequently found as part of the normal oral and respiratory flora in cats.

Pathophysiology

B. bronchiseptica is especially well adapted to colonize the respiratory tract. Systemic infection is rare. In all species, *B. bronchiseptica* colonizes the ciliated respiratory epithelial cells in the trachea and nasal cavity. Both endotoxins and exotoxins are released and these, together with other injury, cause stasis of respiratory cilia, significantly compromising clearance mechanisms (mucociliary apparatus).

Clinical presentation

The predominant clinical signs include cough, fever, sneezing, purulent nasal discharge, and regional lymphadenomegaly (**Figures 21.38, 21.39**). Clinical

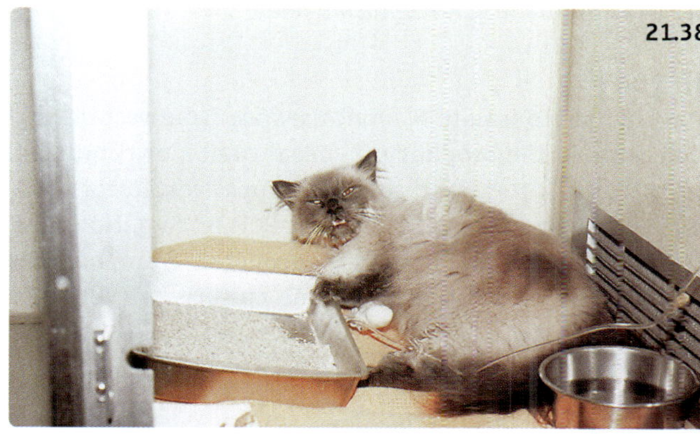

Figure 21.38 The upper respiratory signs associated with *Bordetella* infection are difficult to distinguish from other causes of feline infectious respiratory disease such as feline calicivirus or feline herpesvirus. (Courtesy M. Schaer and C. Steers)

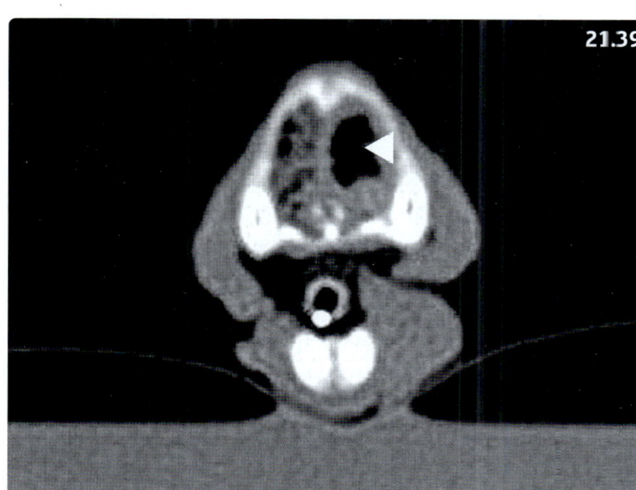

Figure 21.39 CT of the nasal and sinus areas of a Siamese cat with chronic rhinosinusitis and positive bacterial culture results for *Bordetella* spp. Note the absence of turbinates, perhaps due to the destructive nature of a primary feline herpesvirus infection , which is particularly visible on the right side (arrowhead). (Courtesy M. Schaer)

signs are reported to resolve within 10 days, assuming co-infections and/or complications of pneumonia do not develop. Kittens appear to be most prone to developing bronchopneumonia associated with feline bordetellosis. Clinical signs include dyspnea, cyanosis, and death. Coughing is more likely to be reported in kittens with bordetellosis than in adults.

Differential diagnosis

Clinical illness associated with bordetellosis is characteristically associated with other respiratory pathogens such as feline calicivirus (FCV) or feline herpesvirus (FHV). Other differential diagnoses include cleft palate associated with aspiration pneumonia and bacterial pneumonia (e.g. *Mycoplasma felis*).

Diagnosis

It is possible to isolate *B. bronchiseptica* from respiratory secretions in the oropharynx, nasal cavity, or conjunctival sulcus of kittens and cats with upper respiratory disease, either by bacterial culture or PCR testing. However, *B. bronchiseptica* is commonly recovered from healthy cats; therefore, positive bacterial culture or PCR test results, or a positive antibody titer, do not constitute diagnostic confirmation.

Management

B. bronchiseptica is susceptible to commonly used disinfectants. In a multi-cat household or shelter, stress management, including reduction of overcrowding to reduce disease transmission and thorough cleaning and disinfection to reduce fomite transmission of upper respiratory pathogens, should be instituted.

Treatment/prognosis

Several antimicrobial agents are appropriate for use in kittens and cats with clinical signs associated with *B. bronchiseptica*. Considering the potential for kittens concurrently infected with viral upper respiratory infection (e.g. FCV or FHV), antimicrobial therapy is justified in affected kittens to prevent development of bronchopneumonia. Doxycycline (5–10 mg/kg PO q12–24h, with 5 ml water to follow; permanently stained dentition is a possible adverse effect in young kittens), amoxicillin–clavulanate (62.5 mg/kg PO q12h) and pradofloxacin (10 mg/kg PO q24h for 7 days) all have published efficacy in the treatment of feline bordetellosis. In both dogs and cats, *B. bronchiseptica* can persist for as long as 12 weeks following the initial infection. Extended treatment durations of 4 weeks or longer are not unusual.

Prevention

In the USA, a live, avirulent *B. bronchiseptica* vaccine has been licensed for topical (intranasal) administration in cats and kittens. Considering the overall low incidence of clinical disease and the difficulty in documenting infections attributable to *B. bronchiseptica* in kittens, it is currently recommended that this vaccine be limited to use in multi-cat households where there are documented clinical infections with *B. bronchiseptica*, either as a single pathogen, or as a comorbid infection with FHV and/or FCV. Currently, there appears to be little indication for the routine vaccination of adult cats against feline *B. bronchiseptica* (**Tables 21.8** and **21.9**).

Public health implications

Although there are limited reports of *B. bronchiseptica* infections occurring in people, some of which included exposure to dogs, there is no evidence to support direct transmission from cats to humans. However, transmission between cats and dogs has been documented using molecular techniques.

MYCOPLASMA FELIS INFECTION

Definition/overview

Mycoplasma felis has been isolated from the upper respiratory tracts of cats with clinical signs of upper respiratory tract disease and also from healthy cats. Whether acting as a primary pathogen or secondary opportunistic invader, *Mycoplasma* spp. are important infectious agents in feline upper respiratory tract disease.

Etiology

Mycoplasma spp. are degenerate, obligatory parasitic intracellular bacteria, bound by a single limiting cell membrane. *Mycoplasma* spp. have been recovered from the normal flora of the upper respiratory tract, conjunctiva, and genital tract of cats. In addition, *M. felis* has also been implicated as the cause of upper respiratory tract disease, conjunctivitis, and polyarthritis.

Pathophysiology

Mycoplasma infections are generally spread by direct contact or fomite transmission. They often act as opportunistic pathogens where cats are stressed or overcrowded, or when there are comorbid infections.

Clinical presentation

The most common clinical signs are upper respiratory and ocular: sneezing, nasal discharge, conjunctivitis, and/or ocular discharge. Pyrexia and inappetence can occur.

Table 21.8 Initial vaccination of cats/kittens (based on the 2013 AAFP Feline Vaccination Advisory Panel Report)

Core vaccines	Administration	First booster
MLV panleukopenia + MLV herpesvirus + MLV calicivirus. **Note:** When feasible, avoid the use of killed (adjuvanted) vaccines in cats	Primary kitten (≤16 weeks of age) series: administer 1 dose as early as 6 weeks of age, then every 3–4 weeks until 16 weeks of age. Can give an additional dose at 20 weeks of age where risk of exposure is high. Primary adult (>16 weeks of age): administer 2 doses 3–4 weeks apart	Not later than 1 year following the last dose in the initial series. **Note:** Annual booster of cats against FHV-1 and FCV may be recommended in cats housed in high risk environments
Recombinant rabies (nonadjuvanted) (now available as 1-year and 3-year products) or killed rabies (adjuvanted) (available as 1-year and 3-year products)	Single dose usually given at 12–16 weeks of age. (State/Local/Provincial law applies)	Administer a single dose 1 year following administration of the initial dose. (State/Local/Provincial law applies)
Noncore vaccines	**Administration**	**Booster recommendations**
Recombinant feline leukemia virus (nonadjuvanted); also available as killed feline leukemia virus (adjuvanted)	'Highly recommended' for all kittens Give 2 doses at 12 and 16 weeks of age followed by a booster 1 year after completion of the initial series	Where risk of exposure exists administer a single dose annually thereafter. (Some authors recommend revaccination every 2 years for cats considered to be at 'low risk' for exposure)
Killed feline immunodeficiency virus (only available as a killed-adjuvanted vaccine). **Note:** This vaccine is not recommended by the World Small Animal Veterinary Association	3 initial doses, 2–4 weeks apart, if indicated	**Note:** Initial vaccination can cause a false-positive FIV test result on ALL commercial FIV tests for several years. Kittens having nursed from a vaccinated cat may also have a false-positive test result if tested prior to 6 months of age
Feline *Bordetella bronchiseptica* (attenuated live intranasal (nonadjuvanted vaccine)	A single dose, administered intranasally, as early as 4 weeks of age, if indicated	Booster annually where there is documented risk of exposure Indications for use of this product are limited
Chlamydia felis (both nonadjuvanted and adjuvanted products are available)	2 initial doses 3–4 weeks apart, if indicated	Booster annually where there is documented risk of exposure Indications for use of this product are limited
Virulent systemic calicivirus (killed-adjuvanted)	2 initial doses 2–4 weeks apart, if indicated	Disease prevalence is considered low, even within high-density housing environments (e.g. shelters)

AAFP, American Association of Feline Practitioners; MLV, modified live virus.

Note:

- Unless specifically indicated for intranasal administration, all feline vaccines should be administered by the SC route.
- The feline infectious peritonitis vaccine has been recategorized as noncore.
- The World Small Animal Veterinary Association (Vaccine Guidelines Group) does not recommend administration of either the feline infectious peritonitis or the feline immunodeficiency virus vaccine, on grounds of low to no demonstrated efficacy.
- Inactivated (killed), adjuvanted vaccines are only indicated for administration to pregnant queens, and retrovirus (FeLV or FIV) infected cats.

Table 21.9 Booster recommendations for adult cats.

- Core vaccines (MLV panleukopenia + herpesvirus + calicivirus): administer a single dose every 3 years following completion of the initial kitten series and the first booster.
- Recombinant (nonadjuvanted) rabies: a 1-year product and a 3-year product are currently available; administer in accordance with State, Local, or Provincial law.
- (Alternative) killed (adjuvanted) rabies: administered in accordance with State, Local, or Provincial law.
- Noncore vaccines (FeLV): recommended every 1 (or 2) years if risk is sustained (i.e. outdoor cats with reasonable risk of encounter with other cats). The parenteral recombinant FeLV (rFeLV) vaccine is not adjuvanted; all other FeLV vaccines contain adjuvant. (**Note:** Recommendations for booster intervals of FeLV vaccine in adult cats vary from 'annually' to 'every 3 years', regardless of the product used. Consult individual vaccine manufacturers for further brand-specific information and details of post-vaccination support provided.)
- Other noncore vaccines are seldom administered and should be considered only after assessing and defining a clear risk of exposure. All other noncore vaccines are recommended for annual administration as long as the risk of exposure persists.

Lower respiratory infections have also been reported, accompanied by coughing, bronchopneumonia, and/or suppurative bronchitis.

Differential diagnosis

The most common pathogens causing upper respiratory tract disease in cats are FHV-1, FCV, *M. felis*, *Bordetella bronchiseptica*, and *Chlamydia felis*. Other causes of feline pneumonia include bacterial, fungal, and parasitic pathogens, aspiration pneumonia, and neoplasia.

Diagnosis

Commercially available PCR testing is thought to be the most sensitive diagnostic tool available and it specifically detects *M. felis*, thereby avoiding false-positive results due to the presence of other *Mycoplasma* spp. Because of their fastidious nature and limited ability for survival outside the host, bacterial culture of *Mycoplasma* spp. is challenging, requiring rapid transport, special culture techniques, and prolonged incubation periods of up to 3 weeks.

Management

Stress management is paramount to environmental control, and special attention should be given to reducing overcrowding to reduce disease transmission. Thorough cleaning and disinfection is required to reduce fomite transmission of upper respiratory pathogens. *M. felis* is susceptible to routine disinfectants.

Treatment/prognosis

Doxycycline (5–10 mg/kg PO q12–24h; 5 ml water should be administered after every dose; permanently stained dentition is a possible adverse effect in young kittens) is the treatment of choice. Prolonged courses (up to 6 weeks) might be necessary to reduce pathogen load to undetectable levels using quantitative PCR testing, but clinical resolution of infection typically occurs in 1–2 weeks. *M. felis* also has published *in-vitro* and *in-vivo* susceptibility to fluoroquinolones such as marbofloxacin (5 mg/kg PO q12–24h for 6 weeks).

There are no antimicrobial regimens that are proven to clear infection and *M. felis* persists in the host for extended periods, resisting clearance using intracellular localization, immunomodulatory effects, and surface antigen variations. For this reason, clinical resolution might be more important than achieving negative PCR results post-treatment.

Prevention

Population management is the main prevention tool in multi-cat environments. There are currently no vaccines available for the prevention of *M. felis* infection.

Public health implications

There have been isolated case reports of human infections with *M. felis*, but the vast majority of human *Mycoplasma* infections have been due to *Mycoplasma* spp. not found in cats or dogs.

FELINE CHLAMYDIOSIS (FELINE 'PNEUMONITIS')

(See also Chapter 19: Ocular manifestations of systemic diseases.)

Definition/overview

Feline chlamydiosis is caused by the obligate intracellular gram-negative organism *Chlamydia felis*. The organism, which is relatively unstable outside the host, is associated with upper respiratory and ocular (conjunctival) infections. Limited studies suggest that chlamydiosis infection comprises approximately 5% of upper respiratory infections in cats in the USA. In the UK, it is estimated that up to 30% of respiratory disease in cats is associated with *C. felis* infection.

Etiology

Genomic classification of Chlamydiaceae had divided this family into two genera: *Chlamydophila* and *Chlamydia*. However, full genome sequencing has resulted in a recommendation to revert to a single genus, *Chlamydia*.

Pathophysiology

There is still limited information on the pathogenesis of this infection in cats; however, chronic infections, particularly among households of cats, have been documented. *C. felis* has been isolated from experimentally infected cats for periods of up to 18 months, suggesting the development of a carrier state subsequent to recovery.

Clinical presentation

Despite the common name, feline 'pneumonitis', *C. felis* infection in cats is most commonly associated with unilateral or bilateral conjunctivitis and chemosis (**Figure 21.40**). Occasional sneezing (much less than that associated with viral upper respiratory disease) is also reported. Although the organism can disseminate and has been found in the GI and reproductive tracts, clinical signs associated with dissemination are not reported. Currently, there is no known direct association between *C. felis* infection and feline reproductive disease.

Differential diagnosis

Infections with FHV, FCV, *Bordetella bronchiseptica*, and/or *Mycoplasma felis*; conjunctival injury.

Diagnosis

PCR detection of *C. felis* from conjunctival swabs is the preferred method of diagnosis. Since the organism is intracellular, it is important to submit swabs that contain sufficient cellular material. Cotton swabs with plastic stems should be used; plain sterile tubes without transport medium are required for transport. Cats suspected of having chlamydiosis could also be tested for FeLV and FIV infection.

Direct cytologic examination of conjunctival swabs for basophilic intracytoplasmic inclusions has been previously described. However, specimens are only likely to be positive early in the infection, so false-negative cytologic findings are common. Confusion with other causes of basophilic inclusions can also occur resulting in false-positive results.

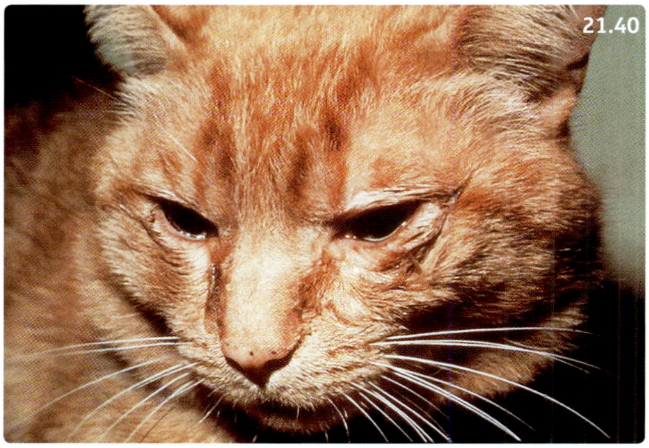

Figure 21.40 Bilateral conjunctivitis in a 2-year-old cat with chlamydiosis.

Management

Treatment/prognosis

Tetracyclines are regarded as the most effective antibiotics for use against *C. felis* infection in cats. Because this organism is known to disseminate, both topical and systemic treatment are recommended. For conjunctivitis, tetracycline ophthalmic drops are preferred over chlortetracycline ophthalmic drops. Both eyes should be treated four times daily for 7–10 days. Oral doxycycline (5–10 mg/kg q24h for at least 4 weeks, or at least 2 weeks after clinical resolution, whichever is longer) can also be given. Oral doxycycline should be followed with 5 ml of water when administering this antimicrobial to cats. Azithromycin treatment has not been shown to completely eliminate *C. felis* infection and is not currently recommended.

Prevention

The most effective means of preventing chlamydiosis in cats is to limit exposure of susceptible kittens and cats to any cat with signs of respiratory or conjunctival disease. However, within catteries, animal shelters, and boarding catteries, preventing contact with infected carrier cats may be difficult or impossible to achieve. Currently, all available *C. felis* vaccines approved for use in cats must be administered parenterally (**Tables 21.8** and **21.9**); accidental ocular inoculation of modified live vaccines against *C. felis* can result in typical signs of infection. These vaccines appear to give reasonable protection against clinical signs of disease, but not against infection. The current recommendation for administration of *C. felis* vaccine is limited to those cats with known or suspected risk of exposure. The vaccine is recommended for administration to cats with documented risk of exposure to *Chlamydia*.

Public health implications

C. felis is generally regarded as a pathogen unique to the cat. Isolated reports of human infection with feline *C. felis* have raised concern regarding its potential as a zoonotic infection. However, the few reports of human infection are limited to minor, self-limiting conjunctivitis. *C. felis* is not regarded as an important zoonotic disease. Human *Chlamydia psittaci* infections are generally acquired from birds rather than cats or dogs.

HEMOPLASMAS (HEMOTROPIC MYCOPLASMAS)

(See also Chapter 16: Hematologic disorders.)

Definition/overview

Mycoplasma haemofelis (formerly *Haemobartonella felis*) belongs to a genus of gram-negative, non-acid-fast, epicellular parasites of red blood cells (RBCs). Acute infections are characterized by rapid-onset hemolytic anemia, hence the name 'infectious anemia'. While chronic *M. haemofelis* infection is characterized by episodes of fluctuating parasitemia, clinical anemia does not usually occur in the absence of comorbidities. Persistent Coombs-positive autoagglutination by antibodies bound to RBCs can be found in cats with acute anemia due to *M. haemofelis* infection.

Other variants of hemoplasmas known to infect cats are *Candidatus* Mycoplasma 'haemominutum' and *Candidatus* Mycoplasma 'turicensis'. However, infections with these species appear to be subclinical in cats; infections with more than one hemoplasma species are relatively common. Retrovirus (FeLV and FIV) infection appears to be a risk factor for hemoplasma infection and co-infections with retroviruses are likely to increase the clinical severity of disease.

Etiology

The disease is thought to be transmitted predominantly by fleas, although conclusive evidence has not yet been published. Older, male nonpedigree cats are at higher risk of infection and outdoor roaming and the presence of cat fight abscesses has also been associated with infection. Direct cat-to-cat infection by casual contact, such as mutual grooming, is thought to be unlikely, while transfusion of blood from apparently healthy carrier cats is an effective means of transmitting *M. haemofelis*.

Pathophysiology

Acute *M. haemofelis* infection is associated with significant morbidity and can be fatal if left untreated. Cats that ultimately recover from acute infections remain chronically infected for years. Depending on the intrinsic immunologic and phagocytic responses, chronic carrier cats may manifest small numbers of organisms on the surface of RBCs, or may manifest no evidence of infection until stressed (e.g. chronic corticosteroid therapy, FeLV/FIV-positive status). Sequestration in the spleen or liver at times of low circulating organism numbers has not been demonstrated.

Clinical presentation

While acute infections are often associated with significant anemia, many cats with chronic infections experience only mild anemia and manifest few, if any, clinical signs. When clinical signs are present, they are most likely related to anemia (i.e. weakness, lethargy, pallor, and splenomegaly). Cats are only occasionally noted to be icteric (**Figure 21.41**).

Differential diagnosis

Immune-mediated hemolytic anemia, erythroid hypoplasia, or aplasia, in addition to FeLV and FIV, are not only important differential diagnoses, but each may occur concurrently with *M. haemofelis* infection.

Diagnosis

Hematologic changes are the most important laboratory findings in clinical hemoplasmosis. Significant anemia (hematocrit 0.2 l/l [20%] and frequently <0.1 l/l [10%]) and associated lethargy are characteristic. Organisms are recognized in stained blood films in only about 50% of cats during the acute phase of infection. Leukocyte and platelet counts are usually normal. The bone marrow myeloid to erythroid ratio is typically normal (1:1) during the early stage of the disease, but may decrease later. RBC autoagglutination may be observed in anticoagulated whole blood during acute hemoplasmosis. A direct Coombs test may also be positive at this time.

Definitive diagnosis of *M. haemofelis* infection is based on the demonstration of organisms in peripheral blood (**Figure 21.42**). A blood film stained with a Romanowsky-type stain (e.g. Wright, Giemsa, Diff-Quik®) is recommended. Since organisms can detach themselves from erythrocytes during storage, it is recommended that blood

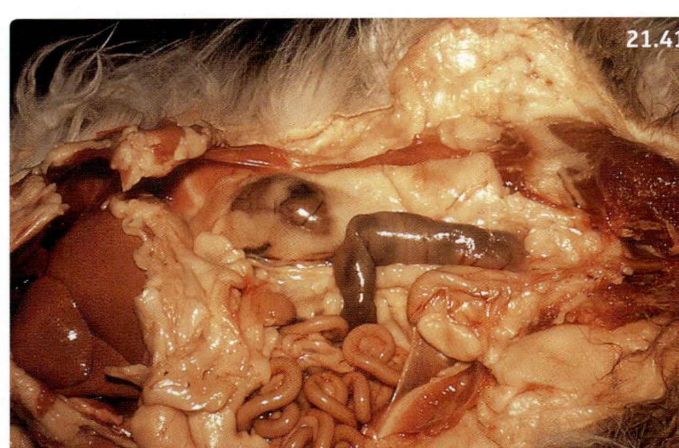

Figure 21.41 Necropsy of a 1-year-old cat with severe hemolytic anemia associated with severe acute *Mycoplasma haemofelis* infection. Icterus was marked and was accompanied by hepatic lipidosis.

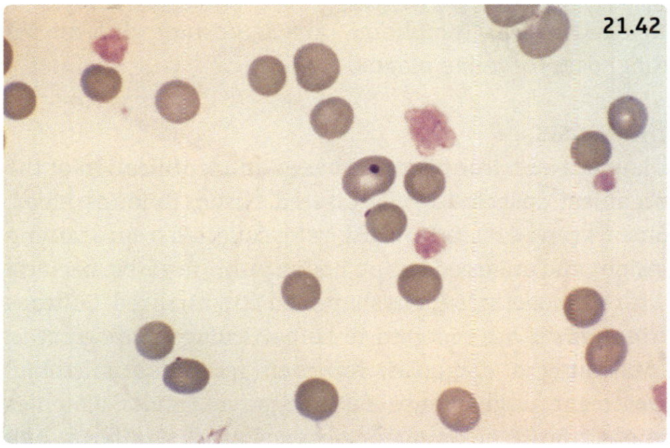

Figure 21.42 Peripheral blood smear from a cat demonstrating faint staining *Mycoplasma haemofelis* on the red blood cell surface.

smears be made immediately upon collection. Artifacts such as Howell–Jolly bodies and other hemotropic organisms, such as *Candidatus* Mycoplasma 'haemominutum' or *Candidatus* Mycoplasma 'turicensis', might be interpreted as *M. haemofelis* on visual examination of stained blood smears, resulting in false-positive results. It is not possible to differentiate between hemoplasma species cytologically. However, PCR assays based on 16S rRNA gene detection can enable speciation and be either conventional (nonquantitative; PCR) or real-time (qualitative; qPCR).

Management

Treatment/prognosis

Transfusion of whole blood is generally recommended in cats with hematocrits <0.15 l/l (15%). This is particularly important in cats with clinical signs associated with acute-onset anemia.

Both doxycycline (5 mg/kg PO q12h for 2–6 weeks, followed at each administration by 5 ml water) and fluoroquinolones (marbofloxacin 2 mg/kg PO q24h for 4 weeks; pradofloxacin 10 mg/kg PO q24h 21 days) have been recommended for the treatment of *M. haemofelis* infection in cats. Because of the highly fluctuating nature of *M. haemofelis* parasitemia, a reduction in organism load on qPCR cannot be interpreted as response to treatment. Pradofloxacin can also be used for refractory cases or when reduction in circulating load needs to be maximized. Since no treatment regimen has been shown to clear infection, the treatment of subclinically infected cats is not currently recommended. As a means of reducing the immune-mediated components of clinical disease, administration of prednisolone (1–2 mg/kg PO q12h for at least 7–10 days) might be indicated to augment resolution of anemia due to hemophagocytosis. However, there is no published evidence for the efficacy of glucocorticoid treatment and some case reports have shown efficacy with antimicrobial treatment alone.

The prognosis for uncomplicated *M. haemofelis* infection in cats is good, assuming that treatment can be administered and is tolerated by the cat. However, the correlation of clinical hemoplasmosis with retrovirus infection justifies routine testing of anemic cats for FeLV and FIV.

Prevention

Since fleas are thought to be involved in the transmission of feline hemoplasmosis, a flea control program should be instituted. Additionally, prevention of cat fight abscesses might also reduce risk. There is currently no vaccine available for cats or dogs against hemoplasmosis.

Public health implications

Infection is unique to the cat and, as such, does not pose any health risk to humans.

PLAGUE

Definition/overview

Plague is an uncommon infection of cats caused by the facultative anaerobic, gram-negative bacterium *Yersinia pestis*. The organism has been sustained for centuries by chronic bacteremia in wild rodents, including rock squirrels, ground squirrels, and prairie dogs. In the USA, reported cases of plague have a seasonal distribution, corresponding to the period when rodents and fleas are most active and humans are most likely to be outdoors (February to August). *Xenopsylla cheopis* fleas are considered efficient vectors, while *Ctenocephalides* species are not as likely to transmit *Y. pestis*.

Although infections in domestic animals are uncommon, the fact that both domestic and feral cats are susceptible to *Y. pestis* infection, and that cats are a documented source of human infection, means that plague must be regarded as a significant zoonotic infection of cats. Although dogs can become infected, their susceptibility is considerably less than cats.

Etiology

Transmission of the bacterium to susceptible hosts occurs predominantly through flea bites or the ingestion of infected rodents or lagomorphs; humans, dogs, and cats are usually accidental hosts and are not responsible for the transmission of infection. However, infection can also be transmitted directly through contact with broken skin or by inhalation of infectious microdroplets from cats or humans infected with the pneumonic form of plague.

Pathophysiology

The incubation period depends on the route of entry of the organism: 2–6 days with flea bites; 1–3 days after inhalation or ingestion. Typically, there is evidence of neutrophilic leukocytosis with a left shift and lymphopenia, and hyperglycemia, azotemia, hypokalemia, hypoalbuminemia, hyperglobulinemia, hypochloremia, hyperbilirubinemia, and elevated SAP and ALT.

Clinical presentation

Three clinical forms of *Y. pestis* infection have been recognized in cats: bubonic (most common), septicemic, and pneumonic. Following ingestion of infected rodents, cats that become infected typically develop fever, necrotic stomatitis and lymphadenomegaly, particularly around the head and neck (**Figure 21.43**). Lymph nodes may rupture and drain through to the skin surface. Subsequently, septicemia may develop in a small number of cats (septicemic plague). Fever, shock, DIC, and pneumonitis are short-lived signs that precede death. Hematogenous spread of the organism to the lungs in cats culminates in pneumonic plague, which is particularly likely to be fatal.

Within endemic areas (particularly the southwestern USA and western coastal states), cats presented with persistent fever, lymph node enlargement, tonsillar enlargement, necrotic stomatitis, facial ulceration, or abdominal distension should be evaluated for plague.

Differential diagnosis

Any cat living in, or from, a plague-endemic area should be considered suspect if presented for stomatitis, chronic respiratory disease, and/or lymphadenomegaly. Feline frontal sinusitis/rhinitis, sepsis, neoplasia, toxemia, pyometra, and lymphoma are important differential diagnoses for feline plague.

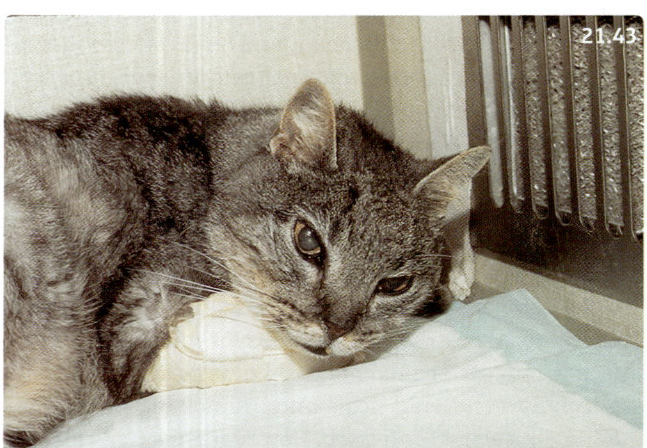

Figure 21.43 Feline plague can cause signs of other more familiar syndromes such as the severe frontal sinusitis shown in this cat. (Courtesy M. Schaer)

Diagnosis

Diagnosis of feline plague is based on identification of the organism collected from cultured tissue, fluid, or blood. Smears can be made from aspirates collected from draining lesions and enlarged lymph nodes; gram-negative bacteria with a bipolar safety pin shape can be visualized. Cultures from tonsils are reported to be particularly important in confirming a diagnosis; however, recent antimicrobial treatment might cause false-negative results. Colonies might take 48 hours to appear; they are a significant biohazard and should be sent to recommended laboratories obtained on the advice of local public health authorities. Acute and convalescent antibody titers can also be used to document infection. Since the incubation period is relatively short (1–6 days), seronegative results can occur initially in infected cats. A four-fold rise in antibody titer over 3–4 weeks is necessary to distinguish active disease from prior exposure. Because of the zoonotic potential of feline plague, attempts to culture the organism in a veterinary practice are discouraged. IFA testing can be performed on heat fixed slides of tissue aspirates or on impression smears collected at necropsy and submitted to recommended testing facilities. Specimens should not be shipped to routine veterinary diagnostic laboratories; local public health authorities should be contacted regarding approved testing laboratories and specific shipping instructions.

Management

Treatment/prognosis

Because of the time delay involved in confirming a diagnosis, treatment is typically initiated prior to establishing a diagnosis. The medical management of cats suspected of having plague includes treatment for fleas, flushing abscesses or draining lymph nodes, and administering antimicrobial therapy for a minimum of 10 days. It is particularly important that all cats suspected of having plague be handled by persons wearing full personal protective equipment, including examination gloves, gowns, and a surgical mask and goggles or a full face mask. Extreme care should be taken when working with cats that manifest signs of pneumonia. All suspect cases should be isolated for at least the first 3 days of antimicrobial therapy and the number of people in contact with the case should be reduced to the bare minimum.

Although several antimicrobials have been effective against *Y. pestis* in cats, drug resistant strains are being isolated with increasing frequency. Administration of doxycycline (10 mg/kg IV or PO q24h 10 days; administer

IV diluted in 100 ml of lactated Ringer's solution over 2 hours) is recommended. Parenteral treatment is recommended for at least the first 72 hours to avoid contact with the oral cavity of infected cats. Alternatively, gentamicin (5–8 mg/kg IV, IM, or SC q24h for 10 days) can be administered. Chloroamphenicol (25–50 mg/kg PO q12h for 10 days; 12–30 mg/kg IV, IM, or SC q12h for 10 days) and trimethoprim–sulfamethoxazole (30 mg/kg PO q12h for 10 days) also have efficacy against *Y. pestis*. Cats that have been exposed to plague may be treated prophylactically with doxycycline (10 mg/kg IV or PO q24h for at least 7 days). The prognosis for cats with clinical signs associated with plague depends on treatment status. Up to 75% of infected cats may die if untreated, but >90% cats treated with appropriate antimicrobial therapy survive.

Prevention

Since it is impractical to control the wild rodent population within endemic areas, and a plague vaccine is not available for use in animals at risk, effective flea control is the best means of preventing infection. In addition, dogs and cats should be restricted from hunting and access to carcasses of dead rodents or rabbits.

Public health implications

The risk of human exposure to plague appears to be greatest in the western USA, particularly California, Arizona, and New Mexico. Because human plague infection, particularly pneumonic plague, has a significant mortality rate, veterinarians working in endemic areas should be particularly alert to potential infections in cats. Because feline and canine cases are now relatively rare, underrecognition could be problematic. Furthermore, there appears to be an increased risk of exposure when maintaining and treating nondomestic cats living in endemic areas. Attempts should be made to limit exposure to these potential carriers.

VIRAL INFECTIONS

FELINE INFECTIOUS PERITONITIS

Definition/overview

Feline infectious peritonitis (FIP) is a common disease in cats caused by a virulent mutation of feline enteric coronavirus (FECV). During the process of mutation from FECV to FIP virus (FIPV), the virus loses its tropism for enterocytes and gains tropism for macrophages, enabling it to replicate inside a specific population of precursor monocytes/macrophages with an affinity for the endothelium of venules in the serosa, omentum, pleura, meninges, and uveal tract. At least three types of mutations in FECVs are currently under study in the transition of FECV to FIPV, two in the spike protein and one in the accessory 3c genes. Clinical FIP is characterized by widespread immune-mediated vasculitis and/or pyogranulomas, manifesting as an effusive form, with high-protein effusions in body cavities, or a noneffusive form characterized by tissue granulomas. While the disease course from the onset of clinical signs until death can be variable, ranging from weeks to months and, rarely, years, it is usually shorter in younger cats and those with effusive disease. The mortality rate is extremely high and one study reported a 1-year survival rate of 5%.

Etiology

Coronaviruses are large enveloped RNA viruses and are the most common pathogen isolated from the feces of cats. Infection with FECV is typically acquired by kittens or young cats in multi-cat households from exposure to chronically shedding cats via the fecal–oral and oral–oral routes. Mutation from FECV to FIPV is thought to occur at some point after FECV infection, between viral replication in enterocytes and replication in macrophages. Direct transmission of FIPV between cats is thought to be extremely rare, since FIPV is found inside macrophages.

Pathophysiology

Initially, the virus replicates in oropharyngeal tissues and in the enterocytes at the tips of the intestinal villi. The manifestation of infection depends on several predisposing factors, including the immunocompetence of the host and the strain and dose of virus. A vigorous cell-mediated immune response is required for protection from FIP, while antibodies produced in response to infection enhance the uptake and replication of FIPVs in macrophages and contribute to the immune-mediated vasculitis seen in effusive cases. If the antibody-mediated immune response predominates, effusive FIP results, but if an intermediate cell-mediated immune response occurs, noneffusive FIP results. The noneffusive (dry) form of the disease is limited to relatively small numbers of FIPV-infected macrophages in pyogranulomas in specific target organs. Experimental infections resulting in the noneffusive form have demonstrated brief episodes of effusive disease before the dry form predominates and conversely, in the terminal stages of the dry form, the immune system can be overwhelmed and the effusive form results.

Clinical presentation

There are two predominant clinical manifestations of FIP recognized in domestic cats: the effusive, or 'wet', form characterized by a viscous, high protein-content fluid in

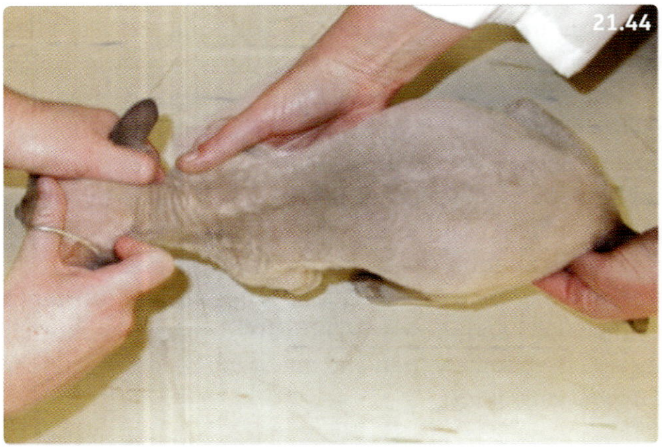

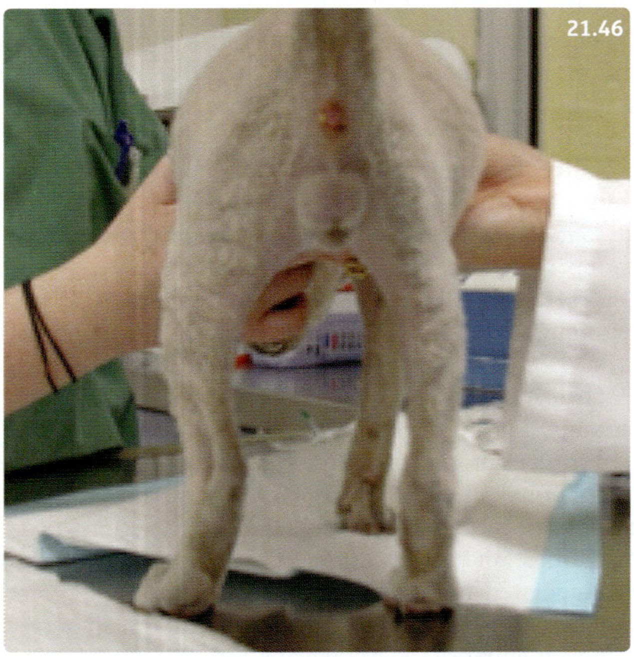

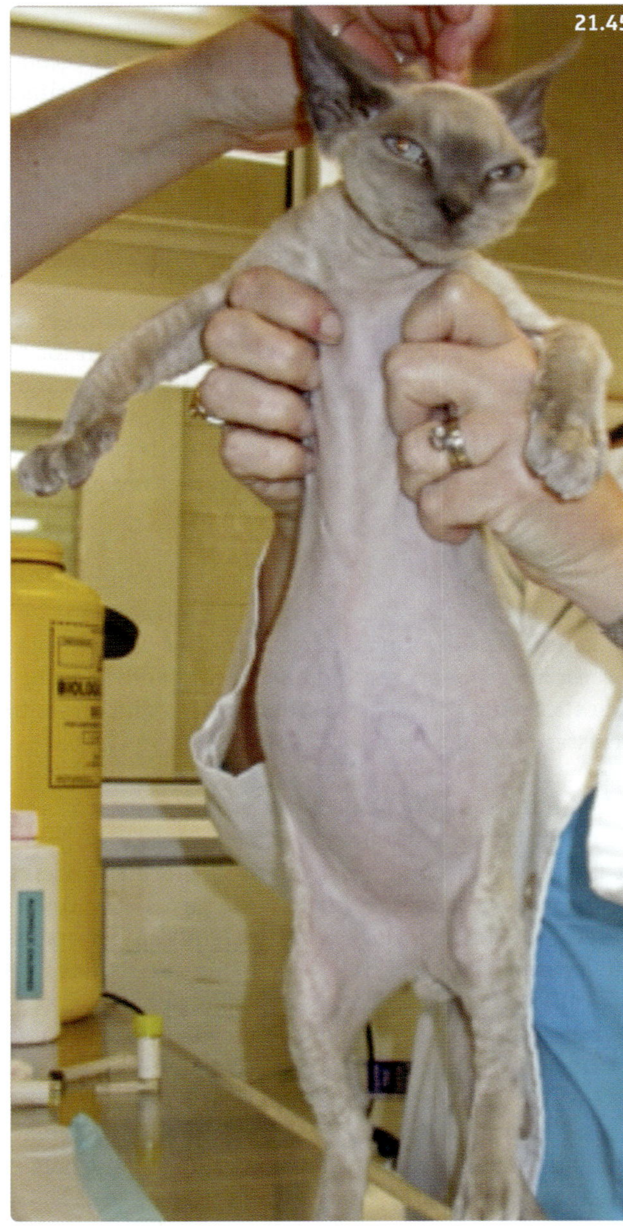

Figures 21.44–21.46 Eight-month-old neutered male Siamese cat with effusive FIP. (21.44, 21.45) Note the abdominal distension due to the peritoneal effusion. (21.46) Note the scrotal effusion.

the abdominal or, less often, the pleural cavity; and the noneffusive, 'dry', form characterized by pyogranulomatous lesions seen predominantly in the abdominal cavity, but also occurring in the thorax, eyes, or CNS. Although infections are most common amongst cats 2 years of age and younger, cats of any age are susceptible.

The effusive form of FIP is readily diagnosed by examination of fluid recovered from any body cavity (**Figures 21.44–21.46**). The highly viscous effusion is classified as an inflammatory exudate; it contains a high protein content (>35 g/l [3.5 g/dl]) and has a high specific gravity (**Figure 21.47**). Cytologic evaluation of the fluid usually reveals a relatively hypocellular (<5,000 nucleated cells/μl) fluid comprised of low to moderate numbers of neutrophils and macrophages and some lymphocytes (**Figure 21.48**). Abdominal swelling with a fluid wave is typically described, although fluid can accumulate in the pleural space, scrotum, and/or pericardium.

The absence of fluid accumulation, combined with the wide spectrum of clinical signs associated with this form of the disease, makes noneffusive FIP considerably more difficult to diagnose than the effusive form. The most common sites for lesions to occur are in the abdominal cavity, particularly in the liver, mesenteric lymph nodes, and spleen, and the CNS. Ocular signs of FIP include anterior uveitis, hyphema, hypopyon, keratic precipitates

(**Figure 21.49**), retinal detachment, perivascular cuffing, hemorrhage, and retinitis (see **Figures 19.20–19.23**). A variety of neurologic signs can develop, depending on the particular site within the CNS in which the lesions occur. The most commonly reported CNS signs of FIP are seizures and posterior paresis.

Interestingly, FIP is not regarded as a cause of 'fading kitten' syndrome (severe illness and death occurring between birth and weaning), perhaps because of maternally derived immune protection in young kittens. It has been shown that isolating kittens from all other cats by the age of 5 weeks and keeping them in small groups is an effective strategy for protecting kittens born into endemically infected households. However, FIP remains a relatively common cause of death due to infection among weaned kittens.

Differential diagnosis

Differential diagnoses for cats with the effusive form of FIP include ascites (hepatic or cardiac origin), cholangiohepatitis, peritonitis, neoplasia, and pregnancy. Among cats with significant accumulation of pleural fluid, neoplasia, diaphragmatic hernia, heart failure, exudative pleuritis (pyothorax), and chylothorax are reasonable differential diagnoses that should be considered.

The noneffusive form of FIP includes an extensive list of differential diagnoses depending on the organ system(s) involved (e.g. neurologic/ocular signs [seizures, posterior paralysis, toxoplasmosis, neoplasia, idiopathic encephalomyelitis/meningitis, feline spongiform encephalopathy, retinitis with or without retinal detachment, uveitis ± keratic precipitates and hyphema]).

Diagnosis

Clinical diagnosis is based predominantly on clinical signs and selected laboratory abnormalities. Analysis of effusion can be used to support a clinical diagnosis of FIP:

- Viscous effusion; clot may form when fluid is exposed to air.
- High protein-content effusion (usually >35 g/l [3.5 g/dl).
- Albumin:globulin ratio of effusion is usually <0.45.
- Cytology: relatively hypocellular (<5,000 nucleated cells/µl); pyogranulomatous fluid consisting of neutrophils and macrophages and low numbers of lymphocytes.

The Rivalta test (**Figure 21.50**), which involves placing drops of effusion fluid into a tube containing weak acetic acid and watching for characteristic clots to appear, showed promise, but positive results can occur with

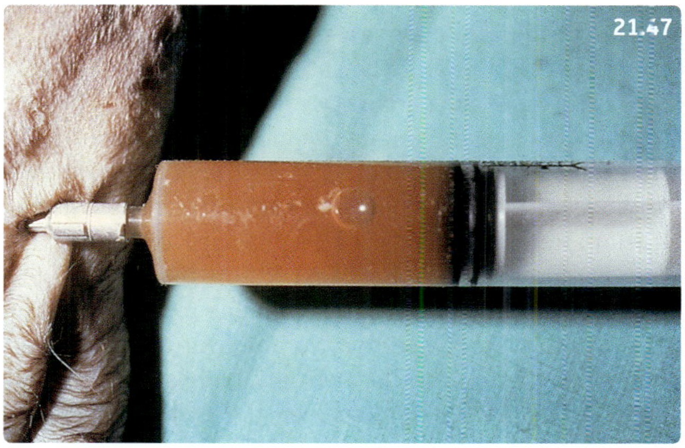

Figure 21.47 Abdominocentesis in a cat with effusive FIP reveals the characteristic viscous, high specific gravity exudate. Note that in some cases the globulin concentration of the fluid is sufficiently high that the sample might clot when exposed to air.

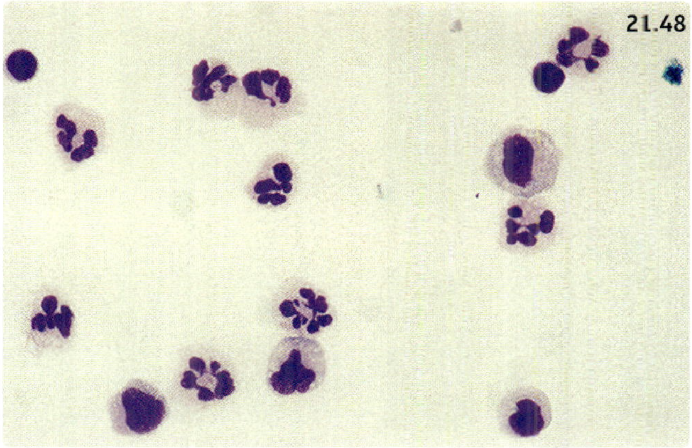

Figure 21.48 Cytopathology of abdominal fluid from a cat with the effusive form of FIP is characterized as a relatively hypocellular fluid containing a mixture of neutrophils and macrophages (pyogranulamatous effusion).

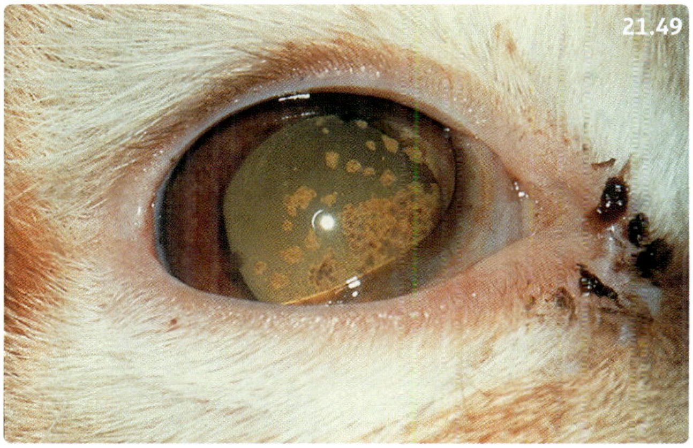

Figure 21.49 Keratic precipitates in the right eye of a cat with the noneffusive form of FIP.

effusions collected from cases of lymphoma or bacterial infections. Additionally, the subjective nature of the test reduces its diagnostic accuracy.

Serologic tests are among the most commonly utilized and frequently criticized tests undertaken to establish a diagnosis of FIP, particularly in cats presenting without effusion. However, it must be emphasized that currently there is no reliable serologic test for the diagnosis of FIP virus infection. Serologic tests available to veterinarians are limited to the detection of coronavirus antibody only and do not distinguish between antibodies against FIPV and those against FECV. However, the magnitude of the antibody titer can be of some use clinically, in that healthy cats exposed to FECV are likely to have titers of 1:100–1:400, a titer of 1:1600 is suspicious for FIPV, and a titer of at least 1:3,200 is highly suggestive of FIP. False-negative antibody titer results can occur in the terminal stages of FIP because of antigen–antibody binding. Antibody titers are also linked to the likelihood of fecal shedding of FECV, with titers of 1:100 or less denoting a low likelihood of fecal shedding, while cats with titers of at least 1:400 are usually shedding FECV in the feces.

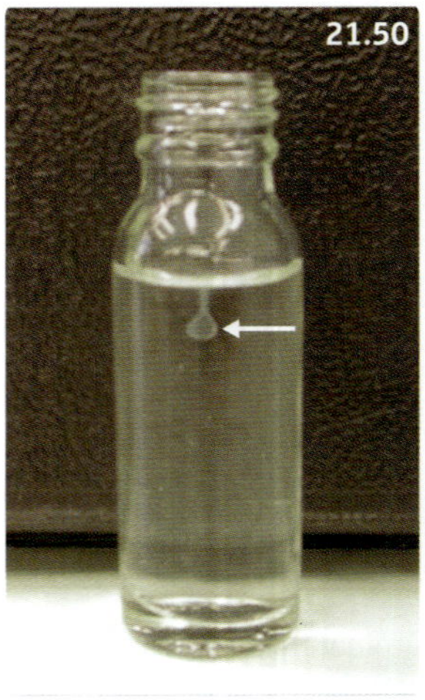

Figure 21.50 Positive Rivalta's test from a cat with effusive FIP showing clotted droplet of effusion in weak acetic acid (arrow).

A number of direct detection methods using PCR to detect FIP virus, rather than FECV, in blood, effusions, and feces have been developed over the last 20 years, but problems with diagnostic sensitivity and specificity have inevitably emerged after more widespread clinical use. More recently, a PCR test designed to differentiate between FECV and FIPV, based on detection of the spike protein, has become commercially available. Test results from 186 cats that were either healthy or had FIP confirmed on biopsy, produced a calculated sensitivity of 98.7% and a specificity of 100%. The preferred specimens are pleural or abdominal effusions, but PCR can also be performed on tissue aspirates, or fresh tissues. Whole blood in EDTA is not recommended, as often the level of viremia is too low to permit biotyping.

The only reference standard method for diagnosing FIP antemortem is immunohistochemistry on biopsy specimens. While this test is highly specific, it cannot be used to rule out a diagnosis of FIP and its accuracy is dependent on specimen selection and the expertise of the microscopist reading the slides. Additionally, cases suspect for FIP often have clinical signs and laboratory abnormalities that do not make them good surgical candidates. A stressful event, such as anesthesia and surgery, has been known to result in clinical progression of disease.

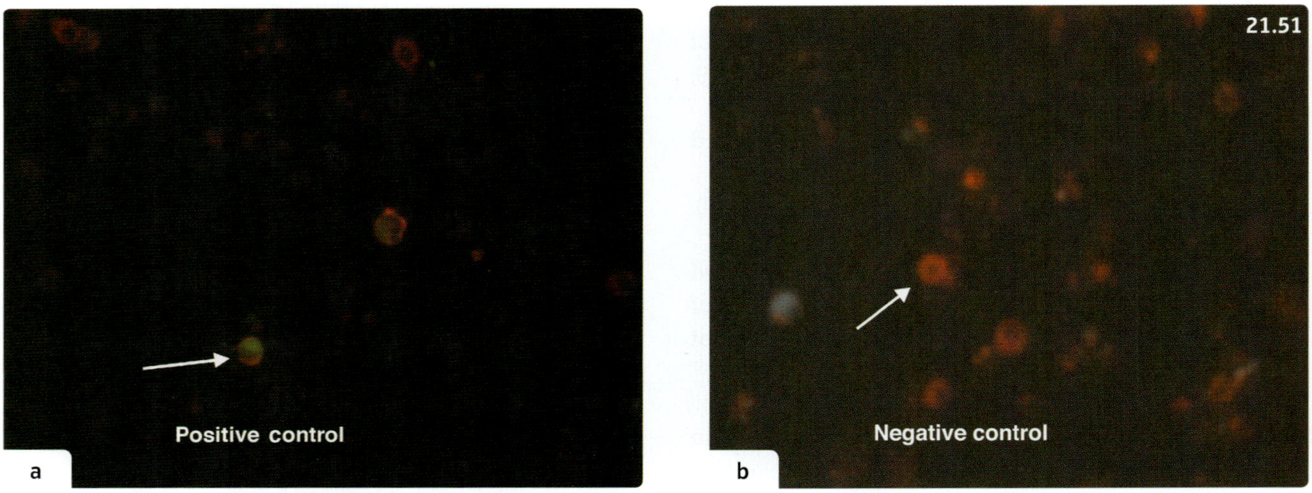

Figures 21.51a, b (a) Direct immunofluorescence staining of feline abdominal effusion – positive control specimen (arrow). (b) Direct immunofluorescence staining of feline abdominal effusion – negative control specimen (arrow).

Direct immunofluorescence staining detects intracellular FIPV in macrophages in effusions from cats with FIP and is widely used in Europe and Australia (**Figures 21.51a, b**). This was once thought to be a confirmatory test, but a recent publication reported its specificity to be 71.4%, relegating it to the ranks of contributory evidence rather than a reference standard test.

Routine hematology often shows mild, chronic nonregenerative anemia; leukocytosis with absolute neutrophilia and lymphopenia is frequently reported. Elevated serum bilirubin and bilirubinuria are also common in cats with FIP and up to 70–75% have elevated serum protein. Assessment of albumin and globulin typically reveals a slight decrease in the albumin fraction and a significant, sometimes dramatic, increase in the globulin fraction. When FIP disease prevalence is low, a high A:G ratio can rule out FIP, but a low A:G ratio does not confirm a diagnosis of FIP.

Characteristically, a polyclonal hypergammaglobulinemia can be documented in cats with hyperproteinemia. Serum protein electrophoresis provides a graphic portrayal of the serum proteins; however, this test does not provide definitive diagnostic information, since other chronic infections (e.g. FeLV and FIV) may also produce similar findings on electrophoresis (**Figure 21.52**).

A diagnosis of FIP can be confirmed with histopathology, which identifies pyogranuloma formation and/or vasculitis, and/or immunohistochemistry to identify FIPV (**Figure 21.53, 21.54a, b**). This usually takes place at necropsy.

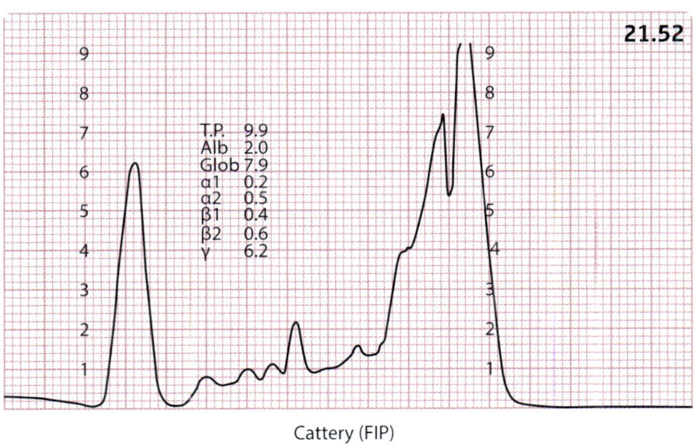

Figure 21.52 Serum protein electrophoresis (densitometer tracing) from a cat with hyperglobulinemia and hypoalbuminemia associated with noneffusive FIP.

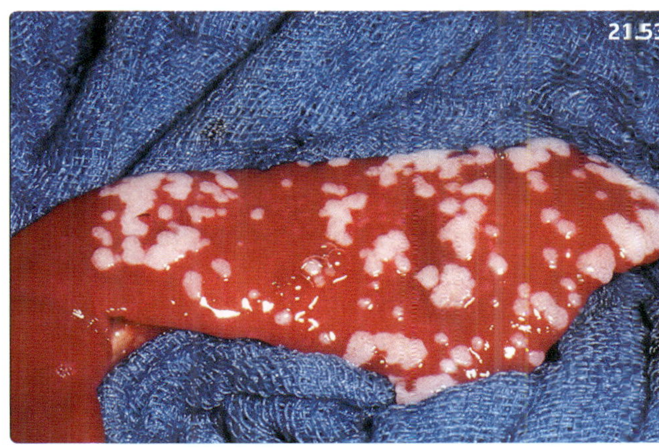

Figure 21.53 Splenic pyogranulomas in a cat with noneffusive FIP.

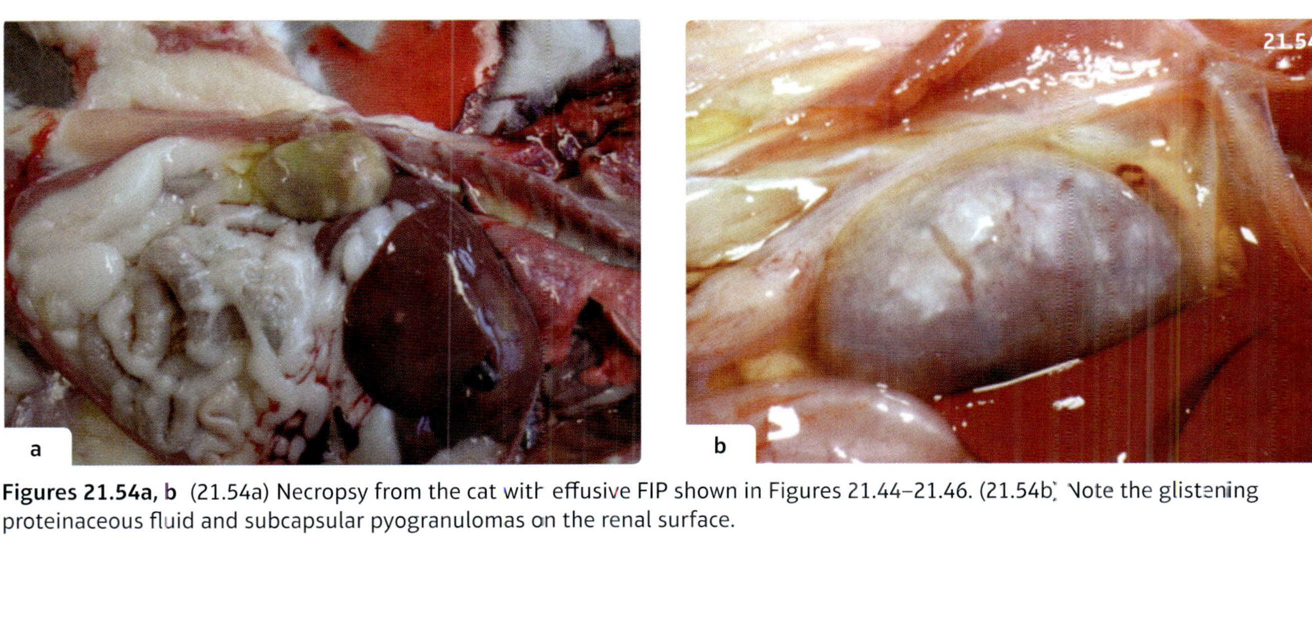

Figures 21.54a, b (21.54a) Necropsy from the cat with effusive FIP shown in Figures 21.44–21.46. (21.54b) Note the glistening proteinaceous fluid and subcapsular pyogranulomas on the renal surface.

Management

Treatment/prognosis

Despite efforts to assess the value of various antiviral, anti-inflammatory, immunosuppressant, and immunostimulant drugs, there is still no definitive treatment for cats with clinical FIP. Although some cats may survive for several months or years with supportive treatment, antiviral therapy is not available. Cats with effusive disease usually live days to weeks after diagnosis. The long-term prognosis for cats with FIP is grave. A variety of anti-inflammatory and immunosuppressive treatments have been recommended (e.g. prednisolone, 2–4 mg/kg PO q24h, with gradually reducing doses every 10–14 days, as needed, to control signs). However, no treatment is known to extend the life of an infected cat.

Prevention

Although a modified live FIP vaccine is commercially available, husbandry and management of kittens in multi-cat households are significantly more important in the prevention of FIP among susceptible cats. Kittens that derive maternal antibodies from coronavirus-shedding queens should be protected until they are 5–6 weeks of age. When possible, early weaning by 5 weeks of age and permanent separation of kittens from the queen and other potentially FECV-shedding cats are particularly valuable management tools in minimizing coronavirus transmission from queens to kittens.

Although most authors agree that the modified live FIP virus vaccine is safe to administer to cats, the efficacy of the vaccine has been challenged. Furthermore, the manufacturer's recommendation to administer the first dose of vaccine (intranasally) at 16 weeks of age may be too late to protect susceptible kittens from infected queens.

Public health implications

FIP poses no known public health risk.

FELINE LEUKEMIA VIRUS

Definition/overview

FeLV is a single-stranded RNA virus (oncornavirus) belonging to the retrovirus group. FeLV is a highly fatal, oncogenic (tumor-producing) virus that replicates within numerous tissues in cats, including bone marrow, salivary glands, and respiratory epithelium.

Etiology

The virus is spread both vertically (to offspring *in utero* or to neonates through milk) and horizontally (from cat to cat). Subtypes A, B, C, and T exist; the FeLV-A subtype is ubiquitous and present in all infections. The virus has worldwide significance and is among the most important infectious diseases affecting cats.

Pathophysiology

The biology of FeLV infection in cats is highly complex. After infection, usually by the oronasal route after constant exposure to chronically shedding cats, the virus travels via the lymphocytes to the bone marrow. Viral RNA integrates into the host cells to replicate, producing proviral DNA that can be detected by PCR testing. Viremia ensues and the virus infects the salivary glands and GI epithelium; viral shedding is via saliva and feces. In a household endemically infected with FeLV, in which no control measures are instituted, there are four possible outcomes of infection:

- Abortive infection. These cats were formerly called 'regressor cats'. They mount an effective humoral and cell-mediated immune response on exposure to low doses of FeLV. They do not test antigen positive on p27 ELISA tests or on provirus PCR blood tests at any stage.
- Regressive infection. These cats were formerly classified as 'transiently viremic followed by latent infection'. After infection, FeLV reaches the bone marrow and viral integration occurs; the cat temporarily tests p27 ELISA positive; the cat's blood is provirus PCR positive and viral shedding occurs, mainly in the saliva. An immune response ensues and within 3-16 weeks of initial infection, the cat tests p27 ELISA negative. FeLV-positive status persists on proviral PCR blood testing, but viral load is low. Since active viral replication is needed for the clinical effects of FeLV to develop, the risk of clinical disease is relatively low. However, there is a potential risk of reactivation, especially in the first year of infection.
- Progressive infection. These cats are persistently viremic (antigen positive on p27 ELISA tests and high viral loads are detected on provirus PCR blood tests).
- Focal or atypical infection. This is rare in naturally infected cats and is characterized by anatomically localized viral replication (e.g. in the bladder, eyes, mammary glands) that can result in intermittent antigenemia, with accompanying positive p27 ELISA test results. Weak positive, discordant, or fluctuating positive/negative p27 ELISA results can occur.

In progressive or reactivated infection, integration can culminate in malignant transformation, especially hemopoietic neoplasia (lymphoma or leukemia).

Myeloproliferative disorders can also occur, but these are rare and are not always FeLV associated. However, the most common outcome of infection is profound immune deficiency. Nonregenerative anemia, opportunistic infections, and malignancy represent the predominant causes of death among infected cats.

Susceptibility to FeLV infection is greatest in kittens under 4 months of age and vertical transmission is relatively common. Transmission of infection usually occurs through 'friendly' contact, such as mutual grooming, but can also occur through bites. Regressively infected queens do not usually transmit the virus to their kittens *in utero*, but individual kittens from a litter can become infected after they are born. Embryonic deaths and stillbirths are common among progressively infected viremic queens, and if live kittens are born, they can become viremic and die while they are still neonates. Older cats can have significant natural resistance to infection, probably associated with maturation of the immune response in older cats. Additionally, FeLV infection can be sustained for months to years before culminating in physical deterioration and death. The ability of persistently infected cats to shed virus in high concentrations in saliva results in rapid and effective transmission of virus via grooming and oronasal contact to susceptible kittens, particularly in cluster households. There is no sex or breed predilection to FeLV infection.

Clinical presentation

The clinical signs of FeLV infection are highly variable and potentially involve any organ system. FeLV-infected cats are at risk of developing solid tumors (e.g. lymphoma) or leukemia. In addition, bone marrow suppression involving white cells, leukocytes, and erythrocytes is commonly encountered in clinical practice. Compromise of cell-mediated immunity culminates in increased susceptibility to bacterial, viral, and/or fungal infections. Immune complex disease affecting renal function and causing polyarthritis has also been documented, as have a number of reproductive and CNS disorders.

Differential diagnosis

Cats presenting with any chronic, debilitating illness, fever, or weight loss should be tested for FeLV, regardless of age. Chronic upper respiratory infection, stomatitis, gingivitis, and periodontitis are common respiratory/oral signs that justify antigen testing. Since FeLV has oncogenic potential, cats with neoplasia, especially lymphoid tumors, should be tested for FeLV. Hematologic abnormalities such as nonregenerative anemia, lymphoblastic leukemia, leukopenia, thrombocytopenia, or thrombocytosis (>1 million platelets/mm^3) can be associated with FeLV infection.

Diagnosis

Because of the nonspecific nature of clinical signs associated with FeLV infection, it is essential that FeLV testing is performed on sick cats presented for evaluation. The most commonly used point-of-care tests detect FeLV p27 antigen in the blood of infected cats and are highly sensitive and specific. However, it should be remembered that disease prevalence affects the positive and negative predictive value of any diagnostic test, so false-positive results are more likely in low prevalence areas and cats with low risk of infection. IFA testing detects FeLV in leukocytes and is a highly specific test. However, false-negative results can occur if there is leukopenia or if only a few peripheral leukocytes are infected; IFA-positive cats are usually progressively infected. If initial testing with point-of-care screening tests is inconclusive for any reason, testing should be repeated, preferably by a veterinary diagnostic laboratory, using IFA and/or PCR for FeLV provirus. There is no commercial test routinely available for FeLV antibody testing.

Management

Treatment/prognosis

Specific treatment modalities for FeLV-infected cats are directed at the clinical manifestation of illness. Several immunomodulatory and antiretroviral treatments have been attempted (**Table 21.10**). Results of treatment are highly variable and have not yet been subjected to controlled studies. As in FIV-infected cats, azidothymidine (AZT), phosphonylmethoxyethyladenine (PMEA), and human recombinant alpha-interferon have been used in an attempt to treat FeLV-infected cats. The dosage regimens recommended for these products are outlined in **Table 21.10**. Lymphoma is the most common solid tumor associated with FeLV infection. Several chemotherapeutic combinations have been recommended to manage tumors. Administration of corticosteroids is minimally effective as a single agent treatment modality for FeLV-induced cancer. CHOP (cyclophosphamide, hydroxydaunorubicin [doxorubicin], Oncovin [vincristine], and prednisone) and CHOP-based protocols are widely used in cats diagnosed with lymphoma. In most cases, only cats that achieve complete remission after induction chemotherapy go on to have long-term disease-free status. In cats with mediastinal or multicentric lymphoma, complete remission rates of up to 90% and 1-year survival rates of up to approximately 55% have been reported. Those with aggressive GI lymphoma do not fare as well; about one-third to two-thirds of cats will achieve a complete remission, and 1-year survival is approximately 20–40%. FeLV and FIV status does not affect initial response to therapy, but positive retroviral status negatively affects long-term

Table 21.10 Treatment protocols in the management of clinical signs in feline FeLV and/or FIV infections.

Immunomodulation therapy
• Staphylococcal protein A (SPA, Kabi Pharmacia, Inc) (10 µg/kg IP twice weekly). Continue as needed. The drug has been used in cats for periods of up to 8 weeks. No improvement in humoral immunity has been documented
• Acemannan (Carrisyn, Carrington Laboratories) (2 mg/kg IP once weekly for 6 weeks). No improvement in clinical outcome or CD4/CD8 ratios was documented following 8 weeks of treatment
• *Propionibacterium acnes* (Immunoregulin, ImmunoVet) (0.5 ml per cat IV once or twice weekly as needed). Clinical improvement has been anectodally reported
• Human recombinant interferon-alpha (rHuIFN) (Roferon-A, Hoffmann LaRoche). (The availability of this drug varies.) Various dosing regimens are described:
  ◦ High dose: 1,000–10,000 U/kg IM q24h for 3–7 weeks. Treatment beyond this period is associated with anti-interferon antibody
  ◦ Low dose: 30 U PO q24h for life

Antiviral therapy • Azidothymidine (formerly called AZT; now, Retrovir, GlaxoSmithKline) (5 mg/kg PO q8h for periods of up to 4–6 weeks depending on degree of bone marrow toxicity [anemia]). Alternatively, administered at 15 mg/kg PO q12h • 9-(2-Phosphonylmethoxyethyl) adenine (PMEA) (2.5 mg/kg SC q12h [duration not stipulated]). Availability is limited

FeLV-associated lymphoma/lymphosarcoma
Single-agent glucocorticoids are minimally effective and, therefore, are reserved for palliative management. Combination drug therapy is recommended:
• Induction (weeks 1–4):
  ◦ Cyclophosphamide (Cytoxan, Bristol-Myers) (300 mg/m^2 PO given once on weeks 1 and 4 only);
  ◦ plus vincristine (Oncovin, Eli Lily) (0.75 mg/m^2 IV given once weekly on weeks 1, 2, 3, and 4);
  ◦ plus prednisone (2 mg/kg PO q24h for 4 weeks)
• Maintenance (beyond 4 weeks):
  ◦ Discontinue the cyclophosphamide and vincristine
  ◦ Continue the prednisone daily as outlined above. Once the cat is determined to be in remission, the drug dose is gradually reduced over 3 weeks then stopped
  ◦ Beginning with week 7, administer doxorubicin (25 mg/m^2 IV once every 3 weeks) until it is determined the cat is in remission

Cytopenia • Human recombinant erythropoietin (100 IU/kg SC q48h for 2 weeks or until the desired hematocrit is reached) Anti-erythropoietin antibody may develop against exogenous and endogenous erythropoietin • Granulocyte-colony stimulating factor (G-CSF) (5 µg/kg SC q12h 1–2 weeks)
Stomatitis • Metronidazole (5 mg/kg PO q8h 2–4 weeks as needed) • Clindamycin (12.5 mg/kg PO q8h 2–4 weeks) • Prednisone (5 mg per cat PO q12h 2–4 weeks) • Bovine lactoferrin (available from chemical suppliers only) (40 mg/kg applied directly to the oral mucosa, q24h as needed)

survival, mostly because of the occurrence of other FeLV- and FIV-related disorders.

Cats with myelosuppressive disease have a particularly poor prognosis and are best managed with administration of whole blood as needed to resolve the anemia. However, the value of this treatment is limited by the expense and the consequences of administering multiple blood transfusions. Recombinant human erythropoietin (rHuEPO) (100 U/kg SC q48h) can also be used in cats with clinical signs associated with anemia (hematocrit usually <0.2 l/l [20%]). At least 3–4 weeks of treatment may be required before a response is observed. It is estimated that between 20% and 30% of cats treated with rHuEPO develop anti-erythropoietin antibodies 6–12 months into therapy. Cats that initially respond but then fail to respond to rHuEPO may be transiently discontinued and restarted on the drug 1–2 months later. The target of rHuEPO therapy is a hematocrit of 0.3 l/l (30%) or greater. Recombinant omega interferon of feline origin has also been used to treat FeLV-related disease (1 million units/kg SC q24h for 5 days; three separate 5-day treatments performed at day 0, day 14, and day 60), although it is not available in the USA.

In cats that develop persistent FeLV-related neutropenia, recombinant human granulocyte colony-stimulating factor (filgrastim), may be indicated (5 μg/kg SC q24h until neutrophil count exceeds 3.0 x 10^3/μl for 2 days). Cost and the development of antibodies might limit the use of this agent.

Healthy FeLV-infected cats should be housed indoors and kept away from other cats to limit the risk of disease transmission; veterinary checks should be performed at least 6-monthly. The prognosis for infected cats is highly variable, depending on the specific disease manifested during the course of infection and the availability of supportive treatment for secondary infections. Although a small percentage of FeLV-positive cats may remain healthy for several years, the prognosis for persistently FeLV-positive cats is poor. Most persistently infected cats living within cluster households are expected to die within 3 years from the time of diagnosis. Persistently infected single household cats afforded supportive medical care could potentially have longer survival times.

Prevention

Currently, several vaccine types are on the market that offer relatively good protection against FeLV. Killed whole virus (adjuvanted), killed sub-unit (adjuvanted), and recombinant (adjuvant-free) vaccines are available (**Tables 21.8** and **21.9**). Routine testing, as well as vaccination of cats determined to be at risk, are key factors in FeLV prevention. Vaccine-associated sarcoma (VAS) in cats has been associated with vaccination against FeLV and also a wide variety of other vaccines and injections; conflicting accounts of differential risk by vaccine type have been reported. Extensive studies have shown that VAS in cats is not the result of vaccine virus reverting to a virulent state and causing tumor. A familial predisposition among certain families of cats to develop tumors has also been suggested. Kittens are clearly the most susceptible to FeLV infection following exposure, while adult indoor cats are among the least susceptible to infection. As with any vaccination decision, risk assessment for infection should be made on an individual basis, based on lifestyle factors and local prevalence. None of the currently available FeLV vaccines will cause false-positive tests for FeLV antigen on either IFA or ELISA tests. However, FeLV testing should be performed before FeLV vaccination to establish FeLV infection status. Routine vaccination with core (nonFeLV) vaccines should not be avoided in FeLV-infected cats, although inactivated (killed) vaccines are recommended.

Public health implications

FeLV has been the subject of extensive studies pertaining to its zoonotic potential. Although there are studies available to suggest that human infection with FeLV might be possible, no human has ever been known to become infected with FeLV nor has human leukemia ever been traced to FeLV antigen. Currently, FeLV in cats is not regarded as a human health hazard.

FELINE IMMUNODEFICIENCY VIRUS

Definition/overview

First described in 1987, FIV is an RNA retrovirus (lentivirus) infection unique to cats. The major risk factors for infection are male gender, intact status, free roaming/outdoor access, and clinical signs of ill health.

Etiology

Transmission among cats occurs primarily through bite wounds. Transfusion of blood from an infected cat is also a highly effective means of transmitting the disease. Vertical transmission of FIV has been reported, but is much less likely in naturally infected cats than in experimental infections.

Pathophysiology

FIV is a lentivirus and, therefore, shares many properties with other retroviruses such as HIV. Because of this, FIV infection in cats has been used extensively in the study of HIV infection. Many cats are subclinically infected, but clinical FIV infection is characterized by chronic, variable illness, immunosuppression, decreased CD4+ lymphocytes (T-helper lymphocytes), and a reduced CD4+:CD8+ (cytotoxic lymphocytes) lymphocyte ratio.

Clinical presentation

Cats infected with FIV manifest a wide variety of nonspecific clinical signs. Dermatitis, stomatitis, ocular disease, renal insufficiency, lower urinary tract infections, neurologic abnormalities, and opportunistic infections have been reported in infected cats (**Figures 21.55, 21.56**). FIV infection is significantly associated with the development of lymphoma. However, many cats with FIV infection manifest no clinical signs for weeks to years following infection and can eventually die of unrelated causes. In addition, laboratory findings in cats with FIV infection are equally nonspecific and contribute little to establishing a diagnosis of FIV infection. Mild, nonregenerative anemia, neutropenia, lymphopenia, and hypergammaglobulinemia characterized on biochemistry profile as hyperproteinemia are commonly found on routine hematology and serum biochemistry.

Differential diagnosis

Any adult cat presented for chronic or debilitating illness, fever, or weight loss should routinely be

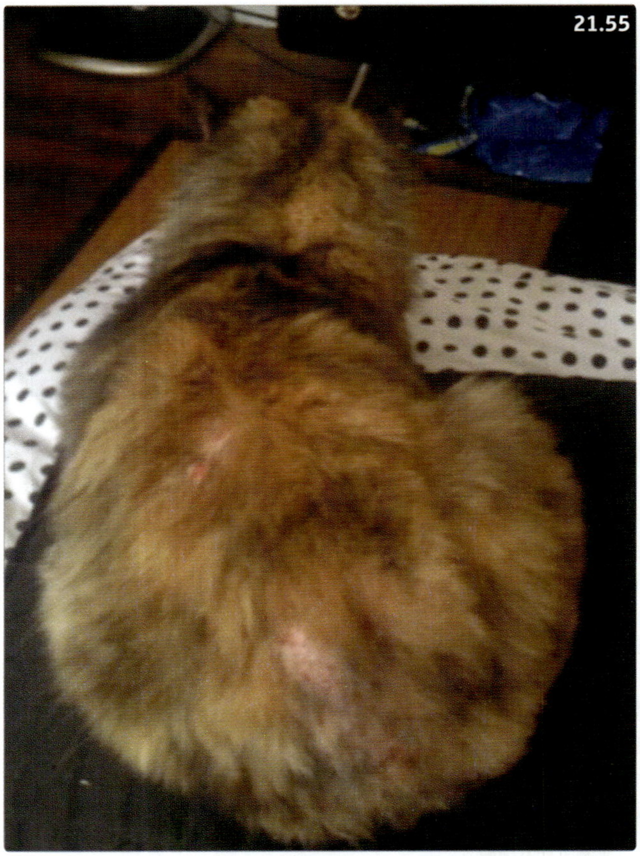

Figure 21.55 Chronic inflammatory skin disease is sometimes diagnosed in cats infected with FIV.

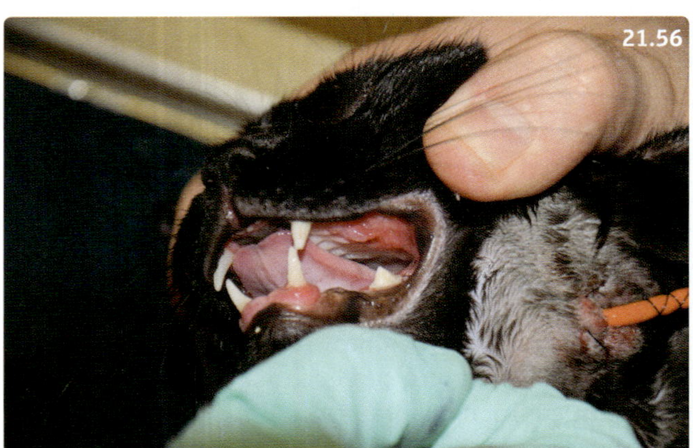

Figure 21.56 Chronic stomatitis in a cat.

tested for FIV as well as FeLV. Cats with anemia, neutropenia, stomatitis, glossitis, lymphoma, or chronic upper respiratory infection should be evaluated for FIV infection. FIP is an important differential diagnosis among FIV-infected cats with significant hypergammaglobulinemia.

Diagnosis

Detection of FIV-specific antibodies in blood or serum is the most widely accepted means of establishing a diagnosis. Point-of-care tests are highly specific and sensitive for the detection of anti-FIV antibodies. The presence of antibodies in blood or serum denotes exposure as well as infection. Interpretation of a positive antibody test in kittens under 6 months of age is complicated by the fact that maternal antibody from an infected queen may be transferred via the colostrum to kittens. FIV antibody-positive kittens must be retested after 6 months of age. FIV PCR testing to detect FIV antigenemia is commercially available, and a positive result is regarded as confirmation of positive FIV status. However, negative FIV PCR results do not necessarily mean that the cat is not infected, as the primers used in the test might not detect all field strains. Cats vaccinated against FIV, using the commercially available inactivated (killed) vaccine, also remain ELISA positive for years after vaccination. PCR testing does not detect vaccine virus and cats that test positive on initial point-of-care screening tests and are also PCR positive are regarded as infected, even if there is a history of vaccination, as infection can occur while the cat is fully vaccinated.

Management

Treatment/prognosis

There is currently no FIV-specific antiviral therapy available. The use of nucleoside analogs such as AZT and PMEA has produced some short-term clinical improvement and increased CD4+:CD8+ ratio in a small number of published studies, but significant side-effects, particularly anemia, can occur subsequent to the use of either of these drugs. Human recombinant alpha-interferon has also been used to treat immunodeficient cats subsequent to retrovirus infection. Treatment is inexpensive and clinical improvements have been reported over the first 2 months of treatment. While the life span of treated cats exceeded that of placebo-treated cats, there was no change in CD4+:CD8+ ratio or other hematologic parameters. Additionally, none of the treatments listed in **Table 21.10** will convert an FIV-positive status to a negative status.

FIV-positive cats can be susceptible to a number of chronic inflammatory and secondary infections. Supportive treatment is indicated and may, in those cats that respond to treatment, extend the life of the clinically infected cat for several months or years. There is no published evidence of increased rates of adverse effects after administration of modified live virus vaccines in FIV-positive cats. Most authors agree that routine vaccination is indicated, assuming significant risk of exposure exists.

Prevention

The most effective means of preventing FIV infection is to limit exposure to, and agonistic encounters with, FIV-infected cats that could result in biting. A number of published studies have demonstrated that casual contact between harmoniously cohabiting FIV-positive and FIV-negative cats over years has not resulted in viral transmission, despite mutual grooming, minor episodes of aggression, and sharing food and water dishes, litter pans, and bedding. However, careful management is required when cats are first introduced to one another, as the potential for agonistic interactions that could result in FIV transmission is increased. Because of this, it is important to determine FIV status before cats are introduced to one another and then to observe interactions until the likelihood of aggression resulting in penetrating bite wounds is remote. If there is a reasonable suspicion that such agonistic interactions will occur when the cats are unobserved, FIV-positive and FIV-negative cats should be segregated from one another.

There is currently only one FIV vaccine licensed for use in cats (**Table 21.8**). Availability of the vaccine is limited to countries where the manufacturer has received approval. The vaccine is dual-clade (FIV sub-groups A and D viruses are present in the product). The efficacy of vaccination against FIV is the subject of some debate. Post-vaccination FIV-positive ELISA status can persist for many years and places vaccinated cats under some risk of potential misclassification as FIV infected. It is also possible for vaccinated cats to subsequently become infected, severely confounding the interpretation of FIV diagnostic testing. If vaccination is deemed necessary, veterinarians are strongly encouraged to use microchip identification in an attempt to avoid incorrect clinical choices in cats that subsequently test FIV ELISA positive. A method of differentiating infected from vaccinated cats, based on CD4%:CD8(low)% T-lymphocyte ratio, has recently been reported.

Public health implications

FIV poses no known health risk to humans.

FELINE PANLEUKOPENIA (FELINE PARVOVIRUS)

Definition/overview

Feline panleukopenia (FPL) is caused by a small, single-stranded DNA parvovirus recognized in cats worldwide. Once a common fatal viral infection, feline panleukopenia virus (FPV) infection is a rare disease among vaccinated pet cats. However, FPV infection regularly occurs in cats housed in animal shelters. One published study indicated that only about one-third of free roaming cats had protective antibody titers when tested in a trap–neuter–return program.

Etiology

Like CPV infection, FPV infection is transmitted by contact with the feces, saliva, and/or secretions of infected cats, or by fomite transmission. Droplet infection can occur via sneezing, especially if there is concurrent upper respiratory tract disease. Virus is shed in the urine and feces for up to 6 weeks (usually 2–3 weeks) following recovery from clinical disease. The virus is capable of persisting in the environment, outside the host, for periods of at least 1 year. Some unvaccinated adult cats can acquire natural immunity subsequent to subclinical infection via low-level viral exposure to infected cats or fomites. Kittens are more likely to become infected (**Figure 21.57**), but once clinical infection occurs, both kittens and adults have similar mortality rates.

Pathophysiology

The virus requires rapidly multiplying cells for replication, so it has a tropism for those tissues with a high mitotic rate (e.g. bone marrow, lymphoid organs, and the intestinal crypts). Cellular depletion and immunosuppression occur when lymphoid tissue is infected and myeloid cell populations are depleted by bone marrow infection; panleukopenia results. Rapidly dividing intestinal crypt cells are also a site of infection, resulting in malabsorption, increased permeability, and hemorrhagic diarrhea. Fetal and neonatal infection targets the CNS, including the cerebrum, cerebellum, retinae, and optic nerves. Fetal death, fetal absorption, abortion, or mummified fetuses

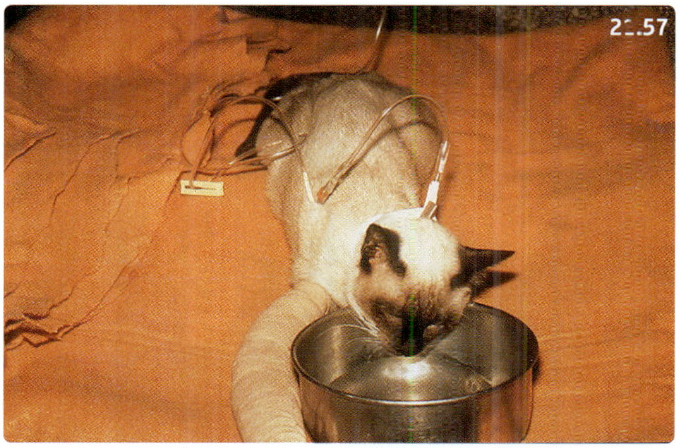

Figure 21.57 This young Siamese kitten had marked vomiting, diarrhea, and fever caused by feline panleukopenia virus. It was an unvaccinated cat that was hospitalized for a fracture repair. (Courtesy M. Schaer)

can occur in infected pregnant queens. Blindness and cerebellar hypoplasia (**Figure 21.58**), manifesting as non-progressive hypermetria and ataxia, are common among kittens infected as neonates.

Clinical presentation

Following FPV exposure, clinical disease is more likely to develop in unvaccinated kittens under 5 months of age, as they are less likely to have protective antibody titers. It should be remembered that vaccinated kittens can be infected, as maternally derived antibodies can interfere with the response to vaccination. Kittens suckling queens with high antibody titers are likely to receive large amounts of anti-FPV antibodies, prolonging interference with the immune response to vaccination, sometimes until 16–20 weeks of age. When clinical disease does develop, the onset is acute and may culminate in death within 12 hours, sometimes without apparent clinical signs of disease. FPV infection, therefore, is frequently included in the differential diagnosis list for fading kitten syndrome. Infected cats generally present with clinical signs including fever, lethargy, anorexia, vomiting, diarrhea, and/or dehydration. Death can result from shock, DIC, secondary bacterial infections, and/or profound dehydration. One retrospective study reported that clinical recovery most often occurred approximately 5 days after the onset of clinical signs (range 1–9 days), while in fatal cases, death occurred approximately 1 day after the onset of clinical signs (range 0–9 days). Cerebellar hypoplasia is a clinical finding among kittens born to queens infected during pregnancy. Affected kittens ambulate with a characteristic broad-based stance and manifest hypermetric movements. Intention tremors of the head may occur when food is offered to affected kittens. One or more of a litter of kittens may be affected. The condition is not progressive, so affected cats can make good pets if their clinical signs allow good quality of life.

One study reported that low leukocyte counts (<1 x 10^3 leukocytes/µl), hypoproteinemia (less than 30 g/l [3 g/dl]) and hypokalemia (<4 mmol/l) were poor prognostic indicators in FPV-infected cats.

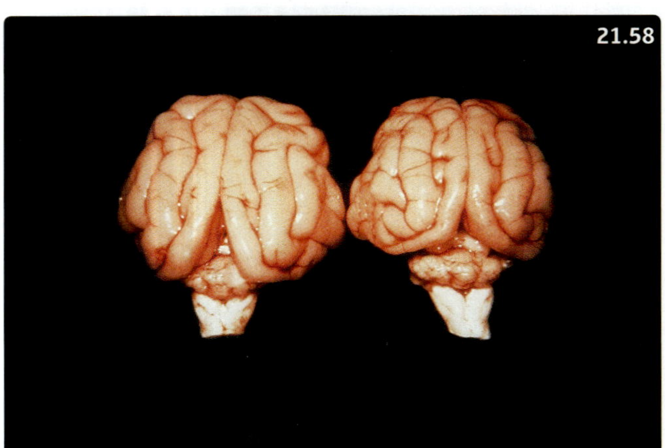

Figure 21.58 Brain from a normal kitten (right) compared with the brain of a kitten with cerebellar hypoplasia associated with feline panleukopenia virus infection.

Differential diagnosis

Intestinal parasitism, including coccidiosis, infectious enteritis, intussusception, and poisoning, are consistent with acute, enteric FPV infection, particularly in young cats. *Salmonella* infections can cause hemorrhagic diarrhea and panleukopenia. Sepsis and enteric foreign body may also be considered. Neurologic signs associated with cerebellar hypoplasia may be consistent with acute head trauma.

Diagnosis

Infected cats usually have a history of possible exposure to FPV and risk factors for infection, such as lack of a vaccination history and/or age less than 16 weeks. The point-of-care canine ELISA fecal antigen test has been validated for use in cats and a positive test result is considered confirmation of infection. However, a negative test result does not rule out infection, since viral shedding is intermittent. False-positive results can occur 1–14 days after vaccination, although these are rare. The hallmark laboratory finding in kittens with FPV infection is a leukocyte count between 50 and 3,000 cells/µl, and this can be determined in practice with microscopic examination of a simple blood smear. Thrombocytopenia is occasionally reported. Biochemical profiles are of little value in establishing a diagnosis of FPV infection. Although serologic testing and virus isolation are effective means of diagnosing the disease, these procedures are not routinely available in clinical practice. A full necropsy should be performed on any cat suspected to have succumbed to FPV infection. The most important tissue to submit for histopathology is the intestinal tract. Neonatally infected cats may have cerebellar hypoplasia or retinal degeneration.

Point-of-care FPV antibody tests are commercially available to determine protection status during outbreaks, but they have relatively low levels of sensitivity and specificity, making them unreliable for use in clinical or shelter practice.

Management

Treatment/prognosis

There is no specific antiviral therapy available for the treatment of FPV-infected cats. While feline recombinant interferon-ω has been used successfully to treat CPV, one feline study using the agent as a preventive measure before an FPV outbreak was unable to demonstrate improved outcomes in treated kittens. Intensive supportive therapy and nursing care offer the only reasonable means of treating clinically affected cats. A single dose of serum from an immune cat can be administered through a filter either IV or intraperitoneally, to cross-matched, exposed, unvaccinated kittens (2 ml in kittens <12 weeks; 4 ml in kittens >12 weeks). Only one dose can be administered, to prevent subsequent anaphylaxis, and vaccination against FPV should be delayed in treated kittens by 3–4 weeks to prevent antibody interference with the immune response. Once recommenced, the course of vaccination should continue 2–4 weeks longer than usual (up to 18–24 weeks old).

Parenterally administered balanced electrolyte solutions, such as lactated Ringer's solution, are of utmost importance in replacement of electrolytes and fluids; hetastarch or plasma could be considered in hypoproteinemic cats. Antimicrobial therapy is indicated, since secondary bacterial infections and sepsis are common complications resulting from viral injury to the intestinal mucosa. As with antiemetic and fluid therapy, all antimicrobials should be administered parenterally. Parenteral ampicillin sodium/sulbactam sodium (50 mg/kg [combined] IV q8h) is a good empiric choice. Parenterally administered maropitant citrate (1 mg/kg IV or SC q24h) is an effective antiemetic. Appetite stimulants, such as mirtazapine (3–4 mg per cat PO q72h) or cyproheptadine (2–4 mg/cat q12–24h) can be used during the recovery phase.

Prevention

Several excellent vaccines are available for immunization of kittens against FPV (**Table 21.8**). Although maternal antibody interferes with vaccination, most cats can be effectively immunized by 16–20 weeks of age. Cats that do recover from natural infection probably derive lifelong immunity. Recent resurgence of FPV in shelter-housed cats in the USA has prompted a change in initial vaccine recommendations for owned pet cats to commence at 6 weeks of age, with boosters every 3–4 weeks until 16–20 weeks of age, followed by a booster 1 year following the last vaccine in the initial series. Shelter-housed kittens should be vaccinated using modified live vaccine from 4 weeks of age, every 2–3 weeks, until 16–20 weeks old.

Both modified live virus (MLV) and killed (adjuvanted) virus vaccines are available. Vaccines are administered by the subcutaneous route. At least one manufacturer in the USA does market an intranasal (combined with FHV-1 and FCV) vaccine but this may not be as effective for the prevention of FPV infection as subcutaneous MLV. Although MLV vaccines are used predominantly in clinical practice and in shelters, they should not be administered to kittens <4 weeks of age or pregnant queens, as vaccine virus may replicate in the cerebellum of unborn kittens and kittens <6 weeks old and may cause neurologic signs after birth.

FPV is long lived in the environment and quaternary ammonium disinfectants are not usually effective. Bleach (1:32 solution, used within 24 hours of dilution and protected from light) or accelerated hydrogen peroxide- or potassium peroxymonosulfate-based disinfectants should be used with a contact time of at least 10 minutes, after thorough cleaning to remove all organic material.

Public health implications

FPV poses no risk to human health.

FELINE RABIES

(See also Chapter 14: Disorders of the nervous system and muscle.)

Definition/overview

Feline rabies virus infection, although similar to that described in the dog, has worldwide importance, particularly in the USA, where the incidence of feline rabies has been greater than that in the dog since the mid-1980s. This is considered to be associated with cats' nocturnal behavior and encounters with wildlife vectors and probable lower rabies vaccination rates. It is also known that younger cats, as well as dogs, are more susceptible to rabies virus infection than adult animals. The high concentration of rabies virus in the saliva of infected cats poses a particular threat to humans because of their popularity as companion animal pets and their ability to penetrate skin with their teeth. It has been estimated that <20% of domestic cats in the USA are ever vaccinated against rabies. This fact, combined with the increasing incidence of wildlife rabies in the mid-Atlantic and northeastern USA, justifies efforts to promote feline rabies vaccination.

Etiology

Rabies is caused by an RNA virus of the Rhabdoviridae family. In areas with good pet vaccination programs, wildlife tend to be the major reservoirs and vectors, whereas in areas with poor programs, domesticated animals are the major reservoirs and vectors.

Pathophysiology

After inoculation into the subcutaneous tissues and muscle, the virus replicates in muscle cells at the bite site for weeks to months before attaching to peripheral nerve endings and undergoing retrograde migration up nerve axons to the CNS. Rabies virus replicates in the spinal ganglia, from where it disseminates throughout the CNS and continues replicating. The virus is then transported out of the CNS to other body tissues, including the salivary glands, through peripheral, motor, and sensory nerves. An animal is infectious when the salivary glands are affected. Infectious virus may be shed in saliva for up to 13 days before clinical signs of illness are manifest.

Clinical presentation

The incubation period for rabies is from just over 1 week to 6 months, and is shorter if the site of inoculation is close to the CNS. Clinical rabies infection in cats, like dogs, is divided into two general categories: furious and paralytic. A prodromal phase can also occur before the furious stage, but it is often subclinical. Prodromal clinical signs, if they occur, include vague neurologic and behavioral changes, irritation at the site of viral inoculation, fever, and increased agitation lasting for 1–2 days.

As the disease progresses, about two-thirds of affected cats manifest the furious type of disease, which lasts up to 7 days. Affected cats become particularly aggressive towards humans as well as other animals and inanimate objects. They are described as having an anxious appearance and will make vicious attempts to bite or scratch at any moving object. Affected cats may run or pace continuously until they collapse. In contrast to dogs, cats with rabies frequently manifest increased vocalization and a change in the pitch of voice. The clinical signs of furious rabies progress to paralytic disease in those cats that survive this long. Affected cats manifest flaccid ascending paraparesis, which often involves the site of inoculation, incoordination, paralysis, coma, and death.

Differential diagnosis

Kittens and cats infected with and shedding rabies may not manifest clinical signs, at least during the early stages of infection. (**Note:** Any cat with unexplainable neurologic and/or behavioral changes should be considered suspect for rabies.) Neoplasia, spinal or head trauma, and poisoning or toxicity are important differential diagnoses for feline rabies. In the USA, the use of killed and recombinant rabies vaccines in cats has eliminated vaccine-induced signs of rabies.

Diagnosis

No specific changes are characteristic of rabies infection on hematology, serum biochemistry, or CSF analysis. Serum tests to detect anti-rabies virus antibodies in infected animals are often negative. Direct IFA staining or immunohistochemistry of nervous tissue collected at necropsy is the most common and recommended method of confirming rabies infection in both dogs and cats (**Figure 21.59**). Reverse transcriptase (RT)-PCR is a sensitive and specific test that can provide fast (within hours) results when neural tissues and/or saliva are submitted for testing. However, attempts to make antemortem diagnoses of rabies in animals are not recommended and a negative RT-PCR test performed on saliva cannot be used to rule out rabies. The proper procedure for handling specimens from suspect rabies cases has been outlined earlier (see Canine rabies).

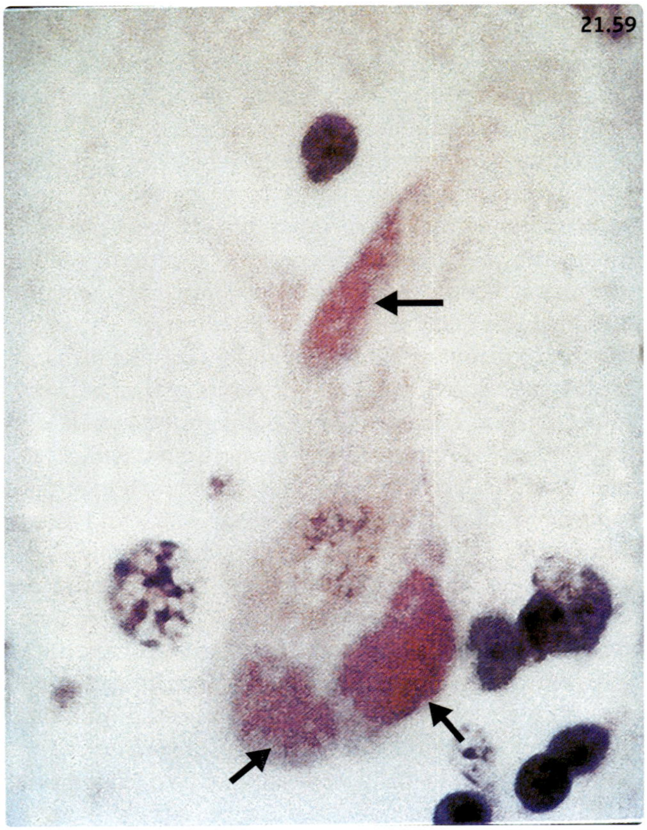

Figure 21.59 Rabies causes characteristic microscopic Negri bodies (arrows) in the brains of affected animals. (From Kassira JP (1997) (ed.) *Images in Clinical Medicine*. Selections from the *New England Journal of Medicine*, with permission.)

Management

Treatment/prognosis

The zoonotic threat posed by rabies virus infection in cats justifies strict isolation and quarantine of cats suspected of or known to be infected. Treatment should not be attempted. The prognosis for recovery from the clinical infection is grave.

Prevention

Killed (adjuvanted) virus vaccines (1-year and 3-year) and a feline recombinant (adjuvant-free) rabies vaccine are available for use in cats. Current standards for vaccination of cats against rabies are outlined in **Tables 21.8** and **21.9**. Where feline rabies vaccine is mandated by law, the first dose of vaccine can be given as early as 3 months of age. A second dose, administered 1 year following the date of the initial rabies vaccine, is required. Today, there is considerable variation among states and countries as to the frequency of booster vaccinations in adult cats. It is recommended that rabies vaccinations should be administered as low as possible on the right hindlimb, so that if a sarcoma develops subsequent to vaccination, there is a history of the type of vaccine used at the site. Vaccination intervals range from 1 to 3 years depending on the specific product used. While rare, there have been cases of rabies in vaccinated animals when vaccinations have been allowed to lapse.

Public health implications

As with dogs, any human exposed to the saliva of a cat suspected of having rabies should be considered exposed and immediate isolation and treatment should be instituted. Treatment of a bite wound in a person caused by any domestic or feral cat must be treated aggressively by washing thoroughly as soon after the injury as possible. Irrigation of the wound with large quantities of a 20% aqueous soap solution or quaternary ammonium solution (e.g. benzalkonium chloride) is recommended. Humans who receive unprovoked bite wounds from feral or free-roaming cats have the highest risk of exposure. In addition to local wound treatment, these individuals are justifiably treated according to standard post-exposure prophylaxis, which includes administration of human rabies immune globulin and diploid cell vaccine. Rabies virus is quickly inactivated outside the host and susceptible to routine disinfectants.

FELINE VIRAL UPPER RESPIRATORY INFECTION

Definition/overview

Feline viral upper respiratory infection is generally attributable to either or both of two viruses: FHV-1 and FCV. It is important to acknowledge that bacterial upper respiratory tract infections with *Bordetella bronchiseptica*, *Chlamydia felis*, *Mycoplasma felis*, *Staphylococcus* spp. and/or *Streptococcus* spp. may concurrently infect cats with FHV-1 or FCV, thereby complicating the course of clinical disease.

FHV-1 is a double-stranded enveloped DNA virus that is extremely labile outside the host. Capable of surviving for only up to 18 hours in a damp environment, FHV-1 is highly susceptible to common disinfectants. FCV, on the other hand, is a small, single-stranded unenveloped RNA virus that can survive outside the host and is not susceptible to some commonly used disinfectants, such as quaternary ammonium compounds. While FHV-1 causes fairly uniform clinical disease, several strains of FCV have been identified and are known to vary in their clinical effects, anatomic localization, virulence, and antigenicity. Despite widespread vaccination against FHV-1 and FCV, these viruses still occur very frequently in the domestic cat population, particularly in multiple cat households and animal shelters.

Etiology

Transmission from infected to susceptible cats occurs most commonly by direct contact and through fomites; airborne transmission is not thought to be important, although sneezed droplets can spray over 1–2 meters. Cats living in high-density populations are known to be particularly susceptible to infection because crowding facilitates viral transmission and immune function in stressed cats can be suboptimal. In addition, kittens that recover from the acute infection are likely to develop a chronic carrier state with either FHV-1 or FCV. This chronic carrier state usually persists for months to years (likely for life in the case of FHV-1 carriers) and contributes significantly to the persistence of the virus within cat populations, particularly in multi-cat environments. FHV-1 shedding by carriers is intermittent, but can be precipitated by stress or immunosuppressive therapy; FCV shedding is usually constant, but can fluctuate in individuals.

Pathophysiology

After initial infection, FHV-1 is carried as a latent virus. Intermittent periods of shedding may occur for 1–2 weeks following a 'stressful' episode (e.g. boarding, general anesthesia, corticosteroid therapy). During this time cats may manifest mild clinical signs, but they are capable of shedding virulent virus.

It has been reported that 50% of FCV-recovered cats develop a carrier state and shed virus for at least 75 days after infection. Although chronic FCV carriers may shed virus for weeks to possibly years following the initial infection, they shed virus continuously from conjunctival, nasal, and oral secretions and, as such, pose a significant risk to susceptible kittens and adults.

Clinical presentation

The hallmark clinical sign of acute viral upper respiratory infection is sneezing, frequently accompanied by a serous to mucopurulent nasal and ocular discharge, dehydration, anorexia, and varying degrees of chemosis (**Figures 21.60, 21.61**). Oral ulceration can be common among FCV-infected cats, but is relatively uncommon in FHV-1 infections. Epiphora, keratitis, dendritic ulceration (**Figure 21.62**), corneal sequestra, symblepharon, and profound chemosis are more likely to occur in cats with FHV-1 than with FCV (see **Figures 19.10–19.19**). Acute, recrudescent FHV-1 infection is most likely to manifest signs consistent with traumatic keratitis (edema, neovascularization) or conjunctivitis, with or without corneal ulceration. Chronic ocular signs associated with viral infection can be unilateral or bilateral. Polyarthropathy and pyrexia (febrile limping syndrome) can occur in juvenile cats infected with FCV (**Figure 21.63**), but has not been reported in association with FHV-1. However, attempting to distinguish one viral infection from another on the basis of clinical signs is particularly difficult. Clinical signs and history are usually sufficient to make a clinical diagnosis of viral upper respiratory infection. Given the treatment options available, it is not always important to distinguish one viral infection from another, although environmental disinfection requires compounds capable of inactivating enveloped viruses in FCV outbreaks.

FHV-1 carrier cats may manifest chronic, secondary bacterial rhinitis and sinusitis because of permanent viral turbinate osteolysis. Clinical signs characteristically resolve during periods of antimicrobial administration, only to reappear following discontinuation of the drug. FCV has also been implicated in the development of chronic plasmacytic–lymphocytic stomatitis, faucitis, and gingivitis.

Differential diagnosis

Ocular signs of acute viral upper respiratory infection in kittens, such as severe conjunctivitis and chemosis, may be consistent with *C. felis* infection, although the viral infection is characteristically associated with more severe respiratory signs. *B. bronchiseptica* may cause

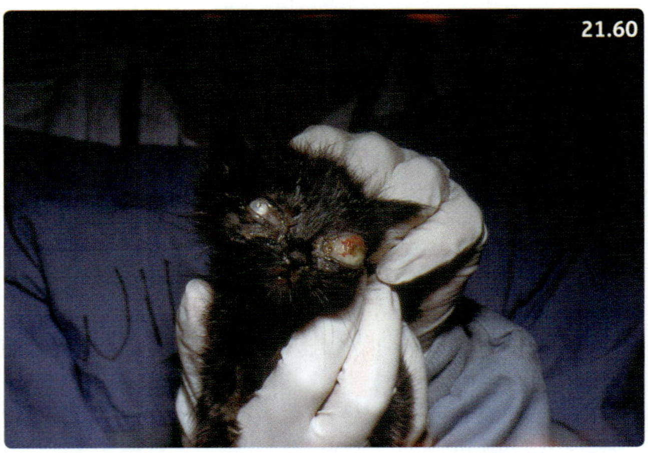

Figures 21.60 Bilateral conjunctivitis in a kitten caused by an upper respiratory virus. (Courtesy M. Schaer)

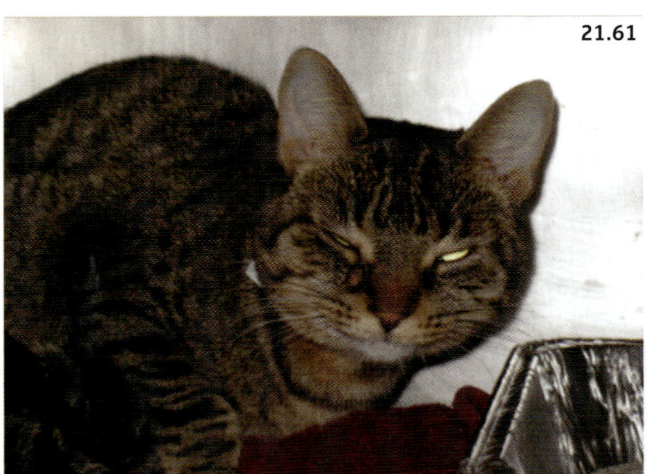

Figure 21.61 Cat with unilateral conjunctivitis and photophobia due to feline herpesvirus.

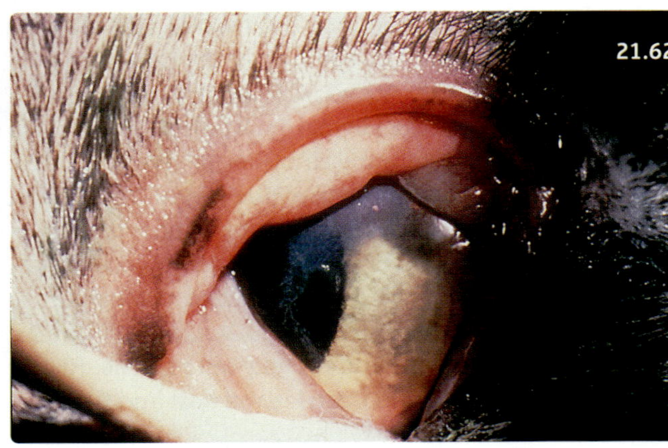

Figure 21.62 Keratoconjunctivitis and dendritic ulcer in an adult cat with recrudescent feline herpesvirus infection.

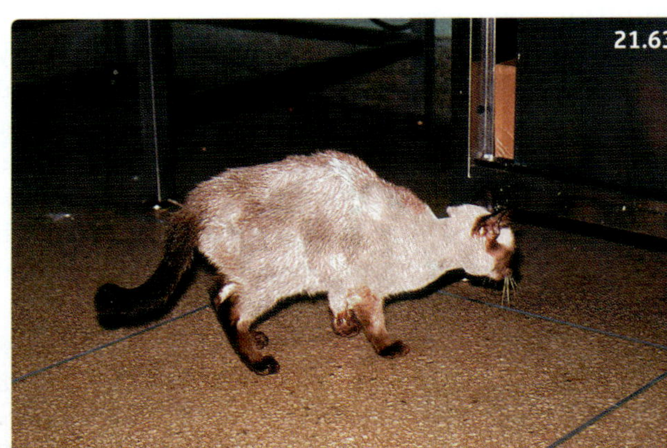

Figure 21.63 Siamese cat with a hunched posture associated with diffuse polyarthropathy caused by feline calicivirus. (Courtesy M. Schaer)

opportunistic infections culminating in pneumonia and sudden death among kittens with acute viral respiratory disease. *M. felis* infection can cause acute upper respiratory and/or ocular signs, and is a cause of bacterial pneumonia in cats.

Diagnosis

Commercial veterinary laboratories offer PCR testing for feline upper respiratory tract pathogens, including FHV-1, FCV, *C. felis*, *B. bronchiseptica*, and *M. felis*. A sterile cotton-tipped swab with a plastic (not wooden) stem is used to collect specimens from the conjunctival sac, oropharynx, and/or nostrils, although fine swabs with wire stems are required to fit inside small feline nostrils. The swab should be transported in a plain sterile tube that does not contain transport medium. Because of the high number of vaccinates and the frequency of chronic carrier cats, serology has not been a valuable aid. A highly sensitive and specific commercially available point-of-care ELISA test is available for the detection of protective antibody titers against FHV-1 and FCV, but since strong cell-mediated immunity is also required for protection from infection, protective antibody titers can only prevent severe clinical signs. Conversely, a cat with negative antibody titers against FHV-1 and/or FCV is not necessarily susceptible to infection, since test results only reflect the humoral arm of the immune response.

Management

Treatment/prognosis

The focus of treatment for cats with viral upper respiratory infection, whether it be FHV-1 or FCV, centers around the ability to provide good nursing care, calories, fluid and electrolyte replacement, and antimicrobial therapy to combat secondary bacterial infection. Doxycycline is a good empiric choice, as it is also effective against *C. felis*, *B. bronchiseptica*, and *M. felis*. Dehydration results from reduced food and fluid intake and losses via secretions, which can be copious. In severe cases, dyspnea can occur. Placement of a nasoesophageal feeding tube facilitates the administration of fluids and calories to affected cats (**Figure 21.64**).

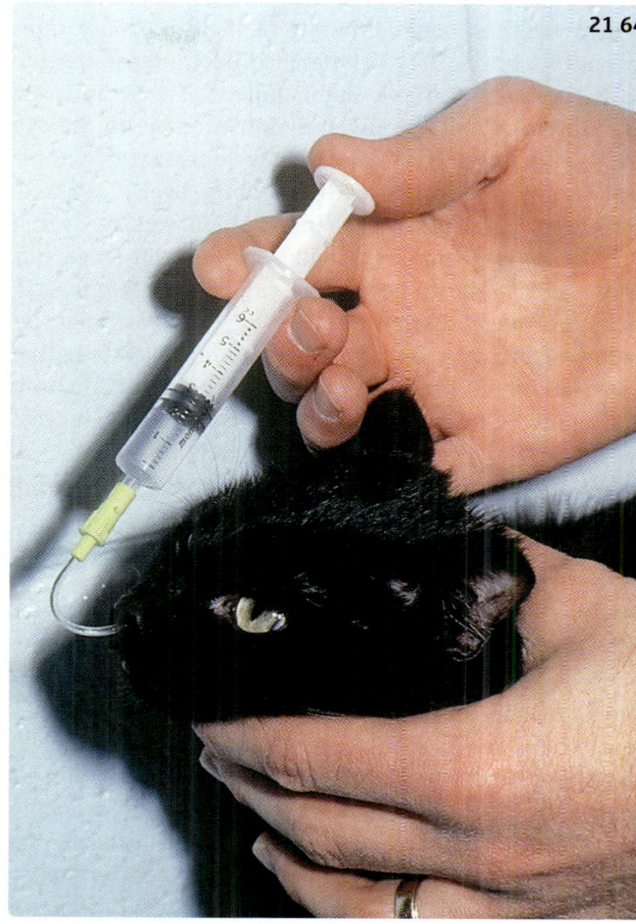

Figure 21.64 A nasoesophageal tube being used to provide fluids and calories to an anorexic cat with acute viral upper respiratory tract infection.

There is no antiviral therapy registered for use in FHV-1- or FCV-infected cats. The popular antiherpesvirus drug used in human herpesvirus infection, acyclovir, has been studied in cats and shown not to be effective against FHV-1. It can cause leukopenia and anemia, which are reversible when therapy is discontinued. There have been promising reports of favorable responses to treatment with famciclovir in cats naturally infected with FHV-1, but these have mostly been anecdotal or the result of uncontrolled studies. Dose and dose frequency are critical with this drug and the cost of therapy at the currently recommended dose rate of 90mg/kg q12h is prohibitive in most cases. However, in cats with ulcerative keratitis associated with FHV-1, ophthalmic trifluridine (1% solution) can be administered topically at 4–6-hour intervals until 1 week beyond resolution of clinical signs. The use of oral L-lysine, which competitively inhibits the growth-promoting effects of arginine on FHV-1, has been controversial. However, a number of recent studies have not supported its efficacy in infected cats, and one study even showed that oral L-lysine led to increased severity of disease compared with placebo-treated cats.

The prognosis for recovery from acute viral upper respiratory infection is excellent if supportive care is provided and the cat housed to avoid known risk factors for clinical disease, such as stress due to overcrowding. In the absence of treatment, most infections are self-limiting in 10–14 days. However, secondary bacterial infections can become severe. Complicating pneumonia is especially devastating in kittens, particularly if *B. bronchiseptica* is involved, and may culminate in high mortality rates among litters of affected kittens. The long-term prognosis is dependent on the establishment of a chronic carrier state and, potentially, anatomic damage to the eye and turbinates (FHV-1) or the development of chronic oral conditions, which are thought to be FCV related. Associated clinical signs of infection in cats recovered from acute infection are usually intermittent (sneezing, ocular and nasal discharge), but can be continuous (ocular and/or nasal discharge, sneezing, gingivostomatitis). Following recovery from acute infection, development of a carrier state is common for both viruses. It is thought that many FCV-infected cats will develop a carrier state for months to years following infection, and almost all FHV-1 infected cats develop a carrier state following recovery that will persist for the life of the cat.

Prevention

Both parenteral (killed and modified live) and topical (intranasal/intraocular) vaccines are commercially available. Vaccination helps protect cats from the severe effects of clinical disease if vaccinations are kept current. Vaccination of kittens is particularly important and should commence at 8 weeks of age, with boosters given every 3–4 weeks until 16–20 weeks old in privately owned cats. In shelter-housed kittens, vaccination should start as early as 4–6 weeks old, followed by boosters every 2–3 weeks until 16–20 weeks of age. Although parenteral vaccine is used predominantly in clinical practice, intranasal vaccination has recently been shown to offer a clinical advantage and reduced post-vaccinal viral shedding if administered concurrently with parenteral vaccine in an experimental FHV-1 challenge study in kittens. Another study of intranasal FHV-1 vaccination demonstrated cross-protection against *B. bronchiseptica* infection in a 7-day challenge model in kittens. Intranasal vaccination should only be administered with a vaccine approved for use by this route, and mild sneezing is common for 3–5 days after vaccination. However, severe clinical upper respiratory signs can occur if injectable vaccines are administered intranasally. The 2013 American Association of Feline Practitioners Feline Vaccination Advisory Panel Report recommends that boosters are administered every 3 years from 1 year after the primary series.

Public health implications

Despite concerns that human infection can result from contact with an infected cat, the infections must be considered independent. Neither FHV-1 nor FCV is considered to be a human pathogen and, as such, poses no risk to human health.

VIRULENT SYSTEMIC CALICIVIRUS INFECTION

Definition/overview

Since 1998, a small number of infectious disease outbreaks in the UK and the USA within cluster households of cats has been associated with a virulent systemic feline calicivirus (VS-FCV). Initially reported as 'hemorrhagic feline calicivirus', the limited number of infections caused by this emerging pathogen has resulted in mortality rates of up to 67% in previously healthy adult cats. Prior vaccination with a combination FHV-1/FCV vaccine for the prevention of upper respiratory infections may not provide cross-protection against the VS-FCV, because in every outbreak of VS-FCV, a genetically distinct strain of FCV has been involved.

Etiology

Caliciviruses comprise a large group of genetically diverse viruses. Infections are reported in a variety of species. The ability of FCV to infect cats, whether or not they are vaccinated, and for infected cats to develop a chronic carrier state associated with persistent shedding from the nasopharynx, explains the high prevalence of calicivirus in the general cat population. Although each VS-FCV has been associated with a separate mutation of one of the feline caliciviral strains, similar clinical presentations have been reported. Outbreaks have been reported among both vaccinated and unvaccinated cats. Index cases from all reported outbreaks have come from crowded, high-stress environments, such as shelters, rescues, and sometimes veterinary clinics. This highly contagious virus is transmitted by infected cats and their fomites; just a few hairs have acted as fomites and transmitted infection in some outbreaks.

Pathophysiology

Changes in the capsid gene of FCV, or in virus–host interactions, are thought to be responsible for VS-FCV infection. Affected cats develop acute systemic vascular compromise and hemorrhagic fever-like signs. Physical findings are likely to be associated with viral invasion of epithelium and endothelium, host cytokine responses, and cytolysis. Unlike the usual field strains of FCV, adult cats are particularly affected by VS-FCV, perhaps because the immune response to the virus is responsible for some of the clinical manifestations of disease.

Clinical presentation

Initially, the infection may present as moderate to severe upper respiratory infection. However, the disease rapidly progresses, and clinical signs include fever, facial and limb edema, and ulceration and crusting of skin on the face, muzzle, feet, and pinnae. Viral invasion of both epithelium and endothelium occurs and visceral involvement (lungs, pancreas, liver) can occur. DIC can ensue and mortality rates are high, especially among adult cats. Laboratory findings are nonspecific. Necropsy findings include necrosis of major organs such as the liver, spleen, pancreas, lung, and GI tract. Laboratory testing cannot distinguish VS-FCV from regular field strains of FCV and carriage rates for FCV are high (approximately 25–30%) among the general feline population.

Differential diagnosis

The differential diagnosis includes sepsis, vasculitis, systemic toxicity, envenomation, cutaneous neoplasia, or severe viral upper respiratory infection. Systemic signs may include laboratory and clinical evidence of acute pancreatitis or acute liver failure (e.g. jaundice). Feline panleukopenia virus is a differential diagnosis for sudden death, and can also be a comorbid infection, especially in shelter outbreaks.

Management

Treatment/prognosis

Because of the high morbidity and mortality associated with outbreaks, deaths usually occur over a relatively short initial period, followed by prolonged clinical recovery for severely ill but surviving cats. If an outbreak can be contained within a population, spread of the virus is typically limited. However, VS-FCV is extremely easily transmitted to other cats by fomites (hands, hair, clothing, food dishes); therefore, strict control procedures, including isolation, quarantine, thorough disinfection with appropriate agents, and the use of disposable personal protective equipment by all personnel in contact with infected or exposed cats, must be implemented in order to effectively contain an outbreak. Supportive care is indicated, although the rapid course of infection may not yield effective patient care and long-term survival. Because of vasculitis associated with VS-FCV, fluid therapy might be more effectively administered orally than IV. If possible, infected cats should be cared for on an out-patient basis, by the minimum number of staff. Ideally, catteries, rescues, shelters, and veterinary hospitals should be closed to prevent disease transmission until the outbreak is under control.

Prevention

Population management by reduction of overcrowding in multi-cat housing and adoption of healthy cats into low density homes reduces the risk of a VS-FCV outbreak. Vaccines have been introduced into the UK and the USA for the prevention of VS-FCV infection (**Tables 21.8** and **21.9**). However, every reported outbreak of VS-FCV has been due to a genetically distinct viral strain. Additionally, protection is not provided until at least 2 weeks after the second vaccination with VS-FCV vaccines because they are inactivated.

Public health implications

VS-FCV poses no known threat to human health.

FUNGAL AND PROTOZOAL INFECTIONS

FELINE CRYPTOCOCCOSIS

Definition/overview

Cryptococcosis is an important fungal disease of cats worldwide and infection is usually via inhalation of cryptococcal basidiospores from the environment. Eight genotypes exist, with varying geographical distribution, pathogenicity, and antimicrobial susceptibility. Infection is usually in the nasal cavity, although CNS signs can occur if infection breaks through the cribriform plate; pulmonary infections are rare. Dermatologic infections with ulcerative cutaneous lesions can also occur, as can disseminated infections, which are associated with clinical signs including lethargy, cachexia, meningoencephalomyelitis, uveitis, chorioretinitis, osteomyelitis and polyarthritis, systemic lymphadenitis, or multi-organ involvement, including renal infection.

Etiology

Cryptococcus spp. are encapsulated yeasts and most feline infections are due to *C. neoformans* and *C. gattii* (formerly *C. neoformans* var. *gattii*). *C. neoformans* is usually associated with avian feces, particularly pigeon guano, but has also been isolated from decaying vegetation such as eucalyptus leaves. Asymptomatic colonization of the respiratory tract is the most usual outcome of environmental exposure.

Pathophysiology

The cryptococcal yeast capsule contains protective factors that can inhibit phagocytosis, so infection can be disseminated via infected macrophages and neutrophils. There is debate in the published literature regarding the possible role of immunosuppression in clinical infection. The incubation period varies from months to years and fungal factors, such as infective burden, genotype, and virulence factors, as well as the host immune response, determine the outcome of exposure. Once established in the nasal cavity or lung, hematogenous spread can occur to the lymph nodes, eye, skin, and CNS.

Clinical presentation

Cats with nasal cryptococcosis usually present with a chronic unilateral nasal discharge, often accompanied by unilateral or bilateral swelling that can be followed by ulcerative nasofacial lesions (see **Figures 21.28–21.30**). Submandibular lymph nodes are usually enlarged. Nasopharyngeal granulomas can sometimes protrude from the nostrils, causing dyspnea and open-mouth breathing. Blindness can result from ocular infection and if the cribriform plate is breached, intracranial neurologic signs, including blindness from optic neuritis, and/or chorioretinitis, can ensue (**Figure 21.65,** see **Figures 19.28–19.31**). Dermatologic infection presents as single or multiple ulcerated or non-ulcerated cutaneous masses.

Differential diagnosis

Cryptococcal rhinitis can cause similar signs to infections with FHV-1, FCV, *Chlamydia felis, Bordetella bronchiseptica, Mycoplasma felis,* or *Aspergillus* spp; neoplasia (e.g. nasal lymphoma), foreign bodies (e.g. plant awns), and oronasal fistulae should also be considered. Ocular and CNS signs could also be caused by neoplasia (e.g. lymphoma, meningioma), toxoplasmosis, FIP, or bacterial meningitis. The differential diagnosis for the cutaneous form in cats includes other deep mycoses, mycobacteriosis, nocardiosis, neoplasia (e.g. squamous cell carcinoma) herpetic dermatitis, and eosinophilic granuloma complex.

Diagnosis

The latex cryptococcal antigen agglutination test (LCAT) to detect capsular antigen in serum, CSF, or urine is the diagnostic test of choice. Diagnostic accuracy can be improved by pre-treating samples with heat and a proteinase (pronase, often included in commercial diagnostic kits), since false-negative results can occur. Cytology, histology, and culture should be performed in suspected cryptococcal cases that are LCAT negative. Cytologic examination of tissue aspirates, infected body fluids, or impression smears of cutaneous lesions or biopsies, stained with Romanowsky-type stains (Wright, Giemsa, Diff-Quik®), usually reveal pink to violet round or budding extracellular *Cryptococcus* organisms with thick unstained capsules (see **Figure 21.34**). Histopathology can also be performed on biopsy specimens. Cryptococcal culture can be performed using Sabouraud dextrose agar or on bacterial standard media after incubation for 10 days; the addition of antibiotics to media might prevent overgrowth by secondary bacterial isolates from contaminated sites such as the nasal cavity. Diagnostic imaging, including radiography and advanced imaging (CT and MRI) when appropriate, should be performed for further evaluation of clinical signs.

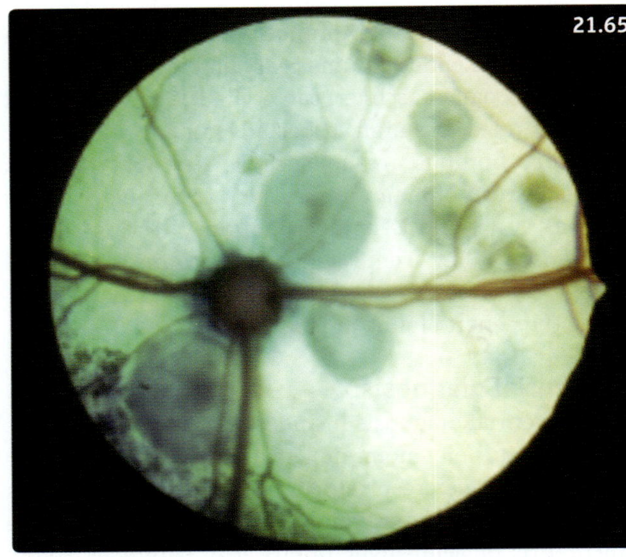

Figure 21.65. A funduscopic view showing cryptococcal chorioretinitis in a cat. (Courtesy D. Brooks)

Management

Published prospective controlled studies do not exist for the treatment of cryptococcal infections. Sinonasal disease is often treated with a combination of debulking therapy followed by prolonged courses of azole therapy (itraconazole 50–100 mg/cat PO q24h; fluconazole 50 mg/cat PO q24h; or ketoconazole 10 mg/kg PO q12h), sometimes in combination with amphotericin B. Regular (1–2 monthly) liver enzyme testing should be performed for possible azole-related hepatotoxicity and treatment should continue until the LCAT titer is zero. A 4–5-fold reduction in LCAT titer indicates an adequate response; LCAT titers should be repeated every 3–6 months thereafter so that recrudescent infections can be diagnosed early. Amphotericin B is the most efficacious anti-cryptococcal drug and can be administered as amphotericin deoxycholate (0.5 mg/kg per cat of 5 mg/ml stock solution diluted in 350 ml of 0.45% NaCl with 2.5% dextrose SC two or three times weekly to a cumulative dose of 10–15 mg/kg; nephrotoxicity can occur) or as liposomal amphotericin B (1–1.5 mg/kg IV q48h to a cumulative dose of 12–15 mg/kg; administer as a 1–2 mg/ml solution in 5% dextrose by IV infusion over 1–2 hours; this is less nephrotoxic than amphotericin B deoxycholate, but azotemia can occur). Monotherapy with 5-flucytosine should not be used because of the potential for drug resistance to develop, but it is synergistic with amphotericin B (25–50 mg/kg PO q6h). The combination of flucytosine and amphotericin B is recommended for feline CNS infections or cats that fail azole therapy. Fluconazole can be substituted for 5-flucytosine in CNS infections if 5-flucytosine is unaffordable, as it can penetrate the blood–brain barrier.

Localized cutaneous disease can often be treated successfully with fluconazole (10 mg/kg PO q12h) until lesions are completely resolved and cryptococcal LCAT titer reduces to zero. As with sinonasal or CNS infections, a 4–5-fold reduction in LCAT titer indicates an adequate response and LCAT titers should be repeated every 3–6 months thereafter so that recrudescent infections can be diagnosed early.

Prevention

Avoidance of exposure to environmental sources can usually be achieved by indoor only housing; however, cases have occurred in indoor only cats in endemic areas.

Public health implications

Infection is acquired from direct exposure to contaminated environmental sources such as avian guano and rotting vegetation, such as eucalyptus bark and leaves. Since there is no aerosolization of cryptococcal organisms from infected tissues, infection is not transmitted between animals or from infected animals to people.

FELINE ASPERGILLOSIS

(See also Chapter 4: Respiratory disorders.)

Definition/overview

Although aspergillosis does occur in the cat, the incidence of infection is far less than that in the dog. There are two anatomic forms of upper respiratory tract aspergillosis in cats and both commence in the nasal cavity: sinonasal aspergillosis and, more commonly (65% cases), invasive sino-orbital aspergillosis. This is in contrast with the dog, in which 99% of cases are noninvasive and sinonasal. Disseminated aspergillosis is typically associated with immunosuppression and while it has been reported in the cat, it is rare. Invasive focal (nonupper respiratory tract) infections have also been the subject of rare feline case reports.

Etiology

Aspergillosis is caused by several species of fungus of the genus *Aspergillus*, which occurs in rotting vegetation, moldy hay, and sewage. Animals become infected through inhalation of airborne spores. *A. fumigatus* and *A. niger* are most commonly associated with sinonasal aspergillosis, while *A. felis*, a newly described *A. fumigatus*-like fungus, is the most common isolate responsible for sino-orbital aspergillosis.

Pathophysiology

Colonization is usually prevented by a local immune response to inhaled spores involving mucociliary clearance, macrophages, and dendritic cells that recognize specific fungal epitopes. Infection usually occurs in young to middle aged cats, and brachycephalic breeds, such as Himalayans, are predisposed to upper respiratory tract aspergillosis.

Clinical presentation

Cats with upper respiratory tract aspergillosis can present with sneezing, stertor, unilateral or bilateral serous to mucopurulent nasal discharge, mild ipsilateral mandibular lymphadenopathy, and clinical signs relating to periorbital involvement such as exophthalmos. Epistaxis, pyrexia, and/or a discharging sinus or soft tissue mass involving the nasal bone or frontal sinus are less commonly seen.

Differential diagnosis

Differential diagnoses include viral upper respiratory disease (FHV-1 and/or FCV), nasal cryptococcosis or other fungal infection (e.g. sporotrichosis, phaeohyphomycoses), nasal neoplasia (e.g. lymphoma, squamous cell carcinoma), nasal foreign body, penetrating bite wound, tooth root abscess, oronasal fistula, trauma to the nasal cavity or frontal sinus, or congenital abnormalities such as choanal atresia or palatine defects.

Diagnosis

Diagnostic tools include serology, radiography, advanced imaging (CT and/or MRI), rhinosinuscopy, cytology, histology, fungal culture, and molecular identification. Identification of fungal hyphae on cytology or histologic examination of biopsy specimens or sinonasal fungal plaques can confirm aspergillosis. Ventrodorsal radiography with the animal's mouth open usually reveals major lysis of the turbinates and increased radiolucency. CT scanning has become the imaging technique of choice for sinonasal aspergillosis because it shows clearly the destruction of the turbinates, increased soft tissue attenuation in the nasal cavity, and fluid or soft tissue accumulation in the frontal and sphenoid sinuses; signs are usually bilateral. MRI is preferred for assessment of intracranial soft tissue. In sino-orbital aspergillosis a ventromedial orbital mass with dorsolateral displacement of the globe and lytic lesions in the paranasal bones are also visualized. The cribriform plate should be inspected for integrity before topical antifungal treatment is considered. Nasopharyngoscopy, rhinoscopy, and/or sinuscopy usually reveals white to greenish-gray colonies, which are typical of nasal aspergillosis. Hematology is unremarkable, and a stress or inflammatory leukogram with eosinophilia can be found; mild to severe hyperglobulinemia on serum biochemistry is relatively common.

Management

Evidence-based treatment protocols from prospective controlled studies are not currently available for feline aspergillosis. However, before treatment commences, the fungal isolate and its susceptibility should be identified and the integrity of the cribriform plate should be determined on CT examination. Endoscopy and saline irrigation should be used to débride fungal plaques from the nasal cavity and frontal sinuses. Pre-treatment assessment of renal and liver function should be undertaken because of the hepatotoxic and nephrotoxic nature of the systemic therapies used.

For noninvasive sinonasal infections (intact cribriform plate), topical 1-hour intranasal infusions with 1% clotrimazole or enilconazole can be administered under general anesthesia. Polyethylene glycol must be used as the vehicle for clotrimazole, since polypropylene glycol can cause severe mucosal edema and ulceration. The head should be tilted to ensure drainage of the infusion at the end of the procedure.

For invasive sinonasal infections (paranasal soft tissue infiltration and orbital involvement, and/or interruption of the cribriform plate), systemic antifungal therapy using itraconazole (10 mg/kg PO q24h with food; hepatotoxicity can occur), or posaconazole (2.5–3.75 mg/kg q12h with food; hepatotoxicity can occur), perhaps combined with amphotericin B deoxycholate (0.5 mg/kg per cat of 5 mg/ml stock solution diluted in 350 ml of 0.45% NaCl with 2.5% dextrose SC two or three times weekly to a cumulative dose of 10–15 mg/kg; nephrotoxicity can occur) or liposomal amphotericin B (1–1.5 mg/kg IV q48h to a cumulative dose of 12–15 mg/kg; administer as a 1–2 mg/ml solution in 5% dextrose by IV infusion over 1–2 hours; this is less nephrotoxic than amphotericin B deoxycholate, but azotemia can occur), are the preferred therapeutic options for feline sinonasal aspergillosis.

Treatment of sino-orbital aspergillosis is based on systemic therapy with itraconazole or posaconazole, combined with amphotericin B, as described above. At least 6 months of therapy is required and reinfections or relapses can occur.

A minimum of a 2–3-month course of systemic antifungal therapy should be administered. *Aspergillus* spp. are intrinsically resistant to fluconazole therapy. Treatment should be continued for at least 1 month beyond cessation of clinical signs. The prognosis for feline sinonasal aspergillosis is generally favorable, while sino-orbital aspergillosis has a poor prognosis, although there are only a handful of published case reports. Pre-treatment surgical débridement should be considered on an individual case basis.

FELINE TOXOPLASMOSIS

Definition/overview

Feline toxoplasmosis is caused by infection with the obligate intracellular coccidian parasite *Toxoplasma gondii*. Infections are known to occur on a worldwide basis, with estimates of up to approximately 30% of clinically ill cats having serologic evidence of exposure; seroprevalence is lowest in areas of low humidity. The organism is capable of infecting virtually all species of warm-blooded animals, including humans, although cats are the definitive hosts for the parasites.

Etiology

Infection among cats can occur subsequent to ingestion of infectious oocysts, or transplacentally or via transmammary transmission among kittens born to infected queens. While infection via ingestion of sporulated oocysts in cat feces is possible, this is thought to be a rare source of infection because of fastidious elimination habits in cats. Cats with outdoor access are especially at risk of exposure subsequent to hunting and ingesting *T. gondii* cysts in the tissues of intermediate hosts or mechanical vectors such as cockroaches, earthworms, and rodents; indoor only cats can also have access to some of these intermediate hosts. In addition, feeding raw meat to cats has been associated with infection. Tissue cysts (bradyzoites) are likely to persist lifelong in infected cats and dogs; therefore, serum antibodies indicate current infection.

Pathophysiology

As the cat is the definitive host of *T. gondii*, it is the only species where the parasite undergoes the enteroepithelial cycle, where infection in intestinal cells undergoes asexual and sexual phases to produce oocysts, which are passed in the feces. After primary infection, cats shed unsporulated oocysts in the feces for 3–21 days. Oocysts sporulate and become infective in 1–5 days under suitable environmental temperature and humidity conditions before being ingested by warm-blooded intermediate hosts. Oocyst shedding after the primary infection in cats is rare, even in immune suppressed cats. Clinical abnormalities associated with the enteroepithelial cycle are rarely identified in cats. Self-limiting small bowel diarrhea of 1–2 weeks' duration has been reported in approximately 10–20% of cats.

In the cat and all other mammals, extraintestinal infection occurs. After contact with cat feces containing sporlated oocysts, or ingestion of bradyzoites in infected tissues, sarcocysts penetrate the intestinal wall and develop into an actively replicating phase (tachyzoites) in infected tissues. As the host immune system responds, parasitic replication slows and bradyzoites are formed in tissue cysts.

Clinical illness subsequent to the ingestion of tissue cysts or oocysts, or reactivation of latent infection (extraintestinal infection), is relatively uncommon in cats. The reason that some cats develop significant clinical disease while many others do not is most likely dependent on parasite virulence factors and the immune response of the host. Immunosuppression due to high-dose corticosteroid therapy and FIV infection has been associated with recrudescent *T. gondii* infection. Disseminated toxoplasmosis has been reported in association with FIV, FeLV, or FIP and after chronic immunosuppressive doses of cyclosporine.

Clinical presentation

Clinical signs of extraintestinal toxoplasmosis, if present, are likely to include fever, ocular inflammation, ataxia, seizures, muscle pain, and dyspnea, depending on the anatomic location of infection. Hepatitis (occasionally with icterus), pancreatitis, myocarditis with associated arrhythmia, encephalitis (**Figures 21.66, 21.67**), and a variety of ocular signs such as uveitis, chorioretinitis, glaucoma, and retinal detachment have also been reported (see **Figure 19.27**). Cardiac arrhythmia may be associated with sudden death in some cats. Among kittens, ocular disease, fading kittens, and stillbirths are commonly associated with transplacental infection

Differential diagnosis

Bacterial pneumonia with respiratory distress is the most important differential diagnosis for clinical pulmonary toxoplasmosis in cats. In addition, sepsis, pancreatitis, hepatitis, and cardiomyopathy should also be considered, depending on the localization of tissue cysts. *Neospora caninum* infection is uncommon, but has been reported to manifest signs similar to toxoplasmosis in cats. Among kittens, sudden death may be reported, so FPL virus infection should be considered. FeLV and FIV testing are indicated and these viral infections may be an important underlying disorder.

Diagnosis

A variety of hematologic and biochemical changes are reported in cats with extraintestinal *T. gondii* infection. However, the inconsistency with which these changes occur diminishes their diagnostic value. Mild anemia, leukocytosis, and eosinophilia are reported. In addition, hypoalbuminemia in the presence of polyclonal hyperglobulinemia has been reported in cats with chronic toxoplasmosis. Depending on the degree of hepatic necrosis associated with infection, liver enzymes and serum bilirubin may be dramatically increased. Creatine kinase is elevated if tachyzoites cause myocyte necrosis. Infected cats with radiographic evidence of pneumonia may demonstrate evidence of *T. gondii* on fine-needle

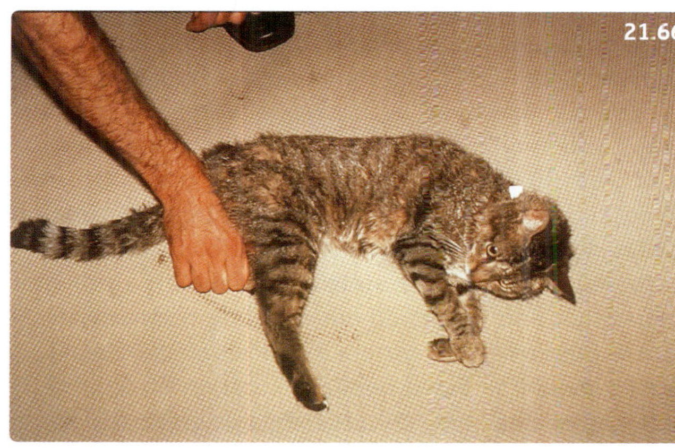

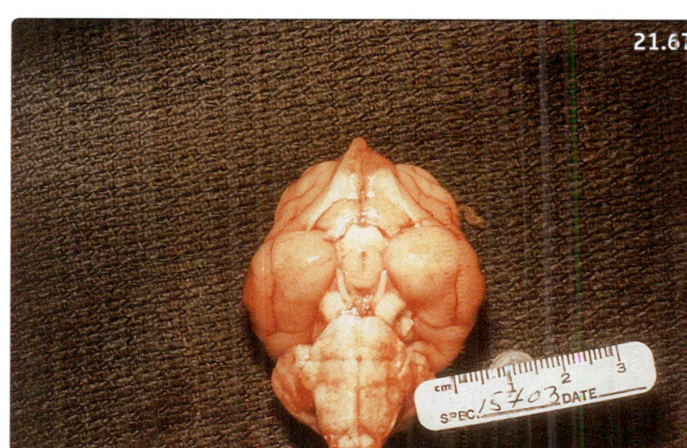

Figures 21.66, 21.67 This 4-year-old Domestic Shorthair cat has diffuse *Toxoplasma* encephalitis (21.66). The cat was euthanized and the diagnosis confirmed on necropsy. The ventral view of the brain (21.67) shows swelling of the piriform processes associated with the temporal lobes. (Courtesy M. Schaer)

aspiration of the lung. Tachyzoites can also be recovered from peritoneal and thoracic fluids of infected cats.

Routine fecal examination of cats suspected of having toxoplasmosis is rarely successful in confirming a diagnosis, as most cats are no longer shedding oocysts by the time clinical signs of extraintestinal infection occur. Following primary infection, cats usually shed *T. gondii* oocysts for less than 3 weeks (usually 1–2 weeks) and repeat oocyst shedding is rare, even in immune suppressed cats. Furthermore, the extremely small size of the oocysts (10 × 12 μm) and the lack of experience of most personnel in recognizing *T. gondii* oocysts justifies alternative diagnostic studies. Fecal PCR assays are available for *T. gondii*, but the test has poor predictive value for the same reasons given for fecal flotation.

Since infected cats harbor *T. gondii* tissue cysts for life, it is possible to detect IgM and IgG class antibodies in feline sera. Anti-*T. gondii* IgM antibodies are usually associated with recent or recrudescent extraintestinal infection (from 2–4 weeks until 16 weeks after infection; persistent IgM titers can occur in FIV-infected cats), but positive results do not correlate with active disease. Anti-*T. gondii* IgG antibodies generally indicate infection of at least 10 days' duration, but again, positive results do not correlate with active disease. Serum agglutination assays are designed to detect all antibody classes, but can give false-negative results when only IgM antibodies are present and results do not correlate with active disease. A tentative antemortem diagnosis of toxoplasmosis in cats should be based on a combination of: (1) an IgM titer higher than 1:64; (2) a four-fold or greater increase in IgG titer; (3) clinical signs consistent with extraintestinal toxoplasmosis; and (4) positive response to treatment for toxoplasmosis. On necropsy, cats that have died from toxoplasmosis are most likely to manifest evidence of tissue inflammation and necrosis in the liver, mesenteric lymph nodes, pancreas, and lungs.

Management

Treatment/prognosis

Cats with extraintestinal toxoplasmosis can be treated with clindamycin (10–15 mg/kg PO q12h for 4 weeks) or trimethoprim/sulfa combination antimicrobial drugs (15 mg/kg PO q12h for 4 weeks). Clinical improvement is expected within 7 days following onset of therapy. If clinical response does not occur with one drug within 7 days, therapy with the other drug can be tried. Cats with clinical uveitis associated with toxoplasmosis may be treated with topical or systemic corticosteroids, to prevent secondary lens luxation and glaucoma. Cats with hepatic, CNS, or pulmonary disease, and those with concurrent FeLV or FIV, carry a significantly poorer prognosis with treatment. Complete resolution of signs might not occur in neurologic infections after clinical resolution.

Prevention

No drug has been shown to eliminate extraintestinal *T. gondii* infection in cats or dogs, and reactivated infection is always possible. Although an oral vaccine against toxoplasmosis has been demonstrated to reduce oocyst shedding in infected cats under research conditions, no such vaccine is commercially available at this time. Preventing kittens and cats from hunting (including ingesting transport hosts such as cockroaches) and feeding only commercially prepared cat food, without raw meat supplements, is a highly effective means of preventing exposure. Meat that has been frozen prior to feeding can harbor infectious tissue cysts.

Public health implications

Since the cat is a definitive host for *T. gondii* and is capable of excreting oocysts in feces during the enteroepithelial phase of infection, the cat does represent a potential threat to human health, although oocyst excretion is very rare after the primary infection. Administration of clindamycin (20 mg/kg PO q24h) can reduce the period of oocyst shedding if it is demonstrated in an individual cat. Additionally, because of fastidious grooming habits, cats are unlikely to harbor infective oocysts on their hair coat. However, during the period of initial oocyst excretion in the feces, cats are unlikely to manifest any clinical signs of disease. Excreted oocysts are not infectious until they have undergone sporulation (approximately 48 hours at room temperature, although reduced sporulation times can occur at higher environmental temperatures), and oocysts are resistant to disinfectants. Sporulated oocysts are more environmentally resistant than unsporulated oocysts.

Cat owners who are regarded as being at risk of infection, such as immunocompromised individuals or seronegative pregnant women, with *T. gondii* can take basic precautions to avoid exposure. If possible, at-risk individuals should not have access to litter pans; however, cleaning litter boxes at least every 24 hours will minimize the chance of exposure to sporulated oocysts. Since sporulated oocysts have demonstrated their ability to survive in a wide range of environmental temperatures and humidity (up to 18 months or more), avoiding locations where cats are likely to defecate or wearing gloves while working in soil can minimize the risk of exposure to humans. To clean contaminated litter pans, boiling water is superior to liquid disinfectants. Steam cleaning can be used to decontaminate hard, impervious surfaces.

The cat is a rare source of direct infection to people, since infective oocysts are only passed during the primary infection in cats, infected oocysts are unlikely to be found on the hair coat during primary infection, and cats bury their feces. Most human infections are acquired by eating undercooked meat containing tissue cysts, and the prevalence of protective antibody titers against *T. gondii* is high in people who eat meat. Human infection can result in mild self-limiting malaise, fever, and lymphadenopathy, and is commonly misdiagnosed. Primary infection during pregnancy can result in clinical toxoplasmosis in the fetus, with stillbirths, CNS, and ocular disease. Toxoplasmic encephalitis from reactivated infections occurs in approximately 10% of people with HIV/AIDS as CD4+ T cell counts decline. Assessment of human risk of infection is best carried out by determination of anti-*T. gondii* antibody protection status, as protection rates are very high in most populations.

RECOMMENDED FURTHER READING

Ettinger SJ, Feldman EC (2010) (eds.) *Textbook of Veterinary Internal Medicine*, 7th edn. Elsevier Saunders, St. Louis.

Greene CE (2011) (ed.) *Infectious Diseases of the Dog and Cat*, 4th edn. Elsevier Saunders, St. Louis.

Plumb DC (2011) (ed.) *Plumb's Veterinary Drug Handbook*, 7th edn. PharmaVet Inc, Stockholm.

Sykes JE (2013) (ed.) *Canine and Feline Infectious Diseases*. 1st edn. Elsevier Saunders, St. Louis.

Chapter 22

Immunologic disorders

Michael J. Day

INTRODUCTION

The immune system interfaces with virtually all other body systems and consequently almost all diseases have an immunologic aspect. For example, the immune system will respond appropriately to the presence of infectious or neoplastic disease, or the existence of a chronic disease state may lead to secondary immunosuppression. More importantly, there is a wide range of diseases that have an immunopathological basis and these are the focus of this chapter. In order to fully understand these primary immunologic disorders, a solid working knowledge of the immune system is required. This chapter will briefly overview current knowledge of the immune response and immunopathology, and then discuss the four major categories of immune-mediated disease: (1) allergic disease; (2) autoimmune disease; (3) primary immunodeficiency disease; and (4) immune system neoplasia. Many of the key diseases within these groups are discussed in the individual systems-based chapters of this book. These will be cross-referenced from this chapter, and only selected immunologic disorders not covered elsewhere will be presented here.

THE IMMUNE RESPONSE

The immune system may be fundamentally considered in terms of innate and adaptive immunity. Innate immunity encompasses the more primitive, nonspecific defense mechanisms of the body, while adaptive immunity is antigen-specific, considerably more potent, and encompasses the phenomenon of immunologic memory. It is now known that activity within the innate immune system directs the nature of the subsequent adaptive response. The key cell that links these two systems is the dendritic antigen presenting cell (APC).

Innate immunity

The innate immune system is most dominant at the mucocutaneous barriers of the body, which are the front line of exposure to pathogens. The microanatomic aspects of these barriers themselves are considered part of the innate immune system and are represented by structures such as:

- The thick, keratinized epidermis of the skin, which is coated by antimicrobial secretions of the sebaceous and sweat glands (**Figure 22.1**).
- The mucociliary escalator of the lower respiratory tract.
- The peristaltic motion of the intestinal tract, coupled with the rapid turnover of enterocytes and secretion of a wide range of enzymatic and antimicrobial substances.

Similarly, the natural microflora of many of these surfaces provides powerful competitive exclusion to pathogens and may also be considered an innate protective feature.

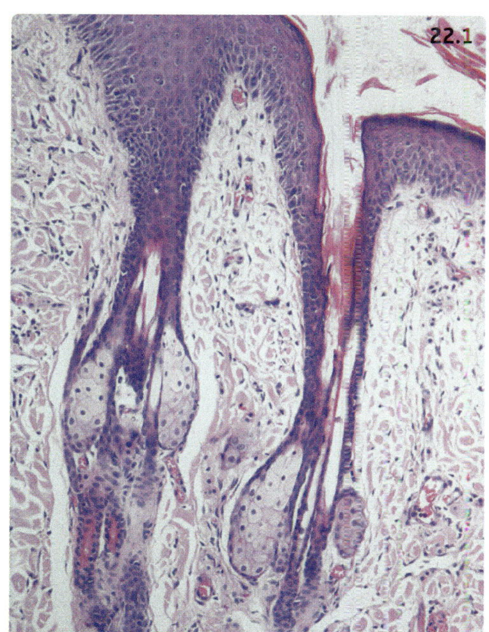

Figure 22.1 Section of skin from a cat displaying features of the innate immune system including the keratinized epidermal barrier, sebaceous gland secretions, and resident leukocytes within the epidermis and superficial dermis.

These barrier functions are supported by the soluble and cellular constituents of the innate immune system. The former include secreted immunologic molecules such as components of the alternative complement pathway, antimicrobial peptides such as the 'defensins', selected proinflammatory cytokines (such as interleukin [IL]-1, IL-6, and tumor necrosis factor [TNF]-α), and polyreactive IgA and IgM. The cellular components of the innate immune system include nonspecific phagocytic cells (neutrophils and macrophages), the natural killer (NK) cells, which undertake cytotoxic destruction of target cells (e.g. virally infected cells or tumor cells) in a less specific fashion than T lymphocytes, and the specialized subset of T lymphocytes that express an antigen-specific T-cell receptor (TCR) comprised of a γ and δ chain (γδ TCR).

These components of innate immunity work together to provide immediate protection following exposure to a potential pathogen. Although a relatively less effective means of immune defense, the innate immune system is crucial for the provision of this protective cover until the adaptive response is activated, mobilized, and recruited to the site of pathogen exposure.

22.2

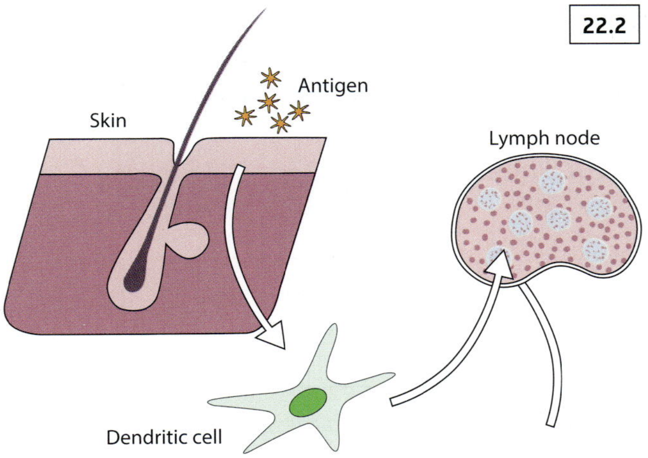

Figure 22.2 The dendritic cell is the key link between the innate and adaptive immune systems. In this example, percutaneously absorbed antigen is taken up by an epidermal Langerhans cell and translocated to regional lymphoid tissue via the dermal lymphatic drainage.

The dendritic cell; link between innate and adaptive immunity

The dendritic APC provides the link between innate and adaptive immunity. Dendritic cells are widely distributed throughout the tissues of the body, and are particularly prominent at the mucocutaneous barriers. Some of the best characterized dendritic cells are those of the skin, and these include the epidermal Langerhans cell and the dermal dendritic cells. The primary role of the dendritic cell is the capture of foreign antigen as it penetrates these barriers, the 'processing' of this antigen to a form which can stimulate adaptive immunity, and the translocation of antigen from the peripheral point of exposure to the regional draining lymphoid tissue for induction of the adaptive immune response (**Figure 22.2**).

The initial encounter between foreign antigen and dendritic cell involves a series of dendritic cell receptor molecules termed 'pattern recognition receptors' (PRRs) or 'Toll-like receptors' (TLRs). These PRRs are expressed either on the surface membrane of the dendritic cell or within the cytoplasm. They interact with ligands that are derived from foreign antigen (e.g. pathogenic microorganisms) or damaged body cells. These ligands are termed 'pathogen-associated molecular patterns' (PAMPs) or 'microbe-associated molecular patterns' and include structural antigens expressed on the surface of microbes (e.g. lipopolysaccharide) or their internal constituents (e.g. portions of microbial DNA). Ligands derived from altered tissue cells are referred to as 'damage-associated molecular patterns'. The interaction between PRR and PAMP permits the foreign antigen to be internalized into the cytoplasm of the dendritic cell where it may enter one of two distinct intracellular antigen-processing pathways. The first of these pathways involves the enzymatic degradation of the antigen within a cytoplasmic membrane-enclosed compartment. Within this compartment, the complex antigenic structure is degraded into small peptide constituents (of the order of 25 amino acids in length), which become associated with molecules that line the inner surface of the compartment. These are the class II molecules of the major histocompatibility complex (MHC), which are pivotal to the generation of the immune response. Following this 'processing' event, the combination of MHC class II and peptide becomes re-expressed on the surface of the dendritic cell, such that the dendritic cell is now 'presenting' the antigen–MHC complex (thus the terminology 'antigen-presenting cell').

The second intracellular antigen-processing pathway involves degradation of antigen within a distinct cytoplasmic compartment known as the proteasome. Within the proteasome, slightly smaller peptide fragments (10 amino acids in length) are generated, which are then translocated into the cytoplasmic Golgi apparatus where they become associated with class I molecules of the MHC. These complexes of class I MHC and antigenic peptide are also then expressed on the surface of the dendritic cell.

Which of these intracellular processing pathways is activated is determined by the nature of the foreign antigen and, therefore, which of the dendritic cell PRRs become engaged. Broadly speaking, the majority of antigens that are derived from outside of the body (exogenous antigens) and require phagocytosis or pinocytosis enter the MHC class II expression pathway. In contrast, antigens that are derived from within tissue cells (endogenous antigens [e.g. viral antigens synthesized in the cytoplasm from viral genetic material within the cell] or tumor antigens expressed by a tissue cell) are processed by the class I pathway. These pathways are not mutually exclusive, so it is possible for an antigen to be processed by both routes ('cross-presentation').

The antigen-processing procedure involves not only expression of MHC–peptide on the surface of the dendritic cell, but the upregulation of other (co-stimulatory) molecules on the dendritic cell surface and the secretion of soluble intercellular messengers (cytokines) by the activated APC (**Figure 22.3**). Again, the nature of these co-stimulatory molecules and the type of cytokines are directed by the nature of the inciting antigen and the intracellular signaling pathways triggered when that antigen binds to particular dendritic cell PRRs. All of these outcomes of antigen processing (e.g. presentation by MHC I or II, the nature of co-stimulatory molecules and cytokines) will in turn determine the type of adaptive immune response that is made to the antigen. Thus, the dendritic cell truly is the link between innate and adaptive immunity and the key factor determining the quality of the adaptive immune response.

All of the events described above occur within the dendritic APC, but the second major role of this cell is in translocation of antigen from the site of exposure (e.g. at a mucocutaneous surface) to the regional draining lymphoid tissue. This procedure involves the antigen-laden dendritic cell entering the tissue lymphatics where it travels to the lymph node and enters the T-cell area (paracortex) of the node.

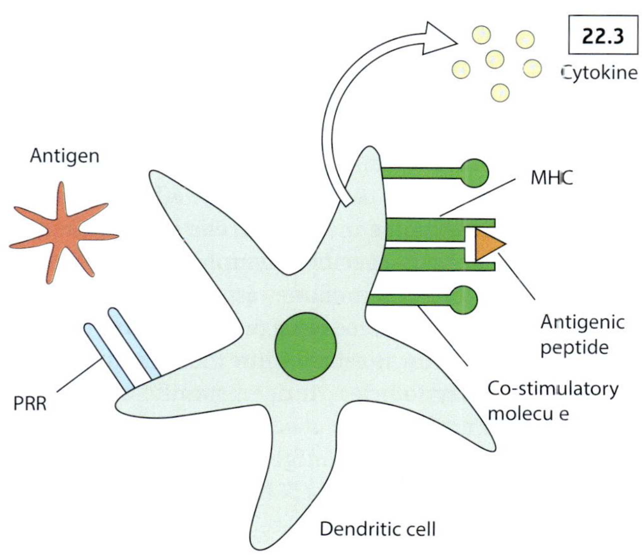

Figure 22.3 The APC (dendritic cell) engages foreign antigen via surface PRRs. The antigen is internalized, processed, and re-presented on the surface of the cell associated with a class II MHC molecule. The dendritic cell also upregulates the expression of co-stimulatory molecules and secretes co-stimulatory cytokines.

The adaptive immune response

Once the antigen-laden dendritic cell arrives in the lymph node paracortex it remains relatively stationary, while numerous T lymphocytes approach it to 'test out' whether their TCRs are designed to be able to bind to the combination of antigenic peptide and MHC expressed by the APC. These T cells express a receptor comprised of an α and β chain, the antigen-binding capacity of which has been predetermined by gene rearrangements within the cell. The T- and B-cell populations of the body between them bear an enormous range of receptor specificities (the receptor 'repertoire'), which are designed to be able to interact with any foreign antigen that may ever be encountered by that individual. In order to maximize the potential for any one T or B cell to encounter the antigen that they are 'pre-programmed' to recognize, the lymphoid cells of the body continually recirculate through a complex pathway involving the tissues, lymphatics, and vascular circulation ('immune surveillance'). The recirculating T cells within the lymph node paracortex may or may not be relevant to a particular antigen expressed by any one dendritic cell at any time. *In-vivo* video microscopy of labeled T cells and dendritic cells has shown that an APC within the paracortex might be expected to be approached by up to 500 different T cells each hour.

Possibly the most amazing feature of the immune response is that such interactions between APCs and T cells do occur and result in generation of the adaptive immune response. For antigens that have never before been encountered by the individual, the 'naïve' T cell that associates with the APC is not yet committed to generating an adaptive immune response of any particular type. Again, it is the dendritic cell that now determines the nature of this adaptive response by the way in which it signals the naïve T cell.

Dendritic cells expressing antigenic peptide primarily associated with MHC class II are most likely to stimulate that subset of T cells bearing the CD4 ('cluster of differentiation' molecule number 4) molecule (T helper [Th] cells), whereas class I-peptide expression is more likely to activate the CD8-expressing T-cell subset (T cytotoxic [Tc] cells). There are a number of key functional subpopulations of $CD4^+$ T cells and which of these is preferentially activated by activation of the naïve CD4⁺ T cell precursor by the dendritic cell determines the functional nature of the ensuing adaptive immune response.

Signaling of the naïve CD4⁺ T cell, involving release of APC-derived cytokines such as IL-12, IL-18, and IL-27 and activation through the T-cell intracellular signaling pathway STAT 4, results in differentiation of the naïve cell into a mature Th1 cell. The Th1 cell is defined functionally by production of the cytokines IL-2 and interferon (IFN)-γ and by the initiation of an adaptive immune response dominated by cell-mediated immunity (CMI). CMI involves the activation of cytotoxic CD8⁺ T cells and NK cells for destruction of virally infected or neoplastic target cells, or the activation of macrophages to permit destruction of an intracellular pathogen such as *Leishmania*, *Salmonella*, or *Mycobacterium*. The Th1-driven immune response features only limited antibody production of those IgG subclasses that might be involved in opsonization or antibody-dependent cell-mediated cytotoxicity. Consequently, the antigens that induce this form of immune response are largely exogenous pathogens of the type listed above (**Figure 22.4**).

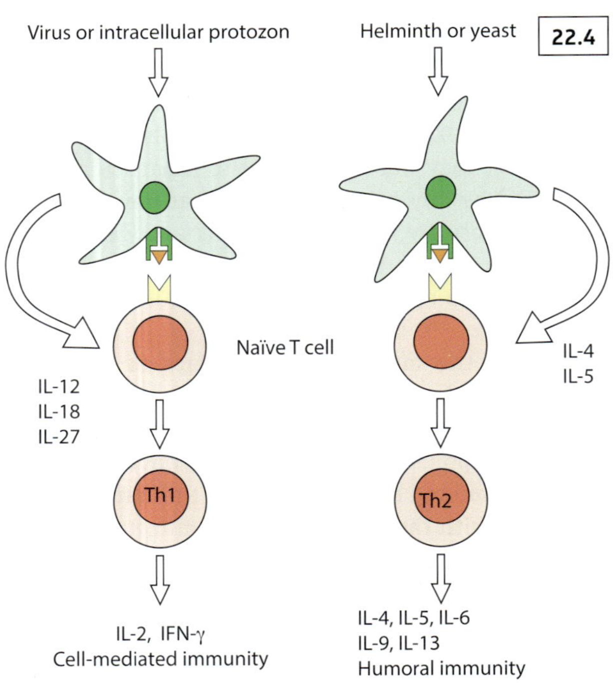

Figure 22.4 Processed antigen is presented by the dendritic cell to naïve CD4⁺ T lymphocytes. The nature of the inciting antigen determines the type of stimulatory signal provided by the dendritic cell and thus the pathway of differentiation of the T cell. Differentiation towards Th1 promotes a cell-mediated effector immune response, whereas the Th2 subpopulation induces a humoral effector response.

By contrast, signaling of the naïve CD4⁺ T cell, involving release of APC-derived cytokines such as IL-4 and activation through the T-cell intracellular signaling pathway STAT 6, results in differentiation of the naïve cell into a mature Th2 cell. The Th2 cell is defined functionally by production of the cytokines IL-4, IL-5, IL-6, IL-9, and IL-13 and by the initiation of an adaptive immune response dominated by humoral (antibody-mediated) immunity. Such antibody responses (involving production of alternative IgG subclasses to those above, IgA and IgE) might be required in adaptive immune responses driven by the presence of pathogens such as yeasts, *Escherichia coli*, or helminth parasites (**Figure 22.4**).

Activation of the naïve CD4⁺ T cell via the STAT 3 pathway and APC-derived IL-6, IL-23 or transforming growth factor (TGF)-β results in differentiation into a Th17 cell. Th17 cells are defined by their production of IL-17 and have a key role in the defense against bacterial and fungal infections.

Although less well understood, the dendritic cell–T cell encounter is also likely to control the differentiation of the subsets of CD4⁺ T cells that are involved in suppression (or 'downregulation') of the immune response. The major suppressive populations include the CD4⁺CD25⁺ 'natural suppressor cells', which are constitutively present in the body, the CD4⁺ IL-10 producing 'induced suppressor cells' (T regulatory cells [Tregs]), which are induced following antigen exposure, and the Th3 cells that are important in the regulation of mucosal immune responses and defined by the production of TGF-β.

The activation of T cells by interaction with APCs involves not only determination of the qualitative nature of the adaptive immune response, but the expansion of antigen-relevant clones of T cells via the process of clonal proliferation. This generates large numbers of antigen-specific T cells that mediate the effector immune response. At least some of these T cells are required for activation of antigen-specific B lymphocytes, which will undertake the humoral immune response.

B-cell activation proceeds in a different fashion to that described for T cells. B cells within the lymphoid tissue reside in primary follicles. Antigen-specific B cells similarly require a combination of activation signals. The first of these comes from the antigen itself, which is recognized by the B-cell receptor (BCR) or surface membrane immunoglobulin. The naïve B cell expresses the combination of IgD and IgM receptor molecules of identical, genetically determined, antigen specificity. The BCR recognizes a large, conformational determinant of antigen (rather than an MHC-associated peptide fragment). This antigenic determinant may be present in soluble form in the B cell environment or may be physically delivered on the surface of an APC. Again, only those B cells bearing antigen-relevant BCRs will be able to recognize antigen, and continual B-cell recirculation is important to maximize the chance of this occurrence. For the majority of (T-dependent) antigens, B-cell activation requires T-cell help. It is now known that following Th cell activation (as described above), some of these cells migrate from the paracortex into the margins of primary follicles, where they encounter B cells carrying receptors for the same stimulating antigen (**Figure 22.5**).

Following BCR–antigen recognition, the B cell internalizes these surface molecules into a cytoplasmic compartment where there is antigen processing and association with MHC class II molecules as described for the dendritic cell. The B cell also presents these MHC–antigen complexes on its surface membrane. T-cell help for B-cell activation takes the form of:

- TCR binding MHC–peptide on the B-cell surface.
- The interaction of other co-stimulatory molecules on the surface of each cell.
- The release of co-stimulatory cytokines from the T cell (e.g. IL-4, IL-5), which bind cytokine receptors on the B-cell surface (**Figure 22.6**).

B-cell activation also results in clonal proliferation, which in the case of a B cell is shown by the formation of a secondary follicle with a blastic germinal center and surrounding mantle zone of small lymphocytes. Additionally, the stimulated B cells undergo the 'immunoglobulin class switch', which involves genetic recombination to permit expression of a single immunoglobulin class (generally IgG, IgA, or IgE). The type of immunoglobulin is determined by the type of Th cell (Th1 versus Th2) and in turn by the nature of the stimulating antigen (see above). For example, an intestinal helminth parasite is most likely to stimulate Th2 activation and IgE class switching within the mesenteric lymph node. The end stage of B-cell activation is transformation of that B cell into a plasma cell, which can actively secrete immunoglobulin of the predetermined class and antigen specificity.

Having expanded antigen-specific T- and B-cell populations within the regional lymphoid tissue, the next (effector) phase of the immune response necessitates these cells leaving the node within efferent lymph, which eventually drains into the vascular circulation. The antigen-specific lymphocytes circulate in the blood until they encounter modified endothelial cells bearing molecules ('vascular addressins') that bind to ligands on the circulating cells ('homing receptors') and enable the

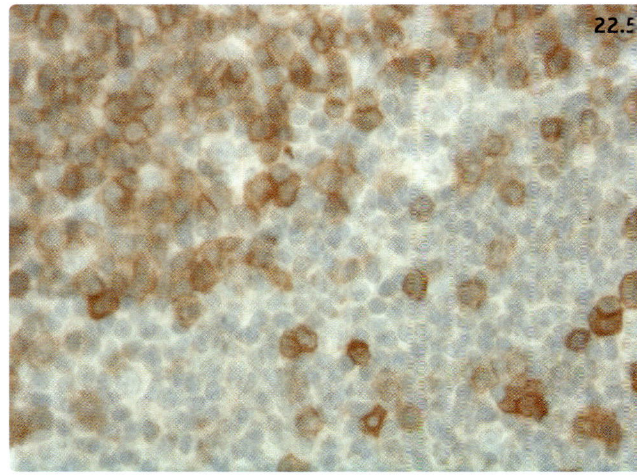

Figure 22.5 Canine lymph node labeled to show expression of the T-cell marker CD3. The image includes the junction between paracortex and a primary lymphoid follicle. Scattered T cells are found within the follicular (B cell) area. These helper cells will provide co-stimulation for antigen-activated B cells and generation of a secondary lymphoid follicle.

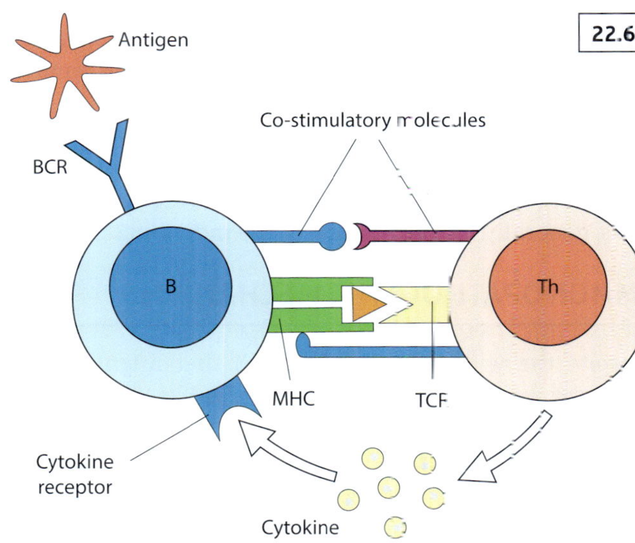

Figure 22.6 Provision of T-cell help for activation of a B cell. The B lymphocyte recognizes intact antigen through surface immunoglobulin (the B-cell receptor). The B cell internalizes the antigen, processes it, and re-presents a peptide fragment of antigen associated with an MHC class II molecule. The T helper cell physically interacts with the B cell through the TCR and engagement of co-stimulatory molecules expressed on the surface of each cell. In addition, the T cell releases co-stimulatory cytokine that binds cytokine receptor on the target B cell.

circulating lymphocytes to be arrested in their flow and to diapedese between endothelia into the tissue containing the inciting antigen. Having attained this position, these lymphocytes of the adaptive immune system are now able to reinforce the innate immunity that has, to date, dealt with the initiating pathogen. The nature of this effector immune response is determined by the nature of the pathogen and those aspects of the immunologic armory that are best able to eliminate it. For example, the cutaneous immune response to *Leishmania* would best be served by the action of Th1 lymphocytes producing IFN-γ, which may stimulate parasitized macrophages and allow them to destroy the pathogen that was replicating within their cytoplasm. Concurrently, the activation of IgG-secreting plasma cells would provide antigen-specific antibody that might bind and neutralize free amastigotes that were released from ruptured parasitized cells. In this instance, a Th2 response with dominant humoral immunity would not be protective, which is exactly the situation that arises in susceptible dogs that succumb to the infection.

The final stage of the adaptive immune response involves suppression of the response when it is no longer required (i.e. when antigen is eliminated). Such suppression is an active event, and primarily involves the range of Tregs described above. Through either physical contact or inhibitory cytokine production, or both, suppressor cells are able to inhibit the function or physically remove (by induction of apoptosis) the effector populations. The antigen-stimulated cells are never entirely removed, as for each immune response that is made, a residual population of long-lived memory T and B lymphocytes persists, generally for the lifetime of the individual.

IMMUNOPATHOGENIC MECHANISMS

Despite the wide array of antigens that might potentially be encountered by an individual (e.g. infectious agents, allergens, tissue alloantigens, autoantigens, tumor antigens), the immune system generally responds to stimulation by using one or more of a series of well-defined immunopathogenic mechanisms. These were defined many years ago by Gell and Coombs as types I to IV hypersensitivity, and this classification still provides a useful framework for consideration of immune effector function. These are best considered as 'immunopathogenic mechanisms' rather than 'hypersensitivity mechanisms' because while they do form the basis for allergic (hypersensitivity) disease, the same mechanisms are involved in other immune-mediated diseases (e.g. autoimmune disease) and in beneficial immune responses to foreign antigens (for which reason they probably evolved initially).

Type I (immediate) hypersensitivity

Type I hypersensitivity follows exposure to antigens that selectively trigger Th2 lymphocytes and the production of IgE antibodies. These antibodies bind specific receptor molecules on the surface of basophils and tissue mast cells, and when the sensitized individual is re-exposed to antigen there is binding and cross-linking of these cell-bound IgE molecules. This results in rapid (within 15–20 minutes, thus 'immediate' hypersensitivity) mast cell or basophil degranulation, with the release of a wide range of proinflammatory mediators that lead to the well-recognized clinical effects of such reactions, which may be localized or generalized (anaphylactic) (**Figures 22.7, 22.8**). These effects include:

- Vasodilation with tissue edema and egress of plasma protein and leukocytes.
- Bronchoconstriction via contraction of smooth muscle.
- Cutaneous pruritus caused by interaction with neurologic pathways.

The type I reaction probably evolved to provide protective immunity in the case of intestinal helminth parasitism, but it is now most widely recognized as the mechanism underlying the range of allergic diseases of the skin, conjunctivae, respiratory tract, and gastrointestinal tract of the dog and cat.

22.7

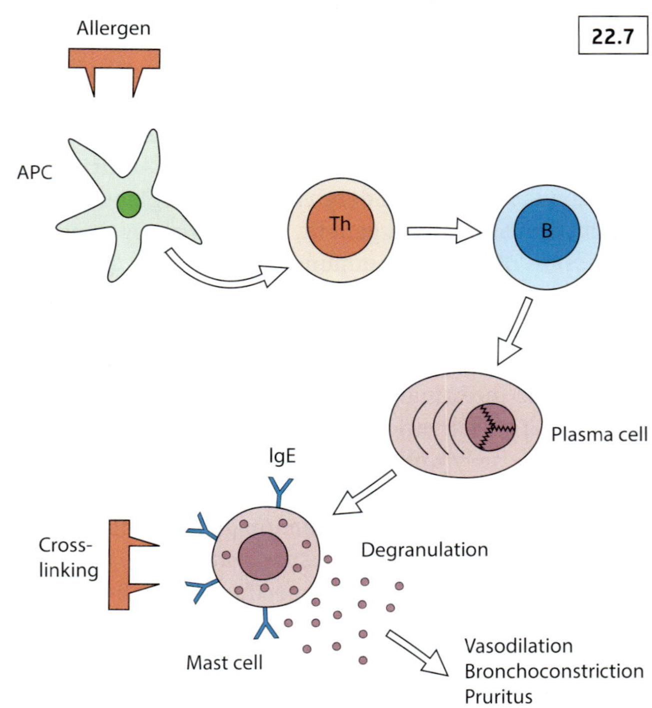

Figure 22.7 The type I hypersensitivity reaction. Presentation of allergen by dendritic cells results in stimulation of Th2 immunity, with the generation of allergen-specific IgE antibodies that coat mucocutaneous mast cells. On re-exposure to allergen there is mast cell degranulation, which mediates the classical clinical features of this reaction.

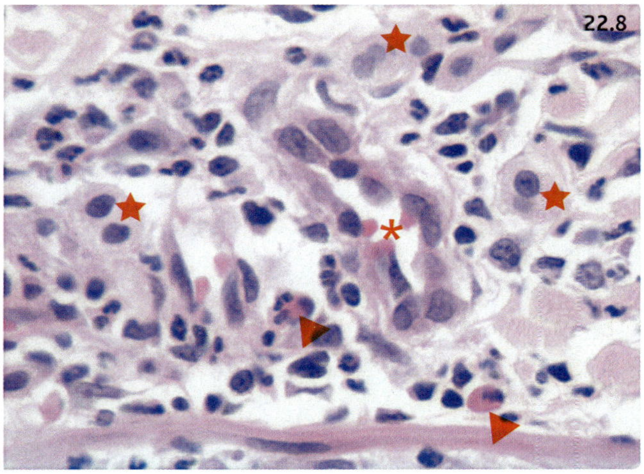

Figure 22.8 Skin biopsy from a 5-year-old Domestic Shorthair cat with pruritus and miliary dermatitis. The histopathologic features are characteristic of a type I hypersensitivity reaction. There is a mixed inflammatory infiltration surrounding the superficial dermal vessel (asterisk), which includes small clusters of mast cells (stars) and eosinophils (arrowheads).

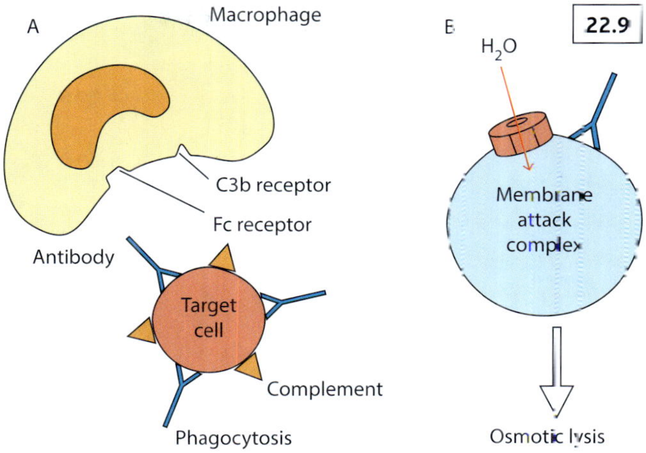

Figure 22.9 The type II hypersensitivity reaction. Immunologic sensitization leads to production of antibody that coats a target cell and activates complement deposition via the classical pathway. (A) The target cell is thus opsonized for phagocytosis by a macrophage bearing Fc and C3b receptors. (B) Alternatively, the membrane attack complex of complement inserts through the cell membrane, creating an ionic imbalance and resulting in a net influx of water into the target cell cytoplasm with subsequent lysis of the target.

Type II (antibody-mediated) hypersensitivity

In this reaction, the individual is sensitized to produce antibody that attaches to the surface of a target cell and subsequently activates the classical pathway of the complement system. The deposition of complement molecules onto the target cell surface leads to destruction of that target via either formation of the membrane attack complex of complement with osmotic lysis of the cell or phagocytosis of the immunoglobulin and complement opsonized target (**Figure 22.9**). The classical target cell for this type of reaction is the erythrocyte, and type II hypersensitivity is the immunopathogenic mechanism that underlies diseases such as immune-mediated haemolytic anemia (IMHA) or blood transfusion reactions. Also included in this category are disorders involving the interaction of antibody with receptor molecules, classically causing either receptor blockade (e.g. antibody to the neuromuscular acetylcholine receptor [AChR] in myasthenia gravis) or receptor activation (e.g. stimulation of the thyroid stimulating hormone receptor by antibody in human Grave's disease).

Type III (immune complex) hypersensitivity

This immunopathogenic mechanism has two distinct subtypes defined by the relative proportions of antigen and antibody involved in the reaction. In antibody excess type III hypersensitivity, the individual is sensitized to mount a marked antibody response to antigen. On re-exposure to that antigen, the high concentrations of antibody that may be found at the site of antigen entry immediately bind to the antigen at the site of exposure. The antigen–antibody interaction results in local formation of insoluble immune complexes, with subsequent activation of complement and production of inflammatory mediators and local recruitment of inflammatory cells. The classical example of such a reaction is the human 'Arthus reaction' involving exposure to inhaled antigens (of an occupational nature), with the development of pulmonary disease post exposure in a sensitized individual. Such reactions are rarely documented in the dog and cat.

In antigen excess type III hypersensitivity there are higher concentrations of antigen than antibody, resulting in the formation of small, soluble immune complexes that circulate in the bloodstream. Depending on the nature of the antigen and antibody involved and vascular factors (e.g. endothelial damage, turbulent flow), these complexes may become lodged in the walls of small capillaries in predilection sites such as the renal glomerulus, synovium, uveal tract, and cutaneous basement membrane zone. The ensuing local inflammation (vasculitis) may lead to thrombosis and ischemic necrosis of the tissue supplied by the vessel (**Figure 22.10**). This form of type III reaction is not uncommon in dogs and cats and, although the inciting antigens are rarely identified, they are often presumed to be of infectious origin and such type III reactions to be post-infectious immune sequelae. A classical example of such a reaction is immune complex glomerulonephritis secondary to *Leishmania* or *Borrelia*

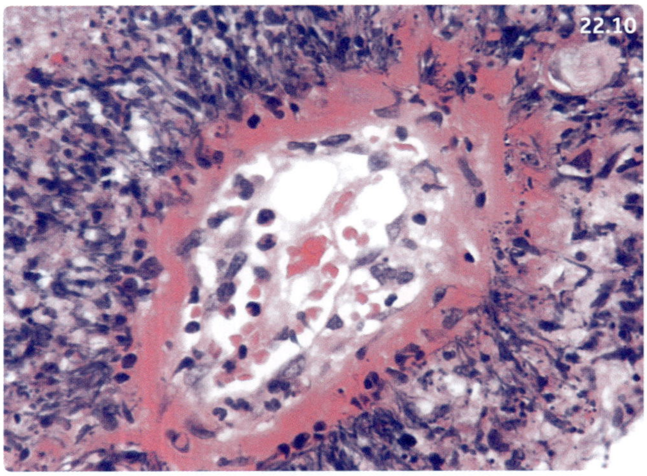

Figure 22.10 Cutaneous vasculitis in a dog. This is one of multiple affected dermal blood vessels in biopsy samples taken from ulcerative lesions on the flanks and scrotum of an 11-year-old dog. There is deposition of fibrin in the remains of the wall of this vessel, together with numerous apoptotic neutrophils within the wall and within the surrounding dermal collagen. The cause of this presumptive type III hypersensitivity reaction was not ascertained.

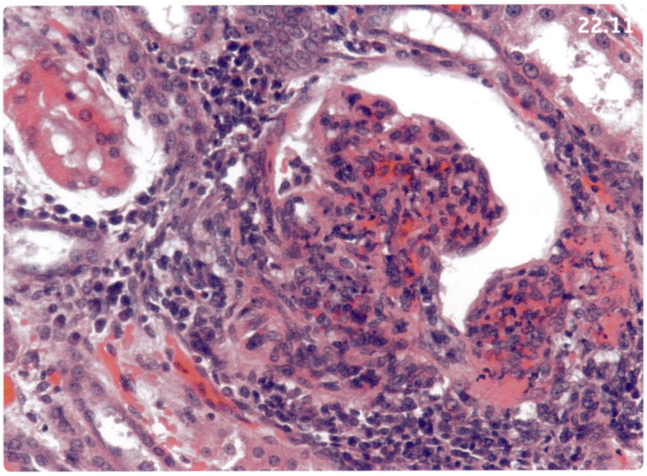

Figure 22.11 Section of kidney from a dog with leishmaniasis. There is mononuclear cell infiltration of the interstitium, with distortion and inflammation of the glomerular tuft. Arterial vessels in this section had clear evidence of leukocytoclastic vasculitis. The pathogenesis of these lesions likely involves the deposition of immune complexes containing IgG antibody and *Leishmania* antigen.

infection in the dog (**Figure 22.11**). Such reactions are also likely to have a role in diseases such as cutaneous lupus erythematosus (CLE), immune-mediated polyarthritis, and immune-mediated uveitis.

Type IV (delayed) hypersensitivity

This hypersensitivity reaction involves cellular rather than humoral immunopathologic mechanisms. The response to local tissue re-exposure to antigen in a sensitized individual is the activation of memory T cells, with the recruitment of mononuclear cells (chiefly macrophages, CD4$^+$, and CD8$^+$ T cells) into the site of antigenic exposure via activation of endothelia that permits this site-specific migration. Local tissue damage is mediated by the infiltrating cells and the cytokines that they produce (**Figure 22.12**). The activation of T-cell memory and recruitment of mononuclear cells takes some time to occur (classically 72 hours), leading to the description of this reaction as 'delayed type hypersensitivity'. This type of immunopathologic mechanism is the classical manifestation of a protective Th1 response to a range of tissue pathogens but, when used inappropriately, it forms the basis of the contact hypersensitivity reaction or autoimmune reactions involving cellular infiltration (e.g. immune-mediated polyarthritis, lymphocytic thyroiditis, granulomatous meningoencephalitis).

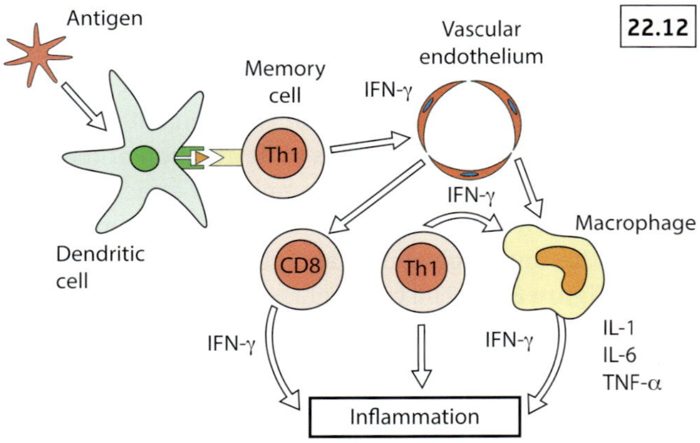

Figure 22.12 In type IV hypersensitivity, re-exposure to the sensitizing antigen leads to local activation of memory Th1 cells. These secrete IFN-γ, which activates vascular endothelium and permits recruitment of further T cells (Th1 and CD8$^+$) and macrophages. These in turn secrete further cytokines, which mediate the local inflammatory reaction.

IMMUNE-MEDIATED DISEASES

Immune-mediated diseases arise when the range of immunologic mechanisms described above are activated inappropriately to produce tissue pathology and clinical signs. This is clearly the case in the range of allergic diseases where there is an inappropriate and excessive immune response (involving combinations of type I and IV reactions) to allergens (e.g. aeroallergens, arthropod-derived allergens) to which a clinically normal individual might be exposed but fail to respond. The allergic diseases are of immense clinical significance in both human and veterinary medicine, and consequently are widely researched and relatively well characterized in terms of their immunopathogenesis.

ALLERGIC DISEASES

There are clear genetic predispositions to the development of allergy in human families and breeds and pedigrees of dog, yet the genetic basis of allergy is not well characterized. Several genome-wide association studies searching for single nucleotide polymorphisms in genes that might be associated with canine atopic dermatitis have produced conflicting data. Whatever the genetic basis, it is clear that some individuals (human and canine) have a predisposition to make high IgE responses to ubiquitous environmental allergens. Such individuals also have reduced effectiveness of immunoregulation, and the allergic state correlates with lack of induced regulatory T cell function (e.g. IL-10-producing Tregs). In addition to genetic and immunologic factors, there are clear environmental influences over the development of allergic disease. This may be as simple as environmental exposure, and reduction of exposure levels to causative allergens is one part of the clinical management of such disorders. In human medicine, much research has focused on the 'hygiene hypothesis', which links the high incidence of juvenile allergy and autoimmune disease to lack of exposure to infectious microbes and intestinal parasites in early childhood. Such exposure to infectious agents, particularly those present at the intestinal mucosa, is critical for generating Tregs.

AUTOIMMUNE DISEASES

The second major group of immune-mediated disorders are the autoimmune diseases. These too involve an inappropriate and excessive induction of type II, type III, or type IV hypersensitivity to self-antigens (autoantigens) in the presence of reduced effectiveness of natural Tregs, which would normally prevent such reactions. Clinically normal humans and animals (including dogs) harbor, as part of their lymphocyte repertoire, T and B cells bearing receptors able to recognize self-antigens. These autoreactive cells are normally kept in check by a range of immunoregulatory mechanisms, including:

- Deletion of autoreactive T cells as part of intrathymic development or within the body tissues after thymic emigration.
- Exposure to autoantigen but failure to activate (anergy).
- Failure to expose to autoantigen by lack of antigen presentation or physical sequestration of antigen (immunologic ignorance).
- The activity of natural Tregs.
- Failing to provide autoreactive B cells with T-cell help.

When these control mechanisms fail (leading to loss of immunologic tolerance to autoantigens), an autoimmune reaction with tissue pathology and clinical signs may arise.

As for allergic disease, there is a clear genetic predisposition to autoimmunity in dogs, but such predispositions (for allergic or autoimmune disease) are not well-recognized in feline medicine. The strongest genetic linkages are with specific allotypic variants of the genes encoding MHC molecules. Associations with class II MHC gene haplotypes are now described for a range of canine autoimmune diseases, including rheumatoid arthritis, IMHA, lymphocytic thyroiditis, hypoadrenocorticism, necrotizing meningoencephalitis, diabetes mellitus, and breed-associated chronic hepatitis.

While it was once considered that autoimmunity involved a spontaneously arising immunologic defect in a genetically predisposed individual, there is now recognition that autoimmune diseases have many defined predisposing and trigger factors. Predisposing factors include age (autoimmunity is generally a phenomenon of middle to old age), gender, and lifestyle (e.g. stress exercise, diet). A recent study has shown that neutered dogs are more likely to die from immune-mediated diseases. Trigger factors are largely environmental and include exposure to drugs, vaccines, and infectious agents. In fact, most autoimmune disease is now considered to be a post-infectious phenomenon and in humans, the active infection may precede onset of the autoimmune disease by months or years. Finally, other chronic disease states (particularly neoplasia or chronic inflammatory disease) may sufficiently disturb immune homeostasis to result in secondary autoimmunity.

This growing concept of recognized trigger factors for autoimmune disease has reshaped the way in which we think about these disorders in companion animal medicine. One example of this changing trend has been the impact of molecular diagnostic methodology for the range of arthropod-transmitted infectious agents that are generally unculturable and may remain cryptic within an infected animal ('stealth pathogens'). The use of molecular diagnostics increasingly allows us to attribute 'idiopathic' disease to an infectious agent, and modify management protocols accordingly.

PRIMARY IMMUNODEFICIENCY DISORDERS

The third category of immune-mediated diseases includes the primary immunodeficiency disorders. Instead of being an inappropriate excess of immunity (as in allergy or autoimmunity) this is the reverse scenario, which means that there is an inability to mount a protective immune response due to a congenital, inherited genetic mutation in a gene encoding a key immunologic molecule. Such defects may occur at different levels of immunologic development and consequently lead to clinical disease of varying severity. For example, some defects mean that the animal fails to develop adequate T and B lymphocytes (e.g. X-linked severe combined immunodeficiency; X-SCID), with severely impaired immunity and death during early life. By contrast, a more subtle immunodeficiency (e.g. selective IgA deficiency) may not lead to clinical disease or produce only mild changes. A wide range of primary immunodeficiency disorders is documented in humans and for many the precise genetic mutation is known. A similarly wide range of disorders is suggested to have an immunodeficiency basis in numerous breeds of dog, but only a few of these have been defined at the molecular level. Thus, many of this group of canine diseases should only be considered putative immunodeficiencies at this time. Of note is the fascinating dichotomy between cat and dog in this regard; primary immunodeficiency is extremely rare in the cat, with only a handful of reported cases.

IMMUNE SYSTEM NEOPLASIA

The final group of immunologic disorders comprises those of immune system neoplasia. Although not classically an 'immune-mediated' pathology, these tumors are clear manifestations of an abnormal immune system and can impair the remaining immune function of an animal, thus leading to immunocompromise. These disorders include lymphoma, lymphoid leukemia, plasmacytoma, and multiple myeloma, and arguably might also include neoplasia affecting adjunct immune cells such as dendritic cells (the range of histiocytic neoplasia) and mast cells. There are many gaps in our knowledge of the factors that underlie the development of this range of tumors. In cats, retroviral infection has a role, although these diseases still occur in geographical areas with a low prevalence of feline leukemia virus infection or where vaccination and testing programs have reduced the prevalence of infection. There are some well-documented genetic associations for canine lymphoma (e.g. Boxer) and histiocytic neoplasia (e.g. Bernese Mountain Dog, Flat-coated Retriever) and limited epidemiological studies have suggested a role for various environmental carcinogens (e.g. cigarette smoke and feline lymphoma, pesticides and radiation for canine lymphoma).

Although these disorders may be considered as individual entities, there is some linkage between them, as they are all manifestations of disturbed immune system homeostasis. It is possible for more than one type of immunologic abnormality to exist in any one patient at any one time, and a number of such associations are recognized, including:

- Thymoma and myasthenia gravis.
- IgA deficiency and autoimmunity.
- Inflammatory bowel disease and immune-mediated thrombocytopenia (IMTP) or IMHA.
- Lymphoma or leukemia and IMHA.

Similarly, different types of autoimmune disease may be recognized concurrently (e.g. combinations of IMHA, IMTP, and immune-mediated neutropenia; IMNP) or may present as multisystemic autoimmune disease (e.g. systemic lupus erythematosus, SLE).

LABORATORY DIAGNOSIS OF IMMUNE-MEDIATED DISEASE

Allergic disease

Key to the diagnosis and management of allergic disease is identification of the causative allergen. This may be addressed through obtaining a detailed exposure history or by determining whether there is clinical improvement following dietary trial, parasiticidal treatment, or following removal of the animal from the normal environment. For aeroallergens and arthropod-derived allergens (e.g. flea saliva), the generally accepted 'gold standard' diagnostic procedure remains the intradermal test, and some experimental studies have described efficacy of patch testing for demonstration of late-phase responses. Intradermal or percutaneous challenge has not proven reproducible for the diagnosis of food allergy. The use of serologic testing has increased, and many specialists now use these tests in parallel with traditional methodology.

Serologic tests are designed to demonstrate the presence of circulating allergen-specific IgE and/or IgG antibodies. Such tests are almost all based on the ELISA, but vary in the technology used for immunoglobulin detection. Most involve coating test allergens onto the plastic wells of the plate and subsequent incubation with patient serum and then an enzyme-linked detecting reagent (**Figure 22.13**). The most novel detection technology involves the application of a recombinant version of the IgE Fc receptor molecule. Serologic testing can be informative, but it does not necessarily correlate with intradermal test results, which measure cutaneous mast cell-bound IgE (rather than free antibody in the circulation).

At the research level (but not clinically available), tests such as *in-vitro* mast cell degranulation, blood lymphocyte

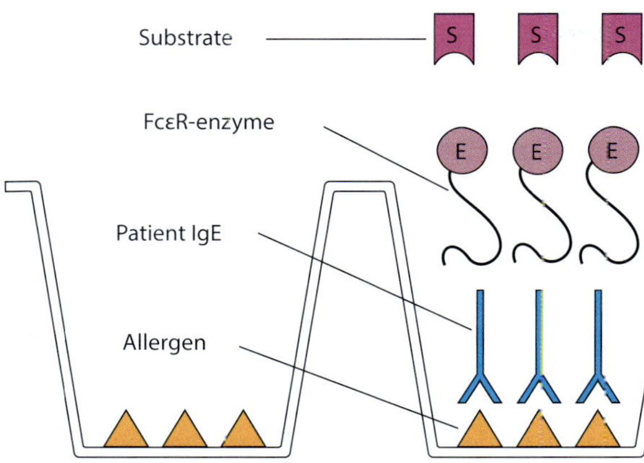

22.13

Figure 22.13 Serologic testing for allergen-specific IgE antibody. The wells of a microtitration plate are coated with allergen and subsequently incubated with patient serum. Serum allergen-specific IgE binds to the target and this interaction is visualized by the detection reagent (recombinant Fcε receptor conjugated to alkaline phosphatase) and enzyme substrate.

allergen stimulation (with measurement of cytokine gene transcription), and western blotting for fine definition of the serologic response, have been employed.

Autoimmune disease

The aim of immunodiagnostic testing in autoimmunity is to confirm an autoimmune pathogenesis by demonstrating circulating or cell- or tissue-bound antibody (and/or complement) relevant to the clinical presentation of the animal. Although a number of autoimmune diseases involve cell-mediated immunopathogenesis, it is not possible at present routinely to investigate these aspects of clinical disease. The key to logical application of these tests is to become familiar with the purpose and limitations of each. For example, there is little rationale in selecting a Coombs test to support the diagnosis of a dog with putative immune-mediated polyarthritis unless that animal is concurrently anemic.

Coombs test

The most widely available immunodiagnostic test for autoimmunity is the Coombs test. This is indicated to support the diagnosis of IMHA in an animal with appropriate clinical and hematologic features. The aim of the test is to demonstrate the presence of IgG/IgM/complement C3b on the surface of patient erythrocytes as presumptive evidence that these immunoreactants are involved in the hemolytic reaction (**Figure 22.14**). There are numerous reasons for false-positive and false-negative Coombs tests, but the most common reason for the latter is that a complete test has not been performed. Many commercial laboratories offer a simple Coombs test using only a polyvalent Coombs reagent, with minimal titration at a single incubation temperature. A full Coombs test (which is more likely to provide a positive result) should use a combination of polyvalent and specific antisera (for IgG, IgM, and complement C3) that are fully titrated in a microtiter system at both 4° and 37°C. An alternative approach to diagnosis using flow cytometry to detect red cell-bound antibodies is not widely available.

22.14

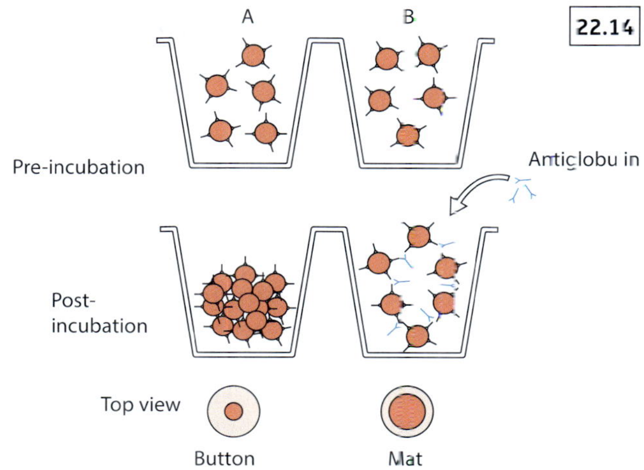

Figure 22.14 Coombs test. Wells A and B of a microtiter plate contain a suspension of washed erythrocytes from an animal with IMHA. The patient red cells are coated with antibody *in vivo*. An antiglobulin reagent (e.g. one of polyvalent canine Coombs reagent, anti-dog IgG, anti-dog IgM or anti-dog complement C3) is added to well B only. After a period of incubation the wells are examined for gross evidence of agglutination. In well B, the antiglobulin has cross-linked Ig molecules on the patient erythrocytes to form a lattice-like structure that appears as a diffuse mat of red cells that covers the base of the well (agglutination). In well A, no antiglobulin has been added, so the erythrocytes settle to the base of the well by gravity, forming a tight 'button' of packed red cells. In a complete Coombs test, the different antiglobulin reagents would be fully titrated and the test performed in duplicate at both 4° and 37°C.

Antiplatelet and antineutrophil antibody detection

The detection of antiplatelet antibody in IMTP or antineutrophil antibody in IMNP is rarely available outside of specialist laboratories. A range of approaches to the detection of platelet-bound Ig has been attempted including immunofluorescence, ELISA-based, and radioimmunoassay-based tests. The most sensitive modality has proven to be flow cytometric detection using fluorochrome-labeled antibodies, but this is not widely available. Older test methodologies, such as the platelet factor 3 test and megakaryocyte immunofluorescence, can no longer be recommended. One limitation of direct testing for platelet-bound Ig is the fact that thrombocytopenic animals are often so markedly thrombocytopenic that it is difficult to harvest sufficient cells for analysis. IMNP has only recently been well-documented as a disease and although flow cytometric testing is feasible, availability is limited.

Serum antinuclear antibody detection

The detection of serum antinuclear antibody (ANA) is widely available. The most commonly employed test involves the layering of diluted patient serum onto substrates of nucleated cells grown in monolayers on a sectored microscope slide. ANA bound to the nucleus is subsequently detected by use of an anti-IgG reagent coupled to a fluorochrome or enzyme (**Figures 22.15, 22.16**). The test is read by microscopic examination for the pattern of nuclear labeling and determination of the titer. Classically, the ANA test is used to support the diagnosis of SLE, but it may also be present in animals with other autoimmune diseases. The key to interpretation is the titer, as many clinically normal animals and animals with chronic inflammatory, infectious, or neoplastic disease may have low-titered ANA as a reflection of cell turnover.

Rheumatoid factor tests

Serum or synovial fluid rheumatoid factor (RF) may be tested in order to support a diagnosis of immune-mediated polyarthritis. Ideally, both RF and ANA would be requested in such patients as either autoantibody may be present, despite the fact that RF is classically reported to be associated with erosive rheumatoid arthritis. RF is an IgM (or rarely IgA) autoantibody with specificity for an IgG molecule that in turn is bound to an undefined antigen (**Figure 22.17**). RF may have a role in the pathogenesis of polyarthritis, and is thought to be formed in the synovium and leak into the circulating blood. RF may be detected by ELISA, in which target IgG is coated to the wells of a microtitration tray, or via the Rose Waller test in which the target IgG is affixed to the surface of erythrocytes and the RF causes cross-linking of target IgG and therefore agglutination of these cells.

Other autoantibody tests

Other commonly used autoantibody tests include those for thyroglobulin autoantibodies in dogs with hypothyroidism attributed to lymphocytic thyroiditis, and for AChR autoantibodies in dogs with putative myasthenia gravis. Thyroglobulin autoantibody testing is widely available, but only one laboratory internationally offers the AChR autoantibody test.

Immunohistochemistry

For some autoimmune diseases (e.g. autoimmune skin disease, immune complex glomerulonephritis), immunohistochemistry or immunofluorescence testing has been employed in order to demonstrate the presence of immunoglobulin and/or complement within lesional tissue (**Figure 22.18**). Such testing is not particularly sensitive, but it can be helpful in supporting a diagnosis where histopathology is equivocal.

Immunodeficiency disease

The diagnosis of immunodeficiency disease is one of the great frustrations of clinical veterinary medicine. At the research level, it has proven possible to assess the competence of all aspects of the immune system (i.e. immunoglobulin, complement, phagocytic cell and

22.15

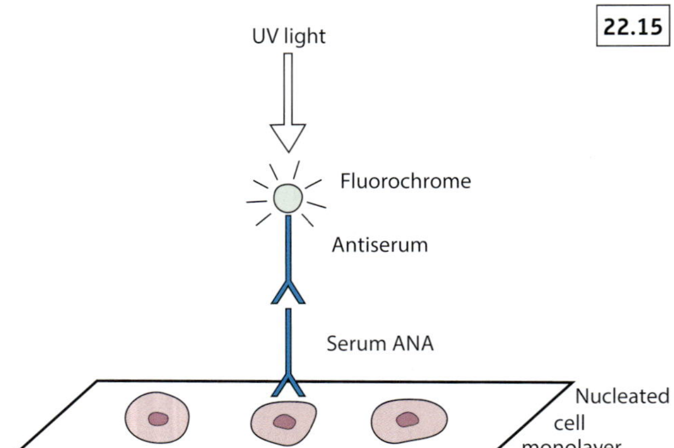

22.16

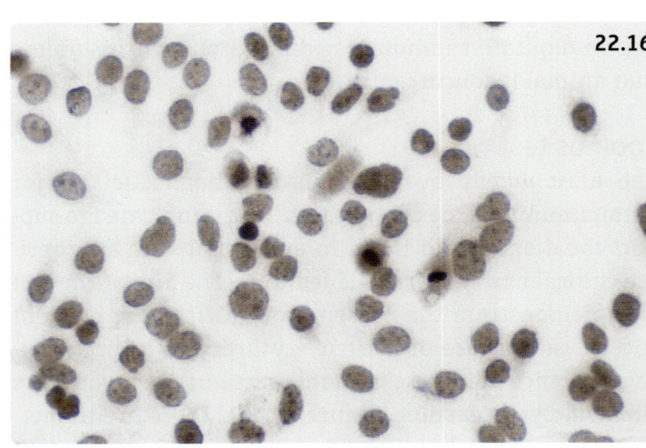

Figures 22.15, 22.16 The antinuclear antibody (ANA) assay. (22.15) Serial dilutions of patient serum are incubated with a source of nucleated cells to permit any ANA to bind to target antigens. Binding is visualized by subsequent incubation with an antiserum coupled to either a fluorochrome (for examination under UV light) or an enzyme (for reaction with substrate for light microscopic examination). (22.16) Positive ANA reaction as shown by immunoperoxidase labeling of nuclei within the target cell line.

22.17

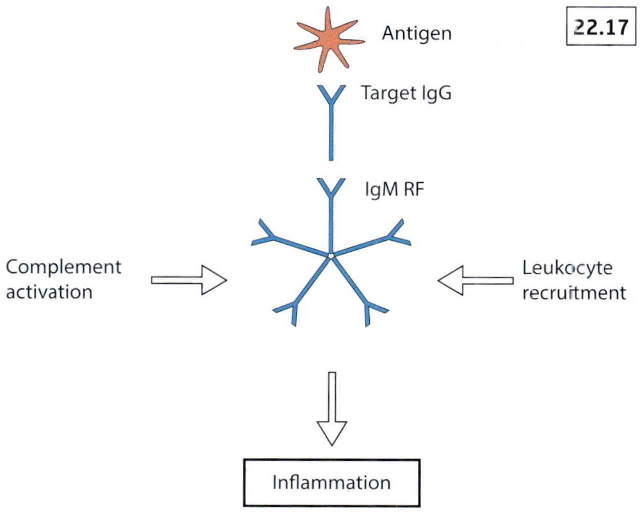

Figure 22.17 Rheumatoid factor (RF). An undefined synovial antigen is complexed with an IgG antibody, which in turn forms the target for the IgM RF. Binding of RF leads to activation of the classical pathway of complement and subsequent recruitment of leukocytes. RF may thus have a role in the pathogenesis of polyarthritis in addition to being a useful serologic marker of disease.

22.18

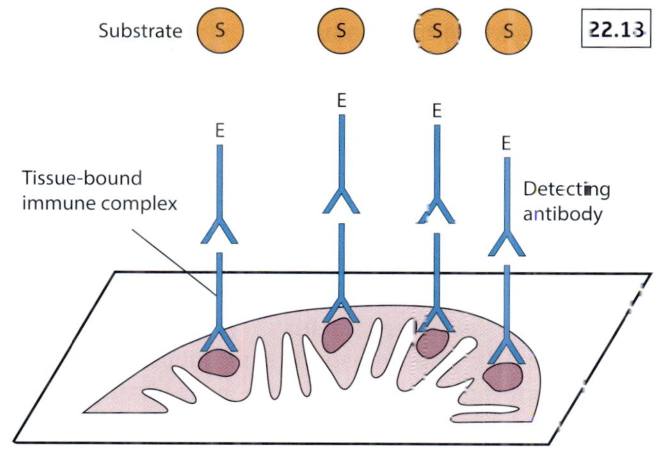

Figure 22.18 Immunohistochemistry. The microscope slide displays a section of kidney with suspected immune complexes localized to the glomerular capillaries. The immunoglobulin component of these complexes is detected by overlaying the section with an enzyme-linked antiserum (e.g. anti-dog IgG). On application of the appropriate substrate, there is a color change at the site of antibody binding, confirming the presence of immune complex.

lymphocyte function, cytokine production), but such testing is not available commercially. Consequently, the diagnosis of primary immunodeficiency largely relies on simple measures of immune system assessment (e.g. hematology, serum protein electrophoresis, lymphoid tissue histopathology) together with characterization of any secondary infection. The only readily available immunodiagnostic test is determination of serum immunoglobulin concentration by single radial immunodiffusion (SRID) (**Figure 22.19**). For the dog, the serum concentrations of IgG, IgM, and IgA can be determined, but there are few reference ranges for animals of different age and breed. Specialist laboratories that have flow cytometry may offer blood lymphocyte phenotyping, generally to determine the relative proportions of $CD4^+$ and $CD8^+$ T cells and $CD21^+$ B cells amongst the circulating lymphoid population. These percentages should be related back to absolute lymphocyte number (as for a differential leukocyte count). At present there is relatively sparse information about how such changes correlate with disease, but marked decreases might be predicted in some immunodeficiency states. Finally, for a limited number of canine immunodeficiencies, molecular diagnostic tests have been developed after elucidation of the genetic mutation underlying the disease. These include tests for X-SCID, canine leukocyte adhesion deficiency (CLAD), the trapped neutrophil syndrome in Border Collies, and cyclic hematopoiesis in the gray Collie dog.

22.19

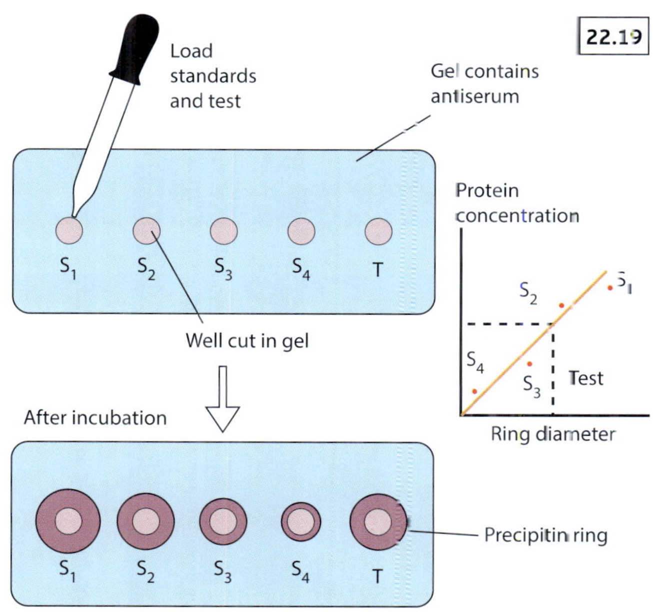

Figure 22.19 Single radial immunodiffusion. This test is used to determine the concentration of immunoglobulin in patient serum. An agarose gel is poured within which is mixed an antiserum (e.g. anti-dog IgG). Wells are cut into the gel and loaded with a precise volume of standards of known concentration and the patient sample. During an overnight incubation, IgG diffuses from the wells into the gel matrix where it encounters antiserum that precipitates the IgG. The higher the concentration of IgG, the larger the diameter of the precipitin ring obtained. A standard curve derived from the four samples of known value is used to determine the concentration in the test sample.

Immune system neoplasia

The front line for diagnosis of immune system neoplasia is clinical and imaging examination, hematology and bone marrow analysis, cytology, and biopsy. In recent years there has been wide uptake of tissue immunohistochemistry for confirmation of the phenotype of round cell neoplasia. Following routine light microscopic diagnosis, most pathology laboratories are able to apply antisera in order to determine whether the neoplasm is of T cell, B cell, or histiocytic origin (**Figures 22.20, 22.21**). In similar fashion, some laboratories offer immunocytochemical or flow cytometric testing of cellular suspensions derived from a fine-needle aspirate, which provides a similar (but more rapid) outcome. Flow cytometric testing has also become available for the determination of the nature of leukemia, and a range of lymphoid and myeloid markers are generally employed to phenotype such neoplastic populations. The most recent advance in this area of diagnosis has been the development of 'clonality testing'. This molecular test can determine whether a population of lymphoid cells is clonal (and therefore neoplastic) by examining restriction in rearrangements in TCR and BCR genes. Such testing is of particular benefit in distinguishing between a reactive and a neoplastic lymphoid infiltration (for example in the intestinal mucosa) or for monitoring the presence of residual neoplastic cells in blood or tissue throughout chemotherapy. These new

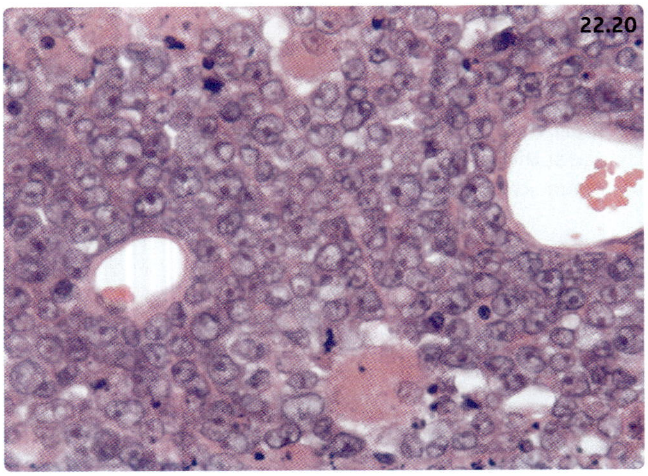

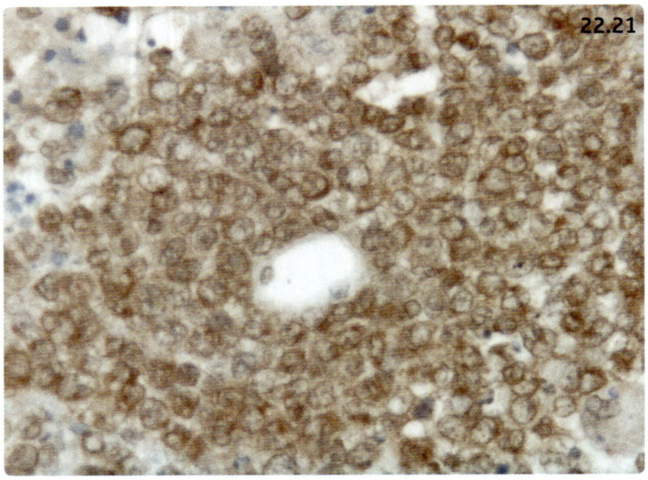

Figures 22.20, 22.21 Lymphoma immunophenotyping. Section of skin from a dog with dermal lymphoma. (22.20) The H&E-stained section reveals a closely packed population of blastic cells with a vesicular, cleaved nucleus, with central prominent nucleolus and minimal cytoplasm. (22.21) Immunolabeling with anti-CD79a reveals this to be a B-cell lymphoma.

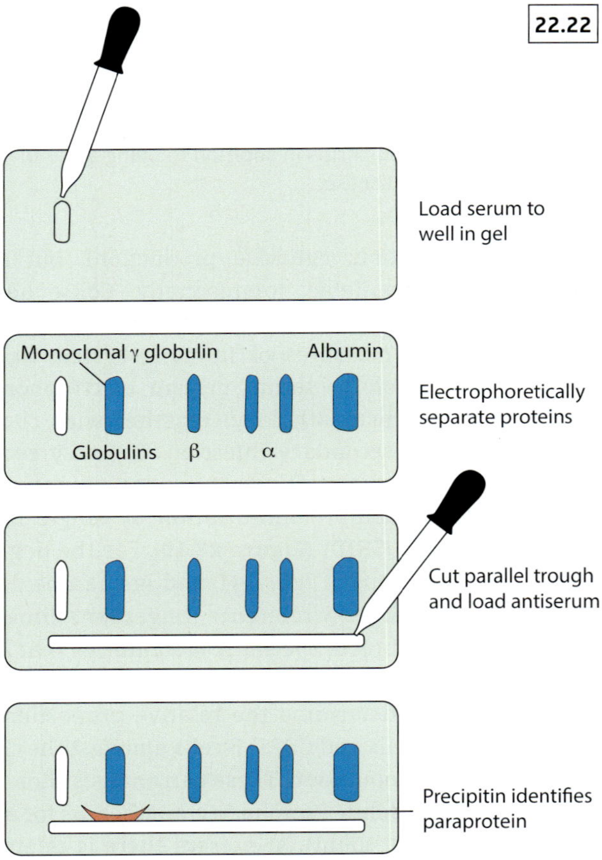

Figure 22.22 Immunoelectrophoresis. Serum from a patient with suspected paraproteinemia is separated electrophoretically in a gel matrix. Following this, a trough is cut into the gel parallel to the separated proteins and loaded with antiserum (e.g. anti-dog IgG γ heavy chain). During a period of incubation, the antiserum diffuses from the trough to react specifically with the paraprotein and form an arc of precipitation. The position of this arc relative to that produced with normal serum immunoglobulin indicates that the paraprotein carries altered charge and is thus structurally altered.

diagnostic approaches to tumor classification have helped to refine prognosis for canine lymphoma. Two recent studies have shown the longest median survival time (or event-free survival time) for low-grade T-cell lymphoma, the shortest survival time for high-grade T-cell lymphoma, and intermediate survival for dogs with B-cell lymphoma.

Multiple myeloma is characterized in part by serum paraproteinemia, resulting in a monoclonal gammopathy identified by serum protein electrophoresis. The immunodiagnostic work-up in this disease entails more detailed analysis of this paraprotein. The traditional means of achieving this is via immunoelectrophoresis (**Figure 22.22**) in which the identity of the paraprotein (class of Ig) is determined together with demonstration of altered electrophoretic mobility confirming the abnormal physicochemical properties of the molecule. Similar information can be derived from immunofixation or western blotting studies, although in reality, typing of paraprotein is not routinely performed in cases satisfying the diagnostic criteria for this disease.

MAJOR IMMUNE-MEDIATED DISEASES

This section will review the major immune-mediated disorders of companion animals. Where these are described elsewhere in this book by body system, a cross-reference to the appropriate chapter will be given. Significant features of diseases that are not discussed elsewhere will be described in this chapter; however, this list is not exhaustive, and less common entities are not included.

ALLERGIC DISEASES

ATOPIC DERMATITIS

See Chapter 18: Dermatologic disorders.

FLEA ALLERGY DERMATITIS

See Chapter 18: Dermatologic disorders.

FOOD ALLERGY

See Chapter 18: Dermatologic disorders, and Chapter 8: Digestive diseases (pharynx to anorectum).

FELINE EOSINOPHILIC GRANULOMA COMPLEX

See Chapter 18: Dermatologic disorders.

ALLERGIC RHINITIS

See Chapter 4: Respiratory disorders

FELINE ASTHMA

See Chapter 4: Respiratory disorders.

CANINE EOSINOPHILIC BRONCHOPNEUMOPATHY

See Chapter 4: Respiratory disorders.

ALLERGIC CONJUNCTIVITIS

Definition/overview

Allergic conjunctivitis may occur as a distinct entity or in conjunction with cutaneous allergy. The likely mechanism is type I hypersensitivity.

Clinical presentation

The clinical features include conjunctival erythema and edema, pruritus, and ocular discharge. There may be secondary bacterial infection, and blepharitis and keratitis may also occur. Conjunctival lymphoid follicular hyperplasia may be visible grossly or on biopsy.

Diagnosis

Diagnosis may involve cytologic examination (eosinophils and mast cells may be expected) and the investigation of concurrent cutaneous hypersensitivity.

CONTACT HYPERSENSITIVITY

See Chapter 18: Dermatologic disorders.

AUTOIMMUNE AND IDIOPATHIC IMMUNE-MEDIATED DISEASES

IMMUNE-MEDIATED HEMOLYTIC ANEMIA AND PURE RED CELL APLASIA

See Chapter 16: Hematologic disorders.

IMMUNE-MEDIATED THROMBOCYTOPENIA

See Chapter 16: Hematologic disorders, and Chapter 17: Disorders of hemostasis.

IMMUNE MEDIATED-NEUTROPENIA

See Chapter 16: Hematologic disorders.

RHEUMATOID ARTHRITIS

See Chapter 15: Bone and joint disorders.

IMMUNE-MEDIATED POLYARTHRITIS

See Chapter 15: Bone and joint disorders.

PEMPHIGUS FOLIACEUS

(See also Chapter 18: Dermatologic disorders.)

Definition/overview

Pemphigus foliaceus is the most common of the pemphigus disorders that are characterized by the formation of autoantibody specific for the desmosomal intercellular adhesion molecules that join together the epidermal keratinocytes. Less common pemphigus variants include pemphigus vulgaris, pemphigus erythematosus, and panepidermal pustular pemphigus (pemphigus vegetans).

Pathophysiology

Autoantibody binding leads to physical disruption of these junctions and local activation of the complement and plasminogen–plasmin pathways. Vesicles form within the epidermis, and these contain the separated keratinocytes (acanthocytes). There is chemotactic attraction of neutrophils and/or eosinophils into these spaces to form sterile pustules.

Clinical presentation

Classically, in pemphigus foliaceus the pustules are subcorneal in location, which is likely related to the distribution of the target autoantigen (**Figure 22.23**). Direct immunohistochemistry may be used to demonstrate the intercellular deposition of immunoglobulin and/or complement (**Figure 22.24**). Clinically, intact vesicles or pustules are rarely observed and the predominant lesion is of crusting affecting the face, feet, and trunk.

Diagnosis

Diagnosis is by skin biopsy.

Management

Treatment involves immunosuppressive doses of oral glucocorticoid.

BULLOUS PEMPHIGOID

Definition/overview

Bullous pemphigoid is an autoimmune disease in which autoantibody targets structures within the hemidesmosome that anchors the basal keratinocytes into the basement membrane zone between epidermis and dermis.

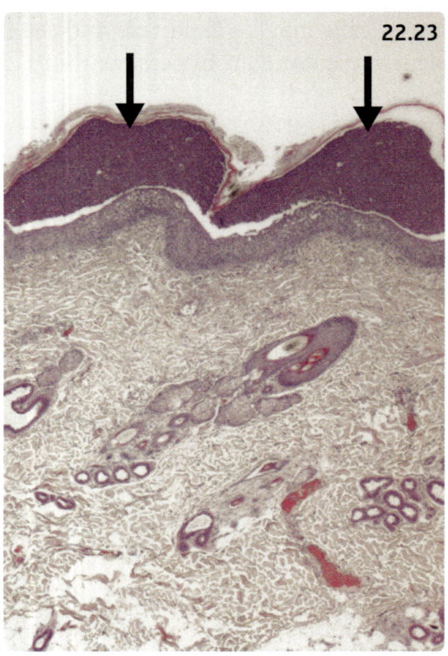

Figure 22.23 Skin biopsy from a 10-year-old Collie-cross dog with a generalized pustular and crusting dermatosis. There is a large, intact subcorneal pustule filled by nondegenerate neutrophils and acanthocytes (arrows). These features are consistent with pemphigus foliaceus.

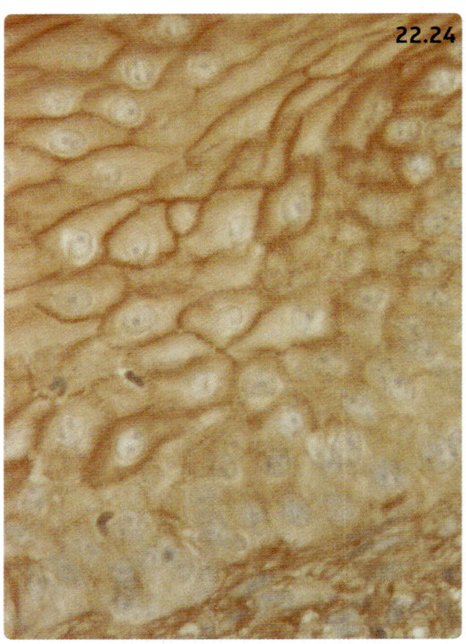

Figure 22.24 Skin biopsy from a 9-year-old German Shepherd Dog with pemphigus foliaceus confirmed histologically. This biopsy is labeled to detect IgG, which is present associated with the desmosomes of the mid to superficial level keratinocytes. Note there is no intercellular deposition associated with the basal cells.

Bullous pemphigoid variants include epidermolysis bullosa acquisita, linear IgA bullous disease, and mucous membrane pemphigoid.

Pathophysiology

Disruption of this adhesion results in separation of the epidermis from the dermis, with formation of a cleft lined by the basal keratinocytes (uppermost) and basement membrane (lowermost). This space may become filled with fluid and/or inflammatory cells.

Clinical presentation

Clinically, the bullous lesions are often disrupted and the presentation is of ulceration that particularly affects the oral mucocutaneous junctions, axilla, groin, and footpads.

Diagnosis

Diagnosis is by biopsy and immunohistochemistry may be used to demonstrate the deposition of immunoglobulin/complement within the basement membrane zone.

Management

Treatment is by immunosuppression, and adjunct immunosuppression may be required in addition to oral glucocorticoid.

CUTANEOUS LUPUS ERYTHEMATOSUS

(See also Chapter 18: Dermatologic disorders.)

Definition/overview

CLE is the name given to a group of immune-mediated skin diseases with a common pathogenesis. The prototype disorder of this group is discoid lupus erythematosus, which is now termed 'nasal planum CLE'. Other diseases within the CLE group include oral cavity or mucocutaneous CLE, generalized CLE, vesicular CLE of Collies and Shelties, exfoliative CLE of German Shorthaired Pointers, and lupoid onychodystrophy.

Pathophysiology

CLE has a complex pathogenesis, which in part involves infiltration of the basement membrane and epidermis by lymphocytes ('interface dermatitis') that target and destroy individual keratinocytes by induction of apoptosis (**Figure 22.25**). Additionally, there is deposition of immunoglobulin/complement at the basement membrane zone, although this may be an 'epiphenomenon' rather than having a direct role in pathogenesis. Exposure to ultraviolet (UV) light is thought to play a role in the triggering of this disease.

Diagnosis

Diagnosis is by skin biopsy and immunohistochemistry may be used to demonstrate the local deposition of immunoreactant (**Figure 22.26**).

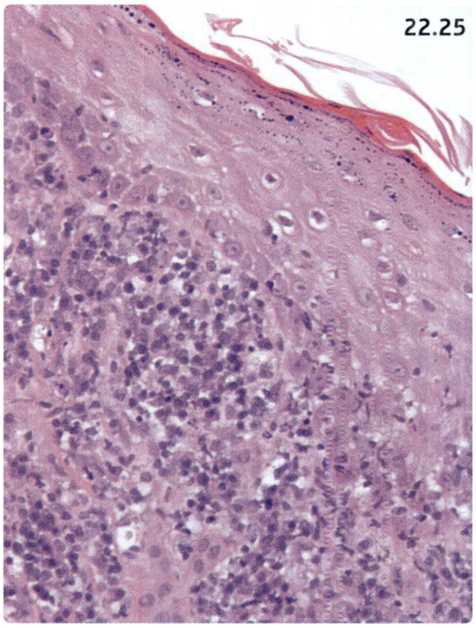

Figure 22.25 Skin biopsy from a 16-year-old German Shepherd Dog with depigmentation and loss of 'cobblestone' pattern to the nasal planum. There is a lymphoplasmacytic interface dermatitis with prominence of the basement membrane and mild hydropic degeneration of the basal keratinocyte layer. The other key feature of 'nasal planum cutaneous lupus erythematosus' not present in this field is individual keratinocyte apoptosis at higher levels.

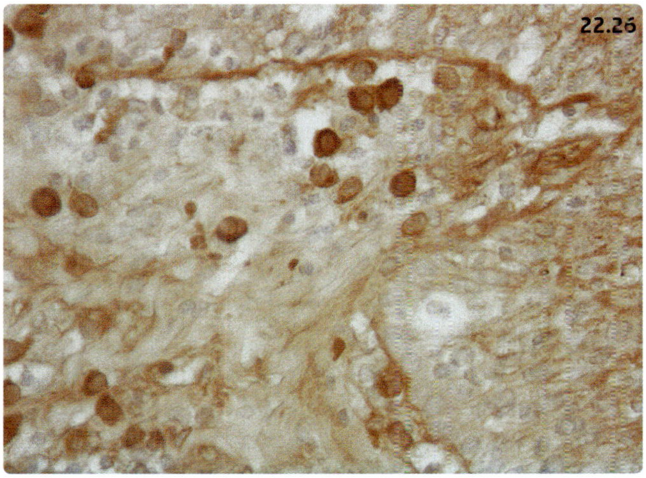

Figure 22.26 Skin biopsy from an 8-year-old male Norfolk Terrier with histopathologic evidence of interface dermatitis. The slide is immunolabeled to demonstrate the presence of IgG. There is a linear deposit of this immunoglobulin at the basement membrane zone between epidermis and dermis, and the cytoplasm of IgG^{+} plasma cells within the dermal infiltrate is also labeled.

Management
A range of therapeutic options is proposed, most commonly involving the use of combination tetracycline (doxycycline) and niacinamide, topical glucocorticoid, or oral glucocorticoid at anti-inflammatory (rarely immunosuppressive) doses.

DERMATOMYOSITIS

Definition/overview
This immune-mediated disorder primarily occurs in Collies and Shelties and is inherited as autosomally dominant with variable expression.

Pathophysiology
The pathogenesis is poorly defined, but is thought to involve immune complex deposition, as elevation in circulating immune complexes is documented before the onset of clinical signs. UV light and estrus are suggested trigger factors.

Clinical presentation
This disease affects young dogs (under 6 months of age). They develop alopecic, erythematous, scaling, crusting, or ulcerative lesions that target the face, oral mucocutaneous junctions, pinnae, limbs, footpads, and tail tip. Concurrent muscular involvement particularly affects facial and limb muscle groups and these have inflammation and atrophy on biopsy and display electromyographic abnormalities. Megaesophagus may also occur. The outcome is variable; some dogs may show spontaneous resolution of disease, in others it may be cyclical, and in others progressive.

Management
Treatment options include immunosuppressive oral glucocorticoids, vitamin E, and pentoxifylline.

ERYTHEMA MULTIFORME/TOXIC EPIDERMAL NECROLYSIS

Definition/overview
These disorders are found at each end of a spectrum of entities defined on the basis of their severity: erythema multiforme (EM) minor, EM major, Stevens–Johnson syndrome (SJS), SJS–toxic epidermal necrolysis (TEN) overlap syndrome, and TEN.

Pathophysiology
These diseases may be triggered by drug administration or infection and involve an interface inflammatory infiltration of lymphocytes that induce cytotoxic apoptosis in small groups of keratinocytes (EM), through to full-thickness epidermal necrosis and ulceration (TEN) (**Figure 22.27**).

Clinical presentation
Lesions may be localized or generalized and affect cutaneous and/or mucocutaneous surfaces. The lesions of EM are relatively mild erythematous macules, papules, or confluent plaques, which may regress spontaneously following removal of the trigger. By contrast, TEN is a severe disease due to loss of fluid, electrolytes, and colloid from the ulcerated lesions, with high potential for secondary bacterial infection.

Management
Standard immunosuppressive glucocorticoid regimes are often ineffectual in these diseases, but IV administration of human immunoglobulin has proven beneficial.

PANNUS

Definition/overview
Pannus (chronic superficial keratitis/keratoconjunctivitis) is a putative immune-mediated disorder of the cornea that particularly affects German Shepherd Dogs and may be triggered by UV light exposure.

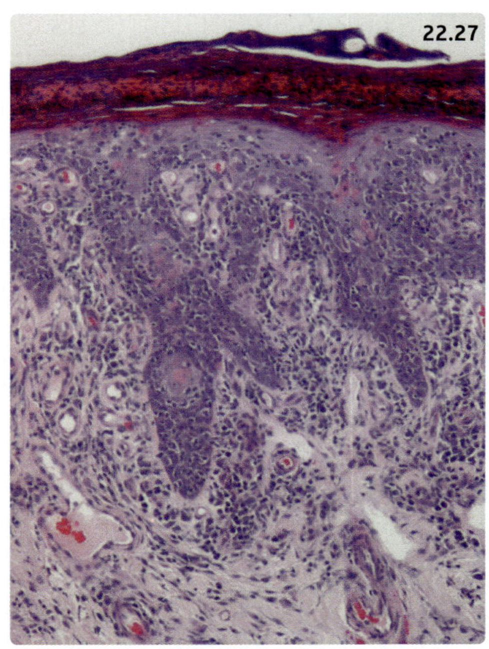

Figure 22.27 Skin biopsy from a 10-year-old West Highland White Terrier with severe, generalized crusting dermatosis. There is interface dermatitis with clusters of apoptotic keratinocytes within the epidermis associated with the infiltrating lymphocytes ('satellitosis'). These features are consistent with erythema multiforme.

Pathophysiology

There is lymphocytic infiltration, vascularization, and fibrosis of the superficial corneal stroma, which extends from the limbus.

Management

Application of topical cyclosporine has proven efficacious in management of this disease.

KERATOCONJUNCTIVITIS SICCA/SJÖGREN'S SYNDROME

See Chapter 19: Ocular manifestations of systemic diseases.

UVEODERMATOLOGIC SYNDROME

See Chapter 19: Ocular manifestations of systemic diseases.

IDIOPATHIC UVEITIS

See Chapter 19: Ocular manifestations of systemic diseases.

LYMPHOCYTIC THYROIDITIS

See Chapter 11: Endocrine disorders.

DIABETES MELLITUS

See Chapter 11: Endocrine disorders.

INFLAMMATORY BOWEL DISEASE

See Chapter 8: Digestive diseases (pharynx to anorectum).

ANTIBIOTIC-RESPONSIVE DIARRHEA

See Chapter 8: Digestive diseases (pharynx to anorectum).

EXOCRINE PANCREATIC INSUFFICIENCY

See Chapter 10: Pancreatic disorders.

IMMUNE COMPLEX GLOMERULONEPHRITIS

See Chapter 12: Nephrology/urology.

MYASTHENIA GRAVIS

See Chapter 14: Disorders of the nervous system and muscle.

POLYMYOSITIS

See Chapter 14: Disorders of the nervous system and muscle.

MASTICATORY MUSCLE MYOSITIS/ EXTRAOCULAR MUSCLE MYOSITIS

See Chapter 14: Disorders of the nervous system and muscle.

GRANULOMATOUS MENINGOENCEPHALITIS

See Chapter 14: Disorders of the nervous system and muscle, and Chapter 19: Ocular manifestations of systemic diseases.

STEROID-RESPONSIVE MENINGITIS ARTERITIS

See Chapter 14: Disorders of the nervous system and muscle.

SYSTEMIC LUPUS ERYTHEMATOSUS

Definition/overview

SLE is a rare disease of the dog and even less common in the cat. SLE is the prototype multisystemic autoimmune disease and is defined by strict diagnostic criteria. The simplest of these criteria are:

- The animal must show multisystemic disease involving at least two distinct body systems.
- The disease affecting these body systems must be compatible with an immune-mediated process and laboratory evidence of an immunologic pathogenesis for these changes must be obtained.
- The animal must have a high-titered serum ANA.

Although these criteria are simple, they are generally very difficult to satisfy; therefore, in many cases a diagnosis of an 'SLE-overlap' syndrome (with partial fulfilment of the criteria) is made.

Pathophysiology

The most common clinicopathologic manifestations of canine SLE include IMHA, IMTP, immune complex glomerulonephritis, polyarthritis, and immune-mediated skin disease. In endemic areas it is important to rule out arthropod-transmitted infectious disease (particularly leishmaniasis), which can mimic the clinical presentation of SLE. SLE has also been induced by drugs and may arise secondary to underlying lymphoid or myeloid neoplasia. SLE may be inherited and early research demonstrated that it was possible to establish breeding lines in which there were dogs with serologic and clinical abnormalities of autoimmunity (but with no clear mode of inheritance).

Diagnosis
Multiple diagnostic and immunodiagnostic procedures may be required to support the diagnosis of SLE.

Management
Treatment is generally by immunosuppressive oral glucocorticoid therapy.

PRIMARY IMMUNODEFICIENCY DISEASE

IgA DEFICIENCY

Definition/overview
Selective IgA deficiency is the most commonly reported canine immunodeficiency disorder and is most often suggested in animals that have chronic, recurrent infectious disease, most often of the mucocutaneous surfaces.

Etiology/pathophysiology
The spectrum of infectious diseases associated with IgA deficiency includes pyoderma, demodicosis, rhinitis, bronchopneumonia, inflammatory bowel disease, and antibiotic-responsive diarrhea. IgA deficiency has been definitively documented in the Shar Pei and in one colony of Beagle dogs. IgA deficiency has been proposed to be part of the pathogenesis in Irish Wolfhounds with chronic, recurrent rhinitis–bronchopneumonia syndrome, but although these dogs have subnormal serum IgA, the concentration of this immunoglobulin in bronchoalveolar lavage fluid is normal to elevated. IgA deficiency has been suggested to predispose to allergic disease, and there is evidence that (as for humans) there is an association with autoimmunity. Some of the IgA deficient Beagle dogs described above had serum RF, and IgA deficiency was widespread in a colony of English Cocker Spaniels in which there was also frequent occurrence of a variety of autoimmune diseases.

IgA deficiency has been proposed to underlie the multiple immunologic, infectious, and inflammatory diseases to which the German Shepherd Dog is predisposed. Although German Shepherd Dogs generally have normal serum IgA, there is increasing evidence for an inability to secrete sufficient mucosal IgA in dogs of this breed, and the IgA deficient phenotype may be particularly associated with inflammatory bowel disease and antibiotic-responsive diarrhea. Dogs have four genetic variants of IgA, and it is of note that all German Shepherd Dogs have a restricted genotype that is homozygous for a single variant.

Diagnosis
Diagnosis of IgA deficiency is not straightforward. In clinical practice the only test that is widely available is SRID for determination of serum IgA concentration. This test is insufficiently sensitive to measure the lower IgA concentrations that are found in secretions. IgA deficiency (in both man and dog) is not a simple genetic mutation in the gene encoding the α heavy chain. Instead, it is a relative immunodeficiency that in dogs is defined as serum IgA concentration persistently lower than 0.22 mg/ml. The serum concentration should be measured on at least two occasions (at least 1 week apart), as there are both day-to-day and diurnal variations in canine serum IgA concentration.

PUTATIVE IgG DEFICIENCY

Definition/overview
Selective IgG deficiency has recently been reported to occur in young Cavalier King Charles Spaniels with pneumonia caused by *Pneumocystis carinii*. Infection with this opportunist organism is a hallmark of immunodeficiency disease, and is also the clinical presentation of a putative immunodeficiency disorder affecting Miniature Dachshunds. These latter dogs may also have subnormal concentrations of serum IgM and IgA and reduced responsiveness of blood lymphocytes to nonspecific stimulation with mitogens. In both breeds this is a relatively subtle immunodeficiency, as affected dogs appear to recover with appropriate antimicrobial therapy, although pulmonary disease may be recurrent. IgG deficiency is also the major immunologic feature of the disorder affecting Weimaraner dogs that is described below.

Diagnosis
IgG deficiency is determined by a consistently low serum concentration (below 10 mg/ml in adult dogs) of this immunoglobulin as determined by SRID.

COMPLEMENT C3 DEFICIENCY

Definition/overview
Deficiency of the third component of complement (C3) has been reported only once, in an experimental colony of Brittanys. Affected dogs were more susceptible to infection and some developed glomerular disease.

WEIMARANER IMMUNODEFICIENCY

Definition/overview

This complex disorder is now recognized in the Weimaraner breed internationally.

Clinical presentation

Affected dogs are young adults (6–12 months of age) that present with chronic recurrent infections of multiple body sites, particularly mucosal and cutaneous surfaces. Another feature is the presence of hypertrophic osteodystrophy (HOD), which is more consistently a feature in affected dogs in the USA (where the disease is known as HOD of Weimaraners [**Figures 22.28–22.30**]). The most consistent immunologic abnormality in affected dogs is subnormal serum IgG, and in patients that are serially monitored this immunoglobulin appears never to attain its normal range. Some dogs also have IgM and/or IgA deficiency and in the USA, neutrophil function defects have also been documented. The most unusual feature of this disorder is that the clinical signs appear to be triggered by vaccination and the disease often has clinical onset around the time of the 12 month booster vaccine.

Management

The prognosis for this disease is variable; some dogs spontaneously recover, others have chronic recurrent disease, and some die during the initial disease outbreak. Anti-inflammatory doses of glucocorticoids appear to provide the best therapeutic outcome.

SEVERE COMBINED IMMUNODEFIENCY

See Chapter 16: Hematologic disorders.

CANINE LEUKOCYTE ADHESION DEFICENCY

Definition/overview

CLAD affects Irish Setters (Red and, rarely, Red and White dogs) internationally.

Pathophysiology

Affected dogs develop chronic recurrent infections of multiple body sites from a young age. This is one of the few examples of a canine immunodeficiency disorder for which the precise genetic mutation and associated pathogenesis have been determined. The gene defect means that affected dogs are unable to express the adhesion molecules CD11b and CD18 on the surface of granulocytes. Consequently, these cells are unable to interact with ligands on vascular endothelium to mediate exocytosis from blood into tissue. These dogs therefore develop severe infection of tissues (without pus formation) associated with a striking blood neutrophilia.

Diagnosis

A molecular diagnostic test is available to determine the carrier status of Irish Setters (the disease is autosomal recessive in inheritance) and with the cooperation of the breed association, this trait has been virtually eliminated. This can be regarded as one of the great success stories of veterinary immunology.

Management

As immunodeficiency disorders are untreatable (except experimentally – see below), testing and genetic counseling offer the most practical approach to management.

CYCLIC HEMATOPOIESIS

(See also Chapter 16: Hematologic disorders.)

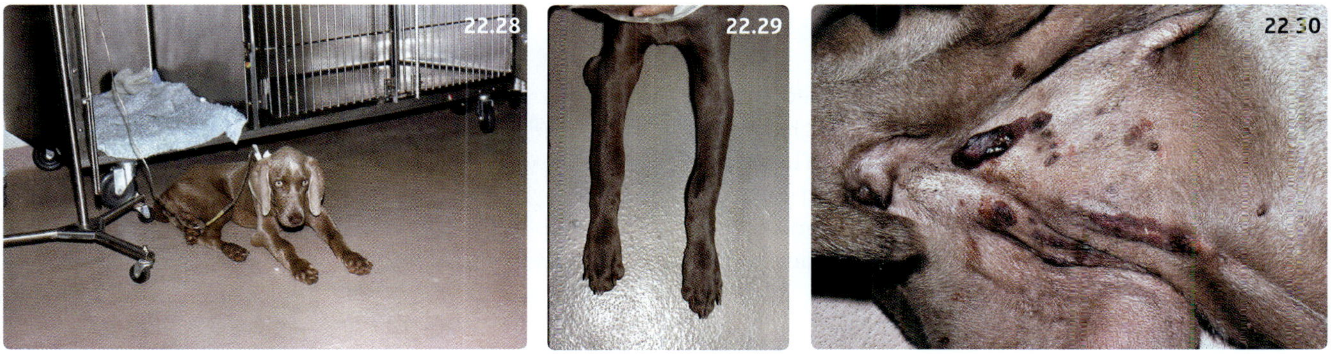

Figures 22.28–22.30 This 3-month-old Weimaraner puppy (22.28) had severe debilitating hypertrophic osteodystrophy that was complicated by bacterial sepsis. The dog was hospitalized in intensive care in order to receive parenteral fluid support and antibiotics. Besides having severe metaphyseal swelling (22.29), the puppy also became septic and developed hemorrhagic skin bullae (22.30) from which bacteria were isolated. It also had meningitis and several abscesses that were found on postmortem examination. (Courtesy M. Schaer)

Definition/overview

Recent experimental studies (using this canine disease as a model for the human equivalent) have identified the precise genetic mutation of this disorder, which lies in the gene encoding the adaptor protein complex 3 β subunit, the effect of which is to disrupt the intracellular movement of neutrophil elastase.

Management

Gene replacement therapy has been developed in an experimental setting.

THYMIC HYPOPLASIA AND HYPOTRICHOSIS OF BIRMAN CATS

Definition/overview

This is one of the few documented primary immunodeficiency disorders of cats, and was reported in a single litter of kittens. The association between hairlessness and thymic development is also well-recognized in particular inbred experimental strains of 'nude' rats and mice, and is also likely to affect the Mexican Hairless Dog.

IMMUNE SYSTEM NEOPLASIA

LYMPHOMA

See Chapters 8 (Digestive disorders [pharynx to anorectum]), 18 (Dermatologic disorders), and 19 (Ocular manifestations of systemic diseases).

LYMPHOID LEUKEMIA

See Chapter 16: Hematologic disorders.

PLASMACYTOMA

Definition/overview

This benign plasma cell tumor is documented in both dogs and cats, and generally presents as a single nodular mass arising on the face (lip), ears, and feet. The plasma cells may display considerable pleomorphism histologically (**Figure 22.31**), but these tumors do not recur after excision and only rarely progress to multiple myeloma.

MULTIPLE MYELOMA

Definition/overview

Multiple myeloma is a malignant plasma cell tumor that targets the bone marrow in dogs and soft tissue (particularly liver and spleen) in cats, although a range of sites may be affected in both species (**Figure 22.32**).

Pathophysiology

The proliferating plasma cells are associated with two distinct paraneoplastic effects. The first relates to the production of parathyroid hormone-like peptide, which leads to osteoclastic resorption of bone and the development of focal 'punched-out' osteolytic lesions. The second is the characteristic secretion of a structurally abnormal immunoglobulin (paraprotein), which appears as a monoclonal gammopathy on protein electrophoresis.

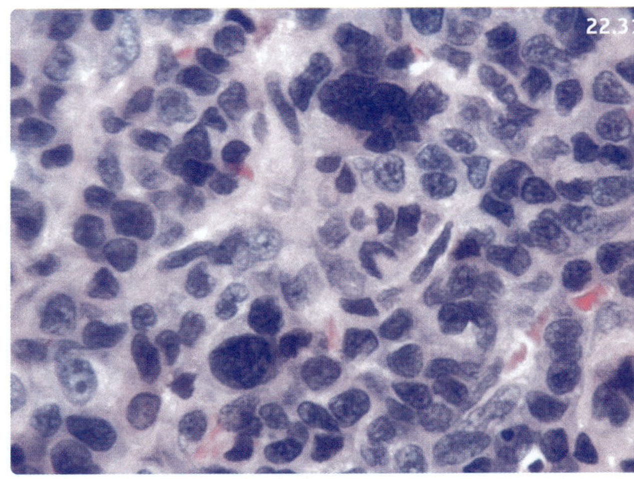

Figure 22.31 Section from a discrete nodular mass excised from the pinna of an 8-year-old male Dachshund. The tumor comprises a closely packed sheet of plasmacytoid cells, with scattered examples of multinucleate cells and cells with giant nuclei (both represented here). Although cytologically this appears to be an aggressive neoplasm, these are generally benign lesions that do not recur following excision.

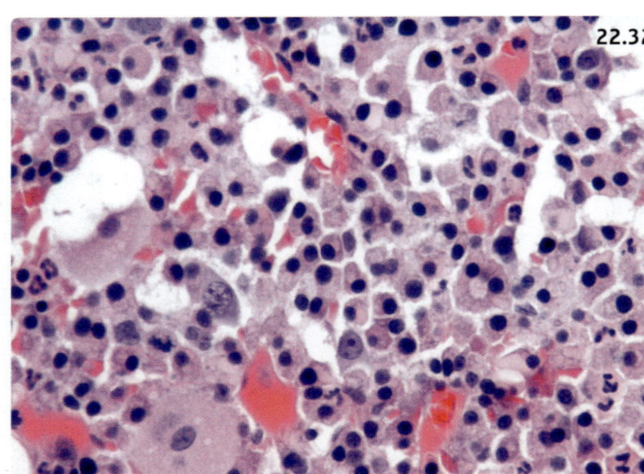

Figure 22.32 Bone marrow core biopsy from a 12-year-old neutered female Golden Retriever with monoclonal gammopathy identified on serum protein electrophoresis. The medullary cavity is filled by well-differentiated neoplastic plasma cells, which have virtually excluded the hemopoietic lineages in this field. The large cell at the base of the image is a megakaryocyte.

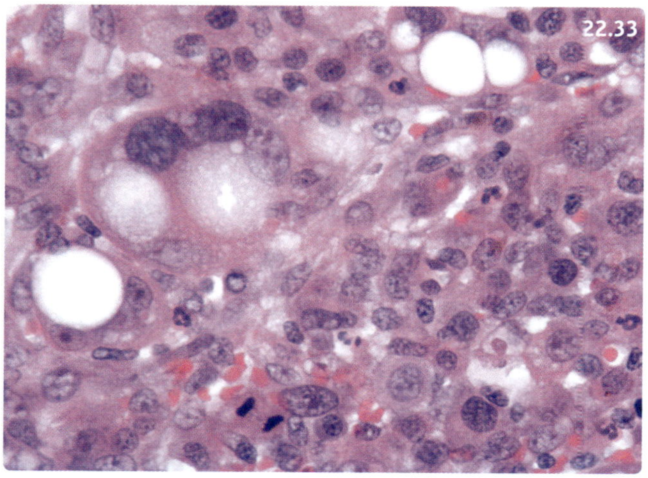

Figure 22.33 Section from a pulmonary mass taken at necropsy from a 6-year-old neutered female Bernese Mountain Dog. The mass comprises a sheet of highly pleomorphic histiocytic cells with abundant eosinophilic to mildly vacuolated cytoplasm and a round, pale nucleus with chromatin clumps. There are both multinucleate cells and cells with giant nuclei present. A mitotic figure is present at the lower edge of the image. The sternal lymph nodes of this dog were also infiltrated.

These paraproteins are more commonly IgG than IgA or IgM, and rarely may take the form of free heavy or light chains that are not assembled into an immunoglobulin structure. Free light chains are of sufficiently low molecular weight to pass through the glomerular filter and be present in urine as 'Bence Jones protein'. IgA and IgM paraproteins may be associated with serum hyperviscosity and a range of secondary effects related to this.

Diagnosis

Diagnosis of multiple myeloma relies on identification of characteristic clinical and radiographic features and the presence of monoclonal gammopathy. Further immunodiagnostic investigation of this gammopathy is discussed above. Important differentials for monoclonal gammopathy include particular infectious diseases such as ehrlichiosis and leishmaniasis in the dog and feline infectious peritonitis virus infection in the cat. A range of tests may be applied to the identification of Bence Jones proteinuria.

Management

Chemotherapeutic protocols are described for management of this disease.

HISTIOCYTIC NEOPLASIA

(See also Chapter 18: Dermatologic disorders.)

Definition/overview

A spectrum of histiocytic neoplasia is documented in the dog and it has a particular predilection for Bernese Mountain Dogs and Flat-coated Retrievers.

Pathophysiology

Immunohistochemical studies have defined this group of tumors as being of dendritic cell origin. The disorders range from the benign and spontaneously regressive histiocytoma of young dogs through to the reactive disorders (cutaneous and systemic histiocytosis) and the malignancies (localized and disseminated histiocytic sarcoma) (**Figure 22.33**).

Diagnosis

Diagnosis is by biopsy, and immunohistochemical confirmation is now widely applied.

MAST CELL TUMOR

See Chapter 18: Dermatologic disorders.

RECOMMENDED FURTHER READING

Day MJ (2011) *Clinical Immunology of the Dog and Cat*, 2nd edn. Manson Publishing, London.

Day MJ, Schultz RD (2014) *Veterinary Immunology: Principles and Practice*, 2nd edn. CRC Press, London.

Hoffman JM, Creevy KE, Promislow DEL (2013) Reproductive capability is associated with lifespan and cause of death in companion dogs. *PLoS ONE* **8**:e61082.

Nuttall T (2013) The genomics revolution: will canine atopic dermatitis be predictable and preventable? *Vet Dermatol* **24**:10-18.

Whitley N, Day MJ (2011) Immunomodulatory drugs and their application to the management of canine immune-mediated disease. *J Small Anim Pract* **52**:70–85.

Part 4

Elements of therapy

Chapter 23 **Fluid therapy**
Gareth Buckley & Travis Lanaux

Chapter 24 **Pain management**
Steven M. Fox

Chapter 25 **Nutrition of the critically-ill dog and cat**
Justin Shmalberg

Chapter 26 **Management of the obese dog or cat**
Alexander J. German

Chapter 23

Fluid therapy

Gareth Buckley & Travis Lanaux

INTRODUCTION

Fluid therapy is one of the most commonly employed therapies in veterinary medicine. Treatment of a variety of diseases may employ some form of fluid therapy. Fluids are drugs and have many potential benefits and possible side-effects. It is important to tailor a specific fluid plan to each individual patient. The goals of this chapter are to introduce the types of fluids available, describe the characteristics of different fluid types, develop a fluid plan, and discuss specific clinical situations that present particular challenges in using fluids.

CRYSTALLOIDS

Crystalloids are the most commonly encountered class of fluids. Crystalloids are solutions of salt. There are various ways to describe categories of crystalloids including tonicity or osmolality, whether the fluid is balanced, and the type of buffer contained. Sodium and potassium concentrations are often the major determinants of crystalloids for descriptive purposes.

Tonicity is determined by the number of impermeant solutes in a solution, meaning the number of solutes that do not freely diffuse across cellular membranes. Similar to tonicity is osmolality. Osmolality refers to the number of osmotically active particles in a particular solution. Water will diffuse across a membrane and try to balance the relative ratio between water molecules and impermeant solutes on either side of a membrane. As an example, if a large amount of an impermeable solute is added to one side of a membrane, water will move across the membrane from the lower solute concentration to the higher solute concentration to dilute the side with higher number of solutes (**Figures 23.1a–d**).

When describing the tonicity or osmolality of a crystalloid, it is often described in reference to normal plasma. Often, sodium is the major electrolyte determining the tonicity of crystalloid solutions. Therefore, crystalloids are generally categorized as hypotonic, isotonic, or hypertonic based on sodium concentration. However, it should be noted that dextrose will also significantly contribute to tonicity of a fluid and some of the lower sodium preparations that contain dextrose may actually be isotonic or even hypertonic. Plasma sodium concentration in most species is around 140 mEq/l (140 mmol/l). As a generalization, fluids absent of dextrose with a sodium concentration less than 125 mEq/l are typically considered hypotonic fluids. Isotonic fluids typically have a sodium concentration in the 130–150 mEq/l range. Hypertonic fluids typically have a sodium concentration greater than 160 mEq/l.

Another common way to describe crystalloid solutions is whether the solution is a maintenance or a replacement fluid:

- Maintenance fluids. Typically low in sodium compared with normal plasma. Many maintenance fluids also contain higher potassium concentrations. The term maintenance is in regard to the normal losses associated with the patient that occur during the day. Usually, water and electrolytes are lost through respiration, urination, defecation, sweating, and other insensible losses. These secretions are generally low in sodium and high in potassium. Maintenance fluids are intended to account for these regular losses and are usually administered at lower 'maintenance' rates to maintain a normal state of hydration and euvolemia. Most maintenance fluids have a sodium concentration in the 40–80 mEq/l range and a potassium concentration in the 10–20 mEq/l (10–20 mmol/l) range. Examples of maintenance fluids, such as half strength (0.45%) saline, PlasmaLyte-M, and Normosol-M, are listed in **Table 23.1**. It is extremely important to realize that maintenance fluids and hypotonic fluids may be dangerous to bolus or administer at high rates. Administration of water or a hypotonic fluid intravenously (IV) may cause a rapid shift of water into the red blood cell (RBC), leading to cell lysis. Dextrose is often added to maintenance fluids to supply calories to the patient. The addition of dextrose will also make the fluid isotonic to hypertonic and safer in case of an accidental rapid administration of the fluid.

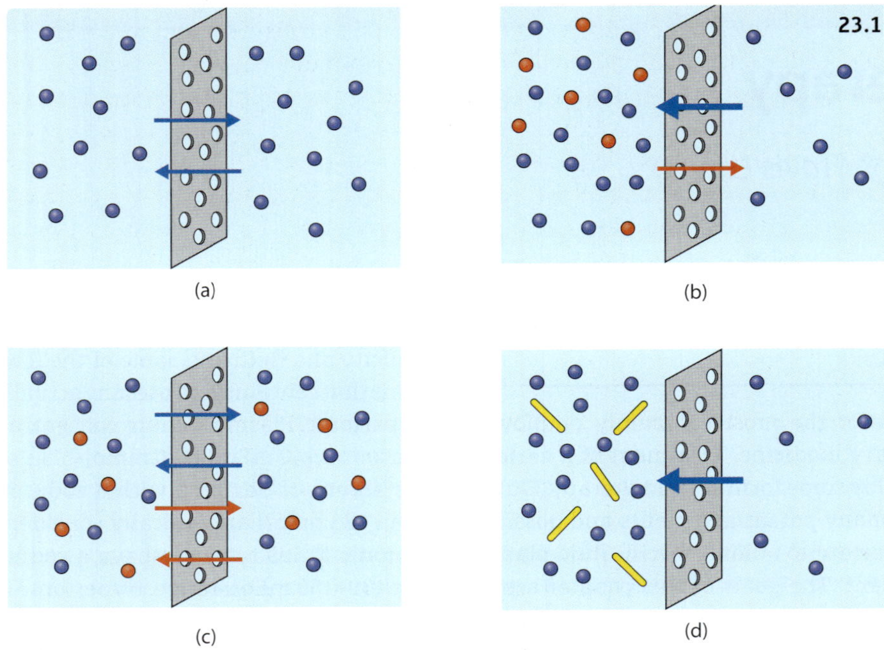

Figures 23.1a–d (a) A chamber separated by a semipermeable membrane. The dark blue dots represent freely permeable water molecules. (b) Sodium ions (red dots) are added to the left side. Sodium is able to slowly diffuse across the semipermeable membrane. Initially, water will be drawn to the left side due to the osmotic activity of sodium. As sodium diffuses across the membrane the water will also re-equilibrate as shown in 23.1c. (d) Large impermeable molecules (yellow bars) are added to the left side of the chamber. Water will be drawn to the left side of the membrane and an osmotic gradient will be maintained.

Table 23.1 Composition of maintenance fluids.

Fluid	Na^+ (mEq/l)	K^+ (mEq/l)	Glucose (g/l)	Cl^- (mEq/l)	Ca^{2+} (mEq/l)	Mg^{2+} (mEq/l)	Buffer	Osmolarity (mOsmol/l)
0.45% NaCl	77	0	0	77	0	0	0	155
2.5% Dextrose in 0.45% NaCl	77	0	25	77	0	0	0	280
Normosol-M in 5% dextrose[t]	40	13	50	40	0	3	Acetate	363
Plasma-Lyte 56	40	13	0	40	0	3	Acetate	111
Plasma-Lyte 56 in 5% dextrose[ʃ]	40	13	50	40	0	3	Acetate	363

[t] Hospira, Inc. Lake Forest, IL. [ʃ] Baxter Healthcare Pty Ltd. Toongabbie, NSW.
Note: For Na^+, K^+, and Cl^-: 1 mEq/l = 1 mmol/l; for Ca^{2+} and Mg^{2+}: 1 mEq/l = 0.5 mmol/l.

- Replacement fluids. Have sodium and potassium concentrations closer to those of normal plasma. Replacement fluids are isotonic and typically have potassium concentrations similar to that of normal plasma (4.0 mEq/l or mmol/l). Replacement fluids may generally be administered at much higher rates than maintenance fluids and are intended to 'replace' a missing volume of plasma. In veterinary medicine, replacement fluids are often used in a maintenance setting due to the fact that most patients with normally functioning kidneys will excrete the excessive sodium load supplied by a higher sodium replacement fluid. However, in patients who may be more sensitive to sodium loading, such as those with heart disease, end-stage liver disease, or kidney disease with reduced glomerular filtration rates, extreme caution should be used with replacement fluids. Examples of replacement fluids, such as 0.9% NaCl, lactated Ringer's solution, and Normosol-R, are listed in **Table 23.2**. **Note:** 0.9% NaCl is an acidic solution because of the extra chloride it contains; some clinicians no longer recommend using it as a resuscitating solution because of its adverse effects on the cellular environment.

Another common descriptor applied to crystalloids is whether the solution is a balanced solution. A balanced solution refers to the different electrolytes added to the fluid. Balanced solutions have common electrolytes supplemented in concentrations similar to those of plasma. Other types of electrolytes found in plasma include calcium, magnesium, and phosphorus. Examples of balanced crystalloid solutions include lactated Ringer's solution, Normosol, and Plasma-Lyte. Conversely, 0.45% and 0.9% saline are examples of fluids not containing additional electrolytes. Balanced solutions are often preferred except in certain circumstances in which a patient may have an electrolyte disturbance; for example, patients with hypercalcemia or when co-administration with other treatments such as blood products is required.

A buffer may also be added to the crystalloid solution to help maintain a more neutral pH. The chloride anion found in most crystalloid solutions has an acidifying effect within the patient. Many crystalloid solutions have a buffer to help counteract this effect and maintain a more neutral pH in the patient. Commonly used buffers include lactate, acetate, gluconate, and bicarbonate. These compounds are weak acids or bases depending on the pH. Ideally, in dogs and cats a pH of 7.3 to 7.4 would be considered normal. Buffers found in commonly used products can be found in **Tables 23.1** and **23.2**. There are some instances in which a specific buffer may influence the fluid choice for a patient. Lactate is converted within the liver and should be avoided in patients with end-stage liver failure. Lactate buffered solutions do not need to be avoided in patients with type A lactic acidosis. Lactic acidosis will be discussed in more detail later in this chapter. Caution should be used with acetate-containing fluids when administering rapid, large volume IV boluses due to reports of refractory hypotension, mostly in cats.

Hypertonic saline and mannitol are examples of hypertonic or hyperosmotic crystalloid solutions. The most common preparations of hypertonic saline are 3%, 5%, and 7.2% sodium chloride in solution. Hypertonic saline has become more widely used for initial resuscitation strategies for an array of diseases and management of patients with head trauma. The high tonicity of hypertonic saline preparations will draw water out of the interstitial and intracellular spaces into the vasculature. Hypertonic saline has a rapid onset of effect for intravascular expansion, but the duration is often limited to 15–30 minutes. When 7.2% hypertonic saline is used in resuscitation strategies, other fluid types are often administered in conjunction with this solution. Another commonly employed use for hypertonic saline is for the management of cerebral edema and head trauma. When used for the management of cerebral edema, hypertonic saline may be used alone or independent of other fluids. Hypertonic saline (7.2%) is usually administered as IV boluses of 2–4 ml/kg body weight over a period of 5–10 minutes.

Mannitol is an example of a hyperosmotic solution. Unlike the other crystalloids, it has no sodium chloride

Table 23.2 Composition of replacement fluids.

Fluid	Na^+ (mEq/l)	K^+ (mEq/l)	Glucose (g/l)	Cl^- (mEq/l)	Ca^{2+} (mEq/l)	Mg^{2+} (mEq/l)	Buffer	Osmolarity (mOsmol/l)
0.9% NaCl	154	0	0	154	0	0	0	308
Lactated Ringer's solution	130	4	0	109	3	0	Lactate	280
Normosol-R[ŧ]	140	5	0	98	0	3	Acetate, gluconate	294
Plasma-Lyte 148[ʃ]	140	5	0	98	0	3	Acetate	294

[ŧ] Hospira, Inc. Lake Forest, IL. [ʃ] Baxter Healthcare Pty Ltd. Toongabbie, NSW.
Note: For Na^+, K^+, and Cl^-: 1 mEq/l = 1 mmol/l; for Ca^{2+} and Mg^{2+}: 1 mEq/l = 0.5 mmol/l.

contained within the preparation. Mannitol is a crystalline sugar that is dissolved in sterile water. Mannitol has a tendency to form microcrystalline particles, especially at room temperatures or below. Mannitol should generally be warmed to body temperature and administered through a filter to prevent embolization of the crystalline precipitation particles in the patient. Mannitol is another agent used for management of cerebral edema, intracranial hypertension, and acute glaucoma. Mannitol is usually administered as an IV infusion of 0.5–1.5 g/kg body weight of patient over 15–30 minutes.

COLLOIDS

Colloids are suspensions containing large molecules. There are normally a large number of circulating proteins in the plasma. Examples of these proteins include albumin, immunoglobulins, and enzymes. Similar to sodium and the osmotic effect, these molecules will draw water, producing a colloid oncotic effect. There are two properties determining the oncotic effect of a particular colloid in solution: the number of particles and the net charge of the molecule. For example, albumin is the major determinant of colloidal oncotic pressure within the vasculature. One particle of a colloid is theoretically equal to one sodium ion in solution in the ability to attract water molecules. However, albumin's net negative charge allows it to draw more water than would be predicted if only the number of molecules in suspension were considered. This is referred to as the Bohr effect and occurs because the negatively charged albumin will attract positively charged ions (mainly sodium) to maintain electroneutrality on either side of a semipermeable membrane. Water will diffuse across the membrane to balance the concentrations between the numbers of particles on each side of the membrane.

Ernest Starling described an equation to help better understand fluid dynamics within the body. Simply stated, he said that the changes in hydrostatic and oncotic pressures across a membrane help determine the net flux of fluid across that membrane. There are other intrinsic properties of the membrane itself, such as permeability to water and proteins, which may also modify how much hydrostatic pressure difference and oncotic pressure difference contribute to fluid flux in that particular tissue. Development of peripheral limb edema or cavitary transudate effusions in severely hypoalbuminemic patients without development of pulmonary edema is a clinical example of this concept. Within the lung, there is easy passage of large molecules across the alveolar capillary membranes. This means that colloids exert very little effect and the colloid oncotic pressure is minimal in determining fluid flux within the lung. The major determinant of fluid flux within the lung is the difference in hydrostatic pressure across the capillary membrane, as in congestive heart failure. An increased left atrial pressure leads to increased pulmonary capillary pressures causing fluid leakage out of the capillary into the interstitial and alveolar spaces, leading to development of pulmonary edema.

Colloids are typically used for low volume resuscitation strategies or in the management of hypoproteinemic patients. Large molecules have more difficulty leaking out of the vasculature into the interstitial space than sodium. The proposed benefit is that colloid solutions will remain within the intravascular space longer than crystalloid solutions and will pull fluid from the interstitial space into the vascular space, maintaining intravascular volume. There are two broad categories of colloid solutions: natural colloids and synthetic colloids.

Albumin is the major contributor to oncotic pressure in states of health. Approximately 80% of the intravascular colloid oncotic pressure is due to albumin. The natural colloids are albumin-containing products and include whole blood, plasma, and concentrates of albumin. Whole blood and plasma are examples of weak colloids; because the albumin concentration is similar to that of a normal patient, it takes very large transfusion amounts to make a significant change in the patient's albumin, making plasma or whole blood transfusions impractical for purposes of increasing colloidal oncotic pressure in anything but very small patients. However, whole blood and plasma products are often useful for supplying clotting factors in animals with coagulopathies.

Another example of natural colloid preparations are the albumin concentrates. Lyophilized canine albumin is currently not available, but 5% and 25% human albumin products may be purchased commercially. Human albumin is relatively inexpensive and may be diluted to a desired concentration and administered to correct a calculated albumin deficit (**Box 23.1**).

Human albumin should be used with extreme caution in veterinary patients. It should never be used in a relatively healthy animal or in a patient that has received a human albumin transfusion in the past. Human albumin transfusions should be reserved for critically-ill patients where other colloidal options have been exhausted. Client education as to the risks versus benefits should be of pre-eminence. Human albumin has been shown to cause acute anaphylaxis, delayed hypersensitivity reactions, and even death in healthy animals, animals with no known exposure to human albumin, and especially in animals with previous human albumin exposure.

Box 23.1. Calculating the albumin deficit.

The albumin deficit can be calculated using the equation below:

$$\text{albumin deficit (g)} = 10 \times (\text{desired albumin [g/dl]} - \text{patient albumin (g/dl)}] \times \text{body wt (kg)} \times 0.3$$

It is important to check and change units to accurately determine transfusion amounts needed.

For example, increasing the albumin by 1 g/dl in a 20 kg dog with an albumin concentration of 1.5 g/dl requires 60 g of albumin.

$$\text{albumin deficit (g)} = 10 \times (2.5\ \text{g/dl} - 1.5\text{g/dl}) \times 20 \times 0.3 = 60\ \text{g}$$

If fresh frozen plasma (FFP) is used and an average albumin concentration of 3.0 g/dl is assumed, then 1 liter of FFP would have 30 g of albumin. This dog would require 2 liters of FFP (i.e. approximately 7 units of plasma!).

Canine albumin seems to have less risk of severe adverse reactions in the limited veterinary research currently available on the product. However, lyophilized canine albumin was not commercially available during the development of this text due to a manufacturing issue.

Hydroxyethyl starches, dextrans, and gelatins are examples of synthetic colloids. Hydroxyethyl starches are the most commonly used synthetic colloid solutions in veterinary medicine and will be the focus of this chapter. The dextrans are rarely used anymore due to higher risk of kidney injury. Gelatins are available in Europe and the most commonly reported adverse effects are hypersensitivity reactions.

Hydroxyethyl starches are produced from hydrolysis of amylopectin. They are described based on the degree of substitution and the average molecular weight of the solution (**Table 23.3**). Hydroxyethyl starch solutions are polydisperse solutions (i.e. the solution contains numerous different size particles in suspension). This is in contrast to albumin, which is highly preserved across species and generally has a molecular weight around 69 kDa. The degree of substitution refers to the number of glucose moieties that have been substituted for hydroxyethyl groups and is usually reported as a number between 0 and 1. A tetrastarch with four substitutions would be given a designation of 0.4, whereas a pentastarch with five substitutions would be given a designation of 0.5. The molecular weight reported for a hydroxyethyl starch solution is a calculated number based on the number of different size particles and percentage of those sizes within the solution. In general, higher molecular weight hydroxyethyl starch solutions tend to be more substituted, but this is not an absolute rule. Commercial hydroxyethyl starch solutions are generally prepared using 0.9% saline or lactated Ringer's solution. The degree of substitution and molecular weight are important in determining the properties of the hydroxyethyl starch solutions. The size of a molecule does not determine the oncotic force generated; smaller molecules of hydroxyethyl starch generate the same oncotic force as a larger molecule. However, larger molecules persist in the vasculature longer and take longer to be degraded by the body. Hydroxyethyl starches are commonly administered as rapid IV infusions; however, in veterinary medicine it has become common practice to give prolonged infusions of synthetic colloids over 24–48 hours, especially in patients with hypoalbuminemia. Currently, there is little to no evidence-based medicine supporting the use of hydroxyethyl starch in this way.

Maximum recommended daily dosages of hydroxyethyl starches (**Table 23.3**) are often based on the risk of developing adverse reactions; in particular development of a coagulopathy. There are several possible mechanisms by which hydroxyethyl starch may interfere with the coagulation system. The most likely proposed mechanisms of hydroxyethyl starch interference in coagulation include platelet dysfunction and weakening of clot formation due to incorporation into the fibrin clot. Adverse effects on coagulation seem to be directly related to the degree of substitution and not the molecular weight of the hydroxyethyl starch solution. Higher substituted hydroxyethyl starches tend to have a greater effect on coagulation. The clinical significance of hydroxyethyl starch on *in-vitro* coagulation testing and how it relates to *in-vivo* effects is a popular area of interest in current veterinary research.

Other reported adverse effects of hydroxyethyl starches include acute kidney injury (AKI), fluid overload, and anaphylaxis. In human medicine, there is a trend away from synthetic colloid use due to the risk of AKI and higher rates of mortality in certain types of disease processes. There is little to no evidence providing a clear benefit of the use of a synthetic colloid over a crystalloid. There is some evidence supporting the use of human albumin in certain disease processes such as sepsis; however, in veterinary medicine, there are limitations with availability of safe natural colloid products especially canine albumin preparations. There is very little data regarding incidence of AKI in veterinary patients receiving hydroxyethyl starch solutions. As with any therapy,

Table 23.3 Characteristics of common hydroxyethyl starch solutions.

Hydroxyethyl starch solution	Molecular weight (kDa)	Degree of substitution	Base solution	Suggested maximum daily dose
Hextend[1]	670	0.75	Lactated electrolyte solution	20 ml/kg
Hespan[2]	670	0.75	Lactated Ringer's solution	20 ml/kg
Hetastarch (6% Hetastarch in 0.9% saline)	450	0.7	Saline	20 ml/kg
VetStarch[3]	130	0.4	Saline	20 ml/kg
Voluven[4]	130	0.4	Saline	50 ml/kg

[1] B. Braun Medical Inc. Bethlehem, PA, USA
[2] BioTime, Inc. Berkeley, CA, USA
[3] Abbott Laboratories. North Chicago, IL, USA
[4] Fresenius Kabi Norge AS, Halden, Norway

the risk to benefit ratio should always be considered by the clinician before instituting a therapy.

DEVELOPING A FLUID THERAPY PLAN

There are several considerations when developing a fluid therapy plan. It is vital to tailor therapy to the individual patient. Considerations include pre-existing hydration status, expected normal losses, ongoing abnormal losses, and pre-existing comorbidities. The most important part of any fluid plan is reassessment of the patient frequently and making changes accordingly.

Determining the hydration status may not always be simple based on physical examination parameters alone. Serial physical examinations are better at determining hydration status than a single examination. An estimation of hydration status may be made based on certain examination findings. Indicators of dehydration include tacky mucous membranes, decreased skin turgor, sunken eyes, and many others. It is important to remember that a well hydrated cachectic patient will have decreased skin turgor because of the loss of normal skin elasticity (**Figure 23.2**). Obese patients, on the other hand, can have moderate dehydration with normal skin turgor because of the increased resiliency provided by subcutaneous fat. A more quantitative method to estimate hydration in a hospitalized patient is to weigh the patient daily while noting that a liter of water weighs 1.0 kg and any weight loss or gain within any 24-hour period will likely represent an addition or loss of body water. **Table 23.4** helps summarize physical examination findings and correlate them to hydration status. It is also vital to realize the difference between dehydration and hypovolemia. Hypovolemia represents a loss of plasma volume, whereas dehydration represents a loss of interstitial fluid volume. Hypovolemia should be corrected rapidly, whereas dehydration is generally corrected more slowly over 6–24 hours. Clinical markers of hypovolemia and poor perfusion include tachycardia, weak or bounding pulses, pallor (**Figure 23.3**), cold extremities, and alteration of certain biochemical assays such as elevated serum lactate concentration.

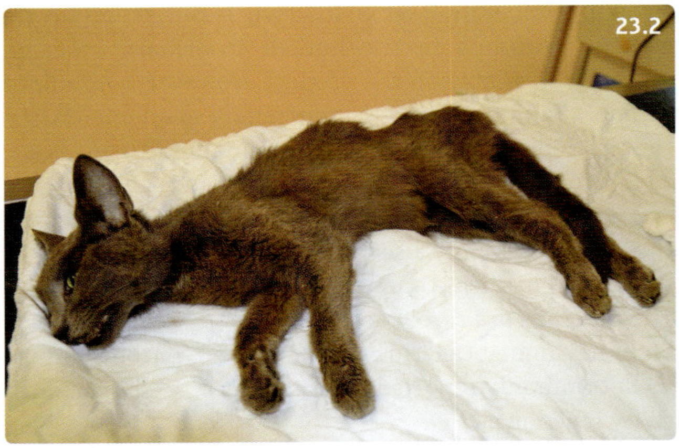

Figure 23.2 This very cachectic cat would have a loss of skin resiliency, which might exaggerate its true degree of dehydration. (Courtesy M. Schaer)

Table 23.4 Estimation of hydration status.

Estimated hydration status	Physical examination findings	Presence of hypoperfusion
Overhydration	Serous nasal discharge, chemosis, pitting edema, jugular venous distension, increasing respiratory rate and effort	N/A
<5% dehydration	No detectable abnormalities	Unlikely
6–8% dehydration	Mild decrease in skin elasticity (<2 sec), tacky/sticky mucous membranes	Unlikely
8–10% dehydration	Mild lethargy, decreased skin elasticity (>3 sec), tacky/sticky mucous membranes, eyes may appear to be slightly sunken in orbits, slight prolongation of capillary refill time	Possible
10–12% dehydration	Marked lethargy, loss of skin elasticity (skin tent persists), dry/cold mucous membranes, eyes appear to be sunken in orbits, prolongation of capillary refill time	Likely
>12% dehydration	Recumbent/moribund, loss of skin elasticity (skin tent persists), dry/cold mucous membranes, eyes appear to be sunken in orbits, prolongation/absence of capillary refill time	Definite

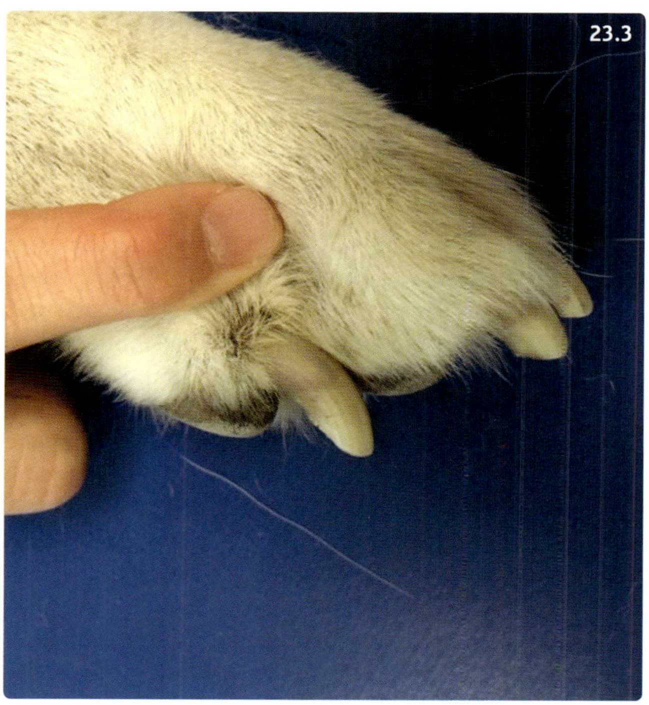

Figure 23.3 The paw in this picture shows poor perfusion, as shown by the digital pallor. (Courtesy M. Schaer)

Once the hydration and perfusion status of the patient is determined, it is important to approximate the expected normal daily losses of a patient. This is often referred to as the maintenance requirement portion of the fluid therapy plan. In simplistic terms, this is the amount of fluid required to maintain a normal hydration status in a patient that is not eating or drinking. It is important to realize that maintenance requirements vary between patients based on factors such as body size, life stage, and comorbidities such as kidney disease. Several methods of approximating daily maintenance fluid requirements for veterinary patients are shown in **Boxes 23.2** and **23.3**. However, these are approximations and the actual needs of the patient may vary greatly from the calculated values. For example, a pet with chronic kidney disease may require a much greater volume of fluid to maintain hydration than a pet with normally functioning kidneys that is able to concentrate urine, making frequent serial evaluations and reassessment of the patient the most important part of any fluid plan.

Clinical example of a simple fluid therapy plan

A 2-year-old castrated male mixed-breed dog weighing 7 kg is presented for acute vomiting and diarrhea. While obtaining a history, it is revealed that the client's grandfather is visiting and fed the patient a slice of pepperoni pizza with extra cheese a couple of hours prior to the onset of vomiting and diarrhea. The patient had four episodes of emesis over the last 12 hours, each time vomiting approximately 2–3 teaspoons of liquid. He also had a single bout of approximately one cup of watery brown diarrhea. Based on your physical examination findings you determine the patient to be approximately 7% dehydrated. His vitals are within normal reference ranges and he has good femoral pulse quality. The patient has no significant abnormalities on a complete blood count, chemistry profile, or serum lactate concentration.

Box 23.2. Common methods of estimating daily water requirements.

Calculation based on daily resting energy requirement equations:

$$(30 \times BW[kg]) + 70 = ml/kg/24 \text{ hours}$$
$$70 \times BW^{0.75} = ml/kg/24 \text{ hours}$$

Quick estimates of daily water requirements:

- 80–100 ml/kg/24 hours for neonates
- 60 ml/kg/24 hours for small dogs
- 50 ml/kg/24 hours for medium dogs and cats
- 40 ml/kg/24 hours for large breed dogs
- 30 ml/kg/24 hours for giant breed dogs

Once the approximate maintenance requirements for a patient are determined, the clinician must also address the abnormal ongoing losses of fluid from the patient. Examples include vomiting, diarrhea, and exudative wounds. Collection of fluids and measuring these losses by direct means or calculating fluid volumes through changes in weight of soiled bedding may help to quantify and better approximate these losses. Some common useful conversions are listed in **Box 23.3**.

A clinical example: if fresh bedding weighed 1.8 kg prior to being soiled and increased to 2.3 kg after the patient vomited on the bedding, there is a net gain of 0.5 kg. This means that the patient vomited approximately 0.5 liters of fluid based on the concept that 1 liter of water weighs 1 kilogram.

Combining the calculated requirements together to make a basic fluid therapy plan, the following equation can be used:

Estimated percent dehydration + estimated maintenance requirements + plus estimated ongoing losses = predicted total volume of fluid.

Box 23.3. Helpful fluid conversions.

- One liter of water weighs one kilogram
- One teaspoon is approximately 5 ml
- One tablespoon is approximately 15 ml
- One cup is approximately 237 ml

The first step is to calculate the estimated percent dehydration and decide how rapidly you wish to correct the patient's hydration status. The estimated percent dehydration should be converted to decimal point form and multiplied by the bodyweight as below:

The patient is estimated to be 7% dehydrated = 0.07
$0.07 \times 7 \text{ kg} = 0.49 \text{ kg}$

This would equate to a 0.49 liter (490 ml) loss of body water.

You wish to correct the patient's hydration over a 10-hour period. Therefore, for the first 10 hours of your fluid therapy plan you will add 49 ml/hour to the estimated maintenance and ongoing losses.

The second step is to estimate the patient's maintenance requirements. You decide to use the calculated resting energy requirement (RER) formula as demonstrated below:

$$RER = 70 \times (7 \text{ kg})^{3/4} = 301 \text{ kcal/day or } 301 \text{ ml/day}$$

Therefore, divide 301 ml by 24 hours and the estimated maintenance fluid rate will be 12.5 ml/hour.

The third step in developing a fluid therapy plan is to estimate the ongoing abnormal fluid losses. The ongoing losses are often much more difficult to estimate. Some clinicians prefer to use a multiple of the predicted maintenance fluid requirements as a starting point, such as 2 or 3 times the calculated maintenance rate. Alternatively, you can estimate losses based on history. For example, the client reported that the patient vomited 2–3 teaspoons of liquid each time emesis occurred and the patient had four episodes of emesis over the last 12 hours. He had a single bout of approximately one cup of watery brown diarrhea within that time. His estimated losses over the 12 hour period would then be:

One teaspoon equals 5 ml, therefore each emesis was approximately 15 ml of fluid; the patient had four episodes over 12 hours, equaling approximately 60 ml. The patient was also estimated have one cup of liquid diarrhea, which is equal to approximately 236 ml of fluid. Adding the losses together, you calculate that the patient's ongoing losses are 296 ml of fluid per 12 hours or 25 ml per hour.

The fourth step is combining all the calculations together:

Correction of estimated percent dehydration + estimated maintenance requirements + plus estimated ongoing losses = predicted total volume of fluid.
49 ml/hour + 12.5 ml/hour + 25 ml/hour = total fluid rate of 86.5 ml/hour for the first 10 hours of therapy

The fifth and most important step is frequently reassessing the patient, as a large volume of fluid will be administered over a 10-hour period. It is important the patient is reassessed every 1–2 hours and the fluids adjusted accordingly. A couple of hours after beginning therapy, the patient stops vomiting and only has one more episode of small volume diarrhea. You determine that the patient's hydration status is improving and decide to decrease the fluid rate to account only for continued correction of hydration status and calculated estimated maintenance rate (49 ml + 12.5 ml). The fluid rate is therefore decreased to 62 ml/hour, rounding to the nearest whole number. The patient's body weight should hold steady once all of the fluid deficits are replaced and maintenance fluids are continued.

FLUID RESUSCITATION

Fluid resuscitation strategies are employed when there is evidence of hypovolemia and reduced intravascular volume. In general, the aim of treatment is to identify then correct the volume deficit safely and rapidly. This is different to the strategies described previously in this chapter for correction of mild–moderate dehydration or provision of maintenance requirements, as fluids to correct hypovolemia are usually delivered as a bolus over a short period of time (15–20 minutes) rather than over several hours or days.

Identification of hypovolemic shock

Physical examination, cardiovascular monitoring, and point-of-care laboratory testing can be used in the assessment of volume status. Patients with hypovolemic shock typically go through two distinct phases: compensated or 'hyperdynamic' and decompensated or 'hypodynamic' shock (**Table 23.5**). Patients in compensated shock are hypovolemic; however, the cardiovascular system is able to compensate for the loss in volume by increasing heart rate and increasing cardiac contractility. In these patients, cardiac output may actually be increased. As hypovolemia progresses, the compensatory mechanisms are unable to keep up with the loss of intravascular volume, and life-threatening decompensated shock occurs.

Table 23.5 Signs of hypovolemic shock in dogs.

Compensated	Decompensated
Tachycardia	Tachycardia
Injected mucous membranes	Pale mucous membranes
Rapid CRT	Prolonged CRT
Bounding pulses	Weak/thready pulses Weakness/collapse Reduced consciousness Low rectal temperature

Physical examination findings in compensated shock are reflective of an increase in cardiac output. These patients are typically tachycardic with bounding or 'tall, narrow' pulses, slightly injected mucous membranes, and a rapid capillary refill time (CRT) (normal <2 seconds). They are usually mentally aware, ambulatory, and with a normal rectal temperature. As patients progress to decompensated shock, they develop signs of reduced perfusion. They usually remain tachycardic until they enter a terminal phase, peripheral pulses become difficult to feel or palpate as 'thready', mucous membranes become pale, and CRT becomes prolonged (**Figure 23.4**). Weakness or collapse is common and the level of consciousness will begin to decline in severely affected patients. Rectal temperature in dogs is often normal or slightly low.

Cats usually enter a phase of hypodynamic shock much earlier than dogs. Typical signs of hypovolemia in a cat include lethargy, bradycardia, and low rectal temperature.

Cardiovascular monitoring can be helpful to confirm physical examination findings. The most commonly used technique is noninvasive measurement of blood pressure. Dogs will maintain their blood pressure until they are markedly hypovolemic, so a normal blood pressure does not rule out hypovolemic shock. Often, dogs in

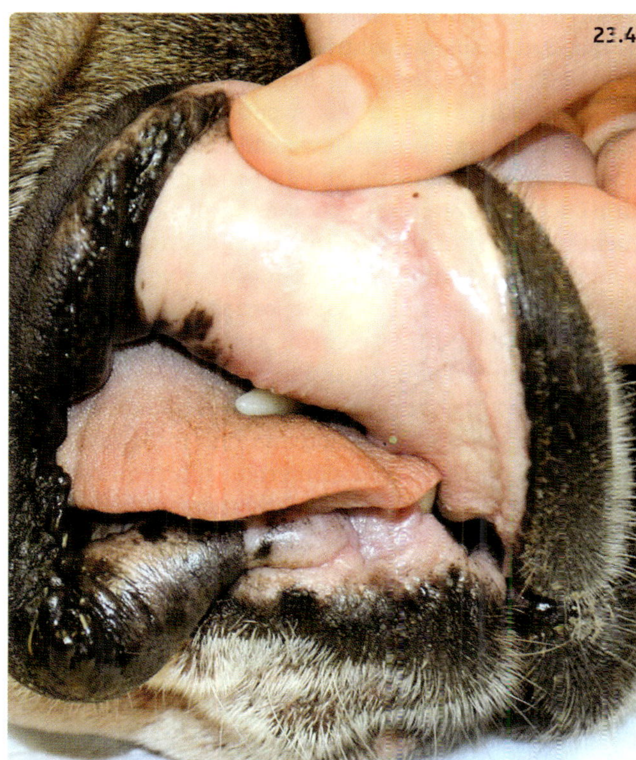

Figure 23.4 The lip pallor illustrates this dog's delayed capillary refill time. (Courtesy M. Schaer)

decompensated shock will have a blood pressure below normal (systolic <90 mmHg, mean <65 mmHg). As discussed above, cats will enter a hypodynamic phase of shock with associated low systolic and mean arterial blood pressure much earlier than dogs. Urine output can also be monitored. Normal urine output (>2 ml/kg/hour) usually indicates adequate renal perfusion if the kidneys are able to concentrate urine. Another commonly used monitoring technique for assessing volume status is bedside echocardiography, using cardiac chamber size as a measure of preload. Central venous pressure, which has been widely used for many years as a method of assessing preload and hence volemic status, has been widely discredited in more recent studies and cannot be recommended as an accurate indication of volume status. Other more advanced techniques, such as cardiac output monitoring, pulse pressure variation, and microperfusion scanning, may be excellent indicators of volume status but are rarely used due to the need for specialized equipment and training.

Some basic laboratory testing can be extremely helpful in the assessment of hypovolemia. Measurement of packed cell volume (PCV) and total solids (TS), combined with physical examination findings, can indicate the presence of volume loss and often directs the clinician to the cause of the volume loss. For example, an acutely hemorrhaging patient would be expected to have low TS, but due to splenic contraction might have a normal or high PCV. With ongoing hemorrhage, the PCV will also eventually begin to fall. A patient that has severe dehydration leading to hypovolemia will be hemoconcentrated, resulting in a high PCV and high TS. A patient with massive protein loss, such as in hemorrhagic gastroenteritis (see Chapter 8: Digestive diseases [pharynx to anorectum]), will often present with a very high PCV but a low TS, suggesting a disproportionate loss of plasma water over RBCs. Assessment of kidney function using blood urea nitrogen (BUN) and creatinine combined with urine specific gravity can also be helpful. A patient that is developing a prerenal azotemia due to hypovolemia and subsequently reduced glomerular filtration rate will often have a high BUN with slightly increased or normal creatinine and concentrated urine.

Point-of-care lactate measurement can be extremely helpful in the assessment of hypovolemia; lactate in a normal patient at rest is usually <2 mmol/l. Lactate is formed during anaerobic metabolism and so will increase in situations where oxygen demand is outstripping supply, as seen in hypovolemic shock. Normal vigorous exercise and pathologic conditions that cause excessive muscle movement, such as grand mal seizures and tremor syndromes, can cause elevations in lactate without hypovolemia being present. Additionally, certain conditions without hypovolemia can cause what is known as a type B hyperlactatemia; these include cancer, sepsis, severe liver disease, and certain drugs such as epinephrine. Lactate measurement can be especially helpful in detecting hypovolemia in critical situations such as a busy emergency room, and in detecting hypovolemia where physical examination signs are subtle or contradictory. Lactate can be measured using an inexpensive handheld device similar to a glucometer or using handheld or bench top blood gas analyzers. The smaller handheld devices tend to be less accurate at low ranges (<3 mmol/l); however, moderate to severe elevations in lactate, indicating significant hypovolemia, can be easily detected.

Treatment of hypovolemia

The different types of fluids available for fluid resuscitation have been discussed at length earlier in the chapter. There are, broadly, two approaches to fluid resuscitation. These should be varied according to the underlying cause of the hypovolemia (if known) and the severity of the condition. Examples of different clinical scenarios will be discussed later in the chapter. The most commonly employed approach is conventional resuscitation. This involves using relatively large IV boluses of isotonic crystalloids, usually 15–30 ml/kg at a time for dogs and 10–15 ml/kg for cats, repeated to effect. Each bolus is usually delivered over 15–20 minutes before reassessment of volume status and clinical response to the bolus. This is probably the method of choice for patients with large water losses, such as animals with severe vomiting and diarrhea or hypovolemia secondary to dehydration. The advantages of this technique are that the fluids used are inexpensive, familiar to all practitioners, and widely available. The disadvantage is that use of large volumes of crystalloids can dilute out blood components such as clotting factors. This is especially important when managing patients with severe hemorrhage (see Severe hemorrhage).

The 'myth' of shock dose fluids

Many texts advocate providing 'shock dose' fluids to patients with signs of hypovolemic shock. The volumes quoted are usually 90 ml/kg (dog) and 60 ml/kg (cat); this actually represents the entire blood volume of the animal. Clinically, it is rarely necessary to administer this large a volume of crystalloid fluids and so fluids should be administered in smaller aliquots (15–30 ml/kg for dogs and 10–15 ml/kg for cats) and titrated to effect (see Knowing when to stop: endpoints in fluid resuscitation). Over-resuscitation can be as harmful as under-resuscitating the patient (**Figures 23.5a–d**). Occasionally, extremely large volumes of crystalloids are necessary, such as in patients with massive gastrointestinal losses of fluid. In these cases fluid therapy can be continued until endpoints are reached with careful monitoring of the patient's clinical response and laboratory values.

The second major strategy is low volume resuscitation. This usually involves using hypertonic fluids, commonly 7.2% saline. A normal dose range is 2–4 ml/kg administered IV over 5–10 minutes. The mechanism of action of these fluids has been discussed above. Hypertonic saline is low cost and, as a low volume is administered, it can allow for more rapid correction of hypovolemia than using conventional fluid resuscitation, especially in large breed dogs. Use of hypertonic saline in resuscitation should be avoided where the patient has significant pre-existing dehydration and/or hypernatremia. Sometimes, hypertonic saline is combined with artificial colloids such as hetastarch at a dose of 5 ml/kg; this will prolong the action of the hypertonic fluid but may carry some of the disadvantages of artificial colloids as discussed above.

Knowing when to stop: endpoints in fluid resuscitation

How to figure out when to stop fluid resuscitation can be more challenging than initial identification of hypovolemia. In straightforward cases, such as gastrointestinal loss, the parameters used to diagnose hypovolemia can be used to assess response to treatment; this includes normalization of heart rate and pulse quality, mucous membrane color, CRT, mental status, correction of hypotension, and restoration of urine output. Remember that in some cases other strategies will be needed and sometimes it will not be possible to achieve these endpoints. For example, in trauma patients or patients with acute abdominal disease, pain may be a confounding factor and will increase heart rate independent of volemic state. In patients with distributive shock (e.g. those with gastric dilatation-volvulus or sepsis), correction and treatment of the underlying disease, along with fluid resuscitation, will be required to normalize physical examination parameters. Patients with septic shock present one

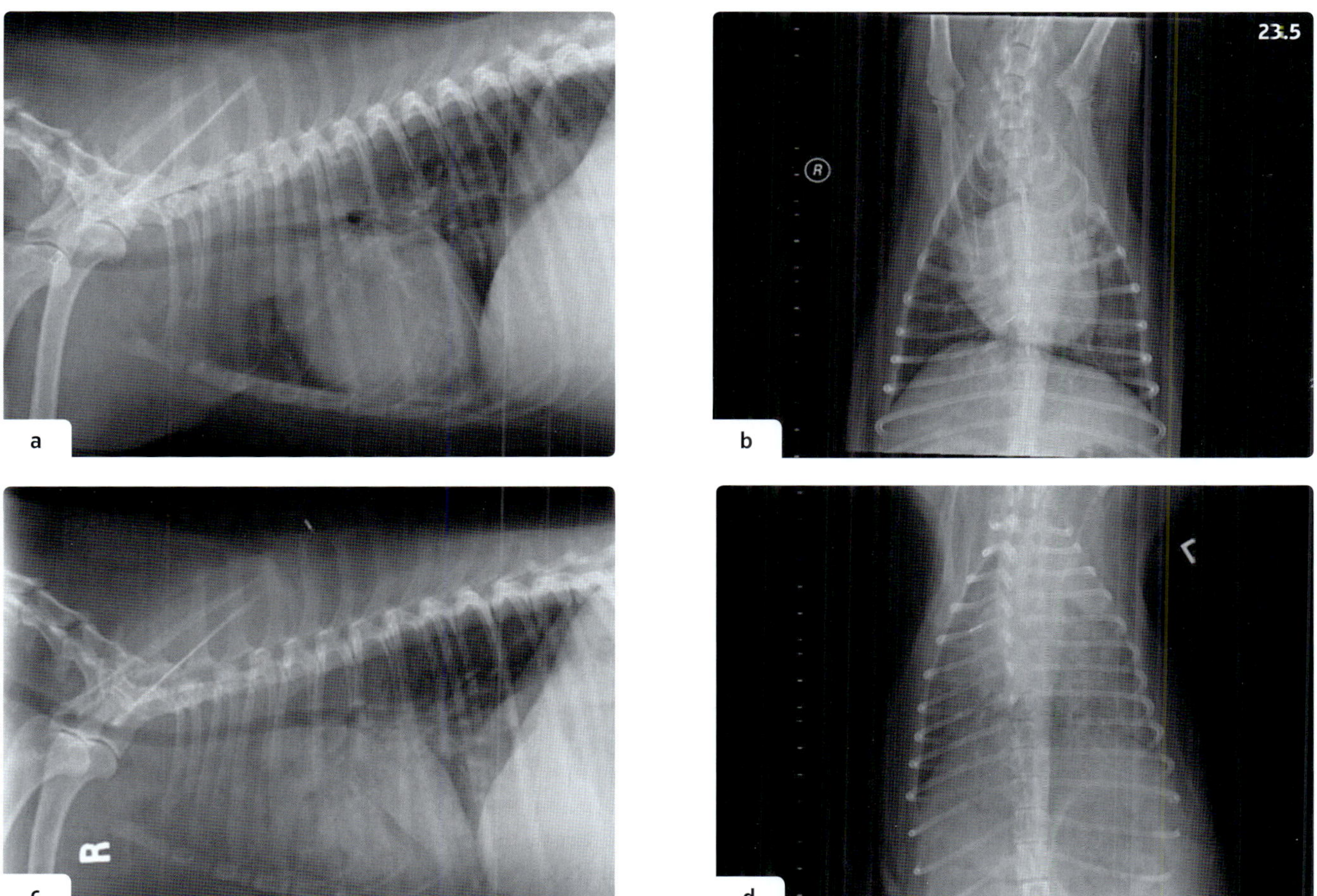

Figures 23.5a–d These four radiographs illustrating intravenous overload are from a dog taken at the time of admission (a, b) and after 2 days of intravenous fluids (c, d).

of the biggest challenges in assessing endpoints of fluid resuscitation. For these more complex situations, assessment of lactate clearance and use of more advanced techniques such as echocardiography and cardiac output monitoring can be helpful. The key factor overall is continuous reassessment of the patient to ensure adequate but not excessive fluid resuscitation.

Specific scenarios in fluid resuscitation

Severe hemorrhage

Hemorrhagic shock is a major challenge in small animals; it can be caused by trauma or by spontaneous bleeds, for example in a coagulopathic state (e.g. anticoagulant rodenticide toxicity) or from rupture of benign or neoplastic masses. Severe external bleeding can be easily recognized and often temporarily controlled during stabilization; however, internal bleeding, especially into the abdominal cavity, can be more challenging to recognize promptly. In veterinary medicine, rapid emergency surgery is not always readily available and so it is important for veterinarians to have a strategy for medical stabilization of acute hemorrhage (**Box 23.4**).

The aim of fluid resuscitation in acute hemorrhage is to replace just enough intravascular volume to restore oxygen delivery to the tissues, but to avoid some of the major pitfalls of giving large amounts of fluids to a hemorrhaging patient. These complications include dilution of clotting factors by vigorous fluid resuscitation and increasing blood pressure to supranormal values. Furthermore, certain fluid choices, such as artificial colloids, can directly induce coagulopathy and enhance further bleeding. It can be thought of as a vicious cycle; the more the patient bleeds, the more fluids they require for resuscitation, the more they are resuscitated, the more they bleed. Additionally, the fluids used in conventional resuscitation (isotonic crystalloids) do not have any oxygen carrying capacity, so if large volumes of isotonic crystalloids are being used, clinicians should be aware that they are replacing RBCs and plasma with a plain crystalloid fluid. For this reason, conventional resuscitation (see above) is probably not the best approach to an acutely hemorrhaging patient.

Low volume resuscitation using hypertonic fluids (see above) is commonly used as it provides a method of resuscitation that avoids large fluid volumes and can be rapidly delivered. There are additional benefits for patients with polytrauma (see Raised intracranial pressure).

Hemostatic resuscitation is an emerging technique for fluid resuscitation of patients with severe hemorrhage. These are patients that have severe, ongoing hemorrhage where the clinician anticipates a requirement to administer multiple blood transfusions during stabilization. The principle of hemostatic resuscitation is to replace what is lost. In hemorrhagic shock, blood is being lost and so the patient is resuscitated using blood products, typically either fresh whole blood or a combination of packed RBCs and FFP. This approach appears effective in minimizing development of iatrogenic coagulopathy and of further bleeding. The disadvantages of hemostatic resuscitation include needing immediate access to blood products, cost, and the risk of transfusion reactions (see Chapter 16: Hematologic disorders). This can be combined with conventional or low volume resuscitation.

Traditional endpoints of resuscitation can be used. Blood pressure monitoring is important in these cases; a mean arterial pressure of 60 mmHg and a systolic pressure of 90 mmHg are recommended to minimize the risk of re-bleeding following resuscitation.

> **Box 23.4.** 'Recipe' for a 30 kg dog with severe hemorrhage (30%+ blood loss).
>
> Dog will appear extremely tachycardic, may become bradycardic in terminal phase, pulses will be very weak/undetectable, mucous membranes will be very pale or white with a prolonged or absent CRT. Blood pressure will be low.
>
> Place a peripheral IV catheter. Give a bolus of 4 ml/kg 7.2% hypertonic saline over 5–10 minutes. Can follow with 500–1,000 ml isotonic crystalloids while blood products are being prepared. Transfuse 2 units packed RBCs with one unit of FFP rapidly. If further packed RBC units are required, transfuse in a ratio of 1:1 with FFP.

Raised intracranial pressure

Clinicians confront the challenge of treating patients with raised intracranial pressure (ICP) regularly; head trauma, inflammatory diseases, and space occupying lesions can all contribute to raising of ICP and the risk of brain herniation. Recognition of this problem is crucial in appropriate management and is discussed elsewhere in this book (see Chapter 14: Disorders of the nervous system and muscle). There are two main considerations for fluid therapy management of a patient with raised ICP: the first is to ensure that the brain is adequately perfused with blood to allow for healing and to reduce the risk of secondary brain injury; the second is to use fluids that either lower ICP or at least do not exacerbate the problem.

Cerebral perfusion pressure can be calculated using the equation below:

Cerebral perfusion pressure = mean arterial pressure (MAP) – intracranial pressure (ICP)

Using this equation, it can be deduced that a patient must have at least an adequate MAP to overcome the increase in ICP, otherwise the brain will not be perfused. During fluid resuscitation in a brain injured patient, it is recommended to achieve a systolic blood pressure of at least 100 mmHg and a MAP of at least 80 mmHg. In human medicine, ICP monitoring is used to guide therapy. This is currently impractical in most veterinary institutions and so the guidelines above give us a reasonable approximation.

Fluid choices become important – in the injured brain, large volumes of isotonic crystalloids can worsen cerebral edema, even as they correct hypotension. For this reason, low volume resuscitation with hyperosmolar agents such as 7.2% hypertonic saline is preferred, as described previously. Hypertonic saline, in addition to providing volume resuscitation and restoration of blood pressure, also has the potential to reduce cerebral edema and hence lower ICP. Mannitol, another hyperosmolar agent, typically dosed at 1–1.5 g/kg IV, can be effective at lowering ICP; however, it will induce a marked osmotic diuresis and so should be avoided in patients with concurrent hypovolemia, as it could lead to worsening hypotension and reduced cerebral perfusion.

Overall, fluid therapy should be targeted to clinical signs and to blood pressure. Vigorous resuscitation with large volumes of isotonic crystalloids should be avoided for fear of worsening edema; however, fluids should not be withheld from patients with raised ICP as the risk of leaving the brain underperfused and leading to secondary brain injury is high.

Pulmonary disease

In general, the principles of fluid therapy for the pulmonary patient are similar to those for other conditions; however, it is imperative to avoid administration of excessive amounts of fluids. The lungs of dogs and especially cats are prone to development of edema in response to increases in hydrostatic pressure. This effect is amplified in the diseased lung, especially in inflammatory conditions such as acute lung injury and in patients with pulmonary contusions. Isotonic crystalloids are generally used; fluid boluses should be smaller (15–20 ml/kg for dogs and used cautiously, if at all, in cats) with continuous reassessment of the patient. Fluid resuscitation should be stopped once endpoints are (or are almost) met. Artificial colloids should be avoided in patients with severe pulmonary disease because of the risk of colloid particles leaking into the interstitial space and thereby worsening the edema. The take home message in treating patients with lung disease is to err on the side of caution with fluid resuscitation; it is easy to give more but harder to take away. Provide enough fluids to maintain adequate perfusion and hydration (**Table 23.6**).

SUMMARY

Regardless of the disease being treated or the technique being used, it is recommended to attempt to recognize and correct hypovolemic shock rapidly. Reassess the patient early and often and look for achievement of endpoints. Remember that lactate can be a useful tool in

Table 23.6 Comparison of fluid resuscitation strategies.

Conventional	Low volume	Hemostatic
Description		
Large fluid volume, isotonic crystalloids	Small fluid volume, hypertonic crystalloids +/- colloids	Variable volume, blood products
Advantages		
Inexpensive, widely available	Inexpensive, widely available, minimize dilutional coagulopathy, rapid resuscitation	Provides O_2 carrying capacity, minimizes coagulopathy
Disadvantages		
No O_2 carrying capacity, dilutional coagulopathy, formation of edema	No O_2 carrying capacity, cannot use in dehydrated patients	Not widely available, expensive, risk of transfusion reaction

addition to physical examination parameters for both identification of hypovolemia and assessing response to treatment. Fluid therapy is often essential but is not always benign. Certain conditions, especially uncontrolled hemorrhage or pulmonary disease, have the potential to be worsened by inappropriate or overly aggressive fluid therapy. In these cases, the use of small increments of fluids along with regular patient reassessment will provide the opportunity to titrate the dose of fluids to effect and hopefully avoid the pitfalls associated with cardiopulmonary fluid overload.

RECOMMENDED FURTHER READING

DiBartola SP (2006) *Fluid, Electrolyte, and Acid–Base Disorders in Small Animal Practice*, 3rd edn. WB Saunders, Philadelphia.

Silverstein DC, Hopper K (2015) *Small Animal Critical Care Medicine*, 2nd edn. Saunders Elsevier, St. Louis.

Chapter 24

Pain management

Steven M. Fox

INTRODUCTION

Pain management has become one of the most inspiring contemporary issues in veterinary medicine. It is an area of progressive research, revealing new perceptions on an almost daily basis. Accordingly, 'current' insights into pain management is a relative term. In some respects the management of pain, especially in companion animal practice, is more thorough than in human medicine. It is worth noting that most pain in humans is managed based on rodent data, while considerable direction for managing pain in animals is based on human data. This is because many physiologic systems are similar across species, and large population studies often conducted in human medicine require resources prohibitive in veterinary medicine. Therefore, evidence-based veterinary pain management will likely always be under some degree of scrutiny.

The frontier of discovery for treating pain is founded on an understanding of physiology. Physiologic mechanisms underpin the quality of evidence supporting treatment protocols and provide insights for new drug development. An overview of pain physiology is intellectually intriguing but extensive. Therefore, the following synopsis is selected to gain an appreciation of the complex mechanisms underlying pain and to encourage lateral thinking with regard to treatment modalities. To paraphrase Albert Einstein: "some things can be made simple, but only so much so before they lose meaning".

UNDERSTANDING THE PHYSIOLOGY OF PAIN

Nociception is the transduction, conduction, and central nervous system (CNS) processing of signals generated by a noxious insult. The conscious, cognitive processing of nociception results in pain (i.e. pain infers consciousness). It is reasonable to assume that a stimulus considered painful to a human, that is damaging or potentially damaging to tissues, and evokes escape and behavioral responses would also be painful to an animal, because anatomic structures and neurophysiologic processes leading to the perception of pain are very similar across species.

The pain pathway

The pain pathway (**Figure 24.1**) suggests reference to the simplistic nociceptive pathways of a three-neuron chain, with the first-order neuron originating in the periphery and projecting to the spinal cord, the second-order neuron ascending the spinal cord, and the third-order neuron projecting into the cerebral cortex and other supraspinal structures. 'For every complex issue, there is an answer that is simple, neat… and wrong!' Pain is not a stimulus. There are no 'pain fibers' in nerves and no 'pain pathways' in the brain. The experience of pain is the final product of a complex information-processing network.

The existence of a specific pain modulatory system was first clearly articulated in 1965 by Melzack and Wall in the gate control theory of pain (**Figure 24.2**). This was the first theory to propose that the CNS controls nociception. The basic premises of the gate control theory of pain are that activity in large (non-nociceptive) fibers can inhibit the perception of activity in small (nociceptive) fibers and that descending activity from the brain can also inhibit that perception.

Transcutaneous electrical nerve stimulation (TENS) is a clinical implementation of the gate theory. TENS is thought to act by preferential stimulation of peripheral

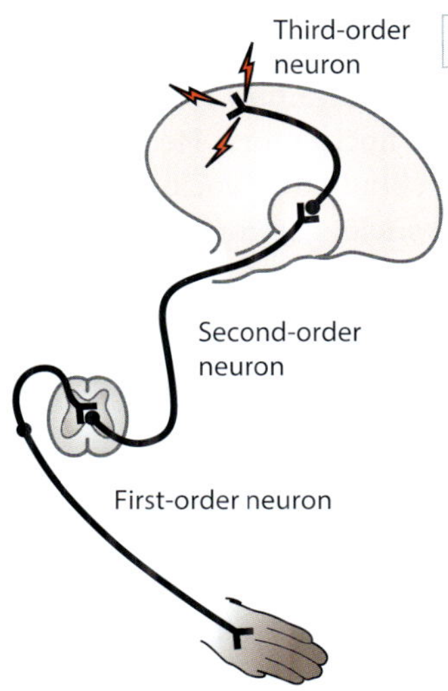

Figure 24.1 Simplified representation of the afferent pain pathway. (Adapted from Tranquilli WJ, Grimm KA, LA Lamont (2000) *Pain Management for the Small Animal Practitioner*. Teton New Media, Jackson.)

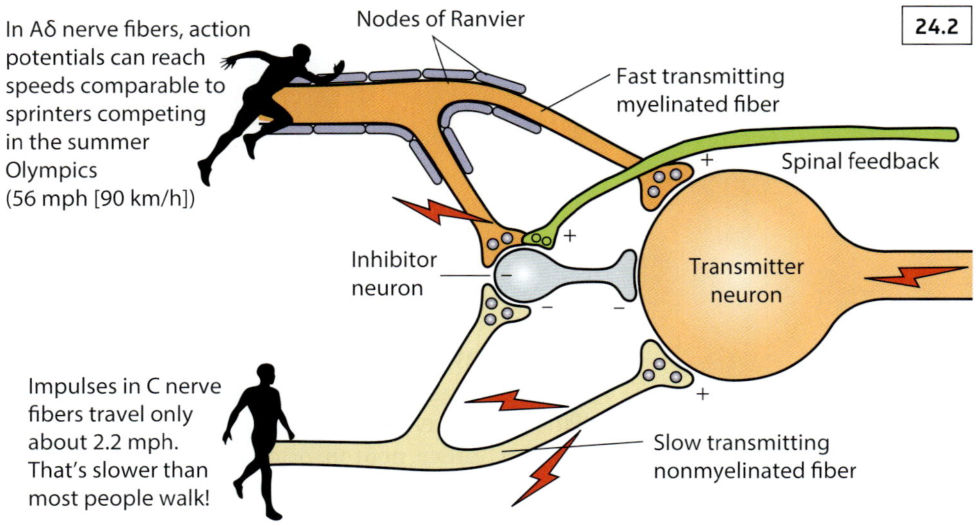

Figure 24.2 Melzack and Wall's Gate Theory of pain. Signals conducted through the fast-transmitting myelinated fiber reach the inhibitor neuron faster than signals from the slow-transmitting unmyelinated fiber. The inhibitor neuron then shuts down the transmitter neuron, rendering the signal from the slow-transmitting unmyelinated fiber ineffective.

somatosensory fibers, which conduct more rapidly than nociceptive fibers. This results in a stimulation of inhibitory interneurons in the second lamina of the posterior horn (substantia gelatinosa) that effectively blocks nociception at the spinal cord level. Furthermore, the gate theory may explain why some people feel a decrease in pain intensity when skin near the pain region is rubbed with a hand, and how a local area is 'desensitized' by rubbing prior to insertion of a needle.

Hyperalgesia

Peripheral neural mechanisms of pain from noxious stimuli are only one aspect of pain sensibility. There is an additional dynamic plasticity of great biological importance that relates to stimulus intensity and sensation: the phenomenon of hyperalgesia.

Hyperalgesia is defined as a leftward shift of the stimulus–response function that relates magnitude of pain to stimulus intensity (**Figure 24.3**) and is a consistent feature of somatic and visceral tissue injury and inflammation. Hyperalgesia to both heat and mechanical stimulus that occurs at the site of an injury is due to sensitization of primary afferent nociceptors. Mechanisms of the phenomenon have been studied in various tissues including the joint, cornea, testicle, gastrointestinal (GI) tract, and bladder. Hyperalgesia at the site of injury is termed primary hyperalgesia, while hyperalgesia in the uninjured tissue surrounding the injury is termed secondary hyperalgesia.

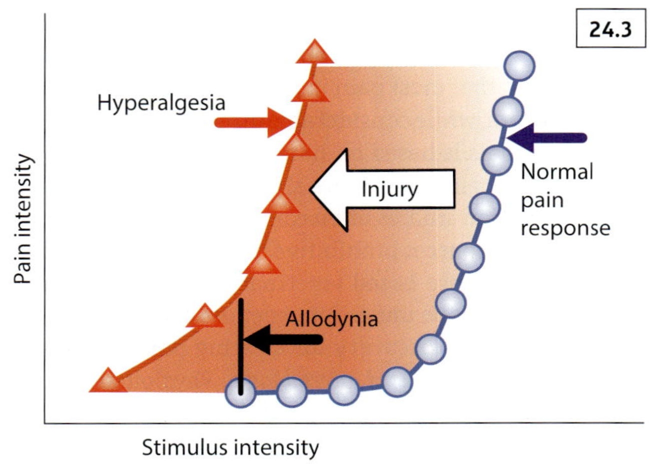

Figure 24.3 Hyperalgesia is a leftward shift of the stimulus/intensity curve.

WHY DOES IT KEEP HURTING?

An important tenet underlies enhanced response of the CNS to mechanical stimuli of cutaneous injury: 'the peripheral signal for pain does not reside exclusively with nociceptors; under pathologic circumstances, other receptor types, which are normally associated with the sensation of touch, acquire the capacity to evoke pain'. This principle applies to secondary hyperalgesia, as well as to neuropathic pain states in general. Central sensitization is the term denoting augmentation of responsiveness of central pain-signaling neurons to input from low-threshold mechanoreceptors; it is central sensitization that plays the major role in secondary hyperalgesia, not peripheral sensitization. This underlines the value of local anesthetic blocks. When the CNS is spared the input of nociceptors at the time of the acute insult, the hyperalgesia does not develop.

Injured nerve fibers develop ectopic sensitivity. A substantial proportion of C fiber afferents are nociceptors, and abnormal spontaneous activity has been observed in A fibers and C fibers originating from neuronal-resultant nerve transections. In patients with hyperalgesic neuromas, locally anesthetizing the neuroma often eliminates the pain.

Nociceptor activity induces increased sympathetic discharge. In certain painful patients, nociceptors acquire sensitivity to noradrenaline released by sympathetic efferents. Pain dependent on activity in the sympathetic nervous system is referred to as sympathetically maintained pain. In human studies of stump neuromas and skin, it is concluded that apparently sympathetically maintained pain does not arise from too much adrenaline, but rather from the presence of adrenergic receptors that are coupled to nociceptors. In sympathetically maintained pain, nociceptors develop α-adrenergic sensitivity such that the release of noradrenaline by the sympathetic nervous system produces spontaneous activity in the nociceptors. This spontaneous activity maintains the CNS in a sensitized state. Therefore, in sympathetically maintained pain, noradrenaline that normally is released from the sympathetic terminals acquires the capacity to evoke pain. In the presence of a sensitized central pain-signaling neuron (second order), pain in response to light touch is signaled by activity in low-threshold mechanoreceptors – allodynia. Alpha-1 adrenergic antagonists would lessen the nociceptor activity and the resultant hyperalgesia.

The predominant neurotransmitter used by all primary afferent fibers is glutamate, although other excitatory transmitters, notably adenosine triphosphate (ATP), act to depolarize dorsal horn neurons directly or on presynaptic autoreceptors to enhance glutamate release during action potential firing. Primary afferents, unique in their capacity to release neurotransmitters peripherally and so underlie neurogenic inflammation, convey information to the CNS. In the dorsal horn, peptides such as substance P impact on postsynaptic dorsal horn neurons, thus setting the gain or magnitude of the nociceptive response.

Following thermal, mechanical, or chemical stimulation of primary afferents, the excitatory event must initiate a regenerative action potential involving voltage-gated sodium, calcium, or potassium channels, culminating in neurotransmitter release if sensory information is to be conveyed from the periphery to the spinal cord dorsal horn. Within the dorsal horn, the CNS 'decides' if the message lives or dies. The hypersensitization of windup is testimonial that the CNS dorsal horn is dynamic, and the important role of these voltage-gated ion channels makes them attractive targets for novel and selective analgesics.

Windup

Windup is a form of activity-dependent plasticity characterized by a progressive increase in action potential output from dorsal horn neurons elicited during the course of a train of repeated low-frequency C fiber or nociceptor stimuli. Repetitive discharge of primary afferent nociceptors results in co-release of neuromodulators such as substance P and calcitonin gene-related peptide (CGRP), together with glutamate (the main neurotransmitter used by nociceptors synapsing with the dorsal horn) from nociceptor central terminals. These neuropeptides activate postsynaptic G-protein-coupled receptors, which leads to slow postsynaptic depolarizations lasting tens of seconds. Resultant cumulative depolarization is boosted by recruitment of N-methyl-D-aspartate (NMDA) receptor current through inhibition of Mg^{2+} channel suppression.

The most involved receptor in the sensation of acute pain, alpha-amino-3-hydroxy-5-methyl-isoxazole-4-proprionic acid (AMPA), is always exposed on afferent nerve terminals. In contrast, those most involved in the sensation of chronic pain, NMDA receptors, are not functional unless there has been a persistent or large scale release of glutamate. Repeated activation of AMPA receptors dislodges magnesium ions, which act like stoppers in transmembrane sodium and calcium channels of the NMDA receptor complex (**Figure 24.4**). Calcium flowing into the cell activates protein kinase C, the enzyme needed for nitric oxide (NO) synthase production of NO. NO diffuses through the dorsal cell membrane and synaptic cleft into the nociceptor and stimulates guanyl synthase-induced closure of K^+ channels. Since endorphins and enkephalins inhibit pain by opening these channels, closure induces opioid resistance. NO also stimulates the release of substance P, which by binding to neurokinin-1 receptors in the dorsal horn membrane, triggers c-fos gene expression and promotes neural remodeling and hypersensitization. Accompanying this windup, less glutamate is required to transmit the pain signal and more antinociceptive input is required for analgesia. Endorphins cannot keep up with their demand and essentially lose their effectiveness. The clinical implications are underappreciated. Inadequately treated pain is a much more important cause of opioid tolerance than use of opioids themselves. NMDA activation can also cause neural cells to sprout new connective endings.

The dorsal horn of the spinal cord is organized into lamellae comprised of dorsal horn neurons and the inhibitory and excitatory synaptic connections they receive and make (**Figure 24.5**). Non-neural glial cells – the oligodendrocytes, astrocytes, and microglia – modulate the operation of these neuronal circuits. A key feature of the somatosensory system, modifiability or plasticity, resides in the dorsal horn. Neuronal information processing is not fixed, but is instead dynamic, changing in a manner that is dependent on levels of neuronal excitability and synaptic strength, profoundly diversifying for either a short period (seconds) or prolonged periods (days),

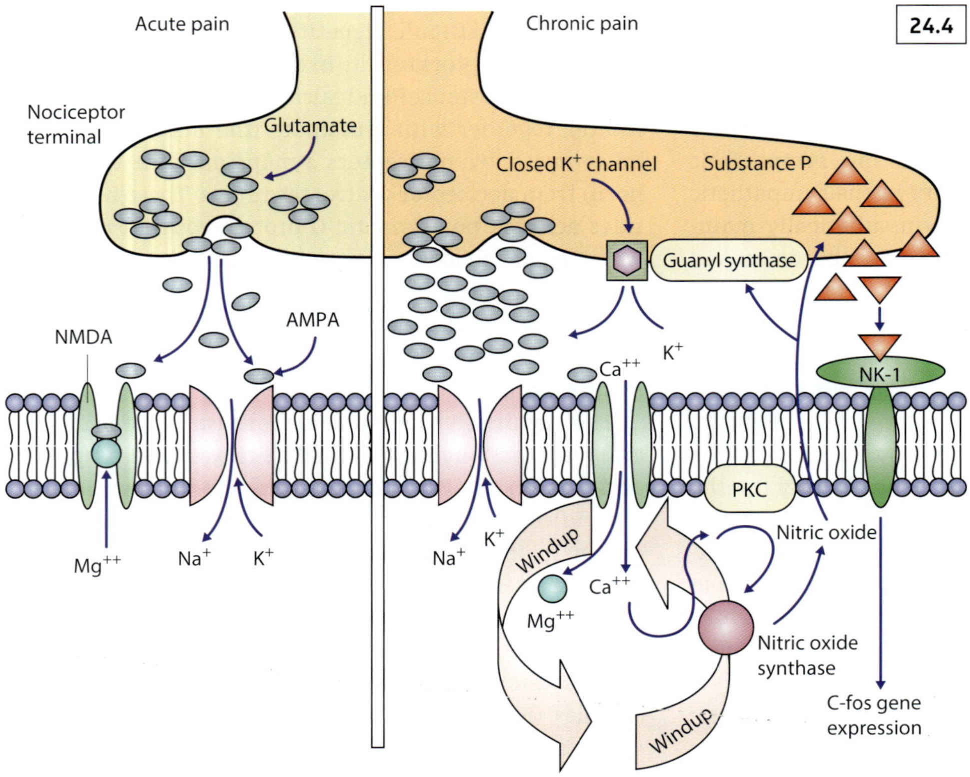

Figure 24.4 The NMDA receptor is a primary player in CNS 'windup'. In chronic pain, which involves the massive release of glutamate, the magnesium plug of the NMDA receptor is dislodged, allowing an intercellular increase of calcium, which stimulates the cell to a heightened state of transmission.

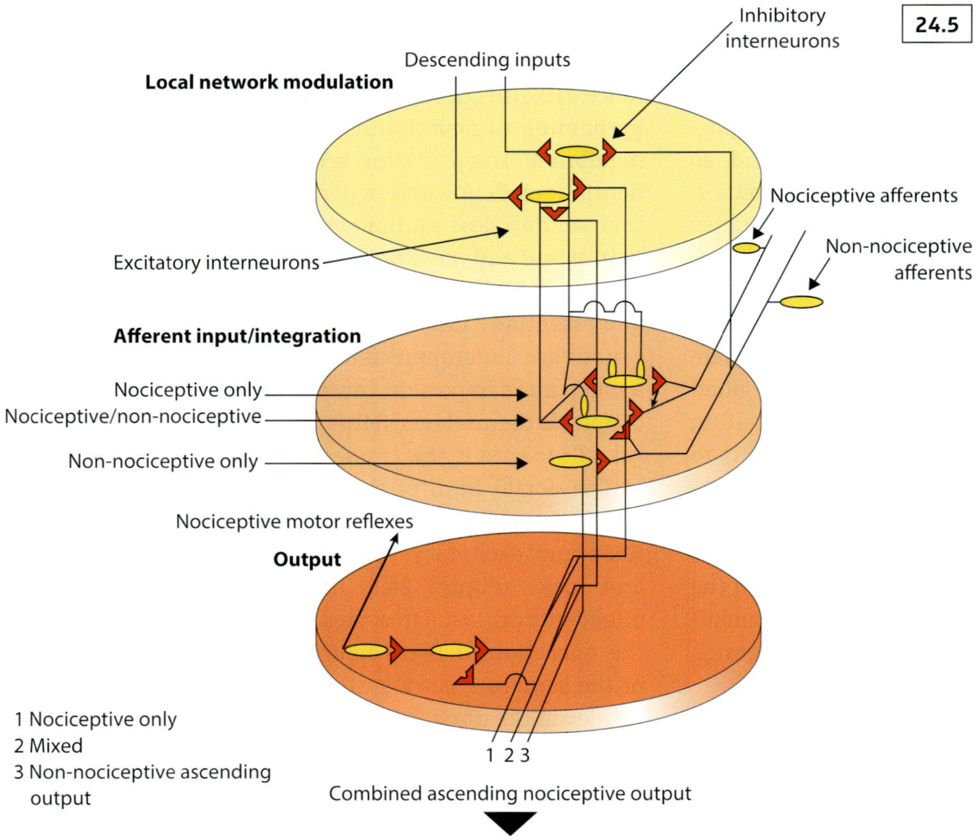

Figure 24.5 Schematic organization of dorsal horn input, output, and local modulatory networks.

or perhaps indefinitely. Spinal cord transmissions work as a binary response: low-intensity stimuli interpreted as innocuous or nonpainful (e.g. touch vibration or hair movement) versus high-threshold stimuli producing pain. Different responses are elicited depending on whether low- or high-threshold afferents have been activated, because of the different central circuits engaged.

Contributing to CNS plasticity is its capacity for structural reorganization of synaptic circuitry. Neurons may die, axon terminals may degenerate or atrophy, new axon terminals may appear, and the structural contact between cells at the synapses may be modified. This can result in the loss of normal connections, formation of novel abnormal connections, and an alteration in the normal balance between excitation and inhibition. Structural reorganization and its functional sequelae can result in changed sensory processing long after the initial injury has healed.

TYPES OF PAIN

Nociceptive pain

Everyday acute pain, or 'nociceptive pain,' occurs when a strong noxious stimulus (mechanical, thermal, or chemical) impacts the skin or deep tissue. In response to these stimuli, nociceptors, a special class of primary sensory nerve fibers, fire impulses that travel along the peripheral nerves, past the sensory cell bodies in the dorsal root ganglion (DRG), along the dorsal roots, and into the spinal cord (or brainstem).

Thereafter, the conscious brain interprets these transmissions from populations of second- and third-order neurons of the CNS. Acute pain is purposeful. It protects us from potentially severe tissue injury by noxious insults from everyday activities. Acute pain is also short acting and relatively easy to treat. Examples of nociceptive pain would be contact with a hot object, a painful toe pinch, or a chemical burn.

Postoperative, incisional pain

Postoperative, incisional pain is a specific and common form of acute pain. Studies in rodents have characterized the primary hyperalgesia to mechanical and thermal stimuli. Primary hyperalgesia to mechanical stimuli lasts for 2–3 days, while hyperalgesia to heat lasts longer – 6 or 7 days after plantar incision. The secondary hyperalgesia is present only to mechanical, not thermal stimuli. Conversion of mechanically insensitive silent nociceptors to mechanically responsive fibers is thought to play an important role in the maintenance of primary mechanical hyperalgesia, while release of ATP from injured cells is considered to play an important role in the induction of post-skin incision mechanical allodynia. The incision-induced spontaneous activity in primary afferent fibers helps to maintain the sensitized state of wide dynamic range neurons of the dorsal horn, in contrast to other forms of cutaneous injury where hyperalgesia is NMDA dependent.

It is important to note that adequate levels of general anesthesia with a volatile drug such as isoflurane do not prevent central sensitization. The potential for central sensitization exists even in unconscious patients who appear to be clinically unresponsive to surgical stimuli (**Figure 24.6**). This has been validated in the dog where

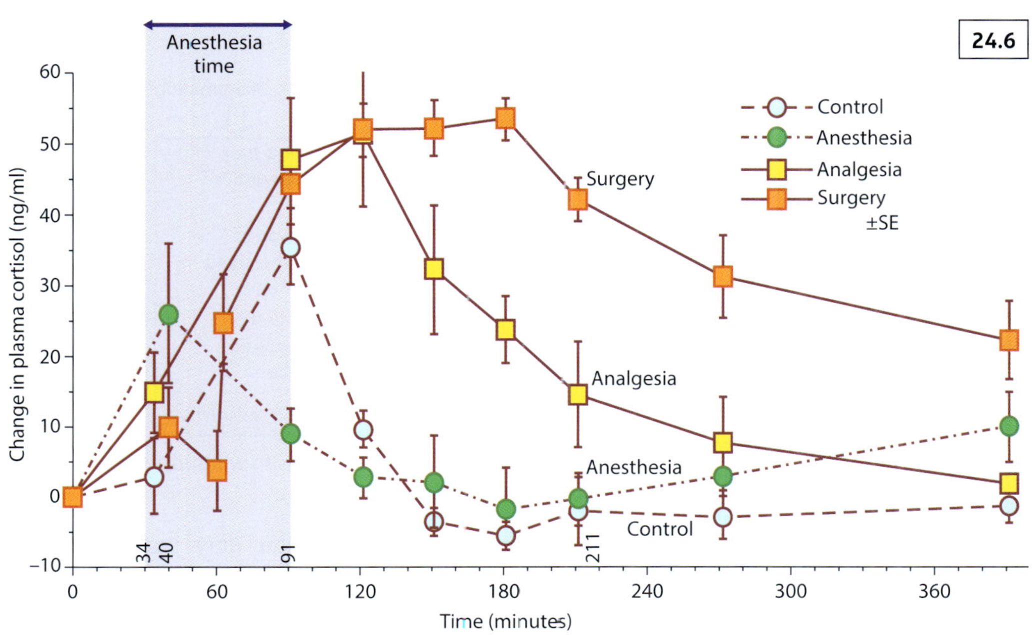

Figure 24.6 Changes in plasma cortisol concentrations from pretreatment values. Although dogs may be at a surgical plane of anesthesia, the noxious stimuli of surgery are still conducted, as assessed by pain-induced cortisol responses. (Adapted from Fox SM, Mellor DJ, Firth EC *et al.* (1994) Changes in plasma cortisol concentrations before, during and after analgesia, anaesthesia and anaesthesia plus ovariohysterectomy in bitches. *Res Vet Sci* **57**:110–118.)

cortisol spikes in response to ovariohysterectomy noxious stimuli occur during the anesthetic period.

Inflammatory pain

Inflammatory pain, often classed along with acute pain as 'nociceptive,' refers to spontaneous pain and tenderness felt when the skin or other tissue is inflamed, hot, red, and swollen (e.g. infection). The inflammatory process is mediated and facilitated by the local release of numerous inflammatory mediators. When there is tissue injury and inflammation, the firing threshold of the Aδ and C nociceptive afferents in response to heating of the skin is lowered into the non-noxious range. This is a result of prostaglandin production from cyclo-oxygenase (COX) activity in the arachidonic acid cascade, which acts directly on the peripheral terminals of the Aδ and C fibers, lowering their threshold to thermal (but not electrical) stimuli.

Release of substance P and nerve growth factor (NGF) into the periphery causes a tissue reaction termed neurogenic inflammation, which can occur in any neuropathic pain state (**Figure 24.7**). Neurogenic inflammation is driven by events in the CNS and does not depend on granulocytes or lymphocytes, as with the classic inflammatory response to tissue trauma or immune-mediated cell damage. Cells in the dorsal horn release chemicals that cause action potentials to fire backwards down the nociceptors. The result of this dorsal root reflex is that nociceptive dendrites release substance P and CGRP into peripheral tissues, causing degranulation of mast cells and changing vascular endothelial cell characteristics. The resultant outpouring of potent inflammatory and vasodilatating agents causes edema and potentiates transmission of nociceptive signals from the periphery.

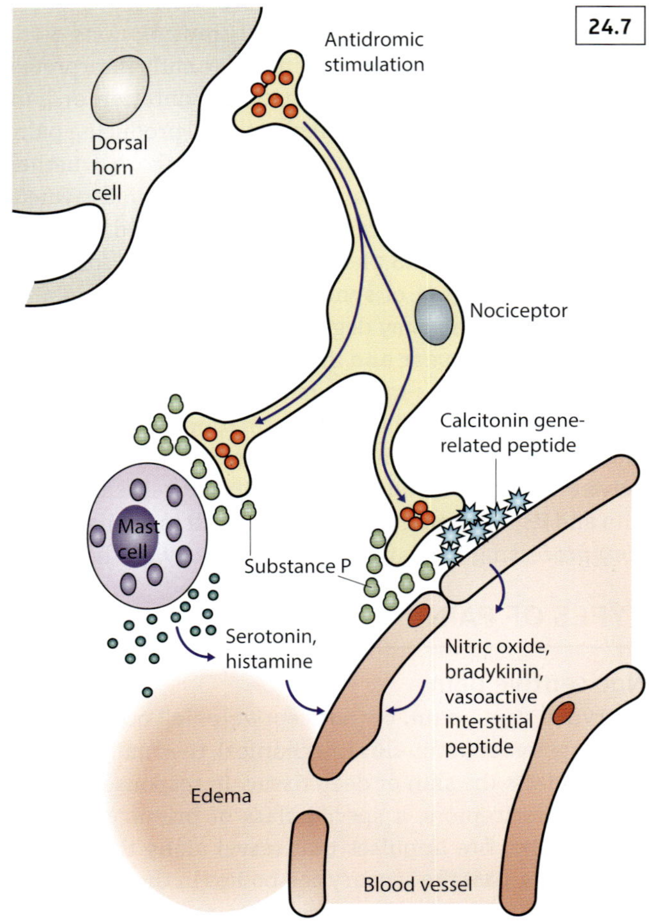

Figure 24.7 Neurogenic inflammation involves an antidromic firing of neurons (action potentials fire backwards down the nociceptors). Packets of chemicals located at the peripheral terminals are released. Thereafter, pain signals from peripheral nerves are heightened and the cycle of chronic pain is continued.

CHRONIC PAIN

Chronic pain can result from sustained noxious stimuli, such as ongoing inflammation, or it may be independent of the inciting cause (**Figure 24.8**). Regardless of its etiology, chronic pain (e.g. osteoarthritis, cancer, or chronic otitis) is maladaptive and offers no useful biologic function or survival advantage. The nervous system itself actually becomes the focus of the pathology and contributes to patient morbidity. Effective treatment for chronic pain can be an enigma. A number of studies have shown that the longer a pain lingers, the harder it is to eradicate. This is because pain can reconfigure the architecture of the nervous system it invades (**Figure 24.9**).

In contrast to acute pain, where the pain stops quickly after the noxious stimulus has been removed, the pain

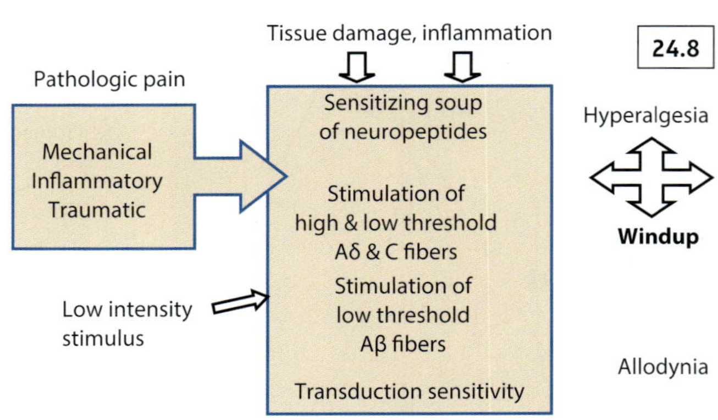

Figure 24.8 Chronic pain often leads to windup, with hyperalgesia and allodynia.

and tenderness of inflammation may last for hours, days, months, or years. Recognition of the potential peripheral mediators of peripheral sensitization after

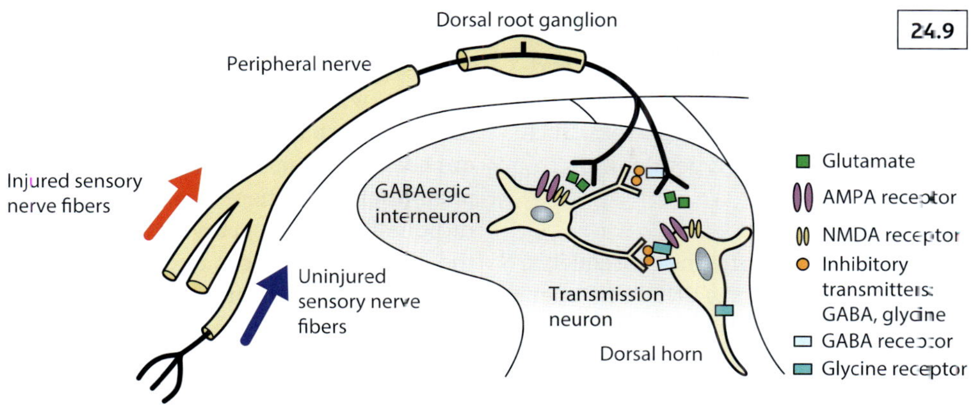

Figure 24.9 Peripheral nerve injury leads to a number of changes in the peripheral nervous system as well as the central nervous system. Peripheral nerve injury causes (1) spontaneous activity in primary sensory afferents; (2) changes in the production and distribution of membrane receptors and ion channels; (3) phenotypic shift of sensory neurons; (4) shrinkage and loss of distal nerve stump; (5) sprouting of sympathetic nerve fibers; (6) invasion and activation of immune cells. In the spinal cord peripheral nerve injury causes (1) central sensitization; (2) synaptic reorganization; (3) loss of GABAergic inhibition; (4) downregulation of rapid receptors; (5) activation of microglia.

inflammation gives an insight as to the complexity of this process. A second type of persistent, or chronic, pain is neuropathic pain, which arises from injury to the peripheral nervous system (PNS) or CNS. Neuropathic pain can be a sequela to any pain state, especially pain that has been allowed to 'windup' the CNS. Chronic pain appears to have no purpose, is characterized by extended duration, and is frequently difficult to treat.

ACUTE TO CHRONIC PAIN

Normally, a steady state is maintained in which there is a close correlation between injury and pain. However, long-lasting or very intense nociceptive input or the removal of a portion of the normal input can distort the nociceptive system to such an extent that the close correlation between injury and pain can be lost. A progression from acute to chronic pain might be considered as three major stages or phases of pain, proposing that different neurophysiologic mechanisms are involved depending on the nature and time course of the originating stimulus (**Figure 24.10**). These three phases are: (1) the processing of a brief noxious stimulus; (2) the consequences of prolonged noxious stimulation, leading to tissue damage and peripheral inflammation; and (3) the consequences of neurologic damage, including peripheral neuropathies and central pain states.

Phase 1: acute nociceptive pain

Mechanisms underlying the processing of brief noxious stimuli are fairly simple, with direct route of transmission centrally toward the thalamus and cortex

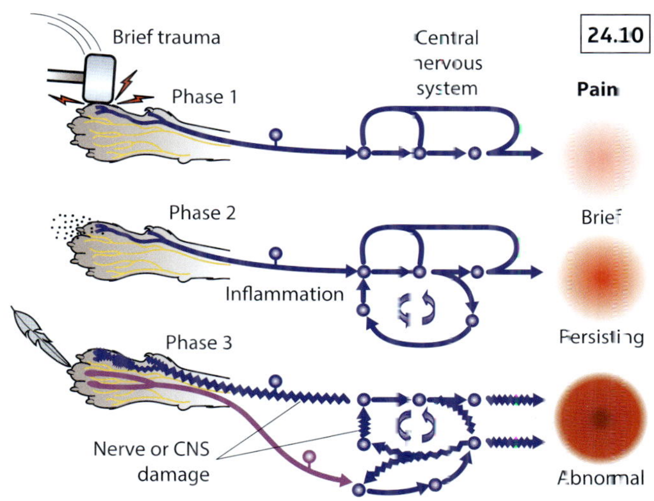

Figure 24.10 The three major stages or phases of pain.

resulting in the conscious perception of pain, with the possibility for modulation occurring at synaptic relays along the way. It is reasonably easy to construct plausible and detailed neuronal circuits to explain the features of phase 1 pain.

Phase 2: inflammatory pain

If a noxious stimulus is very intense or prolonged, leading to tissue damage and inflammation, it might be considered phase 2 pain, as influenced by response properties of various components of the nociceptive system changing. These changes signify that the CNS has moved to a new, more excitable state as a result of the noxious input generated by tissue injury and inflammation. Phase 2 is characterized by its central drive, a drive that is triggered and maintained by peripheral inputs. Patients experience spontaneous pain and sensation changes evoked by stimulation of the injured and surrounding areas. Such change is known as hyperalgesia (see Hyperalgesia).

Phase 3: neuropathic pain

Phase 3 pain is abnormal pain, generally the consequence of damage to peripheral nerves or to the CNS itself, characterized by a lack of correlation between injury and pain. Clinically, phase 1 and 2 pains are symptoms of peripheral injury, whereas phase 3 pain is a symptom of neurologic disease. These pains are spontaneous, triggered by innocuous stimuli, or are exaggerated responses to minor noxious stimuli. A particular combination of mechanisms responsible for each of the pain states is likely unique to the individual disease or to a particular subgroup of patients. Phase 3 pain may involve genetic, cognitive, or thalamic processing that has yet to be identified. Activation of these mechanisms may be abnormally prolonged or intense due to abnormal input from damaged neurons, or simply because the regenerative properties of neurons are very poor or 'misdirected'. Healing may never occur.

NEUROPATHIC PAIN

The International Association for the Study of Pain defines neurogenic pain as 'pain initiated or caused by a primary lesion or dysfunction or transitory perturbation in the peripheral or central nervous system'. Due to potential vagaries within this definition, simplistically, neuropathic pain can be identified as pain due to a primary lesion of the PNS or CNS. Neuropathic pain is divided from diseases with demonstrable neural lesions in the PNS and CNS and conditions with no tangible lesion of major nerves. Therefore, there are ambiguities in identifying neuropathic diseases and currently no tests are available that can unequivocally diagnose neuropathic pain. Nevertheless, a large body of evidence validates the physiologic process of neuropathic pain.

The relative role of peripheral and central mechanisms in neuropathic pain is not well understood and likely reflects different disease states and genetic differences; however, the abnormal input of neural activity from nociceptor afferents plays a dynamic and ongoing role in maintaining the pain state. Two key concepts are central to an understanding of neuropathic pain: (1) inappropriate activity in nociceptive fibers (injured and uninjured); and (2) central changes in sensory processing that arise from these abnormalities.

CANCER PAIN

Because we are practicing better medicine in more patients, our patients are living longer. Consequently, we are seeing a higher prevalence of cancer in our patient population, and there is an increased focus on improving quality of life. Many patients present with pain as the first sign of cancer, and 30–50% of all human cancer patients will experience moderate to severe pain. Life-altering cancer-induced pain will be experienced by 75–95% of human patients with metastatic or advanced cancer. Insights from cancer pain in humans are valuable because animals cannot talk. Recently, the first animal model of cancer pain has been developed. This is the mouse femur model, where bone cancer pain is induced by injecting murine osteolytic sarcoma cells into the intramedullary space of the femur.

Tumor cells and tumor-associated cells secrete a variety of factors that sensitize or directly excite primary afferent neurons (i.e. prostaglandins, endothelins, interleukins 1 and 6, epidermal growth factor, transforming growth factor, and platelet-derived growth factor). Identification of these factors provides potential blocking strategies for treatment. One such strategy is treatment with selective COX-2 nonsteroidal anti-inflammatory drugs (NSAIDs). COX-2 inhibitors (coxib-class NSAIDs) are currently used to inhibit inflammation and pain. Further, experiments suggest that coxibs may have the added advantage of reducing the growth and metastasis of the cancer.

Endothelin-1 is a second pharmacologic target for cancer pain. Clinical studies in humans have shown a correlation between prostatic cancer pain and plasma levels of endothelins. Similar to prostaglandins, endothelins that are released from tumor cells are also thought to be involved in regulating angiogenesis and tumor growth.

A hallmark of tissue injury is local acidosis, and tumor cells become ischemic and apoptotic as the tumor burden exceeds its vascular supply. Transient receptor potential vanilloid-1 (TRPV1) and acid-sensing ion channel (ASIC)-3 are expressed by nociceptors and are sensitized by the acidic tumor environment. This is likely accentuated by osteolytic tumors where there is a persistent extracellular microenvironment of acidic pH at the osteoclast and mineralized bone interface. Studies have shown that osteoprotegerin and a bisphosphonate, both of which induce osteoclast apoptosis, are effective in decreasing osteoclast-induced bone cancer pain.

To appreciate the complexity of cancer pain is to understand that the biochemical and physiologic status of sensory neurons is a reflection of factors derived from the innervated tissue, and therefore changes in the periphery associated with inflammation, nerve injury, or tissue injury influence changes in the phenotypes of sensory neurons. NGFs and glial-derived neurotrophic factor influence such changes. The medley of growth factors to which the sensory neuron is exposed will change as the growing tumor invades the peripheral tissue innervating the neuron. With the potential for changing phenotype and response characteristics, it is understandable that the same tumor in the same individual may be painful at one site of metastasis but not at another. It follows that different patients with the same cancer may have vastly different symptoms.

As the tumor state progresses, changing factors may complicate the cancer pain state. In the mouse model of bone cancer, as the tumor cells begin to proliferate, pain-related behaviors precede any noticeable bone destruction. This is attributed to pro-hyperalgesic factors such as active nociceptor response in the marrow to prostaglandins and endothelins released from growing tumor cells. At this point, pain might be attenuated by a coxib-class NSAID or endothelin antagonist. With continued tumor growth, sensory neurons innervating the marrow are compressed and destroyed, giving rise to neuropathic pain, possibly responsive to gabapentin. Once the tumor becomes invaded by osteoclastic activity, pain might be largely blocked by anti-osteoclastogenic drugs such as bisphosphonates or osteoprotegerin. As the intramedullary space becomes filled with dying tumor cells, generating an acidic environment, TRPV1 or ASIC antagonists may attenuate the pain. In the later stages of bone destruction, antagonists to the mechanically gated channels and/or ATP receptors in the highly innervated periosteum may alleviate movement-evoked pain. This scenario illustrates how a mechanistic approach to designing more effective therapies for cancer pain should be created, based on an understanding of how different stages of the disease impact on tumor cell influence on nociceptors, and how phenotypes of nociceptors and CNS neurons involved in nociceptive transmission change with the course of the disease process.

Clearly, the mechanisms associated with pain are complex. However, only through an understanding of these mechanisms can we best manage our patient's pain with an evidence-based confidence.

PRE-EMPTIVE ANALGESIA

Pain memories imprinted within the CNS, mediated by NMDA receptors, produce hyperalgesia and contribute to allodynia (**Figure 24.11**). In several animal experiments, c-fos expression (the c-fos gene serves as a marker for

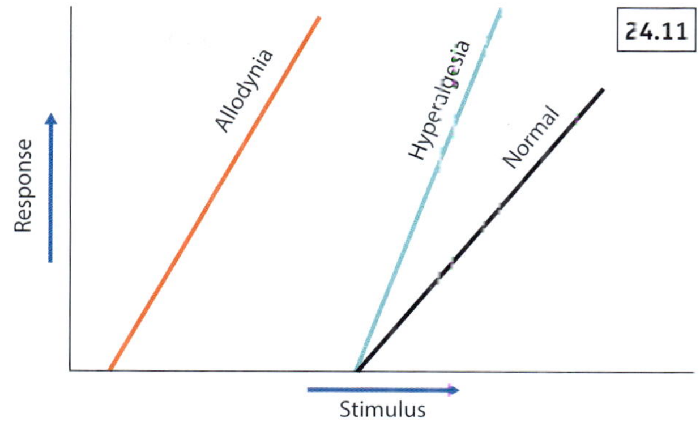

Figure 24.11 Graphic representation of normal pain, hyperalgesia, and allodynia showing response relative to stimulus.

cellular activation [i.e. nociception]), central sensitization, and windup do not occur if nociceptive blockade is applied prior to the nociceptive event. Such findings suggest that presurgical blockade of nociception may prevent postsurgical wound pain or pain hypersensitivity in clinical surgery (i.e. pre-emptive analgesia, as advocated by the eminent pain physiologist Patrick Wall). Successful pre-emptive analgesia must meet three criteria: (1) deep enough to block all nociception; (2) wide enough to cover the entire surgical area; and (3) prolonged enough to last throughout surgery and even into the postoperative period.

Professor Wall introduced the concept of pre-emptive analgesia to clinicians in his editorial in the journal *Pain* in 1988. The emphasis of pre-emptive analgesia is to prevent sensitization of the nervous system throughout the perioperative period. Pain can be expected from an initial surgery and the hypersensitivity that subsequently develops. Analgesia administered after sensitization may decrease pain somewhat, but it has little long-term benefit in addressing the pain resulting from postsurgical inflammation. Analgesia administered before surgery limits the pain from that stimulus and decreases subsequent hypersensitivity; however, the most effective pre-emptive analgesic regimen is initiated before surgery and continued throughout the postoperative period (**Figure 24.12**) (i.e. 'preventive analgesia'). A review of pre-emptive analgesia, with inclusion of suggested drugs and dosage, has been provided elsewhere (see Recommended further reading). A logical pre-emptive drug protocol would include an opioid alpha-2 agonist ± an NMDA antagonist and an NSAID. The implementation of perioperative NSAID therapy is controversial based on their antiprostaglandin effect, which, in the face of hypotension, might enhance the potential for acute kidney injury. This is why perioperative fluid support is such an important consideration.

However, anti-inflammatory drugs play a substantial role in perioperative pain management because surgery cannot be performed without subsequent inflammation, and reducing the inflammatory response in the periphery, and thereby decreasing sensitization of the peripheral nociceptors, should attenuate central sensitization. It has also been recognized for some time that NSAIDs synergistically interact with both mu-opioid and alpha-2 adrenoceptor agonists. In human medicine the use of NSAIDs has reduced the use of patient-controlled analgesic morphine by between 40 and 60%.

PAIN ASSESSMENT

Pain management is a cardinal example of integrating the science of veterinary medicine with the art of veterinary practice. New graduate veterinarians are well schooled in the science, whereas the art comes only with experience. This is particularly true in managing pain, because pain is a subjective phenomenon. In humans, pain is what the patient says it is, whereas in animals, pain is what the assessor says it is! Because pain is subjective, an abstract, multi-attribute construct similar to intelligence or anxiety, pain management does not lend itself to a 'cookbook' approach. For example, following surgery, if the dog is lying quietly in its cage, is it doing so because it is very content, or because it is too painful to move? Furthermore, trained as scientists, veterinarians are schooled to assess responses based on the mean ± standard deviation, yet effective pain management suggests we target the least respondent patient within the population, so as to ensure no patient is denied the relief it needs and deserves.

There are many clues the attentive assessor may note that will suggest that an animal is in pain (**Table 24.1**).

As a rule of thumb, any change in behavior can signal pain; however, the most reliable indicator of pain is response to an analgesic. Physiologic parameters including heart rate, respiratory rate, blood pressure, and temperature are not consistent or reliable indicators of pain.

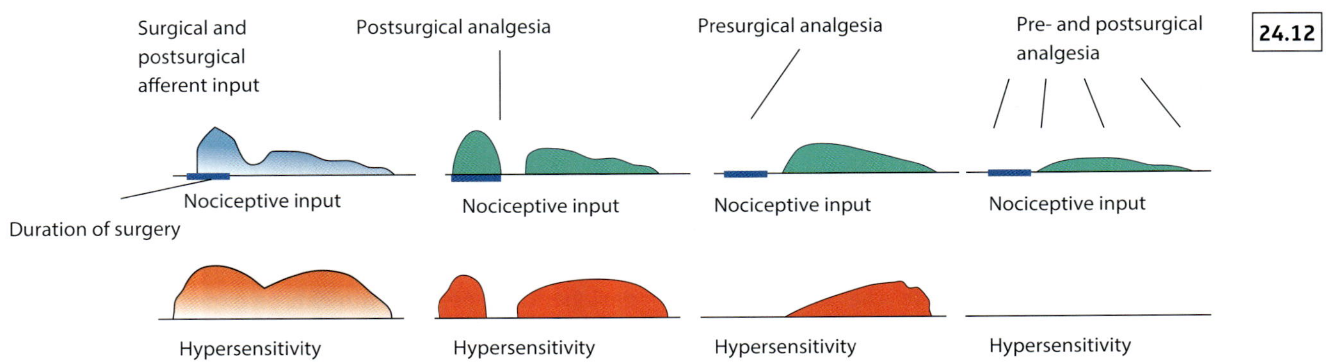

Figure 24.12 The benefits of pre-emptive analgesia are best appreciated when it is implemented as part of a perioperative analgesia protocol.

Table 24.1 Characteristics associated with pain in cats and dogs. (Modified from Mathews KA (2000) Management of pain. *Vet Clin North Am Small Anim Pract* **30(4)**:729–752.)

Characteristic	Example
Abnormal posture	Hunched up guarding or splinting of abdomen. 'Praying' position (forequarters on ground, hindquarters in air) Sitting or lying in an abnormal position. Not resting in a normal position
Abnormal gait	Stiff No to partial weight bearing on injured limb Slight to obvious limp
Abnormal movement	Thrashing Restless Inactivity when awake Escape behavior

Table 24.1 Characteristics associated with pain in cats and dogs. (Modified from Mathews KA (2000) Management of pain. *Vet Clin North Am Small Anim Pract* **30(4)**:729–752.)

Characteristic	Example
Vocalization	Screaming Whining Crying None
Miscellaneous	Looking, licking, or chewing at painful area Hyperesthesia or hyperalgesia Allodynia Failure to stretch or 'wet dog shake' Failure to yawn Failure to use litterbox (cat)
*May also be associated with poor general health	Restless or agitated Trembling or shaking Tachypnea or panting Weak tail wag Low carriage of tail Depressed or poor response to care giver Head hangs down Not grooming Decreased or picky appetite Dull Lying quietly and not moving for long durations Stupor Urinates or defecates without attempt to move Recumbent and unaware of surroundings Unwilling or unable to walk Bites or attempts to bite care givers
May also be associated with apprehension or anxiety	Restless or agitated Trembling or shaking Tachypnea or panting Weak tail wag Low tail carriage Slow to rise Depressed Not grooming Bites or attempts to bite care giver Ears pulled back Restless Barking or growling Growling or hissing Sitting in back of cage or hiding (cat)
May be normal behavior	Eye movement, but reluctance to move head Stretching when abdomen touched Penile prolapse Licking a wound or incision
Physiologic signs that may be associated with pain	Tachypnea or panting Tachycardia Dilated pupils Hypertension Increased serum cortisol and epinephrine

Various acute pain assessment measures have been used by researchers to quantify pain. These include verbal rating scales, simple descriptive scales, numeric rating scales, and visual analog scales, all of which have their limitations. The historical limitation of scales used to assess pain has been assessment of pain on intensity alone. Such limitation has led to the development of multidimensional scales, taking into account the sensory and affective qualities of pain in addition to its intensity. The 'Glasgow Pain Scale' is such a multidimensional scheme and although it is detailed, its ongoing refinement may result in greater utilization. Currently, there are no 'scales' to assess chronic pain. Several investigators have suggested exploring this area of interest through the creation of novel questionnaires as an instrument for measuring chronic pain in dogs through its impact on health-related quality of life.

Current methods of classifying pain are considered unsatisfactory by some for several reasons. Foremost is that pain syndromes are identified by parts of the body, duration, and causative agents, rather than the mechanism involved. The argument holds that anatomic differences should be disregarded in favor of mechanisms that apply to either particular tissues or all parts of the body, rather than a particular part of the body. For example, the term cancer pain relates only to the disease from which the patient suffers, not the mechanism of any pain the patient may experience. A mechanism-based approach is likely to lead to specific pharmacologic intervention measures for each identified mechanism within a syndrome. Advances in pain management are, therefore, contingent on first determining the symptoms that constitute a syndrome and then finding mechanisms for each of these. The clinical approach for a mechanism-based classification of pain is shown (**Figure 24.13**). This illustrates how a patient with pain could be analyzed from a pain mechanism perspective. It is the mechanism that needs to be the target for novel drugs rather than particular disease state. Herein lies the greatest potential for advancement in pain management (**Table 24.2**).

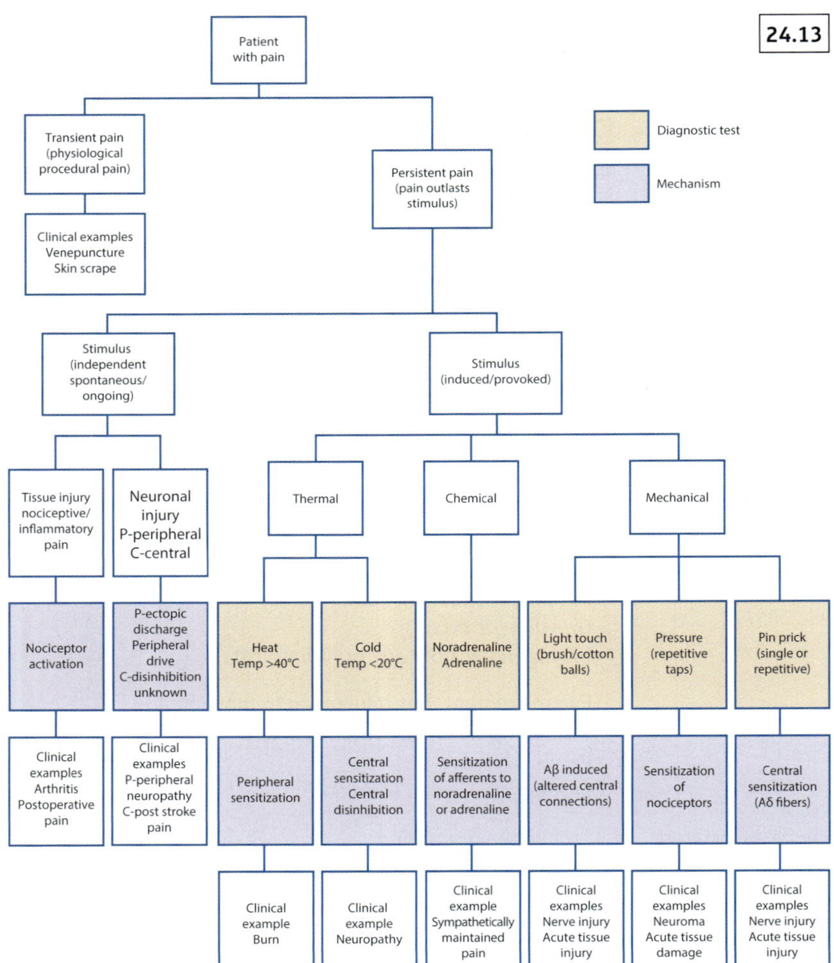

Figure 24.13 Clinical approach for a mechanism-based classification of pain.

Table 24.2 Characterization of various pain states.

Pain categories	Pain conditions	Pain mechanisms	Potential drug/ targets	Animal models	Proof-of-concept
Transient stimulus-induced pain (nociceptive pain)	Procedural pain (injections/minor injuries)	Nociceptor activation	VRs, Na+ -TTXs, MOR, nAChR	Thermosensitivity, mechanosensitivity, chemosensitivity	Minor surgical procedures
Tissue damage (inflammatory pain); spontaneous and provoked pain	Trauma/ postoperative pain; arthritis/infection	Nociceptor activation. Peripheral sensitization. Central sensitization. Phenotype switch	COX-2, EPR, 5-HTR, P_{2x}, BKR, IL-β, TNF-α, TrkA, TrkB, Na+-TTX-R, ASIC, α_2, MOR, DOR, A1, N-Ca^{2+}, NK1, nAChR, NMDA-R, GluR5, mGluR, PkCγ	Chemical irritants: capsaicin, mustard oil, formalin. Experimental inflammation: carageenan, UVB, Freund's adjuvant, cytokines/growth factors	Dental postoperative pain. Abdominal postoperative pain. Thoracotomy. Joint replacements. Osteoarthritis
Injury: primary afferent (neuropathic pain); spontaneous and provoked pain	Peripheral nerve injury; diabetic neuropathy (human); toxic neuropathy; postherpetic neuralgia (human)	Ectopic activity. Phenotype switch. Central sensitization. Structural reorganization. Disinhibition	Na+-TTXr/TTXs, α_2, NMDA-R, N-Ca^{2+}, PKCγ NGF/GDNF, GABA, AEAs, gabapentin, TCA, SNRIs	Peripheral nerve section. Partial nerve section. Loose ligatures. Experimental diabetes. Toxic neuropathies	Diabetic neuropathy (human). Postherpetic neuropathy (human). Radicular pain
Injury: central neuron (neuropathic pain); spontaneous and provoked pain	Spinal cord injury; stroke (humans)	Secondary ectopic activity. Disinhibition. Structural reorganization	GABA-R, Na+-TTXs, AEAs, TCA, SNRIs	Spinal cord injury. Ischemia. Central disinhibition (e.g. strychnine/ bicuculline)	Spinal cord injury
Unknown mechanism	Irritable bowel syndrome; fibromyalgia (humans)	? Altered gain	COX-2, NMDA-R, Na+ channels		Irritable bowel syndrome/ fibromyalgia

VRs, vallinoid receptors; Na+-TTXs, tetrodotoxin-sensitive sodium ion channels; MOR, μ-opiate receptors; nAChr, nicotine acetylcholine receptor; COX-2, inducible cyclo-oxygenase inhibitors; EPR, prostaglandin receptors; 5-HTR, serotonin receptors; P_{2x}, ligand-gated purino receptors/ion channels; BKR, bradykinin receptors; IL-β, interleukins; TNFα, tumor necrosis factor; TrkA, TrkB, high-affinity eurotrophin tyrosine kinase receptors; Na+-TTX-R, tetrodotoxin-resistant sodium ion channels; ASIC, acid-sensitive ion channels; α_2, adrenergic receptors; DOR, delta opiate receptors; A_1, adenosine receptors; N-Ca^{2+}, voltage-gated calcium ion channels; NK1, neurokinin receptors; NMDA-R, N-methyl-D-aspartic acid receptors; GluR5, kainate receptors; mGluR, metabotropic glutamate receptors; PKCγ, protein kinase C; NGF/GDNF, nerve growth factor, glial derived neurotropic factor; AEAs, antiepileptic agents, GABA-ergic compounds; TCA, tricyclic antidepressants; SNRIs, serotonin and norepinephrine reuptake inhibitors.

DRUG CLASSES

OPIOIDS

The World Health Organization's (WHO) proposed method for relief of cancer pain was originally published in 1986, with an update in 1996. The guidelines contain the WHO analgesic ladder, a simple yet effective method for controlling cancer pain, which, when used as described, can provide substantial relief of pain in 75–90% of human cancer patients. The WHO ladder advocates the use of three classes of analgesics: nonopioid, adjuvant, and opioid. This ladder has been embraced by many for treating pain in veterinary patients.

The analgesic effects of opium have been known for more than 5,000 years. Unfortunately, opioid abuse is limiting its use. Society has attempted to find a balance between licit and illicit use, therapeutic versus adverse effects, and medical needs and legal issues. Regardless of the legal, administrative, and social interference issues, no other class of drugs has remained in use for the treatment of pain for as long as opioids.

In common with spinal and supraspinal opioid receptors, the binding of opioid agonists results in K^+ channel-mediated neuronal hyperpolarization, attenuation of Ca^{2+} entry through voltage-gated Ca^{2+} channels, and reduced cAMP availability, with resultant reduction in nociceptor activity. However, morphine and other opioids do not have fixed actions, but operate on receptor mechanisms that are subject to alterations by other transmitters and receptors.

Knockout mice studies suggest that three opioid receptor types regulate distinct pain modalities:

- Mu receptors (OP3) influence responses to mechanical, chemical, and supraspinal thermal nociception.
- Kappa receptors (OP2) modify spinally-mediated nociception and chemical visceral pain.
- Delta receptors (OP1) increase mechanical nociception and inflammatory pain.

Although controversial, studies suggest that neuropathic pain due to peripheral nerve damage more often than not shows reduced sensitivity to opioids. This is attributable to a reduction of spinal opioid receptors, nonopioid receptor-expressing Aβ fiber-mediated allodynia, increased cholecystokinin antagonism of opioid actions, and NMDA-mediated dorsal horn neuronal hyperexcitability, likely requiring a greater opioid inhibitory counteraction.

Opioids are probably the best drugs available for small animal pain control, and one might argue that 'serious pain control' cannot be implemented without them. Morphine, oxymorphone, fentanyl, hydromorphone, and meperidine are opioid agonists acting mainly at the mu receptor, where they have a high affinity. The agonist–antagonists (butorphanol, nalbuphine, buprenorphine, pentazocine) are able to reverse some of the effects of the pure agonists, but they can produce analgesia. Buprenorphine is a kappa antagonist, with high affinity for mu receptors and classified as a partial agonist, while butorphanol acts at the kappa receptor and acts as a mu antagonist. Opioid antagonists, which include naloxone, naltrexone, and nalmefene, reverse the actions of both mu and kappa agonists. The 'potency' of different opioids can be misleading in that relative ranking is based on affinity of the specific drug for binding to the receptor. The most common side-effects seen with opioids include respiratory depression, nausea and vomiting, histamine release, constipation, and central excitement. Urine production may be decreased for several hours following morphine administration.

Oral administration yields low (20–60%) bioavailability because opioids are metabolized in the liver. Codeine has the highest bioavailability, approaching 60%, and is often administered in combination with acetaminophen. (**Note:** Acetaminophen is lethal in cats.) Although morphine and hydromorphone are available as suppositories, there is little difference in efficacy or bioavailability (~20%) from oral administration; however, this delivery form is an option if oral administration is unavailable. The available oral/rectal preparations of morphine (for human use) in the USA are listed in **Table 24.3**.

The highly lipid-soluble opioid fentanyl lends itself to transdermal delivery and is available in a patch containing a drug reservoir. An ethylene-vinyl acetate copolymer membrane controls the rate of delivery to the skin. Due in part to the differences in dermal vascularization, drug uptake varies between the dog and cat. Studies suggest it takes 12–24 hours to reach peak effect in the dog, whereas peak values in the cat are reached sooner (2–18 hours). Fentanyl patches certainly have their place; however, they are not without concerns (e.g. classified drug in many countries, expense, difficulty sticking, variable absorption, possible skin reaction, requires skin preparation and optimal location). Following

Table 24.3 Available oral/rectal preparations of morphine (for human use) in the USA.

Duration of action	Preparation	Dosage formulation
Immediate release	Tablet/capsule	1.5 mg, 30 mg
	Soluble/ sublingual	10 mg
	Solution	10 mg/5 ml; 10 mg/2.5 ml; 20 mg/5 ml; concentrate 20 mg/ml
	Suppository	5, 10, 20, 30 mg
Controlled/ sustained release	MS Contin	15, 30, 60, 100, 200 mg
	Oramorph SR	15, 30, 60, 100 mg
	Kadian (food sprinkles)	20, 30, 50, 60, 100 mg
	Avinza (food sprinkles)	30, 60, 90, 120 mg

discharge, if a pet at home shows hyperexcitability, the pet owner cannot differentiate if the behavior is due to uncontrolled pain or opioid overdose. Patches may have their optimal use in chronic conditions such as cancer. For postoperative pain, one might consider a patient requiring opioid administration as an in-house hospital patient who can be closely monitored and treated with cost-effective morphine, discharging the patient only when appropriate pain management can be provided by oral medication (e.g. an NSAID). In the year 2012, topical fentanyl was introduced into the USA for postoperative pain associated with surgical procedures in dogs. This unique formulation provides 4 days of analgesic effect from a single dose of 2.7 mg/kg.

Morphine is also used for intra-articular analgesia. Several investigators suggest that morphine works best in combination with bupivacaine; however, local anesthetics are recognized to be chondrotoxic. With recognition that there are opioid receptors in the spinal cord, opioids are applied directly to these receptors by epidural or intrathecal administration. This takes advantage of smaller doses to minimize systemic effects.

Opioids are relatively safe. Potential side-effects include:

- Sedation or CNS depression.
- Excitement or dysphoria.
- Bradycardia.
- Respiratory depression.
- Panting.
- Laryngeal reflex depression.
- Histamine release (particularly with IV administration).
- Vomition and defecation (nausea).
- Constipation (longer-term use).
- Urinary retention (more common with epidural administration).

Opioids at-a-glance (see also Table 24.4)

Meperidine (pethidine)

- Less sedation than morphine.
- More likely to cause histamine release; IV use discouraged.
- Anticholinergic effects associated with structural similarity to atropine.
- In humans, the metabolite normeperidine is a neurotoxic CNS stimulant associated with adverse reactions.
- Very short acting.

Oxymorphone

- Does not cause histamine release.
- May induce panting.

Table 24.4 Classification of various opiates/opioids by the World Health Organization.

Weak opioids	Full agonists
Codeine	Morphine
Dihydrocodeine	Fentanyl
Dextropropoxyphene	Hydromorphone
Tramadol	Codeine
	Methadone
Strong opioids	Tramadol
Morphine	Meperidine (pethidine)
Methadone	
Fentanyl	**Partial agonists**
Hydromorphone	Buprenorphine
Meperidine (pethidine)	Pentazocine
Oxycodone	Butorphanol
Buprenorphine	
Levorphanol	**Agonists–antagonists**
Dextromoramide	Nalbuphine
	Nalorphine
	Full antagonists
	Naloxone
	Naltrexone
	Alvimopan

Methadone

- Does not cause histamine release.
- Higher bioavailability than morphine.
- NMDA and serotonin reuptake inhibitor (SRI) activity.

Hydromorphone

- More sedation than oxymorphone, but shorter duration.
- No histamine release with IV administration.

Fentanyl

- Rapid onset of action (2–3 minutes).
- Short duration of action.

Butorphanol

- Agonist–antagonist.
- Weak analgesic, with analgesic ceiling effect.
- Short duration of analgesia (~40 minutes in the dog)

Buprenorphine

- Agonist (strong for mu receptor)–antagonist (kappa receptor).
- Less analgesia than morphine, ceiling effect.
- Slow onset (40–60 minutes), long acting (8–12 hours).
- Affinity for mu receptor makes reversal more difficult.
- Most popular opioid used in small animal practice in the UK.
- Oral transmucosal administration very effective in the cat.
- Considered by some to be the best opioid investigated in the cat.

Codeine

- 'International standard' weak opioid.
- Approximately 9% of Caucasians lack enzyme to provide analgesia – relevance in animals unknown.
- Substantially improves analgesia of nonopioids (e.g. NSAIDs).

Tramadol

- 40% activity at the mu receptor, 60% as serotonin and noradrenaline neuronal reuptake inhibitor (monoaminergic).
- Reduces synovial fluid concentrations of substance P and interleukin-6 in human patients with knee osteoarthritis.
- Augments analgesia of opioids and NSAIDs.
- Bioavailability is about 65%, with a short half-life (<1.7 hours) in dogs; 62% (4.8 hours) in cats.
- Simulated oral dosing regimens at 5 mg/kg q6h and 2.5 mg/kg q4h are predicted to produce tramadol and M1 levels consistent with analgesia in humans.
- No safety or efficacy data are available for use in dogs or cats.

ALPHA-2 AGONISTS

The prototypical alpha-2 adrenergic agonist used in veterinary medicine has been xylazine. Since its introduction in 1962, xylazine has been used, mostly in ruminants, as an anesthetic or anesthetic adjuvant. The newer alpha-2 adrenergic agonist medetomidine has gained acceptance in companion animal practice. Medetomidine is an equal mixture of two optical enantiomers, of which dexmedetomidine is a potent alpha-2 agonist, while levomedetomidine is pharmacologically inactive. Medetomidine has a high affinity for the alpha-2 receptor, with an alpha-2/alpha-1 binding ratio of 1,620, compared with ratios of 260, 220, and 160 for detomidine, clonidine, and xylazine, respectively. Currently, administering large doses of alpha-2 agonists as monoanesthetic agents is uncommon, but it is commonly accepted that low doses are very useful when used as adjuncts in a balanced analgesic protocol.

Since its USA launch in 2007, medetomidine has been phased out (in the USA) and replaced by dexmedetomidine. Dexmedetomidine is the dextrorotary enantiomer of the racemic mixture medetomidine (**Figure 24.14**). It is approximately twice as potent as medetomidine in terms of its ability to produce sedation and analgesia. Dexmedetomidine is supplied as a 0.5 mg/ml solution, which allows clinicians to use the same injection volume as medetomidine because the dexmedetomidine dilution has the same potency as medetomidine.

One mechanism of alpha-2 agonist action is the inhibition of adenylate cyclase. Decreased availability of intracellular cAMP attenuates the stimulation of cAMP-dependent protein kinase and, hence, the phosphorylation of target regulatory proteins. In addition alpha-2 adrenoceptor activation of G-protein-gated potassium channels results in membrane hyperpolarization, causing a decrease in the firing rate of excitable cells in the CNS.

Presynaptic alpha-2 adrenoceptors secrete noradrenaline, which binds with postsynaptic adrenoceptors to stimulate target cell response governing autonomic functions.

Alpha-2 agonists produce rapid sedation by selectively binding to alpha-2 adrenoceptors in the neuron, inhibiting the release of noradrenaline necessary for neurotransmission (**Figure 24.15**).

Dense populations of alpha-2 adrenoceptors are concentrated in the mammalian spinal cord dorsal horn, both pre- and postsynaptically, on non-noradrenergic nociceptive

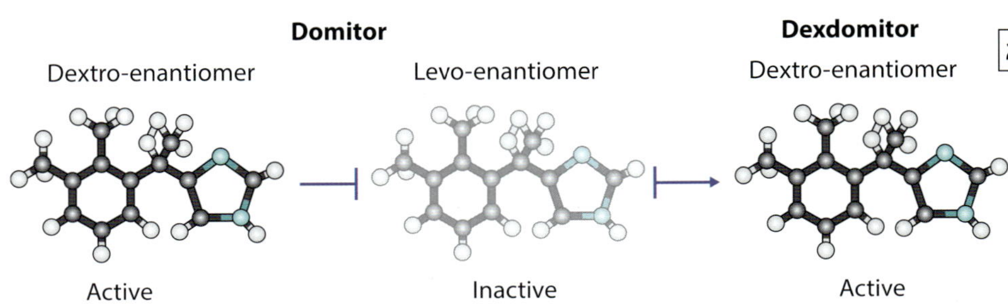

24.14

Figure 24.14 Dexmedetomidone provides sedation and analgesia using only the active enantiomer of medetomidine.

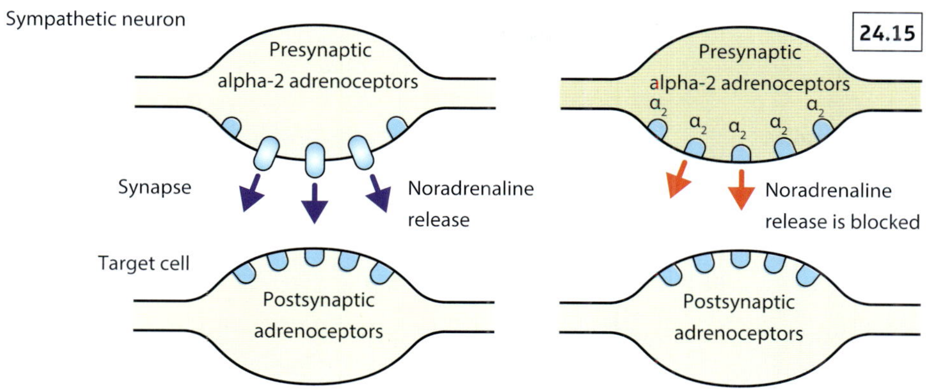

Figure 24.15 Noradrenaline release is inhibited by alpha-2 agonist administration.

neurons. On presynaptic alpha-2 adrenoceptors, when G_0 proteins are activated, a decrease in calcium influx is mediated, leading to decreased release of neurotransmitters and/or neuropeptides, including glutamate, vasoactive intestinal peptide, CGRP, substance P, and neurotensin. At postsynaptic alpha-2 adrenoceptors, G_i protein-coupled potassium channels produce neuronal hyperpolarization that dampens ascending nociceptive transmission, thereby producing postsynaptically-mediated spinal analgesia. The sedative–hypnotic effects are apparently mediated by activation of supraspinal alpha-2 adrenoceptors located in the brainstem, where there is a relatively high density of alpha-2 agonist binding sites.

Potential side-effects include:

- Sedation, muscle relaxation, and anxiolysis.
- Short-duration hypertension accompanied by a compensatory baroreceptor-mediated reflex bradycardia.
- Decreased respiratory rate, but with a maintained arterial pH, PaO_2, and $PaCO_2$.
- Both cats and dogs will vomit: cats (90%) more than dogs (20%).
- GI atony with possible gas accumulation.
- Increased urinary output.
- Transient hypoinsulinemia and hyperglycemia have been reported in dogs.

The data in **Table 24.5** are from an educational demonstration in a live dog, demonstrating the physiologic responses to the α_2-agonist medetomidine, the anticholinergic atropine, and the reversal agent antipamezol.

Alpha-2 agonists at-a-glance

- Not first-line analgesic agents, but excellent analgesic adjuncts.
- At low dosages, both sedation and analgesia are dose dependent.
- Ceiling effect at higher dosages.
- Co-administration with anticholinergics is controversial.
- Inclusion in a premedication protocol markedly reduces the required dose of induction agents.
- Up to 20% of dogs and 90% of cats will vomit after administration.
- Increased urine output is reported in both dogs and cats.
- Transient hypoinsulinemia and hyperglycemia are reported in dogs.
- Alpha-2 agonists are sedative–analgesics, not anesthetics; therefore, under their influence, caution the possibility that the animal may still bite.
- Reflex bradycardia and bradyarrhythmias are not uncommon. Heart rate may decrease by 50%.
- Blood pressure may fall by one-quarter to one-third and cardiac output may decrease by one-third to one-half of baseline value.
- Should be avoided in animals with compromising cardiovascular disease.

MEMBRANE STABILIZERS (LOCAL ANESTHETICS, TRICYCLIC ANTIDEPRESSANTS, SEROTONIN REUPTAKE INHIBITORS)

It is likely that an individual patient has neuropathic pain as a result of many underlying mechanisms. However, there may be a dominant mechanism that, when treated, reduces pain to a tolerable level. For example, if it can be demonstrated that ectopic impulse generators (due to abnormal sodium channel activity and located in injured or abnormally functioning primary afferent fibers) are generating increased traffic entering CNS pathways, treatment with a Na^+ channel-blocking agent that reduces ectopic firing may dramatically reduce pain. Mechanism-based pain management is an area of intense research. This includes reducing transmitter release in pro-nociceptive neurons by opiates or $\alpha 2\delta$ calcium channel-binding drugs, by inhibiting postsynaptic excitatory

Table 24.5 Data demonstrating the physiologic responses to the alpha-2 agonist medetomidine, the anticholinergic atropine, and the reversal agent antipamezol.

	Heart rate (bpm) [70–110]	Mean BP (mmHg) [60–100]	Cardiac output (l/min) [2.5–6]	O_2 saturation (%) [95–100]	Mucous membrane color [pink, CRT 1–3 sec]	PaO_2 (mmHg) [500–600]	$PaCO_2$ (mmHg) [40–55]	Resp rate (breaths/min) [6–20]
Baseline (1.1% isoflurane)	91	76	2.95	98	Pink, fast	575	52	20
Medetomidine administration (10 mcg/kg IM)								
+ 5 min	49	96	1.33	93	Pale, slow	630	55	24
+ 15 min	50	90	1.36	95	Pinker, slow	563	54	18
Anticholinergic (atropine) administration (0.04 mg/kg IV)								
+ 3 min	77	125	1.45	100	Pink, faster	602	59	13
Antipamezol administration (50 mcg/kg IM)	77	125		100				
+ 1 min	86	147	1.56	99	Pink, fast	X	X	15
+ 5 min	89	96	2.3	98	Pink, fast	597	54	12

Note: Numbers in square brackets represent the normal reference intervals for each parameter.

receptors such as the NMDA or AMPA/kainate receptors, by potentiating inhibitory transmitters through reduced transmitter uptake or by agonist administration, and by use-dependent Na^+ channel-blockers.

Trafficking, upregulation and downregulation, and even functional modulation of Na^+ channels, constitute major modes of action in neuropathic membrane remodeling and hyperexcitability, with K^+ channels playing an important role. Many drugs that block Na^+ channels are available for clinical use. Local anesthetics are most widely used (e.g. lidocaine and bupivacaine). The inflammatory phase of wound healing typically lasts approximately 72 hours and this is the period that has been recommended as the minimum amount of time analgesics should be provided following surgery; however local, infiltrative lidocaine typically lasts no more than 120 minutes and bupivacaine no more than 360 minutes. Recognizing the need for a long-acting local anesthetic, a bupivacaine liposomal injectable suspension has been developed (Aratana Therapeutics) that is promising to provide 72 hours of local analgesic efficacy following intraoperative tissue infiltration. When applied at high concentrations to a nerve, impulse conduction and pain stop when the impulse originates distal to the application site. This is effective for both nociceptive and neuropathic pain. Low concentrations of lidocaine (two to three orders of magnitude lower than those required to block normal impulse propagation) selectively suppress subthreshold oscillations and ectopic neuroma and DRG discharge, with similar CNS activity. Such sensitivity to sodium channel blockage is the basis for these drugs to be given systemically without serious toxicity from failure of normal neuronal conduction of the cardiovascular and nervous systems.

A problem with systemic lidocaine is its short duration of action and the need for it to be administered IV. This first issue is solved by anticonvulsants, whose mode of action is sodium channel blockade. Another option is tricyclic antidepressants (TCAs). For many years, drugs with a characteristic tricyclic structure (**Figure 24.16**) have been used to treat depression. Imipramine was among the first in its class and only a few years after its introduction in 1958, its analgesic properties were identified. Nowadays, TCAs are the mainstay for treatment of neuropathic pain. Although treatment of neuropathic pain with TCAs in humans is evidence based, it is not clear how these drugs actually relieve pain. Most research is based on their ability to inhibit presynaptic reuptake of norepinephrine and serotonin, but these drugs also act as NMDA-receptor antagonists and apparently block ion channels. Amitriptyline is best known as an inhibitor of catecholamine reuptake, although it is also a strong local anesthetic and is likely to relieve neuropathic pain by suppressing ectopic discharge.

Anticonvulsants are a category of medications grouped together based only on their ability to suppress epileptic seizures. Anticonvulsants together with antiarrhythmics can be looked on as sodium channel or other channel neuronal activity regulators. Evidence firmly supports that anticonvulsants and local anesthetic drugs relieve neuropathic pain. Based on number needed to treat (NNT) calculations, gabapentin is comparable with TCAs for neuropathic pain and is used more frequently than any other anticonvulsant for human chronic pain. Gabapentin has demonstrated analgesic efficacy for human patients with painful diabetic neuropathy and postherpetic neuralgia, with NNT calculations of 3.8 and 3.2, respectively. Gabapentin was developed as an analog of the neurotransmitter gamma-aminobutyric acid (GABA), but it has since been shown not to interact with either $GABA_A$ or $GABA_B$ receptors. Although not a sodium channel-blocker, gabapentin depresses ectopic discharge by suppression of Ca^{2+} conductance. Its mode of action is associated with binding to the α2δ site on voltage-gated calcium channels (**Figure 24.17**).

The newer nontricyclic antidepressants, such as selective SRIs, antidepressants that alter both serotonergic and noradrenergic neurotransmission, and noradrenaline (a selective antidepressant), have preferential use in human medicine because of better tolerability; however, their efficacy for neuropathic pain relief is not convincing. Apparently, anticonvulsants that act synaptically (e.g. barbiturates) are nonanalgesic, while membrane stabilizing anticonvulsants are effective analgesics. Corticosteroids also have membrane stabilizing properties, which may be a major mechanism of pain control when depot form corticosteroids are injected.

Topical forms of the TCA doxepin, gabapentin, lidocaine, and bupivacaine are now available on the human market, as well as ketamine.

24.16

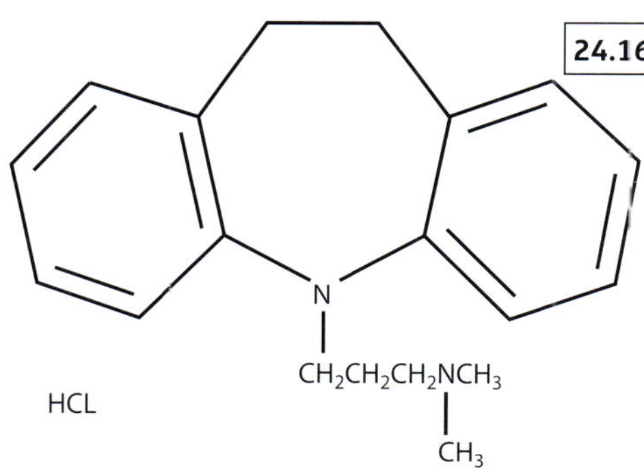

Figure 24.16 Typical structure of tricyclic antidepressants.

Membrane stabilizers at-a-glance (selected agents)

Local anesthetics

- The amide link (lidocaine, bupivacaine) or ester link (procaine, benzocaine) for the different local anesthetics determines the drug disposition within the body:
  - Metabolism of ester-linked local anesthetics is primarily by enzymatic hydrolysis in the plasma of nonspecific pseudocholinesterases.

24.17

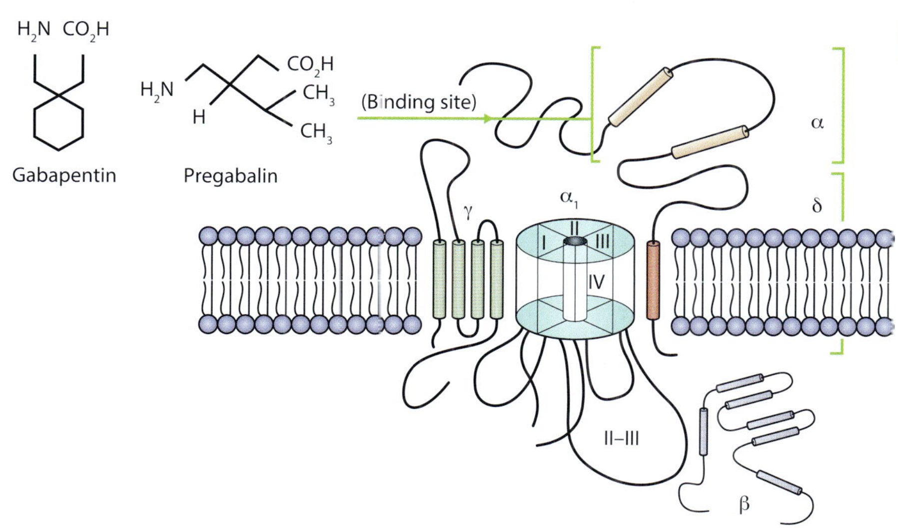

Figure 24.17 The gabapentin-specific binding site is the α2δ subunit of voltage-dependent calcium channels, with the highest affinity for $α2δ_1$ subtype. Gabapentin can inhibit high-threshold calcium currents in cultured sensory neurons and inhibits excitatory amino acid release through its interaction with the calcium channels. Gabapentin also interacts with the NMDA receptor complex at the glycine site.

    - Amide local anesthetics are metabolized primarily in the liver.
- Local anesthetics are weak bases, and the predominant form of the compound in solution at physiologic pH is the ionized or cationic form.
- At clinical doses vasodilation is present, whereas at low concentrations local anesthetics tend to cause vasoconstriction.
- Adding a vasoconstrictor to the local anesthetic decreases local perfusion, delays the rate of vascular absorption, and prolongs anesthetic action. Epinephrine (5 μg/ml or 1:200,000) is commonly used for such a response.
- Bupivacaine extended-release injectable suspension for managing postoperative pain in cats and dogs following surgery has been developed. This product consists of multivesicular liposomes encapsulating aqueous bupivacaine that is gradually released over 96 hours. Administration can be associated with mild granulomatous inflammation of adipose tissue at the injection site.
- There are currently no data to enlighten the concept of mixing local anesthetics (e.g. short onset and duration agent with a different agent of long onset and duration).
- Harmful side-effects are usually associated with accidental IV administration or vascular absorption of large amounts of anesthetic after aggressive regional administration. (**Note:** Always aspirate before injecting. Bupivacaine can cause cardiac dysrhythmias and ventricular fibrillation if injected IV.)
- Clinical applications:
    - Local infiltration – soaker catheters.
    - Topical anesthesia.
    - Intravenous block.
    - Epidural block.
    - Spinal (supra-arachnoid) block.
    - Peripheral nerve block.

NMDA-antagonists (ketamine, tiletamine, amantadine, methadone, dextromethorphan)

- Ketamine acts both centrally and peripherally at multiple receptor sites, including NMDA, opioid, AMPA, kainate, and $GABA_A$ receptors.
- Oral administration of ketamine produces few adverse effects and may be more effective than SC administration.
- Microdoses of ketamine have few if any side-effects, and its best use is with an analgesic such as an opioid.
- Amantadine was originally developed as an antiviral drug for use in humans and is available as an oral preparation. It is well absorbed in the GI tract and excreted relatively unchanged in urine.
- The pharmacology of amantadine in dogs and cats has not been well established.
- In humans, amantadine has been used for neuropathic pain.
- Amantadine is used in veterinary patients for allodynia and opioid tolerance, allowing lower opioid doses and complementing the opioid analgesia.
- Amantadine is available as 100 mg capsules and a 10 mg/ml elixir.
- The feline toxic dose of amantadine is 30 mg/kg.
- As an NMDA-antagonist, amantadine does not alter nociceptive thresholds; therefore, it does not produce analgesia, but assists other drugs analgesic response by blocking 'facilitation' (**Figure 24.18**).
- Behavioral side-effects from amantadine in dogs and cats begin at 15 mg/kg PO.
- Methadone and dextromethorphan are opioid derivatives. Both are weak, noncompetitive NMDA antagonists.
- Methadone also functions as a norepinephrine reuptake inhibitor.
- Parenteral formulations of dextromethorphan are currently unavailable.
- Methadone is commonly used for cancer pain in human patients because of its high oral bioavailability, rapid onset, and time to peak analgesic effect, as well as the relatively long duration of activity.

Gabapentin

- Originally introduced as an antiepileptic drug.
- Has no analgesic effect at GABA receptors.
- Well suited for neuropathic pain.
- Is highly bioavailable in dogs.
- Is metabolized by the liver and excreted almost exclusively by the kidneys. $T_{1/2}$ is approximately 3–4 hours.

NONSTEROIDAL ANTI-INFLAMMATORY DRUGS

In most respects NSAIDs can be characterized as a class; however, there are molecule-specific characteristics. NSAIDs manifest their mode of action in the arachidonic acid (AA) cascade (**Figure 24.19**). AA is a ubiquitous substrate derived from the continual degradation of cell membranes. Corticosteroids act at this step. Because corticosteroids have their mode of action at a location higher in the arachidonic cascade than NSAIDs, it is redundant to use them concurrently; doing so markedly increases the potential for adverse reactions.

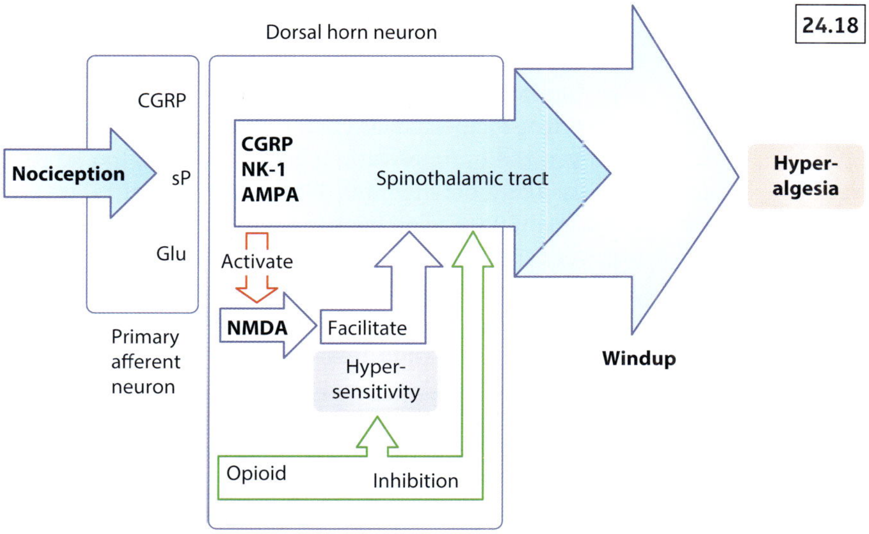

Figure 24.18 NMDA-mediated windup facilitates the underlying nociceptive signaling, resulting in a state of hyperalgesia. Therefore, NMDA-antagonists (amantadine) are administered as 'adjuncts' to a baseline protocol for optimal results.

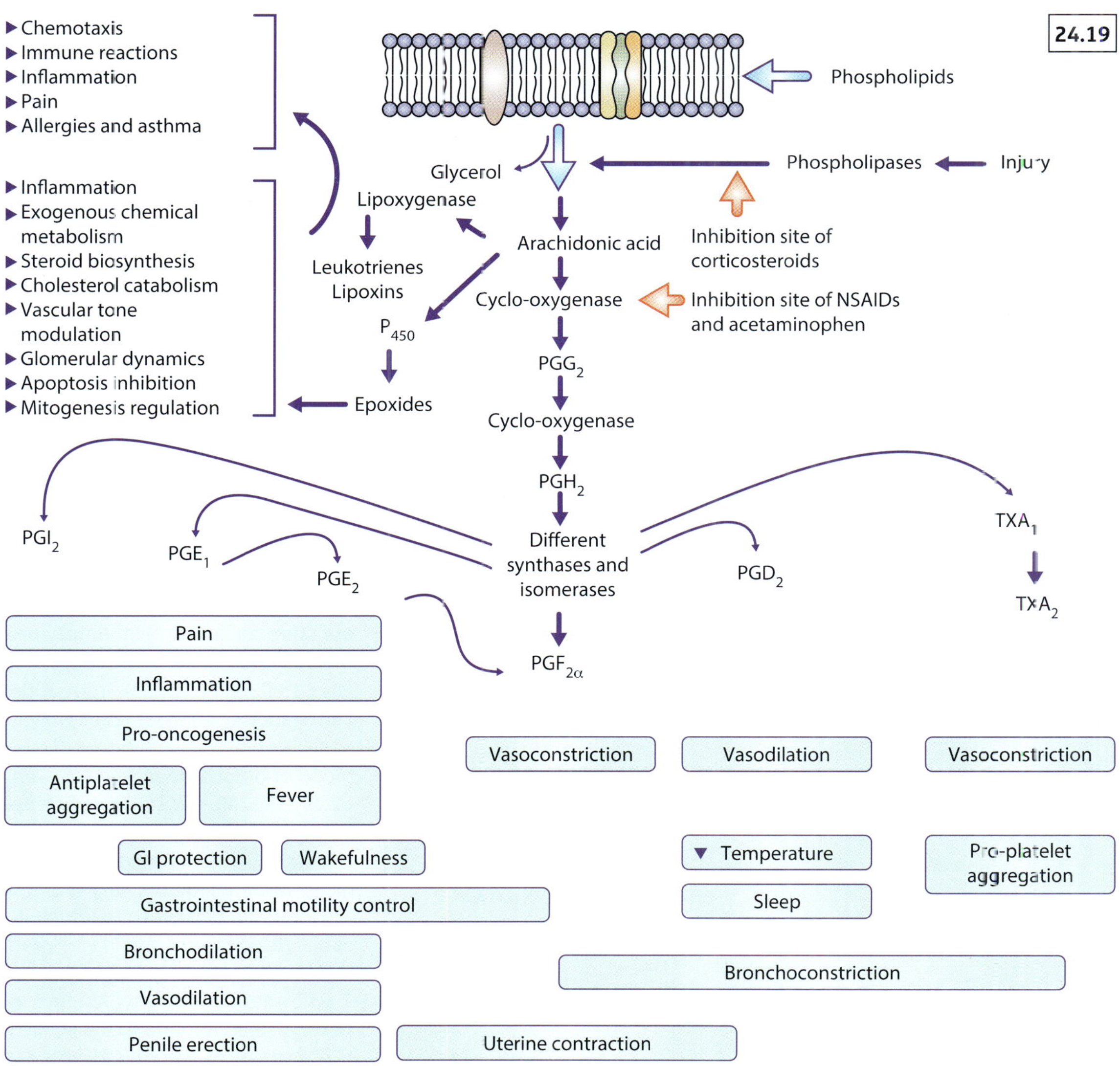

Figure 24.19 Arachidonic acid cascade.

Approximately 20 years following discovery of the AA pathway as the mode of action for aspirin, it was discovered that the COX enzyme exists in the form of at least two isoenzymes: COX-1 and COX-2 (**Figure 24.20**). Early thinking was that COX-1-mediated prostaglandins were constitutively physiologic and should be retained, while COX-2-mediated prostaglandins were pathologic and should be eliminated for the control of inflammation and pain. COX-2-selective NSAIDs were designed with this in mind (i.e. the selective suppression of COX-2-mediated prostaglandins) (**Figure 24.21**).

COX-1:COX-2 ratios vary depending on laboratory techniques and although finite ratios may vary among investigators, relative ratio standings provide an insight as to a drug's expected COX activity (**Figures 24.22-24.25**). However, the optimal ratio is unknown, and too large a ratio is likely detrimental. While the clinical relevance of optimal COX-2 selectivity is open to debate, the importance of COX-1-sparing is well established.

COX ratios are also species dependent (i.e. ratios in the dog cannot be applied to the cat). Furthermore, all marketing information relative to COX data carries the

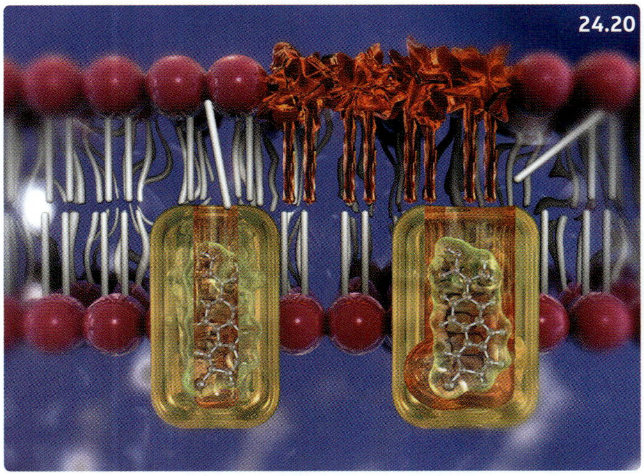

Figure 24.20 The COX-1 receptor site (left) differs from the COX-2 receptor site (right) by only a couple of amino acids; however, the COX-2 site has a larger entry port and a characteristic side pocket. Small, traditional NSAIDs fit into both sites, blocking both COX-1- and COX-2-mediated prostaglandin production from arachidonic acid (white sticks), hence the term nonselective NSAIDs.

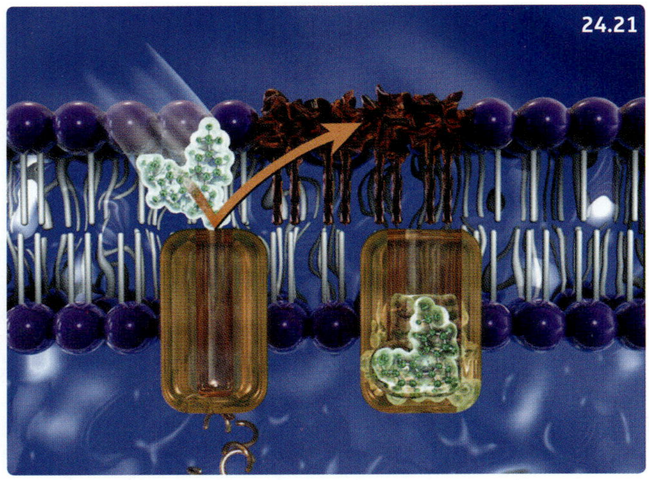

Figure 24.21 Coxib-class NSAIDs were designed to be too large for the COX-1 receptor site (at labeled dose); however, they fit hand-in-glove within the COX-2 receptor site. These drugs spare COX-1-mediated prostaglandin production and block COX-2-mediated prostaglandin production (i.e. they are COX-1 sparing and COX-2 selective).

24.22

Drug	Ratio of IC_{50} COX-1/COX-2
Meloxicam	12.2
Carprofen	1.8
Ketoprofen	0.4

24.23

Drug	Ratio of IC_{50} COX-1/COX-2
Meloxicam	10
Carprofen	9
Ketoprofen	6.5

24.24

Drug	Ratio of IC_{50} COX-1/COX-2
Meloxicam	2.7
Carprofen	16.8
Ketoprofen	0.2
Aspirin	0.4

24.25

Drug	Ratio of IC_{50} COX-1/COX-2
Carprofen	5
Celecoxib	6.2
Deracoxib	36.5
Firocoxib	155

Figures 24.22–24.25 COX-1:COX-2 ratios. (24.22) From Kay-Mugford P, Benn SJ, LaMarre J *et al.* (2000) *In vitro* effects of nonsteroidal anti-inflammatory drugs on cyclooxygenase activity in dogs. *Am J Vet Res* **61**:802–809. (24.23) From Brideau C, Van Staden C, Chan CC (2001) *In vitro* effects of cyclooxygenase inhibitors in whole blood of horses, dogs, and cats. *Am J Vet Res* **62**:1755–1760. (24.24) From Streppa HK, Jones CJ, Budsberg SC (2002) Cyclooxygenase selectivity of nonsteroidal anti-inflammatory drugs in canine blood. *Am J Vet Res* **63**:91–94. (24.25) From Li J, Lynch MP, DeMello KL *et al.* (2005) *In vitro* and *in vivo* profile of 2-(3-di-fluoromethyl-5-phenylpyrazol-1-yl)-5-methanesulfonylpyridine, a potent, selective, and orally active canine COX-2 inhibitor. *Bioorg Medicinal Chem* **13**:1805–1809.

disclaimer, 'clinical relevance undetermined'. This is because all these data are determined *in vitro*. One study reported an assessment of the *in-vivo* action of NSAIDs in the region of the GI tract, which appears to be at greatest risk for ulceration in the dog. Findings from this study suggest that different NSAIDs reduce protective prostanoid production to a different degree in the canine pylorus and duodenum, and this appears to relate to their COX selectivity.

Some authors suggest a COX-1:COX-2 ratio of <1 would be considered COX-1 selective, a ratio of >1 as COX-2 preferential, a ratio of >100 as COX-2 selective, and a ratio of >1,000 as COX-2 specific. Selectivity nomenclature is used loosely and comparative ranking has not been associated with clinical relevance.

It is now recognized that the 'good-guy COX-1', 'bad-guy-COX-2' approach is naïve; COX-2 is needed constitutively for reproduction, CNS nociception, renal function, and GI lesion repair. In fact, the physiologic functions associated with COX activity overlap. Accordingly, there is a limit as to how COX-2 selective an NSAID can be without causing problems (e.g. inhibiting the repair of a gastric lesion). However, this limit is not known. In addition, it is logical to avoid a COX-1-selective NSAID (ratio <1) perioperatively so as not to enhance bleeding. Coxib-class NSAIDs were not designed to be more safe for either hepatic or renal function. They were designed specifically to provide an improved GI safety profile over traditional NSAIDs, particularly in high-risk patients, and this has been demonstrated in human studies. Finally, it is fortunate that dogs are not a risk for coxib-class NSAID cardiovascular problems, primarily because they are not a species that experiences atherosclerosis. It may well be that the canine is the optimal target species for this class of drugs.

Safety

The comparative safety of different NSAIDs in dogs is difficult to determine. Such a query compares the incidence of problems with one NSAID with that for a second NSAID. Incidence is a ratio consisting of the number of dogs with problems (numerator) over the number of dogs treated with that drug at a given point in time (denominator). Not all adverse drug events (ADEs) are reported and not all reported events are directly causal, therefore the numerator is unknown. The denominator is also unknown, because it is impossible to determine the number of dogs on a drug at any given time. For these reasons, accurate comparative data are unobtainable. Accordingly, most NSAID manufacturers can state with credibility, that 'no NSAID has been proved safer than (fill in the blank)'. Nevertheless, all ADEs should be reported to the appropriate authority and drug manufacturer so that general trends can be tracked.

ADE reports to the US Food and Drug Administration (FDA) Center for Veterinary Medicine provide some insights as to why ADEs from NSAID use might be so high:

- 23% of owners: veterinarian never discussed any adverse effects of the medication.
- 22%: veterinarian did not issue client information sheet provided by pharmaceutical company.
- 14%: dispensed NSAID in other than original packaging.
- 4%: preadministration blood analyses not performed.

As a class of drug, NSAIDs are most commonly associated with adverse reactions in the GI tract (**Table 24.6**), renal system, and liver. GI problems associated with NSAIDs can be as benign as regurgitation or as serious as gastric ulceration and perforation. Vomition has been identified as the most frequent clinical sign associated with gastric perforation. Owners should be informed that if their pet experiences vomiting while taking an NSAID, the drug should be stopped and the patient rechecked. This is a conservative approach since dogs are considered a 'vomiting species' and some NSAIDs are associated with more vomiting than others.

Gastric perforations are most frequently found near the gastric pylorus and have a poor prognosis if not discovered early and treated aggressively. Risk factors identified with NSAID-associated gastric ulceration are most

Table 24.6 Gastrointestinal adverse events reported in clinical trials for US Registration.

Drug	Vomiting	Diarrhea
Carprofen	3.1% (3.8)	3.1% (3.8)
Etodolac	4.3% (1.7)	2.6% (1.7)
Deracoxib	2.9% (3.8)	2.9% (1.9)
Tepoxalin	2.0% (4.8) at 7 days 19.6% at 28 days	4.0% (0) at 7 days 21.5% at 28 days
Meloxicam	25.5% (15.4)	12.1% (7.4)
Firocoxib	3.9% (6.6)	0.8% (8.3)

* Values represent mean of test article (placebo).

** Data sourced from drug inserts. Caution should be used in comparing adverse events among different drugs because of differences in study populations, data collection methods, and reporting methods.

commonly seen with inappropriate use: (1) overdosing; (2) concurrent use of multiple NSAIDs; and (3) concurrent use of NSAIDs with corticosteroids. 'Postmarketing' data suggests that 70–80% of NSAID ADEs can be eliminated by 'responsible' NSAID use.

COX-2-selective NSAIDs have been embraced in an effort to gain greater NSAID safety (greater suppression of pain and inflammation (COX-2), but with COX-1-sparing); however, it is now appreciated that COX-2 can be associated with some level of constitutive homeostasis, specifically in the GI tract. This renders the selection of any contemporary NSAID an unknown quantity relative to GI risk. For example: COX-2-mediated prostaglandins are important in the repair of gastric ulcers, supressing ulcer progression to perforation. Therefore, placing a dog on a COX-2-selective/specific NSAID could exacerbate the risk for an adverse response in the event that the dog had an ulcer at risk for perforation. GI perforations can be life-threatening and dogs predisposed are virtually impossible to diagnose, especially given an underappreciation of stress related to hospitalizations and treatments.

Mechanism-based investigation as to the clinical manifestation of pain subsequent to nociceptor response to prostaglandin E_2 (PGE_2) has revealed four receptor subtypes for PGE_2: EP1–4. EP4 has been identified as a major player in the pain pathway. In 2013, the WHO defined a newly recognized class of drug that acts as a prostaglandin receptor antagonist (PRA) – the piprant class. A first-in-class selective EP4 PRA, analgesic, and anti-inflammatory has recently been developed. This drug is proposed to suppress pain and inflammation, while sparing other homeostatic, COX-dependent physiologic functions.

Washout

Since NSAID manufacturers (and the US FDA) warn against concurrent NSAID administration, practitioners switching patients from one NSAID to another often find themselves addressing the issue of 'appropriate washout' between different NSAIDs. There are no published peer-reviewed scientific studies that define what constitutes an adequate washout period when switching a dog from one NSAID to another. In the absence of scientific evidence, some pharmacologists offer washout guidelines that are based on NSAID serum half-life data (i.e. 5–10 half-lives of the drug). However, an NSAID's tissue effect may not mirror its serum half-life, therefore such guidance should be taken with caution.

Reasons for changing NSAIDs fall into two classes: lack of efficacy and drug intolerance. When efficacy is the issue, a short washout (perhaps five half-lives) may be acceptable, bridging the interval with other class drugs. When switching NSAIDs because of intolerance, an extended washout period may be necessary, the minimum period being resolution of the clinical signs associated with the intolerance. Decisions regarding washout duration must be tailored to individual patients and include the following factors:

- Patient health status.
- Concurrent medications.
- Previous NSAID experience.
- Personalized benefit versus risk assessment.

It is important to involve the owner in the patient's benefit:risk assessment, ensuring that the owner understands:

- What to expect from the medication.
- Medication dose and dosing interval.
- Potential side-effects.
- Inappropriate concurrent medications (e.g. aspirin and other over-the-counter medications).
- What action to take if side-effects are seen.

Such information should be provided to the owner verbally and in writing and documented in the patient's medical record.

Aspirin

Aspirin presents unique risk factors to the canine patient. Aspirin is both topically (to the GI mucosa) and systemically toxic (even at low doses of 5 mg/kg q24h), chondrodestructive, causes irreversible platelet acetylation, and is potentially associated with GI bleeding of approximately 3 ml/day. The American Medical Association reports that 16,500 people die each year associated with aspirin toxicity (**Table 24.7**), yet pet owners often consider it benign because it is available over-the-counter and the media suggest it is safe. Even low-dose aspirin has consistently been associated with GI petechiation and hemorrhage. In most countries, aspirin does not have a license for use in the dog. In theory, since aspirin causes GI lesions, it would be inappropriate to sequentially progress from aspirin to a strongly COX-2-selective NSAID (which might restrict the COX-2 necessary for repair) without an adequate washout period following the aspirin. It is also dangerous to use aspirin together with another NSAID or corticosteroid.

Development of gastric mucosal hemorrhage, erosion, and ulceration associated with the administration of aspirin is largely attributed to reduction of prostaglandin E

Table 24.7 Risk factors for NSAID-induced complications (humans).

		Estimated increased risk
Established	Prior clinical GI event (ulcer/complication)	2.4–4 times
	Advanced age (65+)	2–3.5 times
	Concomitant anticoagulation therapy	3 times
	Concurrent corticosteroid use	2 times
	High-dose NSAID or multiple NSAID use	2–4 times
	Major co-morbidity (e.g. heart disease)	variable
Probable	Long-term NSAID use	
	Coexisting *H. pylori* infection	
	Dyspepsia caused by an NSAID	

synthesis in the gastric mucosa. In addition, aspirin can cause direct cellular toxicosis independently of the inhibition of PG synthesis. Standard formulations of buffered aspirin have been shown not to provide sufficient buffering to neutralize gastric acid or to prevent mucosal injury. Enteric-coated aspirin causes less gastric injury in humans compared with that from administration of unbuffered or buffered aspirin, but absorption is quite variable. Complications of administering aspirin together with another NSAID/corticosteroid reside in the suppression of aspirin-triggered lipoxin, an endogenous protective mechanism in both humans and dogs, with resultant enhancement of systemic toxicity.

Gastrointestinal protectants

One goal of anti-ulcer treatment is to lower intragastric acidity in order to prevent further destruction of the GI tract mucosa (**Table 24.8**); this enhances ulcer repair. Cimetidine (a histamine, H2-receptor blocker) is commonly used, although its inhibition of the CYP 450 enzyme system may preclude its use in some cases. Cimetidine requires dosing 3–4 times daily and it is not effective in preventing NSAID-induced gastric ulceration. The adverse reactions of cimetidine mimic those of gastritis and ulcerations.

Table 24.8 Pharmacologic agents for NSAID gastrointestinal prophylaxis and treatment.

Group	Generic name	Brand name	Dose
Proton pump inhibitors	Omeprazole	Prilosec	Canine: 0.7 mg/kg PO. (**Note:** Dose for omeprazole is 0.7–1.0 mg/kg PO q12–24h – see Chapter 8: Digestive diseases [pharynx to anorectum].)
	Lansoprazole	PrevAcid	
	Rabeprazole	AcipHex	
	Pantoprazole	Protonix	
	Esomeprazole	Nexium	
Prostaglandin analog	Misoprostol	Cytotec	Canine: 2–5 μg/kg PO q8h
H2 blockers	Cimetidine	Tagamet	Canine/feline: 10 mg/kg PO, IV, or IM q8h; feline: 3.5 mg/kg PO q12h or 2.5 mg/kg IV q12h
	Ranitidine	Zantac	Canine: 2 mg/kg PO or IV q8h
	Famotidine	Pepcid	Canine/feline: 0.5 mg/kg PO, IV, IM, or SC q24h or 0.25 mg/kg PO, IV, IM, or SC q12h
	Nizatidine	Axid	Canine: 2.5–5 mg/kg PO q24h
Mucosal sealant	Sucralfate	Carafate	Canine: 0.5–1 g PO q8–12h; feline: 0.25 g PO q8–12h

Omeprazole is a substituted benzimidazole that acts by inhibiting the hydrogen–potassium ATPase (proton pump inhibitor) responsible for production of hydrogen ions in the parietal cell. It is 5–10 times more potent than cimetidine in inhibiting gastric acid secretion and has a long duration of action. Omeprazole may be useful in decreasing gastric hyperacidity, but it has minimal effect on ulcer healing.

Misoprostol is a synthetic prostaglandin E_1 analog used to prevent gastric ulceration. It decreases gastric acid secretion, increases bicarbonate and mucus secretion, increases epithelial cell turnover, and increases mucosal blood flow. Misoprostol requires dosing 3–4 times daily and its adverse reactions mimic those of gastritis and ulcerations.

NSAIDs with other agents

Drugs and agents that may be influenced by the concurrent administration of NSAIDs are listed in **Table 24.9**. Because pet owners tend to be using more and more 'natural' products (**Table 24.10**), some of which can potentially

Table 24.9 NSAIDs: potential drug interactions.

Drug	May increase the toxicity of	May decrease the efficacy of	Toxicity may be increased by
Classical NSAIDs (clinically significant COX-1 inhibition)	Warfarin, methotrexate, valproic acid, midazolam, furosemide, spironolactone, sulfonylureas, heparin	Furosemide, thiazide, ACE inhibitors, beta-blockers	Aminoglycosides, furosemide, cyclosporine (renal), glucocorticoids (GI), heparin, gingko, garlic, ginger, ginseng (hemorrhage)
Coxibs and relatively COX-2 selective agents	Warfarin, methotrexate, valproic acid, midazolam, furosemide, spironolactone, sulfonylureas	Furosemide, thiazides, ACE inhibitors, beta-blockers	Aminoglycosides, furosemide, cyclosporine (renal), glucocorticoids (GI)
Phenylbutazone, acetaminophen	Warfarin, sulfonylureas		Phenobarbital, alcohol, rifampin, metoclopramide

(Modified from Trepanier LA (2005) Potential interactions between non-steroidal anti-inflammatory drugs and other drugs. *J Vet Emerg Crit Care* **15(4)**:248–253.)

Table 24.10 Potential herb–drug interactions.

Herb	Interacting drugs	Results
St. John's Wort	Cyclosporine, fexofenadine, midazolam, digoxin, tacrolimus, amitriptyline, warfarin, theophylline	Decreased plasma drug concentrations
Ginko	Warfarin, heparin, NSAIDs	Bleeding
	Omeprazole	Decreased plasma concentrations
Ginseng	Warfarin, heparin, NSAIDs	Bleeding Falsely elevated serum digoxin levels (laboratory test interaction with ginseng)
	Opioids	Decreased analgesic effect (laboratory test interaction with ginseng)
Garlic, chamomile, ginger	Warfarin, heparin, NSAIDs	Bleeding

(Modified from Goodman L, Trepanier L (2005) Potential drug interactions with dietary supplements. *Comp Contin Educ Pract Vet* **27(10)**:780–789.)

influence the concurrent use of an NSAID, owners should be asked to supply a complete listing of everything they are giving their pet per os.

NSAID caution in cats

Salicylate toxicity in cats is well established. Cats present a unique susceptibility to NSAID toxicity because of slow clearance and dose-dependent elimination. Acetaminophen toxicity in cats results in methemoglobinemia, liver failure, and death. Cats are particularly susceptible to acetaminophen toxicity due, in part, to defective conjugation of the drug and conversion to a reactive electrolytic metabolite.

Minimizing adverse drug events

The following guidelines will minimize risk factors for NSAID ADEs:

- Proper dosing.
- Administer minimal effective dose.
- Dispense in approved packaging together with owner information sheets.
- Avoid concurrent use of multiple NSAIDs and NSAIDs with corticosteroids.
- Refrain from use of aspirin.
- Provide pet owners with both oral and written instructions for responsible NSAID use.
- Conduct appropriate patient chemistry/urine profiling.
- Conduct routine check-ups and chemistry profiles for patients on chronic NSAID regimens. Do not fill NSAID prescriptions without conducting patient examinations.
- Caution pet owners regarding supplementation with over-the-counter NSAIDs.
- Administer GI protectants for high-risk patients on NSAIDs.
- Avoid NSAID administration in puppies and pregnant animals.
- NSAIDs may decrease the action of angiotensin-converting enzyme inhibitors and furosemide, a consideration for patients being treated for cardiovascular disease.
- Geriatric animals are more likely to be treated with NSAIDs on a chronic schedule, therefore their 'polypharmacy' protocols and potentially compromised drug clearance should be considered.
- Provide sufficient hydration to surgery patients administered NSAIDs.
- Report ADEs to the product manufacturers and regulatory authorities.

Recent NSAID developments

Meloxicam

Meloxicam is a member of the oxicam family of NSAIDS, and is both COX-1-sparing and COX-2-selective. The elixir presentation is a highly palatable, honey-based presentation.

Since 2003, the oral (liquid) formulations of meloxicam have been licensed in the USA for use in dogs only, with the January 2005 product insert specifically warning in bold-face type: "Do not use in cats." An injectable formulation for use in dogs was approved by the FDA in November 2003, with a formulation for cats, for surgical use only, approved in October 2004.

In the USA, per the manufacturer's clinical instructions as of July 2010, injectable meloxicam is indicated for operative use in felines as a single, one-time dose only, with specific and repeated warnings not to administer a second dose. In June 2007, a new oral version of meloxicam was licensed in Europe for the long-term relief of pain in cats. As of June 2008, meloxicam is registered for long-term use in cats in Australia, New Zealand, and throughout Europe.

The liquid oral formulation is available as both 1.5 mg/ml and 0.5 mg/ml, while the SC injectable solution is available as 5 mg/ml.

Along with the introduction of new pain management drugs over the past several years, has also come the development of new delivery forms. Meloxicam transmucosal oral spray (OroCAM/RevitaCAM: Abbott Laboratories) is such an example. This product is bioequivalent to the oral suspension, but is sprayed onto the buccal and/or gingival mucosal surfaces. Dosage for the control of pain and inflammation associated with osteoarthritis in dogs is 0.1 mg/kg q24h. The product is supplied in three vial sizes containing 6 ml, 11 ml, and 33 ml of meloxicam solution. Each vial has a different metered dose pump delivering a dose of 0.25 mg, 0.5 mg, or 1.075 mg meloxicam per spray, respectively.

In pharmacokinetic studies, maximum concentration (C_{max}) was achieved 2 hours after dosing, with a secondary peak or shoulder seen at 8 hours. Many characteristics of the product are similar to the oral solution; however, the T_{max} is 31% less. It is purported that the IC_{50} for plasma would be exceeded within 15 minutes after administration, contrasting with 30–60 minutes for oral dosing with the oral suspension. This product feature demonstrates how first-pass metabolism by the liver can be avoided by mucosal mist application.

Given the innovative delivery form of this popular NSAID, with its COX-2 selectivity, COX-1-sparing features, and short time to plasma C_{max}, the transmucosal oral spray will find its place in clinical practice. Dog owner acceptance of the oral spray will dictate commercial success.

More recent NSAIDs

Mavacoxib, a triangular-shaped chewable tablet, was introduced to the European Union (EU) market in late 2009. The approved indication is 'for the treatment of pain and inflammation associated with degenerative joint disease in dogs in cases where continuous treatment exceeding 1 month is indicated'. This NSAID has focused on the concept of 'stronger–longer'. Mavacoxib is a monthly treatment (2 mg/kg), where the initial dose is given, repeated 14 days later, and then monthly dosed for up to a maximum of 7 consecutive doses (6.5 months). The most common side-effects noted in the European Medicines Agency (EMEA) submission dossier were loss of appetite, diarrhea, and vomiting (consistent with the NSAID class of drugs).

In dogs mavacoxib is intermediately specific to COX-2, with a COX-2:COX-1 ratio of 21.2. Mavacoxib tablets are COX-sparing at recommended doses in dogs. The majority of the product is excreted in the feces. The tablet contains an artificial beef flavor (soybean origin) with desiccated pork liver powder. An investigation into the population pharmacokinetics of mavacoxib in osteoarthritic dogs reported that their model predicts a typical $T_{½}$ of 21 days in 1-year-old, 10 kg laboratory dogs. The model also predicts that young adult laboratory Beagle dogs (1–2 years of age) will have a $T_{½}$ that is typically 29–39% shorter than that of an identically sized, 10-year-old osteoarthritic patient.

Robenacoxib is a NSAID of the coxib class that selectively inhibits COX-2 (**Figure 24.26**). The active substance, robenacoxib, is a structural analog to diclofenac (**Figure 24.27**). Robinacoxib is approved in the EU for both cats and dogs, while it is approved only for the cat (as of 2011) in the USA. Within the EU, robinacoxib is available as tablets and as a solution for injection, while in the USA it is available only as tablets for cats.

The approved EU indications are:

- Tablets:
  - Cats: treatment of acute pain and inflammation associated with musculoskeletal disorders at a once daily dose of 1 mg/kg body weight for up to 6 days.
  - Dogs: treatment of pain and inflammation associated with chronic osteoarthritis at a once daily dose of 1 mg/kg body weight as long as required (as directed by the veterinarian).

24.26

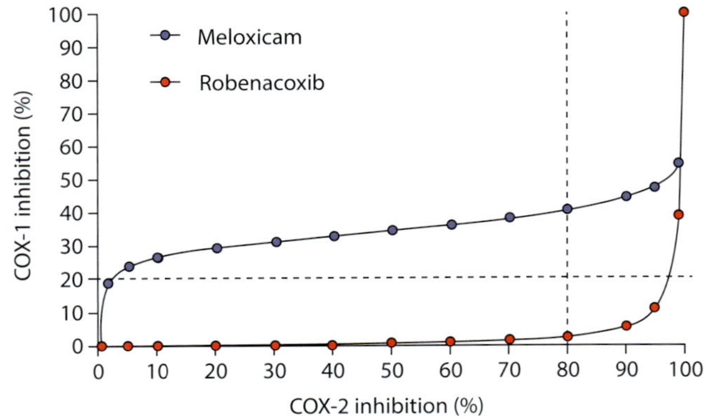

Figure 24.26 Inhibition percentages of COX-2 and corresponding inhibition percentages of COX-1 for a range of concentrations of robenacoxib in the cat. Dotted lines indicate cut-off values for inhibition of COX-1 (20% inhibition of COX-1 = percentage above which a risk of side-effects is assumed) and COX-2 (80% inhibition for COX-2 = percentage above which a good therapeutic effect is expected). Data for meloxicam, generated in a previous investigation, are included for comparison. (From Giraudel JM, Toutain PL, King JN *et al.* (2009) Differential inhibition of cyclooxygenase isoenzymes in the cat by the NSAID robenacoxib. *J Vet Pharmacol Ther* **32:**31–40.)

24.27

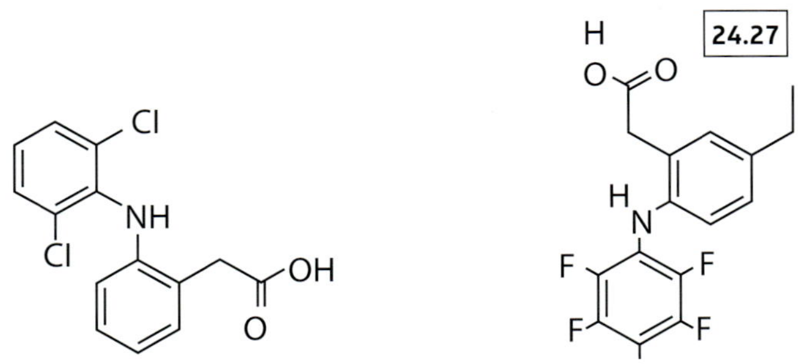

Figure 24.27 Molecular structure of diclofenac (left) and robenacoxib (right).

- Solution for injection (single SC dose of 2 mg/kg, both dog and cat):
  - Cats: treatment of pain and inflammation associated with soft tissue surgery.
  - Dogs: treatment of pain and inflammation associated with orthopedic or soft tissue surgery.

The approved USA indication is:

- Tablets:
  - Cats: treatment for the control of postoperative pain and inflammation associated with orthopedic surgery, ovariohysterectomy, and castration in

cats ≥5.5 lbs (2.5 kg) and ≥6 months of age; 1 mg/kg once daily for up to a maximum of 3 days.
    - Preoperatively: administer approximately 30 minutes prior to surgery.
    - Postoperatively: tablets may be given with or without food.
  - Dogs: not approved in the USA.
- Solution for injection: not approved in the USA.

No antimicrobial preservative is added to the injectable multidose preparation. Ethanol is present to enhance the preservative efficacy. The artificial beef flavor is only contained in the dog formulation and is sourced from desiccated pork liver powder and not of ruminant origin, associated with a risk of spongiform encephalopathy. T_{max} for the cat is 1 hour and 0.5 hours for SC injection and oral administration. The same is true for the dog. The systemic bioavailability of robenacoxib tablets is 49% in cats without food. In dogs, the average systemic bioavailability of robenacoxib tablets is 62% with food and 84% without food. Bioavailability was 88% after SC injection. The drug is rapidly metabolized by the liver in both cats and dogs. Robenacoxib is excreted predominately via the biliary route (65–70%) in both dogs and cats, with the remainder via the kidneys. Consistently, robenacoxib has shown no inferiority to meloxicam, with a suggestion of improved safety based on inhibition of COX-1.

Radiosynoviorthesis

In the USA alone, there are an estimated 16.6 million dogs with some degree of osteoarthritis (OA), the most common canine musculoskeletal disease. The first choice and most efficacious therapy is use of NSAIDs by the oral route. However, most NSAIDs require daily dosing and are primarily symptom-modifying agents. Injection into synovial joint spaces with therapeutic chemicals is a well-established therapeutic modality in equine medicine and human health that utilizes corticosteroids, local anesthetics, hyaluronic acid, and other compounds for inflammation reduction and symptom control. An ideal treatment for OA would be cost-effective, require few or a single administration, be administered locally (avoiding side-effects resulting from systemic administration), be administered in the veterinary clinic (eliminating compliance issues), modify the disease rather than simply improve symptoms, and provide prolonged relief.

Radiosynoviorthesis is a well-accepted therapeutic procedure outside the USA, involving the injection of a radioisotope into the joint synovial space, targeting inflammatory mediators to reduce inflammation and pain. All previously existing isotopes have limitations: (1) adjacent tissue damage; (2) joint leakage resulting in systemic distribution and distant adverse effects; (3) costly, with difficulty in manufacturing and shipping restrictions; and (4) lack of USA approval for any condition. R-NAV proprietary homogeneous tin-117m colloid technology is free of these limitations, with a mode of action that eliminates the macrophages contributing to the inflammation associated with rheumatoid arthritis and OA.

SUMMARY (SEE ALSO TABLE 24.11)

Opioid analgesics have provided the most consistent and effective analgesia for many years and are still the best drugs available for pain control in small animals. It is frequently said that one cannot implement 'serious' pain management without the availability of opioids. Opioids are the cornerstone of perioperative pain management, where they are commonly supplemented with other classes of drugs such as alpha-2 agonists and NSAIDs. The actual agents administered within these classes of drugs are patient-dependent. Selection criteria include the patient disease state, concurrent drug administration, delivery form, duration of effect, potential for side-effects, drug familiarity of the prescriber, and cost.

Whereas opioids are the cornerstone for 'severe' and perioperative pain, NSAIDs are the cornerstone for 'lesser' pain states treated longer term. This is because of the NSAID characteristics as anti-inflammatories, analgesics, and antipyretics. Furthermore, the ease of administration and side-effects of NSAIDs are less than for extended-use opioids. The WHO has suggested an approach to pain management (**Figure 24.28**), progressing from NSAIDs to opioids.

As veterinary medicine becomes more sophisticated in pain management, drug profiles from human medicine are being considered (and often implemented) for veterinary application. Consequently, a number of drugs administered in human medicine are being used in veterinary medicine based on an anthropomorphic approach and empirical or hearsay support. However, considering that veterinary clinical trials with many of these drugs (e.g. tramadol, amantadine, and gabapentin) are presently nonexistent, the use of such drugs may have a role in veterinary medicine provided (1) the drug's mode of action is understood, and (2) the presumption that there is similar physiology between humans and the veterinary target species is correct.

Neuropathic pain can be thought of as the 'progressed pain state', potentially resulting from any significant

Table 24.11 Commonly used drugs with doses and characteristics.

	Dose	Species	Route	Duration	Comments
Opioids					
Morphine	0.5–1.0 mg/kg	Canine	IM, SC	3–4 hours	Caution with IV administration: histamine release
	0.05–0.1 mg/kg	Feline	IM, SC	3–4 hours	
	0.2 mg/kg loading dose, then 0.1–0.5 mg/kg/hour	Canine	IM then CRI		
	0.2 mg/kg loading dose, then 0.05–0.1 mg/kg/hour	Feline	IM then CRI		
	0.1 mg/kg preservative free	Canine/feline	Epidural	12–24 hours	
	1–5 mg in 5–10 ml	Canine	Intra-articular		
Meperidine	3–5 mg/kg	Canine/feline	IM, SC	1–2 hours	
Methadone	0.1–0.5 mg/kg	Canine/feline	IM, SC	2–4 hours	NMDA antagonist activity
Oxymorphone	0.05–0.1 mg/kg	Canine	IM, IV, SC	3–4 hours	Minimal histamine release
	0.03–0.05 mg/kg	Feline	IM, SC	3–4 hours	
Hydromorphone	0.1–0.2 mg/kg	Canine	IM, IV, SC	2–4 hours	Minimal histamine release
Fentanyl	5 μg/kg initial dose, then 3–6 μg/kg/hour	Canine	IV then CRI		
	2–3 μg/kg initial dose, then 2–3 μg/kg/hour	Feline	IV then CRI		
Fentanyl patch	25 μg/hour	Canine 3–10 kg body weight		1–3 days	24 hours to reach peak concentrations
	50 μg/hour	Canine 10–20 kg body weight		1–3 days	
	75 μg/hour	Canine 20–30 kg body weight		1–3 days	
	100 μg/hour	Canine >30 kg body weight		1–3 days	
	25–50 μg/hour	Feline		≤6 days	6 hours to reach peak concentrations
Butorphanol (10 mg/ml)	0.1–0.2 mg/kg	Canine/feline	IM, IV, SC	Dog 1 hour; cat 2–4 hours	Low oral bioavailability
	0.2–0.4 mg/kg, then 0.1–0.2 mg/kg/hour	Canine/feline	IV then CRI		

Table 24.11 Commonly used drugs with doses and characteristics.

	Dose	Species	Route	Duration	Comments
Pentazocine	1–3 mg/kg	Canine/feline	IM, IV, SC	2–4 hours	
Nalbuphine	0.03–0.1 mg/kg	Canine/feline	IM, IV, SC	2–4 hours	
Buprenorphine	5–20 μg/kg	Canine/feline	IM, IV, SC	4–10 hours	15–30 minute onset. Excellent buccal mucosa absorption in cats
Tramadol	2–10 mg/kg	Canine	PO	12–24 hours	Non-scheduled. Mu agonist activity. Serotonin and norepinephrine reuptake inhibitor. NMDA antagonist at lower doses, GABA receptor inhibitor at high concentrations
Codeine	1–2 mg/kg	Canine	PO		
Alpha-2 agonists					
Medetomidine (1.0 mg/ml)	2–15 μg/kg	Canine	IM, IV	0.5–1.5 hours	Sedation, bradycardia, vomition. For dexmedetomidine use one-half the dosing recommendations made for medetomidine
	5–20 μg/kg	Feline	IM, IV	0.5–1.5 hours	
	1 μg/kg, then 0.0015 mg/kg/hour	Canine/feline	IV then CRI		
	1–5 μg/kg	Canine/feline	Epidural		
	2–5 μg/kg	Canine/feline	Intra-articular		
Xylazine (antagonist), yohimbine (antagonist), atipamezol	0.1–0.5 μg/kg	Canine/feline	IM, IV	0.5–1.0 hours	
	0.1 mg/kg IV; 0.3–0.5 mg/kg IM	Canine/feline	IV, IM		
	0.05–0.2 mg/kg	Canine/feline	IV		2–4 times the medetomidine dose
NMDA antagonists					
Ketamine	0.5 mg/kg, then 0.1–0.5 mg/kg/hour	Canine/feline	IV then CRI		
Amantadine	3–5 mg/kg	Canine/feline	PO	24 hours	Neuropathic pain
Dextromethorphan	0.5–2 mg/kg	Canine	PO, SC, IV		D-isomer of codeine; weak NMDA antagonist
Methadone	0.1–0.5 mg/kg	Canine/feline	IM, SC	2–4 hours	Opioid derivative

(Continued)

Table 24.11 Commonly used drugs with doses and characteristics. (*Continued*)

	Dose	Species	Route	Duration	Comments
Tricyclic antidepressant					
Amitriptyline	1.0 mg/kg	Canine	PO	12–24 hours	
	0.5–1.0 mg/kg	Feline	PO	12–24 hours	
Ca^{2++} channel modulator					
Gabapentin	5–10 mg/kg	Canine/feline	PO	12–24 hours	
Adjunct					
Acepromazine	0.025–0.05 mg/kg	Canine	IM, IV, SC	8–12 hours	3 mg maximum total dose; used to potentiate or prolong analgesic drugs
	0.05–0.2 mg/kg	Feline	IM, SC	8–12 hours	
Diazepam	0.1–0.2 mg/kg	Canine/feline	IV	2–4 hours	Used to potentiate or prolong analgesic drugs
	0.25-1.0 mg/kg	Canine/feline	PO	12–24 hours	
Local anesthetics					
Lidocaine (1–2%)	≤6.0 mg/kg	Canine	Perineural	1–2 hours	Onset 10–15 minutes. Maximum dose: 12 mg/kg (canine); 6 mg/kg (feline)
	≤3.0 mg/kg	Feline	Perineural	1–2 hours	
	2–4 mg/kg, then 25–80 mcg/kg/minute	Canine	IV then CRI		
	0.25–0.75 mg/kg, then 10–40 mcg/kg/minute	Feline	Slow IV then CRI		
Bupivacaine (0.25–0.5%)	≤2.0 mg/kg	Canine	Perineural	2–6 hours	Onset 20–30 minutes. Maximum dose: 2 mg/kg (canine or feline)
	≤1.0 mg/kg	Feline	Perineural	2–6 hours	
Mepivacaine (1–2%)	≤6.0 mg/kg	Canine	Perineural	2–2.5 hours	
	≤3.0 mg/kg	Feline	Perineural	2–2.5 hours	

noxious insult. It is much easier to identify in humans than in other animals. Although not evidence based, a logical approach to managing the progressive pain state is suggested (**Figure 24.29**). In this approach the protocol of pain management is a multimodal scheme, with drug classes added rather than substituted. The doses are empirical, and one could debate the order of implementation from bottom to top. The merit of this approach is the addition of agents from different drug classes in an attempt to block as many of the 'pain pathways' (transduction, transmission, modulation, and perception) as possible.

The real mandate of medical care is not the saving of lives, but the dispensing of comfort. We cannot expect to

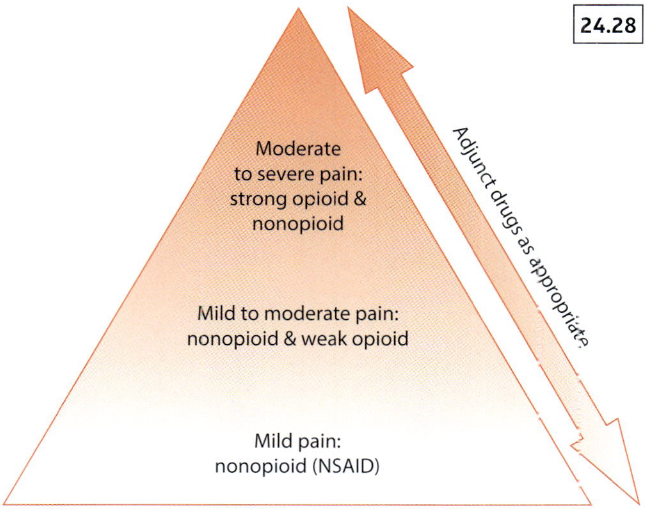

Figure 24.28 An approach to pain management as suggested by the World Health Organization.

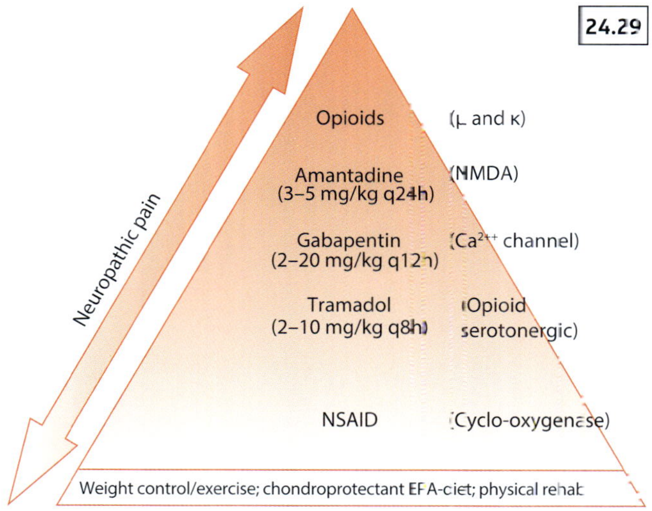

Figure 24.29 A logical approach to managing the progressive pain state.

extend life forever, but we can hope to extend lives free of suffering. When treating pain, knowledge is still the best weapon.

RECOMMENDED FURTHER READING

Bianchi M, Broggini M, Balzarini P *et al.* (2003) Effects of tramadol on synovial fluid concentrations of substance P and interleukin-6 in patients with knee osteoarthritis: comparison with paracetamol. *Int Immunopharmacol* **3:**1901–1908.

Fox SM (2009) *Chronic Pain in Small Animal Medicine*. Manson Publishing, London.

Fox SM (2014) *Pain Management in Small Animal Medicine*. CRC Press, Boca Raton.

Fox SM, Mellor DJ, Firth EC *et al.* (1994) Changes in plasma cortisol concentrations before, during and after analgesia, anaesthesia and anaesthesia plus ovariohysterectomy in bitches. *Res Vet Sci* **57:**110–118.

Honore P, Luger NM, Sabino MA *et al.* (2000) Osteoprotegerin blocks bone cancer-induced skeletal destruction, skeletal pain and pain-related neurochemical reorganization of the spinal cord. *Nat Med* **6(5):**521–528.

Kukanich B, Papich MG (2004) Pharmacokinetics of tramadol and the metabolite O-desmethyltramadol in dogs. *J Vet Pharmacol Ther* **27:**239–246.

Lascelles BDX, Blikslager AT, Fox SM *et al.* (2005) Gastrointestinal tract perforations in dogs treated with a selective cyclooxygenase-2 inhibitor: 29 cases (2002–2003). *J Am Vet Med Assoc* **27(7):**1112–1117.

Lee VC, Rowlingson JC (1995) Pre-emptive analgesia: update on nonsteroidal anti-inflammatory drugs in anesthesia. *Adv Anesth* **V12:**69–110.

Liu SK, Tilley LP, Tappe JP *et al.* (1986) Clinical and pathologic findings in dogs with atherosclerosis: 21 cases (1970–1983). *J Am Vet Med Assoc* **189(2):**227–232.

Mannix K, Ahmedazai SH, Anderson H *et al.* (2000) Using bisphosphonates to control the pain of bone metastases: evidence-based guidelines for palliative care. *Palliative Med* **14:**455–461.

Robertson SA, Lascelles BDX, Taylor PM *et al.* (2005) PK-PD modeling of buprenorphine in cats: intravenous and oral transmucosal administration. *J Vet Pharmacol Ther* **28:**453–460.

Shafford HL, Lascelles BDX, Hellyer PW (2001) Preemptive analgesia: managing pain before it begins. *Vet Med* **6:**478–491.

Singh G, Fort JG (2006) Celecoxib versus naproxen and diclofenac in osteoarthritis patients: SUCCESS-I Study. *Am J Med* **119:**255–288.

Souter AJ, Fredman B, White PF (1994) Controversies in the perioperative use of nonsteroidal anti-inflammatory drugs *Anesth Analg* **79:**1178–1190.

Wooten JG, Blikslager AT, Ryan KA *et al.* (2008) Cyclooxygenase expression and prostanoid production in pyloric and duodenal mucosae in dogs after administration of nonsteroidal antiinflammatory drugs. *Am J Vet Res* **69:**457–464.

Chapter 25

Nutrition of the critically-ill dog and cat

Justin Shmalberg

INTRODUCTION

Nutrition is increasingly recognized as an essential component of veterinary evaluation and treatment. The provision of adequate calories and nutrients in critically ill patients has received significant attention in recent years. Nevertheless, controversy and varying quality of evidence persist. Non-interventional retrospective studies demonstrate that critically-ill patients are less likely to be fed to meet estimated caloric requirements and are also more likely to have extended hospital stays. However, the retrospective nature of these studies limits the ability to draw a clear link between caloric deficit and patient outcome. Such studies do document a failure by clinicians to provide specific nutritional orders, suggesting that nutrition is often overlooked regardless of clinician opinion on the merits of nutritional support. One controlled study of early enteral nutrition in puppies hospitalized for parvovirus infection did document an earlier clinical improvement in those patients fed through a nasoesophageal tube. Therefore, specific critical patients are likely to benefit from voluntary and assisted enteral nutrition.

CURRENT EVIDENCE

Critical care veterinary nutrition has been poorly studied in hypothesis-driven research. Consequently, nutritional evidence from human nutritional research often guides interventions in clinical practice. Acute illness in both humans and other animals is characterized by a reduction in appetite and increased catabolism of endogenous reserves of protein. These effects are mediated by a complex milieu of cytokines including tumor necrosis factor-alpha, interleukin (IL)-6, IL-1B, hormones such as cortisol, epinephrine, glucagon-like peptide 1, changes in resting metabolic rate, and the immune response. The decline in lean body mass secondary to protein catabolism has been associated with prolonged hospital stay and rehabilitation in human patients. Provision of protein and/or essential amino acids has decreased the magnitude of muscle loss in some studies. Such data have not been collected for veterinary patients, but are thought to be similar. Fasting may have protective effects, however, on some aspects of recovery. Starvation is associated with increases in protein recycling through the ubiquitin–proteasome pathway, which processes damaged or potentially toxic proteins. Other studies in human subjects determined that delivery of the full calculated nutritional requirement was associated with increased morbidity compared with those patients receiving more conservative nutritional interventions. Therefore, the timing and type of nutritional intervention in critical patients is still the subject of much debate.

Human nutritional studies in acute or hospitalized patients are often characterized by small sample sizes and differing patient populations, making meta-analyses challenging. The paucity of data in the veterinary literature makes definitive conclusions even more elusive. Experience with hospitalized human subjects suggests that nutritional best practices may vary with different diseases; recommendations for patients with acute kidney injury (AKI) or chronic kidney disease (CKD) are quite different, for example. As such, veterinary patients likely also experience different condition- and individual-specific requirements for nutrients and for calories. The level of sophistication of evidence-based interventions in veterinary medicine is therefore poor. Interestingly, dogs display increased adaptability to starvation compared with humans, and are evolutionarily programed for significant post-prandial fasting. Cats, conversely, have constitutive upregulation of gluconeogenesis and a lower gastric volume, suggesting adaptability to frequent feedings. Future studies are needed to better refine clinical knowledge, and the guidelines contained herein should be critically evaluated in such a context.

CLINICAL EVALUATION

Nutritional intervention relies on a complete and thorough clinical examination. Specific attention must be paid to body condition score (BCS), muscle condition, visible markers of nutritional status such as dermis and coat, and appropriate identification of co-morbidities. A detailed diet history is equally critical. The initial diet history may be complicated by triage and stabilization of the patient as well as owners' focus on other critical aspects of their animal's care. However, historical diet information should be obtained at the earliest opportunity. This permits detection of chronic malnutrition due to hyporexia, chronic gastrointestinal (GI) abnormalities, or previous dietary deficiencies. The provision of nutrition should ideally be tailored to the individual based on the clinician's subsequent synthesis of owner input and examination findings.

History

A diet history is a commonly overlooked aspect of nutritional assessment. Historical information can provide information about a patient's caloric requirements, feeding habits, recent caloric intake, and food preferences. The latter is especially important in cats, who may be neophobic, especially during acute hospitalization. An awareness of recent calorie consumption can determine the timing of nutritional intervention. For example, a hospitalized cat with several weeks of marked hyporexia should receive nutritional support sooner to prevent hepatic lipidosis, compared with a cat with acute anorexia. Some individual dogs may receive food in the home environment at an amount close to the resting fed energy requirement used for hospitalized patients. Dogs of some breeds, such as Labrador Retrievers, Newfoundlands, and Corgis, commonly consume less than calculated with predictive equations. Such factors are critical when individualizing care.

A thorough diet history may not be possible at a patient's initial presentation. However, technicians or the supervising clinician should try to obtain this information following triage. The diet history should include:

- The type of food commonly fed, including brand, type, and flavor.
- The type and quantity of treats and supplemental foods.
- Specifics regarding dietary supplements.
- Feeding habits (free-choice, meal fed).
- Food allergies, aversions, or preferences.

Clients may need to investigate packaging at home before providing pertinent details given the diversity of foods on the market and the distracted focus of many owners during their pet's illness. Such detailed information is necessary to determine the caloric content and nutrient profile of various foods. Dietary supplements are increasingly encountered, and the potential for toxicity and interactions between herbs and drugs has been reported. Knowledge of feeding habits can provide useful information regarding the likelihood of a patient eating on a particular schedule. Some dogs, with small breeds appearing overrepresented, are accustomed to being fed free-choice and may not be accustomed to the scheduled feeding initiated during hospitalization. Food allergies and intolerance are frequently reported by owners; regardless of the merits of these claims, care should be taken to avoid significant dietary changes in order to prevent acute GI signs. A diet history form can be designed to incorporate these questions and be tailored to a particular practice; such forms can also be employed during therapeutic weight loss.

Body weight and condition

Body weight is frequently measured in clinical patients, primarily for assessing fluid status. Acute changes are most likely fluid related, but repeated measures in chronically treated patients can suggest inadequate nutritional intake. Ideal body weight is also the basis for predictive caloric requirement equations. Patients with effusions, edema, and extensive neoplasia are more reliably assessed by BCS and muscle condition score (MCS) than by body weight.

Body condition scoring provides an assessment of energy reserves, primarily adipose tissue. A 9-point system of scoring has been objectively validated, with 4–5/9 representing ideal body weight (**Figure 25.1**). This is characterized by a clearly visible waist, an 'abdominal tuck' when viewed from the side, and minimal fat covering over the ribs. Many sighthounds display a normal body condition of 3/9. Some breed standards and purebred dog owners may regard 6/9 as ideal for the breed, but unlike sighthounds, there is no physiologic advantage to this preference.

Ideal body weight is calculated for overweight dogs (BCS 6–9/9) using simple conversions. Assessments of patient adiposity demonstrate that each BCS over 5 represents 10–15% over a patient's ideal body weight in dogs. For example, a 40 kg dog with a BCS of 8/9 is 30–45% over ideal weight; using the upper end of this range, the dog's measured body weight is 145% of ideal body weight and therefore ideal body weight is equal to (40 kg)/(145%) or about 28 kg.

The ideal weight of most cats can be estimated by visual assessment. Most cats should be between 3 and 5 kg, so mathematical formulas are unnecessary. Overweight cats are predisposed to a number of conditions encountered in critical care medicine, including hepatic lipidosis, lower urinary tract obstruction, and diabetes mellitus.

Muscle condition

Protein catabolism and loss of lean body mass is poorly assessed with body condition scoring. A separate score has been developed to assess muscle, which is the primary source of amino acids in catabolic animals. Multiple methods of scoring are available, and some may be referred to as a cachexia score. The author uses a 3-point scale where 3/3 indicates normal muscle mass,

25.1

5 Point	Cat	Description	Dog	9 Point
1/5	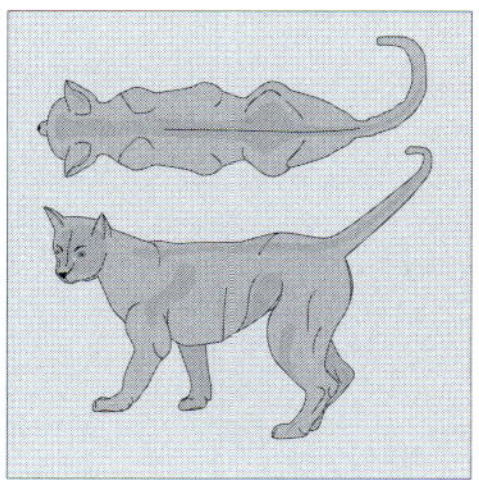	Dogs: Ribs, lumbar vertebrae, pelvic bones, and all bony prominences evident from a distance. No discernible body fat. Obvious loss of muscle mass. Cats: Ribs visible on short-haired cats; no palpable fat; severe abdominal tuck; lumbar vertebrae and wings of ilia obvious and easily palpable.	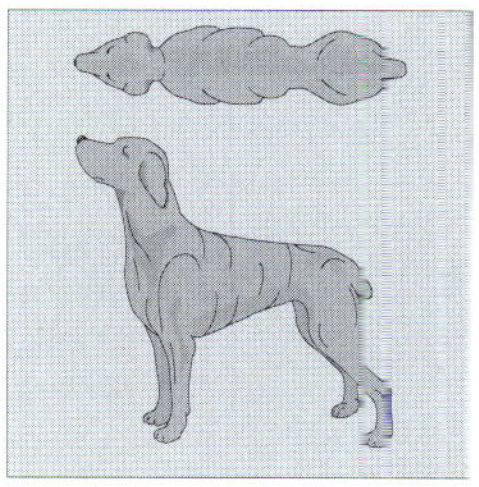	1/9
1.5/5		Dogs: Ribs, lumbar vertebrae and pelvic bones easily visible. No palpable fat. Some evidence of other bony prominence. Minimal loss of muscle mass. Cats: Shared characteristics of BCS 1 and 3.		2/9
2/5	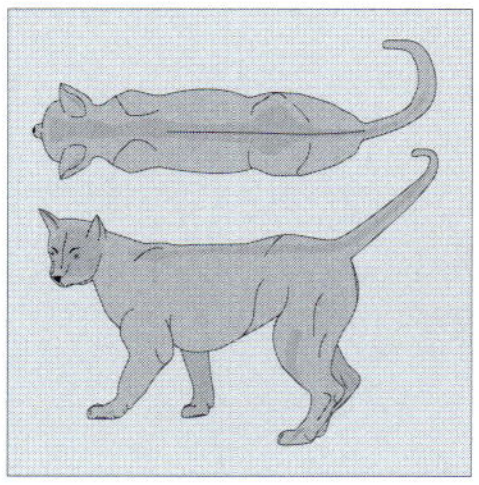	Dogs: Ribs easily palpated and may be visible with no palpable fat. Tops of lumbar vertebrae visible. Pelvic bones becoming prominent. Obvious waist. Cats: Ribs easily palpable with minimal fat covering; lumbar vertebrae obvious; obvious waist behind ribs; minimal abdominal fat.	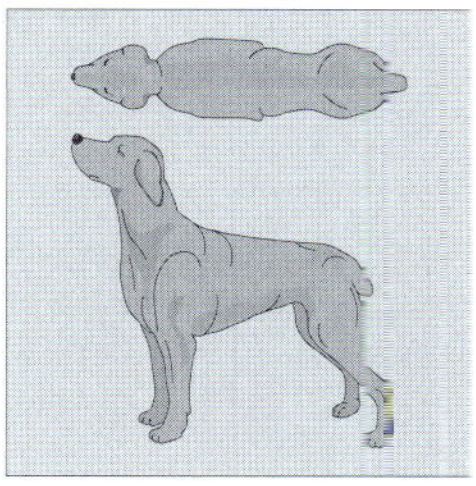	3/9
2.5/5		Dogs: Ribs easily palpable, with minimal fat covering. Waist easily noted, viewed from above. Abdominal tuck evident. Cats: Shared characteristics of BCS 3 and 5.		4/9
3/5	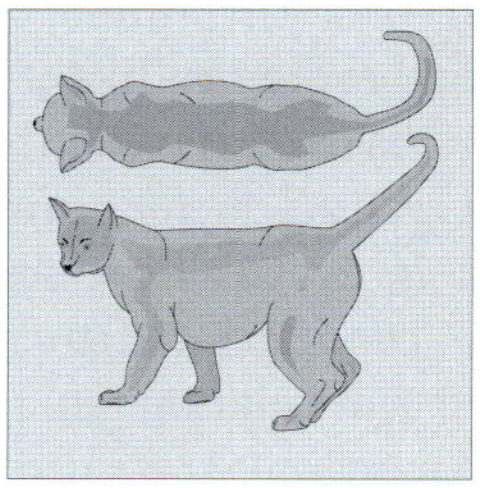	Dogs: Ribs palpable without excess fat covering. Waist observed behind ribs when viewed from above. Abdomen tucked up when viewed. Cats: Well proportioned; waist observed behind ribs; ribs palpable with slight fat covering; abdominal fat pad minimal.	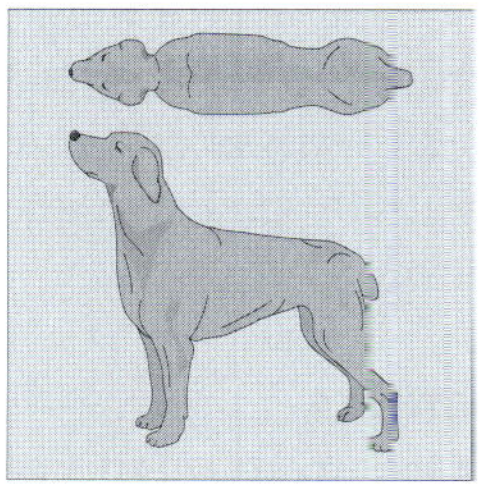	5/9

(Continued)

5 Point		Description		9 Point
3.5/5		Dogs: Ribs palpable with slight excess fat covering. Waist is discernible viewed from above but is not prominent. Abdominal tuck apparent. Cats: Shared characteristics of BCS 5 and 7.		6/9
4/5	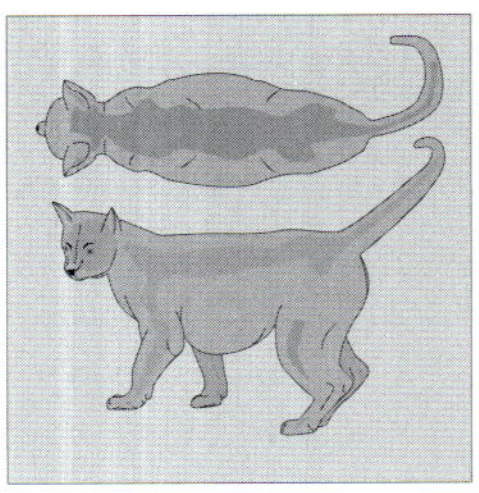	Dogs: Ribs palpable with difficulty; heavy fat cover. Noticeable fat deposits over lumbar area and base of tail. Waist absent or barely visible. Abdominal tuck may be present. Cats: Ribs not easily palpable with moderate fat covering; waist poorly discernible; obvious rounding of abdomen; moderate abdominal fat pad.	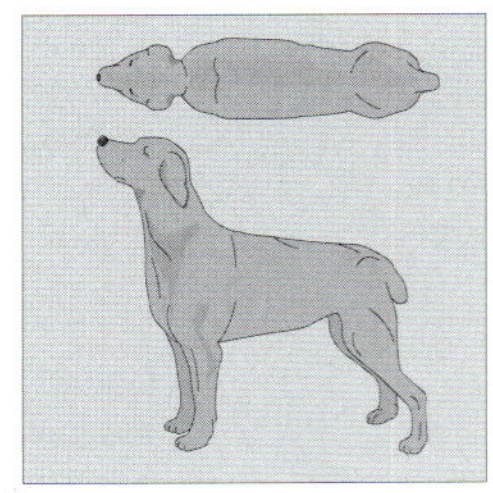	7/9
4.5/5		Dogs: Ribs not palpable under very heavy fat cover, or palpable only with significant pressure. Heavy fat deposits over lumbar area and base of tail. Waist absent. No abdominal tuck. Obvious abdominal distension may be present. Cats: Shared characteristics of BCS 7 and 9.		8/9
5/5	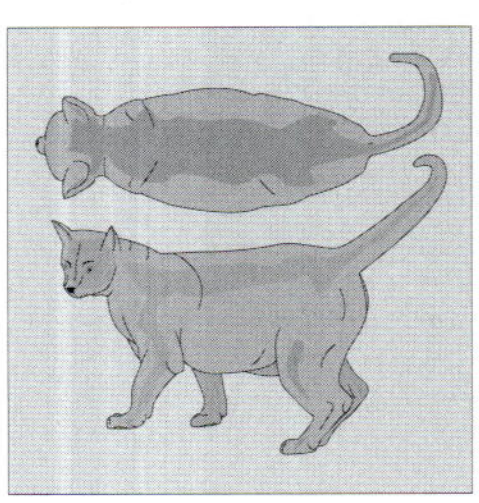	Dogs: Massive fat deposits over thorax, spine, and base of tail. Waist and abdominal tuck absent. Fat deposits on neck and limbs. Obvious abdominal distention. Cats: Ribs not palpable under heavy fat cover; heavy fat deposits over lumber area, face, and limbs; distension of abdomen with no waist; extensive abdominal fat pad.	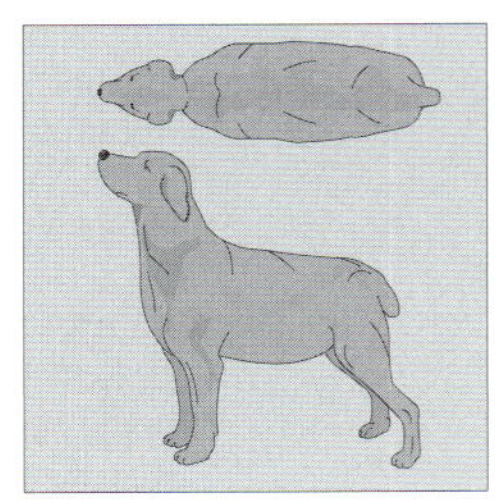	9/9

Figure 25.1 Body condition score (BCS).

2/3 mild muscle wasting, 1/3 moderate, and 0/3 marked (**Figure 25.2**). The high rates of weight loss (>2% per week) seen in prolonged anorexia are characterized by loss of lean body mass as well as adipose stores. Therefore, a decline in both muscle condition and body condition is a sign of malnutrition.

Laboratory markers

Laboratory values from significantly malnourished animals are often within normal limits. Biochemical profiles and complete blood counts are unreliable indicators of nutritional status. Severe hypoalbuminemia, for example, is rarely encountered with prolonged starvation as production is prioritized by the animal; patients presenting with this condition are more likely to have decreased production or increased loss from another cause. Specialized diagnostic testing, such as amino acid profiles and vitamin levels, is available at some academic research laboratories. The extended turnaround times and limited published information on many of these tests in critical care settings limit their use to those cases where clinical suspicion of nutrient deficiency is high, such as in dilated cardiomyopathy in dogs fed lower protein diets or in suspected thiamine deficiency in cats.

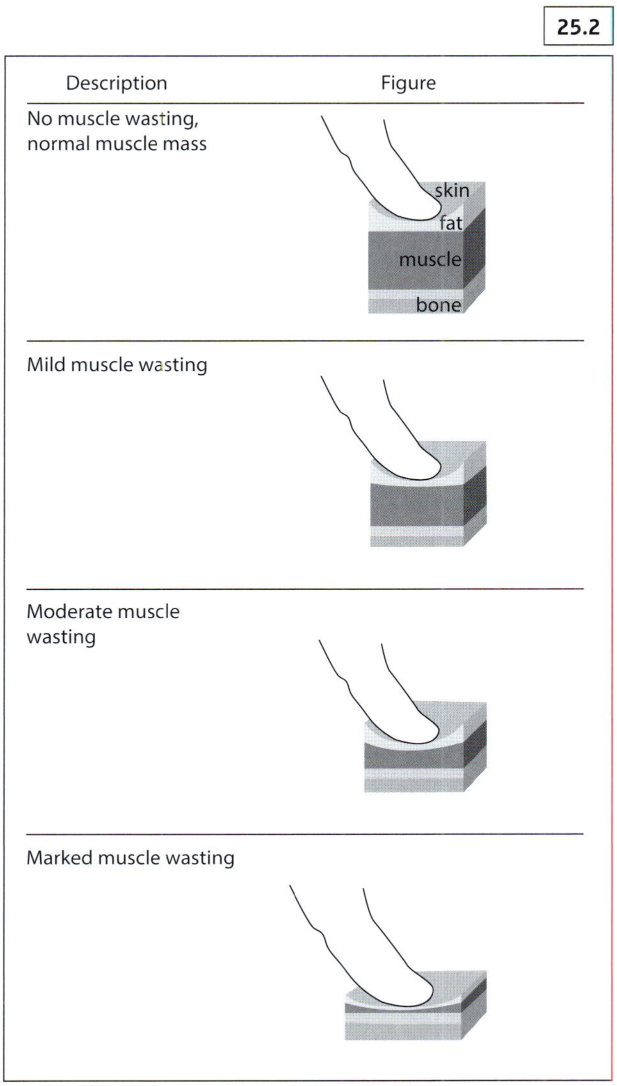

Figure 25.2 Muscle condition score.

TIMING OF NUTRITIONAL SUPPORT

The decision-making rubric for when to intervene with nutritional support is the most contested aspect of critical care nutrition. Current clinical guidelines in humans promote early enteral feeding, and in the event of severe or lengthy caloric deficits, parenteral nutrition (**Figure 25.3**). The trials that suggested a survival benefit for early enteral nutrition were small and contained interventions in the control group, such as parenteral nutrition, which could have worsened survival. The only comparable controlled study in veterinary medicine enrolled puppies with parvovirus infection. All dogs in that study survived, so the statistically significant outcome measure was a 1-day reduction in clinical signs in dogs fed a liquid diet via a nasoesophageal tube. Dogs are documented to survive longer with complete starvation compared with people, suggesting an adaptive ability to tolerate extended fasting. Dogs also display higher rates of fatty oxidation at rest and may therefore be uniquely suited to accommodating for increased lipolysis and beta-oxidation. Nutritional support is often provided earlier in the course of disease in cats due to concerns about hepatic lipidosis. However, only 1 of 12 cats experimentally receiving 25% of their energy requirements developed hyperbilirubinemia after 1 month, and provision of a high-protein diet at this reduced intake decreased hepatic lipid concentration. Early interventional nutrition at low caloric intakes may be protective against complications during illness, but further work is required and species-specific studies may not be translational to other animals. A simplified algorithm for veterinary patients is suggested in the absence of definitive information (**Figure 25.4**).

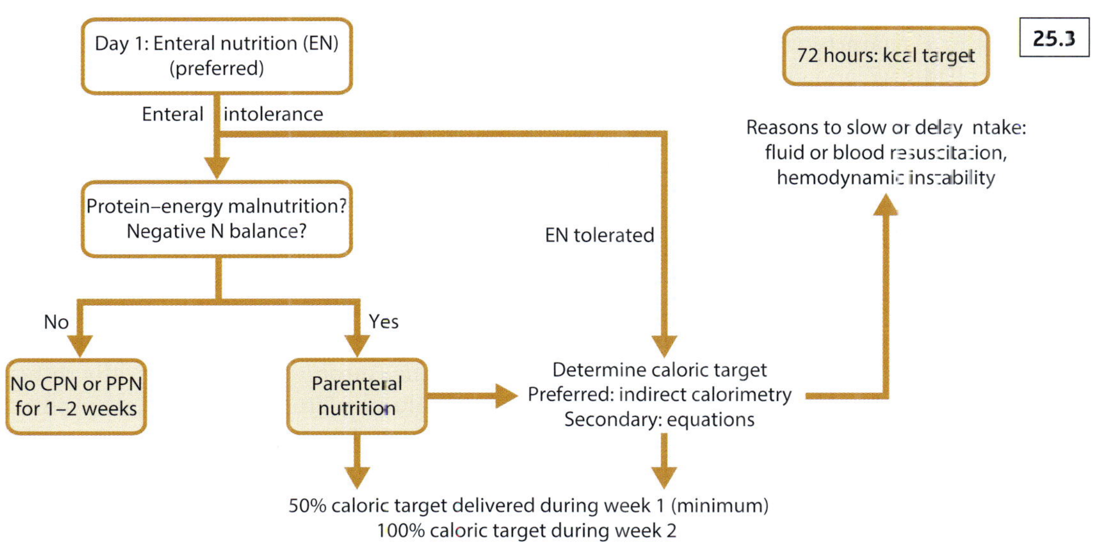

Figure 25.3 Human nutritional intervention rubric. (Adapted from American Society for Parenteral and Enteral Nutrition Guidelines.) N, nitrogen; CPN, central parenteral nutrition; PPN, peripheral parenteral nutrition.

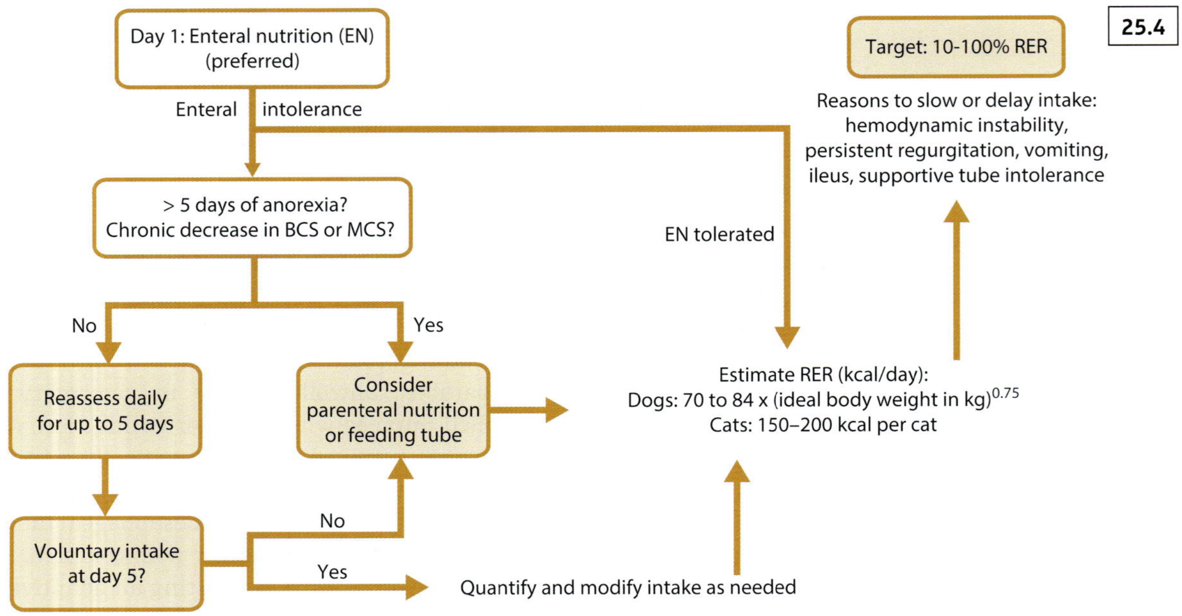

Figure 25.4 Proposed veterinary nutrition decision tree for critically-ill patients. BCS, body condition score; MCS, muscle condition score; RER, resting energy requirements.

NUTRITIONAL AND CALORIC REQUIREMENTS

Dietary nutrient percentages or concentrations define a food's composition, but knowledge of the amount of food fed is critical to determining the dose of nutrients to be administered. Therefore, calculation of caloric needs and an accurate assessment of intake are critical in nutritional support. The hospitalized animal is generally less active than when at home, with the exception of some cats who may be less active during daily routines. The resting energy expenditure (REE) is commonly used as an assessment of fasting, resting land mammals in thermoneutral environments, which characterizes most hospitalized patients. The so-called Kleiber equation ($70 \times [\text{ideal body weight in kg}]^{0.75}$) is used to calculate this figure. The logarithmic component explains why small animals consume more calories per unit of mass than large animals. For dogs between 5 and 25 kilograms, a simplified linear equation ($[30 \times \text{ideal body weight in kg}] + 70$) kcal/day is employed. Ideal body weight is calculated from current body weight in obese patients to prevent overfeeding, as adipose tissue is less metabolically active than lean body mass.

Patients receiving nutritional support are not fasting, and therefore resting fed metabolic rate is more appropriate than REE. The digestion and conversion of nutritional substrates requires energy, generally about 10–20% more than in fasting animals. The dramatic differences in energy expenditure between animals largely negate the benefits of using this higher amount, which requires a more complex formula or a second multiplication step. Clinicians historically also applied illness factors for specific conditions thought to be associated with increased metabolic rate (e.g. burns, sepsis, neoplasia). However, studies suggest that these factors are unnecessary and overestimate true caloric needs.

Cats, unlike dogs, present with relatively homogeneous ideal body weights of between 3 and 5 kilograms. Most resting cats, which includes both those hospitalized and indoor pets, should consume 200–250 calories per day. Equations are unnecessary in cats, and the author typically uses an estimate of 150 kcal/day for a small cat and 200 kcal/day for a larger cat. Most owners dramatically overfeed domestic cats, which could be detrimental if continued during treatment.

The percentage of energy requirements met with nutritional support is likely to affect morbidity and possibly mortality. Human energy requirements can be guided by indirect calorimetry, whereby a medical device measures oxygen consumption to determine the actual instantaneous metabolic rate of that individual. Such measurements are technically difficult and expensive. Human studies relying on predictive equations, similar to those used in veterinary medicine, produced hyperalimentation in some patients, which may increase overall morbidity. Conversely, in studies examining permissive underfeeding, where the intentional provision of caloric intake is less than the calculated or measured requirements, the results generally show favorable or better outcomes compared with those receiving full caloric intake.

Parenteral nutrition in humans, when compared with fasting for up to a week, has in some studies produced poorer outcomes. The complications of IV nutrition include hyperglycemia, secondary infections, activation of the reticuloendothelial system, hyperlipidemia, and thrombophlebitis. Hyperglycemia is the most commonly reported complication in the dog, but this is likely related to provision of high concentrations of dextrose. Dogs and cats appear to tolerate low dextrose, high amino acid, and high-fat diets better than human patients. It is therefore unclear if comparisons of enteral and parenteral nutrition in humans accurately reflect the clinical picture in small animals. Further research in veterinary medicine is necessary to compare fasting, permissive underfeeding, and feeding to meet calculated requirements.

DIET EVALUATION AND COMPARISON

Commercial pet foods are difficult to evaluate and to compare using product packaging. Most veterinarians are interested in nutrient comparisons, and generally turn to the guaranteed analysis on the product label to identify critical nutritional information. The label itself, which is generally modeled after Association of American Feed Control Officials suggested guidelines in the USA, may be misleading. Firstly, the amounts listed are the minimum or maximum 'guaranteed' to be present and the percentages are 'as fed,' which includes the dietary moisture. Canned diets, containing approximately 80% water, have lower listed nutrient percentages than dry foods containing 10% moisture or less. Secondly, conversion to dry matter percentages overcomes the moisture variable, but there are other nutrients that add weight to the food but not calories, including fiber and ash. Nutritionists and veterinarians therefore should only compare foods on a caloric basis, commonly expressed as the grams of a particular nutrient per 1,000 calories (kcal), or 1 Mcal.

The caloric basis for commercial pet foods can be calculated using the guaranteed analysis and caloric density located on the bag. Specific simplified formulas are available (**Figure 25.5**). Some diets with low fat percentages on the label are not in fact fat restricted and therefore inappropriate for the long-term management of chronic active pancreatitis. Many weight loss diets appear restricted in nutrients on the label due to the inclusion of large amounts of fiber, but when fed at an appropriate number of calories, are often higher in nutrients. The caloric basis in many product guides is now readily available to veterinarians. Current nutrient profiles for diets encountered in many critical care centers are provided (see **Table 25.1**).

NUTRIENT CONSIDERATIONS

Water

Water is an important essential nutrient, the requirement for which is directly related to caloric requirements. Dogs generally require 1 ml of water per kcal consumed, and cats only about 0.6 ml of water per kcal consumed. Careful attention should be paid to voluntary water intake, and hydration should be frequently assessed to determine if intervention is needed.

Protein

Many acute illnesses increase the rate of skeletal muscle proteolysis and contribute to a decrease in lean body mass. Dietary protein can ameliorate some of this protein loss and is generally well-tolerated, with the common exceptions of severe renal disease or hepatic encephalopathy. In addition, if a patient's food intake is reduced, then a higher protein concentration in the diet is required to meet daily minimums. A hyporexic patient with AKI often should not consume a protein-restricted renal diet, for example, because it may be insufficient in the amount consumed to replace amino acid losses.

Specific amino acids have been discussed as an adjunct to nutritional therapy in the critically ill patient. Glutamine, a non-essential amino acid, is a nitrogen donor produced by skeletal muscle to provide substrate for amino acid production in critical tissues such as the GI mucosa and liver. Decreased glutamine levels have been documented in hospitalized human patients, but data on supplemental doses of glutamine have been mixed. Clinical studies in dogs are lacking, but a research study of fasted dogs suggested some positive effects on GI glutathione status. Most foods contain glutamine, especially animal protein sources, so the provision of dietary protein is likely more important than glutamine supplementation. Arginine, an essential amino acid in the dog and cat, is a precursor to nitric oxide and an intermediate in the urea cycle. Clinical utility in immunomodulation has been suggested, and one therapeutic diet administered to lymphoma patients includes elevated levels. However, patient selection for supplementation in human subjects is unclear, and no information is available for dogs and cats. Nevertheless, it is prudent to meet minimal requirements.

25.5

TABLE 1. STEP BY STEP: ESTIMATING NUTRIENT CONCENTRATION ON A CALORIC BASIS

Step 1	• Add 1.5% to protein percentage from pet food label • Add 1% to fat percentage from pet food label
Step 2	Divide kcal/kg by 10,000
Step 3	Divide estimated protein % and fat % by number obtained in Step 2

TABLE 2. COMPARISON OF PET FOODS BY CALORIC BASIS

Canine Diets	**NRC RA*** (g/1000 kcal)	**Low** (g/1000 kcal)	**Moderate** (g/1000 kcal)	**High** (g/1000 kcal)
Protein	25	< 60	60–90	> 90
Fat	13.8	< 30	30–50	> 50
Carbohydrate	n/a	< 50	50–90	> 90
Feline Diets	**NRC RA*** (g/1000 kcal)	**Low** (g/1000 kcal)	**Moderate** (g/1000 kcal)	**High** (g/1000 kcal)
Protein	50	< 80	80–120	> 120
Fat	22.5	< 40	40–60	> 60
Carbohydrate	n/a	< 35	35–70	> 70

*National Research Council recommended allowance[2]

TABLE 3. CONVERSION OF GUARANTEED ANALYSES + COMPARISON OF TWO COMMERCIAL DOG FOODS

Ingredient	**PET FOOD 1 (DRY)**	**PET FOOD 2 (WET)**
GUARANTEED ANALYSIS		
Crude protein (min)	25%	8%
Crude fat (min)	15%	5%
CALORIE CONTENT		
kcal/kg	3606	1198
CONVERSION		
Protein	**1.** 25% + 1.5% = 26.5% **2.** 3606 kcal/kg /10,000 = 0.3606 **3.** 26.5 / 0.3606 = **74 g/1000 kcal**	**1.** 8% + 1.5% = 9.5% **2.** 1198 kcal/kg/ 10,000 = 0.1198 **3.** 9.5 / 0.1198 = **79 g/1000 kcal**
Fat	**1.** 15% + 1% = 16% **2.** 3606 kcal/kg / 10,000 = 0.3606 **3.** 16 / 0.3606 = **44 g/1000 kcal**	**1.** 5% + 1% = 6% **2.** 1198 kcal/kg / 10,000 = 0.1198 **3.** 6 / 0.1198 = **50 g/1000 kcal**
FINAL RESULT	**Moderate protein / moderate fat**	**Moderate protein / high fat**

References

1. Hill RC, Choate CJ, Soott KC *et al.* (2009) Comparison of the guaranteed analysis with the measured nutrient compostion of commercial pet foods. *JAVMA* **234(3):**347-351.
2. National Research Council Ad Hoc Committee on Dog and Cat Nutrition (2006) *Nutrient Requirements of Dogs and Cats.* National Academies Press, Washington DC

Figure 25.5 Caloric basis calculations and comparisons. (Reprinted from Shmalberg J (2013) Beyond the guaranteed analysis: comparing pet foods. *Today's Veterinary Practice* **3(1):**43, with permission.)

Table 25.1 A selection of commercial liquid diets administered to dogs in the USA.

Nutrient density	Abbot Ensure Plus	Abbot Clinicare	Abbot Jevity 1.5	Nestle Vivonex Plus
Protein (g/Mcal)	37	82	43	45
Fat (g/Mcal)	31	51	33	7

Note: Consult product guides for current specifications.

as with all amino acids. The recommended allowance for protein is 25 grams and 50 grams per Mcal, respectively, for dogs and cats. Hospitalized animals may consume less than average pets, and therefore a provisional minimal concentration of 50 grams of protein in dogs and 75 grams of protein per Mcal in cats is recommended.

Fats

Fats and protein are essential macronutrients; there is no requirement for dietary carbohydrate. Glucogenic amino acids can form glucose, but fatty acids cannot and must be processed through beta-oxidation. Many fasting animals have higher rates of beta-oxidation than when fed, and small animals, especially the dog, may be distinctly adapted to high-fat diets during starvation. Fats are also more than twice as energy dense as protein and carbohydrate. The recommendations for dietary fats for maintenance are 13.8 and 22.5 grams per Mcal in dogs and cats, respectively. As with protein, dietary concentrations should be increased for reduced intake; values of 30 grams and 40 grams, respectively, are advised. The type of fat may also modulate response to disease. Polyunsaturated fatty acids of the omega 3 and 6 fatty acid series are converted to inflammatory mediators in the prostaglandin and leukotriene classes as well as thromboxanes. In general, omega 3 fatty acids, such as eicosapentaenoic acid (EPA) and docosahexaenoic (DPA) found in marine sources such as fish, produce less potent inflammatory mediators, whereas omega 6 fatty acids such as linoleic acid produce more potent mediators. A therapeutic dose of 1–3 mg of EPA+DHA per calorie has been suggested as an adjunct measure in the treatment of renal disease in order to increase glomerular filtration rate, osteoarthritis due to a reduction in intra-articular cytokines, and in neoplasia likely due to chemosensitization. European markets license a parenteral lipid solution with elevated omega 3 fatty acids, while the American forms are primarily omega 6 fatty acids. The influence of these various lipid types when administered parenterally in clinical veterinary patients is not yet known.

Vitamins

Fat-soluble and water-soluble vitamins are commonly added to commercial pet foods. Water-soluble vitamins are of greatest concern in acute disease given the limited storage pools and the effect of diuresis on vitamin loss. B vitamins are the most common conditional deficiencies and broadly function as cofactors to cellular metabolism. Vitamin B12 deficiency requires chronic deficiency. The lack of intrinsic factor production by the pancreas in cats (as opposed to the pancreas and stomach in dog) with chronic pancreatitis, or with impaired absorption due to severe ileal disease in either species, could warrant prophylactic supplementation of B12. Injectable B complex can be used to provide other B vitamins. Thiamine deficiency in cats causes anorexia, postural changes including ventroflexion, short seizures, and death, if untreated. Clinical supplementation is warranted if these symptoms are encountered, especially in cats historically fed canned or unprocessed fish-based diets. In most clinical situations, supplementation of vitamins A, D, E, and K is not advised.

Minerals

Many minerals are stored in sufficient quantity by tissues so that acute supplementation is not needed except with obvious deficiencies. Adult dogs and cats, for example, have accessible calcium stores in bones. Conditions that cause acute electrolyte shifts, however, may prompt supplementation. Re-feeding syndrome has been reported in cats and humans; it has been theorized to occur in dogs but is poorly documented. The mechanism of re-feeding syndrome in severely emaciated patients is thought to be due to a rapid infusion of carbohydrate into the duodenum, which stimulates a large release of insulin, triggering intracellular electrolyte shifts and resulting in severe hypokalemia, hypophosphatemia, and hypomagnesemia. Fatal sequelae are possible. Therefore, diets given to emaciated animals should be replete in minerals and ideally high in protein and fat while low in carbohydrate; kitten and puppy foods generally provide suitable diets. Supplementation of other minerals, such as zinc for effects on immune function and selenium as a component of the intracellular antioxidant glutathione, has been recommended but poorly supported.

ROUTES OF ADMINISTRATION

Voluntary intake

Voluntary food intake by hospitalized or acutely ill patients is ideal given the low cost and the ability of the animal to control the rate of feeding. Interventional nutrition is generally associated with a greater potential for iatrogenic harm than voluntary intake, except in those patients that have refractory vomiting or regurgitation despite normal appetite. Ideally, the animal's previous diet should be offered during hospitalization, especially for cats. Only if necessary should a single new and sacrificial diet be offered. Therapeutic diets intended for long-term feeding should not be offered during hospitalization or acute illness so as to avoid the development of food aversion. Similarly, offered foods should not be left in a cage with an animal unless that animal has a history of free-choice feeding and clinical suspicion is high that they will voluntarily consume food. The constant smell of a particular diet within the cage during a period of illness has been hypothesized to also trigger aversion. Ideally, voluntary intake should be precisely quantified to determine the percent of caloric requirement being met. Weighing of the food may be necessary for smaller animals.

Assisted enteral feeding

The decision to provide assistive support is guided by the patient's diet history, clinical assessment, and interventional logarithms (see **Figure 25.4**). Selection of the appropriate assistive strategy is critical for ensuring the best patient outcome.

Nasoenteral feeding tubes (**Figures 25.6a–g**)

Nasoenteral feeding tubes are generally employed for short-term inpatient feeding. These tubes can be placed without anesthesia or special equipment. The measurement of the tube before placement varies based on the intended location of the distal aspect of the tube. Nasoesophageal tubes should be measured from the tip of the nose to ribs 7 to 9. Nasogastric tubes are measured from the tip of the nose to the last rib. Nasojejunal tubes are reported, but require a weighted tube and fluoroscopy for accurate placement. Nasoenteral tubes are usually of 3–8 French size, and are placed ventromedially in the nasal cavity following intranasal administration of a local anesthetic gel or topical ophthalmic solution. Entry into the ventral meatus permits passage of the tube through the nasal cavity into the esophagus. Animals should ideally be monitored for swallowing as the tube is passed. The distance from the nose to the medial canthus can be marked on the tube to guide when a swallow should be observed. The tube is passed to the measured length determined above. Tubes are generally affixed to one of the nares with suture (a 22-guage needle can be inserted first with suture passed through the sharp end of the needle and then the needle removed leaving the suture in tissue). Adhesive 'super' or tissue glue may also be used, but removal of the tube can be more difficult and is presumably more painful for the patient. The tube is affixed in one or two additional sites in order to place it away from the eyes and for additional security. Placement is confirmed with a two-view thoracic radiograph. Negative pressure should be present if the tube is placed in the esophagus, and administration of sterile saline should not elicit a cough. Nasogastric tubes have been theorized to cause irritation of the lower esophageal sphincter and increased regurgitation or vomiting, but there have been no documented differences in complication rates. Nasogastric tubes facilitate assessment of residual gastric volumes, but large residual volumes are not associated with increased GI signs and therefore routine monitoring and removal cannot be recommended. Complications of nasoenteral tubes include rhinitis, transient epistaxis, patient intolerance, and tracheal placement or feeding. Only liquid diets can be administered, either as a continuous infusion or in bolus feedings. Bolus feedings using nasojejunal tubes have been successful in clinical studies.

Esophagostomy tube (**Figures 25.7a–m**)

Esophagostomy tubes are a convenient means of short- or long-term nutritional support that are well-tolerated and free of significant side-effects, with the exception of possible abscess formation around the tube site. The tube is most easily placed in the left mid-cervical region with the patient anesthetized and in right lateral recumbency. A red rubber catheter or a commercially available feeding tube with a size greater than or equal to 5 French is measured from rib 7 to 9 to the anticipated exit point, and that measure is marked on the tube. For large dogs requiring significant volumes of food, stallion urinary catheters can be used to provide a greater diameter tube. Curved hemostats or Carmalt forceps are placed in the mouth following aseptic preparation of the lateral neck. The instrument tip is placed in the proximal esophagus, and lateral pressure is applied to 'tent' the skin over the esophagus using the curved aspect of the forcep. An incision through all the tissue overlying the instrument tip is made until the instrument tip is exteriorized. The instrument handle is then opened and the tip of the catheter clamped firmly over the distal end of the tube. The tube is withdrawn aborally and the tip redirected orally into the esophagus as the tube is slowly withdrawn at the level of the skin until it 'turns' and advances down the esophagus until the previous mark is reached. Two-view thoracic radiographs should be obtained in order to confirm placement. The tube can be used following anesthetic recovery, and both canned and liquid diets can be administered.

Gastrostomy tube

Gastrostomy tubes are generally reserved for planned long-term nutritional support when esophageal bypass is clinically necessary due to megaesophagus, esophageal stricture, cervical disease, or for large volume feedings. 'Low-profile' gastrostomy tubes may also be better tolerated than chronic esophagostomy tubes in some patients that require months to years of assisted feedings. Gastrostomy devices have a larger lumenal diameter (18–24 French) than esophagostomy tubes, allowing for a larger volume of fluid or food to be more easily administered. Tubes can be placed percutaneously, with or without endoscopic support, or surgically. The left side of the patient is aseptically prepared 1–2 cm caudal to the last rib and about one-third of the distance from epaxial muscles to ventral midline. Endoscopic insufflation of air permits endoscopic visualization of the stomach and allows for closer contact between the stomach and the abdominal wall. The endoscope permits tactile and visual (due to the light source) assessment of the position of the stomach to facilitate needle penetration (18 gauge, 1.5 inch) into the gastric lumen. A sterile flexible stylet or suture is then passed through the needle, grasped with endoscopic forceps in the stomach, and removed through the patient's oral cavity. A gastrostomy

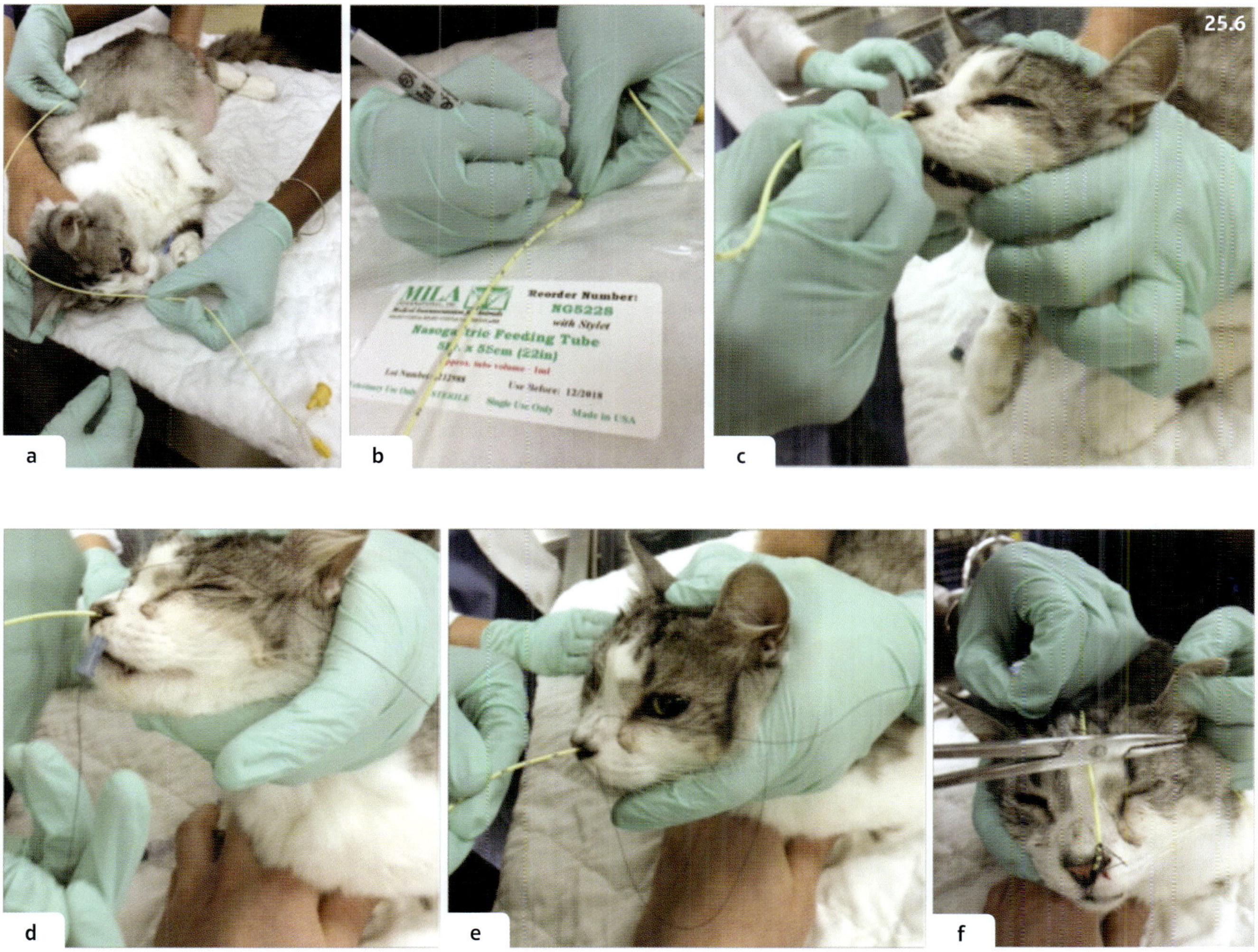

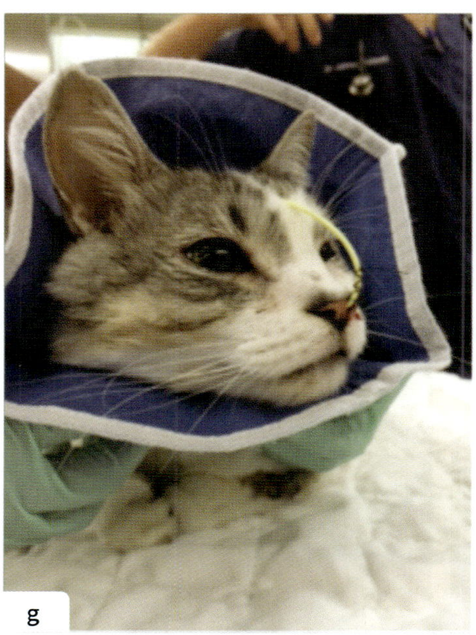

Figures 25.6a–g Nasoesophageal tube placement. (a) The nasoenteral tube is positioned for measurement. Rib 13 is used as a landmark for nasogastric tubes and ribs 7–9 for nasoesophageal tubes. (b) The desired length is marked with permanent ink. The distance from the naris to the medial canthus can also be marked to provide visual feedback as to when to monitor for a swallow response. (c) The tube is placed ventromedially to facilitate entry into the esophagus. Topical local anesthetic is recommended. (d, e) The tube is passed to the previous mark, and the tube affixed with a Chinese finger trap suture pattern, a skin staple, or glued to the fur near the lateral aspect of the naris. (f) One or two additional affixing sutures are placed to position the tube between the eyes so that the feeding end of the tube is caudal to the head. (g) An Elizabethan collar is placed to prevent the patient from dislodging the tube. Radiographs should confirm appropriate placement following placement. The aspiration of negative pressure and a lack of a cough with sterile saline administration can provide additional confirmation, but may be inaccurate as the sole method of assessing placement.

tube is then attached to the suture and the suture pulled orally until the tube exits the abdominal wall. A balloon or other device at the end of the tube prevents it from pulling through the abdominal wall, but the position of the tube should be marked to allow easy assessment of migrating tubes. A retainer flange is used to provide apposition of the gastric mucosa and the abdominal wall. Alternatively, the blind technique usually involves a special curved device, which is sized for the patient and passed orally into the stomach to provide visual assessment for needle penetration. Appropriate placement of blindly inserted tubes can be confirmed with liquid contrast and radiographs. Surgical techniques, described in greater detail in surgical texts, have the advantage of direct visualization of the tissues along with the ability to place intra-abdominal appositional sutures to prevent leakage of gastric contents due to separation of the peritoneal wall and gastric surface.

Gastrostomy tubes are generally well-tolerated by small animals. However, Elizabethan collars must be employed in the first 2 weeks following placement and animals should always be carefully monitored for licking or attempts at tube removal. Prevention of bacterial contamination in the tissues around the skin is critically important, as abscessation or chronic dermatitis can force premature removal of the tube. Both esophagostomy and gastrostomy tubes should be replaced as quickly as possible if inadvertently removed, as natural closure will rapidly occur.

Jejunostomy tube

Jejunostomy tubes are reserved for patients that require gastric or duodenal bypass feeding. Such circumstances include severe pancreatitis, persistent vomiting or regurgitation, gastric or duodenal neoplasia, gastric hypomotility, or gastric outflow obstruction. Surgical placement

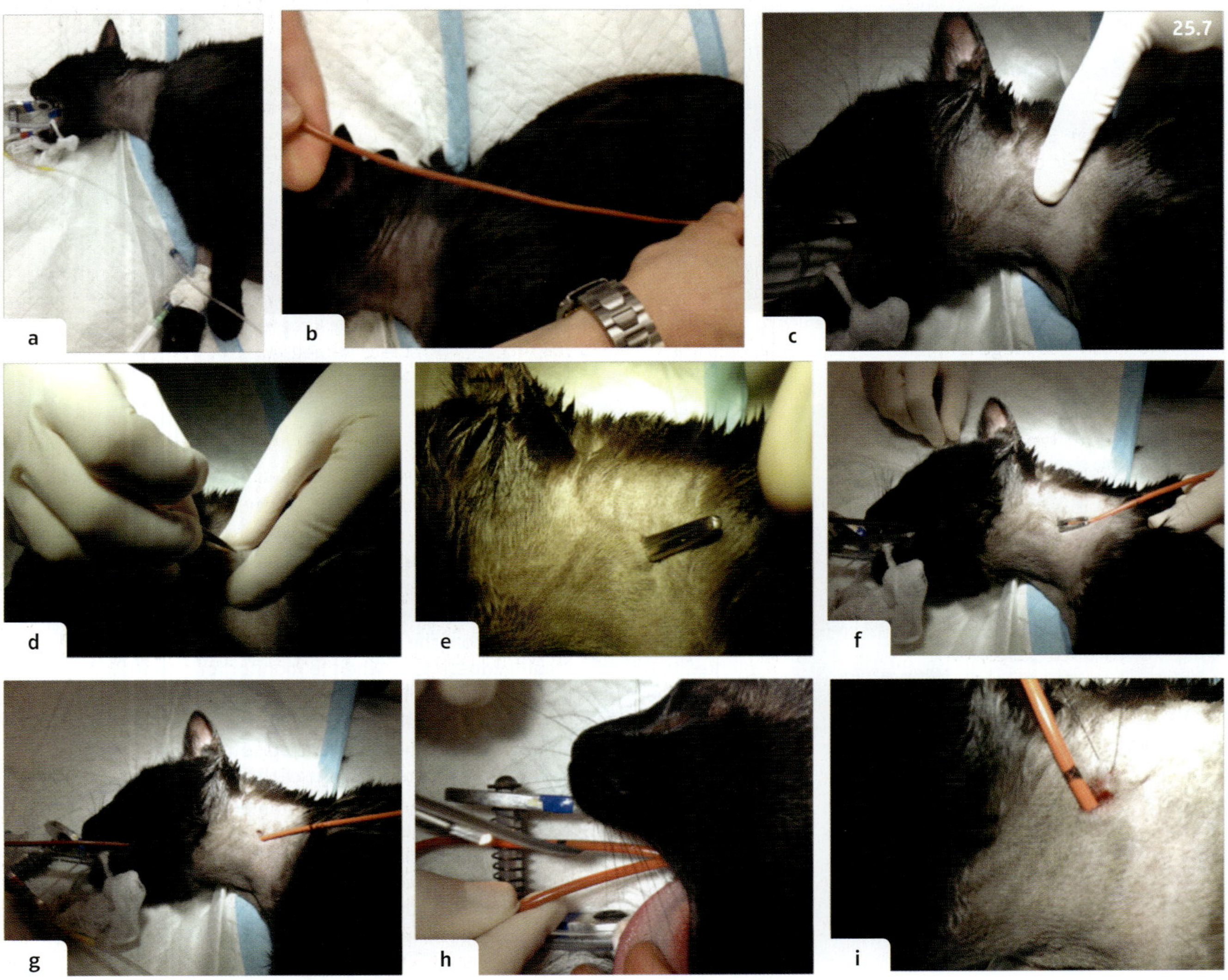

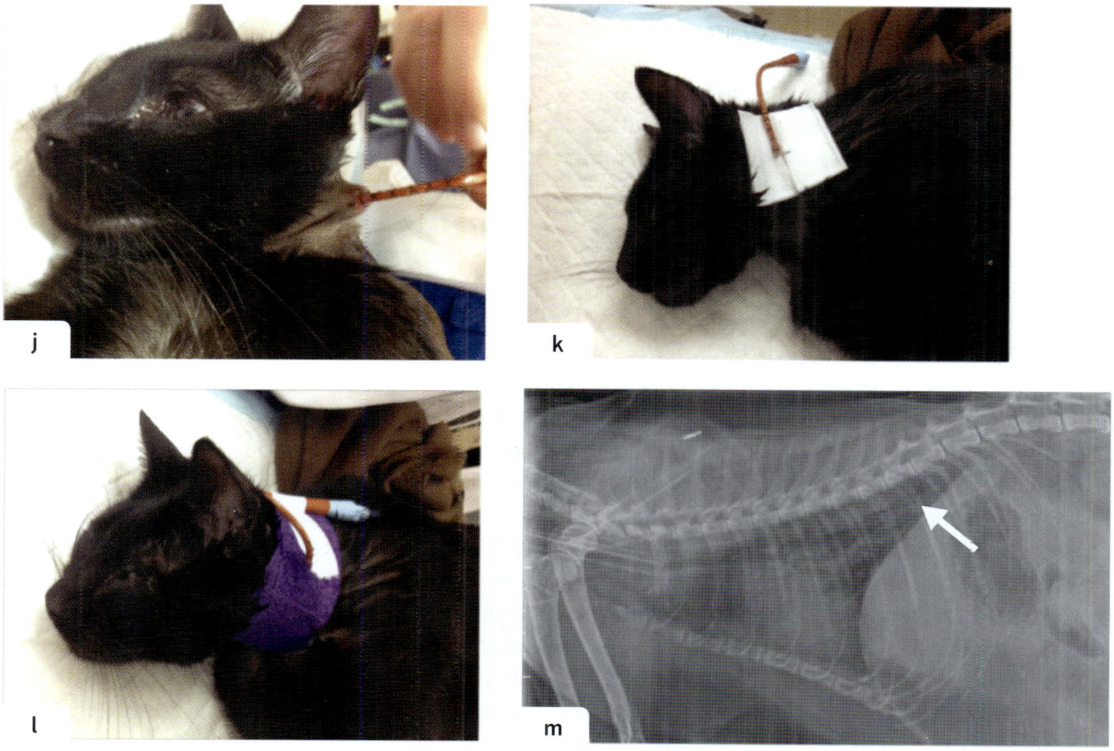

Figures 25.7a–m Esophagostomy tube placement. (a) The left lateral neck is aseptically prepared. (b) The esophagostomy tube is measured from the expected point of insertion to rib 7–9, and that distance marked on the tube with permanent ink. (c) A curved instrument is passed orally into the esophagus and lateral pressure is applied until the instrument tip is palpated. (d) A stab incision is made over the tip of the instrument. (e) The curved instrument tip is moved laterally to exit the incision. (f) The distal end of the tube is grasped with the instrument. (g) The tube is pulled aborally with gentle traction. (h) The end of the tube is passed orally back into the esophagus while slowly pulling laterally on the syringe end of the tube in order to facilitate movement of the tube into the distal esophagus. (i) The tube is inserted to the level of the previous mark. (j) Chinese finger trap sutures are used to secure the tube to the dermis. (k) Antibiotic ointment and/or gauze is applied over the esophagostomy site. The catheter end of the tube is capped. (l) A nonocclusive bandage is applied to protect the area and to secure the tube. (m) A thoracic radiograph confirms appropriate placement. (The arrow indicates the tip of the esophagostomy tube in front of the lower esophageal sphincter.)

with or without laparoscopy is generally required. Tubes cannot be removed for 7–14 days following insertion as creation of a stoma is required to prevent septic peritonitis, the most catastrophic of jejunostomy tube complications. Jejunostomy tubes may also be placed through a gastrostomy tube, but endoscopic or intraoperative guidance of the tube into the intestinal lumen is usually required. In both cases, tube diameter limits feeding to liquid enteral diets, and such diets are most commonly administered as a continuous infusion. However, three bolus feedings per day were not associated with increased adverse effects in one study. Dogs and cats also clinically appear to tolerate liquid diets of varying composition.

Tube management

Tube feedings can be complicated by obstructions within the tube caused by saponification of fat, improperly mixed diets, pH changes, incompatible medications, and similar substances. Tubes are commonly flushed with warm water before and after each use, with an amount consistent with the volume of the tube. Carbonated beverages and pancreatic enzyme solutions may also prove helpful if obstructions do not respond to water alone.

Water is first administered following placement of an assistive feeding tube. Nasoenteral and esophagostomy tubes may be used shortly following recovery from any sedation or anesthesia. Other tubes that critically rely on stoma formation, such as gastrostomy or jejunostomy tubes, should be tested with water 12 hours after placement, and food can be administered about 24 hours after insertion. Esophagostomy and jejunostomy tubes should be wrapped when not being used and cleaned daily with disinfectant solution.

Dietary options for feeding tubes are dictated by the size of the feeding tube and the required caloric density. Clinical veterinary and human liquid diets with caloric densities of 1–1.5 kcal/ml are used for small diameter tubes such as nasoenteral and jejunostomy tubes (**Table 25.1**). Human enteral diets should not be used in cats, given the more stringent nutritional requirements of this species, including an obligatory need for taurine and arachidonic acid, and higher protein intakes compared with dogs and humans. Canned diets can be employed in most other assistive feeding devices. Any canned diet is theoretically an option, but high-fiber diets have a very low caloric density when mixed with sufficient water. High-calorie, low-fiber, moderate to high protein and fat diets facilitate the highest caloric densities (~1 kcal/ml) (**Table 25.2**). Many 'recovery' diets are commercially manufactured to permit ease of administration through a feeding tube.

Animals with feeding tubes may require frequent feedings. No significant differences in continuous infusions as opposed to bolus feedings have been identified. Aspiration and measurement of gastric residual volumes is not beneficial in most cases. Gastric volume is the limiting factor in determining the number of feedings. Clinical experience suggests that cats tolerate about 60 ml/feeding when administered over 10–15 minutes and therefore require about four feedings per day. Dogs display much greater gastric expansion with sufficient time. A figure of 50 ml/kg is commonly employed as an estimate of tolerated volume, but dogs are known to consume about 10% of body weight in a single meal. Many dogs can be fed on routine twice daily schedules with feeding tubes. Owners should be instructed that less frequent feedings may be possible, but will require additional time at each feeding.

Parenteral nutrition

IV administration of nutrients is reserved for those cases with documented or anticipated periods of prolonged hyporexia or anorexia. However, patients with low BCSs or MCSs may benefit from earlier intervention with parenteral nutrition. This method of nutritional support may be appropriate for animals with prolonged ileus, those receiving ventilator support, and those who display diffuse refractory GI symptoms. Parenteral nutrition requires specialized techniques and solutions that may not be available at all practices. The cost to feed patients with this method can be substantially higher than with enteral feeding.

IV nutrition can be administered through a central line (central parenteral nutrition) or through a dedicated peripheral catheter (peripheral parenteral nutrition). The terms total and partial parenteral nutrition are no longer used, as most veterinary parenteral nutrient mixtures do not meet the total nutrient requirements for patients. Frequent complications of parenteral nutrition include hyperglycemia and thrombophlebitis. Lowering the dextrose content of the solution can reduce the risk of the former and the latter is reduced by placement of a central line. Peripheral parenteral nutrition solutions should have an osmolality no greater than 650 mOsm/l. Infection, possibly leading to sepsis, is theoretically possible, as some components of parenteral nutrition, such as IV lipid, could serve as a bacterial media. However, the high osmolality of parenteral nutrition solutions and careful technique usually prevent contamination of the fluid itself. Most parenteral nutrition-related infections occur due to migration of bacteria around the catheter site, so aseptic catheter technique is critically important. Only a dedicated catheter or a dedicated port on a multi-lumen catheter should be used. Injections should not be given through the same port as parenteral nutrition.

Parenteral mixtures generally contain carbohydrate, fat, and protein in the forms of dextrose, lipid emulsion, and amino acids (**Table 25.3**). Carbohydrate is not required in the formulation, and both cats and dogs have been managed with mixtures of only lipid emulsion and amino acids. The concentration of dextrose appears related to the incidence of hyperglycemia. IV lipid emulsions have been reported to impair reticuloendothelial

Table 25.2 Commercial diets marketed for tube feeding critical patients in the USA.

Diet	Protein (g/1,000 kcal)	Fat (g/1,000 kcal)	Fiber (g/1,000 kcal)	Carbohydrate (g/1,000 kcal)
Royal Canin Recovery	107	67	7	4.7
Science Diet A/D	92	63	3	32
Iams Maximum Calorie	72	64	5	21.5
Purina CN	79	74	1.5	15

Note: Consult product guides for current specifications.

Table 25.3 Common components of parenteral nutrition.

Component	kcal/ml	mOsm/l
50% dextrose	1.7	2525
5% dextrose	0.17	253
20% lipid	2.0	260
8.5% amino acids without electrolytes	~0.57	~700
8.5% amino acids with electrolytes	~0.57	~920

Note: Peripheral solutions should be limited to less than 650 mOsm/l. The addition of electrolytes may increase osmolality. Hypertonic saline provides 1.2 mEq of sodium and chloride per ml and contains 2.4 mOsm/ml.

Table 25.4 A general parenteral nutrition solution for peripheral administration.

Component	Volume (ml)
8.5% amino acids without electrolytes	500
20% lipid	250
5% dextrose	250
50% dextrose	25
Hypertonic (7.2%) saline	40
Heparin (1,000 units/ml)	1

Note: The calorie distribution of nutrients is 23% protein (56 g/Mcal), 12% carbohydrate (30 g/Mcal), and 66% as lipid (73 g/Mcal). The caloric density is 0.71 kcal/ml, and the calculated osmolality is 600 mOsm/l. Electrolyte composition is 61 mEq/l sodium, 46 mEq/l chloride, and 4 mEq/l phosphorus. Additional electrolytes, minerals, and vitamins should be added as the patient's status dictates.

Table 25.5 A general parenteral nutrition solution for central administration.

Component	Volume (ml)
8.5% amino acids without electrolytes	1,000
20% lipid	250
5% dextrose	500
Hypertonic (7.2%) saline	60
Heparin (1,000 units/ml)	1.8

Note: The calorie distribution of nutrients is 20% protein (50 g/Mcal), 50% carbohydrate (125 g/Mcal), and 30% as lipid (33 g/Mcal). The caloric density is 0.93 kcal/ml, and the calculated osmolality is 1,200 mOsm/l. Electrolyte composition is 58 mEq/l sodium, 41 mEq/l chloride, and 2 mEq/l phosphorus. Additional electrolytes, minerals, and vitamins should be added as the patient's status dictates.

system function in other species, which could have implications for their use in septic patients. Such solutions could also worsen hyperlipidemia and have been hypothesized to worsen pancreatitis. However, the effect of IV lipid on canine and feline pancreatitis is rarely reported, and both species have been managed for this condition with high-fat solutions. Peripheral parenteral nutrition solutions commonly contain increased lipid compared with centrally administered solutions, as lipid possesses a lower osmolality compared with other constituents (**Tables 25.4** and **25.5**). The higher basal rate of fatty acid oxidation has prompted some authors to advocate the use of lipid concentrations higher than those used in human nutrition.

Multiple amino acid solutions are available, each with a different blend of essential and nonessential amino acids. Products are produced with or without electrolytes; electrolyte-containing products generally require supplemental potassium and phosphorus, especially in animals that have experienced prolonged anorexia or tissue catabolism. Insulin release causes both an intracellular shift of potassium and an increased cellular phosphate utilization related to the increased production of energy stores, such as adenosine triphosphate or creatine phosphate. Phosphorus is typically added to achieve a concentration of 5–10 mmol/l. Electrolyte-free amino acid solutions can be modified to include sodium and chloride at rates consistent with maintenance or replacement fluids as required through the addition of hypertonic (7.2%) saline.

Provision of water-soluble vitamins supports normal energy metabolism by providing essential cofactors in metabolic reactions. Some IV B complex solutions are low in vitamin B12, so this should be administered SC if deficiency is predicted. Fat-soluble vitamins may be added and are included in some multivitamin combinations designed for parenteral nutrition, but substantial reserves are likely present in many patients. Trace elements for parenteral administration are available but controversial.

The amount of protein, in the form of amino acids, to administer is controversial. Protein requirements may be expressed as a percentage of calories in some resources or as an amount in grams to be fed per day. Protein may also be given on top of the calculated caloric requirement

(200 kcal for most cats, 70 × [ideal body weight in kg]$^{0.75}$ kcal for dogs) by some clinicians. The theory is that protein, when given above the calorie needs of an animal, will be more likely used for anabolic reactions rather than for ketogenesis or gluconeogenesis. The provision of dietary protein only partially reverses catabolism in many disease states characterized by high rates of nitrogen turnover and suspected protein loss. Provision of 20% of calories as protein (50 g/1,000 kcal) is adequate for most patients, although encephalopathy may warrant values as low as 40 g/1,000 kcal, and patients with other conditions with high protein requirements can be given solutions up to 28% of calories (70 g/1,000 kcal). Patients fed less than their expected caloric requirements need a solution with greater amino acid or fat concentrations to maintain a consistent 'dose'. Administration of low concentration amino acid solutions (3%) is unlikely to prevent muscle catabolism, especially in the absence of other macronutrients, as most of the amino acids would be converted to energy. Therefore, protein without adequate caloric intake is unlikely beneficial.

Parenteral nutrition requires special monitoring and careful administration. Parenteral nutrition solutions should be refrigerated and kept for no longer than 7–10 days after mixing. Vitamins, if administered, should be added just before hanging a bag to prevent degradation during storage. Careful aseptic techniques should be employed when connecting parenteral nutrition, and a new fluid line should be used with each new bag. Sterile gloves are used when spiking each bag and when connecting a new line to the patient's catheter. Injection ports can be disinfected and covered with sterile gauze, as can all connections between the bag and patient. Some vitamins degrade with ultraviolet light, and when exposure is likely, the bag and line should be covered with special amber sleeves, bandage material, or aluminum foil. The patient should be disconnected from parenteral nutrition only once daily. The bags can be wrapped and taken outside with the patient if necessary. Parenteral solutions may benefit from the inclusion of 1 unit of heparin per ml of mixture to prevent local thrombosis formation and prevent the need for periodic flushing with heparinized saline. Recommended monitoring includes electrolytes twice daily along with a hematocrit/total protein and a visual check of the serum for hyperlipidemia. Most patients can receive parenteral nutrition at one-half of the calculated energy requirements during hospitalization over the first 6–12 hours, with an increase to the full calculated rate thereafter, assuming that the patient tolerates the volume and is unlikely to suffer severe electrolyte shifts secondary to re-feeding.

Nutritional reassessment

Nutritional reassessment is difficult in critically-ill patients, as many commonly measured laboratory parameters are unreliable indicators of malnutrition. Electrolytes should be closely monitored during any nutritional intervention as feeding can create and correct potential abnormalities. Body weight is affected by fluid status, and both body condition and muscle condition scoring systems are unlikely to change during a hospitalization period of 1 week or less. Frequent monitoring of compliance to nutrition orders is preferred, as patient procedures, anesthetic events, failure to follow treatment sheets, and other factors may influence daily caloric intake. Tolerance to feeding plans should also be assessed because persistent vomiting, regurgitation, or diarrhea may warrant alterations to the nutrition orders.

Disease-specific considerations

A number of conditions encountered in critically-ill patients may benefit from specific nutritional strategies. Each patient should be evaluated as an individual, but general recommendations exist for a variety of conditions.

Pancreatitis

Dietary triggers for acute and chronic active pancreatitis are well described, with ingestion of foods high in fat being the most common. Hyperstimulation of cholecystokinin has been hypothesized as a possible mechanism in combination with other patient factors, such as elevated cortisol, obesity, or hyperlipidemia. Evidence-based data on the nutritional treatment of acute pancreatitis are lacking. Many practitioners argue that withholding enteral nutrition in favor of fasting or parenteral nutrition decreases pancreatic stimulation and therefore reduces premature activation of pancreatic enzymes. However, pancreatic responses to nutrition may be abnormal in pancreatitis, so that enzyme activation is actually decreased in response to lumenal nutrition. Jejunostomy tube feeding in dogs and in humans has been tolerated in both species. Humans display lower morbidity when fed through such a tube compared with parenteral nutrition, but it is unclear if this is due to worsened outcome with total parenteral nutrition rather than a beneficial effect of enteral nutrition alone. Luminal nutrition is associated with reductions in the systemic inflammatory response and in preservation of the mucosal barrier, thereby reducing bacterial translocation. The ideal timing of enteral nutrition is unclear. Studies in canine parvovirus infection showed that early enteral nutrition improved outcome and that feeding was well-tolerated irrespective of whether patients were vomiting or regurgitating.

Additional studies are required before definitive recommendations are made on the timing and type of feeding in canine pancreatitis. Dogs with chronic pancreatitis, however, do benefit from low-fat diets (<30 g/Mcal) following discharge. Most therapeutic diets labeled for pancreatitis meet this criterion. Clinicians should consider the expected caloric intake of a patient before making a dietary recommendation. Patients consuming large amounts of food to maintain an ideal body weight would require a lower concentration of fat than dogs consuming a very small amount. Access to high-fat treats and prepared diets intended for consumption by the owner should be restricted.

Serum triglycerides are an important aspect of patient monitoring as free fatty acids, very-low-density lipoprotein, and low-density lipoprotein increase in this condition. A decrease in lipoprotein lipase, causing a subsequent increase in triglyceride and chylomicrons, has been observed in humans but not yet in dogs. Low-fat diets reduce the hypertriglyceridemia in many cases, and provision of omega 3 fatty acids (EPA, DHA) could have an additive benefit along with niacin.

Feline pancreatitis displays many features distinct from those observed in dogs. Concurrent hepatobiliary or inflammatory bowel disease is commonly identified in cats affected with this condition. Premature activation of trypsinogen has been postulated as the mechanism, but the etiology is unclear. Cats presenting with pancreatitis display less vomiting than dogs, and enteral feeding is therefore less complicated. Supportive enteral feeding tubes (nasoenteral, esophagostomy) are often recommended for feline pancreatitis, as hepatic lipidosis (discussed below) is a common clinical sequela in anorectic cats. Jejunostomy tubes are only rarely required. Fasting should be avoided. There is no evidence that dietary fat restriction is necessary in cats, which is in stark contrast to the evidence and clinical experience in dogs. Cats should receive parenteral vitamin B12 injections because intrinsic factor, the requisite cofactor for B12 absorption, is produced only in the pancreas in cats as opposed to both the stomach and pancreas of dogs.

Chronic gastrointestinal disease

Acute gastroenteritis and colitis often respond to fasting, and no specific nutritional interventions are required. Patients may present with chronic GI complaints requiring stabilization. Such patients may suffer from malabsorption, protein-losing enteropathy, maldigestion, and reduced total and lean body mass. Many animals will have concurrent anorexia, and therefore consideration of assistive feeding devices is recommended. Feeding tubes appropriate for at-home use should be prioritized, as a protracted period of stabilization may be required while the underlying disease is managed. Food allergy or intolerance is a common differential for chronic GI disease, and diagnosis or exclusion of these conditions requires a strict food trial. Such trials are best started following patient discharge and only if an animal is voluntarily eating, as food aversion can develop due to perceived associations between diet and disease. Animals with a feeding tube can begin the diet immediately. Some authors advocate the routine use of hydrolyzed diets in the theory that food allergy may develop in patients with a compromised GI barrier. Novel protein diets are the other class of diets used to assess food allergy, but their use requires collection of a thorough diet history to exclude the possibility that an animal has previously received a particular protein source. Previously rare dietary protein sources such as rabbit, kangaroo, and venison are now available over the counter. Diet trials should last 12 weeks, and no other proteins, treats, or flavored medications should be given.

Chronic colitis may respond to hydrolyzed or novel protein diets. Dietary fiber and probiotics are additional considerations. Dietary fiber is generally classified as soluble or insoluble. Soluble fiber sources, such as gums and beet pulp, provide substrates for bacterial fermentation. Insoluble fibers, such as cellulose and peanut hulls, increase fecal bulk. Fiber modification influences intestinal transit, stool consistency, bacterial flora, and fecal moisture. Psyllium supplementation of foods has gained considerable attention. Psyllium, a partially fermentable fiber, contains mucilage that absorbs water and helps to normalize GI transit. It is frequently employed in the dietary management of feline megacolon. Probiotics, living microorganisms administered for health effects, may influence immune responses and nutrient absorption in the colon. Several veterinary specific probiotics have been shown to reduce the duration of diarrhea. However, product quality has been poor for many probiotic products marketed for animal use. The benefits of probiotics in patients receiving concurrent antibiotics are unclear.

Hepatic lipidosis

Excessive accumulations of triglycerides in the hepatocytes of some anorectic, generally overweight cats produce hepatic dysfunction and cholestasis. The occurrence of this condition in cats, but not in dogs, is likely related to the metabolic peculiarities of the cat, a true carnivore. Cats display significant mobilization of triglycerides during fasting, which are transported to the liver for use as energy. In lipidotic cats, however, the rate of mobilization exceeds the rate of clearance. Carnitine complexes with fatty acids to facilitate transport across the mitochondrial membrane, and deficiency of this compound has been proposed as a cause in some cats. Oxidative stress may also be increased, and some B vitamins may be decreased as a function of prolonged anorexia or the condition itself. A variety of nutraceuticals have been recommended, such as carnitine (250 mg daily), SAMe (100–200 mg daily), B complex vitamins (added to fluids), and vitamin B12 (0.5–1 ml [500–1,000 µg] SC daily). Administration of caloric needs is likely more important than supplementation. Supportive feeding measures should be pursued as soon as possible in the disease course. Fat restriction is unnecessary. Despite the intrahepatic lipid accumulation, fat ingestion, when combined with other nutrients, decreases the release of peripheral lipid stores due to the action of insulin. High-protein diets (>90 g/Mcal) are commonly recommended as they may support tissue regeneration. Severely affected cats may display hepatic encephalopathy, and in these rare cases, the protein concentration of the diet should be reduced.

Hepatic encephalopathy

Hepatic encephalopathy warrants immediate nutritional modification following initial stabilization. In addition to lactulose, which converts ammonia to ammonium, thus preventing absorption, neomycin, which decreases ammonia-producing urease-positive bacteria, and the correction of alkalosis, which prevents worsening of encephalopathy, dietary protein restriction is indicated in most patients. Estimates suggest that one-third of blood ammonia is from bacterial production and the remainder from dietary protein intake, because encephalopathic patients lack adequate urea cycle activity to convert ammonia to blood urea nitrogen. Therefore, most dogs with average caloric intake ($90 \times BW^{0.75}$ kcal/day) should receive enough protein to prevent muscle catabolism and provide maintenance requirements, approximately 40–50 g/Mcal. Cats, with higher protein requirements, should receive around 70 g/Mcal. Protein-restricted diets may also be restricted in purine content as the crude protein of the diet is derived from measurement of nitrogen, which includes amino acids, purines, and pyrimidines. Impaired conversion of purines to allantoin results in increased uric acid excretion, predisposing to urate uroliths. Most therapeutic hepatic diets are appropriate for encephalopathic patients; however, patients consuming few calories may be fed a normal diet. Renal diets are not commonly recommended for extended feeding of the encephalopathic patient, as such diets tend to be alkalinizing, which worsens clinical signs. In addition to the standard therapies listed above, soluble fiber has been suggested in the management of encephalopathy, mainly due to lactulose-like effects on lowering intestinal pH.

Renal disease (see also Chapter 12: Nephrology/urology)

Most patients with AKI or CKD do not require immediate dietary modification. Azotemia may predispose to anorexia and nausea, and attempts to administer a new diet can result in profound food aversion. The role of nutrition in AKI is unclear, but it is generally accepted that such patients have high rates of protein catabolism and may therefore benefit from normal maintenance diets. If animals consume little food during hospitalization, high-protein diets may even be appropriate to prevent loss of lean body mass. CKD patients can typically be fed their historical diet during hospitalization. The effects of diet in CKD are well studied in both dogs and cats and directly impact survival when fed for extended periods. Advanced stages of renal disease may require assistive feeding tubes, primarily esophagostomy or gastrostomy, in order to facilitate owner administration of calories and sufficient water.

The features of most diets designed for CKD include reduced phosphorus and protein, elevated omega 3 fatty acids, reduced sodium, and increased caloric density. One diet fed to dogs with stage 3 and 4 CKD permitted a median survival time of about 600 days compared with 200 days in the control group. Similar findings of a feline diet marketed for renal disease were reported: 633 days versus 264 days. Another study of a different feline diet found a median survival time of 750 days. Commercially available kidney diets and calcitriol administration in dogs are in fact the only interventions for which grade I evidence exists. Different diets labeled for use in renal disease contain different ingredients and nutrient concentrations; therefore, product guides should be carefully reviewed if a patient requires more or less of a certain nutrient or if one particular product is refused. The amount of protein to administer to patients with renal failure is controversial, and should probably be increased to the amount needed to maintain muscle condition. Protein does not appear as toxic to renal tubules in dogs and cats as in rodents, but protein frequently contains a large percentage of dietary phosphorus, which is reduced to prevent renal secondary hyperparathyroidism. No clinical studies exist that compare protein modification independent of phosphorus concentration. Animals who consume little food may benefit from higher protein diets. Those patients in stage 4 renal disease (www.iris-kidney.com) may require feeding tubes if voluntary

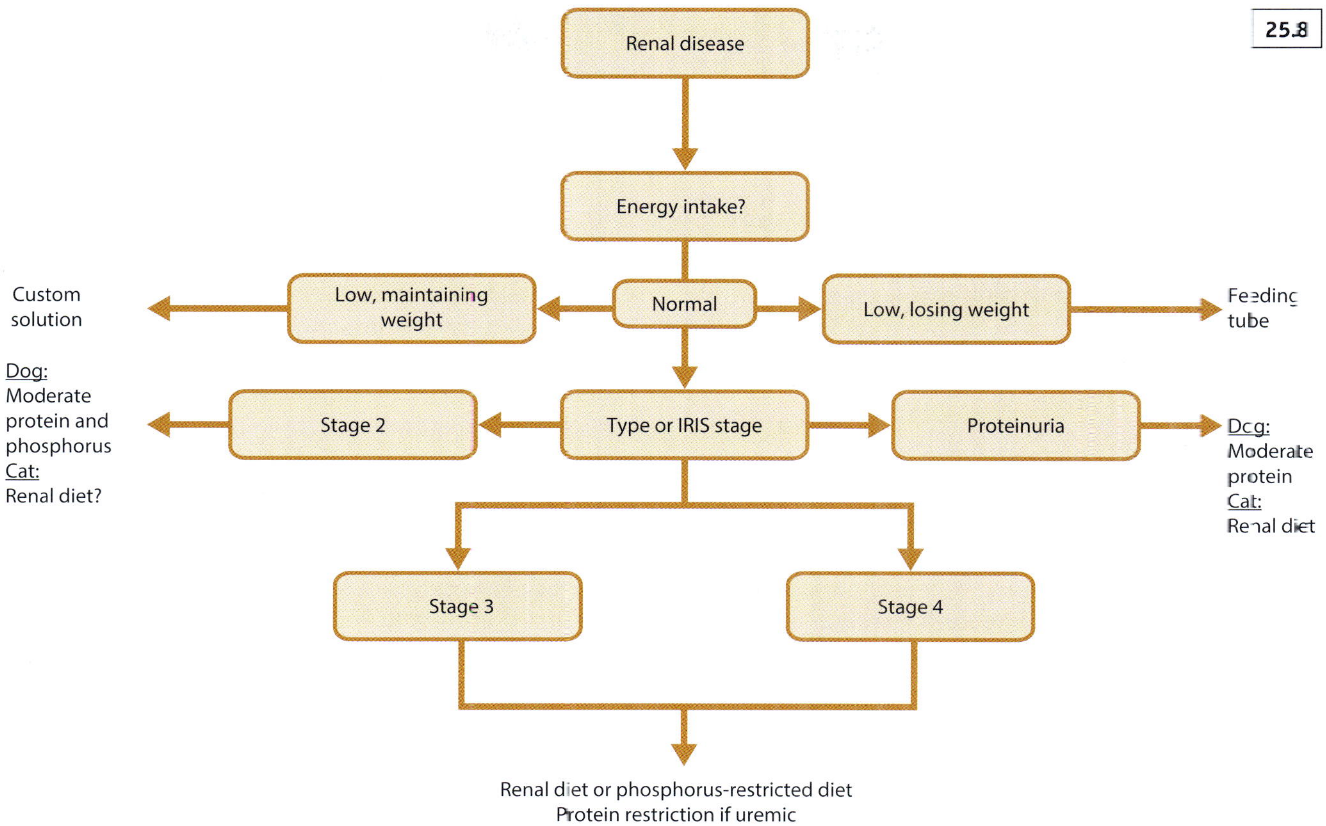

Figure 25.8 An algorithm for nutritional management of patients with renal disease.

intake is insufficient to maintain body weight. Therefore, interventions should be tailored to the patient's caloric intake and International Renal Interest Society (IRIS) stage (**Figure 25.8**).

CONCLUSION

Critical care patients benefit from frequent nutritional assessments during hospitalization. Controversies exist regarding when, how, and what to feed critically-ill patients. However, most conditions benefit from a methodical approach to nutritional support. Those animals with significant anorexia, hyporexia, or reduction in MCS or BCS may require earlier interventions compared with animals who present with acute illness and adequate tissue reserves. Certain conditions such as sepsis may benefit from permissive underfeeding. In many conditions, the provision of some calories is preferred compared with no calories or caloric excess. Specific attention should be given to patients presenting with GI disease, pancreatitis, hepatic encephalopathy, hepatic lipidosis, and renal disease, as these conditions have well-defined nutritional considerations. Additional randomized controlled trials are needed to better characterize the influence of nutrition on patient outcome.

RECOMMENDED FURTHER READING

Brunetto MA, Gomes MO, Andre MR *et al* (2010) Effects of nutritional support on hospital outcome in dogs and cats. *J Vet Emerg Crit Care* **20**:224–231.

Casaer MP, Van den Berghe G (2014) Nutrition in the acute phase of illness. *New Engl J Med* **370:**1227–1236.

Desai SV, McClave SA, Rice TW (2014) Nutrition in the ICU: an evidence-based approach. *Chest* **140:**1148–1157.

Fascetti AJ, Delaney SJ (2012) (eds.) *Applied Veterinary Clinical Nutrition*. Wiley-Blackwell, Ames.

Han E (2004) Esophageal and gastric feeding tubes in ICU patients. *Clin Tech Small Anim Pract* **19**:22–31.

Kirk C (2006) (ed.) Dietary management and nutrition. *Vet Clin North Am Small Anim Pract* **36:**1183–1410.

Mohr AJ, Leisewitz AL, Jacobson LS *et al.* (2003) Effect of early enteral nutrition on intestinal permeability, intestinal protein loss, and outcome in dogs with severe parvoviral enteritis. *J Vet Intern Med* **17:**791–798.

National Research Council Subcommittee on Dog and Cat Nutrition (2003) *Nutrient Requirements of Dogs and Cats*. National Academies Press, Washington DC.

Pibot P, Biourge V, Elliot D (2006) *Encyclopedia of Canine Clinical Nutrition*. Aniwa SAS, Aimargues.

Pibot P, Biourge V, Elliot D (2008) *Encyclopedia of Feline Clinical Nutrition*. Aniwa SAS, Aimargues.

Queau Y, Larsen JA, Kass PH *et al.* (2011) Factors associated with adverse outcomes during parenteral nutrition administration in dogs and cats. *J Vet Intern Med* **25:**446–452.

Schuetz P, Bally M, Stanga Z *et al.* (2014) Loss of appetite in acutely ill medical inpatients: physiological response or therapeutic target. *Schweiz Med Wochenschr* **144:**w13957.

Yu MK, Freeman LM, Heinze CR *et al.* (2013) Comparison of complication rates in dogs with nasoesophageal versus nasogastric feeding tubes. *J Vet Emerg Crit Care* **23:**300–304.

Chapter 26

Management of the obese dog or cat

Alexander J. German

DEFINITION AND OVERVIEW

Human obesity

In humans, obesity is defined as a disease in which adipose tissue has been accumulated to the point that health can be adversely affected. There are various methods of quantifying adiposity in people, the most common of which is the body mass index (BMI; weight [in kg] divided by height^2 [in m]). Although not perfect, for the majority of the human population, this measure approximates to body fat mass. Epidemiologic studies have suggested that the optimal BMI for adult Caucasians is 20–25, and have further demonstrated that disease and mortality risk progressively increase when BMI exceeds this. Increased BMI has been categorized into 'overweight' (BMI 25–30), 'obese' (BMI 30–40), and morbidly obese (BMI >40), with each representing a progressive increase in disease and mortality risk. Some recent work has questioned whether people with an overweight BMI are genuinely at an increased risk of mortality and developing concurrent disease. This phenomenon might be explained by confounding, since some people with an ideal BMI have a concurrent disease that has caused them to lose weight. There has been a dramatic increase in the prevalence of this disease in the human population. According to the Centers for Disease Control in the USA, more than a third (35%) of adults are obese. However, this is not a problem that is limited to the westernized world and, indeed, the Overseas Development Institute has recently highlighted a growing concern in developing countries, with almost a billion adults now being classed as obese. Thus, obesity truly is an epidemic of global proportions.

Canine and feline obesity

As with humans, excess adiposity in companion animals can be categorized either as overweight or as obese, depending on the degree with which current weight exceeds ideal weight. Rather than using a measure equivalent to the BMI, most veterinarians will classify on the basis of the body condition score (BCS) (see **Figure 25.1**). The WSAVA Global Nutrition Committee has recently recommended using the 9-integer unit BCS, with BCS 4/9–5/9 being ideal, 6/9–7/9 being overweight, and 8/9–9/9 being obese. Given that beyond 5/9 each integer unit represents ~10–15% of excess weight, overweight animals are typically up to 20% above their ideal weight, while obese dogs are >20% above ideal. As in humans, various studies have suggested that adverse health effects can arise when dogs and cats are not maintained in optimal body condition. A number of recent international studies have determined the prevalence of excess body weight in dogs and cats: for dogs, 29–39% are defined as overweight and 5–20% as obese, while, for cats, 19–29% are defined as overweight and 8–10% as obese. Differences represent variations in the populations studied and methodology. Furthermore, as with human obesity, prevalence is increasing, with recent reports suggesting a 37% and 90% increase in prevalence over the last 5 years for dogs and cats, respectively.

ETIOLOGY AND PATHOPHYSIOLOGY

Etiology

For body weight to remain stable, energy intake in food must match expenditure from basal metabolic rate, activity, and thermoregulation. When energy intake exceeds expenditure, usually as a result of a number of risk factors, the net energy gained is stored in body fat. Adipose tissue can expand both by hypertrophy and/or hyperplasia: in some individuals, the response to energy imbalance is adipocyte hypertrophy while for others hyperplasia predominates, with a lesser degree of hypertrophy. Differences in the degree of hyperplasia to hypertrophy have recently been shown to be associated with the metabolic derangements that manifest as a result of obesity. Intriguingly, recent research has demonstrated that some cats can maintain a stable weight despite *ad-libitum* feeding, likely by self-regulating intake. However, others are unable to do this and, if excess intake remains unchecked, weight gain develops gradually.

Thus, slow and insidious energy imbalance is a major factor, perhaps explaining why obesity is most prevalent in middle aged dogs and cats.

Pathophysiology

The clinical significance of obesity relates not to the accumulation of adipose tissue *per se*, but to the effect this has on the function of other organs. There are two proposed mechanisms for such effects: 'mechanical' and 'endocrine'. Mechanical effects can occur from excessive weight of adipose tissue, and this can cause excessive loading of structures of the musculoskeletal system. Alternatively, effects may arise from the excess volume of the tissue and the effect this has on compressible structures, for instance of the respiratory (affecting breathing function) or urinary (causing incontinence) system. In addition, the excess volume and weight can affect the ability to groom, while the insulating effect of adipose tissue can create problems with reduced heat dissipation.

However, in addition to these mechanical problems, there may be effects due to derangement of the endocrine functions of white adipose tissue. A range of cytokines, chemokines, and other inflammation-related proteins, collectively termed 'adipokines', are now known to be synthesized, suggesting that adipose tissue can influence the function of a variety of organ systems (**Figures 26.1a, b**). When there is expansion of adipose tissue, it can become hypoxic, causing derangement in adipokine synthesis and release. This can lead to a body wide state of chronic mild inflammation and, ultimately, to a range of end effects. In humans, increases in the production of certain inflammatory adipokines (e.g. leptin, tumor necrosis factor α, interleukin 6, plasminogen activator inhibitor 1, and haptoglobin) have been causally linked to the development of metabolic syndrome and other disorders linked to the obese state. As mentioned above, adipose tissue can expand both by hypertrophy (through increased cell size) and hyperplasia (through synthesis of new cells from preadipocytes). Individuals that predominantly react by adipocyte hypertrophy have greater hepatic fat deposition and more marked metabolic disturbances than those who do not. It is thought that these differences may arise through mitochondrial dysfunction, since the same studies demonstrated that mitochondrial gene expression pathways are downregulated, while inflammatory pathways are upregulated in the adipose tissue of affected individuals.

Inflammatory adipokine gene expression has been documented in both canine and feline white adipose tissue, and studies are now highlighting their effects in these species. As with humans, metabolic derangements are most evident. Increased plasma leptin concentrations have been shown to be independently associated with insulin sensitivity in lean and overweight cats. Other studies indicate decreased circulating adiponectin in obese dogs and cats, and this is also linked to insulin resistance. Furthermore, low serum adiponectin has been associated with failure of a subsequent weight loss program and excessive lean tissue loss during weight

26.1

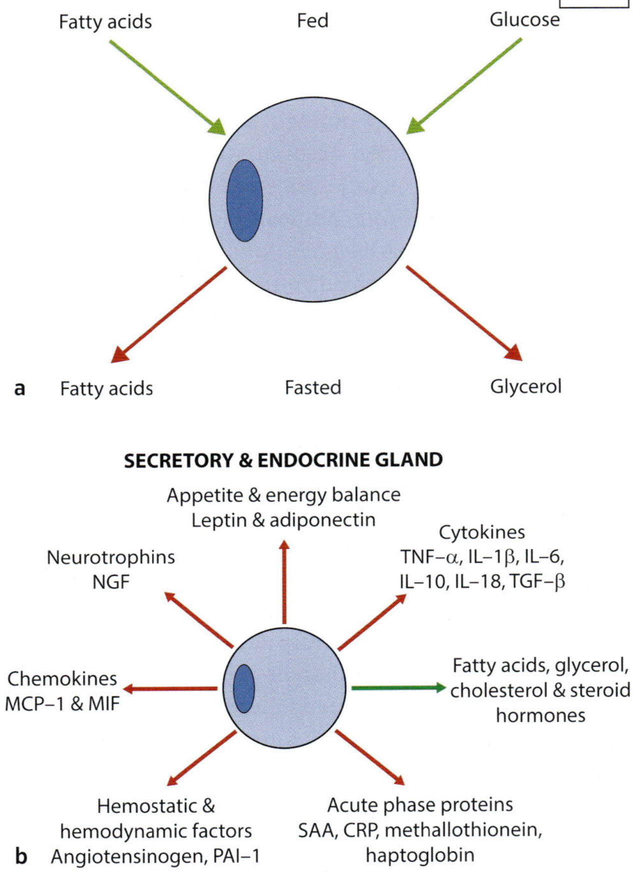

Figures 26.1a, b Evolving views of the biological functions of adipose tissue. (a) Adipocytes were previously considered to be inert storage depots releasing fuel as fatty acids and glycerol at times of fasting or starvation. (b) Recently, however, it has become increasingly clear that adipocytes are endocrine cells, which secrete important hormones, cytokines, vasoactive substances, and other peptides. This figure outlines the range of such proteins secreted from adipose tissue. CRP, C-reactive protein; IL, interleukin; MCP-1, monocyte chemoattractant protein-1; MIF, macrophage migration inhibitory factor; PAI-1, plasminogen activator inhibitor-1; SAA, serum amyloid A; TGF-β, transforming growth factor-β; TNF-α, tumor necrosis factor-α. (From German AJ, Ryan VH, German AC *et al.* (2010) Obesity, its associated disorders and the role of inflammatory adipokines in companion animals. *Vet J* **185**:4–9, reprinted with permission.)

management. Increases in serum paraoxanase 1 have also recently been demonstrated and, once again, this is associated with insulin resistance. Further work is ongoing to better characterize these effects.

Risk factors for the development of obesity

A number of risk factors are known to predispose to the development of obesity in dogs and cats, as outlined below.

Co-existing health problems

Some diseases, such as hyperadrenocorticism, can cause polyphagia, and if the animal is allowed to consume more food, weight gain can occur. Other diseases can reduce energy expenditure, for instance by decreasing physical activity or slowing the basal metabolic rate. Orthopedic diseases that lead to lameness are a classic example of a disease that decreases activity, while hypothyroidism is, perhaps, the best example of a disease predisposing to weight gain by decreasing metabolic rate. Although thought to be a common endocrinopathy, relatively speaking, hypothyroidism is actually an uncommon cause of obesity in dogs. In this respect, the prevalence of hypothyroidism is reported to be <1%, and less than half are overweight (see Chapter 11: Endocrine disorders), while the current prevalence of dogs that are above their ideal weight is much greater (typically 34–59%); thus, only a minority of the overweight dogs attending veterinary practices are likely to have concurrent hypothyroidism. Furthermore, given that hypothyroidism is extremely rare in cats, it is a negligible cause of obesity in this species.

Beyond this, some therapeutic interventions can predispose to weight gain. One example is the use of drugs that stimulate appetite (e.g. glucocorticoids or anticonvulsants), but not energy requirement; here weight gain can occur if the owner provides more food. A second example is surgical sterilization (spaying/neutering), which alters behavior by decreasing physical activity while increasing food-seeking behavior.

Rapid early-life weight gain

In humans, overly rapid gain of weight during the early years of life predicts the likelihood of being obese during adulthood. A similar phenomenon has recently been identified in cats. Although the reason for this phenomenon is not yet known, genetic factors are suggested to play a role. Armed with such knowledge, a simple comparison of the ratio of bodyweight between 2 months (i.e. 2nd vaccination) and 12 months of age (first annual booster) could be used to identify at-risk cats, enabling preventive strategies to be implemented (see below).

Age

As mentioned above, the prevalence of both canine and feline obesity gradually increases throughout life, with the condition being most prevalent in middle aged animals. However, some individuals can become overweight even during growth. The prevalence of overweight and obesity decreases in senior animals, possibly due to the onset of various chronic diseases associated with the aging process.

Sex and neutering

Some canine studies have suggested that female dogs are predisposed, while a recent feline study suggested males to be overrepresented. More importantly, neutering is an important risk factor for obesity in both species, with studies suggesting that this is the result of behavioral alterations rather than a direct effect on metabolism. In this respect, the hormonal changes produced by obesity lead to an increased food intake, decreased physical activity, or both. Given that neutering is typically an elective procedure, unwanted post-neutering weight gain is arguably preventable if body weight is monitored closely and food intake adjusted accordingly (see below).

Breed

On rare occasions, single gene disorders can cause obesity in humans, but polygenic effects are more common with a number of predisposing genes recently identified. At the current time, no single-gene disorders have been described in either dogs or cats. Since there are a number of known breed predispositions in both dogs (e.g. Cocker Spaniels, Beagles, Labrador Retrievers, Golden Retrievers, Shetland Sheepdogs, Rottweilers, and mixed-breed dogs) and cats (e.g. Domestic Shorthair), genetic influences remain likely, although these are more likely to be due to polygenic effects. Gene mapping studies are underway to characterize the genetic influences in these companion animals.

Environment and activity

Dogs and cats that live indoors are reportedly at greater risk of developing obesity than those who go outside. Similar findings have also been seen for indoor cats, including those that are apartment dwelling. Furthermore, cats that live with one or two other cats or with a dog may also be at increased risk.

Dietary factors

Some published studies have suggested associations between companion animal obesity and diet type, but others have not. In one study, no difference in obesity prevalence was observed between dogs fed commercial food versus those fed a homemade diet. However, the cost of food might play a role, with inexpensive ('grocery store') diets more likely to have been fed to obese dogs compared with more expensive foods; in contrast, obese cats are more likely to have been fed a premium food. Although, there have been many anecdotal suggestions that feeding a high carbohydrate diet to cats predisposes to obesity and diabetes mellitus, there is no evidence to support this assertion. In fact, increased dietary fat rather than carbohydrate predisposes to weight gain in cats. Furthermore, obese cats more commonly have free choice of food intake. For dogs, obesity is correlated with the number of meals and snacks, the feeding of table scraps, and the animal being present when owners prepared or ate their own meal.

Owner factors and behavior

The owners of overweight dogs have a lower income than dogs of ideal weight, but this is not the case for cats. Owners of obese dogs also tend overhumanize them, and this is also the case for cats, where owners often utilize their cat as a substitute for human companionship. Owners of overweight cats also spend less time playing with their pet, and reward with food rather than extra play. Owners of both overweight cats and dogs are more likely to be overweight themselves, less interested in preventive health, and to observe their pet more closely during feeding.

Some studies have suggested that there may be behavioral influences on the development of feline obesity, including anxiety, depression, failure to establish normal feeding behavior, and failure to develop control of satiety. The human–animal relationship is also of importance, and appears to be more intense in owners of obese cats. Cat owners usually feed their cats two meals per day, even though the wild ancestors of domestic cats are 'trickle feeders' and eat many small meals each day. Misinterpretation of feline behavior on the part of the owner is a critical factor in feline obesity, with owners misreading behavior signals with regard to eating. In this respect, domestic cats prefer to eat alone and have no requirement for social interaction during this time. Thus, when a cat initiates contact, this would not normally be for food-related reasons. However, owners often mistakenly believe their cat to be hungry and asking for food; if they give food at this point, the cat will quickly learn that initiating contact results in a food reward. Another misconception is that it is only young cats that need play activity, but this is needed throughout life. Therefore, most cat owners do not bother to play with their cat once it has reached adulthood.

PATHOLOGICAL CONSEQUENCES OF OBESITY

Obesity-associated disorders in humans (Table 26.1)

Obesity is known to have a number of significant effects on the human body, the most notable of which is metabolic syndrome, whereby metabolic and vascular derangements develop that predispose the individual to type II diabetes mellitus and cardiovascular disease. As fat mass increases (especially within the abdomen), so does the severity of insulin resistance and, ultimately type II diabetes mellitus. Given this close association, it is not surprising that the prevalence of type II diabetes mellitus has increased at an equivalent rate to that of obesity. Obesity, through metabolic syndrome, also leads to cardiovascular disease, with an associated increased prevalence of coronary heart disease, atherosclerosis, hypertension, and dyslipidemias in people who are overweight. Most notably, metabolic syndrome is a predictor of a future vascular event and, therefore, its presence should prompt interventions aimed at reducing the risk of such problems.

Other obesity-associated co-morbidities include respiratory disorders (especially sleep apnea and asthma), kidney disease (especially diabetic nephropathy), and osteoarthritis. Obesity is now the most important cause of liver disease, given the increased likelihood of affected patients developing steatosis, cirrhosis, and hepatocellular carcinoma. Obesity also increases the risk of certain types of cancer, most notably affecting the breast, prostate, ovary, colon/rectum, kidney, and esophagus.

Obesity-associated disorders in companion animals (Table 26.1)

Life span

In a long-term prospective study, restricting caloric intake (by approximately 25%) in dogs was shown to maintain optimal body condition (BCS 4.5/9 vs. 6.8/9), and extend life span (based on time to euthanasia) by almost 2 years. In the same study, the restricted dogs were less likely to develop hip dysplasia (during growth) and osteoarthritis later in life (especially of the hip and shoulder joint). Finally, these dogs had improved glucose tolerance and lower circulating triglyceride

Table 26.1 Diseases associated with overweight and obesity in humans, dogs, and cats. (From German AJ, Ryan VH, German AC *et al.* (2010) Obesity, its associated disorders and the role of inflammatory adipokines in companion animals. *Vet J* **185:**4–9, reprinted with permission.)

Disease category	Species		
	Human	**Dog**	**Cat**
Endocrine and lipid	Type II diabetes, metabolic syndrome, dyslipidemias	Hypothyroidism, hyperadrenocorticism, diabetes mellitus, insulin resistance, metabolic syndrome (experimental)	Diabetes mellitus, hepatic lipidosis
Cardiorespiratory	Coronary heart disease, atherosclerosis, hypertension, obstructive sleep apnea, asthma	Tracheal collapse, expiratory airway dysfunction (experimental), hypertension (of doubtful clinical significance), portal vein thrombosis, myocardial hypoxia	
Orthopedic and impaired mobility	Osteoarthritis, musculoskeletal pain, gout	Osteoarthritis, cruciate ligament disease, humeral condylar fractures, intervertebral disk disease, hip dysplasia	Increased lameness
Oncological	Various cancers including: breast (post-menopausal), renal, endometrial, prostatic, esophageal, colonic/rectal, hepatocellular carcinoma	Variable neoplasia risk: transitional cell carcinoma, mammary carcinoma (some but not all studies)	Increased neoplasia risk
Urogenital	Diabetic nephropathy	Urinary tract disease, urethral sphincter mechanism incompetence, calcium oxalate urolithiasis, transitional cell carcinoma, glomerular disease (experimental), dystocia	Increased risk of urinary tract disease
Alimentary	Pancreatitis, hepatic steatosis, cirrhosis	Pancreatitis	Increased oral cavity disease and gastrointestinal disease
Other	Depression, postoperative complications, various dermatologic diseases	Immune function	Increased risk of dermatoses

concentrations compared with the *ad libitum* fed and overweight dogs.

Quality of life effects

In a recent study, health-related quality of life was assessed in obese dogs before and after weight loss. Quality of life was worse than for dogs at optimal weight, but improved as a result of successful weight loss. These effects were most notable for 'vitality' factors, which improved dramatically, and there was also less evidence of factors indicating chronic pain and emotional derangements. Moreover, the more body fat the dog lost, the greater the improvement in vitality. Dogs that failed to complete their weight loss program had worse quality of life at the outset than those successfully losing weight, most notably worse vitality and greater emotional disturbance.

Orthopedic disorders

Of all disease associations the link between obesity and orthopedic disease is most important in dogs. An increased prevalence of a variety of orthopedic disorders has been noted including cranial cruciate ligament rupture, intervertebral disk disease, humeral condylar fractures, hip dysplasia, and osteoarthritis. Based on force plate analysis, weight reduction in obese dogs with osteoarthritis can lead to a substantial improvement in mobility.

As with dogs, obesity may be a risk factor for feline orthopedic disease. One study suggested that obese cats were five times more likely to be lame than normal condition cats, although not all studies confirm this finding. Further work is required to determine whether obesity truly has a causal effect on feline orthopedic disorders and, if so, what diseases specifically.

Endocrine and metabolic diseases

In dogs, associations between obesity and diabetes mellitus, hypothyroidism, and hyperadrenocorticism have been demonstrated; for cats, the only association is with diabetes mellitus. Cats most often suffer from a form of diabetes mellitus resembling human 'type II' diabetes, with insulin resistance being a major factor. Successful weight loss improves insulin sensitivity, significantly reducing the requirement for exogenous insulin therapy.

In diabetic dogs, there is progressive beta cell loss and absolute insulin deficiency, meaning that an affected dog will always need lifelong insulin therapy. The pathogenesis of beta cell loss is poorly understood, and might not be the same as human type I diabetes. Putative causes include pancreatitis and autoimmune-mediated beta cell destruction. Furthermore, a large scale epidemiological study in dogs demonstrated an association between obesity and diabetes mellitus. Since obese dogs are also prone to pancreatitis, it might be that concurrence of this condition provides the causal link with diabetes mellitus. However, insulin resistance may also play a role because it is known to occur in experimental models of canine obesity. Indeed, a recent study of naturally occurring obesity in dogs has demonstrated that the percentage of body fat correlates with the degree of insulin resistance, and insulin sensitivity is improved significantly on successful weight loss.

Obesity can have marginal effects on thyroid homeostasis, but the changes are not biologically significant and are unlikely to affect the interpretation of thyroid function tests. In this respect, obese dogs have slightly greater total thyroxine (T4) and triiodothyronine (T3) concentrations than ideal weight dogs, but generally remain within the reference interval, and free T4, thyroid stimulating hormone (TSH), and TSH tests are not significantly different.

Hyperlipidemia and dyslipidemia

Feline obesity has long been known to predispose to hepatic lipidosis, and epidemiological studies have confirmed this link. Experimental studies in obese dogs have demonstrated mild (but likely clinically insignificant) hypercholesterolemia, hypertriglyceridemia, and increased circulating phospholipid concentrations. In contrast, experimental studies of canine obesity have demonstrated increased plasma nonesterified fatty acid and triglyceride concentrations (increased very-low-density lipoprotein and high-density lipoprotein; decreased high-density lipoprotein cholesterol), which associate with insulin resistance.

Respiratory function

A number of studies have now demonstrated that excessive body fat can adversely affect respiratory function in dogs, and the same is likely to be true in cats. Such effects are similar to those seen in humans, and may help to explain the link between obesity and certain respiratory diseases in dogs, most notably tracheal collapse, laryngeal paralysis, and brachycephalic airway obstruction syndrome. The exact nature of the effects on respiratory function differs depending on the study. In one experimental study, airway resistance was markedly increased during hyperpnea but not when breathing normally. A second study demonstrated that obese dogs had a decreased tidal volume and increased respiratory rate, as well as increased airway reactivity. In a further study, obesity had a significant effect on oxygenation but not on oxygenation indices, being most closely negatively associated with thoracic fat percentage. Finally, in a further study, obesity was shown to negatively effect cardiopulmonary function, as determined by the 6-minute walk test. The human term 'Pickwickian syndrome' is sometimes used to describe respiratory impairment in morbidly obese pet animals. This s taken from Charles Dickens' character Mr. Pickwick, who showed the signs that the syndrome is named after.

Cardiac function

In dogs, obesity is known to affect cardiac function, as demonstrated by alterations in cardiac rhythm and increases in left ventricular volume; there is no evidence of a similar association in cats. However, overweight cats with heart failure have reduced survival times compared with cats in normal body condition. Mild hypertension does occur in canine obesity, but the effect has not yet been shown to be as clinically significant as in humans.

Finally, obesity in dogs may be associated with portal vein thrombosis and myocardial hypoxia.

Neoplasia

Although epidemiological studies have demonstrated an association between obesity and the presence of neoplasia in both dogs and cats, such a link has not been confirmed in all studies. Other studies have examined associations with specific cancer types and, although not conclusive, links have been suggested with transitional cell carcinoma and mammary carcinoma.

Renal system function and disease

In experimental dogs, the onset of obesity is associated with glomerular pathology and changes in function, including increased plasma renin and insulin concentrations, mean arterial pressure, and renal blood flow. In a more recent study, a number of renal biomarkers were assessed in obese dogs with evidence of subclinical decreases in renal function, which improved after weight loss. However, it is unclear as to the significance of these changes and, most importantly, whether or not they may predispose to renal disease, as in humans. Associations have also been demonstrated between obesity and urethral sphincter mechanism incompetence, while obese animals have an increased risk of dystocia.

Other disorders

Epidemiological studies have demonstrated associations between feline obesity and oral cavity disease, dermatologic disorders, and diarrhea. However, the reasons for such an association are not known.

CLINICAL PRESENTATION

Obesity is typically a disorder that develops insidiously and is most commonly seen in early middle age, with peak prevalence occurring in 6–10-year-old dogs and 5–11-year-old cats. In both species, prevalence declines in old age, and is also less in growing dogs. The disease can be seen in dogs and cats of either sex and typically (but not always) they are neutered. Any breed may be affected, although there are certain predispositions including Cocker Spaniels, Beagles, Labrador Retrievers, Golden Retrievers, Shetland Sheepdogs, Rottweilers, and mixed-breed dogs.

Clinical signs vary depending on how overweight the dog or cat is and the extent of obesity-associated diseases. Common signs directly attributable to the obesity include lethargy, exercise intolerance, increased respiratory rate and effort, abnormal respiratory tract sounds (e.g. stertor and stridor, often commonly while recumbent or sleeping), and altered gait (typically due to the mechanical effects of excessive truncal and limb fat deposition). Appetite can be variable; while some dogs are polyphagic and scavenging, some owners may report that their dog has a picky appetite and does not eat all of the food in its bowl. The latter is thought to be due to owners providing food vastly in excess of requirements and, often, giving significant numbers of food-based rewards. This means that the dog or cat can still overeat despite not eating everything they are given. Examples of clinical signs include lameness (orthopedic disease), abdominal pain (pancreatitis), vomiting (pancreatitis, hepatic lipidosis), icterus (hepatic lipidosis), polydipsia and polyuria (diabetes mellitus), coughing (respiratory disease), and incontinence (urethral sphincter mechanism incompetence).

On physical examination, altered body shape is always readily apparent, most easily determined using body condition scoring (see below). There may be signs of an associated disease, for instance abdominal pain with pancreatitis or pain on joint manipulation. Poor skin and coat condition is often present, and cats that are markedly obese often have fecal soiling of the perineum due to inability to groom. In dogs with concurrent hypothyroidism or hyperadrenocorticism, alopecia and other typical skin changes may also be evident. Auscultation and abdominal palpation can be problematic given excess truncal fat deposition, both subcutaneously and within both body cavities. Likewise, while a pulse is usually palpable, it can be more difficult to determine pulse quality due to excess subcutaneous fat in the inguinal region. Thoracic auscultation can be muffled because of intra- and extrathorasic fat deposits.

DIFFERENTIAL DIAGNOSIS

In addition to body fat mass accumulation, other possible reasons for weight gain include changes in hydration status (usually iatrogenic) and intracavitary fluid accumulation (e.g. ascites). In such cases, the weight change is rapid and other signs are expected. Thus, they can be readily distinguished from weight gain due to obesity. In male cats, gradual weight gain can also arise secondary to acromegaly, although weight gain results from increases in muscle mass, organomegaly, and increased bone mass, in addition to adipose tissue. Therefore, this can usually be distinguished on physical examination; however, this might be counteracted by co-existing diabetes mellitus.

Therefore, if weight gain is gradual, obesity is the most likely cause and the aim of the clinician is to distinguish 'simple obesity' (due to energy imbalance) from cases that have arisen secondary to another disease, most notably hyperadrenocorticism or hypothyroidism (dogs). Other than this, possible differential diagnoses relate to the presence of other signs that may have developed secondary to associated diseases. Such lists can sometimes be extensive, given that the signs associated with obesity can be both diverse and nonspecific, and the diagnosis of simple obesity can only be made once other possibilities have been adequately excluded. Therefore, the differential diagnosis list needs to be tailored to the individual case. For example, in cases presenting with respiratory tract signs, consideration should be given to other possibilities that present insidiously in middle age such as upper respiratory tract diseases (e.g. laryngeal paralysis, brachycephalic airway disease), airway diseases (e.g. chronic airway disease), pulmonary disease (e.g. pulmonary neoplasia), and other intrathoracic diseases. In a similar manner, tailored differential diagnosis lists should be created when there are signs of lameness, vomiting, abdominal pain, and incontinence.

DIAGNOSIS

The overall aim is to confirm that the weight gain is the result of increased adipose tissue mass, determine which risk factors are present, and determine whether there is evidence of an underlying cause (e.g. endocrinopathy, iatrogenic weight gain) and whether other concurrent diseases might be present. In addition, the clinician should aim to determine current health status (which will influence how the case is investigated and managed) and quantify the degree of obesity. With regard to health status it is critical to identify all concurrent diseases, whether or not they are likely to be directly related to the obesity. This will then enable the clinician to determine the most appropriate plan for weight management, determine both the ideal weight and an appropriate target weight, and also to decide on the safest and most effective approach for weight loss. The exact tests that are required in the individual case can then be decided.

History and physical examination

The first stage of diagnosis is to obtain a history, including diet history, and perform a physical examination. In addition to a standard medical history (including any prior or current therapy), the history should include details of diet, exercise, environment, the family unit (pets and people), lifestyle, and neuter status. Physical examination should focus on quantifying the obesity and determining the presence of associated diseases that are either causing or contributing to weight gain or presenting as incidental findings.

Body weight measurement

The dog or cat should be weighed on electronic scales that, ideally, have been calibrated for precision and accuracy, as well as being serviced regularly (e.g. annually). If test weights are not available, an item of known weight can be used instead (e.g. bag of dry dog food). It is advisable for the practice always to use the same set of electronic weigh scales for weight measurements, since this will minimize errors from readings obtained with different sets of scales. Adopting a practice policy of weighing all animals at every visit throughout life is recommended, combined with regular BCS assessment (see below); given that most cases of obesity develop later in life, there may be a historical record of an early adult weight (i.e. 1 year for cats, 2 years for dogs), where the animal was in ideal condition. This can be used to estimate the ideal weight of the patient (see below).

Clinical assessment of body shape and composition

Body condition scoring

The most widely accepted clinical method of assessing body composition is body condition scoring. BCS schemes assess adipose tissue mass through visual assessment and palpation. Although a number of methods are available, including a modification called the body fat index, the WSAVA Global Nutrition Committee has recently recommended the use of the 9-integer unit system, with an additional assessment for muscle mass (as + or –) (see **Figures 25.1, 25.2**). This ensures consistency amongst clinicians.

Systems for determining BCS are the simplest indirect measures of body composition currently available. Such systems are repeatable when used by trained individuals, and correlate well with body fat mass measured by dual-energy X-ray absorptiometry (DEXA), although owners tend to underestimate the shape of their dogs. BCSs can also be used determine how overweight a patient is, with each point (for a 9-unit system) correlating with ~10–15% of excess total body weight. This will enable the degree of obesity to be determined, and will enable the ideal weight to be estimated (**Box 26.1**). BCSs should also be used periodically during the weight program to check on progress and adjust target weight if required. However, this should not be done too frequently, as changes in body composition are relatively insensitive

Box 26.1 Calculations for estimating ideal weight in obese cats and dogs.

In published studies, each unit on a 9-point BCS scheme approximates to 10% of excess body weight. Therefore, a simple equation can be used to estimate the ideal weight of a dog or cat from current body weight and BCS:

Current weight = 50 kg

↓

Current condition score = 9/9 (~40% overweight)

↓

Ideal weight = 50 kg – (50 × 40/100) = 30 kg.

Note: While this is a reasonable guide, due to individual variability, this equation can over- or underestimate ideal weight. If necessary, as weight loss progresses, adjustments to the estimated ideal weight may be needed.

with, on average, a 10% change in body weight being required to change scores.

Zoometry

Various zoometric approaches have been described, usually performed with a tape measure. Measurements that correlate with overall 'stature' (e.g. head, thorax, and limb length) are combined with measures that correlate with adiposity (e.g. body weight and body [thorax, abdomen, or neck] circumference). Equations are then used to predict body fat mass from these measurements. An early example was the Feline Body Mass Index™ while, more recently, a new zoometric system (Hill's Healthy Weight Protocol) was reported, which used a combination of four (dog) or six (cat) measurements. Both of these systems correlate well with body fat mass measured by DEXA. However, while these may be more objective than traditional BCS assessment, it is arguable as to whether or not they offer any real advantage. In this respect, they are more complicated to perform and require greater patient compliance. In addition, they may be more prone to errors of inaccuracy amongst investigators (who may measure differently) or to small patients (where minor errors in measurements could have a profound effect). Finally, the accuracy of such measurements decreases as patients become leaner.

Bioimpedance is another noninvasive method potentially applicable to first-opinion practice. However, handheld machines designed for dogs can be unreliable, and are inferior to body condition scoring. Finally, photographs can provide a subjective means of demonstrating longer term changes in body weight to clients, thus highlighting success (**Figures 26.2a–f**). Techniques for indirect body condition assessment from photographs have also been described.

Further investigations

Routine hematologic examination, clinical biochemistry, and urinalysis can provide general information on health, but are not essential in all cases. Such procedures are more commonly performed in older animals or in animals where there are concerns about concurrent disease (based on the historical and physical examination findings). Depending on the case and the judgment of the attending clinician (i.e. if there is a suspicion of an associated disease), additional investigations may be required in some circumstances, with the exact tests required being at the discretion of the clinician. For instance, some cases may require measurement of blood pressure, assessment of thyroid and adrenal gland function in dogs, pancreatic enzyme measurement, fructosamine measurement for diabetes mellitus, survey radiography for possible orthopedic and respiratory disease, abdominal ultrasonography (most commonly to assess pancreas, liver, adrenal glands, kidneys, and lower urinary tract), fine-needle aspiration cytology, and/or liver biopsy (for suspected hepatic lipidosis). Bacterial culture of urine, bladder ultrasonography, and radiographic contrast studies might also be needed for cases presenting with lower urinary tract diseases.

Other investigations

Advanced body composition measurement

Body composition can be assessed in various ways. DEXA is precise and reliable, and has been used extensively in research studies and in referral clinical practice (**Figures 26.3a–c**). It can help to determine ideal body weight, and also be used to monitor progress with weight loss (i.e. determining loss of lean tissue). However, it is a specialist procedure, so is not needed in first opinion practice, where simpler methods suffice. Instead, such procedures should be considered for problem cases where weight loss has been problematic despite instigating a weight management regime (see below).

Other advanced techniques, which have been validated for use in dogs and cats, include CT and MRI. Such techniques are arguably better at determining regional body fat mass distribution than DEXA. However, they are more expensive and again are limited to referral institutions and have limited availability; once again, therefore, they are more appropriate for referral rather than primary care cases. Finally, assessment of total body water

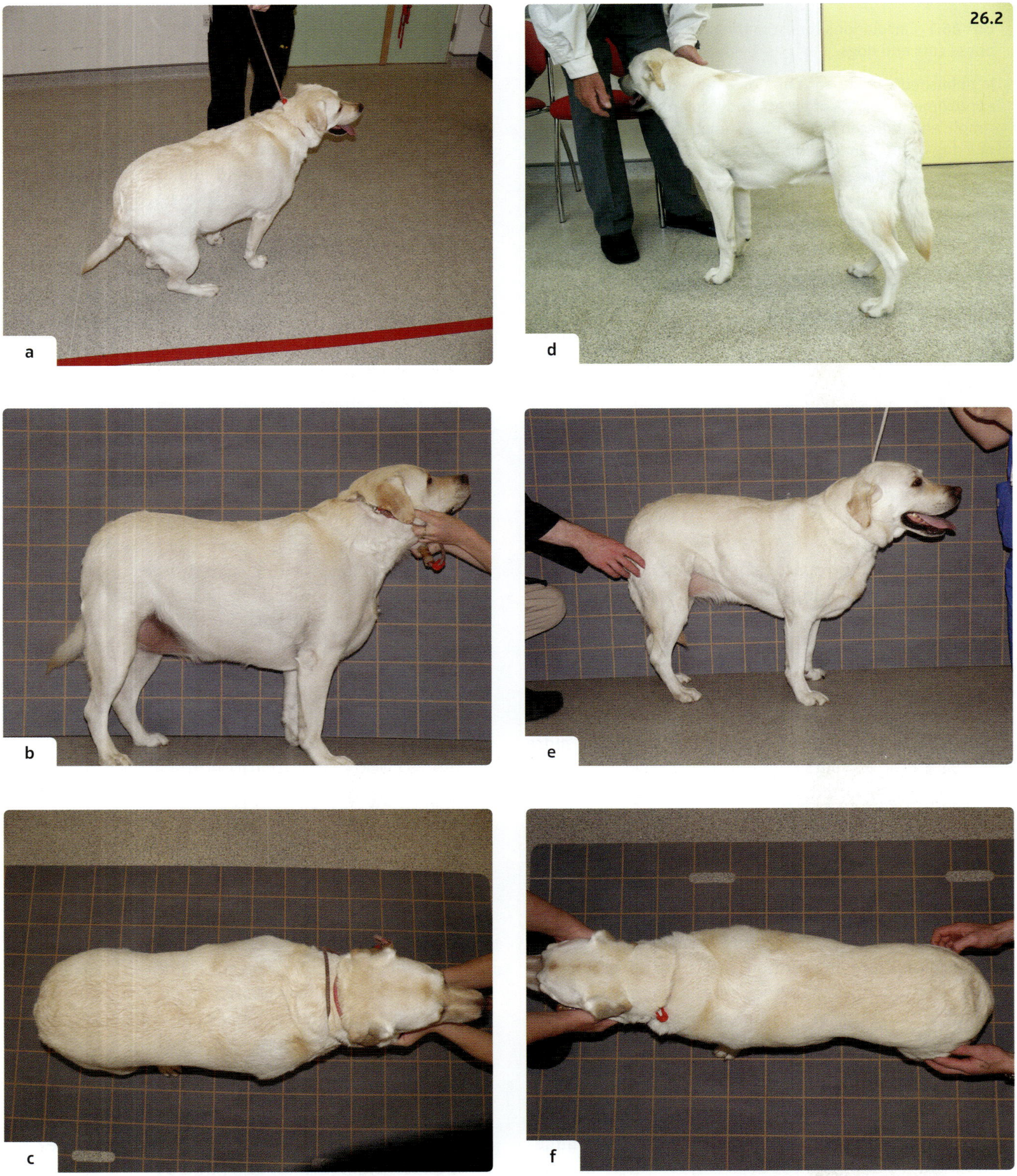

Figures 26.2a–f (a–c) Photographs of an obese 5-year-old neutered female Labrador Retriever, weighing 49.0 kg (108.0 lb), and with a body condition score of 9/9. (d–f) Photographs of the same dog, 268 days later, after successful weight loss on a high-protein high-fiber diet. Body weight had decreased to 33.6 kg (74.1 lb), and condition score was 5/9. Total weight lost was 31% of starting body weight, at a rate of 0.8%/week.

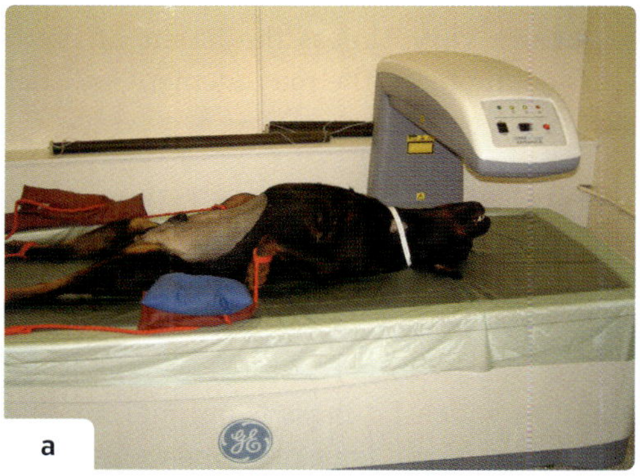

a

26.3

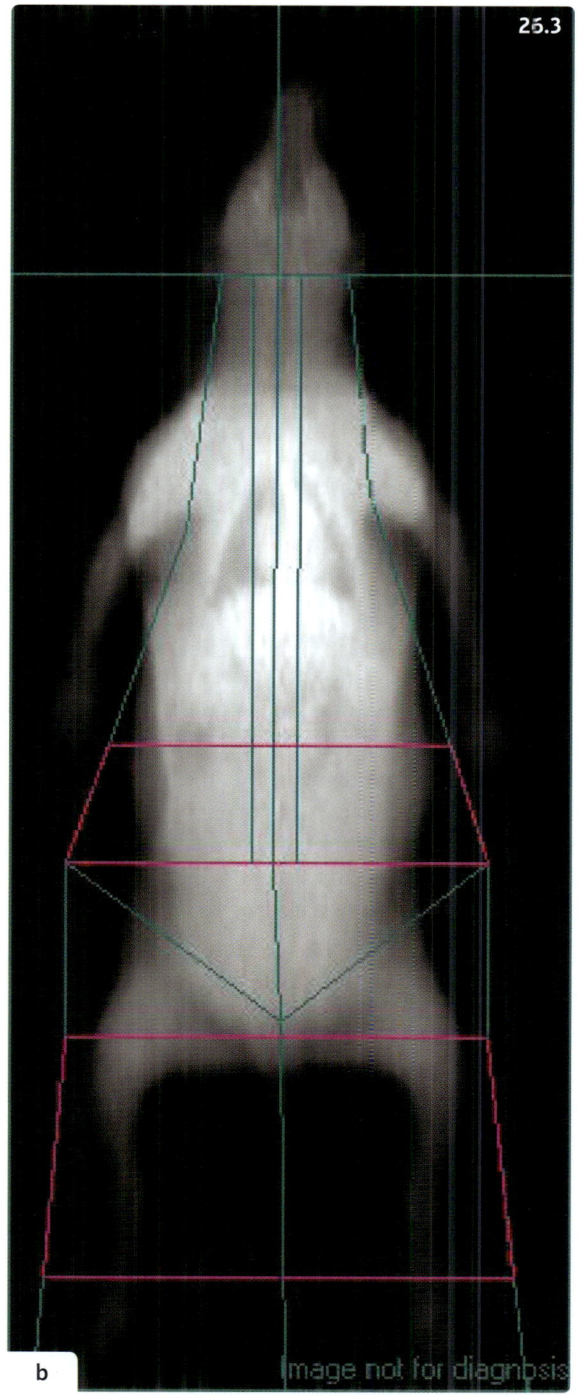

b

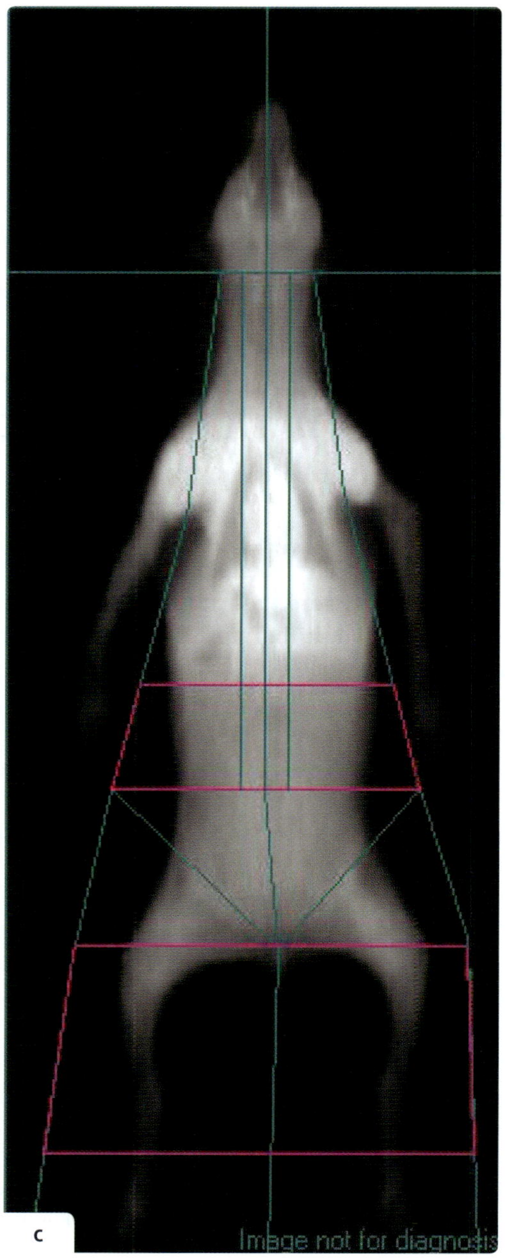

c

Figures 26.3a–c Dual-energy X-ray absorptiometry (DEXA) as a noninvasive means of determining body composition. (a) A fan-beam DEXA machine. (b) Image from a pre-weight-loss DEXA scan performed on the dog featured in Figure 26.2; body fat mass was estimated to be 51%. (c) Post-weight-loss DEXA scan from the dog featured in Figure 26.2 demonstrating that body fat mass had declined to 36%. Based on the DEXA figures, the estimated composition of the body tissue lost was 83% fat and 17% lean.

(typically using isotope studies) has been used extensively in a research setting for determining body composition in dogs and cats. However, such methods have not yet found a clinical application.

Assessment of metabolizable energy requirements and energy expenditure

For success in weight management, it is usually necessary to estimate the metabolizable energy requirement to maintain body weight (a.k.a. maintenance energy requirement [MER]). The most common method of determining MER is to use predictive equations, but such equations represent little more than an educated guess and, even in healthy individuals, may miss actual requirement by 50%. Research methods for determining MER include feeding experiments, while methods for determining energy expenditure (EE) (a proxy measure for MER) include indirect calorimetry and tracer studies such as double-labeled water. Arguably, indirect calorimetry is most applicable to the clinic; it has been widely used in human patients including for the determination of EE in the morbidly obese. Indirect calorimetry can provide reliable measurements of EE in healthy dogs, trauma cases, and cancer patients. However, this technique has not yet found a clinical application for obesity management. Portable indirect calorimeters have recently been developed for human patients and, once validated for dogs and cats, might provide a useful tool to help in weight management.

MANAGEMENT

In humans, the most successful approach to achieve weight loss is through bariatric surgery, but this is not likely to be either practical or ethically justifiable in companion animals. Dietary therapy is the most widely accepted method of weight management, although drug therapy (using microsomal membrane transfer protein [MTP] inhibitors) is also approved for the weight loss phase in dogs but not cats. The weight loss phase can be variable in length, but is typically 6–18 months and occasionally prolonged (i.e. over 2 years).

Weight management in cats and dogs involves two stages: the weight loss phase whereby there is steady fat mass loss, and weight maintenance, which involves stabilizing body weight and preventing rebound. The fundamental aims of weight management are to improve quality of life and reduce associated disease risk. In so doing, you aim to change the relationship between pet and owner to one that promotes a healthy lifestyle. Thus, the amount of weight loss that you recommend and the target weight can vary. Unless the habits of the owner change for the long term, the management will fail, and weight regain will occur.

Target weight, ideal weight, and tailoring the individual plan

In setting a weight loss plan, it is essential to know the ideal weight, since this will be used to set the initial caloric intake (see below). The ideal weight is defined as the weight at which fat mass is optimal for that animal. In reality, there will be a range of weights that are deemed to be ideal, rather than a single weight (typically body fat <20% for domestic cats and <35% for dogs). If a historic weight measurement is available (e.g. an early adult weight), where the animal was in optimal condition, that weight corresponds to the animal's ideal. If such a weight is not available, an alternative approach is to determine ideal weight from the current weight and BCS. In this regard, each unit on the scale between 5/9 and 9/9 approximately corresponds to 10–15% of excess weight. Therefore, with a simple calculation, the ideal weight can be calculated (see **Box 26.1**).

Although often used interchangeably, the terms target weight and ideal weight are not the same. The target weight is defined as the weight that the clinician determines to be an appropriate end-point for weight loss. For some animals, the target weight and ideal weight may be equivalent, while for others target weight is greater. The main benefits of aiming for ideal weight (as your target) is that the greatest beneficial effects on disease prevention and life span extension might be expected. Such an approach would be most beneficial for young animals with a long expected life span and free from concurrent disease. However, such benefits diminish in older cats and dogs, where remaining life span is shorter and concurrent diseases may already exist. Instead, weight management should focus on improving quality of life, and it may not be necessary to achieve ideal weight to achieve this. In fact, a study in dogs has revealed that reductions in severity of disease typically occur with modest (i.e. >5%) reductions in weight. Therefore, aiming for partial weight loss would be more realistic, quicker, and, arguably, more appropriate in older animals, especially those with concurrent disease. In humans, an 'obesity paradox' has been identified. In this respect, being overweight increases the risk of developing certain diseases, but once that disease develops, increased BMI can improve survival. Examples of a similar obesity paradox have also been seen in animals with chronic kidney disease and cardiac disease, with a recent study demonstrating longer survival times in overweight cats. In such cases, only a modest weight reduction (of 5–10%) would be recommended, but aiming to maintain the patient within its overweight range. Such a weight loss protocol will not lead to significant loss of lean tissue, but can improve quality of life.

Expected rate of weight loss

The recommended rate of weight loss is controversial, since initial recommendations of 1–2%/week were based on obese dogs managed in a colony setting, and not client-owned dogs. While such rates can be achieved early in the weight loss process (i.e. first 1–2 months), it becomes increasingly difficult to maintain this over the long term. Instead, an average rate of weight loss of 0.5–1.0%/week is more realistic and appears to be safe. Overly rapid rates of weight loss (>2%/week) are not recommended since there is a potential to cause problems (e.g. excessive lean tissue loss or hepatic lipidosis [cats only]). However, in reality such rates are rare. Slower rates of weight loss (<0.5%/week) might be acceptable, although the whole process will likely take longer and might be a source of owner frustration.

Dietary management

Diet formulation

Purpose-formulated weight loss diets are recommended because energy content is reduced. This helps to promote weight loss because rate is principally determined by energy intake. Weight loss diets are also supplemented with protein (amino acids) and micronutrients, relative to their energy content, and this ensures that deficiency states do not arise despite energy restriction. A recent study has demonstrated that, despite often marked energy restriction, nutrient deficiencies are not observed. While supplementing protein, relative to energy content, does not speed up the rate of weight loss, it ensures that lean tissue loss is minimized, and also has beneficial effects on satiety (see below). L-carnitine facilitates transport of fatty acids in mitochondria, assisting their oxidation, and supplementation in a weight loss diet also assists with maintaining lean tissue mass during weight loss, while supplementation of micronutrients, relative to energy content, ensures that deficiency states do not arise.

Altering the macronutrient content of a weight management diet can also improve satiety, and the most common approach is to supplement fiber content. However, in dogs, supplementing both protein and fiber provides an additive benefit, and such diets improve the outcome of weight loss by speeding up the overall rate, increasing the likelihood of reaching target weight, and preserving lean tissue. The situation is more complex for cats, since protein content is a key determinant of voluntary food intake and incorporating more can increase rather than decrease voluntary food intake. Furthermore, incorporating too much fiber can make the diet unpalatable. Therefore, for cats, the greatest effect on satiety occurs when fiber and protein are both moderately, rather than markedly, supplemented.

Energy intake during weight loss

There are various approaches to calculating the energy intake required for controlled weight loss. Some clinicians recommend first calculating resting energy requirements for the current body weight (i.e. for dogs: 70 kcals × body weight$^{0.75}$/day), and then feeding 80% of this amount. While this has the benefits of simplicity, it does not take into account the degree of excess body weight and the initial response may be more variable. Adjustments may be required in the early weeks to determine the correct energy intake for the individual case.

The author prefers an approach whereby energy intake is, instead, based on ideal body weight and not the current weight. Arguably, this approach enables the clinician to produce a more precise starting point for the energy intake required for weight loss because the magnitude of excess weight is better factored in. Ideal weight can be estimated in various ways (see above). Exact recommendations on energy intake are then varied depending on the species, gender, neuter status, and presence of co-existing (especially orthopedic) disease. In dogs, a recent study suggested that a typical starting allocation for weight loss should be approximately 60 kcal/kg metabolic body weight (MBW) at target weight$^{0.75}$, with neutered dogs requiring less energy than entire dogs and female dogs less than male dogs. However, while this initial allocation might be sufficient during the first few weeks of the weight loss program, energy intake often needs subsequently to be modified, as and when weight loss slows. Typically, small adjustments (of up to 5%) are made on each occasion. Indeed, in the canine study described above, mean energy intake over the entire weight loss period was 57 kcal/kg MBW at target weight.

Calculating energy intake for weight loss is simpler in cats, where a linear equation is suitable. In one study, an average starting allocation of 40 kcal/kg target weight was successful in most cats, with mean energy intake over the whole of weight loss being 32 kcal/kg. With this degree of restriction, the mean rate of weight loss is 0.8% body weight/week.

Whatever the method of determining food intake, precision in portioning is absolutely critical in order to ensure success. Use of measuring cups should be avoided since portion sizes are imprecise and variable (usually being overestimated). Instead, electronic kitchen scales to weigh out food portions are strongly recommended. If at all possible, owners should not give any additional food (e.g. table scraps or treats) and care should be taken to prevent the patient from scavenging. If desired, food can be given in two, or more, meals per day, preferably providing more food at times when the owner is with the pet (since this is when begging is most likely to occur). However, use of an interactive feeding device is preferred (e.g. puzzle feeding toy or modified feeding bowl). These devices have the effect of slowing food intake, thereby improving satiety.

Occasional treats may be sanctioned (preferably some of the weight management food or a dog treat of known caloric content [e.g. dental treat]), but it is essential to take them into account so that they are included in the overall allocation and provide <5% of total daily requirements.

Pharmaceutical therapy and weight loss

Two drugs have been licensed for use in dogs (but NOT cats): mitratapide and dirlotapide. Although they have now been available for a number of years, and there is reasonable evidence of efficacy, they have not been used widely in a clinical setting. Both of these drugs are MTP inhibitors and have a local effect on the intestinal epithelial cell, blocking the assembly and release of lipoprotein particles into the bloodstream. Dietary caloric intake is decreased both by decreasing lipid absorption and by decreasing appetite (the latter thought to be due to release of a satiety signal that acts centrally on the appetite center). The efficacy of these drugs declines if they are administered in conjunction with a low-fat (<10%) diet. In Europe, both mitratapide and dirlotapide are licensed, but only dirlotapide is licensed in North America.

Mitratapide is only licensed for short-term use (i.e. 8 weeks) and was designed to kick-start a conventional weight loss program. In contrast, dirlotapide is licensed for continuous use for up to 12 months, which is sufficient for many, but not all, weight loss programs. Weight loss occurs at a steady rate (0.75%/week on average), but periodic increases in dose are required to maintain weight loss.

The most common side-effects are vomiting and diarrhea, and these are observed in up to 20% of patients. If owners are forewarned that it may occur, then it is usually better tolerated. Anorexia can also occur. While these drugs can be successful in promoting weight loss, appetite returns rapidly when they are discontinued and so other strategies (feeding and behavioral) must also implemented to be successful. Without this, a rapid and predictable rebound occurs.

Lifestyle management

Increasing physical activity is also recommended for most affected animals since it can assist in lean tissue preservation and, possibly, help to prevent the rapid regain in weight that can occur after a period of successful weight loss. It is also rewarding for owners since it represents an alternative to giving food-based rewards. Suitable exercise strategies in dogs include lead walking, swimming, hydrotherapy, and treadmills. Cats can be encouraged to increase their activity through regular play sessions with cat toys (e.g. fishing rod toys), motorized units, and puzzle feeders (see above). Ideally, daily exercise should be taken and, for dogs, 30 minutes or more is preferred. For cats, short periods of play activity are used, typically 1–2 minutes at a time two or more times per day. The exercise program should be tailored to the individual, and take account of any concurrent medical concerns.

Monitoring weight loss

Regular weight checks should be scheduled during weight loss. At the start of the program, it is best to book reweigh sessions at 2-week intervals, since this is the time when the owner is becoming accustomed to dramatic changes in lifestyle, and adjustments to the plan may be required if weight loss is progressing too quickly or too slowly. Thereafter, in patients where weight loss is progressing steadily, the interval between checks can be increased, but should not, ideally, exceed 4 weeks. More frequent checks may be needed in cases where weight loss is slow or stalls regularly. It is usually best if a dedicated member of staff takes charge of weight management. That way, they can get to know the client, and build up a trusting relationship, improving the likelihood of success. Given that some clients require intensive support throughout the program, it is advisable for staff to be trained in owner counseling.

Once the target weight is reached, food intake is increased gradually (typically in increments of up to 5%), until body weight stabilizes. Thereafter, weight checks should continue but the frequency can be gradually decreased. It is essential to continue to monitor body weight after ideal weight has been achieved to ensure that weight that was lost is not regained. Weight regain is a recognized phenomenon in humans who diet, although the reasons are still unclear. The most likely explanation is that when obese humans are returned to a lean state, their resting metabolic rate slows. Studies in dogs have also demonstrated a tendency for weight regain, although it affects fewer patients and rarely do dogs regain all the weight lost. Other studies have demonstrated that, as in humans, the MER is less after weight loss. In a recent study examining follow-up after successful weight loss, almost half of the dogs regained weight. Critically, when the diet was switched from the purpose-formulated weight management diet to a different diet (typically a standard maintenance diet), dogs were 20 times more likely to regain weight. Thus, owners should be strongly recommended to continue to feed the weight management diet, albeit to maintain weight rather than achieve further weight loss. In a similar study in cats, weight regain was again identified, and the problem was of a similar magnitude to dogs. However, the most notable factor associated with weight regain was age, with younger cats (<9 years of age) more likely to rebound.

PROGNOSIS

When an animal is predisposed to obesity, both through individual and environmental factors, many of these predispositions will remain after weight loss. Further, the post-weight loss MER is significantly less than it was prior to weight loss. For these reasons, obesity can only be managed and never cured, and the prognosis for long-term success is guarded. In the author's experience, most (80–90%) cats and dogs lose at least 10% of weight on a program, with approximately two-thirds reaching their target weight. Recent work by the author has identified that initial body fat mass is negatively associated with the likelihood of reaching the target weight. Furthermore, dogs fed a dry weight management diet were more likely to succeed than those fed either wet food or a combination of wet and dry food. The remaining dogs and cats fail to lose significant weight, and are commonly lost to follow-up. Owners of these animals often decide not to return to the clinic and become noncontactable. Thus, the exact reasons for discontinuing the program are difficult to determine.

PREVENTION

Given the variable outcome of weight management diets, prevention of obesity is likely to have a more significant beneficial effect on the health and welfare of all dogs and cats, rather than by treating once the problem has developed. Advice on correct nutrition and exercise should be included in all puppy and kitten consultations and continued throughout the life of the animal. Body weight and BCS should be assessed at every consultation and also during the annual health check. Regularly monitoring body weight and BCS throughout life can enable subtle changes (e.g. ±5%) to be identified and rectified before the problem worsens. Veterinarians should also be alert to the weight gain that can occur as a consequence of neutering. It is advisable to schedule 2–3 checks for weight and BCS in the first 6–12 months after neutering to identify those patients that gain excessive amounts of weight at this time.

Finally, knowledge of pet ownership styles could ultimately be used to help in obesity prevention. If certain ownership styles were known to predispose to weight gain and obesity, then targeted owner education could be applied to owners with such styles. A recent study has identified that different populations of cat exist that respond differently to long-term *ad-libitum* feeding. Some cats are unable to regulate their food intake, leading to gradual lifelong weight gain, while others maintain stable weight and optimal body condition lifelong, presumably by regulating intake. Therefore, this work suggests that different groups of cats have different feeding styles; some are regulators, while others tend to overeat. When it comes to preventing weight gain, attention should be paid to matching pet ownership style to feeding style. For example, an owner with an indulgent feeding style would be a bad match for a cat that overeats, but is likely to be fine if they were to own a cat that self-regulates intake.

RECOMMENDED FURTHER READING

German AJ (2006) The growing problem of obesity in dogs and cats. *J Nutr* **136:**1940S–1946S.

German AJ, Holden SL, Morris PJ *et al.* (2012) Long-term follow-up after weight management in obese dogs: the role of diet in preventing regain. *Vet J* **192**:65–70.

German AJ, Holden SL, Wiseman-Orr ML *et al.* (2012) Quality of life is reduced in obese dogs but improves after successful weight loss. *Vet J* **192:**428–434.

German AJ, Ryan VH, German AC *et al.* (2010) Obesity, its associated disorders and the role of inflammatory adipokines in companion animals. *Vet J* **185:**4–9.

Kealy RD, Lawler DF, Ballam JM *et al.* (2002) Effects of diet restriction on life span and age-related changes in dogs. *J Am Vet Med Assoc* **220:**1315–1320.

Kopelman PG (2000) Obesity as a medical problem. *Nature* **404:**635–643.

Lund EM, Armstrong PJ, Kirk CA *et al.* (2005) Prevalence and risk factors for obesity in adult cats from private US veterinary practices. *Int J Appl Res Vet M* **3:**88–96.

Lund EM, Armstrong PJ, Kirk CA *et al.* (2006) Prevalence and risk factors for obesity in adult dogs from private US veterinary practices. *Int J Appl Res Vet M* **4:**177–186.

Trayhurn P, Wood IS (2004) Adipokines: inflammation and the pleiotropic role of white adipose tissue. *Brit J Nutr* **92:**347–355.

Appendix: Clinical cases

CASE 1: HEPATITIS – ROBERT ARMENTANO

Signalment/history

A 6-year-old neutered male Cocker Spaniel presents for a 1-week history of acute onset of polyuria, polydipsia, mild inappetence, lethargy, and intermittent vomiting.

Clinical examination and initial diagnostics

The dog is quiet, alert, and responsive. Physical examination is unremarkable apart from icteric sclera, skin, and mucous membranes. Body condition score is 2/5. The dog resides in a wooded area in the Midwest USA with access to standing water. There is one other dog in the household who is clinically normal.

Minimum database tests. Serum chemistry: ALP = 1,263 U/L (reference interval [RI], 5–160); ALT = 2,562 U/L (RI, 18–121); AST = 755 U/L (RI, 16–55); total bilirubin = 4.5 mg/dl (RI, 0.0–0.3). Urinalysis: urine SG 1.012; 3+ bilirubinuria. Other serum chemistry, CBC, and urinalysis values are unremarkable.

Differential diagnosis

Common differential diagnoses in a middle aged dog with a severe hepatopathy include toxicity, drug-induced hepatitis, bacterial hepatitis (including leptospirosis), obstructive biliary disease, autoimmune/inflammatory hepatitis (chronic active hepatitis), copper-associated hepatitis, and neoplasia.

Recommended diagnostic testing

Abdominal radiographs, abdominal ultrasound, leptospirosis serology, urine PCR, liver biopsy.

Test results

Abdominal radiographs show mild microhepatica, abdominal ultrasound is unremarkable, and leptospirosis serology is negative (serologic titers <50, urine PCR negative). Laparoscopy reveals a diffusely mottled liver (**Figure 1.1**). Liver histopathology shows a moderate, widespread portal lymphoplasmacytic infiltrate. Copper stains are negative, aerobic and anaerobic cultures are negative.

Histopathologic diagnosis

Chronic active hepatitis.

Treatment recommendations

Chronic active hepatitis is an inflammatory hepatopathy of unknown etiology. If primary causes such as drug-induced, bacterial, and copper-associated hepatopathy are excluded, then the diagnosis is consistent with an idiopathic, autoimmune condition. Common breeds predisposed to this disease include the Dobermann, Cocker Spaniel, and Labrador Retriever, but it can occur in any breed. The mainstay therapy includes glucocorticoids with other immunosuppressive medications such as azathioprine, if indicated. Additional therapy includes antioxidant medications such as S-adenosylmethionine, silybin, and vitamin E as well as a low-protein diet. Monitoring and treating for portal hypertension (ascites),

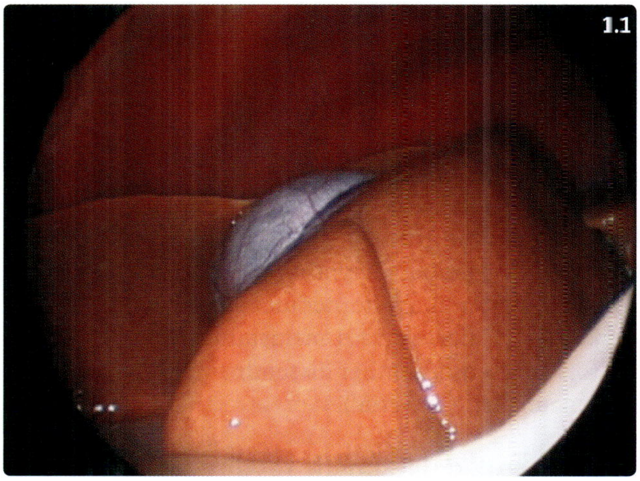

Figure 1.1 Moderately, diffusely mottled liver with normal appearing gallbladder.

as well as hepatic encephalopathy are crucial in managing patients with progressive disease leading to fibrosis and end-stage cirrhosis.

Conclusions

Chronic hepatopathies can present with acute signs requiring a thorough diagnostic work up. Early diagnosis is invaluable as the liver can regenerate if treatment is implemented. The prognosis for cirrhosis is considered guarded to poor.

CASE 2: BLASTOMYCOSIS – ROBERT ARMENTANO

Signalment/history

An 8-year-old neutered male Labrador Retriever presents for a 1-week history of a nonproductive cough, hyporexia, and lethargy, and a 24-hour history of hemoptysis.

Clinical examination and initial diagnostics

The dog is quiet, depressed, and responsive. Temperature is 104.8°F (40.4°C), heart rate is 120 bpm, and respiratory rate is 60 breaths per minute. On physical examination there are increased bronchovesicular lung sounds in all lung fields, with no crackles or wheezing. The remainder of the physical examination is unremarkable. The mucous membranes are pink with a CRT <2 seconds. Body condition score is 2.5/5. The dog resides in a wooded area in Wisconsin, USA.

Minimum database tests. CBC: neutrophilia of 16.5 k/µl (RI, 2.95–11.64); PCV = 38.7% (RI, 37.3–61.7); platelet count = 205 k/µl (RI, 148–484). Coagulation profile: prothrombin time = 12 seconds (RI, 12–17), partial thromboplastin time = 80 seconds (RI, 70–102). Serum chemistry profile was unremarkable, as was urinalysis. Pulse oximetry: SpO_2 = 95% (RI, 95–100). Urine SG = 1.030 with an inactive sediment. Thoracic radiographs are shown (**Figures 2.1, 2.2**).

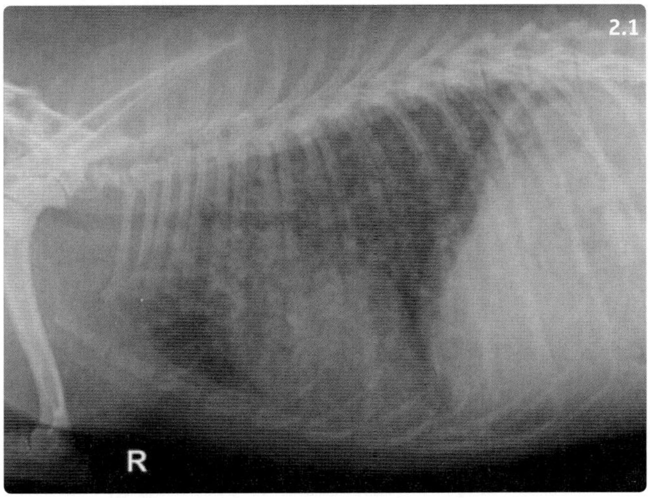

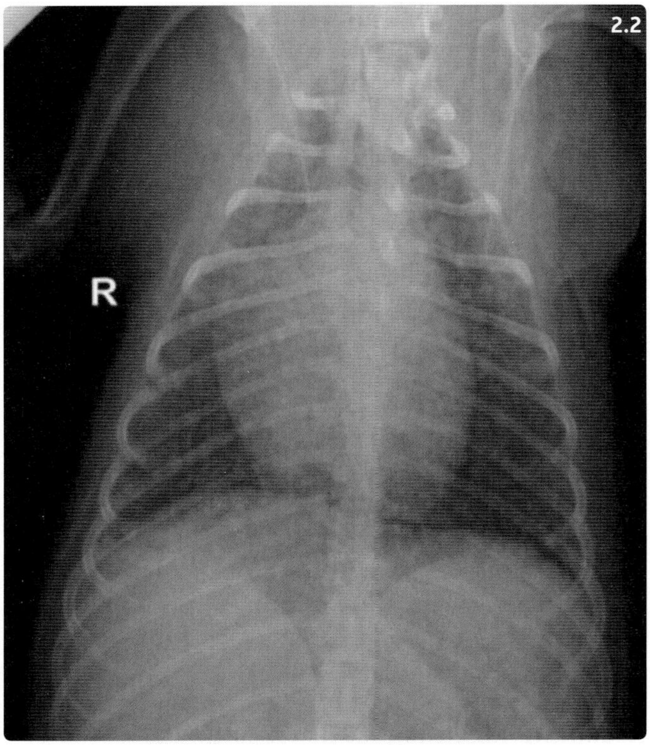

Figures 2.1, 2.2 Lateral and ventrodorsal thoracic radiographs demonstrating a diffuse military to nodular lung pattern.

Differential diagnoses

Common differential diagnoses in a middle aged dog with a diffuse miliary to nodular lung pattern include neoplasia (primary versus metastatic), fungal pneumonia (blastomycosis or other disseminated fungal disease), and pneumonia (bacterial).

Recommended diagnostic testing

Abdominal radiographs, abdominal ultrasound, urine blastomycosis antigen testing, lung fine-needle aspirate with cytology or biopsy.

Test results

Abdominal radiographs and ultrasound examinations were normal. The urine blastomycosis antigen test had an antigen titer of 11.61 ng/ml (RI, 0.2–14.7). Lung cytology via an ultrasound guided lung nodule fine needle aspirate is shown (**Figure 2.3**).

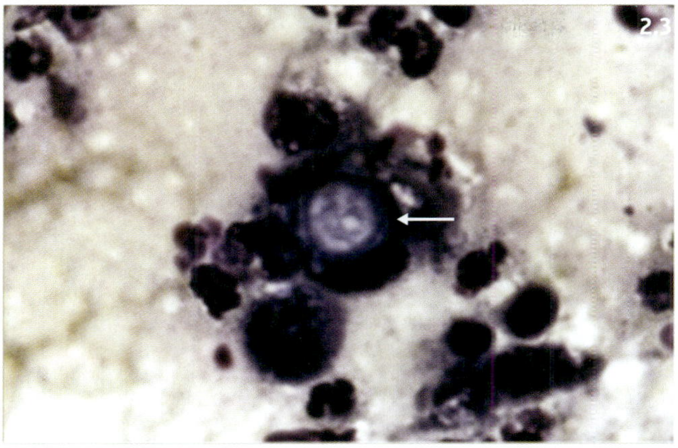

Figure 2.3 *Blastomyces dermatitidis* spore (arrow) obtained by fine needle aspiration and cytology. Diff-Quik®, ×100.

Treatment

The preferred medication is with a triazole antifungal agent, with itraconazole recommended as the best initial medication. Fluconazole has also been shown to be effective.

Conclusions

Canine blastomycosis most commonly presents as a respiratory disorder with the main clinical signs including increased respiratory rate and coughing. Blastomycosis can involve any organ system, including the eye, bone, and skin. The most common thoracic radiographic lesion is a diffuse interstitial to nodular pattern; however, in up to 50% of cases the lung pattern can include a nondiffuse infiltrate, alveolar pattern, or thoracic mass. The most effective diagnostic test for blastomycosis is either cytology evaluation or urine antigen testing, while histopathology and culture are also acceptable. Sensitivity for urine antigen testing ranges from 93.5% to 100%, thus serving as an excellent screening test. This test is also effective in monitoring remission of disease.

The prognosis for systemic blastomycosis is favorable (about 20% overall mortality) with multiple months of treatment. Reported negative prognostic factors include: severity of lung disease, oxygen dependency, as well as central nervous system and/or ocular involvement.

CASE 3: IMPACTED TOOTH – ERIN P. RIBKA & BROOK A. NIEMIEC

Signalment/history

A 7-year-old spayed female Maltese was referred for evaluation of missing teeth noted during routine dental prophylaxis approximately 3 months earlier.

Clinical examination

The dog was bright, alert, responsive, and hydrated. Heart and lungs auscultated within normal limits. Preanesthetic laboratory work was unremarkable. Conscious oral examination revealed missing right (105) and left (205) maxillary first premolars, left mandibular canine (304) and first premolar (305), right mandibular first incisor (401), and a partially erupted right mandibular canine (404) (**Figure 3.1**). During anesthetized examination and probing, the left maxillary second molar (210) and the right and left third molars (311, 411) were also discovered to be missing. In addition, the right maxillary second incisor (102) was mobile and discolored, the left mandibular incisors (301–303) were mobile, and the remaining right mandibular incisors (402, 403) were crowded. Scant or mild tartar was noted throughout the mouth. The left mandibular first molar (309) was partially erupted and a 4 mm periodontal pocket was probed at this tooth.

Differential diagnosis

Missing tooth: congenitally missing permanent tooth; previously extracted tooth; fracture below the gingiva; impacted tooth. Partially erupted teeth: congenital, developmental.

Provisional diagnosis

Impacted tooth with possible dentigerous cyst formation; partially erupted permanent mandibular canines

Diagnostic testing

Intraoral radiographs of the entire mouth were obtained. The left mandibular canine and first premolar teeth were impacted and an associated dentigerous cyst was seen

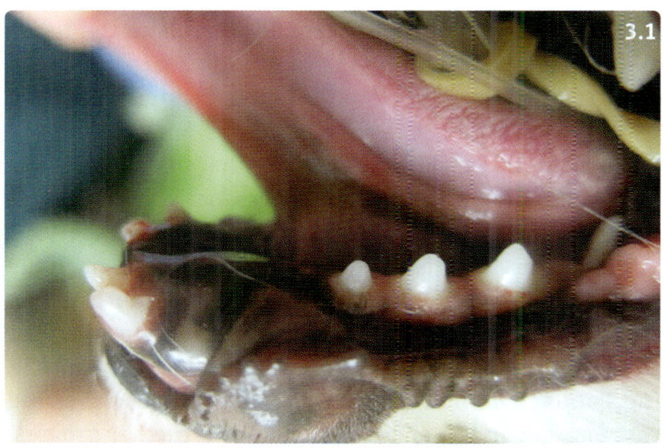

Figure 3.1 Photograph of the rostral left mandible. The left mandibular canine (304) and first premolar (305) are missing.

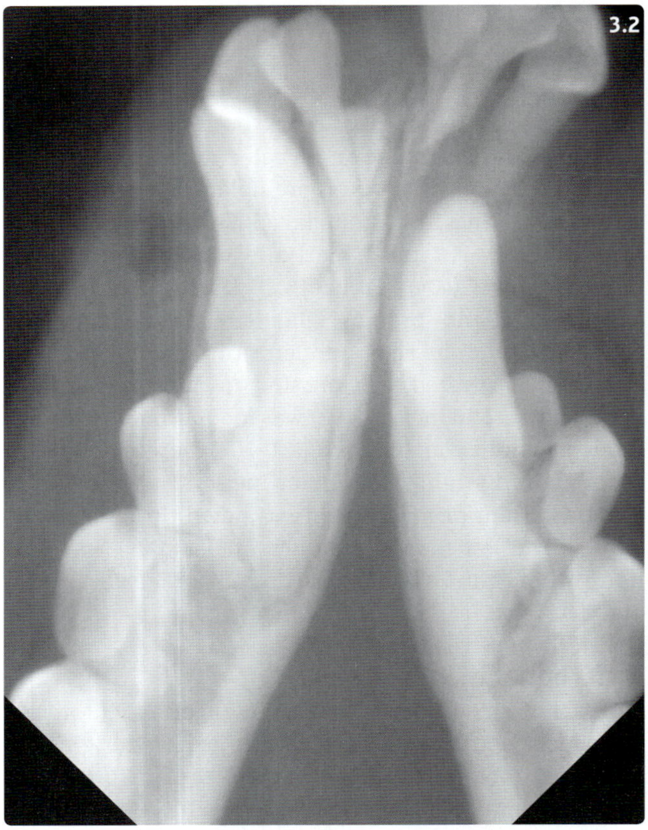

Figure 3.2 Radiograph of the rostral mandibles. Note the minimal amount of bone adjacent to the impacted left canine (304) compared with the right (404).

radiographically. (**Figure 3.2**). Intraoral dental radiographs are a necessity for proper diagnosis of 'missing' teeth.

Treatment

Full dental prophylaxis (i.e. scaling and polishing) was performed. A gingival incision was made over the area of the missing canine and premolar teeth and the tissue gently elevated from the bone with periosteal elevators to create a large envelope flap. Bone was carefully removed using a 701 cross-cut taper fissure bur on a high-speed air driven hand-piece to expose the impacted teeth. Gentle luxation and elevation were performed to ease the teeth out of the mandible so as not to damage vital structures or fracture the jaw (**Figure 3.3**). The partially erupted right mandibular canine was treated with an apical repositioning flap to expose the enamel, lengthen the crown of the tooth, and prevent future periodontal pocketing. The left mandibular first molar was treated with closed root planing and a perioceutic to prevent further progression of periodontal disease. All of the mandibular incisors were removed as well as the right maxillary second incisor, which was found to have an unstable root fracture on radiography.

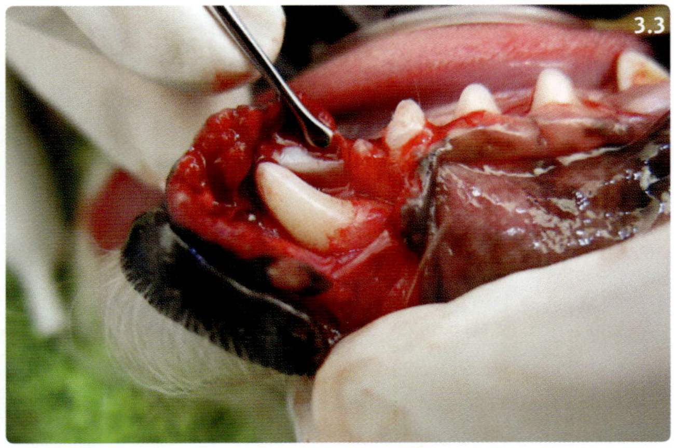

Figure 3.3 Intraoperative photograph showing the impacted left mandibular canine (304) and first premolar (305).

Conclusion

Impacted teeth are frequently diagnosed, particularly in small breed and brachycephalic dogs, and should always be radiographed. Dentigerous cysts are fairly common sequelae of impacted teeth and, if left untreated, can lead to serious consequences such as pathologic jaw fracture. Partially erupted teeth can lead to development of periodontal disease and should be treated with appropriate periodontal surgical techniques.

CASE 4: TOOTH RESORPTION – ERIN P. RIBKA & BROOK A. NIEMIEC

Signalment/history

An 11-year-old spayed female Chesapeake Bay Retriever was presented for extraction of a left maxillary 4th premolar (208).

Clinical examination

The patient had a reputation for being snappish and the referring veterinarian advised that previous examinations had to be performed under mild sedation. The dog was bright, alert, responsive, and hydrated on presentation. A severe tooth resorption lesion of 208 was obvious on careful conscious examination (**Figure 4.1**). An uncomplicated crown fracture of 108 was also noted. No abnormalities were noted on auscultation of heart and lungs and preanesthetic CBC, chemistry panel, and thoracic radiographs performed by the referring veterinarian were unremarkable.

Anesthetized oral examination revealed gingivitis and widespread early periodontal disease evidenced by pockets 4–6 mm deep in many teeth. Uncomplicated crown fractures were confirmed in the right maxillary fourth premolar (108) and also in the left mandibular

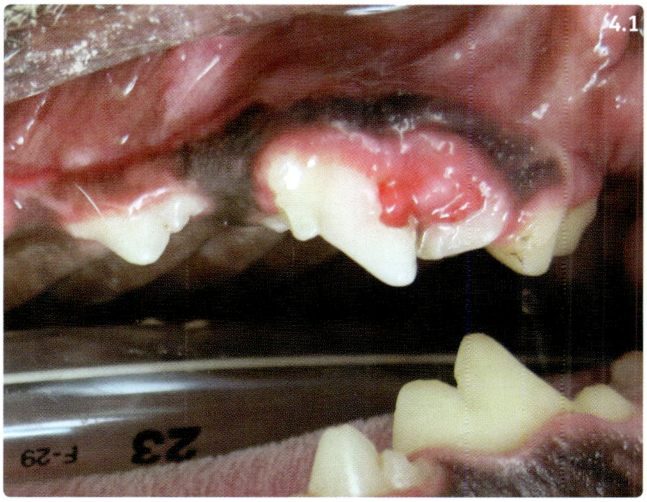

Figure 4.1 Photograph of left maxillary 4th premolar (208) with gingival overgrowth.

second premolar (306) and right mandibular third incisor (403). Abrasive wear was noted on the occlusal surfaces of all molar teeth. The tooth resorption of the left maxillary fourth premolar (208) was seen to be extensive, invading well into the pulp chamber (**Figure 4.2**).

Differential diagnosis

Tooth resorption, complicated crown fracture, periodontal disease, neoplasia.

Provisional diagnosis

Tooth resorption.

Diagnostic testing

Intraoral dental radiographs were obtained of the affected tooth (**Figure 4.3**).

Treatment

Full dental prophylaxis was performed. An envelope flap was made by sharp incision of the interdental gingiva and buccal gingival attachment of the affected tooth. The flap was gently elevated with a periosteal elevator to expose the buccal alveolar bone and furcation of the tooth. A cross-cut taper fissure bur (#701L) on a high-speed, water-cooled dental hand-piece was used to section all three tooth roots, from the furcation to the coronal aspect of the crown. Buccal alveolar bone was carefully removed (using the same bur) to better visualize and elevate the roots. The roots were carefully and gently luxated to fatigue the periodontal ligament, elevated from the bone, and extracted completely. The remaining edges of bone were smoothed with a coarse diamond bur and the sockets were curetted gently to remove debris, granuloma

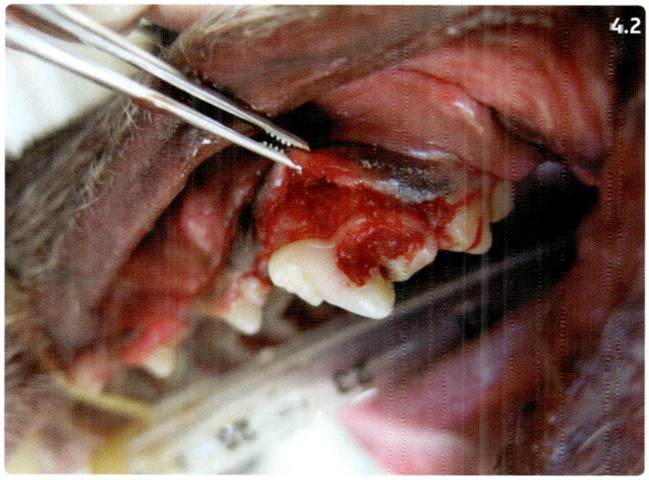

Figure 4.2 Same tooth as shown in Figure 4.1 after the removal of the excess gingiva and creation and elevation of an envelope flap, revealing a large tooth resorption of the buccal surface of 208.

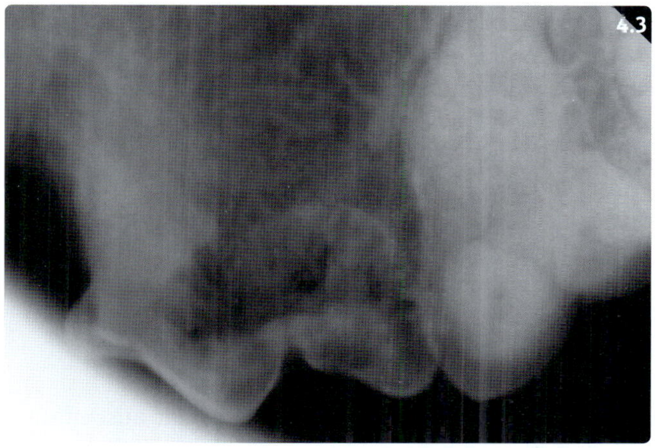

Figure 4.3 Dental radiograph of the same tooth. Note the obvious radiolucency of the affected crown.

tissue, and any small fragments of bone or root. The flap was closed without tension using 4-0 poliglecaprone 25 on a reverse cutting needle in a simple interrupted pattern. Complete extraction of all roots and fragments was confirmed with dental radiographs.

Conclusion

Although generally considered to be a feline disease, tooth resorptions can and do occur in dogs as well. These very painful lesions should be dealt with definitively as early as possible to minimize discomfort and possible behavioral changes (as seen in this case). At the 2-week recheck, the patient was visibly more comfortable and her owner was very pleased with the improvement in her demeanor and greater energy and activity level after tooth extraction. Dental radiography is essential to properly diagnose and plan treatment and to ensure that extraction is complete.

CASE 5: PULMONARY FIBROSIS – CÉCILE CLERCX & ELODIE ROELS

Signalment/history

An 11-year-old West Highland White Terrier (WHWT) presented with chronic cough, progressive exercise intolerance, and tachypnea. Previous treatment with steroids improved the cough, but the treatment induced polyphagia, polydipisa, and weight gain.

Clinical examination

Body condition score was 8/9. A severe restrictive dyspnea was noted, with increased respiratory rate and increased expiratory effort. Ausultation revealed diffuse inspiratory crackles, easily audible in both lung fields, but no heart murmur. Mucous membranes were congested. Clinical examination failed to reveal any other abnormality. The abdomen was distended and hepatomegaly was palpated.

Differential diagnosis

Causes of chronic cough, exercise intolerance, tachypnea, and syncope include lower airway disease (pulmonary fibrosis, chronic bronchitis, tracheobronchial collapse, neoplastic pulmonary disease), cardiac disease, thromboembolic disease, or a combination of diseases.

Provisional diagnosis

Since the dog is a WHWT, and since cardiac auscultation failed to reveal any murmur, the crackles were thought to be due to pulmonary fibrosis. Cushing's disease was suspected but was possibly iatrogenic.

Blood work (**Table 5.1**) revealed thrombocytosis, neutrophilic leukocytosis, and elevated alkaline phosphatase and cholesterol, possibly related to steroid administration. Thoracic radiographs (**Figures 5.1a, b**) showed generalized interstitial pattern, right cardiomegaly, and a redundant tracheal membrane. Echocardiography confirmed the absence of a primary cardiac disease. Doppler-echocardiographic evidence of mild pulmonary hypertension (PH) was noted, with systolic pressure gradient estimated at 37 mmHg (RI, <31.4 mmHg). Blood gas analysis revealed severe hypoxemia (64 mmHg, RI, 85–100) and elevated Aa gradient (23 mmHg, RI, <15). Bronchoscopy showed a grade 1 tracheal collapse and severe bronchomalacia (**Figure 5.2**). Bronchoalveolar lavage fluid analysis was unremarkable. Fecal analysis (Baerman) failed to reveal any parasites.

Table 5.1 Blood parameters: hematology and biochemistry. (Abnormal values in bold.)

	Day 1	After 6 months	Units	Reference interval
Hematology				
Hematocrit	53	**60**	%	37–55
White blood cells	**29.0**	13.47	10^9/l	6.0–15.0
Neutrophils	**27.9**	10.53	10^9/l	3.0–11.4
Platelets	**675**	378	10^9/l	200–500
Biochemistry				
Total proteins	73	71	g/l	52–62
Albumin	38.04		g/l	27–32
BUN	6.8	15	mmol/l	1.66–18.21
Creatinine	76.16	55.69	μmol/l	<133
Sodium	152	147	mmol/l	140–155
Potassium	5.6	5.3	mmol/l	3.6–5.6
ALT	39.30	25.00	U/L	5–62
ALP	**834**	243	U/L	27–74
Bilirubin	2.68		μmol/l	1–6
Cholesterol	**10.69**		mmol/l	<7.8

Therefore, primary canine idiopathic pulmonary fibrosis (CIPF) was suspected, with secondary tracheal collapse, bronchomalacia, and pulmonary arterial hypertension. High-resolution tomography of the thorax was proposed in order to raise the index of suspicion and revealed lesions compatible with CIPF (**Figure 5.3**). Although histopathology of lung tissue is considered as the gold standard to confirm diagnosis, it was not performed ante mortem in the present case.

Treatment, prognosis, follow up

To date, and despite a huge amount of investigation in this field, no treatment is able to cure pulmonary fibrosis, either in humans or in dogs. Acetylcysteine seems to slow down the progression of fibrosis in human PH without significant side-effects, presumably through an antioxidant activity, therefore it was prescribed for

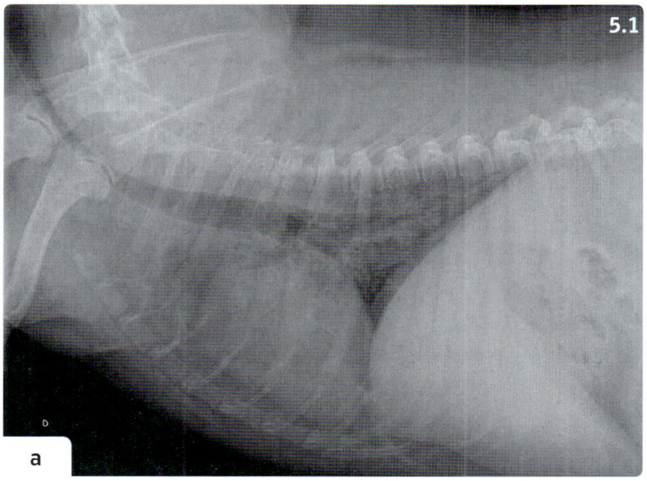

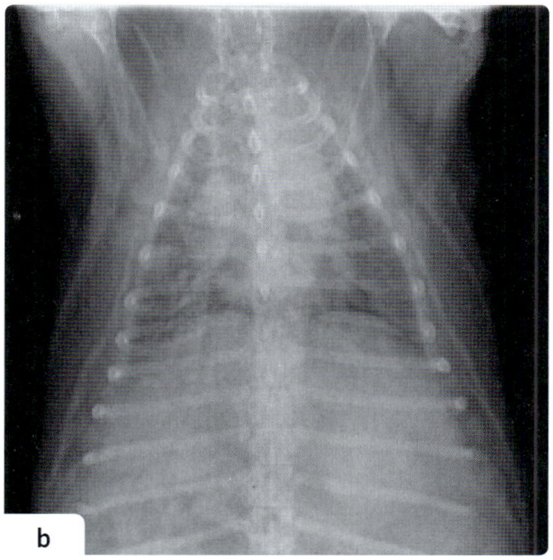

Figures 5.1a. b Thoracic radiographs (right lateral and dorsoventral views) showing generalized interstitial pattern, right cardiomegaly, and a redundant tracheal membrane.

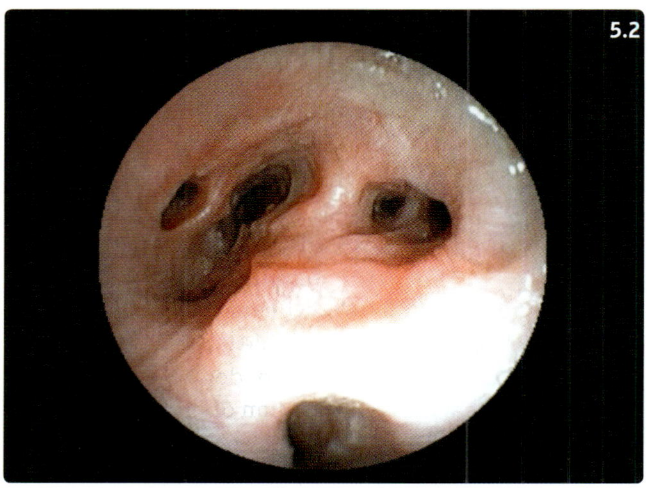

Figure 5.2 Bronchoscopic examination showing bronchomalacia.

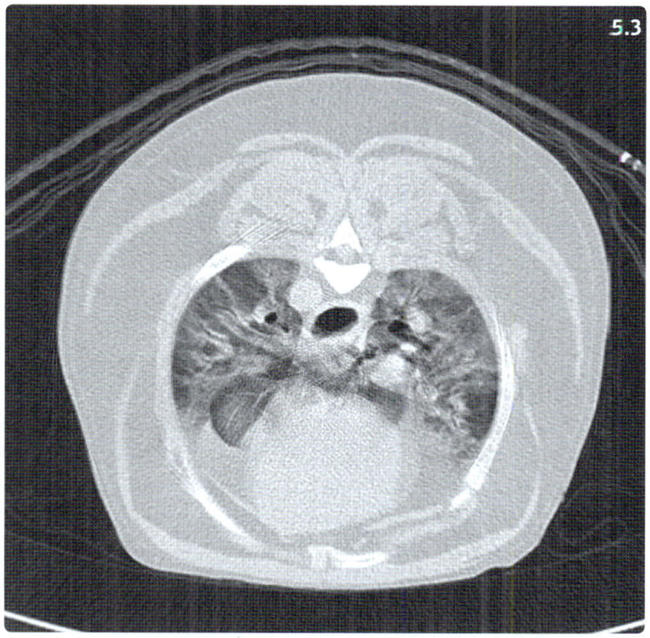

Figure 5.3 Transverse thoracic pre-contrast high-resolution CT image (lung window) at the level of the caudal lung lobes. Scan reveals a generalized ground-glass opacity in a patchy distribution, resulting in a mosaic attenuation pattern, in addition to parenchymal bands and bronchovascular thickening.

this dog (15 mg/kg q12h). In order to manage the cough, at least partly related to chronic bronchitis and tracheal collapse, oral steroid therapy was progressively replaced by inhaled therapy with fluticasone. Theophylline (10 mg/kg q12h) was added, with the hope of improving ventilation. Sildenafil (1 mg/kg q12h) was prescribed to manage the pulmonary arterial hypertension. Last but not least, since obesity has a negative impact on ventilation performance, a diet was advised to reduce the body weight.

Treatment improved the quality of life of the patient, despite the persistence of some cough and exercise intolerance. Six-minutes-walking distance increased and CT and echocardiographic findings were stable up to 9 months after diagnosis.

CASE 6: RESPIRATORY WORMS – CÉCILE CLERCX

Signalment/history

A 5-month-old male Pomeranian weighing 1.7 kg, recently acquired and originating from an eastern European country, was presented with cough, exercise intolerance, and tachypnea of 2 weeks' duration. The dog was presumed to be up-to-date with his vaccination.

Previous treatment with antibiotics had not helped resolve the signs.

Clinical examination

Body condition score was 5/9. Rectal temperature was normal. The dog was alert. A slight expiratory effort was noted, with increased respiratory rate (80 breaths per minute). Auscultation revealed increased lung sounds but no crackles and no heart murmur. No other abnormality was revealed.

Differential considerations

Lower airway disease of infectious origin was suspected. Since the dog was young, originated from an eastern European country (poor transport conditions, poor vaccination, and parasite control), was in good general condition, and failed to respond to antibiotics, the most likely differentials included parasites (e.g. enteric worms or lung worms [*Crenosoma vulpis*, *Filaroides osleri*, *Angiostrongylus vasorum*]), toxoplasmosis, kennel cough (mainly *Bordetella bronchiseptica*), and infection with mycoplasmas or *Pneumocystis carinii*. Distemper was less likely in the absence of systemic signs and immune deficiency can always occur.

Diagnosis

Blood work revealed moderate neutrophilic leukocytosis with a moderate left shift. Thoracic radiographs (**Figures 6.1a–c**) showed a generalized bronchointerstitial pattern and an alveolar pattern in peripheral areas of both left and right caudal lung lobes, as well as ventrally in the left cranial and right middle lung lobes. These findings were

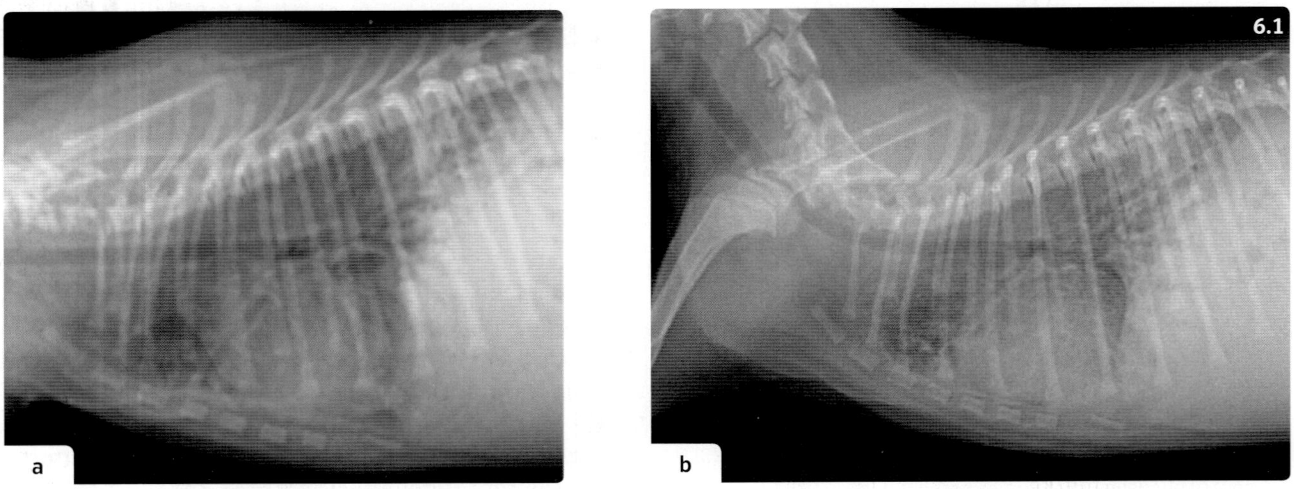

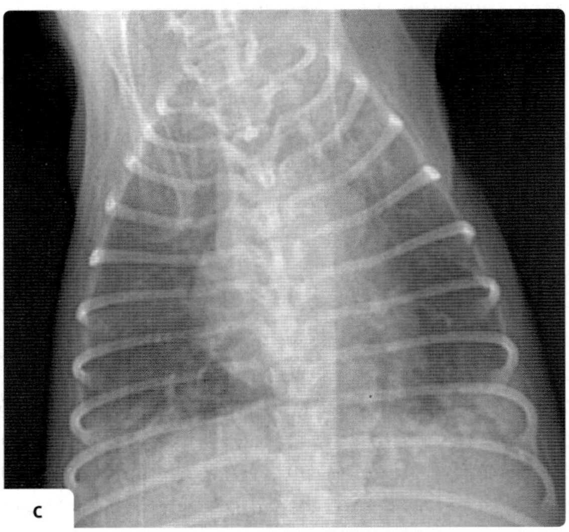

Figures 6.1a–c Left lateral (a), right lateral (b), and ventrodorsal (c) thoracic radiographs.

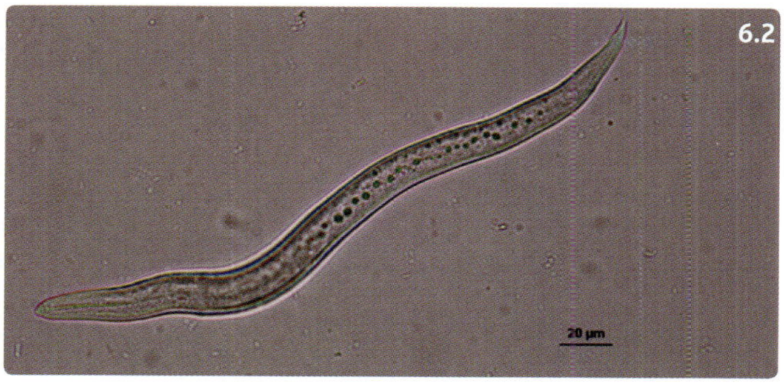

Figure 6.2 Baermann analysis of feces showing a larva of *Crenosoma vulpis*.

compatible with an atypical bronchopneumonia (*A. vasorum*) embolism.

Bronchoalveolar lavage fluid was used for RT-PCR assessment of organisms. Moderate levels of *A. vasorum* were detected, while *B. bronchiseptica*, distemper, *Mycoplasma cynos* and *M. cani* were negative. Fecal analysis revealed the presence of *Uncinaria* and *Toxocara canis* (floatation) and *Crenosoma vulpis* (Baermann, **Figure 6.2**).

Therefore, parasitic tracheobronchopneumonia (mainly due to *A. vasorum* or *C. vulpis*, or possibly to *Uncinaria*, *T. canis* and *Toxoplasma*) was diagnosed.

Treatment

The dog was treated with fenbendazole (50 mg/kg PO q24h for 20 days) and amoxicilline + clavulanic acid (20 mg/kg q12h for 8 days) as well as clindamycin (12.5 mg/kg PO q12h for 2 weeks) against potential toxoplasmosis. The condition of the dog worsened after 48 hours, the cough increased and a severe dyspnea appeared, supected to be due to massive destruction of respiratory parasites. Prednisolone (0.4 mg/kg PO q12h for 3 days then 0.5 mg/kg q24h for 2 days, then 0.5 mg/kg every other day) was added; the dog quickly improved, was discharged, and had no more clinical signs.

CASE 7: TRACHEAL TEAR – JESSICA BULLOCK

Signalment/history

A 10-year-old spayed female Chihuahua is examined for evaluation of a 10-day history of progressive cough and a 5-day history of progressive subcutaneous emphysema. The history revealed normal blood work prior to a dental cleaning performed 10 days ago at another clinic.

Clinical examination

The dog is bright, alert, anxious, and breathing, with moderately increased respiratory rate and effort. There is marked subcutaneous emphysema extending from the carpi to the tarsi with 2–3 cm of emphysema between the skin and body wall dorsally. The remainder of the physical examination is unremarkable.

Differential diagnoses

Trauma to the trachea, body wall, or mediastinum; tracheal injury secondary to neoplasia or infection.

Provisional diagnosis

The most likely diagnosis is tracheal injury secondary to recent endotracheal intubation based on the recent clinical history and normal status prior to the dental procedure. However, given the patient's signalment, other possible causes for tracheal injury should be ruled out.

Emergency treatment

The patient was allowed to rest quietly in oxygen at 40% and sedatives were administered as needed. Acepromazine (0.01–0.04 mg/kg IV q4–6h) and butorphanol (0.1–0.3 mg/kg IV q4–6h) are commonly recommended in such situations to help decrease respiratory anxiety. Acepromazine can induce hypotension and is contraindicated in hypotensive patients.

Diagnostic testing

- Blood gas analysis showed a mild respiratory alkalosis with normal serum electrolytes; this is expected with the increased respiratory rate and excess loss of CO_2. The patient had a mild azotemia and a urine SG from a free-catch sample was 1.040; mild dehydration with prerenal azotemia was presumed.
- Blood pressure was slightly elevated at 150 mmHg and assumed to be caused by increased anxiety.
- Thoracic radiographs (taken after mild sedation) showed severe subcutaneous emphysema, moderate pneumomediastinum, mild pneumothorax, and mild pneumoretroperitoneum. There was no evidence of neoplasia or other type of lung pathology (**Figure 7.1**).

Recommended procedures

Although the large majority of tracheal injuries can be managed medically with rest time and medications, this patient's condition was deteriorating rather than improving. Due to the severity of the patient's symptoms and the progressive nature of the signs, tracheoscopy was performed for a more detailed evaluation of the trachea. This study showed that nine tracheal rings were linearly ruptured in a 3-cm stretch – the esophagus had fortuitously partially occluded the tear. The rent was surgically repaired, and the dog recovered and convalesced uneventfully.

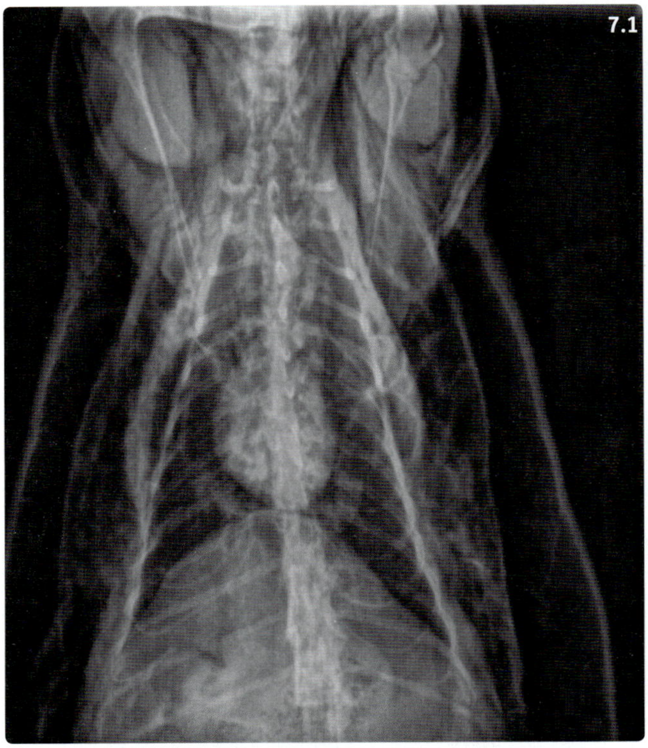

Figure 7.1 A ventrodorsal thoracic radiograph showing marked subcutaneous emphysema associated with a tracheal tear.

CASE 8: KIDNEY DISEASE – JESSICA BULLOCK

Signalment/history

A 7-year-old neutered male Domestic Shorthair cat is examined for a 2–3-day history of lethargy and decreased appetite. The patient is a historically healthy outdoor cat, and all vaccinations are current.

Physical examination

The cat is quiet, alert, responsive, and approximately 7% dehydrated. There are no other significant findings. A hemogram was normal. Serum chemistry abnormalities: BUN = 310 mg/dl (RI, 16–36); creatinine = 20 mg/dl (RI, 0.8–2.4); phosphorus = 20 mg/dl (RI, 3.1–6.0); potassium = 6.0 mEq/l (RI, 3.5–5.8). Urine SG = 1.012.

Differential diagnosis

Acute kidney injury (AKI) due to toxin ingestion (ethylene glycol, lily, various human medications, others); infection (leptospirosis, ascending bacterial infection); neoplasia (lymphoma, although there was no renomegaly); urinary obstruction (urethral, ureteral, combination); acute exacerbation of underlying chronic kidney disease.

Provisional diagnosis

The provisional diagnosis is AKI due to toxin ingestion or chronic kidney disease (fibrosis or pyelonephritis) based on normal abdominal palpation and lack of observed lower urinary tract signs.

Additional diagnostic testing

- Ethylene glycol screening tests (serum testing and urine sediment examination) are recommended as intoxication with ethylene glycol at the stage of marked azotemia is uniformly fatal unless immediate dialysis is possible – it then still carries a grave prognosis. Urine sediment examination was unremarkable in this cat.
- Urine culture to rule out urinary tract infection (UTI). Although a simple UTI is both statistically unlikely and unlikely to cause these symptoms, it could contribute as a co-morbidity and is less likely to be identified on screening tests due to the low urine SG. Urine culture was negative in this cat.
- Abdominal ultrasound is an excellent screening modality to help characterize renal changes, specifically looking for evidence of neoplasia (confirmed with fine-needle aspirates or biopsies), pyelectasia (potentially indicative of pyelonephritis or obstruction, confirmed with cultures), and/or hydronephrosis (indicative of current or previous obstruction, confirmed as needed with contrast studies). In this case, abdominal ultrasound was unremarkable.

Initial treatment

This cat was treated with 100 ml/kg/day of lactated Ringer's solution IV, ampicillin/sulbactam (30 mg/kg IV q8h), antinausea medication (maropitant 1 mg/kg SC q24), and a gastroprotectant (famotidine 1 mg/kg q24h). After 3 days of treatment, the kidney values had only mildly improved to a BUN 196 mg/dl and a creatinine of 14.9 mg/dl. The cat had gained 0.5 kg body weight, respiratory rate was increasing, and he was still inappetent and lethargic.

Other recommended procedures

Dialysis is recommended in cases of severe azotemia that become unresponsive to traditional medical management and in certain cases of known acute intoxications. At this author's institution, approximately 50% of the acute kidney injury patients treated with dialysis leave the hospital improved after 2–3 weeks of treatment.

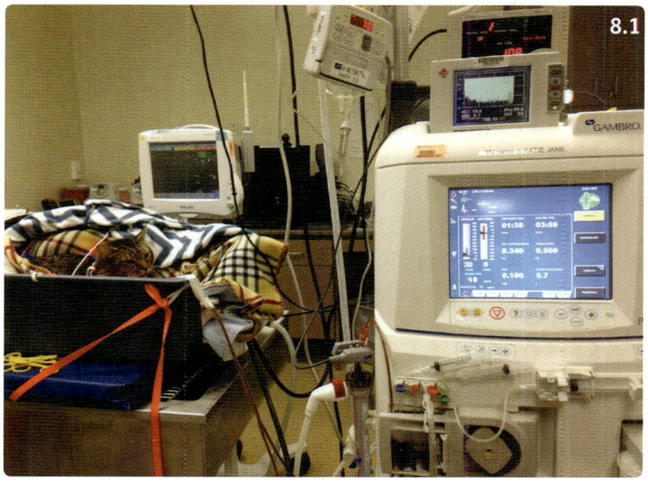

Figure 8.1 The cat being treated with hemodialysis.

Although expensive, this treatment option can be very beneficial to the patient. Prior to dialysis treatment, testing for leptospirosis should also be considered. Although this condition is rare in cats, diagnosis could alter treatment and prognostic recommendations. This cat was treated with dialysis (**Figure 8.1**) over a 2-week period, hospitalized for 1 additional week to gradually reduce his fluid needs, and recovered uneventfully. He was discharged from hospital with the recommendation that he be fed a high-quality protein ('renal') diet, which he ate well. His water intake was adequate. After 3 months, his BUN and creatinine concentrations stabilized at 40 mg/dl and 2.2 mg/dl, respectively, showing mild continued azotemia.

Recommended reading

Creighton KJ, Koenigshof AM, Weder CD *et al.* (2014) Evaluation of two point-of-care ethylene glycol tests for dogs. *J Vet Emerg Crit Care* 24(4):398–401.

CASE 9: CYCAD PLANT CAUSING ACUTE LIVER FAILURE – JESSICA BULLOCK

Signalment/history

A 2-year-old neutered male Labrador crossbreed dog is examined because of a 2–3-day history of vomiting and inappetence. The vomitus initially contained food and plant material (small amounts of fibrous bark-like material and grass-like material), but progressively became clear to bilious. The dog has a long history of eating foreign objects, trash, and plants. His owners are avid gardeners and their backyard contains oleanders, coontie palms, fruit trees, lilies, azaleas, hibiscus, and lantanas. The vomiting began a few hours after the owners saw him eating bits of plants from a trimmings pile that was only unguarded for a brief period of time. This has happened before, but the dog has always seemed to recover uneventfully in the past. He is current on his vaccines and preventive care.

Clinical examination

The dog is quiet, alert, and responsive. He is approximately 7% dehydrated, has a mildly tense abdomen on palpation, and is slightly icteric. Other physical examination findings are normal.

Differential diagnoses

Although many possibilities exist for causing nausea, few also cause icterus: toxin (cycad, xylitol, aflatoxin, blue-green algae, acetaminophen, others); extrahepatic biliary duct obstruction (pancreatitis, inflammation, neoplasia); infection (leptospirosis, cholangitis, cholangichepatitis, cholecystitis, combination); neoplasia (lymphoma, hepatocellular carcinoma); foreign body/gastrointestinal obstruction.

Which plants are potentially toxic?

The plants listed are known to be potentially toxic to dogs if ingested. Cycad palms are constantly increasing in popularity and use in the USA, and pet owners should be made aware of their potential lethal consequences. All portions of the plant (stem, leaves, flowers, and especially seeds) are highly toxic, even in small quantities.

Diagnostic testing

- CBC: normal
- Chemistry panel: abnormals listed: ALT = 5,210 U/l (RI, 32–83 U/l); ALP = 3,568 U/l (RI, 11–60); total bilirubin = 5.4 mg/dl (RI, 0.3–0.9); BUN = 35 mg/dl (RI, 8–29); creatinine = 2.0 mg/dl (RI, 0.6–2.0).
- Urine SG is >1.050.
- Abdominal radiographs are normal.
- Abdominal ultrasound shows no abnormalities.
- PCR and/or serology testing for leptospirosis are recommended.

Presumed diagnosis: cycad palm ingestion

Ingestion of cycads (sago palms, coontie palms, fern palms, cardboard palms) can cause acute liver failure and death (**Figures 9.1, 9.2**). All parts of the plant are toxic. Prognosis is guarded for short-term recovery, and long-term complications, such as cirrhosis, can occur. The laboratory test results have no influence on prognosis. If recent ingestion has occurred, routine decontamination efforts are recommended (induction of emesis/gastric

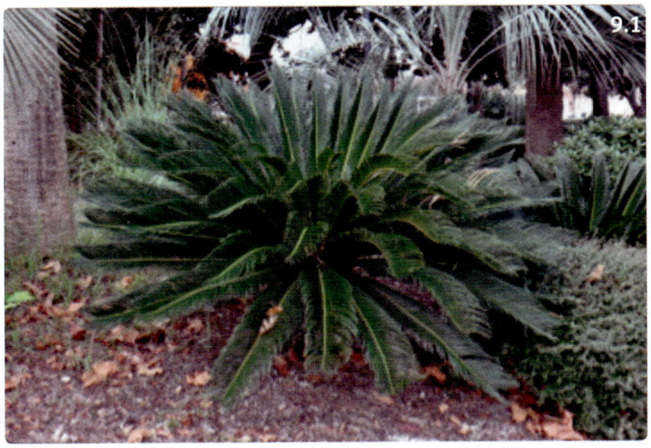

Figure 9.1 A cycad plant.

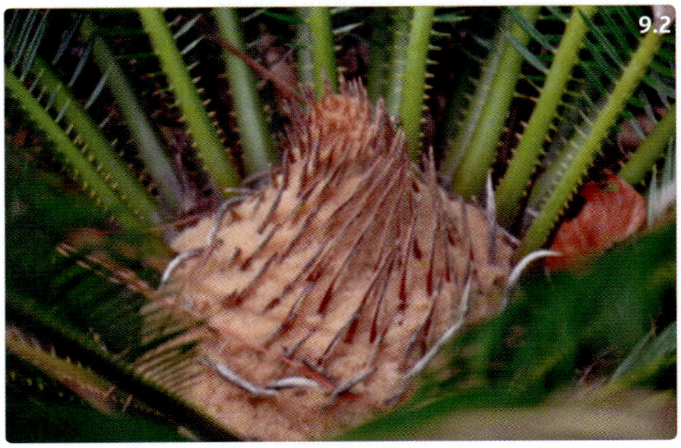

Figure 9.2 Fruit of a cycad plant.

lavage, administration of repeated doses of charcoal due to significant enterohepatic recirculation). Recovery often requires 3–7 days of supportive care, but can exceed 10 days in more severe cases.

Treatment

Initial supportive care

- IV crystalloids at 120 ml/kg/day until rehydrated, then decreased to approximately 60 ml/kg/day.
- Ampicillin/sulbactam (30 mg/kg IV q8h) to treat possible leptospirosis while test results are pending.
- Maropitant (1 mg/kg SC) as an antinausea medication.
- Gastroprotectants: famotidine (1 mg/kg q24h), or pantoprazole (1 mg/kg IV q12h), or omeprazole (1 mg/kg PO q24h).
- Liver supportive care: N-acetylcysteine at 140 mg/kg initially, followed q6h by 7 doses of 70 mg/kg IV or PO, as tolerated; S-adenosylmethionine at 18 mg/kg PO once daily and/or silymarin at 20–50 mg/kg PO once daily for at least 30 days.
- Outcome: the dog responded well to treatment and was discharged without any subsequent complications.

Other recommended procedures

Placement of a nasogastric or nasoesophageal feeding tube is often beneficial in cases of cycad ingestion. While primarily used to deliver nutrition to inappetent patients, it can also provide an easier delivery method for medications and fluids when encouraging home care for longer recoveries.

CASE 10: CONGESTIVE HEART FAILURE – ROMAIN PARIAUT & CARLEY SAELINGER

Signalment/history

A 9-year-old neutered male Cavalier King Charles Spaniel. Previously healthy with exception of intermittent cough; last night developed inappetence, lethargy, and increased respiratory rate, which has worsened overnight.

Clinical examination

The dog is dyspneic and tachypneic with a respiratory rate of 52 breaths per minute. He is also tachycardic (160 bpm). A grade 4/6 left apical systolic murmur is auscultated. Lung auscultation reveals fine crackles throughout the left hemithorax. Lung sounds are diffusely harsh. The dog is mildly hyperthermic (102.7°F [39.3°C]).

Differential diagnosis

Left-sided congestive heart failure; degenerative valve disease; infectious endocarditis; congenital defect; pneumonia; pulmonary thromboembolism; pulmonary hypertension.

Diagnostic tests

Thoracic radiographs show generalized cardiomegaly with moderate to severe left atrial enlargement, distended pulmonary vasculature, and an interstitial-to-alveolar pattern in the perihilar region and right middle and caudal lung lobes (**Figure 10.1**). A serum biochemistry profile and complete blood count are within normal limits.

Diagnosis

Left-sided congestive heart failure.

Initial treatment

The dog is placed in oxygen and a CRI of furosemide is started at 0.5 mg/kg/hour after an initial bolus at 4 mg/kg IV. Pimobendan is administered at 0.25 mg/kg PO, and scheduled to be given every 12 hours. The dog's respiratory rate decreases to 36 breaths per minute and the heart rate decreases to 100 bpm over the next 6 hours.

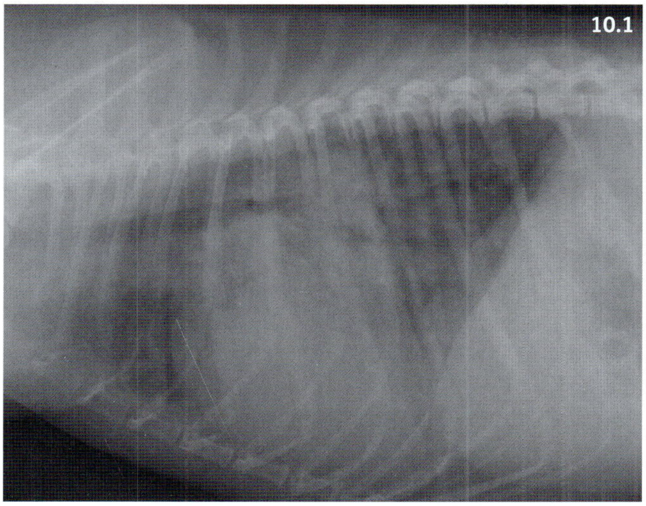

Figure 10.1 Left heart enlargement and pulmonary edema.

An echocardiogram shows a thickened mitral valve with secondary severe mitral valve regurgitation and moderate to severe left atrial enlargement. The underlying cause of the left-sided congestive heart failure is degenerative mitral valve disease. Thoracic radiographs are repeated 24 hours after initial hospitalization and show cardiomegaly with normal pulmonary parenchyma and pulmonary vasculature. The animal is therefore ready to be released from the hospital.

Long-term treatment

Furosemide (2 mg/kg PO q12h), pimobendan (0.25 mg/kg PO q12h), enalapril (0.5 mg/kg PO q12h). Renal values should be rechecked 1–2 weeks after initiation of therapy. A mild azotemia should be tolerated as long as the patient is not showing any clinical signs (nausea, vomiting, inappetence, lethargy). The owner should be instructed to carefully monitor the resting respiratory rate at home. It should be <40 breaths per minute. If it increases more than 25% over 3 days or if it is >40 breaths per minute, the owner should be instructed to seek veterinary care. Long-term monitoring should include renal values every 3–6 months and annual thoracic radiographs and echocardiogram to assess for disease progression.

CASE 11: ARRHYTHMOGENIC CARDIOMYOPATHY – ROMAIN PARIAUT & CARLEY SAELINGER

Signalment/history

A 6-year-old neutered male Boxer was presented for evaluation of syncope noted during exercise.

Clinical examination

The dog is bright, alert, and responsive. Intermittent paroxysms of tachycardia up to 270 bpm and a grade 2/6 left apical systolic heart murmur are noted on thoracic auscultation. Pulses are fair with intermittent deficits. Physical examination is otherwise unremarkable.

Differential diagnosis

Tachycardia: ventricular tachycardia; supraventricular tachycardia; sinus tachycardia. Murmur: mitral valve insufficiency secondary to arrhythmogenic cardiomyopathy; mitral valve insufficiency secondary to degenerative valve disease; mitral valve insufficiency secondary to endocarditis. Syncope: tachyarrhythmia secondary to arrhythmogenic cardiomyopathy; poor cardiac output due to systolic dysfunction when exercising secondary to arrhythmogenic cardiomyopathy or aortic stenosis; pulmonary hypertension; pericardial effusion.

Provisional diagnosis

The provisional diagnosis is arrhythmogenic cardiomyopathy given the breed (Boxer), tachyarrhythmia, murmur, and historical syncope.

Diagnostic tests

Electrocardiogram reveals paroxysms of sustained and nonsustained ventricular tachycardia (**Figure 11.1**). Lidocaine IV bolus administered during sustained ventricular tachycardia converts to normal sinus rhythm.

An echocardiogram reveals moderate left ventricular dilation in diastole and systole. The mitral leaflets are not thickened. Left ventricular enlargement and mitral annulus dilation result in displacement of the leaflets and incomplete closure, and secondary regurgitation. Mild right atrial and right ventricular dilation is present.

11.1

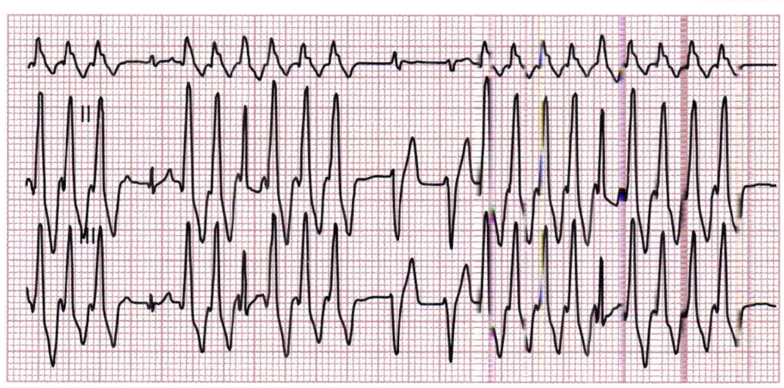

Figure 11.1 Ventricular tachycardia of right ventricular origin.

Thoracic radiographs show moderate to severe generalized cardiomegaly with normal pulmonary parenchyma and vasculature.

Conclusion

After administration of an IV bolus of lidocaine, a CRI was started. Oral sotalol (2 mg/kg q12h) was also administered for long-term management of ventricular arrhythmias. Congestive heart failure was not present, so other cardiac medications were not prescribed at this time. This patient is at risk for sudden death and congestive heart failure.

CASE 12: ARTERIAL THROMBOEMBOLISM – ROMAIN PARIAUT & CARLEY SAELINGER

Signalment/history

An 8-year-old neutered male Domestic Shorthair cat presented for acute onset paraplegia. He was found next to the bed vocalizing, nonambulatory, and open-mouth breathing. He was previously healthy.

Clinical examination

On presentation, the patient was agitated, vocalizing, and open-mouth breathing. T = 98.3°F (36.8°C), heart rate = 190 bpm, respiratory rate = 80 breaths per minute, mucous membranes were pink and moist with a normal CRT. A fixed gallop was present with no murmur or arrhythmia. Bronchovesicular sounds were increased but otherwise normal. Motor activity, spinal reflexes, and deep pain were negative in the hindlimbs and femoral pulses were absent. The distal hindlimbs were cool with cyanotic nail beds when compared with the forelimbs.

Differential diagnosis

Arterial thromboembolism (ATE) is the most common cause (approximately 80–90%) of acute limb paresis/paralysis in feline patients. Other differentials that should be considered: primary neurologic disease (spinal trauma, intervertebral disk disease, fibrocartilagenous emboli [reported in dogs], neoplasia), neoplasia (neoplastic emboli or paraneoplastic thrombocytosis/hypercoagulability), aortic/arterial foreign body (rare).

Diagnostic tests

The diagnosis of ATE is primarily clinical. 'Quicking' a toenail to assess bleeding (typically no or only a minimal amount of dark colored blood), assessing blood flow with Doppler ultrasound, and obtaining a differential glucose or lactate between an affected and an unaffected limb support the diagnosis. Angiography provides a definitive diagnosis but is not commonly performed clinically. Ultrasound at the level of the distal aortic bifurcation may identify a thrombus or reduced blood flow but is highly user dependent. Thoracic radiographs reveal cardiomegaly in 90% of cases and congestive heart failure (CHF) in approximately 50% of cases. Therefore, chest radiographs should always be obtained to determine if the signs of tachpnea or dyspnea result from pain only or from pulmonary edema. Serum biochemistry may show elevated ALT, AST, and CPK due to ischemic muscle damage/necrosis and azotemia associated with poor perfusion or thromboembolism proximal to the renal arteries. An echocardiogram will determine the presence and type of cardiac disease. Additional findings may include an enlarged left atrium, decreased systolic function, spontaneous echo contrast ('smoke'), or a thrombus within the left atrium (**Figure 12.1**). An ECG is appropriate if an arrhythmia is present.

Treatment, prognosis, complications

Treatment is primarily palliative and supportive care. No specific treatment has shown improved outcome over cage rest alone. Opioids are the analgesic of choice and pain management is the most important aspect of acute treatment. Appropriate treatment of acute CHF is indicated if present. Cautious fluid therapy may be indicated in patients with poor perfusion that are not eating or drinking provided active CHF is not present. Medications to reduce clot extension and for long-term thromboprophylaxis may be used including heparin, low molecular weight heparin, aspirin, and clopidogrel. Thrombolytics have been shown to reduce time to spontaneous perfusion

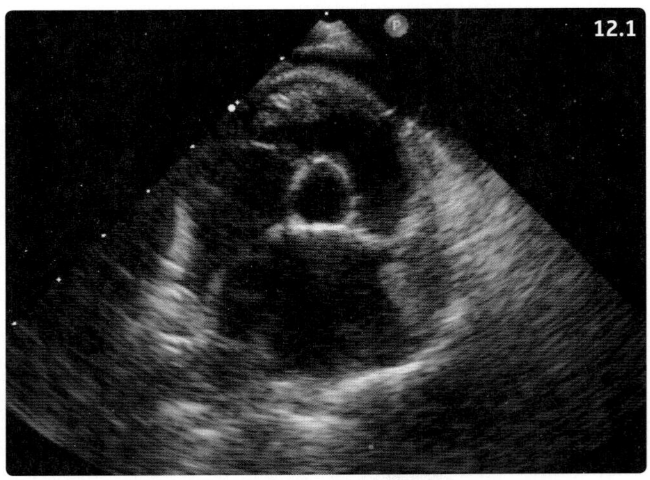

Figure 12.1 Echocardiogram showing left atrial enlargement and a possible thrombus.

and functional use of limbs; however, they increase risk of complications and have not proven effective in improving outcome or survival. Standard wound and nursing care of nonambulatory patients is important. Approximately 33–40% of patients survive the acute period with long-term survival ranging from 3 months to 6 years (median of 6 months). Complications include re-thrombosis, reperfusion syndrome, ischemic necrosis, muscle contracture, and permanent loss of function.

CASE 13: WEAKNESS IN A CAT – AMANDINE LEJEUNE & MICHAEL SCHAER

Signalment/history

A 13-year-old neutered male Domestic Shorthair cat weighing 8 kg was taken to an emergency veterinary hospital when the owners noticed him unable to greet them when they came home from work that evening.

Clinical and laboratory examinations

Pertinent clinical findings included generalized muscular weakness. The cat's blood pressure ranged from 220 to 260 mmHg. Abnormal serum chemistry findings included sodium 159 mEq/l (RI, 146–160) and serum potassium 2.1 mEq/l (RI, 3.6–5.4). The urine SG was 1.009 with other parameters being normal. He was referred for further evaluation for possible aldosteronoma.

At the time of referral, the abnormal physical examination findings included mental dullness while able to relate to his environment, generalized muscle weakness, and flaccid ventral cervical flexion (**Figure 13.1**). There was a small retinal hemorrhage in his right eye. The rest of the physical examination was unremarkable.

Differential diagnosis

With major complaints of progressive muscular weakness, hypertension, and right retinal hemorrhage, the following differentials should be considered: primary myopathy; metabolic abnormality(ies) such as renal and electrolyte disorders including hypokalemia and hypernatremia); endocrine abnormalities such as hyperaldosteronism and pheochromocytoma.

Diagnostic evaluation

The serum electrolyte abnormalities were persistent. Because of the clinical findings being compatible with hyperaldosteronism, a serum sample for aldosterone determination was submitted to an outside laboratory and the aldosterone concentration was 3,032 pmol/l (RI, 194–388). Chest radiography was normal. An echocardiogram was done in order to search for any cardiac abnormality because of the sustained hypertension; this showed left ventricular concentric hypertrophy and papillary muscle hypertrophy. An abdominal ultrasound evaluation showed left adrenal gland enlargement (**Figure 13.2**). The right adrenal gland was visible. CT (axial) showed a normal thorax and an enlarged left-sided adrenal gland with no evidence of nearby tissue invasion or metastasis.

Medical and surgical treatment

Preoperative treatment consisted of IV fluids with potassium chloride supplementation (60 mEq/l), spironolactone (1 mg/kg PO q12h), and amlodipine (1.25 mg PO q24h). The cat's muscular strength and the serum potassium concentration gradually improved over the next 8 days. Surgery was performed and a solitary enlarged left adrenal gland was removed without complication. The cat required 6

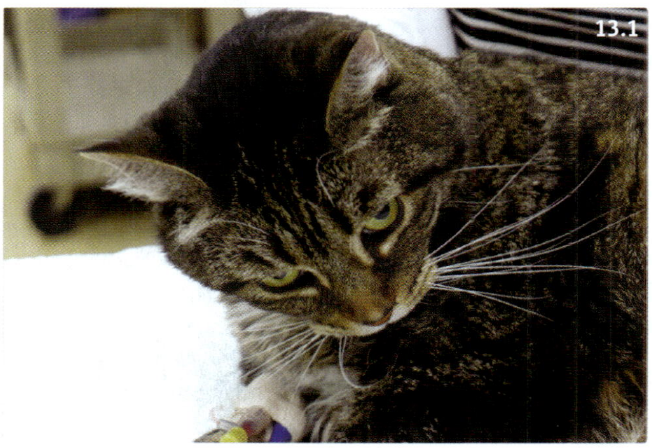

Figure 13.1 The cat is showing ventral cervical flexion typical of hypokalemic myopathy.

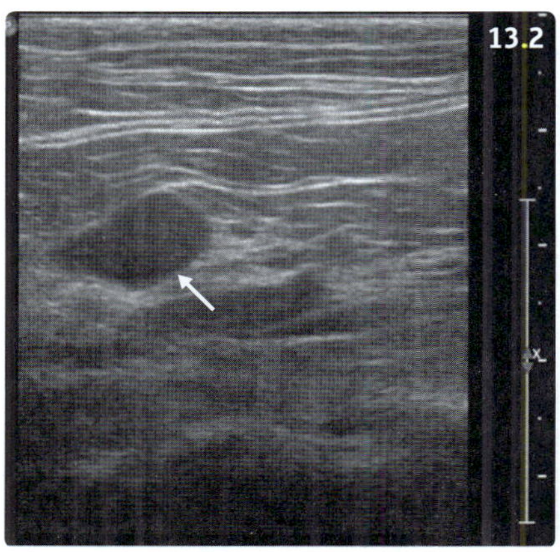

Figure 13.2 Abdominal ultrasound examination showing left adrenal gland enlargement (arrow).

days of continued medical support with oral potassium gluconate. The histopathology results showed adrenocortical adenoma and the cat went on to recover well.

Comments

Hyperaldosteronism in the cat is not a rare condition. It can be caused by adrenocortical hyperplasia affecting the zone glomerulosa or by an adrenocortical tumor that can be either an adenoma or an adenocarcinoma. The tumor can be endocrinologically functional and produce excessive amounts of either aldosterone and/or cortisol. If the tumor is secreting excessive cortisol, it is possible for the contralateral adrenal gland to become inactive because of negative feedback inhibition. The patient with adrenocortical hyperplasia is treated medically with aldosterone antagonist and hypotensive drugs, while the adrenal tumor is preferably treated surgically, if possible. Prognosis varies from good to grave depending on the etiology. The cat in this report had a benign tumor that was successfully treated with combined medical and surgical options as described.

CASE 14: MUSCLE ATROPHY IN A DOG – SHEILA JUSTIZ-CARRERA

Signalment/history

A 10-year-old neutered male Labrador Retriever weighing 36 kg was seen by its veterinarian for the primary complaints of head muscle atrophy and difficulty with eating. At that time, atrophy of the left side of the head was noted and the dog was referred to a neurologist.

Clinical examination

At the time of referral, there was marked atrophy of the left temporalis and masseter muscles (**Figure 14.1**). There was enophthalmia of the left eye and elevation of the third eyelid. There was absent corneal sensation in the left eye. The menace response was normal bilaterally, but the palpebral reflex was absent in the left eye, although the patient would blink on his own. The remaining physical examination parameters were normal.

Abnormalities

Left masticatory muscle atrophy: cranial nerve (CN) V (mandibular nerve). Absent corneal sensation left eye: CN V (ophthalmic nerve). Absent left facial sensation with intact motor: CN V (maxillary nerve). Left enophthalmia, likely secondary to atrophy of pterygoid muscles: CN V (mandibular nerve). Left elevation of the third eyelid, likely secondary to enophthalmia.

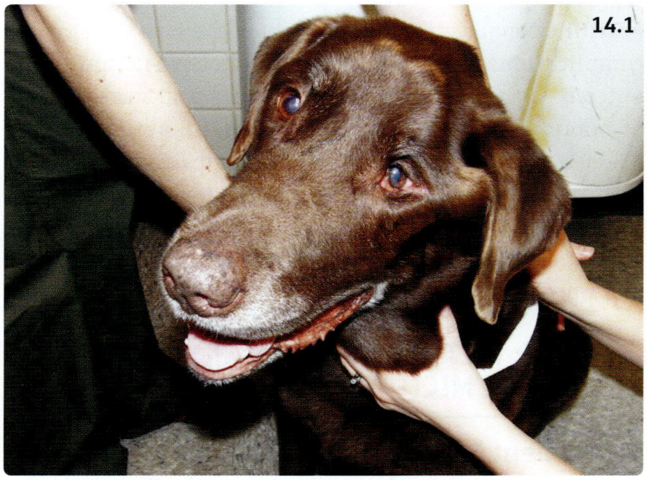

Figure 14.1 Labrador Retriever showing left-sided temporal and masseter muscle atrophy and enophthalmos compatible with left-sided trigeminal nerve pathology.

Neurolocalization

Left trigeminal nerve lesion.

Differential diagnosis

Trigeminal nerve neoplasia: peripheral nerve sheath tumor vs. lymphoma; trigeminal neuritis: inflammatory vs. infectious (*Neospora canis*).

Diagnostic evaluation

CBC and serum chemistry panel were unremarkable. Thoracic radiographs were unremarkable. MRI of the brain showed a markedly enlarged and abnormal left trigeminal nerve that was compressing the left brainstem. The mass could be tracked out of the skull. There was marked atrophy of all the left masticatory muscles. These changes are consistent with a trigeminal nerve tumor. Differential diagnoses include a malignant peripheral nerve sheath tumor, lymphoma or, less likely, a meningioma. Cerebrospinal fluid analysis was unremarkable, making lymphoma a less likely diagnosis, although it is still possible.

Medical and surgical treatment

Treatment options to consider include medical palliative therapy and radiation therapy. Surgical resection of these lesions is not often recommended, as often it is not possible to resect most of the lesion. Palliative therapy for this patient included anti-inflammatory doses of prednisone (0.5 mg/kg/day) and ophthalmic lubricant ointment (left eye, at least q8h). Radiation therapy was recommended, but declined by the owners.

Comments

Nerve sheath tumors can affect any peripheral nerve, but the trigeminal nerve is the most commonly affected cranial nerve. Any of the three branches can be affected and clinical signs will vary accordingly, although most dogs show severe masticatory muscle atrophy corresponding to mandibular branch disease. Long-term prognosis is grave with survival after diagnosis ranging from 5 to 21 months with a median of 12 months.

CASE 15: A VERY SWEET DOG! – LEO LONDOÑO

Signalment/history

An 11-year-old spayed female mixed breed dog is examined for evaluation of a 3-day history of generalized weakness, anorexia, and dark-tarry diarrhea. The dog had originally presented to the primary veterinarian 2 weeks ago for evaluation of lethargy, polydipsia, and polyuria. The dog was started on amoxicillin (250 mg PO q12h). A urine sample was sent to the laboratory and the results showed a large amount of glucose (1,000 mg/dl) and ketonuria (2+), with inactive sediment and a urine SG of 1.031. Based on these results, the primary veterinarian recommended further diagnostics and treatments for suspected diabetic ketoacidosis, but the owner declined at that point. The dog's condition continued to deteriorate despite antibiotic therapy, and she was brought to the emergency service for further evaluation. The dog was previously diagnosed with sudden acquired retinal degeneration syndrome 2 years ago and became blind. She was also diagnosed with hyperadrenocorticism around the same time, based on an ACTH stimulation test, but no treatment was started due to lack of major clinical signs. Otherwise the dog is current on vaccines and receives monthly flea and heartworm prevention (spinosad + milbemycin oxime) as well as daily glucosamine/chondroitin supplementation.

Clinical examination

The dog is initially quiet, alert, and responsive. Body weight is 5.89 kg, BCS is 6/9, and temperature is 101.3°F (38.5°C). She is bilaterally blind with absent pupillary light reflexes, dazzle, and menace responses in both eyes. The dog is ambulatory with mild generalized weakness and muscle tremors. Heart rate is 124 bpm with a grade 2/6 left systolic, apical heart murmur; synchronous and bounding femoral pulses are also detected. Respiratory rate is 18 breaths per minute and the lung sounds are clear. Mucous membranes are pale pink and tacky with a CRT of 2 seconds. The dog has sunken eyes and there is prolonged skin tenting, giving an estimated 10% dehydration. The abdomen is pendulous and nonpainful, and hepatosplenomegaly is detected with abdominal palpation. Rectal examination yields soft feces with melena. Peripheral lymph nodes are soft, small and symmetrical.

Initial diagnostics (abnormalities listed only)

Biochemistry

ALP = 508 U/L (RI, 8–114); albumin = 1.5 g/dl (RI, 2.9–3.8); calcium = 7.2 mg/dl (RI, 8.9–10.8); phosphorus = 8.0 mg/dl (RI, 2.7–5.6); creatinine = 4.7 mg/dl (RI, 0.6–1.7); BUN = 94 mg/dl (RI, 8–25); glucose = 1,196 mg/dl (RI, 79–120); sodium = 125 mEq/l (RI, 142–153); potassium = 6.7 mEq/l (RI, 3.5–5.2); chloride = 90 mEq/l (RI, 107–115); anion gap = 35.7 mEq/l (RI, 14–24).

Hematology

WBCs = 32,050/µl (RI, 5,000–13,000); neutrophils = 26,080/µl (RI, 2,700–8,900); bands = 2,900/µl; toxicity, 2+; monocytes = 3,410/µl (RI, 100–800); RBCs = 3.68 × 10^6/µl (RI, 5.7–8.3); hemoglobin = 7.6 g/dl (RI, 14–20); PCV = 21% (RI, 40–56); MCV = 60.3 fl [RI, 64–74]; MCHC = 34.1 g/dl (RI, 33–38); platelets = 9.2 × 10^5/µl (RI, 1.3–3.9).

Urinalysis

SG = 1.018; glucose = 2,000 mg/dl; ketones = 40–80 mg/dl; blood, trace; pH = 5.5; dipstick: protein, 2+; SSA protein, 1+; WBCs, 4–8/HPF; RBCs, 0–3/HPF; bacteria (many monomorphobacilli); crystals, occasional amorphous. Sediment evaluation also revealed budding yeast and pseudohyphae.

Venous blood

pH = 7.12 (RI, 7.335–7.446); pCO_2 = 25.5 mmHg (RI, 35–40); HCO_3 = 8.4 mEq/l (RI, 18–27).

Problem list

Severe hyperglycemia; moderate azotemia; moderate hyponatremia; mild hyperkalemia; severe hypoalbuminemia; severe metabolic acidosis; severely elevated anion gap; moderate leukocytosis with left shift and toxicity; severe microcytic, normochromic anemia; severe thrombocytosis; glucosuria, ketonuria, pyuria, bacteriuria and yeast infection; severe dehydration; heart murmur; melena; hepatosplenomegaly.

Case discussion

This dog has been diagnosed with diabetic ketoacidosis. The hyperglycemia in this case is severe and raises the concern for hyperglycemic hyperosmolar syndrome

(HHS). The diagnostic criteria in veterinary medicine for HHS include a serum glucose concentration >600 mg/dl (30 mmol/l), absence of urine ketones, and osmolality >350 mOsm/kg. The human guidelines for HHS are more extensive, but the presence of small quantities of urine ketones does not exclude HHS. Osmolality can be measured by freezing-point depression or calculated with the formula (using conventional values):

$Osm_{(serum)}$: $2(Na^+) + (BUN/2.8) + (GLU/18) \rightarrow 2(125) + (94/2.8) + (1196/18)$: *350 mOsm/kg*

Due to the equilibration of BUN across cell membranes, using the effective osmolality formula may provide a better estimate of osmolality:

Effective $Osm_{(serum)}$: $2(Na^+) + (GLU/18) \rightarrow 2(125) + (94/2.8)$: *316 mOsm/kg*

Based on the estimated effective osmolality and presence of ketones in the urine, this patient is not considered to have pure HHS, although the dog can have a combined hyperosmolar ketoacidosis disorder. The blood work results also had moderate azotemia (with relatively dilute urine in light of the degree of dehydration) as well as moderate hyperkalemia and hyperphosphatemia. These results are consistent with acute kidney injury (AKI) and reduced glomerular filtration rate, which may worsen the hyperglycemia and lead to HHS syndrome in the future. Other possible causes of AKI in this patient are: pyelonephritis secondary to ascending bacterial and fungal urinary tract infections; thromboembolism secondary to thrombocytosis and previously diagnosed Cushing's syndrome; and hypotension due to marked dehydration and potential hypovolemia. The severity of the metabolic acidosis and increased anion gap are consistent with accumulation of lactic acid, secondary to poor tissue perfusion, uremic acids, and ketoacids. The expected compensation for the metabolic acidosis can be calculated by using:

0.7 mmHg decrease in pCO_2 per 1 mEq/l decrease in $[HCO_3^-]$ +/- 3:

0.7 mmHg × (22 mEq/l – 8.4 mEq/l) : *9.5*

In this case the primary respiratory compensation is appropriate, as the pCO_2 in this dog is approximately 10 mmHg lower than the low end of the reference interval. Other electrolyte abnormalities included moderate to severe hyponatremia and hypochloremia. The low sodium in this dog is consistent with spurious hyponatremia secondary to the osmotic pull of water into the vasculature by the high levels of glucose. Corrected sodium can be calculated as follows:

$Na^+_{(corr)}$: $Na^+_{(measured)}$ + 1.6 ([measured glucose - normal glucose]/100)

$Na^+_{(corr)}$: 125 + 1.6 ([1196 - 100]/100) : *142.5 mEq/l*

The hyperkalemia is explained by the renal impairment interfering with excretion and the effects of hyperosmolality on the serum potassium concentration where cellular potassium is drawn into the plasma space.

The dog had a leukocytosis characterized by a neutrophilia with a left shift and toxicity, likely secondary to the bacterial and fungal infections of its urinary system, in addition to diabetic ketoacidosis, which can impair leukocyte destruction of infectious organisms. The nonregenerative anemia based on red blood cell indices (microcytic, normochromic) is likely secondary to chronic inflammation, but at this point chronic kidney disease and/or bleeding from the GI tract (melena) with no time for regeneration have to be considered. The newly identified heart murmur in this dog can be physiologic secondary to anemia and dehydration, but a primary cardiomyopathy and vegetative endocarditis cannot be ruled out. The low albumin levels in this patient can be attributed to several factors including loss from GI bleeding, renal loss, decreased production (negative phase protein), decreased intake from anorexia, and/or translocation from endothelial dysfunction.

Conclusion

Diabetic ketoacidosis can lead to severe systemic illness leading to a myriad of electrolyte, acid–base, and hematologic disorders. A thorough analysis of serum biochemistry results and ample knowledge of pathophysiology will prevent the clinician from misdiagnosing patients with hyperosmolar syndromes, as well as misinterpreting various forms of hyponatremia.

CASE 16: SEVERE NECROTIZING PANCREATITIS – LEO LONDOÑO

Signalment/history

A 7-year-old spayed female mixed breed dog is referred for evaluation of vomiting and anorexia over the past few days. Four days prior, the dog vomited after being fed dinner and continued to vomit a mixture of food and bile throughout the night. The next day she stopped eating and was hiding in a corner, appearing painful. She was taken to her veterinarian where blood work and abdominal radiographs were done. The blood test results showed an elevated BUN, decreased protein and albumin, and increased amylase. Radiographs were interpreted as normal. She was hospitalized with supportive treatment including IV fluid therapy, penicillin, dexamethasone, and butorphanol/tramadol for pain management. Blood tests were repeated 2 days later and showed a further increase in BUN and decreased albumin, along with severe leukocytosis characterized by a mature neutrophilia. On the day of referral, the dog remained anorectic and began to regurgitate. She also developed black-tarry feces and her mentation deteriorated.

Clinical examination

The dog is alert, responsive, and ambulatory. She is febrile with a body temperature of 103.6°F (39.8°C), body weight is 13.2 kg, and BCS is 6/9. The dog has tachycardia with a heart rate of 180 bpm with bounding and synchronous femoral pulses. Thoracic auscultation is normal and the dog is eupneic. Abdominal palpation showed that she had a mildly tense abdomen with nonlocalizing discomfort. Rectal examination produced melena. Mild to moderate pitting edema was identified over the hocks and inguinal region. The rest of the physical examination was normal.

Diagnostics

Radiography

Diffuse absence of peritoneal detail with a nodular appearance (**Figures 16.1a–c**). Diagnostic interpretation was consistent with suspected carcinomatosis with peritoneal effusion. Normal thorax.

Abdominal ultrasound

Moderate amount of anechoic free fluid; hyperechoic mesentery with multiple hypoechoic nodules throughout (**Figure 16.2a**); pancreas is enlarged and hypoechoic (**Figure 16.2b**); duodenum is corrugated. Diagnostic interpretation was consistent with possible carcinomatosis with peritoneal effusion and steatitis, pancreatitis, or pancreatic neoplasia such as adenocarcinoma, as well as duodenitis.

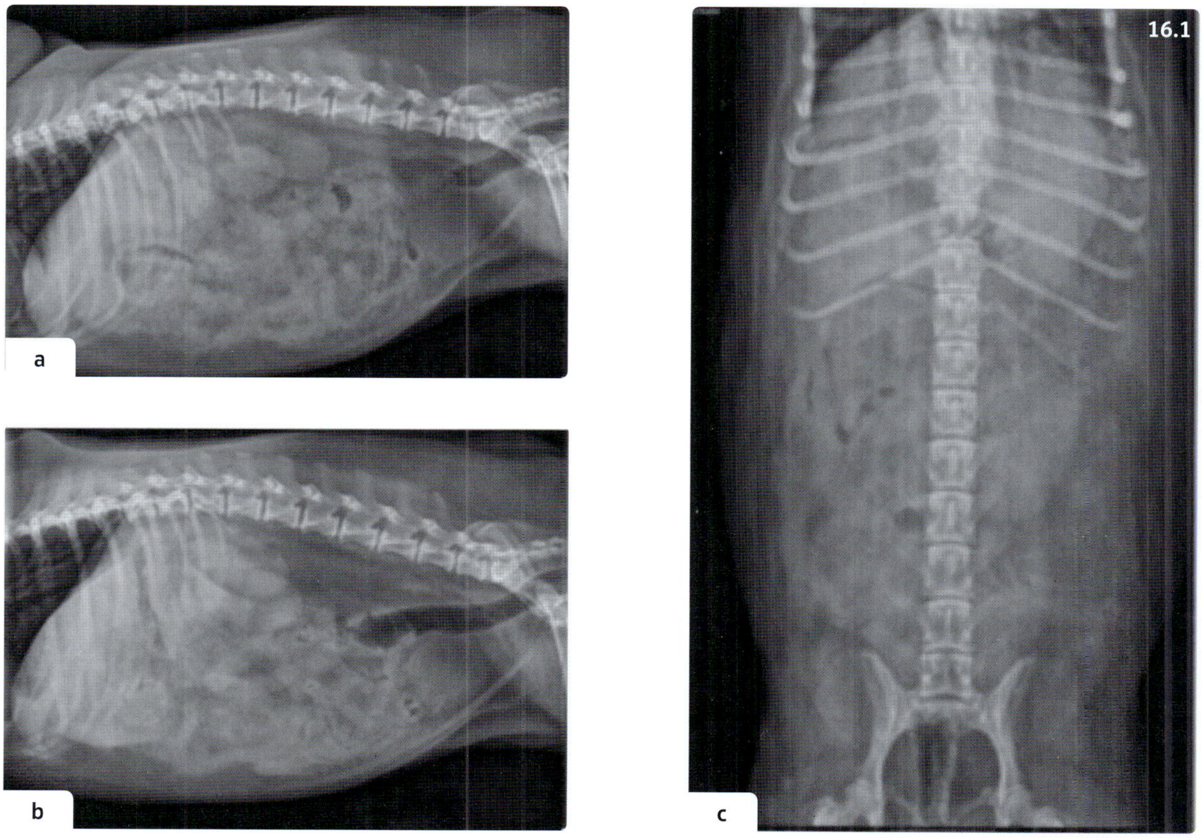

Figures 16.1a–c Abdominal radiographs showing diffuse loss of detail due to abdominal effusion.

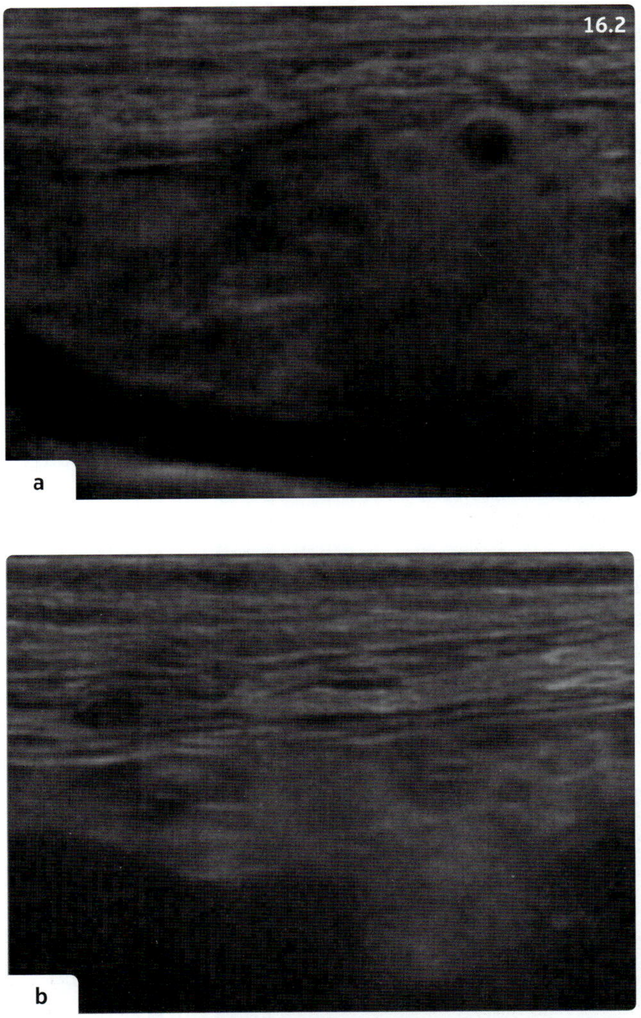

Figures 16.2a, b (a) Ultrasonogram showing abnormal pancreas. (b) Ultrasonogram showing abnormal mesentery.

Abdominal effusion cytology and biochemical analysis

Exudate; degenerative neutrophils without presence of intracellular bacteria; rare extracellular bacilli present. Glucose = 44 mg/dl (RI, 79–120); lactate = 2.1 mmol/l (RI, <2.5).

Pancreas cytology

Suppurative inflammation and evidence of mineralization. Mildly atypical pancreatic epithelium is suggestive of reactive pancreatic epithelium. The degree of inflammation and the mild atypia of pancreatic epithelial cells are most consistent with pancreatitis. However, the less likely consideration of an inflamed pancreatic carcinoma cannot definitely be excluded on the basis of this aspirate.

Biochemistry

ALP = 379 U/L (RI, 8–114); ALT = 113 U/L (RI, 18–64); AST = 244 U/L (RI, 15–52); total bilirubin = 0.9 mg/dl (RI, 0.1–0.4); total protein = 2.9 g/dl (RI, 5.6–7.5); albumin = 0.9 g/dl (RI, 2.9–3.8); calcium = 7.3 mg/dl (RI, 8.9–10.8); phosphorus = 8.1 mg/dl (RI, 2.7–5.6); creatinine = 3.5 mg/dl (RI, 0.6–1.7); BUN = 77 mg/dl (RI, 8–25); glucose = 52 mg/dl (RI, 79–120); sodium = 163 mEq/l (RI, 142–153); potassium = 4.7 mEq/l (RI, 3.5–5.2); chloride = 126 mEq/l (RI, 107–115); lactate = 0.9 mmol/l (RI, <2.5).

Clinical recommendations

The patient was treated with Plasma-lyte 56 and 5% dextrose solution IV, human albumin 25% (100 ml IV/2 hours), ampicillin–sulfabactam (50 mg/kg IV q8h), enrofloxacin (15 mg/kg IV q24h), maropitant (10 mg/kg q24h), and methadone (0.2 mg/kg IV q6h). Due to the dog's deteriorating condition, presence of an abdominal exudative effusion with evidence of extracellular bacilli, along with glucose and lactate differentials of the effusion vs. peripheral blood, the dog was sent to surgery for an abdominal exploratory because of a suspect septic abdomen. Surgery showed multifocal plaque-like nodules diffusely distributed through the greater omentum, body wall, and mesenteric fat, and scattered plaques on the diaphragm and visceral surfaces of the spleen, liver, and pancreas. The pancreas was surrounded by moderately thickened fat and had a small area of mild thickening on the right lobe. During the dog's recovery from surgery, she became more painful and her fever increased to 104°F (40°C). The dog was started on a fentanyl IV CRI (5 μg/kg/hour), lidocaine IV CRI (25 μg/kg/minute), and ketamine IV CRI (10 μg/kg/minute). The dog was monitored overnight and the next day she developed cardiopulmonary arrest. Closed-chest cerebrocardiopulmonary resuscitation was instituted but discontinued at the owners' request. The dog's body was submitted to necropsy (**Figures 16.3a, b**).

Necropsy report

- Pancreatitis: necrotizing, diffuse, marked, subacute to chronic, with saponification of fat and necrotizing steatitis.
- Hepatitis: lymphoplasmacytic and neutrophilic, chronic.
- Fibrous adhesions: multifocal, moderate, subacute to chronic, omentum and spleen.
- Peritonitis: fibrinous, locally extensive, mild to moderate.

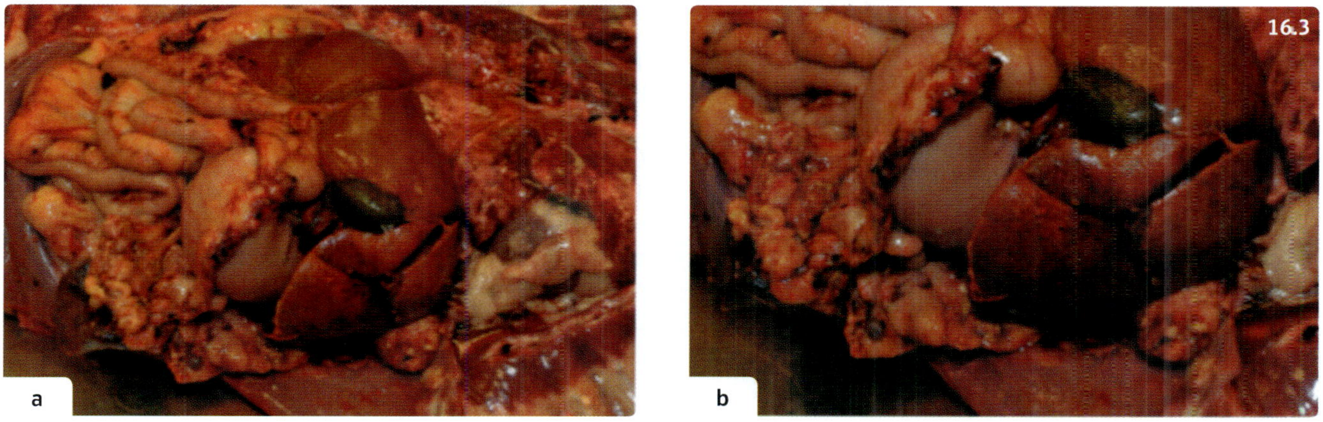

Figures 16.3a, b Necropsy findings.

- Peritoneal and pleural effusion: hemorrhagic, mild (thorax) to moderate (abdomen), with lipid droplets.
- Petechial hemorrhages: multifocal to coalescing, mild, acute, ventral abdominal skin.

Conclusion

Necrotizing pancreatitis is an acute and devastating syndrome that may progress to systemic inflammatory response syndrome, DIC, and sepsis, as suspected in this case. Mortality rates in humans can reach up to 30% in cases complicated by multiple organ dysfunction. Surgical intervention is indicated for those cases in which infected necrosis or abscess is documented. Despite surgical intervention, these patients carry a poor prognosis.

CASE 17: SYSTEMIC HISTOPLASMOSIS – KATIE M. BOES & ROSE E. RASKIN

Signalment/history

A 2-year-old indoor/outdoor spayed female Domestic Shorthair cat is presented for a 3-week history of weight loss and lethargy.

Clinical examination

The cat is quiet, alert, responsive, and mentally dull with normal vital signs. There are general signs of ill thrift, including dull hair coat, poor BCS (2/9), and mild muscle atrophy of the hindlimbs. Mucous membranes are pale and the cat is estimated to be 8% dehydrated. A grade 2/6 systolic heart murmur is auscultated.

Provisional hematologic abnormalities

Pale mucous membranes suggest anemia. Since icterus is not observed, hemolytic anemia is less likely. There is no evidence of external hemorrhage (e.g. trauma, external parasitism), internal hemorrhage (e.g. distended abdomen), or GI hemorrhage (e.g. perineal blood). Therefore, likely causes for the anemia are decreased RBC production and occult GI hemorrhage. The murmur is secondary to the anemia.

Differential diagnosis

Causes of chronic disease, ill thrift, and anemia in a young cat include: viral (FeLV, FIV, feline panleukopenia virus) infection; intestinal parasites; systemic fungal infection; lymphoma; mycoplasmosis; chronic or congenital kidney disease.

Laboratory tests

A FeLV/FIV SNAP test was negative. A serum chemistry panel was consistent with stress (glucose = 184 mg/dl: RI, 71–165), inflammation (albumin = 2.8 g/dl [RI, 3.0–4.0]; globulins = 5.4 g/dl [RI, 3.0–5.2]), and minimal cholestasis (GGT = 2 U/L [RI, 0–1]; total bilirubin = 1.3 mg/dl [RI, 0.0–0.4]). A CBC (**Table 17.1**) and blood smear review (**Figure 17.1**) were also performed.

Blood smear review: few schistocytes and acanthocytes; nRBCs are metarubricytes; many neutrophils with Döhle bodies and foamy cytoplasm; rare small ovoid yeast forms within monocytes.

Interpretation

The moderate to marked normocytic hypochromic anemia is primarily due to decreased production since it is nonregenerative, there is other evidence of hematopoietic hypoplasia (thrombocytopenia), and bone marrow injury is suspected (inappropriate metarubricytosis). Anemia of chronic disease may be contributing to the anemia, but is not expected to cause this severity of anemia by itself. The schistocytes, acanthocytes, and thrombocytopenia raise concern for concurrent

Table 17.1 Hemogram results.

Test	Result	Reference interval (from author's lab)
RBC	3.70×10^6/µl	7.28–11.36
Hemoglobin	5.3 g/dl	12.1– 6.7
Hematocrit	17.1%	33.7–47.5
MCV	46.2 fl	38.4–49.2
MCHC	31.0 g/dl	34.1–37.0
Reticulocytes	15,400/µl	13,050–71,570
nRBCs	6/100 WBCs	0–1
WBCs	5,302/µl	4,250–11,360
Segmented neutrophils	3,287/µl	2,272–9,639
Band neutrophils	212/µl	0–0
Lymphocytes	1,750/µl	804–9,240
Monocytes	53/µl	0–952
Platelets	97,000/µl	148,700–531,600

17.1

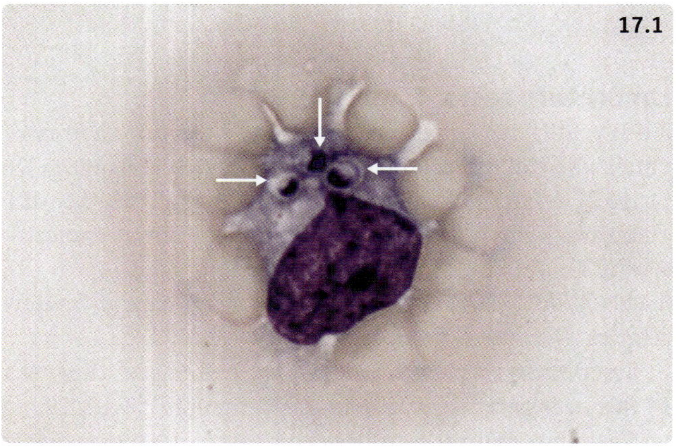

Figure 17.1 Three small, ovoid yeasts (arrows) in the cytoplasm of a monocyte.

microangiopathic hemolysis and platelet consumption secondary to DIC. There is no evidence of blood loss anemia, such as increased BUN relative to creatinine or panhypoproteinemia. The left shift and toxic neutrophils (Döhle bodies and foamy cytoplasm) denote inflammation. The cause for the hematologic changes is present on the blood smear as intracytoplasmic yeast consistent with *Histoplasma capsulatum*.

Clinical diagnosis

The diagnosis is systemic histoplasmosis with probable bone marrow infection and DIC.

Case outcome

The cat was given a guarded prognosis for recovery, and the owners elected to euthanize the cat. A necropsy was not performed, but the owners authorized aspiration of the bone marrow after euthanasia. Cytologic evaluation of the bone marrow confirmed granulomatous fungal myelitis resulting in erythroid hypoplasia, myeloid hyperplasia, and megakaryocytic hypoplasia.

CASE 18: ANTICOAGULANT RODENTICIDE INGESTION – BOBBI CONNER

Signalment/history

A 3-year-old neutered male domestic cat is presented for sudden onset lethargy and inappetence. He is a primarily indoor cat, but does have occasional access to the outdoors.

Clinical examination

The cat is moderately mentally depressed on examination. Vital signs are: temperature 99.3°F (37.4°C), heart rate 240 bpm, respiratory rate 24 breaths per minute. Mucous membranes are pale pink with a CRT of 2 seconds. Lung sounds are clear bilaterally and no abnormal heart sounds are heard. Femoral pulses are normal and synchronous with the heart rate. The cat is uncomfortable on gentle palpation of the right forelimb, and a soft tissue swelling is noted in the area of the proximal right humerus. A mild, weight-bearing lameness is noted on the right forelimb.

Differential diagnosis

Given this cat's age, onset of signs, and exposure to the outdoors, trauma and toxin exposure should be strongly considered. Infectious causes of possible anemia should also be contemplated.

Shaving of the fur over the right shoulder reveals severe bruising associated with the soft tissue swelling (**Figure 18.1**). PCV/TS (27%, 4.8 g/dl) are consistent with blood loss anemia. Radiographs rule out a fracture. No other sources of bleeding are identified.

Provisional diagnosis

Given the new information, the presumptive diagnosis is ingestion of an anticoagulant rodenticide. On laboratory testing, PT and PTT are both severely prolonged (a stable clot never forms). Platelet count was estimated to be normal on a peripheral blood smear.

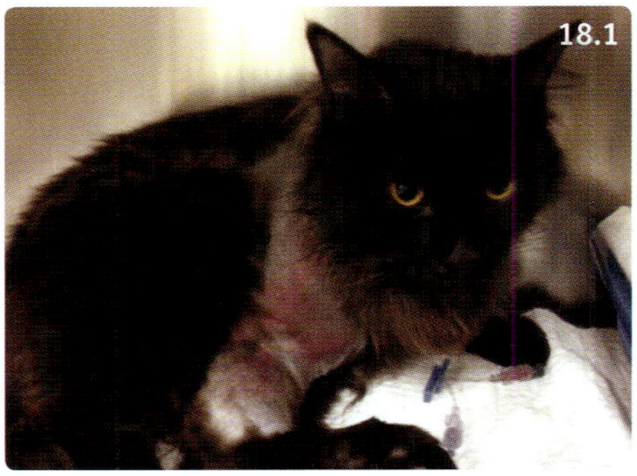

Figure 18.1 Severe bruising and swelling over the right shoulder.

Treatment, follow up

Treatment with fresh frozen plasma (10 ml/kg IV over 2 hours) and vitamin K1 supplementation (5 mg/kg IV given slowly once over several hours) are initiated. Two hours after completion of the plasma transfusion, the PT and PTT times are normal. The cat becomes brighter and begins eating. The cat is discharged the following morning on vitamin K1 at 3 mg/kg/day PO for 4 weeks. Three days after discontinuing vitamin K1 supplementation, the cat's PT and PTT are still normal. No additional rechecks are recommended.

Conclusion

This cat was treated presumptively for anticoagulant rodenticide ingestion and confirmation was achieved by favorable response to therapy. In some cases, testing for proteins induced by vitamin K absence or antagonism may be helpful; however, results of this test are not immediately available and treatment must be started prior to receiving results in clinically bleeding animals. This cat was presented with bleeding in an atypical location, and possible exposure to toxins and his young age increase the suspicion of intoxication. Additionally, the degree of bleeding seen in the absence of other signs of severe trauma (i.e. fracture) increased suspicion for a coagulation abnormality.

Editors' note: A rapid IV injection of vitamin K1 as a bolus can cause an anaphylactoid reaction. This can be avoided by administering the vitamin K1 SC or IV slowly over 12 or more hours; however, anaphylactoid reactions can still occur with slow administration techniques, albeit uncommonly.

CASE 19: SKIN HYPERSENSITIVITY – DIANE T. LEWIS

Signalment/history

A 7-year-old neutered male Domestic Shorthair cat (**Figure 19.1**) is presented with a 6-month history of progressive erosion, ulceration, alopecia, and severe pruritus of the face. The cat lives indoors with four unaffected cats. The owner has been applying a corticosteroid cream twice daily. Lesions are limited to the head.

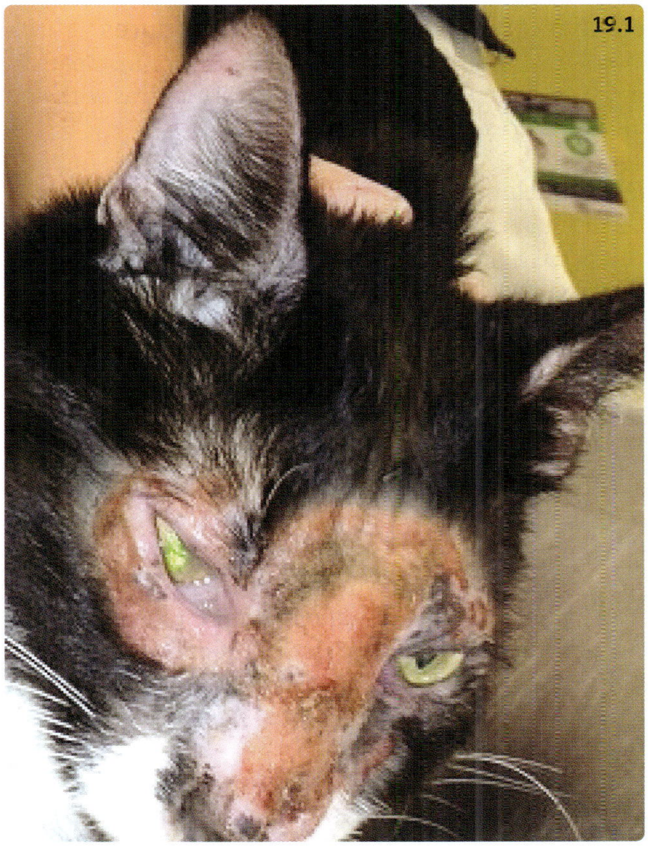

Figure 19.1 The cat on presentation.

Laboratory tests

Skin scrapings and fecal floatation are negative, a dermatophyte culture is pending, and surface cytology of the erosions yields occasional *Malassezia* yeasts and coccoid bacteria.

The bacteria and yeast are likely secondary to an underlying disease but contributing to the pruritus.

Initial treatment

Amoxicillin–clavulanate (PO q12h), itraconazole (PO, once daily, two consecutive days/week), and selamectin (topically every 2 weeks) are initiated. An Elizabethan collar is placed.

Four weeks later, there is no improvement in the pruritus and the facial lesions are progressing. Surface cytology is negative; dermatophyte culture indicates saprophytic contaminants. Three doses of selamectin have been applied to the skin of the dorsal neck.

Further laboratory diagnostic procedures

Two 6 mm skin specimens are submitted for histopathology. Results indicate an eosinophilic dermatitis with epidermal necrosis and serocellular crust.

Differential diagnosis

Differential diagnoses include food hypersensitivity, cutaneous adverse drug reaction, allergic contact dermatitis, severe mosquito bite hypersensitivity, feline herpesvirus, and irritant contact dermatitis.

Further considerations

- Review the systemic drug and vaccine history (there is no oral medication or vaccine history in this cat in the 6 months preceding lesion development).
- Review use of topical products (owner is requested to bring in and discontinue use of any and all topical medications used on the cat).
- A novel protein food elimination diet was planned pending review of topical medications.

Case update

Medications brought in by the owner included an over-the-counter neomycin–bacitracin ointment. The owner began applying the ointment 6 months previously when a single papule was noted on the cat's dorsal muzzle. Within 2 weeks of discontinuation of all topical products (including the neomycin ointment), the cat was notably less pruritic and the lesions were less erythematous. Six weeks after discontinuation of topical products, the cat was not pruritic and re-epithelialization of the skin of the face was occurring. The lesions healed with extensive scarring (**Figure 19.2**) of the muzzle, but not of the periocular areas.

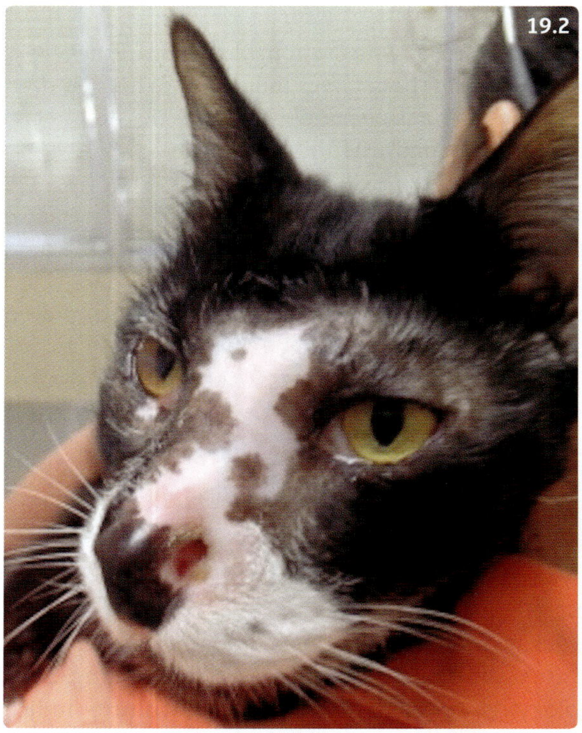

Figure 19.2 The cat post treatment showing extensive scarring of the muzzle.

Editors' note: Neomycin is a known cause of skin hypersensitivity, making a thorough history of utmost importance, as seen in this case.

CASE 20: HYPERVISCOSITY SYNDROME SECONDAY TO IGM MACROGLOBULINEMIA – DENNIS E. BROOKS

Signalment/history

A 9-year-old, male fawn Great Dane. The dog presented with a history of intermittent epistaxis, anorexia with weight loss, possible seizures, and progressive loss of vision over the past 3 months. The left eye became red and painful 2 weeks prior to examination.

Initial clinical findings

Physical examination revealed a quiet, thin dog in no apparent distress. Vital signs were within normal limits. Ophthalmic examination demonstrated severe visual deficits. A weak right direct pupillary light reflex (PLR) was present. No other PLRs could be detected. Schirmer tear test values were 15 and 18 mm/minute in the right eye and left eye, respectively. Intraocular pressure (IOP) by applanation tonometry was 12 and 65 mmHg in the right eye and left eye, respectively. Examination of the left eye revealed buphthalmos, slight blepharospasm, epiphora, conjunctival hyperemia and chemosis, episcleral congestion, and superficial and deep circumferential corneal neovascularization. Generalized corneal edema prevented further examination of the left eye (**Figure 20.1**). A mydriatic pupil, total retinal detachment in a 'morning glory'-type pattern, and areas of retinal thinning were present in the right eye (**Figure 20.2**). The retinal veins were slightly distended with intraretinal hemorrhages noted near the right optic nerve head.

Differential considerations

Retinal detachments (RDs) can be congenital and associated with retinal dysplasia and multiple congenital anomalies. They may also be acquired. Acquired RD can be exudative or be caused by vitreal traction. Exudative or bullous RD can be associated with infection, including

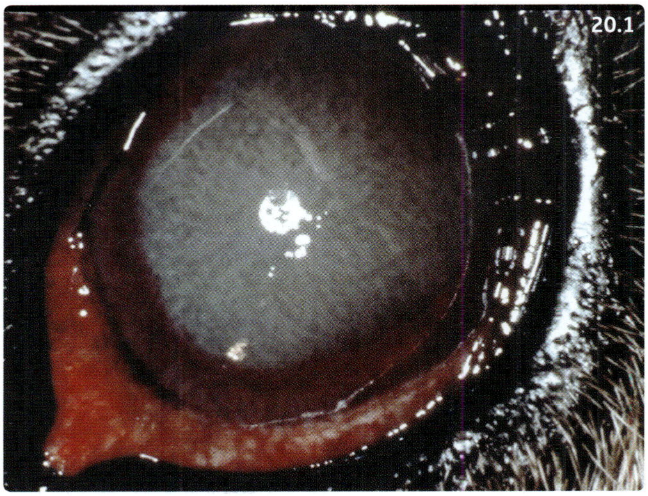

Figure 20.1 Generalized corneal edema and neovascularization in the glaucomatous left eye.

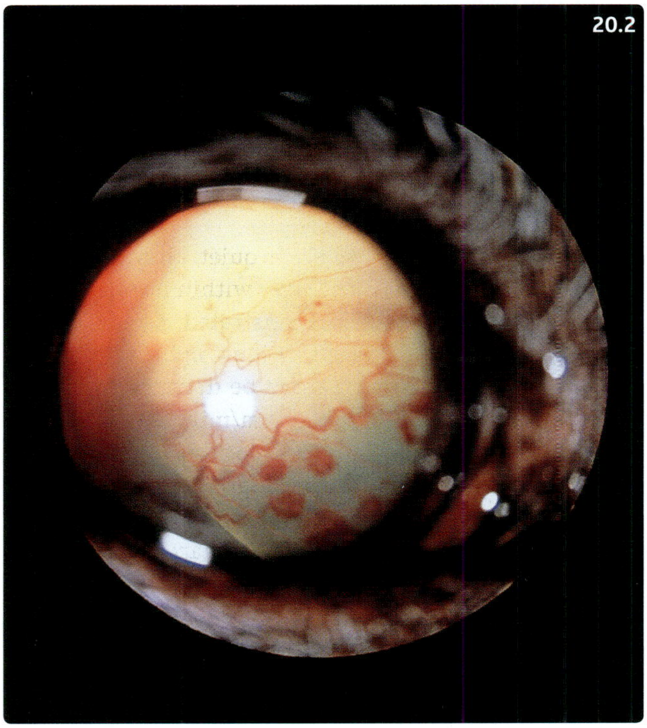

Figure 20.2 Bullous retinal detachment with many intraretinal hemorrhages. Right eye.

blastomycosis, cryptococcosis, toxoplasmosis, geotrichosis, protothecosis, and coccidioidomycosis, or be from neoplasia such as lymphosarcoma, multiple myeloma, fibrosarcoma, or reticulosis. RD can be associated with vascular diseases such as hypertension or hyperviscosity syndrome. Sometimes the cause is idiopathic. Traction RD from vitreal degeneration can result from vitreal hemorrhage or uveitis. Rhegmatogenous RD from tears or holes in the retina can result from retinal degeneration, myopia, glaucoma, intraocular surgery, vitreous degeneration, and trauma. The glaucoma in this case could be primary but was most likely secondary to uveitis.

Laboratory diagnostic tests requested and results

The results of the diagnostic work up are summarized here and listed in **Tables 20.1** and **20.2**:

- Hematology. Moderately severe normocytic/normochromic nonregenerative anemia (PCV = 21%) and slight leucopenia (WBC = 4,200/µl). Hyperproteinemia (8.8 g/dl), slight hypofibrinogenemia, and marked rouleaux formation were reported.
- Serum chemistry panel. The most striking findings were hypoalbuminemia (1.2 g/dl) with hyperglobulinemia (7.5 g/dl). There was also mild elevation of the renal parameters.
- Urinalysis. Isosthenuric urine with 4+ proteinuria was present. Many bacteria and WBCs were noted on sediment examination. Culture and sensitivity yielded a 4+ growth of *E. coli* sensitive to cephalosporins.
- Radiography. There were no radiographic abnormalities of the thorax and abdomen. In particular, there were no osteolytic lesions and no apparent neoplastic masses.
- Ultrasonography. RD, right eye; no significant finding, left eye.
- Cytology. Bone marrow core samples revealed a hypoplastic bone marrow with small clusters of malignant looking lymphocytes noted in a few samples.
- Serum protein electrophoresis. Revealed a monoclonal gammopathy in the gamma region.
- Immunoelectrophoresis. Nearly all (90%) of the immunoglobulin was IgM. Normal is <10%.
- Urine electrophoresis. High albumin levels. Heat test for Bence-Jones proteins was negative.
- Serum viscosity. 5.2, with normal in the author's laboratory being <3.

Initial treatment and rationale

The history, ocular changes, and hematologic data were consistent with a diagnosis of hyperviscosity syndrome secondary to IgM macroglobulinemia. Alleviation of the hyperviscosity syndrome by decreasing IgM production by the abnormal lymphocytes was attempted with alternate day melphelan (2 mg PO) and prednisone (25 mg PO) therapy, and weekly vincristine (0.65 mg IV). The owner refused plasmapheresis therapy. Cephalexin was prescribed to treat the urinary tract infection.

No treatment of the right RD was attempted due to the severity of the lesions. The primary aim of therapy in the left eye was to minimize pain associated with the elevated IOP. Vision was thought to be lost. A carbonic anhydrase inhibitor, methazolamide (100 mg PO q8h), to decrease aqueous humor formation, and topical 2% pilocarpine/ 1% epinephrine (q8h, left eye) to increase aqueous outflow and decrease aqueous formation, were prescribed. Progress of therapy was monitored by weekly CBCs, serum protein electrophoresis, and IOP measurement.

Progress report

The dog's initial response to therapy was favorable. He began to eat and was more active. The IOP 24 hours following initial therapy was 15 and 9 mmHg in the left eye and right eye, respectively. The left eye was less painful. The IOP in the left eye remained at a level of 12–15 mmHg over the next 3 months. The left cornea became progressively pigmented and the left globe phthisical. Follow-up laboratory work (**Tables 20.1** and **20.2**) indicated little improvement of the systemic disease. WBC counts remained low, viscosity measurements were the same, and lgM levels remained elevated. A repeat bone marrow biopsy 2 months following examination revealed hypocellularity with a large percentage of immature lymphoid cells. The dog developed severe diarrhea after 3 months of therapy and was euthanized.

Histopathology revealed a multifocal lymphocytoid neoplasia of the spleen and bone marrow, and chronic, diffuse membranoproliferative glomerulonephritis. The right retina was detached with a large amount of PAS-positive subretinal fluid present. Intraretinal PAS-positive deposits, retinal vessel dilatation, and retinal pigment epithelium hyperplasia were noted (**Figure 20.3**). The left globe was reduced in size with marked corneal and scleral thickening, corneal neovascularization and pigmentation, fibrous tissue proliferation in the anterior and vitreal chambers, peripheral anterior synechiae, intravitreal hemorrhage, and severe retinal disorganization.

Table 20.1

	Initial	Weeks post therapy			
		2	3	4	12
Serum chemistries					
SGPT (U/L)	16				
ALP (U/L)	34		35		
Ca (mg/dl)	9.5		10.3		
Cl (mEq/l)	116		110		
P (mg/dl)	5.4		4		
Na (mEq/l)	154		150		
Creatinine (mg/dl)	1.2		2.1		2.7
Glucose (mg/dl)	125		79		
BUN (mg/dl)	33		24		
Albumin (g/dl)	1.2		1.4	1.6	1.1
Globulin (g/dl)	7.5		8.1	7.8	8.1
Total protein (g/dl)	8.8		9.5	9.4	9.2
Serum viscosity	5.2	See Table 20.2			

	Initial	Weeks post therapy			
		2	3	4	12
CBC					
RBC (×10⁶/µl)	3.2		5.24		
WBC (/µl)	4,200	4,500	3,900	4,400	4,000
Hemoglobin (g/dl)	7.7		12.5		
PCV (%)	21	30	34.6	32	35
MCV (fl)	67		66		
MCHC (g/dl)	34		35		
MCH (pg)	24		24		
Diff. bands (%)	1.5		3		
Neutrophils (%)	80.5		79		
Lymphocytes (%)	10		4		
Monocytes	8		4		
Fibrinogen (mg/dl)	100		100		
Plasma protein (g/dl)	8.8				
Platelets (×10⁵/µl)	300,000		200,000		250,000
Urinalysis					
Urine SG	1.027		1.034		1.025

Note: Refer to cases 15 and 16 for general RIs. Serum viscosity RI = 1.57–1.69 mPas.

Table 20.2

	Initial	Weeks post therapy				
		1	2	3	8	12
IgM levels (mg/ml)	9.35	9.4	9.4	9.2	9.1	8.9
Viscosity	5.2	5.0	5.1	5.1	5.5	5.2

Note: IgM RI = 100–400 mg/dl; serum viscosity RI = 1.57–1.69 mPas.

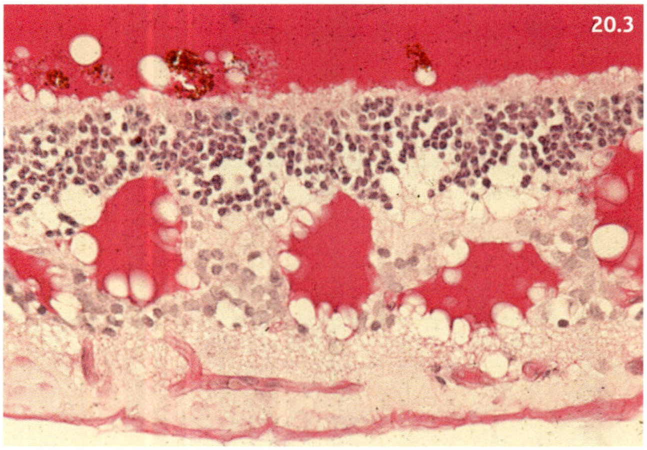

Figure 20.3 Note the PAS-positive subretinal exudate in the left eye. PAS, ×250.

Clinical diagnoses

- RD in right eye secondary to hyperviscosity syndrome associated with Waldenström's macroglobulinemia.
- Secondary glaucoma and phthisis bulbus – left eye.
- Glomerulonephritis.

Summary

Waldenström's macroglobulinemia is a malignant proliferation of B lymphocytes that secrete IgM into the serum. Serum viscosity increases due to the large size and shape of the IgM molecule.

Hyperviscosity is believed to be the primary cause of clinical symptoms in this and other monoclonal gammopathies, as infiltration of ocular structures by neoplastic cells is an unusual feature. Lethargy, weakness, congestive heart failure, neural and renal disease, bleeding diastheses, and ocular changes have been reported in human and canine patients with Waldenström's macroglobulinemia. Ophthalmic disease is reported in 60–70% of human patients.

Intravascular hyperviscosity in Waldenström's macroglobulinemia produces a pattern of retinal changes including vessel distension, 'string of sausages' appearance of vessels, intraretinal hemorrhages, retinal and optic disk edema, and serous RD. Retinal hemorrhages result from compromise of the retinal vasculature and platelet dysfunction produced by coating of platelets with IgM. Reversal of hyperviscosity-related retinopathy has been documented in humans and dogs, but was not possible in this case due to the severity of the lesions. The pathophysiology of the RD seen in this case and in a human patient with Waldenström's macroglobulinemia may be unique. A recent report in a human patient showed the presence of IgM surrounding the photoreceptors. These authors postulated that a transretinal pigment epithelium route for Ig deposition in the subretinal space would increase the osmotic pressure to cause serous elevation of the retina. The intraretinal PAS-positive deposits seen in a human patient have been shown to contain IgM. The presence of such deposits in this case suggest a similar etiology for the right RD, but immunoperoxidase and immunofluorescent studies on formalin fixed sections to detect IgM were negative. Retrospectively, had Michel's fixative been used, a positive result might have been obtained.

Keratoconjunctivitis and secondary glaucoma have been reported in humans with Waldenström's macroglobulinemia. No explanation for the glaucoma was suggested, but intraocular inflammation or hemorrhage associated with the syndrome could have compromised the iridocorneal angle.

Plasmapheresis is the therapy of choice in syndromes of serum hyperviscosity, as most IgM molecules are located in the intravascular compartment and their removal eliminates the hyperviscoisty and ameliorates the clinical signs if performed early enough. Cytotoxic drugs are believed to be an effective alternative to plasmapheresis for treating concurrent hyperviscosity syndrome and lymphoproliferative disease if the hyperviscosity syndrome is not severe. The permanent ocular changes, the dog's initial positive response to medical therapy, and the risk of infection and possibility of defective hemostasis associated with plasmapheresis dissuaded the owner from choosing this mode of therapy.

CASE 21: ONION TOXICITY – LISA A. MURPHY & KENNETH J. DROBATZ

Signalment/history

An otherwise healthy 3-year-old spayed female Wirehaired Fox Terrier is presented by her owners with a concern for bloody urine. The dog had been acting fine otherwise and the owners left this morning for work and returned this evening and fed her as they normally do. When they took her for a walk the dog urinated bloody urine. There was no stranguria or pollakiuria noted. All her other body systems are reportedly fine, and the dog is not receiving any medications. There is no history of any previous medical problems, and the dog has never had any urinary problems prior to today.

Clinical examination

The dog is bright, alert, responsive, and appears clinically well hydrated. Temperature, pulse, and respiration are all within normal limits. Heart and lungs auscult normally and the abdomen is soft and nonpainful. Rectal examination is unremarkable and the stool appears normal in color and consistency. The rest of the clinical examination was normal.

Differential diagnosis

Common causes of bloody urine in dogs and cats include urinary tract infection, cystic calculi, renal hemorrhage, urinary tract vascular abnormality, neoplasia, coagulopathy (including thrombocytopenia or thrombocytopathia), trauma, and pigmenturia.

Laboratory tests

Urinalysis revealed grossly dark red urine, SG of 1.035 (RI, 1.015–1.045), and 4+ blood on a urine dipstick, but was otherwise unremarkable. Urinary sediment examination was also unremarkable, but the supernatant remained dark red after centrifugation. The normal sediment and failure of the urine supernatant to clear with centrifugation suggested that the abnormal color was consistent with pigmenturia, most likely hemoglobinuria.

A peripheral blood PCV and a blood smear were obtained. The PCV was within reference interval (37–55%), but the plasma was pink colored, indicating red blood cell hemolysis. A blood smear was performed **(Figure 21.1)**.

The red cell morphology findings are consistent with eccentrocytes and Heinz bodies. These are a result of oxidant injury to the red cell membranes and hemoglobin.

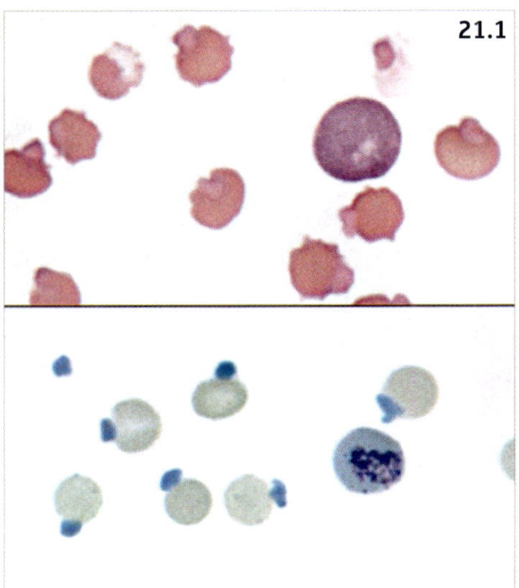

Figure 21.1 Peripheral blood smear shown stained with Diff-Quick® (top) and new methylene blue (bottom).

This injury can result in hemolysis of the red cells and subsequent hemoglobinuria.

Conclusion

The owners were asked about potential exposure to any zinc-containing metals or onions. They remembered that the dog had got into the trash that morning and eaten a plateful of deep-fried onions. The case history, exposure to onions, and the red cell morphology all support a clinical diagnosis of onion toxicity. The dog was given supportive care with IV fluid diuresis, and monitoring of vital signs and PCV. The PCV decreased over the first 12 hours but never dropped below 37%. She was discharged 48 hours after admission without ever needing a blood transfusion.

CASE 22: CORAL SNAKE ENVENOMATION IN A CAT – RACHEL B. DAVY

Signalment/history

An 8-year-old spayed female Domestic Shorthair cat weighing 3.56 kg was presented to an emergency facility for vomiting and ataxia progressing to tetraplegia approximately 6 hours after playing with a coral snake in the yard.

Clinical examination

On arrival at the emergency facility, the cat was in cardiopulmonary arrest. She was intubated and CPR was performed for approximately 2 minutes, which resulted in return of spontaneous circulation. On physical examination post arrest, she was comatose, had generalized lower motor neuron paralysis, and required manual ventilation. One vial of Coralmyn® coral snake antivenom was slowly administered over 30 minutes, at the end of which the cat began having an anaphylactic reaction characterized by facial swelling. She was administered epinephrine (0.03 mg/kg SC and 0.006 mg/kg IV) and dexamethasone sodium phosphate (0.22 mg/kg IV). She was then transported while being hand-ventilated to a referral facility and placed on a mechanical ventilator.

Diagnostic tests

CBC showed a mild thrombocytopenia (139,000/µl; RI, 160,000–502,000/µl). Serum chemistry panel showed a moderately elevated ALT (423 U/L; RI 32–83), a moderately elevated AST (207 U/L; RI, 13–43), a moderate hypocalcemia (7.6 mg/dl; RI, 8.2–10.4), a moderate hypophosphatemia (2.2 mg/dl; RI, 3.1–6), and a mild hyperglycemia (196 mg/dl; RI, 70–140). These findings are consistent with what has been previously reported in cats with coral snake envenomation. In one study involving three cats, one of the patients was hypophosphatemic, all three patients were hypokalemic and hyperglycemic, two had an elevated AST, and all three had an elevated creatinine kinase.

Treatment

Although normal on presentation, the cat's sodium fell precipitously by the third day on the ventilator. Her sodium fell from 153 mEq/l (RI, 148–156) on day 2 to 128.8 mEq/l 24 hours later, at which point her fluid therapy was changed from lactated Ringer's solution to 0.9% NaCl. When her sodium continued to drop, reaching 122.9 mEq/l 9 hours later, the fluid therapy was changed to 3% saline, which resulted in normonatremia.

Since the cat was not displaying any outward signs of fluid overload suggesting a hypervolemic hyponatremia, syndrome of inappropriate antidiuretic hormone secretion (SIADH) was suspected. The primary stimulus for release of ADH is plasma hyperosmolality or hypovolemia. Therefore, the definition of SIADH is an excess of ADH in the absence of hyperosmolality or hypovolemia. This leads to water retention by the kidneys and a dilutional hyponatremia. Specifically in patients that are receiving positive pressure ventilation, especially in those that are on high levels of positive end expiratory pressure (PEEP) ventilation, there is decreased production of atrial natriuretic peptide (ANP) due to decreased venous return. Since ANP normally inhibits ADH secretion, a lack of ANP results in increasing levels of ADH, thus resulting in SIADH.

When the cat's endotracheal tube was replaced as part of her daily care, mucopurulent exudate was noted around the end of the tube. Cytology of this showed intracellular rods and a culture showed scant to moderate growth of *Pasteurella multocida* ssp. *multocida*. Antibiotics (ampicillin/sulbactam, 50 mg/kg IV q8h) were initiated after identifying bacteria on cytology. Thoracic radiographs taken 2 days later showed increased soft tissue opacities in the left cranial and right middle lung lobes, suspected to be secondary to atelectasis from prolonged recumbency; however, aspiration pneumonia was not excluded.

Additional treatment consisted of pantoprazole (1 mg/kg IV q24h). Enteral nutrition was started via nasogastric tube feedings on day 4; a metoclopramide CRI (1 mg/kg/day IV) was also initiated at that time.

The cat remained on the ventilator for a total of 77 hours. After weaning her off mechanical ventilation, she slowly regained normal motor function, initially restricted to tail movements, but gradually progressing to limb movements and eventually standing and walking the fourth day off the ventilator. She was discharged with oral amoxicillin/clavulanate treatment for her suspected aspiration pneumonia.

Discussion

Coral snakes belong to the family Elapidae, which also includes cobras, mambas, kraits, brown snakes, and tiger snakes. Geographically, the Eastern coral snake (*Micrurus fulvius fulvius)* ranges from eastern North Carolina to the southern tip of Florida and then westward to Louisiana. The venom of the Eastern coral snake is primarily neurotoxic, capable of causing a lower motor neuron paralysis and CNS depression. The venom also has hematologic effects, causing hemolysis in dogs, but this has not been noted in cats. This is thought to be due to the dog's red blood cell membrane showing greater sensitivity to the lipoprotein lipase in the coral snake venom. The venom causes only minimal tissue reaction and pain. Due to the lack of tissue inflammation, it can be initially challenging to identify which exposed, asymptomatic patients are actually envenomated. Additionally, the time of onset of clinical signs can range from minutes to as long as 36 hours, which makes it difficult to determine which exposed patients will develop severe signs of envenomation. Current recommendations at our facility for exposed pets include in-hospital monitoring for 48 hours with serial neurologic evaluations and monitoring of serum and urine every 12 hours for evidence of hemolysis (in dogs). Antivenom should be administered at the first sign of envenomation or before the onset of clinical signs if the chances of being bitten were high (i.e. if the pet was found with the snake in its mouth; **Figure 22.1**).

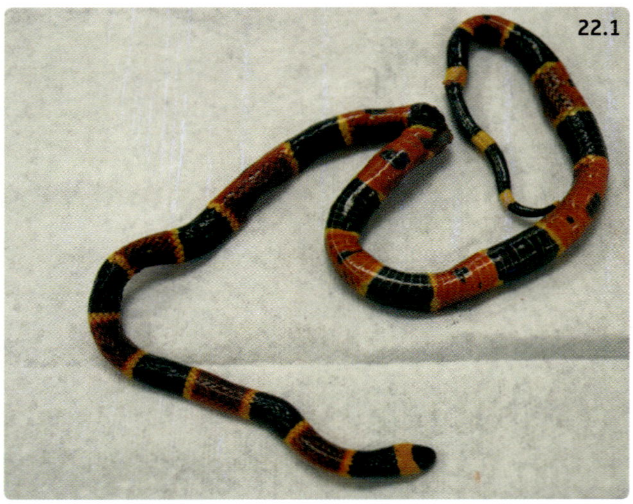

Figure 22.1 A dead Eastern Coral snake following its encounter with a dog. Any patient having this type of close contact with a coral snake is a candidate for antivenom treatment.

Early treatment is recommended in an attempt to avoid the onset of respiratory paralysis and the need for ventilatory support.

Coral snake envenomation should be included in the differential diagnosis when the geographic locale and clinical signs are compatible with this diagnosis. Any dog in the Southeastern USA with the combined signs of hemolysis with lower motor neuron weakness is strongly suspect for coral snake envenomation.

Further reading

Arce-Bejarano R, Lomonte B, Gutierrez JM (2014) Intravascular hemolysis induced by the venom of the Eastern coral snake, *Micurus fulvius,* in a mouse model: identification of directly hemolytic phospholipases A2. *Toxicon* **90:**26–35.

Chrisman CL, Hopkins AL, Ford SL *et al.* (1996) Acute, flaccid quadriplegia in three cats with suspected coral snake envenomation. *J Am Anim Hosp Assoc* **32(4):**343–349.

Perez ML, Fox K, Schaer M (2012) A retrospective evaluation of coral snake envenomation in dogs and cats: 20 cases (1996–2011). *J Vet Emerg Crit Care* **22(6):**682–689.

CASE 23: IMMUNE-MEDIATED HEMOLYTIC ANEMIA AND IMMUNE-MEDIATED THROMBOCYTOPENIA – MICHAEL J. DAY

Signalment/history

A 3-year-old female English Cocker Spaniel had a litter of pups several months ago and was in estrus 2 weeks ago. The bitch is now presented with a 7-day history of weakness and lethargy. The owner reports recent intermittent diarrhea, although at present there are no signs of this problem.

Clinical and laboratory examination

The main finding on clinical examination is pallor of the mucous membranes. Hematologic and serum biochemical examinations are performed and the results are given below.

Examination of the blood smear (**Figure 23.1**) reveals anisocytosis ++, polychromasia ++, spherocytosis +++, macrothrombocytes +, and 1–2 platelets per high-power field (hpf).

The serum biochemistry profile is unremarkable apart from mild hypoalbuminemia (25.7 g/l; RI, 32–38) with normal globulin concentration (33.6 g/l; RI, 20–35) and normal A:G ratio (0.77; RI, 0.6–1.5). There is also an elevation in total bilirubin (13.5 µmol/l; RI, 0–10 µmol/l).

Parameter	Patient	Reference interval
Hematocrit	6.6%	35–55
Hemoglobin	2.41 g/dl	12–18
RBC count	0.74×10^{12}/l	5.4–8.0
MCV	89.1 fl	65–75
MCHC	36.5 g/dl	34–37
MCH	22.5 pg	22–25
Nucleated RBCs	0.6×10^9/l	
Platelets	6×10^9/l	170-500
WBCs (corrected)	14.2×10^9/l	5.5–17.0
Neutrophils	11.4×10^9/l	3.0–11.5
Lymphocytes	0.29×10^9/l	0.7–3.6
Monocytes	0.57×10^9/l	0.1–1.5
Eosinophils	0.43×10^9/l	0.2–1.4

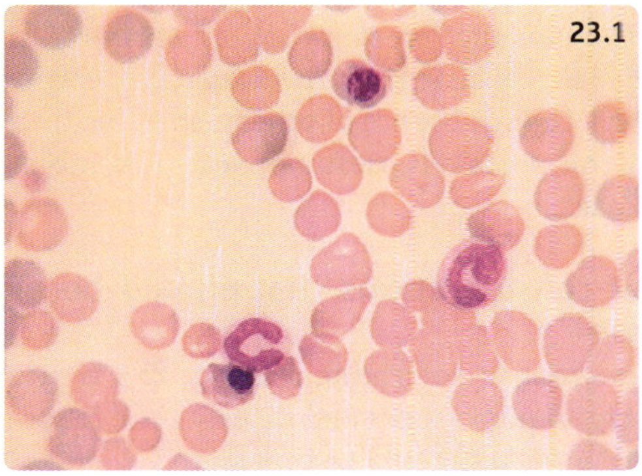

Figure 23.1 Blood smear.

Interpretation of hematologic data

The dog has a severe macrocytic, normochromic anemia. The anemia is strongly regenerative as indicated by the elevated MCV and the presence of nucleated erythrocytes. The presence of marked spherocytosis suggests immune-mediated hemolysis. There is an accompanying thrombocytopenia with evidence of regeneration (macrothrombocytes). The machine platelet count may be artificially low, but the number of platelets/hpf is subnormal (5–10 platelets/hpf would be expected). The leukogram is within normal limits.

The clinical history and hematologic data suggest an immune-mediated hemolytic anemia (IMHA). Although there is no clinical evidence of hemorrhage, the presence of thrombocytopenia would be consistent with concurrent immune-mediated thrombocytopenia (IMTP, Evans' syndrome).

Other laboratory diagnostic procedures

A Coombs test and (if available) testing for the presence of antiplatelet antibody. Antinuclear antibody testing might be considered, but was not performed in this case.

There was no evidence of cold autoagglutination of red cells in this case. The Coombs test was positive for polyvalent canine Coombs reagent (titer 160 at 37°C and 80 at 4°C) and anti-dog IgG (titer 640 at 37°C and 320 at 4°C). Tests for IgM and complement C3 were negative at both temperatures. A test for antiplatelet antibody was not available. A coagulation screen was also performed and revealed a PT of 8.0 seconds (control 7.6 seconds), APTT of 13.8 seconds (control 14.4 seconds), and D-Dimer concentration of 0.4 mg/l (RI, 0.1–0.5).

Presumptive diagnosis

The result of the Coombs test confirms the presence of IMHA and the presence of a warm-reactive IgG antibody is consistent with dominant extravascular hemolysis. In the absence of other causes for thrombocytopenia, this process is presumptively immune-mediated in this case.

Further considerations that should be made in this case

It is important to determine whether this is primary or secondary immune-mediated disease. The following key underlying causes should be considered:

- Recent administration of drugs (no history in this dog).
- Recent administration of vaccine (no history in this dog).
- Infectious disease, particularly arthropod-borne infections (e.g. *Babesia, Ehrlichia, Leishmania*). This dog lives in a nonendemic area for these diseases (the UK) and there is no history of recent travel to an endemic area.
- Neoplastic disease. There is no clinical or laboratory evidence that this relatively young dog has cancer.
- Inflammatory disease. The recent history of intermittent diarrhea and hypoalbuminemia might justify further exploration. Inflammatory enteropathy can underlie IMHA and IMTP in the dog.

In the absence of recognized underlying factors, it is likely that this dog has primary, idiopathic immune-mediated disease (Evans' syndrome). The disease may have been triggered by recent estrus, which is a recognized trigger factor for IMHA.

Treatment

This dog received a whole blood transfusion and was started on combination immunosuppressive therapy with oral prednisolone and azathioprine.

CASE 24: NUTRITIONAL MANAGEMENT – JUSTIN SHMALBERG

Signalment/history

A 9-year-old neutered male Domestic Shorthair cat is presented postoperatively for nutritional management of idiopathic chylothorax, intermittent constipation, and anorexia.

Clinical examination

The cat was quiet and alert with normal respiratory effort and rate. Cardiac sounds were audible and a chest tube was present, through which moderate amounts of serosanguineous fluid were aspirated (15–25 ml q2h). Abdominal palpation was unremarkable and no feces were palpated within the colon. The patient was normotensive and normothermic. The patient's body condition score (BCS) was 6/9 with a body mass of 6.3 kg. Concurrent therapies included fentanyl (2 mcg/kg/hour CRI), cefazolin (20 mg/kg IV q6h), and IV fluids (15–30 ml/hour with rate adjusted based on hydration status).

Pertinent laboratory tests

Triglyceride concentration in thoracic fluid (preoperative) = 469 mg/dl; triglyceride concentration in serum (preoperative) = 41 mg/dl; heartworm antibody, FeLV antigen, FIV antibody: negative; serum chemistry: ALP = 54 U/L (RI, 10–46); total T4: within normal limits; CBC: lymphocytes = 300/µl (RI, 2–7.2); eosinophils = 190/µl (RI, 300–1,700).

Pertinent preoperative imaging

Thoracic radiographs: severe pleural effusion with atelectasis and rounding of the lobar margins, consistent with pleural fibrosis (**Figure 24.1**). Thoracic ultrasound: severe pleural effusion (**Figure 24.2**). Echocardiogram: normal cardiac appearance and function. Thoracic CT: no evidence of neoplasia

Surgical intervention

No masses or structural anomalies were identified during surgery. A subtotal pericardectomy, thoracic duct ligation, and bilateral cranial lung lobectomy due to severe pleural fibrosis are elected.

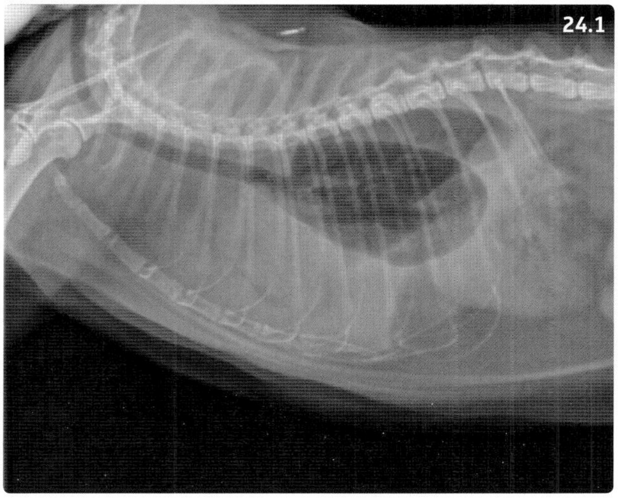

Figure 24.1 Initial thoracic radiograph demonstrating pleural effusion.

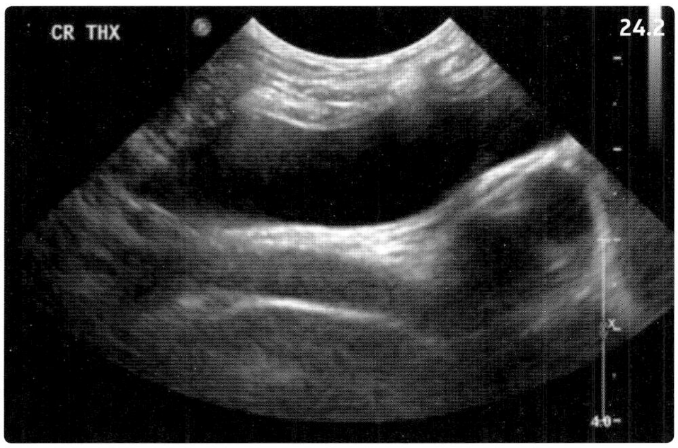

Figure 24.2 Thoracic ultrasound confirming effusion.

Problem list at time of nutritional intervention

Anorexia; lymphopenia; eosinopenia; elevated ALP; historical chylothorax.

Lymphopenia is a common clinical finding in cats with chylothorax, and the eosinopenia is unlikely to be of clinical significance. ALP is liver-specific in cats and therefore not commonly associated with stress. Cholestatic disease is a concern, and given the patient's signalment and presentation, hepatic lipidosis is a differential diagnosis. Elevated ALP is a common clinical finding in affected cats before overt clinical signs manifest. The referring veterinarian reported that the cat had decreased in weight from 7.2 kg to 6.3 kg (12%) in the 2 months prior to presentation, which is consistent with rates in experimentally induced lipidosis.

Assessment of estimated metabolic rate

The patient is 10–15% over ideal body weight with a BCS of 6/9. The patient's ideal body weight is calculated as 6.3 kg/1.10, or 5.7 kg. Published equations give values for daily caloric requirements of 230–273 kcal/day. Average cats should receive 200–250 calories per day, so calculations and general estimates are in agreement. Illness factors are unnecessary in almost all animals.

Nutritional intervention

Immediate enteral feeding is necessary given the cat's acute anorexia, chronic hyporexia, dramatic weight loss, and possible biomarkers for hepatic lipidosis. A nasoesophageal tube is placed in order to avoid additional anesthesia. Cats have higher rates of protein oxidation, decreased downregulation of gluconeogenesis, and possibly elevated requirements during recovery. As a result the minimal protein requirement for cats (40 g/1,000 kcal) is insufficient, and a higher protein diet should be selected. Dietary fat restriction is also a goal of nutritional therapy. Long-chain triglyceride intake may increase chyle flow. Chyle is thought to be irritating to the pleura and could have contributed to the pleural fibrosis in this cat. Previous reports of fat restriction in cats with chylothorax are variable, but diets with <35 g/1,000 kcal are considered. A liquid diet is the only option for a nasoesophageal tube. Two diets are fed to approximate the desired nutrient composition. The combined average diet contains 61 g protein and 26 g fat per 1,000 kcal, with 1 kcal/ml. One hundred and twenty calories are delivered in four bolus feedings in the first 24 hours, with double that amount given in the following 3 days. The patient's previous dry diet is offered before discharge, but anorexia persists.

Nutritional discharge and follow up

The patient is discharged with the recommendation to offer both the previous diet and a high-protein, low-fat diet containing 116 g protein and 27 g fat per 1,000 kcal to assess voluntary intake when in a more familiar location. The patient is presented 48 hours following discharge, as instructed, for persistent anorexia, recurrent constipation, and dehydration. No changes in BCS or muscle mass are evident. Esophagostomy tube placement is recommended to the owners, and the tube is placed using standard techniques. Thoracic radiographs demonstrate appropriate placement and a reduction in effusion (**Figures 24.3, 24.4**). A canned diet is given containing 102 g protein and 25 g fat with a moderate amount of soluble fiber to provide 220 calories over four feedings. Lactulose is given to

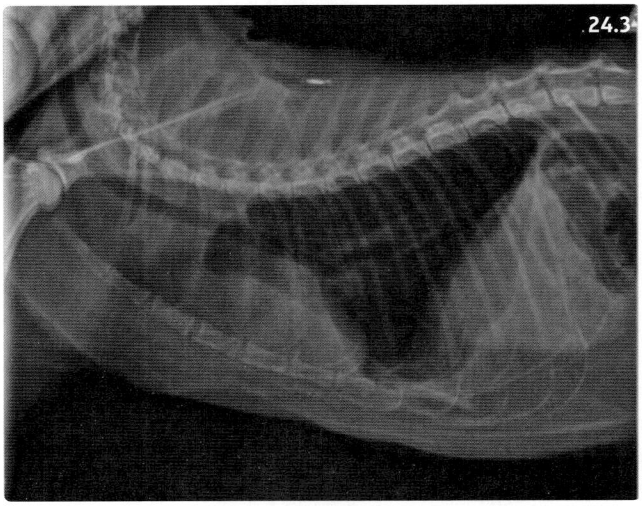

Figure 24.3 Recheck thoracic radiograph demonstrating resolution of effusion.

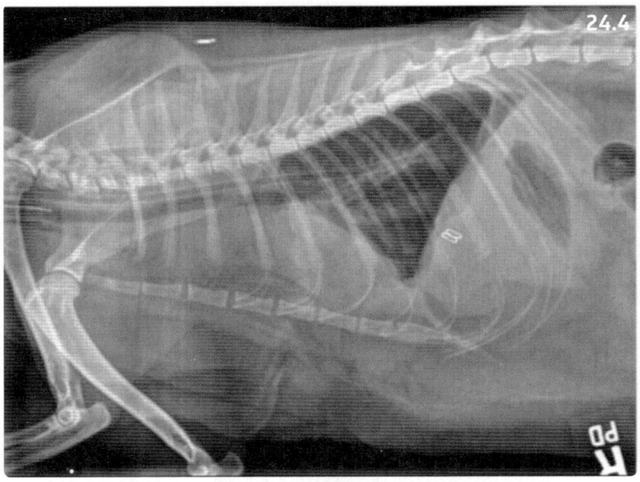

Figure 24.4 Thoracic radiograph after esophagostomy tube placement demonstrating appropriate positioning.

increase fecal moisture and to stimulate colonic motility. Additive water (60–80 ml after each feeding) is given the first day to replace fluid deficit.

Recheck examination and conclusion

Nausea is reported during the week of esophagostomy tube feedings. BCS is decreased to 5/9. A reduction in food volume is desired, so a kitten food and powdered enteral diet are mixed together with water, yielding a diet with 2.6 kcal/ml and 70 g protein and 26 g fat per 1,000 kcal. Feedings are well-tolerated for the following week and the patient begins to eat about 20 calories of the high-protein diet recommended at discharge. The feeding tube is removed, and monitored free-choice feeding is recommended. The patient consumes an average of 260 calories per day, maintains weight and body condition, and displays no recurrence of chylothorax. Lactulose is discontinued and fecal quality remains normal.

Index

Note: Page numbers in *italic* refer to figures, tables, or boxes

abdominal distension
  cardiac disease 196
  FIP 960
abdominal masses
  differential diagnosis *518*
  radiography 516–18
abdominal radiography
  abdominal wall 512–13
  adrenal glands 525, 528
  anal sac tumor 329
  anterior vena caval thrombosis *760*
  cholelithiasis 351
  colon 323, *324*, 541–2, *543*
  dietary indiscretion *293*
  extra-abdominal structures 512–13
  foreign bodies *280*, 539–41
  in hyperadrenocorticism 424–5
  intestinal pythiosis 301, *302*
  lead ingestion 902, *903*
  liver *354*, *355*, *359*, 518–20
  mass effects 516–18
  pancreas 542–3
    pancreatitis *363*, *369*, *370–2*, 1113
  peritoneal space 513–18
  reading 512
  reproductive tract 528–31
  retroperitoneal space 522–4
  small intestines *297*, 538–41
  spleen 520–2
  stomach 282, 283, *284*, 534–8
  technique and positioning 511–12
  urinary tract
    bladder 439, 532
    lower 531–3
    upper 524–5, *526–8*
  urolithiasis 497
abdominocentesis 210, 960, *961*
abscesses
  liver 342–3, 520
  prostatic 71, 531
  subcutaneous 783
  tooth root *86*
acanthocytes *697*, 701
acanthomatous ameloblastoma 96, *97*
acepromazine *1056*
acetaminophen
  efficacy in osteoarthritis *640*
  interactions *1050*
  toxicity 695, 710, 893–5
acetate tape preparations *774–5*
acetazolamide 550, 551
acetylcholine 879, *880*
acetylcholine receptor (AChR) antibodies 624, 625
acetylcholinesterase 879, *880*
acetylcysteine 710–11, 895, 1106
achalasia 253
achondroplasia 646
acidosis, renal disease 462–3
acne, feline 799
acral lick dermatitis 803–4
acromegaly *239*, 391–3
actinic dermatitis 808–9
Actinomyces spp. 143, 144, 948
actinomyces-like bacteria 143
actinomycosis, feline 948–50
activated charcoal 458
acute hemorrhagic diarrhea syndrome (AHDS) 43–4, 294–5
acute kidney injury (AKI) 450–9
  clinical case 1104–5
  clinical presentation 451
  diagnosis 451–5
  differentiation from CKD 449–50
  drug dosages 457
  Easter lily ingestion 891
  ethylene glycol ingestion 451, 454–5, 899–901
  etiology 25–6
  grape/raisin ingestion *451*, 891–2
  management 455
  nutritional support 1076–7
  pathophysiology 450–1, *452*
acute lymphoblastic leukemia (ALL) 737–8
acute myeloblastic leukemia 741
acute myeloid leukemia (AML) 742–3
acute myelomonocytic leukemia 743
acute respiratory distress syndrome (ARDS), in pancreatitis 370, *372*
acyclovir 829, 975
Addison's disease 414–19, 713–14
adenocarcinoma
  colon *543*
  gastric 283, *285*, *537*
  larynx 121
  nasal/olfactory bulb *558*
  pancreas 383–5
  perineal 332
  small intestines 313, 314
adenoma
  parathyroid gland 410, *411*, *412*
  perineal 332
adenosine diphosphate (ADP) *745*
adenovirus-1, canine (CAV-1) 825, 923–5
adenovirus-2, canine (CAV-2) 910
  vaccination 912, 924
'adipokines' 1080
adipose tissue, biological functions 1080–1
adrenal glands
  enlargement/hyperplasia 426, 434, 1109
  physiology 411–13
  radiography 525, 528
  tumors 421, 425, 426, *427*, 432–3, 434, 528
    pheochromocytoma 435–7
adrenalectomy 432–3

adrenocortical insufficiency, idiopathic 414
adrenocorticotropic hormone (ACTH) 389, 412–13
  deficiency 419
  excessive secretion 419–20
  plasma endogenous concentration *429*
adrenocorticotropic hormone (ACTH) stimulation test *35*, 417, *418*, 427, *428*, 430–1
aflatoxins *49*
agar gel immunodiffusion 108, 919
age-related behavior changes 553–4
air bronchogram 187, 189, *190*
airway sampling 54
alanine transaminase (ALT) 48–9, *50*, 334, 335, 350
albaconazole 232
albumin
  bilirubin binding 47
  intravenous fluids 1014–15
  serum 309, 311, 373–4
albumin deficit 1014
aldose reductase 858–9
aldosterone 412, 413
  excess secretion 433–5
aldosterone antagonists *478*, 479
alfacalcidol *408*
algal disease, protothecosis 840
alkaline phosphatase (ALP) 48–9, *50*, 334
  hepatic lipidosis 335
  hepatitis/hepatocellular degeneration 344
  hyperadrenocorticism 423–4
  isoenzyme 423–4
  steroid hepatopathy 356
allantoin 496
allergen-specific immunotherapy (ASIT) 791–2
allergic bronchitis, feline 12–13, 136–7
allergic contact dermatitis 794–5
allergy testing 994–5
  intradermal *776*, 994
  serologic *776*, 994–5
Allium spp., toxicity 905–6
allodynia 1030, 1033
allopurinol 500
alopecia
  atopic dermatitis *791*, *793*
  congenital hypopituitarism 389
  demodicosis 786
  feline psychogenic 804–5
  hyperadrenocorticism 421, 423
  hypothyroidism 398, *399*
  sebaceous adenitis 811
alpha-2 adrenergic agonists 1040–1, *1042*
  doses and characteristics *1055*
alpha-adrenergic agonists 485
alpha-adrenergic receptor blockers *240*, *478*, 479
alpha-amino-3-hydroxy-5-methyl-isoxazole-4-propionic acid (AMPA) 1027
alpha-mannosidosis 726–7, 875
aluminum carbonate 465
aluminum hydroxide 465
alveolar pulmonary pattern 187, 189–91
amantadine 1044, *1045*, *1055*
amatoxins 892
Amblyomma americanum 699
Amblyomma maculatum 730
amikacin *508*, 949
amino acid solutions 1073
amino acid supplementation 348
amino acids 1065–7
aminocaproic acid 591
aminoglycosides 287
  ototoxicity 575–6
aminophylline 244
amiodarone 250, *251*
amitraz 786, *787*
amitriptyline 493, *792*, 1043, *1056*
amlodipine *209*, *240*, *478*, 479
ammonium biurate crystals 358, *359*
ammonium chloride 509
amoxicillin *274*, 296
  feline actinomycosis 949
  leptospirosis 921
  Lyme disease *916*
  UTIs 500, *508*
amoxicillin–clavulanate 129, *508*, *778*, 950, 952
amphotericin 566, 835, 836, *947–8*, 978–9, 980
ampicillin 500, *508*, 554, 971
amylase, serum 371
amyloidosis 468–74
anal furunculosis 329–30
anal sac disorders 328–9
anal sphincter incontinence 327–8
Anaplasma phagocytophilum 934
anaplasmosis 934–6
Ancylostoma caninum 290–1
Ancylostoma tubaeforme 290–1
anemia 681
  aplastic 705
  in CKD 466–7
  classification of general causes 684–5
  clinical presentation 78, *79*, 681–2
  diagnosis 682–5
  ehrlichiosis 934–5
  FeLV-asociated 706–7
  hemolytic 688–99
    acetaminophen toxicity 695, 893–4
    alloimmune 692–3
    babesiosis 694–5
    drug-induced 692
    hemoplasmosis 693–4, 956–7
    hereditary nonspherocytic 698
    immune-mediated (IMHA) 49, 688–92, 1125–6
    microangiopathic 696–7
    oxidant-induced 695–6
    phosphofructokinase deficiency 698
    pyruvate kinase deficiency 697–8
    uncommon causes 698–9
  management 686–7
  nonregenerative *79*, 699–707
    chronic kidney disease 700–1
    endocrine disease 701–2
    immune-mediated 703–4
    inflammatory or chronic disease 700
    iron deficiency 702–3
    liver disease 701
  ocular signs 847–8
  protein-losing nephropathy 470
Angiostrongylus vasorum 131–2, 241, 1102–3
angiotensin II 206–7, 413
angiotensin-converting enzyme (ACE) inhibitors 208, *209*, 210, *240*
  CKD 466
  feline cardiomyopathy *229*
  hypertension 478–9
  mitral valve disease 220
  protein-losing nephropathy 473
anodontia 90
anorexia, in CKD 467
antebrachium, deformities 648–50
anterior uveitis 868–9
  bartonellosis 822
  clinical presentation 868
  diagnosis 869

etiologies *826*, 868
FeLV 830–1
FIV infection 831–2
lymphoma *857*
protothecosis *840*
thrombocytopenia 847–8
UVD syndrome 853, *854*
anterior vena cava, thrombosis *760*
anthelmintics
diarrhea 44, 45
gastric parasites 271
heartworm 242
respiratory parasites 1103
whipworm infestation 316
antibiotic-responsive diarrhea (ARD) 45
antibiotics
acute diarrhea 44–5
acute pancreatitis 377
AHDS 295
bacterial pneumonia 129
broad-spectrum, hemorrhagic gastroenteritis 295
Campylobacter infections 289
canine chronic enteropathy 306
FUO 67
osteomyelitis 664–5
otitis media/interna 575
ototoxic 575–6
parvovirus infection 287, 931
pyothorax 144
resistance 782
urolithiasis *498*, 499–500
UTIs 508
anticholinergics 503
anticholinesterase drugs 266, 625
anticholinesterase insecticides 879–81
anticoagulant rodenticides 755–7, 886–8
anticonvulsants 1043, 1044
antidepressants 1042–3, *1056*
antidiuretic hormone (vasopressin/ ADH) 206–7, 394
response test *34*, *35*, *36*, *395*, *396*
antiemetics *28*, 30, 287, 296, 375, *457*
antifibrinolytics 757, 760
antifreeze ingestion 899–901
antigen-presenting cell (APC/dendritic cell) 986–7
antihistamines *792*
antihypertensive drugs 478–9
antinuclear antibody (ANA) 996
antioxidants 340
antipamezol *1042*
antiprotozoal drugs 293
antithrombin III 474
antithrombotic drugs 229, 474, *762*
antitussives 55, 124
aortic arch
enlarged 183, 185
right persistent (PRAA) 219
aortic thrombosis (saddle thrombus) 583–4, 760–2
aortic valve, vegetative lesions *221*, *222*
aortography 213
apex beat 197
aplastic anemia 705
appetite
increased 421
stimulating 467
aqueous humor, lipemic 846–7
arachidonic acid (AA) cascade 1044, *1045*
arachnoid cyst, intracranial 551–2
arachnoid diverticula (subarachnoid cysts) 602–3
arginine 1065
arrhythmogenic right ventricular (Boxer) cardiomyopathy 224–5, 1107–8
arterial thrombosis 229, *230*, 760–2, 1108–9
arthritis 666–9
degenerative 638–40
erosive 667
rheumatoid 666–9
septic 667–9
arthroscopy 680
ascarids 292
ascites 48
liver disease 338, *339*, 345
pancreatic 368
protein-losing enteropathy *309*
ascorbic acid 895
aspartate transaminase (AST) 48–9, *50*, 334, 335
aspergillosis
canine sinonasal 105–10, 936–40
feline 110, 979–80
ocular 339–40
Aspergillus spp., diskospondylitis 611, 613, *666*
Aspergillus felis 979
Aspergillus fumigatus 106–7, 936, 937, 979
Aspergillus niger 979
aspiration pneumonia 129, 265 *266*, 267
aspirin 311, 474, *640*, *762*, *1046*
GI adverse effects 1048–9
asthma, feline (feline bronchial syndrome) 135–7
astrocytoma *558*
atelectasis 165, *166*, 189, *191*
atenolol *209*, 212, *229*, *249*, 250, *251*, *478*
atlantoaxial instability 603–5
atopic dermatitis
canine 791–3
feline 793
atrial enlargement *202*
atrial fibrillation (AF) 247–9
'lone' 247, 248
atrial premature contraction (APC) *202*
atrial septal defect (ASD) *211*, 217
atrial standstill 247, *489*
atrioventricular (AV) block 245–6
atropine 124, *244*, 246, 699, 881, *1042*
auscultation, cardiac 197–9
autoantibodies
acetylcholine receptor (AChR) 624, 625, 991
detection 995–6
thyroglobulin (TgAA) 402
autoimmune diseases 995
dermatologic 799–802, 1000–2
laboratory diagnosis 995–6
MMM 256–7
polyglandular 414
avermectins, toxicity 883
azathioprine
dermatologic disease *801*
IMHA 691
inflammatory bowel disease *308*
in protein-losing nephropathy *473*
azidothymidine (AZT) 965, *966*, 968
azithromycin 116, 222, 289, 300, *778*, *916*, 950
azotemia 449
postrenal 449
prerenal 416, 449
renal 449

B cells 988–9
B-cell receptor (BCR) 988–9
B-type natriuretic peptide, nonbiologically active (NT-proBNP) 205–6, 228
Babesia canis 694, 940
Babesia felis 694

Babesia gibsoni 694, 940
babesiosis 694–5, 940–1
Bailey chair 266, *267*
Balisascaris procyonis 844
balloon dilatation, esophageal stricture 261, *262*
balloon valvuloplasty 212–13, 214
barium-impregnated polyethylene spheres (BIPS™) 282
Bartonella henselae 101, 230, 822, 950
bartonellosis
  endocarditis 221, 222
  feline 950–1
  ocular signs 822
basophilia 715
Batten's disease 869
batteries, ingestion 901–2
Baylisascaris procyonis 292
Beck's triad 233
benazepril *209*, *240*, 473
  feline cardiomyopathy *229*
  hypertension *478*, 479
Bence-Jones proteinuria 738, 1007
benznidazole 232
beta-adrenergic receptor blockers *209*, 212, 225, *240*
  feline cardiomyopathy *229*
  hypertension *478*, 479
bethanechol 266–7
bicarbonate, serum 461
bicarbonate therapy 440–1, *457*, 463
bile, in vomit 29
bile acids, hepatic lipidosis 336
bile duct, rupture 352
bile peritonitis 352, *353*
biliary obstruction, extrahepatic 350–1
bilirubin 47, 344
bilirubinuria 23, *24*, *26*, 47, *48*, 350
bioflavonoids 147
bioimpedance 1087
biopsies
  colonic 320
  intestinal mucosa 305, *306*
  liver 336, *338*, *339*, 342
  lung 126–7
  muscle 21, 619
  renal 471–2
  skin
    CLE 1001
    erythema multiforme 1002
    pemphigus foliaceus 1000
  temporalis muscle *257*
  thyroid 402
  urethral 501
Birman cats
  abnormal neutrophil granulation 727–8
  thymic hyperplasia and hypotrichosis 1006
bisacodyl *326*
bismuth subsalicylate *274*
bisphosphonates 411
bite wounds, rabies transmission 932, 934
bladder
  atonic 71–2
  calculi 72, *73*, *425*, 531–2
  filling and emptying phases 480–1
  gas 439, 532
  innervation 480, *481*
  masses 484
  neoplasia 73, *74*, 501–3, *524*
  pelvic *480*, 482, 484, 487
  radiography 531–2
  trauma 72
Blastomyces dermatitidis 943
blastomycosis *193*, 836–9, 943, 1096–7
  clinical signs 943, *946*
  etiology 836
  ocular disease 837, *838–9*, 944
  treatment protocols *947–8*
bleaches, ingestion 898–9
blepharitis 866–7
blepharoconjunctivitis *866*
blepharospasm *867*
blindness, sudden onset *841*
blood cell dysplasia 707–9, 724–5, 734
blood culture, FUO 66
blood gas analysis 21
blood loss
  acute 687–8, 751
  fluid resuscitation 1022
blood pressure
  CKD 461–2
  measurement 239, 476–8
  normal canine and feline 474
  in protein-losing nephropathy 474
  regulation 475
blood smears
  abnormal neutrophil granulation 727, *728*
  aplastic anemia 705, *706*
  babesiosis 940
  canine distemper virus 929
  chronic lymphocytic leukemia 737
  ehrlichiosis 729, 936
  feline Chédiak–Higashi syndrome 728
  IMHA 689–91
  infectious diseases 728–32
  inflammatory left shift *725*
  lead poisoning 708, *709*
  lymphoma 735
  methemoglobinemia *894*
  Mycoplasma haemofelis 693, *694*, 956–7
  myelofibrosis 706
  neutrophil toxicity 726, *727*
  oxidant-induced hemolytic anemia 695–6
  Pelger–Huët anomaly *725*
blood transfusion 751
  DIC 764
  hemolytic reactions 692–3
  massive 687, 751
  principles 686–7
  rodenticide toxicity 888
blood typing 686
blood urea nitrogen (BUN) 275, 454, 461
body condition score (BCS) 1060, *1061–2*
  icteric patient 48
  obesity 1079, 1086, *1088*, 1093
body language 3
body mass index (BMI) 1079
body temperature, regulation 61
body weight 1060
  and cough 55
  calculation of ideal 1086, *1087*, 1090
  loss in cardiac disease 196
  loss in diabetes mellitus 438
  loss in obese animal *1088*, 1090–3
bone cysts 671–2
bone disease 638
  iatrogenic 669–70
  idiopathic 670–3
  inflammation 664–9
  metabolic 651–7
  nutritional 663–4
  toxicity 673–4
  traumatic 674–6
  tumors 657–63
bone lesions, lytic 738
bone marrow
  dyscrasia of Poodles 707–8
  fibrosis 706, *707*, 742
  hypoplasia *720*
  infiltrative disease (myelophthisis) 705–6

bone marrow evaluation
acute lymphoblastic leukemia 737, *738*
histoplasmosis 732
procedures 684, *685*
bones, ingestion 259, 260
Bordetella bronchiseptica 127–8, 135, 909–10
canine infection 909–10
feline 951–2
human infection 913
vaccination *912*, *953*
Borrelia burgdorferi 913, 914, 915
borreliosis (Lyme disease) 821, 913–17
vaccination *912*
botulinum toxin A 254
botulism 623, 917–18
Bowen's disease 815–16
Boxer cardiomyopathy 224–5
brachial plexus avulsion 587–91
brachycephalic airway obstructive syndrome (BAOS) 117–19
brachycephalic dogs 117–19
bradyarrhythmias 243–7
bradycardia 243
brain disorders 545–72
degenerative 552–3
developmental 548–52
hemorrhage 546
inflammatory infectious 559–66
inflammatory noninfectious 566–8
intracranial arachnoid cyst 551–2
metabolic 554–5
neurodiagnostic investigation 545–6
nutritional 568–9
trauma 569–72
tumors 556–9, *865*
vascular 546–8
bromethalin 888
bronchial collapse 122
bronchial pulmonary pattern 193, *194*
bronchiectasis 135, 193, *194*
bronchitis
chronic in dogs 53–4, 55, 133–4
feline (feline bronchial syndrome) 12–13, 136–7
bronchoalveolar lavage (BAL) 125–6
bacterial pneumonia 129
chronic bronchitis 134
feline bronchial syndrome 136–7
bronchodilators 124, 134, 137
bronchoesophageal fistula (BEF) 267–8
bronchopneumonia, bacterial 128–30
bronchopneumopathy
eosinophilic in dogs *125*, 132–3
parasitic in dogs (angiostrongylosis) 131–2, 1101–3
bronchoscopy 125–6
Brucella canis 918
brucellosis 821, 918–19
budesonide 308
bulla *770*
bulla osteotomy 575, 811
bullous pemphigoid 1000–1
bupivacaine 1042, 1043–4, *1056*
buprenorphine *377*, 1038, 1040
dose and characteristics *1055*
burr cells 700, *701*
butorphanol 123, 124, *377*, 1039, *1054*

cachexia 196, *309*, 1016
caffeine 906
calcinosis cutis 422–3, 425, 816, *817*
calcitonin 889
calcitonin gene-related peptide (CGRP) 1027, 1030
calcitriol *408*, 410, 463–4, 495
exogenous therapy 466
calcium
serum
ionized 311, 371, 408–9
total 409, 411
urolithiasis 495
supplementation 408
urinary 495
see also hypercalcemia; hypocalcemia
calcium acetate 466
calcium channel blockers *209*, *240*, 248, 456, *478*, 479
calcium EDTA 708, 904
calcium gluconate *408*, 411, *457*
calcium oxalate uroliths *453*, 899, *900*
etiology 494–6
management 500
calcium soap deposits *364*, 368, *369*
calculi, *see* gallstones; urolithiasis
calicivirus, feline, *see* feline calicivirus (FCV)
Campylobacter jejuni 288–9, 622
cancer pain 1032–3
canine adenovirus 1 (CAV-1) 825, 923–5
canine adenovirus-2 (CAV-2) 910
Canine Chronic Enteropathy Clinical Activity Index (CCECAI) *304*
canine coronavirus (CCV) 926–7
canine distemper virus (CDV) 552–3, 705, *706*, 928–30
aplastic anemia 705, *706*
clinical presentation 928–9
diagnosis 929–30
management 930
myelitis 615
neurologic disease 615, 928, *929*
ocular disease 823–5, 928, *929*
vaccines 930
canine infectious hepatitis (CIH) 825–6, 924
canine infectious respiratory disease (CIRD) 53, 127–8, 909–13
Canine Inflammatory Bowel Disease Activity Index (CIBDAI) *304*
canine influenza virus (CIV) 910, 925–6
vaccination *912*, 926
canine juvenile cellulitis 809–10
canine leukocyte adhesion deficiency (CLAD) 725, *726*, 1005
canine oral papillomavirus (COPV) 927
canine parainfluenza virus (CPiV) 910
vaccination *912*
canine teeth
'lance' 88
persistent deciduous *90*
capillary refill time (CRT) 78, 196, 688, 1019
carbamate insecticides 879–81
carbimazole 407, 408
carboxypeptidase *362*
cardiac biomarkers 205–6
cardiac catheterization 212–13, 237
cardiac index 362
cardiac murmurs 198–9
causes and location *198*
DCM 223
grading 199
VSD 216
cardiac output 77–8, 475
cardiac tamponade 187, 233, 234
cardiac troponin I (cTNI) 206, 232, 618
cardiac tumors 226, 233, 234, 235
cardiomegaly 178–9
generalized 181, 183, 1106, *1107*
left-sided 180–1, *183*
right-sided 179–80, *183*
cardiomyopathy
arrhythmogenic right ventricular 224–5, 1107–8
canine 222–6
feline 226–30

cardiomyopathy – *contd*
in hyperthyroidism 405, 406
hypertrophic obstructive (HOCM) *197*
cardiovascular disorders
causing pallor 78, *79*
congenital 211–19
ECG 199–202
history and physical examination 195–9
thoracic radiography *159*
carnitine 1076
carprofen *640*, *1046*, *1047*
carpus, deformation 648, *649*
cartilage, degeneration 638, *639*
cartilage core, retained 650–1
casts, urine 453
cat scratch disease (CSD) 950, 951
cataracts
in anterior uveitis 868, *869*
diabetic 858–9
Ehlers–Danlos syndrome 867
hypoparathyroidism 409
cauda equina syndrome 597–9, 644–5
caval syndrome 241, 242
cecum, diseases 315
cefadroxil *778*
cefovecin *778*, *916*
cefpodoxime *778*
celecoxib *1046*
celiotomy 278, *306*
cellulitis 783
canine juvenile 809–10
central core myopathy (inherited myopathy in Great Danes) 629
central sensitization 1026, 1029–30
central venous pressure (CVP) measurement 455, *456*
centronuclear myopathy 628–9
cephalexin *508*, *778*
drug reaction *818*
cerebellar hypoplasia 970
cerebral edema 569, 1023
cerebral perfusion pressure 1023
cerebrospinal fluid (CSF)
analysis 545
bacterial encephalitis 562
brain tumors 557
CDV infection 930
Chiari-like malformation 602
CNS inflammatory disease 560
FIP 564, 616
GME 567
indications 21
neuromuscular disorders 619
protozoal myelitis 616, *617*
SRMA 613, 614
collection 581–2
obstruction of flow 550, 551
cerebrovascular disease 546–8
ceroid lipofuscinosis, neuronal (Batten's disease) 869
cervical spine disorders
atlantoaxial instability 603–5
clinical signs 580–1
fractures 585, *588*
spondylomyelopathy (wobbler syndrome) 595–7
cetirizine *792*
Chagas disease 230–3
chamomile *1050*
Chédiak–Higashi syndrome, feline 728
chemodectoma 233
chemoreceptor trigger zone (CRTZ) 27
chemosis *827*, *828*
chemotherapy
brain tumors 557–8
'CHOP' protocols 736, 965, *966*
chronic lymphocytic leukemia 737
FeLV-associated lymphoma 965, *966*
lymphoma 736
transitional cell carcinoma 503
chest tube placement 141–2
Cheyletiella spp. *775*, *787*, 789–90
Chiari-like malformation syndrome (CLMS) 550–1, 601–2
chiggers 790–1
Chlamydia felis 954–6
clinical signs 843–4
diagnosis 955
management 955–6
ocular disease 843–4, 955
vaccination *953*, 955
Chlamydophila felis 115, 117
chlorambucil *308*, 312, 340, *473*, *801*
chloramphenicol *508*, *778*, 936, 959
chlorothiazide 396
chlorpheniramine *792*
chlorpromazine *28*, 923
chlorpropamide 395–6
choanal atresia 113
chocolate ingestion 906–7
cholangiohepatitis *803*
cholangitis, feline 337–40
cholecalciferol 663
rodenticides *451*, 458, 889
cholecystitis 352
cholelithiasis 351–2
cholestasis 335, 350–1
cholesterol levels 399–400, 424
chondrodystrophia fetalis 646
chondrosarcoma 162, 659
chorioretinitis 870–1
aspergillosis *839*
blastomycosis 837, *838*
canine distemper *824*
clinical presentation 870, *871*
cryptococcosis 834, 978
etiology *825*, 870
FIP 829, *830*
granulomatous 834, *835*, *836*, *838*, *839*, 840
choroid plexus tumors 556
chronic idiopathic large bowel diarrhea (CIBLD) 322
chronic inflammatory demyelinating polyneuropathy (CIDP) 621
chronic kidney disease (CKD) 459–68
anemia 700–1
clinical presentation *34*, *35*, 461
congenital 459, *460*
diagnosis 461–2
differentiation from AKI 449–50
management 462–8
nutritional support 1076–7
pathophysiology 460
retinal detachment 847
staging 462
chronic lymphocytic leukemia (CLL) 736–7
chronic myelomonocytic leukemia 741
chylothorax *139*, *140*, 145–8, *165*
nutritional intervention 1126–8
chyluria 23
chymotrypsin *362*
cidofovir 829
ciliary body tumor *864*
ciliary dyskinesia, primary 130–1
cimetidine 895, 1049
ciprofloxacin, dermatologic disorders *778*
cirrhosis 344–6
macronodular *354*
cisapride 264, 266, *283*
cisplatin 503, 657, 658
clarithromycin *274*, *778*, 949
cleaning agents, ingestion 896–8
clemastine *792*
clindamycin 565, *778*, 941
clinic surroundings 4

clinical cases
  arrhythmogenic cardiomyopathy 1107–8
  arterial thromboembolism 1108–9
  blastomycosis 1096–7
  congestive heart failure 1106–7
  coral snake envenomation 1123–5
  cycad palm toxicity 1105–6
  diabetic ketoacidosis 1111–12
  hepatitis 1095–6
  hyperviscosity syndrome 1118–22
  immune-mediated hemolytic anemia and thrombocytopenia 1125–6
  kidney disease 1104–5
  masticatory muscle atrophy 1110–11
  nutritional management of chylothorax 1126–8
  onion toxicity 1122–3
  pulmonary fibrosis 1100–1
  respiratory worms 1101–3
  rodenticide ingestion 1116–17
  severe necrotizing pancreatitis 1112–15
  skin hypersensitivity 1117–18
  systemic histoplasmosis 1115–16
  tooth impaction 1097–8
  tooth resorption 1098–100
  tracheal tear 1103–4
  weakness in cat 1109–10
clomipramine *792*
clonality testing 998–9
clopidogrel *229*, 311, 474, 762
clostridial infections 289–90, 294, 316, 821
Clostridium botulinum 623, 821, 853, 917
Clostridium difficile 289–90
Clostridium perfringens 289–90, 294, 316
Clostridium tetani 821, 922
clotrimazole 110, 939
co-infection 909, 910
coagulation 746–7
coagulopathy
  liver disease 765–6
  of trauma (CoT) 766–7
  sepsis 764–5
cobalamin
  deficiency 307–8, 311, 336, 704
  subcutaneous injections *308*, 311
Coccidioides immitis 233, 835
coccidioidomycosis 236, 835, 943–8
codeine 1038, 1040, *1055*
cognitive disorder 553–4
colchicine 472
cold agglutinin disease 689
colitis *41*
  acute idiopathic 316–17
  diet-responsive 318
  fungal and oomycetal 317
  granulomatous 319–21
  inflammatory 318–19
  nutritional support 1075
  parasitic 315–17
collagen *745*
Collies, cyclic hematopoiesis 721
colloids 569, 1014–16
colon
  anatomy and physiology 314–15
  displacement 542
  distension 542, *543*
  impaction 322–4
  inflammatory disease 318–19
  neoplasia 326–7, 542, *543*
  obstruction 321–2
  radiography 541–3
colonoscopy 319, 320
color Dopper, VSD 216
coma, diabetic 438
comedones 422, *786*
common bile duct (CBD), obstruction *51*
communication skills 4–8
complement C3 deficiency 1004
complet blood count (CBC), in protein losing nephropathy 470
compression radiography 515–16
computed tomography (CT) 679–80
  brain 426, *427*, 546, 549, 557, *558*
  diaphragmatic herniation 151, *153*
  head trauma 570, *571*
  lung lobe torsion 148, *149*
  lymphangiography 146, *147*
  musculoskeletal disorders 679–80
  otitis media/interna 573
  pneumothorax 140, *141*
  skull 108, *109*, 114, *115*
  spinal 582, 586, *587*, 592–3, 599, 612
  thoracic neoplasia 154, *155*
congenital heart diseases 211–19
congestive heart failure (CHF) 186–8, 206–11
  canine 14
  classification *209*
  clinical cases 1106–7, 1108–9
  clinical presentation 207–8
  cough 53, 195, 207
  diagnosis 208
  differential diagnosis 208
  feline 12–13
  left-sided 186–7, *188*, 207–8
  management 208–10
  pathophysiology 206–7
  prognosis 210–11
  radiography 136–7, *188–9*, 1107
  right-sided 186, *189*, 208
  signs in hyperthyroidism 405
  thrombosis 1108–9
conjunctivae
  lymphosarcoma *857*
  signs of systemic disease 865
conjunctivitis
  allergic 999
  blastomycosis *838*
  chlamydial 843–4, 955
  feline calicivirus 823, 973–4
  feline viral upper respiratory infection *974*
  herpesvirus 826, *827–8*, *974*
  mycoplasma infections 822–3
constipation 322–5
  management in cats 324–5, *326*
consultation 3–8
  clinic setting 4
  communication skills 4–8
  structure and organization 8
continuous renal replacement therapy 459
Coombs test 691 956, 995
Coonhound paralysis 621
copper toxicity familial 348–9
coral snake envenomation 1123–5
cornea
  edema ('blue eye') 825, *856*
  lipidosis 398, *399*, *845*, 865–6
  sequestrum *827*
  ulceration 826, *827–8*
coronavirus, canine respiratory (CRCoV) 910, 926–7
corticosteroid-induced eosinopenia 722
corticosteroid-induced lymphopenia 722–3
corticosteroid-induced monocytosis 717
corticosteroid-induced myopathy 625–6
corticosteroid-induced neutrophilia 712

corticosteroids
acute pancreatitis 377
brain disorders
CLMS 551
hydrocephalus 550
dermatologic disease *801*
feline enteropathy 312
feline inflammatory liver disease 340
hypoadrenocorticism 418–19
inflammatory bowel disease 307, *308*
insulinoma 447
MMM 257
corticotropin-releasing hormone (CRH) 412–13
cortisol:creatinine ratio, urinary *428*, 429
cortisol, plasma, in surgery 1029–30
cough 53–5
airway sampling 54
cardiac disease 53, 195, 207, *211*
cats 53, 136
chronic 134
definition 53
diagnostic algorithm *54*
diagnostic imaging 54
etiology/pathophysiology 53
'goose honk' 910
'kennel' (canine infectious respiratory disease) 53, 127–8, 909–13
lower airway diseases *106*
management 55, 124, *211*
nocturnal 53
physical examination 53–4
upper airway disease *106*
tracheal collapse 122, 124
cough medications (over-the-counter) 895–6
cough reflex 53
cough suppressants 55, 124, *211*
coumarins 755
cranial cruciate ligament rupture 676–9
cranial drawer test 678–9
cranial nerve disorders 572–80
facial nerve (CN VII) 579–80
trigeminal nerve (CN V) 576–8, 1110–11
craniectomy 557, *559*
craniomandibular osteopathy 653–4
creatine kinase 618, 628
creatinine *423*, 429, 453, 461, 469, 473
Crenosoma vulpis 1103
cricopharyngeal dysphagia 253–4
cross-matching 686
Crotalus atrox, vaccine *912*
crust *771*
cryptococcosis 110–11, 565–6
clinical signs *946*
CNS 565–6
CSF cytology *560*
diagnosis 565–6, 978
feline 977–9
management 566, 978–9
ocular disease 65, 833–5, 978
treatment protocols *947*
Cryptococcus gattii 977
Cryptococcus neoformans *945*, 977
cryptosporidiosis 299–300
Cryptosporidium canis 299
Cryptosporidium felis 299
crystalloid fluids 1011–14
crystalluria 23, 358, *359*
calcium oxalate *453*, 899, *900*
cystine *498*
struvite *498*
urate *498*
Ctenocephalides spp. 957
Ctenocephalides felis felis 793
Cushing's disease *239*, 419–33, 626, 656–7
cutaneous (discoid) lupus erythematosus (CLE) 800–2, 1001–2
cutaneous larva migrans 292
cutaneous T-cell lymphoma 812, *813*
cutaneous trunci (panniculus) reflex 581
cyanosis 196
cycad palm toxicity 1105–6
cyclic hematopoiesis 721, 1005–6
cyclophosphamide *473*, 691, 965, *966*
cyclosporine 103, *308*, 312, 330, 340, *473*, 691, *801*
cyproheptadine *792*, 971
cystadenocarcinoma, common bile duct *350*
cysterna chyli, ablation 147
cystine uroliths *498*, 501, 531–2
etiology 496–7
management 501
cystitis 71
emphysematous 72, 439, 532
feline idiopathic (FIC) 487–8
cystocentesis 72
cystography 73, *74*
cystometry 74, 484
cystoscopy 74, *488*
cysts
arachnoid 551–2
bone 671–2
prostatic 531
renal 503–4
spinal synovial 600, *601*
subarachnoid 602–3
Cytauxzoon felis 699
cytauxzoonosis 699
cytokines 61, 712, 724, 988

D-dimers 748
dacryocytosis 706, 742
dalteparin *762*
DAMNIT acronym 637
danazol 691–2
dantrolene 634
dapsone *801*
darbepoetin alfa 467
deciduous teeth
eruption times 84
persistent 89–90
decubital ulcers 586, *588*
deferoxamine *23*
degenerative joint disease (DJD) 638–40
radiosynoviorthesis 640, 1053
degenerative myelopathy 590–1
dehydration 78
estimating degree *455*, 1016–17
Demodex canis 786–7
Demodex cati 787–8
Demodex gatoi 787, 788
demodicosis 786–8, *866*, 867
dendritic (antigen-presenting) cell 986–7
dental formulae 83–4
dental plaque 86
dentin 84, 92
depigmentation 812, 853–5
L-deprenyl (selegiline hydrochloride) 432
deracoxib *640*, *1046*, *1047*
Dermacentor spp. 623, 699
Dermacentor variabilis 699, 940
dermatitis
acral lick 803–4
actinic (solar) 808–9
allergic contact 794–5

atopic 791–3
feline miliary 805–6
in FIV infection 967, *968*
Malassezia 785–6
pyotraumatic 779, *780*
dermatologic disorders
anti-inflammatory/immunosuppressive therapy *801*
antibiotic therapy *778*
antihistamine therapy *792*
autoimmune 799–802, 1000–2
examination 769–73
fungal and yeast infections 784–6
hepatocutaneous syndrome 346–7
history taking 769
hyperadrenocorticism 422–3
investigations *773–6*
lesion classification *770–2*
metabolic 802–3
parasitic 786–91
psychogenic 803–5
tumors 812–16
dermatomyositis 817, *818*, 1002
dermatophytosis 784–5
dermatosis, feline idiopathic ulcerative 816–17
desmopressin 395, 753
desoxycorticosterone pivalate 418
detergents, ingestion 896–8
detrusor instability *480*, 482, 484, 487
dexamethasone 418, 691, 752, *801*
dexamethasone suppression tests 427–9
dexmedetomidine 1040
dextromethorphan 55, *1055*
diabetes insipidus *34*, *35*, *36*, 394–7
diabetes mellitus 437–45
in acromegaly 391
in acute pancreatitis 378, 379
cataracts 858–9
classification 438
clinical presentation *34*, *35*, 438
complications *441*
neuropathy 620
concurrent illnesses 441
diagnosis 439
etiology 437
exocrine pancreatic insufficiency 382
incidence 438
investigation of instability 443–5
management 439–45
obesity 1084
pathophysiology 437–8
diabetic ketoacidosis
case study 1111–12
management 439–41
dialysis 459, 468
diaphragm
herniation *139*, 149–51, *152–4*
radiography 163
rupture 165, 167
diarrhea
acute 43–5
acute hemorrhagic syndrome 294–5
bloody *39*, *40*, *43*, 286, 294
canine coronavirus infection 926
chronic 44, 45, *46*
clinical approach to 44–5
clinical signs 39, *40–1*
differential diagnosis 41–4
large intestinal disease *39*, 45, *46*, 322
pathophysiology 41
small intestinal disease *39*
diazepam 548, 881, 885, 886, 890
doses and characteristics *1056*
diazoxide 447–8
diclofenac *1052*
dicyclomine *485*
diet
canine chronic enteropathy 305, 307, 308
cirrhosis 346
in CKD 467
commercial pet foods 1065, *1066*
diabetes management 441–2
feeding tubes 1071–2
feline idiopathic cystitis 492
fiber supplementation 319, *323*, 1075
gastric emptying disorders 282
gastric ulceration 276
hyperthyroidism management 407
'hypoallergenic' *45*
idiopathic chylothorax 1127–8
insulinoma 447, *448*
in megaesophagus 266
obesity management 1091–2
protein-losing enteropathy 310
renal disease 463, 473–4, 492, 1076–7
urolithiasis 500
see also nutritional support
diet history 1060
dietary indiscretion *40*, 293–4
N,N-diethyl-M-toluamide (DEET) 884
digoxin *209*
dihydrostreptomycin 919
dihydrotachysterol *408*, 410
dilated cardiomyopathy (DCM) 222–4
diltiazem *209*, *240*, 248, 456
dimercaptosuccinic acid (succimer) 904
dimethyl sulfoxide (DMSO) 472
diminazene aceturate 699, 941
dioctyl sodium succinate *326*
diphenhydramine *792*
diphenoxylate 294
diphenoxylate hydrochloride 124
Dipylidium caninum 794
direct antiglobulin (Coombs) test 691, 956
dirlotapide 1092
Dirofilaria immitis 240, 696, 713
microfilaria *696*
ocular 844, *868*
dirofilariasis 696
disinfectants
feline panleukopenia virus 971
giardiasis 299
parvovirus management 237
diskospondylitis 611–13, 665–6, 918
disseminated intravascular coagulation (DIC) 751, *760*, 762–4
distemper virus, *see* canine distemper virus
diuresis, postobstructive *34*
diuretics
in AKI 456
causing polydipsia/polyuria *34*
diabetes insipidus 396–7
heart failure *209*, 210
hypercalcemia 411
osmotic 570–1
systemic hypertension *240*
dobutamine *209*, 210
docosahexaenoic acid (DPA) 1067
dog erythrocyte antigens (DEAs) 686, 692
Döhle bodies *727*
dolasetron *28*, *457*
Doppler flow detector 476–8
doramectin 264–5
dorsal horn 1027–9
dorsal laminectomy 594–5
doxapram hydrochloride 120
doxepin *792*
doxorubicin 736
doxycycline
brucellosis 919
canine ehrlichiosis 730, 936
CIRD 128, 911, 913
dermatologic disorders *778*

doxycycline – *contd*
feline actinomycosis 949
feline bartonellosis 950
feline bordetellosis 952
feline chlamydiosis 955
feline plague 958–9
feline URT disease 115, 117
FUO 67
heartworm 241
leptospirosis 921
Lyme disease 915, *916*
Mycoplasma felis 954
RMSF 942
drawer test 678–9
dropped jaw 576–7
drug reactions 817, *818*, 1117–18
drug-induced hemolytic anemia (DIIHA) 692
drugs
causing blood cell dysplasia 734
causing GI ulceration *274*
causing liver injury 344, 349
causing pigmenturia 23
ingestion of over-the-counter 895–6
dual-energy X-ray absorptiometry (DEXA) 1086, 1087, *1089*
ductus arteriosus
normal closure 214
patent (PDA) 185, *186*, 196, *197*, *211*, 214–16
DUMBELS mnemonic 879
dwarfism
chondrodystrophia fetalis 646
pituitary 388–91
dynamin 1 gene 631
dysbiosis, intestinal 303, 305–6
dyschezia 321, 326
dyserythropoiesis 704
dysphagia 27, 253–4
dyspnea *106*
cardiac disease 195, 207
pneumothorax 140
typical causes in cats 12–13
typical causes in dogs *12*, 13–15
dystocia, radiography 530
dystrophin deficiency 627–8
dysuria 69–70
etiology 70–2
investigations 72–5

ear disorders, *see* otitis externa; otitis media/interna
ear margin dermatosis 798
ear mites *787*, 789
ear tip necrosis *689*, *819*
Easter lilies *451*, 891
ecchymotic hemorrhages 749, *750*, *887*
echocardiography 202–5, *206*
animal positioning 203
canine heartworm 241
cardiac chamber evaluation 204–5
DCM 223, *224*
Doppler 205, *206*
endocarditis 222
feline cardiomyopathy 228, *230*
indications 202–3
left atrial thrombus 1108
M-mode *204*
mitral valve disease 220, *221*
pericardial effusion 234
pulmonary hypertension 237, 237–8, *238*
pulmonic stenosis 213–14
subaortic stenosis 212
transducer selection 203–4
transthoracic windows 203
VSD 216, *217*
echothiophate iodide 853
ectopic ureters *480*, 481–2, 483
correction 485–7
ectrodactyly 645–6
edema
facial *894*
laryngeal 121–2
pulmonary 189, 191, 207, 208
subcutaneous *309*
edrophonium response 21, 625
EGC, *see* eosinophilic granuloma complex
Ehlers–Danlos syndrome 867
Ehrlichia canis 705, 716, *729*, 841–2, 934
ehrlichiosis 716, 728–30, 934–6
clinical presentation 729, 935
diagnosis 729–30, 935–6
etiology 728, 934
management and prevention 730, 936
ocular signs 841–2
pathophysiology 728–9, 934–5
eicosapentaenoic acid (EPA) 1067
Eisenmenger's physiology 214
elastase *362*
elbow
dysplasia 646–8, *670*
luxation 649, *650*, *675*
synovial cell sarcoma *662*
electrocardiogram (ECG) 199–202
addisonian crisis *417*
ambulatory (Holter monitoring) 199, *200*, 225
arrhythmogenic right ventricular cardiomyopathy 225, 1107
atrial standstill 247, *489*
AV block 245–6
cardiac tamponade 234
DCM 223, *224*
features in normal dog/cat *200*
feline cardiomyopathy 228, *229*
hyperkalemia *417*, 455, *457*, *489*
hyperthyroidism 405
indications 199–200
interpretation 201, *202*
methods 200–1
sick sinus syndrome 243
syncope/episodic weakness 18
ventricular tachycardia 250
electroencephalogram (EEG) 545–6
electrolyte disturbances 555–6
in AKI 456, *457*
phosphate 336, 409, 463, 465, 889
potassium
hyperkalemia 416, *417*, 456, *457*
hypokalemia *34*, *35*, 433–5
sodium 416, 419, 555–6
electromyography (EMG) 21, 616, 618, 625
electrophoresis, serum protein 963
electrophysiologic testing 618, *619*
emesis, *see* vomiting
emetic center 27
empyema, spinal 614–15
enalapril *209*, *229*, *240*, 473, *478*
enamel, dental 84
hypoplasia 928, *929*
tetracycline staining *911*
encephalitis
bacterial 562
necrotizing meningo(leuko) encephalitis 567–8
Toxoplasma 981
encephalopathy, hepatic 333–4, 335, 346, *357*, *358*, 554, 1076
endocarditis, bacterial 221–2
endochondral cartilage core, retained 650–1
endocrine disease
anemia 701–2
causing syncope/episodic weakness 18, *20*, 1109–10

  myopathies 625–7
  neuropathies 620–1
  and obesity 1081, *1083*, 1084
  see also named diseases
endophthalmitis, blastomycosis *839*
endorphins 1027
endothelial dysfunction 753
endothelin-1 1032
enemas 324, *326*
energy expenditure 1090
energy requirements 1018, 1064–5, 1090
enilconazole 110, 938–9
enophthalmos 578
enoxaparin *762*
enrofloxacin 129, 287, 296, 320, *508*, *778*
  retinopathy 873–4
enteral feeding, assisted 1067–72
enteritis
  bacterial 288–90
  dietary indiscretion *40*, 293–4
  granulomatous *306*
  nutritional support 1075
  parasitic 290–3, 296, 298–300
  use of probiotics *289*
  viral 286–8, 931
enteropathy
  antibiotic-responsive 45
  chronic canine 302–9
  chronic feline 311–12
  diet-responsive *40*, 293–4, 318
  protein-losing 309–11
envenomation 763, 1123–5
environmental enrichment (cat) 489–92
eosinopenia 721–2
eosinophilia 713–15
eosinophilic bronchopneumopathy (dogs) *125*, 132–3
eosinophilic enteritis 306
eosinophilic granuloma complex (EGC) 102–3
  feline 806–8
eosinophilic plaque, feline 806–7
eosinophils, gray 713
ependymomas 556
epidermal collarette *772*
epidural space, empyema 614–15
epidurography 582
epinephrine 58, 711, *745*, 1044
epiphyseal ossification, delayed 399, *400*
epiphysis, disorders 638
epistaxis 57–9, *750*
epsilon aminocaproic acid (EACA) 757
epulis 96
equine influenza A virus (H3N8) 925
erythema multiforme 1002
erythrocytosis 709–10
  primary 741–2
  relative 709
  secondary absolute 709–10
erythroid dysplasia 707–9
erythroid hypoplasia/aplasia, selective 700
erythroleukemia, acute 743
erythromycin 266, *283*, *778*
erythropoietin (EPO) 709
  deficiency 700–1
  human recombinant 467, 700–1, 966
Escherichia coli 128, 319–20, 562, 783
esmolol *249*, *251*
esophageal disorders
  clinical signs *258*
  diverticulum *175*, 267
  fistula 267–8
  foreign bodies 174, 259–60
  masses/neoplasia 175, 261
  rupture 170
  stricture 260–1, *262*
esophagitis 258, 261, 263–5
  secondary in hiatal hernia 269
esophagoscopy 261, *262*, *263*
esophagostomy tube 462, *464*, *1028*, 1068, *1069–70*, 1127, *1128*
esophagram, positive contrast 268
esophagus
  anatomy 258
  normal function 258
  radiography 172–5
estriol 485
estrogen supplementation 481, 485
ethanol 901
ethylene glycol toxicity 899–901
  clinical signs 451, 899
  diagnosis *453*, 454–5, 899–900
  management 458, 900–1
  pathophysiology *451*, 899
etodolac *640*, *1047*
Eutrombicula alfreddugesi 790
Eutrombicula cinabaris 790
Evan's syndrome 690
examination room 4
excoriations *771*, *793*
exercise intolerance 17, 421
exercise testing, muscle disorders 617
exercise-induced collapse (Labrador Retrievers) 631–2
exertional rhabdomyolysis 633–4
exocrine pancreatic insufficiency 380–3
exophthalmos 578, 862, *863*, 864, *865*
exostoses, multiple cartilaginous 672–3, *674*
expectorants 129
extrahepatic bile duct obstruction (EBDO) 47, 48
extraocular muscles, myositis 862–3
exudates *165*
eye disease, *see* ocular disease
eyelid disease 866–7

face mask, oxygen therapy 11
facial edema *894*
facial paralysis 579–80
factor IX deficiency 753–5
factor VIII deficiency 747, 753–5
factor X 747
factor XII (Hageman factor) deficiency 747, 753–5
'fading kitten' syndrome 961, 970
famciclovir 975
familial sensory neuropathies 620
famotidine *272*, *274*, 375, *457*, 467, *1049*
Fanconi syndrome 453, 461
fasting
  dietary indiscretion 294
  in diarrhea 44
fat pad, infrapatellar 677–8
fats, dietary 1066–7
fecal flotation 316
fecal incontinence 327–8
fecal testing
  acute diarrhea 44
  exocrine pancreatic insufficiency 381, 382
  giardiasis 298, *299*
feeding
  ad-libitum 1079, 1093
  in acute gastritis 270
  management in megaesophagus 266
  see also diet; nutritional support
feeding tube placement 1068–72
  esophagostomy 462, *464*, *1028*, 1068, *1069–70*, 1127, *1128*
  gastrostomy tube 1068, 1070
  jejunostomy tube 1070–1
  nasoenteral 1068, *1069*
  tube management 1071–2

feline acne 799
feline bronchial syndrome 12–13, 136–7
feline calicivirus (FCV) 101, 823, 973–6
  vaccination *953*, 976
  virulent systemic infection 976–7
feline central retinal degeneration (FCRD) *873*
feline dysautonomia (feline dilated pupil syndrome) 853
feline enteric coronaviruses (FECVs) 959
feline herpesvirus-1 (FHV-1) 101, 826–9, *953–4*, 973–6
  diagnosis 975
  management 975–6
  ocular disease 826–9, 973–4
  respiratory disease 973–6
  vaccination 976
feline idiopathic cystitis (FIC) 487–9, 492–493
feline immunodeficiency virus (FIV) 101, 967–9
  clinical presentation 967–8
  diagnosis 968
  etiology and pathophysiology 967
  management 968
  ocular disease 831–2
  prevention 969
  vaccination *953*, 969
feline infectious peritonitis (FIP) 563–4, 959–64
  clinical presentation 959–61
  CNS 563–4, 615–16
  diagnosis 961–3
  etiology 959
  management 964
  ocular disease 564, 615, 616, 829–30, 960–1
  pathophysiology 959
  prevention/vaccination 964
feline leukemia virus (FeLV) 964–7
  anemia 706–7
  association with AML 742–3
  clinical presentation 965
  diagnosis 965
  differential diagnosis 965
  etiology 964
  management 965–7
  ocular disease 830–1
  pathophysiology 964–5
  vaccination *953*, 967
feline lower urinary tract disease (FLUTD) 487–93
  clinical presentation 488
  diagnosis 488–9
  etiology 487
  management 489–92
  pathophysiology 487–8
feline panleukopenia virus (FPL/feline parvovirus) 831, 969–71
  vaccination *953–4*, 971
feline plague 957–9
feline psychogenic alopecia 804–5
feline sarcoma virus 832
female reproductive tract, radiography 528–30
femoral condyle, osteochondrosis 677
femoral head
  aseptic necrosis (Legg–Calvé–Perthes disease) 670–1
  DJD *639*
  luxation *641*
femoral pulse 196
femoropatellar luxation 674–6
fenbendazole 44, 45, 132, 291, 298, 299, 316, 1103
fenoldopam 456
fentanyl
  intravenous *1054*
  transdermal *377*, 1038–9, *1054*
fetus, radiography 528, 530
fever of unknown origin (FUO) 61–7
  differential diagnosis *62–4*
fexofenadine *792*
fiber, dietary 319, *323*, 441, 1075
fibrin 747, 763
fibrinolysis 747–8
  disorders 757–8, 763
  in liver disease 765, 766
fibrocartilaginous embolic myelopathy 582–3
fibrosarcoma 97, 261, 661
  retrobulbar *864*
fibrotic myopathies 632–3
filariasis, ocular 844, *868*
fine-needle aspirate, liver *51*
fipronil *787*
  toxicity 881
firocoxib *640*, *1042*, *1047*
fistulas
  bronchoesophageal 267–8
  perianal 329–30
  urorectal *480*, 482, 484–5
  urovaginal *480*, 482, 484–5
flavoxate *485*
fleas
  feline plague transmission 957
  hypersensitivity to 793–4
flow cytometry 998
flow-by oxygen 11
fluconazole 566, 835, 938, 978, 979
  systemic mycoses *947–8*
5-flucytosine 835, 978–9
fludrocortisone acetate 418–19
fluid overload 455
fluid therapy
  AKI 455–6
  cholecalciferol toxicity 458
  diabetic ketoacidosis 439, *440*
  head trauma 570, 1022–3
  hypoadrenocorticism 417–18
  hypovolemic shock 1019–22
  pancreatitis 373, 375
  parvovirus infection 287
  protein-losing nephropathy 474
  pulmonary disease 1023
  raised ICP 1022–3
  severe hemorrhage 1022
  subcutaneous in CKD 462, *463*
  therapy planning 1016–19
fluids
  colloids 569, 1014–16
  crystalloids 1011–14
flukes, liver 337
fluorescent in situ hybridization (FISH) 320
fluoroquinolones 287, 289
5-fluorouracil, ingestion 896
fly larva, ocular (ophthalmomyiasis) 871–2
folate deficiency 704
folliculitis
  pyotraumatic 779, *780*
  staphylococcal 781–2
food hypersensitivity *781*, *782*, 795–6
foods
  causing urine coloration 23
  commercial pet foods 1065, *1066*
  toxic *451*, 458–9, 891–2, 905–7, 1122–3
foot pads
  in aortic thromboembolism 761
  ulceration 346–7
foreign bodies (FBs)
  causing pericarditis 235–6
  colorectal 321
  esophagus 173–4, 259–60

hairballs 29, *30*, *279*
ingested 29–30, 535–6
inhaled 143
metal 902–5
nasal 57, 58, 112–13
pharyngeal 255
small intestines 296, *297*, 539–41
stomach *272*, 278–9, *280–1*, 535–6
urethral *75*
fractures
jaw 94–5
skull *571*
spinal 584–7
fragmented coronoid process 646–8
fresh frozen plasma 756, 764, 766, 888
fucosidosis 553, 869–70
funduscopy, cryptococcosis *65*, 978
fungal culture *774*
furosemide
feline cardiomyopathy *229*
heart failure *209*, 210
hypercalcemia 411
in AKI 456
systemic hypertension *240*
furunculosis
anal 329–30
staphylococcal 782–3
Fusobacterium spp. 783

G-cells 269, *270*
gabapentin 55, 551, 602, 1033, 1043, 1044
dose and characteristics *1056*
gait abnormalities, neuromuscular disorders 617
galactocerebrosidosis 875
gallbladder, mucoceles 352–3
gallstones 351–2
gamma-aminobutyric acid (GABA) blockade 881
gamma-glutamyltransferase (GGT) 48–9, *50*, 334
gangliosidosis 553, 727, 875
GM1 875
GM2 *552*, 875
garlic *1050*
gas
bladder 439, 532
esophagus 172–3, *174*
free peritoneal 514–15
spleen 521
gastric acid production 269, *270*
inhibitors *272*
gastric dilatation and volvulus (GDV) 30, 277–8, 521, 536–7, *538*
radiography 536–7, *538*
secondary changes 537
gastric lavage 888
gastric outlet obstruction 278–81, 534–5
gastrin (CCK type 2) receptors 269, *270*
gastrinomas 274
gastritis
acute 270
chronic 270–2
eosinophilic 271
gastrointestinal (GI) decontamination 756, 888, 903
gastrointestinal (GI) protectants *272*, 276–7, *457*, 1049–50
gastrointestinal (GI) tract
disorders causing vomiting *28*
motility 41, 281–2, 312
motility modifiers *283*, 931–2
radiography 534–43
colon 541–3
small intestines 538–41
stomach 534–8
ulceration 274–7
gastropexy 278
gastroscopy
acute NSAID toxicosis 276
Helicobacter spp. infection 273
gastrostomy tube 1068, 1070
gentamicin *508*, 919, 959
ghost cells 690, 695, *696*
Giardia duodenalis 298
giardiasis 298–9
GIF-Tube 462, *463*
ginger *1050*
gingivitis 86, 87
ginkgo *1050*
ginseng *1050*
Glasgow Coma Scale (GCS), modified 545, 570
glaucoma, secondary *854*
gliomas 556, *558*
globoid cell leukodystrophy (Krabbe's disease) 875
glomerular filtration rate (GFR) 450, 457
glomerular membrane 450, *452*, 468
glomerulonephritis 468, 471–4
glomerulosclerosis 460
glossopharyngeal nerve 258
glucagon, intravenous 446–7
glucocorticoids
brain tumors 557
causing polydipsia/polyuria 34
eosinophilic bronchopneumopathy 133
feline bronchial syndrome 137
hepatopathy 355–6, 518
in cough 55
inhaled 55, 124, 137
laryngeal edema 122
see also corticosteroids
glucose
blood 378, 439
high (hyperglycemia) 424, 439, 444
low (hypoglycemia) 445–8, 554–5
monitoring in insulin therapy 439, 442–5
urinary 453
glucose tolerance, acromegaly 391
glutamate 1027
glutamine 1065
glutathione 340
glycated proteins 443
glycopyrrolate *244*
glycosaminoglycans (GAGs) 488, 553
goblet cells 314, *315*
goiter 405
gracilis myopathy 632
granulocyte colony-stimulating factor (G-CSF) 712, 724
human recombinant 932
granulocyte/macrophage colony-stimulating factor (GM-CSF) 712, 724
granuloma, eosinophilic 102–3, 806–8
granulomas
aspergillosis *939*
cryptococcal *944*
histoplasmosis *944*
granulomatous colitis 319–21
granulomatous enteritis *306*
granulomatous meningoencephalitis (GME) 566–7, 855–6
grapes, toxicity *451*, 458–9, 891–2
grapiprant 640
grass awns, migrating 235–6
'gray Collie syndrome' 721
Great Danes, inherited myopathy 629
great vessels, enlarged 183–5
Greyhounds, canine influenza 925
grooming (self-grooming), lack of 101
growth deformities 648–50

growth hormone (GH) 388, 389
  excess secretion (acromegaly) 391–3
  inadequate secretion 388–91
  stimulation test *390*
  therapeutic 391
growth plates
  delayed ossification 399, *400*
  lead deposition *903*
  premature closure 648–50
growth retardation
  differential diagnosis *389–90*
  hypopituitarism 388–9

Hageman factor (factor XII) deficiency 747, 753–5
hair coat
  in hyperadrenocorticism 423
  in hyperthyroidism 405
  in hypopituitarism 389
  in hypothyroidism 398, *399*
hairballs, feline 29, *30*, *279*
hard-pad disease, *see* canine distemper virus
harvest mite 790
head tilt 572–4
head trauma 569–72, 1023
heart
  auscultation 197–9
  palpation 197
  radiography 178–83
  size evaluation 178
heart sounds 197–8
  muffled 78
heartworm
  canine 240–2
  drug resistance 242
  feline 242–3
  French 131–2, 241, 1101–3
  prophylaxis 242
  radiography 193, *194*
heartworm associated respiratory disease (HARD) 242, 243
Heinz bodies 695, *696*, 710, *894*, 905
Helicobacter spp. 272–3
  eradication *274*
hemangiosarcoma 660–1
  cardiac *155*, *156*, 233, 235
hematemesis *30*, 275, *750*
hematochezia *39*, *40*, *43*, 321
hematocrit (Hct)
  calculation 682
  polycythemia vera 742
hematoma, thoracic wall 163
hematuria 23, *24*, *26*, 69
heme protein 24
Hemerocallis toxicity *451*
hemilaminectomy 594, *595*
hemivertebrae 605
hemodialysis 459, 468
hemoglobin 682
  oxygen saturation 78, *79*
hemoglobinuria 23, 24, *26*, 894, *895*
hemolysis
  acetaminophen-induced 894, *895*
  see also anemia, hemolytic
hemophilias 747, 753–5
hemoplasmas 693–4, 956–7
hemorrhage
  acute 687–8, 751
  blood transfusion 751
  fluid resuscitation 1022
  nasal (epistaxis) 57–9
hemorrhagic gastroenteritis, *see* acute hemorrhagic diarrhea syndrome
hemostasis
  primary 745–6
    disorders 748–52
  secondary 746–7
    disorders 753–7
hemostatic resuscitation 1022
hemostatins 763
hemothorax *140*, *165*
heparins 759, *762*
hepatic encephalopathy 333–4, 335, 346, *357*, *358*
  management 554
  nutritional support 1076
hepatic lipidosis
  canine *333*, 356–7
  feline 334–7, 1075–6
  management 1076
hepatitis
  acute 343–4
  canine chronic 340–2, 1095–6
  canine infectious (CIH) 825–6, 924
hepatocellular carcinoma 354
hepatocellular degeneration/necrosis 343–4
hepatocutaneous syndrome 346–8, 802
hepatocytes, damage/toxicity 344
hepatojugular reflux 196–7
hepatomegaly 354, 424–5, 518–19
  classification 518
  focal 519
  nodular 519
hepatopathy, vacuolar and steroid 355–6, 518
hepatotoxicity 344, 349, 765
Hepatozoon americanum 730
Hepatozoon canis 730
hepatozoonosis 730–1
herb–drug interactions *1050*
hereditary nonspherocytic hemolytic anemia 698
hernia
  diaphragmatic *139*, 149–51, *152–4*
  hiatal 175, 268–9
  perineal 330–2
herniorrhaphy, diaphragm 151, *154*
herpesvirus
  canine 823
  feline (FHV-1) 101, 826–9, *953–4*, 973–6
Heterobilharzia americana 296–7
heterotopic bone 192–3
hiatal hernia 175, 268–9
hindlimbs
  hyperextension 616
  muscle atrophy 598, 626
hip dysplasia 640–2
histamine type 2 (H2) receptor blockers *272*, 276–7, *457*, 467, 1049
histamine type 2 receptors 269, *270*
histiocytic neoplasia 1007
histiocytoma 812–13
Histoplasma capsulatum 300, 731–2, 835, 944, *945*, 1115–16
histoplasmosis 317, 731–2
  clinical signs 943–4, *946*
  intestinal 300–1
  ocular 835–6, *837*
  systemic 943–8, 1115–16
  treatment protocols *947*
history taking 3–8
Holter recording 199, *200*, 225
homeopathic nosodes 913
hookworms 290–2
horizontal beam radiography 514–15
Horner's syndrome 574, 575, 589, 607, 852
  clinical presentation 852
  diagnosis 852
  etiology and pathophysiology 852
household management, for cats 489–92
Household Resource questionnaire *490–2*

human disease
  Bordetella bronchiseptica 913
  cat scratch (CSD) 950, 951
  toxoplasmosis 982–3
  see also public health
humeral head, osteochondrosis *653*
hydralazine *209*, *240*
hydration status 1016–17
hydrocephalus, congenital 548–50
hydrochlorothiazide *209*, 210, *240*, 396
hydrocortisone sodium succinate 418
hydromorphone 1039, *1054*
hydronephrosis 487, 504–5
hydroxycobalamine *23*
hydroxyethyl starches 1015–16
hydroxyurea 559
hydroxyzine *792*
hyperadrenocorticism (Cushing's disease) *239*, 419–33
  adrenal-dependent 420, 432–3
  bone disease 656–7
  clinical presentation 420–3, 656
    polydipsia/polyuria *34*, *35*, 421, 424
  diagnosis 423–9, 656–7
  etiology 656
  hepatopathy 355–6, 518
  management 430–3
  myopathy 626
  pituitary-dependent 393–4, 419–20, 430–2, 657
hyperaldosteronism, primary 433–5, 1109
hyperalgesia 1025, 1029, 1030, 1033
hyperbilirubinemia 47
hypercalcemia
  causes of canine *495*
  differential diagnoses *411*
  hyperparathyroidism 411, *412*
  hypoadrenocorticism 416
  ocular signs 844
  polydipsia/polyuria *34*, *35*
  rodenticide toxicity 756, 889
  treatment 889
hypercalciuria 495
hypercholesterolemia 399–400, 424
hypercoagulation, *see* thrombosis
hypereosinophilic syndrome, cats 714–15
hyperfiltration 460
hypergammaglobulinemia, polyclonal 963
hyperglycemia 439
  cataract formation 858–9
  in hyperadrenocorticism 424
  insulin-induced 444
hyperkalemia 416, *417*, 456, *457*, 489
  ECG *417*, 455, *457*, *489*
  management *457*
hyperkeratosis *772*, 798–9
hyperlipidemia
  obesity 1084
  ocular signs 845–7, 865–6
  pancreatitis *366*
hypernatremia 555–6
hyperparathyroidism 410–11
  primary 410
  renal secondary 463, 465
  skeletal disease 654–5
hyperphosphatemia 409, 463, 465, 889
hyperpigmentation *772*, *786*, *791*, 817, *818*
hypersensitivities
  Arthus-type reaction 825
  cutaneous 791–7
  eosinophilia 713
  feline indolent ulcer 808
  food *781*, *782*, 795–6
  mosquito bite 796–7
  neomycin 1117–18
  type I (immediate) 990, *991*
  type II (antibody-mediated) 991
  type III (immune complex) 991–2
  type IV (delayed) 992
hypertension 474–9
  arterial 461, 475, 848, *849–51*
  clinical presentation 475–6
  diagnosis 476–8
  in protein-losing nephropathy 474
  ocular disease 475, *475*, 847, 848, *849–51*
  pathophysiology 475
  systemic 238–40, 433–4, 435, 474–5
hyperthyroidism *34*, *35*, 404–8
hypertrophic cardiomyopathy (HCM)
  canine 225–6
  feline 226–30
  in hyperthyroidism 405, 406
  thrombus 761
hypertrophic obstructive cardiomyopathy (HOCM) *197*
hypertrophic osteodystrophy 655–6
hyperviscosity *239*
  syndrome 844–5, 1118–22
hypervitaminosis A 663–4
hyphema *750*
  anemia *847*
  etiologies *842*
  hyperlipidemia *846*
  hypertension *849*, *851*
  uveitis *869*
hypoadrenocorticism
  anemia 701–2
  eosinophilia 713–14
  lymphocytosis 716–17
  polydipsia/polyuria *34*, *35*, 421
  primary (Addison's disease) 414–19, 713–14
  secondary 419
hypoalbuminemia 309, 311, 334
hypocalcemia 408, 409, 444
hypochondroplasia 646
hypochlorite bleach, ingestion 898–9
hypodontia 90–1
hypoglobulinemia 305
hypoglycemia 554–5
  clinical signs 446, 555
  in hypoadrenocorticism 416
  insulinoma 445–6
  management 447–8, 555
hypoglycemic agents 395–6
hypokalemia *34*, *35*, 433–4, 463
  differential diagnosis of feline *434*
  management 435
  myopathy 629–30, 1109
hyponatremia 416, 419, 556
hypoparathyroidism 409–10
hypophosphatemia 336, 698
hypophysectomy 432
hypopituitarism, congenital 388–91
hypoproteinemia 373–4
hypothalamic–pituitary–adrenal axis 411–13
hypothalamus 387, *388*
  thirst center 36
hypothyroidism *366*, 397–404
  anemia 701–2
  clinical presentation 398–9, 620
  congenital (cretinism) 397–8, 398–9
  diagnosis 399–402
  etiology 397–8
  management 402–3
  myopathy 625–7
  myxedema 403–4
  ocular signs *866*
  secondary 389, 391

hypovolemic shock
  fluid resuscitation 1020–2
  identification 1019–20

ibotenic acid 892
icterus 47–51
  anemia 681
  clinical approach 48–51
  etiology 47, 681
  hepatic *49*
  hepatic lipidosis 334–5
  imaging 49–51
  leptospirosis 920
  posthepatic 49
  prehepatic 49
idiopathic pulmonary fibrosis (IPF) 134–5, 1100–1
idoxuridine 829
ileocolic junction 314
ileus
  functional 293, 541
  gastric 535
  paralytic 312
iliopsoas fibrotic myopathy 632
imidacloprid, toxicity 882
imidacloprid–moxidectin 786, *787*
imidocarb dipropionate 699, 941
imipramine 1042–3
immune response
  adaptive 987–90
  innate 985–7
immune-mediated diseases 992
  allergic 993
  autoimmune 993
  causing FUO 61, *62*, *63*
  laboratory diagnosis 994–9
  neoplasia 994, 1006–7
    diagnosis 998–9
immune-mediated hemolytic anemia (IMHA) 49, 688–92
  clinical case 1125–6
  clinical presentation 689
  diagnosis 689–91
  management 691–2
  nonregenerative 703–4
  pathophysiology 689, 991
immune-mediated thrombocytopenia 690, 751–2, 1125–6
immunodeficiency
  feline viral, *see* feline immunodeficiency virus
  primary 993–4, 1004–6
  severe combined 723–4, 994
  Weimaraner 1005
immunoelectrophoresis *998*, 999
immunoglobulin A (IgA), deficiency 1004
immunohistochemistry 313, 314, 962–3, 996, *997*
immunomodulation therapy *966*
immunophenotyping 998
immunosuppression
  cyclosporine 330
  feline inflammatory liver disease 340
  inflammatory bowel disease 307, *308*
  in protein-losing nephropathy 473
impetigo 779–80
inborn errors of metabolism 552–3
incontinence, *see* fecal incontinence; urinary incontinence
indolent ulcer, feline 808
inflammatory bowel disease (IBD)
  colonic 318–19
  small bowel *40*, 302–9
influenza, canine 925–6
infraspinatus myopathy 632
inhaled medications, steroids 55, 124, 137
inotropes, positive *209*
insecticide, toxicity 879–85
insulin, inhibition 447–8
insulin resistance 445, 1084
insulin therapy
  diabetes
    uncomplicated 441
    unstable 443–5
  diabetic ketoacidosis 439–40
  hyperkalemia *457*
  pancreatitis 378
insulin-like growth factor-1 (IGF-1) *390*
insulinoma 18, 445–8, 555, 620–1
interferons
  dermatologic disorders *801*
  feline panleukopenia virus 970–1
  herpesvirus infection 829
interleukins (IL) 988
International Renal Interest Society (IRIS), staging of CKD 462
intertrigo 776–9
intervertebral disk disease 642–4
  clinical presentation 643
  diagnosis 643
  etiology 642
  Hansen type I 591–4, 642–3
  Hansen type II 594–5, 642–3
  management 593–4, 644
  osteomyelitis/diskospondylitis 611–13, 665–6, 918
intervertebral stenosis, lumbosacral *72*, 73
intestinal lymphangiectasia, primary idiopathic *307*, 309, 310
intestinal motility
  abnormal 41, 281–2, 312
  modifiers *283*, 931–2
intestinal mucosa 41, 285, 286
  biopsies 305, *306*
intracranial pressure (ICP)
  head trauma 569–70
  lowering 545, 570, 572
  raised 545, 874, 1022
    fluid therapy 1022–3
intradermal allergy test (IDAT) *776*, 791, 794
intrapleural pressure gradient 140
intravenous catheters, thromboembolism 758–9
intussusception 295
iodine
  dietary 407
  radioactive therapy 408
ion channels, muscle 630–1
iridocyclitis, *see* anterior uveitis
iris
  color change *854*, 868, *869*
  hyperpigmentation *831*
  lymphosarcoma *856–7*
  neovascularization *822*, *829*, *868*
iron
  deficiency 78, 702–3
  toxicity 904–5
islet cell tumors, functional (insulinomas) 18, 445–8, 555, 620–1
isoproterenol *244*
isosorbide dinitrate *209*
Isospora spp. 292–3
itraconazole 108, 111, 302, 566, 938
  cryptococcosis 978
  feline aspergillosis 980
  histoplasmosis 836
  systemic mycoses *947–8*
ivermectin
  causing chorioretinitis 870, *871*
  demodicosis 786, *787*
  heartworm 242
  nasal mites 113

sensitivity testing 786
toxicity 883
Ixodes spp. 623, 914, 934, 935, 950

jaundice, *see* icterus
jaw
dropped 93, 576–7
fractures 94–5
length discrepancy *88*
jejunum, mucosa 285, 286
joint disease
degenerative 638–40
see also arthritis
'joint mice' 653
jugular veins, examination 196–7

kallikrein *362*
kanamycin *508*
Kartagener's syndrome 130
'kennel cough', *see* canine infectious respiratory disease (CIRD)
keratic precipitates, 'mutton fat' 829, *830*
keratitis, herpesvirus *827*, 828, *974*, 975
keratoconjunctivitis sicca (KCS) 823, *824*, *825*, 860
keratopathy
calcific band 865
lipid 865–6
keratosis, zinc-responsive 867
keratouveitis, leishmaniasis 832
ketamine 1044, *1055*
ketoconazole 108, 330, 432, 835, 836, 978
ketoprofen *1046*
Key–Gaskell syndrome (feline dysautonomia) 853
kidneys
biopsy 471–2
cystic disease 503–4
displacement 528
drug excretion 457
enlarged (renomegaly) 524, *526*
histoplasmosis *944*
polycystic 524
radiography 524–5, *526–8*
small irregular 524, *526*
tumors 505–6
uroliths 524–5, *527*
'kissing lesion' 117, *118*
Klebsiella spp. 128, 562
Kleiber equation 1064
Krabbe's disease (globoid cell leukodystrophy) 875
kyphosis, thoracolumbar pain 592

Labrador Retrievers
exercise-induced collapse 631–2
myopathy (centronuclear myopathy) 628–9
lacrimal system disease 860–1
lactulose *326*, 331, 554
laminectomy 594–5
'lance' canines 88
Langerhans cells 986
lanthanum carbonate 466
large intestines
anatomy and physiology 314–15
diarrhea *39*, 45, *46*, 322
inflammatory disease 318–19
neoplasia 326–7, 542, *543*
see also colon
larva migrans
cutaneous 292
ocular 344
laryngeal collapse 117, *119*
laryngeal edema 121–2
laryngeal paralysis
cats 120–1
dogs 119–20, 619–20
laryngeal tumors 121
laryngoscopy 117, *118*, *119*
latex cryptococcal antigen agglutination test (LCAT) 978
laxatives *326*, 331
lead poisoning 673–4, *675*, 708–9, 902–4
leflunomide *801*
left atrium
echocardiography 205
enlargement 181, *182*
thrombus 229, *230*, 1108–9
left atrium to aortic ratio (LA/Ao) 205
left bundle branch block *202*
left ventricle
echocardiography 204
enlargement 181
outflow tract obstruction (LVOTO) 226
left ventricular internal diameter in end-diastole (LCIDd) 204–5
Legg–Calvé–Perthes disease 670–1
leiomyoma 261
leiomyosarcoma 312–13
leishmaniasis 731, 832
Leptospira interrogans serovars 920
leptospirosis 821, 919–22
acute kidney injury *451*, 457
diagnosis 454
vaccination *912*, 921–2
Leptotrombidium subquadratum 790
leukemias
acute lymphoblastic 737–8
chronic lymphocytic 736–7
myeloid 739–43
leukocyte adhesion deficiency, canine (CLAD) 725, *726*, 1005
leukocytes
abnormal nuclear morphology 724–8
infectious agents 728–32
leukocytosis 711–18
leukogram, stress 423
leukopenia 718–24
levetiracetam 554
lichenification *772*, *791*
lidocaine *249*, 250, *251*, 1042, 1043–4
doses and characteristics *1056*
life span, factors in 1082–3
lifestyle, and obesity 1082, 1092
Lilium spp., toxicity *451*, 458–9, 891
limb deformities 648–50
lime sulfur *787*
lincomycin *773*
lipase *362*, 372
lipemia 424
lipemia retinalis 846
lipid emulsions, IV 383
lipidosis
canine hepatic *333*, 356–7
corneal 398, *399*, *846*, 865–6
feline hepatic 334–7, 1075–6
lipoma, thoracic wall 162
lipoprotein lipase deficiency 846
listening skills 7
liver
abscesses 342–3, 520
enlargement 354, 424–5, 518–19
imaging 49–51, 518–20
toxins 344, 349, 765
liver biopsy
canine chronic hepatitis 342
feline hepatic lipidosis 336
feline inflammatory liver disease *338*, *339*
liver disease
acute hepatitis/hepatocellular degeneration 343–4
anemia 701

liver disease – *contd*
canine chronic hepatitis 340–2, 1095–6
canine infectious hepatitis 825–6, 924
causing polydipsia/polyuria *34*, *35*
cirrhosis 344–6
clinical signs 333–4
coagulation abnormalities 765–6
cycad palm toxicity 1105–6
drug-induced 349
familial copper toxicity 348–9
feline inflammatory 337–40
icterus 48–51
iron intoxication 904, *905*
lipidosis 334–7, 356–7, 1075–6
masses/tumors *51*, 353–5, 519
metabolic alterations 333
nutrition 1075–6
liver enzymes 34, 48–9, 335
liver flukes *49*, 337
lobar sign *180*, 189
lobster claw deformity (ectrodactyly) 645–6
local anesthetics 1042, 1043–4
doses and characteristics *1056*
lomustine *801*
loperamide 44, 294
loratadine *792*
low-grade alimentary lymphoma (LGAL) 313–14
low-molecular-weight heparin (LMWH) 759, *762*
lower airway disease, diagnosis 125–7
lufenuron, toxicity 883–4
lumbosacral stenosis, degenerative (cauda equina syndrome) 597–9, 644–5
lung sounds 78
lungs
biopsy 126–7
lobe torsion *139*, 148–50
lobectomy 130, 142, 148
metastases 15, *192*, 425
nodules 191, 193
radiography 187, 189–94
size 189
lupoid onychitis 819
luxation 674–6
elbow 649, *650*, *675*
femoral head *641*
femoropatellar 674–6
patellar 674–6
TMJ 93–4
Lyme disease 913–17
nephropathy 914–15
ocular signs 821
vaccination *912*
lymph flow, alteration 723
lymph nodes
gastric *284*
mediastinal 175, *176–7*
sublumbar 523–4
lymphangiectasia, primary intestinal *307*, 309, 310
lymphangiosarcoma *146*
lymphoblast 735
lymphocytes, granular 716, 729
lymphocytic–plasmacytic cholangitis 337, *338*
lymphocytosis 715–17
chronic inflammatory 716
chronic lymphocytic leukemia 737
physiologic (excitement/shift) 715
lymphoid hypoplasia 723
lymphoid neoplasia 734–9
lymphoma 734–6, 994
alimentary 312–14
cutaneous T-cell 812, *813*
diagnosis 998
gastric 282–4
hepatic *51*, 354–5
in FIV/FeLV 965, *966*
intraocular 856–8
mediastinum *176–7*
nasal (cats) 112
renal 505–6
spinal 610–11
tonsillar 254, *255*
lymphopenia 423, 722–4
lymphoplasmacytic enteritis *306*, 307
lymphosarcoma
intraocular 830–1, 856–8
myocardial infiltration 226
L-lysine 975
lysosomal storage diseases 552–3, 726–7, 874–5

macrocyclic lactones 242
macroglobulinemia, IgM 1118–22
macrothrombocytopenia 733
macules *770*, *794*
magnetic resonance imaging (MRI) 679
brain
bacterial encephalitis *562*
cerebrovascular disease 546–7
CLMS 551
cryptococcosis 565, *566*
FIP 564
GME 567
hydrocephalus 549
intracranial arachnoid cyst 551
necrotizing meningoencephalitis 567
pituitary mass *392*, *394*
thiamine deficiency 568, *569*
trauma 570, *571*
tumors 557, *558*
musculoskeletal disorders 679
peripheral nerve sheath tumors 578, 607, *608*
spinal 582
arachnoid diverticula 602–3
cervical spondylomyelopathy 596, *597*
Chiari-like malformation 602
diskospondylitis 612
fibrocartilaginous embolus 583
fractures 586, *587*
IVDD 593
lumbosacral stenosis 599
lymphoma 611
nephroblastoma 610
synovial cysts 600, *601*
main pulmonary artery, enlargement 183, *184*
maintenance energy requirement (MER) 1090
major histocompatibility complex (MHC) 986–7, 989
Malassezia pachydermatis 774, 785–6, *810*
male reproductive tract
radiography 530–1
see also prostate gland
malignant hyperthermia (MH) 633–4
malignant melanoma, oral 97
malnutrition
laboratory markers 1062
muscle wasting 1061–2, *1063*
malocclusion 88–9
mandible
fibrosarcoma *661*
fractures 94–5
osteopathy 653–4
mandibular brachygnathism *88*
mannitol 456, 545, 570–1, 888, 1023
contraindications 456
mannosidosis 726–7, 875
marbofloxacin *778*, 950, 954

maropitant *28*, 55, *296*, 375, *457*, 574, 971
mast cell tumors 274, 276, 813–14, *867*
mast cells 718, 990, *991*
masticatory muscles
  atrophy 577–9, 1110–11
  myositis (MMM) 256–7, 861–2
mastocytemia 718
mavacoxib 1052
maxilla, fractures 94, 95
mean cell hemoglobin concentration (MCHC) 682
mean cell volume (MCV) 682–3
meclizine 574
medetomidine 1040, *1042*, *1055*
mediastinum
  gas (pneumomediastinum) 170
  lymph nodes 175, *176–7*
  masses 165, *166*, 171, *174*
  radiography 168–77
  shift 170, *171*
medroxyprogesterone acetate 391
megacolon 323, *324*
megaesophagus 172–3, *174*, 265–7, 624
megaloblastosis 740
melarsomine dihydrochloride 241
melena *39*, *40*, 275, *750*
meloxicam *1046*, *1047*, 1051–2
  relative efficacy *640*
  transmucosal oral spray 1051–2
membrane stabilizers 1041–4, *1056*
membranoproliferative glomerulonephritis (MPGN) 469, *470*
membranous nephropathy (MN) 469, *471*
meningiomas 556–9, 606, *864*
meningitis, FIP 615–16
meningitis–arteritis, steroid-responsive (SRMA) 613–14
meningoencephalitis
  bacterial 562
  granulomatous (GME) 566–7, 855–6
  necrotizing 567–8
meperidine (pethidine) 1039, *1054*
mepivacaine *1056*
2-mercaptoethanol rapid slide agglutination test (ME-RSAT) 919
mesenteric venous portography *359*
mesothelioma
  cardiac 235
  pleural *154*, *156*
metabolic acidosis
  in AKI 456–7
  in CKD 462–3
metabolic disorders
  and obesity 1084
  bone 651–7
  brain 554–5
  causing vomiting *28*
  causing weakness *20*
  dermatologic 802–3
  storage diseases 552–3, 726–7, 874–5
metal foreign bodies 902–5
metaldehyde toxicity 885–6
metaphyseal osteopathy (hypertrophic osteodystrophy) 655–6
metastases
  liver 354
  pulmonary 15, *192*, 425
  spinal 73, 608–9
  vertebral body 608–9
methadone 1039, 1044, *1054*, *1055*
methemoglobinemia 710–11, 893–4, 905
methenamine hippurate 508–9
methimazole 349, 407, 408
methocarbamol 885, 886, 890
methylene blue 23, 895
methylprednisolone 312, *801*
methylpyrazole 458, 901
methylsulfonylmethane (MSM) 472
methylxanthines 906–7
4-methylypyrazole 458, 901
metoclopramide *28*, 264, *283*, *296*, 375, *457*, 932
metronidazole *274*, 296, 299, 306, 311, 324–5, 554, 923
  toxicity 576
mexiletine 225, 250, *251*
microangiopathic hemolytic anemia 696–7
microbiota, intestinal 303, 305–6
microcardia 187, 416, *417*
microfilariae 240, 241, *696*
microhepatica 358, *359*, 519
microscopic agglutination test (MAT) 454, 921
Microsporum canis 784–5
milbemycin 113, 132, 242, 316, *787*
miliary dermatitis, feline 805–6
milk thistle exract (silymarin) 340
mineral oil *326*
minerals 1067
minimum inhibitory concentration (MIC) test 507
minocycline *778*, *916*, 936
miosis 852
mirtazapine 467, 971
misoprostol *272*, 277, 458, *1049*, 1050
mites
  Cheyletiella spp. *775*, *787*, 789–90
  Demodex spp. 786–8, *866*, 867
  ear *787*, 789
  nasal 113
  scabies *787*, 788–9
  Trombiculidae (chiggers) 790–1
mitotane 394, 414, *415*, 430–2, 433
mitoxantrone 657
mitral valve disease *182*, *188*
  degenerative 219–21
  dysplasia *211*, 217–18
mitratapide 1092
monocytosis 717–18, 741
monoplegia, forelimb 589
morphine 1038, 1039, *1054*
mosapride *283*
mosquitoes
  heartworm transmission 240
  hypersensitivity 796–7
mothballs, ingestion 902
motor deficits
  forelimb 580
  hindlimb 581
mouth, difficulty/pain on opening 257
moxidectin 316
moxifloxacin *778*
mucoceles
  gallbladder 352–3
  salivary glands 255–6
mucociliary clearance, impairment 130–1
mucocutaneous pyoderma 780–1
mucolipidosis II 875
mucolytics 116
mucopolysaccharidoses (MPS) 553, 726–7, 875–6
mucosa
  intestinal 41, 285, 286
    biopsy 305, *306*
  stomach 274–5
mucous membranes
  cyanosis 195
  dark red 740, *741*
  discoloration 23
  pale 681
mucus, feces 41

multiple myeloma 738, 1007
  diagnosis 999
  pathophysiology 1006–7
muscarine 892
muscimol 892
muscle atrophy
  hepatic lipidosis 335
  hindlimb 598, 626
  inherited myopathy in Great Danes 629
  masticatory muscles 577–9, 1110–11
  muscular dystrophy 627–8
  steroid myopathy 625–6
muscle biopsies 21, *257*, 619
muscle condition scoring 1061–2, *1063*
muscle relaxation, in tetanus 923
muscular dystrophy 627–8
musculoskeletal disorders 637–9
  advanced diagnostics 679–80
  anomalies 645–6
  degenerative 638–40
  history and examination 637–8
  idiopathic 670–3
  inflammation 664–70
  metabolic 651–7
  neoplastic 657–63
  nutritional 663–4
  toxic and traumatic 673–9
mushroom toxicity 892–3
myasthenia gravis (MG) 18, 624–5
  clinical presentation 624–5
  diagnosis 21, 625
  focal 265–7
  management 266, 625
  pathophysiology 624
mycobacteria, atypical (opportunistic) 816
Mycobacterium spp. *729*
Mycobacterium smegmatis 784
mycophenolate *473*, *801*
Mycoplasma spp., ocular disease 822–3
Mycoplasma felis infection 952–3
Mycoplasma haemocanis 694
Mycoplasma haemofelis 693–4, 956–7
mycoses, systemic 943–8
mycotic rhinosinusitis 105–10
myelitis
  canine distemper virus 615, 928, 930
  feline infectious peritonitis 615–16
  protozoal 616–17
myeloblasts 743
myelodysplastic syndrome 739–40
myelofibrosis 705–6, *707*, 742
myelography 582, 643
myelopathy
  degenerative 590–1
  fibrocartilaginous embolic 582–3
myelophthisis 705–6
myeloproliferative neoplasia (MPN) 740–2
myocarditis 230–3
  canine parvovirus 931
  clinical presentation 231–2
  diagnosis 232
  etiology 230
  management 232–3
  pathophysiology 230–1
  Trypanosoma cruzi 231–3
myocardium
  depressed contractility *79*
  fibro-fatty replacement 224
myoglobinuria 23, 25, *26*, 618, 633–4
myopathies *20*, 625–35
  dystrophic 627–8
  endocrine 625–7
  fibrotic 632–3
  hypokalemic 629–30, 1109
  immune-mediated 634–5
  infectious 634
  inherited in Great Danes 629
  nondystrophic congenital 628–31
myosin binding protein C (MyBPC3) gene 227
myositis
  extraocular muscles 862–3
  masticatory muscles 256–7, 861–2
myotonia, hyperadrenocorticism 421–2
myotonia congenita 630–1
myxedema 403–4
  of skin 398, *399*

N-methyl-D-aspartate (NMDA) antagonists 1044, *1045*
  doses and characteristics *1055*
N-methyl-D-aspartate (NMDA) receptor 1027, *1028*
nalbuphine *1055*
naphthalene 902
nares
  hyperkeratosis 107, *108*
  stenosis 105, *108*
nasal adenocarcinoma *558*
nasal bleeding (epistaxis) 57–9
nasal catheters 11–12
nasal cavity disorders
  aspergillosis 107, 937
  clinical signs 105, *106*
  foreign body 57, 58, 112–13
  tumors 111–12, *558*
nasal planum
  CLE 1001
  erosion in aspergillosis 937
  hyperkeratosis 107, *108*
nasodigital hyperkeratosis 798–9
nasoenteral feeding tubes 1068, *1069*
nasopharyngeal polyps 113–14, 575
nasopharyngeal stenosis 113, *114*
nasopharyngeal tube 975
natriuretic peptides 205–6, 228
natural killer (NK) cells 988
neck
  stabilization 604
  ventroflexion 433, 434, *569*, 630
  see also cervical spine disorders
necrolytic migratory erythema (NME) 802–3
necrotizing meningo(leuko) encephalitis 567–8
Negri bodies *972*
neomycin 554, 1117–18
neonatal isoerythrolysis (NI) 692–3
neoplasia
  adrenal 421, 425, 426, *427*, 432–3, 434
  anal sacs 328–9
  bladder 484
  bone 657–63
  brain 556–9, *865*
  cardiac 226, 233, 234, 235
  causing FUO *62*, *64*, 65
  colorectal 326–7, 542, *543*
  esophagus 261
  gastric 274, 282–4, *285*, *537*
  immune system 994, 1006–7
    diagnosis 998–9
  larynx 121
  liver 353–5
  lymphoid 734–9
  nasal/paranasal 111–12, *558*
  obese animals 1085
  ocular 856–8
  oral 96–8
  orbital 858, 863–5
  pancreas 383–5, 445–8
  perineal 332
  pituitary 392, 393–4

prostate gland 530–1
pulmonary 165, *166*, 191–3
renal 505–6
salivary glands 256
skin 812–16
small intestines 312–14, 539
spinal 606–11
spleen *522*
thoracic *139*, 151, 154–6
thoracic wall 161–2
thyroid 404
trachea 125
trigeminal nerve 578, 1110–11
urinary tract 501–3
vertebral body 608–9
Neospora caninum 564
neosporosis
brain 564–5
myelitis 616–17
myopathy 634
neuritis 622–3
neostigmine 625
Neotrombicula autumnalis 790
nephroblastoma, spinal 609–10
nephrocalcinosis 525, *527*
nephropathy
hypercalcemic 411, *412*
Lyme 914–15
membranous (MN) 469
protein-losing (PLN) 468–74
nephrotic syndrome 847
nerve biopsy 619
nerve growth factor (NGF) 1030
nerve root tumors 608–9
nerve sheath tumors 578, 606–8, 1110–11
neuritis, protozoal 622–3
neurodegenerative disease 552–3
neurodiagnostic investigations
brain disorders 545–6
neuromuscular disorders 617–19
spinal disorders 581–2
neurologic disease
causing dysuria 71–2
causing syncope/weakness *21*
causing vomiting *28*
hyperadrenocorticism 423
hypothyroidism 398, *399*
in CDV infection 928, *929*
in FPL infection 970
liver disorders 333–4, 335, 346, *357*, *358*
Toxoplasmosis 981
neuromuscular disorders *20*, *435*, 617–25
clinical signs 617
inflammatory 621–3
lesion localization 617
myasthenia gravis 624–5
neurodiagnostic investigation 617–19
toxic 623–4
neuropathies
breed-related 619–20
CIDP 621
endocrine 620–1
neurotransmitters 1027
neutering
and obesity 1081
and urinary incontinence *480*, 481, 483, 485
neutropenia 719–21
neutrophilia 423, 711–13
physiologic (excitement/shift) 711–12
neutrophilic enteritis *306*
neutrophils
abnormal granulation in Birman cats 727–8
band 724, *725*
hypersegmentation 726, *740*
inflammatory left shift 724
toxicity 726
niacinamide *801*
nictitans protrusion 578, *852*, *865*
nifurtimox 232
nitazoxanide 300
nitenpyram, toxicity 884
nitrates *209*
nitrofurantoin *508*
nitroglycerin *209*
nitroprusside *209*, 210, *240*
nizatidine *283*, *1049*
Nocardia spp. 143, 144, 948
nocardiosis, feline 948–50
nociception 1025–6
nodule *770*
nonsteroidal anti-inflammatory drugs (NSAIDs) 1044–53
acute kidney injury *451*, 458
acute toxicosis 276
antipyresis 67
caution in cats 1051
changing agents 1048
COX-1:COX-2 ratios 1046–7
COX-2 selective 1032, 1048
GI protection 276–7, 1049–50
GI ulceration 274
interactions 1050–1
mechanism of action 1044–7
minimizing adverse effects 1051
perioperative use 1034
recent drug developments 1051–3
relative efficacy in DJD *640*
safety 1047–8
washout 1048
noradrenaline 1027, 1040, *1041*
nosodes 913
Notoedres spp. *773*, *787*
nucleus pulposus herniation 591, 642
nutraceuticals 147, 340, 1076, 1106
nutritional assessment 1059–63
laboratory markers 1062
nutritional disorders
feline retinal degeneration (taurine retinopathy) 872–3
of bone 663–4
thiamine deficiency 568–9
nutritional support
assisted enteral feeding 1067–72
calculation of requirements 1064–5
diet evaluation and comparison 1065
disease-specific
chronic gastrointestinal disease 1075
chylothorax 1126–8
hepatic encephalopathy 1076
hepatic lipidosis 336–7, 1075–6
pancreatitis 377 1074–5
renal disease 1076–7
evidence supporting 1059
nutrients 1065–7
nutritional reassessment 1074
parenteral 336, 377, 1065, 1072–4
re-feeding 336, 1067
timing 1063, *1064*
voluntary food intake 1067
nystagmus 572

obesity
clinical presentation 1085
diagnosis 1086–90
differential diagnosis 1085–6
etiology 1079–80
feline 334
human 1079, 1082
ideal/target weight 1086, *1087*, 1090
management and prognosis 1090–3
pathological consequences 1082–5

obesity – *contd*
pathophysiology 1080–1
risk factors 1081–2
oclacitinib *801*
octreotide 448
ocular disease
algae (protothecosis) 840–1
diabetes mellitus 858–9
filariasis 844, *868*
fungal infections 833–40
aspergillosis 839–40
blastomycosis 836–9, 944
coccidioidomycosis 835
cryptococcosis 65, 833–5, 978
histoplasmosis 835–6
hemorrhagic retinopathy 848–52
hyperlipidemia 845–7, 865–6
in anemia 847–8
in bacterial infections 821–3
in hypertension 475, *475*, 848, *849–51*
in protozoal infections 831, 832–3, 981, 982
in rickettsial infections 841–4, 955
in viral infections 823–32
CAV-2 924
CDV 823–5, 928, *929*
FCV/FHV-1 823, 826–9, 973–4
FIP 564, 615, 616, 829–30, 960–1
hyperviscosity syndrome 844–5
lymphosarcoma 830–1, 856–8
renal disease 847, *849*
retina and optic nerve 869–74
uvea 868–9
odansetron *28*, *296*
odontogenic fibroma, peripheral 96
olfactory bulb tumor *558*
oligodendroma *558*
oligodontia 90
oligosaccharides, urinary 553
oliguria, acute kidney injury 450–1, *452*
Ollulanus tricuspis 271
olsalazine 319
omega 3 fatty acids 1067, 1076
omeprazole 264, *272*, 377, *457*, 550, 551
ondanretron 375, *457*
onion toxicity 905–6, 1122–3
onychitis, lupoid 819
onychodystrophy *819*
open-chest biopsy 126–7
ophthalmomyiasis 871–2
opioid receptors 1038
opioids 1037–40
bioavailability 1038
doses and characteristics *1054–5*
in cough 55
side effects 1038
WHO classification *1039*
optic nerve, meningioma *864*
optic nerve head, swelling 874
optic neuritis 874
canine distemper *824*
clinical presentation 874
diagnosis 874
etiology and pathophysiology *625*, 874
GME 855, *856*
hypertension *849*
oral examination 84–5
oral masses 96–8
orbit, neoplasia 858, 863–5
orellanine 892
organic acids, urinary 553
organophosphates (OPs) 879–91
ormetoprim/sulfadimethoxine *778*
orogastric intubation 278
Ortolani sign *642*
oscillometric devices 476–8
osmolality
plasma 394, *395*
urine 395
osteoarthritis 638–40
radiosynoviorthesis 640, 1053
osteochondrodysplasia 646
osteochondromatosis 672–3, *674*
osteochondrosis 646, 652–3, 677
osteodystrophy, hypertrophic 655–6
osteomalacia 663
osteomas, pulmonary 192–3
osteomyelitis
suppurative 664–5
vertebral 611–13, 665–6
osteopathy, secondary hypertrophic (pulmonary osteopathy) 672
osteophytes *648*, *677*
osteoporosis 656, 657
osteosarcoma 658–9
mandible/maxilla 98
orbital 864
parosteal in cat 657–8
telangiectatic *660*
otitis externa 574, 810–11
otitis media/interna 573, 574–5
CNS infection 562
Otodectes spp. *787*, 789
ototoxicity 575–6
overbite (overshot) *88*
owners
and pet obesity 1082, 1093
household management for cats 489–92
veterinary consultation 3–8
oxacillin resistance 782
oxidative agents
inducing hemolytic anemia 695–6
methemoglobinemia 710
oxybutinin *485*
oxygen delivery 77–8, *79*
oxygen supplementation
bacterial pneumonia 129
head trauma 572
techniques 11–12
oxymorphone 1039, *1054*

P-glycoprotein 882
pacemaker 244–5
wandering *201*
packed cell volume (PCV) 78
in AHDS 294, 295
in CKD 467
myeloproliferative disorders 740, 742
pain
acute to chronic 1031–2
assessment 1034–7
cancer 1032–3
gate control theory 1025, *1026*
inflammatory 1030
mechanism-based classification 1036, *1037*
neuropathic 1032, 1053, 1056
nociceptive 1029
physiology 1025–9
types postoperative, incisional 1029–30
pain management
adjuncts *1056*
alpha-2 agonists 1040–1
drug doses and characteristics *1054–6*
in osteosarcoma 658–9
in pancreatitis 377
logical approach to progressive pain 1056–7
membrane stabilizers 1041–4, *1056*
NSAIDs 1044–53
opioids 1037–40
pre-emptive 1033–4

pallor 77–9, 681
  differential diagnoses *79*
  digital 1016, *1017*
pamidronate 458, 889
pancreas
  phlegmon formation *366*, *378*
  pseudocyst 374
  radiography 542–3
  tumors 383–5, 445–8
pancreatic enzymes 284, 285, *362*
  characteristics *362*
  therapy 382
pancreatic exocrine insufficiency *41*, 380–3
pancreatic lipase immunoreactivity (PLI) tests 351, 372, 373, 385
pancreatitis *51*, 361–80
  acute 350, 351
    clinical presentation 366–9
    clinicopathology 371–3
    complications/long-term care 379, *380*
    diagnosis 370–1, *372–3*, 543
    etiology 361, *366*
    feline 367, *368*, 372, 373
    management 373, 375, 377–9
    pathophysiology 361–6, *367*
  chronic active *365*
  nutritional support 377, 1074–5
  severe necrotizing 1112–15
  severity scoring *369*
panniculitis *784*, 816–17, *818*
panniculus (cutaneous trunci) reflex 581
pannus 1002–3
panosteitis 651, *652*
pantoprazole *272*, 377
panuveitis 853, *854*
papilledema 874
papillomatosis
  cutaneous *813*, 814–15
  oral 96–7, 814, 927–8
papillomaviruses 814, 927
papules *799*
paracetamol, *see* acetaminophen
paradichlorobenzene 902
paralysis
  arterial thromboembolism 1108–9
  Coonhound 621
  IVDD 586, *588*, 592
  laryngeal 119–21, 619–20
  tick 623–4
paraneoplastic eosinophilia 714
paraneoplastic neutrophilia 712
paraplegia 586, *588*, 592
paraproteins *998*, 999, 1006–7
parasites
  bronchopulmonary 131–2, 1101–3
  causing colitis 315–16
  causing eosinophilia 713
  causing esophagitis 263–4
  dermatoses 786–91
  ear mites 789
  gastric 271
  intestinal *42*, *43*, *44*, *45*, 290–3, 296, 298–300
  nasal 113
parathyroid glands
  disorders 409–11, *412*
  physiology 408–9
parathyroid hormone (PTH) *35*, 408–9, 463, 465, 495, 654
  inadequate production/secretion 409–10
  increased production/secretion 410–11
parathyroid hormone-related peptide (PTHrP) 495
parathyroidectomy 411, *412*
parenteral nutrition 336, 377, 1065, 1072–4
paresis, cardiac disease 196
parietal cells 269, *270*
paromomycin 300
partial thromboplastin time (PTT) 746, 747
  prolongation of 754
parvovirus infection 930–2
  clinical presentation 931
  diagnosis 287
  enteritis 43, 44, 286–8, 931
  feline, *see* feline panleukopenia virus
  management 287–8, 931–2
  myocarditis 931
  prognosis 288, 932
  vaccines 932
Pasteurella multocida 128, 783
patch testing *776*, 994
patellar luxation 674–6
patent ductus arteriosus (PDA) 185, *186*, 196, *197*, *211*, 214–16
pathogen-associated molecular patterns (PAMPs) 986
pathologic fractures 94, 95
pattern-recognition receptors (PRRs) 986, 987
PDE-5 inhibitors, *see* phosphodiesterase-5 inhibitors
Pelger–Huët anomaly 724–5
pelvic bladder *480*, 482, 484
pemphigus foliaceus *775*, 799–800, 867, 1000
  skin biopsy 1000
D-pencillamine 349
penicillin G *508*, 921, 923, 949
penicillin V *508*
Penicillium spp. 106, 937
pentazocine *1055*
pentobarbital 886, 890, 923
pentoxifylline *301*
percussion, thoracic 125
perfusion status 1016–17
perianal fistulae 329–30
pericardial effusion 151, 187, *188*, *189*, 233–6
  idiopathic 235
  malignant *155*
pericardiocentesis 235
pericarditis
  constrictive 233, 236
  infectious 235–6
perineal hernia 330–2
perineal tumors 332
perinephric pseudocyst 524, *526*
periodontal disease 85–8
periodontal pocket *86*, 87
periodontitis 86, 87
peripheral nerve injury 1030–1
peripheral nerve sheath tumors (PNSTs) 578, 606–8, 1110–11
peripheral vestibular diseases 572–5
peritoneal effusion 513, 524, 950
peritoneal lavage 373–9
peritoneopericardial diaphragmatic hernia (PPDH) 233–4
peritonitis
  bile 352, *353*
  feline infectious, *see* feline infectious peritonitis (FIP)
periuria 487
persistent right aortic arch (PRAA) 219, 261, *263*
  breed predisposition *211*
Perthes disease 670–1
pet foods, commercial 1065, *1066*
petechiae 749, *750*
pharyngeal dysphagia 253, 254
pharyngitis 254–5
phenamidine isethionate 941

phenobarbital 548
phenothiazines 923
phenoxybenzamine 437
phentolamine 437
phenylbutazone *1050*
phenylephrine 58
phenylpropanolamine 485
pheochromocytoma *239*, 435–7
pheromones, cats 493
phlegmon, pancreatic *366*, *378*
phosphate
  serum 336, 409, 461, 463, 465, 698, 889
  supplementation 336, 440
phosphate-binding agents 465–6
phosphodiesterase-5 (PDE-5) inhibitors *209*, 210, 238
phosphofructokinase deficiency 698
phospholipase A_2 *362*
phosphonylmethoxyethyladenine (PMEA) 965, *966*, 968
phosphorus, dietary 1076
phrenic nerve 581
Physaloptera spp. 271
physostigmine 853
phytonadione (vitamin K1) 336, 339, 756–7, 887, 888
pigmenturia 23–6, 69
pilocarpine 853
pimobendan *209*, 210, *229*
pinna
  mast cell tumor 814
  sebaceous adenitis 811
  vasculitis 819
pinnal–pedal scratch reflex 773
piprant class drugs 640
piroxicam 503, *801*
pituitary gland
  neoplasia 392, 393–4, 426, *427*, 557
  physiology 387–8
pituitary-dependent hyperadrenocorticism 393–4, 419–20
plague, feline 957–9
plants, toxic 891, 1105–6
planum nasale, *see* nasal planum
plaque
  dental 86
  dermal *770*
  eosinophilic 806–7
plasma, icteric *48*
plasma cell myeloma 738–9
plasma cell pododermatitis 817, *818*
plasma osmolality *395*
plasma therapy 373, 375, 756, 764, 766, 888
plasmacytoma 739, 1006
plasmin 748
plasminogen 748
platelet activating factor (PAF) *745*
platelets
  abnormalities of function 752–3
  activation and aggregation 745–6
  consumption/loss 751
  giant (macrothrombocytopenia) 733
  immune-mediated destruction 690, 751–2
  increased (thrombocytosis) 732–3
  non-neoplastic disorders 732–3
  reduced production 748–51
Platynosum concinum 334
pleural effusion
  acute pancreatitis *364*
  heart failure 208
  malignant 151
  radiography 163–7
  types and causes *140*, 164, *165*
pleural fibrosis 147
pleural fluid, chylous 146, 1126–8
pleural hemorrhage *887*
pleural lavage 144
pleural space disease *79*, *106*, *159*
  chylothorax 145–8, 1126–8
  diaphragmatic herniation *139*, 149–51, *152–4*
  feline 13
  lung lobe torsion 148–50
  masses 151, 154–6, 167
  pneumothorax 139–43, 168
  pyothorax 143–5
  radiography 163–5
Pneumocystis carinii 135
pneumomediastinum 170
pneumonia 14
  aspiration 129, 265, *266*, 267
  bacterial 128–30
  granulomatous 191
  mycotic 945
  parasitic 131–2, 1101–3
'pneumonitis', feline (feline chlamydiosis) 843–4, 954–6
Pneumonyssoides caninum 113
pneumoperitoneum 514–15
pneumothorax 139–43
  closed 168
  open 168
  radiographic signs 168, *169*
  spontaneous 14, 142, 168
podocytes 468
pododermatitis
  food hypersensitivity *795*
  Malassezia 785
  plasma cell 817, *818*
polyarthritis 666–9
polycystic kidney disease (PKD) 503–4
polycythemia 219, *239*
  relative 406
polycythemia vera (PV) 740–2
polydipsia 33–6
  psychogenic *35*, 36, *395*
polydipsia–polyuria 33–6
  clinical signs 33, *35*, 36
  diabetes insipidus *35*, 394
  diabetes mellitus *35*, 438
  differential diagnosis *394*
  etiology 33, *34*
  hyperadrenocorticism *34*, *35*, 421, 424
polyethylene glycol (PEG) 324, *326*
polymyositis, idiopathic 634–5
polyneuropathy, chronic inflammatory demyelinating 621
polyps, nasopharyngeal 113–14, 575
polyradiculoneuritis 621–3
polyuria 33–6
ponazuril 293
Porphyromonas spp. 783
portosystemic vascular anomalies 357–9
posaconazole 980
posterior vena cava, pheochromocytoma 436
pot-bellied appearance 421, 425
potassium 413, 629–30
  excessive secretion 433–4
  low serum (hypokalemia) *34*, *35*, 433–4, 629–30, 1109
  raised serum (hyperkalemia) 416, *417*, 455, 456, *457*, 489
  serum, in CKD 463
  supplementation 435, 440, 463, 630
potassium bromide 554
potassium citrate 463, 500, 501
potassium gluconate 463
pradofloxacin, dermatologic disorders *778*
pralidoxime chloride (2-PAM) 881
praziquantel 298
prazosin *240*, *478*, 479, 493

precordial thrill 197
prednisolone 232, 307–8, 312, 340, 418, 447–8, *801*
prednisone 133, 302, 307, *308*, 330, 550
pregabalin 602
primary ciliary dyskinesia (PCD) 130–1
probiotics *289*, 1075
Problem Oriented Medical Record 637
procainamide *249*, 250, *251*, 631
prochlorperazine *28*
progestogen therapy 391
prokinetic drugs *283*, 931–2
proligesterone 391
propantheline 503
propofol 886
propranolol *209*, *240*, *478*
prostaglandin analogs *1049*, 1050
prostaglandin receptor antagonists 640
prostaglandins 361–2
prostate gland
abscesses 71, 531
benign hypertrophy 530, *531*
neoplasia 73, *75*, 530–1
radiography 530–1
protamine zinc insulin 442
proteasome 986
protein
catabolism 1059
dietary requirements 1065–6
renal excretion 469
protein C 747, 764
protein-losing enteropathy (PLE) 305, 307, 309–11
protein-losing nephropathy (PLN) 468–74
proteins induced by vitamin K antagonism/absence (PIVKA) 336, 756
proteinuria 466, 469
prothrombin time (PT) 754, 887
proton pump inhibitors (PPIs) *270*, *272*, 276, 375, 377, *1049*, 1050
protopam chloride 881
protothecosis 840
prucalopride *283*
pseudocoprostasis 323
pseudocysts
pancreatic 374
perinephric 503–4, 524, *526*
pseudoephedrine 895–6
psilocybin 892
psychogenic disorders
dermatologic 803–5
polydipsia *35*, 36, *395*
psyllium *323*, *326*, 1075
ptyalism 357, *358*
public health
actinomycosis and nocardiosis 950
B. bronchiseptica 913, 952
brucellosis 919
canine ehrlichiosis 936
cryptococcosis 979
feline bartonellosis 950, 951
feline leukemia virus 967
feline plaque 959
leptospirosis 922
Lyme disease 917
Mycoplasma felis infections 954
rabies 934, 973
RMSF 942–3
toxoplasmosis 982–3
Pug encephalitis 567–8
pulmonary artery, enlarged 183, *184*
pulmonary artery pressure (PAP) 237
pulmonary bullae 139, *142*
pulmonary contusions 135–6
pulmonary edema 189, 191
and fluid therapy 1023
cardiogenic *188*, *191*, 207, 208, 1107
noncardiogenic *191*
pulmonary exchange capacity *140*
pulmonary fibrosis 15, 134–5, 1100–1
pulmonary function tests 127
pulmonary hemorrhage *887*
pulmonary hypertension (PH) *211*, 236–8
pulmonary lobectomy 130, 142, 148
pulmonary metastases 15, *192*, 425
pulmonary nodules 191–3
pulmonary osteoarthropathy 672
pulmonary osteomas 192–3
pulmonary pattern
alveolar 187, 189–91
bronchial 193, *194*
interstitial 191–3
pulmonary thromboembolism (PTE) 15, *191*, 236, 238, 758–9
pulmonary veins, enlarged 185–6
pulmonic stenosis *182*, *211*, 213–14
pulses 196, *197*, 223, 233
pulsus alternans *197*
pulsus bigeminus *197*
pulsus bisferiens (bifid) *197*
pulsus paradoxus *197*, 233
pulsus parvus et tardus *197*
pumpkin, canned *323*
pupil
dilated 824, 834, *845*, 853, 871, 874
miotic 852
pupillary reflexes, abnormal 831, *841*, 875
pure red cell aplasia (PRCA) 703, 707
purines, dietary 496, 500, *501*
pustule cytology *775*
pyelectasia 462
pyloric antral hypertrophy 279–81
pyloric outflow obstruction 535
pyoderma
deep 782–3
mucocutaneous 780–1
puppy (impetigo) 779–80
skin fold (intertrigo) 776–9
pyometra *34*, *35*, *529*
pyothorax *139*, *140*, 143–5
pyotraumatic dermatitis 779, *780*
pyrantel pamoate 291
pyrethrins/pyrethroids *787*
toxicity 884–5
pyridostigmine 266, 625
pyrogens 61
pyruvate kinase deficiency 697–8
Pythium insidiosum (pythiosis) 271
esophageal 264, 265
gastric 271
intestinal 301–2, *303*
treatment 265, 301–2

quality of life, and obesity 1083
quaternary ammonium compounds, ingestion 897
quinidine 631
quinuronium sulfate 941

R2A anomaly 213
rabies 560–1
canine 561, 932–4
feline 561, 971–3
ocular signs 823
public health 934, 973
vaccines *912*, 933–4, *953–4*, 972–3
panniculitis 817, *818*
raccoon roundworm 292
radiation, pituitary gland 393
radiation therapy, brain tumors 557
radio-ulnar synostosis 669–70
radioactive iodine 408

radiography
abdominal, *see* abdominal radiography
compression 515–16
elbow dysplasia 647
horizontal beam 514–15
nasal cavity 937, *938*
spinal 581, *586*
cauda equina syndrome *645*
intervertebral disk disease 643
stress 599
thoracic, *see* thoracic radiography
urinary tract 73, *74*, *75*
radiosynoviorthesis 640, 1053
radius, deformities 648–9
raisins, toxicity 458–9, 891–2
ranitidine *272*, *283*, *1049*
ranula 255–6
Rathke's pouch, cystic dilatation 388
re-feeding syndrome 336, 1067
rectal prolapse 325–6
rectal stricture 321–2
red blood cells (RBCs)
antigens 686
disorders 681–711
reflex dyssynergia 72
regurgitation 27, 260
differentiation from vomiting *258*
renal biopsy 471–2
renal carcinoma 505–6, 524, *672*
renal disease
hyperthyroidism 406
leptospirosis 920
nutritional support 1076–7
obese animals 1085
systemic hypertension 239
see also acute kidney injury (AKI); chronic kidney disease (CKD); urolithiasis
renal pelvis dilatation (pyelectasia) 462
renal therapy, advanced 459, 467
renal transplantation 467–8
renal tubules
obstruction 450, *452*
oxalate deposits 899, *900–1*
renin 206, 413
renin–angiotensin–aldosterone system (RAAS) 210, 413, 434, 848
reproductive tract, radiography 528–31
respiratory disease 105
acute feline upper tract 115
canine infectious (CIRD) 53, 127–8, 909–13
clinical signs *106*
feline viral upper tract 973–6
lower airways 125–37
radiography *158–9*
upper airways 105–25
respiratory distress 11
respiratory function, obese animal 1084
resting energy expenditure (REE) 1064
resting energy requirement (RER) 1018
restrictive cardiomyopathy (RCM), feline 227
retching 27
reticulocyte counts 683–4
retinal abscess *838*
retinal detachment (RD)
diagnosis 871
ehrlichiosis *841*
etiology *841*, 871
histoplasmosis *837*
hypertension *475*, *850*, *851*
hyperviscosity syndrome 844, *845*
in infectious disease 821
lymphosarcoma *857*
management 871
pathophysiology 871
systemic vascular disease 847
retinal dystrophy, Briard dog 870
retinal hemorrhage
etiology *842*
FeLV 830, *831*
FIP 829, *830*
histoplasmosis *836*
hypertension *849*, *850*
hyperviscosity syndrome 844, *845*
Rocky Mountain spotted fever *843*
toxoplasmosis 833
retinal vessels, 'box carring' *850*
retinopathy
diabetic 858
enrofloxacin 873–4
hemorrhagic 848–52
hypertensive 848, *849–51*
taurine deficiency 872–3
retrobulbar mass *864*, *865*
retroperitoneal effusion 523
retroperitoneal space, radiography 522–4
rhabdomyolysis, exertional 633–4
rhabdomyoma 121
rhabdomyosarcoma *663–4*
rheumatoid arthritis (RA) 666–9
rheumatoid factor (RF) test 996, *997*
rhinitis
idiopathic lymphoplasmacytic (dogs) 115–16
parasitic (nasal mite) 113
recurrent infectious (dogs) 114–15
rhinoscopy *107*, 108, *109*, 111, *112*, *114*, 937–8
rhinosinusitis
feline idiopathic 116–17
mycotic 105–10
Rhipicephalus sanguineus 730, 934, 940
rickets (osteomalacia) 663
rickettsial disease 941
ehrlichiosis 716, 728–30, 934–6
ocular signs 841–4, 955
Rocky Mountain spotted fever 842–3, 941–3
rifampin *23*, *778*
right atrium
echocardiography 205
enlargement 179
right bundle branch block *202*
right ventricle
echocardiography 205
enlargement 180, *182*
right ventricular end-systolic pressure (RVESP) 237
ristocetin *745*
Rivalta test 961–2
robenacoxib 1052–3
Rocky Mountain spotted fever (RMSF) 842–3, 941–3
'rodent' ulcer 103
rodenticide toxicity 886–91
anticoagulants 755–7, 886–8, 1116–17
bromethalin 888–9
cholecalciferol-based rodenticides *451*, 458, 889
hypercalcemia 756, 889
strychnine 889–90
zinc phosphide 890–1
ronidazole 318
rouleaux formation 690
roundworms 292
rubeosis iridis *822*, *829*, *868*

S-adenosylmethionine (SAMe) 340, 895, 1076, 1107
saddle thrombus 583–4, 760–2

St. John's wort *1050*
saline test 690
salivary gland disorders 255–6
salmon calcitonin 889
Salmonella spp. infections 290
Salmonella cholerasuis subsp.
    arizonae 729
salt supplementation 419
sarcoma
  histiocytic causing pharyngitis 255
  synovial cell 661–3
sarcoma virus, feline 832
Sarcoptes scabiei var. *canis* 788
Sarcoptes spp. *787*
scabies, canine *787*, 788–9
scale *771*, *790*
scar *771*
Schiff–Sherrington posture 581,
    585, *586*
Schirmer tear test 860
schistocytes *697*
schistosomiasis, canine 296, 298
sciatic neuropathy 620
scissors bite *88*
sclera, icteric *48*
scratch reflex 773
scratching, 'phantom' 550–1, 601
sebaceous adenitis 811
seborrhea, canine 797
sedation, alpha-2 adrenergic agonists
    1040–1
seizures
  canine brain tumors 557
  CDV infection 928, *929*
  hepatic encephalopathy 554
  hypoglycemia 446
  insecticide toxicity 881
  metaldehyde toxicity 886
  strychnine toxicity 890
selamectin 113, 242, *787*
  toxicity 882
selegiline hydrochloride
    (L-deprenyl) 432
sepsis 764–5
septic arthritis 667–9
serotonin *745*
serum amyloid A (SAA) 469, 472
severe combined immunodeficiency
    723–4
  X-linked 994
shock
  hemorrhagic 1022
  hypovolemic 1019–22
short-chain fatty acids (SCFAs) *323*
shunt
  portosystemic 357–9
  ventriculoperitoneal 550
sialadenitis 256
sialocele 255–6
sick euthyroid syndrome 401
sick sinus syndrome 243–5
sildenafil *209*, 210, *211*, 238
silocin 892
silymarin 340, 1106
single radial immunodiffusion
    (SRID) 997
sinonasal aspergillosis
  cats 110
  dogs 105–10
sinus arrhythmia, respiratory *201*
situs inversus 130
Sjögren's-like syndrome 860–1
skin
  barrier functions 985
  elasticity 422, 1016, *1017*
skin scrapings *773*, *787*
skull
  abnormalities of development
    548, *549*
  fracture *571*
SLUD mnemonic 879
small intestines 284–314
  adhesions 367, *369*
  diameter assessment 538
  foreign bodies 296, *297*, 539–41
  inflammatory disease *40*, 302–9
  mechanical obstruction 539–41
  neoplasia 312–14, 539
  normal anatomy and
    function 285–6
  obstruction 295–6, *297*
  radiography *297*, 538–41
snake bites 763, 1123–5
sneezing 105, *106*, 116
soaps, ingestion 896–8
sodium:potassium ratio 416
sodium, serum 416, 419,
    555–6, 556
sodium ascorbate (vitamin C) 711
sodium bicarbonate 440–1,
    457, 463
sodium chloride, ingestion *34*
solar (actinic) dermatitis 808–9
Somogyi overswing 444
sorbitol dehydrogenase 858–9
sotalol 225, *249*, 250, *251*
spaying
  and obesity 1081
  urinary incontinence following *480*,
    481, 483, 485
sphingolipidoses 875
spinal cord
  compression, vertebral body
    tumor 609
  infarction 582–3
  inflammatory diseases 615–17
spinal disorders
  causing dysuria *72*, 73
  causing urinary incontinence 483
  clinical signs 580–1
  degenerative 590–601
  inflammatory diseases 611–17
  intervertebral disc disease
    591–5, 642–4
  neoplastic 73, 605–11
  neurodiagnostic investigations 581–2
  synovial cysts 600, *601*
  trauma 584–90
  vascular 582–4
  vertebral column
    malformations 603–6
spinal radiography 581, *586*, 643, *645*
spinal stability, assessment 586, *588*
spinal stenosis 605–6
  degenerative lumbosacral 597–9
Spirocera lupi (spirocercosis) 263–5
  treatment 264–5
spironolactone *209*, 210, *240*, *478*,
    479, 630
spleen *365*, 520–2
splenitis 521, *523*
spondylosis deformans 599–600
squamous cell carcinoma (SCC) 657,
    813, 815–16
  esophagus 261
  multicentric in situ (Bowen's disease)
    815–16
  oral 98
  orbital *865*
Staphylococcus pseudintermedius
    781, 783, *800*
Staphylococcus schleiferi coagulans 781
Staphylococcus schleiferi schleiferi 781
Starling equation 1014
steatorrhea 331, 332
stent
  trachea 124
  ureter 497, *498*
  urethra 503

steroid hepatopathy 355–6, 518
steroid myopathy 625–6
steroid-responsive meningitis-arteritis (SRMA) 613–14
stertor 105, *106*
stomach
  acid and enzyme production 269, *270*
  anatomy 269
  bleeding 275
  distension 29, 534–6
  foreign bodies *272*, 278–9, *280–1*, 535–6
  Helicobacter spp. infection 272–3, *274*
  malpositioning 30, 277–8, 521, 535–7, 536–7, *538*
  motility 269
  mucosal barrier 274–5
  neoplasia 274, 282–4, *285*, *537*
  nonobstructive emptying disorders 281–2
  opacity alterations 537–8
  outflow obstruction 278–81, 534–5
  parasites 271
  radiography 534–8
stomatitis
  feline caudal 101–2
  in FIV *966*, 967–8
storage diseases 552–3, 726–7, 874–5
strabismus 548–9
stranguria 69
Streptococcus spp. 562
Streptococcus equi subsp. *zooepidemicus* 910
stress
  and blood pressure measurement 478
  and FLUTD 487–8, 492
striae 422
strictures
  esophageal 260–1, *262*
  rectal 321–2
stroke 546–8
struvite uroliths 494, 497, *498*, 499–500
strychnine toxicity 889–90
stunting, *see* growth retardation
subaortic stenosis (SAS) *197*, 211–13
  breed predisposition *211*
subarachnoid cyst 602–3
subpleural blebs 139
substance P 1027, 1030
succimer (dimercaptosuccinic acid) 904
sucralfate 264, 267, *272*, 276, *457*, *1049*
sulfadimethoxine 293
sulfasalazine 319
sulfisoxazole *508*, 949
sulfonylureas 395–6
'sulfur' granules 949
sunlight exposure 657, 808, 809
superoxide dismutase 1 (*SOD*) gene 590
surgery
  perioperative pain management 1033–4
  postoperative/incisional pain 1029–30
swallowing, physiology *253*
sweeteners, artificial 906
symblepharon, herpesvirus *828*
symmetric dimethylarginine (SDMA) 461
syncope 17–21
  algorithms *19*
  diagnostic tests 18, 21, *195*
  differential diagnosis *20–1*
  in cardiac disease *211*
syndactyly *645*
synostosis 669–70
synovial cell sarcoma 661–3
synovial cysts, spinal 600, *601*
syringomyelia 550, 551, 601–2
systemic lupus erythematosus (SLE) 667–9, 1003–4
systemic vascular resistance 475

T helper (Th) cells 987–8
T lymphocytes 987–8
T regulatory cells (Tregs) 988
tachyarrhythmias 247–51
tachycardia 78, 207, 405
tachypnea 11, 195, 207
tail tone, decreased 598
tapetum, hyperreflective 928, *929*
tarsometatarsal joint, synovial cell sarcoma *662*
taurine retinopathy 872–3
tears, lack of 860
teeth
  dental formulae 83–4
  eruption times 84
  extraction
    feline caudal stomatitis 102
    periodontal disease 87–8
    persistent deciduous tooth 90
  fractures *85*, 91–3
  impacted 91, 1097–8
  in acromegaly 392
  malocclusion 88–9
  'missing' 90–1, 1097
  numbering systems 83–4
  persistent deciduous 89–90
  resorptions 98–101, 1098–100
  root abscess *86*
  structure 84
temporalis muscle, myositis 256–7
temporomandibular joint (TMJ)
  in craniomandibular osteopathy 654
  luxation 93–4
tenesmus 316, 321
tepoxalin *640*, *1047*
terbinafine 302
terbutaline 137
  sick sinus syndrome 244
tetanus 922–3
tetracycline *508*, *778*, *801*, 942, 955
  enamel staining *911*
tetralogy of Fallot *211*, 218–19
theobromine 906–7
theophylline *244*
thiamine deficiency 568–9, 1067
thiazide diuretics 396, 500
third eyelid protrusion 578, *852*, *865*
thirst center 36
thoracic duct
  injury 145
  ligation *147*
thoracic radiography 54
  anticoagulant rodenticide ingestion *887*
  blastomycosis *943*
  chylothorax 146, 1126, *1127*, 1128
  congestive heart failure 186–7, *188–9*, 1107
  diaphragm and cranial abdomen 163
  diaphragmatic herniation 151, *152*
  eosinophilic bronchopneumopathy 132, 133
  esophageal foreign body 259
  esophagus 172–5
  extrathoracic structures 161–3
  heart 178–87, *188–9*
  heartworm disease 241
  hiatal hernia 268
  hyperadrenocorticism 425
  hypertrophic cardiomyopathy 406
  hypoadrenocorticism 416, *417*
  indications *158–9*
  laryngeal collapse 122, *123*
  lungs 187, 189–94
    alveolar pulmonary pattern 187, 189–91

    bronchial pulmonary pattern 193, *194*
    interstitial pulmonary pattern 191–3
    lobe torsion *149*
    vascular pulmonary pattern 193, *194*
  mediastinum 168–77
  megaesophagus 265, *266*, 624
  neoplasia 154, *155*
  pericardial disease 234
  pleural space 163–8
  pneumonia 129
  pneumothorax 140, *141*
  reading 158–61
  respiratory worms 1102
  systemic mycoses 945
  technique and positioning 157–8
  trachea 171–2
thoracic trauma 14
thoracic wall, abnormalities and masses 161–2
thoracolumbar spine
  injuries 584–5
  intervertebral disk disease 591–4
  tumor of young dogs (spinal nephroblastoma) 609–10
thoracoscopy *142*, 144, *145*
thoracostomy tube 140–2, 144–5
thorax, percussion 125
thrombin *745*, 747
thrombocythemia, essential 742
thrombocytopathia 752–3
thrombocytopenia 748–52
  immune-mediated 690, 751–2, 1125–6
  ocular signs 847–8
  platelet consumption/loss 751
  platelet destruction 751–2
  with giant platelets (macrothrombocytopenia) 733
thrombocytosis, reactive 732–3
thromboelastography 765, *766*, 767
thromboembolism
  glomerulonephropathy 474
  in PLE 311
  pulmonary 15, *191*, 236, 238, 758–9
thrombolytic agents 1108–9
thrombomodulin 747
thrombosis 758–62
  antithrombotic drugs 229, 311, 474, *762*
  arterial 229, *230*, 760–2, 1108–9
  venous 758–60
thromboxane *745*
thymic hyperplasia and hypotrichosis, Birman cats 1006
thymoma *155*, 175, *177*, 624
thymus 175
thyroglobulin autoantibodies (TgAA) 402
thyroid disease
  anemia 701–2
  lymphocytic thyroiditis 397, *398*
  tumors 397, 404
  see also hyperthyroidism; hypothyroidism
thyroid function tests 400–2, 406–7
thyroid gland
  biopsy 402
  imaging 406–7
  physiology 397
thyroid hormones
  obese animal 1084
  replacement 402–3
thyroid stimulating hormone (TSH) 397, 424, 1084
  measurement 402
  stimulation test *401*, 402
thyroidectomy 407–8
thyroiditis, lymphocytic 397, *398*
thyrotoxicosis 404–8
thyrotropin 397
thyrotropin releasing hormone (TRH) 397, 424
  stimulation test *401*, 402
L-thyroxine 402
thyroxine (T4) 397, 400–1, 424, 1084
  replacement 402–3
tick paralysis 623–4
tick-borne diseases
  anaplasmosis 934–6
  babesiosis 694–5, 940–1
  cytauxzoonosis 699
  ehrlichiosis 728–30, 934–6
  hepatozoonosis 730–1
  Lyme disease 821, *912*, 913–17
ticks
  American dog 699, 940
  brown dog 934
  Ixodes spp. 623, 914
  limiting exposure to 916
tissue factor (TF) 746, 747
tissue-plasminogen activator (tPA) 748
tobramycin *508*
Toll-like receptors (TLRs) 303, 986
tomcat catheter *490*
tongue, necrosis in AKI *453*
tonsillitis 254–5
torsemide *209*, 210
torsion
  lung lobe *139*, 148–50
  spleen 521, *523*
toxic epidermal necrolysis (TEN) 1002
toxicities
  acetaminophen 695, 710, 893–5
  acute kidney injury *451*
  batteries 901–2
  bleaches 898–9
  botulism 623, 917–18
  causing diarrhea *42*
  causing icterus *49*
  ethylene glycol 899–901
  familial copper 348–9
  grapes and raisins *451*, 458–9, 891–2
  hepatotoxins 344, 349, 765
  human foods 891–2, 905–7
  insecticides 879–85
  iron 904–5
  lead 673–4, *675*, 708–9, 902–4
  metaldehyde 885–6
  metronidazole 576
  moth balls 902
  mushrooms 892–3
  onions 905–6, 1122–3
  ototoxic agents 575–6
  over-the-counter medications 695, 710, 893–5, 893–6
  plants 891, 1105–6
  rodenticides 78, 755–7, 886–91, 1116–17
  soaps and detergents 896–8
  topical medications 896
  zinc 904
Toxocara canis 292
Toxocara cati 292
Toxoplasma gondii 564–5, 616–17, 622, 832–3, 980–1
  CSF cytology *617*
toxoplasmosis 729
  CNS 564–5, 931
  feline 980–3
  human disease 982–3
  myelitis 616–17
  myopathy 634
  neuritis 622–3
  ocular signs 832–3, 981, 982

trachea
causes of narrowing *172*
collapse 14, 53, 122–4, 171, *172*
elevation 180, *182*
extrathoracic 168
hypoplasia *119*
injuries 124, 1103–4
normal diameter *172*
radiography 171
tumors 125
tracheal stripe sign 172
tracheal wash 126
tracheobronchopneumonia, parasitic 1101–3
tracheoscopy 123, *124*
tramadol 55, 1040, *1055*
tranexamic acid (TXA) 757, 767
transcutaneous electrical nerve stimulation (TENS) 1025–6
transforming growth factor-β (TGFβ) 988
transitional cell carcinoma 73, *74*, 501–3
transthoracic needle biopsy 126
transudates *165*
trauma
brachial plexus 587–91
coagulopathy 766–7
diaphragmatic herniation 150
diaphragmatic rupture 165, 167
head 569–72
jaw fractures 94–5
spinal 584–90
teeth *85*, 91–3
thoracic 135
thorax 14
trachea 124
urinary tract 72
tremor, insecticide intoxication 881, 885
Triadan numbering system, modified 83, *84*
'triaditis' 338
triamcinolone 261, *801*
trichobezoars 29, *30*, *279*
Trichomonas foetus 317–18
Trichuris vulpis 315–16
tricuspid valve disease *211*, 218, 237
tricyclic antidepressants (TCAs) 1042–3, *1056*
trientine hydrochloride 349
trifluorothymidine 829
trifluridine, ophthalmic 975
trigeminal nerve (CN V)
idiopathic neuritis 576–7
tumor 578, 1110–11
triglycerides, serum 1075, 1084
triiodothyronine (T3) 397, 401, 1084
reverse (rT3) 402
trilostane 394, 414, 430, 657
trimeprazole–prednisolone *792*
trimethoprim–sulfadiazine *508*, *778*
trimethoprim-sulfamethoxazole 959
trimethoprim–sulfonamide 565
trismus 578
trombiculosis 790–1
trophozoites 298, 299, 317–18
Trypanosoma cruzi 230–3
trypsin *362*
trypsin-like immunoreactivity (TLI) test 372, 382
tube agglutination test (TAT) 919
tubulointerstitial fibrosis 460
tylosin 45, 300, 306, 311
tympanic membrane, rupture 575

ulcerative dermatosis, feline 816–17
ulcers
aural 810
cornea 826, *827–8*
decubitus 586, *588*
feline indolent 808
foot pads 346–7
GI tract *274*, 276
'rodent' 103
skin *771*
ultrasonography
abdominal 283, *284*
adrenal gland enlargement 1109
adrenal gland tumor 426, *427*
biliary obstruction 350, *351*
cholelithiasis 352
hyperadrenocorticism 425–6
icteric patient 49–51
necrotizing pancreatitis 1113–14
pancreatic insulinoma 446, *447*
pancreatitis 370–1, *373*, *374*
pheochromocytoma 436
protein-losing enteropathy 305
pythiosis 301, *302*
hydrocephalus 549
parathyroid glands 411, *412*
thoracic 125, 146
urinary tract *71*, 74–5
bladder 484
kidneys *412*, 454, 462, 505, *506*
ultraviolet (UV) light exposure 657, 808, 809
Uncinaria stenocephala 290
undershot *88*, *89*
ununited anconeal process 646–8, *670*
upper airway obstruction 13–14
brachycephalic syndrome 117–19
radiographic signs *172*
urate calculi 531–2
etiology 496
management 500–1
urease, bacterial 494, *495*
urease test 273
ureters
ectopic *480*, 481–2, 483, 485–7
radiography 525, *527*
stent 497, *498*
uroliths 525, *527*
urethra
innervation *481*
obstruction 71, *75*, 487, 488, 499
radiography 532–3
stent 503
transitional cell carcinoma 501–3
urethral occluder, hydraulic 485, *486*
urethral 'plug' 487
urethral pressure profile 74, 483
urethral sphincter incompetence *480*, 481, 485
urethral suction biopsy 502
urethroscopy 74, 498, *499*
urinalysis
AKI 453, *454*
CKD 461
diabetes mellitus 439
dysuria 72, *75*
protein-losing nephropathy 469
storage diseases 553
urinary catheter, feline 489, *490*
urinary cycle 480–1
urinary incontinence 479–87
urinary tract
radiography 531–3
trauma 72
ultrasonography *71*, 74–5
urinary tract infections (UTIs) 483, 487, 499
diagnosis 506–7
management 508–9
urination, difficulty, *see* dysuria
urine
acidification 508–9
alkalinization 500–1

bilirubin 23, *24*, *26*, 47, *48*, 350
calcium oxalate crystals *453*, 899, *900*
color 23–6
cortisol:creatinine ratio *428*, 429
crystal sediments 23
ammonium biurate 358, *359*
myoglobin 633, *634*
osmolality 395
pH 494, *495*, 500–1
protein:creatinine (UPC) ratio 453, 461, 469, 473
urine culture 72, *75*, 454
urine specific gravity (USG) *35*, 36, *37*
bilirubinemia 47
diabetes insipidus 395, *396*
diabetes mellitus 439
hyperadrenocorticism 424
urolithiasis 500
urobilinogen 47
urokinase 748
urolithiasis 493–501
bladder 72, *73*, *425*, 531–2
calcium oxalate *453*, 494–6, 500, 899, *900*
cats *494*
cystine 496–7, 501, 531–2
diagnosis 497
dogs *493*
management 497–501
renal 524–5, *527*
struvite 494, 497, *498*, 499–500
urate 496, 500–1
ureters 525, *527*
urethral 533
urorectal fistula *480*, 482, 484–5
urovaginal fistula *480*, 482, 484–5
ursodeoxycholic acid 340
uterus, radiography 528, 530
uveodermatologic syndrome, canine 853–5

vaccination
Bordetella *912*, *953*
borreliosis *912*
CAV-2 *912*, 924
CDV *912*, 930
Chlamydia felis *953*, 955
CIRD 911–13
CIV *912*, 926
Crotalus atrox *912*
FCV *953*, 976
FeLV *953*, 967
FHV-1 976
FIP *953–4*, 971
FIV *953*, 969
FPL *953–4*, 971
guidelines for cats *953–4*
guidelines for dogs *912–13*
leptospirosis *912*, 921–2
Lyme borreliosis 916
parvovirus 932
rabies *912*, 933–4, *953–4*, 972–3
vagus nerve 258
valgus deformities 648, *649*
varus deformities 648, *649*
vascular disease
cerebral 546–8
spinal 582–4
vascular endothelial dysfunction 753
vascular ring anomalies 174–5, 219
esophageal obstruction 261
PRAA 219, 261, *263*
vascular tumors, bone 660–1
vasculitis 753, 819
drug-induced 667
vasoconstriction 78, *79*
vasodilators *209*, 238, *240*
vasopressin, *see* antidiuretic hormone
vena cava
anterior, thrombosis *760*
enlargement 185
posterior, pheochromocytoma 436
venous thrombosis 758–60
ventricular premature contraction (VPC) *202*
ventricular septal defects (VSDs) 216–17
breed predisposition *211*
ventricular tachycardia 249–51
ventriculoperitoneal shunts 550
ventroflexion 433, 434, *569*, 630, 1109
vertebral body, tumors 608–9
vertebral column malformations 603–6
vertebral heart scale (VHS) 178
vesicle *771*
vestibular disease 572–4
central 572–4, 576
idiopathic 574
peripheral 574–5
vestibular system, function 572
vestibulocochlear nerve (CN VIII) 579
veterinarian
communications skills 4–8
physical appearance 4–5
veterinary health care team 3
video footage 618
video-assisted thoracic surgery 142, 148, *150*
video-assisted thoracoscopy 127
villous atrophy 236, 285, 286, 305
vincristine 965, *966*
viral infections, causing FUO *63*
vitamin A, excess 663–4
vitamin B group, feline hepatic lipidosis 336
vitamin B12 (cobalamin)
deficiency 307–8, 311, 336, 704, 1067
subcutaneous injections 308, 311, 1076
vitamin C 711
vitamin D 311
deficiency 663
supplementation 410, 411
vitamin E 340
vitamin K
antagonists 78
cycle 755
K1 336, 339, 756–7, 887, 888
K2 756–7
vitamins 1067
vitreal haze *839*, *840*
Vogt–Koyanagi–Harada (VKH)-like syndrome 853–5
volvulus
gastric 30, 277–8, 521, 536–7, *538*
intestinal 295
vomiting 27–31
acute gastritis 270
chronic/intermittent 30
clinical approach to 29–30, *31*
common causes *28*
control *457*
differential diagnoses 27–8
differentiation from regurgitation *258*
foreign bodies 29–30
gastric tumors 283
GI motility disorders 282
in AKI 457
pancreatitis 366–7
parvovirus infection 286, 287
pathophysiology 27
treatment (antiemetics) *28*, 30, 287, *296*, 375

von Willebrand disease (vWD) 752–3
von Willebrand factor (vWF) 745, 752, 753
vulva, involuted 499, 508

Walchia americana 790
Waldenström's macroglobulinemia 1122
warfarin 755, *762*
water deficit 555–6
water deprivation test *35*, 36, *37*, 395
  protocol *396*
water requirements 1065
  estimating daily 1017, *1018*
weakness
  differential diagnosis *20–1*
  endocrine disease 18, *20*, 433–4, 1109–10
  episodic 17, *19*, 435–7
  hypokalemia 433, 434, 629–30, 1109–10
  neuromuscular disorders 617, 624
weight, *see* body weight
Weimaraner immunodeficiency 1005
wheal *770*
wheat bran *326*
whipworms 315–16
'white coat effect' 478
windup 1027–9, 1030–1
wobbler syndrome 595–7
Wolbachia spp. 240, 241
Wood's lamp *774*, 899
World Health Organization (WHO), analgesic ladder 1037, *1057*
wound healing, impairment 422
wry bite *88*

xanthine uroliths 500
Xenopsylla cheopis 957
xerophthalmia 860, 861
xerostomia 861
xylazine 1040, *1055*
xylitol toxicity 906

Yersinia pestis 957–9
yohimbine *28*

zinc phosphide, toxicity 890–1
zinc toxicity 904
zinc-responsive keratosis 867
zoometry 1087